EDITION

Introduction to Medical-Surgical Nursing

Adrianne Dill Linton, PhD, RN, FAAN
Professor Emeritus and Former Chair, Department of Family and Community Health Systems
The University of Texas Health Science Center at San Antonio School of Nursing
San Antonio, Texas

ELSEVIER

ELSEVIER
SAUNDERS

3251 Riverport Lane
St. Louis, Missouri 63043

INTRODUCTION TO MEDICAL-SURGICAL NURSING, SIXTH EDITION

ISBN: 978-1-4557-7641-2

Notices

Library of Congress Cataloging-in-Publication Data

Linton, Adrianne Dill, author.
Introduction to medical-surgical nursing / Adrianne Dill Linton.—6th edition.
p. ; cm.
Includes bibliographical references and index.
ISBN 978-1-4557-7641-2 (hardcover : alk. paper)
I. Title.
[DNLM: 1. Nursing Care. 2. Nursing Process. WY 100.1]
RT41
617'.0231–dc23

2014020551

Content Strategist: Nancy O'Brien
Content Development Manager: Ellen Wurm-Cutter
Content Development Specialist: Heather Rippetoe
Publishing Services Manager: Deborah L. Vogel
Senior Project Manager: Brandilyn Flagg
Designers: Karen Pauls, Renee Duenow

Printed in Canada

Last digit is the print number: 9 8 7 6 5 4 3 2 1

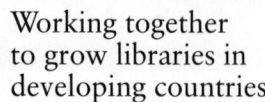

Dedicated to my mother, Margie Crouch Dill (April 15, 1926 – July 11, 2014),
who was a forward-thinking woman before that was fashionable.

Adrianne Dill Linton

Acknowledgments

The sixth edition of *Introduction to Medical-Surgical Nursing* is the product of multiple teams of amazing people. Before revisions began, chapters from the previous edition were reviewed by experienced LVN/LPN educators and content experts. The input of these individuals ensured readability, accuracy, appropriateness for the LVN/LPN student, and timeliness. Using the reviews and extensive literature searches, chapter authors crafted new manuscripts that reflect the best practices known to us as of the publication date. Once again, reviewers were invited to provide feedback on the new manuscripts.

The incredible Elsevier staff managed this entire process and then pulled all the pieces together to create this fine edition. I particularly wish to acknowledge the following individuals who each brought unique knowledge and skills to the production process. Jacqueline Kiley and Heather Rippetoe have worked to develop and carry this edition to publication with great skill and creativity. The Elsevier team included Nancy O'Brien, Senior Strategist; Kate Odem, Marketing Manager; Karen Pauls and Renee Duenow, Book Designers; Debbie Vogel, Production Services Manager; and Brandi Flagg, Senior Project Manager. Behind the scenes are many other individuals involved in the development of the ancillary materials. One of those is Dr. Nancy Maebius who continues to be a strong force in the development of this text and remains the author of the Study Guide. As an LVN educator, her insights and guidance are vital.

I am grateful to my family for their support, encouragement, and patience as I immersed myself in this labor of love once again. Thanks to my husband, Ken; my daughter, Leigh; and my son-in-law, Paul.

Contributors and Reviewers

CONTRIBUTORS

Elizabeth Anderson RN, MSN, OCN
Clinical Instructor
School of Nursing
Health Restoration and Care Systems Management
University of Texas Health Science Center at San Antonio
San Antonio, Texas

Victoria Dittmar, ADN, BSN, MSN
Assistant Professor
School of Nursing
Health Restoration and Care Systems Management
University of Texas Health Science Center at San Antonio
San Antonio, Texas

Amanda Flagg, PhD, RN, ACNS-BC, CNE
Assistant Professor
School of Nursing
Middle Tennessee State University
Murfreesboro, Tennessee

Carl Flagg, ADN, RN
Clinical Specialist
AngioDynamics
Albany, New York

Lark A. Ford, MSN, MA, RN
Assistant Professor, Clinical
School of Nursing
University of Texas Health Science Center at San Antonio
San Antonio, Texas

Margit B. Gerardi, PhD, WHCNP, PMHNP-BC
Assistant Professor
Family and Community Health Systems
University of Texas Health Science Center at San Antonio
San Antonio, Texas

Mary L. Heye, BSN, MSN, PhD
Adjunct Associate Professor
Health Restoration and Care Systems Management
University of Texas Health Science Center at San Antonio
San Antonio, Texas

Lisa Hooter, MSN, RN-BC
Hospital Education Coordinator
LifeCare Hospitals of San Antonio
San Antonio, Texas

Maria Danet Sanchez Lapiz-Bluhm, BSc, BSN, BScHons, PhD
Assistant Professor
Family and Community Health Systems
University of Texas Health Science Center at San Antonio
San Antonio, Texas

Cheryl Ann Lehman, PhD, RN
Clinical Associate Professor
School of Nursing
University of Texas Health Science Center at San Antonio
San Antonio, Texas

Judy L. Maltas, BSN, MSN
Clinical Associate Professor
Health Restoration and Care Systems Management
School of Nursing
University of Texas Health Science Center at San Antonio
San Antonio, Texas

Mary Ann Matteson, BSN, MSN, PhD
Professor Emerita
School of Nursing
University of Texas Health Science Center
San Antonio, Texas

Mark A. Meyer, PhD, RN
Dean of Nursing
Brookhaven College
Dallas, Texas

Barbara Owens, RN, PhD, OCN
Instructor
Nursing
Houston, Texas

Linda Porter-Wenzlaff, PhD, MSN, MA, BSN
Clinical Associate Professor, Distinguished Teaching Professor
Health Restoration and Care Systems Management
University of Texas Health Science Center at San Antonio
San Antonio, Texas

Kathleen A. Reeves, MSN, BSN
Clinical Associate Professor
Health Restoration and Care Systems Management
School of Nursing
University of Texas Health Science Center at San Antonio
San Antonio, Texas

Catherine Robichaux, PhD, RN, CCRN, CNS
Assistant Professor, Adjunct
Health Restoration and Care Systems Management
University of Texas Health Science Center at San Antonio
San Antonio, Texas

Mary Stephens, BA, BSN, MSN
Charge nurse
Intermediate Intensive Care Unit
Metropolitan Methodist Hospital
San Antonio, Texas

Mary Walker, ASN, BSPA, BSN, MSN
Clinical Assistant Professor (Retired)
Health Restoration and Care Systems Management
University of Texas Health Science Center at San Antonio
San Antonio, Texas

Sherry Dawn Weaver, MSN, RN, CNS
Academic Success Liaison
Academic Administration
Galen College of Nursing
San Antonio, Texas

Stacey Young-McCaughan, RN, PhD
Professor
Psychiatry
University of Texas Health Science Center at San Antonio
San Antonio, Texas

REVIEWERS

Cindy Anderson, MSN, RN-BC
Practical Nursing Instructor
Meridian Community College
Meridian, Mississippi

Janice Ankenmann-Hill, RN, MSN, CCRN, FNP-C
Professor
Napa Valley College
Napa, California

Kristen Bagby
Saint Louis University
Saint Louis, Missouri

Terry Bichsel, RN, BSN
Practical Nursing Coordinator
Moberly Area Community College
Moberly, Missouri

Joy Boyd, MSN, RN
Associate Professor of Nursing
Jackson State Community College
Jackson, Tennessee

Jacqueline Rosenjack Burchum, DNSc, FNP-BC, CNE
Associate Professor, College of Nursing
University of Tennessee Health Science Center
Memphis, Tennessee

Barbara Carrig, RN, MSN, APN-C
Program Coordinator/Instructor
Passaic County Technical Institute
Wayne, New Jersey

Susan A. Carzo, RN, BSN, CNOR (RNFA)
RN Staff Nurse/RNFA
Winchester Hospital
Winchester, Massachusetts

Penny C. Fauber, RN, BSN, MS, PhD
Associate Professor, Director, Practical Nursing Program
Dabney S. Lancaster Community College
Clifton Forge, Virginia

Leeanna K. Gardner, MSN, CNP, RN
Surgical Nurse Practitioner
Ohio Health, Dublin Methodist Hospital
Dublin, Ohio

Alison M. Gray, RN, BSN
Adjunct Faculty
Macomb Community College
Macomb Township, Michigan;
Oakland University Riverview LPN
Detroit, Michigan

Sherry Herrington, RN, BSN
Faculty/VN Program
Texas State Technical College West Texas
Breckenridge, Texas

Alice Hildenbrand, RN, MSN, CNE
Department Chair of Nursing, Jasper Campus
Vincennes University
Jasper, Indiana

Margaret Donnelly Hoefel, BSN
Legal Nurse Consultant
Certified Inpatient Obstetric RN
St. Louis, Missouri

Beth Ellen Hopper, ASN, BSN
Lead Practical Nursing Instructor
Paris, Tennessee

Tiffany Jakubowski, RN
Adjunct Instructor
Front Range Community College
Longmont, Colorado

Tracey Jensen, RN, MBA, MMIS, MSN
Vice President/COO
WestMed College
La Jolla, California

Laura Bevlock Kanavy, RN, MSN
Practical Nursing Instructor
Career Technology Center of Lackawanna County
Practical Nursing Program
Scranton, Pennsylvania

Frances A. Koubek, RN, MSN
Clinical Instructor
Fortis College of Nursing
Centerville, Ohio

Lauralee S. Krabill, MBA, RN-BC, CNOR
Director
Sandusky Career Center School of Practical Nursing
Sandusky, Ohio

Leanna Krabill, CNP, RN, MSN
Certified Nurse Practitioner
Dublin Methodist Hospital
OhioHealth
Dublin, Ohio

Carol Lynch, MSN, RN
Instructor, Nursing Department
Triton Community College
River Grove, Illinois

Ruth S. Martin, RN, MSN
Professor, Nursing
Somerset Community College
Somerset, Kentucky

Deborah Milling, MSN, RN
Division Chair, Health Sciences
J. F. Drake State Technical College
Huntsville, Alabama

Martha Olson, MSN, MS, RN
Professor of Nursing
Iowa Lakes Community College
Emmetsburg, Iowa

Trisha Otts, RN
Vocational Nursing Instructor
Texas State Technical College West Texas
Breckenridge, Texas

Nancy Pares, RN, MSN
Director of Nursing Programs
Metro Community College
Omaha, Nebraska

Terri Peterson, RN, BSN, MSN, Ed
Professor
Bauder College
Atlanta, Georgia

Jennifer Ponto, BSN, RN
Faculty
Vocational Nursing Program
South Plains College
Levelland, Texas

Chad Rogers, MSN, RN
Assistant Professor of Nursing
Associate Degree Nursing Program
Morehead State University
Morehead, Kentucky

Kristin M. Ruiz, RN, MN
Practical Nursing Faculty
Southeast Community College
Beatrice, Nebraska

Annette M. Saint, RN, BSN
PN Nursing Instructor
North Central Kansas Technical College
Beloit, Kansas

Russlyn A. St. John, RN, MSN
Professor and Coordinator, Practical Nursing
Practical Nursing Department
St. Charles Community College
Cottleville, Missouri

Billie J. Shelton, RN, MSN
Associate Professor, Nursing
Somerset Community College
Albany, Kentucky

Holly Stromberg, RN, MSN, CCRN
ADN Nursing Faculty
Allan Hancock College
Santa Maria, California

Elizabeth A. Summers
Coordinator of PN Program
Cass Career Center
Harrisonville, Missouri

Laura Travis, MSN, RN
Director Practical Nursing
Tennessee College of Applied Technology – Dickson
Dickson, Tennessee

Anne Van Landingham, RN, BSN, MSN
Instructor
Medical Careers Magnet Program
Apopka High School
Apopka, Florida

Andrea L. Wilkins, RN, BSN
Nursing Instructor
Bauder College
Atlanta, Georgia

LPN Advisory Board

Tawne D. Blackful, RN, MSN, MEd
Instructor, Associate Degree Nursing
Blinn College
Bryan, Texas

Nancy Bohnarczyk, MA
Adjunct Instructor
College of Mount St. Vincent
New York, New York

Sharyn Boyle, MSN, RN-BC
LPN Instructor
Passaic County Technical Institute
Wayne, New Jersey

Dolores Cotton, RN, MSN
Practical Nursing Coordinator
Meridian Technology Center
Stillwater, Oklahoma

Shelly R. Hovis, RN, MS
Director, Practical Nursing
Kiamichi Technology Centers
Antlers, Oklahoma

Dawn Johnson, RN, MSN, Ed
Practical Nurse Administrator and Nurse Educator
Erie Business Center PN Program
Erie, Pennsylvania

Patty Knecht, PhD, RN, ANEF
Director of Practical Nursing
Practical Nursing Program and West Grove Satellite
Chester County Intermediate Unit
Downingtown, Pennsylvania

Nancy Maebius, PhD, RN
Community Relations Liaison & Education Consultant
Galen College of Nursing
San Antonio, Texas

Hana Malik, RN, MSN, FNP-BC
Academic Director
Illinois College of Nursing
Lombard, Illinois

Toni L.E. Pritchard, RN, BSN, MSN, EdD
Department Head and Professor, Nursing and Allied Health
Central Louisiana Technical Community College
Leesville, Louisiana

Barb Ratliff, RN, MSN
Associate Director of Health Programs
Butler Technology and Career Development Schools
Hamilton, Ohio

Russlyn A. St. John, RN, MSN
Professor and Coordinator, Practical Nursing
Practical Nursing Department
St. Charles Community College
Cottleville, Missouri

Faye Silverman, RN, MSN/Ed, PHN, WOCN
Director of Nursing
Kaplan College
North Hollywood, California

Fleur de Liza S. Tobias-Cuyco, BSc, CPhT
Dean, Director of Student Affairs, and Instructor
Preferred College of Nursing
Los Angeles, California

To the Instructor

The first five editions of this text were designed to provide practical and vocational nursing students with accessible, comprehensive coverage of the nursing care of adults with disorders that require medical, surgical, and psychiatric management. The needs of older adults and residents of nonacute care settings received special attention. This sixth edition has maintained that focus. To keep pace with the rapidly evolving field of nursing, we have added useful and exciting new features, many of which were suggested by instructors and students.

ORGANIZATION

Unit I explores patient care concepts, including the health care system, patient care settings, legal and ethical considerations, leadership, the nurse-patient relationship, cultural aspects of nursing care, the nurse and the family, health and illness, nutrition, developmental processes, the older patient, and the nursing process and critical thinking. Chapter 1 has been extensively revised to reflect the increased emphasis on quality and safety in health care. The 2010 health care reform bill (Patient Protection and Affordable Care Act) received more extensive coverage, as it is now being implemented. **Unit II** focuses on physiologic responses common to many disorders: inflammation, infection, and immunity; imbalances of fluids and electrolytes; and pain. **Unit III** covers first aid, emergency care, and disaster management; shock; general care of the surgical patient; and intravenous therapy. Detailed coverage of cardiopulmonary resuscitation and choking response are not included because the guidelines are likely to change within the lifetime of this textbook. Therefore the reader is referred to the American Heart Association for the latest guidelines. The in-depth coverage of topics in Units II and III provides both a foundation for understanding many disorders and a scientific basis for many aspects of nursing care. This approach avoids repetition of content such as common electrolyte imbalances that are encountered in numerous conditions.

As LVN/LPNs are the backbone of nursing care in settings that serve older adults, **Unit IV** provides comprehensive coverage of four clinical problems (falls, incontinence, confusion, and immobility) and end-of-life care. The last of the introductory units, **Unit V**, takes a broad look at the nursing care of patients with cancer and patients with an ostomy. This overview creates a foundation on which the student can build when studying a variety of systems and disorders. Care of patients with specific types of cancer is addressed in later chapters. **Units VI** through **XVI** follow a systems approach to medical-surgical disorders. For each system, a thorough nursing assessment, age-related considerations, diagnostic tests and procedures, drug therapy, and other common therapeutic measures are discussed. The specific role of the LVN/LPN in data collection for focused assessments is emphasized. Common therapeutic measures are intended not to replace a fundamentals text but, instead, to provide a limited summary or review of key aspects of nursing care. Specific aspects are covered, including pathophysiology, signs and symptoms, complications, diagnosis, and medical treatment. Nursing care is organized in the traditional nursing process format with current NANDA nursing diagnoses, outcomes, and evaluation criteria. Sample nursing care plans illustrate the application of the nursing process in realistic patient scenarios. For continuity, the chapter on Nose and Sinus Disorders was moved to the section with other respiratory disorders. **Unit XVII** consists of three chapters that address psychosocial responses to illness, psychiatric disorders, and substance use disorders and addiction. This unit can eliminate the need for a separate mental health nursing textbook.

KEY FEATURES

Introduction to Medical-Surgical Nursing has been received enthusiastically by both students and instructors. They told us which features were most helpful to them and we listened.

Accessible Language

The text is straightforward and direct, avoiding the cumbersome third person. What's more, we have continued to improve consistency and to standardize the reading level throughout.

Key Terms with Phonetic Pronunciations

Complex medical, nursing, and scientific words can be tricky to understand and pronounce. A Key Terms list at the beginning of each chapter shows students how to pronounce important terms they may encounter as nurses. All phonetic pronunciations have been reviewed by a specialist in English as a Second

Language (ESL). Key terms appear in color in the text and are defined.

Nursing Diagnoses, Goals, and Outcome Criteria

Nursing care is the heart of this text, which is organized according to the steps of the nursing process. For each major disorder covered, nursing diagnoses, goals, outcome criteria, and relevant interventions are presented.

Key Points

To succeed in the fast-paced world of health care, the nurse must be able to put it all together. Each chapter brings students a few steps closer by summarizing the most important points in a succinct and memorable way.

Boxed Features Content

Number features described in the Student Introduction highlight important points such as pharmacology alerts, cultural considerations, and complementary and alternative therapies. These features emphasize and reinforce chapter content. Content that warrants specific safety tips is marked with a red exclamation point.

OTHER FEATURES

UPDATED CONTENT THROUGHOUT

Instructors and students trust *Introduction to Medical-Surgical Nursing* because it has led the way in presenting innovative, accurate, and up-to-date content. Every chapter has been updated and reviewed by content and clinical experts.

MULTIPLE-CHOICE, MULTIPLE-RESPONSE, AND SHORT ANSWER REVIEW QUESTIONS

These are provided at the end of each chapter for immediate reinforcement of chapter content. Answers and rationales for these questions are located on Evolve Student Resources. Like NCLEX® items, these questions are in multiple-choice format with single and multiple correct answers as well as in short answer format. Items with more than one correct answer direct the student to "Select all that apply." See page xii for additional key features within the text.

ANCILLARIES

FOR THE INSTRUCTOR

Evolve Resources

- ExamView Test Bank with NCLEX ®–style questions and answers and separate test bank in Word for alternate format questions; approximately 1700 questions total. Each question in the test bank includes topic, nursing process step, objective, cognitive level, correct answer, rationale, and text page number references
- Open-book quizzes (approximately 550 questions)
- Suggestions for working with English as a Second Language (ESL) students
- Image collection
- TEACH Instructor Resource
- Lesson Plan Manual based on textbook chapter learning objectives, which provides a roadmap to link and integrate all parts of the educational package
- PowerPoint Presentation including Audience Response Questions (approximately 3300 slides)

FOR STUDENTS

Study Guide

Practical and student-friendly, this useful study guide, based on the textbook chapter objectives, is designed to help students master the content presented in the text. It includes the following:

- Learning activities (including listing, matching, and labeling exercises) and multiple-choice questions

Virtual Clinical Excursions 3.0

This interactive workbook and online program package complements the textbook and guides students through a multifloor virtual hospital in a true-to-life, hands-on clinical learning experience. Students can collect and analyze data to assist in making nursing diagnoses, planning interventions, prioritizing, and implementing and evaluating care. NCLEX®–style review questions provide immediate testing of clinical knowledge.

Evolve Resources

- Answer Keys—In-text NCLEX Review Questions, Put on Your Thinking Cap Questions, and Nursing Care Plan Critical Thinking Questions, as well as the Study Guide.
- Appendixes—Laboratory Reference Values and Helpful Phrases for Communicating in Spanish
- Spanish/English Glossary
- Review Questions—NCLEX-PN ® Examination
- Review Questions—Prioritization and Delegation Exercises
- Fluid & Electrolyte and Pharmacology Tutorials

To the Student

KEY FEATURES

Designed with the student in mind, *Introduction to Medical-Surgical Nursing*, 6th edition, has a visually appealing and easy-to-use format that will help you to master medical-surgical nursing.

Following are some of the numerous special features and aids that will help you as you study.

READING AND REVIEW TOOLS

Objectives introduce the chapter topics and **Key Terms** are listed, with difficult medical, nursing, or scientific terms accompanied by simple phonetic pronunciations. Key terms are presented in color the first time they appear in the narrative and are briefly defined in the text, with complete definitions in the Glossary.

Each chapter ends with a section called **Get Ready for the NCLEX® Examination! Key Points** follow the chapter objectives and serve as a useful chapter review. An extensive set of **Review Questions for the NCLEX® Examination** provides an immediate opportunity to test your understanding of the chapter content. **Answers** are located on Evolve Student Resources.

ADDITIONAL LEARNING RESOURCES

The online **Evolve Student Resources** at **http://evolve.elsevier.com/Linton/medsurg** gives you access to even more review questions for the NCLEX® Examination, animations, and much more.

CHAPTER FEATURES

Nursing Care Plans, with critical thinking questions at the end of each care plan, encourage students to synthesize key concepts. Answer guidelines are given on the Evolve Student Resources site.

Nursing Diagnoses Goals, and Outcome Criteria are screened and set apart in the text in a clear, easy-to-understand format to help you learn to participate in the development of a nursing care plan.

! Safety Alert! icon indicates potential risks that will carry over into clinical practice.

Drug Therapy tables developed for specific disorders provide quick access to action, dosage, side effects, and nursing considerations for commonly used medications.

Diagnostic Tests and Procedures tables in the systems chapters provide quick references to relevant drugs and tests.

Health Promotion boxes highlight timely wellness and disease prevention topics.

Patient Teaching boxes appear frequently in the text to help develop awareness of the vital role of patient and family teaching in health care today.

Coordinated Care boxes help nurses to prioritize tasks and assign them safely and efficiently.

Complementary and Alternative Therapies boxes provide a breakdown of specific nontraditional therapies, along with precautions and possible side effects.

Cultural Considerations boxes explore select specific cultural preferences and how to address the needs of a culturally diverse patient and resident population when planning nursing care.

Nutrition Considerations boxes emphasize the role that nutrition plays in disease and nursing care.

Pharmacology Capsule boxes alert students to important precautions, interactions, and adverse effects of medications.

Home Care Considerations boxes discuss the issues facing patients and caregivers in the home setting.

Put on Your Thinking Cap! boxes encourage analysis of content for application to clinical situations.

Contents

UNIT XI UROLOGIC DISORDERS, 890

42 Urologic Disorders, 890

UNIT XII MUSCULOSKELETAL DISORDERS, 939

43 Connective Tissue Disorders, 939

44 Fractures, 971

45 Amputations, 990

UNIT XIII ENDOCRINE DISORDERS, 1005

46 Pituitary and Adrenal Disorders, 1005

47 Thyroid and Parathyroid Disorders, 1036

48 Diabetes Mellitus and Hypoglycemia, 1058

UNIT XIV REPRODUCTIVE DISORDERS, 1088

49 Female Reproductive Disorders, 1088

chapter 1

The Health Care System

http://evolve.elsevier.com/Linton/medsurg

Objectives

1. Describe the organization of the health care system in the United States.
2. Identify the health care issues addressed by the Patient Protection and Affordable Care Act.
3. Describe the focus of the Public Health Service.
4. Discuss the financing of health care in the United States, including Medicare and Medicaid programs.
5. Describe the components of the health care system that provide both outpatient and inpatient care and the types of service that each system provides.
6. Describe the impact of cost containment measures on the delivery of care.
7. Discuss the contribution that nurses can make to cost containment.
8. Explain the potential benefits of a national health information infrastructure.
9. Describe the six aims of health care.
10. Define the QSEN quality and safety competencies for nurses.

Key Terms

Diagnosis-related group (DRG)
Extended care
Health maintenance organization (HMO)
Long-term care facility
Managed health care
Medicaid
Medicare
Older Americans Act
Patient Protection and Affordable Care Act
Preferred provider organization (PPO)
Skilled nursing facility

The health care system in the United States is very complex. Fueled by the increase in the older adult population, with a resulting rise in the number of people with chronic illness and expensive medical technology, costs have risen alarmingly. Government officials, health care providers, and consumers now face the hard issues of deciding who is to receive care, what type of care should be provided, and how to pay for it. Health care reform is a major issue for government officials and the American people, all of whom are interested in the provision of equitable health care to all Americans.

ORGANIZATION OF THE HEALTH CARE SYSTEM

The health care system is made up of the patient, the patient's family, the community, governmental agencies, health care providers, and insurance companies. Although insurance covers a significant amount of health care expenses for enrolled members, many health-related services are funded with financial assistance from government or private agencies. Unfortunately, not all citizens of the United States are able or willing to obtain private insurance, and they may not be eligible for government funds. In addition, government funding and private insurance frequently do not cover all costs of health care. Therefore many people cannot afford and may not receive the services they need. In the United States, 15.7% of the population is uninsured, which equals 48.6 million uninsured Americans. While ensuring care for older adults and children is of great concern, young adults actually comprise the age group least likely to be covered. Recent changes in the law require insurers to permit parents of adult children up to age 26 to keep those children on family insurance policies. This change has decreased the number of uninsured young adults. Disparities exist in insurance coverage by race and ethnicity. The uninsured population includes 30.7% of Hispanic persons, 14.5% of non-Hispanic African-American persons, and 11.7% of Caucasian persons.

Numerous problems are driving the support for reform of our health care system. In addition to financing problems, the existing system has no overall philosophy or plan for health care. Critical care and the treatment of illness have long received more attention than health promotion and disease prevention. Standards to ensure quality of care are inadequate and consumer participation in decision making is low. Coordination of services is lacking and communication among service providers is poor.

The health care system is now dominated by managed care. **Managed health care** is intended to provide comprehensive health care at a reasonable cost through enrollment in a **health maintenance organization (HMO)**, **preferred provider organization (PPO)**, or similar plan that includes incentives to reduce costs. Managed care has stimulated increased interest in wellness and prevention, increased outpatient and home health care, and increased cost sharing. Managed care organizations often follow business models and are responsible to shareholders and investors who expect a strong profit margin. Thus the money obtained through cost savings are not solely reinvested in health care delivery, further limiting the resources that health care organizations and providers have available to support their services. This circumstance fuels the ongoing struggle to balance the delivery of efficacious care with a demand to produce a profit.

HEALTH CARE REFORM

The **Patient Protection and Affordable Care Act** (commonly referred to as "Obamacare"), which was signed into law in 2010, has the potential to dramatically alter the financing and delivery of health care in the United States. The law is intended to address many of the deficiencies in the current system. When fully implemented in 2019, it is designed to expand insurance coverage to millions of uninsured Americans, prevent insurance companies from denying care on the basis of preexisting conditions, and expand Medicare and Medicaid benefits.

ADMINISTRATION

The U.S. Department of Health and Human Services (HHS) is the principal federal agency responsible for protecting the health of Americans and providing essential services, especially for those who cannot help themselves. Specific programs are administered by three human services agencies and the Public Health Service. The human service agencies are the Centers for Medicare and Medicaid Services (CMS), Administration for Children and Families (ACF), and the Administration for Community Living (ACL). CMS administers the services that provide health insurance for older and disabled Americans. These services provided by Medicare and Medicaid are discussed later in this chapter. ACF directs programs that promote economic and social well-being of children, families, and communities; it also administers the Head Start program for preschool children. ACL provides services to enable older adults and disabled persons to remain independent.

The Public Health Service agencies include the National Institutes of Health, the U.S. Food and Drug Administration, the Centers for Disease Control and Prevention, the Indian Health Service, Health Resources and Services Administration (HRSA), Substance Abuse and Mental Health Services Administration, the Agency for Healthcare Research and Quality, and the Agency for Toxic Substances and Disease Registry (ATSDR). The major activities of the Public Health Service agencies are to:

- Support medical research
- Support research on health care systems, health care quality and cost issues, access to health care, and the effectiveness of medical treatments
- Ensure the safety of foods and cosmetics
- Ensure the safety and efficacy of drugs and medical devices
- Monitor and prevent disease outbreaks
- Provide health services to Native Americans and Alaska Natives
- Provide access to essential health care services for low-income uninsured persons with limited access to health care
- Improve substance abuse prevention, addiction treatment, and mental health services

Public Health

Public health is concerned with the improvement of health at the level of communities and aggregates (collections of people) rather than the individual (see the *Cultural Considerations* box). The main goals of public health intervention are to protect and improve the health of populations at risk in the community and to prevent disease and disability. The focus of public health is usually directed to the levels of prevention traditionally classified as primary, secondary, and tertiary.

Primary Prevention. Primary prevention aims to improve health and prevent disease and injury. Examples of health promotion activities are exercise programs to improve strength and cardiovascular fitness, campaigns in schools to discourage smoking, and efforts to encourage people to wear seat belts.

Secondary Prevention. Secondary prevention focuses on early detection and treatment of disease to improve patient outcomes. Papanicolaou ("Pap") smears and screening mammograms are examples of secondary prevention activities.

Tertiary Prevention. Tertiary prevention aims to prevent disease recurrences or complications. The use of physical therapy to prevent contractures in a stroke patient and teaching proper diet and foot care to people with diabetes are examples of this third level of prevention activities.

Cultural Considerations

The U.S. Department of Health and Human Services offers Medicare and Medicaid publications in English, Spanish, Chinese, Korean, Russian, Tagalog, and Vietnamese.

Put on Your Thinking Cap!

You have a friend who has limited income and no health insurance. She is a single mother with two small children. She has been advised to apply for Medicaid and she asks you to help her. Find out the qualifications for Medicaid and how to make an application. Obtain an application form and complete it. Discuss the implications of the application process for persons with low reading levels, poor vision, poor hearing, no personal transportation, or no telephone.

COMPONENTS OF THE HEALTH CARE SYSTEM

Components of the health care system can be categorized into outpatient (ambulatory) care and inpatient care. Outpatient care is provided for patients who do not need hospitalization. Services may involve health promotion and disease prevention, the diagnosis of disease, or the treatment and follow-up of disease processes. Outpatient care settings include physicians' offices, clinics, day surgery centers, adult day centers for handicapped or disabled persons, patients' homes, and hospices.

Inpatient settings include acute care hospitals, transitional and subacute hospitals, emergency rooms, psychiatric hospitals, rehabilitation centers, and long-term care facilities. The number of persons in inpatient settings is decreasing as the length of hospitalizations is reduced and as services are shifted to outpatient settings.

Within acute care settings, various specialty units may exist. Specialty units designed for older adults include geriatric evaluation and management (GEM) units and acute care for elders (ACE) units. These units have demonstrated positive effects on patient mortality, lower rates of discharge to nursing homes, improvement in functional status, and other important outcomes. ACE units are designed to promote mobility and safety and provide patient-centered care. They conduct frequent interdisciplinary rounds and begin discharge planning on admission.

NICHE (Nurses Improving Care for Healthsystem Elders) is a program designed by nurses to help hospitals and other health care facilities to provide sensitive and exemplary care to older adults. Hospitals that meet certain standards of elder care can achieve the NICHE designation.

Cost containment measures are driving a shift from inpatient care so that more services are offered in outpatient settings. The term *community-based care* is sometimes used to describe the variety of services, both inpatient and outpatient, provided to meet the changing needs of patients in various states of health. The term also implies the provision of services based on the needs of individual communities.

OUTPATIENT CARE

Physicians' Offices

Many people, especially elderly adults, receive their primary medical care in physicians' offices. Older people have more office visits per year than younger people, especially since the enactment of Medicare and Medicaid. The cost of visits to physicians' offices is covered, in part, by some forms of private health insurance and by Medicare Part B. Physicians may practice in individual or group settings. Many group practices are now made up of various medical specialties so that clients may have all of their health care needs managed in one location. The focus of medical care traditionally has been on the diagnosis and treatment of specific conditions rather than on health promotion and preventive services. However, medical education has begun to place increased emphasis on health maintenance.

Clinics

Outpatient clinics may be associated with community hospitals, teaching hospitals, or public health departments (Fig. 1-1). They usually focus on providing care for people with chronic illnesses, such as diabetes or heart disease, but people with acute illnesses also may be seen. The goal of care in clinics is to diagnose and treat the current illness.

Clinics offer many services, including physician services, nursing services, rehabilitative services, prenatal care, well-baby checkups, immunizations, preventive dental and eye care, and laboratory and diagnostic

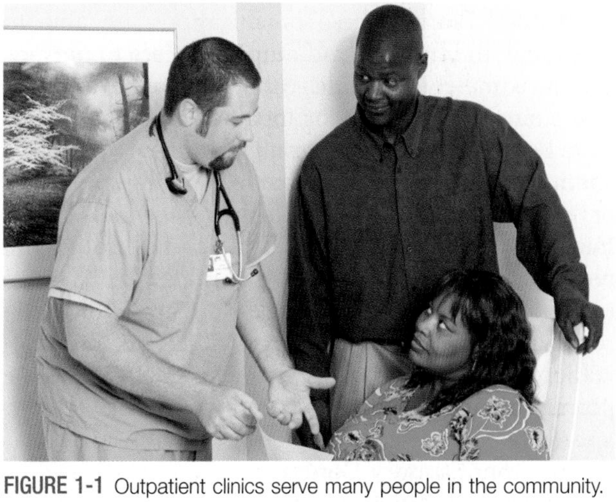

FIGURE 1-1 Outpatient clinics serve many people in the community. (From Potter P, Perry A, Stockert P, Hall A: *Basic nursing*, ed 7, St. Louis, 2011, Mosby.)

services. In large hospitals, clinics are usually organized according to medical subspecialties, such as urology, neurology, and orthopedics. For many people, especially older adults, specialty clinics can be a problem because they have many chronic illnesses and are seen in many different clinics. This circumstance makes the coordination of care more difficult than if the patients were seen in a facility with one set of health care providers.

Health Maintenance Organizations

HMOs provide health care and services through group practice. The principles on which HMOs are based include group practice with prepayment, voluntary enrollment, a combination of hospital and outpatient facilities, an emphasis on health promotion and prevention of illness, and physician responsibility for direction of patient care. The membership fee covers all health care services. Depending on the plan, an additional small charge, called a *copayment,* may be levied for services. The copayment is paid at each visit.

Because HMOs collect only a set fee from clients, they have an interest in promoting health and maintaining wellness. Healthy clients do not need as many services as sick ones and therefore are less expensive to treat. HMOs employ physicians, nurses, and other health care providers; they also have a broad group of specialists available for referral. Clients are required to use only the services of the health care providers and hospitals associated with the HMO.

In 1973 the federal government enacted the Health Maintenance Organization Act. The purpose was to help private agencies develop new methods of health care delivery in an effort to control the accessibility, quality, and cost of health care. This Act helped to stimulate the development of HMOs throughout the United States. The first HMO in the United States was the Kaiser Permanente Medical Care Program.

HMOs are considered to be one way to stop rising health care costs and have become very popular in the United States. These organizations are able to provide both inpatient and outpatient care to persons at approximately the same cost that commercial insurance companies charge for inpatient care only. Costs have been contained as a result of utilization reviews conducted by the HMO, discharge planning, and home or "step-down" care. Utilization review entails examining how resources are used and how health care money is spent. It is the process of reviewing resource utilization based on an external standard. Utilization reviews have resulted in decreased rates of hospitalization, shorter lengths of stay (by up to 45%), and the promotion of preventive care and wellness.

Ambulatory Surgery Centers (Outpatient or Day Surgery)

An alternative to inpatient surgery is outpatient or day surgery. Increasingly, surgical procedures are being performed in ambulatory settings. Ambulatory surgery centers may be located in hospitals, freestanding clinics, health care centers, and physicians' offices. Many procedures, such as cataract extraction, hernia repair, tonsillectomy, and the removal of foreign objects, that once required hospitalization are now often managed in outpatient facilities. Most forms of insurance cover the expenses. In addition, urgent care centers provide 24-hour service for patients with minor injuries or illnesses such as lacerations or influenza.

Ambulatory surgery is less costly than inpatient surgery and allows people to recover in the familiar surroundings of their own homes. Preoperative assessments and laboratory tests are usually performed on an outpatient basis several days ahead of the procedure and then the patient reports to the setting early on the morning of surgery. After recovery from anesthesia, the patient is discharged home, usually on the same day.

The primary criticism of outpatient surgery is that patients may be at increased risk for postoperative complications in the absence of professional monitoring. This system makes the role of the nurse in patient and family teaching a critical one; it also requires that the patient have appropriate support at home.

Home Health Agencies

History of Home Health Care. Home health nursing has a long and distinguished history that began when St. Vincent de Paul organized the Daughters of Charity in 1617. Members went from house to house, bringing food, education, and health care to the sick in their homes. This facility was one of the first organized groups to provide health education to the poor and to help people help themselves.

In the mid-1800s, William Rathbone, a wealthy English businessman, was impressed with the skill of the nurses who cared for his dying mother at home. Convinced that visiting nurses could help the poor and ill of Liverpool, he organized the first district nursing organization. This experiment was so successful that he then opened the first training school for visiting nurses in 1859. Rathbone is often called the Father of the Visiting Nurse Associations because he was the first to employ the district nursing concept.

In the United States, Lillian Wald is considered to be the forerunner of the modern public health nurse. She came from a wealthy family and studied nursing at New York Hospital in 1891. Her experiences teaching bedside nursing to women in the poor sections of New York City had a profound impact on her and led to the founding of Henry Street Settlement House in 1893. The facility was a place where the poor could come for care and was supported by funds from wealthy benefactors. Wald believed that all people had the right to direct access to the services of a nurse. She also maintained that nurses should live in the area where their patients lived, to gain insight into the complexity of health care problems and their probable causes. Many of Wald's beliefs about people and nursing find expression today in Nursing's Agenda for Health Care Reform, in which community-based services and access to care are key issues.

Focus of Home Health Care. Home health services are provided to individuals and families in their homes or in assisted living centers to promote, maintain, or restore health or to minimize the effects of illness and disability (Fig. 1-2). As hospitals strive to reduce inpatient days, the demand for professional home health care is rising in all age groups. Fewer people are being admitted to hospitals and they are being discharged sooner, with more need for special care. The necessary services may include medical and dental care, nursing care, physical and occupational therapy, speech therapy, enterostomal and wound care therapy, social work, nutrition counseling, transportation, laboratory services, provision of medical equipment and supplies, and the assistance of home health aides and homemakers. Home health care is provided by hospitals, private for-profit and nonprofit agencies, and public agencies such as public health and social service departments.

Funding of Home Care Services. Home care services may be short term, long term, or intermittent. Services are funded by individual payment, by private insurance, by Medicare, and by Medicaid. To be covered by Medicare, the agencies must adhere to regulations put forth by the federal government. Most nursing services that are paid for by Medicare must be skilled care, with strict governmental guidelines defining the skilled care that must be provided. Regulations vary from state to state but are generally patterned after federal governmental regulations. The registered nurse is the case manager of services provided by health care workers in the home. Federal Medicare regulations for home care identify standard duties of the licensed vocational nurse/licensed practical nurse (LVN/LPN), which include furnishing health services, preparing progress notes, assisting the registered nurse in special procedures, and assisting the patient in learning self-care techniques.

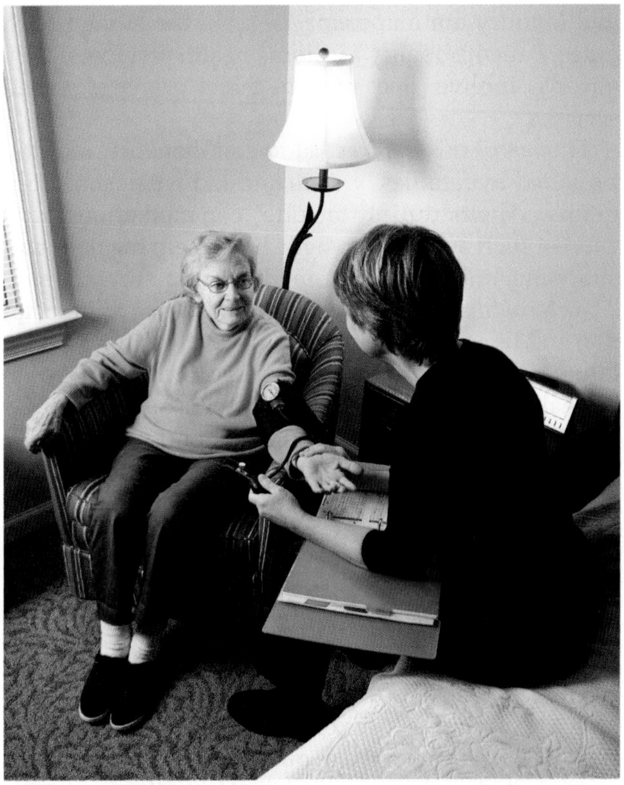

FIGURE 1-2 A nurse takes the blood pressure of a resident in an extended care facility. (Copyright ThinkStockPhotos.com. All Rights Reserved. Item #147048655.)

Types of Home Care Agencies. Several types of home care agencies exist: voluntary, official, proprietary, and hospital-based agencies. Some agencies specialize in specific care, such as intravenous therapy or ventilator management. These entities include hospital-based, private for-profit, nonprofit, and Medicare-certified agencies.

Voluntary Agencies. Voluntary agencies were the first to deliver nursing care in the home. They were financed by wealthy philanthropists in the community and their mission was to care for the sick poor. Today the Visiting Nurse Associations are the most common examples of voluntary agencies. These associations are usually governed by a community board of directors that determines service delivery policies and assists with fund-raising. Because board members are drawn from different areas and social strata within the community, services often reflect community needs. Funding for voluntary agencies usually comes from a variety of sources, including Medicare, Medicaid, the United Way, private insurance, endowments, donations, and patients themselves. Once the primary provider of home care services, Visiting Nurse Associations saw their share of the home care market dwindle with the growth of proprietary (for-profit) agencies during the 1990s. However, the 1997 Balanced Budget Act put a limit on the amount of money spent on a patient's home health care regardless of diagnosis or needs. This payment limitation was a factor in the closing of many home health agencies.

Official Agencies. Official agencies are those supported by tax dollars and are authorized by law to deliver services to a defined area or community. Traditionally, state, regional, and local health departments have been assigned the responsibility of providing health promotion and disease prevention services, as well as communicable disease investigation and environmental health protection. The nursing divisions of state, regional, and local health departments are usually tasked with delivering nursing services to populations at risk. In most states, maternal and child services, sexually transmitted disease clinics, tuberculosis surveillance and treatment, and other health services are included, as funds permit.

Thirty years ago, home health services were often delivered by local health departments, as well as by voluntary agencies. As the concept of public health became more defined, caring for the sick in the home was no longer seen as a public health role. Gradually, more and more health departments dropped home health services. By the 1980s, competition from proprietary and hospital home health agencies had reduced the number of official home health agencies to a handful.

Proprietary Agencies. Proprietary agencies are organized to make a profit on their operation. They may or may not participate in Medicare but most of these agencies do. Proprietary agencies may be owned by individuals or by corporate chains. Their sources of revenue are often private insurance, private-pay clients, Medicare, and Medicaid.

The prospective payment system contributed substantially to the growth of home health care. Much of this growth was in the number of proprietary and hospital-based home health agencies. As noted earlier, the limitations imposed by the 1997 Balanced Budget Act affected the profitability of proprietary agencies and many have closed.

Hospital-Based Agencies. Institution-based home health agencies increased in number during the 1990s. Hospitals that were losing money under the prospective payment system saw the opportunity to recoup lost profits by opening home health agencies. These agencies are usually governed by the hospital's board of directors. The hospital-based agency usually gets most of its referrals from the hospital itself. Philosophy and policies are usually consistent with those of the parent institution. Some hospital-based agencies closed when profits declined.

Home Health Care Services. Three primary skilled services are available in home health care: (1) nursing, (2) physical therapy, and (3) speech therapy. Secondary services include occupational therapy (which may be a primary service under certain conditions), social work services, and home health aide services. The role of the nurse in home health is discussed in detail in Chapter 2. An overview of other services is provided here.

Physical Therapy. Home health patients recovering from health problems that affect mobility, such as hip fractures and strokes, are common candidates for physical therapy. Physical therapists assess the need for assistive devices such as walkers, wheelchairs, and grab bars and work with patients and their families on therapies to regain strength and mobility. To receive these services in the home, the patient must be homebound.

Speech Therapy. Speech therapists work with patients who have speech or swallowing disorders. A common indication for speech therapy is aphasia. As with all home health services, to receive speech therapy in the home that is reimbursed by Medicare, all of the criteria for Medicare must be met.

Occupational Therapy. Patients who have conditions that impair movement of the upper extremities are prime candidates for occupational therapy. People with arthritis or strokes may benefit from assistive devices for dressing and other daily personal care and household activities. Occupational therapists also provide muscle reeducation, splinting, and improved control of fine-motor movement. Timely occupational therapy interventions can help the patient to become safer and more independent in the home setting.

Social Work Services. Social workers can provide valuable assistance to families that are trying to manage chronic illness in the home. Typically, social workers work with families to identify problems that arise in managing illness at home and recommend referrals to community resources. They also may provide information about financial assistance and help families with applications for community services such as Meals on Wheels and respite care.

Home Health Aide Services. The home health aide is a valuable member of the home care team. Home health aides provide personal care for the patient in the home, such as bathing, ambulating, transferring, skin care, and oral hygiene; they also may measure and record vital signs and perform other basic, nonskilled tasks. Incidental homemaking, such as making the bed and straightening the client's room, are common home health aide tasks. General housecleaning, shopping, and laundry are inappropriate tasks for home health aides. Patients qualify for home health services if they already receive one of the three primary skilled services.

Homemaker Services. Homemakers are usually provided by families or state and local assistance programs. Their duties include common household chores, such as cooking, light housekeeping, laundry, shopping, and picking up medications.

Enterostomal and Wound Care Therapy. Enterostomal and wound care therapists are employed by many large home health agencies. These professionals are specialists in the care of all types of wounds, such as pressure ulcers, surgical wounds, and ostomies. They provide care to patients and consultation to nurses on how to manage wounds; they also have extensive knowledge of skin care products and ostomy appliances.

Other Home Health Care Services. Dietitians, nurse practitioners, and psychologists may deliver services in the home.

Specialty Home Care Services. Prospective payment systems and the use of diagnosis-related groups (DRGs) have provided a stimulus for the development of specialty home care, especially for pediatric, psychiatric, and terminally ill patients. In addition, insurance companies, faced with the rising costs of intravenous and ventilator therapies in the hospital setting, have recognized the potential cost savings of delivering these therapies in the home. In the past few years, the use of high technology in the home has increased dramatically. Patients using these technologies most commonly are those who need intravenous therapy or those who are ventilator dependent. Pediatric home care and mental health home care are also specialties.

Pediatric Home Care. Since the late 1980s the number of sick children cared for in the home has increased. This increase is largely the result of advances in technology that have enabled the medical community to save many newborn infants who otherwise would not have survived. These same technological advances have produced the equipment necessary to provide adequate care in the home environment. Small compact pumps, ventilators, and monitors have enabled children with cancer, respiratory disease, and cerebral palsy to live more normal lives at home.

Pediatric home care provides a better quality of life for young patients but it also contributes to strain and role overload for parents and other caregivers. Many pediatric home care services are funded by Medicaid and state children's services. Private insurance companies are becoming more interested in funding pediatric home care because of the potential cost savings over hospital treatment.

Mental Health Home Care. Another growing area of home health care is the delivery of mental health services in the home. Nurses in this role have advanced training in psychiatric disorders; they provide medication monitoring and teaching and perform mental status examinations and suicide assessments. They often provide consultation to other home care nurses on mental health problems that arise in patients with nonpsychiatric problems.

Hospice

Hospice is a concept of caring that originated in fifteenth-century Europe as the provision of respite and comfort for travelers. Later, this concept was extended to the dying in both hospitals and home settings. Families and hospital personnel collaborated to provide palliative care to dying family members.

During the early part of the twentieth century, the dying experience in the United States gradually shifted from the home to the hospital. Instead of being surrounded by family and friends in familiar settings, the dying found themselves in unfamiliar settings and being cared for largely by strangers. The first hospice in America was established in Connecticut in 1974 and provided both home care and inpatient care. Today, many more freestanding and hospital-based hospices all over the country deliver around-the-clock services to the dying.

Hospice services may be delivered in the home, acute care hospital, or extended care facility. Requirements for admission to hospice care include:

- A diagnosis of a terminal illness
- A prognosis of less than 6 months to live
- Informed consent by the patient to elect hospice care
- A physician's order

The purpose of hospice is to enable terminally ill patients to live as full a life as possible, with skilled personnel managing the pain, discomfort, and other symptoms associated with the illness. In addition, hospices assist families during the bereavement process. Some hospices are associated with hospitals whereas others are associated with home health agencies. Most of them are independent organizations in the community.

Hospice services are provided by the Medicare statute. Under law, hospice services are granted for a total of 210 days. If the patient elects hospice services, he or she must waive the traditional home health services. All criteria for the home health care benefit must be met except for the homebound requirement. In return, the patient is eligible for the following services:

- Nursing, home health aide, social worker, and therapist visits, as determined by the team
- Other services, including pastoral care, dietary counseling, and respite care
- Prescription drugs related to symptom management, including pain control
- Durable medical equipment as required

Hospice care is a worthwhile alternative for the terminally ill person and provides a more natural and humane approach to the dying process. The team method is used to meet a variety of physical, psychologic, social, and spiritual problems encountered by the terminally ill and their families. A multidisciplinary team of professionals and volunteers contributes collective efforts to provide a better quality of life for the dying and their families.

Adult Day Centers

Adult day centers provide a structured program of activities related to health and socialization for selected populations. The activities are most often directed toward elderly and mentally ill persons. Day centers may be associated with hospitals or nursing homes or they may function independently. Older people benefit from day services because they can continue to live in the community and have supervision during the day while family members work. For many families, it also provides a welcome respite from constant caregiving. The centers provide all kinds of health-related services, health promotion programs, nutritional meals, and social activities. Most services are provided on a sliding scale fee basis or without charge.

Many of the services provided at day centers are funded through the **Older Americans Act**, which was originally passed in 1965. The goals of the Older Americans Act are to ensure that elderly persons have adequate income and suitable housing, physical and mental health services, community services, and the opportunity to pursue meaningful activities.

Mental health services are also offered through day centers. People who need counseling, follow-up care after hospitalization, and rehabilitation related to chemical dependence may benefit from day center programs. Most of these services are covered by private insurance for a limited period.

INPATIENT CARE

Hospitals

Hospitals vary greatly in size, shape, and organization throughout the United States. Some are small 20-bed rural hospitals, some are intermediate-sized community hospitals, and others are large urban university medical centers. Some hospitals are public and financed by the local, state, or federal government; others are private and owned by churches, businesses, corporations, or charitable organizations. Hospital care accounts for approximately 40% of personal health care expenditures in the United States. In 2005, hospitals billed approximately $875 billion for 39.2 million inpatient stays. The average length of stay was 4.6 days. The cost of hospitalization varies greatly with the diagnosis. Among the most expensive hospitalizations are those for sepsis, chest pain, respiratory failure, and back pain. The predominant sources of payment for hospital services are Medicare, Medicaid, and private insurance. Approximately 5% of all hospitalizations are not covered by any type of insurance.

Among the most frequent reasons for hospitalization are infant delivery, newborn care, cardiovascular disease, pneumonia, and depression. Hospitals are major providers of health and related services to elderly adults. People age 65 and older, while comprising only 13% of the U.S. population, account for 36% of all hospital stays. In addition, older people tend to account for more hospital stays than other age groups (Fig. 1-3).

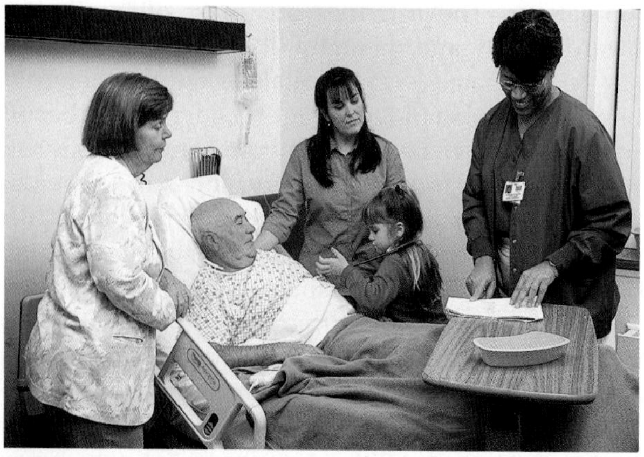

FIGURE 1-3 A large number of patients in the hospital setting are older adults. (From Potter PA, Perry AG, Stockert P, Hall A, editors: *Fundamentals of nursing*, ed 8, St. Louis, 2013, Mosby Elsevier.)

The DRG system has had a great impact on hospital care and length of stay for patients. Because hospitals receive only a fixed amount of money, physicians are now discharging patients as early as possible to reduce costs. As a result, admissions to nursing homes and the use of home health agencies are increasing to care for people who are not leaving the hospital as fully recovered as those who have had longer hospital stays. Therefore the demand for high-technology services such as respiratory therapy and intravenous therapy at home and in nursing homes is increasing. In addition, many health care providers believe now that a "revolving door syndrome" exists, meaning that patients return to the hospital for care after discharge because they did not fully recover at home.

Transitional and subacute facilities are intended to provide intermediate levels of care when needed after hospital discharge. Transitional hospitals receive patients with acute but stable conditions who will need a lengthy minimal stay (often 25 days). Examples of patients who might need such a service are those with spinal cord injuries, those with severe diabetes who have had amputations, and those who are ventilator dependent. DRG requirements for Medicare patients are waived for transitional care. Some transitional hospitals lease space in acute care hospitals and contract for some of the acute care facility's services, such as laboratory and radiology services.

Subacute care units provide care for patients who need more intensive care than what is usually provided in a skilled nursing facility but who no longer need acute care. When DRG days are used up, patients may be transferred from acute care hospitals to subacute care units.

Psychiatric Hospitals

Psychiatric patients may be treated in specialty areas of regular acute care hospitals or separate hospitals may be designated specifically for mentally ill patients. These facilities provide inpatient and outpatient treatment for individuals with acute psychiatric illnesses, with a focus on helping clients to control their behavior or restore their behavior to what it was before entering the hospital.

Psychiatric hospitals may be private nonprofit organizations that are sponsored by organized churches or may be operated by the local, state, or federal governments. The cost of care is covered by most private insurance companies but only for 30 to 60 days.

Rehabilitation Centers

The aim of rehabilitation is either to restore individuals to their former level of functioning or to maintain or maximize remaining function (Fig. 1-4). Rehabilitation can and should be carried out in all health care settings by a variety of health care professionals with the active involvement of patients and their families. Most formal

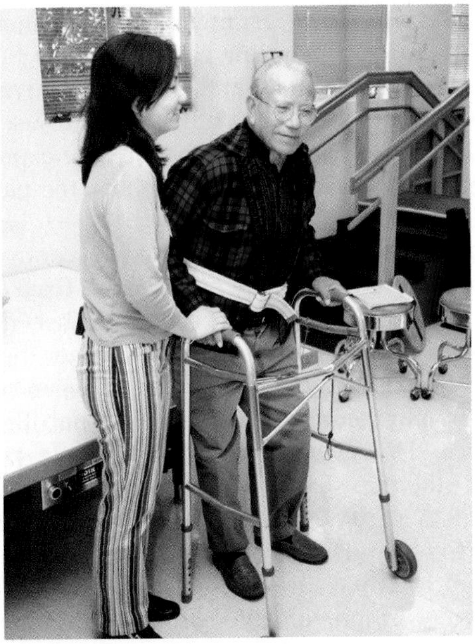

FIGURE 1-4 A patient is assisted with ambulation in a rehabilitation center. (From Ignatavicius DD, Workman ML: *Medical-surgical nursing: patient-centered collaborative care*, ed 7, St. Louis, 2013, Saunders.)

rehabilitation centers are located either within the hospital or nursing home or in a freestanding residential institution.

Rehabilitation may focus on physical problems, such as those caused by stroke, spinal cord injury, or amputation, or on mental health problems, such as drug dependency or mental illness. To restore affected persons to their highest level of functioning, the rehabilitation process attempts to meet psychologic, social, and physical needs. Therefore the rehabilitation team includes many health professionals, including physicians, nurses, social workers, physical and occupational therapists, and speech therapists. Conducting a rehabilitation program is difficult without a team effort.

Long-Term Care Facilities

The term **long-term care facility** was originally used to describe institutions that were attached to hospitals for the purpose of recovery from acute illness. The term is now used to describe several different kinds of institutions, such as nursing homes, convalescent homes, and some residential institutions, the primary purpose of which is to care for people with chronic illnesses and physical impairments. The focus of care is on those who do not need hospitalization but who are unable to care for themselves.

Modern long-term care for elderly and disabled persons had its beginnings in nursing home care, which dates back at least to the turn of the twentieth century. Ill and elderly persons who had no families to care for them were housed in publicly funded homes or boarding homes. The care provided was largely custodial and included housing, food, and personal care. These homes were not licensed and standards were few. Quality depended on the good graces of those providing the care. Later, nursing home care became tied to the medical care system and the nursing home increasingly became a place for patients needing skilled nursing and social services. The range of services now available for people requiring some level of assistance is expanding to provide a variety of options. Examples include independent living retirement centers, boarding and personal care homes, assisted living facilities, special care units for patients with dementia, intermediate care nursing homes, and skilled nursing homes. Independent living retirement centers commonly offer levels of care that permit the resident to access the level of care needed at a given point in time. Boarding and personal care homes typically provide a room and meals and, in some cases, minimal assistance and supervision. Residents of these facilities usually come and go as they please. Assisted living facilities permit a high degree of independence but usually have limited access to nursing care. Help with medications and some treatments may be provided. Although residents often have kitchens, some group meals are typically provided. The intermediate care skilled nursing facility provides care from a licensed nursing staff, including rehabilitative care for people who have the potential to regain function. Services include medical and nursing care; physical rehabilitation; long-term ventilator care; wound care; pharmaceutical, dietary, and social services; dental care; and recreational activities. Federal regulations require a registered nurse to serve as director of nursing and a licensed nurse to be on duty for at least 8 hours a day in an intermediate care facility. This level of care is also called **extended care**.

To receive Medicare benefits in a **skilled nursing facility**, residents must be in need of nursing care that consists of observation during an acute or unstable phase of an illness, administration of enteral (tube) feedings or intravenous fluids, bowel and bladder retraining (for a limited period), administration of intramuscular or intravenous medications, or changing of sterile dressings. Persons who do not fit into any of these categories are deemed to be in need of custodial care and thus are ineligible for skilled nursing care benefits under Medicare. These facilities must have skilled health professionals available around the clock. The care of patients in these settings requires physician supervision and the services of a registered nurse, physical therapist, or speech therapist. Even so, research has found that most resident care is provided by nursing assistants. The average resident receives 30 minutes of care daily by registered nurses, 38 minutes by LVNs/LPNs, and 2 hours and 18 minutes by assistants.

FINANCING HEALTH CARE

An overview of health care financing is essential in light of the astronomical rise in expenditures. The health care system in the United States is the most expensive in the world. In 2011, $2.7 trillion, equal to 17.9% of the country's gross domestic product, was spent on health care, as compared with 5% in 1960. CMS predicts an average growth in health care expenses of 5.7% per year between 2011 and 2021. The largest component of health care costs is hospital care followed by professional services. Prescription drug expenditures contribute approximately 10% to overall health care costs. In 2012, Americans spent $325.7 billion on prescription drugs. Approximately one half of these drug costs were paid out of pocket by patients or their families.

In an effort to contain the rapidly rising costs of health care, the government has established rules and regulations aimed at controlling costs. *Cost containment* occurs when the rate of increase is controlled rather than costs being reduced. As a result, private spending for health care is growing rapidly to fill the gap between the contained or controlled reimbursement provided by government and insurance agencies and the real costs of goods and services provided.

Many different approaches to health care financing are used in the United States. HMOs, PPOs, and governmental agencies all affect the way in which health care is delivered. Historically, health care systems have operated on a fee-for-service basis. This model means that the patient pays a fee to the provider for specific services, after which the patient may seek reimbursement from an insurance company. Although this traditional system of payment is changing rapidly, some private-pay insurance options are still available that support fee-for-service activities. Such coverage tends to be costly, typically requires deductions and copayments, and has limits that may not cover actual costs. However, it permits the patient to choose care providers rather than being assigned to them. Many employers provide group health care insurance for employees. A type of coverage that blends multiple options is the point-of-service (POS) arrangement. POS includes a variety of options, including HMO and PPO participation. Each option has advantages and disadvantages. Enrollees select which option they want to use. When health insurance pays for the health care expenses of members enrolled in health care plans, the payments are called *third-party reimbursements*.

Capitation is a strategy designed to control costs. With capitation, HMOs pay physicians a fixed amount of money each month for each member (patient) enrolled in the plan, regardless of whether the physician sees the patient that month. If physician costs are below the payment amount, the physician keeps the difference. However, if costs exceed the payment amount, the physician does not receive additional payment. A variety of HMOs receive capitated payments from enrollees to cover a variety of services, such as preventive care and acute care. PPOs are fee for services at previously negotiated reduced rates with health care providers in return for the numbers of clients the PPO brings to the physician or health care system. Physicians and hospitals must balance the economy of scale they can realize with increased volumes of clients with the costs to provide services at reduced rates. Similar arrangements are increasingly being made with hospitals and health care systems, whereby HMOs and PPOs representing large numbers of clients use volume of care incentives to negotiate very tight contracts that afford little profit margin for the hospitals involved. This process transfers the risk for cost overruns from the HMOs and PPOs to the health care provider.

Most health care agencies are funded through a combination of government funds, private insurance, and other third-party payers, such as HMOs and PPOs. Out-of-pocket fee-for-service funding is a stronger influence in hospitals with more affluent clients than in those serving less affluent clients in which uncompensated care is a significant reality. The major means of government funding are Medicare and Medicaid, which are overseen by the Health Care Financing Administration (HCFA) (Table 1-1). Increasingly, all but out-of-pocket fee-for-service payers are moving

Table 1-1 Comparisons of Medicare and Medicaid

	MEDICARE	MEDICAID
Funding	Monthly premium from paycheck; funds matched by government	Federal, state, and local taxes
Eligibility	All persons older than 65 years, persons with permanent kidney failure, plus disabled persons younger than 65 years who qualify for Social Security benefits	Needy, low-income, and disabled persons younger than 65 years and their dependent children
How administered	Federal government	Both federal and state governments
Benefits	Physician services, hospital expenses, home health care, and outpatient services; geared toward acute, short-term care	Same health benefits as Medicare plus nursing home care

toward capitation. With hospitals competing for capitation contracts, new budget-cutting procedures have been implemented and the opportunity for profit is increasingly limited.

MEDICARE

Established in 1965, **Medicare** is a health insurance program administered by the U.S. government (CMS) as part of the Social Security Act. Medicare helps to pay for health care for anyone age 65 and older, persons of any age with permanent kidney failure, and individuals younger than age 65 who qualify for Social Security disability benefits. Medicare insures more than 42 million older and disabled Americans. A monthly premium is deducted from each worker's paycheck and the funds are matched by the federal government. Medicare insurance provides two types of coverage. Part A, hospital insurance, helps to pay for inpatient care in a hospital or skilled nursing facility and certain home health services. Part B, medical insurance, helps to pay for physician services and other services not covered by Part A. The list of services covered varies from time to time, depending on changing governmental regulations. Medicare benefits are geared toward acute, short-term care. Coverage in a skilled care facility is usually limited to a period of 100 days and patient eligibility is based on the need for skilled care services on a daily basis. Medicare does not cover long-term care, such as nursing home care, over an extended period. The *Health Promotion* box describes how nurses can access information related to Medicare.

Health Promotion

Helping Patients to Access the Medicare Prescription Drug Benefit

Patients may ask nurses in community settings about the Medicare prescription drug benefit. Health care providers and consumers can obtain information by contacting Medicare at 1-800-MEDICARE or by accessing https://www.medicare.gov/part-d/index.html.

Pharmacology Capsule

The Medicare prescription drug benefit covers insulin and diabetes-testing supplies, such as syringes, needles, and swabs.

Since 1983, hospitals have been paid for care under a system called *prospective payment*. Under the prospective payment system, patients are grouped according to diagnoses that account for similar amounts of resources, or **diagnosis-related groups (DRGs)**. Hospitals are reimbursed a flat fee for a specified number of days based on a predetermined fee schedule for a diagnosis. If the patient gets better faster, the hospital makes money; if the patient requires a longer stay, the hospital loses money. When first implemented, this change in Medicare financing caused the early discharge of thousands of patients and stimulated growth in transitional and community-based health care services.

MEDICAID

Similar to Medicare, **Medicaid** was established in 1965 as part of the Social Security Act. It is the governmental insurance program for persons of very low income. Unlike Medicare, which is administered only by the federal government, Medicaid is funded by federal, state, and local taxes and is administered by both federal and state governments on a partnership basis. States develop and operate the Medicaid programs within federal guidelines, so benefits vary from state to state.

Medicaid benefits are provided for needy, low-income, disabled individuals under age 65 and their dependent children. Individuals older than age 65 who are below a specified income level may also receive benefits, including services that Medicare does not cover. Services covered by Medicaid include inpatient and outpatient care, maternal and child health care, skilled nursing home care, physicians' fees, medications, laboratory work, diagnostic imaging, equipment, and home health care. Medicaid is more likely to cover long-term care than Medicare. Medicaid provides health coverage for nearly 45 million persons.

Persons with Medicare Part A or Medicare Part B (or both) can enroll in a prescription drug plan by paying a monthly premium. Once a person is enrolled, a deductible must be met, after which Medicare typically will pay approximately one half of the individual's annual drug costs. Once prescription drug expenditures exceed a certain amount in a year ($4700 in 2013), most of the excess is covered by Medicare for the remainder of that year. Persons with limited income and resources may qualify for additional coverage of drug costs.

Medicare and Medicaid have been strained because costs have risen much more quickly than anticipated. Some instances of fraud and abuse related to these programs have been reported. The goals of providing comprehensive health care for persons over age 65 and for the indigent have not yet been achieved. The impact of the Patient Protection and Affordable Care Act cannot be assessed at this time.

NURSING'S ROLE IN COST CONTAINMENT

Perhaps more than any other health care provider, the nurse feels the impact of cost containment most fully. Because of the direct, comprehensive, and ongoing nature of our patient contact, we experience with them the reality of the limitations placed on care and services. Nurses also experience firsthand the organizational decisions made to control spending. In both cases, the nurse often works to bridge the gaps in services and to provide quality care with limited personnel and material resources. This effort often leaves nurses feeling overworked, frustrated, and at odds with the institutions in which they work, which is counterproductive for all involved. Given the reality of health care financing today, nurses must recognize the critical role they have in the fiscal viability of their organizations. No other professional group is closer to the care delivery process or more able to identify opportunities to streamline care, save resources, maximize quality, and generally enhance the use of the resources that are available. Being leaders in this process is the nurses' collective responsibility because nursing has the most to gain from it. Because of the significance of the cost of nursing salaries to organizations, nurses are often seen as necessary financial liabilities instead of valuable partners. Our attention to cost saving will not only benefit our systems financially, but also enhance our ability to influence the system decisions being made that affect our circumstances and our practice.

QUALITY AND SAFETY IN HEALTH CARE

The National Academy of Sciences (NAS) is a private, nonprofit society of distinguished scholars that advises the federal government on scientific and technical matters. The NAS established the Institute of Medicine (IOM) to enlist appropriate professionals to address issues related to the health of the public. In recent years, NAS and IOM have taken a prominent role in addressing the quality of health care in the United States. A series of publications has been especially powerful in bringing attention to the flaws in our health care system and making recommendations for improvement.

The first of these publications was *To Err Is Human: Building a Safer Health System* (IOM, 2000). This report startled the public and the health care community by stating that as many as 98,000 people in the United States die each year as a result of preventable medical errors. The majority of these errors were attributed to problems in systems, processes, and conditions rather than to individual carelessness. The report stresses the importance of identifying and correcting the flaws that led to the error instead of blaming or punishing the individual who made the error. Based on the findings and recommendations of the report, a variety of efforts designed to decrease medical errors have been implemented.

One major aspect of safety is medication use. The potential for medication errors exists when the drug is obtained, prescribed, dispensed, and administered, and after administration when drug effects should be monitored. Some sources estimate that 1.5 million preventable adverse drugs effects occur in the United States each year. The following recommendations by the IOM (2006) are intended to help prevent medication errors:

- Medication prescribers should educate and work with patients to enable the patients to take more responsibility for monitoring their medications and recognizing and reporting adverse effects.
- Health care providers should use information technologies to access drug information and submit prescriptions electronically. E-prescription systems can detect drug duplications, drug interactions, and specific patient contraindications.
- Drug labels and information sheets should be redesigned to serve as effective means of communication for patients and providers.
- Research is needed to identify strategies that effectively reduce medication errors.

Another significant publication was *Patient Safety: Achieving a New Standard for Care* (NAS, 2004). It includes recommendations for a national health information infrastructure that would both prevent errors and learn from errors when they do occur. The new system would maintain complete patient databases, as well as tools, to aid in making clinical decisions in all health care settings. A patient database (electronic health record or EHR) can reduce the risk of duplications and contraindications in diagnostic and therapeutic procedures, including medications. Rapid dissemination of information about best practices, as well as warnings, could greatly improve the quality of practice.

Recognizing that safety is only one requirement for quality care, the IOM (2000) issued the following broader recommendations to improve patient safety:

- Establish a national focus to create leadership, research, tools, and protocols to enhance the knowledge base about safety
- Identify and learn from errors by developing a nationwide public mandatory reporting system and by encouraging health care organizations and practitioners to develop and participate in voluntary reporting systems
- Raise performance standards and expectations for improvements in safety through the actions of oversight organizations, professional groups, and group purchasers of health care
- Implement safety systems in health care organizations to ensure safe practices at the delivery level

The second important IOM report was *Crossing the Quality Chasm* (2001), which focuses on a broader view of quality health care than in the past. Citing fragmentation, lack of clinical information systems, overuse of some services, duplication of other services, long waiting times, and additional costs imposed by medical errors, the committee called for restructuring of the health care system to apply information technology advances to support both administrative and clinical processes. The authors proposed that the aims of the health care system in the twenty-first century should

Box 1-1 Aims for the Twenty-First Century Health Care System

Health care should be:
- Safe: avoiding injuries to patients from the care that is intended to help them
- Effective: providing services based on scientific knowledge to all who could benefit and refraining from providing services to those not likely to benefit (avoiding underuse and overuse, respectively)
- Patient centered: providing care that is respectful of and responsive to individual patient preferences, needs, and values and ensuring that patient values guide all clinical decisions
- Timely: reducing waits and sometimes harmful delays for both those who receive and those who give care
- Efficient: avoiding waste, including waste of equipment, supplies, ideas, and energy
- Equitable: providing care that does not vary in quality because of personal characteristics such as gender, ethnicity, geographic location, and socioeconomic status

From *Crossing the quality chasm: a new health system for the 21st century,* 2001, by the National Academy of Sciences. Courtesy of the National Academies Press, Washington DC.

be safe, effective, patient-centered, timely, efficient, and equitable care (Box 1-1).

Having presented persuasive support for the need for change, the IOM next addressed the education of health care providers in *Health Professions Education: A Bridge to Quality* (2003). This report stresses the need for health professionals to be proficient in five core competency areas: (1) delivering patient-centered care, (2) working as part of interdisciplinary teams, (3) practicing evidence-based medicine, (4) focusing on quality improvement, and (5) using information technology. To meet this challenge in nursing education, the Robert Wood Johnson Foundation funded *Quality and Safety Education for Nurses (QSEN),* a project designed to "reshape professional identity formation in nursing to include commitment to quality and safety competencies for nursing" (2007). The QSEN faculty has identified the knowledge, skills, and attitudes to be developed in nursing education. The competencies are listed in Box 1-2. The QSEN website (www.qsen.org) shares ideas and strategies to promote the development of quality and safety competency in nursing.

Box 1-2 QSEN Quality and Safety Competencies and Definitions

- Patient-centered care: Recognize the patient or designee as the source of control and full partner in providing compassionate and coordinated care based on respect for the patient's preferences, values, and needs.
- Teamwork and collaboration: Function effectively within nursing and interprofessional teams, fostering open communication, mutual respect, and shared decision making to achieve quality patient care.
- Evidence-based practice: Integrate the best current evidence with clinical expertise and patient and family preferences and values for delivery of optimal health care.
- Quality improvement: Use data to monitor the outcomes of care processes, and use improvement methods to design and test changes to improve continuously the quality and safety of health care systems.
- Safety: Minimize the risk of harm to patients and providers through both system effectiveness and individual performance.
- Informatics: Use information and technology to communicate, manage knowledge, mitigate error, and support decision making.

From Cronenwett L, Sherwood G, Barnsteiner J, et al: Quality and safety education for nurses. *Nurs Outlook* 55(3):122–131, 2007. http://qsen.org/competencydomains/competencies_list. Accessed October 19, 2008.

Get Ready for the NCLEX® Examination!

Key Points

- The health care system is made up of patients, families, the community, governmental agencies, health care providers, and insurance companies.
- Despite a complex health care system, some people in the United States still do not receive the services they need.
- The Patient Protection and Affordable Care Act includes provisions to expand insurance coverage through numerous mechanisms.
- One effect of *managed health care* is an increasing focus on wellness and prevention.
- HSS is charged with organizing the various health and welfare agencies in the federal government.
- The purpose of the Public Health Service is to provide better health services by reviewing health care, providing grants and conducting research, raising public awareness of health problems, operating hospitals for national health problems, providing health science training grants, and publishing vital statistics.
- The health care system includes outpatient and inpatient services.
- Increasingly, more health care services, including surgery, are being carried out in ambulatory settings and the number and length of hospitalizations are decreasing.
- Outpatient services are provided in physicians' offices, clinics, ambulatory (day) surgery facilities, and adult day centers.
- Hospice services may be delivered to terminally ill patients who meet certain criteria in their homes, in acute settings, or in extended care facilities.

- Inpatient services are provided in acute care hospitals, in psychiatric hospitals, in rehabilitation centers, and in long-term care facilities.
- Home health care grew rapidly during the 1990s as fewer people were admitted to hospitals and those admitted were discharged sooner with special needs for health care services.
- The Balanced Budget Act of 1997, which limited the total amount that can be spent on a patient's home health care regardless of diagnosis, resulted in the closure of many home health agencies.
- Long-term care facilities include nursing homes, skilled nursing facilities, and intermediate care (extended care) facilities.
- Financing of health care is a complex system made up of insurance companies, HMOs, PPOs, and governmental systems.
- Medicare is a federal health insurance program that is geared toward acute, short-term care for people age 65 and older and for disabled people of any age, including those with permanent kidney failure.
- Medicaid provides health care benefits for needy, low-income, and disabled people and their dependent children.
- Cost increases have created stresses in the health care system and have resulted in a variety of approaches to contain costs.
- Nurses can play an important role in cost containment by streamlining care, saving resources, maximizing quality, and enhancing the use of available resources.
- The majority of preventable medical errors have been attributed to problems in systems, processes, and conditions rather than to individual carelessness.
- To reduce medication errors, the IOM recommends improved patient education, use of information technologies, better drug labeling and information sheets, and research to identify effective strategies to reduce errors.
- A national health information infrastructure that maintains a complete patient database (EHR) and rapidly disseminates information about best practices, as well as warnings, would both prevent errors and learn from errors when they do occur.
- According to the IOM in *Crossing the Quality Chasm,* health care should be safe, effective, patient centered, timely, efficient, and equitable.
- Nursing quality and safety competencies, as identified in the QSEN project, include patient-centered care, teamwork and collaboration, evidence-based practice, quality improvement, safety, and informatics.

Additional Learning Resources

SG Go to your Study Guide for additional learning activities to help you master this chapter content.

evolve Go to your Evolve website (http://evolve.elsevier.com/Linton/medsurg) for the following learning resources and much more:

- Interactive Prioritization Exercises
- Fluid & Electrolyte Tutorial
- Pharmacology Tutorial
- Review Questions for the NCLEX® Examination

Review Questions for the NCLEX® Examination

1. An LVN/LPN enrolls in a managed care program for her health care. The nurse knows that one outcome of managed care has been:
   1. Decreased cost sharing
   2. Increased emphasis on inpatient care
   3. Decreased use of home health care
   4. Increased focus on wellness

   NCLEX Client Need: Health Promotion and Maintenance
2. A nurse who is interested in working in the Public Health Service will find opportunities to work in which agencies? (Select all that apply.)
   1. Indian Health Service
   2. Administration for Children and Families
   3. Centers for Medicare and Medicaid Services
   4. Substance Abuse and Mental Health Services
   5. Administration on Aging

   NCLEX Client Need: Health Promotion and Maintenance
3. A patient tells the clinic nurse: "I won't have to pay for any more health care now that I have Medicare coverage." The nurse should advise the patient that Medicare coverage includes:
   1. Inpatient care in a hospital or skilled nursing facility
   2. Unlimited nursing home care
   3. No eligibility requirements for skilled nursing care
   4. Private nursing care when needed

   NCLEX Client Need: Safe and Effective Care Environment: Coordinated Care
4. The husband of a patient with advanced cancer asks if hospice is an option for his wife as her need for care increases. The nurse informs the couple that the criteria for admission to hospice care includes:
   1. A prognosis of less than 1 year to live
   2. A diagnosis of a terminal illness
   3. Cooperation of the patient's family
   4. Inability to pay for care in a hospital

   NCLEX Client Need: Safe and Effective Care Environment: Coordinated Care
5. A patient comments: "When my mother had hip surgery years ago, she stayed in the hospital for 3 weeks. Now they want me to go home just a few days after surgery." The nurse knows that earlier discharge of patients from hospitals is the result of:
   1. Decreased Medicare/Medicaid funding
   2. Balanced Budget Act of 1997
   3. The implementation of DRGs
   4. Improved medical and surgical care

   NCLEX Client Need: Safe and Effective Care Environment: Coordinated Care
6. After several medication errors occur on a nursing unit, the staff discusses the need to address the root of the problem. According to the IOM, most medication errors are caused by:
   1. Lack of concern
   2. Individual carelessness
   3. Failure of patients to follow directions
   4. Problems in systems, processes, and conditions

   NCLEX Client Need: Safe and Effective Care Environment: Safety and Infection Control

7. As reported in *Crossing the Quality Chasm,* the aims of twenty-first century health care should be which of the following? (Select all that apply.)
   1. Patient centered
   2. Efficient
   3. Safe
   4. Effective
   5. Inexpensive
   6. Equitable

   NCLEX Client Need: Safe and Effective Care Environment: Safety and Infection Control
8. If a nursing home Committee on Quality and Safety uses the QSEN quality and safety competencies as a framework for a self-assessment, which competencies will be included? (Select all that apply.)
   1. Evidence-based practice
   2. Equality
   3. Teamwork
   4. Informatics
   5. Quality control

   NCLEX Client Need: Safe and Effective Care Environment: Safety and Infection Control
9. A nursing staff meeting is called to discuss recent budget cuts in a health care facility. An LVN/LPN asks if there is anything nurses can do to help contain costs. The best reply is:
   1. "Nurses can identify ways to streamline care and save resources while maximizing quality of patient care."
   2. "Nurses in administrative roles can require staff to decrease costs on their units."
   3. "Nurses can become involved in the political process to seek more resources."
   4. "Nurses can refuse to work in settings that limit the materials and resources available."

   NCLEX Client Need: Safe and Effective Care Environment: Coordinated Care
10. A speaker at a professional nurses meeting is explaining the intended benefits of a national health information infrastructure, which include: (Select all that apply.)
    1. Rapid dissemination of best practices
    2. Prevention of errors
    3. Education of the public
    4. Improved access to health care
    5. Less duplication of diagnostic procedures

    NCLEX Client Need: Safe and Effective Care Environment: Safety and Infection Control

chapter

2 Nursing in Varied Patient Care Settings

http://evolve.elsevier.com/Linton/medsurg

Objectives

1. Describe the role of the LVN/LPN in long-term care settings, community-based and home health care, and rehabilitation facilities.
2. Differentiate community health nursing and community-based nursing.
3. Describe the types of specialty care that may be provided in home health care.
4. Describe the principles of rehabilitation.
5. List the four levels of disability.
6. Identify the goals of rehabilitation.
7. Discuss legislation passed to protect the rights of disabled persons.
8. Identify the roles and responsibilities of the members of the interdisciplinary rehabilitation team.
9. Describe the types of long-term care facilities.
10. Discuss the effects of institutionalization on the elderly person.
11. Describe the principles of nursing care in long-term residential facilities.

Key Terms

Disability
Handicap
Impairment
Rehabilitation

Chapter 1 briefly introduced the most common settings in which health care is delivered. Throughout this book, the care of patients in acute care settings is covered in detail. As the health care system changes, however, licensed vocational nurses/licensed practical nurses (LVNs/LPNs) are finding a variety of opportunities for employment in community, rehabilitation, long-term care, and other settings. This chapter provides a more complete description of nursing in the more common employment settings.

COMMUNITY AND HOME HEALTH NURSING

Community health nursing and home health nursing are specialized areas of nursing practice that are often considered as being similar. This viewpoint probably comes from defining community health nursing as anything that occurs outside the hospital setting. However, despite sharing common historic roots, these two practice areas have significant differences.

COMMUNITY HEALTH NURSING

For both humane and economic reasons, keeping people healthy is better than waiting until disease or disability occurs. Traditional community health nursing focuses on (1) improving the health status of communities or groups of people (called *aggregates*) through public education, (2) screening for early detection of disease, and (3) providing services for people who need care outside the acute care setting.

Community Health Nursing Roles

The following example demonstrates typical community health nursing roles.

> A community health nurse notices a rise in blood pressure, an increase in weight, and a general lack of fitness in members of a senior citizen high-rise in her district. Her assessment shows that no recreational facilities are available nearby, the meals served at the high-rise tend to be high in fat and sodium, and social activity is generally lacking at the facility. On the positive side, a residents' organization exists, although it has never been very active. By working with the residents' organization and a local church, the nurse initiates a group exercise program to improve the strength, cardiovascular fitness, and weight control of the elderly residents. By working with the management of the high-rise and the residents' association, the nurse gets the building manager to serve healthier meals. The nurse also asks a local school of nursing to hold a monthly blood pressure and health education clinic for the residents.

In this example, the community health nurse not only gave direct service to individual clients, but also worked with three existing community groups to provide a significant number of services designed to enhance the health of the senior citizen group. Community health nurses often work with many different individuals and groups to create or modify systems of care to improve the health of a defined group. This function requires the nurse to assume several roles to accomplish care goals. The roles listed in the example include case finder, care manager, teacher, advocate, and coalition builder. To perform all aspects of the community health nurse role requires at least a bachelor's degree in nursing. However, the LVN/LPN is increasingly visible in community health settings such as clinics, retirement/senior centers, and schools.

Community-Based Nursing

The term *community-based nursing* has been used in several contexts but should not be confused with community health nursing. Community-based nursing may be described as the delivery of health care services that meet the needs of citizens at various levels of wellness and illness based on identified community needs. In a more general sense, the term is sometimes used to describe the provision of various levels of care in traditional and nontraditional community settings.

HOME HEALTH NURSING

Home health nursing blends direct nursing care and community health nursing. The main difference between home health nursing and traditional public health nursing is that home health nursing provides more direct care to patients. The main difference between home health nursing and nursing in an institution is the increased emphasis on the family and the environment in the home.

Home health nursing requires careful consideration of the family and its role in the care of the ill family member. Although giving direct care to an individual is an important part of home health care, a more important nursing role is to teach the patient and family to care for themselves (Fig. 2-1). This important role is similar to that of the rehabilitation nurse, for whom the goal is the independent functioning of the patient and family. The LVN/LPN who works in home health settings must be aware of the legal scope of practice in his or her state, as well as agency policies. LVNs/LPNs must recognize their limitations and inform the supervisor if they are not prepared to perform the tasks or activities required in a particular patient's home.

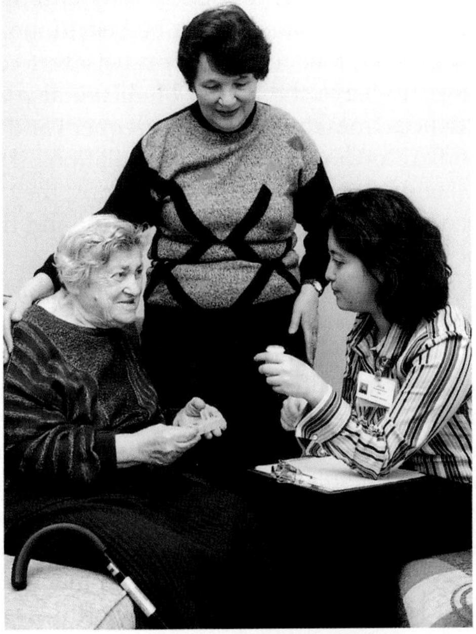

FIGURE 2-1 Home health agencies deliver the services of a variety of professionals. (From Maurer FA, Smith CM: *Community/public health practice*, ed 5, St. Louis, 2013, Saunders.)

The environment in which home health nursing is practiced is very different from the hospital practice environment. Homes often have only a fraction of the resources of the hospital. Small bedrooms, low beds, inadequate climate control, and limited space are common. Maintaining asepsis can be challenging because of inconvenient or absent hand washing facilities and the lack of biohazard disposal devices. Families are often overwhelmed by the task of caring for ill loved ones. They need instruction not only in the care of the patient but also in how to perform the care within the context of daily family activities in a home that was not designed for that purpose.

Home health nurses must collect data for the plan of care about the patient, the family, and the environment. Ongoing data collection is critical because the home health nurse often sees the patient more frequently than other care providers and can detect problems early. For example, the observation of weight gain and ankle edema alerts the nurse to possible heart failure in the cardiac patient. Prompt intervention may prevent serious consequences. The use of technology in the delivery of health care to patients is increasingly common. Examples include videoconferencing, patient examination cameras, video otoscopes, and remote electrocardiogram (ECG) and vital sign monitoring. The nurse must become familiar with tools that permit patient communication and assessment from the home.

To illustrate the importance of collecting data about the family and the environment, consider the patient who requires wound care. In the home setting, decisions that need to be made include: Who can do the care? What does that person need to know? What supplies are needed and where can they be obtained? What is the best way to dispose of soiled dressings? Addressing these questions requires the home health nurse to be resourceful, knowledgeable, skillful, and creative.

Reimbursement Realities in Home Health Nursing

Medicare, though not the sole source of home health care funding, is probably the most important source. Reimbursement by the Medicare program depends on documentation that four basic conditions have been met: (1) the physician has determined the need for home care and has made or authorized a plan for home care; (2) the patient needs intermittent skilled nursing care, or physical or speech-language therapy, or continued occupational therapy; (3) the patient is homebound; and (4) the agency providing the care is Medicare certified. The number of hours per day and days per week that Medicare will cover are limited. Medicare will not pay for 24-hour care at home, meals delivered to the home, or personal care given by home health aides if this is the only care needed. The patient may be required to pay a portion of the cost of Medicare-covered medical equipment, such as oxygen equipment. Private insurance companies may have different eligibility requirements and benefits for home care.

Physician Must Design or Authorize a Plan of Care. All home care treatment must be authorized by a physician. A plan of care must include pertinent diagnoses, results of mental status evaluations, identification of the types of services needed, the supplies and equipment required, frequency of visits, prognosis, rehabilitation potential, functional limitations, nutritional requirements, medications, and treatments. This plan also must include safety measures to protect against injury and plans for discharge from home care.

In practice, the initial referral usually includes the patient's name, address, and telephone number, as well as the major medical diagnoses and a list of medications and treatments—not unlike a physician's orders in a hospital. On the first visit, the admitting nurse usually formulates the plan of care, adding all other required elements. This plan is sent to the physician for review and signature. Because the care provided in the home is predominately *nursing* care, it is appropriate that the nurse has a major role in developing the plan of care. The LVN/LPN's role is to participate in patient data collection and contribute to the development and revision of the care plan. If assistive personnel are involved in the home care, the LVN/LPN may assign appropriate tasks, verify the staff member's abilities and limitations, and evaluate the staff member's performance. Disabled and frail persons may not be able to defend themselves and may have little contact with others besides the health care team. Therefore, the home nurse must report evidence of abuse, neglect, and violation of rights according to agency policy.

Care Must Be Skilled, Intermittent, Reasonable, and Necessary. Medicare reimburses nursing care in the home provided that the care given is "skilled." This stipulation means that the care delivered must be the kind that only a nurse trained in that kind of care could be expected to do. However, not all care provided by a nurse qualifies as skilled care. Skilled nursing care is discussed below with the types of home health services.

Nursing is one of three primary home health care services considered to be skilled. The others are physical therapy and speech therapy. Occupational therapy may be considered skilled, depending on the complexity of the patient's problems. Social work and home health aide services are not considered skilled in themselves but may be reimbursed if the patient has qualified for one of the three primary skilled services. These home care services are discussed in more detail later in this chapter.

The preceding definition of skilled care is an interpretation of the Medicare law. Some nursing activities that require the skill of a nurse may not be recognized as skilled under Medicare. Medicare law does not prevent nurses from giving the care they judge necessary; it only defines what care is *reimbursable* under that law.

Medicare reimbursement requires that the nursing visits be intermittent in nature, meaning that visits occur periodically and usually do not exceed 28 hours per week. Under normal circumstances the patient is not seen daily. However, situations exist in which daily visits are justified. These situations usually indicate the need for family members to be trained in daily procedures such as diabetic care or dressing changes. Under these circumstances, Medicare will reimburse daily visits for 2 or 3 weeks. These instances are considered special cases and reimbursement depends on clear and accurate documentation of the need for daily visits. Otherwise, visiting frequency can range from three to four times per week to monthly.

To demonstrate that care is reasonable and necessary, objective clinical evidence clearly justifying the type and frequency of services is required. The nurse must clearly document functional losses and goals for care. Ongoing progress or lack of progress toward treatment goals must be documented. Poor documentation not only jeopardizes patient care, but also often results in denial of the agency's claim for payment because the documentation did not prove that the care given was "reasonable and necessary."

Patient Must Be Homebound. This criterion does not mean that the patient must be bedridden. It does mean, however, that the patient must exert considerable effort to leave the home. Medicare also requires that absences from the home be infrequent and of short duration. According to Medicare regulations, if patients are well enough to leave home frequently, they are able to visit a physician's office for treatment and therefore are not in need of home care.

Home Health Agency Must Be Medicare Certified. Medicare-certified home health agencies can be located by using the telephone directory, by referral from a health care provider or other persons who have used these services, or from a list of Medicare-approved agencies on www.medicare.gov. The list is found under "Home Health Compare." A home health agency can decline to accept a patient if it cannot meet the patient's needs.

Types of Home Health Services

The primary skilled services in home health care are (1) nursing, (2) physical therapy, and (3) speech therapy. Secondary services include occupational therapy (which may be primary under certain conditions), social work services, and home health aide services.

Skilled Nursing. According to Medicare regulations, skilled nursing includes skilled observation and assessment, teaching, and performing skilled procedures.

Skilled Observation and Assessment. The phrase *skilled observation and assessment* implies that the skills of a nurse are required to observe a patient's progress, to assess the importance of signs and symptoms, and to decide on a course of action. For example, good assessment skills and judgment are needed to detect the signs and symptoms of congestive heart failure early enough to prevent rehospitalization. LVNs/LPNs commonly perform focused assessments, meaning that they collect specified data related to specific health areas. The information obtained by the LVN/LPN can become part of the registered nurse's comprehensive assessment and help guide the nursing care plan.

Teaching. Teaching is considered a skilled task because to teach effectively the nurse must identify the patient's and the family's current level of knowledge, determine their learning style, relay information at an appropriate level and pace, and evaluate the results of the teaching.

Teaching is the most important skill in home care. Much care in the home must be done by the patient and caregiver. Good patient teaching should begin in the acute care setting, but newly discharged patients may need considerable teaching to manage their care at home. When high-technology therapies are involved, teaching is even more important.

Families that have difficulty understanding complex medical issues or high-technology equipment may be anxious when the nurse is not there to help or to answer their questions immediately. Skilled nurses understand this problem and ensure that their teaching is thorough and addresses precisely what the family needs to know to care successfully for their loved one at home. To accomplish this task, the nurse must identify the exact nature of the problem. A family member's difficulty in administering an injection may arise from a lack of knowledge of the procedure, a fear of needles, an inability to read the markings on the syringe, or a denial of the disease process. Identifying the specific learning need is critical to successful patient teaching. In teaching high-technology care, keeping instructions as simple and specific as possible is especially important. Each step in the procedure should be written down and reviewed with the patient. The skill should be demonstrated several times, asking the family caregiver to cue the nurse for each step. After this task is performed a few times, the caregiver should perform a return demonstration of the skill.

Family caregivers must understand exactly what should be done in an emergency. Any questions about the family's ability to manage their portion of the care should be immediately referred to the home care nurse responsible for establishing the care plan and managing the case.

Performing Skilled Procedures. Skilled procedures include dressing changes, Foley catheter insertions, and venipunctures. However, after certain nursing procedures are taught to the family, they are no longer considered skilled procedures and are not reimbursable under Medicare. For example, injecting insulin is not considered skilled because most diabetics can inject insulin themselves. Teaching how to draw up the insulin and inject it properly, however, is considered skilled because teaching is considered a skilled activity. Once the injection skill is learned, the injection itself is no longer a skilled activity according to the Medicare definition. Also, procedures such as enema administration, unsterile dressing changes, care of small wounds, and administration of eye drops are not usually considered skilled because they can be performed safely by most people.

Specialty Home Care

In the past few years, the number of high-technology cases in the home has increased dramatically. In most instances, patients need intravenous therapy or are ventilator dependent.

Intravenous Therapy. Rising hospital costs and the development of reliable intravenous pumps have stimulated the growth of intravenous therapy in the home. The most common intravenous therapies provided in the home are hydration, antibiotics, pain control, total parenteral nutrition, and chemotherapy. Many different types of intravenous lines may be used. Nurses should be familiar with the devices commonly used in their communities. Chemotherapy drugs are almost always given through central lines by registered nurses. LVNs/LPNs must know their role and limitations in relation to all intravenous therapy.

High-technology therapies add to the complexity of home health care. Home care may be more cost effective than a hospital stay but it also significantly increases the risk to the client and the liability of the home health agency. Agency policies and procedures should be current and specific enough to guide the nurse in managing the provision of intravenous therapy in the home. These policies protect not only the agency and the patient but also the nurse.

The safe and successful provision of any high-technology therapy in the home depends on the commitment of everyone involved. Families must be capable of understanding what is required and have the time to participate fully in the patient's care. Nurses delivering this type of care must be thoroughly trained in the procedures and use of equipment required in these therapies. Agencies must have appropriate staff to provide care at any time if needed, including days, evenings, nights, and weekends. The pharmacy or intravenous therapy company must provide high-quality products and support to both the nurse and the family. Finally, physicians must be closely involved and available to respond to emergency problems.

The nurse's role in the delivery of high-technology care in the home includes skilled observation and assessment, the performance of skilled procedures, and teaching. Skilled observation and assessment in the delivery of intravenous therapy includes determining the adequacy of the home environment and the patient's and the family's knowledge regarding care procedures. The intravenous access site must be inspected for swelling and redness. Any side effects of the treatment should be noted, along with the family's level of comfort with performing specific procedures.

Skilled procedures with home intravenous therapy include changing access-site dressings and performing venipunctures. Because home care nurses are not instantly available 24 hours a day, some procedures must be taught to the family.

Ventilator Therapy. Ventilator-dependent patients are increasingly being cared for in the home setting. This type of care is complex and should be provided only by nurses and caregivers specifically trained in the use of necessary equipment and procedures. In many instances, the care of ventilator-dependent patients in the home is coordinated by the respiratory therapist. The home care nurse seeing the patient should be aware of policies and procedures followed by the respiratory therapy company, be familiar with respiratory therapy equipment, and be certified in cardiopulmonary resuscitation.

Initial assessment of the home environment includes an assessment of all factors important in other high-technology therapies, with the addition of an assessment of the electrical and structural condition of the home. This information is important to ensure proper functioning of the equipment and necessary backup generators.

As with intravenous therapy, committed family members or other caregivers must be available. In this case, the commitment is for around-the-clock observation. Physicians and respiratory therapists must be on call for any problems.

Communication Between Home Health Care Team Members

The importance of the team approach in home health care cannot be overemphasized. Quality home care requires the collaboration of several disciplines. Because these disciplines may provide their services in the home at different times, communication among health care team members is necessary if effective collaboration is to occur. Interdisciplinary communication is accomplished through clear, detailed documentation and case conferences.

Documentation. In any interdisciplinary work, the actions of one discipline often depend on the actions of another. A nurse's discovery of an unused walker in the corner of a room may prompt the physical therapist to recommend strengthening exercises and gait training. A social worker's attempts to find funding for a patient's medications may reveal that the patient is fearful of taking pain medications, which can be addressed by the nurse. If these concerns are not communicated, however, they will not be addressed. Most quality-of-care problems in home health care can be attributed to failure to communicate patient care problems. Most of the time, this results from either incomplete documentation or failure to keep the nursing case manager informed. Documentation of nursing care should be accurate, complete, and submitted in a timely manner.

As mentioned earlier, reimbursement for home health nursing visits depends on clear documentation of the patient's homebound status, the skilled nature of the services provided, and the medical need for the services. Failure to provide such documentation often results in denial of reimbursement by Medicare. Denials of reimbursement have serious consequences for the patient, family, and home health agency and, when excessive, denials have resulted in agencies going out of business.

Case Conferences. Clear documentation of interdisciplinary case conferences can go a long way toward preventing reimbursement denials based on lack of medical necessity. These conferences often provide detailed information about the complexity of problems that justifies increased visits.

Usually, a home health nurse must report to a patient's case manager, who is responsible for admitting the patient, establishing the plan of care (including visit frequencies), and coordinating the efforts of other disciplines. The case manager schedules periodic formal case conferences in which all disciplines work together to solve clinical problems. The details of these conferences are documented in the patient's record.

In addition to these regularly scheduled conferences, the case manager should be kept informed of any changes in the response of the patient or family to the plan of care. For example, significant changes in vital signs, weight, and wound parameters are important physiologic indications for a call to the case manager. A change in the home environment, such as an absence of family caregivers, deterioration in sanitation, or signs of patient neglect or abuse, should also prompt a call to the case manager.

Communication by the case manager is also important. Field nurses have the right to expect clear and current information regarding recent changes in physicians' orders, current laboratory information, and the availability of documentation by other nurses and disciplines. High-quality patient care cannot be accomplished without meticulous communication from all disciplines involved in the care of the patient.

REHABILITATION

The acute phase of many illnesses is often followed by a prolonged chronic phase, which may last from days to years and may involve the delivery of a number of health care services in a variety of settings, such as rehabilitation centers, long-term care facilities, outpatient facilities, group residential homes, and, increasingly, the patient's own home. Rehabilitation focuses on restoring maximal possible function after illness or injury.

REHABILITATION CONCEPTS

Rehabilitation Is a Process of Restoration

Rehabilitation is the process of restoring an individual to the best possible health and functioning after a physical or mental impairment. The type of assistance provided allows people to care for themselves as much as possible. Inherent in this process is a commitment by the caregiver to provide the care and support that foster the client's independence.

Impairment Is a Disturbance in Functioning

Impairment refers to a disturbance in functioning that may be either physical or psychologic. An example of physical impairment is paralysis of an arm or leg as the result of a stroke. Mental impairment such as loss of memory may occur as a result of Alzheimer disease. In either case, a loss of function occurs.

Disability Is a Measurable Loss of Function

The term **disability** generally refers to a measurable loss of function and is usually delineated to indicate a diminished capacity for work. For example, individuals with an injured back may be classified as 50% disabled, meaning that they are incapable of doing 50% of their jobs. This type of measurable loss of function allows for specific reductions in work responsibility or may indicate how much compensation to which a worker may be entitled.

Handicap Is an Inability to Perform Daily Activities

The term **handicap** means that an individual is not able to perform one or more normal activities of daily living (ADL) because of a mental or physical disability. For example, the person who experienced a stroke may be handicapped in driving a car because of the related paralysis.

Remember that disability and handicap are not the same things. A person can be moderately disabled but still manage to perform routine daily activities. People who were born without arms are often able to perform all essential ADL by using their feet and certain assistive devices. Although these people are disabled, they are not handicapped. Impairments and their resulting disabilities may not be reversible but handicaps often can be prevented or reduced with modifications of the environment and a community attitude that seeks to promote the abilities of the disabled (see the *Cultural Considerations* box).

Cultural Considerations

What Does Culture Have to Do with Minorities with Disabilities?

Research shows that minority groups in the United States are more vulnerable to health problems, including disabilities. Health care providers and agencies are working to raise awareness and to learn more about the physical health of minorities with disabilities, their ability to access health care, the process of becoming disabled among people in minority groups, and barriers to using rehabilitation facilities and other resources.

LEVELS OF DISABILITY

A disability is often classified by level to determine its impact on an individual's quality of life and appropriate levels of compensation:

- Level I: slight limitation in one or more ADL; usually able to work
- Level II: moderate limitation in one or more ADL; able to work but the workplace may need modifications
- Level III: severe limitation in one or more ADL; unable to work
- Level IV: total disability characterized by nearly complete dependence on others for assistance with ADL; unable to work

GOALS OF REHABILITATION

Rehabilitation aims to return the disabled individual to the highest possible level of functioning. The specific goals are to promote self-care, maximize independence, restore and maintain optimal function, prevent complications, and encourage adaptation. The rehabilitation team must treat the "whole" patient, meaning that it must consider not just the patient's physical condition, but also the emotional state and psychologic and social needs of both the patient and the family.

Return of Function

The goal of return of function includes the restoration of as much function as possible in traditional ADL, such as bathing, dressing, eating, toileting, and walking. Ideal functioning includes independence in the instrumental activities of daily living (IADL) as well, such as preparing meals, shopping, doing laundry, and using the telephone. The ultimate goal of rehabilitation is to live independently. Full independence implies a return to employment status. Not all patients can be restored to their previous state but they can learn to adapt to the changes they have experienced, which requires emphasis on abilities rather than disabilities. Instead of focusing on what is lost, the patient and the care providers must focus on what remains.

Prevention of Further Disability

Rehabilitation also involves the prevention of further disability (secondary disability) that may potentially be caused by the patient's primary disability. Examples include prevention of problems in stroke patients such as pneumonia, decubitus ulcers, and limb contractures, which are often caused by lack of mobility. Attention to safety concerns also reduces the risk of further disability. For example, a walker and environmental modifications may be advised for a poststroke patient who is at risk for falls and fractures. The nurse plays an important role in the prevention of secondary disability.

Rehabilitation is a long-term process that requires the commitment of both the patient and the family. The process is often difficult and marked by periods of progress followed by occasional relapses in functional disability. These relapses can be frustrating to everyone involved and require determination on the part of the family, as well as patience and understanding by the nurse. The rehabilitation process can place additional burdens on family members when roles once filled by the disabled family member must be filled by other family members. Attention is frequently focused on the disabled member, leaving other family members feeling neglected. Ongoing family problems may intensify during this time, making the rehabilitation process even more difficult.

An important aspect when caring for a disabled patient is to be aware of the attitudes and behaviors of all family members. In many instances, families can be assisted in adjusting to role changes that occur during the rehabilitation process. The more consistently patients and family are involved in the process, the more likely it is that success will occur. Involvement in goal setting and a clear explanation of patient and family roles in daily rehabilitation activities help families to understand better the challenges of the process. This approach gives a sense of control and increases family strength.

LEGISLATION

Public attitudes toward people with disabilities play a significant role in the degree of handicap experienced by the disabled. Lack of knowledge about a disability often causes the public to react negatively to people who appear disabled. Individuals who are blind are sometimes treated as though they are deaf as well. People with conditions such as cerebral palsy that affect speech and muscle control are often treated as though they have decreased intelligence. Some employers are reluctant to hire disabled workers, fearing an increase in insurance rates or negative reactions from their customers (see the *Health Promotion* box).

Health Promotion

Help Disabled Patients Understand Their Employment Rights Under the Americans with Disabilities Act (ADA)

- Nurses and other providers should understand basic laws that affect their patients' well-being even after they leave the health care setting. One of the most important pieces of health care legislation to be passed in recent decades is the Americans with Disabilities Act of 1990.
- Title 1 of the Act prohibits private employers with 15 or more employees, state and local governments, employment agencies, and labor unions from discriminating against qualified individuals with disabilities. An employer is required to accommodate the disability of a qualified applicant or employee if doing so would not impose an undue hardship on the employer's business. However, an employer is not required to lower quality or production standards to make an accommodation. The employer is also not obligated to provide personal use items such as glasses and hearing aids.
- Employers may not ask job applicants about the existence, nature, or severity of a disability. They are allowed to ask applicants about their ability to perform specific job functions. A job offer may be made on the condition that the applicant passes a medical examination but only if the examination is required for all newly hired employees in similar jobs. These medical examinations must be job related and consistent with the employer's business needs. To learn more, visit www.eeoc.gov.

The federal government has passed laws over the years to protect the rights of the disabled. The first law passed to aid the rehabilitation of World War I servicemen was the Vocational Rehabilitation Act of 1920. This law provided job training for injured veterans. The Social Security Act of 1935 provided additional aid to states for both direct relief and vocational rehabilitation. The Rehabilitation Act of 1973, however, provided a comprehensive approach to problems experienced by the disabled. This Act not only expanded available resources for vocational training, but also defined services to be included in rehabilitation programs. It also began affirmative action programs to assist in the employment of the disabled and prohibited discrimination against the disabled in programs receiving federal funds. In 1990 the Americans with Disabilities Act (ADA) was passed. This law extended the protection given to the disabled in the public sector by the Rehabilitation Act of 1973 to the private sector as well. It was designed to give the disabled full access to housing, employment, transportation, and communications. As a result of this law, any business endeavor designed to serve the public must ensure that its services are accessible to the disabled. In many cases, this requirement involves the installation of wheelchair ramps, the construction of restrooms that can accommodate wheelchairs, and the provision for communication services for the hearing and speech impaired. Public transportation authorities must ensure that buses, train cars, and concession shops are all accessible to the disabled. Businesses with fewer than 15 employees are currently exempt from many of the law's provisions. This law has prompted significant progress toward improving the quality of life of many disabled people.

REHABILITATION TEAM

Nurses who care for disabled clients must consider the whole person when planning interventions. Difficulties in physical functioning may affect many aspects of a person's life and require the coordinated services of a significant number of health care professionals to enable the individual to stay well and prevent complications or injuries.

The case of Mr. T. provides a good example of the kinds of expertise and the number of services that may be required during rehabilitation.

Mr. T., age 72, suffered a left-sided brain hemorrhage 3 weeks ago. Because of this injury, he was unable to speak or use his right arm or leg. He was also incontinent of urine and exhibited some right-sided facial paralysis. After 5 days in the hospital, care providers determined that Mr. T's condition had stabilized and he was transferred to a rehabilitation facility to continue the rehabilitation process. At this time, his speech had returned but was slurred and halting. He had minimal movement in his right arm and leg but was still unable to walk or feed himself. The incontinence of urine persisted and he had several reddened areas on his right hip and coccyx. Before his injury, Mr. T had been living with only his wife of 50 years, who also was in poor health. They had no family living in the state and she was quite concerned about how she would care for him once he was sent home.

When trying to comprehend all that is involved in helping Mr. T. to return to full functioning (if that is possible), the nurse should first imagine a typical day in the T. household and identify all the ADL and IADL competencies required to get through the day. Next, the types of people and services that may be necessary to prevent further injury and to increase functioning should be considered. At a minimum, the rehabilitation team will consist of the patient's wife, personal physician, rehabilitation physician, and rehabilitation nurse. Other likely members include the physical therapist, who assists the patient in all aspects of mobility from regaining strength and function in the extremities to the use of assistive devices such as crutches and walkers; the occupational therapist, who assists the patient with regaining fine-motor skills necessary for dressing, eating, and grooming; the speech therapist, who assists the patient in regaining swallowing or speaking functions; and the social worker, who may assist with coordinating resources for placement in the home or a convalescent facility after discharge. In other situations, the rehabilitation team might also include a clinical nurse specialist in rehabilitation nursing, a psychologist, a recreational therapist, and a vocational counselor.

The nurse's concern at this time should be that of becoming an effective member of the rehabilitation team. The successful resolution of rehabilitation problems often depends on the ability of health care workers to consider how the individual functions within the family and to work closely with other health professionals toward a common goal. If this goal is to be achieved, good communication skills are essential, which entail clear, specific documentation of the patient's functional deficits and abilities and active participation in multidisciplinary conferences to resolve patient problems.

APPROACHES TO REHABILITATION

Perhaps the most important goal of successful rehabilitation of a disabled person is independence. This fact is sometimes forgotten when a caregiver sees the slow, agonizing attempts to move an arm or a leg. The tendency is to do for patients that which is difficult for them to accomplish on their own. Occasionally, patients need to be helped to complete a task, especially when they become increasingly frustrated. However, caregivers who intervene too soon encourage dependence and delay rehabilitation. Rehabilitation patients should be cheerfully encouraged to do as much as possible for themselves. Praise for accomplishing a task should be given promptly and caregivers should reflect continuing optimism about the patient's progress.

Health professionals frequently plan comprehensive programs of rehabilitation without much thought as to how the program will be implemented once the patient returns home. To be effective, the program should commence immediately after an injury and should involve the patient and family from the outset. Failure to involve the family in establishing goals and strategies often produces family dependence, just as doing too many things for the patient produces individual dependence.

Rehabilitation nurses undertake several roles, all designed to assist the patient and family in returning to a high level of functioning. These roles include care planner, teacher, caregiver, counselor, coordinator, and advocate.

In the home setting, nurses can best assist patients and families by helping them to adjust their activities to accommodate the disability (Fig. 2-2). Even though families may have been taught care routines in a previous setting, routines must often be adapted to the new setting and prioritized differently. In this role, the nurse is an expert caregiver and teacher. Problem-solving sessions often identify ways in which care routines can be adapted to the realities of the home setting. Caregivers may not have thought through changes in

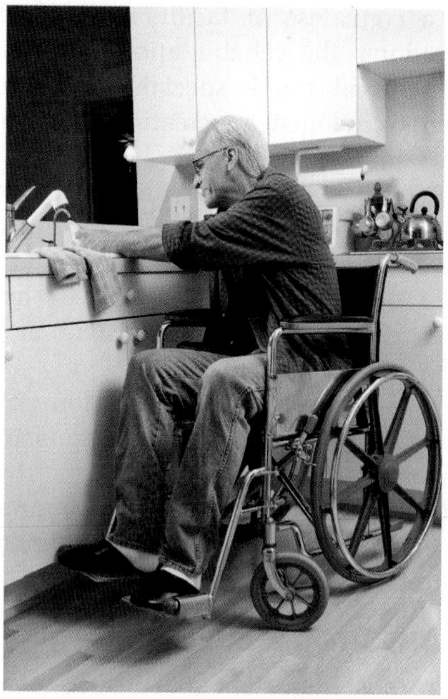

FIGURE 2-2 An important nursing role in home health care is to teach patients to care for themselves. (Copyright ThinkStockPhotos.com. All rights reserved. Item #86538777.)

sleeping arrangements, how they will transport the patient for follow-up office visits, or how to plan for periodic relief from their caregiver role. Nurses can help families to anticipate these predictable stress points and plan realistically for how they will handle them.

Nurses should also be prepared to handle a wide variety of patient and family emotions, ranging from extreme optimism to depression. At these times, families need a great deal of support and may need the assistance of outside community support systems. Local support groups can often be very effective in helping families to respond appropriately to the stresses of a disabled family member. Professional organizations such as the Association of Rehabilitation Nurses can be an invaluable resource to nurses working in the rehabilitation field.

LONG-TERM CARE

Long-term care is provided in a variety of settings, such as personal homes, board and care homes, assisted living centers, continuing care retirement communities, and nursing homes. In the United States, approximately 16,000 nursing homes have been certified by both Medicare and Medicaid to provide residential skilled nursing care. The great majority of these are freestanding facilities, with the others being hospital-based entities. Several thousand other nursing facilities exist that are not certified or are certified only by either Medicaid or Medicare. After an acute care hospitalization of at least 3 days, Medicare covers 100 days per event in a skilled nursing facility.

The United States population in certified nursing homes is approximately 1.3 million people. Many people think only of elderly persons in institutional settings when they think of long-term care settings. Long-term care services, however, are required by people of all ages who are temporarily or permanently unable to function independently. Fourteen percent of nursing home residents are ages 31 to 64 years. Thus long-term care refers to a range of services that address the health, personal care, and social needs of all people who lack some ability necessary for self-care. The number of elderly persons who live in institutions actually comprises a relatively small percentage of elderly persons; many more live with extended families or by themselves. Unfortunately, a significant number of elderly adults who live alone are poor and live in inadequate housing, often without adequate heat, ventilation, food, or telephones. Eventually, problems with mobility and mental functioning force many older adults into long-term care.

RISKS FOR INSTITUTIONALIZATION

Government statistics indicate that only 1% of people ages 65 to 74 reside in nursing homes. This figure rises to 6% for ages 75 to 84 and to 20% for those ages 85 and over. The main reason for institutionalization, however, is not age. The best indicator of who will need nursing home placement is ADL dependency. As the number of ADL limitations increases, the likelihood of residing in a nursing home rises; half of elderly persons with five or six ADL limitations reside there. This figure highlights the fact that if home care services were available to assist elderly adults in meeting more ADL needs, costly residential care might be delayed. Individual characteristics associated with increased risk of nursing home residency include age 85 and older, female gender, Caucasian race, cognitive impairment, functional dependence, and reliance on Medicaid. The long-term care resident today has more medical diagnoses and functional limitations than in the past. This trend has important implications for staffing these facilities. Among long-term care residents, the most common medical diagnoses are heart disease, stroke, diabetes mellitus, depression, and dementia.

Other factors bearing on who requires nursing home care include financial resources, whether the person lives alone or with family, the presence of mental illness, the type of disease process, and the degree of social support.

LEVELS OF CARE

Modern long-term residential care consists of four levels: (1) domiciliary care, (2) personal care homes, (3) intermediate care, and (4) skilled care. In many instances, one type of facility will offer more than one level of care (usually skilled and intermediate); however, in most states, institutions must have approval for whatever levels of care they plan to provide.

Domiciliary Care Homes

Facilities providing basic room, board, and supervision are sometimes called domiciliary care homes. In this arrangement, 24-hour care is not provided and residents usually come and go as they please.

Personal Care Homes

Personal care homes provide medically ordered medications and treatments, supervise residents in self-medication, and provide three or more personal services. Two types of personal care homes have been established. A personal care home *with nursing* (nursing care home) must employ at least one registered or licensed nurse; no more than one half of the residents receive nursing care. A personal care home *without nursing* has no residents who are receiving nursing care.

Intermediate Care Facilities

Intermediate care facilities provide custodial care at a level usually associated with nursing homes. Patients at this level often need assistance with two to three ADL (Fig. 2-3). Facilities offering this level of care must have personnel available 24 hours a day. They are not considered by the government to be medical facilities and thus receive no reimbursement under Medicare. Many of these facilities do, however, receive the bulk of their financing under Medicaid. Federal regulations require a registered nurse to serve as director of nursing and an LVN/LPN to be on duty for at least 8 hours a day.

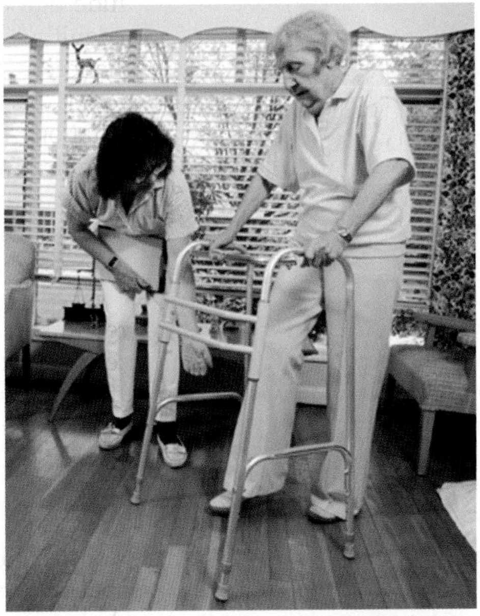

FIGURE 2-3 Patients in intermediate care facilities often need assistance with activities of daily living. (From Potter P, Perry A, Stockert P, Hall A, editors: *Fundamentals of nursing*, ed 8, St. Louis, 2013, Mosby Elsevier.)

Skilled Nursing Facilities

Skilled nursing facilities must have skilled health professionals present around the clock. The care of patients in skilled nursing facilities must be supervised by a physician and requires the services of a registered nurse, physical therapist, or speech therapist.

IMPACT OF RELOCATION

Relocation to a long-term care facility is rarely easy. In the best of circumstances, patients, families, and health professionals anticipate the possible future need for long-term care, set aside funds for that purpose, and make plans that are acceptable to everyone involved. Then, when patients cannot make sound decisions for themselves, families seek help from extended family members and professionals in making decisions for long-term care placement. More commonly, however, the situation is quite different. A crisis situation often precipitates the decision. A sole caregiver may become ill, leaving the care of the disabled elder to the extended family members who may be either unable or unwilling to continue care. Patients may suddenly become physically or mentally incapable of caring for themselves or making their own decisions. Family members frequently feel guilty for considering institutional care. Few know very much about modern long-term care facilities and have not investigated potential placement.

In this situation, home health nurses, social workers, and other health professionals must work closely with the family to defuse the crisis situation and provide realistic options from which the family may choose. This time is when families need the utmost support and acceptance. Simply clarifying the situation, affirming the family's caring and concern, and pointing out realistic options will often return a family to effective functioning.

If relocation to a long-term care facility is the only logical choice, the patient and family must be prepared for the move. Research has shown that the more prepared the patient is, the better the adjustment will be. Preparation includes providing as much choice as possible for the patient and responding to patient questions and concerns. If possible, choices of facility, room location, types of personal belongings, and room decor are helpful, as are tours of the facility before entering. Also helpful is a professional staff member who can check on the new patient frequently during the first few weeks. Patients should be introduced to other residents with similar interests and invited or assisted to participate in appropriate activities.

EFFECTS OF INSTITUTIONALIZATION

The response to institutionalization varies with the individual resident. Positive effects can include improved nutrition, socialization, and management of medical problems. With support and assistance, the resident's overall function may improve. Other effects of institutionalization are predictable and must be considered in helping the new nursing home resident adjust to the surroundings. Frequently observed effects include depersonalization, indignity, redefinition of "normal," regression, and social withdrawal.

Depersonalization

Depersonalization plays a major part in institutional life. Caregivers often know little of a resident's life history and therefore treat individual residents in light of their diagnosis or dysfunctional behavior patterns. The case study (Box 2-1) about Herman and Kristina illustrates this point.

One way to help see the resident of a long-term care facility as a whole person with past relationships, accomplishments, and interests is to ask family members to bring in photographs. The photographs may have been taken on significant occasions, such as on graduation or wedding days, or they may be simple family pictures that depict the older person's place in the family or community. The photographs can be mounted on poster board or placed on a bulletin board in the resident's room. This effort helps caregivers to see more than a frail, weak, older person and can open up conversation that encourages reminiscing, which is a therapeutic means of dealing with one's past life and preparing for death.

Indignity

Indignity is another effect of institutionalization. Routine activities such as toileting and obtaining food and drink must be requested. The prompt fulfillment of the request sometimes depends on the relationship between the patient and the caregiver. Residents of long-term care facilities may be exposed unnecessarily, especially when caregivers enter rooms without knocking. Simple courtesies such as using a person's title and last name, knocking before entering the room, and draping during care activities help the resident to maintain dignity. A useful exercise would be to consider: "How would I want to be treated if I were weak and frail and could not do the things that I can do for myself now?"

Assistive personnel are important members of the nursing care team in long-term care. Because they provide much personal care, the LVN/LPN should know what tasks can be assigned to them. Also, the LVN/LPN must verify the skills of assistive personnel, provide guidance as needed, and participate in their evaluation.

Redefinition of "Normal"

Behaviors that were considered normal in one's home may be labeled abnormal or be unacceptable in a long-term care facility. Watching television at 3:00 AM, loud singing, or sexual activity may be frowned upon, depending on the residence's rules and routines. Although consideration of others is important, giving residents of long-term care facilities some flexibility and some measure of control in their daily lives is also important.

Box 2-1 Case Study

I don't think I truly understood what depersonalization was until I met Herman. Herman and his wife, Kristina, lived alone in a small house in a northwestern city. Herman was 62 years old and had Alzheimer disease. I met them while working as a home health nurse. I was asked to look into respite services to help relieve Kristina of the strain of caring for Herman. I remember my first impression of Herman, formed after reading his chart and talking to the staff nurse about his care problems. He was starting to neglect his personal appearance. The staff nurse said he often put soup on the stove for lunch then went out to the garden to tend his flowers, forgetting about the soup. This and other images of his functioning created in me a picture of an incompetent and helpless old man.

Over a period of weeks, Kristina shared many stories with me about who this man was, what he cared about, how they had met, and her deep devotion to her husband of 35 years. Gradually, I was able to see the distorted image I held. Herman was an Olympic gold medal skier from Austria who came to this country as a young man. He held several jobs as a ski instructor and repaired ski equipment until he met and married Kristina and moved to the northwestern United States to become the owner and manager of a small ski resort. He was tall and muscular, with an easy smile and a kind word for everyone. He was admired by many in the community for his skill as a skier and his friendliness. He was a good father and family man who was known as "the rock" because all of his family and friends relied on him for advice and assistance.

Over a period of 5 years, Herman became more and more forgetful, less talkative, and often preoccupied with household tasks that he would start but not complete. He also failed to recognize many of his close friends and, at times, would wander off downtown without knowing why or where he was going. Throughout this, Kristina remained fiercely devoted to Herman, though the strain of the caregiver role was beginning to affect her health. "He cared for us for so many years. Now it is my turn to care for him."

I was surprised at how my view of Herman changed as I learned more about him. I was seeing him as dependent, helpless, and a burden to his small and frail wife—a view created by my observations of his behavior and what I knew of the Alzheimer disease process and a view that changed radically once I knew more about Herman. I doubt I will ever minimize the importance of learning about the whole patient.

Regression

Over time, a resident's physical, mental, and social abilities may be lost because of disuse. If people are left in bed for a greater part of the day, it soon becomes impossible for them to walk. If visits from friends and relatives are few, the skill of conversation may also be lost. Encouraging independence and social interaction as much as possible is important. Avoid infantilizing older patients. Although simplifying language and activities for those who are cognitively impaired may be necessary, avoid baby talk.

Social Withdrawal

If a resident never leaves the nursing home or if family visits are few and include little discussion of the outside world, the institution can become a barrier, cutting off interest and participation in the outside world. If this situation is allowed to continue, life in the facility becomes, for many patients, their entire world. They tend to withdraw into the boundaries of their own room (see the *Cultural Considerations* box). Nurses can help by conversing with residents about events inside and outside the nursing home. When you know your patients well, you can bring up news that you expect will be of interest to them. Discussion of current events in small groups can broaden the resident's horizons.

> **Cultural Considerations**
>
> **What Does Culture Have to Do with Social Withdrawal?**
>
> Most facilities are dominated by a single culture that is reflected in mealtimes, social mores, religious services, and holiday traditions. Consider how a person from a different culture might feel in this setting.

PRINCIPLES OF LONG-TERM RESIDENTIAL CARE

Long-term residential care has been called *custodial care*. This term invokes passive images such as maintenance, warehousing, or waiting to die. Some people have called such facilities "heaven's waiting rooms." Publicized abuses by some nursing homes are at least partly responsible for negative stereotypes of long-term residential care. However, long-term care facilities in general have changed substantially in recent years. Although some continue to provide care of questionable quality, many excellent facilities do exist.

Modern facilities care for individuals with a wide array of medical and surgical problems. People who reside in long-term care facilities are commonly referred to as residents rather than patients. Not all residents are admitted for permanent stays in the facility. In many communities, the nursing home has become a convalescent hospital for elderly persons who have recently undergone surgical procedures, such as repair of a fractured hip. These acute cases often strain already limited resources. Many individuals are admitted for short stays that are prompted by care demands that temporarily overwhelm the family. Illness of a family caregiver also can result in temporary admission to the facility. When the home situation has stabilized, these residents often return home. Increasingly, those admitted for long stays are elderly and suffer from mental health problems. In these cases, the family has exhausted most of its physical, emotional, and financial resources and home care is no longer feasible.

When a person is admitted to a long-term care facility, the care delivered should be based on three principles: (1) promotion of independence, (2) maintenance of function, and (3) maintenance of autonomy.

> **Put on Your Thinking Cap!**
>
> If you have a clinical experience in a long-term care facility, interview a resident there. Specifically, ask:
>
> 1. What circumstances brought you here to live?
> 2. What are the benefits and disadvantages of living in this type of facility?
> 3. What advice would you give to a new resident here?
> 4. What can nurses do to make adjustment to living here easier?
>
> Discuss the resident's responses in relation to the effects of institutionalization and implications for nurses.

Promotion of Independence

Successful relocation to a long-term care facility depends, in part, on the ability of patients to do things for themselves and on the involvement of families to keep the elderly family member in contact with the outside world. Feeding residents rather than spending time encouraging residents to feed themselves may be tempting for institutional caregivers. When the workday is a never-ending series of tasks, doing things quickly often takes priority over promoting independence. Watch for this type of behavior and try to restructure assignments of nursing assistants to reward the promotion of independence. This effort can be accomplished by setting specific goals for each resident that encourage independent functioning. Then, explain to the staff members how their efforts can contribute to the goal. Involvement of staff in this way often produces results.

Maintenance of Function

In many cases, loss of function prevents an elderly person from staying at home. Health professionals who are disease oriented often concentrate on the disease process at the expense of a functional assessment. An incontinent resident may be incorrectly perceived as having a complication of the aging process. This kind of thinking fosters an emphasis on maintenance care, leading to efforts to prevent skin breakdown by frequent changes of clothing and linens. A more thorough assessment would begin with the determination of possible causes of the incontinence. A functional assessment explores factors that might be responsible for the incontinence. Immobility may be the basic problem. Questions to ask include: Is the resident normally mobile? If so, does the room have a light that facilitates locating the bathroom? Is the resident able to manage clothing for independent toileting? Are the side rails normally up or down? Viewing this problem as a functional problem may lead to simple solutions, such as placing a light in the room at night or a urinal next to the bed. Interventions, whenever possible, should focus on restoring and preserving function.

Maintenance of Autonomy

Most people value control over their lives. Successful relocation to a long-term care facility depends on preserving as much autonomy as possible. Elders who participate in selecting the facility adjust better than those who have no choice in the matter.

Allowing as much flexibility as possible in establishing a routine for the new resident is also important. Choices in activities, such as when to have a bath or how late to watch television, go a long way toward preserving the autonomy and self-esteem of the elderly resident. As much as possible, encourage the resident to assist in establishing care goals. For example, the frequency and duration of exercise and goals for weight loss or gains require the facility resident's commitment. Mutually established goals are more likely to be achieved than those selected for the resident.

Families also have a role in maintaining autonomy in the elderly member. Autonomy depends on knowing one's place in the world and what roles one still holds in the family structure. Families who relate to their elder members by stressing their importance in the family and keeping them up to date on family happenings and decisions reinforce the idea that the elder remains a valued family member who simply resides at another address.

Put on Your Thinking Cap!

Identify one thing you can do to achieve each of the following: (1) maintain autonomy, (2) maintain function, and (3) promote independence in:

a. The long-term care facility resident
b. The hospitalized patient

ASSISTED LIVING

Assisted living facilities provide an alternative to nursing home care. These facilities are residences that provide self-contained living units for individuals who live independently but have on-site access to support if needed at any time. Typical services include congregate meals, recreation, housekeeping and laundry, social services, transportation, help with ADL (but not full-time nursing care), and some health-related services such as medication management. Medicare and Medicaid do not pay for assisted living care.

CONTINUING CARE RETIREMENT COMMUNITIES

Continuing care retirement communities (CCRCs) usually have various living options ranging from independent quarters, to assisted living, to skilled nursing units. As residents age, they may need to move from one level of care to another. Residents pay an entry fee as well as monthly fees that may vary as the level of care changes. Medicare and Medicaid do not pay for CCRCs, except in the skilled nursing areas.

OTHER PATIENT CARE SETTINGS

The settings addressed in this chapter represent many of those that traditionally employ licensed nurses. Other employment settings include clinics, physicians' offices, and schools, as well as adult day centers, respite care, hospice, and correctional facilities. Each setting presents unique experiences and challenges. In some of these settings, the LVN/LPN may be the only licensed nursing professional on site. Therefore the nurse's responsibilities must be clearly defined and consistent with legal functions.

Get Ready for the NCLEX® Examination!

Key Points

- The changing health care system has greatly increased the number and types of health care settings.
- Community health nurses work with individuals and aggregates (groups) to improve the health of the entire community.
- The main difference between home health care nursing and public health nursing is that home health care is more focused on providing direct care to patients.
- A major nursing function in home health care is teaching patients and families to care for themselves so as to promote independent functioning.
- Medicare is a major source of home health care funding.
- To receive Medicare reimbursement for home health care, four conditions must be met: (1) the physician has determined the need for home care and has made or authorized a plan for home care; (2) the patient needs intermittent skilled nursing care, or physical or speech-language therapy, or continued occupational therapy; (3) the patient is homebound; and (4) the agency providing the care is Medicare certified.
- Specialty home care services include high-technology interventions (the provision of intravenous therapy and

ventilator therapy), hospice services, pediatric care, and mental health care.
- Rehabilitation is the process of restoring an individual to the best possible health and functioning following a physical or mental impairment and the prevention of further disability.
- Caring for disabled patients requires the coordinated services of a large number of health care professionals to help patients stay healthy and prevent complications or injuries.
- As an effective member of a multidisciplinary rehabilitation team, the nurse is a care planner, teacher, caregiver, counselor, coordinator, and advocate.
- Health care workers must consider the way in which a disabled individual functions within the family, and the patient and family should be involved from the outset in determining the plan of care.
- Government statistics indicate that only 1% of people ages 65 to 74, 6% of people ages 75 to 84, and 20% of people age 85 and over reside in nursing homes.
- Dependence in activities of daily living is the best indicator of who will need nursing home placement.
- Modern long-term residential care exists in four levels: (1) domiciliary care, (2) personal care homes, (3) intermediate care, and (4) skilled care. Care delivered in a long-term care residential facility is based on three principles: (1) promotion of independence, (2) maintenance of function, and (3) maintenance of autonomy.
- Alternatives to nursing home care include assisted living facilities and continuing care retirement communities.
- The LVN/LPN's responsibilities must be clearly defined and consistent with legal functions regardless of the employment location.

Additional Learning Resources

SG Go to your Study Guide for additional learning activities to help you master this chapter content.

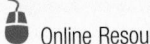

Online Resource
- http://www.medicare.gov/Publications/Pubs/pdf/10153.pdf

evolve Go to your Evolve website (http://evolve.elsevier.com/Linton/medsurg) for the following learning resources and much more:
- Interactive Prioritization Exercises
- Fluid & Electrolyte Tutorial
- Pharmacology Tutorial
- Review Questions for the NCLEX® Examination

Review Questions for the NCLEX® Examination

1. A home health nurse performed all of the following activities listed with Medicare patients. Which activities are reimbursable? (Select all that apply.)
   1. Used sterile technique to clean and dress a large wound
   2. Took a frail older couple for a short walk to provide exercise
   3. Performed a venipuncture to obtain a blood sample for laboratory tests
   4. Taught a patient with recently diagnosed diabetes how to inject insulin
   5. Removed outdated food from the refrigerator and pantry

   NCLEX Client Need: Safe and Effective Care Environment: Coordinated Care
2. Which nursing activity might commonly be provided by community health nurses but not by home health nurses? (Select all that apply.)
   1. Conducting health education programs in a senior citizen residence
   2. Monitoring the recovery of a postoperative patient at home
   3. Arranging blood pressure screening at a community shopping center
   4. Seeing patients in a clinic to monitor problems related to chronic illness
   5. Administering influenza vaccines at a public location

   NCLEX Client Need: Safe and Effective Care Environment: Coordinated Care
3. LVN/LPN students are discussing the difference between community health nursing and community-based nursing. They correctly identify an example of *community-based nursing* as:
   1. Meeting with residents of low-income housing to identify their health needs
   2. Telephoning patients at home after discharge from the hospital
   3. Asking nurses to identify the health services lacking in their communities
   4. Developing a hospital-based home health care service

   NCLEX Client Need: Safe and Effective Care Environment: Coordinated Care
4. The LVN/LPN in a long-term care facility is caring for a patient who is unable to feed or dress herself independently because of a neurologic disease. Her status is most accurately described as:
   1. Impaired
   2. Handicapped
   3. Disabled
   4. Disadvantaged

   NCLEX Client Need: Physiological Integrity: Basic Care and Comfort
5. A nurse who has been diagnosed with a chronic illness, a nursing school applicant with hearing impairment, and a patient with cancer are all protected from discrimination in employment because of their health problems by the:
   1. Social Security Act
   2. Americans with Disabilities Act
   3. Rehabilitation Act of 1973
   4. Vocational Rehabilitation Act

   NCLEX Client Need: Safe and Effective Care Environment: Coordinated Care

6. A patient who is being discharged from a rehabilitation facility is applying for Medicare coverage for home health nursing care. The LVN/LPN knows that Medicare will reimburse nursing care in the home only if the care meets which criteria? (Select all that apply.)
   1. Short-term
   2. Necessary
   3. Skilled
   4. Reasonable
   5. Intermittent

   NCLEX Client Need: Safe and Effective Care Environment: Coordinated Care
7. A patient who has suffered a head injury is feeding herself with considerable difficulty. In terms of rehabilitation, what is the most appropriate nursing response?
   1. Offer to feed her so that she will not be embarrassed by her handicap
   2. Order a liquid diet so that she will not have to use eating utensils
   3. Point out that the sooner she can feed herself, the sooner she can go home
   4. Ensure that her food is accessible and compliment her efforts at self-feeding

   NCLEX Client Need: Physiological Integrity: Basic Care and Comfort
8. A patient's record indicates that he is able to perform only 25% of his usual job activities since his motorcycle accident. This information is a measure of the extent of his:
   1. Handicap
   2. Disability
   3. Incapacity
   4. Impairment

   NCLEX Client Need: Physiological Integrity: Physiological Adaptation and Psychosocial Integrity
9. A nursing home resident has his name printed neatly on the door to his room. The interior of the room is decorated in masculine colors. One wall is covered with pictures of the resident at various occasions in his personal and professional life. In one corner is a leather recliner with a reading lamp and table. This room best reflects an effort to:
   1. Prevent depersonalization
   2. Maintain the resident's dignity
   3. Prevent regression
   4. Prevent social withdrawal

   NCLEX Client Need: Psychosocial Integrity
10. At a health class for older adults, one participant comments: "I guess we will all end up in a nursing home one day." The LVN/LPN can inform the group that the *best* indicator of who will need nursing home placement is:
    1. The medical diagnosis
    2. The availability of family caregivers
    3. Dependence in activities of daily living
    4. Financial resources

    NCLEX Client Need: Safe and Effective Care Environment: Coordinated Care

chapter 3

Legal and Ethical Considerations

http://evolve.elsevier.com/Linton/medsurg

Objectives

1. Define ethics, bioethics, values, morality, and moral or ethical dilemma.
2. Explain the principles of ethics: autonomy, justice, fidelity, beneficence, and nonmaleficence.
3. Explain how values are formed.
4. Explain how values clarification is useful in nursing practice.
5. Discuss the relationship between culture and values.
6. Describe the following philosophical bases for ethics: deontology, utilitarianism, feminist ethics, and ethics of care.
7. Describe the steps in processing ethical dilemmas.
8. Describe the role of institutional ethics committees.
9. Explain the role of the licensed vocational nurse/licensed practical nurse (LVN/LPN) in relation to informed consent.
10. Explain examples of intentional, quasi-intentional, and unintentional torts.
11. Use the NCSBN Model Nursing Practice Act and Standards of LVN/LPN Responsibilities to identify the role of the LVN/LPN in patient care.
12. Employ the NAPNES Standards for Nursing Practice to describe the LVN/LPN's range of capabilities, responsibilities, rights, and relationship to other health care providers.

Key Terms

Autonomy (ăh-TĂWN-ō-mē)
Beneficence (be-NEF-i-sens)
Bioethics (bī-ō-ĔTH-ĭks)
Confidentiality
Deontology (dē-ŏn-TŎL-ō-jē)
DNR (do not resuscitate) orders
Ethical dilemmas
Ethics
Ethics of care
Ethnocentrism (ĕth-nō-SĔN-trĭsm)
Feminist ethics
Informed consent
Justice (JŬS-tĭs)
Malpractice
Nonmaleficence (nŏn-mă-LĔF-ĭ-sĕns)
Risk management
Statutory laws (STĂCH-ū-tōr-ē)
Tort
Utilitarian (ū-tĭl-ĭ-TĀR-ē-ĕn)
Values
Values clarification
Veracity (vĕ-RĂ-sĭ-tē)

Nursing practice is guided by both ethical and legal principles. These topics are usually addressed in fundamentals but their importance merits a review in this text as we begin to address serious and often complicated medical-surgical and psychiatric conditions.

ETHICS

Ethics deals with values relevant to human conduct that are specific to a group. For example, nurses have professional codes of ethics. Ethics is concerned with defining what actions are right and wrong and whether the motives and outcomes of those actions are good or bad. If choices were simply two opposite actions, with one clearly good and one clearly bad, ethical decision making would be simple, but all choices are not simple. The choices are often shades of gray, not black and white, or a choice must be made between two good or two bad options. **Ethical dilemmas** are perplexing situations because ethics does not prescribe one right answer. Rather, ethics defines formal processes to explore what is proper conduct. **Bioethics** is concerned with the ethical questions that arise in the context of health care.

The concept of morality is closely related to ethics because moral beliefs provide a personal foundation for rules of action. Whereas ethics is prescribed by a given group, morals are the views of right and wrong held by an individual. For example, a patient might choose to discontinue renal dialysis knowing that he will die from renal failure. As a professional, the nurse knows that the patient has a right to make that decision. However, the nurse's personal moral beliefs might include the view that life should be preserved at all costs. Conflicts sometimes arise between the ethics of the profession and the nurse's personal beliefs or moral code. When no single solution seems to be satisfactory because of conflicting morals or ethical principles, an ethical dilemma exists. Nurses may feel powerless because their moral beliefs cannot be followed as a result of institutional or other barriers. These experiences are believed to be one reason that some nurses leave nursing, others experience "burnout," and still others seem to stop caring about their patients.

Put on Your Thinking Cap!

Describe a specific patient-care situation in which a nurse is likely to feel an ethical or moral dilemma. How might repeated similar incidents lead to job burnout? What can a hospital, clinic, or other institution do to help prevent such burnout?

PRINCIPLES OF ETHICS

When facing decisions that have no easy answers, nurses can consider options against each of the principles of health care ethics. The principles are autonomy, justice, fidelity, beneficence, and nonmaleficence (http://www.nursingworld.org/MainMenuCategories/EthicsStandards/CodeofEthicsforNurses/Code-of-Ethics.pdf). Respect for the rights of persons to make decisions about their own health and health care, such as accepting or refusing blood transfusions or medications, is based on the principle of **autonomy**. Recognition of autonomy is inherent in the concept of informed consent and in advance directives. **Beneficence** is another core value in nursing. To act with beneficence means that the nurse behaves in the patient's best interest. Beneficence incorporates actions to promote good, prevent harm, or remove the patient from harm. The problem with promoting *good* is to define what is good, recognizing that the patient, the family, the nurse, and the physician all may define it differently. An example of preventing harm is reporting a co-worker who is impaired or incompetent. **Justice** is concerned with fairness, equity, and appropriateness of treatment when considering what is due to a person. An important aspect of justice is the recognition that goods and services are limited so that giving to some means that others will not receive those goods or services (or both). An important role of the government is to devise and implement policies for the fair and equitable distribution of scarce resources. Decisions about who will receive limited resources can be based on various philosophies and might use the criteria of equal distribution; individual need, merit, social contribution, rights, or effort; or serving the greatest good for the greatest number of individuals. The principle of **nonmaleficence** requires that nurses "do no harm." Of course, instances occur when therapeutic interventions are uncomfortable but the benefits must be judged to justify the discomfort. A patient getting out of bed for the first time after surgery will likely experience some pain but the benefits of mobilization far outweigh temporary discomfort. Fidelity, or faithfulness, is a commitment to carry through on promises. Such promises may be spoken or implied. Patients in health care settings have the right to expect that staff will be committed to their care and will not abandon them. Another aspect of fidelity is the duty of the nurse to practice within the legal definition of the profession and to remain competent.

Nursing and other professions have sets of ethical principles that are accepted as basic to the profession. These principles may be set forth as a *code of ethics*, which defines expectations of conduct. Several documents define ethical codes for nurses but their common themes are accountability, responsibility, advocacy, confidentiality, and veracity. Nurses are accountable to themselves, their patients, their employers, the profession, and society. Adherence to standards of care is one way that nurses demonstrate accountability for their actions. A responsible nurse knows right from wrong and carries out duties in a knowledgeable and careful manner. Nurses demonstrate advocacy when they provide information to help the patient make an informed decision or when they speak up for the patient's wishes or rights. The **confidentiality** of patient information must be protected. Patients have the right to control who has access to personal information. Nurses must guard against the careless, accidental, or deliberate sharing of private information. **Veracity** (truth) requires that nurses be honest not only with patients, but also in documentation and communication with colleagues.

The code of ethics for the licensed vocational nurse/licensed practical nurse (LVN/LPN) as defined by the National Association for Practical Nurse Education and Service (NAPNES) is presented in Box 3-1.

VALUES

Values are specific beliefs and attitudes that are important to a person and that influence the choices the person makes on a daily basis. For example, one person may value kindness and honesty whereas another values financial success and material possessions. Our values affect our choice of friends, mates, and professions.

Values are learned as a result of cultural, social, and personal experiences. The family provides the foundation for values formation. Ideas about children and child rearing reflect not only how children are valued, but also what values will be rewarded. As the child's experiences extend beyond the family, some values are reinforced, some are challenged, and some new values are formed through contacts with peers, the church, schools, and the media. Modes by which values may

Box 3-1 National Association for Practical Nurse Education and Service (NAPNES) Code of Ethics for LVNs/LPNs

The LVN/LPN shall:

1. Consider as a basic obligation the conservation of life and the prevention of disease.
2. Promote and protect the physical, mental, emotional and spiritual health of the patient and the patient's family.
3. Fulfill all duties faithfully and efficiently.
4. Function within established legal guidelines.
5. Accept personal responsibility (for his or her acts), and seek to merit the respect and confidence of all members of the health team.
6. Hold in confidence all matters coming to his or her knowledge, in the practice of his or her profession, and in no way and at no time violate this confidence.
7. Give conscientious service and charge just remuneration.
8. Learn and respect the religious and cultural beliefs of his or her patient and of all people.
9. Meet his or her obligation to the patient by keeping abreast of current trends in health care through reading and continuing education.
10. As a citizen of the United States of America, uphold the laws of the land and seek to promote legislation that will meet the health needs of its people.

be acquired include copying role models (modeling), moralizing by authority figures, personal exploration, and experiences that are rewarded or punished. Values that have been identified as essential for professional nurses include altruism, equality, esthetics, freedom, human dignity, justice, and truth (American Association of Critical-Care Nurses, 1986).

Values Clarification

Professional education is an example of an experience that can profoundly influence a person's values. To help nursing students with acquiring values of the profession, the faculty encourages them to become aware of their personal values and how those values affect their behavior. This process is one of self-discovery, called **values clarification**. The value of this process is that a person learns to make choices from alternatives and to determine whether those choices were made carefully. Values clarification enables nurses not only to understand themselves better, but also to understand their patients and to help patients explore what is important to them. Nurses need to be aware of the tendency toward **ethnocentrism**—the belief that one's own culture (and its values) is superior to others (see the *Cultural Considerations* box).

Cultural Considerations

What Does Culture Have to Do with Values?

Ethnocentric beliefs about issues such as drug use and sexual orientation can influence a nurse's attitude toward patients so subtly that he or she might not even be aware of it. Values clarification helps nurses to be aware of their own values and to respect the values of others so that the patient receives optimal care regardless of a nurse's personal convictions.

Values Conflicts

The term *values conflict* is used when the values of individuals or institutions, or both, are different. In this situation, a risk exists that the patient's values may not be recognized or respected. As a nurse, you can recognize values conflicts by being aware of your own values and learning about those of your patients. A positive response to values conflicts is to try to understand the other person's views and to find common ground. Nurses sometimes experience values conflicts with employers who institute cost saving measures that nurses believe negatively affect the quality of care.

PHILOSOPHICAL BASES FOR ETHICS

Determining what is right or wrong (good or bad) is no simple task. The conclusions reached in various situations may vary depending on the philosophy that forms a base for a person's values. Some examples of philosophies that help to shape ethical principles are deontology, utilitarianism, feminist ethics, and ethics of care. **Deontology** defines right and wrong based on whether an action meets the criteria of fidelity, veracity, autonomy, beneficence, and justice. The consequences of the action are not considered. A limitation of deontology is apparent when an action represents conflicting values. For example, controlling the activity of a confused person may prevent harm (a good thing!) but may also interfere with autonomy (a bad thing?). From a **utilitarian** point of view, the "right" action is that which produces the greatest good for the greatest number of people. The challenge here is to come to agreement on what the "greatest good" is. Among human beings, there are bound to be differences in opinion as to what constitutes a good outcome. **Feminist ethics** focuses on inequalities among people, particularly based on gender, and places value on relationships. Closely related to feminist ethics is **ethics of care**, a theoretical viewpoint that care is a central activity of human behavior. This theorist would ask how particular actions reflect caring. The emphasis on relationships and patients' stories that reveal their uniqueness is quite different from theories that rely on universal principles.

STEPS IN PROCESSING ETHICAL DILEMMAS

Because of the emotional component in many ethical dilemmas, a guide for addressing them is recommended. The initial task is to decide whether the situation actually constitutes an ethical problem. An ethical problem has one or more of the following characteristics (Curtin, 2004, in Potter, Perry, Stockert, & Hall, 2013):

- Scientific information alone does not provide the answer.
- The problem is perplexing; that is, the answer is not simple.
- The solution is profoundly relevant to several areas of human concern.

During the data gathering process, participants need to consider their own values in relation to the problem or issue. Once it is agreed that the problem is an ethical one, the problem must be stated clearly so that all can agree on it. Next, possible courses of action and consequences are outlined. Options should be discussed in an atmosphere of mutual respect until agreement is reached. Action is then taken and the outcome is evaluated (Box 3-2).

Put on Your Thinking Cap!

Give an example of an ethical problem related to patient care that has been in the news recently. How does the issue or situation meet the three-part definition of an ethical problem?

INSTITUTIONAL ETHICS COMMITTEES

Health care providers deal with ethical issues frequently and are usually able to resolve problems with patients, families, and the health care team. Sometimes, however, formal help is needed. Most institutions have committees to process ethical dilemmas. The membership is usually multidisciplinary and seeks input from patients, families, professionals, and administrators. The functions of the ethics committee typically include education, policy recommendation, oversight of policy implementation, and consultation on specific cases.

Box 3-2 Key Steps in the Resolution of an Ethical Dilemma

- **Step 1:** Ask the question, is this issue an ethical dilemma? If a review of scientific data does not resolve the question, if the question is perplexing, and if the answer will have relevance for areas of human concern, an ethical dilemma probably exists.
- **Step 2:** Gather information relevant to the case. Patient, family, institutional, and social perspectives are important sources of relevant information.
- **Step 3:** Clarify values. Distinguish among fact, opinion, and values.
- **Step 4:** Verbalize the problem. A clear, simple statement of the dilemma is not always easy, but it helps to ensure effectiveness in the final plan and facilitates discussion.
- **Step 5:** Identify possible courses of action.
- **Step 6:** Negotiate a plan. Negotiation requires a confidence in one's own point of view and a deep respect for the opinions of others.
- **Step 7:** Evaluate the plan over time.

From Ecker, M: Ethics and values. In Potter PA, Perry AG, Stockert PA, Hall AM (eds): *Fundamentals of nursing*, ed 8, St. Louis, 2013, Mosby Elsevier.

LEGAL IMPLICATIONS FOR NURSING PRACTICE

The law defines the boundaries of nursing practice. Nurses are obligated to know their legal functions and limitations to protect both their patients and themselves. A nursing license is granted only to persons who have met specific educational standards and demonstrated the minimal required level of knowledge as assessed by an examination. The state board of nursing can revoke or suspend the license of a nurse who violates the provisions of the licensing statutes. The scope of LVN/LPN practice is outlined in the National Council of State Boards of Nursing (NCSBN) Model Nursing Practice Act (see the *Coordinated Care* boxes).

Coordinated Care

NCSBN Model Nursing Practice Act

Boards of Nursing publish standards of nursing care to communicate broad expectations and to guide nurses for safe and effective practice. Professional and specialty organizations may develop more detailed, specific standards intended to promote excellence in clinical practice. According to the National Council of State Boards of Nursing (2011):

- Practice as a LPN/VN means a directed scope of nursing practice, with or without compensation or personal profit, under the supervision of an RN, advanced practice registered nurse (APRN), licensed physician, or health care provider authorized by the state; is guided by nursing standards established or recognized by the BON [Board of Nursing]; and includes, but is not limited to:
- Collecting data and conducting focused nursing assessments of the health status of individuals.

  A focused assessment* is an appraisal of an individual's status and situation at hand, contributing to comprehensive assessment by the RN, supporting ongoing data collection, and deciding who needs to be informed of the information and when to inform.**
- Planning nursing care episodes for individuals with stable conditions.
- Participating in the development and modification of the comprehensive plan of care for all types of clients.
- Implementing appropriate aspects of the strategy of care within a client-centered health care plan.

Coordinated Care—cont'd

- Communicating and collaborating with other health care professionals.
- Providing input into the development of policies and procedures.
- Other acts that require education and training as prescribed by the BON, commensurate with the LPN/VN's experience, continuing education and demonstrated LPN/VN competencies.

Each nurse is accountable to clients, the nursing profession and the BON for complying with the requirements of this Act and for ensuring the quality of nursing care rendered, for recognizing limits of knowledge and experience, and for planning for the management of situations beyond the nurse's expertise.

From National Council of State Boards of Nursing: *Model Nursing Practice Act.* www.ncsbn.org/Model_Nursing_Practice_Act_March 2011.pdf. Accessed March 19, 2013.

*The first step in the nursing process assessment is the basis for nursing decisions and interventions. The subcommittee believes that the first step is implemented in much the same way across jurisdictions, but that it is described and discussed very differently. The subcommittee members believe that both LPN/VNs and RN assess, but the members identified a significant difference in the breadth, depth, and comprehensiveness of the assessments conducted by the two levels of licensed nurses. These differences are reflected in the term "focused assessment" to describe the LPN/VN role in the first step of the nursing process and the term comprehensive assessment to describe the role of the RN. An alternative for BONs that have difficulty with the term assessment is to not use the term with either LPN/VN or RN practice, but rather describe what is expected of the level of licensee for the first step of the nursing process.

**Additions to the LPN/VN scope of practice are based on analysis of the various elements that make up this scope, as evidenced by the most recent LPN/VN job analysis. This remains a directed scope of practice.

Coordinated Care

Standards Related to LVN/LPN Professional Accountability

The National Council of State Boards of Nursing (2011) details specific standards that relate to professional accountability, membership on an interdisciplinary health care team, and nursing practice implementation. Standards related to LVN/LPN professional accountability include the following:

- Practices within the legal boundaries for practical nursing through the scope of practice authorized in the Model Nursing Practice Act (MNPA) and rules governing nursing
- Demonstrates honesty and integrity in nursing practice
- Bases nursing decisions on nursing knowledge and skills, the needs of the clients, and the expectations delineated by the Board of Nursing (BON)
- Accepts responsibility for individual nursing actions, competence, decisions, and behavior in the course of practical nursing practice
- Maintains continued competence through ongoing learning and application of knowledge in the client's interest

From National Council of State Boards of Nursing: NCSBN Model Nursing Practice Act and Model Nursing Administrative Rules. https://www.ncsbn.org/Model_Nursing_Practice_Act_March2011.pdf. Accessed March 19, 2013.

Coordinated Care

Standards Related to LVN/LPN Responsibilities for Nursing Practice Implementation

The LVN/LPN, practicing under the direction of an RN, advanced practice registered nurse (APRN), licensed physician, or other authorized licensed health care provider:

- Conducts a focused nursing assessment, which is an appraisal of the client's status and situation at hand that contributes to ongoing data collection
- Plans for episodic nursing care
- Demonstrates attentiveness and provides client surveillance and monitoring
- Assists in identification of client needs
- Seeks clarification of orders when needed
- Assists in the evaluation of the impact of nursing care. Contributes to the evaluation of client care
- Recognizes client characteristics that may affect the client's health status
- Obtains orientation/training for competency when encountering new equipment and technology or unfamiliar care situations
- Implements appropriate aspects of client care in a timely manner:
  - Provides assigned and delegated aspects of client's health care plan
  - Implements treatments and procedures
  - Administers medications accurately
- Documents care provided
- Communicates relevant and timely client information with other health team members
  - Client status and progress
  - Client responses or lack of response to therapies
  - Significant changes in client condition
  - Client needs
- Participates in nursing management:
  - Assigns nursing activities to other LVNs/LPNs
  - Delegates nursing activities for stable clients to assistive personnel

Continued

Coordinated Care—cont'd

- Observes nursing measures and provides feedback to the nursing manager
- Observes and communicates outcomes of delegated and assigned activities
- Takes preventive measures to protect client, others, and self
- Respects the client's rights, concerns, decisions, and dignity (This standard includes respecting the client's concerns regarding end-of-life care.)
- Attends to client or family concerns or requests
- Promotes a safe client environment
- Maintains appropriate professional boundaries
- Assumes responsibility for the nurse's own decisions and actions

From National Council of State Boards of Nursing. NCSBN Model Nursing Practice Act and Model Nursing Administrative Rules. https://www.ncsbn.org/Model_Nursing_Practice_Act_March2011.pdf. Accessed March 19, 2013.

Coordinated Care

Standards Related to LVN/LPN Responsibilities as a Member of an Interdisciplinary Health Care Team

- Functions as a member of the health care team, contributing to the implementation of an integrated health care plan
- Respects client property and the property of others
- Protects confidential information unless obligated by law to disclose the information

The Model Nursing Practice Act (MNPA) includes delegation of tasks and functions by LVNs/LPNs in specified settings but acknowledges that some states do not authorize LVN/LPN delegation. In states that permit delegation, the MNPA notes that delegated tasks, functions, or activities must be "appropriate to the skill of the nursing assistive personnel and within the range of functions as defined by the board of nursing for the level of nursing assistive personnel." Nursing assistive personnel include the medication assistant/medication aide and nursing assistant/nurse aide. Chapter 4 addresses delegation in greater detail.

From National Council of State Boards of Nursing. NCSBN Model Nursing Practice Act and Model Nursing Administrative Rules. https://www.ncsbn.org/Model_Nursing_Practice_Act_March2011.pdf. Accessed March 19, 2013.

Coordinated Care

NAPNES Standards for Nursing Practice

The standards for nursing practice and educational competencies of graduates of LVN/LPN programs as defined by the National Association for Practical Nurse Education and Service (NAPNES, 2009) define the LVN/LPN's range of capabilities, responsibilities, rights and relationship to other health care providers. It addresses the standards as Professional Behaviors, Communication, Assessment, Planning, Caring Interventions, and Managing.

NAPNES STANDARDS OF PRACTICE AND EDUCATIONAL COMPETENCIES OF GRADUATES OF PRACTICAL/VOCATIONAL NURSING PROGRAMS

Professional Behaviors

Professional behaviors, within the scope of nursing practice for a practical/vocational nurse, are characterized by adherence to standards of care, accountability for one's own actions and behaviors, and use of legal and ethical principles in nursing practice. Professionalism includes a commitment to nursing and a concern for others demonstrated by an attitude of caring. Professionalism also involves participation in lifelong self-development activities to enhance and maintain current knowledge and skills for continuing competency in the practice of nursing for the LP/VN, as well as individual, group, community and societal endeavors to improve health care.

Upon completion of the practical/vocational nursing program the graduate will display the following program outcome:

Demonstrate professional behaviors of accountability and professionalism according to the legal and ethical standards for a competent licensed practical/vocational nurse.

Competencies which demonstrate this outcome has been attained:

1. Comply with the ethical, legal, and regulatory frameworks of nursing and the scope of practice as outlined in the LP/VN nurse practice act of the specific state in which licensed.
2. Utilize educational opportunities for lifelong learning and maintenance of competence.
3. Identify personal capabilities, and consider career mobility options.
4. Identify own LP/VN strengths and limitations for the purpose of improving nursing performance.
5. Demonstrate accountability for nursing care provided by self and/or directed to others.
6. Function as an advocate for the health care consumer, maintaining confidentiality as required.
7. Identify the impact of economic, political, social, cultural, spiritual, and demographic forces on the role

Coordinated Care—cont'd

of the licensed practical/vocational nurse in the delivery of health care.

8. Serve as a positive role model within health care settings and the community.
9. Participate as a member of a practical/vocational nursing organization.

Communication

Communication is defined as the process by which information is exchanged between individuals verbally, nonverbally, and/or in writing or through information technology. Communication abilities are integral and essential to the nursing process. Those who are included in the nursing process are the licensed practical/vocational nurse and other members of the nursing and health care team, client, and significant support person(s). Effective communication demonstrates caring, compassion, and cultural awareness, and is directed toward promoting positive outcomes and establishing a trusting relationship.

Upon completion of the practical/vocational nursing program the graduate will display the following program outcome:

Effectively communicate with patients, significant support person(s), and members of the interdisciplinary health care team, incorporating interpersonal and therapeutic communication skills.

Competencies which demonstrate this outcome has been attained:

1. Utilize effective communication skills when interacting with clients, significant others, and members of the interdisciplinary health care team.
2. Communicate relevant, accurate, and complete information.
3. Report to appropriate health care personnel and document assessments, interventions, and progress or impediments toward achieving client outcomes.
4. Maintain organizational and client confidentiality.
5. Utilize information technology to support and communicate the planning and provision of client care.
6. Utilize appropriate channels of communication.

Assessment

Assessment is the collection and processing of relevant data for the purpose of appraising the client's health status. Assessment provides a holistic view of the client which includes physical, developmental, emotional, psychosocial, cultural, spiritual, and functional status. Assessment involves the collection of information from multiple sources to provide the foundation for nursing care. Initial assessment provides the baseline for future comparisons in order to individualize client care. Ongoing assessment is required to meet the client's changing needs.

Upon completion of the practical/vocational nursing program the graduate will display the following program outcome:

Collect holistic assessment data from multiple sources, communicate the data to appropriate health care providers, and evaluate client responses to interventions.

Competencies which demonstrate this outcome has been attained:

1. Assess data related to basic physical, developmental, spiritual, cultural, functional, and psychosocial needs of the client.
2. Collect data within established protocols and guidelines from various sources, including client interviews, observations/measurements, health care team members, family, significant other(s), and review of health records.
3. Assess data related to the client's health status, identify impediments to client progress, and evaluate response to interventions.
4. Document data collection, assessment, and communicate findings to appropriate members of the health care team.

Planning

Planning encompasses the collection of health status information, the use of multiple methods to access information, and the analysis and integration of knowledge and information to formulate nursing care plans and care actions. The nursing care plan provides direction for individualized care and assures the delivery of accurate, safe care through a definitive pathway that promotes the client's and the support persons' progress toward positive outcomes.

Upon completion of the practical/vocational nursing program the graduate will display the following program outcome:

Collaborate with the registered nurse or other members of the health care team to organize and incorporate assessment data to plan/revise patient care and actions based on established nursing diagnoses, nursing protocols, and assessment and evaluation data.

Competencies which demonstrate this outcome has been attained:

1. Utilize knowledge of normal values to identify deviation in health status to plan care.
2. Contribute to formulation of a nursing care plan for clients with noncomplex conditions and in a stable state, in consultation with the registered nurse, and, as appropriate, in collaboration with the client or support persons, as well as members of the interdisciplinary health care team, using established nursing diagnoses and nursing protocols.
3. Prioritize nursing care needs of clients.
4. Assist in the review and revision of nursing care plans with the registered nurse to meet the changing needs of clients.
5. Modify client care as indicated by the evaluation of stated outcomes.
6. Provide information to client about aspects of the care plan within the LP/VN scope of practice.
7. Refer the client, as appropriate, to other members of the health care team about care outside the scope of practice of the LP/VN.

Caring Interventions

Caring interventions are those nursing behaviors and actions that assist clients and significant others in meeting their needs and the identified outcomes of the plan of care. These interventions are based on knowledge of the natural sciences, behavioral sciences, and past nursing experiences. Caring is the "being with" and "doing for" that assists clients to achieve the desired outcomes. Caring behaviors are nurturing, protective, compassionate, and person-centered. Caring creates an environment of hope and trust where client choices related to

Continued

Coordinated Care—cont'd

cultural, religious, and spiritual values, beliefs, and lifestyles are respected.

On completion of the practical/vocational nursing program the graduate will display the following program outcome:

Demonstrate a caring and empathic approach to the safe, therapeutic, and individualized care of each client.

Competencies which demonstrate this outcome has been attained:

1. Provide and promote the client's dignity.
2. Identify and honor the emotional, cultural, religious, and spiritual influences on the client's health.
3. Demonstrate caring behaviors toward the client and significant support persons.
4. Provide competent, safe, therapeutic, and individualized nursing care in a variety of settings.
5. Provide a safe physical and psychosocial environment for the client and significant others.
6. Implement the prescribed care regimen within the legal, ethical, and regulatory framework of practical/vocational nursing practice.
7. Assist the client and significant support persons to cope with and adapt to stressful events and changes in health status.
8. Assist the client and significant others to achieve optimum comfort and functioning.
9. Instruct the client regarding individualized health needs in keeping with the licensed practical/vocational nurse's knowledge, competence, and scope of practice.
10. Recognize the client's right to access information and refer requests to appropriate persons.
11. Act in an advocacy role to protect client rights.

Managing

Managing care is the effective use of human, physical, financial, and technological resources to achieve the client identified outcomes while supporting organizational outcomes. The LP/VN manages care through the processes of planning, organizing, and directing.

Upon completion of the practical/vocational nursing program the graduate will display the following program outcome:

Implement patient care, at the direction of a registered nurse, licensed physician, or dentist, through performance of nursing interventions or directing aspects of care, as appropriate, to unlicensed assistive personnel (UAP).

Competencies which demonstrate this outcome has been attained:

1. Assist in the coordination and implementation of an individualized plan of care for clients and significant support persons.
2. Direct aspects of client care to qualified UAPs commensurate with abilities and level of preparation and consistent with the state's legal and regulatory framework for the scope of practice for the LP/VN.
3. Supervise and evaluate the activities of UAPs and other personnel as appropriate within the state's legal and regulatory framework for the scope of practice for the LP/VN as well as facility policy.
4. Maintain accountability for outcomes of care directed to qualified UAPs.
5. Organize nursing activities in a meaningful and cost-effective manner when providing nursing care for individuals or groups.
6. Assist the client and significant support persons to access available resources and services.
7. Demonstrate competence with current technologies.
8. Function within the defined scope of practice for the LP/VN in the health care delivery system at the direction of a registered nurse, licensed physician, or dentist.

As approved and adopted by NAPNES Board of Directors, May 6, 2007. http://napnes.org/drupal-7.4/sites/default/files/pdf/standards/standards_read_only.pdf. Accessed March 20, 2013.

TYPES OF LAW

Laws that guide nursing practice are derived from three types of law: statutory, regulatory, and common law. Laws created by elected legislative bodies, including nurse practice acts, are **statutory laws**. The legal boundaries of nursing practice in a given state are defined and described in nurse practice acts. Statutory law is classified as either civil or criminal. Criminal laws are concerned with preventing or punishing harm to society, whereas civil laws protect individual rights. Crimes are classified as felonies or misdemeanors. A felony is a serious crime and a misdemeanor is a crime that is less serious than a felony. Administrative bodies such as state boards of nursing create regulatory laws in the form of rules and regulations that address the conduct of nurses. Common law is the result of judicial decisions made when individual cases are decided in the courts.

Tort

A civil wrong against a person or property is called a **tort.** Torts are classified as intentional, quasi-intentional, or unintentional. *Intentional torts* are willful acts that violate a person's rights. Examples are assault, battery, false imprisonment, and defamation of character. Nursing students may be surprised to learn that some nursing actions can be considered torts. For example, assault is a threat of some contact without the patient's consent. If a nurse threatens to restrain or medicate a person against his or her wishes, the patient can claim assault by the nurse. If the patient is actually touched in an offensive or harmful manner without consent, the nurse can be accused of battery. For both assault and battery, the key issue is whether the patient consented to the action. False imprisonment occurs when a person is restrained or restricted to an area without justification and without legal warrant. The individual must be aware of the confinement.

Examples of *quasi-intentional torts* are invasion of privacy and defamation of character. Patients have the right to be protected against unwanted intrusion into their private affairs. When that right is violated, the patient can claim invasion of privacy. Examples of invasion of privacy can include improper release of medical information, publication of patient photographs, and distributing information or images through social media. If false information that might damage a person's reputation is released, a charge of defamation of character can be made. If the information is spoken, it is called *slander;* if written, it is called *libel*.

Unintentional torts include negligence and malpractice. Negligent conduct is that which falls below the standard of care. Professional negligence is called **malpractice**. To be found liable for malpractice, the following conditions must be met: The nurse owed a duty to the patient, the nurse did not carry out that duty, the patient was injured, and the injury was caused by the nurse's failure to carry out the duty. Examples of common negligent acts are listed in Box 3-3.

The nurse's best protection against negligence and malpractice is to adhere to standards of care. Other measures are to provide competent care; communicate with other members of the health care team; fully document assessments, interventions, and evaluations; and establish good relations with patients (Potter, Perry, Stockert, & Hall, 2013).

Student nurses are held to the same standards of care as are licensed nurses. Students should never perform care for which they have not been prepared. When nursing students are employed as nursing assistants, they must perform only tasks that are within the job description of the nursing assistant, even if they have acquired additional skills as nursing students. For more information on scope of practice, standards of care, and professional responsibility and accountability for LVNs/LPNs, see the *Coordinated Care* boxes.

Box 3-3 Common Negligent Acts

- Failure to assess and/or monitor
- Failure to monitor in a timely fashion
- Failure to use proper equipment to monitor the patient
- Failure to document the monitoring
- Failure to notify the health care provider of problems
- Failure to follow orders
- Failure to follow the six rights of medication administration
- Failure to convey discharge instructions
- Failure to ensure patient safety, especially that of patients who have a history of falling, are heavily sedated, have disequilibrium problems, are frail, are mentally impaired, get up in the night, and are uncooperative.
- Failure to follow policies and procedures
- Failure to properly delegate and supervise (as permitted within state laws)

Adapted from Durbin CR: Legal implications in nursing practice. In Potter PA, Perry AG, Stockert PA, Hall AM (eds): *Fundamentals of nursing*, ed 8, St. Louis, 2013, Mosby Elsevier.

Malpractice Insurance

Health care institutions commonly provide malpractice insurance for nurses they employ. This coverage generally covers legal fees and awards if a nurse is sued for professional negligence or medical malpractice. However, if the act in question occurs outside the place of employment, the agency insurance does not cover the nurse. Therefore nurses need to decide whether to carry personal liability insurance as well. Seeking legal advice regarding this decision is wise (Durbin, 2013).

At times, nurses administer assistance at the scene of accidents. As long as nurses' actions are within accepted standards, Good Samaritan laws protect them from liability. Because state laws vary, nurses should acquaint themselves with the laws in their states of residence (Durbin, 2013).

LEGAL CONSIDERATIONS IN SPECIFIC SITUATIONS

Confidentiality

Nurses have access to volumes of extremely private information that must be protected. Patients have a right to expect that their personal information, including medical diagnoses and treatment, be kept confidential. Therefore you must protect the privacy of patient records and avoid public discussion of patient information. Never copy or remove any part of a patient's record. If you make notes about patients or write care plans for nursing school assignments, do not include identifying information such as the patient's name, initials, or Social Security number. Such assignments should be shared only with your instructor. The Health Insurance Portability and Accountability Act (HIPAA) laws that went into effect in 2003 have made health care providers acutely aware of the actions needed to protect patient confidentiality. Your employing agency should have written policies for informing patients of their rights and how their health care information can be used (Box 3-4).

Put on Your Thinking Cap!

A pregnant patient's partner accompanies her to an appointment with her obstetrician. Later that afternoon, the partner calls the clinic to ask a question about the woman's care. Can you discuss her medical record with the partner? Is your answer the same if the partner's name is noted in the patient's record as being the father of the child?

Consent

The ethical principle of autonomy mandates that patients have the right to make decisions about their own care and that caregivers should not impose care against the patient's wishes. The term **informed consent**

Box 3-4 What Does the Health Insurance Portability and Accountability Act (HIPAA) Mean?

- Written permission is required to disclose protected health information if it is not for treatment, payment, or health care operations.
- Clinics or offices can have patients register on a "sign-in" sheet if no sensitive data are available for others to see.
- With the patient's permission, you can inform clergy that a church member is in the facility.
- Informal consent may be obtained to include patient names and condition in a provider directory.
- Do not post names with medical diagnoses, surgical procedures, or any other protected information where it can be seen by persons not involved in the patient's care.
- Do not give health care information to a patient's family or other persons without the patient's permission.
- Visit the US Department of Health and Human Services for more information (http://www.hhs.gov/ocr/privacy/).

Adapted from Brooke PS: Understanding HIPAA compliance, *LPN* 1(4):37–39, 2005; and US Department of Health and Human Services: Summary of the HIPAA Privacy Rule. http://www.hhs.gov/ocr/privacy/hipaa/understanding/summary/index.html.

means that health care providers must provide sufficient information for the patient to make an informed decision. The essential elements of informed consent are patient decision-making capacity, sufficient information, and voluntary agreement.

State law defines who can give consent, including who can give consent for minors or persons who are not capable of making their own decisions. Remember that a confused or sedated person cannot give consent even if that person is usually capable of making decisions. Therefore signatures on consent forms must be obtained before administering sedating drugs such as preoperative medications. For the patient to have sufficient information for informed consent, the person must have been advised of risks, benefits, alternatives, and consequences of refusing the treatment. A patient has the right to have all questions answered. Consent must be voluntary; real or implied coercion cannot be used. That is, the patient must be making the decision freely without fear of retaliation for refusal or because of expectation of some real or implied reward beyond the medical benefit.

In various health care settings, you should know the agency policies regarding procedures requiring signed consent forms. They are required for hospital admission, surgery, some treatments, and research participation. The physician is responsible for obtaining informed consent. Nurses may obtain patient signatures and serve as witnesses to the signature as agency policy permits. The nurse should ask the patient if he or she understands the procedure. If the nurse suspects the patient lacks decision-making capacity or does not fully understand the implications of the consent form, the physician should be contacted and the supervisor notified. When a nurse signs the consent form as a witness, that nurse is confirming that the patient gave voluntary consent, that the patient's signature is authentic, and that the patient appears competent to consent.

Physicians' Orders

Legal, appropriate physicians' orders should be carried out. If the nurse believes that an order is erroneous or inappropriate, the physician should be contacted for confirmation or correction. If the physician confirms the order and the LVN/LPN still believes that the order is inappropriate, the nurse should contact the supervisor to intervene. The nurse may share legal responsibility for harm that follows implementation of an inappropriate order. Verbal orders increase the risk for error; follow agency policy regarding verbal orders.

DNR (Do Not Resuscitate) Orders

Sometimes a decision is made by the patient or other decision maker in consultation with the health care team that resuscitation will not be initiated if a patient ceases to breathe or the heart stops. Once such a decision is made, **DNR (do not resuscitate) orders** should be written and they should be reviewed regularly in case the patient's status changes. Nurses are encouraged to talk with patients and, if appropriate, with patients' families to help them understand the practical and legal implications of a DNR order. In many states, in the absence of a written order, the assumption is that resuscitation is appropriate.

Put on Your Thinking Cap!

What are some reasons a mentally competent person might choose to sign a DNR order in the event that his or her breathing ceases or his heart stops?

Short Staffing

When nurses believe that staffing is inadequate to provide competent care, the supervisor should be notified. A written protest should be submitted when a nurse is required to accept an assignment without adequate staffing. Walking out or refusing an assignment might be viewed as patient abandonment. Nurses should know their state regulations and agency policies for such situations. For example, the Texas Nurse Practice Act focuses on the nurse's duty to the patient and emphasizes that "the nurse's duty is not defined by any single event such as clocking in or taking report." Actions that might be interpreted as patient abandonment include sleeping on the job, leaving in the middle of a shift without notifying anyone, failing to show up or complete an agreed-upon assignment in a home setting, and leaving the patient care area and remaining unavailable such that patient safety may be compromised. In some settings, a nurse may be able to invoke "safe harbor" if given an assignment that the nurse believes violates his or her duty to the patient. Safe harbor protects nurses from actions against their license when they notify the supervisor at the time the assignment is made. Again, agency policies and state law must be considered by the individual nurse.

Floating

Nurses are obligated to inform supervisors if they lack the skill to care for particular patients. Nurses who float to new units must be oriented to the setting and trained for the new area.

Coordinated Care

The National Council of State Boards of Nursing (NCSBN): A Resource for LVNs/LPNs

More detailed information about the legal roles and responsibilities of the LVN/LPN are available at the website of the National Council of State Boards of Nursing (www.ncsbn.org) and from individual state licensing bodies. The following is a sampling of what you will find on the NCSBN website:

- A list of legal requirements for becoming a licensed LVN/LPN, including an NCLEX® candidate bulletin and fact sheet
- Complete, current contact information for the board of nursing in your state, including a link to the board's website
- Information about the progress of the NCSBN in developing continued competence assessments for nurses
- The NCSBN's position statements on the issue of working with nursing assistive personnel (NAP), also known as unlicensed assistive personnel (UAP)
- A delegation decision-making tree and grid, as well as a concept paper that outlines practical guidelines for delegating responsibilities
- The Five Rights of Delegation

Right to Refuse Treatment

Patients have the right to refuse medical treatment, including life-sustaining care. When patients are not competent to make their own decisions, an effort is made to determine what the person would have wanted. Advance directives help to define the patient's wishes. Highly publicized cases, such as that of Theresa Schiavo, have increased public awareness of the importance of making one's wishes known in writing while still able to make decisions. See Chapter 24 for a more complete discussion of legal and ethical issues related to death and dying.

RISK MANAGEMENT

Risk management aims to identify potential hazards and eliminate them before harm occurs. Organizations usually have a formal structure to identify actual or potential risks, analyze the risks, take action to reduce the risks, and evaluate the effectiveness of the actions taken. To illustrate, four residents in a nursing home have fallen in the past week. Risk management processes can be employed to analyze the falls to determine contributing factors. Preventive measures would be identified and implemented. The effectiveness of the interventions would be measured weekly and revised as needed. To analyze actual or potential risks, accurate documentation of events such as falls or medication errors is essential. Agencies have occurrence reports, also called incident reports, to provide a record of the incident. Occurrence reports are submitted in accordance with agency policy and are retained separate from the patient record. The nurse would document the event in the patient record but would not include the information that an occurrence report was completed (Durbin, 2013).

SUMMARY

Patient care is much more than simply the management of the effects of illness or injury. The clinical decision-making process must continually screen decisions against the guidelines for ethical conduct. Understanding values, ethics, legal constraints, and the process of resolving ethical dilemmas will facilitate the LVN/LPN in providing care that is not only safe, but also ethical.

Get Ready for the NCLEX® Examination!

Key Points

- Ethics deals with values relevant to human conduct that are specific to a group (e.g., professional ethics).
- Morality is an individual's set of principles, judgments, and beliefs about what is right and wrong. When moral or ethical principles conflict, an ethical dilemma exists.
- Informed consent and advance directives give patients autonomy (self-determination) by allowing them to make their own health care decisions.
- A core nursing value is beneficence, or acting in the patient's best interest. Another core value is justice, or fair, equitable, and appropriate treatment in the setting of scarce goods and services.
- The principle of nonmaleficence requires that the nurse not harm the patient, but this idea must weigh the patient's short-term discomfort against long-term treatment goals.
- Fidelity, or faithfulness, is a spoken, written, or implied commitment to provide appropriate, competent patient care within the professional's scope of practice.
- Accountability and responsibility are key aspects of nurses' professional code of ethics. In addition, nurses

must provide advocacy for their patients' needs, protect the confidentiality of patients' medical records, and maintain veracity (truthfulness) in written and spoken communication with patients and colleagues.

- Values are the beliefs and attitudes that underpin our personal and professional choices. Sometimes, our values tend to be ethnocentric, or biased toward our own religious and cultural belief systems.
- Professional education and training can assist in the process of values clarification, which allows us to discover how our values affect our behavior.
- Philosophical frameworks that provide the basis for various ethical belief systems include deontology, utilitarianism, feminist ethics, and ethics of care.
- Ethical problems are complex, cannot be resolved with scientific information alone, and are broadly relevant to other areas of human endeavor.
- Nursing practice is governed by laws that define nurses' functions for their protection and that of their patients.
- Tort law is a specific kind of civil law that classifies violations into intentional, quasi-intentional, and unintentional torts. Malpractice, or professional negligence, is an unintentional tort.
- Informed consent means that a nonsedated adult patient who is sufficiently able to make voluntary decisions is given the information necessary to agree to a procedure or course of treatment.
- A written, legally binding DNR order ensures that a patient will not be resuscitated against his or her wishes.

Additional Learning Resources

SG Go to your Study Guide for additional learning activities to help you master this chapter content.

evolve Go to your Evolve website (http://evolve.elsevier.com/Linton/medsurg) for the following learning resources and much more:

- Interactive Prioritization Exercises
- Fluid & Electrolyte Tutorial
- Pharmacology Tutorial
- Review Questions for the NCLEX® Examination

Review Questions for the NCLEX® Examination

1. Nursing students are discussing the role of ethics in nursing practice. Which statements are true regarding ethics in nursing? (Select all that apply.)
   1. It deals with issues of human conduct.
   2. It is concerned with defining right and wrong actions.
   3. It does not consider whether motives are good or bad.
   4. It prescribes the right answer when an ethical dilemma is present.
   5. It defines processes to explore factors that constitute proper conduct.

   NCLEX Client Need: Safe and Effective Care Environment: Coordinated Care
2. Nursing staff are discussing an ethical dilemma related to one of their patients. The LVN/LPN reminds them that an ethical choice is one that promotes good, prevents harm, and/or removes the patient from harm. This guideline reflects which core nursing value?
   1. Malfeasance
   2. Beneficence
   3. Autonomy
   4. Veracity

   NCLEX Client Need: Safe and Effective Care Environment: Coordinated Care
3. Which choice suggests that a situation poses an ethical dilemma?
   1. A personal injury attorney has filed a lawsuit.
   2. Scientific information alone does not provide the answer.
   3. Government agencies have been unable to agree on a course of action.
   4. Legislation has been proposed but not enacted into law.

   NCLEX Client Need: Safe and Effective Care Environment: Coordinated Care
4. Nursing students are discussing their clinical experiences. Their instructor reminds them that the confidentiality of patient information is protected by which law?
   1. NAPNES Code of Ethics for LVNs/LPNs
   2. Patient Protection and Affordable Care Act (ACA)
   3. Health Insurance Portability and Accountability Act (HIPAA)
   4. Model Nursing Practice Act (MNPA)

   NCLEX Client Need: Safe and Effective Care Environment: Coordinated Care
5. An LVN/LPN is caring for all of the preoperative patients described here. Which one of these patients is able to give legal consent to his or her own treatment?
   1. A 17-year-old honor student who has been accepted to the nursing program at a local college
   2. A 70-year-old recently retired man who is showing unexplained signs of confusion
   3. A 25-year-old immigrant whose husband says that she understands the procedure although she does not speak English
   4. A 35-year-old pregnant woman who says that she *does* understand the proposed procedure, benefits, and risks

   NCLEX Client Need: Safe and Effective Care Environment: Coordinated Care

6. A new patient's admission orders include a DNR order. Which statement(s) about DNR orders is/are true? (Select all that apply.)
   1. The orders should be reviewed regularly in case the patient's status changes.
   2. Even if a written order exists, the physician on call may legally choose to resuscitate a patient if he or she thinks survival is likely.
   3. If a patient is especially ill or is an older adult, the health care team may decide not to resuscitate even when there is no DNR order.
   4. The health care institution cannot be held liable for ignoring DNR orders if staffing falls below a predetermined minimal level.
   5. Individual nurses must decide whether to honor the DNR based on personal beliefs.

   NCLEX Client Need: Safe and Effective Care Environment: Coordinated Care
7. According to the NAPNES Standards of Practice and Educational Competencies of Graduates of Practical/Vocational Nursing Programs, graduates of LVN/LPN programs are able to: (Select all that apply.)
   1. Incorporate interpersonal and therapeutic communication skills
   2. Collect comprehensive assessment data from multiple sources
   3. Independently plan or revise patient plans of care
   4. Demonstrate a caring and empathic approach to the care of each client
   5. Demonstrate professional behaviors according to legal and ethical standards

   NCLEX Client Need: Safe and Effective Care Environment: Coordinated Care
8. An LVN/LPN performs a focused assessment on his patients. According to the NCSBN Model Nursing Practice Act, which option or options correctly describe how a focused assessment should be used? (Select all that apply.)
   1. To support ongoing data collection
   2. To yield a comprehensive evaluation of all available patient data
   3. To substitute for the registered nurse's assessment
   4. To appraise an individual's status and situation at hand
   5. To collect data needed by other health care team members

   NCLEX Client Need: Safe and Effective Care Environment: Coordinated Care
9. In a state where the law permits LVNs/LPNs to delegate to nursing assistive personnel, what factor or factors determine the tasks, functions, or activities that can be delegated? (Select all that apply.)
   1. The willingness of the nursing assistive personnel to perform the task
   2. The knowledge and skill of the nursing assistive personnel
   3. Nursing assistive personnel functions as defined by the board of nursing
   4. Patient consent for the nursing assistive personnel to perform the task
   5. The previous work experience of the individual nursing assistive personnel

   NCLEX Client Need: Safe and Effective Care Environment: Coordinated Care
10. All of the following were observed in patient care settings. According to HIPAA, which violates a patient's privacy?
    1. In a long-term care facility, patients' names are written on a card by their door.
    2. A nurse provides information about a patient's status to a relative with the patient's permission.
    3. Patients in a clinic sign in on a sheet of paper with no sensitive information.
    4. A surgical schedule including patients' names and diagnoses is posted where staff and visitors can see it.
    5. On the patient's request, the nurse notifies a patient's clergyman of the patient's admission.

    NCLEX Client Need: Safe and Effective Care Environment: Coordinated Care

chapter 4

The Leadership Role of the Licensed Practical Nurse

http://evolve.elsevier.com/Linton/medsurg

Linda Porter-Wenzlaff

Objectives

1. Differentiate leadership from management.
2. Describe leadership styles and theories.
3. Discuss contemporary leadership challenges.
4. Discuss management theories and processes.
5. Discuss the processes involved in managing safe, evidence-based, patient-centered care.
6. List effective management tips to achieve quality outcomes.
7. Describe the role of the LVN/LPN as team leader and interprofessional team member.

Key Terms

Assignment
Autocratic leadership
Chaos
Delegation
Democratic leaders
Laissez-faire leadership (lā-sā-FĀR)
Leadership
Management
Multicratic leader
Participative leadership (păr-tĭs-ĭ-PĀ-tĭv)
Patient-centered care
Quality care outcomes
Theory X
Theory Y
Transformational leadership
Transitions in care

Licensed vocational nurses and licensed practical nurses (LVNs/LPNs) manage the care of patients in many health care settings, including hospitals, clinics, home health care, and long-term care, where they may also manage other care providers. However, we are entering a new era in care delivery with the 2009 passage of the Patient Protection and Affordable Health Care Act (ACA). Focus is rapidly shifting from reimbursement for volume of care and items billed to increasingly specified **quality care outcomes**, client satisfaction, and safety for groups of patients. Greater access to care and a focus on prevention and health maintenance means that more care will be delivered outside of hospitals. This will require community engagement and greater management of **transitions in care**, or patients receiving care across multiple health care settings. In response, the LVN/LPN is now expected to have additional skills not only as a manager, but also as a leader. To move from a focus on tasks for a specific patient to a focus on facilitating the care process, the LVN/LPN will need to collaborate with others and influence people and decisions in new ways.

A variety of factors are contributing to this evolution. Historically, the health care delivery system was predictable, with one generally accepted "right way to do things." Over the past 3 decades, the system became increasingly chaotic (disordered) as we embraced rapid change in information and technology and struggled unsuccessfully to contain costs. With the advent of the ACA we are now challenged to restructure health care delivery, which will result in even greater change, complexity, and uncertainty. Vicenzi (1997, p. 26) defines **chaos** as "the apparently irregular, unpredictable behavior of deterministic, non-linear systems." In other words, our health care systems are changing quickly as they struggle to maximize quality and control costs, and they are doing so in many creative and varied ways. In chaos lies the opportunity to discover new and more effective ways to provide care. Finding answers to these opportunities will be critical to the survival of our health care organizations and to our patients' well-being. This challenge is shared by all employees in, and across, organizations. Because nurses are so closely involved in the business of health care (that is, in providing the actual care that organizations exist to provide), they are in a critical position to meet this challenge. Providing safe, quality **patient-centered care** (care driven by client input) in and across systems will increasingly demand rapid, patient-specific decision making at the point of care where nurses are most engaged. We can create order out of chaos. As our health care systems transition from payment for volume to reimbursement for value and work to realign services, job responsibilities will be reevaluated and nursing roles will change and expand. Nurses at all levels are being called on to add new skills and functions. Cost control measures seek to maximize the contribution of each member of the health care team. LVNs/LPNs bring valuable knowledge and skills to many practice arenas and are positioned to be both leaders and strong collaborative followers in managing and providing care. They are critical players in addressing direct care quality, client satisfaction, and continuity of care. The increase in long-term residential care required by the growing older adult population and the movement of care increasingly into the community will shift the focus and demand for LVNs/LPNs.

Long-term care homes are frequently staffed by LVNs/LPNs and nursing assistants, who often provide the bulk of the "hands-on" care. LVNs/LPNs have traditionally filled leadership or management positions in long-term care, often as team leaders and charge nurses. Because LVNs/LPNs are managers of care for the patients to whom they are assigned and often provide the planning connection between their care facility and others as patients move across systems, LVNs/LPNs need to have a working knowledge of leadership, management, and safe health care delivery. As access to care, focus on prevention and health maintenance, and care coordination expand, LVNs/LPNs will be assuming new leadership and management roles. Thus we are seeing a shift to LVNs/LPNs who not only must manage their assigned patients, but also must plan, organize, direct, coordinate, and control care provided by others. As changes evolve, LVNs/LPNs must stay informed of the laws that define their practice in the state where they are employed. State nurse practice acts vary and respond over time to changes in their citizens' health needs. They address scope of practice to protect the public.

LEADERSHIP VERSUS MANAGEMENT

The terms **leadership** and **management** are sometimes used interchangeably but, in fact, they have different meanings. Leadership is a broader and more future-oriented role whereas management is more local and task focused. A leader creates a vision that energizes others to follow; a manager is assigned or appointed to the role and focuses on the day-to-day work of the organization. Leadership is a difficult concept to define but it generally means *guidance* or showing the way to others. Leaders clarify and punctuate unifying values for groups that, when combined with vision, create a mission for the group to work toward. Formal leaders hold formal leadership positions (e.g., your boss is a formal leader). Informal leaders (persons without official titles to whom people listen) also influence systems. Leaders inspire people to strive to accomplish particular goals by doing the right thing. They see beyond the here and now, perhaps beyond the organization's current status, to what might be and are internally driven toward that vision. In contrast, management is the effective use of selected methods to accomplish current organizational goals. Managers are generally driven by external organizational rewards. Management provides the means to achieve the organization's goals by doing the thing right. Managers get things organized so the leader's vision can be achieved. Leadership is often considered the inspiration and management the perspiration. Ideally, leadership and management complement and build on each other.

Both leaders and managers must have certain characteristics to be effective. First, they must be competent. They must have the respect of the people who work with them. Second, they must be able to communicate with others. People in leadership and management positions work well with other people. Success or failure in interactions depends on their ability to communicate. Finally, leaders and managers must be able to motivate others. They must determine what other people consider important and why they behave as they do. Leaders motivate through values and vision and manage through organizational benefits, such as merit raises and recognition. Use of both leadership and management skills reinforces motivation and enhances positive outcomes for everyone. Many people are motivated in multiple ways. Astute leaders and managers provide multiple motivators, as well as personally modeling the value-driven behaviors they desire.

Good leaders and managers seem to have certain characteristics in common, such as setting realistic goals, trying out new ideas, and thinking positively. The *Coordinated Care* box lists the characteristics of good leaders and managers.

Coordinated Care

Characteristics of Leaders and Managers

A good leader and manager:

- Sets realistic goals and works to achieve them
- Seeks and tries new ideas and methods
- Is a positive thinker
- Is accountable for actions
- Is willing to make decisions and take risks
- Is competent in performing work
- Is an effective communicator
- Is assertive; refuses to be manipulated
- Accepts responsibilities of leadership and delegation
- Is emotionally mature; exercises self-control
- Is committed to providing quality patient care
- Recognizes worth of co-workers and welcomes suggestions; answers their questions
- Is not selfish; is willing to share information

Continued

Coordinated Care—cont'd

- Is able to use self-criticism; gives constructive criticism to others
- Has a sense of humor; is able to laugh at self, never at others
- Is loyal to co-workers
- Is self-confident
- Is never self-satisfied; recognizes the need for continued improvement
- Is a facilitator

Adapted from Corona DF: Followership: the indispensable corollary to leadership. In Hein EC, Nicholson MJ (eds): *Contemporary leadership behavior: selected readings*, Boston, 1982, Little, Brown.

LEADERSHIP STYLES

Many different leadership styles are used in various situations. The four basic types of traditional leadership are (1) autocratic, (2) democratic, (3) laissez-faire, and (4) multicratic. As an LVN/LPN, you need to understand your predominant style and how to reinforce it or change it, depending on how effective your style is in a given situation. You also need to understand the styles and approaches of others. Leadership styles vary according to degrees of freedom and control, the identity of the decision makers, leader activity level, assumption of responsibility, output of the group, efficiency, and the situation (Table 4-1). Other factors that influence which leadership style will be most effective are the maturity of the group and of the group's leader, the skills of the leader and group members, the cohesiveness of the group, and the predictability of the work to be done. These factors may also determine who the leader should be. The recent application of chaos and quantum theory to leadership suggests a *transformational style of leadership* in which all members of a group may assume leadership and followership roles in various circumstances based on their unique skills and talents.

AUTOCRATIC LEADERSHIP

Autocratic leadership is also known as *authoritarian, directive,* or *bureaucratic*. Individuals who practice this type of leadership achieve their goals by setting objectives and having them carried out without input or suggestions from others on how to do so. They believe that they have complete authority that should not be questioned. Autocratic leaders do not encourage individual initiative or cooperation among employees; instead, they are task oriented, making decisions independently and issuing orders. Autocratic leaders generally do not demonstrate human consideration in their actions. When an autocratic leader hires an autocratic manager, a power struggle is likely to occur.

Although autocratic leadership does not work well in many situations, this type of leadership is necessary in other situations. For example, during an emergency, one person must take charge because no time is available for group conferences on the best plan of action. Autocratic leadership may also be justified when the leader obviously knows more or has more experience than anyone else in the group. In this situation, group members often need or want someone to tell them what to do and how to do it.

DEMOCRATIC LEADERSHIP

Democratic leaders achieve their goals through the participation of group members by focusing on the individual abilities and attributes of each member. People are encouraged to provide input and decisions are often made through group consensus. Everyone in the group is informed of the goals and direction of the

Table 4-1 Comparison of Traditional Leadership Styles

	AUTHORITARIAN	DEMOCRATIC (INCLUDING PARTICIPATIVE)	LAISSEZ-FAIRE	MULTICRATIC
Degree of freedom	Little freedom	Moderate freedom	Much freedom	Little to moderate freedom
Degree of control	High control	Moderate control	No control	Moderate to high control
Decision making	By the leader	By the leader and group	By the group or by no one	By the leader with group input
Leader activity level	High	High	Minimal	High
Assumption of responsibility	Primarily by the leader	Shared	Abdicated	Primarily by the leader
Output of the group	High quantity, good quality	Creative, high quality	Variable, may be poor quality	High quality, high quantity
Efficiency	Very efficient	Less efficient than the authoritarian leader	Inefficient	Efficient

Modified from Tappen RM: *Nursing leadership and management: concepts and practice*, ed 2, Philadelphia, 1989, FA Davis.

organization so that input has a direct relationship to attaining the goals. Instead of power struggles, democratic leaders turn problems over to the group to manage. The resulting group process takes time and thus may not be feasible in all situations. The term **participative leadership** could be seen as a type of democratic leadership. Sources that differentiate the two types describe participative leadership in terms of less freedom for group members, more leader control, and a higher level of responsibility than in the democratic model.

The primary role of the leader is to keep the group headed in the right direction. Democratic leaders lead by suggestion rather than by domination. They support individual human contributions to the whole. They persuade and teach rather than rule. Most people who work with a democratic leader have a feeling of satisfaction because they have a part in managing their work situation.

LAISSEZ-FAIRE LEADERSHIP

The opposite of autocratic leadership is **laissez-faire leadership**. A laissez-faire leader provides little or no direction. Individuals working in this environment are allowed to do anything they want. The result is that people often do not share common goals, or care about what they are supposed to do, and thus lose all sense of initiative and desire for achievement. The organization then gradually disintegrates into a muddle of confusion. Individuals motivated by goal achievement and recognition generally have great difficulty working under this leadership style. However, laissez-faire leadership may work well with a highly motivated, focused group, especially if members are able to reach group-identified goals.

MULTICRATIC LEADERSHIP

Multicratic leaders are crosses between autocratic and democratic leaders. They are sometimes called *situational leaders*. They present their own personal views to group members, who provide criticism and comments. The multicratic leader analyzes feedback from the group and then makes all final decisions. Multicratic leaders work well within a group and in emergency situations, when events need to be handled quickly. Group members assist the multicratic leader with setting goals, thereby achieving for themselves a sense of empowerment and control. This process reinforces their contributions and their value.

TRANSFORMATIONAL LEADERSHIP

Quantum theory tells us that collectively we seek order in our lives and our work but that many possibilities for that order exist. In other words, we may deal with the same situation in many different ways, each of which may work; some may work better than others, depending on the context or the people involved. One person cannot see or act on all potential possibilities with equal clarity and skill. Experience, personal values, individual personality, maturity, and education all may influence how one sees a situation, as well as what solutions are identified. **Transformational leadership** suggests that, in a well-functioning group that shares a common vision, leadership will flow among the members based on the task or problem at hand and the members' individual skills. Thus all members of the group are both leaders and followers. This style of leadership may not replace reporting lines or formal job responsibilities but it may be very effective in identifying the best option at the moment and in energizing others to take action. This is an increasingly important style of leadership as we seek to provide patient-centered care that maximizes quality outcomes and client satisfaction.

Put on Your Thinking Cap!

Think of a person in your class whom you consider to be a leader. Write down the characteristics that led you to this conclusion. Compare your class leader's characteristics with the identified characteristics in this chapter. Identify the person's leadership style. Remember a time when you influenced another's actions. What type of leadership style did you use?

CLASSIC MANAGEMENT THEORIES

Management theories attempt to explain what motivates people to work, which helps nurses to determine the best management style for their work setting. The classic management theories are labeled X and Y. Numerous other types of theories exist. These theories are briefly described in Table 4-2.

THEORY X

In 1957, Douglas McGregor developed two theories, which he labeled **theory X** and **theory Y**, to explain the nature of people and their relationship to the work environment. Theory X assumes that people in the workplace:

- Find no pleasure in work
- Dislike responsibility
- Are naturally lazy and prefer to do nothing
- Work mainly for money
- Work only because they fear being fired
- Are basically childlike and enjoy being told what to do
- Do not want to think for themselves
- Are not capable of making decisions for themselves

According to theory X, people have these general characteristics and therefore want to be directed and controlled.

Leaders who adhere to the X theory of management usually have an autocratic style.

Table 4-2 Major Leadership Theories

CLASSIFICATION OF THEORIES	CHARACTERISTICS	COMMENTS
Trait	Leaders are those who have specific traits, such as the "right" social background, assertiveness, initiative, or charisma. The *great man theory* proposes that leaders are born, not made.	No traits have been identified that are present in all leaders, although leaders often are above average height and weight, energetic, well-educated, and self-confident, and have good judgment and interpersonal skills.
Attitudinal	A leader's behavior is shaped by his or her attitude toward employees and production.	The leader may be production oriented or employee oriented.
Situational	A leader's effectiveness is affected by the environment and specific situation.	The leader may be described as being the right person in the right place at the right time.
Contemporary	Effective leadership results from the characteristics (traits) of the leader, the leader's attitude, the situation in which leadership is required, and the characteristics of the followers.	Without followers, no leaders would exist. A leader's vision and ability to communicate and move toward that vision is emphasized.

Data from Grossman SC, Valiga TM: *The new leadership challenge: creating the future of nursing*, ed 2, Philadelphia, 2005, FA Davis.

THEORY Y

According to theory Y, people are dynamic, flexible, and adaptive. Believers assume in this theory that people:

- Are active and enjoy setting their own goals
- Work for rewards other than money, such as doing the job well and working with others
- Are productive because of their own personal goals rather than because of goals set for them
- Are mature and responsible
- Are self-directed
- Accept responsibility
- Care about what they are doing
- Are constantly striving to grow

According to theory Y, people are thought to like their work when they know what is expected of them and when their work gives them satisfaction. Leaders who adhere to the Y theory of management usually have a democratic style.

Employees will respond to different leadership styles, depending on their comfort with them. Individuals are motivated variously based on their personal and professional needs, values, and perceptions. Managers seeking to maximize employee productivity and satisfaction will work to provide specific things that connect with the intrinsic motivators of their employees. One can look at the literature on human development and nursing theory to identify specific motivators that may be effective with individual employees. An example is the human need for security identified by Abraham Maslow. In difficult economic times, job security may take precedence over belonging to a commodious work group.

Put on Your Thinking Cap!

You are the charge nurse in a long-term care facility. The nurse manager has asked you to explain the increasing use of disposable items on your shift. Explain how you would approach this problem using X and Y theories of management. What potentials are there in this challenge to address care efficiencies?

FUNCTIONS IN THE MANAGEMENT PROCESS

Management is a problem-oriented process similar to the nursing process. The major functions of management are planning (what is to be done), organizing (how it is to be done), directing (who is to do it), coordinating (who is doing what), and controlling (when and how the task is done).

PLANNING

Planning is the first step in the management process. Planning entails deciding in advance what needs to be done. To provide effective care for patients, a good plan for carrying out their care must be developed. Effective planning is as important for individual patient care as it is for a group of patients.

Two important components of planning are *decision making* and *problem solving*. Decision making is the process of selecting one course of action from alternatives. Problem solving is a part of the decision-making process.

The first step in decision making is to identify a problem. The problem is sometimes quite obvious but at other times underlying issues make the real problem less obvious. When the outcome is low risk and of small consequence, a quick decision may be fine. For larger or more consequential concerns, you should go on a *fact-finding mission* to explore all aspects of the situation to identify the real problem. Seek answers to such questions as who, how, when, and why. You want to solve the problem, not just its symptoms.

Once the real problem has been identified, all possible solutions should be explored. This analysis is a creative process during which brainstorming sessions are often held to obtain input from a variety of sources, including extended members of the health care team as well as patients and family members.

The next step in the decision-making process involves choosing the most desirable action to solve the problem. To select the best solution, you must consider whether the action is likely to accomplish the objectives of the organization and support safe, quality patient outcomes. In addition, it is important to determine whether the action increases the effectiveness and efficiency of the organization and whether implementation is realistic. After the decision has been made, it can be implemented. The decision should be communicated to other people who are involved in the organization to gain their support for carrying out the action. The communication should be expressed in such a way that other individuals become supportive of the decision rather than antagonistic toward it. Antagonism and negative feelings can be avoided in many cases when others are involved in the decision-making and problem-solving processes from the beginning. Interdisciplinary teamwork and collaboration are often essential to efficient, effective outcomes.

The final step in the decision-making process is to determine how the results will be evaluated. An evaluation can be carried out in many ways. Written tools such as audits or checklists may be used, as may verbal or written feedback from individuals in the organization or from patients who are receiving the care. If the chosen solution to the problem is not satisfactory, another alternative can be selected and tried, followed by another evaluation. The *Coordinated Care* box lists the steps in the decision-making process.

Coordinated Care

Steps in the Decision-Making Process

PROCESS	HOW TO ACCOMPLISH
• Identify a problem	• Go on fact-finding mission: who, how, when, why
• Explore possible solutions	• Involve others: brainstorm
• Choose most desirable action	• Determine whether action is realistic and can achieve organization's objectives
• Implement action	• Communicate decision to others
• Plan the evaluation	• Identify evaluation methods and processes (audits, feedback, etc.)

ORGANIZING

Organizing is the second step in the management process. When planning has been completed, a formal structure must be in place to ensure that individuals can carry out actions in an efficient and effective manner. Organizing also helps to develop order, promote cooperation among workers, and foster productivity.

Part of organizing is developing objectives. Objectives help guide the process of planning and organizing. Another part is establishing policies and procedures to provide guidelines for carrying out objectives. The most qualified people should be assigned to carry out the specific activities and tasks that will best achieve the objectives. Making appropriate staff assignments may involve the development of job descriptions, performance standards, and staffing patterns to provide the best patient care possible. Flexibility should be built in to the organization. Census variations, episodic staffing issues, and client demands sometimes change rapidly and the system must be ready to respond. Various staffing models, as well as diversity in staff roles and skills, should be developed prospectively to address these potentialities.

DIRECTING

The third step in the management process is directing. Directing involves making **assignments** and directing people to carry out these assignments. It also involves explaining what is to be done, how it is to be done, and why it is to be done. Attention is paid to ensuring that assignments match the competencies of those assigned and that all activities fall within the state's nurse practice act. Regulatory agencies are paying increased attention to documented competencies of all care providers. This task is especially challenging when agency staff and staff pulled from other areas are involved.

In nursing, making assignments is related to patient care. Assignments should be made carefully so that the skills of assigned personnel match patient needs. Estimating the difficulty of the task and the time needed to complete the care is important. Help or additional instruction should be provided whenever necessary.

Only one person should be responsible for making assignments, especially with team nursing. Assignments must be specific, easily understood, and posted where everyone can see them. Staff members should be helped to understand their assignments and the importance of each task.

Directing people to carry out their assignments requires good communication skills and assertive behavior, as well as complete and understandable directions. Providing written directions increases understanding and compliance. It is also helpful to give directions in a clear, logical order and to limit the number of directions given at any one time.

The manner in which directions are given is also important. Directions are usually given in the form of a request, such as "Will you help Mrs. Smith with her bath today?" Requests encourage cooperation and tend to result in more being accomplished. This approach implies that the individuals who are giving directions are *working with* people rather than having people *work for* them.

COORDINATING

The fourth step in the management process is coordinating. Coordinating helps to pull together various activities to achieve a goal. It ensures that all important activities are being carried out and helps to identify overlap, duplication, and omissions. In nursing, coordinating involves personnel and services. You must be sure that proper nursing care is given by the appropriate people.

The coordination process may be carried out within a single nursing unit or among units and departments in a hospital, in a long-term care facility, or across community agencies. For example, the nurse may want to be sure that medications are being given by designated team members on a unit. The advent of electronic health records is becoming integral to this process. Coordinating involves skill and experience in problem solving and decision making; it also requires good communication skills and an ability to resolve conflicts. To be a good coordinator, you should be able to assess what all individuals and groups in the organization are doing and recognize the value in all parts of the organization functioning effectively for the good of the whole.

Coordination is a prime vantage point from which cost and time saving opportunities may be identified; it is also where quality enhancements may be recognized. Nurses involved in the details of day-to-day operations are often in the best position to recognize both system-wide and local direct care inefficiencies and offer better alternatives. This circumstance is particularly true with direct patient care processes and resulting client outcomes.

CONTROLLING

Controlling, or evaluation, is the last step in the management process. It is an ongoing process in which activities of the organization are analyzed to ensure that plans are being carried out. Both the efficiency and the effectiveness of the organization are evaluated in the controlling process. The purposes of control in nursing service are to determine whether enough staff and supplies are available, whether the operation is economical, and whether the desired objectives have been achieved. Controlling is basically a form of evaluation and includes:

1. Establishing standards (desired outcomes) and objectives
2. Measuring performance and comparing the results with the standards (desired outcomes)
3. Making corrections or adjustments to remedy any deficiencies in the caregiving operations

Continuous Quality Improvement

Quality assurance (QA), *continuous quality improvement* (CQI), and *total quality management* (TQM) are terms frequently used in relation to control. All of these processes measure quality of care and are increasingly influenced by research. QA measures performance against set standards and expectations (outcomes) and alerts the organization when an action or an outcome falls below the standard. Specific standards are set in three areas: structure, process, and outcomes. *Structure standards* address specific things that exist to support efficacious quality care. Job descriptions, policies and procedures, and defined documentation expectations are examples of structure standards. *Process standards* address care delivery activities. Observation of direct care to ensure adherence to established procedures is an example here. *Outcome standards* address what the client is expected to experience as a result of established structure and process standards. Nosocomial infection rates, client satisfaction surveys, and skin integrity measures are examples of outcomes that might be measured. Most agencies have QA committees that set standards for care and evaluate compliance. They may be identifying the best way to achieve desired outcomes or translating current research into best practices. The American Nurses Association, the American Hospital Association, and The Joint Commission are organizations that set standards for nursing practice and medical care. Agencies are evaluated to ensure that objectives and standards are being met and recommendations for necessary change are made. The purpose of CQI is to continually seek new ways to improve nursing outcomes. CQI is carried out through TQM and moves the organization to higher performance than QA alone will. The expectation is that continuous nursing and interdisciplinary processes for evaluating and addressing quality care and that use current automated data to allow for sophisticated analysis and timely response will be in place. Specific quality indicators for nursing care have been identified for monitoring and for focused CQI. These indicators include patient falls, pressure ulcers, nosocomial infections, and nurse staffing. Additionally, in 2006 the Institute of Medicine published a report on preventing medication errors that has moved us to a more systemic focus on medication safety. Reimbursement is increasingly based on a variety of quality indicators such as adverse events, infection rates, readmissions, and satisfaction scores. These indicators are public, so systems depend on nursing to assure strong scores and outcomes to protect their business.

CONFLICT RESOLUTION

Dealing with conflict is an important part of the manager's role. Conflicts arise from differences in many factors, such as beliefs, knowledge, values, personalities, culture, and age. It may also be caused by unclear roles; multiple, shifting, or conflicting priorities; and competition for scarce resources. Current issues may be exacerbated by prior unresolved conflict. When a conflict occurs, it creates stress and negative feelings that can adversely affect the work situation. A conflict may be within an individual (intrapersonal conflict), between two or more people (interpersonal conflict), or between individuals and organizations (organizational conflict).

Conflict is a process with four stages:

1. **Frustration:** People believe that their goals are being blocked; they feel frustrated. Individuals may become angry or resigned to the situation.
2. **Conceptualization:** Each party formulates a view of the basis for the conflict. Conflicts typically center on perceived differences in facts, goals, how to achieve goals, and the values on which goals are based.
3. **Action:** The conflict leads to various behaviors that may or may not help resolve the conflict.
4. **Outcomes:** Outcome follows the action; goals may be reformulated so that they are acceptable to all parties; one party may "win," the other "lose"; emotions may be positive or negative.

Identifying the root cause of the conflict and related prior history is beneficial before beginning the resolution process.

There are multiple approaches to conflict resolution, each with various advantages and disadvantages. The positive and negative consequences of each are summarized in Table 4-3. The leader must select the best approach in each situation. To understand how each of these approaches works in a "real" situation, consider the following scenario: You are the charge nurse on a 30-bed unit in a long-term care facility. Nursing assistants (NAs) are assigned to equal numbers of

Table 4-3 Modes of Conflict Resolution

MODE	POSITIVE OUTCOMES	NEGATIVE OUTCOMES	WHEN TO USE
Accommodation	Agreement is reached	Differences are suppressed; resentment	You are wrong The other person really has a better idea The issue is more important to the other party than to you You are outnumbered or outranked
Collaboration	Generates commitment to work together; focuses on shared higher goals such as good patient care, not on individual immediate needs Builds understanding and empathy	Wastes time if used for resolution of trivial issues or when the outcome has already been decided	To build understanding To find creative solutions that accommodate higher common goals To address difficult issues that affect productivity
Compromise	Can produce mutually acceptable solutions Both parties have achieved something they wanted	The compromised solution may not be the best even though it "keeps the peace"	When time pressures require quick solution When each party is firmly committed to different views A compromise can produce acceptable outcomes
Avoidance	Temporarily defuses highly charged, emotional disagreement Allows both parties to "cool off" until a reasonable approach can be considered	The conflict is not resolved Neither party is satisfied	To deal with trivial issues when more important issues are waiting To delay a decision until parties are calmer, more information has been obtained, etc. When one party's demands cannot possibly be met When others could resolve the issue more readily
Competition	Reflects a strong stance to defend important principles and protect vulnerable parties Person in power takes responsibility for a decision	Can generate bad feelings Creates a winner and a loser May generate behaviors that block the actions of the "winner"	When a quick decision is essential To implement unpopular nonnegotiable actions To defend important principles, individual rights, and group welfare

residents in adjacent rooms. During report, one NA, Alice, complains that her assignment is unfair because all but two of her residents require almost total care. She says that all of the other NAs have easier assignments. Using various strategies, here are possible solutions:

- *Accommodation:* You shift the care of two residents to other NAs.
- *Collaboration:* You reassess the needs of each group of assigned residents. Recognizing that Alice is correct, you work with the NAs to identify more equitable distribution of assignments to ensure good patient care.
- *Compromise:* You tell Alice that you will alternate NAs assigned to that group of residents.
- *Competition:* You tell Alice that everyone has some residents who require a lot of care and the assignment will stand.
- *Avoidance:* You tell Alice that you have more important things to deal with right now and go to your office.

For each of these "solutions," think about the positive and negative outcomes. Again, realize that the best solution will vary with the situation. The art of management is to select the best approach for the situation.

TIPS FOR EFFECTIVE MANAGEMENT

Managing health care workers is a complex task. Some strategies you may use to improve your management skills are to (1) take an active approach to planning, avoiding conflict before it happens; (2) have a clear vision, communicate it well, listen, and stay focused; (3) emphasize the importance of documentation as part of management; (4) treat other health care workers or team members as you would like to be treated yourself; (5) keep confidential information confidential; (6) make employees accountable for their actions and be accountable for yours; and (7) seek help and support from a variety of sources. LVNs/LPNs are frequently asked to assume responsibilities for the care that other staff members give to patients. You may have nursing assistants, unlicensed assistive personnel, technicians, or other practical nurses reporting to you. Your role is not simply to tell them what to do; you must be both a leader and a manager.

LICENSED PRACTICAL NURSE AS A LEADER

TEAM NURSING

Team nursing was introduced during the 1950s when the medical community encountered a shortage of professional nurses and an abundance of auxiliary nursing staff. The team functions by using the skills and knowledge of the professional nurse to direct the care provided by a diverse staff through group action. All members of the team are expected to have input into the nursing care process. Our definition of teams is expanding to include other professionals as we realign care and seek higher quality outcomes. The LVN/LPN role in these teams is currently being explored.

ROLE OF THE TEAM LEADER

The functions of the team leader are to plan, set priorities for, supervise, and evaluate patient care. The role of the team leader was traditionally carried out by a registered nurse (RN) because the thought was that only RNs were prepared to plan nursing interventions, provide supervision, make independent decisions, and evaluate nursing care or the work of team members. However, in many cases an LVN/LPN is assigned to the position of team leader, especially in long-term care settings. In these cases, the job description must differentiate between the practice of an RN team leader and that of an LVN/LPN team leader.

Team leaders are responsible for the ongoing collection of data about each patient and for assisting in the determination of appropriate nursing interventions. They must be sure that medical orders and plans are carried out and documented. Team leaders initiate discharge planning, identify referral needs, and facilitate patient education. They are also responsible for documenting the nursing care provided. In addition, team leaders are responsible for team collaboration and reporting changes to the RN supervisor. An LVN/LPN who assumes the position of team leader can carry out these responsibilities under the supervision and guidance of an RN.

ISSUES RELATED TO TEAM LEADERSHIP

Specific issues such as making assignments and delegation, accident prevention and safety, and accountability concern the team leader.

Making Assignments

You cannot do everything for all patients. To be effective, you must be able to assign tasks to others who are hired to perform them and make sure that those tasks are carried out. **Delegation** allows nurses to accomplish nursing care for more clients than one individual could provide alone. Before you make assignments or delegate as a team leader, you must consult your state's nurse practice act. Delegation, as defined by the National Council of State Boards of Nursing (NCSBN), is "the act of transferring to a competent individual the authority to perform a selected nursing task in a selected situation." (*To assign* is to direct an individual to do activities within an authorized scope of practice.) Among nurses working in clinical settings, delegation involves "working with and through others" and assignment describes "the distribution of work that each staff member is to accomplish in a given work period" (NCSBN, 2005, p. 1). In this book, delegation refers to "working through others" and assignment describes what a person is asked to do. Delegating tasks is specified in your job description; you are delegating some of your responsibilities according to your state's nurse practice act. Currently, however, there is no clear consensus among the states regarding who and what may be delegated, so it is critical that LVNs/LPNs know and follow their state regulations.

The assignment is used in many work settings by LVNs/LPNs. Making assignments involves identifying specific tasks needed to provide care for a specific person. You usually assign the care of several patients to each staff member. Before you can make assignments, you must know what care each patient requires and you must know the strengths and weaknesses of staff members. Assignments are based on your duty to maintain patient safety and on patient needs, available staff, job descriptions, scope of practice for licensed nurses, and scope of functions for nursing assistants (NCSBN, 2006). Although state delegation regulations vary, LVNs/LPNs can assist RNs in the management process. Following delegation by an RN to unlicensed personnel, LVNs/LPNs may assist in the supervision of unlicensed personnel, may assist in training unlicensed personnel, and may verify competencies of unlicensed assistive personnel. In many states, the delegating RN remains accountable for this process, given that RNs are accountable for the tasks delegated to unlicensed persons. Effective delegation requires delegating a clearly identified task and related time frames to a person with appropriate knowledge and skills, validating understanding, identifying patient needs, empowering the staff person to carry out activities to complete the task, monitoring staff performance, and documenting outcomes.

Essential elements of effective delegation include knowing your state nurse practice act statements on delegation and your institution's policies and procedures, knowing the training and background of persons to whom you delegate tasks, deciding which tasks can be delegated safely, and evaluating the patient's response. You must delegate only tasks to unlicensed personnel; you may not delegate nursing processes to unlicensed personnel. The nursing practice functions of assessment, planning, evaluation, and nursing judgment cannot be delegated. Delegation is specific to each client. An unlicensed person who completes a task for one patient cannot do the same task for all patients. Delegation is also situation specific. You delegate a task for one patient in one situation.

Put on Your Thinking Cap!

You are working with two unlicensed assistive personnel (UAP), one with only 3 months of experience and one with 8 years of experience, on your unit. Describe how you would approach the delegation of feeding and ambulating a patient with a stroke to each UAP. How would you identify if you have the authority to delegate these actions?

Accident Prevention and Safety

Every health care facility must meet minimum safety regulations established by law in addition to those adopted by the agency to meet its unique needs. All staff members, particularly the team leader, should learn these regulations during orientation to the job. The team leader should know the regulations and be sure that staff members are aware of them. Everyone must understand the procedures to follow in case of disasters such as fires, tornadoes, or hurricanes. In addition, everyday safety issues related to handling equipment, using proper procedures, and working with potentially dangerous drugs must constantly be addressed to ensure that knowledge and skills are up to date. Organizations are responsible for providing timely information as changes in standards occur and new procedures are developed. Each nurse is accountable for knowing them and leaders are accountable for ensuring adherence. Medication safety and infection control measures are increasingly complex challenges of primary focus on the national health care agenda.

Accountability

Team leaders must demonstrate accountability for their actions, as well as for the actions of the staff they are directing. Accountability means that a person is answerable for his or her actions and may be called on to explain or justify them. Team leaders also are legally responsible for all nursing care and documentation. Ensuring that proper and accurate charting is carried out for all nursing assessments, interventions, and evaluations is the responsibility of the RN team leader. This is increasingly critical as we transition to electronic health records shared across systems to drive increasingly enhanced client outcomes.

Accountability also involves communicating patient needs to others. A common form of communication is the report "handoff" given at the end (or beginning) of every shift. The LVN/LPN is usually responsible for reporting to the RN in charge but may also be indirectly responsible for the report. Guidelines for a clear and complete handoff are as follows:

- Organize information before beginning.
- Give the patient's room number, name, age (if appropriate), diagnosis, and physician.
- Provide a brief, objective account of the patient's condition, including new or changed orders.
- Refer to clinical information as relevant, include deviations from patient or expected norms (vital signs, orientation, intake and output, etc.). Note pain medication, dosage, prescribed frequency, time of last administration, and patient response.
- Review preoperative or preprocedure checklist items. Report postoperative time of arrival from the operating or recovery room; general condition; vital signs; intravenous fluids required (e.g.,

Table 4-4 SBAR

PROCESS STEP	ACTION
Situation	Identify yourself, patient, location, diagnosis, and specific current situation
Background	Explain significant medical history and overview of current treatment
Assessment	Provide current vital signs and critical current assessment data, your clinical impression, and any concerns
Recommendation	Make suggestions; clarify expectations; make recommendations as appropriate to ensure client safety and satisfaction, care continuity, and best outcomes

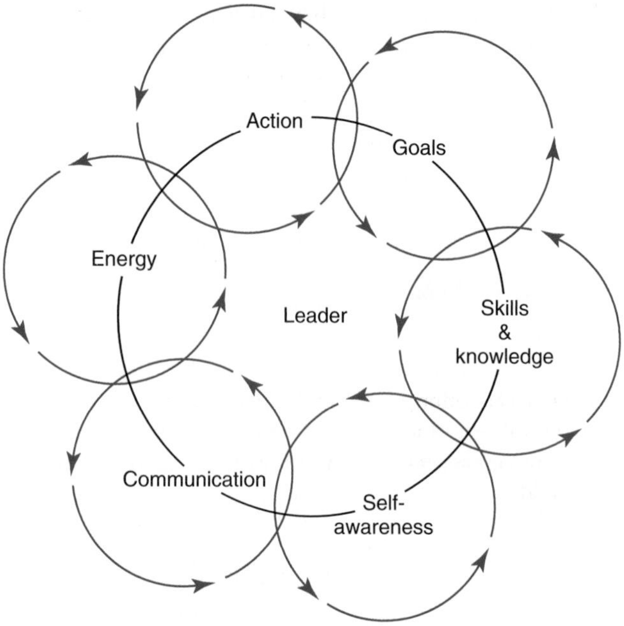

FIGURE 4-1 Components of effective team leadership. (Modified from Tappen RM: *Nursing leadership and management: concepts and practice*, ed 2, Philadelphia, 1989, FA Davis.)

kind, rate of flow, fluids to follow); dressings; voiding; diet; nature of breathing; coughing; type, location, and patency of tubes; and pain medication.
- Share patient/family's specific requests, concerns, etc.

Handoffs occur in a variety of ways. The key to success is clear, concise, and thorough communication.

SBAR (Situation, Background, Assessment, Recommendation; Table 4-4) is a systematic communication process that facilitates the exchange of important information among professionals. It may be used to alert physicians, RNs, and other care providers to changes in condition, to seek new care orders, and for shift handoffs or transfers within and across systems. SBAR provides an excellent foundation for accurate, effective communication in support of enhanced continuity and quality outcomes.

Characteristics of an Effective Team Leader

Effective team leaders must have skills in leadership, management, and supervisory techniques. They should be able to communicate effectively, both orally and in writing. Effective team leaders are able to work well with others and show that they value others' input and suggestions regarding patient care. Figure 4-1 illustrates components of effective team leadership. The leader's possession of these qualities leads to greater satisfaction among the staff and a higher quality of patient care.

To be a good team leader, you must also understand how to build an effective team. A team is more than just a group of people. It is a group of people who need to work together to achieve a goal or task (in this case, delivery of care to patients). Strategies to build an effective team include the following:

- **Establish a clear purpose.** All team members must understand and value their purpose.
- **Listen actively.** Active listening requires genuine interest in understanding another's message, not just waiting for your turn to speak.
- **Be compassionate.** Recognize stress and distress in team members; show genuine concern.
- **Be honest.** Take ownership of your opinions and attitudes; provide constructive feedback.
- **Be flexible.** Recognize that good ideas can come from any team member; invite input and be willing to consider other suggestions and viewpoints.
- **Be committed to conflict resolution.** Resolve to find creative solutions that leave all involved in agreement.

CHARACTERISTICS OF AN EFFECTIVE TEAM

Characteristics of an effective team include clear goals, good communication, a result-driven structure, competent team members, a unified commitment, a collaborative climate, standards of excellence, external support and recognition, and effective leadership.

LICENSED PRACTICAL NURSE AS CHARGE NURSE

Whether an LVN/LPN can assume the role of charge nurse depends on the LVN/LPN's state nurse practice act as well as institutional policy. Filling this role is common for LVNs/LPNs in long-term care. Most states require the LVN/LPN to have written protocols and procedures and to work under the general supervision of an RN. Furthermore, the LVN/LPN who is placed in a charge position is expected to have adequate preparation to perform competently. This situation usually requires education, training, or experience or any combination beyond the basic LVN/LPN educational program. To function as charge nurse, the LVN/LPN should be able to assign patient care, assess patients, delegate or assign tasks (as permitted by state laws), receive and give shift reports, and handle common workplace issues.

Get Ready for the NCLEX® Examination!

Key Points

- LVNs/LPNs often make up the primary staffing and management of long-term care homes.
- Leadership is defined as guidance, or showing the way to others.
- Management is defined as the effective use of selected methods to accomplish goals.
- Leaders and managers must be competent, must have the respect of the people with whom they work, and must be able to motivate others.
- Four basic types of leadership are autocratic, democratic, laissez-faire, and participative.
  - Autocratic leaders are authoritarian, meaning that they act without input or suggestions from others.
  - Democratic leaders achieve their goals through participating, encouraging others to provide input, and making decisions through group consensus.
  - Laissez-faire leaders allow group members to do anything they want, with no direction from administration.
  - Multicratic leaders have a mixture of autocratic and democratic characteristics, soliciting input from group members but making the final decisions themselves.
- Leadership styles are based on leaders' assumptions about workers' motivations.
- Leadership and management are critical LVN/LPN skills as value-based care focuses on patient-centered care, specific quality outcomes, heightened patient satisfaction, and smooth care transitions.
- The major functions of management are planning, organizing, directing, coordinating, and controlling.
- Planning, the first step in the management process, involves decision making and problem solving.
- Organizing provides a structure for carrying out the plan.
- Directing involves making assignments and directing people to carry out the assignments.
- Coordinating pulls various activities together to achieve a goal.
- Controlling includes establishing standards, measuring performance by the standards, and making corrections to remedy deficiencies.
- Strategies for conflict resolution include accommodation, compromise, competition, avoidance, and collaboration.
- The most appropriate strategy for conflict resolution depends on the situation.
- Team nursing was designed to use the skills and knowledge of the licensed nurse to direct the care provided by a diverse staff through group action.
- Team leaders conduct ongoing assessments of patients and determine appropriate nursing interventions.
- Teams may include members of other professions who share responsibility for care delivery and outcomes.
- A good team leader is skilled in leadership, management, and supervisory techniques.
- To build an effective team, the leader must establish a clear purpose; listen actively; be compassionate, honest, and flexible; and be committed to resolution of conflicts.

Additional Learning Resources

SG Go to your Study Guide for additional learning activities to help you master this chapter content.

evolve Go to your Evolve website (http://evolve.elsevier.com/Linton/medsurg) for the following learning resources and much more:

- Interactive Prioritization Exercises
- Fluid & Electrolyte Tutorial
- Pharmacology Tutorial
- Review Questions for the NCLEX® Examination

Review Questions for the NCLEX® Examination

1. An LPN has been offered a position as a charge nurse in a nursing home. How can the LPN best determine the legal limits of practice in this role?
   1. Ask the nursing home administrator what the charge nurse is expected to do
   2. Review a textbook that discusses the LPN as charge nurse
   3. Ask other LPNs who have experience as charge nurses
   4. Contact the state board of nursing

   NCLEX Client Need: Safe and Effective Care Environment
2. Which leadership style is demonstrated when a charge nurse makes the following statement during report: "I don't care how you organize your work, as long as you finish your assignments on time"?
   1. Autocratic
   2. Democratic
   3. Laissez-faire
   4. Multicratic

   NCLEX Client Need: Safe and Effective Care Environment

3. Which description about employees best illustrates the assumption of a manager who believes theory Y?
   1. Find no pleasure in their work
   2. Work mainly for the money
   3. Are mature and responsible
   4. Have similar abilities and status

   NCLEX Client Need: Safe and Effective Care Environment
4. The nursing assistants on your unit complain that the workload is unevenly distributed and ask you to try to find a better way to make assignments. What is your most appropriate first step?
   1. Let the nursing assistants work out their own assignments
   2. Identify and explore the nature of the problem
   3. Adjust tasks so that all nursing assistants have the same number of tasks
   4. Inform the nursing assistants that they need to do the work as assigned

   NCLEX Client Need: Safe and Effective Care Environment
5. Which direction by the team leader is most likely to encourage cooperation among nursing assistants?
   1. "I expect you to pitch in and help each other."
   2. "Since you have finished your morning care, go help Mary to catch up."
   3. "Whoever finishes morning care first can take the first lunch break."
   4. "Ed, would you please help Mary by taking vital signs on her newly admitted patient?"

   NCLEX Client Need: Safe and Effective Care Environment
6. What is the most important factor an LVN/LPN team leader must consider when assigning a task to a nursing assistant?
   1. Institutional policies regarding nursing assistant functions
   2. The background skill level of the nursing assistant
   3. The nursing assistant's willingness to perform the task
   4. State board of nursing regulations related to nursing assistants

   NCLEX Client Need: Safe and Effective Care Environment
7. Which characteristics describe a leader? (Select all that apply.)
   1. Is future oriented
   2. Creates a vision
   3. Handles day-to-day work
   4. Guides others
   5. Makes all decisions

   NCLEX Client Need: Safe and Effective Care Environment
8. To be effective, BOTH leaders and managers must be able to do which of the following? (Select all that apply.)
   1. Communicate effectively
   2. Set realistic goals
   3. Motivate others
   4. Think positively
   5. Create a vision

   NCLEX Client Need: Safe and Effective Care Environment
9. Which of the following options best describes transformational leadership?
   1. Leaders present their personal views to group members and consider feedback to make final decisions.
   2. All members of the group are both leaders and followers, depending on the problem at hand and individual member skills.
   3. Leaders seek input from the group and decisions often are made through group consensus.
   4. Leaders are task oriented, make decisions independently, and issue orders to those working with them.

   NCLEX Client Need: Safe and Effective Care Environment
10. The Patient Protection and Affordable Care Act has led to an increased focus on which of the following? (Select all that apply.)
    1. Quality outcomes
    2. Volume of care provided
    3. Patient care transitions
    4. Patient-centered care

    NCLEX Client Need: Safe and Effective Care Environment

chapter

5

The Nurse-Patient Relationship

http://evolve.elsevier.com/Linton/medsurg

Objectives

1. Define the holistic view of nursing.
2. Define the concept of *self.*
3. Discuss the use of self in the practice of nursing.
4. Compare the meaning of the terms *patient* and *client.*
5. Describe the meaning of the American Hospital Association's Patient Care Partnership document.
6. List commonly held expectations of patients and families.
7. Describe guidelines for nurse-patient relationships.
8. Describe basic components of communication.

Key Terms

Action
Caring
Client
Empathy
Empower
Holism
Patient
Self
Therapeutic relationship (thăr-ŭh-PYĔW-tĭk rē-LĀ-shŭn-shĭp)
Understanding
Values

Nursing means caring for persons. **Caring** is a process characterized by understanding, action, and concern. **Understanding** is the ability to listen to and relate to others so as to perceive their feelings and the meaning of their words. **Action** denotes responding to others with genuineness, compassion, sensitivity, and self-disclosure to promote their well-being.

In the caring process, a therapeutic relationship develops between patients and nurses. Unlike a social relationship, a **therapeutic relationship** is goal directed and focuses on one individual (the patient). To develop therapeutic relationships, nurses must value and accept patients as unique individuals. In addition, nurses must be aware of themselves as individuals. For communication to be effective, nurses must know how their own attitudes, feelings, and beliefs affect others. A nonjudgmental attitude of caring is essential to the practice of nursing.

HOLISTIC VIEW OF NURSING CARE

Holism is a way of viewing people as whole individuals. According to the holistic theory, people are complex beings made up of many parts. Each part interacts with the other parts and the sum of the parts forms a unified whole. Holistic health care is a system of comprehensive patient care that considers the physical, emotional, social, economic, and spiritual needs of individuals and families. The importance of the family to the individual and the role of the nurse in working with families are discussed in Chapter 7.

Individuals are composed of mind, body, and spirit. Caring for one part is impossible without considering how the other parts are affected. Thus a nursing plan of care must consider physiologic, psychologic, sociologic, and spiritual dimensions (Fig. 5-1). For example, a surgical patient has many physical needs, such as pain management, fluid replacement, and wound healing, but these needs reflect only the physical component. The patient may also be frightened about the surgery itself or fearful that he will not be able to return to work. Perhaps he needs education so that he can care for himself after discharge, or perhaps he needs help locating appropriate social services. If he has a chronic or life-threatening illness, his spiritual needs may become more prominent.

USE OF THE SELF IN NURSING

Many tools are used in the process of providing nursing care, including stethoscopes, sphygmomanometers, and thermometers. However, the most important tool that you bring to each patient encounter is the use of self. **Self** is a term used to describe one's personhood: the knowledge, experience, values,

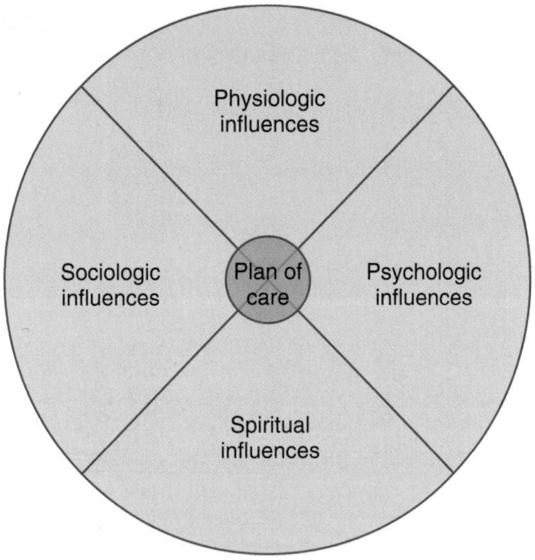

FIGURE 5-1 Physiologic, psychologic, sociologic, and spiritual influences on individual behaviors become integrated into a plan of care.

beliefs, perceptions, strengths, and weaknesses that make each individual unique. As a nurse, your attitudes, beliefs, self-esteem, and feelings become a part of the patient's therapeutic environment, just as those of the patient become a part of your environment. With your assistance, individuals and their families may find meaning in their experience and may achieve a harmonious state of health.

VALUES, BELIEFS, AND ATTITUDES

Self-awareness involves knowing one's own values, beliefs, and attitudes. You should be able to answer the questions "Who am I?" "What do I believe?" and "What is important to me?" so that you can help others to answer these questions about themselves. Almost every day, you will encounter situations that require value judgments. You must make certain choices related to patient care, respond to requests for help and guidance, and provide emotional and spiritual support. Your values, attitudes, and beliefs are outwardly expressed in your behavior as you interact with patients.

As discussed in Chapter 3, **values** can be defined as principles or standards shared by members of a society that determine what is desirable or worthwhile. A value is reflected in the worth you give to an idea or action. A *belief* is a conviction or opinion. *Attitudes* are reactions that flow from values and beliefs. An attitude indicates a feeling toward persons or things. Values and personal beliefs are developed in many ways. They may be acquired from religious education, from examples set by authority figures such as parents and teachers, or from peers. Acquiring values and beliefs is a lifelong process that is affected by one's life experience. As people age, they generally have a fairly fixed set of values, but even older people are able to grow and change.

KNOWLEDGE

Knowledge is a component of self that is acquired through experience or study. The safe practice of nursing is dependent on one's knowledge base and nursing education provides a basic introduction to the physical and social sciences. Nurses use their knowledge of biologic, psychologic, and social sciences to give the best care possible. This knowledge is often shared with patients, families, and the community to promote health, prevent disease, and cope with illness. Nurses also share their knowledge with colleagues on the health care team. Because knowledge about health care is continually growing and the health care system is changing, you will be challenged to continue to learn and expand your knowledge. For example, greater emphasis is placed on prevention of disease and promotion and maintenance of health than in the past. Nurses must not only be informed about healthy practices, but also act as models of healthy living.

Simply having a collection of facts is not sufficient. As a nursing student, you will be expected to develop your critical thinking skills. Critical thinking enables you to think through problems in an efficient and organized manner. It requires that you seek and use information, not just recite facts. Critical thinking is essential because real-life situations are seldom as "cut and dried" as they are in textbooks. Because each patient is unique, nursing care must be individualized, and this requires critical thinking. Chapter 12 discusses critical thinking in relation to nursing care.

SKILLS

Nursing is a skill-oriented field. Nursing care involves the use of many skills that require efficiency and safety. A nurse must master the skills required to carry out nursing interventions, including the technical skills needed to use sophisticated equipment. Your hands can be instruments of healing when used with compassion, competence, and gentleness. The simple act of giving a bed bath or a back rub can be the best use of self that you offer a suffering patient.

Nurses need *interpersonal skills* to communicate effectively and to establish caring relationships with patients. Through the caring relationship, you are able to build a therapeutic relationship with your patients. Developing therapeutic nurse-patient relationships requires:

- A humanistic system of values
- Ability to instill faith and hope
- Sensitivity to one's self and to others
- Ability to develop helping, trusting relationships
- Ability to express both positive and negative feelings
- Ability to use problem-solving methods for decision making

- Ability to promote interpersonal teaching and learning
- Ability to provide a supportive, protective, and corrective mental, physical, sociocultural, and spiritual environment
- Ability to assist with meeting human needs
- Ability to allow for the uniqueness of individuals and their experiences

PERSPECTIVE OF THE PATIENT

The term **patient** is used to refer to an individual, a family, a group, or a community. Patients may function in independent, interdependent, and dependent roles. As recipients of nursing care, patients may receive nursing interventions related to disease prevention, health promotion, health maintenance, illness management, and end-of-life care.

PATIENT VERSUS CLIENT

Some nurses use the term *client* rather than *patient.* This term evolved from a general belief or attitude about the nurse-patient relationship. Those who prefer the word **client** believe that it denotes a feeling of partnership or working with someone and that the word *patient* has a connotation of doing to or for someone. The word *patient* may also imply that an individual is ill. For some nurses, *client* seems to represent a more accurate view of the roles in the nurse-patient relationship because the nurse values people as individuals, honors their individuality, and helps them to achieve the highest level of wellness possible. However, because *patient* is also used and is accepted by nurses and other health care professionals, and frequently by older adults as well, *patient* and *client* are used interchangeably in this text. The term *patient* has been used for years and is used frequently in this text in support of the long-established tradition of the nurse-patient relationship. Depending on the context, patients may be considered *clients* or *consumers of nursing services.* The term *client* is more commonly used in outpatient settings. Another term, *resident,* is commonly used to refer to persons who reside in long-term care settings.

PATIENTS' RIGHTS

Patients, as participants in nursing care, are entitled to receive quality care in a safe, supportive, and nurturing environment. As the health consumer movement becomes more and more active, greater attention is being paid to the rights of patients. In 1973, the American Hospital Association issued a Patient's Bill of Rights that outlined the rights of hospital patients and incorporated the components of quality care. In 2003, this document was replaced with a pamphlet that advises patients on how they can expect to be treated during hospitalization and what caregivers will need from patients to provide good care. Key topics of this pamphlet are outlined in the *Health Promotion* box. Nurses are in a position to ensure that many of these rights are respected. One very basic way to help patients feel respected as individuals is to address and refer to them by name at all times. Be careful to pronounce the patient's name correctly and introduce the patient by name to other health care providers. Never refer to patients by room number or medical diagnosis.

Health Promotion

The Patient Care Partnership: Understanding Expectations, Rights, and Responsibilities

What to expect during your hospital stay:
- High quality hospital care
- A clean and safe environment
- Involvement in your care:
  - Discussing your medical condition and information about medically appropriate treatment choices
  - Discussing your treatment plan
  - Getting information from you
  - Understanding your health care goals and values
  - Understanding who should make decisions when you cannot
- Protection of your privacy
- Preparing you and your family for when you leave the hospital
- Help with your bill and filing insurance claims

From American Hospital Association: *The patient care partnership: understanding expectations, rights, and responsibilities.* http://www.aha.org/advocacy-issues/communicatingpts/pt-care-partnership.shtml Accessed April 29, 2013.

All patients, no matter what their age or state of mind, deserve to be treated with the same respect. Calling an older patient anything other than Mr. Smith or Mrs. Smith is inappropriate for a nurse, unless the patient has requested it. Terms such as "Pops," "Sweetie," "Gramps," or "Baby" are unprofessional and demeaning to older individuals (Fig. 5-2).

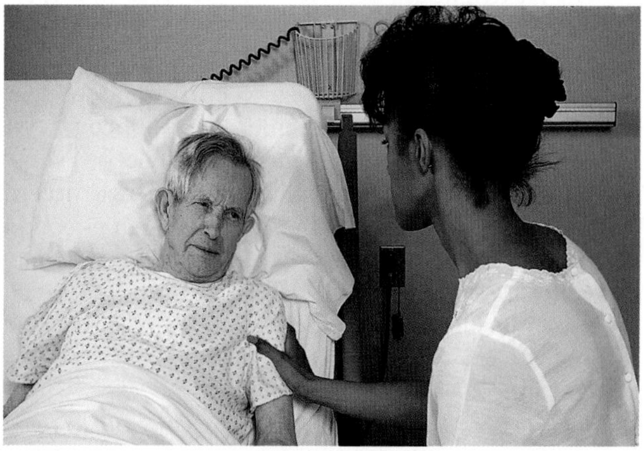

FIGURE 5-2 All people should be treated with respect, regardless of age. (From Potter PA, Perry AG, Stockert PA, Hall AM, editors: *Fundamentals of nursing,* ed 8, St. Louis, 2013, Mosby Elsevier.)

PATIENTS' EXPECTATIONS

Explanation of the Care

The experience of illness and all of the changes in a person's life that it precipitates is very stressful. A method that you can use to help reduce patients' stress and anxiety levels is to **empower** them to participate in their care. To accomplish this task, patients must be given the information they need to be active participants. Patients need and are entitled to an explanation of the care to be given so that they know what to expect and what is expected of them. Patients who are knowledgeable about their care are more likely to be active participants who are better satisfied and less anxious. Explanations and teaching are often left to the nurse. Patients who are not given adequate explanations of what is to be done have been denied their rights as patients and human beings.

With so many technological and medical advances, many options for treatment may be available to the patient. To make informed decisions about their health care choices, patients need to be provided with or have access to the knowledge needed. The nurse may be able to help the patient acquire that information or provide a referral to an appropriate source. Health care information and disease prevention guidelines need to be provided in a way that is individualized to their own personal characteristics and lifestyles.

Patients as Partners in Care

As consumers of health care services, most patients are no longer willing to assume a passive role. They not only want to assume more responsibility for their care, but also expect to do so. Patients who see themselves as partners in their care are more likely to accept responsibility for their care. Their sense of responsibility may improve compliance with the plan of care, thereby preventing needless complications.

The patient can assume an active role from the point of admission. The initial assessment is your first opportunity to set the tone for a relationship that encourages patient participation. You can help patients to understand that their participation is not only wanted, but also needed. You should talk with patients to determine to what extent they wish to participate in their care. The patient's family should also be encouraged to participate in the care whenever possible.

Some patients are more willing than others to accept the role of partner. Factors that may have an effect on patients' decisions to participate in their care are age, ethnicity, personality, social class, educational level, and previous experiences.

Acceptance of Patient Behaviors

Illness is a stressful event and can cause people to react in unusual ways. In many cases, individuals behave differently than they would under normal circumstances and nurses should not take this behavior personally. Patients need to know that nurses and health care providers accept patients' behavior.

For a nurse-patient relationship to be therapeutic, you must be able to see patients' experiences from their perspectives. Encourage patients to share thoughts and feelings freely without fear of being judged. You must be willing to accept unconditionally the patient's values, beliefs, behaviors, and attitudes. Avoid imposing your own values and beliefs on the patient whose values differ from yours. This kind of nurse-patient relationship is a special kind of caring in which the nurse has a high regard for the whole person; it conveys a sense of worth and dignity. Nurses should provide compassionate understanding of their patients' behavior and maintain a therapeutic, accepting environment.

Safety and Security

You have a high degree of responsibility for keeping your patients both physically and psychologically safe while in your care. You must assess a situation quickly, make a decision, and act promptly to solve the problem. A patient needs to feel that a nurse can act quickly and decisively in a crisis to provide the best care possible.

Competence and consistency are two factors that can alleviate stress in patients. Nurses who appear confident and competent help patients to feel more secure. In addition, performing nursing procedures consistently can help to reduce anxiety and build patients' confidence in the nurse. For example, changing dressings in the same step-by-step manner every time helps patients to know what to expect and reassures them of the competence of your care.

GUIDELINES FOR THE NURSE-PATIENT RELATIONSHIP

HELPING ROLE

A helping role occurs when one person reaches out to help another. The goal is to help another individual to grow, mature, cope, and function. A helping relationship is one with genuine caring and compassion.

The following characteristics are necessary for the nurse to assume a helping role:

- Awareness of self
- Ability to analyze own feelings
- Ability to serve as a model to others
- Desire to help others
- Strong sense of ethics and high principles
- Sense of responsibility

Nurses act as helpers by administering direct care to patients, acting as advocates on their behalf, giving psychosocial support, and providing health education and counseling. As a helper, the nurse strives to establish and maintain a therapeutic relationship. The first step in developing a therapeutic relationship is to build trust. Trust develops as the patient begins to feel safe with the nurse. A feeling of safety comes from knowing that the nurse is honest and open and from gaining confidence in the nurse's skill and knowledge. Nurses may use friendly, informal communication initially as a means of putting the patient at ease but eventually the conversation must focus back on the patient. One strategy to build a therapeutic relationship is to encourage patients to share personal stories about their lives.

A helper in the professional sense is different from a friend. The term *friend* connotes intimacy or affection. You must transcend the role of friend to take on a caring role, which requires that the patient's needs take priority over your own. In this way, you can facilitate the health of the patient. Mutual responsibility exists between patient and nurse in a partnership that is different from the responsibilities that friends have toward one another. Friendships with patients can interfere with the therapeutic process but strong authoritarian approaches can interfere also. Including patients and their families in care planning is an example of shared responsibility.

Therapeutic communication is an art and a skill. Maintaining the focus on the patient with genuine warmth and honesty takes time and practice. Self-disclosure refers to the ability to be open and honest about one's feelings. You should not disclose personal information, however, as you would do in a friendship. Table 5-1 notes some differences between a helping person and a friend.

Table 5-1 A Comparison: The Nurse as a Helping Person and the Nurse as a Friend

HELPING PERSON	FRIEND
Responsible to client	Relationship is for friendship or support
Objective of relationship is to meet client's needs	Individuals meet each other's needs
Relationship is goal directed	No plan involved
Attitude is nonjudgmental	Both individuals express feelings, attitudes, and opinions
Does not attempt to influence client to helper's way of thinking	Friends try to influence each other in discussing issues such as religion, politics, and personal philosophy
Does not keep secrets and explains in a direct manner the need to work with the treatment team	Friends may keep secrets
Discourages any sexual overtones in relationship	Sexual overtones or a sexual relationship may develop
Interacts with clients in health care settings	Interaction may occur in any setting
Relationship is time limited	Relationship may continue

Touch can be used to show concern, to let the patient know you are present, or to provide comfort. Giving a bedridden patient a back rub before sleep can stimulate circulation, provide a caring moment, and promote relaxation. However, responses to touch differ from person to person. Some people are more comfortable with touching and being touched than others are. Some patients may mistake touch as an invitation to intimacy (see the *Cultural Considerations* box).

Cultural Considerations

What Does Culture Have to Do with Touch?

Traditional Chinese patients do not like to be touched by strangers but they are accepting of a caregiver working within their personal space.

COMMUNICATION

Communication skills are essential for carrying out the helping role. Communication is the process of exchanging ideas, beliefs, thoughts, and feelings between two or more people. It involves a message, a sender, and a receiver. The sender gives the message to the receiver.

The two types of communicative behavior are verbal and nonverbal language. Verbal language conveys meanings through words whereas nonverbal language conveys meanings through symbols and actions other than words. Examples of nonverbal communication are body position, facial expression, gestures, moaning, crying, laughing, and smiling. Observation of nonverbal language is as important to the communication process as listening is to verbal language. Nonverbal language can indicate a person's thoughts and feelings as well as, if not better than, verbal language can. Nonverbal actions can be in conflict (i.e., incongruent) with the content of what is being said and thus can give clues to true feelings. For example, a patient may claim that everything is all right but may be slumped over and wringing his hands. An astute nurse should recognize that something is indeed wrong even though patients deny it verbally. Language is influenced by the cultural context in which it is used. To interpret the meaning of what is said or done without consideration of cultural context equals stereotyping.

Communication can be assertive or aggressive. Assertive communication is the ability to express oneself *without* violating the rights of another person. Aggressive communication *does* violate the rights of others. Try to express yourself without violating the rights of another person.

Two essential parts of communication are *listening* and *observation.* Listening is an active process that involves trying to understand what is being said. The listener must display genuine interest and concentration to derive meaning from the words. A good listener can provide reassurance, lighten another person's burden, and clarify misunderstandings.

Professional communication refers to the factors that help to create a therapeutic relationship. The nurse demonstrates professional communication by practicing common courtesy, introducing himself or herself to patients and their families, addressing patients respectfully by their last names, maintaining privacy and confidentiality, being trustworthy, and being self-directed and self-assured.

Therapeutic communication is a skill that can be learned through study, observation, and practice. It requires you to be open, honest, and nonjudgmental. Self-awareness is basic to meaningful interactions. Nurses must actively seek to be cognizant of their own thoughts, feelings, values, beliefs, and behaviors. To reach this goal, nurses need to self-explore and assess how the following areas may affect their ability to establish a therapeutic nurse-patient relationship:

- Ethnic, cultural, and socioeconomic background
- Attitudes, values, opinions, and beliefs
- Past unresolved experiences that are still emotionally laden
- Physical and psychologic strengths and weaknesses

To initiate a therapeutic interaction, focus your attention on the patient and listen carefully. Data that will help to obtain a holistic assessment of the patient include the following:

1. Patient's age
2. Patient's cultural background (see the *Cultural Considerations* box)
3. Patient's perception of his or her illness
4. Patient's use of direct eye contact
5. Patient's body language (Is it relaxed or tense?)
6. Quality of the patient's voice (Is it loud or soft?)
7. Patient's use of gestures
8. Patient's emotional tone (or affect) (Is it constant or does it vary? For example, does the patient appear sad, happy, or angry?)
9. Congruence of the verbal message with the patient's body language (For example, is the patient smiling while speaking of a happy event?)

Listening is an active element of therapeutic communication. You must listen and attempt to understand what the patient is saying. Tips for effective listening include the following:

- Make sure you hear what is said; focus on the message and clarify if needed.
- Accept your patient's needs and feelings.
- Pay attention to nonverbal communication.
- Obtain feedback of your understanding by verifying what you have heard.

Understanding is the ability to listen to others to perceive their feelings and the meaning of their words. Some techniques used to facilitate communication are listed in Table 5-2 along with examples of techniques that are generally nontherapeutic. Other suggestions for therapeutic communication include the following:

- Use *I statements.* These statements are sentences that begin with the word *I* and indicate acceptance of responsibility for one's feelings and thoughts (e.g., "I worry less when I know what to expect."). I statements are generally better accepted by the patient than *you statements,* such as "You ought to try getting more sleep."
- Observe the patient's gestures and nonverbal behavior. All behavior has meaning. Try to understand the meaning in the patient's behavior.
- Use open-ended questions. Stay clear of questions that can be answered with a "yes" or a "no." Instead, try questions such as "Tell me about your surgery" or "What was that like for you?"
- Focus the patient on pertinent issues. For example: "Let's talk about your diabetes medications."

Cultural Considerations

What Does Culture Have to Do with Communication?

In Afghanistan, direct eye contact between members of the opposite sex is considered rude whereas people in the United Kingdom look directly at the speaker to indicate interest.

Processing is the act of reviewing a nurse-patient interaction with a trusted teacher, supervisor, or colleague to evaluate content and themes, as well as the techniques that are used. This tool enables the nurse to be critiqued (obtain feedback) and to learn new techniques. Communication is a complex process. "Helping" can occur regardless of one's experience if respect and authenticity are brought to each interaction.

Communication should take place in language that patients understand, without talking down to them. Federal regulations require health care providers who receive federal funding to provide appropriate services to persons with limited English proficiency and those who are deaf or hard of hearing. The patient's language proficiency should be documented at the initial contact by asking what language is spoken at home and how well the person speaks English. Unless the patient reports speaking English very well, an interpreter should be offered. Even though nonmedical personnel and family members may help with everyday conversation, they may not correctly relay information between the nurse and the patient. Therefore an official interpreter should be used to convey health information or obtain informed consent. Even bilingual nursing staff should receive training in the skill and ethics of interpretation.

Failure to use interpreters has been identified as a factor in errors that are made in the health care system. Table 5-3 lists options for oral language assistance.

Table 5-2 Therapeutic and Nontherapeutic Communication Techniques

TECHNIQUE	DESCRIPTION	EXAMPLE
Therapeutic		
Silence	Waiting attentively while the patient speaks or thinks. Allows the patient to think and respond.	Sitting quietly and expectantly when the patient is speaking or gathering his or her thoughts; resisting the urge to fill quiet periods with conversation
Active listening	Attending to the patient's verbal and nonverbal messages. Demonstrates acceptance and respect.	Facing the patient; maintaining an open, relaxed posture; leaning forward; using eye contact
Reflecting	"Mirrors" back to patients what you have heard them say. Provides opportunities for patients to confirm whether they were understood.	"You say you're feeling better since your brother has returned?"
Focusing	Guides the conversation to key elements.	"You have told me about your symptoms; what bothers you the most?"
Summarizing	Reviews the subject matter that the patient has discussed. Ensures common understanding between nurse and patient.	"So you have decided to have surgery but will delay it until after Christmas."
Restating	Repeats information in your own words so the patient can confirm your interpretation.	"I hear you're concerned about your son."
Clarification	Seeks additional information so you can better understand the patient's meaning.	"Do you mean sad when you say upset?"
Sharing observations, feelings	A comment about the patient's behavior or demeanor that may encourage the patient to talk.	"You seem to have more energy today." "This seems to be frustrating for you."
Open-ended statement	A question or comment that requires more than a yes or no answer. Indicates interest but leaves specific details for client to provide.	"Tell me your reactions to your new treatment."
Nontherapeutic		
Premature advice	Offers advice without first encouraging patients to explore their feelings fully. The problem must be explored carefully and potential actions considered before the patient can make a good decision. You cannot decide what is best for the patient.	"The first thing you need to do is make your teenagers help you more."
Assuming truth of statements rather than verifying them	Accepts information without questioning or clarifying. Misunderstandings can persist.	"It's incredible that your doctor didn't tell you when to take this medication."
Commanding	Directing client to do something that creates a power struggle or resistance.	"You must quit smoking immediately."
Communication cutoff	Remark that discourages patient communication. Cliché. Shows lack of effort to understand.	"Try to think positively."
False reassurance	Inappropriately offers personal opinion that the patient should not be concerned about something. Minimizes the patient's feelings. Can lead to feelings of guilt and anger.	"You shouldn't worry about the new treatment."
Arguing	Challenges the patient's perceptions in a negative way.	"I don't see how you could be cold when it is 75 degrees in your room."
Defensiveness	Ignores or dismisses the patient's concerns.	"I am sorry you had to wait but I have other patients to care for also."
Approval or disapproval	Applies the nurse's values or beliefs to the patient's situation.	"Leaving your husband is the best thing to do." "Leaving your husband is the worst thing you could do."

Table 5-3 Options for Oral Language Assistance

OPTION	CONSIDERATIONS
Staff interpreters	Regular employees who are bilingual are trained in interpretation skills and ethics; most useful for non-English languages that are common in the care setting.
Contract interpreters	Professional interpreters may be employed only as needed; often useful for languages that are not commonly encountered in the setting.
Employee language banks	Bilingual individuals throughout the facility are trained in interpretation. A roster is maintained so that appropriate interpreters can be contacted when needed. A disadvantage is that the employee is taken away from his or her usual duties.
Community interpreter banks	Independent agencies maintain lists of trained interpreters in the community. Services are available to any agency or business.
Telephonic services	Twenty-four–hour service using a speaker phone is available to subscribers.
Remote simultaneous interpretation	Wireless remote headsets are used by the patient and the health care provider; an interpreter provides simultaneous interpreting. This is similar to the systems used to address international audiences.

Adapted from Commonwealth of Massachusetts Office of Minority Health: *Best practices recommendations for hospital-based interpreter services* (website): www.hablamosjuntos.org/pdf_files/Best_Practice_Recommendations_Feb2004.pdf. Accessed August 24, 2014.

Put on Your Thinking Cap!

1. During your next clinical experience, listen for therapeutic and nontherapeutic communication techniques used by health care providers in their interactions with patients. Describe and label three examples. Discuss the impact of each statement on the interaction.
2. Describe three things you did in your last patient contact that demonstrated empathy.

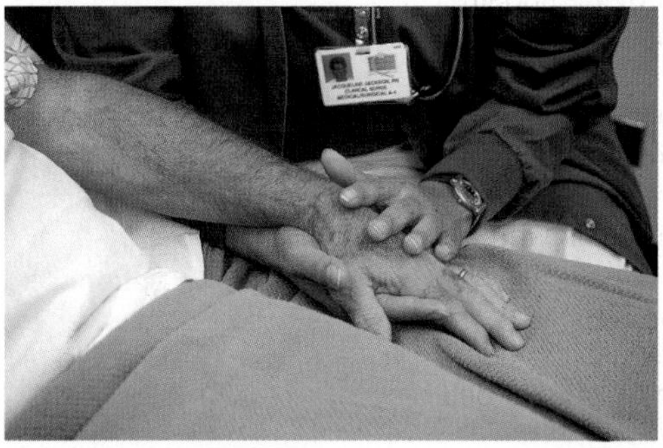

FIGURE 5-3 The judicious use of touch conveys the message that "I care what happens to you and I will help you in every way I can." (From Potter PA, Perry AG, Stockhert PA, Hall AM, editors: *Fundamentals of nursing,* ed 8, St. Louis, 2013, Mosby Elsevier.)

EMPATHETIC RESPONSE

Effective communication requires an empathetic response from a nurse. **Empathy** is the ability to identify with and understand another person's situation, feelings, and motives. An empathetic response requires compassion, understanding, and good therapeutic communication skills. Empathy differs from *sympathy.* When people sympathize with others, they understand another's feelings, but they also become personally involved in the situation. Whatever affects one affects the other. The person who sympathizes can become as distressed as the person getting the sympathy. Empathy, in contrast, is an expression of understanding of another's thoughts and feelings without becoming overly emotionally involved or distressed.

Empathy can be communicated simply through the use of verbal and nonverbal language. You can communicate empathy by telling the patient what to expect, even when the patient is not responsive or is confused. Discussing plans for care, such as treatments or medications, and explaining laboratory studies can provide reassurance to patients who may be frightened. You can also demonstrate your concern to patients and families by sharing your feelings. By sharing feelings, nurses show that they are human and can understand the difficulties of being ill or hospitalized. For example, a nurse might be tearful when a patient is given bad news, or he or she might say, "I was nervous when I had surgery too."

You can show sensitivity nonverbally by respecting confidentiality, allowing the expression of feelings, and respecting patients' privacy. The use of touch is an excellent means of communicating empathy. Holding a patient's hand during a period of anxiety or pain can communicate caring and support and, in many cases, can be more effective than any verbal interaction. The judicious use of touch conveys the message that "I care what happens to you and I will help you in every way that I can" (Fig. 5-3).

When you respond empathetically, you respond with genuineness, warmth, and sensitivity to promote well-being in the patient. This approach is the essence of therapeutic communication.

Get Ready for the NCLEX® Examination!

Key Points

- Caring is a process characterized by understanding and action.
- Action is responding to others with genuineness, warmth, sensitivity, and self-disclosure to promote their well-being.
- Holism views people as complex creatures made up of many parts that interact and form a unified whole.
- The nurse incorporates physiologic, psychologic, sociologic, and spiritual influences into the plan of care.
- Nurses must have awareness of their own values, beliefs, and attitudes and be willing to accept unconditionally the patient's values, beliefs, and attitudes.
- Nurses use their knowledge of physiology, psychology, and social science disciplines, as well as their technical and interpersonal skills, to give the best possible care to patients.
- Nurses can reduce patients' stress and anxiety levels by empowering them to participate in their own care and by demonstrating competence and consistency.
- Patients are the focus of nursing care and are entitled to receive respectful quality care.
- The role of a helper is to assist another to grow, mature, cope, and function.
- Communication is basic to the helping role.
- Individuals who are deaf or hard of hearing or who do not speak English well are entitled to the services of an interpreter.
- Persons who serve as interpreters in the health care system should be trained in interpretation skills and ethics.
- Empathy, genuineness, warmth, sensitivity, and self-disclosure are essentials of therapeutic communication.
- Empathy is the ability to identify with and understand another person's situation, feelings, and motives.

Additional Learning Resources

SG Go to your Study Guide for additional learning activities to help you master this chapter content.

evolve Go to your Evolve website (http://evolve.elsevier.com/Linton/medsurg) for the following learning resources and much more:

- Interactive Prioritization Exercises
- Fluid & Electrolyte Tutorial
- Pharmacology Tutorial
- Review Questions for the NCLEX® Examination

Review Questions for the NCLEX® Examination

1. A patient has asked the nursing student for her phone number. The student declines in order to maintain a therapeutic, rather than a social, relationship. The main difference between social and therapeutic relationships is that therapeutic relationships:
   1. Focus on both the patient and the nurse
   2. Are developed only in inpatient settings
   3. Help the nurse to work through personal problems
   4. Exist to meet patient-centered goals

   NCLEX Client Need: Psychosocial Integrity
2. You are caring for an older adult who has been chronically ill for several years. The patient has decided to discontinue life-sustaining treatment. You believe that life should be maintained at all costs. Which action best reflects acceptance of the patient in a therapeutic relationship?
   1. Asking the patient's family members to try to convince their loved one to continue treatment
   2. Telling the patient that you believe that life is sacred and that it is wrong to refuse available treatment
   3. Telling your nurse manager you cannot continue to care for the patient who refuses treatment
   4. Planning with the patient ways to maintain quality of life for as long as possible

   NCLEX Client Need: Psychosocial Integrity; Safe and Effective Care Environment: Coordinated Care
3. Which behavior is typical of a therapeutic nurse-patient relationship?
   1. The nurse shares feelings honestly.
   2. The nurse spends time with the patient in social settings.
   3. The nurse shares her religious beliefs with her patients.
   4. The nurse assures the patient that any information shared will be kept secret.

   NCLEX Client Need: Psychosocial Integrity
4. All of these statements were made by the nurse when providing morning care to a patient. Which is most likely to facilitate therapeutic communication with a patient?
   1. "Are you in pain now?"
   2. "I am preparing for my daughter's wedding."
   3. "There is nothing to worry about."
   4. "I was nervous before my surgery too."

   NCLEX Client Need: Psychosocial Integrity
5. While a patient is describing a very traumatic accident, he is smiling and making jokes. This is an example of:
   1. Injury
   2. Deceitful communication
   3. False reassurance
   4. Incongruent actions and feelings
   5. Nontherapeutic communication technique

   NCLEX Client Need: Safe and Effective Care Environment: Coordinated Care

6. While collecting data during admission of a new patient, the nurse asked the questions below. Which is the best example of an *open-ended* question?
   1. "How many children do you have?"
   2. "How many hours do you sleep at night?"
   3. "How long have you been taking thyroid replacement drugs?"
   4. "Are you nervous about surgery?"

   NCLEX Client Need: Psychosocial Integrity
7. A patient who is scheduled for a biopsy of a lump in her breast says tearfully, "I am so afraid it will be cancer." The nurse replies, "There is no sense worrying about that until you know for sure." The nurse's response is an example of:
   1. Premature advice
   2. Commanding
   3. False reassurance
   4. Assuming truth of statements

   NCLEX Client Need: Psychosocial Integrity
8. An elderly woman who speaks only Spanish is being admitted to the hospital. Her daughter assures the staff that she can interpret for her mother. What is the most appropriate response by the nurse?
   1. "We do not allow family members to act as interpreters."
   2. "In that case, I will not request our staff interpreter."
   3. "We must provide a trained interpreter for some conversations."
   4. "You will need to stay here around the clock to interpret for her."

   NCLEX Client Need: Psychosocial Integrity
9. A new nursing graduate observes that her preceptor is able to identify with and understand her patient's situation, feelings, and motives. This response to patients is characterized as:
   1. Empathetic
   2. Therapeutic
   3. Sympathetic
   4. Caring

   NCLEX Client Need: Psychosocial Integrity
10. The nursing student is reviewing his interaction with a patient. He finds that he has used all of these communication techniques. Which one is considered nontherapeutic?
    1. Reflecting
    2. Commanding
    3. Silence
    4. Clarification

    NCLEX Client Need: Psychosocial Integrity

chapter 6

Cultural Aspects of Nursing Care

http://evolve.elsevier.com/Linton/medsurg

Objectives

1. Describe cultural concepts related to nursing and health care.
2. Identify traditional health habits and beliefs of major ethnic groups in the United States.
3. Explain cultural influences on the interactions of patients and families with the health care system.
4. Discuss cultural considerations in providing culturally sensitive nursing care.
5. Discuss ways in which planning and implementation of nursing interventions can be adapted to a patient's ethnicity.

Key Terms

Assimilation (ā-sĭ-mĭ-LĀ-shŭn)
Cultural diversity
Culture
Enculturation (ĕn-kŭl-chĕr-Ā-shŭn)
Ethnic group
Subculture
Transcultural nursing

Nurses encounter people of many different backgrounds in their practice. The differences may stem from race, ethnicity, language, or religion. Diverse backgrounds affect the ways in which individuals react to health and illness, hospitalization, and nursing care.

CULTURAL CONCEPTS

CHARACTERISTICS OF CULTURE

Culture is an integrated system of learned values, beliefs, and practices that guides an individual's behavior. Culture includes the arts, beliefs, customs, folk practices, habits, institutions, and all other products of human work and thought created by a people or a group at a particular time. Culture represents the ideas, beliefs, values, and attitudes that a group of people possess. These values and beliefs are the foundation for setting standards and rules of behavior that members of a society consider acceptable and proper. Culture includes learned ways of acting and thinking that are transmitted by group members and that provide solutions for problems. Dietary habits, customs, modes of communication, religion, art, and history are all aspects of culture. Not only does culture affect a person's decisions and actions, but it also affects health care practices.

Cultural diversity is a term used to describe the existence of many cultures in a society. The United States has a rich cultural diversity as a result of the large number of immigrants who have entered the country over the past 200 years. Immigrants to the United States come from all over the world. In 2011, more than 1 million persons attained legal permanent resident status. The greatest numbers were from Asia, North and Central America, and Africa. The states (and district) that received the greatest number of these immigrants were California, New York, Washington DC, Florida, and Texas. America is sometimes called a "melting pot" because many immigrants have been assimilated into their new society. Today, the term *salad bowl* is often used instead to describe the way in which new arrivals seek to maintain individual differences while acclimating to new surroundings. Valuing and respecting the differences among the various cultural groups within our society is important, because each group makes unique contributions to art, science, politics, and health care.

Within certain cultures are groups of individuals who share different beliefs, values, and attitudes from those of the dominant culture. These groups are called **subcultures**. Examples of subcultures in the United States are members of various ethnic groups, such as African Americans, Latinos/Hispanics, Asians, and Native Americans (Fig. 6-1); homosexuals; the military; and religious groups such as the Amish and Mormons. **Transcultural nursing** is the integration of culture into all aspects of nursing care.

Similarities

All cultures share certain basic characteristics: (1) culture is learned; (2) culture is shared; and (3) culture

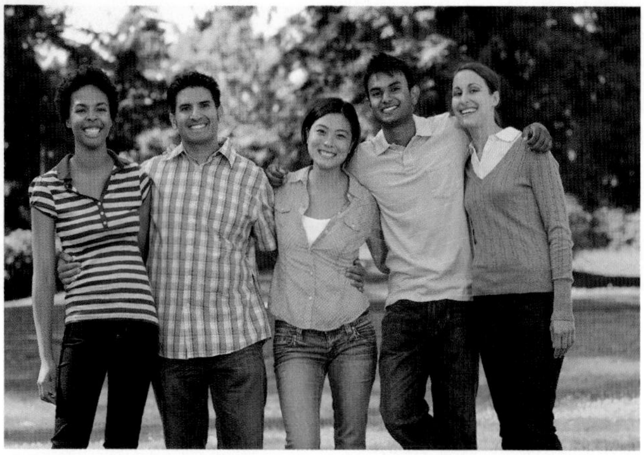

FIGURE 6-1 People living in the United States represent many different subcultures. (Copyright Getty Images. All rights reserved.)

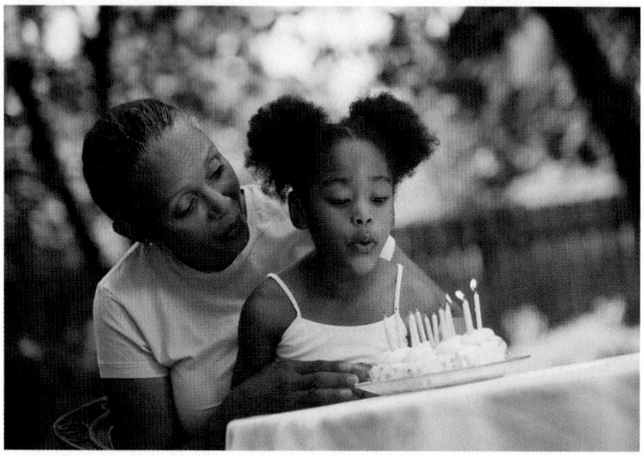

FIGURE 6-2 People of various heritages share a culture as they adopt American practices. (Copyright Jupiterimages. All rights reserved.)

is based on symbols. People *learn* to be a part of a culture as they are growing up, and the learning may continue into adulthood. This process is known as **enculturation**. Cultural learning is passed down from parent to child to grandchild, affecting the personality development of each generation. People learn what is expected of them and how they should behave, dress, and interact on particular occasions. For example, important life events are celebrated differently in different cultures (Fig. 6-2). Weddings and funerals may be quiet, small occasions for introspection or they may be robust, noisy celebrations with a crowd of people in attendance.

Culture also is *shared*. Cultural beliefs, values, and behaviors are shared among individuals within a particular group. Individual behavior does not reflect a particular culture unless it is manifested by other people in the cultural group. From group behavior, the behavior of individuals can then be predicted.

Culture is based on *symbols*. Symbols represent means of communication, spiritual beliefs, economic interactions, and national origins, among other things. Examples of symbols are language (words), religious artifacts (crucifix, Star of David), money (economic interactions), and flags (national origin). Symbols help to convey the beliefs, values, and behaviors of a society or culture.

Differences

Cultural differences may occur among various groups in relation to family, religion, communication, educational background, social class, and economic level. Nurses should be aware of the differences in these areas and recognize how they affect the wellness, illness, and health care practices of their patients.

Family. The family provides a major means for reproducing the population and rearing its children. The family unit is basic to every society. Cultural attitudes, values, and behaviors are transmitted mainly through the family.

The family structure may vary among and within cultures. The traditional nuclear family, consisting of a mother, a father, and children, is becoming less of a standard. Single-parent families made up 29.5% of all households in the United States in 2009. In addition, some cultural groups continue to have extended family members living under the same roof (e.g., grandparents, parents, children, and other relatives). Some families have a strong patriarchal (male, father-dominated) structure whereas others have strong matriarchal (female, mother-dominated) tendencies.

Culture can influence the attitudes and beliefs of families in relation to health care. Behaviors related to health practices, hospitalization, and placement in long-term care facilities can vary among cultures. For example, Latinos and Filipinos are thought to have strong extended family units and family ties; when a person is hospitalized, family members visit frequently. In addition, Latinos and Filipinos have tended to care for their elders in a home setting rather than placing them in residential facilities. Nurses should become acquainted with the various cultural backgrounds of families and how these backgrounds influence behavior, rather than be judgmental about family behaviors.

Religion. Religious beliefs are culturally determined and the way in which individuals fulfill their spiritual needs stems from a lifetime of experience. Religious beliefs and practices can influence perceptions of health and illness, hospitalization, and death and dying. Some patients may observe specific dietary rules and others may have particular practices regarding dress, modesty, daily living habits, or medical interventions. Religious differences also occur in relation to observation of the Sabbath, baptism, the sacrament of the sick, and last rites (Table 6-1).

Communication. Communication involves language. Certain cultural or **ethnic groups** speak different languages, making communication almost impossible without an interpreter. However, subtler forms of miscommunication also exist that can arise because of

Text continued on p. 75

Table 6-1 Religious Beliefs and Practices Affecting Health Care

RELIGIOUS GROUP	BELIEFS AND PRACTICES
	WESTERN RELIGIONS
Judaism	
Orthodox Jews and some Conservative Jewish groups	*Care of women:* A woman is considered to be in a ritual state of impurity whenever blood is coming from her uterus, such as during menstrual periods and after the birth of a child. During this time, her husband will not have physical contact with her. When this time is completed, she will bathe herself in a pool called a *mikvah*. Nurses need to be aware of this practice and be sensitive to the husband and wife because the husband will not touch his wife. He cannot assist her in moving in the bed; therefore the nurse will have to do this. An Orthodox Jewish man will not touch any woman other than his wife, daughters, and mother. *Dietary rules:* (1) Kosher dietary laws include the following: No mixing of milk and meat at a meal; no consumption of food or any derivative thereof from animals not slaughtered in accordance with Jewish law; separate cooking utensils for milk and milk products should be used; if a patient requires milk and meat products for a meal, the dairy foods should be served first, followed later by the meat. (2) During Yom Kippur (Day of Atonement), a 24-hour fast is required, but exceptions are made for those who cannot fast because of medical reasons. (3) During Passover, no leavened products are eaten. (4) May say benediction of thanksgiving before meals and grace at the end of the meal. Time and a quiet environment should be provided for this. *Sabbath:* Observed from sunset Friday until sunset Saturday. Orthodox law prohibits riding in a car, smoking, turning lights on and off, handling money, and using the telephone and watching television. Nurses need to be aware of this tradition when caring for observant Jews at home and in the hospital. Medical or surgical treatments should be postponed if possible. *Death*: Judaism defines death as occurring when respiration and circulation are irreversibly stopped and no movement is apparent. (1) Euthanasia is strictly forbidden by Orthodox Jews, who advocate the strict use of life-support measures. (2) Before death, Jewish faith indicates that visiting of the person by family and friends is a religious duty. The Torah and Psalms may be read and prayers recited. A witness needs to be present when a person prays for health so that if death occurs God will protect the family, and the spirit will be committed to God. Extraneous talking and conversation about death are not encouraged unless initiated by the patient or visitors. In Judaism, the belief is that people should have someone with them when the soul leaves the body, therefore family and friends should be allowed to stay with the patients. After death, the body should not be left alone until buried, usually within 24 hours. (3) When death occurs, the body should be untouched for 8 to 30 minutes. Medical personnel should not touch or wash the body but allow only an Orthodox person or the Jewish Burial Society to care for the body. Handling of a corpse on the Sabbath is forbidden to Jewish persons. If need be, the nursing staff may provide routine care of the body, wearing gloves. Water in the room should be emptied, and the family may request that mirrors be covered to symbolize that a death has occurred. (4) Orthodox Jews and some Conservative Jews do not approve of autopsies. If an autopsy must be performed, all body parts must remain with the body. (5) For Orthodox Jews, the body must be buried within 24 hours. No flowers are permitted. A fetus must be buried. (6) A 7-day mourning period is required by the immediate family. They must stay at home except for Sabbath worship. (7) Organs or other body parts such as amputated limbs must be made available for burial for Orthodox Jews because they believe that all of the body must be returned to earth. *Birth control and abortion:* Artificial methods of birth control are not encouraged. Vasectomy is not allowed. Abortion may be performed only to save the mother's life. *Organ transplants:* Donor organ transplants generally are not permitted by Orthodox Jews but may be allowed with rabbinical consent. *Shaving*: The beard is regarded as a mark of piety among observant Jews. For the very Orthodox, shaving should not be performed with a razor but with scissors or electric razor because a blade should not contact the skin. *Head coverings:* Orthodox men wear skull caps at all times, and women cover their hair after marriage. Some Orthodox women wear wigs as a mark of piety. Conservative Jews cover their head only during acts of worship and prayer. *Prayer:* Praying directly to God, including a prayer of confession, is required for Orthodox Jews. Nurses should provide quiet time for prayer.

Continued

Table 6-1 Religious Beliefs and Practices Affecting Health Care—cont'd

RELIGIOUS GROUP	BELIEFS AND PRACTICES
Reform Jews	*Care of women:* Reform Jews do not observe the rules against touching. *Dietary rules*: Reform Jews usually do not observe kosher dietary restrictions. *Sabbath:* Usually worship in temples on Friday evenings. No strict rules. *Death:* Advocate use of life support without heroic measures. Allow for cremation but suggest that ashes be buried in a Jewish cemetery. *Organ transplants:* Donation or transplantation of organs allowed with permission of a rabbi. *Head coverings:* Generally pray without wearing skullcaps.
Christianity	
Roman Catholic	*Holy Eucharist:* For patients and health care givers who are to receive communion, abstinence from solid food and alcohol is required for 15 minutes (if possible) before reception of the consecrated wafer. Medicine, water, and nonalcoholic drinks are permitted at any time. If a patient is in danger of death, the fast is waived because the reception of the Eucharist at this time is very important. *Anointing of the sick:* The priest uses oil to anoint the forehead and hands and, if desired, the affected area. The rite may be performed on anyone who is ill and desires it. Patients receiving the sacrament seek complete healing and strength to endure suffering. Before 1963, this sacrament was given only to patients at the time of imminent death, therefore the nurse must be sensitive to the meaning this has for the patient. If possible, the nurse calls a priest before the patient is unconscious but may also call when sudden death occurs because the sacrament may also be given shortly after death. The nurse records on the care plan that this sacrament has been administered. *Dietary habits:* Obligatory fasting is excused during hospitalization. However, if no health restrictions exist, some Catholics may still observe the following guidelines: (1) Anyone 14 years of age or older must abstain from eating meat on Ash Wednesday and all Fridays during Lent. Some older Catholics may still abstain from meat on all Fridays of the year. (2) In addition to abstinence from meat, persons 21 to 59 years of age must limit themselves to one full meal and two light meals on Ash Wednesday and Good Friday. (3) Eastern Rite Catholics are stricter than Western Rite Catholics about fasting and fast more frequently than Western Rite Catholics, therefore the nurse needs to know if a patient is Eastern or Western Catholic. *Death:* Each Roman Catholic should participate in the anointing of the sick, as well as Eucharist and penance, before death. The body should not be shrouded until after these sacraments are performed. All body parts that retain human quality must be appropriately buried or cremated. *Birth control:* Prohibited except for abstinence or natural family planning. Referral to a priest for questions about this can be of great help. Nurses can teach the techniques of natural family planning if they are familiar with them; otherwise, this should be referred to the physician or to a support group of the church that instructs couples in this method of birth control. Sterilization is prohibited unless an overriding medical reason exists. *Organ transplants:* Donation and transplantation of organs are acceptable as long as the donor is not harmed and is not deprived of life. *Religious objects:* Rosary prayers are said using rosary beads. Medals bearing the images of saints, relics, statues, and scapulars are important objects that may be pinned to a hospital gown or pillow or be at the bedside. Extreme care should be taken not to lose these objects because they have special meaning to the patient.
Eastern Orthodox	*Holy Eucharist:* The priest is notified if the patient desires this sacrament. *Anointing of the sick:* The priest conducts this in the hospital room. *Dietary habits:* Fasting from meat and dairy products is required on Wednesday and Friday during Lent and on other holy days. Hospital patients are exempt if fasting is detrimental to health. *Special days:* Christmas is celebrated on January 7 and New Year's Day on January 14. This tradition is important to the care of a patient who is hospitalized on these days. *Death:* Last rites are obligatory. This tradition is handled by an ordained priest who is notified by the nurse while the patient is conscious. The Russian Orthodox Church does not encourage autopsy or organ donation. Euthanasia, even for the terminally ill, is discouraged, as is cremation. *Birth control:* Birth control and abortion are not permitted.

Table 6-1 Religious Beliefs and Practices Affecting Health Care—cont'd

RELIGIOUS GROUP	BELIEFS AND PRACTICES
Protestant	
Assemblies of God (Pentecostal)	*Holy Communion:* Notify the clergy if the patient desires. *Anointing of the sick:* Members believe in divine healing through prayer and the laying on of hands. The clergy is notified if the patient or family desires this. *Dietary habits:* Abstinence from alcohol, tobacco, and all illegal drugs is strongly encouraged. *Death:* No special practices. *Other practices:* Faith in God and in the health care providers is encouraged. Members pray for divine intervention in health matters. Nurses should encourage and allow time for prayer. Members may speak in "tongues" during prayer.
Baptist (over 27 different groups in the United States)	*Holy Communion:* The clergy should be notified if the patient desires. *Dietary habits:* Total abstinence from alcohol is expected. *Death:* No general service is provided, but the clergy does minister through counseling, prayer, and Scripture as requested by the patient or family, and the patient is encouraged to believe in Jesus Christ as Savior and Lord. *Other practices:* The Bible is held to be the word of God; therefore the nurse should either allow quiet time for Scripture reading or offer to read to the patient.
Christian Church (Disciples of Christ)	*Holy Communion:* Open communion is celebrated each Sunday and is a central part of worship services. The nurse notifies the clergy if the patient desires it, or the clergy may suggest it. *Death:* No special practices. *Other practices:* Church elders, as well as clergy, may be notified to assist with meeting the patient's spiritual needs.
Church of the Brethren	*Holy Communion:* Usually received within the church, but the clergy will give it in the hospital when requested. *Anointing of the sick:* Practiced for physical healing, as well as spiritual uplift, and is held in high regard by the church. The clergy is notified if the patient or family desires. *Death:* The clergy is notified for counsel and prayer.
Church of the Nazarene	*Holy Communion:* The pastor will administer if the patient wishes. *Dietary habits:* The use of alcohol and tobacco is forbidden. *Death:* Cremation is permitted, and term stillborn infants are buried. *Other practices:* Believe in divine healing but not to the exclusion of medical treatment. Patients may desire quiet time for prayer.
Episcopal (Anglican)	*Holy Communion:* The priest is notified if the patient wishes to receive this sacrament. *Anointing of the sick:* The priest may administer this rite when death is imminent, but it is not considered mandatory. *Dietary habits:* Some patients may abstain from meat on Fridays. Others may fast before receiving the Eucharist, but fasting is not mandatory. *Death:* No special practices. *Other practices:* Confession of sins to a priest is optional; if the patient desires this, the clergy should be notified.
Lutheran (18 different branches)	*Holy Communion:* Notify the clergy if the patient desires this sacrament. The clergy may also inquire about the patient's desire. *Anointing of the sick:* The patient may request an anointing and blessing from the minister when the prognosis is poor. *Death:* A service of Commendation of the Dying is used at the patient's or the family's request.
Mennonite (12 different groups)	*Holy Communion:* Served twice a year, with foot washing as part of the ceremony. *Dietary habits:* Abstinence from alcohol is urged for all. *Death:* Prayer is important at a time of crisis, therefore contacting a minister is important. *Other practices:* Women may wear head coverings during hospitalization. Anointing with oil is administered in harmony with James 5:14 when requested.

Continued

Table 6-1 Religious Beliefs and Practices Affecting Health Care—cont'd

RELIGIOUS GROUP	BELIEFS AND PRACTICES
Methodist (over 20 different groups)	*Holy Communion:* Notify the clergy if the patient requests it before surgery or another health crisis. *Anointing of the sick:* If requested, the clergy will come to pray and sprinkle the patient with olive oil. *Death:* Scripture reading and prayer are important at this time. *Other practices:* Donation of one's body or part of the body at death is encouraged.
Presbyterian (10 different groups)	*Holy Communion:* Given when appropriate and convenient, at the hospitalized patient's request. *Death:* Notify a local pastor or elder for prayer and Scripture reading if desired by the family or patient.
Quaker (Friends)	*Holy Communion:* Because Friends have no creed, personal beliefs are diverse, one of which is that outward sacraments are usually not necessary because of the ministry of the Spirit inwardly in such areas as baptism and communion. *Death:* Believe that the present life is part of God's kingdom and generally have no ceremony as a rite of passage from this life to the next. Personal beliefs and wishes need to be ascertained, and the nurse can then act on the patient's wishes.
Salvation Army	*Holy Communion:* No particular ceremony. *Death:* Notify the local officer in charge of the Army Corps for any soldier (member) who needs assistance. *Other practices:* The Bible is seen as the only rule for one's faith, therefore the Scriptures should be made available to a patient. The Army has many of its own social welfare centers with hospitals and homes where unwed mothers are cared for and outpatient services provided. No medical or surgical procedures are opposed, except for abortion on demand.
Seventh-Day Adventist	*Holy Communion:* Although this is not required of hospitalized patients, the clergy is notified if the patient desires. *Anointing of the sick:* The clergy is contacted for prayer and anointing with oil. *Dietary habits:* Because the body is viewed as the temple of the Holy Spirit, healthy living is essential; therefore the use of alcohol, tobacco, coffee, and tea and the promiscuous use of drugs are prohibited. Some are vegetarians, and most avoid pork. *Special days:* The Sabbath is observed on Saturday. *Death:* No special procedures. *Other practices:* Use of hypnotism is opposed by some. Persons of homosexual or lesbian orientation are ministered to in the hope of correction of these practices, which are believed to be wrong. A Bible should always be available for Scripture reading.
United Church of Christ	*Holy Communion:* The clergy is notified if the patient desires to receive this sacrament. *Death:* If the patient desires counsel or prayer, notify the clergy.
Other	
Christian Science	*Dietary habits:* Because alcohol and tobacco are considered drugs, they are not used. Coffee and tea are often declined. *Death:* Autopsy is usually declined unless required by law. Donation of organs is unlikely but is an individual decision. *Other practices:* Christian Scientists do not normally seek medical care because they approach health care in a different, primarily spiritual, framework. They commonly use the services of a surgeon to set a bone but decline drugs and, in general, other medical or surgical procedures. Hypnotism and psychotherapy are also declined. Family planning is left to the family. They seek exemption from vaccinations but obey legal requirements (e.g., report infectious diseases and obey public health quarantines). Nonmedical care facilities are maintained for those needing nursing assistance in the course of a healing. *The Christian Science Journal* lists available Christian Science nurses. When a Christian Science believer is in the hospital, the nurse should allow and encourage time for prayer and study. Patients may request that a Christian Science practitioner be notified to come.

Table 6-1 Religious Beliefs and Practices Affecting Health Care—cont'd

RELIGIOUS GROUP	BELIEFS AND PRACTICES
Jehovah's Witnesses	*Dietary habits:* Use of alcohol and tobacco is discouraged because these substances harm the physical body. *Death:* Autopsy is a private matter to be decided by the persons involved. Burial and cremation are acceptable. *Birth control and abortion:* Use of birth control is a personal decision. Abortion is opposed based on Exodus 21:22–23. *Organ transplants:* Use of organ transplant is a private decision and, if used, must be cleansed with a nonblood solution. *Blood transfusions:* Blood transfusions violate God's laws and therefore are not allowed. Patients do respect physicians and will accept alternatives to blood transfusions. These alternatives might include use of nonblood plasma expanders, careful surgical techniques to decrease blood loss, use of autologous transfusions, and autotransfusion through use of a heart-lung machine. Nurses should check unconscious patients for Medic Alert cards that state that the person does not want a transfusion. Because Jehovah's Witnesses are prepared to die rather than break God's law, nurses need to be sensitive to the spiritual and the physical needs of the patient.
The Church of Jesus Christ of Latter-Day Saints	*Holy Communion:* A hospitalized patient may desire to have a member of the church priesthood administer this sacrament. *Anointing of the sick:* Mormons are frequently anointed and given a blessing before going to the hospital and after admission by laying on of hands. *Dietary habits:* Abstinence from the use of tobacco; beverages with caffeine such as cola, coffee, and tea; alcohol and other substances that are considered as injurious. Mormons eat meat but encourage the intake of fruits, grains, and herbs. *Death:* Prefer burial of the body. A church elder should be notified to assist the family. If need be, the elder will assist the funeral director in dressing the body in special clothes and give other help as needed. *Birth control and abortion:* Abortion is opposed except when the life of the mother is in danger. Only natural means of birth control are recommended. Artificial means can be used when the health of the woman is at stake (including emotional health). *Personal care:* Cleanliness is very important to Mormons. A sacred undergarment may be worn at all times by Mormons and should only be removed in emergency situations. *Other practices:* Allowing quiet time for prayer and the reading of the sacred writings is important. The church maintains a welfare system to assist persons in need. Families are of great importance, therefore visiting should be encouraged.
Unitarian Universalist Association	*Death:* Cremation is often preferred to burial. *Other practices:* Use of birth control is advocated as part of responsible parenting. Strong support for a woman's right to choice regarding abortion is maintained. Unitarian Universalists advocate donation of body parts for research and transplants.
Unification Church	*Baptism:* No baptism occurs. *Special days:* Sunday mornings are used to honor Reverend and Mrs. Moon as the true parents, and members get up at 5:00 AM, bow before a picture of the Moons three times, and vow to do what is needed to help the Reverend accomplish his mission on earth. *Death:* They believe that, after death, one's place of destiny will depend on his or her spirit's quality of life and goodness while on earth. In the afterlife, one will have the same aspirations and feelings as before death. Hell is not a concern because it will not be a place as heaven grows in size. Persons who leave the Unification Church are warned that Satan may try to possess them. *Other practices:* All marriages must be solemnized by Reverend Moon to be part of the perfect family and have salvation. The church supplies its faithful members with life's necessities. Members may use occult practices to have spiritual and psychic experiences.

Continued

Table 6-1 Religious Beliefs and Practices Affecting Health Care—cont'd

RELIGIOUS GROUP	BELIEFS AND PRACTICES
Islam	
	Dietary habits: No pork is allowed or alcoholic beverages. All *halal* (permissible) meat must be blessed and killed in a special way. This is called *zabihah* (correctly slaughtered). *Death:* Before death, family members ask to be present so that they can read the Koran and pray with the patient. An Imam may come if requested by the patient or family but is not required. Patients must face Mecca and confess their sins and beg forgiveness in the presence of their family. If the family is unavailable, any practicing Muslim can provide support to the patient. After death, Muslims prefer that the family wash, prepare, and place the body in a position facing Mecca. If necessary, the health care providers may perform these procedures as long as they wear gloves. Burial is performed as soon as possible. Cremation is forbidden. Autopsy is also prohibited except for legal reasons, and then no body part is to be removed. Donation of body parts or organs is not allowed because, according to culturally developed law, persons do not own their body. *Abortion and birth control:* Abortion is forbidden, and many conservative Muslims do not encourage the use of contraceptives because this practice interferes with God's purpose. Others believe that a woman should have only as many children as her husband can afford. Contraception is permitted by Islamic law. *Personal devotions:* At prayer time, washing is required, even by persons who are sick. A patient on bedrest may require assistance with this task before prayer. Provision of privacy during prayer is important. *Religious objects:* The Koran must not be touched by anyone ritually unclean, and nothing should be placed on top of it. Some Muslims wear *taviz* (a black string on which words of the Koran are attached). These should not be removed and must remain dry. Certain items of jewelry such as bangles may have religious significance and should not be removed unnecessarily. *Care of women:* Because women are not allowed to sign consent forms or make a decision regarding family planning, the husband needs to be present. Women are very modest and frequently wear clothes that cover all of the body. During a medical examination, the woman's modesty should be respected as much as possible. Muslim women prefer female physicians. For 40 days after giving birth and during menstruation, a woman is exempt from prayer because this period is a time of cleansing for her.
American Muslim Mission	*Dietary habits:* In addition to refusing pork, many will not eat traditional African-American foods such as cornbread and collard greens. *Death:* The family is contacted before any care of the deceased is performed. Special procedures exist for washing and shrouding the body. *Other practices:* Quiet time is necessary to permit prayer. Members are encouraged to use African-American physicians for health care. Because these patients do not smoke, their request for a nonsmoking roommate should be honored.
	EASTERN RELIGIONS
Hinduism	
	Dietary habits: Some sects are vegetarian, believing meats and intoxicants to be too stimulating to the senses. *Belief about illness:* View illness as a result of misuse of the body or a consequence of sins committed in a previous life. They do not oppose medical treatment but view its effect as transitory. Believe that praying for health is the lowest form of prayer. *Death:* See death as a union with Brahman (God) achieved through prayers, ritual, purity, self-control, detachment, truth, nonviolence, charity, and compassion toward all creatures. After death, one will be reborn (reincarnated) into a future life based on the behavior in this life. The record of behavior is called *karma*. Eventually, the process of rebirth stops, which is called *moksha*. A priest may be called at the time of death and may tie a thread around the neck or waist as a blessing. The family washes the body, and it is cremated. *Other practices:* Offer daily worship at a shrine in the home: daily offering to God and morning and evening rites. Society is organized into castes, or strata. People are born into a caste, and the caste shapes one's entire life. Hindus practice a discipline of the mind and body, called *yoga,* to reach God. In the highest state, a meditating yogi does not see, hear, taste, feel, or smell. Beyond good and evil, time and space, the yogi is one with God.

Table 6-1 Religious Beliefs and Practices Affecting Health Care—cont'd

RELIGIOUS GROUP	BELIEFS AND PRACTICES
Buddhism	
	Death: Buddhists believe that salvation depends on one's own right living. They also believe in reincarnation. The person can speed the process toward *Nirvana* (the goal of all humanity's striving) through acts of merit. Meditation, worship, and prayer are some of the acts of merit. Buddhists may drive themselves into more and more ritual or contemplation in the hope that their last moments of consciousness may be filled with thoughts worthy enough to elevate them to a higher existence. Last rights of chanting may be performed at bedside. *Renunciation:* The most important Buddhist feasts. Young boys are taught to despise the world's vanity, and the boy spends a night in a nearby monastery.
Taoism/Confucianism	
	General beliefs: Founded on ethical principles of Confucius. God is not clearly defined as in other religions. Taoism is a mixture of magic and religion. Followers believe that humans and nature are inseparable and that if heaven is upset, earth does not prosper. This relationship is described as *yang* and *yin,* which are two interplaying forces. When yang and yin are in balance, good occurs. *Death:* The dead are remembered in all festivals. The fate of the dead in the afterworld depends not only on the life they led, but also on being properly honored after death; otherwise, they may become demons. Graves are mounds similar to those dedicated to the gifts of the soil. Graves and houses must be in harmony with the universe; otherwise evil will befall the occupants.

From Black JM, Matassarin-Jacobs E: *Luckmann and Sorensen's medical-surgical nursing: a psychophysiologic approach,* ed 4, Philadelphia, 1993, Saunders Elsevier. Modified from Carson VB: *Spiritual dimensions of nursing practice,* Philadelphia, 1989, Saunders Elsevier.

group differences. The speed at which people speak and their tone and inflections vary according to cultural background.

Nonverbal communication is also culturally based. Personal space, eye contact, gestures, displays of emotions, and the amount and meaning of touch that are acceptable are culturally determined. Some cultures find emotional display more acceptable than others. Some are more comfortable with silence than others.

Educational Background and Economic Level. Large differences in educational backgrounds can be found within the United States. Millions of Americans have literacy skills below the eighth grade level, meaning that they have difficulty with reading and writing. One aspect of literacy is *health literacy,* which refers to the ability to obtain and understand basic information needed to make health decisions. Health literacy has been found to be highest among women, Caucasian and Pacific Islander adults, and adults under age 65.

Educational level attained is strongly tied to ethnicity and economic background. School dropout rates appear to be higher among adolescents living in poverty areas. Ethnic groups that are found in large numbers in poverty areas tend to have high dropout rates.

Educational background and economic levels affect the ways in which people perceive the world, health and illness, and the health care system. Teaching about health becomes a challenge because many people with low literacy levels have difficulty reading the materials presented and understanding health care jargon. In addition, people from economically deprived backgrounds may live in crowded, unsafe housing and have inadequate diets. Such conditions make health promotion and disease prevention difficult.

CULTURAL BELIEFS RELATED TO HEALTH AND ILLNESS

Health and illness have different meanings for different people and cultural groups. For some groups, illness is expected as part of life and is out of one's own control. Others believe that illness can be prevented by taking action, such as by eating a proper diet, getting exercise, or scheduling regular physical examinations.

Some groups attempt to attach meaning to illness to explain why it occurs. Many beliefs have developed regarding the onset, course, and cure of disease, as well as the process of death and dying. For example, some people believe that illness is a type of divine punishment for a sin that an individual has committed. Another belief involves an individual's balance with nature. If a person maintains a proper balance, good health results; if a person is not in harmony with the environment, illness occurs.

The "hot" and "cold" theory is an ancient belief about health and illness that is still held widely in many cultures. According to the hot and cold theory, health and illness are influenced by four humors that regulate body functions. The four humors are phlegm, blood, black bile, and yellow bile. The humors are considered either hot (blood and yellow bile) or cold (phlegm and black bile) and an imbalance between the hot and cold areas of the body causes illness. Examples of illnesses that are thought to be caused by cold entering the body are earaches, paralysis, stomach cramps, and arthritis. Examples of illnesses thought to be caused by heat include dysentery, sore throat, abscessed teeth, and kidney disease. Illnesses are treated with herbs, potions, and foods that are considered to be either hot or cold, depending on their effects on the body.

Many ethnic groups use healers who practice health care outside of the formal health care delivery system. Patients may visit a folk healer or use folk remedies along with or in place of conventional treatment. Western societies generally believe that illness has a known cause that can be treated or cured if the cause is identified. Western medicine is also focused on risk reduction and prevention. Generally, non-Western societies believe that illness has supernatural causes and these persons have a more holistic approach to illness. Traditional healers employ forms of healing that may be secular, sacred, or both. The variety of healers depends on the number of health cultures. Examples of traditional healers are *root doctors*, who traditionally practice among urban African Americans, and *curanderos*, who may be consulted by Latinos. They may be sought when mainstream health care is perceived as being too expensive, inconvenient, or unable to provide relief for the problem at hand. The healers provide psychosocial support and counseling in addition to helping with physiologic problems. They use a variety of potions and plants in their practice.

DIMENSIONS OF AMERICAN CULTURE

Despite the "melting pot" of subcultures in the United States, certain characteristics are generally true of American culture. Americans are very time oriented and value being on time, multitasking, and "time-saving" measures. Eager to get tasks done, American health care providers may not take the time to establish rapport with patients. Americans typically embrace change, including the newest technologies and treatments. Americans are likely to believe that people have control over their own destiny rather than attributing outcomes to fate or karma. Self-sufficiency and individualism are highly valued. Reflecting the value of equality and rejection of a social hierarchy, Americans tend to be informal, even with strangers. Americans are described as low-context communicators, meaning that they rely mostly on words and less on nonverbal messages. Americans' direct speech may seem abrupt and rude to others (Carteret, 2011). Nurses need to be aware of these dimensions of American culture and recognize that they may interfere with the nurse-patient relationship. Most important is the need to take time to put patients at ease and listen to what they have to say.

TRADITIONAL HEALTH HABITS AND BELIEFS OF MAJOR ETHNIC GROUPS IN THE UNITED STATES

Although stereotyping individual members of any culture or subculture is inappropriate, various ethnic groups in the United States retain unique, traditional health-culture beliefs and practices. Great variations in beliefs and practices exist not only between, but also within ethnic and subcultural groups. Although individuals vary, a given ethnic group generally has some common ideas and practices regarding health promotion and disease prevention, attitudes and behaviors related to illness, and use of health care resources. One factor that affects the extent to which an individual maintains traditional practices is the extent of enculturation and assimilation into American society that has occurred. **Assimilation** occurs when people change their ways of life and become integrated into another culture. First- or second-generation Americans may have more characteristics associated with their ethnic group than people who have been in the United States for several generations.

Discussed next are examples of traditional health care beliefs and practices of selected ethnic groups. Remember that these examples are included to show a range of possible health customs for selected ethnic groups. They cannot be generalized to all members of the ethnic group or subculture.

CAUCASIANS (EURO-AMERICANS)

As with other racial or ethnic groups, Caucasian Americans are very heterogeneous, even though most descended from European roots. Nevertheless, identifying some values and beliefs common to this group of people is useful. Caucasians generally believe in the work ethic, which values personal achievement, individualism, and competition. These values are apparent in the dimensions of American culture described previously. Values related to health include individual decision making, personal space, and privacy. Illness is viewed primarily as caused by germs in the environment or, among certain religious groups, by divine punishment. The risk of illness can be reduced by eating a proper diet, getting enough exercise, and allowing for adequate rest. In the treatment of illness, the mind, body, and spirit are considered as separate. Caucasians look to science and technology for the treatment of illness.

Caucasian Americans often communicate directly and tend to express feelings of pain openly. Although members of this group tend to use the formal health care system for their medical and nursing needs, they may consult spiritual advisers in times of illness. Traditionally, the health care provider has been seen as the manager of care.

AFRICAN AMERICANS

African Americans value family, community, religion, health, and work. Elders are respected and commonly provide care for grandchildren. When the elder requires care, it is often provided by the family rather than an institution. In addition to an understanding of germs as a cause of illness, some traditional beliefs attribute illness to divine punishment or to an imbalance among body, mind, and spirit. Prevention of illness is thought to be achieved by eating good food, living right, and keeping the system cleaned out. Communication may be direct or indirect and expressions of pain during illness may entail varying degrees of stoicism or vocal outcries to God for assistance. African Americans tend to attempt self-care before consulting a health care professional when they are ill. They also may use folk medicine or consult a root doctor or spiritualist for help.

LATINOS/HISPANICS

People whose heritage is rooted in various parts of South or Central America refer to themselves as Latinos or Hispanics. To reduce repetition, the term *Latinos* will be used in this text. Latinos, particularly those who live in the southwestern United States, are family oriented, value harmony in interpersonal relationships, and tend to defer to those in authority. Traditional beliefs about the cause of illness include magical fright, divine punishment, an imbalance of hot and cold elements in the body, and environmental hazards. Some Latinos believe that illness can be prevented through the use of charms, amulets, or crucifixes. Communication is usually indirect; however, expressions of pain are open and direct. Folk health specialists *(curanderos)* and family members may be consulted along with the formal health care system in times of illness.

ASIANS

Asians value self-respect, self-control, respect for elders, family honor, loyalty, and pride. Holistic health and harmony between the self and the universe are emphasized. There is acceptance of uncertainty in life, so that each day must be taken as it comes. Concepts of time vary among Asians from different countries. Whereas many Asians in the United States use the formal health care system in times of illness, others may favor health care that is provided by herbalists, acupuncturists, and other cultural healers. Communication patterns tend to be indirect, meaning that nonverbal messages are equally as important as words. Smiling may indicate confusion or embarrassment rather than amusement. Pain is endured with varying degrees of stoicism.

NATIVE AMERICANS

Considerable diversity exists among tribes and groups; therefore caution should be used when making generalizations about Native Americans. However, some general characteristics may be noted. Native Americans value family, respect for elders, generosity, and cooperation. They attempt to live in harmony with nature and have deep respect for the environment. Communication is usually indirect, with a great emphasis on nonverbal cues. Pain is usually endured stoically. Traditional health practices emphasize total healing, mental and spiritual renewal, and health maintenance. Ceremonial rituals guided by a *medicine man* may be used to treat illnesses before structured medical care is sought.

MIDDLE EASTERNERS

Like Asians and Latinos, Middle Easterners have roots in many different countries and so nurses must be careful not to generalize without collecting individual patient and family data. One value common among Middle Easterners is a strong need for affiliation characterized by a large network of family and friends. Individuals rely on one another and are attentive to sick friends or family members. Men often speak for their wives, sexual segregation is practiced, and female modesty is important. While the authority of a male physician is not questioned, Middle Eastern patients, especially men, may be uncomfortable with female physicians as authority figures. Middle Easterners are less time oriented than Caucasian Americans and require less personal space. There is a tendency to speak loudly for emphasis and body language is employed to enhance verbal messages. Islam is the most common religion, though other religions are represented. Some Middle Easterners are fatalistic, believing that the outcome of illness is "in Allah's hands" and fearing hospitals as places to die. Although Western medicine is generally respected, some Middle Easterners practice folk beliefs.

Once again, it must be emphasized that the examples given here are intended to convey the wide scope of culturally based practices that may need to be considered when working with individuals from various cultures. The nursing assessment should include gathering information about personal health practices so that the care plan can be individualized.

Put on Your Thinking Cap!

Considering your own race or ethnicity, identify three cultural beliefs related to health that are held by your family. For example, how are you expected to respond to illness or stress? When do you seek medical care and what kind of provider do you see? Do you use any complementary or alternative therapies? What activities are believed to promote health or prevent disease?

CULTURAL INFLUENCES ON PATIENT AND FAMILY INTERACTIONS WITH THE HEALTH CARE SYSTEM

In all health care settings, patients of different cultures may exhibit behavior that is not understood by health care providers from other cultures. The culturally different patients may be labeled *complaining, difficult, uncooperative*, or *noncompliant* when, in reality, they are struggling to adapt to a culture that is foreign to them. Fear of the unknown may result in these behaviors. Culturally congruent care that is in harmony with the patient's values, meanings, beliefs, and practices is urgently needed. Care providers who deliver culturally congruent care are said to be culturally competent. With increasing cultural diversity among all people in the United States, you must consider your patients' cultures and develop culture-specific nursing care.

HOSPITAL HEALTH CARE

The hospital environment is often frightening, even to people who are familiar with it. For individuals who speak different languages, have different eating preferences, and view health and illness differently, adapting to the hospital environment is a formidable task. Admission to the hospital may seem as though traveling to a foreign country where an entirely different language is spoken. Hospital personnel become authority figures and their permission is needed to carry out the most basic activities, such as toileting, eating, and dressing. Patients may feel stripped of their dignity when told to wear hospital gowns that barely cover private parts of the body. Modesty is often ignored, causing humiliation and anxiety.

Not only do people find themselves in a totally new environment but they must also endure separation from their family and friends. Their support systems topple when strict visiting rules are enforced. In some cultures, families expect to advocate for the patient, help with the nursing care, or at least sit with sick people to keep them company and provide support. Nurses and hospital personnel are often uncomfortable with this infringement on their territory. Language barriers may complicate the process of providing care. Hospitals should have access to professional interpretation services. When available, the professional interpreter is recommended because family members and friends may not have the language to convey medical information correctly. Furthermore, information exchanged in the health care setting should be confidential and use of a lay interpreter may violate this confidentiality.

Culture shock associated with hospitalization occurs in three phases. During the first phase, the patient asks questions regarding the hospital routine and the hospital's expectations of the patient. In the second phase, the patient becomes disenchanted with the whole situation and is frustrated, hostile, and then depressed and withdrawn. In the final phase, the patient begins to adapt to the new environment and is even able to maintain a sense of humor during interactions with others.

COMMUNITY AND HOME HEALTH CARE

Community settings in which culturally different individuals interact with the health care system include physicians' offices, outpatient clinics, community mental health centers, home health care, hospices, and day care centers. LVNs/LPNs are increasingly visible in community and outpatient settings. As mentioned earlier, individuals who have different cultural backgrounds may also have their own network of health care, such as spiritualists, *curanderos*, or root doctors. A day's assignment in home health care may include visits to Jewish, Latino, Filipino, and Euro-American homes. Community nursing presents examples of cultural diversity that nurses everywhere are experiencing with the expanded need for home health services.

Many ethnic or cultural minorities have difficulty getting through the maze of health care services, either because of language differences or because of negative attitudes toward health care providers based on past experiences. Minority group members whose financial resources are limited are frequently clinic patients who must wait hours for an appointment only to receive a cursory assessment from the physician or nurse. Their questions about their condition may be left unanswered because of communication barriers, which can affect the ability to follow directions for care. These patients may be labeled *noncompliant* or *difficult*, which only perpetuates a cycle of negative attitudes among patients and health care providers alike.

When entering a patient's home, notice symbolic objects that may indicate cultural identity. Shrines, religious pictures or statues, and special candles are examples of symbols. Ask about your patient's health beliefs and practices that are affected by culture. Patients and their families may have magical, religious, biomedical, or holistic beliefs.

If the patient speaks a different language from yours, a family member is sometimes able to interpret. If no interpreter is available, it may take extra time to teach a procedure to the patient and the family.

LONG-TERM FACILITY HEALTH CARE

The majority of residents in long-term care facilities are Caucasian women. Traditionally, some ethnic groups, including African Americans, Latinos, and Asians, are reluctant to admit older relatives to residential care facilities and prefer to provide care at home.

Many residents of residential facilities suffer from functional impairments (impaired ability to carry out activities of daily living such as bathing and dressing). Individuals from different cultural groups have the added strain of communication problems and extreme changes in lifestyle and dietary practices.

Box 9-1 Fat Content of Some Common Foods

0 GRAMS OF FAT
Most fruits and vegetables
Nonfat milk
Nonfat yogurt
Plain pasta and rice
Angel food cake
Popcorn, air-popped, unbuttered
Soft drinks
Jam, jelly

1–3 GRAMS OF FAT
Popcorn, oil-popped, unbuttered, 1 cup
Low-calorie salad dressing, 1 T
Baked beans, ½ cup
Soup, chicken noodle, canned, 1 cup
Whole wheat bread, 1 slice
Dinner roll, 1
Waffle, frozen, 4-inch, 1
Coleslaw, ½ cup
Flounder or sole, baked, 3 oz
Chicken, without skin, roasted, 3 oz
Tuna, canned in water, 3 oz
Cheese, cottage, 2% fat, ½ cup
Ice milk, soft serve, ½ cup

4–6 GRAMS OF FAT
Low-fat yogurt, 1 cup
Cheese, mozzarella, part skim, 1 oz
Chicken, roasted with skin, 3 oz
Egg, scrambled, 1
Turkey, roasted, 3 oz
Granola, 1 oz
Muffin, bran, 1 small
Pizza, cheese, ¼ of 12-inch pie
Burrito, bean, 1
Brownie, with nuts, 1 small
Margarine or butter, 1 tsp
Popcorn, oil popped, buttered, 1 cup
French dressing, regular, 1 T

7–10 GRAMS OF FAT
Cheese, cheddar, 1 oz
Milk, whole, 1 cup
Bologna, beef, 1 slice
Sausage, 1 patty
Steak, sirloin, broiled, 3 oz
Potatoes, French fried, 10
Chow mein, chicken, 1 cup
Chocolate candy bar, 1 oz
Corn chips, 1 oz
Doughnut, cake type, plain, 1
Mayonnaise, 1 T

15 GRAMS OF FAT
Hot dog, beef, 2 oz
McDonald's Chicken McNuggets, 6 pieces
Peanut butter, 2 T
Pork chop, broiled, 3 oz
Sunflower seeds, dry roasted, ¼ cup
Avocado, ½ medium
Chop suey, beef, and pork, 1 cup
Cinnamon roll, 1

20 GRAMS OF FAT
Lasagna with meat, 1 medium piece
Macaroni and cheese, homemade, 1 cup
Peanuts, dry roasted, ¼ cup
Ground beef, broiled, 3 oz

25 GRAMS OF FAT
Polish sausage, 3 oz
Cheeseburger, large
Pie, pecan, ⅛ of 9-inch pie
Chicken pot pie, frozen, baked, 1 pie
Quiche, bacon, ⅛ pie

From Mahan LK, Escott-Stump S, Raymond JL: *Krause's food and the nutrition care process*, ed 13, St. Louis, 2012, Elsevier/Saunders, p. 40.
oz, Ounce; *T*, tablespoon; *tsp*, teaspoon.

amino acids by a process called *deamination*. Deamination releases amino groups that are used to synthesize several acids. It also yields ammonia, which is transported to the liver where it is converted to urea for excretion by the kidneys. The amino acids are then transported by the blood to the cells, where they can be synthesized into tissue protein, processed to produce adenosine triphosphate, or converted into glucose.

Protein synthesis in the body is controlled by deoxyribonucleic acid (DNA) in the cells. DNA essentially provides a template to link the exact combination of amino acids needed to form a particular protein. An important point to note is that if one or more of the essential amino acids are in short supply or not available at all, nonessential amino acids cannot be used to form a protein. This illustrates the importance of eating a diet that contains all of the essential amino acids, plus enough additional amino acids to allow for synthesis of the nonessential amino acids.

PROTEIN DEFICIENCY

The body cannot store protein; therefore it needs to be eaten each day. Nitrogen in the urine is a good indicator of protein levels in the body. If protein intake is inadequate, nitrogen will be conserved by the kidneys, causing the urine nitrogen to be low. When this adaptive process is no longer adequate, evidence of protein deficiency appears. The signs and symptoms include edema, wasting of body tissues, fatty liver, dermatosis (thickening and hardening of the skin), diminished immune response, weakness, and loss of energy.

EVALUATION OF PROTEIN QUALITY

The average American consumes considerably more than the RDA for protein. The assessment of the adequacy of one's protein should include both the quantity and the quality of the protein consumed. The protein content, by weight, of cooked meat, fish, poultry, and milk solids is between 15% and 40%. The

Box 9-2 Protein Content of Some Foods

0–1 GRAM
Butter, margarine, 1 tsp
Pear, 1 medium
Cake, 1 piece

2–3 GRAMS
Milk chocolate, 1 oz
Cereal, refined, 1 oz
Bread, 1 slice
Corn, canned, ½ cup
Chicken noodle soup, 1 cup
French fries, 1 regular serving

4–6 GRAMS
Cereal, bran, 1 oz
Baked potato, 1 large
Peas, ½ cup

7–8 GRAMS
Navy beans, cooked, ½ cup
Egg, 1 medium
Cheese, 1 oz
Tuna, 1 oz
Tofu, 3½ oz
Milk, 1 cup

9–10 GRAMS
Peanuts, roasted, 1 oz
Macaroni and cheese, ¾ cup
Pizza, cheese, ⅛ of a 12-inch pie

12–15 GRAMS
Taco, 1
Hamburger, 1
Chili with meat, 1 cup

22–26 GRAMS
Meat, lean, 3 oz
Big Mac, 1

From Mahan LK, Arlin M: *Krause's food, nutrition, and diet therapy*, ed 8, Philadelphia, 1992, Saunders.
oz, Ounce; *tsp*, teaspoon.

protein content of cooked cereals, beans, and lentils ranges from 3% to 10%. Ingesting a diet high in animal protein is not necessary and may be too high in fat. Eating a mixture of foods in a meal, if the quantity is sufficient, tends to provide all of the essential amino acids.

More total protein is required in a vegetable protein diet than in a diet of mixed vegetable and animal proteins because more of the lower-quality protein is needed to meet the minimal requirements for amino acids and nitrogen. Also, because of their lower digestibility, vegetable proteins are less available. Box 9-2 gives the protein content of typical foods in the American diet.

Functions of Proteins

The roles of proteins in the body are to:

- Furnish building blocks (amino acids) to build and repair tissue
- Serve as an energy source

Box 9-3 Comparative Kcal of Energy Per Gram

Carbohydrates: 4
Fats: 9
Proteins: 4

- Help to form enzymes, hormones, and other body fluids and secretions
- Assist in the transport of fats, fat-soluble vitamins, and other substances
- Help to maintain osmolarity of body fluids

RECOMMENDED DIETARY ALLOWANCE/ DIETARY REFERENCE INTAKE

The recommended DRI for protein is 56 g/day for men and 46 g/day for women. Protein should contribute 10% to 35% of the macronutrients in the adult diet.

KILOCALORIES OF MACRONUTRIENTS

The kilocalories per gram for carbohydrates, fats, and proteins are noted in Box 9-3.

VITAMINS

Vitamins are organic compounds that the body needs for normal growth and development. They help to regulate metabolic functions within cells; however, only tiny amounts are needed to carry out these functions. Because the body cannot manufacture vitamins, they must be obtained in the diet. As mentioned earlier, vitamins are micronutrients. Most vitamins have multiple forms called *vitamers*. For example, vitamers of vitamin A are retinol, retinal, and retinoic acid.

The use of over-the-counter vitamin supplements is very popular. It is based on the concern that modern diets and processed foods do not provide the daily vitamin requirements. We need to educate our patients about sources of vitamins, daily needs, and the dangers of excessive vitamin intake. Although scientific evidence is lacking, many manufacturers promote "natural" vitamin supplements as being superior to other supplements. In many instances, "natural" products cost more than other supplements but really offer no additional benefits. The use of very large doses of vitamins may be appropriate in certain conditions but generally is not considered beneficial and may be harmful. Vitamins are usually designated by letters and are classified as fat soluble or water soluble.

FAT-SOLUBLE VITAMINS

Fat-soluble vitamins include vitamins A, D, E, and K. Because they dissolve in fat, they are usually absorbed in the body with other lipids. Similar to lipids, fat-soluble vitamins need bile and pancreatic juices for absorption. After entering the body, fat-soluble vitamins attach to lipoproteins and are transported to the liver. If the amount of a vitamin taken in exceeds the amount needed, the extra amount is stored in the fat cells of the body. As stores build up, the excess vitamins can become toxic. Therefore nutrition experts recommend that people avoid taking excessive amounts of these vitamins.

WATER-SOLUBLE VITAMINS

Water-soluble vitamins include the B-complex group (thiamine, riboflavin, niacin, B_6, folate, B_{12}, pantothenic acid, and biotin) and vitamin C (ascorbic acid). Excessive intake of these vitamins is not as dangerous as high intake of fat-soluble vitamins because water-soluble vitamins are readily excreted from the body. Therefore they generally do not accumulate and become toxic. If taken in very large doses, thiamin, niacin, pantothenic acid, vitamin B_6, and vitamin C can have adverse effects, but such doses are unlikely when food is the major source of these vitamins. However, because water-soluble vitamins are readily excreted, they should be replaced daily.

Most of the water-soluble vitamins are components of essential enzyme systems. Many are involved in the reactions that support energy metabolism. They have an essential role in the metabolic processes of living cells, both plant and animal. Table 9-4 gives more information about the sources and functions of vitamins.

MINERALS

Minerals are another group of micronutrients. They are involved in enzyme regulation, maintenance of acid-base balance and osmotic pressure, and maintenance of nerve and muscular irritability. Doubtless, minerals have other functions that are not well understood at this time. Because excess minerals are not readily excreted from the body, the potential exists for toxicity if taken in large amounts.

Minerals are classified based on the daily requirement. Macrominerals (calcium, phosphorus, magnesium, sulfur, sodium, chloride, potassium) are required in amounts of 100 mg/day or more. Microminerals, or trace elements, are required in amounts of less than 15 mg/day (iron, zinc, iodine). Minerals that are required in amounts measured in micrograms (selenium, chromium, copper, manganese, molybdenum, boron, cobalt) are called *ultratrace elements.* Minerals are present in the body in ionized forms (sodium, potassium, etc.) or as constituents of organic compounds (phospholipids, hemoglobin, etc.).

Minerals account for 4% to 5% of body weight. Calcium and phosphorus make up most of this weight. Food sources and functions of minerals are presented in Table 9-5.

WATER

Water is the largest component of the body and body tissues and is essential to all life processes. It provides form and structure to cells and tissues; it is essential to the digestion, absorption, and excretion of metabolic and indigestible wastes; it is a transport medium for nutrients and all body substances; it maintains physical and chemical constancy of intracellular and extracellular fluids; and it regulates body temperature through the process of evaporation of perspiration. The intake of water is controlled by thirst. The sensation of thirst serves as a signal to seek fluids.

Water is ingested through food as well as liquids. The breakdown of food in the body produces water as an end product. Water is lost from the body through the kidneys as urine, through the intestines as part of feces, through the lungs during expiration, and through the skin as evaporated sweat. When an imbalance in the amount of water taken in versus the amount of water lost occurs, the kidneys compensate by conserving more water and excreting less. The amount of water taken in daily should be equivalent to the amount of water lost.

The body is unable to store water; therefore all living things must replenish water daily. Depending on the circumstances, healthy adults can live up to 10 days without water intake. Generally, adults should take in approximately 2700 mL, or a little more than 2.5 quarts, of water per day. More in-depth discussion of fluid balance is provided in Chapter 14.

AGE-RELATED CHANGES

Healthy eating is a lifelong commitment that pays particular benefits in the later years of life. Maintaining a good diet can help middle-aged and older people to maintain a high level of function and reduce the risks of chronic disease. Table 9-6 summarizes changes occurring with aging that are relevant to nutrition.

ENERGY

Because of the normal decline in metabolism and common decrease in physical activity, energy needs are reduced with age. Therefore the older person often reduces the calories taken in per day. This reduction can result in an inadequate intake of other essential nutrients. The recommended daily energy intake for light to moderately active older adults is 30 kcal/kg of body weight. This level reflects a reduction of 600 kcal/day for older men and 300 kcal/day for older women. However, the lifestyle and health status of older adults vary widely and these figures may need adjustment for each individual. Nutrients previously discussed in this chapter, including proteins, carbohydrates, lipids, vitamins, minerals, and water, may need adjustment as people age (Table 9-7). Persons who are less active require less than the usual recommended amounts of thiamine, riboflavin, and niacin. Some experts recommend daily multivitamin-mineral supplements because the average American diet often lacks sufficient amounts of these nutrients. Contrary to popular

Table 9-4 Vitamin Sources and Functions

NAME	SOURCES	COMMENTS
Fat-Soluble Vitamins		
Vitamin A	Liver, kidney, milk fat, fortified margarine, egg yolk, yellow and dark leafy vegetables, apricots, cantaloupe, peaches	Essential for normal growth, development, and maintenance of epithelial tissue. Essential to the integrity of night vision. Helps provide for normal bone development and influences normal tooth formation. Toxic in large quantities.
Vitamin D	Vitamin D–fortified milk; irradiated foods; some in milk fat, liver, egg yolk, salmon, tuna fish, sardines	Essential for normal growth and development; important for formation and maintenance of normal bones and teeth. Influences absorption and metabolism of phosphorus and calcium. Toxic in large quantities.
Vitamin E	Wheat germ, vegetable oils, green leafy vegetables, milk fat, egg yolk, nuts	Is a strong antioxidant. May help prevent oxidation of unsaturated fatty acids and vitamin A in intestinal tract and body tissues. Protects red blood cells from hemolysis. Role in epithelial tissue maintenance and prostaglandin synthesis.
Vitamin K	Liver, soybean oil, other vegetable oils, green leafy vegetables, wheat bran. Synthesized in intestinal tract.	Aids in production of prothrombin, a compound required for normal clotting of blood. Involved in bone metabolism. Toxic in large amounts.
Water-Soluble Vitamins		
Thiamine	Pork, liver, organ meats, legumes, whole-grain and enriched cereals and breads, wheat germ, potatoes	Aids in removal of carbon dioxide from alpha-keto acids during oxidation of carbohydrates. Essential for growth, normal appetite, digestion, and healthy nerves.
Riboflavin	Milk and dairy foods, organ meats, green leafy vegetables, enriched cereals and breads, eggs	Essential for growth. Plays enzymatic role in tissue respiration and acts as a transporter of hydrogen ions.
Niacin	Fish, liver, meat, poultry, many grains, eggs, peanuts, milk, legumes, enriched grains	Aids in transfer of hydrogen and acts in metabolism of carbohydrates and amino acids. Involved in glycolysis, fat synthesis, and tissue respiration.
Vitamin B_6	Pork, glandular meats, cereal: bran and germ, milk, egg yolk, oatmeal, legumes	Aids in the synthesis and breakdown of amino acids and unsaturated fatty acids from essential fatty acids. Essential for conversion of tryptophan to niacin. Essential for normal growth.
Folate	Green leafy vegetables, organ meats (liver), lean beef, wheat, eggs, fish, dry beans, lentils, cowpeas, asparagus, broccoli, collards, yeast	Essential for biosynthesis of nucleic acids; especially important in early fetal development. Essential for normal maturation of red blood cells.
Vitamin B_{12}	Liver, kidney, milk and dairy foods, meat, eggs. Vegans require supplement.	Essential for biosynthesis of nucleic acids and nucleoproteins. Role in metabolism of nervous tissue. Involved with folate metabolism. Related to growth.
Vitamin C (ascorbic acid)	Acerola (West Indian cherrylike fruit), citrus fruit, tomato, melon, peppers, greens, raw cabbage, guava, strawberries, pineapple, potato	Maintains intracellular cement substance with preservation of capillary integrity. Important in immune responses, wound healing, and allergic reactions. Increases absorption of nonheme iron.
Pantothenic acid	All plant and animal foods. Best sources: eggs, kidney, liver, salmon, yeast. Possibly synthesized by intestinal bacteria.	Involved in synthesis and breakdown of many vital compounds; essential for metabolism of carbohydrates, fat, and protein.
Biotin	Liver, mushrooms, peanuts, yeast, milk, meat, egg yolk, most vegetables, banana, grapefruit, tomato, watermelon, strawberries. Synthesized by intestinal bacteria.	Essential component of enzymes. Involved in synthesis and breakdown of fatty acids and amino acids.

Adapted from Mahan LK, Escott-Stump S, Raymond JL: *Krause's food and the nutrition care process*, ed 13, St. Louis, 2012, Elsevier/Saunders, pp. 63–66.

Table 9-5 Minerals in Human Nutrition

MINERAL	LOCATION IN BODY AND SOME BIOLOGIC FUNCTIONS	FOOD SOURCES
Calcium	99% in bones and teeth. Ionic calcium in body fluids essential for ion transport across cell membranes.	Milk and milk products, sardines, clams, oysters, kale, turnip greens, mustard greens, tofu
Phosphorus	About 80% in inorganic portion of bones and teeth. Is a component of every cell as well as of important metabolites, including DNA, RNA, ATP (high-energy compound), and phospholipids. Important to pH regulation.	Cheese, egg yolk, milk, meat, fish, poultry, whole-grain cereals, almost all other foods
Magnesium	About 50% in bone; remainder is almost entirely inside body cells, with only about 1% in extracellular fluid.	Whole-grain cereals, tofu, nuts, meat, milk, green vegetables, legumes, chocolate
Sodium	About 30% to 45% in bone. Major cation of extracellular fluid, with only a small amount inside cell. Regulates body fluid osmolarity, pH, and body fluid volume.	Common table salt, seafood, animal foods, milk, eggs. Abundant in most foods except fruit.
Chloride	Major anion of extracellular fluid, functioning in combination with sodium. Serves as a buffer, enzyme activator; component of gastric hydrochloric acid. Mostly present in extracellular fluid, with less than 15% inside cells.	Common table salt, seafood, milk, meat, eggs
Potassium	Major cation of intracellular fluid, with only small amounts in extracellular fluid. Functions in regulating pH and osmolarity and cell membrane transfer. Iron is necessary for carbohydrate and protein metabolism.	Fruits, milk, meat, cereals, vegetables, legumes
Sulfur	Bulk of dietary sulfur is present in sulfur-containing amino acids needed for synthesis of essential metabolites. Role in oxidation-reduction reactions.	Protein foods such as meat, fish, poultry, eggs, milk, cheese, legumes, nuts
Iron	About 70% is in hemoglobin; about 26% stored in liver, spleen, and bone. Is a component of hemoglobin, which is important in oxygen transfer, and certain enzymes.	Liver, meat, egg yolk, legumes, whole or enriched grains, dark green vegetables, dark molasses, shrimp, oysters
Zinc	Present in most tissues, with higher amounts in liver, voluntary muscle, and bone. Constituent of many enzymes and insulin. Important for nucleic acid metabolism.	Oysters, shellfish, herring, liver, legumes, milk, wheat bran
Copper	Found in all body tissues; mostly in liver, brain, heart, and kidney. Constituent of enzymes and some blood components. May be integral part of DNA and RNA.	Liver, shellfish, whole grains, cherries, legumes, kidney, poultry, oysters, chocolate, nuts
Iodine	Constituent of thyroxine and related compounds synthesized by the thyroid gland. Thyroxine functions in control of reactions involving cellular energy.	Iodized table salt, seafood, water and vegetables in regions without goiter
Manganese	Highest concentration is in bone; also relatively high concentrations in pituitary, liver, pancreas, and gastrointestinal tissue. Constituent of essential enzyme systems.	Beet greens, blueberries, whole grains, nuts, legumes, fruit, tea
Fluoride	Present in bones and teeth. In optimal amounts, reduces dental caries and may minimize bone loss.	Drinking water (1 ppm), tea, coffee, rice, soybeans, spinach, gelatin, onions, lettuce

Adapted from Mahan LK, Escott-Stump S, Raymond JL: *Krause's food and the nutrition care process*, ed 13, St. Louis, 2012, Elsevier/Saunders, pp. 95-97.
ATP, Adenosine triphosphate; *DNA*, deoxyribonucleic acid; *ppm*, parts per million; *RNA*, ribonucleic acid.

Table 9-6 Nutrition-Related System Changes in the Older Adult

SYSTEM/FUNCTION	CHANGES
Sensory	Senses of taste, smell, sight, hearing, and touch are diminished. There are a decreased number of taste buds and a decreased sensitivity to sweet and salty tastes. Patient may experience glossodynia (pain in the tongue).
Gastrointestinal	Changes in appetite response contribute to anorexia. Ill-fitting dentures and periodontal disease make eating painful. Decreased salivary secretion decreases the ability to chew and swallow foods. Decreased acid secretion causes an overgrowth of the bacteria of the gut. Lack of intrinsic factor leads to decreased absorption of vitamin B_{12}. There is an increased incidence of gallbladder disease; decreased motility of intestines leads to constipation.
Metabolic	Decreased tolerance to glucose leads to an increase in plasma glucose levels. Basal metabolic rate decreases by 20% due to decrease in lean body mass.
Cardiovascular	Blood vessels become less elastic. Total peripheral resistance increases. There is an increased risk for hypertension.
Renal	Kidney function diminishes and the acid-base response to metabolic challenges is slowed. There is increased difficulty in handling excessive amounts of protein waste products.
Musculoskeletal	Progressive replacement of lean body mass by fat and connective tissue. Body protein is decreased by 30% to 40%. More fat is deposited on the trunk and around the visceral organs. Bone density is diminished and there is shortening of the spinal column.
Immunocompetence	The immune function declines with age. There is a diminished ability to fight infection.
Psychosocial	Many experience depression as a result of a sense of loss or of loss of loved ones, productivity, a sense of worth, mobility, income, and body image.

Table 9-7 Changes in the Nutritional Requirements for the Older Adult

NUTRIENT	CHANGES IN NEEDS	SPECIAL PROBLEMS
Protein	Need unchanged (0.8 g/kg) unless ill. Needs may increase with infection, altered gastrointestinal function, or chronic diseases that affect metabolism.	Protein-calorie undernutrition may be a special problem for older men who live alone.
Carbohydrate	Need less sugar, more complex carbohydrates. Complex carbohydrates should contribute 55% of calorie intake.	Reduced glucose tolerance, lactose intolerance
Lipid	Same as younger adult (not more than 30% of total kilocalories).	Serum cholesterol levels in men tend to peak during middle age and then drop slightly; levels in women continue to rise with increasing age.
Minerals	The needs for trace elements may be reduced owing to decreased lean body mass; calcium intake of 1000–1500 mg/day for postmenopausal women.	Hypertension is common, which results in the need to decrease sodium and increase potassium and magnesium for those taking diuretics.
Vitamins	Vitamin A is sufficient in the older adult owing to stores in the liver; may require vitamin D supplement if patient is not exposed to sunlight; some require vitamin C supplements; vitamin B_6 and folate are maintained with normal diet; vitamin B_{12} may be deficient owing to loss of intrinsic factor.	A maintenance level multivitamin and mineral supplement may be required. Patient must be monitored closely for overdose.
Water	30–35 mL/kg of ideal body weight.	Dehydration is the most common fluid and electrolyte disturbance. Patient must be monitored closely.

belief, vitamin supplements do not provide energy or slow the aging process. However, there is evidence that patients with macular degeneration and colorectal polyps can benefit from specific supplements. Otherwise, there is not sufficient evidence to claim that supplements prevent various chronic diseases. Psychosocial factors also may lead to poor nutrition in the older person. Depression, cognitive impairment, and loneliness can affect appetite and the intake of food. The term *failure to thrive* has been applied to older adults who are undernourished, depressed, and declining physically and cognitively. Failure to thrive has been attributed to organic and nonorganic factors. This phenomenon is the subject of study to determine how to identify reversible conditions and how best to intervene.

NUTRITIONAL CARE OF THE OLDER ADULT

Dietary Planning

Dietary planning for the older adult is no different from planning for a younger adult. Meals need to be appealing, taking into consideration individual likes and dislikes, and should be tasteful and filling. Planning may be different for older adults with special needs. Some prefer four or five small meals over three large ones. In addition, problems such as difficulty swallowing, dentures that do not fit properly, and arthritis, which makes using utensils uncomfortable, must be considered.

The diet should include all of the food groups. Severely restricted diets such as low-sodium and low-fat diets generally are not advised for older adults. When food is unappetizing, the older person may simply not eat enough to obtain necessary nutrients. The *Patient Teaching* box gives suggestions for teaching older patients about nutrition.

Patient Teaching

Nutrition for the Older Patient

In addition to general information about nutritional requirements, you should share the following with the older adult patient:

- A normal diet typically supplies adequate vitamins; however, a daily multivitamin may be recommended.
- Some dietary supplements can interact with medications.
- Megadoses (very large doses) of vitamins have not been proven to be beneficial and can be harmful.
- "Natural vitamins" are more expensive and there is no evidence that they are better than synthetic vitamins.
- Vitamins do not provide the body with more energy.

Nutrition Programs

Many community-based programs, administered by both public and private agencies, provide hot, nutritious meals to older adults. The meals are served either in a group setting or in the home. Special regulations and conditions must be met to qualify for these programs.

Nutritional Needs during Prolonged Illness

All people have increased nutritional needs during periods of illness. Older adults with chronic diseases such as emphysema and bronchitis, cancer, organic brain disease, cirrhosis, and maldigestion or malabsorption syndromes are at increased risk for protein deficiency and negative nitrogen balance. Individuals at risk need to be monitored very carefully for this condition, which can be prevented by increasing nutritional support. Enteral feedings or parenteral nutrition may be required to meet these increased needs.

Nutritional Care in Institutional Settings

Good nutrition can have a dramatic effect on the physical, mental, and emotional function of your older adult patients. Nurses in long-term care and home health settings must be especially vigilant in monitoring the nutritional status of older adult patients. Age-related changes, chronic and acute conditions, cognitive and emotional disorders, medications, and situational factors can contribute to inadequate nutritional intake, digestion, or elimination. Also, patients who are obese have special needs. Excess body weight makes the task of controlling many chronic conditions more difficult and can greatly interfere with activities of daily living. The nutritional needs of older adults in institutional settings may change over time. Therefore periodic reassessment of nutritional status is critical to avoid imposing unnecessary diet restrictions or missing important nutritional needs.

Assisting older adult patients with meals must be a high priority. How many times have you seen a meal cart with trays that have barely been touched being returned to the kitchen? You should question why patients are not eating and implement nursing measures to improve the situation.

GUIDELINES FOR DIETARY PLANNING

MYPLATE

Over the years, various guidelines have been established in the United States to help in planning for optimal nutrition. The newest program, based on the U.S. Department of Agriculture's *Dietary Guidelines for Americans, 2010*, is MyPlate. The MyPlate icon is a placemat with a simple plate divided into four sections and a glass. The glass represents a dairy serving and the plate divisions represent the recommended proportions of fruits, vegetables, grains, and protein (Fig. 9-1, A). Its intent is to remind Americans to make better food choices. Specific information about food choices is available at ChooseMyPlate.com. See Box 9-4 for key dietary recommendations.

The licensed vocational nurse/licensed practical nurse (LVN/LPN) can promote healthy eating by educating patients and families about sources of accurate information. Individuals can obtain personal dietary plans based on the *Dietary Guidelines for Americans,*

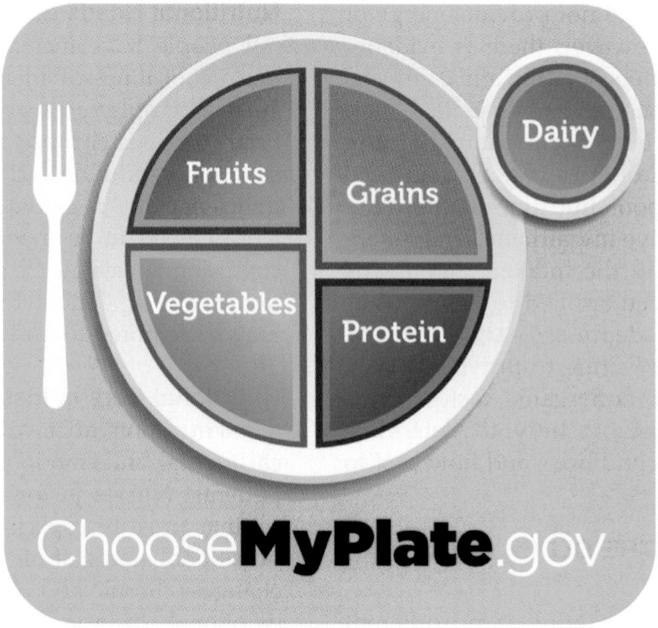

A

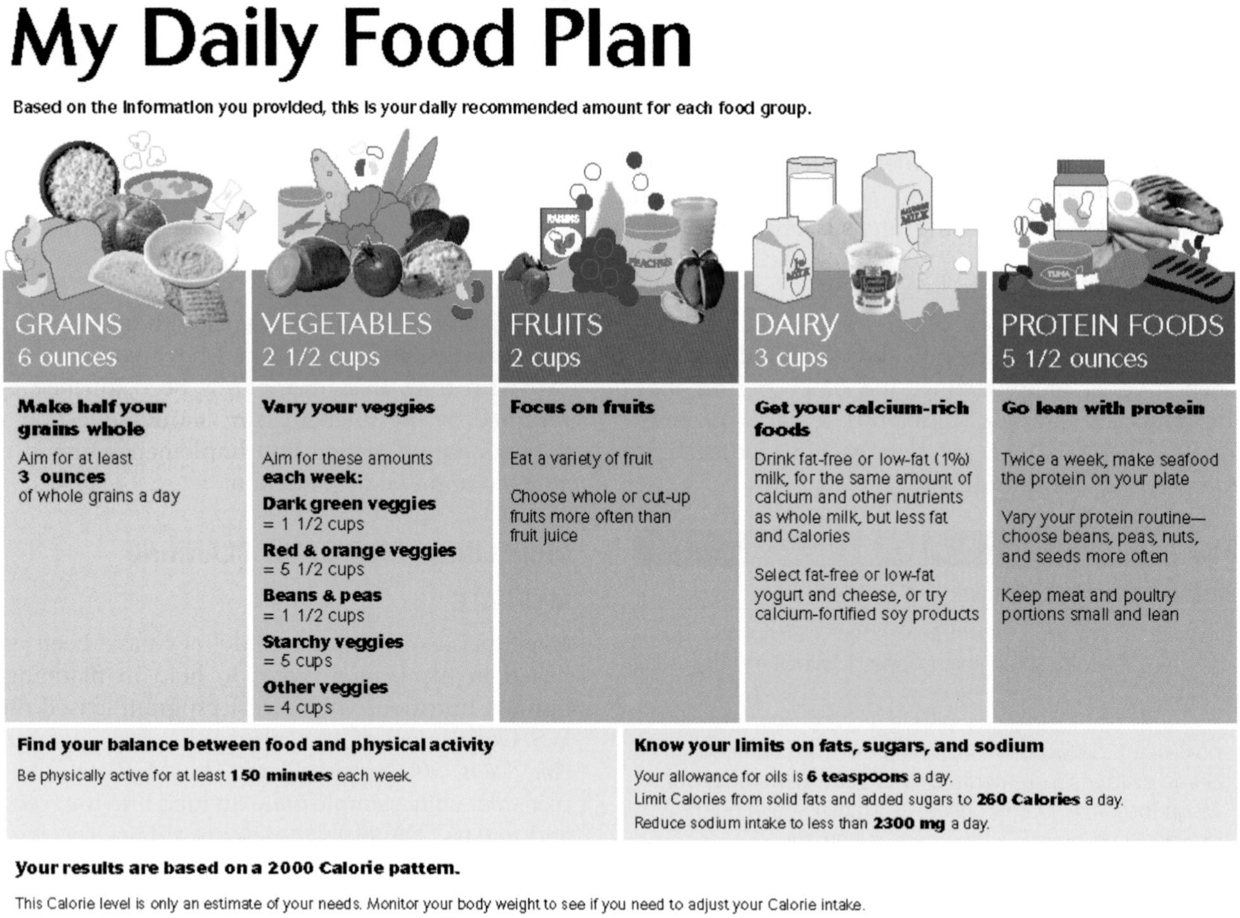
My Daily Food Plan
Based on the information you provided, this is your daily recommended amount for each food group.
GRAINS
6 ounces
VEGETABLES
2 1/2 cups
FRUITS
2 cups
DAIRY
3 cups
PROTEIN FOODS
5 1/2 ounces
Make half your grains whole
Aim for at least 3 ounces of whole grains a day
Vary your veggies
Aim for these amounts each week:
Dark green veggies = 1 1/2 cups
Red & orange veggies = 5 1/2 cups
Beans & peas = 1 1/2 cups
Starchy veggies = 5 cups
Other veggies = 4 cups
Focus on fruits
Eat a variety of fruit
Choose whole or cut-up fruits more often than fruit juice
Get your calcium-rich foods
Drink fat-free or low-fat (1%) milk, for the same amount of calcium and other nutrients as whole milk, but less fat and Calories
Select fat-free or low-fat yogurt and cheese, or try calcium-fortified soy products
Go lean with protein
Twice a week, make seafood the protein on your plate
Vary your protein routine—choose beans, peas, nuts, and seeds more often
Keep meat and poultry portions small and lean
Find your balance between food and physical activity
Be physically active for at least 150 minutes each week.
Know your limits on fats, sugars, and sodium
Your allowance for oils is 6 teaspoons a day.
Limit Calories from solid fats and added sugars to 260 Calories a day.
Reduce sodium intake to less than 2300 mg a day.
Your results are based on a 2000 Calorie pattern.
This Calorie level is only an estimate of your needs. Monitor your body weight to see if you need to adjust your Calorie intake.

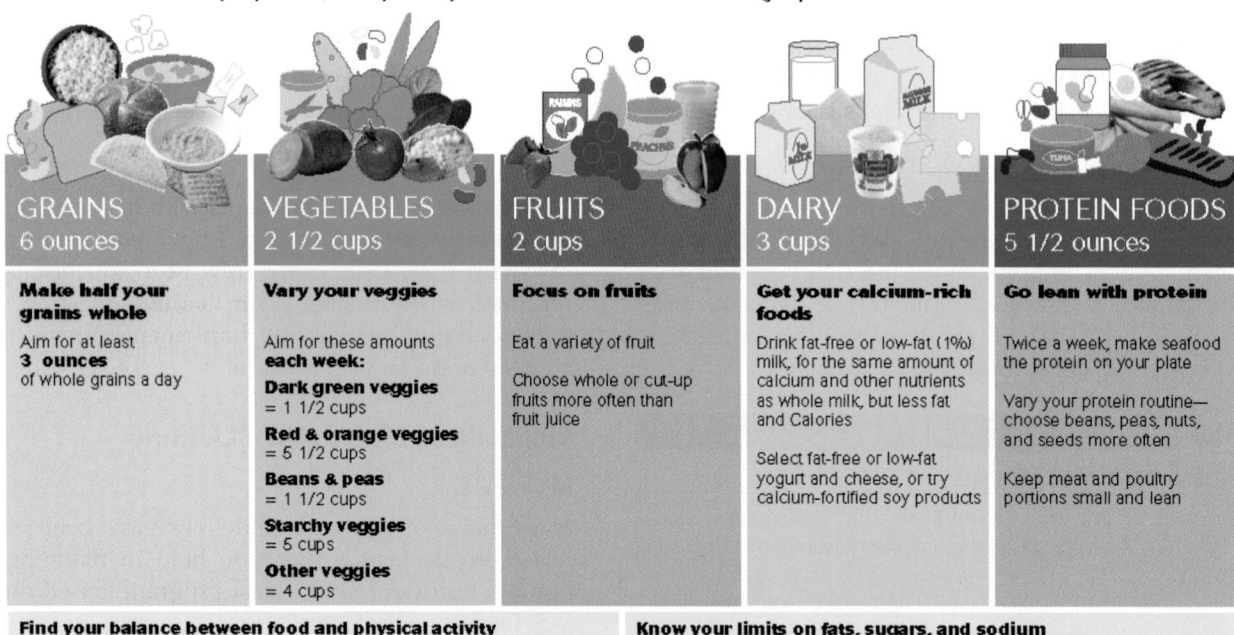

B

FIGURE 9-1 A, U.S. Department of Agriculture's MyPlate. B, Sample individualized meal plan for a 66-year-old female who exercises 60 minutes a day. (Courtesy U.S. Department of Agriculture.)

Box 9-4 ***Dietary Guidelines for Americans, 2010*: Key Recommendations**

BALANCING CALORIES TO MANAGE WEIGHT

- Prevent and/or reduce overweight and obesity through improved eating and physical activity behaviors.
- Control total calorie intake to manage body weight. For people who are overweight or obese, this will mean consuming fewer calories from foods and beverages.
- Increase physical activity and reduce time spent in sedentary behaviors.
- Maintain appropriate calorie balance during each stage of life: childhood, adolescence, adulthood, pregnancy and breastfeeding, and older age.

FOODS AND FOOD COMPONENTS TO REDUCE

- Reduce daily sodium intake to less than 2300 milligrams (mg) and further reduce intake to 1500 mg among persons who are 51 and older and those of any age who are African American or have hypertension, diabetes, or chronic kidney disease. The 1500 mg recommendation applies to about half of the U.S. population, including children, and the majority of adults.
- Consume less than 10% of calories from saturated fatty acids by replacing them with monounsaturated and polyunsaturated fatty acids.
- Consume less than 300 mg per day of dietary cholesterol.
- Keep trans fatty acid consumption as low as possible by limiting foods that contain synthetic sources of trans fats, such as partially hydrogenated oils, and by limiting other solid fats.
- Reduce the intake of calories from solid fats and added sugars.
- Limit the consumption of foods that contain refined grains, especially refined grain foods that contain solid fats, added sugars, and sodium.
- If alcohol is consumed, it should be consumed in moderation—up to one drink per day for women and two drinks per day for men—and only by adults of legal drinking age.

FOODS AND NUTRIENTS TO INCREASE

Individuals should meet the following recommendations as part of a healthy eating pattern while staying within their calorie needs.

- Increase vegetable and fruit intake.
- Eat a variety of vegetables, especially dark green, red, and orange vegetables, and beans and peas.
- Consume at least half of all grains as whole grains. Increase whole-grain intake by replacing refined grains with whole grains.
- Increase intake of fat-free or low-fat milk and milk products, such as milk, yogurt, cheese, or fortified soy beverages.*
- Choose a variety of protein foods, which include seafood, lean meat and poultry, eggs, beans and peas, soy products, and unsalted nuts and seeds.
- Increase the amount and variety of seafood consumed by choosing seafood in place of some meat and poultry.
- Replace protein foods that are higher in solid fats with choices that are lower in solid fats and calories and/or are sources of oils.
- Use oils to replace solid fats where possible.
- Choose foods that provide more potassium, dietary fiber, calcium, and vitamin D, which are nutrients of concern in American diet. These foods include vegetables, fruits, whole grains, and milk and milk products.

RECOMMENDATIONS FOR SPECIFIC POPULATION GROUPS

Women capable of becoming pregnant:

Choose foods that supply heme iron, which is more readily absorbed by the body; additional iron sources; and enhancers of iron absorption such as vitamin C–rich foods.

Consume 400 micrograms (mcg) per day of synthetic folic acid (from fortified foods and/or supplements) in addition to food forms of folate from a varied diet.

Women who are pregnant or breastfeeding:

- Consume 8 to 12 ounces of seafood per week from a variety of seafood types.
- Due to their high methyl mercury content, limit white (albacore) tuna to 6 ounces per week and do not eat the following four types of fish: tilefish, shark, swordfish, and king mackerel.
- If pregnant, take an iron supplement, as recommended by an obstetrician or other health care provider.

Individuals ages 50 years and older:

- Consume foods fortified with vitamin B_{12}, such as fortified cereals, or dietary supplements.

BUILDING HEALTHY EATING PATTERNS

- Select an eating pattern that meets nutrient needs over time at an appropriate calorie level.
- Account for all foods and beverages consumed and assess how they fit within a total healthy eating pattern.
- Follow food safety recommendations when preparing and eating foods to reduce the risk of foodborne illness.

Data from U.S. Department of Agriculture: *Dietary Guidelines for Americans, 2010* (website): www.health.gov/dietaryguidelines/dga2010/recommendations.htm. Accessed June 7, 2013.

*Fortified soy beverages have been marketed as "soy milk," a product name consumers could see in supermarkets and consumer materials. However, the U.S. Food and Drug Administration's regulations do not contain provisions for the use of the term *soy milk*. Therefore, in this document, the term *fortified soy beverage* includes products that may be marketed as soy milk.

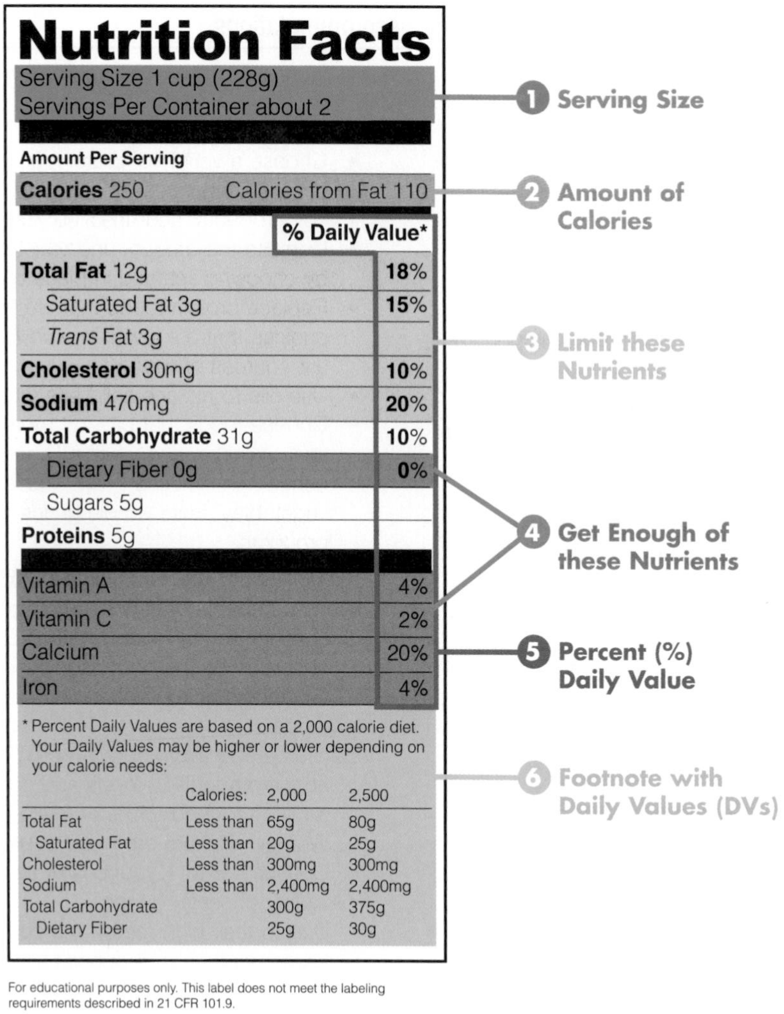
Nutrition Facts
Serving Size 1 cup (228g)
Servings Per Container about 2
Amount Per Serving
Calories 250 Calories from Fat 110
% Daily Value*
Total Fat 12g 18%
Saturated Fat 3g 15%
Trans Fat 3g
Cholesterol 30mg 10%
Sodium 470mg 20%
Total Carbohydrate 31g 10%
Dietary Fiber 0g 0%
Sugars 5g
Proteins 5g
Vitamin A 4%
Vitamin C 2%
Calcium 20%
Iron 4%
* Percent Daily Values are based on a 2,000 calorie diet. Your Daily Values may be higher or lower depending on your calorie needs:
Calories: 2,000 2,500
Total Fat Less than 65g 80g
Saturated Fat Less than 20g 25g
Cholesterol Less than 300mg 300mg
Sodium Less than 2,400mg 2,400mg
Total Carbohydrate 300g 375g
Dietary Fiber 25g 30g
1 Serving Size
2 Amount of Calories
3 Limit these Nutrients
4 Get Enough of these Nutrients
5 Percent (%) Daily Value
6 Footnote with Daily Values (DVs)
For educational purposes only. This label does not meet the labeling requirements described in 21 CFR 101.9.

FIGURE 9-2 Example of a nutrition label. (Courtesy U.S. Food and Drug Administration.)

2010 using www.ChooseMyPlate.gov. Figure 9-1, B, provides a sample plan created for an individual.

Food Labeling

With the increase in public awareness of health and nutrition, many people want information to help them make good food choices. Most foods are labeled so that the average person can make determinations about the quality and quantity of the nutrients consumed. Because of the lack of space available on a package label, the Nutrition Facts table is abbreviated to include essential information to describe the number of nutrients per serving (Fig. 9-2). In addition to calories, calories from fat, and grams of specific nutrients, the label also specifies daily values (DVs). A daily value of 10% means that one serving of the product provides 10% of the recommended daily intake of that nutrient based on a 2000-calorie diet.

VEGETARIAN DIETS

Vegetarian diets are not new but have only gradually gained acceptance as a balanced nutritional option in the United States. Many Americans who call themselves *vegetarians* eat all foods except red meat, although some exclude poultry and fish as well. A *lactovegetarian* diet includes milk, cheese, and other dairy products but excludes meat, fish, poultry, and eggs. A *lacto-ovo-vegetarian* diet includes dairy products and eggs but excludes meat, fish, and poultry. A person who consumes no foods of animal origin is said to be a *vegan*. Only the vegan is at real risk for nutritional deficiencies if the diet is not carefully planned.

Some evidence suggests that vegetarian diets have distinct health benefits, including reduced risks of type 2 diabetes mellitus, breast and colon cancer, and cardiovascular and gallbladder disease. Vegetarians generally consume less protein than nonvegetarians but most still exceed the RDA for protein. Tips for healthy eating for vegetarians are summarized in Box 9-5.

NURSING ASSESSMENT OF NUTRITIONAL STATUS

The areas covered in a nutritional assessment include a dietary history, anthropometric data, laboratory data (if available), and physical examination data.

Box 9-5 Ten Tips: Healthy Eating for Vegetarians

1. **Think about protein.** Your protein needs can easily be met by eating a variety of plant foods. Sources of protein for vegetarians include beans and peas, nuts, and soy products (such as tofu, tempeh). Lacto-ovo vegetarians also get protein from eggs and dairy foods.
2. **Bone up on sources of calcium.** Calcium is used for building bones and teeth. Some vegetarians consume dairy products, which are excellent sources of calcium. Other sources of calcium for vegetarians include calcium-fortified soymilk (soy beverage), tofu made with calcium sulfate, calcium-fortified breakfast cereals and orange juice, and some dark green leafy vegetables (collard, turnip, and mustard greens; and bok choy).
3. **Make simple changes.** Many popular main dishes are or can be vegetarian—such as pasta primavera, pasta with marinara or pesto sauce, veggie pizza, vegetable lasagna, tofu-vegetable stir-fry, and bean burritos.
4. **Enjoy a cookout.** For barbecues, try veggie or soy burgers, soy hot dogs, marinated tofu or tempeh, and fruit kabobs. Grilled veggies are great too!
5. **Include beans and peas.** Because of their high nutrient content, consuming beans and peas is recommended for everyone, vegetarians and nonvegetarians alike. Enjoy some vegetarian chili, three bean salad, or split pea soup. Make a hummus-filled pita sandwich.
6. **Try different versions.** A variety of vegetarian products look—and may taste—like their non-vegetarian counterparts but are usually lower in saturated fat and contain no cholesterol. For breakfast, try soy-based sausage patties or links. For dinner, rather than hamburgers, try bean burgers or falafel (chickpea patties).
7. **Make some small changes at restaurants.** Most restaurants can make vegetarian modifications to menu items by substituting meatless sauces or non-meat items, such as tofu and beans for meat, and adding vegetables or pasta in place of meat. Ask about available vegetarian options.
8. **Nuts make great snacks.** Choose unsalted nuts as a snack and use them in salads or main dishes. Add almonds, walnuts, or pecans instead of cheese or meat to a green salad.
9. **Get your vitamin B_{12}.** Vitamin B_{12} is naturally found only in animal products. Vegetarians should choose fortified foods such as cereals or soy products, or take a vitamin B_{12} supplement if they do not consume any animal products. Check the Nutrition Facts label for vitamin B_{12} in fortified products.
10. **Find a vegetarian pattern for you.** Go to www.dietaryguidelines.gov and check appendices of the *Dietary Guidelines for Americans, 2010* for vegetarian adaptations of the USDA food patterns at 12 calorie levels.

From U.S. Department of Agriculture, Center for Nutrition Policy and Promotion: *DG TipSheet No. 8*, June 2010: www.ChooseMyPlate.gov. Accessed June 8, 2013.

DIETARY HISTORY

While collecting data for the dietary history, observe the patient's physical appearance for signs of malnutrition, obesity, and other factors that may indicate nutritional deficits. The well-nourished person should have shiny and healthy-looking hair, bright and clear eyes, smooth facial skin with good color, smooth lips and tongue, and healthy teeth and gums. Signs of malnutrition include dull, thin, and sparse hair; pale conjunctiva; a swollen or pale face; swollen lips and tongue; teeth with cavities or missing teeth; and bleeding or receding gums.

The dietary history includes physical, psychologic, social, and medical data that may have an impact on nutritional status. Box 9-6 summarizes information you should obtain in the dietary history. Commonly used tools to collect retrospective ("after the fact") data about dietary patterns include the 24-hour recall and the food frequency record. For a 24-hour recall, ask the patient to recall everything eaten during the past 24 hours, usually from the time of awakening until the next morning. Note everything that entered the mouth, including meals, snacks, drinks (especially water), and seasonings (especially salt). The food frequency record uses a list of foods from all food groups to assess how often the patient consumes specific foods. Because neither tool provides perfectly accurate data, using both of them is probably best. From these assessments, general dietary deficits and excesses can be determined.

Anthropometric Data

Anthropometric data include height, weight (including weight patterns), and body composition. Height and weight measurements should be performed correctly to complete an accurate assessment of the patient. Box 9-7 gives guidelines on the proper way to perform these measurements.

Body composition is related to the ratio of fat to lean muscle mass. Determining a person's body composition requires taking several measurements. These measurements include skinfold thickness and hydrostatic weighing. Skinfold thickness is measured by means of calipers that pinch skin over areas of the body that seem to reflect best the fat content of the subcutaneous tissue. These sites include areas over the triceps, over the biceps, below the scapula, above the iliac crest, and on the upper thigh (Fig. 9-3).

A variety of other methods of measuring body composition are available, including bioelectrical impedance analysis, air displacement plethysmography, dual-energy x-ray absorptiometry, and hydrostatic (underwater) weighing. However, these procedures require specific equipment and training so they are not practical for routine assessments. Body mass index (BMI) is a way to evaluate the weight of an adult. BMI

Box 9-6 Dietary History Information

ECONOMICS
Income (frequency and steadiness of employment)
Amount of money for food each week or month and individual's perception of its adequacy for meeting food needs
Eligibility for food stamps and cost of stamps
Public aid recipient?

PHYSICAL ACTIVITY
Occupation (type, hours per week, shift, energy expenditure)
Exercise (type, amount, frequency [seasonal?])
Sleep (hours per day [uninterrupted?])
Handicaps

ETHNIC OR CULTURAL BACKGROUND
Influence on eating habits
Religion
Education

HOME LIFE AND MEAL PATTERNS
Number in household (eat together?)
Person who does shopping
Person who does cooking
Food storage and cooking facilities (stove, refrigerator)
Type of housing (home, apartment, room, etc.)
Ability to shop and prepare food

APPETITE
Good, poor; any changes?
Factors that affect appetite
Taste and smell perception; any changes?

ATTITUDE TOWARD FOOD AND EATING
Disinterest in food
Irrational ideas about food, eating, and body weight
Parental interest in child's eating

ALLERGIES, INTOLERANCES, OR FOOD AVOIDANCES
Foods avoided and reason why
Length of time of avoidance
Description of problems caused by foods

DENTAL AND ORAL HEALTH
Problems with eating
Foods that cannot be eaten
Problems with swallowing, salivation, and food sticking

GASTROINTESTINAL
Problems with heartburn, bloating, gas, diarrhea, vomiting, constipation, and distention
Frequency of problems
Home remedies
Antacid, laxative, or other drug use

CHRONIC DISEASE
Treatment
Length of time of treatment
Dietary modification (physician prescription?, date of modification, education, compliance with diet)

MEDICATION
Vitamin and/or mineral supplements (frequency, type, amount)
Medications (type, amount, frequency, length of time on medication)

RECENT WEIGHT CHANGE
Loss or gain
How many pounds and over what length of time?
Intentional or unintentional?

DIETARY OR NUTRITIONAL PROBLEMS (AS PERCEIVED BY PATIENT)

Data from U.S. Department of Agriculture (website): www.health.gov/dietaryguidelines/dga2005/recommendations.htm. Accessed November 28, 2005.

Box 9-7 Recommendations for the Measurement of Height and Weight

HEIGHT
- Height should be measured without shoes.
- Feet should be together with the heels against the wall or measuring board.
- The subject should stand erect, neither slumped nor stretching, looking straight ahead, without tipping the head up or down. The top of the ear and outer corner of the eye should be in a line parallel to the floor.
- A horizontal bar, a rectangular block of wood, or the top of the stadiometer should be lowered to rest flat on the top of the head.
- Height should be read to the nearest ¼ inch or 0.5 centimeter.

WEIGHT
- Use a beam balance scale, not a spring scale, whenever possible.
- Periodically calibrate the scale for accuracy, using known weights.
- Weigh the subject in light clothing without shoes.
- Record weight to the nearest ½ pound or 0.2 kilogram. Measurements above the 90th or below the 10th percentile warrant further evaluation.

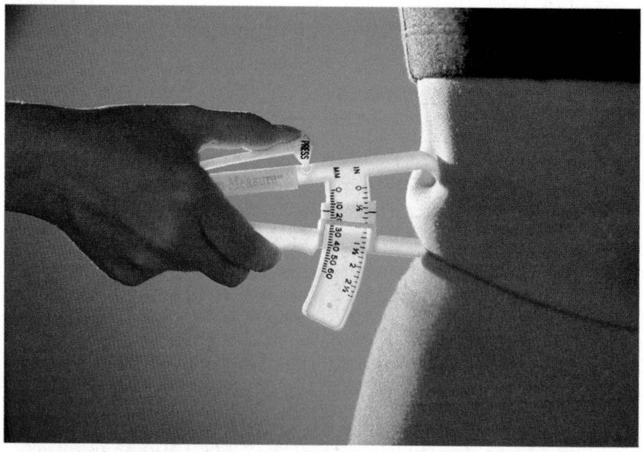

FIGURE 9-3 Skinfold calipers measure in millimeters the thickness of the subcutaneous fat tissue, which gives a rough measurement of adiposity. (Copyright ThinkStockPhotos. Used with permission. All rights reserved.)

is obtained by using the following formula (a value of 20 to 25 is optimal):

$$BMI = Weight\ (in\ kilograms) \div [Height\ (in\ meters)]^2$$

Put on Your Thinking Cap!

Calculate your BMI and determine whether it falls in the optimum range.

Biochemical Assessment: Laboratory Data

Among the laboratory tests that are helpful in assessing nutritional status are:

- *Serum albumin:* Protein depletion is one reason for low serum albumin. The normal serum albumin level is 3.5 to 5.0 g/dL.
- *Total lymphocyte count (TLC):* Protein and calorie deficits interfere with immune function, resulting in a low TLC. The normal lymphocyte count is 2500 mm^3. A count of less than 1500 mm^3 is consistent with protein/calorie malnutrition.
- *Urine creatinine/height index:* Expected urine creatinine, based on the patient's height, provides an estimate of skeletal muscle mass.
- *Nitrogen balance:* Nitrogen balance exists when nitrogen intake and excretion are equal. A patient who is in a state of starvation will excrete more nitrogen in the urine than consumed, creating a negative nitrogen balance.
- *Mean corpuscular volume (MCV):* MCV measures the size of red blood cells (RBCs). With different types of anemia, RBC size varies. Therefore when anemia is present, MCV helps to determine the type of anemia.
- *Transferrin saturation:* Transferrin is a protein that transports iron. Transferrin saturation is normally between 30% and 50%; less than 30% indicates anemia; more than 50% indicates iron overload.

WEIGHT MANAGEMENT AND EATING DISORDERS

Many Americans are on some form of "diet." Dieting may be motivated by health concerns as well as by dissatisfaction with one's appearance. Most people view dieting as deprivation at best and punishment at worst. Changing eating patterns takes motivation, hard work, and the ability to sustain new behaviors over a long period. Most adults have the ability to maintain a constant weight but to do so they must maintain consistent eating and activity patterns on a daily basis. Table 9-8 shows estimated daily energy

Table 9-8 Estimated Calorie Needs per Day by Age, Gender, and Physical Activity Level*

		PHYSICAL ACTIVITY LEVEL†		
GENDER	**AGE (YEARS)**	**SEDENTARY**	**MODERATELY ACTIVE**	**ACTIVE**
Child (female and male)	2–3	1000–1200‡	1000–1400‡	1000–1400‡
Female§	4–8	1200–1400	1400–1600	1400–1800
	9–13	1400–1600	1600–2000	1800–2000
	14–18	1800	2000	2400
	19–30	1800–2000	2000–2200	2400
	31–50	1800	2000	2200
	51+	1600	1800	2000–2200
Male	4–8	1200–1400	1400–1600	1600–2000
	9–13	1600–2000	1800–2200	2000–2600
	14–18	2000–2400	2400–2800	2800–3200
	19–30	2400–2600	2600–2800	3000
	31–50	2300–2400	2400–2600	2800–3000
	51+	2000–2200	2200–2400	2400–2800

From U.S. Department of Agriculture and U.S. Department of Health and Human Services: *Dietary guidelines for Americans, 2010*, ed 7, Washington, DC, 2010, U.S. Government Printing Office.

*Based on Estimated Energy Requirements (EER) equations, using reference heights (average) and reference weights (healthy) for each age/gender group. For children and adolescents, reference height and weight vary. For adults, the reference man is 5 feet 10 inches tall and weighs 154 pounds. The reference woman is 5 feet 4 inches tall and weighs 126 pounds. EER equations are from the Institute of Medicine. Dietary Reference Intake for Energy, Carbohydrate, Fiber, Fat, Fatty Acids, Cholesterol, Protein, and Amino Acids. Washington DC: The National Academies Press; 2002.

†Sedentary means a lifestyle that includes only the light physical activity associated with typical day-to-day life. Moderately active means a lifestyle that includes physical activity equivalent to walking about 1.5 to 3 miles per day at 3 to 4 miles per hour, in addition to the light physical activity associated with typical day-to-day life. Active means a lifestyle that includes physical activity equivalent to walking more than 3 miles per day at 3 to 4 miles per hour, in addition to the light physical activity associated with typical day-to-day life.

‡The calorie ranges shown are to accommodate needs of different ages within the group. For children and adolescents, more calories are needed at older ages. For adults, fewer calories are needed at older ages.

§Estimates for females do not include women who are pregnant or breastfeeding.

needs for both genders and all age ranges based on physical activity level.

OVERWEIGHT AND OBESITY

A person with a BMI of 25.0 to 29.9 is considered overweight whereas obesity is defined as having a BMI of 30 or higher. Obesity is associated with coronary artery disease, lipid disorders, and type 2 diabetes mellitus. It is also considered a risk factor for some kinds of cancer and is associated with joint disease, gallstones, and respiratory problems. Obesity is the result of excessive food consumption in relation to energy expended. However, it is much more complex than that. It is thought to result from various genetic, environmental, and lifestyle factors. Some genes that predispose a person to obesity have been identified. It is possible that lifestyle factors activate these genes. Scientists are studying various other factors that might play a role in obesity. These include inflammation, sleep disturbances and disorders, obesogens (chemicals foreign to the body that disrupt lipid metabolism), and viruses and other pathogens that may stimulate lipid accumulation.

The goal of treatment for obesity is to attain the best weight possible in the context of overall health. Patients tend to have unrealistic goals and may need encouragement to work toward a more modest goal of 5% to 10% body weight loss. For a person with a BMI of 27 to 35, the recommended goal is a weekly loss of 0.5 to 1.0 pounds for a period of 6 months followed by 6 months of maintenance. Lifestyle modifications focus on the patient's environment, nutritional intake, and physical activity. A minimum of 30 minutes of moderate activity each day is advised. In some cases, drug therapy is prescribed along with the lifestyle modifications. In general, drug benefits are described as "modest." Two of these prescribed drugs are sibutramine (Meridia) and orlistat (Alli, Xenical). Sibutramine, which works on the central nervous system to reduce hunger, can cause cardiovascular side effects. Orlistat reduces absorption of fat in the intestines and can cause flatus, fecal urgency, and oily leakage from the anus. Surgical options to treat obesity are addressed in Chapter 40.

UNDERWEIGHT

The underweight person is one whose weight is 15% to 20% or more below accepted weight standards. This circumstance may be caused by food intake insufficient to meet activity needs, excessive activity, poor absorption and use of food consumed, a wasting disease, or psychologic or emotional stress.

EATING DISORDERS

Eating disorders are fairly common, especially among teenaged girls and young women, and may persist into adulthood. Two eating disorders, anorexia nervosa and bulimia nervosa, usually begin in adolescence or early adulthood. A third disorder, binge eating disorder, is not as well documented but represents a significant proportion of people in weight loss programs. Current thinking holds that multiple biologic, psychologic, sociocultural, and spiritual factors influence the development of these conditions. The most common eating disorders are described here. Treatment of eating disorders usually employs a multidisciplinary team that may include a psychiatrist, psychologist, physician, and nutritionist. Depending on the setting of care, the registered nurse (RN) and LVN/LPN may have a role as well.

Anorexia Nervosa

Anorexia nervosa is an eating disorder characterized by self-imposed starvation. Certain features are common in individuals with this disorder. They are generally girls in their midteens, although young adult women and men sometimes develop the disorder. They are often high achievers from educated, middle-class families. The young person with anorexia nervosa is frequently a perfectionist who uses food and exercise as a means of controlling the body.

People with anorexia nervosa become obsessed with weight loss and soon develop a distorted body image, seeing themselves as fat even when their weight is much less than average for their height and age. They experience personality changes, depression, and apathy. Death may occur in as many as 20% of those with anorexia nervosa.

Bulimia Nervosa

Bulimia nervosa is an eating disorder characterized by periods of binge eating followed by purging. This behavior may alternate with periods of fasting as well. The cycle may go as follows: The person may binge several times a week. The episode may last 2 hours or more. The person consumes large amounts of easily ingested calorie-dense foods such as ice cream, candies, cakes, breads, and pastries. The binge is often followed by self-induced vomiting or the use of laxatives, diuretics, or a combination of these.

Bulimia nervosa occurs more frequently than anorexia nervosa and is also seen most often in young women. People with bulimia are usually of normal weight or even overweight. Most are aware that their eating patterns are abnormal. They may experience fear of not being able to stop eating and depression, guilt, and remorse after a binge. Clinical signs of bulimia nervosa may include tooth erosion, calloused knuckles, stomach lacerations, and esophageal infections from excessive vomiting. Electrolyte imbalances may occur, leading to abnormal heart rhythms and injury to the kidneys. Repeated infections of the bladder and kidney may lead to renal failure.

Binge Eating Disorder

Binge eating disorder is characterized by the intake of excessive calories at least twice a week for 6 months. The person eats very rapidly, sometimes consuming as much as 20,000 calories in one sitting. After the binge episode, the person feels guilty, embarrassed, and depressed. Binge eaters are often dieters but may be overweight, underweight, or of normal weight.

NUTRITIONAL SUPPORT WITH SUPPLEMENTAL FEEDINGS

The preferred method of meeting nutritional requirements is through eating a balanced diet. However, when a person's nutritional needs cannot be met by oral feeding, some type of nutritional supplement is required. These supplements can be formulated using liquid or powdered milk, powdered whole eggs, and powdered egg albumin as concentrated protein sources. Commercially prepared products like Ensure and Boost can provide extra nutrients in a convenient way. Liquid feedings can meet the nutritional requirements of patients who are unable to take solid food. Table 9-9 summarizes the situations that might require artificial feeding. Nursing care of patients receiving enteral and parenteral feedings is addressed in Chapter 39.

ENTERAL TUBE FEEDINGS

Patients who are unable to take in supplemental liquid feedings orally may require enteral tube feedings. Enteral feedings bypass the mouth and deliver nutrients directly into the stomach or small intestine through an inserted tube or catheter. Conditions that interfere with taking in liquids orally include oral surgery, GI surgery, dysphagia (difficulty swallowing), unconsciousness, anorexia, or esophageal obstruction. The tubes can be inserted into the stomach, duodenum, or jejunum through the nose or through the abdominal wall (Fig. 9-4).

A variety of formulas are used for enteral feedings. The standard formula provides for the nutritional requirements of most people. Special formulas are available for individuals who require less volume, require extra protein for healing, have poor kidney function or pulmonary disease, or are in critical care. Enteral tube feedings may cause complications such as nasal irritation and erosion, sinusitis, pharyngeal or vocal cord paralysis, nausea or vomiting, diarrhea, GI bleeding, aspiration pneumonia, hyperkalemia (excessive serum potassium), hyponatremia (serum sodium deficit), hyperglycemia (elevated blood glucose), or nutritional deficiencies. Dumping syndrome may occur when hypertonic fluid enters the jejunum; water is drawn into the lumen of the intestine to dilute the fluid, causing a drop in circulating blood

Table 9-9 Nutrition Support Indications and Methods

CONDITION REQUIRING NUTRITIONAL SUPPORT	FEEDING METHODS
Enteral Nutrition	
• Inability to eat • Inability to eat enough • Impaired digestion, absorption, metabolism	• Nasogastric tube • Nasoduodenal tube • Nasojejunal tube • Gastrostomy • Jejunostomy
Parenteral Nutrition	
• Gastrointestinal incompetency • Critical illness with poor enteral tolerance or accessibility	• Peripherally inserted central catheter • "Tunneled" long-term catheter

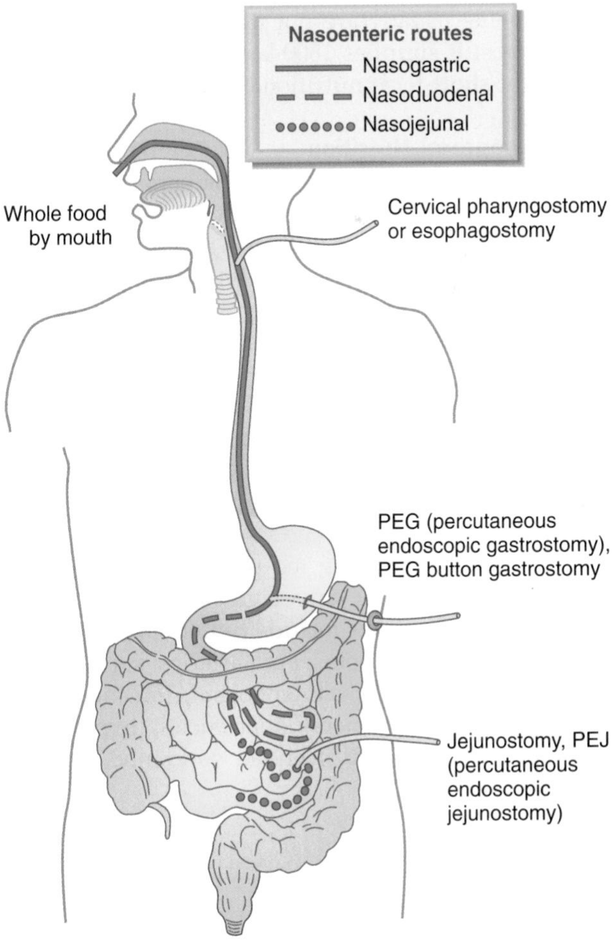

FIGURE 9-4 Diagram of the placement of enteral feeding tubes. (From Mahan LK, Escott-Stump S: *Krause's food and nutrition therapy*, ed 12, St. Louis, 2008, Saunders.)

volume. Tube blockage can occur, most likely caused by viscous formulas with inadequate flushing, crushed medications, and incompatible medications that form clumps.

PARENTERAL NUTRITION

Another method of administering nutrients is through parenteral nutrition, in which nutrients are delivered directly into the bloodstream. The two major types of parenteral nutrition are (1) peripheral parenteral nutrition (PPN) and (2) central parenteral nutrition (CPN) or total parenteral nutrition (TPN). PPN is given through the peripheral veins in the arms and legs and may employ a peripheral venous catheter or a peripherally inserted central catheter. CPN or TPN is given through a central vein, with the catheter usually in the superior vena cava. This method is used for nutrition only if the GI tract cannot be used; it can be lifesaving.

Peripheral Parenteral Nutrition

PPN is the standard intravenous therapy and may be composed of dextrose (5% to 10%), amino acids, vitamins, minerals, and electrolytes. Fat emulsions may be administered peripherally as well. Total nutritional requirements usually are not met with PPN therapy and at most it supplies 1800 kcal/day. It is used primarily for short-term nutritional support.

Total Parenteral Nutrition

CPN or TPN feedings are used for patients who are unable to obtain adequate nutrition enterally or with PPN. They are usually debilitated and malnourished, with a weight loss of 10% of body weight or more.

TPN can meet the high-energy and high-protein needs of burn patients. It can also be used for patients with cancer who have become malnourished as a result of oncologic treatments. TPN can supply up to 4000 kcal/day, which is possible because the solution is administered into the superior vena cava, where the hypertonic solution can be diluted rapidly by the large, fast-flowing volume of blood.

Patients who are being fed parenterally should be monitored closely for any signs of complications. Potential complications include pulmonary complications, injury to the veins and arteries surrounding the TPN catheter site, air embolism, infection, electrolyte imbalance, mineral deficiencies, hyperglycemia, and, if treatment is ended suddenly, rebound hypoglycemia.

TRANSITIONAL FEEDING

When patients are ready to be changed from one of these feeding methods to another, they are ready for transitional feeding. Transitional feeding can be from parenteral nutrition to enteral tube feeding or oral intake, from enteral tube feeding to oral formula or food, or a combination of these.

Transitional feeding should be done gradually and with specific principles in mind. If patients who have been without adequate food for an extended period are given food too quickly, they may develop nutritional recovery syndrome. This syndrome causes hypophosphatemia (deficiency of phosphates in the blood) from the shift of phosphorus from the plasma into the cells. This shift also may affect potassium as it moves into cells with the glucose during refeeding.

Refeeding of the malnourished patient disrupts the adaptive state of starvation and therefore must proceed slowly with close patient monitoring. The ideal early feeding appears to be moderate in carbohydrates, low in sodium, lactose free, and supplemented with phosphorus and potassium.

When moving from parenteral to oral or enteral feeding, continuing the parenteral feeding is important, which allows for maintenance of adequate nutrient and fluid intake as tolerance of enteral feedings is assessed. As the patient is able to tolerate the oral or enteral feedings, the parenteral feedings can be tapered off.

When moving from enteral to oral feedings, the patient may complain of a poor appetite. In making this transition, changing the enteral feeding from a continuous drip to an intermittent feeding may be helpful. In this way the patient has a chance to get hungry between feedings and desire for food may increase.

THERAPEUTIC DIETS

Box 9-8 provides a brief description of various therapeutic diets. Additional information about specific diets is provided in later chapters that address conditions requiring these diets.

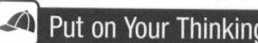

Put on Your Thinking Cap!

Interview an older person (a patient, family member, or other acquaintance) about how his or her eating habits have changed with age. Identify any changes that could lead to inadequate nutrition.

Box 9-8 Diet Progression and Therapeutic Diets

Clear Liquid: clear fat-free broth, bouillon, coffee, tea, carbonated beverages, clear fruit juices, gelatin, fruit ices, popsicles

Full Liquid: As for clear liquid, with addition of smooth-textured dairy products (e.g., ice cream), strained or blended cream soups, custards, refined cooked cereals, vegetable juice, pureed vegetables, all fruit juices, sherbets, puddings, frozen yogurt

Pureed: As for clear liquid, with addition of scrambled eggs; pureed meats, vegetables, and fruits; mashed potatoes and gravy

Mechanical Soft: As for clear and full liquid and pureed, with addition of all cream soups, ground or finely diced meats, flaked fish, cottage cheese, cheese, rice, potatoes, pancakes, light breads, cooked vegetables, cooked or canned fruits, bananas, soups, peanut butter, eggs (not fried)

Soft/Low Residue: Addition of low-fiber, easily digested foods such as pastas, casseroles, moist tender meats, and canned cooked fruits and vegetables; desserts, cakes, and cookies without nuts or coconut

High Fiber: Addition of fresh uncooked fruits, steamed vegetables, bran, oatmeal, and dried fruits

Low Sodium: 4-g (no added salt), 2-g, 1-g, or 500-mg sodium diets; vary from no-added salt to severe sodium restriction (500-mg sodium diet), which requires selective food purchases

Low Cholesterol: 300 mg/day cholesterol, in keeping with American Heart Association guideline for serum lipid reduction

Diabetic: Nutrition recommendations by the American Diabetes Association: focus on total energy, nutrient and food distribution; include a balanced intake of carbohydrates, fats, and proteins; varied caloric recommendations to accommodate patient's metabolic demands.

Regular: No restrictions, unless specified

From Stockert PA: Nutrition. In Potter PA, Perry AG, Stockert PA, Hall AM, editors: *Fundamentals of nursing*, ed 8, St. Louis, 2013, Elsevier/Mosby, p. 1017.

Get Ready for the NCLEX® Examination!

Key Points

- Nutrition is the cornerstone of the healing process. To support and maintain life or fight disease, the body must be supplied with the proper nutrients.
- During the digestive process, enzymes help break down food particles to their simplest form so that the nutrients can be absorbed by the body.
- Regulation of the GI system involves neural control and the secretion of hormones.
- Parasympathetic nerves generally stimulate digestive activity and sympathetic nerves inhibit activity.
- The stomach is normally emptied in 1 to 4 hours, depending on the amount and kinds of foods eaten.
- The primary organ of absorption is the small intestine.
- Fluids, vitamins, and minerals are absorbed through the intestinal mucosa.
- The body makes use of the energy received through the food that is eaten and the largest portion of energy expenditure occurs during rest to carry out the mechanical activities needed to sustain life processes.
- Most of the energy needed to move, perform activities, and live is consumed in the form of carbohydrates, which are converted primarily to glucose for immediate use by the body's cells.
- Although carbohydrates are the body's main source of food energy, fats are the most concentrated source, supplying 9 kilocalories per gram, whereas carbohydrates and protein supply only 4 kilocalories per gram.
- Lipids are a major source of energy for muscle tissue, even when glucose is available.
- The recommended macronutrient proportions for adults are 45% to 65% carbohydrates, 10% to 35% protein, and 20% to 35% fat.
- People should try to eat unsaturated fats, which come from plant sources, rather than saturated fats, which come mainly from animal sources.
- Proteins are made of smaller units called *amino acids*.
- Vitamins and minerals are micronutrients; they are needed in small amounts for good health.
- Water is the largest component of the body and body tissues and is essential to all life processes in the body.
- Maintaining a good diet can help middle-aged and older adults to maintain a high level of function and reduce the risks of chronic disease; however, because of the normal decline in metabolism and physical activity, energy needs lessen with age.
- Most vegetarian diets can provide all nutrients if planned properly.
- Vegans are at risk for megaloblastic anemia if adequate vitamin B_{12} is not added to the diet.
- Most adults have the ability to maintain a constant weight but to do so requires consistent food and exercise patterns on a daily basis.
- Anorexia nervosa, bulimia nervosa, and binge eating disorder are eating disorders that often begin in adolescence.
- Obesity is a complex problem that places a person at risk for numerous health problems.
- Options in the treatment of obesity include lifestyle modifications, drug therapy, and surgical interventions.
- Eating disorders are thought to be caused by multiple biologic, psychologic, sociocultural, and spiritual factors.
- For the patient who cannot take oral feedings, nutritional support may be provided through enteral tube feedings or through peripheral or central intravenous catheters.

Additional Learning Resources

SG Go to your Study Guide for additional learning activities to help you master this chapter content.

Online Resources: Extensive resources about specific nutrient recommendations can be accessed via www.nap.edu:

- Dietary Reference Intakes for Energy, Carbohydrate, Fiber, Fat, Fatty Acids, Cholesterol, Protein, and Amino Acids (2002/2005)
- Dietary Reference Intakes for Water, Potassium, Sodium, Chloride, and Sulfate (2005)
- *Dietary Reference Intakes (DRIs): Estimated Average Requirements* (Updated 2011)

evolve Go to your Evolve website (http://evolve.elsevier.com/Linton/medsurg) for the following learning resources and much more:

- Interactive Prioritization Exercises
- Fluid & Electrolyte Tutorial
- Pharmacology Tutorial
- Review Questions for the NCLEX® Examination

Review Questions for the NCLEX® Examination

1. The nurse anticipates the most serious problems with the absorption of nutrients if the patient has a disorder affecting which part of the digestive tract?
   1. Esophagus
   2. Stomach
   3. Small intestine
   4. Large intestine

   NCLEX Client Need: Physiological Integrity: Basic Care and Comfort
2. The physician has ordered laboratory tests to evaluate a patient's serum lipase and amylase. The nurse knows that lipase and amylase are examples of:
   1. Macronutrients
   2. Metabolic wastes
   3. Carrier proteins
   4. Digestive enzymes

   NCLEX Client Need: Physiological Integrity: Basic Care and Comfort
3. Nursing students are teaching community residents about nutrition. They should inform the participants that energy requirements are greatest during which stage(s) of life? (Select all that apply.)
   1. Infancy
   2. Preschool years
   3. Adolescence
   4. Young adulthood
   5. Middle adult years

   NCLEX Client Need: Health Promotion and Maintenance
4. Excess glucose is stored in the liver as __________.

   NCLEX Client Need: Physiological Integrity: Basic Care and Comfort
5. The LVN/LPN is teaching older adults about the need for adequate dietary fiber. The nurse should note that the functions of dietary fiber include: (Select all that apply.)
   1. Absorb excess gastric acid
   2. Decrease serum cholesterol
   3. Aid in the process of elimination
   4. Decrease fecal bulk
   5. Help form a soft stool

   NCLEX Client Need: Physiological Integrity: Basic Care and Comfort
6. Which of the following is a water-soluble vitamin?
   1. Vitamin E
   2. Vitamin A
   3. Vitamin C
   4. Vitamin D

   NCLEX Client Need: Physiological Integrity: Basic Care and Comfort
7. The nurse is teaching older adults in the community about nutrition. The content should include which of the following? (Select all that apply.)
   1. Older people should eliminate all sodium from their diets.
   2. Older men usually require the same amount of daily calories as younger adults.
   3. Older people who are less active need fewer calories than they did when younger.
   4. Most older people require megavitamins to meet basic requirements.
   5. A moderately active older woman needs 300 fewer calories daily than when younger.

   NCLEX Client Need: Physiological Integrity: Basic Care and Comfort
8. A patient reports that she is lactovegetarian. You know that her diet includes:
   1. Eggs
   2. Fish
   3. Poultry
   4. Milk

   NCLEX Client Need: Physiological Integrity: Basic Care and Comfort
9. When a patient is receiving total parenteral nutrition (TPN), the nurse must monitor for which of the following potential complications?
   1. Vomiting
   2. Air embolism
   3. Hypoglycemia
   4. Aspiration

   NCLEX Client Need: Physiological Integrity: Reduction of Risk Potential
10. A patient is being transitioned from parenteral nutrition to oral nutrition. The nurse should monitor for nutritional recovery syndrome, which is characterized by:
    1. Hypophosphatemia
    2. Hypocalcemia
    3. Hyponatremia
    4. Hypoglycemia

    NCLEX Client Need: Physiological Integrity: Reduction of Risk Potential

chapter 10

Developmental Processes

http://evolve.elsevier.com/Linton/medsurg

Objectives

1. List the developmental tasks for successful adulthood.
2. Identify the health problems specific to the adult age groups.
3. Discuss the health care needs of young, middle-aged, and older adults.

Key Terms

Biologic age
Psychologic age
Social age

Each stage of life has specific developmental processes that must be undertaken and mastered for a person to go on to the next stage successfully. These developmental processes consist of physical, emotional, social, and psychologic changes that present challenges to every living human being. You might think of development as only the process of growing up but adults, as well as children, continue to move through stages of development. Because this book focuses on adults, this chapter addresses the developmental processes associated with young adulthood, middle age, and older age.

Major changes in the stages of development in the life cycle occurred in the past few decades. Americans are marrying later, having fewer children, and living longer than ever before. Certain marker events, such as marriage, childbirth, acquiring a first job, and the departure of young adults from the family home, occur in various developmental stages. Despite the recent changes in the life cycle, broad, general stages of adulthood can still be found, with predictable movement between them. Erik Erikson developed the basis of our view of human growth and development; he introduced the idea that each stage of life is associated with specific developmental tasks (Table 10-1).

YOUNG ADULTHOOD

Young adulthood comes at a time when physical growth ends and social expectations begin. It is considered to occur during a person's 20s, 30s, and 40s; however, these decades are often divided by such terms as *young young adult* (ages 20 to 35) and *old young adult* (ages 35 to 45).

Young adulthood is a time for settling down to a job, raising a family, and taking on new responsibilities. Most people in this age group are expected to leave their parents' home and establish their own home. People in their 20s and early 30s often begin this process by establishing an intimate, lasting relationship with another person in which the physical satisfaction and psychologic security of another are more important than their own. Without the development of an intimate relationship, the young adult can become isolated, lonely, and self-absorbed. In addition, young adults are establishing career goals.

Many young people have extended their education and have prolonged the time in which they continue to live at home; or a job loss, divorce, or other stressor may precipitate a move back home. The entire family then has to adjust to a young adult living at home by redistributing roles and responsibilities, maintaining adequate communication, and reallocating budget and space.

This time may be difficult for parents, who had expected a new time of freedom and independence in their middle years; it is especially difficult if young grandchildren are included in the package.

DEVELOPMENTAL TASKS

The following developmental tasks must be achieved by young adults:

- Accept self and stabilize self-concept and body image.
- Establish independence from parental home and financial aid.
- Assume responsibilities and independent decision making.
- Become established in a vocation or profession that provides personal satisfaction, economic independence, and a feeling of making a worthwhile contribution to society.

Table 10-1 Erikson's Adult Developmental Tasks

DEVELOPMENTAL STAGE	DEVELOPMENTAL TASK	NURSING ASSESSMENT DATA
Young adulthood	Intimacy versus isolation	Assess whether the patient has meaningful, intimate relationships. If the patient has no intimate relationships, ask whether he or she has had one or more in the past. Assess other support systems that the patient may have.
Middle adulthood	Generativity versus self-absorption and stagnation	Assess whether the patient is employed. Ask the patient what he or she does for leisure or recreation. If the patient is not employed or has no regular leisure activity, ask the patient what he or she does during a 24-hour day. Assess for signs of depression, such as excessive sleeping and decreased appetite.
Older adulthood	Ego integrity versus despair	Assess what the patient does each day. Ask about the patient's family and other relationships. Ask the patient if he or she feels lonely; if so, assess for signs of depression.

From Ignatavicius DD, Workman, ML, Mishler, M: *Medical-surgical nursing: A nursing process approach,* ed. 3, Philadelphia, 1999, Saunders.

- Learn to appraise and express love responsibly through more than sexual contact.
- Establish an intimate bond with another, either through marriage or with a close friend.
- Establish and maintain a home and manage a time schedule and life stresses.
- Find a congenial social and friendship group.
- Decide whether to have a family and carry out tasks of parenting.
- Formulate a meaningful philosophy of life and reassess priorities and values.
- Become involved as a citizen in the community.

These developmental tasks focus on marriage, childbearing, and work. However, many young adults are delaying marriage, electing to remain single, choosing cohabitation without marriage, or are divorced. Clearly, a young adult does not have to marry to be well adjusted and achieve the identified developmental tasks.

HEALTH PROBLEMS

Young adults, especially those in their 20s and early 30s, have relatively few health problems. The four most common causes of death in the young adult age group are unintentional injury, homicide, suicide, and malignant neoplasms. Among the youngest members of this age group, the most common cause of unintentional injury is motor vehicle accidents followed by poisoning (drug overdose, carbon monoxide, etc). After age 25, unintentional poisoning causes more deaths than motor vehicle accidents. As young adults progress into their late 40s, the primary causes of death are malignancies and heart disease, followed by accidents and suicide.

Typical health problems are related to stress on the job or in social interactions, lifestyle, and childbearing. These problems include depression; anxiety; complications of pregnancy; cervical and breast cancer; and back, hip, and limb injuries. In the quest for meaningful social relationships and a career that will gain them independence and success, young adults may experience tension and stress and may lack the time to attend to health promotion activities such as a proper diet and nutrition. They may work hard and party enthusiastically. Meals may be eaten on the run and the diet may consist primarily of fast foods. The total number of calories needed is less than during adolescence, given that the adult has completed physical growth. Smoking and alcohol or drug abuse are common. These practices may have a direct bearing on health in the later years (Table 10-2).

As young adults enter their 30s and early 40s, their focus is directed mainly toward raising a family and furthering their careers (Fig. 10-1). This age may be a time to reassess their lives and careers and often major changes are made. Factors that contribute to health problems are stress related to work, marital problems, and stress related to managing a household. Couples who have postponed childbearing may have difficulties with conception and pregnancy.

HEALTH CARE NEEDS

Health care needs are related to promoting optimal health. Having at least one thorough physical examination during the 20s is a good idea. A physical examination should include tests for sexually transmitted infections, hypertension, and elevated blood lipids. During young adulthood, several types of health screening (mammograms, clinical breast examinations, breast and testicular self-examinations, pelvic examinations, and Papanicolaou [Pap] tests) should be initiated and repeated at regular intervals. Women are advised to begin periodic Pap tests to screen for cervical cancer at age 21. The Pap test should be performed every 3 years until age 65, when it is no longer recommended. Women with increased risk of cervical cancer,

Table 10-2 Harmful Health Practices, Effects on Health in the Later Years, and Preventive Measures

HARMFUL HEALTH PRACTICE	POSSIBLE EFFECTS ON HEALTH	PREVENTIVE MEASURES
Lack of physical activity	Diabetes, osteoporosis, heart disease, cancer, obesity, stroke, depression	Increase moderate daily physical activity and reduce sedentary lifestyle.
Obesity	Heart disease, hypertension, type 2 diabetes mellitus, degenerative joint disease, cancer, stroke, atherosclerosis	Maintain ideal weight; maintain low-cholesterol, low-fat, nutritious diet with plenty of vegetables, fruits, and grain products.
Cigarette smoking	Heart disease; cancers of the lung, larynx, pharynx, oral cavity, esophagus, pancreas, and bladder; chronic bronchitis and emphysema	Stop smoking or do not start smoking.
Alcohol and drug abuse	Malnutrition, cirrhosis of the liver, brain damage, mental status changes, homicide, suicide, motor vehicle fatalities	Limit alcohol intake and stop using drugs or do not start; participate in 12-step program for rehabilitation.
Stress	Stress-related conditions such as hypertension and heart disease	Recognize and modify stressors; use a stress management program, such as exercise or biofeedback.

Adapted from U.S. Department of Health and Human Services: *Healthy people 2010, vol 1, With understanding and improving health, vol 2, Objectives for improving health*, ed 2 (Publication No. [PHS] 99-1256), Washington, DC, 1999, U.S. Government Printing Office.

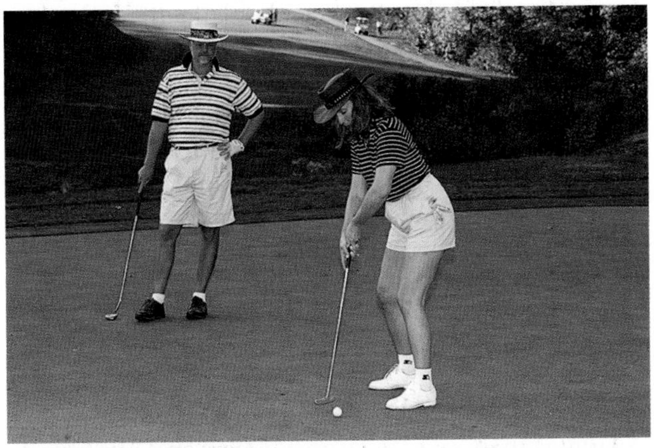

FIGURE 10-1 Middle age is a time of relatively good health, with new opportunities and personal freedom for many individuals. (From Sorrentino S: *Mosby's textbook for nursing assistants*, ed 8, St. Louis, 2012, Mosby.)

such as those with human immunodeficiency virus (HIV) infection, long-term steroid use, organ transplant, or diethylstilbestrol (DES) exposure in utero, may be advised to have more frequent screening. Because of the relationship between the human papilloma virus (HPV) and cervical cancer, an HPV co-test is advised every 5 years for women between the ages of 30 and 65. The HPV co-test is performed along with the cell examination of the Pap test. Women who have had the HPV vaccine should continue Pap tests until age 65. Recommendations related to screening for breast cancer have been controversial in recent years, as research found that breast examinations did not reduce the death rate from breast cancer. At this time, experts agree that mammograms are the best screening tool. The American Cancer Society (ACS) continues to recommend regular professional breast exams as well. The ACS includes breast self-examination as an option. In 2009, the U.S. Preventive Services Task Force recommended that most women wait until age 50 to begin mammograms. This controversial recommendation may or may not result in a change in practice. Some men with high risk factors are advised to have an annual prostate-specific antigen (PSA) test and digital rectal examination to screen for prostate cancer. Whether all men should have regular PSA tests is in question. See Chapter 25, Table 25-6, for additional information about cancer screening.

A tetanus booster should be given if persons have not received one in the past 10 years. The hepatitis B vaccine is recommended for adults at risk of exposure to blood and body fluids. Routine dental and eye examinations should be scheduled. Women who wish to perform breast self-examination (BSE) should be instructed in correct technique. They should also be informed that BSE does not replace periodic professional examinations or mammograms. Young men should be taught to do a testicular examination.

Health counseling in the 20s should focus on health promotion behaviors. Programs may be established to include topics such as nutrition; exercise and leisure; rest and sleep; human sexuality and family planning; and the effects of smoking, drugs, and alcohol.

In the years between ages 30 and 45, especially after age 35, young adults should begin to think about the prevention of chronic illness, particularly cancer and heart disease. They should have periodic physical examinations, usually recommended at ages 30 and 35, and then every 3 years thereafter. The physical examination should include tests for hypertension, anemia, elevated serum lipids, and a cervical Pap test for women. Experts suggest that people in this age group examine their skin and mouth periodically for precancerous lesions. Preventive dental checkups and treatment are usually recommended every 6 months to 2 years.

Health promotion and disease prevention programs have a similar focus as those for people in their 20s. Stress management, effective parenting, proper diet and nutrition, exercise, drug and alcohol awareness, and smoking cessation are appropriate topics for health teaching and counseling.

Put on Your Thinking Cap!

When a young adult is diagnosed with a serious chronic illness, how might developmental tasks be affected?

MIDDLE YEARS

The terms *middle years, middle age,* and *middle adulthood* usually refer to the ages between 45 and 65. However, other factors define middle age, particularly how a person acts and feels. Because life expectancy has increased so dramatically during the last 50 years, middle age is a relatively new concept. What used to be old age is now middle age. In 1900, a person born in the United States had a life expectancy of 47.3 years. In comparison, a child born in 2010 has a life expectancy of 78.7 years (76.2 for men, 81.0 for women). Differences are evident in life expectancy according to race as well as gender: 76.5 years for Caucasian men, 71.8 years for African-American men, and 78.5 for Latino men. Life expectancy for African-American women, is 78.0 compared with 81.3 for Caucasian women and 83.8 for Latina women (National Vital Statistics Reports, 2010).

More than 40 million Americans are considered middle-aged. They earn most of the money, pay most of the taxes, and have most of the power in business and government. Middle age is a time of relatively good health for most. People experience a new personal freedom and enjoy maximal command of themselves and influence over others.

Many people who are in their middle years belong to a group called the "sandwich generation." They may have adolescents and young adults at home and at the same time have ailing, older adult parents to care for. The fact that most middle-aged Americans today still have a living parent is a great change in family dynamics. People who delayed childbearing may have even younger children at home.

Many of today's middle-aged women work outside the home and have developed important careers. Work and family obligations together may require a balancing act for middle-aged women who are trying to maintain continued involvement both at work and at home. In addition to caring for children, the middle-aged woman is the most likely caregiver to older-adult parents. The result can be a great deal of stress and conflict.

DEVELOPMENTAL TASKS

The following developmental tasks should be accomplished by people in their middle years:

- Discover and develop new satisfaction with a mate or significant other by enjoying mutual activities, providing mutual support, and developing a deeper sense of unity and intimacy.
- Help growing and grown children become happy and responsible adults.
- Balance work and other roles; prepare for retirement.
- Accept role reversal with aging parents; prepare emotionally for the eventual death of living parents.
- Achieve mature social and civic responsibilities and give time and resources to the community.
- Accept and adjust to the physical changes of middle age and establish and maintain a healthy lifestyle.
- Continue to formulate a philosophy of life and grow spiritually.
- Develop satisfying leisure activities.
- Recognize the inevitability of death and prepare for one's own eventual death.

Middle-aged persons who successfully master developmental tasks begin to accept their age and gradually come to value the wisdom gained from living and experience rather than the physical power and strength that accompany youth. Emotional and mental flexibility increase the ability to change and adapt to new situations and to be open to others. It is a time of "mellowing out," of accepting what life has to offer.

HEALTH PROBLEMS

People in their middle years continue to be relatively healthy and the same factors that contribute to the deterioration of health habits in the young adult apply to those in middle age. The major cause of death is cardiovascular disease and the most common health problems, along with cardiovascular disease, are cancer, pulmonary disease, diabetes, obesity, alcoholism, anxiety, depression, and glaucoma. Respiratory conditions are a frequent cause of days absent from work among women; injuries are a frequent cause among men. Bone mass begins to decrease in the middle years. Women lose calcium from bone tissue after menopause, leading to an increased risk of osteoporosis. Muscle mass is reduced as a result of decreased muscle fiber. In the 40s, changes in vision typically begin. Age-related farsightedness *(presbyopia)* develops as a result of decreasing elasticity of the lens. The clue to developing presbyopia is that the middle-aged adult begins to hold reading material at a distance to focus on it better. *Presbycusis* (i.e., the common loss of hearing acuity associated with aging) may begin to appear. This life stage is an important time to focus on prevention. Lifestyle changes yield significant benefits in terms of a longer, healthier life.

Put on Your Thinking Cap!

Suppose that a middle-aged adult is diagnosed with a life-threatening illness. What are the effects on family, job, and other roles? How would the middle-aged person's developmental stage affect the response to illness and treatment?

HEALTH CARE NEEDS

The health care goals for middle-aged people are the same as those for younger adults. They are focused on health promotion and disease prevention to preserve and prolong the period of maximal energy and optimal mental and social activity.

During the middle years, regular assessment of health status is important for maintaining good health. Early diagnosis of illness helps to prevent later complications. A complete physical examination is recommended every 3 years and should include routine blood pressure screening and cholesterol and glucose testing. After age 50, the risk of colorectal cancer increases. Depending on the patient's history, a variety of invasive (e.g., sigmoidoscopy, colonoscopy) or noninvasive (e.g., fecal occult blood, fecal immunochemical test) screening procedures may be recommended at intervals.

Annual tests of the PSA have been common practice for some time. An elevated PSA is considered a possible indication of prostate cancer. Evaluation of the benefits of annual PSA testing revealed that elevations often resulted in treatment of slow-growing tumors that were unlikely to lead to serious illness or death. Possible adverse effects of treatment of prostate cancer include urinary incontinence and erectile dysfunction. Therefore the American Urological Association (AUA) recommends routine testing on an individual basis only in men ages 55 to 69 and those with risk factors, including African-American race and family history of prostate cancer.

Women should continue to have mammograms and clinical breast examinations according to the current guidelines in consultation with their physicians. Women with HIV infection, a weak immune system, or a history of DES exposure should continue annual examinations. Proponents of regular BSE believe that it may help with early detection of abnormalities but should not replace medical evaluation. In addition to the recommended mammogram (Centers for Disease Control and Prevention recommends every 2 years for women ages 50 to 74) and clinical breast examination, additional screenings such as magnetic resonance imaging (MRI) may be recommended for women at increased risk for breast cancer.

Women usually enter a perimenopausal period between the ages of 45 and 50. Menopause is preceded by the perimenopausal period (approximately 5 years), during which a gradual decrease in estrogen occurs accompanied by a gradual decrease in menstrual flow. Pregnancy remains possible until the menstrual cycle ceases completely. The permanent cessation of menstruation typically occurs between the ages of 45 and 55. During the menopausal years, women may experience symptoms such as hot flashes, dizziness, headaches, perspiration, palpitations, water retention, nausea, muscle cramps, fatigue, insomnia, or tingling in the fingers and toes. Many women take estrogen to relieve some of the symptoms of menopause. A combination of estrogen and progesterone is safer for the postmenopausal woman who still has her uterus. Estrogen alone increases the risk of endometrial cancer. Menopausal women should be advised to report unexpected bleeding or spotting, which could be signs of endometrial (uterine) cancer.

Health promotion activities during middle age are the same as for young adults. The focus is on proper nutrition; exercise; stress management; and the reduction or elimination of smoking, drug use, and alcohol use.

OLDER ADULTS

Age 65 is commonly considered the beginning of old age. However, many people in their 60s and older do not consider themselves old and they continue to live healthy, productive lives. People are entering old age in better health than in the past. In the United States today, 8 in 10 people will live past their sixty-fifth birthday. Markers that may be more meaningful than chronologic age to define older age include (1) biologic age, (2) psychologic age, and (3) social age. **Biologic age** focuses on the functional capabilities of various organ systems in the body. Many older people, especially those who engage in exercise and other health promotion activities, continue to function well whereas others seem to be prematurely ill and frail. **Psychologic age** refers to the behavioral capacity of the person to adapt to changing environmental demands. The older person's ability to remember, learn, and exercise behavioral control is a factor that affects psychologic age. **Social age** refers to the roles and habits of a person in relation to other members of society, including such aspects as the person's type of dress, language, and social relationships.

As they move through the later years, men and women are required to make many adjustments to physiologic, psychologic, and social changes. Those changes are gradual and vary greatly among individuals. Declines in bodily function, particularly in vision and hearing, and diminished physical strength and resiliency may affect day-to-day functioning. Psychologic changes include a decreased short-term memory, slower performance on cognitive tasks, and longer learning time. Older people retain psychologic skills but those skills usually take longer to accomplish.

Social changes include retirement, a change in living conditions, and loss of spouse and significant others.

Put on Your Thinking Cap!

Consider your own biologic age, psychologic age, and social age. Using examples of family, friends, and acquaintances in your life, think of ways that people can act differently in psychologic and social ages compared to their chronologic ages.

DEVELOPMENTAL TASKS

The following developmental tasks confront older adults:

- Recognize the aging process and adjust to decreasing physical strength and health changes.
- Adjust to retirement; adjust living standards to retirement income.
- Establish satisfactory living arrangements as a result of role changes.
- Maintain emotional satisfaction in relationships with spouse, children, grandchildren, and other living relatives.
- Establish an affiliation with members of one's own age group; maintain an interest in people outside the family and in the community.
- Maintain a maximum level of health; learn to adjust to the loss of physical strength, illness, and one's own mortality.
- Cope with the death of parents, spouse, and friends.
- Learn to combine new dependency needs with the continuing need for independence.

Developmental tasks in older age focus on the redirection of energy and talents to new roles and activities, the acceptance of life with its joys and limitations, and the development of a personal view of death in preparation for this final stage of life.

HEALTH PROBLEMS

The major causes of death in older age are heart disease, cancer, chronic respiratory disease, cerebrovascular disease, Alzheimer disease, diabetes mellitus, influenza and pneumonia, nephritis, and septicemia. Unintentional injuries accounted for more than 41,000 deaths in 2010, making it the ninth most common cause of death in this age group. The most common conditions are arthritis, heart disease, diabetes, and cancer. Benign or malignant enlargement of the prostate is common in older men; breast cancer is common in older women.

HEALTH CARE NEEDS

The health care goals in the older age group are to manage chronic illnesses and to maintain and prolong the period of optimal physical, mental, and social activity. Helping older adults to maintain their independence for as long as possible in the event of one or more chronic illnesses is important.

Physical examinations should be performed yearly and include the same assessment as indicated for middle-aged adults. However, depending on individual risk factors, some screenings can be discontinued after age 65 or 70, or when life expectancy reaches certain limits. Women who have had a total hysterectomy do not require an annual Pap test. If the cervix was left intact after hysterectomy, annual screening should continue until age 65. Dental examinations and treatment should also be continued into older age. As people age, periodic evaluation and treatment of the feet by a podiatrist are recommended to promote mobility. An influenza vaccination is recommended yearly for persons older than 65 years. A single-dose pneumococcal vaccine is recommended, with revaccination every 5 years for people with chronic illnesses. Also, individuals who were vaccinated 5 or more years previously and were younger than age 65 at the time of the first vaccination should have a one-time revaccination.

Health promotion activities should continue into older age. These activities can increase quality of life and, in many cases, prevent many of the chronic illnesses that accompany the later years. Proper nutrition, especially a low-fat, high-fiber diet with a large amount of complex carbohydrates, helps to maintain energy, promote intestinal motility, and decrease susceptibility to some chronic illnesses. Exercise can benefit older adults, even the very old who begin an exercise program for the first time. Walking is the ideal exercise and 20 to 30 minutes, three times a week can help to maintain weight, blood pressure, coordination, and mobility and create a positive outlook on life. Older people also can benefit from counseling for alcohol and drug abuse and smoking cessation. Improving one's health habits can never be done too soon.

Chapter 11 discusses health care issues related to the older adult in greater depth.

Get Ready for the NCLEX® Examination!

Key Points

- In the United States, life expectancy is longest for Latina women and shortest for African-American men.
- Developmental processes are changes that present challenges that must be undertaken and mastered for a person to go on to the next stage successfully.
- Developmental tasks for young adults focus on acceptance of self, independence, intimacy, home and time management, social relationships, community involvement, and formulation of a meaningful philosophy of life.
- Health problems of young adults are related to stress on the job or in social interactions, lifestyle, and childbearing.
- Developmental tasks for middle-aged adults focus on interpersonal relationships, guidance of grown children, creation of a pleasant home, balanced roles, care of aging parents, civic responsibilities, adjustment to physical changes, pursuit of satisfying leisure activities, formulation of a life philosophy, and recognition of death's inevitability.
- Health problems of middle-aged adults include cardiovascular disease, cancer, pulmonary disease, diabetes, obesity, alcoholism, anxiety, depression, and glaucoma.
- Developmental tasks for older adults include adjustment to aging and retirement, establishment of satisfactory living arrangements, maintenance of emotional satisfaction in relationships, affiliation with peers, maintenance of maximal level of health, coping with the deaths of others, and learning to combine new dependency needs with the need for independence.
- Health problems for older adults include cardiovascular disease, cancer, diabetes mellitus, accidents, arthritis, gastrointestinal problems, and respiratory diseases.

Additional Learning Resources

SG Go to your Study Guide for additional learning activities to help you master this chapter content.

evolve Go to your Evolve website (http://evolve.elsevier.com/Linton/medsurg) for the following learning resources and much more:

- Interactive Prioritization Exercises
- Fluid & Electrolyte Tutorial
- Pharmacology Tutorial
- Review Questions for the NCLEX® Examination

Review Questions for the NCLEX® Examination

1. The LVN/LPN is working with young adults who have chronic illnesses. It is important for the nurse to remember that the developmental tasks of the young adult include:
   1. Accepting role reversal with aging parents
   2. Developing satisfying leisure activities
   3. Establishing an intimate bond with another
   4. Achieving mature social and civic responsibilities

   NCLEX Client Need: Psychosocial Integrity
2. Nurses at a community college's Student Health Center are planning interventions to focus on health promotion for students. Which intervention is directed toward reducing the most common cause of death among young adults?
   1. Teach early warning signs of cancer
   2. Encourage cardiovascular fitness
   3. Teach principles of safer sex
   4. Promote safe driving practices

   NCLEX Client Need: Health Promotion and Maintenance
3. Middle-aged adults caring for both children and parents are referred to as the ________ generation.

   NCLEX Client Need: Psychosocial Integrity
4. The Employee Health staff is discussing health promotion programs to reduce the major cause of death for middle-aged adults. Their first priority should be:
   1. Cardiovascular fitness programs
   2. Screening for diabetes mellitus
   3. Driving instruction for older people
   4. Stress management classes

   NCLEX Client Need: Health Promotion and Maintenance
5. Nurses at a long-term care facility are reviewing care plans for older residents. They should consider that a developmental task of older adults is to:
   1. Maintain the pace of middle age despite physical changes
   2. Maintain emotional satisfaction in relationships with others
   3. Decrease one's involvement in social activities
   4. Remain independent regardless of physical and emotional health

   NCLEX Client Need: Psychosocial Integrity
6. A leading cause of death among *both* young adults and older adults is:
   1. Cancer
   2. Accidents
   3. Suicide
   4. Diabetes mellitus

   NCLEX Client Need: Physiological Integrity: Physiological Adaptation
7. The life expectancy of a person born in the United States in 2010 is:
   1. 69.5 years
   2. 72.3 years
   3. 78.7 years
   4. 82.1 years

   NCLEX Client Need: Physiological Integrity: Physiological Adaptation

8. Which of the following statements about life expectancy in the United States is/are true? (Select all that apply.)
   1. Women are expected to live about 5 years longer than men.
   2. Life expectancy has increased by about 30 years over the past century.
   3. African Americans generally are expected to live longer than Caucasians.
   4. African-American men have a shorter life expectancy than African-American women.
   5. Among African Americans, Caucasians, and Latinos, Latina women have the longest life expectancy.

   NCLEX Client Need: Physiological Integrity: Physiological Adaptation

9. To assess a person's progress toward achieving generativity, the nurse should ask:
   1. "Do you often feel lonely or depressed?"
   2. "Who are your main sources of support?"
   3. "How do you spend your spare time?"
   4. "What do you do to stay healthy?"

   NCLEX Client Need: Psychosocial Integrity

10. Which of the following conditions are health risks associated with obesity? (Select all that apply.)
    1. Emphysema
    2. Osteoporosis
    3. Cancer
    4. Atherosclerosis
    5. Hypertension

    NCLEX Client Need: Physiological Integrity: Physiological Adaptation

chapter 11

The Older Patient

http://evolve.elsevier.com/Linton/medsurg

Objectives

1. Describe the roles of the gerontological nurse.
2. Determine the extent to which selected myths and stereotypes about older adults are factual.
3. Describe biologic and psychosocial factors associated with aging.
4. Explain the importance of assessing activities of daily living and instrumental activities of daily living.
5. Explain why drug dosage adjustments may be needed for older persons.

Key Terms

Ageism (ĀJ-ĭzm)
Aging
Cataract (KĂT-ă-răkt)
Conduction deafness (kŏn-DŬK-shŭn DĔF-nĕs)
Gerontological nurse
Gerontology (jĕr-ŏn-TŎ-lŏ-jē)
Glaucoma (glăw-KŌ-mă)
Kyphosis (kī-FŌ-sĭs)
Presbycusis (prĕz-bĕ-KYŪ-sĭs)
Presbyopia (prĕz-bē-Ō-pē-ă)
Sensorineural deafness (sĕn-sō-rē-NYŪ-răl)

The care of older adults can be a richly rewarding experience. As the over-65 population has continued its unprecedented growth, the need for nurses with expertise in the care of older people has grown rapidly. Nursing care of older adults requires specialized knowledge and skills. Indeed, maintaining the best possible quality of life in the presence of aging changes and pathologic processes requires a high level of knowledge, skill, and compassion. This chapter provides an overview of the aging process and the needs of older persons. Nursing care of patients with specific medical conditions is addressed in subsequent chapters.

DEFINITIONS

Aging is the process of growing older or more mature. It is an ongoing developmental process that begins at conception and ends at death (Box 11-1). Defining *old age* is not as simple as it might seem. Most definitions of *old age* refer to having lived for a long time. A child or teenager may define "old people" as persons in their 30s, 40s, or 50s whereas people in their 50s may define old as "at least 10 years older than I am." Most gerontologists agree that old age is not measured in years. Although the age of 65 is commonly used to indicate the onset of old age, this number is clearly arbitrary and a function of social policy. Because the characteristics of individuals between the age of 65 and the end of life are so varied, some gerontologists have divided "old age" into stages. Ages 60 to 74 are considered *young old*, ages 75 to 100 are referred to as *old old*, and individuals over age 100 are *centenarians.*

Gerontology, the study of aging, "encompasses the demography of aging, the biology of aging, the neuropsychology of aging and medical gerontology" (Fillit, Rockwood, & Woodhouse, 2010, p. 1). Geriatrics is the biomedical science of old age and the application of knowledge of aging to the prevention, diagnosis, treatment, and care of older persons.

ROLES OF THE GERONTOLOGICAL NURSE

In 2010, 13% of the U.S. population was age 65 and over. By 2030, estimates predict that 20% of the population will be age 65 and older. These older adults will need health care services to help them maintain their health, prevent disabling and life-threatening diseases and conditions, and manage chronic illnesses. Nurses have always been involved in the care of the aged. Whereas geriatric nursing is the care of sick older adults, gerontological nursing focuses on care of older persons across the health-illness continuum. "Gerontological nursing involves the care of aging people and emphasizes the promotion of the highest possible quality of life and wellness throughout the life span" (Eliopolous, 2014, p. 73).

The term **gerontological nurse** typically refers to professional nurses and advanced-level practitioners, such as nurse practitioners, clinical specialists, and

Box 11-1 An Old Lady's Poem

What do you see, nurse, what do you see?
What are you thinking when you're looking at me?
A crabby old woman, not very wise,
Uncertain of habit, with faraway eyes?
Who dribbles her food and makes no reply
When you say in a loud voice, "I do wish you'd try!"
Who seems not to notice the things that you do,
And forever is losing a stocking or shoe. ...
Who, resisting or not, lets you do as you will,
With bathing and feeding, the long day to fill. ...
Is that what you're thinking? Is that what you see?
Then open your eyes, nurse; you're not looking at me.
I'll tell you who I am as I sit here so still,
As I do at your bidding, as I eat at your will.
I'm a small child of ten ... with a father and mother,
Brothers and sisters, who love one another.
A young girl of sixteen, with wings on her feet,
Dreaming that soon now a lover she'll meet.
A bride soon at twenty—my heart gives a leap,
Remembering the vows that I promised to keep.
At twenty-five now, I have young of my own,
Who need me to guide and a secure happy home.
A woman of thirty, my young now grown fast,
Bound to each other with ties that should last.
At forty, my young sons have grown and are gone,
But my man's beside me to see I don't mourn.
At fifty once more, babies play round my knee,
Again we know children, my loved one and me.
Dark days are upon me, my husband is dead;
I look at the future, I shudder with dread.
For my young are all rearing young of their own,
And I think of the years and the love that I've known.
I'm now an old woman ... and nature is cruel;
'Tis jest to make old age look like a fool.
The body, it crumbles, grace and vigor depart,
There is now a stone where I once had a heart.
But inside this old carcass a young girl still dwells,
And now and again my battered heart swells.
I remember the joys, I remember the pain,
And I'm loving and living life over again.
I think of the years ... all too few, gone too fast,
And accept the stark fact that nothing can last.
So open your eyes, nurses, open and see,
... Not a crabby old woman; look closer ... see ME!

Anonymous. Attributed to an elderly woman who died in a geriatric ward in Scotland. Available at www.carepathways.com.

nurses who hold national certification in the specialty of gerontological nursing. However, some nursing personnel have also demonstrated competencies as a result of on-the-job training. Registered nurses with appropriate knowledge and experience can seek credentialing as a certified gerontological nurse through the American Nurses Credentialing Center. Employment settings for licensed vocational nurses/licensed practical nurses (LVNs/LPNs) have shifted from primarily traditional hospital-bound positions to include a range of community-based, long-term care, and home health care positions. LVN/LPN programs are responding by increasing content and learning experiences to prepare students for this change. Laurie Gunter and Carmen Estes describe gerontological nursing as a health service that incorporates basic nursing methods and specialized knowledge about the aged to establish conditions within the patient and within the environment that (1) increase healthy behaviors in the aged; (2) minimize and compensate for health-related losses and impairments of aging; (3) provide comfort and sustenance through the distressing and debilitating events of aging, including dying and death; and (4) facilitate the diagnosis, care, and treatment of disease in the aged. Dr. Charlotte Eliopolous, a leader in the field, lists the roles of the gerontological nurse as healer, caregiver, educator, advocate, and innovator. Table 11-1 gives examples of the LVN/LPN functions in relation to each of these roles.

AGEISM—MYTHS AND STEREOTYPES

Gerontology is a relatively new science, so we are only beginning to understand aging processes and the lives of older people. In the absence of facts, people rely on "common knowledge" that may or may not be accurate. Many of these "facts" are actually myths that are widely accepted beliefs that have not been proven. Some myths have an element of truth. For example, it is a myth that most old people live in nursing homes. Some old people do live in nursing homes but most do not. When we take a fact about some older people and assume that it applies to all or most older people, we are guilty of stereotyping. When we stereotype, we make assumptions without assessing the individual. Nurses must be knowledgeable about aging and older adults to dispel myths and avoid stereotyping.

Ageism is the systematic stereotyping of and discrimination against people because of their age, most often directed toward older adults. For example, older people may be labeled demented, "set in their ways," asexual, and old-fashioned. Ageism denies the older person's uniqueness. Like other prejudices, ageism influences the behavior of its victims. An older person who believes that retired people are nonproductive may not seek meaningful activity in retirement. Other older adults refuse to conform to this stereotype and seek new interests, activities, or even employment.

MYTHS ABOUT AGING

If myths about aging were true, older people would be unable (or unwilling) to learn, childlike, nonproductive, disengaged, inflexible, and lonely. Even if they were interested in sex, it is assumed that they probably would not be able to perform sexually. Retirement would be a sad state spent in a rocking chair, living in poverty or in a nursing home, and waiting to die. Let's examine these perceptions and see what the facts are.

Some cognitive decline occurs with old age; however, it does not normally impair every day

Table 11-1 The LVN/LPN in Gerontological Nursing Settings

ROLE	LVN/LPN ACTIVITIES
Healer	Consider the individual's physical and psychologic needs. Embrace the philosophy that individuals at every stage of life can have meaning and purpose. Recognize that the physical and emotional environments affect the individual's functioning and well-being. Consider wellness needs even in the frail older person or one with multiple chronic conditions.
Caregiver	Learn about aging and the special needs of older adults. Seek knowledge to provide care based on science rather than tradition. Participate actively in the development of nursing care plans. Because of the amount of time spent with the patient, the LVN/LPN may have information or insights that the RN does not have. Encourage older persons to participate actively in their care and to maintain as much independence as possible.
Educator	Include patient education in care plans. Consider what the older person and/or the significant others want and need to know about health, aging, and management of chronic conditions. Share knowledge about gerontological nursing with colleagues. Explain and demonstrate to assistive personnel appropriate strategies for working with older adults.
Advocate	Participate in organizations that advance causes important to older persons. The National Gerontological Nursing Association welcomes LVN/LPN memberships. Participate in community initiatives that benefit older persons. Speak up for the rights of older adults in your care. Encourage families and other caregivers to hear and consider the patient's wishes.
Innovator	Maintain a questioning attitude. Ask if there is a better way to carry out nursing activities. When you encounter a challenge, engage others in developing novel solutions. Be open to suggestions of others, including patients.

functions. There is some evidence that educational and intellectual experiences actually build *cognitive reserve.* A person who has built a cognitive reserve through the years can continue to function at a higher level despite some decline. Individuals with minimal education and intellectual development will show the effects of decline sooner because they lack cognitive reserve.

Not all cognitive functions decline equally with normal aging. The speed and efficiency of processing and storing information decline. The older person is more readily distracted and less able to focus attention. These changes explain the problem that many healthy older people report with short-term memory. Normal aging does not cause intelligence to plummet. However, there are differences in types of intelligence. Functions related to factual knowledge are retained. On the other hand, the ability to solve complex or novel problems declines.

Dementia is a progressive decline in cognitive function. It is not part of normal aging. Only 5% to 7% of persons older than age 60 have dementia, with the greatest incidence after age 85. Among the many causes of reversible cognitive changes are drug effects, hypoxemia, fluid and electrolyte imbalance, infection, and sensory deficits.

Health Promotion

Encouraging middle-aged and older adults to engage in mentally challenging activities may build cognitive reserve, which provides some protection against future cognitive losses.

Many people, including some older adults, expect sexual interest to fade with age. The idea of older people engaging in sex is a source of endless comedy. That perception may be changing as the baby boomers strive to stay active, view sex as healthy and natural at any age, and seek treatment for sexual dysfunction. In general, older people who have enjoyed sexual activity throughout their lives are likely to retain that interest. Those who were never very interested in sex will probably remain disinterested in later years. Some older people remain interested in sexual activity but either lack a partner or have a partner who is not interested or capable of sexual activity. No doubt, some have been influenced by the stereotype and expect to give up sex in later years.

Older people typically engage in sexual activity less often than younger people. Physical and psychosocial factors may explain this change. The sexual response is slower and less intense in both men and women. Although erectile dysfunction (ED) is not part of normal aging, it is more common in older men. Factors that contribute to ED include diabetes, atherosclerosis, endocrine disorders, and drug therapy. Problems that women often encounter after menopause include vaginal atrophy and dryness, sleep disturbances, and "mood swings." Sexual dysfunction can occur at any age and is usually evidence of some disorder or a result of medication side effects. Baby boomers who grew up with "a pill for every ill" expect medical science to find treatments for everything, including sexual dysfunction.

What really happens when older people retire and no longer have child-rearing roles? First, many people continue to work beyond age 65. In 2012, older persons were heads of 25.1 million households and 81% of those owned their home. More than half of community-dwelling older persons lived with their spouse. More than 8 million older women and 3 million older men lived alone. Institutional settings were home to 1% of persons aged 65 to 74, 3% of persons aged 75 to 84, and 11% of those aged 85 and over. Most older adults have extended family and support networks but still prefer being independent for as long as possible. The majority of older adults are not disabled. Although the percentage was small, 6 million older Americans (14.5%) lived below or near the poverty level in 2012. The highest poverty rates were for Latino and African-American women who lived alone. Many older people are among the wealthiest individuals in the United States. Middle- and upper-income elders have tremendous buying power and disposable income.

The examples cited are only some of the myths that exist about aging and older people. Rather than accepting information as common knowledge, seek the facts from professional sources. Armed with knowledge, you as a nurse can help to dispel many misconceptions.

BIOLOGIC AND PHYSIOLOGIC FACTORS IN AGING

The search for immortality has been a recurrent theme in human history. Medical science has not escaped this quest. Although it has made great strides in conquering many ills, thereby allowing more people live longer, the life span has changed little. Most experts believe that the maximal attainable age is between 115 and 125 years.

How and why do humans age? Why is individual aging so varied? Which of the many theories of aging are valid? Each of these questions represents a fascinating area for scientific exploration. However, despite intense interest in longevity by so many cultures, scientists do not agree on precisely why or how humans age. Knowledge of the underlying mechanisms of aging may enable scientists to slow the aging process. Even if the maximum life span cannot be extended, science may be able to help us remain healthier in the years that we have.

THEORIES OF BIOLOGIC AGING

Numerous theories attempt to explain biologic aging. Most of them can be classified as stochastic or nonstochastic theories. Stochastic theories attribute aging to random events that occur and accumulate over time, resulting in cellular, molecular, and organ malfunction or errors. In contrast, nonstochastic theories assume that aging is the result of a predetermined process governed by some controlling mechanism such as genetic programming, neuroendocrine activity, or immunologic activity. Evolutionary theory approaches aging as a natural selection process.

At this time, no one theory of biologic aging is entirely explanatory or universally accepted. Many experts believe that aging cannot be explained by a single theory but represents multiple processes working simultaneously. Therefore theories about aging continue to evolve in an effort to shed light on this process.

PHYSIOLOGIC CHANGES IN BODY SYSTEMS

Aging occurs slowly and is a complex and dynamic process involving many internal and external influences. It affects every system, organ, and cell in the body to varying degrees. With increasing age, the ability to maintain physiologic functions in the face of challenges is reduced. Common age-related changes are discussed here. However, these changes do not occur at the same rate or to the same extent in all people. For example, wrinkling of the skin is common among older persons but individuals who have had much sun exposure have much more wrinkling. Nurses should consider the implications of common aging changes in planning and providing nursing care.

NERVOUS SYSTEM

Some neurologic changes were discussed earlier in the section titled "Myths about Aging." Brain size is thought to decrease with age due to the loss of neurons (brain cells) that begins in the early 30s. The conduction of impulses slows. This may result in slower responses, problems with short-term memory, and altered learning. Nevertheless, functional ability may not be affected significantly because reserve cells are able to compensate. In the absence of disease, most aged people maintain normal intellectual capability, sound judgment, and creativity.

Atherosclerosis reduces the supply of oxygen to the brain, which may affect the ability to store new information. Short-term memory loss is a frequent complaint of the aged, although long-term memory may remain intact. It may be that old memories are preserved as permanent changes in the structure of the neurons. Consequently, the aged person may experience difficulty remembering planned events for the day but may easily recall childhood experiences. Momentary lapses in memory, such as forgetting a name or misplacing an item, are common examples of normal memory changes.

People who have more persistent memory problems with otherwise normal cognitive function are said to have mild cognitive impairment (MCI). An estimated 40% to 50% of people who develop MCI will develop Alzheimer disease within 3 years; others do not progress to more serious impairment.

Other neurologic functions that are affected by age-related changes include temperature regulation, pain perception, and tactile sensation. The aged individual usually has a low tolerance for extremes in temperature. Changes that may affect maintenance of normal body temperature include deterioration in vascular tone, changes in hypothalamic temperature control, and loss of subcutaneous tissue. Some researchers have found dulling of pain and tactile sensation in older persons but these findings are not consistent. Many diseases and medications can alter sensory perception.

The neurologic changes associated with aging occur gradually; thus the aging person compensates for these changes by using adaptive strategies and modifying behavior. For example, the person may avoid temperature extremes, approach tasks at a slower pace, and attend to one task at a time. Mnemonics and repetition are two strategies that may be used to cope with memory problems. Mnemonics (pronounced *nee-mon-icks*) connects known and unknown information. For example, a person might remember that her grandchildren are named Amy, Brian, and Carl by associating their names with the ABCs. However, stressors such as illness, relocation, or a loss may overwhelm the person's ability to compensate, resulting in a decline in function.

RESPIRATORY SYSTEM

Tests of pulmonary physiology have shown several age-related alterations. Tidal volume is relatively stable with aging; however, residual volume (RV) increases. Forced vital capacity (FVC), forced expiratory capacity in 1 second (FEV_1), forced expiratory volume (FEV), maximal voluntary ventilation (MVV), and vital capacity (VC) are thought to decrease progressively with aging. These alterations are related to atrophy and weakening of the respiratory muscles and changes in the rib cage and spine. Increased curvature of the thoracic spine, called kyphosis, is common. Osteoporosis causes the vertebrae to become more fragile and prone to fracture. The cartilage between the ribs stiffens, which limits chest expansion. Alterations in the lungs include a decreased number of capillaries, thickened capillary walls, and fewer capillaries surrounding the alveoli. The changes in the capillaries affect pulmonary diffusion so that gas exchange is impaired. Pulmonary secretions are handled less effectively. Ciliary action, which normally sweeps secretions from the airway, is less efficient. The cough reflex is frequently less effective because of decreased sensitivity to stimuli and decreased muscle tone. These factors make the older person more susceptible to and less able to recover from respiratory infections. Even though vaccinations and antibiotics are available, influenza and pneumonia are the seventh leading cause of death of Americans ages 65 and older. Chronic pulmonary disease is the third leading cause of death in this age group.

Despite these changes, the healthy older adult usually maintains adequate oxygenation with moderate activity. Problems arise when increased demands are placed on the body, as occurs during periods of extreme exertion or respiratory illness. Exertional dyspnea (shortness of breath with exertion) is a frequent complaint of the older adult. The ability to perform prolonged strenuous work decreases with aging.

Put on Your Thinking Cap!

Considering the many changes in the respiratory system, what nursing care would be especially important when caring for a hospitalized older person?

CARDIOVASCULAR SYSTEM

Resistance to blood flow in many organs increases as people age. In the absence of cardiovascular disease, heart size remains unchanged or decreases slightly. Whitish patches, fibrosis, and sclerosis develop in the endocardium, the inner layer of the heart. The heart becomes increasingly rigid and myocardial contractility is compromised. Coronary blood flow in the aged person may be reduced by as much as 35% because of changes in the vessels. Aortic and pulmonic valves stiffen. If they do not close completely, murmurs result. Aging heart cells have a decreased capacity to use oxygen, which may help to explain the aged person's reduced tolerance for physical work.

The blood vessels of the heart and the systemic circulation, particularly the arteries, undergo age-related changes that may begin as early as the teen years. By age 20, thickening and calcification of the intimal layer of the coronary arteries and aorta are evident. Arteries dilate, lengthen, and become more rigid. The pulse tends to increase in force and the pulse pressure widens. Vascular changes increase the risk for myocardial infarction ("heart attack") and heart failure. In fact, heart disease is the leading cause of death among older adults.

By 70 years of age, the systolic blood pressure commonly increases to approximately 150 mm Hg and the diastolic blood pressure increases to 90 mm Hg for many people. Because of the current guidelines for diagnosis of hypertension, older persons are more likely than younger people to be treated for a blood pressure reading that once was considered normal.

Another cardiovascular change related to aging is a decrease in resting cardiac output, which is the amount of blood pumped by the heart each minute. Between ages 25 and 65, resting cardiac output falls 30% to 40%. This reduced cardiac output reflects a decreased heart rate and a decreased stroke volume. Despite the diminished cardiac output, cerebral blood flow is maintained. However, blood supply to other body systems, notably the liver and kidneys, is diminished. Nevertheless, these organs usually maintain adequate function, partly because of reduced demands.

RENAL SYSTEM

The renal system of healthy older adults functions adequately; however, in the event of injury, disease, or disability, the additional demands may cause the kidneys to fail. By the seventh decade, the number of nephrons in each kidney is reduced by one half to two thirds, with corresponding changes in the glomeruli. The renal filtration rate, plasma flow rate, and tubular reabsorption and secretion all decrease. Blood urea nitrogen tends to increase. The tubules of the aging kidneys are less able to conserve base and eliminate excess hydrogen. Therefore the regulation of acid-base balance is less efficient.

Total body water decreases with age. This is important because it means that the older adult can become dehydrated quickly. The older person's kidneys are less able to compensate for deficient fluid balance by concentrating urine. On the other hand, older persons excrete excess fluid more slowly so they are at risk for overload if given large volumes of fluids quickly.

Additional changes are noted in the ureters, bladder, and urethra as a result of loss of muscle tone. The bladder capacity may be reduced by one half, resulting in frequent trips to the toilet. Furthermore, response to the stretch receptors in the bladder wall that signal the need to void may be delayed until the pressure is high and the bladder is almost full. This condition results in an urgency to urinate, which may be especially problematic for older adults with visual and motor impairment. Urge incontinence, the involuntary passage of urine shortly after the urge to void occurs, is a major health concern for older adults. Poor muscle tone may lead to incomplete emptying of the bladder. The urine that remains after voiding (residual volume) favors bacterial growth, putting the older person at risk for urinary tract infections. Other types of incontinence may appear as a symptom of upper or lower urinary tract dysfunction. For several of these conditions, behavioral treatment may be helpful. Behavioral treatments include scheduled or prompted voiding, environmental adaptation, and pelvic muscle exercises (Kegel exercises). Interventions for incontinence are discussed in Chapter 23.

INTEGUMENTARY SYSTEM

Changes related to aging of the skin include dryness, loss of elasticity, wrinkles, uneven pigmentation and brown spots, roughness, looseness, thinness, and the development of various skin lesions.

One of the first signs of aging is the development of wrinkles. Wrinkles occur when the deep layer of the skin loses moisture and elasticity. Tiny creases and folds are formed. The extent and timing of these wrinkles are determined by genetics and sun exposure. Men and persons in certain ethnic groups that have thicker, oilier skin wrinkle at a slower rate. Skin that is exposed to the sun most often, such as the face, hands, and back of the neck, wrinkles quickly. Older people are encouraged to use sunscreens to prevent excessive dryness and to reduce the risk of skin cancer, which is more common in older persons. The American Academy of Dermatology recommends using a sunscreen with a sun protection factor (SPF) of at least 30.

Pruritus (itching) related to loss of oils in the skin is a common complaint of older persons. Hot baths, harsh soaps, and vigorous scrubbing contribute to dryness. If the patient has generalized itching, inform the registered nurse (RN) or the physician because it may be a symptom of illness such as diabetes, cancer, kidney disease, gallbladder disease, or liver disease.

Most older people can expect some hair loss, hair thinning, and color changes in the hair and nails. Both men and women experience graying and thinning of the hair on the scalp, axilla, and genitalia. Men are more likely to grow bald to varying degrees. Facial and nasal hairs may increase. Gray hair is caused by a slowing of pigment production in the hair follicles. Graying is determined by genetics and tends to be irreversible. Nails tend to become thicker and brittle with longitudinal striations. The most common benign lesions of aging are seborrheic dermatitis, acne, contact dermatitis, drug reactions, pressure ulcers, stasis ulcers, pruritus, herpes zoster, onychomycosis and tinea pedis, and impetigo. Skin cancer is also more common in older people. New lesions or changes in existing lesions should be examined by the physician or nurse practitioner. These conditions are discussed in Chapters 21 and 52.

GASTROINTESTINAL SYSTEM

Changes in gastrointestinal functions occur with normal aging. Changes in the oral cavity include deterioration of the teeth and possibly a decrease in the number or sensitivity of taste buds. The commonly reported dry mouth is probably related to medications, inadequate hydration, and illness states rather than normal aging. Saliva becomes more alkaline and contains less amylase and ptyalin. The muscles associated with chewing weaken, so the patient may avoid foods that require more chewing. These changes may interfere with an older person's ability and desire to eat a nutritious meal.

Muscle contractions of the esophagus weaken, which may explain complaints of reflux symptoms. Gastric emptying of liquids also is slower in older people than in the young. Decreased hydrochloric acid secretion is common in older adults but it is now thought to be caused by *Helicobacter pylori* infection rather than normal aging. With advanced age, calcium and zinc absorption is reduced. This is significant because a calcium deficiency contributes to loss of bone mass. Gallbladder function may decline with aging as well.

Collectively, the changes in the gastrointestinal system caused by aging increase the older person's risk for anorexia, bloating, indigestion, gas, and diarrhea or constipation. Constipation is one of the most frequent gastrointestinal complaints of older adults. Experts tend to agree that constipation is more likely caused by lack of dietary bulk and roughage, disease states, immobility, and drug effects rather than aging changes. Digestive complaints can be signs of more serious disorders. Symptoms that may suggest possible illness are decreased appetite, unexplained weight loss, excessive thirst, blood in the stool, or a change in the usual pattern of bowel movements.

The usual frequency for a bowel movement may range from as many as three movements per day to as few as one bowel movement every 7 days. However, most people have a bowel movement at least every 3 days. The most important factors are the person's usual pattern and whether the stool is passed easily. Constipation may be due to lack of dietary fiber, inactivity, and dehydration rather than normal aging. See Chapter 40 for additional discussion about constipation.

MUSCULOSKELETAL SYSTEM

Of the multiple changes associated with an aging musculoskeletal system, changes affecting mobility are most significant. Age-related changes include decreased muscle strength, endurance, joint range of motion, coordination, bone density, and elasticity and flexibility of connective tissue.

Arthritis is the most prevalent chronic disease in men. However, it is more severe in women and is the leading cause of disability in old age. Osteoarthritis, the most common form of arthritis, is caused by damage to the inside surface of the joint. Age is the primary risk factor for arthritis, with heredity and obesity contributing to its development. The large weight-bearing joints (knees, hips, and spine) are most affected by arthritis. **Kyphosis** is the term applied to the curvature of the thoracic spine and gives rise to the bent-over appearance of some older adults. The loss of bone mass (osteoporosis) increases the risk of fractures, with the most commons sites being the forearm, vertebrae, humerus, pelvis, and hip. Postural instability and low body weight increase the risk of fractures.

Changes in muscle tissue include a gradual decrease in mass accompanied by an even greater decline in strength. The term *sarcopenia* is used to describe the loss of muscle strength. Weight-bearing exercises, particularly resistance strength training, may minimize sarcopenia. Walking, bicycling, and stair climbing also help to maintain bone and muscle mass. Assistive devices such as a walker can help a person to avoid falls if the person is unstable (Fig. 11-1).

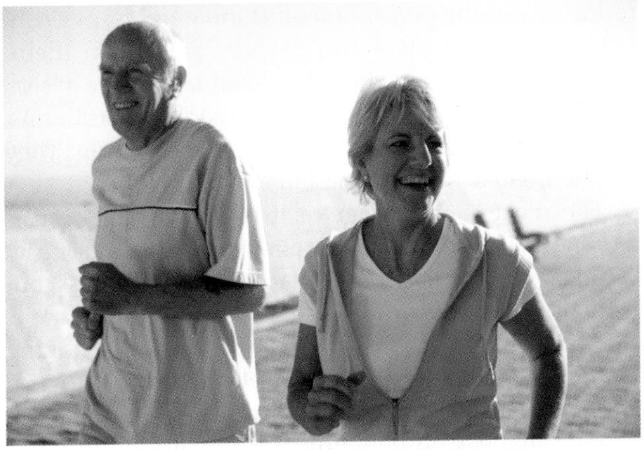

FIGURE 11-1 Regular exercise is an important part of health promotion for the older adult. (Copyright Pixland. All rights reserved.)

SENSORY SYSTEM

Hearing

Because we depend on our five senses for almost everything we do, any loss of sensory ability can greatly affect our quality of life, function, and general well-being. Sensory changes in the older adult also place them at risk for injury and weaken self-confidence.

Presbycusis is the term for hearing loss associated with old age. Age-related causes of presbycusis include atrophic changes in the cochlea, auditory nerve, auditory brainstem pathways, and temporal lobe of the brain.

Basically, two types of hearing loss have been identified. **Conduction deafness** is a blockage of the ear canal caused by impacted cerumen (excessive earwax accumulation), abnormal structures, or infection. This type of loss may be easily treated. The other type of hearing loss is **sensorineural deafness**. It results from damage to nerve tissue as a result of exposure to loud noises, disease, and certain drugs. Hearing aids can often provide significant improvement. Tinnitus, an annoying ringing or buzzing in the ear, is a sensorineural disorder. Some cases of tinnitus can be caused by the use of aspirin or certain antibiotics or diuretics, or by tumors.

Twenty-five percent of adults over age 69 and as many as one half of adults over age 85 are hard of hearing. Older men tend to experience greater hearing loss than women. Many older adults are less able than younger people to hear high-pitched sounds and consonants, particularly *ch, f, g, s, sh, t, th,* and *z.* They can generally hear a lower voice tone better than a high-pitched voice. Not all older adults experience this type of loss and causes other than old age may be involved (e.g., noise exposure, ototoxic drugs). Regardless of the cause, hearing impairment creates a barrier to communication and often is associated with depression and isolation.

Vision

Common vision complaints reported by older persons include floaters, flashers, and dry eyes. Floaters are bits of debris floating in the vitreous that appear as spots moving in the field of vision. Traction on the retina causes the perception of flashing lights, or flashers. Although floaters and flashers are not in themselves harmful, they should be evaluated by a vision specialist as they may be related to serious conditions. Dry eyes occur due to decreased tear production. They can be treated with topical moisturizers.

The most common age-related change in vision is a condition called **presbyopia**, which results from changes in the lens. The shape of the lens is controlled by muscles in the eye. By changing its shape, the lens allows us to change focus when looking from objects that are near to objects that are far. With age, the lens becomes more rigid and less able to change shape. Consequently, reading and other types of close work become difficult. Presbyopia is easily corrected by reading glasses or multifocal lenses. Furthermore, adapting to changes in lighting is also a function of the lenses. Maintaining good lighting in the home, particularly in hallways and around walkways, can help to prevent falls and other accidents. Whether the older person is a candidate for vision-correcting surgeries such as Lasik must be assessed individually.

Whereas presbyopia is considered a normal change, there are pathologic eye conditions that are common in older persons. The leading cause of new cases of blindness in older people is age-related macular degeneration. This condition affects the macula, the part of the eye that is responsible for sharp central vision. The two types are atropic ("dry") and exudative ("wet") macular degeneration. There is no known treatment for the atrophic form. For the exudative form, repeated injections of a monoclonal antibody into the vitreous compartment of the eye are often effective in slowing the progression of macular degeneration. In some cases, a significant improvement in visual acuity has been achieved. Laser surgery offers some benefits but is not the first-line treatment.

Another serious eye disorder that occurs with aging is cataract. **Cataract** is clouding or opacity of the normally transparent lens within the eye. Cataracts are caused by changes in structural lens proteins, by damage to the lens as a result of high levels of blood glucose in people with diabetes, or by other factors. Cataract is treated by surgical removal of the clouded lens. Some type of lens replacements is required. Surgery is highly successful and vision is usually restored in 90% to 95% of cases.

The leading cause of blindness in the United States is glaucoma. **Glaucoma** is characterized by atrophy of the optic nerve, usually associated with elevated pressure of the fluid in the eye. The optic nerve carries visual impulses from the eye to the brain. Therefore damage to the nerve can result in progressive vision loss, described as "tunnel vision."

At present, glaucoma is not curable but is treatable with drugs or surgery. Early detection and effective treatment can slow or halt the disease process and save remaining eyesight. Older adults should receive annual eye examinations and a test for glaucoma.

Taste and Smell

Disorders of the senses involving taste and smell are called *chemosensory disorders*. More than 10 million Americans are affected by these types of disorders. Most of these disorders occur after age 60 and involve the ability to detect and differentiate scents. Men tend to be more affected than women and many causes exist, including nasal obstruction, allergies, and the use of certain drugs. The decline in the sense of smell may be caused by a decrease in olfactory nerve fibers.

Taste perception declines with age, possibly because of changes in the number or sensitivity of taste buds. The ability to detect sweet seems to remain intact while the ability to detect salty and bitter tastes declines. Major changes in the ability to taste are usually caused by diseases or are the side effects of certain drugs. Dentures, decreased saliva, hormonal changes, medications, and changes in chemicals needed to transmit taste are all potential causes of the older person's diminished sense of taste. This loss can affect changes in appetite.

Sensory losses are more than a minor nuisance for older adults. Poor vision and hearing increase a person's risk for falls and other accidents, which are leading causes of accidental death and disability in people over the age of 65. Furthermore, the inability to smell smoke, poisons, or other noxious odors endangers the lives of many older people. Decreased ability to taste food puts the older person at risk for malnutrition. Sensory changes greatly reduce the quality of life. To summarize, many of the physiologic changes associated with aging may reflect the presence of age-related diseases more than aging itself. Research is rapidly expanding and changing our knowledge of aging. Conditions once thought to represent normal aging are now known to be the product of disease. Many of the conditions can be prevented or controlled by good health practices and competent nursing care.

PSYCHOSOCIAL THEORIES OF AGING

Just as biologic changes occur with aging, so do psychosocial changes. Older adults are the products of decades of living that produce unique personalities, coping mechanisms, challenges, and growth. The social network is influential in the aging process and can support the individual in adapting to age-related changes (Fig. 11-2).

The fact that a person has survived to old age is one marker of successful adaptation. The survival of large numbers of relatively healthy older people is a new experience for humankind. The vast majority of older people have adapted adequately. These individuals are able to function independently and maintain a sense of well-being.

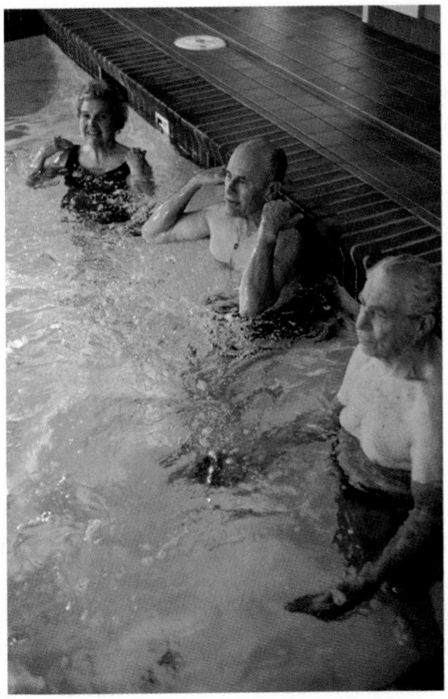

FIGURE 11-2 Most older adults are active and independent. (Photographer: Keith Brofsky. Copyright Getty Images. All rights reserved.)

Maturity is defined as an optimal psychologic, social, and biologic adaptation achieved at some point during the midlife years, arbitrarily set between 45 and 65 years of age. Current thinking asserts that midlife crisis occurs, in part, when the individual in midlife becomes fully aware of his or her mortality.

ERIKSON'S DEVELOPMENTAL TASKS

As explained in Chapter 10, Erik Erikson developed one of the first developmental theories in the area of aging. Erikson identified the developmental task of old age as ego-integrity versus despair. Ego integrity is attained when individuals review their lives and gain a feeling of accomplishment and fulfillment. They remain concerned with life in the face of death and begin to experience the wisdom that they have gained. The opposite of ego-integrity is feelings of despair, in which people feel bitter about their lack of accomplishments in life and tend to regret life as they have lived it. Many people say that they have more regrets about the things they have not done or the risks they have not taken than the mistakes they have made.

Old age involves much more than a psychologic waiting station before death. It represents an important stage of development and coping that occurs between the high points and accomplishments of the middle years and the concerns that are involved as the end of life approaches. Movement toward ego integrity is facilitated when the older person:

- Recognizes and accepts changes in physical and mental capabilities
- Gives up some roles and develops new ones
- Develops new activities that can be carried out successfully with aging
- Develops a different self-concept
- Revises life goals
- Adapts to new lifestyles

In the final stage of development, older persons are faced with a variety of internal and external losses that require coping and adaptation using diminished biologic, psychologic, and social resources. The challenge is to maintain performance in the face of adverse circumstances. A complete discussion of adult developmental tasks is found in Chapter 10.

DISENGAGEMENT, ACTIVITY, AND CONTINUITY THEORIES

Various scientists have studied the way in which social life changes in later years. Disengagement theory predicts the gradual withdrawal of society and older people from each other. The process is described as mutually beneficial, relieving the older person of social responsibilities and making way for younger people to fill the gap. Disengagement theory has lost favor because it has failed to demonstrate mutual appeal and is viewed as disenfranchising older people who still have much to give. Activity theory describes successful aging as remaining mentally and physically active. It assumes that activity is better than inactivity, that happiness is better than unhappiness, and that the older person must decide how successful his or her aging is. In a sense, it actually encourages people to continue their middle-age lifestyle for as long as possible. Continuity theory provided an alternative to disengagement and activity theories. It asserts that old age is part of the life cycle and that old people behave in later years much as they did throughout life. A person who has always been sociable is likely to remain sociable in later years. The individual who preferred a more solitary lifestyle would continue to prefer that lifestyle when older. Other theories that attempt to explain aging from a social perspective include subculture theory, age stratification theory, and person-environment fit theory.

COPING AND ADAPTATION

Old age has been described as the season of losses, including loss of roles, status, and physical abilities, and deep personal losses through the deaths of friends and the disruption of family networks. Loss, whether real, threatened, or imaginary, is a stressor that requires adaptation, flexibility, and resiliency if a person is to cope successfully.

In most respects, older people cope in much the same way as younger people. Differences are largely the result of the different types of stressors experienced. Older people tend to experience more negative and irreversible types of stressors. Given the many losses associated with old age as potential stressors, the older person may cope with these losses in a positive or negative manner. Positive adaptation might include rational action, perseverance, positive thinking (e.g., the lost loved one is now out of pain), intellectual denial (e.g., "I don't want to think about it now"), restraint, drawing strength from adversity, and humor.

Unfortunately, some older individuals are unable to cope effectively with their losses. They lose their sense of personal identity and fulfillment and suffer from deterioration in self-esteem, an altered self-concept, and a loss of meaningfulness in life. A small percentage of older people become seriously depressed. They may lose motivation for working, playing, and living. Depression resulting from loss is a factor in approximately two thirds of the suicides among older people. Suicide is most common among white men ages 85 and older.

FAMILY

With an aging population that needs support and assistance, kinship networks take on added importance. Most of the older persons in the United States occupy a variety of family roles and come from multigenerational units. It is common for a person at age 65 to be married, have at least one living adult child, have at least one living sibling, be a grandparent, and be a great-grandparent. The person over age 65 may also be a child of a much older parent. The kinship network may also include cousins, nieces, and nephews. Of all these roles and relationships, marital relationships and the relationships between parent and child seem to be most important.

In an era when the aged are sometimes labeled as burdens, an important point to recognize is that more financial support flows from the old to the young in the family than in the reverse direction. Although family responsibility is respected by most people, laws exist in many states that can require children to provide financial support for needy parents. However, what is most needed and most often given is emotional support and help in times of illness and disability. Home care for the frail older adult is most often given by a spouse or a child. Typically the caregiver is a daughter, and almost half of these women are also rearing children.

Informal caregivers experience enormous stress and encounter various levels of emotional, physical, financial, and family strain. Caregivers frequently report symptoms of depression, anxiety, helplessness, low morale, and emotional exhaustion. In part because of caregiver stress, more than 1 million older persons are thought to be abused physically and psychologically or are neglected each year by their caregivers. When working with these families, health care providers should acknowledge the stressful impact of caregiving and work with them to identify ways to minimize the burdens on the individuals and the family.

You are in an excellent position to recognize stress, depression, and abuse among caregivers and care recipients. Nurses are obligated to report suspected abuse. The LVN/LPN should work with the RN or other supervisor to handle reporting and interventions in abuse situations. Education for learning positive adaptive behaviors can assist both caregivers and care recipients. Caregivers who feel knowledgeable, useful, productive, and appreciated are usually happier, less stressed, and less prone to be abusive. Nursing care should treat the patient and family as a unit and seek to determine the needs and resources of all members.

FUNCTIONAL ASSESSMENT

Ongoing functional assessments are essential as the needs of the older patient evolve. Although a diagnosis may give you a general idea about a patient's abilities, it does not tell you how well the patient is functioning with that diagnosis. For example, one patient with a medical diagnosis of coronary artery disease might be independent and active whereas another patient might be homebound and on oxygen. The functional assessment should describe both basic and instrumental activities of daily living, noting the amount of assistance, if any, needed to carry out each activity. Activities of daily living include grooming, bathing, dressing, eating, elimination, and mobility. Instrumental activities of daily living (IADL) include the ability to prepare a meal, shop for groceries, use the telephone, negotiate transportation, take medications, and maintain housekeeping and laundry tasks. IADL are less important in institutional settings but are essential for a person to continue or return to independent living.

The LVN/LPN contributes to the functional assessment by collecting data about activities of daily living as well as environmental, financial, family, economic, and community resources.

A variety of tools are available for comprehensive assessments. The Duke Older Americans Resources and Services (OARS) Multidimensional Functional Assessment Questionnaire (MFAQ) is a widely used comprehensive guide for assessing the overall personal functional status and the need for services. A content summary is provided in Box 11-2. In most instances, the nursing home Minimum Data Set incorporates all components of a quality functional assessment. SPICES is a convenient tool that includes six key assessment areas for the older adult patient and can be used for routine focused assessments (Box 11-3).

Put on Your Thinking Cap!

Discuss the importance of functional assessments of older adults who receive home health care. What functions would an older adult need to manage self-care in the home?

Box 11-2 Content Areas of the OARS Multidimensional Functional Assessment Questionnaire

PART A: FUNCTIONAL ASSESSMENT

Social
Living arrangements
Contact with others
Social help from family and kin

Economic
Employment status
Income source, amount, adequacy
Home ownership

Mental
Cognitive and psychiatric status
Mental well-being

Physical
Prescribed medications used
Physical conditions with impairment levels

Activities of Daily Living
Physical and instrumental activities of daily living

Demographics and Administrative
Age, gender, race, education
Location, length of interview
Information source

PART B: SERVICES
Transportation
Social/recreational
Employment
Sheltered employment
Educational, employment related
Remedial training
Mental health
Psychotropic drugs
Personal care
Nursing care
Medical services
Supportive devices/prostheses
Physical therapy
Continuous supervision
Checking
Relocation and placement
Homemaker-household
Meal preparation
Administrative legal and protective
Systematic multidimensional evaluation
Financial assistance
Food, groceries
Housing
Coordination, information, referral

Adapted from Fillenbaum, G.G. *Multidimensional functional assessment of older adults: The Duke Older Americans Resources and Services Procedures.* Erlbaum, Hillsdale, N.J., 1988; updated 1996 (available only from Center for the Study of Aging and Human Development, Duke University Medical Center, Durham, N.C.).

DRUG THERAPY AND OLDER ADULTS

ABSORPTION, DISTRIBUTION, METABOLISM, AND EXCRETION

Medication use by older adults in the U.S. is extremely common. Some sources estimate that 44% of men and 57% of women ages 65 and over take five or more prescription and/or over-the-counter (OTC) medications each week. Twelve percent of both genders take 10 or more medications each week. Imagine the potential for errors and drug interactions with so many medications! Age-related changes affect patterns of drug use and drug effects (Table 11-2). The most important changes involve body composition, the cardiovascular and nervous systems, renal function, tissue sensitivity to drugs, and blood pressure reflex sensitivity.

With aging comes a reduction in body size, with a decrease in lean body mass and body water content and an increase in fat. The serum albumin concentration is reduced, which tends to make additional free drug available to tissues or to permit increasingly rapid elimination of the drug. A gradual decrease in blood flow to the liver and kidneys reduces drug clearance. Drug characteristics also affect distribution of drug molecules in the tissues. For example, a water-soluble drug may result in increased blood concentrations of that drug. However, a highly fat-soluble drug might bind to the increased fat in the aged body and may be stored longer before excretion.

The liver prepares drugs for elimination in the urine or in feces. Age-related changes in the liver, which include decreased size, reduced blood flow, and reduced enzyme activity, affect the metabolism (inactivation) of drugs. When drug metabolism is impaired, drug concentrations in the blood increase and elimination of the drug may be delayed. Because of changes in the kidneys, drugs that are eliminated primarily in

Box 11-3 SPICES Assessment Tool

SPICES
Sleep disorders
Problems with eating or drinking
Incontinence
Confusion
Evidence of falls
Skin breakdown

Table 11-2 Association between Age-Related Physiologic Changes and Drug Effects

AGE-RELATED CHANGES	DRUG EFFECTS
Increased body fat	Increased storage of fat-soluble drugs
Decreased body water	Increased drug/active concentration
Decreased hepatic blood flow	Decreased drug metabolism
Decreased lean muscle mass	Increased drug tissue concentration
Decreased renal function	Decreased drug elimination
Decreased serum albumin	Increased concentration of free drug molecules that bind to protein

the urine may accumulate and have adverse effects. Therefore lower dosages or longer intervals between doses are often indicated to avoid harm.

Put on Your Thinking Cap!

A 75-year-old woman was diagnosed as having a progressive brain disease after she developed urinary incontinence, general mental deterioration, and an inability to walk. She had been taking the fat-soluble drug diazepam (Valium) daily for at least 1 year to treat anxiety. After the drug was discontinued, the patient recovered completely. What might explain this sequence of events?

ADVERSE DRUG REACTIONS

Adverse drug reactions are more common in older people partly because they use more drugs. The risk of adverse drug reactions increases with the number of drugs consumed, dose level, duration of treatment, and severity of illness. Adverse effects may also result when the patient does not take drugs as prescribed.

Some of the common signs and symptoms of adverse drug reactions in the older person are restlessness, falls, depression, confusion, loss of memory, constipation, and urinary incontinence. Older persons tend to be more sensitive than the young to drugs that act on the central nervous system. Therefore drugs for anxiety, pain, or sleep may produce excessive drowsiness and respiratory depression. When patients experience unpleasant side effects, they may not follow the prescribed regimen. Starting new drugs at low doses usually reduces side effects and increases patient cooperation. Some drugs commonly associated with adverse drug reactions in older adults are listed in Table 11-3.

Nurses who work with older adults should be familiar with the Beers Criteria for Potentially Inappropriate Medication Use in Older Adults. This source identifies drugs that are generally problematic in older persons and has a second listing of drugs that are problematic in the presence of specific conditions. Inclusion of a drug in the Beers Criteria does not mean that the drug is absolutely contraindicated but the prescriber should be aware that the drug poses specific risks for the older patient. While the LVN/LPN does not select drugs, he or she should question any drug order that might be harmful and share resources such as the Beers Criteria with other professionals.

Pharmacology Capsule

Copies of the Beers Criteria tables can be obtained at www.americangeriatrics.org/files/documents/beers/2012BeersCriteria_JAGS.pdf.

Because older adults experience a greater number of drug reactions and interactions than younger people and are believed to be more sensitive to some medications, their drug regimens should be monitored carefully. Home care patients should maintain records of data relevant to their medications (e.g., blood pressure, pulse, respiration, drug effect, state of alertness). Such a record could be helpful in making necessary changes. Changing a drug, reducing the dose level, or lengthening the intervals between doses may be necessary to minimize the risk of adverse drug reactions. The nurse is very often in the best position to minimize adverse effects by careful monitoring and notifying the prescriber of concerns. Baseline and continual assessments should include the following:

- The amount, frequency, and purpose of all medications taken
- The older person's ability and willingness to take recommended medications
- The potential for drug interactions and adverse drug reactions

Table 11-3 Drugs Commonly Associated with Adverse Drug Reactions in Older Persons

DRUG CLASS	EXAMPLE	PROBLEM
Analgesics	meperidine	Confusion
Antibiotics	streptomycin	Nephrotoxicity
Anticoagulants	warfarin	Hemorrhage
Antidepressants	amitriptyline	Sedation
Antihypertensives	verapamil	Hypotension
Antiparkinsonians	benztropine	Confusion, psychotic-like symptoms
Antipsychotics	haloperidol	Orthostatic hypotension, sedation, extrapyramidal effects
Diuretics	spironolactone	Hyperkalemia
Nonsteroidal antiinflammatory drugs (NSAIDs)	aspirin, ibuprofen	Bleeding, peptic ulcers
Sedatives/hypnotics	flurazepam	Ataxia, excessive sedation

- The effectiveness of the medication over time
- Whether any of the drugs taken can be discontinued or decreased in dose

Assessment of drug effects and adverse reactions must be documented.

A problem that is sometimes overlooked is the potential for drug interactions between OTC medications and prescription medications taken by older adults. Examples include the use of aspirin, which enhances the effect of anticoagulants, or the use of large amounts of sodium bicarbonate, which counteracts diuretic actions. Botanicals can also interact with prescription and OTC drugs. A second problem is that the older adult may mix older prescription medications with newer ones and fail to discontinue and discard older drugs. Hoarding of medications may be viewed as future savings by an older adult. Having the patient bring all medications to office visits provides an opportunity to review the drugs and identify problems, duplications, or misunderstandings.

THE NURSE AND THE OLDER PATIENT

Nurses who work with older adults have the opportunity to maintain or improve quality of life by providing holistic care that addresses their physiologic and psychosocial needs. The challenges are sometimes daunting but the rewards are huge. This chapter has provided an overview of the aging process and the health care implications of the many changes that occur. Throughout this book, the special needs of older persons will be reinforced. Specific interventions for various health deviations will be addressed in appropriate chapters that cover disease processes in each body system.

Put on Your Thinking Cap!

Recall an older adult who has been discharged from the hospital with some physical or cognitive impairments. What instrumental activities of daily living are likely to be affected in this person?

Get Ready for the NCLEX® Examination!

Key Points

- Aging is an ongoing developmental process that begins at conception and ends at death.
- Gerontology is the study of aging.
- Geriatrics is the biomedical science of old age and the application of knowledge of aging to the prevention, diagnosis, treatment, and care of older persons.
- The roles of the gerontological nurse include healer, caregiver, educator, advocate, and innovator.
- Gerontological nursing aims to increase healthy behaviors in the aged; minimize and compensate for health-related losses and impairments of aging; provide comfort and sustenance through the events of aging; and facilitate the diagnosis, care, and treatment of disease in the aged.
- Health care providers can dispel myths about the older adult and aging that result in stereotyping of and discrimination against older people.
- Aging occurs slowly and is a complex and dynamic process involving many internal and external influences.
- Physiologic changes that are common with aging may reflect the presence of age-related diseases and lifestyle more than the process of aging itself.
- The older adult shows cumulative developmental effects that produce unique personality styles, coping mechanisms, challenges, and growth, all of which occur in a societal context.
- Age-related changes that increase the risk of adverse drug effects include a decreased ability to metabolize and eliminate drugs through the liver and renal system, increased sensitivity to some drugs, and altered body composition.

Additional Learning Resources

SG Go to your Study Guide for additional learning activities to help you master this chapter content.

evolve Go to your Evolve website (http://evolve.elsevier.com/Linton/medsurg) for the following learning resources and much more:

- Interactive Prioritization Exercises
- Fluid & Electrolyte Tutorial
- Pharmacology Tutorial
- Review Questions for the NCLEX® Examination

Review Questions for the NCLEX® Examination

1. The nurse educator in a retirement community is preparing an orientation for new staff about working with older adults. Which statement should be included in the lesson plan?
   1. Many older people continue to enjoy sexual activity.
   2. Older people generally lack family and other support networks.
   3. Almost 50% of people over age 65 have dementia.
   4. Twenty-five percent of the older population resides in nursing homes.

   NCLEX Client Need: Psychosocial Integrity
2. Neurologic changes commonly found in the healthy older adult include: (Select all that apply.)
   1. Impaired short-term memory
   2. Inability to learn new material
   3. Decline in intellectual function
   4. Easy distraction from tasks
   5. Loss of creative abilities

   NCLEX Client Need: Health Promotion and Maintenance and Physiological Integrity: Physiological Adaptation

3. Mr. J. had been a healthy 90-year-old man until he developed pneumonia. While acutely ill with pneumonia, he showed signs of early heart and renal failure. He became weak and his tolerance for physical activity declined. Even though the pneumonia resolved, several months passed before he returned to his previous level of functioning. How would you explain this delay?
   1. At age 90, immune function is severely impaired.
   2. He probably did not seek treatment for his pneumonia soon enough.
   3. Acute illness overwhelmed his already limited cardiac and renal function.
   4. He wanted to continue getting the attention he received when he was acutely ill.

   NCLEX Client Need: Health Promotion and Maintenance
4. Which of the following statements should be included when teaching a group of active older people about skin care? (Select all that apply.)
   1. Sunscreens are recommended to reduce the risk of skin cancer.
   2. Changes in existing skin lesions should be reported to the nurse or physician.
   3. To remove dead skin, take hot baths followed by vigorous towel drying.
   4. Generous use of moisturizers and minimal use of soap prevent skin drying.
   5. Generalized itching may be a symptom of a serious illness.

   NCLEX Client Need: Health Promotion and Maintenance
5. You observe that an older patient's thoracic spine is curved, causing her to bend forward. The term used to describe this condition is ____________________.

   NCLEX Client Need: Physiological Integrity: Physiological Adaptation
6. When a patient has presbycusis, which of the following nursing interventions is most important?
   1. Ensure that room lighting is adequate
   2. Lower the pitch of your voice
   3. Monitor the patient's blood pressure
   4. Implement body fluid precautions

   NCLEX Client Need: Physiological Integrity: Physiological Adaptation
7. Which of these statements by older adults reflects movement toward ego integrity?
   1. "Since I cannot drive now, I rarely get out or see other people."
   2. "After my children grew up and my husband died, I just wasn't needed anymore."
   3. "In my day, when you got married, you stayed married, no matter how bad it was."
   4. "I can't run marathons anymore but I still enjoy a brisk walk around the neighborhood."

   NCLEX Client Need: Psychosocial Integrity
8. Instrumental activities of daily living include which of the following? (Select all that apply.)
   1. Bathing
   2. Cooking
   3. Shopping
   4. Eating
   5. Elimination

   NCLEX Client Need: Physiological Integrity: Basic Care and Comfort
9. An older postoperative patient is receiving pain medications that depress the central nervous system. Based on your knowledge of drug therapy and aging, what adverse effect is most likely?
   1. Respiratory depression
   2. Difficulty sleeping
   3. Vomiting and diarrhea
   4. Agitation

   NCLEX Client Need: Physiological Integrity: Pharmacological Therapies
10. A clinic patient reports that she bruises very easily. She cut herself this morning and the wound continues to ooze blood. An assessment of her medication history reveals that she takes the diuretic spironolactone, verapamil for hypertension, Maalox for heartburn, and aspirin for arthritis pain. Which drug would you suspect is related to her bleeding?
    1. Spironolactone
    2. Verapamil
    3. Maalox
    4. Aspirin

    NCLEX Client Need: Physiological Integrity: Pharmacological Therapies

chapter 12

The Nursing Process and Critical Thinking

http://evolve.elsevier.com/Linton/medsurg

Objectives

1. Describe the components of the nursing process.
2. Explain the role of the licensed vocational nurse/licensed practical nurse (LVN/LPN) in the nursing process.
3. Explain the importance of documentation of the nursing process.
4. Explain the relationship between the nursing process and critical thinking.
5. Describe the characteristics of a critical thinker.
6. Describe how critical thinking skills are used in clinical practice.
7. Describe principles of setting priorities for nursing care.

Key Terms

Assessment
Auscultation (ăw-skŭl-TĀ-shŭn)
Critical thinking
Evaluation
Evidence-based practice
Focused nursing assessment
Implementation
Inspection
Nursing diagnosis
Nursing process
Objective data
Palpation (păl-PĀ-shŭn)
Percussion
Planning
Problem-oriented medical record
Standard of care
Subjective data

The **nursing process** is a systematic method of providing care to patients. It is a problem-solving approach that enables the nurse to provide care in an organized, scientific manner. Specifically, the nurse uses the process to explore the patient's health status, identify actual or potential health care problems, determine the desired outcomes, deliver nursing care, and evaluate the care given. The goal of the nursing process is to prevent, alleviate, or minimize health problems. It enables the nurse to provide care along the entire health-illness continuum.

The nursing process can be applied in any interaction that involves a nurse and a patient or client. (As noted earlier, the terms *patient* and *client* are used interchangeably in this text.) The patient or client can be defined as an individual, a family, a group, a community, or a society. The process can take place in any setting, including a hospital, community setting, private home, or long-term care facility. The nursing process steps and format presented here are more detailed than care plans in health care facilities. However, the process is a tool to demonstrate how the components are related. If you are required to construct original nursing process papers, they will allow your instructor to see how you planned, implemented, and evaluated your nursing care. It also shows the rationale for your decisions.

COMPONENTS OF THE NURSING PROCESS

The five components or steps in the nursing process are (1) **assessment** (the systematic collection of data relating to patients and their problems), (2) **nursing diagnosis** (interpretation of the data for problem identification), (3) **planning** (goals and selected interventions), (4) **implementation** (putting the plan into action), and (5) **evaluation** (assessing the achievement of goals and changing the plan as indicated by current needs). Initially, the steps are followed in sequence. However, after the process has begun, it becomes continuous or cyclic. Each phase of the nursing process is dependent on the others and the interaction among the stages is continuous as the status of the patient changes. The plan must be continually evaluated and revised. As problems are alleviated, new problems may arise, requiring new plans and actions. Licensed vocational nurses/licensed practical nurses (LVNs/LPNs) commonly work in settings in which the nursing process is used. **Standards of care** for registered nurses (RNs) and LVNs/LPNs define the responsibilities of each in relation to the nursing process (see Chapter 3).

The Coordinated Care box describes the LVN/LPN's role in relation to the nursing process.

Coordinated Care

LVNs/LPNs and the Nursing Process

Although the RN has responsibility for developing the nursing process, the LVN/LPN makes important contributions, including:

1. Contributes to an assessment database by collecting patient data using a standardized form, performing basic psychosocial assessment, and taking objective measurements of body functions
2. Assists with the development of nursing care plans and the implementation of the established plan of care
3. Performs basic therapeutic and preventive nursing measures
4. Participates in the evaluation of the care given by reporting observed outcomes and making necessary changes according to the results of the evaluation

ASSESSMENT

The assessment phase of the nursing process involves collecting data about the health status of the patient. An RN must perform the initial admission assessment for each patient; the LVN/LPN collects data through surveillance and monitoring to contribute to the comprehensive assessment and performs focused nursing assessments. A **focused nursing assessment** is defined as "an appraisal of an individual's status and situation at hand, contributing to comprehensive assessment by the RN, supporting ongoing data collection, and deciding who needs to be informed of the information and when to inform" (National Council of State Boards of Nursing, 2006, p. 8).

The word *data* is the plural of *datum* and means information, especially information organized for analysis or decision making. The two types of data are subjective and objective. **Subjective data** consist of information that is reported by the patient and family members in response to direct questioning or in spontaneous statements. Subjective data are usually documented in the patient's own words and include information such as previous experiences and sensations or emotions that only the patient can describe. **Objective data** are items obtained through observation, physical examination, or diagnostic testing. Objective data can be seen or measured (e.g., heart rate, wound condition, laboratory values). Sources of subjective and objective data are the patient, the family and significant others, medical records, and other health care team members.

Subjective Data: Health History Interview

The health history is obtained to collect subjective data by interviewing the patient or significant others, or both. Because of the confidential nature of the content, try to arrange for a quiet, private area. This can be a challenge in a busy nursing unit. Explain the purpose of the interview to the patient and ask whether he or she wishes to have anyone else present. Assure the patient and others included that they can refuse to answer any questions and can add any other information that might be helpful. For information to be accurate and complete, the interview should be purposeful and systematic. The therapeutic communication techniques summarized in Chapter 5, Table 5-2 will facilitate the interview process.

Older patients require special consideration. Never assume that older adults cannot speak for themselves. Even if they request a family member to assist with the interview, be sure to address your questions to the patient. If the patient uses glasses or a hearing aid, ensure that those are in place. Minimize distractions as much as possible. The long-term care patient often has a complex health history and may tire with a lengthy assessment. Several shorter interviews may be more productive.

Various approaches to data collection may be used to ensure that the nursing database is as complete as possible. The traditional nursing health history format includes the following data:

1. Biographic data
2. Source of history and reliability of informant
3. Reason for seeking health care, commonly called the *chief complaint or concern*
4. Present illness or health concerns
5. Past (medical) health history
6. Family history
7. Review of systems
8. Functional assessment of activities of daily living

As you can see, a complete assessment is quite lengthy. Depending on the circumstances and type of service (e.g., urgent care clinic, women's health clinic, hospital emergency department, long-term care facility), not all areas are routinely assessed. Most health care agencies have standardized forms that are used to document essential information in that setting. The health care provider then collects additional specific data as needed. Box 12-1 briefly describes each of these components. Maslow's hierarchy of needs (see Chapter 8, Fig. 8-2) can be used to assess and prioritize needs. The focused assessment is concerned with one very specific problem area, such as pain.

When the interview is complete, review the data with the patient or family members to ensure that the information gathered is correct. Summarizing the data demonstrates interest in the patient and the patient's needs and strengthens the nurse-patient relationship. As the level of trust increases, the patient may add

Box 12-1 Health History

BIOGRAPHIC DATA

Name, address, telephone number, age, birth date, birthplace, sex, marital status, race, ethnic origin, occupation, educational level

SOURCE OF HISTORY

The person or persons who furnish information (patient, family); estimate of reliability of information; special circumstances (e.g., interpreter)

REASON FOR SEEKING CARE

Chief complaint ("What prompted you to seek help now?"); in the patient's own words

- Symptoms—sensations experienced by the individual
- Signs—observable or measureable abnormalities

HISTORY OF PRESENT ILLNESS

Events leading up to the chief complaint or reason for seeking care:

- Location of symptoms (e.g., pain in the chest radiating to the left arm)
- Character or quality (e.g., burning, sharp, or dull pain; sticky, dark- or coffee grounds–colored emesis)
- Quantity or severity (severity of pain interrupts normal daily activities)
- Timing (onset, duration, frequency); when symptoms appeared; how long they lasted; how often they occurred
- Setting (what was happening when symptoms occurred; what brought it on)
- Aggravating or relieving factors (what makes symptoms worse; what makes them better)
- Associated factors (what other symptoms are related, e.g., urinary frequency and burning associated with fever or chills)
- Patient's perception (meaning of symptoms to patient; how they affect daily activities)

PAST HEALTH

Childhood illnesses
Accidents or injuries
Serious or chronic illnesses
Hospitalizations
Operations
Obstetric history
Immunizations
Last examination date
Allergies
Current prescription and over-the-counter medications, herbal products, vitamins

FAMILY HISTORY

Age, health, and cause of death of blood relatives
Family history of heart disease, high blood pressure, stroke, diabetes, blood disorders, cancer, sickle cell anemia, arthritis, allergies, obesity, alcoholism, mental illness, seizure disorders, kidney disease, and tuberculosis
Family tree or genogram to depict members and data under family history

REVIEW OF SYSTEMS

Past and present health state of each body system:

- General overall health state (present weight, weight gain or loss, fatigue, weakness, fever, chills, night sweats)
- Skin (history of skin disease; change in color, pigment, or mole; excessive dryness or moisture; itching; excessive bruising; rash or lesion)
- Hair (recent loss, change in texture; change in shape, color, or brittleness of nails)
- Head (history of head injury, headache, dizziness, or vertigo)
- Eyes (difficulty with vision, including decreased acuity, blurring, blind spots; eye pain; double vision; redness or swelling; watering or discharge; glaucoma or cataracts)
- Ears (earaches, infections, discharge, tinnitus or ringing in the ears)
- Nose and sinuses (discharge, frequent or severe colds, sinus pain, nasal obstruction, nosebleeds, allergies or hay fever, change in sense of smell)
- Mouth and throat (mouth pain, frequent sore throat, bleeding gums, toothache, difficulty swallowing, hoarseness, altered taste)
- Neck (pain, limitation of movement, lumps or swelling, enlarged or tender nodes, goiter)
- Gastrointestinal (history of abdominal diseases [e.g., ulcer, liver or gallbladder, jaundice, appendicitis, colitis], appetite, food intolerance, difficulty swallowing, heartburn, indigestion, abdominal pain, nausea and vomiting, vomiting blood, flatulence, type and frequency of bowel movement, rectal conditions [e.g., hemorrhoids, fistula])
- Breast (pain, lump, nipple discharge, rash, history of breast disease or surgery)
- Axilla (tenderness, lump or swelling, rash)
- Respiratory system (lung diseases [e.g., asthma, emphysema, bronchitis, pneumonia, tuberculosis], chest pain with breathing, wheezing or noisy breathing, shortness of breath, cough, sputum, hemoptysis or coughing up blood)
- Cardiovascular (chest pain, heart palpitation, cyanosis, dyspnea on exertion, orthopnea, nocturia, edema, heart murmur, hypertension, coronary artery disease, anemia)
- Peripheral vascular (coldness, numbness and tingling of extremities, swelling of legs, discoloration of hands or feet, varicose veins, intermittent claudication or pain in legs on exertion, thrombophlebitis, leg ulcers)
- Urinary system (history of kidney disease, kidney stones, or urinary tract infections; frequency of urination; urgency; nocturia or number of times person awakens at night to urinate; painful or difficult urination; oliguria or polyuria; urine color [e.g., cloudy, bloody, straw-colored]; urine odor; incontinence; pain in the flank, groin, suprapubic region, or lower back)
- Male genital system (penile or testicular pain, penile discharge, sores or lesions, lumps, hernia)
- Female genital system (menstrual history [e.g., age at menarche, last menstrual period, cycle and duration, amenorrhea [absence of periods] or menometrorrhagia [bleeding between periods], premenstrual pain or dysmenorrhea [menstrual pain], vaginal itching, discharge and its characteristics, age at menopause, menopausal signs or symptoms, postmenopausal bleeding)

Continued

Box 12-1 Health History—cont'd

- Sexual health (in a relationship involving intercourse, satisfaction, dysfunction, use of contraceptive, exposure to sexually transmitted infection)
- Musculoskeletal system (history of arthritis, gout, back pain, or disk disease; pain, stiffness, or swelling of joints; deformity; limitation of motion; noise with joint motion; muscle pain, cramps, or weakness; problems with gait or coordination; back pain, stiffness, or limitation of motion)
- Neurologic system (history of seizure disorder, stroke, fainting, or blackouts; weakness, tic, or tremor; paralysis or coordination problems; numbness or tingling; cognitive disorder; nervousness, mood changes, depression, or history of mental illness)
- Hematologic system (bleeding tendency, bruises easily, swollen lymph nodes, exposure to radiation or toxins.
- Endocrine system (history of diabetes or diabetic symptoms, or thyroid disease; intolerance to heat and cold; change in skin pigmentation or texture; excessive sweating; relationship between appetite and weight; abnormal hair distribution; nervousness; tremors)

FUNCTIONAL ASSESSMENT

- Self-esteem, self-concept (education, financial status, value-belief system)
- Activity/exercise (daily activities, ability to perform activities of daily living [ADL], use of mobility aids, leisure activities, exercise pattern)
- Sleep/rest (pattern, naps, sleep aids)
- Nutrition/elimination (24-hour recall of food and fluid intake, allergies, food intolerance; usual bowel elimination pattern, use of laxatives)
- Interpersonal relationships/resources (social roles, support system, quality of contact with others)
- Spiritual resources (faith, membership, influence of faith/spirituality on health and self-care, related issues or concerns)
- Coping and stress management (kinds of stresses, strategies used to copy, effectiveness of strategies)
- Personal habits (tobacco, alcohol, street drug use; frequency, amount)
- Environment/hazards (adequacy of housing, occupational exposures, safety hazards)
- Intimate partner violence ("Do you feel safe?"; relationship to violent partner, type of violence, frequency)
- Occupational health

Adapted from Jarvis C: *Physical examination and health assessment,* ed 6, St. Louis, 2012, Saunders.

information that was not included earlier. Some sources recommend recording subjective data in quotation marks whereas others think this is unnecessary. An electronic health record (EHR) is likely to consist of a checklist with space for elaboration as needed.

When the EHR is fully available, the nurse will have access to a complete record of a person's health information so that each visit would require only updates and new information. The EHR will enable all care providers to have access to the same information. Patients will no longer need to provide the same data during every office visit. Diagnostic test and procedure results will be accessible to all providers, avoiding duplications and delays in treatments. When patients are treated by multiple providers, each provider will know what the other has ordered. The electronic system will require a standardized medical vocabulary such as SNOMED Clinical Terms (SNOMED CT). SNOMED CT includes North American Nursing Diagnosis Association International (NANDA-I), Nursing Interventions Classification (NIC), and Nursing Outcomes Classification (NOC) terminologies, with links that guide the nurse in choosing nursing diagnoses, interventions, and outcomes.

Objective Data

Objective data are obtained through physical examination, diagnostic tests, and patient records. Observation is one of the most important means of data collection. Use all of your senses to collect objective data. For example, a patient's disheveled appearance (sight) may indicate an inability to carry out self-care activities. Noisy and labored breathing (hearing) is consistent with respiratory problems. A fruity mouth odor (smell) may be a sign of diabetic ketoacidosis. Cold and clammy skin (touch) may signal that a patient is in shock. When recording observational data, write exactly what is observed (e.g., "The skin is warm and dry"). Avoid words such as *normal, good, bad, better,* or *worse.*

Physical Examination. Physical examination is a systematic way of obtaining comprehensive objective data. Whereas the initial nursing physical examination should be conducted by the RN, some parts of the examination may be performed by the LVN/LPN. In some instances, a complete head-to-toe examination is conducted. At other times, only one or two systems may be examined, as warranted by the patient's symptoms. For example, when a patient is in acute respiratory distress, only the respiratory and cardiovascular systems might be examined initially. A complete examination would be delayed until the patient's breathing improves. Although some aspects of the physical examination require training beyond that of the LVN/LPN, an overview of the complete physical examination process is presented here.

The four methods of examination are (1) inspection, (2) palpation, (3) percussion, and (4) auscultation.

Inspection. Inspection is purposeful observation of the person as a whole and then systematically from head to toe (Fig. 12-1). The observation begins when you first see the patient and continues throughout the examination.

Palpation. Palpation uses the sense of touch to assess various parts of the body and helps to confirm findings that are noted on inspection. The hands, especially the fingertips, are used to assess skin texture, moisture, and temperature or the presence of swelling, lumps, masses, tenderness, or pain (Fig. 12-2). Warm your hands before palpation. When examining the abdomen, palpate lightly at first for surface characteristics, with any tender areas palpated last. Deep palpation for abdominal contents is usually performed only by nurses with advanced skills.

Percussion. Percussion is tapping on the skin of the chest and abdomen to assess the underlying tissues. One hand is placed flat on the skin over the area to be assessed. The tip of the middle finger of the other hand is used to lightly tap the middle finger of the hand that rests on the patient (Fig. 12-3). The sounds that are elicited, called *notes*, tell the examiner whether underlying organs are solid, air-filled, or fluid-filled. Percussion is most often used by advanced practice nurses rather than bedside nurses.

Auscultation. Auscultation is listening to sounds produced by the body, such as heart, lung, and intestinal sounds. Auscultation is performed with a stethoscope (Fig. 12-4), preferably one with a bell and a diaphragm. The diaphragm is best for listening to high-pitched sounds such as the lung and bowel sounds and normal heart sounds. The bell is best for listening to low-pitched sounds such as heart murmurs. Warm the diaphragm by rubbing it against your palm and then place it lightly over the area that is being assessed. If the area is hairy, you may hear a crackling sound similar to abnormal breath sounds. To minimize the problem, press the stethoscope more firmly than usual against the chest or wet the hair with a damp cloth before examination.

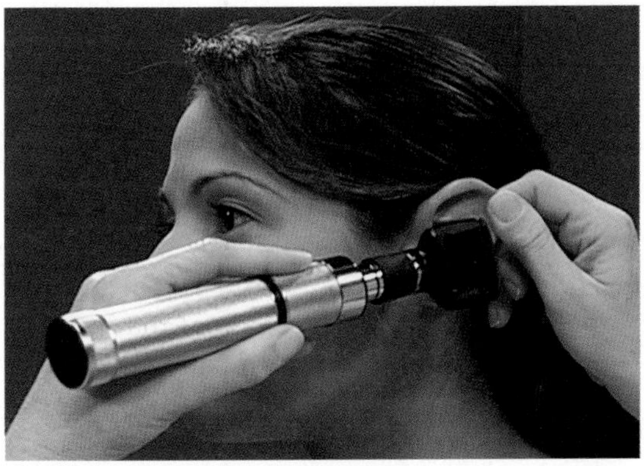

FIGURE 12-1 Inspection. (From Seidel HM et al: *Mosby's guide to physical examination*, ed 7, St. Louis, 2011, Mosby.)

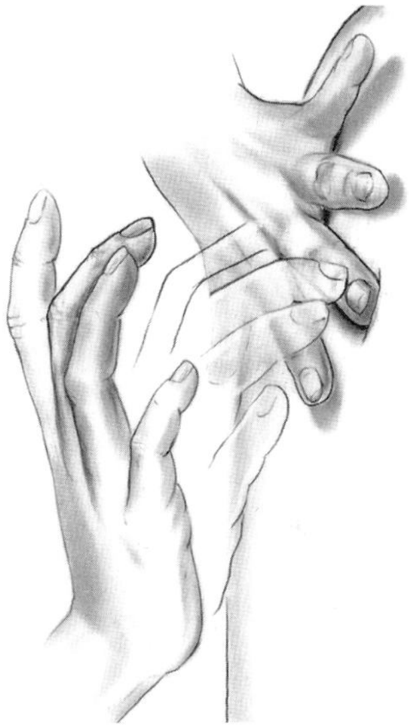

FIGURE 12-3 The striking hand in percussion. (From Jarvis C: *Physical examination and health assessment*, ed 6, St. Louis, 2012, Saunders.)

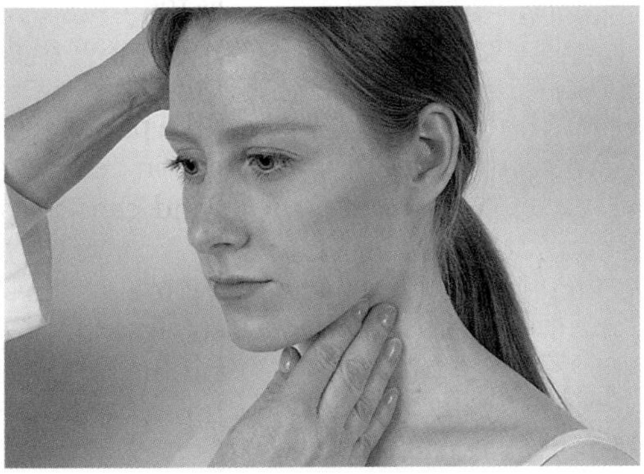

FIGURE 12-2 Palpation. (From Jarvis C: *Physical examination and health assessment*, ed 6, St. Louis, 2012, Saunders.)

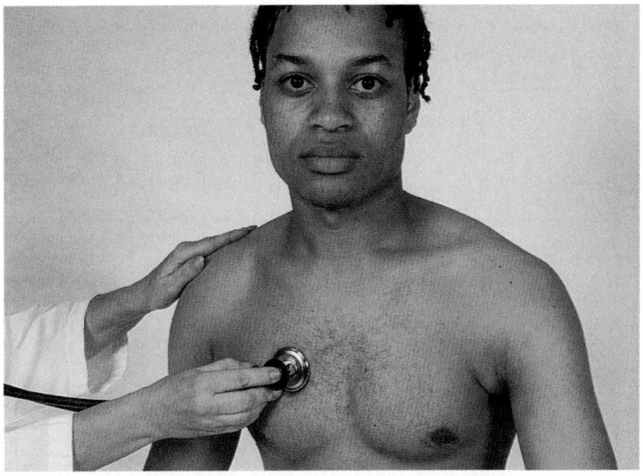

FIGURE 12-4 Auscultation. (From Jarvis C: *Physical examination and health assessment*, ed 5, Philadelphia, 2008, Saunders.)

Box 12-2 presents an overview of the content of a complete physical examination.

Diagnostic Tests. Examples of common diagnostic tests are radiographic studies (x-rays), electrocardiograms (ECGs), magnetic resonance imaging (MRI) scans, computed tomography (CT) scans, positron emission tomography (PET) scans, ultrasound studies, laboratory blood and urine testing, and cultures of possibly infected substances. The information from these tests can be helpful in identifying or validating a nursing or medical diagnosis. Relevant diagnostic tests are addressed with each body system throughout this text.

Patient Records. Patient records provide valuable information regarding the medical history and illness patterns. They can confirm the subjective data and history that the patient and family provide.

When documenting data collected during the assessment, record exactly what was heard, seen, felt, or smelled. This documentation, along with the RN's assessment, provides the basis for making nursing diagnoses. It also makes your findings available to

Box 12-2 Physical Examination

GENERAL APPEARANCE
Age, sex, level of consciousness, skin color, facial features, no signs of acute distress

BODY STRUCTURE
Stature, nutrition (normal weight for height and body build), symmetry, posture, body build (normal proportions), obvious physical deformities

MOBILITY
Gait, range of motion, no involuntary movement

BEHAVIOR
Facial expression, mood and affect, speech, dress, personal hygiene, hair, and makeup

MEASUREMENTS
Height, weight, vital signs

SKIN, HAIR, AND NAILS
Skin (color, general pigmentation, widespread color change, temperature, moisture, texture, thickness, edema, mobility and turgor, hygiene, vascularity or bruising, lesions, tattoos, body piercings)

Hair (color, texture, distribution, scalp lesions)

Nails (shape and contour, consistency, color)

HEAD AND NECK
Head (size and shape of skull, symmetry, expression of face)

Neck (symmetry, range of motion, lymph nodes)

EYES
Central visual acuity, near and far vision, peripheral vision, extraocular muscle function (parallel alignment, nystagmus), external eye structures (eyebrows, eyelids and lashes, eyeballs, conjunctiva and sclera, lacrimal apparatus, cornea, lens, iris and pupils)

EARS
External ear (size and shape, skin condition, tenderness, the external auditory meatus), external canal, tympanic membrane, hearing acuity, vestibular apparatus

NOSE, MOUTH, AND THROAT
Nose (external nose, nasal cavity, sinus area)

Mouth (lips, teeth and gums, tongue, buccal mucosa, palate)

Throat (tonsils)

BREASTS AND REGIONAL LYMPHATICS
General appearance, skin, lymphatic drainage areas, nipple, axilla

THORAX AND LUNGS
Posterior chest (symmetric expansion, fremitus [palpable vibration], lung fields, breath sounds)

Anterior chest (shape and configuration of chest wall, skin color and condition, quality of respirations, symmetric chest expansion, forced expiratory time [number of seconds to exhale])

HEART AND NECK VESSELS
Carotid artery pulse, jugular venous pulse, jugular venous pressure, anterior chest inspection, cardiac rate and rhythm, heart sounds, murmurs

ABDOMEN
Inspection (contour, symmetry, umbilicus, skin, pulsation or movement, hair distribution)

Palpation (surface and deep areas, liver edge, spleen, kidneys)

Percussion (general tympany, liver span, splenic dullness)

Auscultation (bowel sounds, vascular sounds)

PERIPHERAL VASCULAR SYSTEM
Pulses, capillary refill, skin color and temperature, edema, pain

MUSCULOSKELETAL SYSTEM
Joint (size, contour, swelling, warmth, range of motion, crepitus)

Muscles (tone, strength, size)

NEUROLOGIC SYSTEM
Cranial nerves, motor system (muscles, cerebellar function), sensory system (pain, temperature, light touch, vibration, position), reflexes (stretch or deep tendon reflexes, superficial reflexes)

MALE GENITALIA
Penis (lesions, nodules, tenderness, central position of urethra, discharge)

Scrotum (lesions, swelling; testes oval, firm, rubbery, smooth, symmetric, freely moveable)

Inguinal area (hernia, lymph nodes)

FEMALE GENITALIA
External genitalia (skin color, hair distribution, labia majora, labia minora, clitoris, urethral opening, vaginal opening, perineum)

Internal genitalia (cervix, vagina)

ANUS, RECTUM, AND PROSTATE
Perianal area, anus, rectum, stool

other care providers. Baseline data also are used to assess the patient's progress or lack of progress over time.

NURSING DIAGNOSIS

The nursing diagnosis is derived from assessment data and other sources. A nursing diagnosis is different from a medical diagnosis. The medical diagnosis focuses on the etiology (cause) of the dysfunction of a specific organ or system. In contrast, the nursing diagnosis focuses on the patient's physical, psychologic, and social responses to a health problem or potential health problem. Nursing diagnoses provide a basis for planning nursing interventions to prevent, minimize, or alleviate the problem. Although the RN formulates nursing diagnoses, the LVN/LPN assists with the identification of patient needs.

NANDA-I develops and revises nursing diagnoses, which are published every 2 years. NANDA-I's work represents an effort to standardize terminology for nursing diagnoses to be used in all health care settings. Each diagnosis has a definition, defining characteristics, and related factors. Box 12-3 lists NANDA-I nursing diagnoses for 2012 to 2014. Nursing diagnoses are written in a format called PES. *P* stands for the *problem*, *E* stands for the *etiology* or cause of the problem,

Box 12-3 Approved Nursing Diagnoses, North American Nursing Diagnosis Association International, 2012–2014

DOMAIN 1: HEALTH PROMOTION
Class 1: Health Awareness
- Deficient **Diversional Activity**
- Sedentary **Lifestyle**

Class 2: Health Management
- Deficient Community **Health**
- Risk-Prone **Health Behavior**
- Ineffective **Health Maintenance**
- Readiness for Enhanced **Immunization Status**
- Ineffective **Protection**
- Ineffective **Self-Health Management**
- Readiness for Enhanced **Self-Health Management**
- Ineffective Family **Therapeutic Regimen Management**

DOMAIN 2: NUTRITION
Class 1: Ingestion
- Insufficient **Breast Milk**
- Ineffective Infant **Feeding Pattern**
- Imbalanced **Nutrition:** Less Than Body Requirements
- Imbalanced **Nutrition:** More Than Body Requirements
- Readiness for Enhanced **Nutrition**
- Risk for Imbalanced **Nutrition**
- Impaired **Swallowing**

Class 2: Digestion: none at present time
Class 3: Absorption: none at present time
Class 4: Metabolism
- Risk for Unstable **Blood Glucose Level**
- Neonatal **Jaundice**
- Risk for Neonatal **Jaundice**
- Risk for Impaired **Liver Function**

Class 5: Hydration
- Risk for **Electrolyte Imbalance**
- Readiness for Enhanced **Fluid Balance**
- Deficient **Fluid Volume**
- Excess **Fluid Volume**
- Risk for Deficient **Fluid Volume**
- Risk for Imbalanced **Fluid Volume**

DOMAIN 3: ELIMINATION AND EXCHANGE
Class 1: Urinary Function
- Functional Urinary **Incontinence**
- Overflow Urinary **Incontinence**
- Reflex Urinary **Incontinence**
- Stress Urinary **Incontinence**
- Urge Urinary **Incontinence**
- Risk for Urge Urinary **Incontinence**
- Impaired **Urinary Elimination**
- Readiness for Enhanced **Urinary Elimination**
- **Urinary Retention**

Class 2: Gastrointestinal Function
- **Constipation**
- Perceived **Constipation**
- Risk for **Constipation**
- **Diarrhea**
- Dysfunctional **Gastrointestinal Motility**
- Risk for Dysfunctional **Gastrointestinal Motility**
- Bowel **Incontinence**

Class 3: Integumentary Function: none at this time
- Respiratory Function

Class 4: Impaired **Gas Exchange**

DOMAIN 4: ACTIVITY/REST
Class 1: Sleep/Rest
- **Insomnia**
- **Sleep** Deprivation
- Readiness for Enhanced **Sleep**
- Disturbed **Sleep Pattern**

Class 2: Activity/Exercise
- Risk for **Disuse Syndrome**
- Impaired Bed **Mobility**
- Impaired Physical **Mobility**
- Impaired Wheelchair **Mobility**
- Impaired **Transfer Ability**
- Impaired **Walking**

Class 3: Energy Balance
- Disturbed **Energy Field**
- **Fatigue**
- **Wandering**

Class 4: Cardiovascular/Pulmonary Responses
- **Activity Intolerance**
- Risk for **Activity Intolerance**
- Ineffective **Breathing Pattern**
- Decreased **Cardiac Output**
- Risk for Ineffective **Gastrointestinal Perfusion**
- Risk for Ineffective **Renal Perfusion**
- Impaired **Spontaneous Ventilation**
- Ineffective Peripheral **Tissue Perfusion**

Continued

Box 12-3 Approved Nursing Diagnoses, North American Nursing Diagnosis Association International, 2012–2014—cont'd

Risk for Decreased Cardiac **Tissue Perfusion**
Risk for Ineffective Cerebral **Tissue Perfusion**
Risk for Ineffective Peripheral **Tissue Perfusion**
Dysfunctional **Ventilatory Weaning Response**

Class 5: Self-Care
Impaired **Home Maintenance**
Readiness for Enhanced **Self-Care**
Bathing **Self-Care** Deficit
Dressing **Self-Care** Deficit
Feeding **Self-Care** Deficit
Toileting **Self-Care** Deficit
Self-Neglect

DOMAIN 5: PERCEPTION/COGNITION

Class 1: Attention
Unilateral Neglect

Class 2: Orientation
Impaired **Environmental Interpretation Syndrome**

Class 3: Sensation/Perception: none at this time

Class 4: Cognition
Acute **Confusion**
Chronic **Confusion**
Risk for Acute **Confusion**
Ineffective **Impulse Control**
Deficient **Knowledge**
Readiness for Enhanced **Knowledge**
Impaired **Memory**

Class 5: Communication
Readiness for Enhanced **Communication**
Impaired **Verbal Communication**

DOMAIN 6: SELF-PERCEPTION

Class 1: Self-Concept
Hopelessness
Risk for Compromised **Human Dignity**
Risk for **Loneliness**
Disturbed **Personal Identity**
Risk for Disturbed **Personal Identity**
Readiness for Enhanced **Self-Concept**

Class 2: Self-Esteem
Chronic Low **Self-Esteem**
Situational Low **Self-Esteem**
Risk for Chronic Low **Self-Esteem**
Risk for Situational Low **Self-Esteem**

Class 3: Body Image
Disturbed **Body Image**

DOMAIN 7: ROLE RELATIONSHIPS

Class 1: Caregiving Roles
Ineffective **Breastfeeding**
Interrupted **Breastfeeding**
Readiness for Enhanced **Breastfeeding**
Caregiver Role Strain
Risk for **Caregiver Role Strain**
Impaired **Parenting**
Readiness for Enhanced **Parenting**
Risk for Impaired **Parenting**

Class 2: Family Relationships
Risk for Impaired **Attachment**
Dysfunctional **Family Processes**
Interrupted **Family Processes**
Readiness for Enhanced **Family Processes**

Class 3: Role Performance
Ineffective **Relationship**
Readiness for Enhanced **Relationship**
Risk for Ineffective **Relationship**
Parental **Role Conflict**
Ineffective **Role Performance**
Impaired **Social Interaction**

DOMAIN 8: SEXUALITY

Class 1: Sexual Identity: none at present time

Class 2: Sexual Function
Sexual Dysfunction
Ineffective **Sexuality Pattern**

Class 3: Reproduction
Ineffective **Childbearing Process**
Readiness for Enhanced **Childbearing Process**
Risk for Ineffective **Childbearing Process**
Risk for Disturbed **Maternal-Fetal Dyad**

DOMAIN 9: COPING/STRESS TOLERANCE

Class 1: Post-Trauma Responses
Post-Trauma Syndrome
Risk for **Post-Trauma Syndrome**
Rape-Trauma Syndrome
Relocation Stress Syndrome
Risk for **Relocation Stress Syndrome**

Class 2: Coping Responses
Ineffective **Activity Planning**
Risk for Ineffective **Activity Planning**
Anxiety
Defensive **Coping**
Ineffective **Coping**
Readiness for Enhanced **Coping**
Ineffective Community **Coping**
Readiness for Enhanced Community **Coping**
Compromised Family **Coping**
Disabled Family **Coping**
Readiness for Enhanced Family **Coping**
Death Anxiety
Ineffective **Denial**
Adult **Failure to Thrive**
Fear
Grieving
Complicated **Grieving**
Risk for Complicated **Grieving**
Readiness for Enhanced **Power**
Powerlessness
Risk for **Powerlessness**
Impaired Individual **Resilience**
Readiness for Enhanced **Resilience**
Risk for Compromised **Resilience**
Chronic **Sorrow**
Stress Overload

Class 3: Neurobehavioral Stress
Autonomic Dysreflexia
Risk for **Autonomic Dysreflexia**
Disorganized Infant **Behavior**
Readiness for Enhanced Organized Infant **Behavior**
Risk for Disorganized Infant **Behavior**
Decreased **Intracranial Adaptive Capacity**

Box 12-3 Approved Nursing Diagnoses, North American Nursing Diagnosis Association International, 2012–2014—cont'd

DOMAIN 10: LIFE PRINCIPLES
Class 1: Values
- Readiness for Enhanced **Hope**

Class 2: Beliefs
- Readiness for Enhanced **Spiritual Well-Being**

Class 3: Value/Belief/Action Congruence
- Readiness for Enhanced **Decision-Making**
- **Decisional Conflict**
- **Moral Distress**
- **Noncompliance**
- Impaired **Religiosity**
- Readiness for Enhanced **Religiosity**
- Risk for Impaired **Religiosity**
- **Spiritual Distress**
- Risk for **Spiritual Distress**

DOMAIN 11: SAFETY/PROTECTION
Class 1: Infection
- Risk for **Infection**

Class 2: Physical Injury
- Ineffective **Airway Clearance**
- Risk for **Aspiration**
- Risk for **Bleeding**
- Impaired **Dentition**
- Risk for **Dry Eye**
- Risk for **Falls**
- Risk for **Injury**
- Impaired **Oral Mucous Membrane**
- Risk for **Perioperative Positioning Injury**
- Risk for **Peripheral Neurovascular Dysfunction**
- Risk for **Shock**
- Impaired **Skin Integrity**
- Risk for Impaired **Skin Integrity**
- Risk for **Sudden Infant Death Syndrome**
- Risk for **Suffocation**
- Delayed **Surgical Recovery**
- Risk for **Thermal Injury**
- Impaired **Tissue Integrity**
- Risk for **Trauma**
- Risk for **Vascular Trauma**

Class 3: Violence
- Risk for **Other-Directed Violence**
- Risk for **Self-Directed Violence**
- **Self-Mutilation**
- Risk for **Self-Mutilation**
- Risk for **Suicide**

Class 4: Environmental Hazards
- **Contamination**
- Risk for **Contamination**
- Risk for **Poisoning**

Class 5: Defensive Processes
- Risk for **Adverse Reaction to Iodinated Contrast Media**
- **Latex Allergy Response**
- Risk for **Latex Allergy Response**

Class 6: Thermoregulation
- Risk for Imbalanced **Body Temperature**
- **Hyperthermia**
- **Hypothermia**
- Ineffective **Thermoregulation**

DOMAIN 12: COMFORT
Class 1: Physical Comfort
- Impaired **Comfort**
- Readiness for Enhanced **Comfort**
- **Nausea**
- Acute **Pain**
- Chronic **Pain**

Class 2: Environmental Comfort
- Impaired **Comfort**
- Readiness for Enhanced **Comfort**

Class 3: Social Comfort
- Impaired **Comfort**
- Readiness for Enhanced **Comfort**
- **Social Isolation**

DOMAIN 13: GROWTH/DEVELOPMENT
Class 1: Growth
- Risk for Disproportionate **Growth**

Class 2: Development
- Delayed **Growth and Development**
- Risk for Delayed **Development**

and S stands for the *signs* and *symptoms* of the problem. Only actual problems require signs and symptoms; potential problems do not list them. The PES format helps to make the general nursing diagnosis fit a specific patient care problem. The following example shows the application of the general nursing diagnosis "Impaired Skin Integrity" to a specific patient situation. For an older woman who is bedridden and immobilized and has developed a 2-cm pressure ulcer on her sacrum, the nursing diagnosis would be written as follows: Impaired Skin Integrity *(P)* related to immobility *(E)* as evidenced by 2-cm pressure ulcer on sacrum *(S)*.

Although NANDA-I is continually working to define new nursing diagnoses and to standardize nursing diagnoses, these are still not universally used and accepted. Some nursing specialties have developed their own diagnoses. Some references identify collaborative problems as well as nursing diagnoses. Collaborative problems require intervention by multiple members of the health care team. The format for nursing diagnoses in this book states only the problem and the etiology to avoid repetitious lists of signs and symptoms. In an actual patient care plan, the patient's specific signs and symptoms would be included.

PLANNING

The planning phase of the nursing process involves the development of a nursing care plan based on the nursing diagnoses. Nursing care plans are a form of communication with other health care professionals to ensure continuity of care, to prevent complications, and to provide for health teaching and discharge planning. As in the other steps of the nursing process, the comprehensive plan of care is initiated and finalized by the RN. The LVN/LPN may be involved in planning episodic nursing care. In some settings, especially long-term care, LVNs/LPNs may construct a plan that will be approved by the RN.

The steps in planning nursing care are to (1) determine priorities from the list of nursing diagnoses, (2) set long-term and short-term goals to determine outcomes of care, (3) develop objectives to reach the goals, and (4) write nursing orders to direct care to meet the goals. Priorities are usually based on Maslow's hierarchy of needs and on what the patient perceives as important. For example, you should focus on decreased cardiac output (a physiologic need) before addressing disturbed body image (a self-esteem need).

Goals may be short term or long term, meaning that some may be achieved quickly while others will take a longer time period. Goals should be stated in terms of patient outcomes. To continue with our example of the patient with impaired skin integrity, the goal could be stated as "Pressure ulcer over sacrum will be healed within 2 weeks." A classification system for outcomes can be used. The NOC system includes outcomes such as Tissue Integrity: Skin and Mucous Membranes. Each of the nursing-sensitive outcomes (outcomes amenable to nursing intervention) is labeled and defined and includes criteria for assessing the status of the outcome over time.

Nursing orders are the actions or interventions prescribed to help achieve the stated goals and objectives. Nursing orders should include a specific description (what, where, when, how much, and how long) of how the order should be carried out. For example, "Keep off sacrum to promote healing; turn side to side q2h [every 2 hours]. Get OOB [out of bed] twice a day; begin ambulating as tolerated." The NIC is a standardized list of nursing interventions. A NIC intervention consists of a label name, definition, specific nursing activities, and background readings. The NIC currently includes more than 500 interventions divided into 7 domains and 30 classes. To use NIC interventions, the nurse selects the appropriate activities for a specific intervention based on individual patient data. Examples of intervention labels are: Pressure Management, Pressure Ulcer Care, Skin Surveillance, Fall Prevention, and Incision Site Care. Depending on the situation, additional activities might be added. An example of a partial nursing care plan using NANDA-I, NIC, and NOC is available on the Evolve website.

INTERVENTION (IMPLEMENTATION)

Implementation is the actual performance of the nursing interventions in the plan of care. The nursing interventions include direct patient care, health teaching, and carrying out ordered medical treatments such as medications or dressing changes. Nurses provide care to achieve established goals of care. They then communicate the nursing interventions by documentation and report. Some interventions are unplanned because situations arise that demand immediate attention. Thus the care plan must be flexible and responsive to changes in the patient's needs.

EVALUATION

Evaluation is an ongoing process that enables you to determine what progress the patient has made in meeting the goals for care. The outcome criteria provide objective measures for determining the effects of care. Using the previous example of impaired skin integrity, the outcome criteria could be "intact skin" and "absence of redness over bony prominences." Actual outcomes then are compared with expected outcomes of patient care to determine whether the goals have been met, partially met, or not met. If the goal was not met, reassessment is necessary. The plan of care should be reexamined and modified when necessary. Ongoing evaluation is a tool for quality improvement. In the patient care sections of this text, evaluation is not discussed separately.

Evaluation is important in individual patient care and it provides data regarding the quality of care in a health care institution. Quality assurance audits are conducted by individual health care agencies, as well by as The Joint Commission, an organization that requires systematic review of hospitals and other health care organizations. Areas evaluated include the standards of nursing care used, the quality and effectiveness of nursing care, and the organization of the patient care system. Nursing audits are conducted by examining patient records as one method of gathering information to evaluate nursing performance. Documentation of nursing interventions and frequent evaluations of the plan of care demonstrates that the care provided is consistent with the American Nurses Association (ANA) Standards of Care.

Clinical Pathways

Clinical pathways are used in some health care facilities. They are standard care plans developed to set daily care priorities, schedule achievement of outcomes, and reduce length of hospital stays. They include patient outcomes and timelines for the sequence of interventions. Clinical pathways are collaborative and comprehensive in that they are developed jointly by all members of the health care team and they cover many aspects of care rather than just nursing interventions. However, the nursing process will be used to provide the framework for nursing care throughout this text.

Concept Maps

Concept maps are visual plans of care that illustrate the relationships between and among patient data, pathophysiology, signs and symptoms, nursing diagnoses, and collaborative interventions. They are used primarily as learning tools to develop comprehensive plans of care. The visual presentation helps the student, or nurse, to recognize relationships among the clinical data. Nursing diagnoses are derived, followed by identification of interventions and outcomes. An example of a concept map for a patient with hypertension is provided in Figure 12-5.

NURSING DOCUMENTATION

Documentation is an essential component of the nursing process. It should be factual, current, complete, organized, and accurate. Documentation fosters continuity of care because it provides for communication among caregivers and is a record of the patient's progress. The patient record serves as a legal record of the care provided as well as a means to verify services rendered for insurance payments. Failing to document important data can have serious consequences, as it is assumed that "if it was not charted, it was not done."

The following should be documented:

- Patient assessments and observations: subjective and objective data
- Nursing care provided, including treatments, medications, and teaching
- Diagnostic procedures performed at the bedside, on the unit, or inside or outside the facility
- Reaction to therapeutic and diagnostic procedures
- Evidence of changes in physical, psychosocial, and spiritual needs and status
- Any unusual incidents such as falls or injuries that occur during the stay in the health care facility

Principles of documentation using paper charts are addressed in fundamentals textbooks. Increasingly, patient records are entered and maintained in computerized charting systems. Some systems allow documentation at the patient's bedside. Nurses' notes may be composed by selecting from a menu of options related to the plan of care. Advantages of computerized charting include standardization of patient data, ease of retrieving data, and convenient storage. One disadvantage is the risk of information access by unauthorized persons. To reduce the risk of unauthorized access by another person, always log out after completing your entries in the electronic health record and never share your password with anyone else.

DOCUMENTATION FORMATS

Various formats are used for the documentation of patient care, including nurses' notes, flow sheets, and **problem-oriented medical records** (POMRs). Nurses' notes traditionally consisted of pages of narrative recordings containing assessment data, interventions carried out by the nurse, and evaluation data collected. Flow sheets may be graphs of vital signs or tables in which nurses may check or initial boxes indicating activities or care provided.

Examples of charting approaches include focus charting (using key words such as action or response to organize charting), source-oriented charting (charting on separate sheets for different health care workers, such as physical therapy on one page and nurses on another), multidisciplinary charting (charting by different disciplines on the same page), charting by exception (CBE; charting narrative notes only when a change is observed in the patient's condition), and the electronic health record (EHR), which was mentioned above. Health care facilities may combine one or more of these methods.

The POMR is a method of record keeping that focuses on patient problems rather than on medical diagnoses. This method is popular in many clinical areas because it provides an excellent means of communication among the various disciplines that are providing care. Each health care provider involved in the care of the patient charts on the same progress notes in the same format. The data from the history, physical examination, diagnostic tests, and medical diagnoses provide a foundation for problems formulated in the POMR. The problem list consists of active, inactive, potential, and resolved problems. The charting is performed in a SOAPIER format. SOAPIER is an acronym for the components of the charting:

S *Subjective* information, or how the patient perceives the problem
O *Objective* information, or what the nurse observes about the patient
A *Assessment*, or why the patient has the problem
P *Plan*, or how the intervention is to be carried out
I *Intervention*, or what specific care is given
E *Evaluation*, or how effective was the plan or intervention
R *Revision*, or what changes should be made in the original plan of care

In many cases, the SOAPE form is used, omitting the intervention and revision sections. The intervention is closely related to the plan and can be a reiteration of the plan; a revision can be made in the plan simply by revising the original SOAPE notes.

An example of a SOAPE note using our previous example is as follows:

S Feels weak; does "not have the energy to move around."
O Does not turn self in bed; 2-cm stage 2 pressure ulcer on sacrum.
A Pressure ulcer on sacrum related to immobility.
P Turn from side to side q2h. Get out of bed at least twice a day. Begin ambulating as tolerated.
E Turned q2h. OOB twice a day, taking six small steps to and from bed. Pressure ulcer healing; now 1.5 cm.

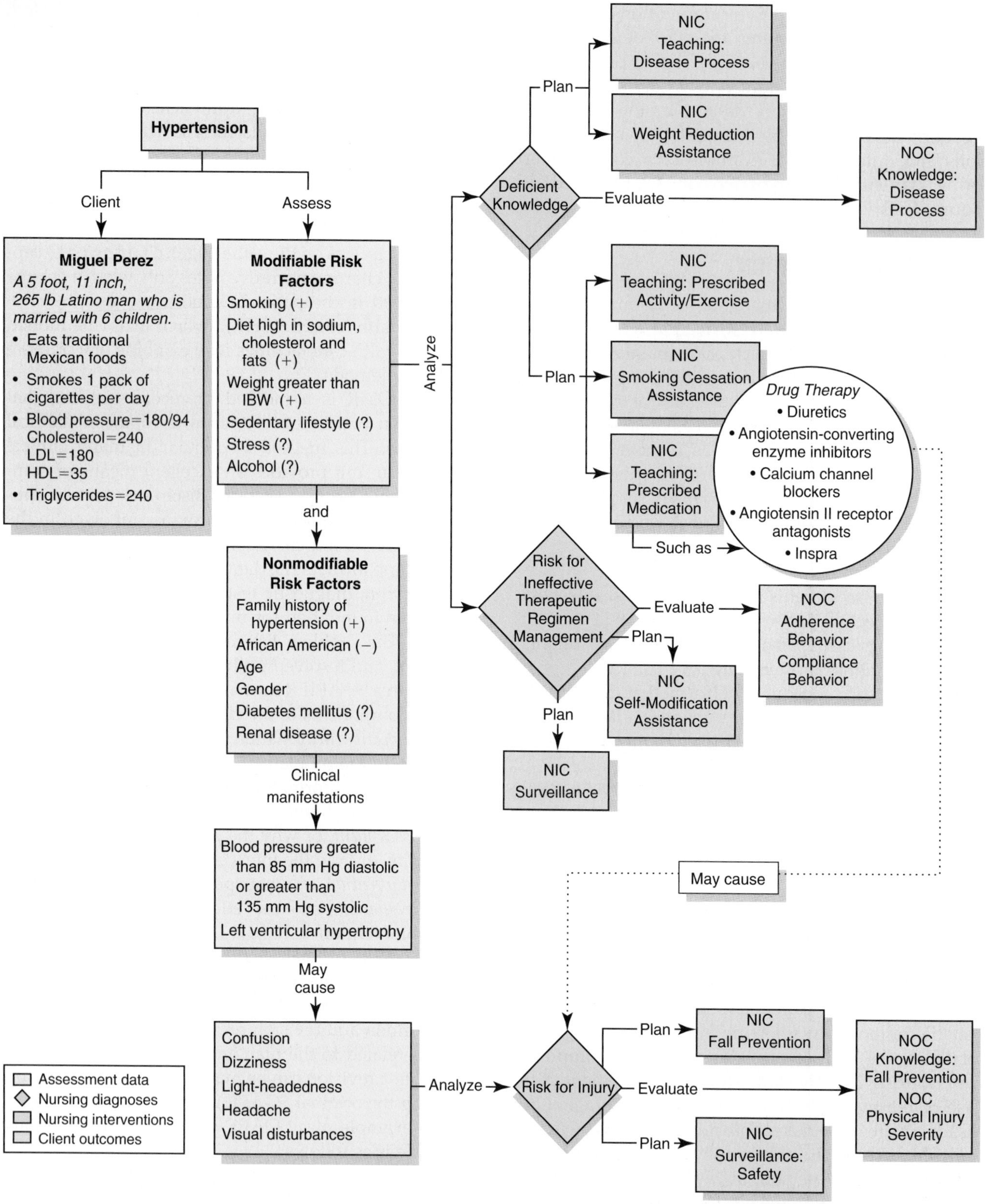

FIGURE 12-5 Hypertension concept map. The concept map is a visual plan that shows the relationships among parts of the plan. (*HDL*, High-density lipoprotein; *IBW*, ideal body weight; *LDL*, low-density lipoprotein; *NIC*, Nursing Interventions Classification; *NOC*, Nursing Outcomes Classification.) (Courtesy Elaine Bishop Kennedy, EdD, RN.)

Another common format is PIE charting, which includes the problem, intervention, and evaluation. An example is as follows:

P Risk for impaired skin integrity related to unrelieved pressure on sacrum.
I Patient informed of need to shift positions and increase ambulation to relieve pressure on sacrum. Assisted to reposition hourly and to get out of bed twice.
E Patient is repositioning herself with occasional prompting. Walked for two 10-minute periods today.

Put on Your Thinking Cap!

Agree with some classmates to observe 5 minutes of the same local television news on a specific date and time. Using objective language, document your observations of the speaker or speakers. Compare your description with that of your classmates. If they have differences, discuss possible explanations for this.

EVIDENCE-BASED PRACTICE

All health providers strive to provide the best care available to their patients. Lifelong learning is essential for nurses because our knowledge of best practices is constantly evolving. Fifty years ago, nurses seated decubitus-prone patients on donut-shaped cushions to relieve pressure from bony prominences. At the time, this action was thought to be an effective intervention. However, later discoveries indicated that the circular cushion actually created pressure around the bony prominence and interfered with blood flow to the vulnerable area. Once this factor was understood, many years were needed for the practice to change accordingly. Whereas research related to nursing interventions was once rare, it is now common and we are questioning many time-honored practices. Many nursing journals are dedicated to research studies that have the potential to improve practice. Nurses have a responsibility to keep up with current knowledge about patient care.

A problem in changing practice has been getting appropriate information to be used at the bedside, largely because bedside nurses may lack the preparation to locate and evaluate the results reported in research studies. **Evidence-based practice** has evolved as a mechanism to convert research findings to useful practice guidelines. To accomplish this task, all research on a given topic is studied to determine the current state of knowledge. The strength of each study is evaluated, evidence supporting a particular intervention is summarized, and the evidence is translated into recommendations for clinical practice and distributed to health care providers. The LVN/LPN can contribute to the application of evidence-based interventions by reading professional journals and taking advantage of professional practice educational opportunities. By bringing information about best practices back to the employment site, every nurse can have a very positive influence on practice.

CRITICAL THINKING

Critical thinking is defined as "reflective and reasonable thinking that is focused on deciding what to believe or do" (Ennis, 1985, p. 45). Although more sophisticated definitions exist, this one is appropriate for our purposes. You will hear a lot about critical thinking during your nursing education. Because you spend a lot of time reading and learning facts, you may assume that critical thinking is just learning many facts. Although facts are indeed important, nursing deals with people in states of change in an environment that is constantly evolving. You will forget many of the facts you learn this year but if you become a critical thinker, you will always have the tools to seek and apply knowledge because nursing and health care are always changing.

RELATIONSHIP OF CRITICAL THINKING TO THE NURSING PROCESS

Why do you need both critical thinking and the nursing process? The nursing process is a framework for developing, implementing, and evaluating a plan of care. It spells out the patient's needs and problems, the goals for care, interventions to achieve goals, and measures to assess goal achievement.

If you have seen a well-written nursing process, you can see how it can be used to guide care. It tells you exactly what to do, right? Unfortunately, the process is not that simple. Suppose that the patient's care plan says he is to be assisted to take a shower for the first time since surgery as part of the plan to promote increasing independence in self-care. However, when you assist the patient out of bed, he becomes dizzy and nauseated. What do you do now? This situation is a simple one that can be used to illustrate how critical thinking is used in nursing. Table 12-1 carries this situation through and outlines the steps of the nursing process along with the critical thinking that occurs at each step. One point to notice is that the nursing process does not flow smoothly from one step to the next; rather, it often moves back and forth between steps. This common scenario illustrates the many decision-making points that can occur in handling a fairly routine nursing situation. Notice that critical thinking was used to determine the focused assessments needed, interventions to be implemented, and evaluation data to collect. The nursing process is a sequence of steps that should be based on critical thinking. That is why your faculty may discourage you from using standardized care plans. Ready-made care plans bypass the vital experience of thinking through

Table 12-1 Analysis of Critical Thinking in a Clinical Situation

Situation: You are assigned to care for Mr. A. today. It is his second postoperative day. One goal for the day is to promote independence in self-care. The nursing care plan notes that you should assist the patient with a shower.

The following table reflects a possible sequence of events when you attempt to implement the plan of care. The steps of the nursing process and the critical thinking skills are identified to illustrate how they are used and interact in a common situation.

SEQUENCE OF EVENTS	NURSING PROCESS STEPS	CRITICAL THINKING TOOLS
When you help Mr. A. stand at the bedside, he becomes dizzy and says that he is nauseated. You ease him back into bed, knowing that he is at risk for falling. Because Mr. A. is nauseated, you anticipate vomiting and reach for an emesis basin.	Intervention Assessment Intervention Planning Intervention	Inference: drawing conclusions Evaluation: assessing possibilities
You collect additional information immediately after Mr. A. lies down. His skin is pale, cool, and moist. His pulse is 110 bpm and faint and his blood pressure is 90/60 mm Hg. When asked how he feels, he replies, "I feel better lying down."	Assessment	Interpretation: clarifying the meaning of events
Knowing that dizziness is associated with hypotension and that the supine position improves blood flow to the brain, you advise him to remain flat in bed for the time being.	Diagnosis Intervention	Inference: drawing conclusions
You reassess Mr. A. after he has spent a few minutes in the supine position. His skin is pink and warm, his pulse rate is 84 bpm and full, and his blood pressure is 114/74 mm Hg.	Assessment	Interpretation: clarifying meaning of data
What do you do now? The care plan says you are supposed to get him up for a shower. You ask yourself what has just happened. You consider a drop in blood pressure related to drug effects, immobility, or dehydration.	Planning	Inference: deriving alternatives Interpretation: clarifying meaning of events
You consider your options: Try again to get him up; give him a bed bath; let him rest for a while and see how he feels later; exercise his legs before helping him stand; notify the physician. These options are all possibilities.	Planning	Inference: deriving alternatives Analysis: examining ideas
How do you choose one option? Think about the possible outcomes (positive and negative) of each action.	Planning	Inference: drawing conclusions
Choose the option that would seem to be safe for the patient without delaying his recovery.	Intervention	—
You think that the patient should remain in bed this morning. However, as a novice nurse you are somewhat unsure of yourself; thus you explain the situation to the charge nurse and request feedback. The charge nurse suggests that you wait and try again later.	Planning Assessment Intervention Evaluation	Self-regulation: recognizing need to make changes, reconsidering conclusions Interpretation: clarifying meaning of data Inference: deriving alternatives

bpm, Beats per minute.

each step to ensure that the care plan is specific and individualized for your patient.

CHARACTERISTICS OF A CRITICAL THINKER

In the situation just described, you (the nurse) demonstrated various characteristics of a critical thinker. Those characteristics include the following:

- *Curiosity:* the desire not just to know, but also to understand how and why to apply knowledge
- *Systematic thinking:* uses an organized approach to problem solving rather than knee-jerk responses
- *Analytical:* applies knowledge from various disciplines, approaches a problem by examining the parts and seeing how they fit together
- *Open-minded:* willing to consider various alternatives
- *Self-confident:* sense of assurance that the problem-solving process produces a favorable conclusion or plan

- *Maturity:* recognition that many variables are at work in patient situations and sometimes the best plans do not work (back to the drawing board!)
- *Truth-seeking:* eager to know, asking questions, seeking answers, reevaluates "common knowledge"

CRITICAL THINKING TOOLS

Just as the critical thinker has certain characteristics, the critical thinker also uses specific tools. These tools include the following:

- *Interpretation:* clarifying meaning of events, data
- *Analysis:* examining ideas, breaking down into components
- *Evaluation:* assessing possibilities, opinions, usual practices
- *Inference:* deriving alternatives, drawing conclusions
- *Explanation:* presenting arguments for views, decisions; justifying
- *Self-regulation:* reconsidering conclusions, recognizing need to make changes

Throughout this text, you will find exercises titled "Put on your Thinking Cap!" As you encounter these features, your first reaction may be to try to find the answer in the chapter. What you will find is that the chapter content provides only the knowledge *base* to answer the question, not the answer itself. A trick question, you say? Not at all. The purpose is to help you develop the essential skills for *critical thinking.*

In closing, the nursing process is a tool—a road map for planning and providing care. Critical thinking is the element that makes the nursing process scientifically sound, appropriate, flexible, and individualized for each patient to whom you provide care.

Get Ready for the NCLEX® Examination!

Key Points

- The nursing process is a problem-solving approach that enables the nurse to provide care in an organized, scientific manner.
- The comprehensive nursing assessment and plan of care are developed by the RN.
- The LVN/LPN assists with collecting data, identifying patient needs, planning care, and evaluating the outcomes of care.
- The steps of the nursing process are assessment, nursing diagnosis, planning, implementation, and evaluation.
- Assessment involves the collection of subjective and objective data about the patient from the patient, family, significant others, medical records, and other care providers.
- The interview is used to obtain an objective picture of the patient's personal and family health history.
- The physical examination uses inspection, auscultation, palpation, and percussion to collect objective data about the patient.
- The nursing diagnosis is a statement of an actual or potential health problem derived from the assessment.
- Nursing diagnoses differ from medical diagnoses in that nursing diagnoses focus on the response of the whole person to the medical problem.
- The parts of a NANDA-I diagnosis are the label, definition of the diagnosis, defining characteristics (signs and symptoms), and related (causative or associated) factors.
- The planning phase of the nursing process involves the development of a nursing care plan for the patient based on the nursing diagnoses.
- The NOC includes standardized outcomes that serve as criteria to judge the results of nursing interventions.
- Planning includes priority setting, goal statements, and nursing interventions to achieve the goals.
- NIC interventions are standardized interventions, each including a label name, definition, list of nursing activities, and background readings.
- Implementation refers to the actual performance of the nursing interventions identified in the plan of care.
- Evaluation is an ongoing process in which the nurse uses outcome criteria to determine what progress has been made toward meeting the goals.
- The value of using systems such as NANDA-I, NIC, and NOC is that they standardize language that describes what nurses do.
- Documentation of data collected, interventions, and evaluation data is an essential aspect of nursing care.
- Evidence-based nursing care is based on evaluation and summarization of the best information available.
- Clinical pathways are standardized, interdisciplinary plans of care that specify the sequence and timing of interventions.
- Critical thinking is defined as "reflective and reasonable thinking that is focused on deciding what to believe or do" (Ennis, 1985, p. 45).
- Critical thinking makes the nursing process appropriate, scientifically sound, flexible, and individualized.
- Critical thinking skills include interpretation, analysis, evaluation, inference, explanation, and self-regulation.
- A critical thinker is curious, open-minded, a systematic thinker, analytical, and truth seeking, and has self-confidence and maturity.

Additional Learning Resources

SG Go to your Study Guide for additional learning activities to help you master this chapter content.

evolve Go to your Evolve website (http://evolve.elsevier.com/Linton/medsurg) for the following learning resources and much more:

- NEW! Case Study from Johnson et al: *NOC and NIC linkages to NANDA-I and clinical conditions*, ed 3, St. Louis, 2012, Mosby.
- Interactive Prioritization Exercises
- Review Questions for the NCLEX® Examination

Review Questions for the NCLEX® Examination

1. Which of the data from the nurse's shift assessment represent subjective data? (Select all that apply.)
   1. Lung sounds clear to auscultation
   2. Urine clear, light yellow
   3. Nauseous and light-headed
   4. Headache and sensitivity to light
   5. Incisional pain rated "5" on 10-point scale

   NCLEX Client Need: Physiological Integrity: Physiological Adaptation
2. "Patient states pain in his neck began when he was wrestling with his brother. The pain radiates across his right shoulder and worsens with movement of the right arm." This statement is an example of:
   1. Biographical data
   2. Chief complaint
   3. Family history
   4. Review of systems

   NCLEX Client Need: Physiological Integrity: Physiological Adaptation
3. Which techniques should the nurse use in a focused assessment of the skin? (Select all that apply.)
   1. Inspection
   2. Auscultation
   3. Percussion
   4. Palpation
   5. Evaluation

   NCLEX Client Need: Health Promotion and Maintenance
4. Which of the following is a complete, correctly stated NANDA-I diagnosis?
   1. Disturbed body image as a result of surgical scars, as evidenced by crying and concealing scars
   2. Decreased cardiac output related to excessive blood loss
   3. Noncompliance evidenced by high blood pressure
   4. Diabetes mellitus related to obesity, as evidenced by high serum glucose

   NCLEX Client Need: Psychosocial Integrity
5. Nursing students wrote the following goals for care of their surgical patients. Which goal is most complete and measurable?
   1. Patient will demonstrate clean wound dressing change before discharge.
   2. Patient will know how to care for wound before leaving the hospital.
   3. Patient will take care of wound himself when he goes home.
   4. Patient will understand the principles of medical asepsis to use during dressing changes.

   NCLEX Client Need: Health Promotion and Maintenance
6. The *primary* purpose of evidence-based practice is to:
   1. Encourage all nurses to participate in research
   2. Explain how to interpret research results
   3. Recruit patients into clinical research studies
   4. Bring research findings into nursing practice

   NCLEX Client Need: Safe and Effective Care Environment: Coordinated Care
7. Which of the following skills is used in critical thinking?
   1. Copy
   2. Recite
   3. Memorize
   4. Analyze

   NCLEX Client Need: Safe and Effective Care Environment: Coordinated Care
8. The nursing team is working on a care plan for a patient who has had several falls despite the usual safety measures. The LVN/LPN says, "Let's see if we can figure out a pattern to his falls. If we can determine contributing factors, we might be able to identify some different interventions." He is demonstrating which characteristics of a critical thinker? (Select all that apply.)
   1. Systematic thinking
   2. Analytical
   3. Open-minded
   4. Self-confident
   5. Maturity

   NCLEX Client Need: Safe and Effective Care Environment: Coordinated Care
9. According to the ANA Standards of Care, the nurse evaluates the patient's progress toward attainment of desired outcomes. What measurement criterion is used for this standard?
   1. Revisions in diagnoses, outcomes, and the plan of care are documented.
   2. Interventions are consistent with the established plan of care.
   3. The plan is developed with the patient, significant others, and health care providers, when appropriate.
   4. Outcomes are realistic in relation to the patient's present and potential capabilities.

   NCLEX Client Need: Safe and Effective Care Environment: Coordinated Care
10. Nursing staff are encouraged to employ evidence-based interventions. The nurses are aware that evidence-based recommendations are determined by what process?
    1. Evaluation and summarization of the best information possible
    2. Consensus based on common practice
    3. Combination of all existing research
    4. Interview of leading experts

    NCLEX Client Need: Safe and Effective Care Environment: Coordinated Care

chapter 13

Immunity, Inflammation, and Infection

Maria Danet Sanchez Lapiz-Bluhm

http://evolve.elsevier.com/Linton/medsurg

Objectives

1. Describe physical and chemical barriers.
2. Describe the immune response.
3. Identify the organs involved in immunity.
4. Compare natural and acquired immunity.
5. Describe how inflammatory changes act as bodily defense mechanisms.
6. Identify the signs and symptoms of inflammation.
7. Discuss the process of repair and healing.
8. Differentiate infection from inflammation.
9. Discuss the actions of commonly found infectious agents.
10. Describe the ways that infections are transmitted.
11. Identify the signs and symptoms of infection.
12. Compare community-acquired and health care–associated infections.
13. Discuss the nursing care of patients with infections.
14. Describe the Centers for Disease Control and Prevention (CDC) Standard Precautions guidelines for infection prevention and control.
15. Describe the CDC isolation guidelines for Airborne, Droplet, and Contact (Transmission-Based) Precautions.
16. Describe the CDC isolation guidelines for a Protective Environment.
17. Differentiate between humoral (antibody-mediated) and cell-mediated immunity.
18. Describe the nursing care of patients with immunodeficiency and of those with allergies.
19. Describe the process of autoimmunity.

Key Terms

Allergen (ĂL-ĕr-jĕn)
Antibodies (ĂN-tĭ-bŏ-dēs)
Antigen (ĂN-tĭ- jĕn)
Autoimmunity (ăw-tō-ĭ-MYŪ-nĭ-tē)
Bacteria (băk-TĒ-rē-ăh)
Communicable disease (kŏ-MYŪ-nĭ-kă-b'l dĭ-ZĒZ)
Contamination
Fungi (FŬN-jī or FŬN-gī)
Health care–associated infection (HAI)
Immunity (ĭ-MYŪ-nĭ-tē)
Immunodeficiency (ĭ-myū-nō-dē-FĬSH-ĕn-sē)
Infection
Inflammation (ĭn-flă-MĀ-shŭn)
Medical asepsis (ā-SĔP-sĭs)
Multidrug-resistant organism (MDRO)
Surgical asepsis (SŬR-jĭ-kăl ā-SĔP-sĭs)
Viruses (VĪ-rŭs-ĕs)

Suppose that you were being attacked. How would you defend yourself? Perhaps you would shout or sound an alarm in some other way. You might even call for reinforcements to help you fight off the attacker, telling them the most direct route to your location. You would probably surround yourself with some sort of barrier either to shield yourself from further harm or to keep the attacker in the area so that he or she would not escape and harm someone else. Then, after the battle was over, you would likely enlist the help of some friends to clean up the debris and return your situation to normal.

Quite remarkably, at a cellular level, the human body protects itself in much the same way. The body relies on many effective barriers to protect itself from injury and disease. However, if these barriers are compromised, several sophisticated processes are triggered to isolate and eliminate the offender. This chapter describes how the body defends itself from injury and disease, what happens when defenses fail, and how good nursing care helps the processes.

PHYSICAL AND CHEMICAL BARRIERS

Intact skin and mucous membranes are the body's first line of defense. They act as a protective covering and secrete substances that inhibit the growth of microorganisms. The sweat glands secrete lysozyme, an antimicrobial enzyme. Sebaceous glands secrete sebum, which has antimicrobial and antifungal properties. Acidic secretions from the skin and the mucosa of the gastrointestinal and genitourinary systems inhibit the growth of many pathogenic organisms. Secretions from the mammary glands and the respiratory and gastrointestinal tracts contain the antibody *immunoglobulin A*, as well as cleanup phagocytes. In addition, skin and mucous membrane surfaces are colonized by "normal" bacterial flora, which prevent pathogens (disease-causing organisms) from gaining access to the body. The cilia in the respiratory tract, the motility of the gastrointestinal tract, and the sloughing of dead skin cells all work to distribute and remove microorganisms, preventing their overgrowth and invasion.

The second line of defense involves two processes: phagocytosis and inflammation. Phagocytosis helps to rid the body of invading microorganisms and debris. White blood cells (leukocytes) are colorless blood cells that have the ability to phagocytose (ingest) bacteria that can cause infection when they invade the body. There are five types of leukocytes: neutrophils, monocytes, eosinophils, basophils and lymphocytes. Neutrophils fight bacterial infections. Monocytes circulate in the blood for approximately 1 day before they enter tissue, where they are called *macrophages*, and ingest many foreign antigens. Eosinophils fight parasitic infections and increase during allergic reactions. Basophils initiate the inflammatory response and release histamine. Measuring the number of these cells gives an indication of the severity of infection and inflammation in the body. B lymphocytes produce antibodies and T lymphocytes increase the body's immune response. Therefore lymphocyte counts provide a measure of immune function. Reticuloendothelial cells are found in the blood, connective tissue, liver, spleen, bone marrow, and lymph nodes. Some reticuloendothelial cells protect the body by digesting and absorbing foreign material, such as old red blood cells, bacteria, and colloidal particles. These cells may also be called *tissue macrophages*.

A more complete description of blood and components of the immune system may be found in Chapters 33 and 34.

IMMUNITY

The immune system is the body's defense network against infection. **Immunity** provides the body with resistance to invading organisms and enables it to fight off invaders once they have gained access. The body is constantly exposed to microorganisms capable of causing disease. If the immune system is intact and functioning properly, adequate protection from most infections and diseases is provided in a healthy individual. When the immune system is not functioning properly, the potential for overwhelming infection exists. Many factors can compromise the immune system, such as disease states, congenital defects, aging, stress, and therapeutic interventions (e.g., drugs, radiation therapy). Understanding the normal immune response and the common immune system disorders will help you to assess patients at risk for infection and provide appropriate interventions.

Any substance that is capable of stimulating a response from the immune system is called an **antigen**. In most cases the antigen is foreign to the body and the body recognizes the antigen as different from itself ("nonself"). Antigens can be microorganisms (bacteria, viruses, fungi, parasites), abnormal or mutated body cells, transplanted cells (from blood transfusions, organ transplants), noninfectious substances from the environment (pollens, insect venom, foods), or foreign molecules from drugs such as penicillin. When healthy, the body protects what it recognizes as self and attempts to destroy that which is nonself. Tissue that is normally recognized as self may be seen as nonself by the immune system if the tissue undergoes change (mutation), is in an abnormal location, or changes structure. Once the body recognizes a substance as an antigen, natural and acquired defenses are put into action to destroy the invader and prevent disease.

Antibodies, also known as *immunoglobulins*, are proteins that are created in response to specific antigens. The formation and function of antibodies are discussed in the "Antibody-Mediated (Immediate) Immunity" section of this chapter.

INNATE (NATURAL) VERSUS ACQUIRED IMMUNITY

Innate (natural) immunity is present in the body at birth and is not dependent on a specific immune response or previous contact with an infectious agent. It may be specific to a species, a race, or an individual. For instance, humans are not as susceptible to distemper as dogs and cats are. Factors such as nutritional status, stress, and environment may influence natural immunity. Nonspecific defense mechanisms that include physical and chemical barriers to infection, phagocytosis (the process of enveloping and destroying foreign matter), and the inflammatory process contribute to natural immunity.

An individual develops acquired immunity after birth as a result of the body's natural immune responses to antigens. Acquired immunity depends on the proper development and functioning of B and T lymphocytes, which are white blood cells that fight infection.

Active acquired immunity is developed after direct contact with an antigen through illness or vaccination. Vaccinations may be prepared by three methods: (1) using dead organisms that can no longer cause disease, as in the diphtheria and pertussis vaccines; (2) destroying bacterial toxins that act as antigens, as in the tetanus toxoid vaccine; and (3) altering the structure of live organisms so that they are unable to cause disease yet maintain their antigenic properties to prevent many viral diseases, such as measles and poliomyelitis vaccines. Once the body has been exposed to an antigen through illness or vaccination, antibodies develop and retain memory for the antigen. If the body is exposed to the same antigen later, the antibodies can react quickly to fight off disease.

When people are injected with immune globulin or antiserum (made from human or animal blood) that contains antibodies to a specific agent, such as for the emergency treatment of snakebite, rabies, or exposure to hepatitis, they receive antibodies or lymphocytes that were produced by another individual. This type of immunity, called *passive acquired immunity*, is temporary and is the kind of immunity that newborns receive from their mothers through the placenta or through ingestion of breast milk (especially colostrum).

Both natural and acquired immunity are necessary for a healthy individual to have protection from disease. Innate and acquired immunity are discussed further in Chapter 34.

CELLS AND ORGANS INVOLVED IN IMMUNITY

A variety of cells work together to provide the body with an adequate defense against injury or disease. Leukocytes (white blood cells) play a key role in immune responses to infectious organisms and other antigens. The two categories of white blood cells are granulocytes and nongranulocytes. Blood cells involved in immune disorders are described in Chapter 33.

Although all parts of the body work together as a whole to resist and fight off disease, several organs are vital to a functional immune system. These organs include the thymus, bone marrow, lymph nodes, spleen, and liver (Fig. 13-1). The thymus and bone marrow participate in the formation and maturation of immune system cells. Located throughout the body, the lymph nodes attack antigens and debris in the interstitial fluid and produce and circulate lymphocytes. The spleen acts as a filter to remove dead cells, debris, and foreign molecules from the blood. The liver filters the blood and plays a part in the production of specific immunoglobulins and other chemicals involved in the immune response.

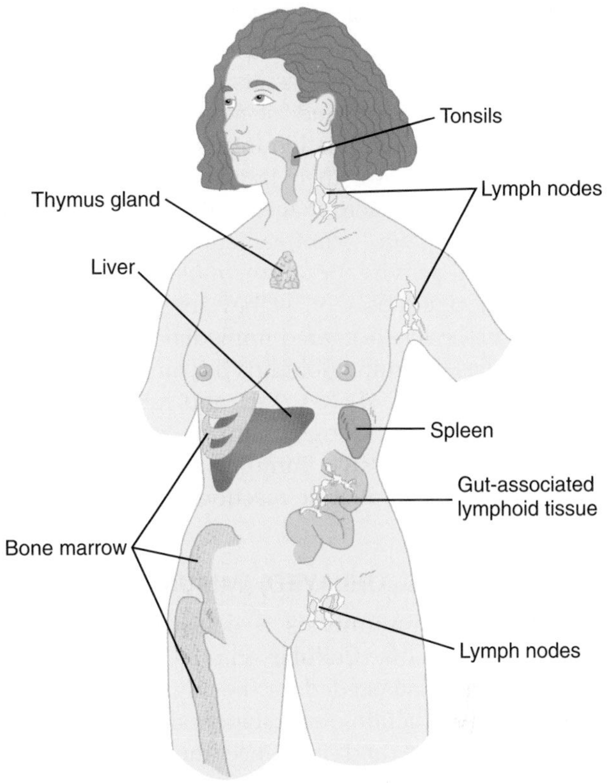

FIGURE 13-1 Organs involved in immunity. (From Black JM, Hawks JH: *Medical-surgical nursing: clinical management for positive outcomes*, ed 8, St. Louis, 2009, Saunders.)

NONSPECIFIC DEFENSES AGAINST INFECTION

Innate (natural) immunity is present at birth and consists of physical and chemical barriers to invasion of the body as well as processes and substances that protect and repair tissues and stimulate the body to fight off disease. Physical and chemical barriers, inflammation, and phagocytosis are nonspecific defenses against infection.

Other nonspecific defenses against infection that protect the body include complement, pyrogen, and interferon. Complement is a series of proteins that enhance the inflammatory process and the immune response. Chemotaxis, phagocytosis, and the activity of antibodies are stimulated by complement. Pyrogen (an eicosanoid) is a substance released in inflammation that causes body temperature to increase. Fever is thought to inhibit the growth of pathogens and slow enzymatic reactions that occur in infectious processes. Another substance, interferon, is produced in viral infections and acts to inhibit the replication of viruses. Interferon (a cytokine) also affects the function of T lymphocytes and is used in the treatment of selected malignancies. Eicosanoids and cytokines are discussed in Chapter 34.

SPECIFIC DEFENSES AGAINST INFECTION—IMMUNE RESPONSE

The immune response is the process by which antigens are recognized as foreign, processed, and destroyed. The two types of immune responses—antibody-mediated (immediate or humoral) and cell-mediated (delayed) responses—function interdependently to provide the immune response.

ANTIBODY-MEDIATED (IMMEDIATE) IMMUNITY

Antibody-mediated (humoral) immunity is immediate. This first-line defense involves B lymphocytes and the production of antibodies in response to specific antigens. The humoral immune response is initiated when an antigen binds to a special receptor on a B lymphocyte. This binding results in the production of antibodies that seek out and "stick to" specific antigens in the body. This combination forms antigen-antibody complexes, which are then targeted for cleanup by neutrophils and macrophages. Formation of these complexes activates complement and intensifies T-lymphocyte activity. Because circulating antibodies bind with antigens as soon as they are recognized, the chemical process is triggered immediately.

Antibodies (immunoglobulins [Ig]) are divided into five classes: IgG, IgM, IgA, IgE, and IgD. IgG is the most abundant immunoglobulin; it crosses the placenta to provide passive immunity for the newborn. IgE is important in allergic reactions and in parasitic infections.

CELL-MEDIATED (DELAYED) IMMUNITY

Cell-mediated immunity is a delayed response to injury or infection. Cellular immunity is delayed because of the time needed for the migration of T cells and for the production of substances that enhance the immune response and influence the destruction of antigens.

T cells include helper cells, suppressor cells, and killer cells. Helper T cells enhance humoral immunity; suppressor T cells help to "turn off" the humoral response. Disease may occur when the normal ratio of helper to suppressor cells (2:1) is altered. In acquired immunodeficiency syndrome (AIDS), for instance, the number of helper T cells is diminished. When the number of suppressor T cells is too high, infections, allergy, or immune disease develop. Killer T cells directly destroy antigens.

Cellular immunity fights most viral or bacterial infections and hinders the growth of malignant cells. This process also launches an attack on transplanted tissue or organs in the body.

INFLAMMATORY PROCESS

The inflammatory process is a series of cellular changes that signal the body's response to injury or infection. Although infection is a common cause of inflammation, this complex phenomenon may be caused by trauma from (1) physical agents (excessive sunlight, x-rays), (2) chemical stimuli (insect venom, other chemicals), and (3) biologic agents (bacteria, viruses).

The word **inflammation** means literally "the fire within." This descriptive phrase illustrates the five signs that indicate local inflammation: (1) rubor (redness), (2) calor (heat), (3) tumor (swelling), (4) dolor (pain), and (5) loss of function. Thinking about the appearance of an insect bite and recalling the redness, warmth, swelling, and pain that it produces would be helpful. These signs are the direct result of several related actions that occur when the inflammatory process is initiated. The actions involve cardiovascular (hemodynamic) changes, increased permeability of membranes, chemical mediators, and hormonal factors.

ACTIONS IN THE INFLAMMATORY PROCESS

Cardiovascular Changes

The first actions of the inflammatory process are the hemodynamic changes (changes in blood vessel diameter). The body initially responds to an injury or infection with dilation of the capillary bed. This dilation brings increased blood flow to the area. The increase in blood flow is responsible for the characteristic warmth and redness at the site of inflammation.

Increased Permeability

The second action is an increased capillary permeability (Fig. 13-2). After the increased blood flow brings leukocytes into the area, chemical mediators cause leukocytes to line the small blood vessel walls near the site of inflammation. This process is called *pavementing*. Gradually, these cells pass through the vessel walls and inhabit the inflamed area. These cells, largely neutrophils and monocytes, are drawn to the site of injury or infection, where they ingest and carry away bacteria and other foreign substances (phagocytosis) (Fig. 13-3). The permeability of these vessels causes protein-rich fluid to flow through the vessel walls into the interstitial space. Some red blood cells may pass through into this area as well. This collection of fluid is responsible for the swelling that is noted when the inflammation site is close to the surface of the skin. This swelling may also produce pain.

Chemical Mediators

The hemodynamic changes and vascular permeability occur with the help of several chemical mediators, including prostaglandins, histamine, and leukotrienes. These powerful substances are found in various body tissues and are liberated during the inflammatory process. Cytokines and eicosanoids, described in Chapter 34, cause blood and blood vessel changes. The kinin system produces bradykinin, which also mediates blood vessel dilation and permeability. It also produces pain, another classic sign of inflammation. In some severe allergic reactions, the inflammatory response is excessive. These reactions cause a massive release of histamine and other substances that produce marked vasodilation, vascular permeability, and smooth-muscle contraction. These cellular changes produce the classic signs of anaphylactic shock: hypotension, swelling, and bronchoconstriction.

Antiinflammation

Cortisol, a hormone produced by the adrenal cortex, is an antiinflammatory substance that slows the release of histamine, stabilizes lysosomal membranes, and prevents the influx of leukocytes. The end result of

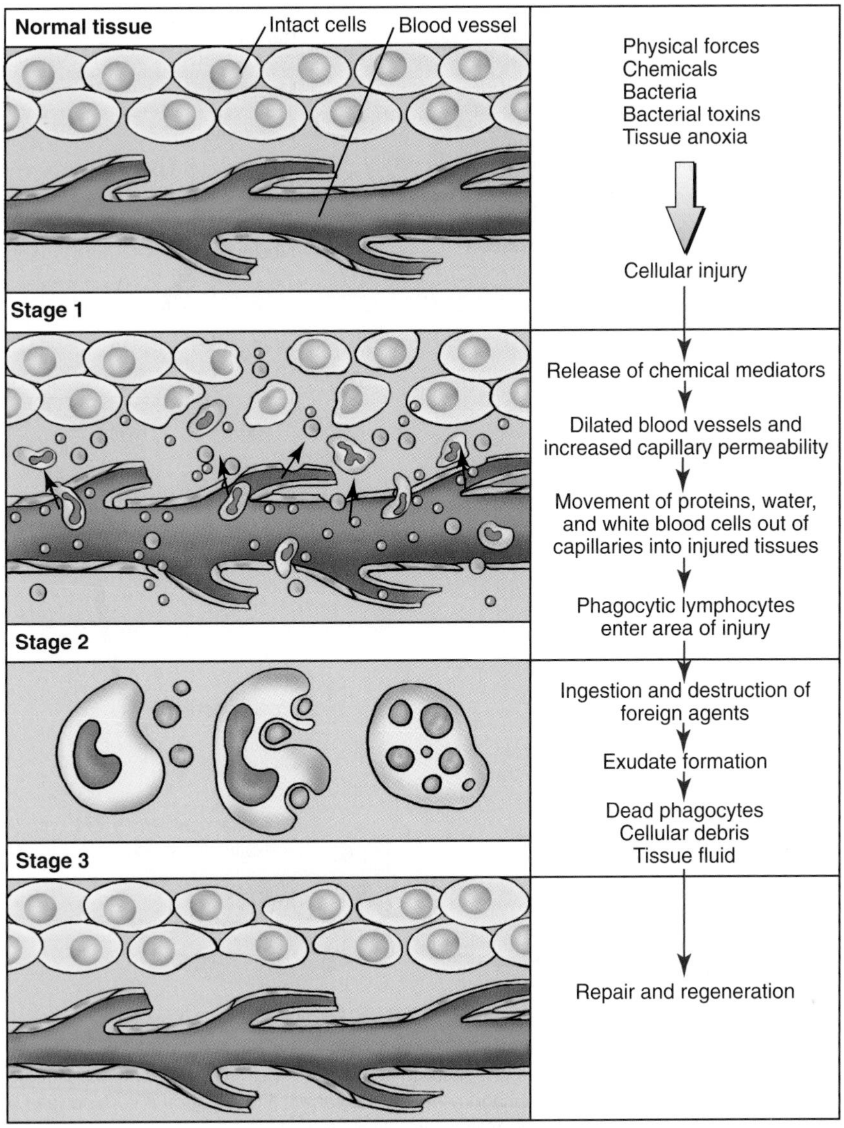

FIGURE 13-2 The inflammatory response after tissue injury. (From Monahan FD, Drake DT, Neighbors M, editors: *Medical-surgical nursing: foundations for clinical practice*, ed 2, Philadelphia, 1998, Saunders.)

these actions is to impede the inflammatory process. By limiting the inflammatory process, cortisol protects the body from the effects of excessive or prolonged inflammation. Drugs (e.g., corticosteroids) that mimic the action of cortisol are often used in the treatment of inflammatory conditions.

SIGNS AND SYMPTOMS OF INFLAMMATION

The signs and symptoms of inflammation vary, depending on whether the reaction is local or systemic. Local inflammation generally produces the classic signs of heat, swelling, redness, and pain, all of which result in loss of function.

Systemic inflammation produces somewhat different reactions. Swelling, redness, and local warmth may not be visible; however, signs of the effects of the chemical mediators may be recognized in other ways. Fever is a common sign of systemic inflammation, probably caused by pyrogens (fever-producing substances) or defense mechanisms that are liberated during phagocytosis, or by bacterial endotoxins, antigen-antibody complexes, and certain viruses. Other symptoms of systemic inflammation include headache, muscle aches, chills, and sweating.

Leukocytosis, a defensive reaction that provides abundant white blood cells for the inflammatory response, is another sign of systemic inflammation. If infection is not present, inflammatory leukocytosis disappears within a few hours.

WOUND HEALING

Repair and regeneration of tissue are set in motion from the very beginning of the inflammatory process. The speed at which this process takes place depends on the type of tissue injured, the severity of the wound, the presence of infection, and the health of the host. At the outset, macrophage cells are produced to clean up inflammatory debris. Fibroblasts begin the repair

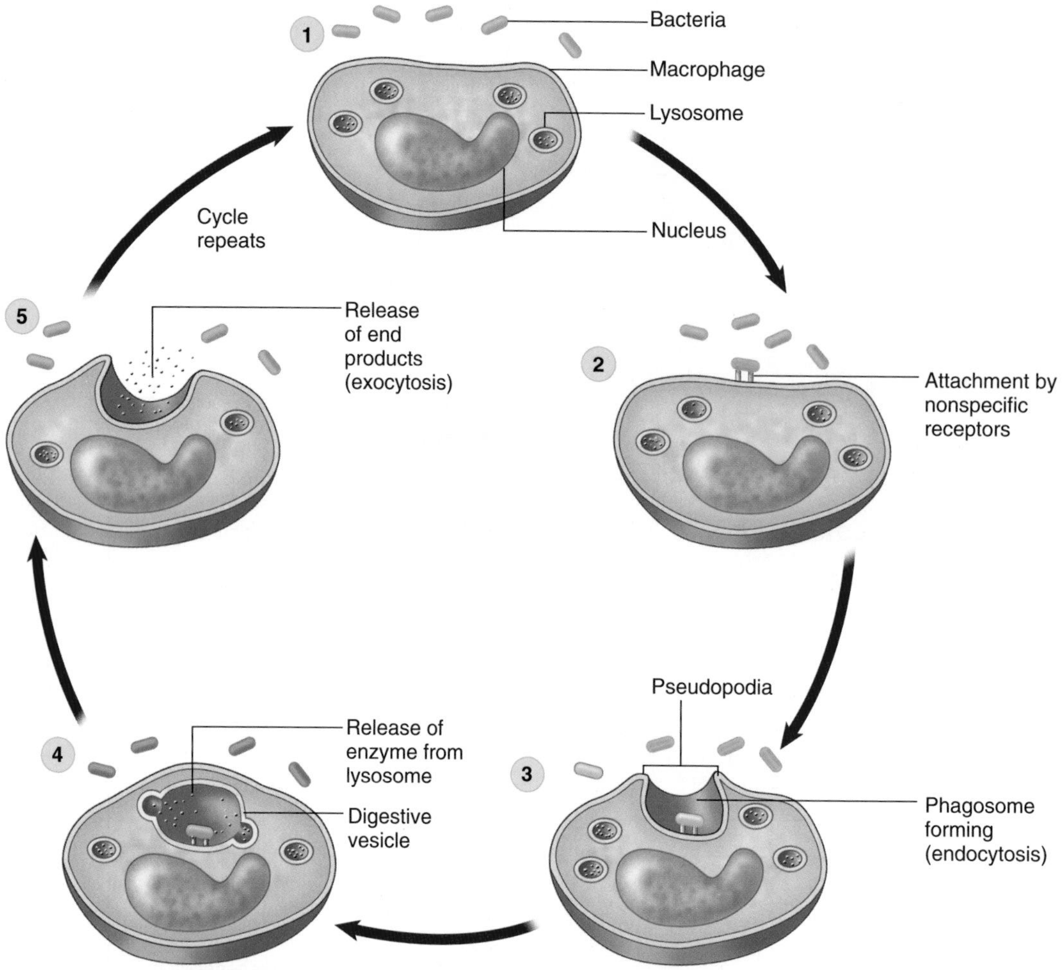

FIGURE 13-3 Phagocytosis. (1) Macrophages migrate to an inflammatory site by chemotaxis. (2) Bacteria attach to macrophages by nonspecific receptors. (3) A phagosome or phagocytic vacuole forms around the microorganisms. (4) Lysosomes attach to the phagosome and release their enzymes, which destroy the microorganisms (5) Breakdown products of phagocytosis are released. (From Patton KT, Thibodeau GA: *Anatomy & physiology*, ed 8, St. Louis, 2013, Mosby, Fig. 24-7, p. 752.)

process by laying down elastin and collagen at the edges of the wound; these substances gradually migrate to the base, forming granulation tissue. Epithelial cells migrate over the wound and under the scab (usually formed of dried blood and fibroblasts). After a few days, the scab falls off. Damaged cells are replaced by new cells of their own composition by the process of regeneration. Some tissue regenerates well whereas other tissue must undergo repair, which may involve the replacement of injured cells with connective tissue that will eventually create a scar. In fact, both types of tissue repair occur in most wounds.

The age and general health of the person affect how rapidly the regeneration and repair processes occur. The healing process can be delayed in the older person as a result of decreased tissue elasticity and decreased blood supply. Deficiencies of vitamin C, zinc, and other important vitamins and minerals can also delay the regeneration and repair processes.

A wound occasionally becomes infected or ulcerated, resulting in tissue loss. Granulation tissue and capillary buds form at the margins of the wound and eventually fill the wound with granulation tissue. The wound bed is sometimes too large for the granulation tissue to fill. In this case, the wound is cleaned and debrided in an effort to enhance healing. The term *delayed primary closure* is used if the wound is sutured closed after the infection has resolved.

INFECTION

Infection is a process involving the invasion of body tissues by microorganisms, the multiplication of the invading organisms, and the subsequent damage of tissue. Infection is different from inflammation in that inflammation is a nonspecific reaction by the body to tissue injury whereas infection refers to a specific process that causes tissue injury. Infection nearly always results in inflammation but inflammation may be caused by processes other than infection. Inflammation precedes infection. Infection is usually the end result of the invasion by organisms. Infection may be caused by a wide variety of microorganisms.

INFECTIOUS AGENTS

The major infectious agents are bacteria, viruses, fungi, protozoa, rickettsiae, and helminths. A limited number of animal and human diseases are caused by prions.

Bacteria

Bacteria are one-celled microorganisms capable of multiplying rapidly within a susceptible host. Bacteria are classified by shape, cluster pattern, whether or not they need oxygen, and their ability to take up and retain stains. Bacteria may be round or rod shaped. Round bacteria are called *cocci*; they are further classified according to how they group or cluster together. Groups of two are called *diplococci* and clusters of cocci are called *staphylococci*. Chains of these microorganisms are called *streptococci*. Rod-shaped organisms, called *bacilli*, can be obligate aerobes or facultative anaerobes.

Bacteria may also be classified according to their ability to grow in the presence of oxygen. Those that grow in the presence of oxygen are classified as *aerobes*; those that do not grow in the presence of oxygen are labeled *anaerobes*.

Bacteria are classified as either gram positive or gram negative, depending on their ability to take up and retain a violet-colored solution called Gram stain. Gram-positive bacteria have a thick covering that retains the stain whereas gram-negative bacteria can be decolorized and counterstained pink. The acid-fast stain is used to identify bacteria such as *Mycobacterium tuberculosis*. Immunofluorescent stains reveal complexes composed of various antigens (bacteria, viruses, fungi, protozoa) and antibodies when exposed to ultraviolet light.

These classifications have a very important purpose. Each classification highlights a characteristic of a microorganism that is considered in the design of an antimicrobial drug to kill or retard the growth of the organism. For example, antimicrobials synthesized to fight gram-positive microorganisms interfere with the formation of that covering, causing the cell wall to be destroyed. Other antimicrobials used to treat aerobic bacteria rely on the ability of the bacterial cell to take up oxygen to produce its effects.

Viruses

Viruses are very small microorganisms that cause significant morbidity (disease) in humans. Viruses cannot be seen with ordinary microscopes but are visible with electron microscopy. They contain a strand of *either* ribonucleic acid (RNA) or deoxyribonucleic acid (DNA), which determines whether they are classified as either DNA or RNA viruses. Viruses are surrounded by a protein capsule but have no cell wall. To replicate, they depend on the resources of the host cell. Viruses cause a variety of illnesses, including the common cold, measles, chickenpox, and several forms of hepatitis. The RNA virus that causes human immunodeficiency virus (HIV) is a retrovirus.

Because replication of the virus occurs within the host cell, killing the virus without harming the host cell is seldom possible. This property explains the relatively few antiviral drugs that are available. Current antiviral and antiretroviral drugs suppress viral reproduction or growth so that they decrease the severity or duration of the infection but they are not curative. Antibiotics do not affect viruses. Prevention (immunizations, hygiene) is still the best way to combat viral illness.

Fungi

Fungi are vegetable-like organisms that exist by feeding on organic matter. Mushrooms and molds are examples of fungal organisms. A few species of fungi are capable of producing disease in humans. Ringworm (tinea corporis) and athlete's foot (tinea pedis) are two examples. Many of these infections are superficial skin infections that rarely produce serious illness. However, systemic fungal infections caused by *Cryptococcus* and *Aspergillus* species can be life-threatening. Patients who have conditions that affect their immune system (e.g., those infected with HIV) are at especially high risk of acquiring opportunistic fungal infections. Fungal infections are called *mycoses*. Because fungi tend to form spores that are resistant to many antiseptics and disinfectants, they are difficult to treat. Both systemic and topical antimycotic drugs are used to treat fungal infections.

Protozoa

Protozoa make up a large group of one-celled organisms. Ones that produce disease in humans include the *Plasmodium* species (malaria), *Entamoeba histolytica* (amoebic dysentery), *Giardia lamblia* (giardiasis, characterized by diarrhea), and *Trypanosoma brucei gambiense* (sleeping sickness). Infections are often spread by food or water that is contaminated by human or animal feces. *Pneumocystis jiroveci* is another protozoal infection that was relatively rare before the onset of the HIV/AIDS epidemic. Lowered immunity with HIV infection is responsible for the dramatic rise in pneumocystic pneumonia.

Rickettsiae

Rickettsiae are microorganisms that are between bacteria and viruses in size. They may appear as rods, cocci, or pleomorphic (varied) shapes. These organisms multiply in the cells of animal hosts, such as rats and squirrels, and are transmitted to humans through the bites of fleas and ticks. Diseases produced by these microorganisms include Rocky Mountain spotted fever and typhus. Diseases caused by *rickettsiae* tend to be more prevalent in areas in which sanitation is poor and rodent and insect populations are not well controlled.

Helminths

Helminths are worms. These parasites are found in soil and water and are generally transmitted from hand to mouth. Infections occur commonly in the gastrointestinal tract and may produce mild abdominal pain and bloating, or they may be asymptomatic. Pinworms are most common, especially in children, and often produce rectal irritation. Tapeworms can be found in the gastrointestinal tract. Weight loss and abdominal pain and bloating may be early signs and symptoms. Hookworms often enter an individual through the soles of the feet and migrate throughout the body, including to the heart and the lungs. Most people infected may have no symptoms. Others may have respiratory symptoms during the migration of the hookworm through the lungs. Others may have gastrointestinal symptoms and anemia due to blood loss when the hookworm attaches to the intestinal wall.

Prions

A prion is an infectious agent composed of protein in a misfolded form. It does not contain any nucleic acids (either RNA or DNA). Although not actually alive, a prion can reproduce by hijacking the functions of living cells. Once transmitted, it can cause brain damage and progressive degenerative diseases of the nervous system. An example of a prion disease in humans is Creutzfeldt-Jakob disease. Bovine spongiform encephalopathy ("mad cow" disease) primarily affects cattle but has been transmitted to humans. Prions typically have a very long incubation period but advance rapidly once the infection becomes active. Prions are not understood as well as diseases caused by other agents. Prions are extremely resistant to standard methods of disinfection.

TRANSMISSION OF INFECTION

Infection is possible only when several factors are present. These factors must occur in sequence for human infectious disease to occur. They include (1) a causative agent, (2) a reservoir, (3) a portal of exit, (4) a mode of transfer, (5) a portal of entry, and (6) a susceptible host. This sequence is known as the *chain of infection*.

Causative Agent

Causative agents are the microorganisms (bacteria, viruses, protozoa, etc.) that are present in sufficient number and virulence to damage human tissue.

Reservoir

Areas in which organisms can pool and reproduce are called *reservoirs*. Reservoirs may be human or animal tissues, as well as any substance such as soil or animal feces, in which microorganisms can pool and multiply. When a reservoir of microorganisms occurs in the tissues of a human, the human is called a *host*.

Portal of Exit

Portal of exit refers to the route by which the infectious agent leaves one host and travels to another. A common route is the gastrointestinal tract, through which bacteria or viruses may escape an infected host. The nose and mouth also are common portals of exit for organisms spread by droplet **contamination** through sneezing or coughing. Fecal-oral transmission also occurs; hepatitis A virus is acquired by ingesting the virus in water contaminated with feces or by direct fecal-oral transmission.

Mode of Transfer

Mode of transfer refers to the means by which a microorganism is transported to a host. Person-to-person transfer may take place in either a direct or an indirect manner. *Direct contact* refers to the transfer of microorganisms directly, as occurs in sexually transmitted infections. *Indirect contact* occurs when pathogens are spread through droplets expelled during a sneeze or a cough or through inanimate objects (e.g., eating utensils on which microorganisms can be transported [fomites]).

Common vehicle transmission occurs when water, food, blood, or air currents contaminated with a pathogen are shared by many people. Air currents, for example, are often the common vehicle for transmission of *Legionella*, the organism responsible for Legionnaires' disease. Vector transmission occurs when microorganisms are transported into a host by a living organism such as a fly or mosquito. Fomites are any items that have been touched or cross-contaminated by the host, such as bed linen, side rails, or hygiene items.

Portal of Entry

Portals of entry are the doorways or pathways into the host. Influenza and cold viruses often enter the body through the mucous membranes of the nose and mouth. Other portals of entry often accessed by bacteria are the gastrointestinal tract and the urethra. Open wounds, intravenous access devices, urinary catheters, and drains also can be portals of entry for bacteria.

Susceptible Host

To produce tissue damage, microorganisms must become implanted in a susceptible host. Not all people exposed to disease-producing microorganisms become ill. Populations adequately immunized against rubella, for example, are not susceptible to measles. Similarly, individuals who have had chickenpox have developed immunity to the virus and do not become ill if exposed a second time.

SIGNS AND SYMPTOMS OF INFECTION

Once an individual becomes infected with a pathogen, symptoms may or may not be apparent. In many instances, a period of subclinical infection or an incubation period occurs during which few, if any, symptoms are present. During this period, asymptomatic persons may be more contagious than those who are exhibiting symptoms. This is especially the case with people infected with such viruses as measles and many cold viruses. Persons recently infected with HIV may feel well but are highly contagious. Persons who have illnesses such as tuberculosis may remain relatively well. Still other persons may remain contagious throughout their convalescence. Asymptomatic carriers, such as patients recovering from typhoid, may go back to their communities and unknowingly infect others.

Signs and symptoms of *localized infections*, such as bacterial infection of a wound, are essentially the symptoms of inflammation: redness, pain, warmth, and swelling. In addition, pus may form.

Patients with *generalized infections* may not show all of the signs that are apparent with localized infections. Redness, for example, may not be visible. Pain may be moderate to severe, depending on the location of the infection. Swelling of infected tissues may produce symptoms ranging from mild to severe, depending on its location. Swelling in a large organ, such as the liver, may produce a dull ache whereas swelling in a small structure, such as an infected appendix, may produce severe discomfort. Warmth is generally expressed as fever in a generalized infection as pyrogens are produced as part of the inflammatory process. Other symptoms that often are present in generalized infections include malaise, anorexia, and prostration.

In some cases, infections in the extremities such as the hands or feet exhibit a faint red line as infection extends upward along the lymphatic channels. Lymph nodes in this chain also are swollen and tender. Prompt antimicrobial treatment is necessary in these cases.

TYPES OF INFECTIONS

Two types of infections are (1) community-acquired and (2) health care–associated infections.

Community-Acquired Infections

Community-acquired infections are acquired in day-to-day contact with the public. Many viral infections are pervasive in society and occur at predictable times of the year. Childhood illnesses are common in September, when children take to school all of the new viruses to which they were exposed during the summer. This sharing of microorganisms is made easier when 20 to 40 children occupy the same classroom. During the fall and winter, people share more indoor activities thus increasing the likelihood that they will share microorganisms with one another.

Poverty, low immunization rates, overcrowding, unsanitary living conditions, and resistant strains of pathogens are at least partially responsible for the increase in infectious diseases that were once well controlled. The resurgence of tuberculosis is an example. This increase was attributed to poverty, the HIV/AIDS epidemic, an increase in the number of infected immigrants, declining public health resources, and the emergence of strains of bacteria that are resistant to multiple drugs. Effective treatment now requires at least two drugs to which a particular tuberculosis bacillus is susceptible.

Foodborne illness is a common community-acquired infectious disease. It is more common in the summer, when picnics and hot weather bring the possibility of food poisoning from *Staphylococcus* and *Salmonella* organisms. Periodic outbreaks of hepatitis A are possible at any time of the year and are the result of poor hygiene by food handlers.

Sexually transmitted infections such as gonorrhea, syphilis, and HIV also are spread in the community. These diseases and many others are required to be reported to public health authorities. The reports are important because they facilitate disease control, make possible the evaluation of disease control programs, and keep track of emerging disease patterns.

Certain communicable diseases must be reported to state health departments. Local laws vary regarding which diseases must be reported. A list of reportable diseases is given in Box 13-1.

Prevention and Control. Prevention and control of **communicable diseases** are possible in several ways. Some childhood infectious diseases can be prevented by ensuring that childhood immunizations are completed. Indifference toward childhood immunizations, as well as parental fear about side effects of vaccination, false information, and belief in alternative medicine, has resulted in the reemergence of several childhood diseases that were once well controlled. Although state laws that require certain immunizations before a child starts school have improved the picture somewhat, large groups of children from 2 to 5 years of age remain susceptible to serious illness. In addition, repeat vaccinations of older schoolchildren may be required to prevent illnesses such as measles. Adult immunizations also help to prevent and control communicable diseases. Immunization schedules for children and adults are available at the Centers for Disease Control and Prevention (CDC) website: www.cdc.gov/vaccines/schedules/.

Although the solution to this problem defies easy answers, at least part of the problem are barriers in the health care system that result in missed opportunities to immunize individuals who are most susceptible. Barriers include such factors as rigid fee schedules; giving immunizations only during regular working hours, Monday through Friday; and giving immunizations only at official, fixed sites such as health departments. Health professionals should take advantage of all possible opportunities to immunize. Schools, primary care providers' offices, shopping

Box 13-1 CDC's Nationally Notifiable and Reportable Diseases, 2014*

Anaplasmosis	Novel influenza A virus infection
Anthrax	Paralytic poliomyelitis
Babesiosis	Pertussis
Botulism	Plague
Brucellosis	Poliovirus infection, nonparalytic
Cancer	Psittacosis (ornithosis)
Chancroid	Q fever
Chlamydia trachomatis infection	Rabies
Coccidiomycosis	Rickettsiosis, spotted fever
Cryptosporidiosis	Rubella (German measles)
Cyclosporiasis	Salmonellosis
Dengue fever	Severe acute respiratory syndrome (SARS)–associated Coronavirus diseases (SARS-CoV)
Dengue virus infections	Shiga toxin-producing *Escherichia coli* (STEC)
Diphtheria	Shigellosis
Ehrlichiosis/anaplasmosis	Silicosis
Escherichia coli, Shiga toxin-producing (STEC)	Smallpox
Foodborne disease outbreaks	Staphylococcus aureus infection
Giardiasis	Streptococcal toxic-shock syndrome
Gonorrhea	*Streptococcus pneumoniae*
Haemophilus influenzae, invasive disease	Syphilis
Hansen disease (leprosy)	Tetanus
Hantavirus pulmonary syndrome	Toxic shock syndrome
Hemolytic uremic syndrome postdiarrheal	Trichinellosis
Hepatitis (all types)	Tuberculosis
HIV infection	Tularemia
Influenza-associated mortality, pediatric	Typhoid fever
Lead, exposure screening test result	Varicella (if hospitalized)
Legionellosis	Varicella (chickenpox)
Leptospirosis	Vibrio cholerae infection (cholera)
Listeriosis	Vibriosis (non-cholera *Vibrio* species infections)
Lyme disease	Viral hemorrhagic fevers
Malaria	Waterborne disease outbreaks
Measles (rubeola)	Yellow fever
Meningococcal disease (*Neisseria meningitides*)	
Mumps	

Adapted from CDC: *Protocol for PublicHealth Agencies to Notify CDC about the Occurrence of Nationally Notifiable Conditions, 2014:* http://wwwn.cdc.gov/nndss/document/NNC_2014_Notification_Requirements_By_Condition.pdf. Accessed July 8, 2014.
CDC, Centers for Disease Control and Prevention.
*Reportable diseases vary among countries and states. Diseases listed have been designated by the Council of State and Territorial Epidemiologists as nationally notifiable and should be reported to the CDC on a regular basis.

malls, and neighborhood health fairs are places where large numbers of children and parents may present themselves for immunization.

Transmission of infectious agents can be interrupted in several ways. First, education of food handlers regarding the importance of hand washing and proper food handling and refrigeration techniques decreases the spread of foodborne illness. Second, diseases such as tuberculosis can be detected through screening and treated early to prevent their spread. Isolation separates the infected individual from the public, thereby breaking the chain of infection. Other examples of measures aimed at interrupting transmission are control of vectors (spraying for mosquitos), administration of antimicrobials to children exposed to *Neisseria* meningitis, and the prompt treatment of streptococcal pharyngitis (strep throat). Sanitation of water supplies helps to prevent the occurrence of waterborne diseases. Cooking meat, eggs, and poultry until well done kills bacteria that can cause serious illness and, in some cases, death.

Personal measures to control the spread of communicable disease include proper hygiene, especially hand washing, and the use of personal barriers such as condoms. Deciding to stay home when symptoms of an infectious disease are present also can help to break the chain of infection.

Health Care–Associated Infections

Health care–associated infections (HAIs) were previously called nosocomial infections. HAIs are an important cause of increased morbidity, prolonged hospitalization, and higher health care costs. These infections occur within a health care facility and may affect both the patient and the health care worker. HAIs are much more serious than those acquired in the community because strains of bacteria in the hospital are usually more virulent and often are resistant to antimicrobials. In addition, the patient's resistance is already compromised from the disorder that led to hospitalization. Recent changes in health care in the United States have seen Medicare and other insurance companies not reimbursing institutions for HAIs such as catheter-associated urinary tract infection and surgical site infections.

A growing number of pathogenic bacteria that are no longer susceptible to previously effective antimicrobials are found in hospital patients. Vancomycin-resistant *Enterococcus* (VRE) is one example; the incidence of vancomycin resistance in patients with health care–associated enterococcal infection is rapidly increasing. The CDC has emphasized the importance of the careful use of antimicrobials and infection prevention and control measures in preventing the spread of VRE. In health care agencies where antimicrobials may be overused or misused, an increase in bacterial resistance is found. Antimicrobials alter the body's normal flora so that resistant strains of enterococci replace susceptible strains.

Bacteria employ a variety of mechanisms to develop resistant strains. Bacterial cells normally develop mutations to survive. Antimicrobials suppress normal forms of the bacteria but the mutations often survive. Chromosomal mutation also permits some bacteria to produce enzymes that deactivate the antimicrobial. Some bacteria are able to alter their metabolic cycles to prevent destruction by antimicrobials. Finally, mutation alters bacterial cell membranes, making antimicrobial penetration more difficult. Newer antimicrobials are then developed to counteract the most resistant strains. As these antimicrobials in turn become more frequently used, resistance again develops and the cycle is repeated.

Microorganisms that are resistant to one or more classes of antimicrobial agents are called **multidrug-resistant organisms (MDROs)**. Examples include methicillin-resistant *Staphylococcus aureus* (MRSA), VRE, some gram-negative bacilli such as *Escherichia coli* and *Klebsiella pneumoniae*, *Acinetobacter baumannii*, and others. Especially among persons with poor resistance, these organisms can produce life-threatening infections.

General practices that can help to impede the development of resistant pathogens include vaccinations for communicable diseases and appropriate use of antimicrobial drugs. Antimicrobials should be reserved for serious bacterial infections. The most appropriate antimicrobial can be selected if based on laboratory studies of infected specimens (wound drainage, body fluids such as urine or blood). Culture and sensitivity tests identify the microorganism and the antimicrobial most likely to be effective. This practice allows the most appropriate therapy to be administered and delays the onset of resistant strains. Efforts are also made to limit the use of antimicrobials that are effective against resistant strains. This practice provides fewer opportunities for the development of strains resistant to the drug. Tables 13-1 and 13-2 present the CDC steps to prevent antimicrobial resistance among hospitalized adults, long-term care residents, and surgical patients.

HAIs are more serious for the hospitalized patient who may have low resistance. These infectious organisms also have been exposed to many antimicrobials so they are more likely to resist therapy. Patients with compromised immune systems are much more susceptible to hospital-acquired infections. These groups include patients with AIDS and patients with cancer who are receiving chemotherapy. Common sites for HAIs in hospitalized patients include surgical wounds, the urinary tract, and the respiratory tract. Patients who have an indwelling urinary catheter are at risk for urinary tract infection. The risk for this infection can be reduced by using proper techniques for catheter insertion and care. Health care workers are also at risk for HAIs. Hepatitis B, for example, may be transmitted through needle punctures. Small, open wounds on the upper extremities may come in contact with resistant strains of *Staphylococcus* or *Pseudomonas* and become infected. In addition, health care workers and patients have developed Legionnaires ' disease when *Legionella* was spread through the facility on air currents from air conditioning systems that became contaminated with infected water. CDC recommendations to prevent transmission of MDROs in health care settings are summarized in Box 13-2.

Iatrogenic infections are caused by the treatment given the patient. For example, iatrogenic infections may be caused by giving immunosuppressive drugs

Table 13-1 12 Steps to Prevent Antimicrobial Resistance: Hospitalized Patients

STRATEGIES	STEPS
Prevent infection	1. Vaccinate 2. Get the catheters out
Diagnose and treat effectively	3. Target the pathogen 4. Access the experts
Use antimicrobials wisely	5. Practice antimicrobial control 6. Use local data 7. Treat infection, not contamination 8. Treat infection, not colonization 9. Know when to say "no" to vanco 10. Stop treatment when infection is cured or unlikely
Prevent transmission	11. Isolate the pathogen 12. Contain the contagion

Data from CDC: *CDC campaign to prevent antimicrobial resistance in healthcare settings*, 2012: www.cdc.gov/getsmart/healthcare/. Accessed July 10, 2013.
CDC, Centers for Disease Control and Prevention; *vanco*, vancomycin.

Table 13-2 Nursing Considerations Related to CDC Recommendations to Prevent Antimicrobial Resistance in Health Care Settings

HOSPITALIZED ADULTS	LONG-TERM CARE RESIDENTS	SURGICAL PATIENTS
Prevent Infection		
1. Encourage patients to have an annual influenza vaccination. 2. Use proper technique for catheter insertion and care.	1. Encourage patients to have a pneumococcal vaccination (usually a one-time vaccination) as well as an annual influenza vaccination. 2. Prevent aspiration and pressure ulcers. 3. Promote good hydration. 4. Use proper technique for catheter insertion and care.	1. Monitor blood glucose and body temperature. 2. Prepare skin with appropriate antiseptic agent and hair removal technique. 3. Use proper technique for insertion and care, such as with urinary catheters and drains. 4. Elevate head of bed 30 degrees or as ordered to reduce risk of health care–associated pneumonia. 5. Avoid contamination of respiratory equipment and medications.
Diagnose and Treat Infection Effectively		
1. Carefully collect specimens for culture to prevent contamination. 2. Consult the agency protocol and infection preventionist for proper precautions and care.	1. Carefully collect specimens for culture to prevent contamination. 2. Promptly report diarrhea in patients on antimicrobials. Cause may be *Clostridium difficile.* 3. Consult the agency protocol and infection preventionist for proper precautions and care. 4. See patient's previous laboratory studies for history of colonization or infection.	1. Carefully collect specimens for culture to prevent contamination. 2. Administer antimicrobials on schedule. 3. Consult the agency protocol and infection preventionist for proper precautions and care as needed.
Use Antimicrobials Wisely		
1. Teach patients that antimicrobials are not always necessary or appropriate for infections. 2. When antimicrobials are prescribed, explain why the entire course should be completed.	1. Question long-term antimicrobial therapy. 2. Document signs and symptoms of infection.	1. Administer preoperative prophylactic antimicrobials within 1 hour before incision is made as ordered.
Prevent Transmission		
1. Use Standard Infection Prevention and Control Precautions for all. 2. Use Airborne, Droplet, and Contact Precautions as needed. 3. Explain precautions to patients, nursing assistants, and visitors. 4. Practice hand hygiene. 5. Stay home when *you* are sick.	1. Use Standard Infection Prevention and Control Precautions for all. 2. Follow specific precautions for patients with multidrug-resistant organisms. 3. Use Airborne, Droplet, and Contact Precautions as needed. 4. Explain precautions to patients, nursing assistants, and visitors. 5. Practice hand hygiene. 6. Stay home when *you* are sick.	1. Use Standard Infection Prevention and Control Precautions for all. 2. Use Airborne, Droplet, and Contact Precautions as needed. 3. Practice hand hygiene. 4. Do not wear artificial nails, tips, wraps, or nail jewelry. Keep nails no longer than ¼ inch from fingertips.

Adapted from CDC: *CDC campaign to prevent antimicrobial resistance in healthcare settings*, 2012: www.cdc.gov/getsmart/healthcare/. Accessed July 10, 2013.
CDC, Centers for Disease Control and Prevention.

to prevent rejection of a transplanted organ, resulting in an infection. Another form of iatrogenic infection can be caused by the treatment of a primary infection. Antimicrobial therapy for one microorganism can permit the overgrowth of a second microorganism that can also cause illness. The term for this process is *superinfection.* It is especially common with treatment using broad-spectrum antimicrobials. An example of this phenomenon is the occurrence of a bowel infection after treatment with oral broad-spectrum antimicrobials. The organism *Clostridium difficile* resides in the gastrointestinal tract of many individuals. It is kept in check by the normal bacterial flora of the gastrointestinal tract. Broad-spectrum antimicrobials can kill enough of the normal flora to allow *C. difficile* to grow out of control, producing severe colitis and diarrhea.

CARE OF PATIENTS WITH INFECTION

Just as controls must be instituted to stop the spread of infections acquired in the community, so must a

Box 13-2 Infection Prevention and Control Precautions to Prevent Transmission of MDROs in Health Care Settings

- Follow Standard Precautions (SP) in all health care settings.
- Use of Contact Precautions (CP):
  - In acute care settings, implement CP for all patients known to be colonized or infected with target MDROs.
  - In long-term care facilities, consider the individual patient's clinical situation and facility resources in deciding whether to implement CP. Consult with the infection preventionist for expert direction.
  - In ambulatory and home care settings, follow SP.
- Masks are not recommended for routine use to prevent transmission of MDROs from patients to health care workers. Use masks according to SP when performing splash-generating procedures, when caring for a patient with an open tracheostomy with potential for projectile secretions, and when evidence has been found for transmission from heavily colonized sources (e.g., burn wound).
- Patient placement in hospitals and long-term care facilities:
  - When single-patient rooms are available, assign priority for these rooms to patients with known or suspected MDRO colonization or infection.
  - Give highest priority to specific patients who have conditions that may facilitate transmission (e.g., uncontained secretions or excretions).
  - When single-patient rooms are not available, cohort patients with the same MDRO in the same room or same patient care area.
  - When possible, cohort staff to minimize the spread of MDROs among patients.

Data from CDC: *CDC management of multidrug-resistant organisms in healthcare settings, 2006*: www.cdc.gov/hicpac/mdro/mdro_0.html. Accessed July 10, 2013.
CDC, Centers for Disease Control and Prevention; *MDRO*, multidrug-resistant organism.

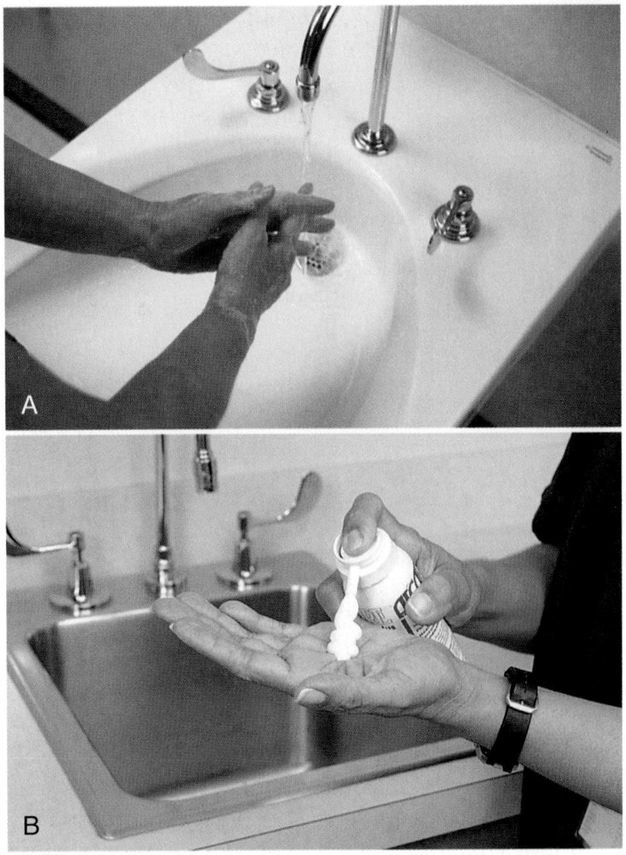

FIGURE 13-4 Hand hygiene is the most basic and effective way to prevent cross-contamination. **A,** Basic hand washing. **B,** Waterless antiseptic. (From Potter PA, Perry AG, editors: *Fundamentals of nursing*, ed 6, St. Louis, 2005, Mosby.)

process be put in place to keep hospitalized patients from acquiring HAIs. The key to preventing the spread of infection is effective medical and surgical asepsis.

MEDICAL ASEPSIS

Medical asepsis means limiting the spread of microorganisms as much as possible. This practice is often called *clean technique* and refers to practices such as changing bed linen, sanitizing bedpans, using individual medication cups for each patient and for each medication administration, and frequent hand hygiene.

Hand Hygiene

Soiled hands are the primary mode of transmission of HAIs. Although everyone agrees in principle with the need for frequent hand hygiene, problems arise when nurses are busy. For example, suppose that a nurse is passing medications and is asked by a patient with pulmonary secretions to hand her the box of tissues. At the same time, the patient's roommate asks the nurse to fill her water glass. After performing this task, the nurse hurries out of the room to pass medications to other patients. This example illustrates how a chain of infection begins. Unless the nurse interrupts the chain with effective hand hygiene, infection is easily spread from one patient to another.

The most basic and effective method of preventing cross-contamination is hand hygiene, which includes hand washing with soap and water, use of an alcohol-based waterless antiseptic, or a surgical scrub. Good hand washing technique includes the use of running water, soap, and friction. The lathered hands should be rubbed together for at least 15 seconds and longer if the nurse works in a high-risk area. The use of antimicrobial soaps is also recommended when working with patients who are more susceptible to infection, such as premature infants or immunocompromised patients. A waterless antiseptic is dispensed into one palm and then the hands are rubbed together to cover all surfaces until the hands are dry. The antiseptic is appropriate for use before and after patient contact. When hands are visibly soiled, they should be washed thoroughly with soap and water (Fig. 13-4). The surgical scrub is reserved for assisting with operative procedures (Fig. 13-5).

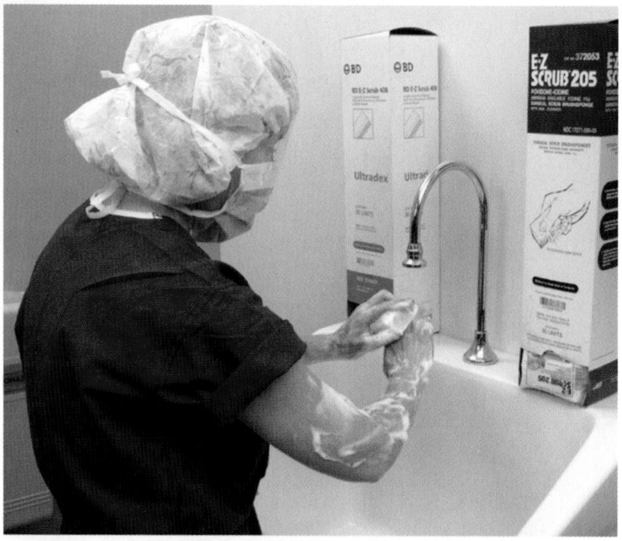

FIGURE 13-5 The surgical scrub uses a topical antiinfective cleanser, takes longer, and is performed in a specific sequence that is different from basic hand washing. (From Perry AG, Potter PA: *Fundamentals of nursing*, ed 8, St. Louis, 2013, Mosby, step 10b, p. 433.)

SURGICAL ASEPSIS

Surgical asepsis, or *sterile technique*, refers to the elimination of microorganisms from any object that comes in contact with the patient. This practice includes care techniques that prevent unsterile surfaces from coming in contact with the patient, such as during surgery or dressing changes.

STANDARD PRECAUTIONS

A set of infection prevention and control guidelines has been developed for hospitals and other health care agencies by the Hospital Infection Control Practices Advisory Committee (HICPAC) and the CDC. Previously the terms *Universal Precautions, Body Substance Isolation Precautions*, and *Disease-Specific Isolation Precautions* were in use. The current guidelines, called *Standard Precautions*, combine the major features of Universal Precautions and Body Substance Isolation Precautions. Standard Precautions are used for the care of all patients in hospitals regardless of their health or medical status. *Transmission-Based Precautions* are disease-specific isolation techniques that are implemented to prevent the spread to others within the agency.

Use Standard Precautions when you perform procedures in which you will have contact with a patient's blood, body fluids, secretions (except sweat), excretions, broken skin, and mucous membranes. In addition, use Standard Precautions when you have contact with materials that are soiled or contaminated with body fluids or blood. Use Standard Precautions with all patients, no matter what their diagnosis or infectious status may be. Guidelines for the use of Standard Precautions are listed in Box 13-3.

Some guidelines under Standard Precautions address specific situations. These precautions are guidelines for Respiratory Hygiene/Cough Etiquette, safe injection practices, and use of masks for insertion of catheters or injections by way of lumbar puncture procedures. Whereas the original Standard Precautions focused on protection of the health care worker, these additional areas focus on patient protection.

Respiratory Hygiene/Cough Etiquette emphasizes education of staff, patients, and visitors to cover the mouth and nose with tissues when coughing, dispose of used tissues promptly, wash the hands after contact with respiratory secretions, and maintain a distance greater than 3 feet from a person who is coughing. Health care providers should wear a mask when giving direct care to patients with a respiratory infection. Health care providers with a respiratory infection should avoid direct patient contact; if unavoidable, the provider should wear a mask. Key points from Safe Injection Practices are noted in Table 13-3.

Box 13-3 Guidelines for Use of Standard Precautions

These precautions are to be used for the care of all patients.

Wear gloves when touching blood, body fluids, secretions, and contaminated objects. Put on clean gloves before touching mucous membranes and nonintact skin.

Wash hands immediately after touching blood, body fluids, secretions, excretions, and contaminated objects, even if gloves were worn.

Wash hands between tasks and procedures on the same patient to prevent cross-contamination of different body sites.

Change gloves after each patient contact, before touching noncontaminated items and environmental surfaces. If patient is allergic to latex, use only nonlatex gloves.

Wear masks, eye protection, or face shields to protect mucous membranes of the eyes, nose, and mouth during procedures that are likely to generate splashes of blood, body fluids, secretions, or excretions.

Wear gowns during procedures that are likely to result in splashes of blood, body fluids, secretions, or excretions.

Handle patient care equipment soiled with blood, body fluids, secretions, and excretions so that skin and mucous membrane exposures, contamination of clothing, and transfer of microorganisms to other settings are prevented.

Place needles and sharp instruments in puncture-resistant containers for disposal to prevent injuries from needles or other sharp items. Do not recap or bend needles or remove them from the syringe.

Perform mouth-to-mouth resuscitation using mouthpieces or other ventilation devices.

Data from CDC: *CDC guidelines for isolation precautions preventing transmission of infectious agents in healthcare settings, 2007*: www.cdc.gov/hicpac/pdf/isolation/Isolation2007.pdf. Accessed July 10, 2013.
CDC, Centers for Disease Control and Prevention.

Table 13-3 Safe Injection Practices

DOs	DON'Ts
• Use aseptic technique when handling sterile injection equipment. • Discard needles, syringes, and cannulas after a single use. • When possible, use single-dose vials for parenteral medications. • If a multidose vial must be used, use sterile equipment (needle/cannula, syringe) every time a dose is accessed. • Discard any multidose vial or injection equipment if sterility is questionable.	• Do not reuse syringes, needles/cannulas; these items are considered contaminated once used to enter or connect a patient's intravenous infusion bag or administration set. • Never use intravenous bags, tubing, and connectors for multiple patients. • Do not keep multidose vials in the immediate patient treatment area. • Do not use containers of intravenous fluids as a common source of supply for multiple patients. • Do not give medications from single-dose vials or ampules to multiple patients. • Do not combine leftover contents of single-dose vials or ampules.

Adapted from CDC: *CDC guidelines for isolation precautions: preventing transmission of infectious agents in healthcare settings 2007*: www.cdc.gov/hicpac/pdf/isolation/Isolation2007.pdf. Accessed July 12, 2013.

Put on Your Thinking Cap!

For one clinical day, note everything you did that represents the use of Standard Precautions.

TRANSMISSION-BASED (ISOLATION) PRECAUTIONS

To prevent the spread of infection in a health care facility, infected patients are sometimes isolated from other patients. Examples of illnesses requiring implementation of Transmission-Based Precautions are listed in Box 13-4. The extent of the isolation depends on the type of infection. The Transmission-Based Precautions were developed to reduce the risk of airborne, droplet, and contact transmission in hospitals. Conditions requiring Transmission-Based Precautions are listed in Box 13-5.

Airborne Infection Isolation Precautions

Use Airborne Infection Isolation Precautions when caring for patients who have diseases that are spread through the air. Examples of diseases that are spread through the air are pulmonary tuberculosis, varicella (chickenpox), and rubeola (measles). Respiratory protection, provided by wearing properly fitted high-efficiency particulate absorption (HEPA) filter respirators or N95 respirators, is indicated when entering the patient's room. A private room is required and the door must be kept closed. Also recommended is a ventilation system that provides a negative pressure and exhausts directly to the outside or through HEPA filtration. In addition, patients with infections spread by airborne transmission must wear surgical masks when leaving their rooms. Surgical masks filter expired air; respirators such as the HEPA filter respirator and the N95 respirator filter inspired air.

Droplet Precautions

Use Droplet Precautions when taking care of patients with infections that are spread by droplets or dust particles containing the infectious agent. Droplets are spread primarily during coughing, sneezing, or talking, and during certain procedures such as suctioning and bronchoscopy. Because droplets usually travel only approximately 3 feet before falling from the air, special air handling and ventilation are not required to prevent droplet transmission, as is the case with Airborne Precautions. The door to the room may be left open. Diseases transmitted by droplets include rubella, mumps, diphtheria, and influenza. Patients should be placed in private rooms. Staff and visitors must wear a surgical mask when within 3 feet of the patient for protection from contaminated droplets.

Contact Precautions

Use Contact Precautions when you are caring for patients who are infected by microorganisms that are transmitted by direct (skin-to-skin) or indirect contact with contaminated equipment. Needles, dressings, stethoscopes, bed rails, and doorknobs may become contaminated. The patient is placed in a private room. Wear gloves when entering the infected patient's room; before leaving the patient's room, remove your gloves and wash your hands. Wear a gown if your clothing will come in contact with the patient, contaminated equipment, or environmental surfaces in the patient's room. A gown is also recommended if the patient is incontinent or has wound drainage. Remove the gown before leaving the patient's room. In addition, use dedicated equipment when treating patients with MDROs. Contact Precautions are used for conditions such as fecal incontinence; infections of the gastrointestinal tract, respiratory tract (including respiratory syncytial virus), and skin (e.g., impetigo, scabies); or wound infections with significant drainage, especially if the infection agent is resistant to multiple antimicrobials. Special contact precautions apply to patients with infections caused by MDROs such as VRE and MRSA. Types of precautions and patients with whom precautions must be used are summarized in Box 13-5.

Box 13-4 Guidelines for Use of Transmission-Based Precautions

AIRBORNE PRECAUTIONS

Use Airborne Precautions with patients who have microorganisms transmitted by droplet nuclei smaller than 5 microns. Patients with tuberculosis, measles (rubeola), and chickenpox (varicella) are in this category.

Patient Placement. Place the patient in a private room with negative air pressure of 6 to 12 air changes per hour. Keep the patient in the room with the door closed. When a private room is not available, place the patient in a room with a patient who has the same microorganism but no other infection (cohort).

Respiratory Protection. Wear respiratory protection when entering the room of patients with tuberculosis. If susceptible persons must enter the room of patients with rubeola or varicella, they should wear respiratory protection.

Patient Transport. Limit patient to essential transport only. If patient must be transported, place a surgical mask on the patient.

Limited Visitation. Visitors who have not had the illness or have not had the appropriate immunization (such as other children) are discouraged and sometimes restricted. This will keep them from becoming ill. If they must visit, they should wear a mask in the room.

DROPLET PRECAUTIONS

Use Droplet Precautions for patients infected with microorganisms that are larger than 5 microns that are spread by coughing, sneezing, talking, or the performance of procedures. Patients with diphtheria, rubella, streptococcal pharyngitis, pneumonia, and mumps are in this category.

Patient Placement. Place the patient in a private room or with a cohort if a private room is not available. The door may remain open and special air handling and ventilation are not necessary.

Mask. Wear a mask when working within 3 feet of the patient; many hospitals require wearing a mask to enter the room.

Patient Transport. Limit the transport of patients to essential trips only. If transport of the patient is necessary, minimize patient spread of droplets by masking the patient.

CONTACT PRECAUTIONS

Use Contact Precautions for patients with microorganisms that can be transmitted by direct contact with the patient (hand or skin-to-skin contact) or indirect contact (touching surfaces or environmental items). Patients with multidrug-resistant organisms, major wound infections, *Shigella*, herpes simplex, and scabies are in this category.

Patient Placement. Place the patient in a private room or with a cohort.

Gloves and Hand Washing. Wear clean gloves when entering the room. Change gloves after contact with infective material. Remove gloves before leaving the patient's room and wash hands immediately.

Gown. Wear a gown into the room if you think your clothing will have contact with the patient or environmental surfaces or if the patient is incontinent or has diarrhea. Remove the gown before leaving the patient's room.

Patient Transport. Limit the transport of patients to essential trips only. If the patient must be transported, ensure that precautions are implemented to reduce transmission of microorganisms.

Patient Care Equipment. Dedicate the use of equipment to a single patient to avoid sharing between patients. If you must use common equipment, clean and disinfect it before use for another patient.

PROTECTIVE ENVIRONMENT

Use a Protective Environment to reduce the risk of fungal infections for vulnerable patients.

Patient Placement. Room should have HEPA filtration of incoming air, directed room air flow, positive air pressure in the room as compared with the corridor, and a ventilator system that changes the room air at least 12 times each hour, and be sealed to prevent air flow from the outside. The room should be easily cleaned (e.g., tile vs. carpet) and may not contain potted plants or live or dried flowers.

Data from CDC: *CDC guidelines for isolation precautions preventing transmission of infectious agents in healthcare settings, 2007*: www.cdc.gov/hicpac/pdf/isolation/Isolation2007.pdf. Accessed July 10, 2013.
CDC, Centers for Disease Control and Prevention; *HEPA*, high-efficiency particulate absorption.

PERSONAL PROTECTIVE EQUIPMENT FOR HEALTH CARE PERSONNEL

Various precautions include the use of equipment designed to protect health care providers from infections. These items include gloves; isolation gowns; face protection including masks, goggles, and face shields; and respiratory protection. Personal protective equipment (PPE) is used along with other types of precautions.

Health care personnel should wear gloves when a possibility exists of exposure to potentially infectious material. When gloves are used in addition to other PPE (gown, mask), the gloves should be put on last. After carefully removing contaminated gloves, hand hygiene should be performed to remove any contaminated material that might have been transferred to the hands.

Isolation gowns protect the health care workers' exposed skin and clothing from contamination by infected material. Gowns, if indicated, are donned before other PPE. They should be discarded in the patient care area to prevent contaminating the environment.

Masks, face shields, and goggles are used to prevent contamination of the mouth, nose, and eyes when a risk exists of facial exposure to infectious materials. They also protect the patient during sterile procedures from infectious material carried in the health care worker's mouth or nose. Personal eyeglasses and

Box 13-5 Types of Precautions and Patients with Whom Precautions Must Be Used

STANDARD PRECAUTIONS

Use Standard Precautions for the care of all patients.

AIRBORNE PRECAUTIONS

In addition to Standard Precautions, use Airborne Precautions for patients known or suspected to have serious illnesses transmitted by airborne droplet nuclei. Examples of such illnesses include the following:

- Measles
- Severe acute respiratory syndrome (SARS)
- Tuberculosis
- Varicella (including disseminated zoster)

DROPLET PRECAUTIONS

In addition to Standard Precautions, use Droplet Precautions for patients known or suspected to have serious illnesses transmitted by large-particle droplets. Examples of such illnesses include the following:

- Invasive *Haemophilus influenzae* type b disease, including meningitis, pneumonia, epiglottitis, and sepsis
- Invasive *Neisseria meningitidis* disease, including meningitis, pneumonia, and sepsis
- Other serious bacterial respiratory infections spread by droplet transmission, including:
  - Diphtheria (pharyngeal)
  - *Mycoplasma pneumoniae*
  - Pertussis
  - Pneumonic plague
  - Streptococcal (group A) pharyngitis, pneumonia, or scarlet fever in infants and young children

SERIOUS VIRAL INFECTIONS SPREAD BY DROPLET TRANSMISSION

- Adenovirus (also Contact Precautions)
- Influenza
- Mumps
- Parvovirus B19
- Rubella

CONTACT PRECAUTIONS

In addition to Standard Precautions, use Contact Precautions for patients known or suspected to have serious illnesses easily transmitted by direct patient contact or by contact with items in the patient's environment. The following are examples of such illnesses:

- Gastrointestinal, respiratory, skin, or wound infections or colonization with multidrug-resistant bacteria judged by the infection prevention and control program, based on current state, regional, or national recommendations, to be of special clinical and epidemiologic significance
- Enteric infections with a prolonged environmental survival, including *Clostridium difficile*
- For diapered or incontinent patients:
  - Enterohemorrhagic *Escherichia coli* 0157:H7, *Shigella*, hepatitis A, or rotavirus
  - Respiratory syncytial virus, parainfluenza virus, or enteroviral infections in infants and young children
- Skin infections that are highly contagious or that may occur on dry skin, including:
  - Diphtheria (cutaneous)
  - Herpes simplex virus (neonatal or mucocutaneous)
  - Impetigo
  - Major (noncontained) abscesses, cellulitis, or decubitus
  - Pediculosis
  - Ritter disease (scalded skin syndrome)
  - Scabies
  - Staphylococcal furunculosis in infants and young children
  - Herpes zoster (disseminated or in the immunocompromised host)
- Viral/hemorrhagic conjunctivitis
- Viral hemorrhagic infections

Data from CDC: *CDC guidelines for isolation precautions preventing transmission of infectious agents in healthcare settings, 2007*: www.cdc.gov/hicpac/pdf/isolation/Isolation2007.pdf. Accessed July 10, 2013.
CDC, Centers for Disease Control and Prevention.

contact lens do not provide adequate protection from infectious material. Before removing a mask, face shield, or goggles, the gloves should be removed and hand hygiene performed. Avoid touching the front of the PPE because doing so is considered contamination.

Respiratory protection from inhalation of infectious particles requires a respirator with N95 or higher filtration. The device must fit the wearer's face securely to prevent air leakage. N95 or higher level respirators are recommended when working with patients who have suspected or confirmed tuberculosis, severe acute respiratory syndrome (SARS), and smallpox. Certain procedures also may mandate the use of a respirator. A single health care worker can reuse a respirator when working with a patient who has tuberculosis as long as the device is clean, uncontaminated, and undamaged and it fits properly.

PROTECTIVE ENVIRONMENT

A Protective Environment (PE) is needed to reduce the fungal spore count in the air and to reduce the risk of invasive environmental fungal infections for vulnerable patients. Components of a PE include HEPA filtration of incoming air, directed room air flow, positive air pressure in the room as compared with the corridor, sealed rooms that prevent air flow from outside, and a ventilator system that changes the room air at least 12 times each hour. In addition, the room should be easily cleaned (e.g., tile vs. carpet), and may not contain potted plants or live or dried flowers.

BIOTERRORISM

So far, we have been discussing infection as a communicable disease that is assumed to be transmitted by unintentional or careless exposure to a pathogen. However, a special situation called *bioterrorism* is the intentional use of microorganisms to cause death or disease. Methods used to spread agents of bioterrorism are varied and might include powders, aerosols, or contamination of food or water. Among the pathogens considered potential biologic weapons are those that cause anthrax, botulism, plague, smallpox, tularemia, and Ebola. In addition to pathogens, bioterrorists may use toxins such as ricin, chemicals such as sarin, and radioactive material released in small explosions ("dirty bombs"). Nurses should be aware of their employing agency's plans for dealing with public exposure to bioterrorism agents, including decontamination procedures and PPE and safety procedures (CDC, 2007).

IMMUNOCOMPROMISED PATIENTS

Immunocompromised patients have decreased immunity to infection and are at increased risk for bacterial, fungal, parasitic, and viral infections. Patients receiving chemotherapy and other patients with low white blood cell counts are at increased risk of infection. Leukemia and aplastic anemia are two examples of disorders that cause low white blood cell counts. The use of Standard Precautions for all patients and of Transmission-Based Precautions for specific situations should reduce the risk of acquiring infections from other persons and from the environment. See Chapter 34 for a discussion of precautions to be used with immunocompromised patients.

❖ NURSING CARE of Patients with Infections

Patients with generalized infections easily become dehydrated because of fever and anorexia. Urge the patient to consume adequate fluids, especially water. For the average adult, fluid intake should be at least 2 liters per day to replace fluids lost through perspiration and respiration. Fluid intake is also important in the transportation of nutrients to the cells to fight infection. Nutrition is very important. Encourage patients to consume a high-protein, high-vitamin diet. Vitamin C is important for wound healing and to promote resistance to future infections. The patient with a poor appetite may benefit from a consultation with a dietitian.

If a patient's infection requires isolation, remember that effective isolation techniques may also isolate the patient from normal human contact. You may be tempted to hasten your work to minimize your chance of becoming infected. Forced seclusion can cause patients, particularly children, to feel lonely, rejected, and depressed. Engage the patient in conversation while giving direct care. Discussing subjects other than the patient's disease may lessen the feeling of being unclean or rejected. Encourage the patient to move about as much as possible to increase stimulation.

Under the current CDC guidelines, some infections and conditions fall into two categories because the microorganisms are transmitted in more than one way. For example, chickenpox can spread through both airborne and contact routes, requiring both Airborne and Contact Precautions.

Laboratory tests used to screen patients for infection include the following:

- White blood cell count—increased in infection
- Erythrocyte sedimentation rate—elevated with inflammation
- Iron level—decreased in chronic infection
- Cultures of urine, blood, sputum, and specimens obtained from the throat or a wound surface. The specimen is placed in a medium that supports growth of microorganisms. Laboratory identification of the organisms that grow in the culture allows the primary care provider to select the most appropriate antimicrobial treatment.
- White blood cell differential count (neutrophils, lymphocytes, monocytes, and eosinophils)—increased; types of increased cells helps to differentiate causes of infection

Examples of nursing diagnoses for patients with infections or who are vulnerable to infections include Risk for Infection, Risk for Injury, Impaired Tissue Integrity, Social Isolation, and Disturbed Body Image. Ineffective Self-Help Management is another related nursing diagnosis. The primary goals in caring for patients with infection are recovery from the infection and prevention of the spread of infection to others.

Antimicrobial drug therapy is the cornerstone of treatment for many infections. Early hospital discharges mean that patients are frequently discharged on a regimen of oral antimicrobial drugs. Many people stop taking antimicrobials once they begin to feel better. This failure to take antimicrobials permits surviving organisms to develop resistance and to thrive, possibly causing a recurrence of illness. Therefore caution patients not to stop taking the medication when they start feeling better. They should continue their antimicrobials until the entire course has been completed or until their primary care provider specifically orders them to stop taking the medication. The emergence of antimicrobial resistance is one important reason why antimicrobial therapy for bacterial infections may fail. Increasingly, bacteria are becoming resistant, often because of the widespread or inappropriate use of antimicrobials, which leads to the killing of susceptible bacteria and allows more resistant strains to multiply.

Patient Teaching

Hyperbaric Oxygen Therapy

- Do not smoke for several hours before and after treatment to decrease lung irritation.
- You can prevent pressure buildup in the ears by swallowing.
- You must wear 100% cotton clothing in the hyperbaric oxygen chamber to prevent static electricity.

Hyperbaric oxygen therapy is an intervention that is used to treat some infections. Breathing 100% oxygen at higher-than-atmospheric pressure in a closed chamber increases the amount of dissolved oxygen transported in plasma. The oxygen-rich environment improves leukocyte phagocytic activity and kills anaerobic bacteria (see *Patient Teaching* box).

During hyperbaric oxygen therapy, the patient must be monitored for the following complications: ear or sinus pain (from pressure buildup), respiratory problems (as a result of oxygen toxicity), seizures (a central nervous system symptom of oxygen toxicity), and bradycardia (reflex response to oxygen toxicity).

Earlier hospital discharges mean that substantial therapy may continue in the home after discharge. Home health care is frequently ordered for infected patients for several reasons. The patient has fewer opportunities to acquire an HAI, opportunities for infection to be spread to other hospitalized patients are reduced, and patients often do better in their own surroundings. If therapy is to be continued at home, teach the patient and other family members how to manage the care. Close coordination between members of the health care team is important to ensure good continuity of care. (Guidelines for infection prevention and control in the home are given in the *Patient Teaching* box.)

Patient Teaching

Infection Prevention and Control When the Patient Is Treated in the Home

Infection control in the home setting is based on Standard Precautions. In the home, adapt the guidelines to the equipment and supplies available.

- *Equipment:* List for the family the activities that require the use of gloves and identify the proper gloves to use. Instruct caregivers to use an apron if clothing is likely to become contaminated and to wear gloves when changing dressings.
- *Hand hygiene:* Demonstrate good hand washing technique and the use of waterless antiseptics to all household members. Tell family members that proper hand hygiene is the most important action they can take to prevent the spread of infection and inform them when hand washing or the use of antiseptics is appropriate.

Patient Teaching—cont'd

- *Sharps disposal:* If a sharps container is not available, tell the family to use a puncture-resistant container such as a detergent bottle or coffee can with the lid securely taped until local regulations on sharps disposal can be initiated.
- *Bandages and linens:* Instruct household members to seal soiled dressings tightly in a plastic bag and dispose of dressings in the trash bag. Clothing and linens with body fluids should be stored in a plastic bag until they are laundered, at which time they should be washed in water as hot as the fabric will tolerate. One cup of bleach is added to the detergent in each load.
- *Spills:* Instruct household members to wear gloves to wash contaminated surfaces with detergent and water and then wash the surfaces with a freshly made solution of 1:10 household bleach. Disposable towels should be used and discarded in a plastic bag.
- *Dishes:* Leftover portions of uneaten food should not be saved. If a dishwasher is available in the home, it should be used for the patient's dishes. Otherwise, soiled dishes should be washed in detergent and hot water immediately after use.

IMMUNODEFICIENCY

CAUSES AND RISK FACTORS

When the body's self-defenses against foreign invasion fail to function normally, a state of immunodeficiency (immunosuppression) exists. In this state, known as an *immunocompromised* or *immunosuppressed state,* the body is unable to launch an adequate immune response and is at great risk for infection. The primary clinical clue to **immunodeficiency**, whatever the cause, is the tendency to develop recurrent infections. Immunodeficiencies can be congenital or, more commonly, acquired and can result from problems with humoral immunity, cell-mediated immunity, vital mediators such as complement, or the process of phagocytosis.

In congenital immunodeficiencies, some part of the immune system fails to develop properly. The result is a defect in the B or T lymphocytes, phagocytes, or complement.

Acquired immunodeficiencies result from factors outside the immune system that render a previously functional immune system inadequate. Some causes of acquired deficiencies are infections, malignancies, autoimmune diseases (systemic lupus erythematosus, rheumatoid arthritis), chronic diseases (diabetes mellitus, renal disease), drugs, aging, stress, and malnutrition.

Stress, whether physical or emotional, alters the body's response to disease. Although the mechanism is not fully understood, the release of hormones plays a part. Stressors include such factors as serious illness, job loss, and divorce; even noise and cold play a part.

The nutritional state of the patient also affects immunity. The malnourished patient is much more susceptible to infection, especially when a protein deficiency exists. People with chronic conditions such as diabetes and renal disease may become debilitated and unable to resist infection fully. Trauma victims, especially those with burns, have diminished immune responses. Many malignant disorders alter the functioning of the immune system. Infectious diseases also cause immunodeficiencies, especially acute viral infections.

Many treatments and interventions aimed at helping patients cause immunodeficiency. Medications often place patients at risk for infection; corticosteroids, antineoplastic drugs (used to treat cancer), and immunosuppressive drugs (used for transplant recipients) are a few.

Surgery, anesthesia, and irradiation for cancer also can alter immune function. In addition, invasive procedures such as urinary catheterization and venipuncture for intravenous therapy or blood work bypass the patient's first line of defense. In the hospitalized patient, all of these factors come into play; disease, stress, nutritional alterations, medications, and invasive procedures all set up the patient for infection.

MEDICAL TREATMENT

Congenital immunodeficiencies are usually treated with replacement therapy of the deficient immune component. Bone marrow transplants or fetal thymus tissue transplants may be used in some cases. Treating an acquired immunodeficiency entails correcting the underlying condition that is causing the problem, such as reducing stressors, correcting malnutrition, and discontinuing medications that alter immunity.

NURSING CARE of the Immunosuppressed Patient

The primary nursing responsibility in cases of immunodeficiency is to prevent infection. Proper hand hygiene by personnel, visitors, and patients themselves is the single most important measure in prevention. Vital signs should be assessed regularly. However, in an immunosuppressed or immunocompromised patient, signs and symptoms of infection are often atypical, masked, or absent. Be aware that a small increase in body temperature in these patients can be significant and should be reported. Avoid rectal thermometers if possible because of the potential for damage to the rectal mucosa. Encourage adequate nutritional intake. Perform effective skin, mouth, perineal, wound, and intravenous site care, with continuous assessment for signs of infection. Encourage patients to turn, cough, and breathe deeply. Protective (compromised host) isolation may be necessary. Flowers or plants may be prohibited because they provide a reservoir for bacterial growth. Fresh produce may be eliminated from the diet if the white blood cell count is too low. Disposable equipment is preferred.

Patient education concerning the risks for and signs of infection should be reinforced. Provide a supportive listening environment because these patients may have anxiety, as well as a high stress level, and feelings of powerlessness are often overwhelming.

HYPERSENSITIVITY AND ALLERGY

CAUSES AND RISK FACTORS

The term *allergy* (or *hypersensitivity*) describes an atypical immune response that is activated by a foreign substance that normally is inoffensive. Although immune responses are usually beneficial, hypersensitivity can be harmful and even deadly. Estimates indicate that 20% to 25% of the U.S. population suffers from allergies of some sort, with allergic rhinitis (hay fever) and asthma occurring most often. Other allergic disorders include allergic contact dermatitis, angioedema (localized swelling that affects the airway if it involves the mouth or tongue), dermatitis, anaphylaxis (severe allergic reaction), gastrointestinal allergies, and urticaria (hives). The tendency to develop an allergy is inherited, although the type of allergy may vary. Someone who is prone to allergies may be called *atopic*. Hypersensitivity as an immune disorder is discussed in Chapter 34.

An antigen that causes a hypersensitive reaction is called an **allergen**. Any substance can act as an allergen to a susceptible person but some of the more common ones are house dust, animal dander, pollens, molds, foods, pharmacologic agents, cigarette smoke, feathers, and insect venoms. Table 13-4 lists common allergies and triggers.

The allergic response begins with sensitization. The first encounter with a specific allergen results in only a small amount of antibody production. With subsequent exposure, however, the body steps up its defense by producing large amounts of antibodies, which circulate in the bloodstream and travel to the affected tissues. This buildup triggers the release of histamine and other chemical agents. Neutrophils arrive at the scene to engulf and destroy the antigens. A cascade of reactions occurs that produces the symptoms typical of an allergic response, although they vary according to the area affected. Local manifestations of allergic reactions include urticaria, pruritus, conjunctivitis, rhinitis, laryngeal edema, bronchospasm, dysrhythmia, gastrointestinal cramps and malabsorption, and angioedema.

MEDICAL TREATMENT

The medical treatment of patients with allergies varies, depending on the specific allergy. However, in any case, care of the airway must be the priority. In general, antihistamines are used to reduce the symptoms caused by histamine release. Many people suffer side

Table 13-4 Common Allergies and Their Triggers

ALLERGIC REACTION	STIMULUS
Allergic rhinitis	Pollens, dust, molds, animal dander
Asthma	Pollens, dust, molds, cigarette smoke, air pollutants, animal dander
Allergic eyes (conjunctivitis)	Pollens, dust, molds, animal dander, cigarette smoke
Anaphylaxis	Antimicrobials (penicillin) Insect venom (bee, wasp stings) Blood transfusions
Hives (urticaria)	Foods, drugs
Atopic dermatitis (eczema)	Soaps, cosmetics, chemicals, fabrics
Allergic contact dermatitis	Plants (poison ivy) Metals (nickel) Chemicals, cosmetics Latex gloves
Gastrointestinal allergies	Foods, drugs

effects from antihistamines, such as dry mouth, nausea, blurred vision, dizziness, and drowsiness. Antihistamines sometimes cause confusion in older patients. For asthma sufferers, bronchodilators, corticosteroids, or both may be prescribed to improve air movement and decrease inflammation in the lungs; oxygen and breathing treatments may also be ordered. Besides antihistamines, topical lotions and ointments may be prescribed to relieve itching associated with urticaria, atopic dermatitis, or allergic contact dermatitis.

Long-term medical treatment of allergies involves testing to determine specific allergens. Testing is performed by injecting small amounts of allergen under the skin (intradermally) or by pricking the surface of the patient's skin and monitoring for the degree of wheal and flare reaction. After the specific agents have been identified, the patient may be desensitized by injections of tiny quantities of the allergen, with the dose gradually increased over a prolonged period. Desensitization is aimed at increasing tolerance to the offending agent and decreasing the severity of the allergic response.

❖ NURSING CARE of the Patient with Allergies

When dealing with the hospitalized patient with allergies, the most important nursing intervention is to document all allergies, the symptoms they cause, and any treatment currently used. Allergies should be posted on the patient's record, on all medication records, on the nursing care plan, and on a patient identification band. Never administer any drug to which the patient reports a previous allergic reaction.

Alert the pharmacy and dietary departments to drug and food allergies. Notify the primary care provider of any allergies that may determine which medications to avoid. For instance, a patient who is allergic to shellfish should not receive drugs containing iodine because an anaphylactic reaction may result. Ensure that patients who have been taking allergy medication, such as inhaler treatments, continue to take these medications when admitted to the hospital. A growing number of patients, as well as health care providers, are reporting latex allergies, necessitating the use of nonlatex gloves.

Patient education is important for all patients with allergies. This area includes knowledge of specific allergens, limiting exposure to or avoiding allergens, the proper use of medications such as inhaled bronchodilators, and the actions and side effects of drugs. Patients who are at risk for life-threatening (anaphylactic) reactions should wear a medical alert bracelet that identifies their allergy. Individuals with insect sting allergies should obtain an emergency sting kit and be taught how to self-inject epinephrine. This kit should be kept readily available at all times.

Nurses should avoid the overuse of perfumes and scented cosmetics while working with patients. Live plants and flowers should not be allowed in the patient's room.

ANAPHYLAXIS

CAUSES AND RISK FACTORS

When an allergen enters the bloodstream, an allergic reaction called *anaphylaxis* can occur throughout the body within minutes. Anaphylaxis is a life-threatening situation that can quickly deteriorate into shock, coma, and death. Histamine released in anaphylaxis causes bronchospasm, vasodilation, and increased capillary permeability throughout the body, which causes fluid to leave the circulation and enter the tissues, causing shock from hypovolemia. Signs and symptoms of anaphylaxis include anxiety, wheezing and difficulty breathing, cyanosis (bluish skin color), hives, facial edema, arthralgia (joint pain), and hypotension (low blood pressure).

Anaphylaxis is an emergency situation and the patient's life depends on rapid intervention. The most common cause of anaphylaxis is the use of antimicrobials, especially penicillin. Other causes include the use of medicines or serum from animal sources, insect venom (especially from bees and wasps), iodinated radioactive contrast media, local anesthetic, and blood products.

MEDICAL TREATMENT

In anaphylaxis, oxygen is given in addition to intravenous epinephrine. Other drugs that might be given are dopamine or a volume expander (or both) to raise the patient's blood pressure, a nebulized bronchodilator to relax the bronchi and improve ventilation, diphenhydramine for antihistamine effects, and corticosteroids to decrease the inflammatory response. Endotracheal intubation, tracheostomy, and mechanical ventilation may be necessary to maintain adequate blood oxygenation.

❖ NURSING CARE of the Patient with Anaphylaxis

The best care is to prevent anaphylaxis whenever possible by obtaining a history of allergies and taking precautions to protect the patient from substances (often drugs) that may trigger this reaction. However, when anaphylaxis occurs, prompt recognition is vital because it is a life-threatening situation. In some settings, nurses have protocols for administering subcutaneous epinephrine in the event of allergic reactions. Nursing interventions are aimed at minimizing the patient's anxiety and, once medical care is initiated, administering prescribed drugs, including oxygen, and monitoring intravenous fluids. Monitor respirations, color, heart rate, and oxygen saturation until the patient is fully recovered.

AUTOIMMUNE DISEASES

CAUSES AND RISK FACTORS

Immune tolerance is the process by which the immune system does not attack an antigen. The body's ability to determine self from nonself is called *natural or self tolerance.* When tolerance is disrupted, the immune system reacts against and destroys its own tissues. This breakdown in tolerance and subsequent damage to self is termed **autoimmunity**. An autoimmune process may be initiated when injury to tissues, infection, or malignancy occurs. The exact causes and pathologic nature of most autoimmune diseases are poorly understood but many of these disorders cause severe illness and death.

Genetic factors appear to be involved because autoimmune diseases tend to be familial. Some autoimmune disorders have apparent causes, such as drug-induced anemia or a low platelet count (thrombocytopenia). Infection is often present before the onset of an autoimmune disease, leading to the conclusion that the disease results as a complication (sequela) of the infection. Autoimmune diseases cause injury in three ways: (1) by the effect of antibodies on cell surfaces, (2) through the deposit of antigen-antibody complexes (particularly in capillaries, joints, and renal tissue), and (3) through the action of sensitized T cells.

Autoimmunity can involve any tissue or organ system. In multiple sclerosis, the white matter of the brain and spinal cord is affected and the myelin sheath that protects nerve fibers is destroyed. Rheumatoid arthritis affects the lining of the joints. In type 1 diabetes mellitus, the pancreatic cells that secrete insulin are attacked. Table 13-5 lists some of the more common

Table 13-5 Autoimmune Disorders and Their Targets

DISORDER	TISSUE AFFECTED
Endocrine System	
Hyperthyroidism (Graves' disease)	Thyroid
Autoimmune thyroiditis	Thyroid
Type 1 diabetes mellitus	Pancreas
Addison disease	Adrenal gland
Central Nervous System	
Multiple sclerosis	Brain and spinal cord
Myasthenia gravis	Neuromuscular junctions
Cardiovascular System	
Rheumatic fever	Heart
Cardiomyopathy	Heart
Gastrointestinal System	
Ulcerative colitis	Colon
Crohn disease	Ileum
Connective Tissue	
Rheumatoid arthritis	Joints
Systemic lupus erythematosus	Multiple tissues
Scleroderma	Multiple tissues
Hematologic System	
Autoimmune hemolytic anemia	Red blood cells
Autoimmune thrombocytopenic purpura	Platelets
Idiopathic neutropenia	Neutrophils
Idiopathic lymphopenia	Lymphocytes
Respiratory and Renal Systems	
Goodpasture syndrome	Lung, kidney
Skin	
Pemphigus vulgaris	Skin
Psoriasis	Skin

Adapted from McCance KL, Huether SE: *Pathophysiology: the biologic basis for disease in adults and children*, ed 9, St. Louis, 2009, Mosby-Elsevier.

autoimmune disorders and the tissues they affect. Probably the most familiar of the autoimmune disorders is systemic lupus erythematosus, which affects multiple organs.

MEDICAL TREATMENT

Medical interventions vary depending on the specific autoimmune disease and the tissues affected as well as on the symptoms. In general, corticosteroids and nonsteroidal antiinflammatory drugs are used to treat inflammation. Immunosuppressive therapies may be tried to moderate the autoimmune response.

❖ NURSING CARE of the Patient with an Autoimmune Disorder

Although nursing interventions vary according to the specific disorder, many nursing diagnoses apply to patients with an autoimmune disease, including:

Risk for Activity Intolerance
Anxiety
Impaired Skin Integrity
Ineffective Breathing Pattern
Impaired Gas Exchange
Deficient Knowledge
Chronic Pain
Fear
Fatigue
Ineffective Coping
Risk for Infection
Imbalanced Nutrition: Less Than Body Requirements

Adequate rest, maintenance of optimal hydration and nutritional status, and prevention of infection are vital in preventing complications in these patients. In addition, a supportive, caring atmosphere is important to enhance the patient's coping skills and promote emotional health. Specific autoimmune disorders are addressed with appropriate systems in this textbook.

Put on Your Thinking Cap!

In your clinical site, locate everything you would need if a patient had an anaphylactic reaction to a drug. What procedure should you use to alert other personnel?

Get Ready for the NCLEX® Examination!

Key Points

- Physical and chemical barriers that shield the body from disease or injury include the skin, the mucous membranes, and various blood cells.
- Many types of leukocytes, especially neutrophils and monocytes, act as nature's cleanup mechanism by migrating to infected or inflamed areas and engulfing and destroying antigens through a process known as *phagocytosis.*
- Reticuloendothelial cells, or tissue macrophages, found in the blood, connective tissue, liver, spleen, bone marrow, and lymph nodes protect the body by digesting and absorbing foreign material such as old red blood cells, bacteria, and colloidal particles.
- The five signs of inflammation are rubor (redness), calor (heat), tumor (swelling), dolor (pain), and loss of function.
- Wound healing begins at the same time that the inflammatory process begins.
- The process of wound healing includes the production of macrophage cells to clean up inflammatory debris, the initiation of the repair process by fibroblasts, the formation of capillaries to provide circulation and nutrients to the new tissue, and the migration of epithelial cells under the scab to form a scar.
- Age and general health affect how rapidly wound healing occurs. Older adults heal more slowly as a result of a decreased blood supply to the tissues, a decrease in tissue elasticity, and poor or inadequate nutrition.
- The major infectious agents are bacteria, viruses, fungi, protozoa, rickettsiae, and helminths.
- Infection, or the invasion of the body by microorganisms, is possible only when a causative agent, a reservoir, a portal of exit, a mode of transfer, a portal of entry, and a susceptible host are present.
- Signs and symptoms of generalized infection are moderate to severe pain, swelling, fever, malaise, anorexia, and prostration.
- Two types of infections are (1) community-acquired infections, acquired through daily contact with the public, and (2) health care–acquired infections (HAIs).
- The most basic and effective method of preventing the spread of infection is hand hygiene.
- The CDC recommends the use of Standard Precautions for all patients, especially those cared for in settings in which exposure to blood or other body fluids is common.
- To reduce MDROs in health care settings, the use of Contact Precautions with infected or colonized patients is recommended.
- In hospitals and long-term care facilities, patients with MDROs should be in single rooms or rooms with others who have the same MDRO.
- The immune system is the body's defense network against infection; it provides the body with resistance to invading organisms and enables it to fight off invaders once they have gained access.
- Antigens are substances that stimulate a response from the immune system. Antibodies, also known as *immunoglobulins*, are proteins that are created in response to specific antigens.
- Innate (natural) immunity is present in the body at birth whereas acquired immunity develops after birth as a result of the body's immune responses to antigens.
- Acquired immunity depends on the proper development of B and T lymphocytes, which are white blood cells that fight infection.
- The two types of immunity—antibody-mediated (humoral) and cell-mediated immunity—function interdependently to provide the immune response.
- Immunodeficiency occurs when the body is unable to launch an adequate immune response, resulting in risk for infection.
- When a normally inoffensive foreign substance stimulates an atypical immune response, allergy or hypersensitivity occurs.
- Anaphylaxis is a life-threatening immune response that requires immediate intervention.
- Autoimmunity occurs when the body fails to recognize itself and the immune system reacts by destroying the body's own tissues.

Additional Learning Resources

SG Go to your Study Guide for additional learning activities to help you master this chapter content.

evolve Go to your Evolve website (http://evolve.elsevier.com/Linton/medsurg) for the following learning resources and much more:
- Interactive Prioritization Exercises
- Fluid & Electrolyte Tutorial
- Pharmacology Tutorial
- Review Questions for the NCLEX® Examination

Review Questions for the NCLEX® Examination

1. A condition in which the body's immune system destroys its own tissues is:
   1. Immunodeficiency
   2. Health care–associated infection
   3. Autoimmunity
   4. Inflammation

   NCLEX Client Need: Physiological Integrity: Physiological Adaptation
2. Bacteria that reside on the skin but do not cause infection serve what purpose?
   1. They stimulate the development of antibodies against pathogens.
   2. They prevent pathogens from gaining access to the body.
   3. They secrete sebum, which inhibits the growth of microorganisms.
   4. They phagocytose pathogenic bacteria that invade the body.

   NCLEX Client Need: Physiological Integrity: Physiological Adaptation
3. The nurse inspects for inflammation at an intravenous infusion site. Which of the following are classic signs of local inflammation? (Select all that apply.)
   1. Heat
   2. Drainage
   3. Redness
   4. Fever
   5. Swelling

   NCLEX Client Need: Physiological Integrity: Physiological Adaptation
4. In the first phase of the inflammatory process, capillary permeability increases. What purpose does this increase serve?
   1. Reduces pain in the inflamed tissue by diluting bradykinin
   2. Draws excess fluid out of inflamed tissue to reduce swelling
   3. Allows monocytes and neutrophils to pass into the inflamed tissue
   4. Counteracts bronchoconstriction in antigen-antibody reactions

   NCLEX Client Need: Physiological Integrity: Physiological Adaptation
5. Why have numerous antibacterial drugs but relatively few antiviral drugs been developed?
   1. Viruses have a more advanced ability to develop resistance to drugs.
   2. Making antibacterial drugs is more profitable because only a few viruses exist.
   3. Very few chemicals that are capable of killing viruses have been developed.
   4. The virus lives inside the host cell and drugs that harm viruses often harm host cells as well.

   NCLEX Client Need: Physiological Integrity: Pharmacological Therapies
6. The last factor in the chain of infection is the:
   1. Portal of entry
   2. Reservoir
   3. Susceptible host
   4. Mode of transfer

   NCLEX Client Need: Physiological Integrity: Physiological Adaptation
7. Characteristics of the incubation period of the infectious process include which of the following?
   1. The infected person is often very contagious.
   2. Signs and symptoms are most severe.
   3. A high fever is usually the only symptom present
   4. The patient is in the recovery phase of the infection.

   NCLEX Client Need: Physiological Integrity: Physiological Adaptation
8. Patients on an infectious disease unit have each of the infections listed. Which is/are health care–associated infection(s)? (Select all that apply.)
   1. Gonorrhea
   2. Hepatitis A
   3. Tuberculosis
   4. Vancomycin-resistant *Enterococcus*
   5. Streptococcal pharyngitis

   NCLEX Client Need: Physiological Integrity: Physiological Adaptation
9. Nurses on an infectious disease unit want to implement measures to reduce bacterial resistance to antimicrobials. Which measure(s) will help to prevent the development of bacterial resistance? (Select all that apply.)
   1. All infections are promptly treated with broad-spectrum antimicrobials.
   2. Antimicrobial selection is based on the results of culture and sensitivity tests.
   3. Antimicrobials are discontinued as soon as symptoms resolve.
   4. Antimicrobials are prescribed only for serious infections.
   5. Vaccinations for infectious diseases are encouraged.

   NCLEX Client Need: Physiological Integrity: Pharmacological Therapies

10. The primary mode of transmission of health care–associated infections is:
    1. Soiled caregiver hands
    2. Direct contact between patients
    3. Organisms brought in by visitors
    4. Faulty sterilization procedures

    NCLEX Client Need: Physiological Integrity: Physiological Adaptation
11. Which statement is true regarding the need to use Standard Precautions?
    1. Standard Precautions are required only when caring for patients who have open wounds.
    2. Standard Precautions are required when caring for any patient in any setting.
    3. Standard Precautions are required only when caring for patients with tuberculosis, hepatitis, or HIV infection.
    4. Standard Precautions are required only when caring for patients who are highly susceptible to infection.

    NCLEX Client Need: Health Promotion and Maintenance
12. The advantage of using HEPA filter respirators rather than surgical masks is that:
    1. Surgical masks are too expensive for routine use
    2. HEPA filter respirators protect the caregiver by filtering inspired air
    3. Surgical masks protect the caregiver against tuberculosis but not other infections
    4. HEPA filter respirators protect the patient but not the caregiver

    NCLEX Client Need: Health Promotion and Maintenance
13. After vaccination for measles, a person will not become ill if exposed to the measles virus. The patient's ability to resist the measles virus is called:
    1. Innate immunity
    2. Nonspecific defense mechanism
    3. Active acquired immunity
    4. Passive acquired immunity

    NCLEX Client Need: Physiological Integrity: Physiological Adaptation
14. The rejection of transplanted organs is the result of:
    1. Passive acquired immunity
    2. Antibody-mediated immunity
    3. Cell-mediated immunity
    4. Innate immunity

    NCLEX Client Need: Physiological Integrity: Physiological Adaptation
15. Nursing care of the immunosuppressed patient should include which of the following?
    1. Take rectal temperatures every 4 hours to detect low-grade fever.
    2. Encourage consumption of fresh fruits and vegetables to increase vitamin intake.
    3. Encourage the family to bring in live plants to increase oxygen in the room.
    4. Emphasize the need for proper hand washing by patients, visitors, and staff.

    NCLEX Client Need: Health Promotion and Maintenance

chapter

14 Fluids and Electrolytes

http://evolve.elsevier.com/Linton/medsurg

Objectives

1. Describe the extracellular and intracellular fluid compartments.
2. Describe the composition of the extracellular and intracellular body fluid compartments.
3. Discuss the mechanisms of fluid transport and fluid balance.
4. Identify the causes, signs and symptoms, and treatment of fluid imbalances.
5. Describe the major functions of the major electrolytes: sodium, potassium, calcium, magnesium, and chloride.
6. Identify the causes, signs and symptoms, and treatment of electrolyte imbalances.
7. List data to be collected in assessing fluid and electrolyte status.
8. Discuss the medical treatment and nursing management of persons with fluid and electrolyte imbalances.
9. Explain why older persons are at increased risk for fluid and electrolyte imbalances.
10. List the four types of acid-base imbalances.
11. Identify the major causes of each acid-base imbalance.
12. Explain the medical treatment and nursing management of acid-base imbalances.

Key Terms

Acid
Acid-base balance
Active transport
Base
Deficient fluid volume
Diffusion (dĭ-FYŪ-zhŭn)
Electrolyte (ĕ-LĔK-trō-līt)
Excess fluid volume
Extracellular fluid (ĕks-tră-SĔL-ū-lăr)
Filtration (fĭl-TRĀ-shŭn)
Homeostasis (hō-mē-ō-STĀ-sĭs)
Intracellular fluid (ĭn-tră-SĔL-yū-lăr)
Osmolality (ŏz-mō-LĂL-ĭ-tē)
Osmolarity (ŏz-mō-LĂR-ĭ-tē)
Osmosis (ŏz-MŌ-sĭs)
Selectively permeable membrane (sĕ-LĔK-tĭv-lē PĔR-mē-ă-b'l MĔM-brān)

Maintaining the correct amount and distribution of body fluids and electrolytes and the correct pH of body fluids is essential for survival. The body constantly makes adjustments to maintain this balance. Unfortunately, many disease processes and medical interventions pose actual or potential threats to patients' fluid and electrolyte balances. Therefore nurses must understand the basic principles of fluid and electrolyte balance to maintain balance and to detect and correct imbalances.

HOMEOSTASIS

Approximately 50% to 60% of the human body is composed of water. To maintain internal balance, the body must be able to regulate the fluids within it. The tendency to maintain relatively constant conditions as in the fluid compartments is called **homeostasis**. All organs and structures of the body are involved in the maintenance of homeostasis.

Homeostasis is necessary for cells to be able to carry out their work. Body fluids are in constant motion, maintaining healthy living conditions for body cells. The process of homeostasis involves the delivery of essential elements such as oxygen and glucose to the cells and the removal of wastes such as carbon dioxide from the cells. When the body does not maintain homeostasis, the cells cannot function properly and illness or death results.

BODY FLUID COMPARTMENTS

Body fluids are classified as intracellular or extracellular, depending on their location. **Intracellular fluid** is fluid within a cell and **extracellular fluid** is fluid outside the cell. Most of the body's fluids are found within the cell.

Extracellular fluids are found in the blood vessels in the form of plasma or serum (called *intravascular fluid*); in the fluid surrounding the cells (called *interstitial*

Table 14-1 Total Body Fluids

	MEN (%)	WOMEN (%)	INFANT (%)
Intracellular	40	36	40
Extracellular	20	18	35
Total body fluids	**60**	**54**	**75**

fluid), including lymph fluid; and elsewhere, such as in digestive secretions, sweat, and cerebrospinal fluid. Extracellular fluid is mainly responsible for the transport of nutrients and wastes throughout the body. The distribution of total body fluids varies by age and gender (Table 14-1).

COMPOSITION OF BODY FLUIDS

WATER

Water makes up the largest portion of the body weight. The percentage of body weight that is water is affected by age, sex, and amount of body fat. A person's percentage of body water usually decreases with advancing age. Women have a lower percentage of body water than men throughout the adult years because women have more fat than men and fat cells contain less water than other cells. Obese people have a relatively lower percentage of body water because of their increased number of fat cells.

SOLUTES

In addition to water, body fluids contain solutes (dissolved substances) such as electrolytes and nonelectrolytes.

Electrolytes

An **electrolyte** is defined as a substance that develops an electrical charge when dissolved in water. Examples of electrolytes are sodium, potassium, calcium, chloride, bicarbonate, and magnesium. When these substances are dissolved in water, they break up into small particles called *ions*, which have either a positive (+) or a negative (−) charge. Ions that have a positive electrical charge are called *cations*. Examples of cations are sodium (Na^+), potassium (K^+), calcium (Ca^{2+}), and magnesium (Mg^{2+}). Ions that have a negative charge are called *anions*. Examples of anions are chloride (Cl^-), bicarbonate (HCO^-_3), and phosphate (HPO^-_4).

Electrolytes maintain a balance between positive and negative charges. For every positively charged cation, a negatively charged anion can be found. In every fluid compartment of the body, the cations and anions combine to balance one another. This process keeps the body cells in homeostasis.

The concentration of an electrolyte in a solution or body fluid compartment is measured in milliequivalents per liter (mEq/L). Milliequivalents indicate the chemical activity or combining power of ions. Hydrogen is used as a standard for comparing chemical activities of electrolytes. One milliequivalent of an electrolyte has the same chemical combining power as 1 mEq of hydrogen.

Table 14-2 Electrolyte Composition of Extracellular and Intracellular Fluids

ELECTROLYTE	EXTRACELLULAR FLUID (mEq/L)	INTRACELLULAR FLUID (mEq/L)
Sodium (Na^+)	130–145	14
Potassium (K^+)	3.5–5.1	140
Chloride (Cl^-)	98–107	4–6
Bicarbonate (HCO^-_3)	24	12
Calcium (Ca^{2+})	5	1–8
Magnesium (Mg^{2+})	1.5–2.5	6–30
Phosphate (HPO^-_4)	2	40–95

Electrolytes can move from one fluid compartment to another. However, the normal concentration of specific electrolytes is different in the two compartments (Table 14-2).

Sodium. Sodium (Na^+) is the most abundant electrolyte in the body and the primary electrolyte in the extracellular fluid. It plays a major role in the regulation of body fluid volumes, muscular activity, nerve impulse conduction, and acid-base balance. To remember the role of sodium in water distribution, think "water goes where sodium is." For example, a person whose sodium level is too high will retain water. We can promote the elimination of excess water by giving a diuretic that promotes excretion of sodium.

Potassium. Potassium (K^+) is found mainly in the intracellular fluid and is the major intracellular cation. Because it is so abundant within the cell, it plays an important role in maintaining fluid osmolarity and volume within the cell. Potassium is essential for normal membrane excitability, a critical factor in the transmission of nerve impulses. It also is needed for protein synthesis, for the synthesis and breakdown of glycogen, and to maintain plasma acid-base balance.

Chloride. Chloride (Cl^-) is an extracellular anion that is usually bound with other ions, especially sodium or potassium. Its major functions are to regulate osmotic pressure between fluid compartments and to assist in regulating acid-base balance.

Calcium. Calcium (Ca^{2+}) is usually combined with phosphorus to form the mineral salts of the bones and teeth. Of the total calcium in the body, 99% is concentrated in the bones and teeth and 1% is in the extracellular fluid. Calcium is ingested through the diet and absorbed through the intestine. Calcium and phosphorus have a reciprocal relationship, meaning that if one falls, the other typically rises; if one rises, the other falls.

In addition to maintaining strong teeth and bones, calcium promotes normal transmission of nerve impulses and helps to regulate normal muscle contraction and relaxation. Constant regulation of calcium levels takes place in the body. If the serum calcium level falls, additional calcium is absorbed in the intestine, reabsorbed through the kidneys, or taken from the bones. If more calcium is needed in the bones, it is taken from the bloodstream and also reabsorbed through the kidneys.

Magnesium. Magnesium (Mg^{2+}) is a cation that is found in bone (50% to 60%), intracellular fluid (39% to 49%), and extracellular fluid (1%). After potassium, magnesium is the most abundant cation in intracellular fluid; therefore it is vital to cellular function. Magnesium plays a role in the metabolism of carbohydrates and proteins, the storage and use of intracellular energy, and neural transmission. Magnesium is important in the functioning of the heart, nerves, and muscles.

Approximately 30% to 40% of magnesium ingested through the diet is absorbed, mainly through the small intestine. Magnesium is excreted through the kidneys and the rate of excretion is regulated by sodium and calcium excretion, extracellular fluid volume, and parathyroid hormone.

Nonelectrolytes

Although most of the solutes in the body are electrolytes, other substances are dissolved in the body fluids as well. Examples are urea, protein, glucose, creatinine, and bilirubin. These solutes do not carry an electrical charge and are measured in milligrams per deciliter (mg/dL).

TRANSPORT OF WATER AND ELECTROLYTES

MEMBRANES

The intracellular and extracellular fluid compartments are separated by **selectively permeable membranes** that control movement of water and certain solutes. Selective permeability maintains the unique composition of each compartment of the body while allowing for the transport of nutrients and wastes to and from cells. For example, selectively permeable membranes surround cells to separate fluid in the cells from fluid in the tissues. Some solutes cross membranes more easily than others. Small molecules and water move freely across membranes whereas larger molecules such as protein move less readily.

TRANSPORT PROCESSES

Water and solutes are transported between intracellular and extracellular fluid compartments by one or more of the following processes: (1) diffusion, (2) active transport, (3) filtration, and (4) osmosis.

Diffusion

Diffusion is the random movement of particles in all directions. The natural tendency is for a substance to move from an area of higher concentration to an area of lower concentration. One example is the movement of oxygen from the alveoli to the pulmonary capillaries. The concentration of oxygen in the alveoli is greater than in the capillaries; therefore oxygen diffuses into the capillaries and is transported through the bloodstream to other parts of the body. The term *facilitated diffusion* is used when a carrier protein transports the molecules through membranes toward an area of lower concentration. This process does not require energy.

Active Transport

Carrier proteins can transport substances from an area of lower concentration to an area of equal or greater concentration. This process, which requires expenditure of energy, is called **active transport**. Many solutes, such as sodium, potassium, glucose, and hydrogen, are actively transported across cell membranes. An example of active transport is the sodium pump. The concentration of sodium is highest in extracellular fluid. Therefore excess sodium cannot leave the cell by diffusion. Active transport "pumps" the excess sodium out of the cell into the extracellular fluid.

Filtration

Filtration is the transfer of water and solutes through a membrane from an area of high pressure to an area of low pressure. This pressure is known as *hydrostatic pressure* and is a combination of pressures from the force of gravity on the fluid and the pumping action of the heart. Filtration is a necessary process for moving fluid out of the capillaries into the tissues and for filtering plasma through the kidneys.

Osmosis

Osmosis is the movement of water across a membrane from a less concentrated solution to a more concentrated solution. It involves the movement of water only but sometimes the force of movement across the membrane carries some solutes along. If a fluid compartment has less water and more sodium, water from another compartment moves to the more concentrated compartment by osmosis to create a better fluid balance.

OSMOLALITY

Osmolality refers to the concentration of a solution determined by the number of dissolved particles per kilogram of water. A higher osmolality means that the concentration of salt, or any other solute, is higher in the water because the solution contains less water. Osmolality controls water movement and distribution in body fluid compartments by regulating the concentration of fluid in each compartment. When solutes such as electrolytes are added to water, the volume is expanded to include both the water and the solutes.

The osmolality of intracellular fluid and extracellular fluid tends to equalize because of the constant shifting of water. A change in osmolality of intracellular fluid affects the osmolality of extracellular fluid and vice versa. The osmolality of intracellular fluid is maintained primarily by potassium and the osmolality of the extracellular fluid is maintained primarily by sodium. The normal range of osmolality of the body fluids is between 280 and 294 milliosmoles per kilogram (mOsm/kg). You will see the term **osmolarity** also used to refer to the concentration of particles in body water. Osmolarity refers to the concentration of particles per liter of solution. For the study of body fluids, measuring liters of fluid is more practical than measuring kilograms; therefore you will see clinical studies of fluids using the term *osmolarity* rather than osmolality.

REGULATORY MECHANISMS

Regulation of fluid balance requires the constant adjustment of fluid volume, distribution, and composition. This process is accomplished by the kidneys and circulatory system, which are influenced by the sympathetic nervous system, specific hormones, and the thirst center.

KIDNEYS

The kidneys are the main regulators of fluid balance. They control extracellular fluid by adjusting the concentration of specific electrolytes, the osmolality of body fluids, the volume of extracellular fluid, blood volume, and pH. Kidney function is delicately controlled by hormones and other coordinating mechanisms (see Chapter 42 for a review of renal structure and function).

The nephron is the functioning unit of the kidney. Each nephron is made up of a glomerulus and tubules. The glomerulus is the filtering portion of the nephron and the tubule is responsible for secretion and reabsorption. The nephrons conduct the work of the kidney through the processes of filtration, reabsorption, and secretion.

Filtration

A primary activity of the kidney is filtration. Blood plasma entering the kidney via the renal artery is delivered to the glomerulus. Approximately 20% of the plasma is filtered into the glomerular capsule. This fluid is called *filtrate.* Most of the remaining plasma leaves the kidney through the renal vein. The filtrate then moves through the tubules, where it is transformed into urine by the processes of tubular reabsorption and secretion.

Tubular Reabsorption

Tubular reabsorption is a process by which most of the glomerular filtrate is returned to the circulation. Water and selected solutes move from the tubules into the capillaries. Waste products remain in the tubules for excretion whereas most water and sodium are reabsorbed into the bloodstream. Tubular reabsorption is important for adjusting the volume and composition of the filtrate and for preventing excessive fluid loss through the kidneys.

Tubular Secretion

Tubular secretion is the last phase in the work of the kidneys. During this phase, the filtrate is transformed into urine. Various substances, among them drugs, hydrogen ions, potassium ions, creatinine, and histamine, pass from the blood into the tubules. This process eliminates some excess substances to maintain fluid and electrolyte balance as well as metabolic waste products.

HORMONES

Hormones that have a major effect on fluid volume and balance are renin, aldosterone, antidiuretic hormone (ADH), and atrial natriuretic factor (ANF). *Renin* is a hormone that is secreted when blood volume or blood pressure falls. Renin activates angiotensinogen, a substance secreted by the liver, to form angiotensin I. Angiotensin-converting enzyme then converts angiotensin I to angiotensin II. Angiotensin II is a potent vasoconstrictor that also stimulates the release of aldosterone, with subsequent sodium and water retention.

Aldosterone is released by the adrenal glands in response to the hormone renin. Aldosterone acts on the kidney tubules to increase the reabsorption of sodium and decrease the reabsorption of potassium. Because the retention of sodium causes water retention, aldosterone acts as a volume regulator. The release of aldosterone from the adrenal gland is stimulated by many factors, including increased potassium levels and decreased sodium levels in the blood.

ADH is produced by the hypothalamus and is secreted into the general circulation by the posterior pituitary gland. It causes the capillaries to reabsorb more water so that urine is more concentrated and less volume is excreted. An increase in plasma osmolality (plasma is more concentrated) stimulates the release of ADH into the bloodstream to replenish needed fluid in the body. Other factors that stimulate the release of ADH are related to stress situations such as hypotension, pain, surgery, and the use of certain medications.

ANF is a hormone released by the atria in response to stretching of the atria by increased blood volume. ANF stimulates excretion of sodium and water by the kidneys, decreased synthesis of renin, decreased release of aldosterone, and vasodilation. The effect of these actions is to reduce blood volume and to lower blood pressure.

Table 14-3 24-Hour Intake and Output of Body Fluids

FLUID GAINS	AMOUNT (mL)	FLUID LOSSES	AMOUNT (mL)
Liquids	1000	Lungs	400
Food (solid)	1200	Skin	400
H_2O of oxidation (metabolic production)	300	Kidneys (urine)	1500
Daily total intake	**2500**	Intestines (feces)	200
		Daily total output	**2500**

THIRST

An additional regulatory mechanism is thirst, which regulates fluid intake. Increased plasma osmolality stimulates osmoreceptors in the hypothalamus to trigger the sensation of thirst. In other words, more sodium and less water in the body make a person thirsty. Additional fluids are consumed and the kidneys conserve water until plasma osmolality returns to normal.

FLUID GAINS AND LOSSES

In a healthy adult, the 24-hour fluid intake and output are approximately equal (Table 14-3). Fluids are gained by drinking and eating and are lost through the kidneys, skin, lungs, and gastrointestinal tract. The usual adult urine volume is between 1 and 2 liters per day (L/day), or 1 milliliter per kilogram of body weight per hour. In the kidneys, water loss varies largely with the amount of solute excreted and with the level of ADH.

Water and electrolyte (sodium, chloride, and potassium) losses through the skin occur by sweating. Water loss through the lungs occurs by evaporation at a rate of 300 to 400 milliliters per day (mL/day). In a hot, dry environment, water loss via the skin and lungs increases. In the gastrointestinal tract, the usual loss of fluid is approximately 100 to 200 mL/day. The bulk of fluid secreted into the gastrointestinal tract is reabsorbed in the small intestine. Water loss through the skin, lungs, and intestinal tract is referred to as insensible loss. Figure 14-1 diagrams the regulation of body fluid volume.

AGE-RELATED CHANGES AFFECTING FLUID BALANCE

Multiple factors place the older person at risk for fluid and electrolyte imbalances. The aging kidney is slower to adjust to changes in acid-base, fluid, and electrolyte balance. The older adult often has a reduced sense of thirst and therefore may be in a state of chronic dehydration because of inadequate fluid intake. Total body water declines with age, with the greatest loss being from the intracellular fluid compartment. Therefore an older person has limited reserves with which to maintain fluid balance when abnormal losses occur.

You must monitor fluid status in the older person and be alert for signs and symptoms of imbalances, including disorientation, confusion, constipation, and falls resulting from postural hypotension. The health history may reveal many chronic conditions, such as heart failure and renal insufficiency, which are more common among older adults and place them at risk for fluid and electrolyte imbalances. Drugs such as antihypertensives, diuretics, and antacids used to treat these and other conditions can also contribute to imbalances. In addition, chronic conditions that affect mobility or mental status may interfere with adequate fluid intake. Some factors that contribute to acute fluid deficits are trauma, infection, fever, influenza or cold, NPO (nothing by mouth) status, and drug therapies (diuretics, antidepressants, sedatives). In addition to the general assessment data, it is especially important to document fluid intake patterns, medications, mental status, and recent weight loss.

Components of the physical examination are described later in this chapter. Note that skin turgor is a less reliable indicator of fluid status in older persons than in younger individuals because some loss of skin elasticity normally occurs with increased age. Assessing turgor on the sternum or forehead is advised for better accuracy in the older person. Serum electrolytes should be the same for all adults, so any abnormalities of such in the older person should be investigated.

Unless contraindicated, fluid requirements for older adults, based on ideal body weight, are 30 mL/kg in persons ages 55 to 65 years and 25 mL/kg in persons ages 65 years and older. Using these guidelines, a 60-year-old person who weighs 150 lb (68.1 kg) would need 2000 mL of fluid daily. A person the same weight at age 70 would require 1700 mL of fluid per day for adequate hydration. Fluid intake should be increased gradually in the older adult because the heart and kidneys adapt more slowly to changes in fluid volume. An individual with cardiac or renal disease sometimes has fluid restrictions because of fluid retention.

Put on Your Thinking Cap!

Measure your fluid intake and output for 24 hours. If they are not equal, list possible explanations for the difference.

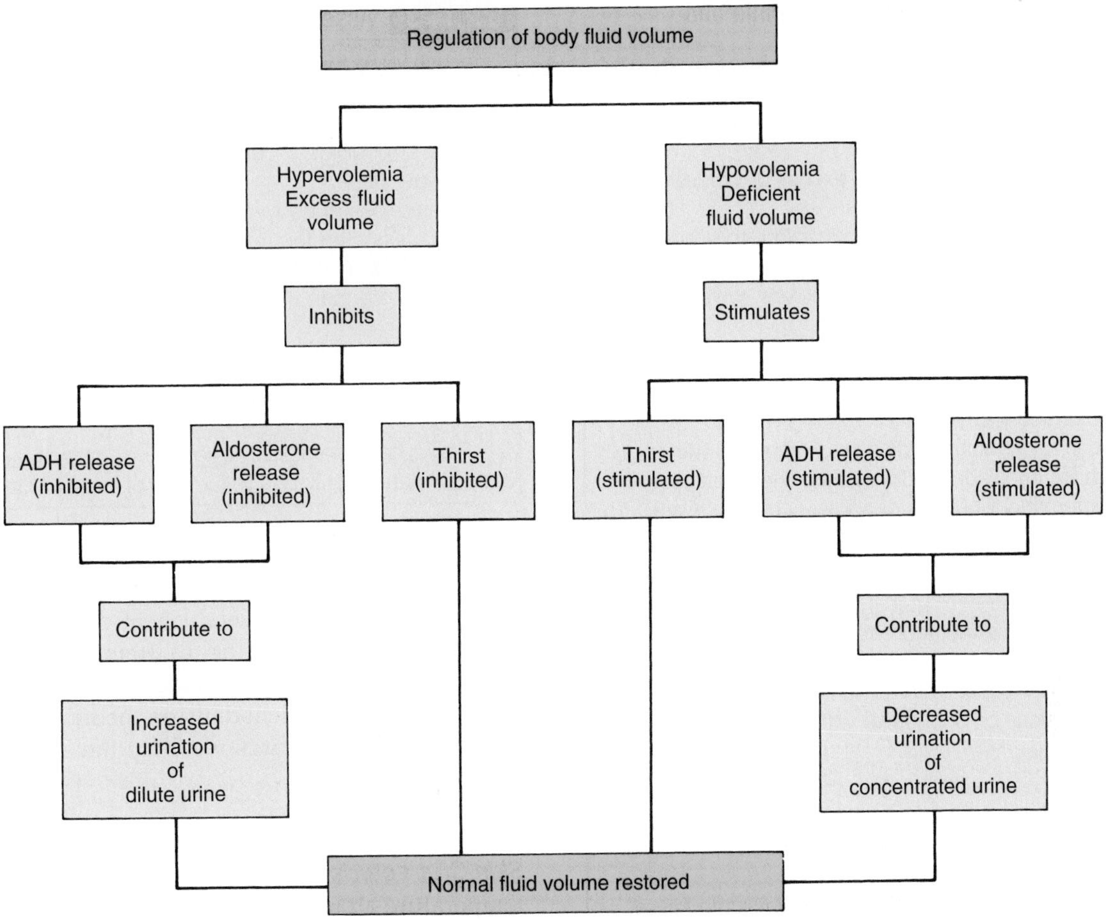

FIGURE 14-1 Regulation of body fluid volume depends on aldosterone, antidiuretic hormone (ADH), and thirst. (From Black JM, Hawks JH, Keene AM: *Medical-surgical nursing: clinical management for continuity of care*, ed 8, Philadelphia, 2009, Saunders.)

ASSESSMENT OF FLUID AND ELECTROLYTE BALANCE

ASSESSMENT

Health History

A complete health history helps to determine whether patients have any conditions that may contribute to fluid or electrolyte imbalances. Conditions that have great potential for disrupting fluid balance are vomiting, diarrhea, kidney diseases, diabetes, salicylate poisoning, burns, congestive heart failure, cerebral injuries, ulcerative colitis, and hormonal imbalances. Other risk factors include the intake of drugs such as diuretics and cathartics and medical interventions such as gastric suctioning. Anticipate fluid and electrolyte imbalances in patients who are at risk. Patient complaints that may be associated with fluid imbalances are fatigue, palpitations, dizziness, edema, muscle weakness or cramps, dyspnea, and confusion. Because electrolyte disturbances produce nonspecific symptoms, they can be confirmed only with laboratory tests.

Vital Signs

Assessment of pulse, respiration, temperature, and blood pressure can detect indicators of changes in both fluid and electrolyte balance, as shown in Box 14-1. Body temperature variations can be associated with excess or deficit fluid volume. Also, fever poses a risk of water and electrolyte loss associated with sweating and an increased metabolic rate. Blood pressure is directly related to blood volume. The pulse rate and quality may change in response to blood volume alterations. Because electrolytes affect the conduction of impulses, electrolyte changes can affect heart rate and rhythm. Respirations are minimally affected by electrolyte changes. However, rapid respirations increase water loss. Also, excess fluid volume can lead to heart failure and pulmonary edema with shortness of breath. Measuring blood pressure with the patient lying, sitting, and standing can detect positional differences that may reflect inadequate blood volume.

Intake and Output

An accurate record of intake and output is essential to determine whether the patient's intake is equal to output. All fluids entering or leaving the body should be noted, as explained in Box 14-2. A changing urine output may reflect attempts by the kidneys to maintain or restore balance or it may reflect a problem that causes fluid disturbances. In addition to urine volume, urine characteristics also give clues to fluid balance.

Box 14-1 Vital Sign Changes with Fluid and Electrolyte Imbalances

PULSE

Increased rate with fluid volume deficit, sodium deficit, or magnesium deficit.

Decreased rate with magnesium excess or potassium deficit.

Weak quality, irregular rhythm, and rapid rate suggest severe potassium excess or sodium deficit.

Bounding quality with fluid volume excess, which often results in circulatory overload.

RESPIRATION

Fluid volume excess can cause pulmonary edema with dyspnea and tachypnea.

Changes in respiratory function are noted also with acid-base imbalances. Slow, shallow respirations with intermittent periods of apnea occur in severe metabolic alkalosis. Deep, rapid respirations indicate metabolic acidosis.

TEMPERATURE

Fever increases the metabolic rate, causing fluid loss; it also increases the respiratory rate, which increases loss of water vapor from the lungs.

Temperature may be subnormal with fluid volume excess.

BLOOD PRESSURE

A fall in systolic pressure of more than 20 mm Hg when the patient changes from the lying to the standing position or from the lying to the sitting position usually indicates fluid volume deficit.

Fluid volume excess that expands blood volume raises the blood pressure.

Box 14-2 Assessment of Intake and Output

- Many serious fluid and electrolyte imbalances can be averted by carefully monitoring records of fluid intake and output.
- If the total intake is substantially less than the total output, the patient is in danger of fluid volume deficit.
- If the total intake is substantially more than the total output, the patient is in danger of fluid volume excess.
- Intake should include all fluids taken into the body: oral fluids, foods that are liquid at room temperature, intravenous fluids, subcutaneous fluids, fluids instilled into drainage tubes or irrigants, tube feeding solutions, water given through feeding tubes, and enema solutions.
- Output measures include urine, vomitus, diarrhea, drainage from fistulas, drainage from suction machines, excessive perspiration, and drainage from excisions; normal adult urine output is 40 to 80 mL/h.

Clear, pale urine in a healthy person suggests the excretion of excess water whereas dark, concentrated urine indicates that the kidneys are retaining water.

Body Weight

Measurement of body weight is a good indicator of fluid loss or retention (Box 14-3). Remember that 1 liter of fluid weighs 2.2 lb. Therefore retention of 1 liter of fluid is reflected as a weight gain of 2.2 lb (1 kg). A patient can accumulate up to 10 lb (4.5 kg) of fluid before pitting edema is evident. To monitor fluid status, weigh the patient daily on the same scale, at the same time of day, and wearing the same type of clothing.

Box 14-3 Assessment of Body Weight

The use of body weight as an accurate index of fluid balance is based on the assumption that the patient's dry weight remains relatively stable. Even under starvation conditions, an individual loses no more than ⅓ to ½ lb dry weight per day.

A rapid loss of body weight occurs when the total fluid intake is *less* than the total fluid output.

A rapid gain of body weight occurs when total fluid intake is *more* than the total fluid output.

	Mild	Moderate	Severe
Rapid loss	2%	5%	8% = deficit
Rapid gain	2%	5%	8% = excess

Rapid gain or loss of 1 kg (2.2 lb) of body weight is approximately equivalent to the gain or loss of 1 liter of fluid.

Skin

Skin Characteristics. Skin color, moisture, turgor, and temperature all reflect fluid balance. Dry, flushed skin is associated with dehydration. Pale, cool, clammy skin is associated with the severe fluid volume deficit that occurs with shock. Moist, edematous tissue, especially in dependent areas, may be seen with excess fluid volume.

Facial Characteristics. The patient who is severely dehydrated usually has a pinched, drawn facial expression. Soft eyeballs and sunken eyes accompany a severe fluid volume deficit. Puffy eyelids and fuller cheeks suggest excess fluid volume.

Skin Turgor. Skin turgor is best measured by pinching the skin over the sternum, the inner aspects of the thighs, or the forehead. In patients who are dehydrated, skin flattens more slowly after the pinch is released. The term *tenting* is sometimes used to describe skin that does not flatten promptly after being gently pinched into a tent shape. The skin of older people generally has a slower return to normal, so assuming a fluid deficit based only on poor skin turgor would be inappropriate in the older person.

Edema. Edema reflects water and sodium retention, which can result from excessive reabsorption or inadequate excretion of sodium, as may occur with kidney failure. Inspect and palpate the skin for edema. Test for edema by pressing the skin that lies over the tibia, fibula, sacrum, or sternum. Edema is described as *pitting* if a depression remains in the tissue after pressure is applied with a fingertip. Pitting edema is evaluated on a four-point scale, ranging from 1+ edema (barely detectable pit) to 4+ edema (deep and persistent pit that is approximately 1 inch or 2.54 cm deep).

Edema can be so severe that pitting is not possible. The tissue becomes so full that fluid cannot be displaced when pressed. Edematous tissue that feels hard is known as *brawny edema*. After a radical mastectomy, brawny edema commonly occurs because the removal of axillary nodes allows fluid to accumulate in the affected arm.

Mucous Membranes

Tongue Turgor. In a normal person, the tongue has one longitudinal furrow. A person with deficient fluid volume has additional longitudinal furrows and the tongue is smaller as a result of fluid loss. Sodium excess causes the tongue to appear red and swollen.

Moisture of the Oral Cavity. A dry mouth may be the result of deficient fluid volume or mouth breathing. Normally, saliva is pooled in the area where the cheek and the gum meet. Dryness in this area usually indicates a true fluid volume deficit. However, dry mouth is a common side effect of many medications.

Veins

The appearance of the jugular veins in the neck and the veins in the hands can suggest either a deficient or excess fluid volume.

Neck Vein Distention. Distention of the jugular veins can indicate excess fluid volume. Inspect the neck veins by having the patient recline with the head of the bed elevated at a 30- to 45-degree angle. If the jugular veins can be seen more than 3 cm above the sternal angle, then excess fluid volume is most likely present.

Deficient fluid volume may be detected by examining the jugular neck veins with the patient lying down. If no distention occurs, then deficient fluid volume is most likely present.

Hand Veins. Observation of hand veins also can be helpful in evaluating the patient's fluid volume. Elevate the hands and then note how long it takes for the veins to empty. Veins usually empty in 3 to 5 seconds. Next, place the hands in a dependent position and note the time needed for the veins to fill. Veins usually fill in 3 to 5 seconds. If the volume is decreased, veins take longer than 3 to 5 seconds to fill. When the fluid volume is increased, veins take longer than 3 to 5 seconds to empty. The nursing assessment of fluid and electrolyte status is summarized in Box 14-4.

DIAGNOSTIC TESTS AND PROCEDURES

A variety of laboratory tests may be performed to assess fluid and electrolyte status and to determine whether they are within the normal range (Table 14-4). Various references report slightly different ranges of normal. Clinical laboratories typically report the normal range along with patient results; therefore you do not need to memorize these ranges.

Box 14-4 Assessment of Fluid and Electrolyte Status

HEALTH HISTORY

Present Illness
Vomiting, diarrhea, burns, head injury

Past Medical History
Renal or cardiac disease, diabetes, inflammatory bowel disease, adrenal or thyroid disease

Current Drugs
Such as diuretics, salicylates, antacids, potassium or calcium supplements

Family History
Diabetes, cardiac disease

Review of Systems
Fatigue, palpitations, dizziness, edema, dyspnea, confusion

Functional Assessment
Change in activity tolerance, mental alertness

PHYSICAL EXAMINATION

General Survey
Alertness, orientation, posture

Vital Signs
Pulse rate/rhythm/quality; respiratory rate/pattern; blood pressure in lying, sitting, and standing positions; temperature

Weight
Present compared with usual

Skin
Color, moisture, turgor, temperature

Facial Characteristics
Expression, firmness of eyeballs, edema of eyelids or cheeks

Edema
Presence, location, pitting or brawny

Mucous Membranes
Tongue turgor, moisture of the oral cavity

Veins
Jugular vein distention, hand vein emptying and refilling time

Urine Studies

Urine pH. The kidneys can change the acidity or alkalinity of the urine by excreting hydrogen (H^+) ions. Urine pH is a measure of hydrogen ions in the urine. It is useful for determining whether the kidneys are responding appropriately to metabolic acid-base imbalances. The normal range is 4.5 to 8.0; however, fresh urine is usually acidic (approximately 6.0). Urine tends to be most acidic in the morning (after a fast) and more alkaline after meals. Diet is a factor in that a person who consumes large amounts of citrus fruits and vegetables tends to have alkaline urine whereas a person who eats a lot of meat tends to have acidic urine. A urine specimen that is not tested within 4 hours of collection may become alkaline; therefore urine pH should be measured within 1 to 2 hours of collection. If the specimen cannot be tested promptly, it should be refrigerated.

Urine Specific Gravity. Urine specific gravity (SpG) is a measure of urine concentration. In most instances, normal urine SpG is between 1.016 and 1.022 in adults.

Table 14-4 Normal Values Related to Fluid and Electrolyte Balance

URINE		BLOOD	
Urine pH	4.6–6.8	Arterial blood pH	7.35–7.45
Urine specific gravity	1.016–1.022	NA	
Urine osmolality (random specimen)	250–1200 mOsm/kg H_2O	Serum osmolality	285–300 mOsm/kg
Urine sodium	40–220 mEq/24 hrs or SI = 40–220 mmol/24 hr	Serum sodium	136–145 mEq/L
Urine potassium	25–125 mEq/24 hr	Serum potassium	3.5–5.1 mEq/L
Urine chloride	40–220 mEq/24 hr or SI: 40–220 mmol/24 hr	Serum chloride	98–107 mEq/L
Urine phosphorus	0.4–1.3 g/24 hr	Serum phosphorus	2.8–4.5 mg/dl
Urine magnesium	6.0–10.0 mEq/L or SI: 3–5 mmol/day	Serum magnesium	Age 21–59 yrs: 1.6–2.6 mg/dL Age 60–90 yrs: 1.6–2.4 mg/dL
Urine creatinine	Male: 1–2 g/day Female: 0.8–1.8 g/day	Serum calcium (total)	Ages 18–60 yrs: 8.6–10.0 mg/dL Ages 60+ yrs: 8.8–10.2
		Serum creatinine	Female: 0.6–1.1 mg/dL Male: 0.7–1.3 mg/dL
		Serum bicarbonate	
		Arterial	21–28 mEq/L
		Venous	24–28 mm Hg or SI: 24–28 mmol/L

From Malarkey, LM, McMorrow, ME: *Saunders nursing guide to laboratory and diagnostic tests*, ed 2, St. Louis, 2012, Elsevier-Saunders.

SpG is a good indicator of fluid balance. A high SpG indicates that the urine is highly concentrated, usually as a result of deficient fluid volume. A low SpG indicates that the urine contains a large amount of water in relation to solutes, usually as a result of excess fluid volume. The SpG also reflects renal function. If the kidneys are not functioning properly, they may fail to concentrate or dilute urine as needed to maintain extracellular fluid balance. The presence of x-ray dyes, glucose, or protein in the urine can cause an increased SpG that may be misleading; that is, the patient may not really have a deficient fluid volume. As people age, their kidneys are less efficient at conserving water by concentrating urine. Therefore the older person may produce relatively dilute urine (low or normal SpG) even when he or she is dehydrated.

Urine Osmolality. Osmolality measures the number of dissolved particles in a solution. This information provides a more precise measurement of the kidney's ability to concentrate urine than does the SpG. For the most accurate interpretation, a serum osmolality should be done simultaneously with the SpG.

Dilute urine has a low osmolality and generally reflects renal excretion of excess water. Low osmolality also is apparent when kidneys are unable to conserve water by concentrating urine. Concentrated urine has a high osmolality and generally indicates renal conservation of water. It can also be present when the kidneys are failing, because the volume of urine secreted declines.

Urine Creatinine Clearance. Urine creatinine clearance tests are used to detect glomerular damage in the kidney. A 24-hour specimen is required. The patient is instructed to void, discard the specimen, record the time, and start collecting all urine thereafter for 24 hours. The specimen must be refrigerated.

During the specimen collection period, the patient should maintain good hydration, should not engage in vigorous exercise, and should avoid high-protein foods, coffee, tea, and cola drinks. Be aware that many drugs, including cephalosporin antibiotics, can alter test results. For best interpretation, serum creatinine clearance should be assessed as well. Also, the laboratory needs to know the patient's height, weight, and age. The normal creatinine clearance for men is 85 to 125 mL/min/1.73 m^2 of body surface area; for women, it is 75 to 115 mL/min/1.73 m^2 of body surface area. The range decreases with age.

Urine Sodium. Urine sodium reflects sodium intake and fluid volume status. When the intake of sodium is high, the kidneys will increase the excretion of sodium in the urine. When large amounts of fluids are taken in or sodium intake is restricted, the urine is more dilute, thus the urine sodium falls. The urinary excretion of sodium is normally highest during the day. The normal urine sodium is 75 to 200 mEq/L. If collected over a period of 24 hours, the normal range is 40 to 220 mEq/24 h or SI = 40 to 220 mmol/24 h.

Urine Potassium. Urine potassium is a measure of renal tubular function. A 24-hour specimen is most meaningful because the urinary excretion of potassium is highest at night and lowest during the day. Therefore a random sample would not truly represent function of the renal tubules. The normal value is 25 to 125 mEq/24 h.

Blood Studies

Serum Hematocrit. The hematocrit is the percentage of blood volume that is composed of red blood cells. An increased hematocrit is seen with deficient fluid volume and dehydration because the blood is more concentrated. A low hematocrit is consistent with excess fluid volume because of dilution. The normal range for hematocrit is 40% to 54% for men and 38% to 47% for women.

Serum Creatinine. Creatinine is a metabolic waste product. The serum creatinine level is a better indicator of renal function than the blood urea nitrogen. A high level of creatinine in the blood indicates poor renal function. The normal range is 0.6 to 1.1 mg/dL for females and 0.7 to 1.3 mg/dL for males. Even small changes in the serum creatinine can be significant.

Blood Urea Nitrogen. Blood urea nitrogen (BUN) provides a measure of renal function. Normal is 5 to 20 mg/dL for adults under age 60 and 8 to 23 mg/dL for adults over age 60 years. A high BUN is associated with deficient fluid volume and possibly impaired renal function; conversely, a low BUN is associated with excess fluid volume.

Serum Osmolality. Serum osmolality is a measure of blood concentration. High serum osmolality is related to a deficient fluid volume and low serum osmolality is related to excess fluid volume. The normal range is 285 to 300 mOsm/kg.

Serum Albumin. Albumin is a plasma protein that helps to maintain blood volume by creating colloid osmotic pressure. The normal range for serum albumin is 3.5 to 5.5 g/dL. Low serum albumin allows water to shift into the interstitial compartment, which reduces blood volume and creates edema.

Serum Electrolytes. Normal values for serum sodium, potassium, chloride, and calcium are shown in Table 14-4.

FLUID IMBALANCES

DEFICIENT FLUID VOLUME

Deficient fluid volume occurs when water is less than normal in the body. The two types of fluid volume deficits are isotonic extracellular fluid deficit (hypovolemia) and hypertonic extracellular fluid deficit (dehydration). A deficient fluid volume may result from decreased intake, abnormal fluid losses, or both. Examples of abnormal fluid losses are the loss of water as a result of excessive bleeding, severe vomiting and diarrhea, and severe burns.

The signs and symptoms of deficient fluid volume vary depending on how suddenly the deficit develops and how severe it is. Symptoms are not as apparent with deficits that are mild and have a gradual onset but the symptoms are quite dramatic when the loss is severe and the onset is abrupt. In general, the body attempts to compensate for fluid volume deficits by decreasing urine output. The heart rate increases in an effort to maintain blood flow to body tissues. The blood pressure may fall because of the reduced blood volume.

Treatment varies somewhat according to the cause of a deficient fluid volume and the severity of symptoms. Nursing care should be based on appropriate nursing diagnoses, which might include the following:

- **Deficient Fluid Volume, Risk for Deficient Fluid Volume** related to inadequate fluid intake, excessive fluid loss, high blood glucose, inadequate ADH production or effect, high fever, altered capillary permeability
- **Acute Confusion** related to decreased cerebral tissue perfusion
- **Constipation** related to excessive reabsorption of water from stool in the colon
- **Fatigue** related to decreased blood volume, decreased tissue perfusion
- **Hyperthermia** related to infectious process, decreased fluid volume
- **Risk for Injury** related to decreased level of consciousness
- **Risk for Impaired Skin Integrity** related to poor tissue turgor
- **Ineffective Peripheral Tissue Perfusion** related to decreased cardiac output secondary to decreased blood volume

The characteristics, causes, assessment findings, treatment, and nursing care for each type of fluid volume deficit are outlined in Table 14-5.

EXCESS FLUID VOLUME

An increase in body water is called **excess fluid volume.** The two types of excess fluid volume are extracellular fluid excess (isotonic fluid excess) and intracellular water excess (hypotonic fluid excess). Excess fluid volume may result from renal or cardiac failure with retention of fluid, increased production of ADH or aldosterone, overload with isotonic intravenous fluids, or the administration of 5% dextrose in water (D_5W) after surgery or trauma. The body attempts to compensate for excess fluid volume by increasing the filtration and excretion of sodium and water by the kidneys and decreasing the production of ADH.

As with deficient fluid volume, the severity of the symptoms in excess fluid volume depends on how quickly the condition develops. Severe excess fluid volume can cause or aggravate heart failure and pulmonary edema.

Nursing care varies somewhat according to the cause of an excess fluid volume and the severity of symptoms. Care should be based on appropriate nursing diagnoses, which might include the following:

- **Excess Fluid Volume** related to fluid retention, excess or hypotonic intravenous fluid administration

Table 14-5 Deficient Fluid Volume

	ISOTONIC EXTRACELLULAR FLUID DEFICIT (HYPOVOLEMIA)	HYPERTONIC EXTRACELLULAR FLUID DEFICIT (DEHYDRATION)
Definition	Deficiency of both water and relative electrolytes	Deficiency of water without electrolyte deficiency
Etiology	Decreased fluid intake related to inability to obtain or ingest fluids Excessive fluid loss related to vomiting, diarrhea Shifting of fluid into interstitial space (third spacing) related to increased capillary permeability	Increased water loss related to high blood glucose as in uncontrolled diabetes mellitus, inadequate ADH production or renal response to ADH, high fever, excessive sweating Decreased fluid intake with continued intake of electrolytes, as with concentrated tube feedings
Assessment Findings		
Blood pressure	Hypotension	Hypotension
Pulse	Weak, rapid	Weak, rapid
Respirations	Rapid	Rapid
Temperature	Decreased	Increased
Weight	Loss	Loss
Tissue turgor	Normal or edema	Poor
Mucous membranes	Moist	Dry
Blood cells	Hgb, Hct, RBCs increased	Hgb, Hct, RBCs increased
Urine output	Decreased	Decreased or increased
Thirst	Normal	Thirsty
Treatment	Correction of underlying cause. Water and electrolyte replacement. Antiemetics, antidiarrheals. Oral and intravenous fluids.	Correction of underlying cause. Water replacement. Oral and intravenous fluids. Hypoglycemic agents, ADH, antipyretics.
Nursing care	Protect edematous tissue with third spacing. Assist with rising and ambulating if patient is dizzy. Keep hourly records of intake and output; expect intake to exceed output at first. Be alert for fluid excess (rising pulse and blood pressure, dyspnea) caused by excessive fluid replacement.	Monitor blood glucose if patient has diabetes. Assist with oral hygiene. Assist with rising and ambulating if patient is dizzy. Keep hourly records of intake and output; expect intake to exceed output at first. Be alert for fluid excess (rising pulse and blood pressure, dyspnea) caused by excessive fluid replacement.

ADH, Antidiuretic hormone; *Hct*, hematocrit; *Hgb*, hemoglobin; *RBCs*, red blood cells.

- **Acute Confusion** related to cerebral edema
- **Activity Intolerance, Impaired Gas Exchange** related to pulmonary edema
- **Risk for Injury** related to decreased level of consciousness
- **Risk for Impaired Skin Integrity** related to edema
- **Ineffective Peripheral Tissue Perfusion** related to reduced cardiac output with heart failure

The causes, assessment findings, treatment, and nursing care of the patient with excess fluid volume are outlined in Table 14-6.

ELECTROLYTE IMBALANCES

The two electrolytes that cause the majority of problems when an imbalance exists are sodium and potassium.

HYPONATREMIA (SODIUM DEFICIT)

Hyponatremia is lower-than-normal sodium in the blood serum. It can be an actual deficiency of sodium or an increase in body water that dilutes the sodium excessively. Causes include excessive intake of water without sodium; excessive loss of sodium, as with vomiting, diarrhea, or diaphoresis with only water replacement; the use of distilled water to irrigate body cavities; and excessive secretion of ADH. Increased ADH secretion is associated with severe stress, some head injuries, and a condition called *syndrome of inappropriate antidiuretic hormone secretion* (SIADH). Other disorders that put the patient at risk for hyponatremia include congestive heart failure, liver cirrhosis, and nephrotic syndrome.

Sodium normally holds water in the extracellular compartment. When serum sodium is low, water can

Table 14-6 Excess Fluid Volume

	EXTRACELLULAR FLUID EXCESS	INTRACELLULAR WATER EXCESS
	Isotonic Fluid Excess	*Hypotonic Fluid Excess*
Definition	Excess of both water and electrolytes. Major symptoms are caused by increased blood volume.	Excess of body water without excess electrolytes. Major symptoms are caused by cerebral edema.
Etiology	Retention of water and electrolytes related to kidney disease; overload with isotonic IV fluids.	Overhydration in presence of renal failure; administration of D_5W after surgery or trauma.
Assessment Findings		
Blood pressure	Increased	Increased systolic
Pulse	Bounding, increased rate	Decreased rate
Respirations	Increased rate, crackles, dyspnea	Increased rate
Weight	Gain	Gain
Edema	Extremities: dependent, pitting Puffy eyelids	Cerebral
Neck veins	Distended	Normal
Mucous membranes	Moist	Moist
Blood	Hgb, Hct, RBCs decreased by dilution	Hgb, Hct, RBCs normal or decreased
Mental status	Irritability, confusion, lethargy	Irritability, confusion, lethargy
Hand vein engorgement	Present	Absent
Pupils	Sluggish response to light with cerebral edema	Sluggish response to light with cerebral edema
Treatment	Correction of underlying cause. Restriction of water and sodium intake. Diuretics to promote fluid elimination, digitalis to improve cardiac output. Renal dialysis if kidney failure is a factor.	Correction of underlying cause. Restricted water intake. IV and oral fluids with electrolytes. Demeclocycline (Declomycin) to decrease kidney response to ADH.
Nursing care	Give drugs and IV fluids as ordered. Monitor for excess diuresis. Explain and enforce fluid restriction. Offer ice chips; use small fluid containers, let patient help design plan for fluid intake. If patient is not confused, allow to swish fluids in mouth and spit out without swallowing. Explain salt restriction; obtain dietary consult for teaching (Box 14-5). Protect edematous tissue: turn and reposition q2h. Inspect for signs of skin breakdown. If dyspneic: Elevate head of bed 30 degrees or for comfort, loosen restrictive clothing, oxygen as ordered.	Give drugs and IV fluids as ordered. Explain and enforce fluid restriction. Offer ice chips, provide oral hygiene, serve only fluids allowed with meal trays, let patient design plan for fluid intake. If patient is not confused, allow to swish fluids in mouth and spit out without swallowing. If confused, take safety precautions: side rails up, bed in low position, call light in reach, check often. Seizure precautions per agency policy.

ADH, Antidiuretic hormone; *D_5W,* dextrose 5% in water; *Hct,* hematocrit; *Hgb,* hemoglobin; *IV,* intravenous; *q2h,* every 2 hours; *RBCs,* red blood cells.

enter cells more freely. This shift of fluids is most significant in relation to brain cells. The accumulation of fluid in brain cells produces the most important physiologic effects of hyponatremia.

Assessment

If hyponatremia is suspected or the patient is at risk, monitor for signs and symptoms, which include headache, muscle weakness, fatigue, apathy, confusion, abdominal cramps, and orthostatic hypotension. Take blood pressures with the patient lying or sitting and then standing to determine whether a drop in pressure is significant. A drop in systolic blood pressure of more than 20 mm Hg indicates orthostatic hypotension.

Medical Treatment

The usual treatment for hyponatremia is restriction of fluids while the kidneys excrete excess water. Intravenous normal saline or Ringer's lactate may be ordered. If sodium falls below 115 mEq/L, hypertonic sodium may be ordered. The diuretic furosemide (Lasix) may be ordered because of its ability to promote water loss that exceeds the sodium loss. A balanced diet usually provides adequate sodium but patients with moderate or severe hyponatremia may need sodium replacement therapy.

If the patient has SIADH, which can be chronic or acute, an effort is made to determine and correct the cause. In addition to fluid management and diuretic therapy, drugs such as tolvaptan (Samsca) and conivaptan (Vaprisol) that block the action of ADH, demeclocycline, or lithium may be ordered. Another pharmacologic option is urea, which induces water loss without excessive loss of sodium.

NURSING CARE of the Patient with Hyponatremia

You can help to prevent hyponatremia in patients with feeding tubes by using normal saline rather than water for irrigation. For patients with hyponatremia, administer prescribed medications and intravenous fluids and monitor the response to these. Measure fluid intake and output, assess mental status, and monitor laboratory test results. If the patient is confused, take safety measures to prevent injury. If the patient who has hyponatremia has low blood pressure or postural hypotension, assist with ambulation.

HYPERNATREMIA (SODIUM EXCESS)

Hypernatremia refers to a higher-than-normal concentration of sodium in the blood. It is a very serious imbalance that can lead to death if not corrected. Hypernatremia can occur alone or in combination with extracellular fluid volume deficit. The high level of sodium in the serum and other extracellular fluids causes water to shift out of the cells, which creates cellular dehydration. Hypernatremia occurs when loss of water or retention of sodium is excessive. Some causes of hypernatremia are vomiting, diarrhea, diaphoresis (profuse sweating), and insufficient ADH. Signs and symptoms of hypernatremia are thirst, a flushed skin, dry mucous membranes, a low urine output, restlessness, an increased heart rate, convulsions, and postural hypotension.

Medical Treatment

Medical intervention focuses on oral or intravenous replacement of water to restore balance. The aim is to restore the fluid balance slowly to prevent cerebral edema resulting from excessive dilution of extracellular fluid. If the patient has an extracellular fluid volume deficit as well, intravenous fluids with decreasing amounts of sodium may be ordered. A low-sodium diet is often prescribed.

NURSING CARE of the Patient with Hypernatremia

Encourage patients with hypernatremia to drink water for hydration. Closely monitor the infusion of intravenous fluids, especially when the patient's cardiac or renal function is abnormal. Patient education is important. Teach the patient with hypernatremia to track daily intake and output and to recognize the signs and symptoms of fluid retention or depletion. Advise patients of any dietary restrictions. If a low-sodium diet is prescribed, patients should avoid foods that are high in sodium: ketchup, monosodium glutamate (Accent), mustard, pickles, olives, ham, most canned foods, artificial sweeteners, laxatives, cough medications, and some antacids. A selection of foods high and low in sodium is found in Box 14-5. Salt substitutes can be used if potassium intake is not restricted, because salt substitutes contain significant potassium.

Box 14-5 Top Ten Categories of High-Sodium Foods

1. Smoked, processed, or cured meats and fish (ham, bacon, corned beef, cold cuts, hot dogs, sausage, salt pork, chipped beef, pickled herring, anchovies, tuna, sardines)
2. Tomato juices and tomato sauce, unless labeled otherwise
3. Meat extracts, bouillon cubes, meat sauces, MSG, and taco seasoning
4. Salted snacks (potato chips, tortilla chips, corn chips, pretzels, salted nuts, popcorn, and crackers)
5. Prepared salad dressings, condiments, relishes, ketchup, Worcestershire sauce, barbecue sauce, cocktail sauce, teriyaki sauce, soy sauce, commercial salad dressings, salsa, pickles, olives, and sauerkraut
6. Packaged mixes for sauces, gravies, casseroles, and noodle, rice, or potato dishes; macaroni and cheese; stuffing mix
7. Cheeses (processed and cheese spreads)
8. Frozen entrees and pot pies
9. Canned soup
10. Foods eaten away from home

From Mahan LK, Escott-Stump S, Raymond JL: *Krause's food and the nutrition care process*, ed 13, St. Louis, 2012, Elsevier-Saunders.
MSG, Monosodium glutamate.
Note: reading labels is most important; some brands are lower in sodium than others.

HYPOKALEMIA (POTASSIUM DEFICIT)

Hypokalemia is low serum potassium. Causes include vomiting, diarrhea, nasogastric suction, inadequate dietary intake of potassium, diabetic acidosis, excessive aldosterone secretion, and drugs such as potassium-wasting diuretics and corticosteroids. Because potassium is necessary for normal cellular function, deficiencies may result in gastrointestinal, renal, cardiovascular, and neurologic disturbances. Most important is the effect on myocardial cells, which tends to cause abnormal, potentially fatal, heart rhythms.

Signs and symptoms of hypokalemia are anorexia, abdominal distention, vomiting, diarrhea, muscle cramps, weakness, dysrhythmias (abnormal cardiac rhythms), postural hypotension, dyspnea, shallow respirations, confusion, depression, polyuria (excessive urination), and nocturia.

Medical Treatment

Potassium replacement by the intravenous or oral route may be prescribed.

NURSING CARE of the Patient with Hypokalemia

When a patient has hypokalemia, monitor for decreased bowel sounds, a weak and irregular pulse, decreased reflexes, and decreased muscle tone. Monitoring the heart rate and rhythm of patients taking digitalis is especially important because hypokalemia increases the risk of digitalis toxicity. Cardiac monitors may be used to detect dysrhythmias.

Administer prescribed oral potassium supplements with a full glass of water or fruit juice to prevent gastrointestinal irritation. Instruct patients to sip slowly. Encourage dietary sources of potassium, particularly fruits and vegetables, such as bananas and oranges or orange juice. A chart of foods high and low in potassium is found in Box 14-6.

Administer intravenous potassium as ordered. ! **Potassium is *always* diluted and never given in concentrated form.** Ideally, it is administered through a central venous catheter; otherwise, the potassium may not be adequately diluted by blood before it reaches the heart. Closely monitor the rate of intravenous infusion because of the risk of cardiac arrest with rapid infusion. Also, inspect the infusion site because potassium salts can cause inflammation of the veins. **Note that potassium is *never* given by intravenous push.**

Check the patient's urine output before starting an intravenous infusion of potassium. When the urine output is low, intravenous fluids without potassium may be given until the urine output is acceptable and then fluids with potassium are started. If you were to administer the intravenous potassium before normal urinary output was restored, the patient could develop hyperkalemia. Urinary output should be no less than 30 mL/h. If it is less than 30 mL/h for 2 consecutive hours, alert the physician, who may order a stop of the infusion.

Box 14-6 Potassium Content in Common Foods

Low (0–100 mg/serving*)	Very High (>300 mg/serving*)
Fruits	***Fruits***
Applesauce	Avocados, ¼ small
Blueberries	Banana, 1 small
Cranberries	Cantaloupe, ¼ small
Lemon, ½ medium	Dried fruit, ¼ cup
Lime, ½ medium	Honeydew melon, small
Pears, canned	Mango, 1 medium
Pear nectar	Papaya, medium
Peach nectar	Prune juice
Vegetables	***Vegetables***
Cabbage, raw	Artichoke, 1 medium
Cucumber slices	Bamboo shoots, fresh
Green beans, frozen	Beet greens, cup
Leeks	Corn on the cob, 1 ear
Lettuce, iceberg, 1 cup	Chinese cabbage, cooked
Water chestnuts, canned	Dried beans
Bamboo shoots, canned	Potatoes, baked, medium
	Potatoes, French fries, 1 oz
	Spinach
	Sweet potatoes, yams
	Swiss chard, cup
	Tomato, fresh, sauce or juice; tomato paste, 2 Tbsp
	Winter squash
	Miscellaneous
	Bouillon, low sodium, 1 cup
	Cappuccino, 1 cup
	Chili, 4 oz
	Coconut, 1 cup
	Lasagna, 8 oz
	Milk, chocolate milk, 1 cup
	Milkshakes, 1 cup
	Molasses, 1 Tbsp
	Pizza, 2 slices
	Salt substitutes, tsp
	Soy milk, 1 cup
	Spaghetti, 1 cup
	Yogurt, 6 oz

Data from Mahan LK, Escott-Stump SE, Raymond JL: *Krause's food and the nutrition care process,* ed 13, St. Louis, 2012, Saunders.

*One serving equals cup unless otherwise specified.

Pharmacology Capsule

Potassium is always diluted before intravenous administration. It is never administered by intravenous push. Rapid infusion of potassium can cause cardiac arrest.

HYPERKALEMIA (POTASSIUM EXCESS)

Hyperkalemia is high serum potassium. Potassium is plentiful in common foods, so taking in adequate amounts is easy for people on normal diets. However, the kidneys do not readily conserve potassium, so continuous replacement is necessary. Patients at risk for hyperkalemia are those with decreased renal function, people in metabolic acidosis, and people taking potassium supplements. Also, patients who have had severe traumatic injuries may develop hyperkalemia because of the loss of potassium from damaged cells into the extracellular fluid.

Hyperkalemia is a serious imbalance because of the potential for life-threatening dysrhythmias. Elevated potassium typically causes first bradycardia, then tachycardia. A risk of cardiac arrest is also present. In the gastrointestinal system, hyperkalemia can cause explosive diarrhea and vomiting. Neuromuscular effects are muscle cramps and weakness and paresthesia (a tingling sensation). Other signs and symptoms of hyperkalemia include irritability, anxiety, abdominal cramps, and decreased urine output.

Medical Treatment

Hyperkalemia is treated by correcting the underlying causes and restricting potassium intake. Polystyrene sulfonate (Kayexalate), a drug that can be given orally or rectally, promotes excretion of excess potassium through the intestinal tract. Intravenous calcium gluconate may be given to decrease the effects of potassium on the myocardium. Temporary effects may be obtained by the intravenous administration of insulin and glucose or sodium bicarbonate to promote the shifting of potassium into the cells.

NURSING CARE of the Patient with Hyperkalemia

Patients with low urine output or those taking potassium-sparing diuretics must be monitored carefully for signs and symptoms of hyperkalemia because decreased renal function can cause hyperkalemia. Patients receiving potassium supplements, especially intravenously, warrant special attention. Carefully monitor the flow rate of intravenous fluids, which should not exceed 10 mEq/h of potassium chloride through peripheral veins. Even when extreme hypokalemia is being treated, no more than 20 mEq/h of potassium chloride should be given and *only* with constant cardiac monitoring. Examine the infusion site because potassium is very irritating to subcutaneous tissues. Extravasation can cause serious tissue damage.

Screen the results of laboratory studies. Because serum potassium levels greater than 5.0 mEq/L can cause cardiac arrest, immediately report the results to the physician and anticipate an order for the patient to be placed on cardiac monitoring and a change in the potassium supplement order. Monitor patients who take potassium supplements for signs and symptoms of abnormal potassium levels. Explain to the patient the importance of frequent blood tests to monitor potassium levels.

CHLORIDE IMBALANCE

Because chloride is usually bound to other electrolytes, chloride imbalances accompany other electrolyte imbalances. High serum chloride, known as *hyperchloremia*, is usually associated with metabolic acidosis. Low serum chloride, known as *hypochloremia*, usually occurs when sodium is lost because chloride is most frequently bound with sodium. Hypochloremia may be caused by vomiting and uncontrolled diabetes.

CALCIUM IMBALANCE

Calcium in the blood is regulated by the parathyroid glands, which secrete parathyroid hormone (PTH). A low serum level of calcium (hypocalcemia) stimulates PTH secretion. PTH enhances calcium retention and phosphate excretion by the kidneys, promotes calcium absorption in the intestines, and mobilizes calcium from the bones to raise the serum calcium level.

Hypocalcemia results from diarrhea, inadequate dietary intake of calcium or vitamin D, multiple blood transfusions (banked blood contains citrates that bind to calcium), and some diseases, including hypoparathyroidism. The most prominent sign of hypocalcemia is neuromuscular irritability manifested by a tingling sensation in the face and hands, muscle twitches, and progressively severe muscle cramps that typically affect the hands, feet, and legs first. Assessment for hypocalcemia is discussed more fully in Chapter 47 (see Fig. 47-3).

Hypercalcemia is the abnormally increased level of calcium in the serum. Causes of hypercalcemia include a high calcium or vitamin D intake, hyperparathyroidism, and immobility that causes stores of calcium in the bones to enter the bloodstream; it is also a complication of certain types of cancer.

MAGNESIUM IMBALANCE

A lower-than-normal concentration of magnesium in the bloodstream is known as *hypomagnesemia*. Hypomagnesemia results from decreased gastrointestinal absorption or excessive gastrointestinal loss, usually from vomiting and diarrhea or from increased urinary loss. Hypomagnesemia often is associated with hypocalcemia and hypokalemia.

A higher-than-normal concentration of magnesium in the bloodstream is known as *hypermagnesemia*. It occurs most often with the excessive use of magnesium-containing medications or intravenous solutions in patients with renal failure or preeclampsia of pregnancy.

ACID-BASE DISTURBANCES

Acid-base balance refers to homeostasis of the hydrogen ion concentration in the body fluids. A solution containing a higher number of hydrogen ions is an **acid**, and a solution containing a lower number of hydrogen ions is an *alkaline* or **base**. The symbol used to indicate hydrogen ion concentration is pH. pH is reported on a scale of 1 to 14, with 1 to 6.9 being acidic, 7 being neutral, and 7.1 to 14 being alkaline.

The hydrogen ion concentration in extracellular fluid is indicated by the pH of the blood. The normal pH of blood is between 7.35 and 7.45, which is slightly alkaline. The normal acid-base balance is maintained by three primary, complex mechanisms: (1) buffers, (2) respiratory control of carbon dioxide, and (3) renal regulation of bicarbonate (HCO^-_3). The principal buffers in renal tubular fluid are the carbonic acid/bicarbonate system, ammonia, and phosphate. Other substances that function as buffers are proteins and hemoglobin. Buffer systems comprise a weak acid and a salt. To maintain body fluids in the normal pH range, the blood buffers circulate throughout the body in pairs, acting as sponges to soak up hydrogen ions. One of the buffers takes away a hydrogen ion if a fluid is too acid and one of the buffers gives an ion if the fluid is too alkaline.

The lungs and kidneys are the next line of defense after the blood buffers for maintaining acid-base balance. The lungs are primarily responsible for the regulation of carbon dioxide in the blood, which is controlled by the rate and depth of respirations. Carbonic acid in the alveolar capillaries breaks down into water and carbon dioxide, which is eliminated through exhalation. Deep, rapid breathing eliminates excess carbon dioxide, thereby reducing extracellular fluid acidity. Shallow, slow respirations reduce the loss of carbon dioxide, thereby increasing extracellular acidity. If the pH of the blood becomes too high or too low, the respiratory center in the brain sends signals to the lungs to increase or decrease respirations to either "blow off" or retain the appropriate amount of carbon dioxide.

The kidneys act as the metabolic regulators of pH by excreting acids or bases as needed. Renal regulation of bicarbonate and excretion of hydrogen ions are the chief means of regulating acid-base balance through the kidneys. Bicarbonate is a major acid buffer in the blood and is reabsorbed and produced through the kidneys.

If the regulatory mechanisms fail, acid-base imbalances occur. The four major types of acid-base imbalances are (1) respiratory acidosis, (2) respiratory alkalosis, (3) metabolic acidosis, and (4) metabolic alkalosis.

ASSESSMENT OF ACID-BASE STATUS

Health History

Note a history of renal, endocrine, or respiratory disease. A history of diabetes mellitus is especially important because acidosis is a complication of diabetes. The nursing assessment focuses on symptoms of acid-base imbalance, which could include very deep or rapid respirations (or both), anxiety, confusion, dizziness, lightheadedness, seizures, and change in weight. List any medications the patient is taking.

Physical Examination

Observe the patient's general appearance in terms of responsiveness. Look for signs of anxiety or other distress. Take the vital signs, and weigh the patient. Pay special attention to the rate, depth, and rhythm of respiration. Test muscle strength and sensory function in the extremities. Evaluate mental status.

In addition to collecting data for the nursing assessment, as described in Box 14-7, note the results of arterial blood gas measurements (Table 14-7).

RESPIRATORY ACIDOSIS

Respiratory acidosis occurs when the respiratory system fails to eliminate the appropriate amount of carbon dioxide to maintain the normal acid-base balance. Carbon dioxide is retained, with a resultant accumulation of carbonic acid and a decrease in blood pH. The body responds to respiratory acidosis by stimulating respirations to eliminate excess carbon dioxide. If that mechanism cannot restore balance, renal compensation begins. The kidneys attempt to help by reabsorbing more bicarbonate to balance the amount of carbonic acid in the blood.

Acute respiratory acidosis is caused by respiratory diseases such as pneumonia, drug overdose, head injury, chest wall injury, obesity, asphyxiation, drowning, or acute respiratory failure. People with chronic pulmonary disease may have elevated carbon dioxide levels but a normal pH as a result of renal compensation. Common clinical signs and symptoms include rapid heart rate, headache, sweating, lethargy, and confusion.

Box 14-7 Assessment of Acid-Base Balance

HEALTH HISTORY

Signs and Symptoms
- Dyspnea, anxiety, confusion, dizziness, seizures, changes in weight, muscle weakness, abnormal sensations (numbness, tingling)

Medical Conditions
- Respiratory impairment, diabetes mellitus, adrenal disorders, cardiac disorders, renal failure

Current Medications

Physical Examination

Height and Weight
- Current compared with previous measurements

Vital Signs
- Pulse rate and rhythm; respiratory rate, depth, and rhythm

Neurologic Function
- Muscle strength, sensation in extremities, mental status

Measures of Oxygenation
- Arterial blood gases

Table 14-7 Arterial Blood Gas Values with Uncompensated Respiratory and Metabolic Acidosis and Alkalosis

CONDITION	CAUSE	PH (7.35–7.45)	HCO^-_3 (21–28 MEQ/L OR SI 21–28 MMOL/L)	$PACO_2$ (35–45 MM HG OR SI 4.7–5.3 KPA)
Respiratory acidosis	Hypoventilation	↓	Normal	↑
Respiratory alkalosis	Hyperventilation	↑	Normal	↓
Metabolic acidosis	Diabetic ketoacidosis Lactic acidosis Diarrhea Renal insufficiency	↓	↓	Normal
Metabolic alkalosis	Vomiting HCO^-_3 retention Volume depletion K^+ depletion	↑	↑	Normal

HCO^-_3, Bicarbonate; *kPa*, kilopascals; *$PaCO_2$*, partial pressure of carbon dioxide in arterial blood.

hypothalamus and secreted by the posterior pituitary gland, promotes water retention.
- ANF is secreted when stretch receptors in atria detect an increase in blood volume. It promotes excretion of water and sodium, decreases renin synthesis, inhibits release of aldosterone and ADH, and causes vasodilation.
- The thirst center creates a desire to drink fluids when extracellular fluid becomes concentrated.
- In a healthy adult, the 24-hour fluid intake and output are approximately equal.
- The body attempts to compensate for deficient fluid volume by increasing the heart rate and conserving water in the kidneys.
- The body attempts to compensate for excess fluid volume by increasing urine output.
- The kidneys are the primary regulators of electrolytes in the blood.
- Two electrolytes that cause the majority of problems when there is an imbalance are sodium and potassium.
- Change in body weight is a good indicator of fluid loss or retention.
- Edema reflects sodium retention, which can result from excessive reabsorption or inadequate secretion because of failing kidney function.
- Potassium excess or deficit can lead to life-threatening cardiac dysrhythmias.
- Because older adults often have a reduced thirst sensation and may not conserve water efficiently, they are at risk for fluid volume deficit.
- Acid-base balance is the homeostasis of the hydrogen ion concentration in the body fluids.
- Mechanisms that maintain acid-base balance are blood buffers, respiratory control of carbon dioxide, and renal regulation of bicarbonate.
- Acid-base imbalances occur when an imbalance in the functioning of the lungs, kidneys, or both exists. The four major acid-base imbalances are (1) respiratory acidosis, (2) respiratory alkalosis, (3) metabolic acidosis, and (4) metabolic alkalosis.

Additional Learning Resources

SG Go to your Study Guide for additional learning activities to help you master this chapter content.

evolve Go to your Evolve website (http://evolve.elsevier.com/Linton/medsurg) for the following learning resources and much more:
- Interactive Prioritization Exercises
- Fluid & Electrolyte Tutorial
- Pharmacology Tutorial
- Review Questions for the NCLEX® Examination

Review Questions for the NCLEX® Examination

1. Fluid surrounding the cells is called ______ fluid.
   NCLEX Client Need: Physiological Integrity: Basic Care and Comfort
2. The largest portion of a person's body weight is contributed by:
   1. Water
   2. Fat
   3. Bone
   4. Muscle

   NCLEX Client Need: Physiological Integrity: Basic Care and Comfort
3. The movement of water across a membrane from a less concentrated solution to a more concentrated solution defines:
   1. Diffusion
   2. Osmosis
   3. Filtration
   4. Active transport

   NCLEX Client Need: Physiological Integrity: Basic Care and Comfort
4. A hormone with physiological effects that decrease blood pressure is:
   1. ADH
   2. Renin
   3. Aldosterone
   4. ANF

   NCLEX Client Need: Physiological Integrity: Basic Care and Comfort
5. A 79-year-old nursing home patient develops severe diarrhea. To plan appropriate care, the nursing staff should understand which of these statements best describes the risk of fluid and electrolyte imbalances in the older adult?
   1. Most older adults can maintain fluid and electrolyte balance just as well as younger adults.
   2. Older adults have limited reserves to maintain fluid balance when abnormal losses occur.
   3. Body water increases with age, putting the older adult at risk for excess fluid volume.
   4. The amount of extracellular fluid declines, leaving the patient with reduced fluid stores.

   NCLEX Client Need: Physiological Integrity: Physiological Adaptation
6. A patient is receiving diuretics to eliminate excess fluid that has been retained in body tissues. In 2 days the patient lost 4.4 lb (2 kg) in body weight. This represents how many liters of fluid loss? ______.
   NCLEX Client Need: Physiological Integrity: Pharmacological Therapies
7. You gently pinch the skin over a patient's sternum. The skin does not flatten right away, leading you to suspect:
   1. Recent weight loss
   2. History of excessive sun exposure
   3. Dehydration
   4. Need for increased diuretics

   NCLEX Client Need: Physiological Integrity: Reduction of Risk Potential

8. When reviewing a patient's laboratory results, the nurse notes that the patient has a potassium imbalance. Which of the following nursing assessments is most important for this patient?
   1. Auscultate bowel sounds
   2. Evaluate muscle strength
   3. Monitor heart rate and rhythm
   4. Assess reflexes

   NCLEX Client Need: Physiological Integrity: Reduction of Risk Potential
9. Arrange the mechanisms that maintain acid-base balance in the correct order of occurrence.
   1. Renal regulation
   2. Buffers
   3. Respiratory regulation

   NCLEX Client Need: Physiological Integrity: Physiological Adaptation
10. What is the physiologic function of deep, rapid respirations in metabolic acidosis?
    1. Eliminates excess carbon dioxide that is formed in the presence of acidosis
    2. Raises the arterial oxygen level, which reduces the pH of the blood
    3. Supplies additional oxygen needed because of the increased metabolic rate
    4. Reduces the $PaCO_2$, resulting in a rise in blood pH and correction of acidosis

    NCLEX Client Need: Physiological Integrity: Physiological Adaptation

chapter

15 Pain Management

http://evolve.elsevier.com/Linton/medsurg

Mary L. Heye, Kathleen A. Reeves

Objectives

1. Define pain.
2. Explain the physiologic basis for pain.
3. Explain the relationships between past pain experiences, anticipation, culture, anxiety, and a patient's response to pain.
4. Identify differences in the duration of pain and patient responses to acute and chronic pain.
5. Identify situations in which patients are likely to experience pain.
6. Explain the special needs of the older adult patient with pain.
7. List the data to be collected in assessing pain.
8. Describe interventions used in the management of pain.
9. Describe the nursing care of patients receiving opioid and nonopioid analgesics for pain.
10. List the factors that should be considered when pain is not relieved with analgesic medications.

Key Terms

Acute pain
Addiction
Analgesia (ăn-ăl-JĒ-zē-ă)
Analgesic (ăn-ăl-JĒ-zĭk)
Anesthesia (ăn-ĕs-THĒ-zhă)
Chronic pain
Neuropathic (nŭ-rō-PĂTH-ĭk)
Nociceptive (nō-sĕ-SĔP-tĭv)
Nociceptor (nō-sĕ-SĔP-tĕr)
Pain
Pain threshold
Pain tolerance
Physical dependence
Referred pain
Tolerance (TŎL-ĕr-ăns)

Pain is one of the most complex experiences to understand and treat. It is also the most common problem that nurses encounter. Research about pain, **analgesics** (drugs that relieve pain), and the mind-body influence is just beginning to filter down to nursing practice. Still, many questions about pain remain unanswered.

Pain is influenced by many variables: the individual experiencing it, the cause of the pain, and the environment. Pain may arise from a new source, from an old injury, or from nerve injury. The cause is sometimes unknown. Pain relief rests primarily with the nurse, who must assess the patient and implement appropriate interventions.

Nurses have many categories of pain-relieving interventions from which to choose yet they frequently administer only analgesics. Most nurses believe that pain is easily managed with analgesic drugs. Patients, however, often report that pain remains moderate to severe despite these medications. Research indicates that nurses fail to assess pain, tend to undermedicate for pain, and have inadequate knowledge of pain relief measures. Because of these findings, The Joint Commission published standards for the management of pain for all patients. Health care facilities are expected to comply with these standards, which include (1) recognizing the right of patients to appropriate assessment and management of pain, (2) screening patients for pain during initial assessment and, when clinically required, during ongoing, periodic reassessments, and (3) teaching patients and families about effective pain management. The purpose of this chapter is to enable the nurse to understand pain, assess pain, and provide the most effective interventions for pain relief.

DEFINITION OF PAIN

Pain is defined in many ways. The International Association for the Study of Pain defines it as an unpleasant sensory and emotional experience associated with actual or potential tissue damage. McCaffery, a nurse and leader in the pain management field, has a more useful definition for nurses. She says, "Pain is whatever the person experiencing it says it is and exists whenever he says it does" (1999, p. 98).

PHYSIOLOGY OF PAIN

The perception of pain involves afferent pathways, the central nervous system, and efferent pathways. Afferent pathways are nerves that carry messages to the brain for interpretation. Efferent (or descending) pathways are nerves that carry messages away from the brain to the rest of the body via the spinal cord.

Afferent pathways are activated by pain receptors called **nociceptors**. These pain receptors are unevenly distributed in muscles, tendons, subcutaneous tissue, and the skin. This distribution may explain why parts of the body are more sensitive to pain than other parts. Pain receptors are sensitive to chemical changes, temperature, mechanical stimuli, and tissue damage. Some receptors are sensitive to more than one type of stimulus. When subjected to repeated stimuli, pain receptors may continue to react even after the stimuli are removed. With repeated stimulation to receptors over time, physical and chemical changes can occur in the pain pathways; thus pain is still perceived after the original painful event or stimulus is removed.

When pain receptors are stimulated, impulses are transmitted to the spinal cord. The impulses then travel up the spinal cord to the brain. In the brain, the cortex interprets the impulses as pain and identifies the location and qualities of the pain. Other structures involved in the interpretation of pain signals activate the stress response and produce the unpleasant qualities associated with pain, such as fear. Once pain is transmitted to the spinal cord and brain, the descending pathway is activated and several substances (e.g., endorphins, serotonin, norepinephrine, gamma-aminobutyric acid, enkephalins) that can inhibit pain transmission to the spinal cord are released.

Endorphins and enkephalins are the body's natural opioid-like substances that block the transmission of painful impulses to the brain. Differences in the amount of endorphins in individuals may explain why some people seem to experience more pain than others. Research suggests that prolonged stress and pain, as well as the prolonged use of morphine and alcohol, decrease endorphin levels. Factors that increase endorphin levels include brief stress and pain, laughter, exercise, acupuncture, transcutaneous electrical nerve stimulation (TENS), massive trauma, and sexual activity.

GATE CONTROL THEORY

Although many theories have been proposed to explain pain, none fully describes the pain experience. One of the best known theories is Melzack and Wall's gate control theory. It assumes that the pain experience reflects both physical and psychosocial factors. Painful impulses are transmitted to the spinal cord through small-diameter nerve fibers in the afferent pathway. When these small-diameter fibers are stimulated, the gating mechanism opens in the spinal cord, which permits the transmission of impulses from the spinal cord to the brain. Consequently the patient perceives pain. Factors that cause the gate to open include tissue damage, a monotonous environment, and fear of pain. These small-diameter fibers end in the spinal cord along with large-diameter fibers. The stimulation of large-diameter fibers can close the gate and interfere with impulse transmission between the spinal cord and the brain. This interference causes diminished pain perception. Large-diameter nerve fibers are stimulated by cutaneous (skin) stimulation through massage, position change, and heat or cold applications. Sensory input such as distraction, guided imagery, and preparatory information also may close the gate. Figure 15-1 shows the structures and mechanisms associated with the gate control theory.

FACTORS INFLUENCING RESPONSE TO PAIN

Consider the following example: Miss Smith and Mrs. Johnson are roommates in Room 200. Miss Smith, age 19, underwent an appendectomy on the previous day, as did Mrs. Johnson, age 67. The nurses discussed the difference in the behavior of each patient: "Miss Smith constantly wants more pain medication. She moans and groans all the time. She won't even turn, cough, or breathe deeply for more than 10 seconds. She always rates her pain as a 9 or a 10 on the pain scale. On the other hand, look at Mrs. Johnson. She's already ambulating. She rarely rates her pain as more than a 2 or a 3 on the pain scale. She usually just complains of aching and she sure doesn't ask for as much pain medication as Miss Smith. You'd never guess they had undergone the same procedure."

This example illustrates that although people may have the same injury or insult (in this case, surgery), they may respond differently. This difference exists because many physical and psychosocial factors affect the response to pain. Health professionals should be nonjudgmental and avoid comparing one individual in pain with another individual in pain.

PHYSICAL FACTORS

Many physical factors influence the pain experience, including the individual's pain threshold, pain tolerance, age, physical activity, nervous system integrity, and, in cases of surgery, the type of surgery performed and the type of **anesthesia** used.

Pain Threshold

The **pain threshold** is the point at which a stimulus causes the sensation of pain. Anger, fatigue, anxiety, insomnia, depression, and uncontrolled pain all lower the pain threshold. With a lower threshold, the person experiences pain more readily with less stimuli. During

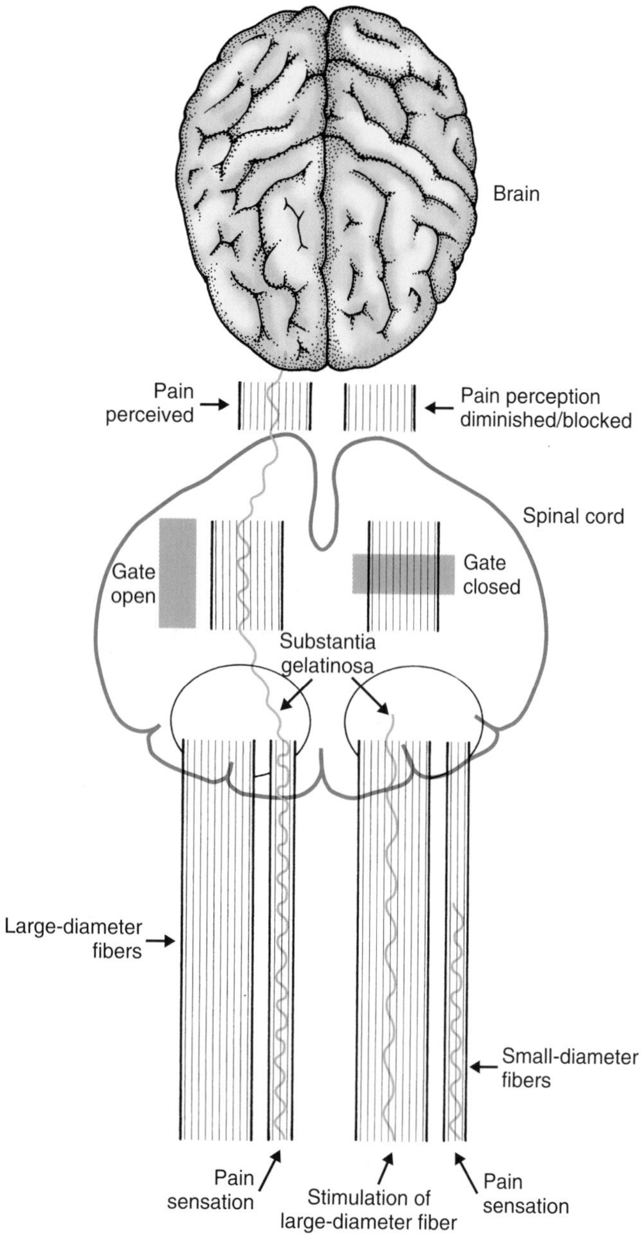

FIGURE 15-1 The gate control theory of pain. (From Ignatavicius DD, Workman ML: *Medical surgical nursing: patient-centered collaborative care*, ed 6, St. Louis, 2010, Saunders-Elsevier.)

hospitalization or illness, a patient may experience anxiety, fatigue, or loss of sleep, all of which can lower the pain threshold or cause the patient to experience pain more easily.

Pain Tolerance

Pain tolerance refers to the intensity of pain that a person will endure. It is another factor influencing response to pain. Pain tolerance varies among patients and varies for an individual patient, depending on the situation. Increasing or prolonged pain may lower the pain tolerance because the patient fears that the pain will not be relieved. Low pain tolerance or high pain tolerance must be respected and must not interfere with adequate pain management.

Age

Age may also influence response to pain. At times, older patients do not report their pain or they report that their pain is much less severe than it really is. Some do not report pain because they are stoic or they have been told incorrectly that pain is a normal part of aging. Some older patients may not want to bother the nurse or they may fear rejection from the caregiver. Pain is *not* a normal part of aging, although older adults often suffer from chronic conditions such as arthritis, cancer, and bone fractures that are associated with pain.

Physical Activity and Nervous System Integrity

Physical activity and the integrity of the nervous system also can influence the reaction to pain. Physical activity may aggravate or precipitate pain. However, with some patients, physical activity may be used to relieve pain. Because pain is perceived and interpreted within the nervous system, the integrity of the system affects the response to pain. For example, patients with diabetic neuropathy may have peripheral nerve damage caused by high glucose levels. As a result, these patients may lose sensation in the extremities and may not feel pain or they may feel burning sensations in their feet and legs at rest or with activity.

Surgery and Anesthesia

In surgical patients, the type of surgery performed and the type of anesthesia used can influence the response to pain. Surgery on the upper thoracic and abdominal regions of the body is thought to be the most painful because of the numerous tissues traumatized during the procedure. Within this group are cardiac, pulmonary, gastric, and gallbladder procedures. The type of anesthetic agent used can influence postoperative pain. For example, ketamine has analgesic properties. Some anesthetic agents injected at the operative site may prolong **analgesia** for 12 to 24 hours after surgery. When these types of agents are used, patients may experience much less pain after surgery than those who do not receive these anesthetic agents.

Surgery or invasive procedures may be performed to relieve pain that is severely debilitating. Rhizotomy and cordotomy are rarely performed surgical procedures that cut or destroy selected nerve tissue to interrupt the pain pathway. Pain relief from these procedures may not be permanent because nerve tissue regenerates. These procedures have been replaced by nerve-deadening procedures performed with localized heating (radiofrequency lesioning) or freezing techniques (cryoanalgesia) by pain specialists usually done in outpatient settings. The goal of these procedures is to provide prolonged pain relief and patients may report tingling or buzzing sensations instead of pain.

Nerve blocks or injections of drugs into specific tissues or joints can reduce pain and improve function for acute pain and chronic pain. Drugs are injected to block the transmission of pain signals. For example, femoral anesthetic nerve blocks may be performed before hip replacement surgery to reduce postoperative pain up to 24 hours after surgery is completed, or a small catheter connected to a container with anesthetic drug may be placed into the surgical wound before closure to provide continuous pain relief in the immediate postoperative period. Acupuncture is another invasive technique that produces anesthesia or analgesia. It is an ancient Chinese practice in which tiny needles are inserted into the skin or subcutaneous tissues at specific points on the body. This technique may be used to relieve acute and chronic pain such as headache, menstrual cramps, and low back pain.

PSYCHOLOGIC FACTORS

Along with physical factors, several psychologic factors can influence the response to pain, including culture, religion, past experiences with pain, anxiety, and situational factors.

Culture, Ethnicity, and Gender

Although studies have been conducted to determine the effect of culture, ethnicity, and gender on people's reaction to pain, you should avoid making judgments based on how you think a person should react or behave. Some persons may deny pain, remain calm and unemotional, or withdraw. Other persons may cry, moan and groan, and involve their families in the painful experience. Be aware of the different ways of expressing pain and respect individual variations in the response to pain.

Religious Beliefs

Religious beliefs also may have an impact on reaction to pain. Some patients may pray and believe that divine intervention will help them to endure the pain. Others may view pain as a punishment for sins. Some individuals believe that suffering is required before pain relief can be obtained.

Past Experiences and Anxiety

Past experiences and anxiety may affect a person's response to current pain. A person may have developed positive coping strategies to deal with previous painful experiences. If, however, previous coping strategies were unsuccessful, the patient may be very anxious and overwhelmed by another painful experience.

Situational Factors

Finally, situational factors may influence response to pain. If the pain is associated with a serious illness such as cancer, the pain may have a greater impact on mood and activity than if the pain were associated with a less serious condition. The pain associated with childbirth is relatively short lived and usually results in a beautiful outcome whereas cancer pain may be chronic and increasing and may be associated with progression of the disease and death.

Cultural Considerations

What Does Culture Have to Do with Pain?

The way a person behaves in response to pain is determined, in part, by cultural norms. Therefore people from some cultures quietly endure pain whereas people from other cultures loudly express their pain. As nurses, we must accept each response and assess and intervene to promote maximal comfort.

RESPONSES TO PAIN

AUTONOMIC NERVOUS SYSTEM

The pain signal is interpreted by the brain as a stressor. The autonomic nervous system activates the fight-or-flight response and certain physiologic responses are initiated. Box 15-1 indicates some of the responses that occur and the associated effects. The patient in pain may exhibit these physiologic responses, along with behaviors such as grimacing, moaning, and verbalizing pain or withdrawing. The nervous system responses can be measured by an increased heart rate, respiratory rate, and blood pressure. These reactions are possible responses to acute pain; however, the pain responses and behaviors will vary from individual to individual and are not reliable indicators of pain. Acute pain and chronic pain elicit different kinds of responses. Table 15-1 lists some differences between acute pain and chronic pain.

ACUTE PAIN

Most pain experienced in the hospital is **acute pain**. Acute pain follows the normal pathway for pain from nociceptor activation to the brain and may be called **nociceptive** pain. Examples are postoperative pain from incisions, renal colic pain from kidney stones, bone fractures, and pain in childbirth. Acute pain is temporary and its cause is known and treatable; it also

Box 15-1 Autonomic Nervous System Responses to Pain

SYMPATHETIC NERVOUS SYSTEM RESPONSES

↑ Blood pressure
↑ Pulse rate
↑ Respiratory rate
Dilated pupils
Perspiration
Pallor

PARASYMPATHETIC NERVOUS SYSTEM RESPONSES

Constipation
Urinary retention

Table 15-1 Differences in Acute Pain and Chronic Pain

CHARACTERISTIC	ACUTE	CHRONIC
Time	Limited, short duration	Lasts 3–6 months, longer duration
Purpose	Sign of tissue injury	No purpose
Verbal	Reports pain, focuses on pain	No report of pain unless questioned
Behavioral	Restless, thrashing, rubbing body part, pacing, grimacing, and other facial expressions of pain	Tired looking, minimal facial expression, quiet, sleeps, rests, attention on other things
Physiologic	Increased heart rate, blood pressure, respiratory rate	Normal heart rate, blood pressure, respiratory rate
Interventions	Responds to analgesics Standard doses effective for pain relief Parenteral or oral route used Additional drugs (adjuvant) seldom needed to manage pain	Less responsive to analgesics Higher doses needed for pain relief Oral route preferred Additional drugs often needed to manage pain

serves as a warning of tissue damage and subsides when healing takes place. Nurses observe behavioral and physiologic signs of acute pain when the patient guards or rubs a body part, wrinkles the brow, bites the lip, and has changes in the heart rate, blood pressure, and respiratory rate. These responses may be absent or lessened in chronic pain.

CHRONIC PAIN

Chronic pain is usually defined as pain that persists or recurs for more than 3 to 6 months; it may last a lifetime. Chronic pain may be nociceptive like osteoarthritis or *neuropathic pain*, which follows an abnormal pathway for processing pain. Review Figure 15-1. **Neuropathic** pain is caused by nerve damage resulting from a wide variety of anatomic and physiologic conditions and underlying diseases. It causes unusual sensations such as burning, shooting pain, and abnormal sensations that occur when no painful stimulus is present. The cause of this pain is often unknown. Treatment may or may not be helpful in relieving the pain. Chronic pain has many classifications. Some chronic pain examples are shown in Table 15-2. Chronic pain is associated with a variety of diagnoses, including cancer, arthritis, peripheral vascular diseases, and traumatic injuries. It usually occurs daily and is not life threatening. *Intractable pain* is another term used to describe pain that cannot be relieved and has no known effective treatment.

Chronic noncancer pain is also defined as persistent pain that interferes with sleep and function, resulting in possible disability and loss of health and normal lifestyle. Although injury often initiates chronic pain, other factors may contribute to ongoing or persistent pain over time. This type of pain is usually best treated by pain specialists and interprofessional health care teams.

Many conditions common in older adults may be associated with chronic pain. Phantom limb pain, in which the patient still feels sensations and pain in the amputated limb, is an example of chronic neuropathic pain. It can be extremely debilitating if it is not recognized and treated early. Phantom limb pain may occur in any related body part that has been amputated or traumatized (e.g., amputation of the breast or leg). Several therapies may be used to reduce this type of pain (e.g., opioids, antidepressants, nerve block, surgical revision, physical therapy).

Table 15-2 Classification of Pain

CLASS	EXAMPLES
Acute pain	Appendicitis Kidney stone Tendonitis
Chronic noncancer pain	Low back pain Rheumatoid arthritis Phantom limb pain Fibromyalgia
Cancer-related pain	Cancer pain syndromes (direct effect of tumor or cancer treatment), postchemotherapy pain, postradiation pain, spinal cord compression

CANCER-RELATED PAIN

Cancer-related pain may be considered acute and chronic pain. Cancer pain may be chronic pain if it lasts longer than 3 to 6 months. Cancer may also cause the development of new nociceptive pain when the cancer causes pressure or damage to tissue or nerves. This type would be acute pain. Pain related to cancer can be very complex because it may include a variety of pain problems that can be nociceptive or neuropathic (or both) and it may be caused by the treatment.

Of the three classes of pain, chronic pain is poorly understood and research-based interventions for various pain syndromes are currently being identified. Some current treatments for chronic pain include opioids, antidepressants, antiepileptics, surgically implanted pumps for drugs, and epidural stimulators that can block pain impulses in the spinal cord.

COMPARISON OF ACUTE PAIN AND CHRONIC PAIN

In contrast to acute pain, which warns of tissue damage and trauma, chronic pain serves no useful purpose. It can have a debilitating and destructive effect on a person's life. Chronic pain can lead to depression, marital difficulties, loss of self-esteem, immobility, and isolation. The patient in chronic pain often does not report pain and shows little facial expression or few physical signs of pain. When pain is chronic, adaptation may occur. The sympathetic nervous system adapts. The heart rate, blood pressure, and respiratory rate may not be elevated and the patient may rest, sleep, or turn attention to other activities despite severe pain.

The nurse may underestimate the severity of the pain or undermedicate a patient with chronic pain. Nursing assessment of pain is essential to identify (1) the characteristics and intensity of pain, (2) whether the pain is chronic or acute, and (3) whether the patient has both acute pain and chronic pain at the same time. The patient who reports pain but shows no pain behaviors or physical symptoms experiences pain but the patient may have learned other ways to deal with the pain or the patient may be taking other medications that block the response of the sympathetic nervous system to pain. For example, some cardiac medications block increases in heart rate and blood pressure.

❖ NURSING CARE of the Patient in Pain

Pain management continues to be a challenge for every nurse. Every individual experiences pain differently and reacts to pain with a variety of physiologic and behavioral responses. Based on an accurate assessment of pain, the physician prescribes treatment and the nurse provides nonpharmacologic and pharmacologic measures together to provide pain relief. The nurse plays a key role by assessing, intervening, and evaluating the patient in pain. Figure 15-2 shows the variety of interventions you can use to relieve pain.

Assessment

Assessment is the first step in pain management. Assessment of pain should be performed on admission and on a regular basis. Anticipate pain as a result of procedures, surgery, or progression of a disease. Accurately record the assessment and compare with previous information. This process permits evaluation of the pattern of pain or the effectiveness of an intervention.

Assessing pain in some patients, especially older adults, can be difficult. Visual, speech, hearing, and motor impairments may limit the ability of older patients to communicate pain or to use scales to rate pain. Patients with cognitive impairment may be unable to report pain or recall pain sensations. Pain can also cause confusion, irritation, and depression in older adults. Consider these aspects when assessing the older adult.

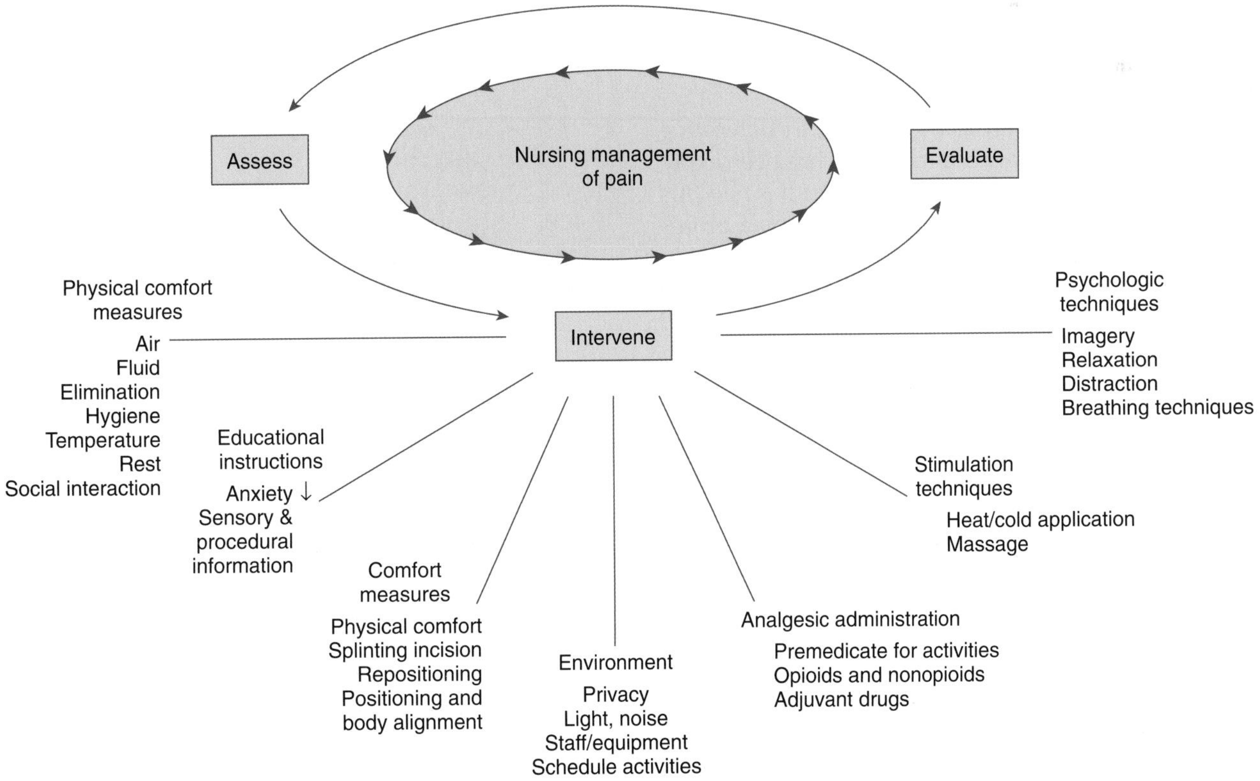

FIGURE 15-2 Nursing management of pain.

When the patient cannot communicate verbally, he or she may be able to point to or direct your attention to a location on a body diagram or pain intensity scale. You may also have to use family observations and patient behaviors to assess pain and pain relief in this type of situation. When the patient cannot report pain, you may have to perform a different assessment that includes observing for usual or unusual behaviors that may indicate pain. These behaviors are not specific to pain; therefore other causes of discomfort, such as fecal impaction or bladder infection, should be assessed as well.

The six steps in pain assessment are listed in Box 15-2 and are discussed in the following sections.

Accept the Patient's Report

The first step in pain assessment is to establish rapport with the patient and accept what the patient says about the pain. When possible, all information about pain should be obtained directly from the patient. The person in pain is the only authority on the pain; no one else can really describe how the pain feels. Accept the report in a nonjudgmental and caring manner. Obtain specific details about the pain and respond positively that action will be taken to relieve the pain.

The assessment of pain requires excellent therapeutic communication skills. Important attitudes are conveyed through verbal and nonverbal behaviors. Listen patiently without interruption, use eye contact, touch the patient, and repeat and clarify information in an unhurried manner to establish trust and obtain information. Do not compare one patient's report of pain with another's report because pain is an individual experience.

Determine the Status of the Pain

The second step in pain assessment is to determine whether the pain is a new occurrence or has been experienced before. Ask the patient if he or she has had this pain before and whether it was diagnosed by a physician. Based on the patient's responses and history, decide whether the pain is chronic in nature or acute pain that needs immediate treatment. For example, a patient who is recovering from a prostatectomy may suddenly have chest pain. The patient identifies this discomfort as the typical angina pain for which he has taken medication in the past. A similar patient with chest pain and no previous cardiac history should be seen by a physician immediately because this pain is a new pain that the patient has not had before. Although both patients need to be evaluated by a physician, an accurate nursing assessment is essential to determine the difference between these two types of pain and consequently the action to be taken.

Describe the Pain

The third step in pain assessment is to describe the pain in terms of its location, quality, intensity, and aggravating and alleviating factors.

Location. Have the patient describe where the pain is and point to the exact location with one finger. If more than one location of pain is described, use a body chart, as shown in Figure 15-3. Have the patient shade in or mark an X at the locations of pain. Then number the various locations on the body chart so that you can refer to the number rather than writing the exact location each time. Also, determine whether the pain is confined to one area or whether it starts at one place and moves to another.

The location identified as painful does not always correspond with the disease or operative site. For example, patients may experience back and neck spasm after surgical procedures. Another example is referred pain. **Referred pain** is often experienced in a location different from its source (Fig. 15-4). To illustrate, pain from appendicitis is usually felt around the umbilicus and is of the aching, cramping type. The

Box 15-2 Six Steps in Pain Assessment

1. Accept the patient's report.
2. Determine the status of the pain.
3. Describe the pain:
   a. Location
   b. Quality
   c. Intensity
   d. Aggravating and alleviating factors
4. Examine the site.
5. Identify coping methods.
6. Record the assessment, interventions, and evaluation of interventions.

(Reassessment after interventions is important to document effectiveness.)

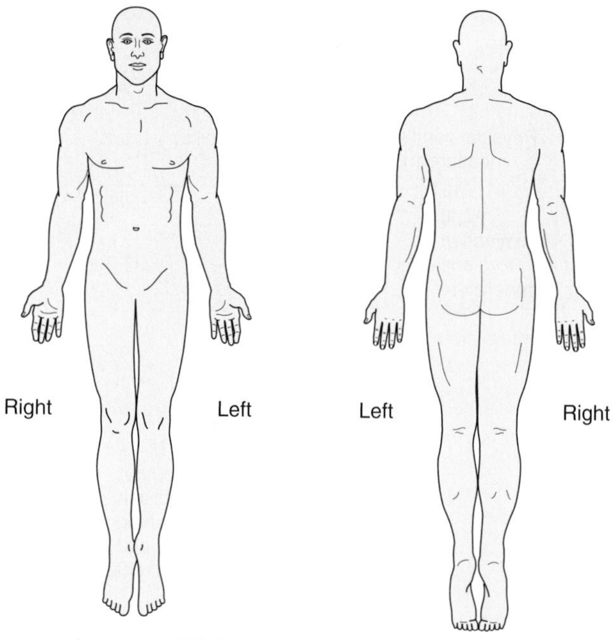

FIGURE 15-3 Body diagram.

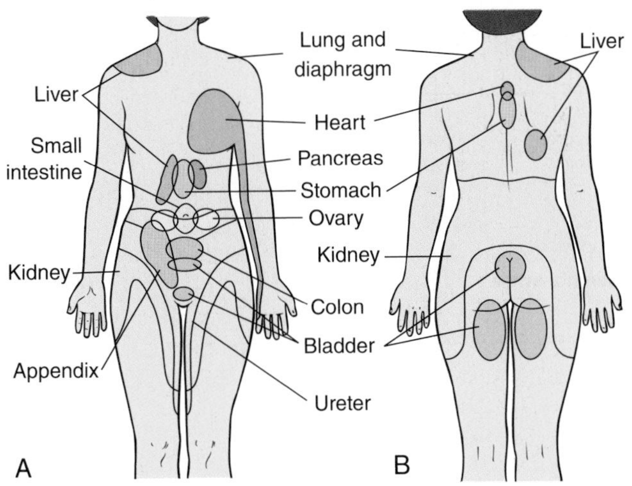

FIGURE 15-4 Anterior and posterior referred pain sites. (From Heuther SE, McCance KL: *Understanding pathophysiology*, ed 5, St. Louis, 2012, Mosby-Elsevier.)

pain impulses come from an inflamed appendix in the right lower quadrant of the abdomen, where sharp pain also may be experienced. Anginal pain is another type of referred pain. It is caused by lack of blood flow to the heart muscle and may be experienced as pain in the jaw, arm, and neck, as well as in the chest.

Quality. Ask the patient: "What words do you use to describe your pain?" or "What would you do to me to have me feel the pain you have?" If the patient has difficulty describing the pain, suggest words. Commonly used words are *sharp, dull, cramping, aching, gnawing, burning, heavy, tender,* and *throbbing*. However, allowing the patient to use his or her own words is best and these exact words should be recorded in the medical record.

Intensity. Because pain is a subjective experience, nurses must have some way to measure the severity of pain. The purpose of asking about intensity is to put the patient's description into an objective term or number. To determine intensity, use one of the scales shown in Figure 15-5. A simple descriptive scale uses words of varying intensity—for example, mild, moderate, or severe. Some patients have difficulty with these words and using words such as "a little pain," "a lot of pain," or "too much pain" may be better. A numeric scale can be 0 to 10 or 0 to 5, with 0 meaning "no pain" and the highest number meaning "the worst pain experienced." A "faces" scale with numbers rating intensity can also be used and some adults prefer to use this type of scale. For example, the Wong-Baker FACES Pain Rating Scale was designed for children but can be used by older adults, some of whom are cognitively impaired. As well, because it has been translated into several languages it may be appropriate for patients of various cultures.

Explain the selected scale to the patient and ask, "Where would you rate your pain right now?" The scale used should make sense to the patient, be easy to use, and be consistently used with the same words or numbers. Remember to explain the scale to the patient each time that pain intensity is assessed. The advantage of using a scale is that it provides a personal measure of the patient's pain and allows evaluation of pain relief using a consistent measure. A scale that is meaningful to the patient and that can be used repeatedly requires less effort for the patient in pain.

For example, a 42-year-old man with multiple fractures in the right arm used the numeric scale from 0 to 10 for rating pain. The patient complained of throbbing in his right arm and a backache. He rated the intensity of both pains at 7 on the scale at 8:00 PM. The nurse applied heat to the lower back as ordered, massaged his back, and administered 10 mg of morphine orally. At 9:00 PM, the patient rated the intensity of both pains at 2 and stated that the pain was slowly going away. The nurse recorded this information and identified that the interventions were effective in relieving the pain in both locations because the pain intensity had decreased from 7 to 2 on the 0-to-10 scale. The nurse also noted that she would reassess the patient's pain every 2 hours. Some hospital policies set a number or "comfort goal" that automatically triggers pain intervention. For example, any pain rating 4 or above on the pain scale requires a nursing intervention for pain relief because research has shown that a pain rating of 4 or above interferes with function and recovery. Pain that is not relieved should be reported to the nurse in charge.

Aggravating and Alleviating Factors. Ask if any event or activity causes the pain or makes it better or worse. Ask: "What were you doing when the pain occurred?" Aggravating factors are those that make the pain worse. Certain positions, temperatures, or times of day or night may cause the pain to be more severe. Similarly, alleviating factors might include specific positions; application of heat, cold, or menthol; or physical activities that reduce pain in specific areas.

Patients can usually identify factors that aggravate or reduce pain and what specific pain relief methods have worked in the past. For example, four patients having abdominal surgery may have arthritic shoulder pain and have four different methods of reducing the pain. The first patient obtained relief with elevation and rest of the right arm. The second applied an analgesic balm, a menthol ointment. The third patient used a heating pad on the area and the fourth increased the antiinflammatory drug dose as prescribed by the physician.

Examine the Site of the Pain

The fourth step in the assessment of pain is to examine the location that the patient states is painful. Assess the area for heat, redness, swelling, tenderness, abnormal position, or other factors that may be causing local irritation.

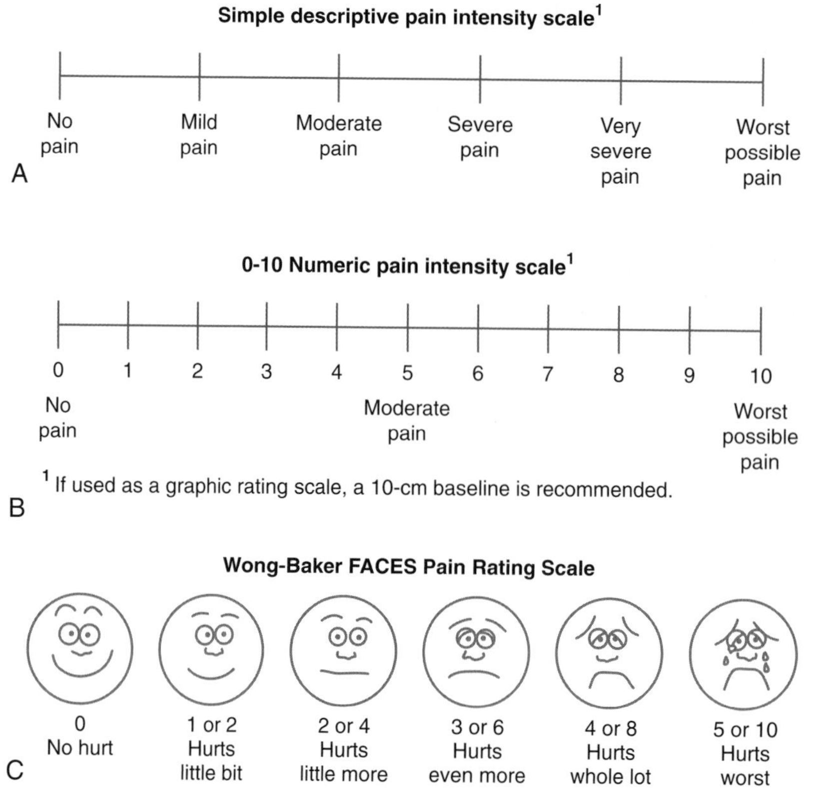

FIGURE 15-5 Examples of pain intensity scales. **A,** Simple descriptive pain intensity scale. **B,** 0–10 numeric pain intensity scale. **C,** Wong-Baker FACES Pain Rating Scale. (A and B, From Acute Pain Management Guidelines Panel: *Acute pain management: operative and medical procedures and trauma. Clinical practice guidelines* (AHCPR Publication No. 92-0052), Rockville, Md, 1992, Agency for Health Care Policy and Research, Public Health Service, U.S. Department of Health and Human Services. C, From Hockenberry MJ, Wilson D: *Wong's nursing care of infants and children*, ed 8, St. Louis, 2015, Mosby. Used with permission. Copyright Mosby.)

Patients may identify a location of pain that is not expected as part of their medical problem. This pain location may be the result of a complication or an injury that was sustained during a procedure or hospitalization. For example, one patient who had undergone orthopedic surgery on the ankle had also sustained a large burn on his back at some time during the procedure. When the nurse examined the pain location, the burn was discovered. Another example is a patient who had undergone abdominal surgery and complained of pain in the right calf. Examination of the right calf revealed a red, firm, tender area that was reported to the physician and diagnosed as thrombophlebitis. When the exact location of the pain was examined, the correct cause of the pain could be identified.

Identify Coping Methods

The fifth step in pain assessment is to identify the patient's coping methods. People develop coping methods to increase control over pain or to relieve pain. Nurses should become aware of the methods that patients use to cope with pain and should support these coping methods. Some patients actively deal with pain. For example, they may complain and get up and move around or perform some other activity. Some patients cope by staying quiet, praying, sleeping, or withdrawing.

Nurses must emphasize to patients and their family that their cooperation and information are critical to achieving pain relief. Some patients expect nurses to know that they are experiencing pain and to know what to do about it. Confirm how the patient copes with pain by discussing observations of the patient's behavior with him or her. You can also suggest other coping methods that could be used to relieve pain (e.g., changing positions, imagery, distraction). Pain in older adults, especially those with cognitive deficits, can be difficult to evaluate. Boxes 15-3 and 15-4 offer guidelines for evaluating pain in cognitively impaired older adults and list common pain behaviors that are likely to be observed in such patients.

Document Assessment Findings and Evaluate Interventions

The sixth and last step in the pain assessment is to record the information in the patient's medical record so that this information can be conveyed to nurses on other shifts and to other health care professionals. Record the location, quality, and intensity of the pain; related factors; and how the patient copes with pain. Document the interventions provided and their

Box 15-3 Evaluating Pain in Cognitively Impaired Older Adults and Observing Pain Behaviors

Ask the patient about pain first. Many patients who appear cognitively impaired may be able to answer yes/no questions about pain or complete a simple descriptive or numeric pain intensity scale.
Ask family members and caregivers what particular behaviors indicate pain for the patient.
Review the medical record to identify a past history of pain or diagnoses that are associated with pain.
Examine the patient physically to identify potential sources of pain or common problems causing pain.
Observe behaviors that may indicate pain for the patient. Observe the behaviors at rest and with activity. Note whether the behaviors change or improve when pain medication is administered. Assess, intervene, and evaluate behaviors again after intervention.

Box 15-4 Common Pain Behaviors in Cognitively Impaired Older Adults

FACIAL EXPRESSION
Frown, grimace, rapid blinking, wince, clenched teeth, narrowed eyes
SOUNDS
Sighing, moaning, groaning, calling out, noisy breathing, cursing during movement
BODY MOVEMENT
Rigid, tense body posture, fidgeting, pacing, gait changes, rocking, rubbing affected area
CHANGES IN INTERACTIONS WITH OTHERS
Aggressive, striking out, resisting care, withdrawn, decreased social interactions
CHANGES IN ACTIVITY PATTERNS OR ROUTINES
Refusing food, appetite changes, sleep or rest pattern changes, increased wandering
MENTAL STATUS CHANGES
Crying, increased confusion, irritability, distress

effectiveness. Include the intensity of the pain after the intervention. If the nursing intervention was not effective in relieving the pain or reducing pain to an acceptable comfort goal, record what intervention was performed and report this to the charge nurse. This reassessment of pain after intervention is an important step in complying with The Joint Commission's standard about pain management.

You may also use the following diagnoses to identify other problems that often accompany pain:

- Activity Intolerance
- Anxiety
- Disturbed Sleep Pattern
- Fatigue
- Impaired Comfort

Put on Your Thinking Cap!

Think of one of your patients who had pain. Discuss with your classmates how you knew that the patient had pain. Compare and contrast how different patients expressed pain, the interventions that were used for pain control, and the effectiveness of these interventions.

Nursing Diagnoses, Goals, and Outcome Criteria: Patients in Pain

Nursing Diagnoses	Goals and Outcome Criteria
Potential or actual **Acute Pain** related to surgery	Pain relief: Patient states pain is relieved, has relaxed manner.
Chronic Pain related to arthritic joint inflammation	Pain reduction or relief: Patient states pain is lessened or relieved, has relaxed manner.

Interventions

Nonpharmacologic Interventions

Nonpharmacologic interventions are those that do not employ drugs. They include a wide range of physical and psychologic interventions for pain relief (Table 15-3). Physical interventions usually involve comfort measures, adjusting the patient's environment, and cutaneous application techniques such as heat or cold. Psychologic interventions include unconditionally accepting the patient's pain report and providing information about pain, analgesics, and procedures or psychologic strategies such as relaxation and imagery. These types of interventions should be used along with analgesics to obtain optimal pain relief.

Physical Interventions

Physical Comfort Measures. These nursing interventions focus on the patient and the environment. Comfort may increase pain tolerance and the patient may experience less pain. Because adequate air, food and fluid, elimination, mobility, hygiene, temperature, and rest and sleep are essential to comfort, monitor these areas for potential problems. For example, patients who are sleep deprived or fatigued may have increased pain. Therefore providing for uninterrupted sleep and periods of rest can enhance pain relief.

For some patients in pain, progressive exercise or immobility may be prescribed as a treatment for pain. The patient with an injury or incision should be moved carefully so that further trauma is avoided. Turning the patient carefully from side to side or supporting an affected extremity during activity can reduce pain. The patient can usually describe which movements or positions increase or decrease the pain.

Administer analgesic medications before painful experiences to reduce the pain intensity and anxiety associated with the event. Aggressively treat pain,

Table 15-3 Nonpharmacologic Interventions

INTERVENTION	COMMENTS
Physical	
Heat, cold, massage, transcutaneous electrical nerve stimulation (TENS)	Increase pain threshold, reduce muscle spasm, and decrease congestion in injured area. Effective in reducing pain and improving physical function. Techniques require skilled personnel and special equipment. May be useful as adjuncts to drug therapy.
Psychologic	
Relaxation	
Jaw relaxation Progressive muscle relaxation	Effective in reducing mild to moderate pain and as an adjunct to analgesic drugs for severe pain.
Simple imagery	Use when patients express an interest in relaxation. Requires 3–5 minutes of staff time for instructions.
Music	Both patient-preferred and "easy listening" music are effective in reducing mild to moderate pain.
Imagery	Effective for reduction of mild to moderate pain. Requires skilled personnel.
Educational instruction	Effective for reduction of pain. Should include sensory and procedural information and be aimed at reducing activity-related pain. Requires 5–15 minutes of staff time.

Adapted from Acute Pain Management Guidelines Panel: *Acute pain management: operative and medical procedures and trauma. Clinical practice guidelines* (AHCPR Publication No. 92-0032), Rockville, Md, 1992, Agency for Health Care Policy and Research, Public Health Service, U.S. Department of Health and Human Services.

nausea, vomiting, loss of appetite, constipation, and other problems. Assist and teach patients how to splint abdominal and thoracic wounds to minimize pain when deep breathing, coughing, and ambulating. A change of bed linen and sheets free of wrinkles can be refreshing and reduce irritation of the skin. Apply ointment to cracked lips and provide ice chips for a dry mouth. Any tubes or equipment attached to the patient should be secure but should not produce tension on the skin. Correct body alignment and frequent changes of position will relieve monotony, increase circulation, and prevent muscle contractures and spasms, which aggravate pain.

Pharmacology Capsule

Analgesics should be administered before painful activities to reduce the pain and anxiety associated with these events.

Environmental Control. Each patient has individual preferences that affect comfort. Some patients prefer an active environment in which they can be distracted from pain. Listening to audio recordings or music on the radio, watching television, working with the hands, walking around, or visiting with others allows a person to focus attention on stimuli other than the pain sensation. On the other hand, the lights, noise, and constant activity of the hospital environment often cause sensory overload for the patient in pain, which can increase pain. In this event, coordinate with staff to promote a quiet environment with nonglaring lights and scheduled rest and activity periods that meet the patient's needs.

Stimulation Techniques. Stimulation of the skin and underlying tissues relieves pain. Various types of skin or cutaneous stimulation can be applied and each type has variable effects. These techniques are not curative; rather, they can decrease the intensity of pain or change the sensation so that it is more acceptable. The exact mechanism for pain relief is unknown but the belief is that superficial stimulation may block the transmission of pain impulses to the brain. Applications of heat, cold, massage, and TENS are examples of cutaneous stimulation. These interventions tend to be most effective for mild to moderate pain, well-localized pain, and acute and chronic pain. The effects of these therapies last as long as or slightly longer than the application.

The physician may prescribe the application of heat or cold for pain. Heat or cold is used to reduce muscle spasm and decrease congestion or swelling in an injured area. Either therapy may be applied to the painful site, at a location beyond the site, between the site and the brain, or on the opposite side of the body. These therapies should be applied intermittently, not continuously. Heat and cold may be alternated. Both therapies should be applied at a temperature that is comfortable for the patient and the patient's skin and circulation should be monitored frequently.

Cold may be applied with ice packs or cooling pads to decrease initial tissue injury and swelling (e.g., with musculoskeletal sprains or orthopedic procedures). Cold is contraindicated for patients with peripheral vascular disease or heart disease because it may cause further vasoconstriction of blood vessels and thus decrease circulation. Cold application should be limited to 15 minutes per session to prevent tissue injury or frostbite.

Moist or dry heat can be applied with heating pads, hot-water bottles, towels, gel packs, or warm tub baths or showers. Superficial heat has been shown to be effective for gastrointestinal cramps and muscle and joint pain. Treatment should be limited to 30 minutes to prevent tissue injury. Heat should not be applied to a site of malignancy, to areas of decreased sensation or circulation, or to patients who cannot communicate their discomfort.

Massage involves rubbing, kneading, manipulating, and applying pressure and friction to the body. Rubbing or massaging an area is a natural response when one has an injury or ache. Massage may be used to promote relaxation and relieve muscle cramps. Massage is commonly applied to the back, neck, and large leg muscles; however, massage of the hands and feet is more easily performed and perhaps more effective. Massage should not be applied to areas with injury, phlebitis, or skin lesions or to patients with bleeding problems.

Cold, heat, and massage are easy to apply, inexpensive, effective, and simple for the patient or family to learn. For each therapy, evaluate whether the method or location of application is effective and monitor for any side effects.

Compared with the therapies just mentioned, TENS is less widely used. It requires a physician's order and the physical therapy department often handles the equipment. The therapy involves external electrical stimulation of the skin and underlying tissues through electrodes attached to a small unit that the patient can carry around. The electrodes are placed over, above, or below painful sites and attached to a battery-operated device that delivers low-voltage electrical currents to block the pain signals.

Psychologic Interventions

Anxiety Reduction. Anxiety, fear of the unknown, and feelings of loss of control may be directly related to the level of pain experienced. The patient who is anxious and uncertain will tend to rate pain high. If the nurse can increase the predictability and control of painful stimuli, pain may be reduced. An important aspect of relieving anxiety associated with pain is the relationship between the nurse and the patient. The nurse can be with the patient, assure the patient that everything possible is being tried, and provide timely and appropriate interventions for pain relief.

Several strategies are used to decrease anxiety and increase control. Telling the patient about events and providing descriptions of the sensations or feelings that may accompany the event can reduce anxiety. However, some patients may prefer not to know this information and their wishes should be respected. Allowing the patient to choose physical comfort measures and the time for treatments or to rearrange items in the room also provides control.

Preoperative teaching should include skills to help patients cope with their pain, such as breathing, relaxation, or imagery techniques. Providing strategies to help the patient cope with pain and anxiety also provides the patient with a sense of control. The *Health Promotion* box describes a sample relaxation exercise, one of the psychologic interventions used for pain relief.

Health Promotion

Sample Relaxation Exercise: Slow, Rhythmic Breathing

1. Breathe in slowly and deeply.
2. As you breathe out slowly, feel yourself beginning to relax; feel the tension leaving your body.
3. Now breathe in and out slowly and regularly at whatever rate is comfortable for you. You may wish to try abdominal breathing. If you do not know how to do abdominal breathing, ask your nurse for help.
4. To help you focus on your breathing and to breathe slowly and rhythmically, do the following:
   a. Breathe in as you say silently to yourself, "in, two, three."
   b. Breathe out as you say silently to yourself, "out, two, three."
   c. Each time you breathe out, say silently to yourself a word such as "peace" or "relax."
5. You may imagine that you are doing this in a position and a place you have found very calming and relaxing, such as lying on a beach in the sun.
6. Perform steps 1 through 4 only once or repeat steps 3 and 4 for up to 20 minutes.
7. End with a slow, deep breath. As you breathe out, say to yourself, "I feel alert and relaxed."

ADDITIONAL POINTS

If you intend to perform this exercise for more than a few minutes, try to get into a comfortable position in a quiet environment. You may close your eyes or focus on an object. This technique has the advantage of being very adaptable in that it may be used for only a few seconds or for up to 20 minutes.

Adapted from McCaffery M, Beebe A: *Pain: clinical manual for nursing practice*, St Louis, 1989, Mosby.

Distraction. Distraction refers to focusing on stimuli other than pain. Distraction may help the patient to gain a sense of control, as well as increase pain tolerance, decrease pain intensity, and alter the quality of pain, but it does not eliminate pain. Because the pain is not eliminated, the patient will usually need analgesics and other methods of pain relief. A patient using distraction such as watching a movie may not appear or behave as if in pain, which may cause other people to doubt that the pain exists. After a patient has used a distraction technique, he or she may once again focus on the pain and experience a heightened awareness of pain.

Distraction techniques are often most helpful with mild to moderate pain or during brief periods of pain associated with painful procedures such as dressing changes, intramuscular injections, and venipunctures. Examples of distraction methods include rhythmic breathing, listening to music, laughing, counting,

Table 15-4 Nonopioid Analgesics: Commonly Used NSAIDs

DRUGS	COMMENTS
Oral NSAIDs	
Acetaminophen (Tylenol, et al)	Lacks the peripheral antiinflammatory activity of other NSAIDs
Aspirin*	The standard against which other NSAIDs are compared. Inhibits platelet aggregation; may cause postoperative bleeding
Choline magnesium (Trilisate)	May have minimal antiplatelet activity; also available as trisalicylate oral liquid
Fenoprofen calcium (Nalfon)	—
Ibuprofen (Motrin, others)	Available in several brand name formulations and as a generic product; also available as oral suspension
Ketoprofen (Orudis)	—
Magnesium salicylate	Many brands and generic forms available
Naproxen (Naprosyn)	Also available as oral liquid
Naproxen sodium (Anaprox)	—
Salsalate (Disalcid, others)	May have minimal antiplatelet activity
Sodium salicylate	Available in generic form from several distributors
Parenteral NSAID	
Ketorolac (Torodol, et al)	IM administration not to exceed 5 days

Adapted from Acute Pain Management Guidelines Panel: *Acute pain management: operative and medical procedures and trauma. Clinical practice guidelines* (AHCPR Publication No. 92-0032), Rockville, Md, 1992, Agency for Health Care Policy and Research, Public Health Service, U.S. Department of Health and Human Services.
IM, Intramuscular; *NSAIDs*, nonsteroidal antiinflammatory drugs.
*Contraindicated in the presence of fever or other evidence of viral illness.
Note: Only the NSAIDs listed in the table have been approved by the U.S. Food and Drug Administration for use as simple analgesics but clinical experience has been gained with other drugs as well.

Opioid Analgesics. Opioid analgesics are generally used for moderate to severe acute pain, chronic cancer pain, and some other types of pain. The opioids vary in potency and duration of action.

Currently, the two types of opioid analgesics are:

- **Opioid agonists.** Examples include codeine, methadone (Dolophine), hydromorphone (Dilaudid), meperidine (Demerol), morphine, and fentanyl.
- **Opioid agonist-antagonists.** Examples include buprenorphine (Buprenex), nalbuphine (Nubain), butorphanol (Stadol), and pentazocine (Talwin).

Both types of opioids relieve pain at the level of the central nervous system. Agonist drugs fit into receptor sites on the cell to "turn on" the site and produce the drug effect. Antagonists are drugs that block drug effects at the receptor sites. Opioid agonists bind to opioid receptors to produce analgesia but also bind to other receptors to produce unwanted side effects such as decreased respiration, drowsiness, and nausea. Opioid agonist-antagonists are drugs designed to produce analgesia and block certain side effects. The agonist-antagonists block some of the effects of the pure opioid agonists in much the same way that naloxone (Narcan) acts to block or reverse the effects of opioids. Drugs classified as agonist-antagonists (e.g., pentazocine, nalbuphine, buprenorphine) produce analgesia but also can block the effects of opioids such as morphine or meperidine if the patient has been receiving these drugs. Thus a patient receiving pure opioid agonists for pain relief should not be given opioid agonist-antagonists because they may block analgesia, precipitate withdrawal symptoms, and increase pain. For example, if a patient has been receiving morphine intramuscularly for several days, administering nalbuphine (Nubain) would not be advisable because it may block some of the analgesic effects of morphine.

Older adults are generally more sensitive to the analgesic effects of opioids because of delayed excretion and slower metabolism. Also, side effects may be more pronounced in older adults. Thus the recommended adult dose should be reduced 25% to 50% initially and then titrated (adjusted) for optimal pain control with minimal side effects. Some older adults are small and thin and weigh less than 100 pounds. In this case, charts with recommended opioid doses for adults and children weighing less than 50 kg or less than 110 pounds are available. Table 15-5 provides guidelines for dosing opioids with adults.

Referring to an equianalgesic (approximately equal analgesia) table is important when changing to a new opioid or a different route. Table 15-5 is such a table, showing approximately equianalgesic oral and parenteral doses. The information in the table helps to estimate the new dose, which should then be modified based on the specific patient reaction and drug. An equianalgesic table shows that oral doses are two to six times larger than parenteral doses of the same drug to achieve the same effect, largely because oral opioids must pass through the liver after absorption, which reduces the amount of medication absorbed. Therefore larger doses of oral opioids must be ordered to provide the same amount of analgesia as parenteral opioids. For example, a patient receives 10 mg of morphine intramuscularly for pain relief and the order is changed to oral morphine. To receive an equianalgesic dose of morphine, the patient should be given 30 mg of morphine orally.

Meperidine or Demerol use for moderate to severe pain has declined. Clinical practice guidelines state that meperidine may cause central nervous system

Table 15-5 Opioid Analgesics: Starting Oral Dose Commonly Used for Severe Pain

	EQUIANALGESIC DOSE (mg)		
NAME	ORAL	PARENTERAL*	STARTING ORAL DOSE ADULTS (mg)
Morphine	30	10	15–30
Hydromorphone (Dilaudid)	7.5	1.5	4–8
Fentanyl	—	0.1	—
Oxycodone	20	—	15–30
Methadone (Dolophine)	10	5	5–10

From American Pain Society: *Principles of analgesic use in the treatment of acute pain and cancer pain*, ed 5, Glenview, Ill, 2003, The American Pain Society.
*These are standard intramuscular doses for acute pain in adults. Equianalgesic doses should be based on the opioid characteristics and patient characteristics such as age, weight, liver and renal function, and reaction to the drug.

toxicity. You should be aware that one of the products of meperidine metabolism is normeperidine, which is a central nervous system stimulant. When this metabolite accumulates in the body, the patient may exhibit anxiety, twitching, tremors, muscle jerking, and generalized seizures. This opioid is contraindicated for long-term administration, specifically over 48 hours, and for patients who have diminished renal function. Because many older adults have decreased renal function, meperidine should be avoided.

Pharmacology Capsule

Older adults are more sensitive to opioid analgesics and should be monitored frequently for side effects.

Misconceptions About Opioid Analgesics. When discussing opioid analgesics, a few terms should be reviewed that are often misunderstood, resulting in undertreatment of pain. Patients, families, nurses, and physicians have misconceptions about **addiction**; therefore the term must be defined and differentiated from the terms **tolerance** and **physical dependence**. Box 15-5 contains information about these terms. When patients take opioids over a period for pain, tolerance and physical dependency may occur. The patient who is tolerant requires higher doses of a drug to achieve an analgesic effect. The patient who is physically dependent on an opioid will experience unpleasant withdrawal symptoms when the opioid is stopped. Both tolerance and physical dependence are normal responses to continued opioid administration for pain relief; they do not lead to a craving for the drug for its mind-altering effects. Fear of addiction is greatly exaggerated and addiction rarely occurs (<1%) in patients taking opioids for pain relief. Remind patients that pain relief is an important goal and they should not worry about addiction. Most patients simply stop taking opioids when the pain stops.

Box 15-5 Characteristics of Tolerance, Physical Dependence, and Addiction

TOLERANCE

Physiologic changes that occur from repeated doses of opioids

Result: Higher doses are needed to achieve pain relief.

PHYSICAL DEPENDENCE

Physiologic changes that occur from repeated doses of opioids

Result: Withdrawal symptoms (e.g., irritability, chills, sweating, nausea) may occur if the opioid is stopped abruptly.

ADDICTION

Psychologic dependence characterized by continued craving for opioid for other than pain relief

Result: Compulsive and continued use for psychic effects despite harm.

Note: Risk of addiction is not a concern in treating acute pain or cancer pain.

Routes of Administration. The opioids can be administered through various routes, depending on the needs of the patient. If tolerated, the oral route is preferred, especially for patients with chronic pain. Oral opioids can control severe pain when given in adequate dose levels.

Although not the recommended route, the intramuscular route may be used to administer opioids for breakthrough pain, that is, pain that occurs between regularly scheduled doses of pain medication. Breakthrough pain would require immediate-acting or short-acting analgesic medication, such as morphine. Consider the drug being administered when selecting appropriate needle-gauge size and administration site for intramuscular medication. For example, to administer 10 mg of morphine intramuscularly, you may need to use at least a 1.5-inch needle to reach the muscle, depending on the patient's size. Some drugs are more irritating to muscle tissue and should be administered deep into the muscle with the Z-track method. You can use the ventrogluteal, deltoid, and vastus lateralis muscles. The intramuscular route is impractical for repeated injections. Absorption is often unpredictable with intramuscular injections, particularly in older adults, who have reduced muscle mass. This route is also painful. An accessible and appropriate site for the intramuscular injection of analgesics is the ventral gluteal muscle, especially in older adults.

A limited number of opioids, such as morphine, hydromorphone, and oxymorphone, may be administered rectally. This route is useful when the patient is nauseated or has difficulty swallowing (e.g., when a patient is dying).

Opioids may also be administered sublingually (under the tongue). Intermittent bolus injections, continuous infusions, and patient-controlled analgesia (PCA) are methods of administering medications subcutaneously. These methods may be used in patients in whom the oral and rectal routes cannot be used and who also have poor intravenous access.

The intravenous route is another method of administering opioids. Intravenous PCA is commonly used postoperatively. With PCA, the patient is able to self-administer doses of analgesics to control pain. Opioids, when administered intravenously, have a rapid onset but shorter duration of action than when given by any other route. Although the registered nurse (RN) is usually responsible for the PCA, the licensed vocational nurse/licensed practical nurse (LVN/LPN) may be responsible for monitoring the patient's response and the effectiveness of the medication. Side effects should be reported to the registered nurse or charge nurse. See the *Patient Teaching* box.

Opioids also can be administered via the spinal route epidurally (in the epidural space) or intrathecally (in the subarachnoid space). The epidural or intrathecal route may be selected in patients with postoperative pain and chronic cancer pain. The LVN/LPN may participate in monitoring the patient. Side effects such as itching, hypotension, nausea, urinary retention, sedation, and respiratory depression may occur more frequently in patients receiving opioids epidurally or intrathecally than by other routes of administration. The older adult who has received a spinal opioid infusion is at increased risk for respiratory depression. If anesthetics such as bupivacaine are used with spinal opioids, the nurse must be alert for the side effects of numbness and motor weakness. Side effects, as well as any adverse effects, should be reported promptly. A sedation assessment scale should be used with patients receiving spinal opioid infusions. Sedation is usually seen before signs of respiratory depression.

Patient Teaching

Patient-Controlled Analgesia (PCA)

Safety features: The pump has a delay feature and a lockout interval that prevents the patient from receiving more than the prescribed amount of medication. Only the patient should push the PCA button.

Patient instructions: Press the PCA button when pain begins to return; then put it down and wait 10 to 15 minutes to evaluate pain relief. If pain returns, push the PCA button again and repeat the process until the pain is relieved.

If pain is not relieved: Notify the RN, who can then recommend changes in the opioid, bolus amount, or lockout interval to the physician to achieve satisfactory pain relief.

Other routes of administration of opioids also are available. Liquid morphine may be administered sublingually. Duragesic or fentanyl transdermal patches are used to treat cancer and chronic pain by producing constant delivery of the opioids for 72 hours through the skin surface. Fentanyl patches can be used only for patients who have developed opioid tolerance. They are applied to a hairless area of the upper torso and pressed for 30 seconds to assure adherence. External heat will increase absorption, so the patient should be instructed not to apply heat in any form over the patch. Used patches must be discarded so that children and pets cannot touch them because they still contain a significant amount of the drug. Intranasal butorphanol is available and may be used preoperatively for sedation and postoperatively for analgesia. Package inserts should be reviewed for doses, precautions, and administration guidelines.

Side Effects. Regardless of the route of administration, opioid analgesics have specific side effects. A common side effect is constipation. Tolerance for this side effect does not develop. Assess the patient for abdominal distention, cramping, and abdominal pain. Stool softeners and laxatives, along with increased fluid intake, exercise, and bulk-containing foods, may prevent this side effect.

Opioids may also cause nausea, with or without vomiting. Some patients develop a tolerance for nausea but may require antiemetic therapy until tolerance develops. At times, the order may need to be changed to a different opioid to relieve this problem.

Sedation is another side effect that may occur initially with opioids but it usually subsides in a few days. In patients who have had unrelieved pain for some time and have been sleep deprived, sudden pain relief may allow the patient to sleep, which may be misinterpreted as sedation. When sedation is noted, however, the dose of the opioid may need to be titrated to a level that does not cause sedation but still provides pain relief. Box 15-6 illustrates a sedation scale that should be used each time an opioid is administered. Patients receiving opioids should be at 1 or 2 on the sedation scale. If a nurse rates the patient as 3 on the sedation scale, notify the registered nurse because the opioid dose should be reduced to prevent progression to respiratory depression. Respiratory depression can occur but does

Box 15-6 Sedation Scale

S	Sleeping but easy to arouse when called or stimulated
1	Awake and alert
2	Slightly drowsy but easily aroused
3	Frequently drowsy, arousable but drifts off to sleep during conversation—alert the RN
4	Somnolent, minimal or no response to physical stimulation—emergency

not occur as frequently as commonly thought. If a patient is easily arousable, respiratory depression is highly unlikely. If severe respiratory depression occurs (fewer than six to eight respirations per minute) and physical stimulation does not awaken the patient, this situation is an emergency. Stay with the patient and call for help. The RN may administer naloxone (Narcan) intravenously if prescribed to reverse the opioid. Be aware that drugs such as promethazine (Phenergan) or lorazepam (Ativan) may be ordered to be given with opioids. These drugs when given with an opioid may contribute to sedation, respiratory depression, and hypotension.

Other side effects may be noted with the use of opioid analgesics. These include confusion, hypotension (especially orthostatic), dizziness, itching, and urinary retention. Nonopioid analgesics given with opioids may allow a decrease in the opioid dose to one that maintains pain control with fewer opioid side effects.

Placebos. Placebos are inactive substances (e.g., saline) used in research or clinical practice to determine the effects of a legitimate drug or treatment. Placebos are appropriately used in studies in which patients consent to participate in the study. Many professional health care organizations take the position that placebos should not be used to assess or manage pain. Nurses have an ethical obligation to ensure that patients are not deceived and that institutional policies related to placebos are followed.

Complementary and Alternative Therapies

Patients who have migraines may be taking feverfew, an herbal supplement, for headache prevention. No evidence of effectiveness in treating other conditions has been found. Advise patients that feverfew can increase the risk of bleeding in patients taking aspirin, warfarin, or heparin.

Put on Your Thinking Cap!

Ask five people (patients, friends, strangers) what helps when they have pain. Compile a list with your classmates and sort the treatment measures into pharmacologic and nonpharmacologic. Include home remedies and herbal remedies.

Pharmacology Capsule

Oral analgesics are preferred for the treatment of chronic pain.

Adjuvant Analgesics and Medications. Drugs that are not usually classified as analgesics may relieve pain in certain situations. For instance, a patient who has undergone back surgery may complain more about muscle spasms than incisional pain. A muscle relaxant may be more effective in relieving pain than an opioid alone. Specific pain syndromes, especially neuropathic pain syndromes, may be controlled with drugs other than the commonly known analgesics. Table 15-6 lists some of the adjuvant drugs and the conditions they treat effectively.

Table 15-6 Adjuvant Drugs and Pain Treatment

DRUG CLASSIFICATON WITH GENERIC AND BRAND NAME EXAMPLES	EXAMPLES OF PAIN AND PAIN-RELATED PROBLEMS
Antidepressants	Neuropathic pain; dull, aching pain
Amitriptyline (Elavil)	Various neuropathic pain syndromes, pain associated with herpes zoster (shingles), headache
Bupropion (Wellbutrin)	Painful diabetic neuropathy, headache, fatigue
Duloxetine (Cymbalta)	Painful diabetic neuropathy, fibromyalgia, depression-associated pain
Muscle Relaxants	Muscular pain, spasms, anxiety
Methocarbamol (Robaxin)	Acute traumatic sprains or strains, myofascial pain syndromes, low back or neck pain
Cyclobenzaprine (Flexeril)	Acute traumatic sprains or strains, myofascial pain syndromes, low back or neck pain
Benzodiazepines	Anxiety
Alprazolam (Xanax)	
Lorazepam (Ativan)	Procedural pain, anxiety
Antihistamines	Nausea, anxiety
Hydroxyzine (Vistaril, Atarax)	
Corticosteroids	Pain syndromes associated with cancer, spinal cord or nerve compression
Methylprednisone (Medrol)	Bone pain, pain related to metastasis
Dexamethasone (Decadron)	Preradiation therapy
Anticonvulsants/Antiepileptics	Neuropathic pain; sharp, shooting, stabbing pain
Carbamazepine (Tegretol)	Neuropathic pain, trigeminal neuralgia
Topiramate (Topamax)	Headache pain, migraine

Continued

Table 15-6 Adjuvant Drugs and Pain Treatment—cont'd

DRUG CLASSIFICATON WITH GENERIC AND BRAND NAME EXAMPLES	EXAMPLES OF PAIN AND PAIN-RELATED PROBLEMS
Gabapentin (Neurontin)	Acute, chronic, and neuropathic pain; acute perioperative pain
Pregabalin (Lyrica)	Acute, chronic, and neuropathic pain; fibromyalgia
Local Anesthetics	Acute, chronic, and neuropathic pain
Lidocaine	Local analgesia, local or regional anesthesia for acute pain
Lidocaine (Topical Lidoderm 5% patch)	Pain associated with herpes zoster, painful diabetic neuropathy, arthritis, back pain
EMLA	Anesthetize tissue prior to needle insertion or superficial skin surgery
Bupivacaine	Local or regional anesthesia for surgery; wound infiltration
Other Adjuvants	
Clonidine (Catapres)	Pain from spinal cord injury, phantom limb pain, peripheral nerve injuries
Capsaicin (Zostrix)	Arthritis pain, postmastectomy pain, myofascial pain, back pain, peripheral nerve pain, painful diabetic neuropathy
Ketamine (Ketalar)	Acute pain, chronic pain
Baclofen (Lioresal)	Pain/spasm from spinal cord injury, multiple sclerosis

Pharmacology Capsule

The adverse effects of opioid analgesics include constipation, nausea, sedation, respiratory depression, confusion, hypotension, dizziness, itching, and urinary retention.

Problem Solving with Pain Medication. Nurses often encounter patients whose prescribed analgesic drugs do not relieve pain. In these situations, use all of the information presented here. Ask questions about the analgesic drug and the "five rights" (right dose, right patient, right time, right route, right analgesic) to determine why the patient is not getting adequate pain relief. Box 15-7 provides a nursing plan of care checklist. Box 15-8 describes a method for problem solving when analgesic drugs do not provide effective pain relief.

The administration of analgesics is simply one intervention in the nursing care of a patient in pain. Nurses should provide many interventions along with analgesics to relieve pain. The *Coordinated Care* box also includes the expected patient outcomes and guidelines for nursing care.

Coordinated Care

Delegation of Pain Assessment

Pain assessment is one of the most important responsibilities for which the nurse is accountable. According to the American Pain Society, one half of all hospitalized patients experience moderate to severe pain during the last days of their lives. Of the 70% of patients with cancer and with significant pain, fewer than one half of them receive adequate relief. Pain may also be caused by postoperative wounds, sickle cell disease, arthritis, and many other conditions.

Pain assessment cannot be delegated to an unlicensed person. However, unlicensed personnel must understand the importance of informing the nurse of any reports of pain from the patient. Although a licensed practitioner with prescribing authority is ultimately responsible for adjusting dosages, both the LVN/LPN and the RN must be able to assess the patient's pain to implement range dose orders. Working within their scope of practice and adhering to applicable organizational policy, nurses must draw on their knowledge, skills, abilities, and experience to execute the pain management plan. They must be aware of the following:

- The medication to be administered
- Dosage and route of administration
- Potential interactions with other medications
- Time to onset and peak effect
- Duration of action
- Potential side effects

If the patient experiences an unacceptable level of pain or has troublesome side effects, the nurse should document the finding and report it to the prescriber so that appropriate pharmacologic or nonpharmacologic interventions can be implemented. Ideally, the patient will take part in achieving safe, effective pain management. Good communication among all members of the health care team is essential to ensure the patient's optimal comfort and well-being.

Box 15-7 Southwest Texas Methodist Hospital Nursing Plan of Care: Pain

NURSING DIAGNOSIS/PATIENT PROBLEM

Pain (Acute/Chronic) related to:
Date/initials
Disease processes/illness
Surgery
Injury/trauma
Diagnostic procedures

Pain Assessment

Type of pain scale
Verbalization of pain/discomfort
Verbalization of spasms (specify bladder, back, muscle)
Facial grimacing
Tense body posture
Rubbing/guarding of body parts
Inability to concentrate
Increased vital signs
Restlessness/difficulty sleeping
Crying, moaning
Withdrawal
Change in appetite
Decreased activity

Pain Evaluation/Goals/Reassessment of Interventions

Patient will verbalize/demonstrate minimal discomfort or absence of pain as evidenced by:

- Statements of pain relief and effectiveness of pain medications and/or other interventions
- Decreased need for pain medication
- Relaxed facial expression and body part
- Increase in voluntary movement, ambulation, and ADL
- Increased ability to concentrate
- Stable vital signs
- Statements or demonstrations of coping behaviors and/or factors that reduce or eliminate discomfort or pain
- Able to sleep/rest
- Increased appetite

NURSING INTERVENTIONS

Accept patient's level/tolerance of pain
Assess pain characteristics to include location, intensity, duration, type, precipitating factors
Provide the patient with prescribed medication as ordered
Provide and teach alternative methods of pain relief based on individual needs and/or physician orders:

- Positioning
- Back rub
- Massage
- Application of heat
- Application of cold
- Diversion/distraction
- Relaxation/imagery
- Exercise/ambulation
- Range of motion
- Other:
- Consults:

Teach patient and/or significant other pain management strategies:

- Use of PCA
- Medications

Explain procedures to decrease/relieve anxiety
Validate patient's understanding/coping
Evaluate effectiveness of interventions and reintervene as necessary

ADL, Activities of daily living; *AEB*, as evidenced by; *PCA*, patient-controlled analgesia.

Box 15-8 Problem Solving with Pain Medication

When the analgesic medication prescribed for pain is not effective in relieving pain, the nurse should take the following steps to solve the problem.

1. Check the analgesic order.
   a. **Right dose:** Is the dose prescribed a recommended starting dose for analgesia or is the dose prescribed less? If a dose range of medication is prescribed, has the maximal dose been administered? If the order states morphine 10–20 mg IM PRN for pain and 10 mg morphine is ineffective for pain relief, has 20 mg been administered? *Solution:* Adjust the dose up as ordered until the pain is relieved without serious side effects or minimal side effects.
   b. **Right patient:** Is the patient experiencing side effects of the analgesic at the present dose? Can the patient tolerate the increase in dose with few side effects?
   c. **Right time:** What are the onset, peak, and duration of the analgesic? Is the analgesic administered around the clock based on the duration or properties of the drug? *Solution:* Evaluate pain intensity periodically to see if correct timing of drug is more effective in relieving pain.

If the patient's pain is still not relieved, the following steps should be taken.

2. Consider an alternative prescription.
   a. **Right patient:** What is the diagnosis or source of pain and what analgesic is most effective for this type of pain? What are patient characteristics to consider (e.g., age, liver or renal problems, NPO status)?
   b. **Right route:** Which route is most appropriate for the patient's condition, severity of pain, and medication prescribed (e.g., IV, IM, PO, or topical administration)?
   c. **Right analgesic:** Which analgesic or adjuvant drug is best for this type of pain? Which analgesic has proven effective for the patient in the past or in a similar condition? Can the opioid or nonopioid prescribed be switched to another drug in the class that may provide more effective pain relief? Have both opioids and nonopioids been prescribed to increase pain relief?

Continued

Box 15-8 Problem Solving with Pain Medication—cont'd

d. **Right dose:** Has the dose of opioid been titrated up or adjusted to a higher dose to reduce the pain? Has the patient been receiving opioids over time and require increased doses of opioids to control pain because of the development of tolerance? If switching opioid drugs, is the correct equianalgesic dose calculated to make sure you have the approximate same level of analgesia?
e. **Right time:** What is the time interval at which the analgesic should be administered or evaluated given its duration of action and patient?

3. Collaborate with the patient, other nurses, pharmacist, and family.
   a. Collect information.
   b. Establish credibility with facts about the patient, analgesics, and written references (articles or drug guides).
   c. Anticipate questions.
   d. Be assertive and keep trying.
   e. Always use other nursing interventions in addition to the analgesic to relieve pain.

Adapted from Walker M, Wong D: A battle plan for patients in pain, *Am J Nur* 91(6):32–36, 1991. Used with permission.
IM, Intramuscularly; *IV*, intravenously; *NPO*, nothing by mouth; *PO*, orally; *PRN*, as needed.

Get Ready for the NCLEX® Examination!

Key Points

- Pain is the most common problem that nurses encounter.
- "Pain is an unpleasant sensory and emotional experience associated with actual or potential tissue damage, or described in terms of such damage" (International Association for the Study of Pain, 1986).
- When pain receptors are stimulated, impulses are transmitted to the spinal cord and then to the brain, where the cortex interprets the signals as pain.
- Endorphins are natural opioid-like substances that block the transmission of painful impulses to the brain.
- According to the gate control theory, stimulation of large-diameter fibers in the spinal cord interferes with the transmission of painful impulses to the brain.
- Physical factors that influence the pain experience are pain threshold, pain tolerance, age, physical activity, nervous system integrity, and, in surgical patients, the type of surgery and anesthesia.
- Psychologic factors that influence the pain experience include culture, religion, past experiences with pain, anxiety, and situational factors.
- Based on the duration and cause, pain is classified as acute, chronic, and cancer-related pain.
- Most chronic pain is neuropathic because of nerve damage.
- Assessment is the first step in pain management.
- Pain can be described in terms of location, quality, intensity, and aggravating and alleviating factors.
- Assessment findings and the effects of pain interventions must be documented.
- Nursing diagnoses for the patient in pain may include Acute Pain, Chronic Pain, Activity Intolerance, Anxiety, Fatigue, Disturbed Sleep Pattern, and Impaired Comfort.
- Examples of nonpharmacologic interventions are comfort measures, control of environmental factors, stimulation techniques, and measures to reduce anxiety.
- Predictable pain is best controlled by ATC analgesics rather than PRN medication.
- The categories of drugs used to relieve pain are nonopioid analgesics, opioid analgesics, and adjuvant drugs.
- Fear of addiction to opioids is greatly exaggerated. Addiction rarely occurs when opioids are taken for pain relief.
- Placebos are inactive substances such as saline that are used as a control to determine the effects of a legitimate drug or treatment.
- Most professional health care organizations take the position that placebos should not be used to assess or manage pain.
- Opioid side effects to monitor and treat include constipation, nausea, sedation, and respiratory depression.

Additional Learning Resources

SG Go to your Study Guide for additional learning activities to help you master this chapter content.

evolve Go to your Evolve website (http://evolve.elsevier.com/Linton/medsurg) for the following learning resources and much more:
- Interactive Prioritization Exercises
- Fluid & Electrolyte Tutorial
- Pharmacology Tutorial
- Review Questions for the NCLEX® Examination

Review Questions for the NCLEX® Examination

1. Pain is *best* defined by the:
   1. Patient
   2. Nurse
   3. Physician
   4. Physiologist

   NCLEX Client Need: Physiological Integrity: Basic Care and Comfort

2. When you cut your finger, which of the following represents the steps involved in your experiencing pain?
   1. Afferent pathways activate nociceptors, which transmit information to the spinal cord for interpretation.
   2. Nociceptors are stimulated and afferent pathways send impulses to the spinal cord and then to the brain.
   3. Efferent pathways stimulate nociceptors, which transmit impulses to the brain.
   4. The brain stimulates nociceptors, which trigger efferent pathways to send impulses to the spinal cord.

   NCLEX Client Need: Physiological Integrity: Basic Care and Comfort
3. Mr. A. and Mr. B. both had back surgery yesterday. Mr. A. has used his PCA regularly. He says that he is "pretty comfortable" and he sleeps most of the time. Mr. B. has used the maximal analgesic permitted by his PCA and has required an additional analgesic twice while continuing to complain of some discomfort. Of the following, which is the most likely explanation for the difference in the pain experience of these two patients?
   1. Mr. B. is a complainer who is seeking attention.
   2. Mr. B. has higher pain tolerance than Mr. A.
   3. Mr. B. has a lower pain threshold than Mr. A.
   4. Mr. B. is more anxious, which has raised his pain threshold.

   NCLEX Client Need: Physiological Integrity: Basic Care and Comfort
4. Autonomic nervous system responses to pain include which of the following? (Select all that apply.)
   1. Decreased respiratory rate
   2. Constipation
   3. Urinary frequency
   4. Increased heart rate
   5. Constricted pupils

   NCLEX Client Need: Physiological Integrity: Basic Care and Comfort
5. A patient says that she has pain whenever she bends over. Which aspect of the pain assessment is she describing?
   1. Location
   2. Alleviating factor
   3. Quality
   4. Aggravating factor

   NCLEX Client Need: Physiological Integrity: Basic Care and Comfort
6. A frail, older adult patient who is being cared for by her family at home says that she finds a heating pad soothing to stiff joints. What patient or family teaching is needed for safe and effective heat therapy? (Select all that apply.)
   1. "It is more effective to use the heating pad intermittently rather than continuously."
   2. "Do not apply heat to any area that lacks normal sensation or circulation."
   3. "Set the heating pad at the highest temperature that the patient can tolerate."
   4. "Heat application is not a safe or effective strategy for pain management."
   5. "Limit heat application to 15 minutes."

   NCLEX Client Need: Physiological Integrity: Reduction of Risk Potential
7. Which statement correctly describes a nonpharmacologic approach to pain control?
   1. Imagery is the use of the patient's imagination to help control pain.
   2. Distraction is most effective in the management of chronic pain.
   3. Relaxation therapy requires that the nurse must be able to hypnotize the patient.
   4. Patient education is usually all that is needed to reduce anxiety.

   NCLEX Client Need: Physiological Integrity: Basic Care and Comfort
8. When preparing to give a nonopioid analgesic, the nurse notes that the patient also takes drugs for hypertension. The nurse knows that nonopioid analgesics must be used cautiously in patients with hypertension because the drugs cause:
   1. Peripheral vasoconstriction
   2. Potassium loss
   3. Sleep disturbances
   4. Fluid retention

   NCLEX Client Need: Physiological Integrity: Reduction of Risk Potential
9. The medication nurse has several patients who take NSAIDs in addition to the drugs listed below. The nurse should question the NSAID order for a patient who is also taking:
   1. Antibiotics
   2. Decongestants
   3. Anticoagulants
   4. Hormone replacements

   NCLEX Client Need: Physiological Integrity: Reduction of Risk Potential
10. When patients take opioid analgesics, the nurse's *first* priority is to assess which of the following?
    1. Bowel elimination
    2. Hydration
    3. Respiratory system
    4. Urinary elimination

    NCLEX Client Need: Physiological Integrity: Reduction of Risk Potential

chapter 16

First Aid, Emergency Care, and Disaster Management

http://evolve.elsevier.com/Linton/medsurg

Mary Stephens

Objectives

1. List the principles of emergency and first-aid care.
2. List the steps of the initial assessment and interventions for the person requiring emergency care.
3. Describe the components of the nursing assessment of the person requiring emergency care.
4. Outline the steps of the nursing process for emergency or first-aid treatment of victims of cardiopulmonary arrest, choking, shock, hemorrhage, traumatic injury, burns, heat or cold exposure, poisoning, bites, and stings.
5. Discuss the roles of nurses and nursing students in relation to bioterrorism and natural disasters.
6. Explain the legal implications of administering first aid in emergency situations.
7. Explain the implications of the Good Samaritan doctrine.

Key Terms

Avulsion (ă-VŬL-zhŭn)
Cardiac tamponade (KĂR-dē-ăk tăm-pōn-ĀD)
Cardiopulmonary arrest (kăr-dē-ō-PŬL-mō-nĕr-ē)
Epistaxis (ep-ĭ-STĂK-sĭs)
Evisceration (ē-vĭs-ĕr-Ā-shŭn)
Flail chest
Hemorrhage (HĔM-ŏr-ĭj)
Hemothorax (hē-mō-THŌ-răks)
Hyperthermia (hī-pĕr-THĔR-mē-ă)
Hypothermia (hī-pō-THĔR-mē-ă)
Pneumothorax (nū-mō-THŌ-răks)
Poison
Respiratory arrest (RĔS-pĕ-ră-tō-rē)
Shock
Sprain
Strain

In the inpatient setting, the nurse is often the first person on the scene when accidents or emergencies occur. Nurses also need to be prepared to act in emergency situations in homes and other community settings. Prompt intervention can make a dramatic difference in patient outcomes. Knowledge of first aid can mean the difference between life and death in many situations. This chapter addresses first-aid interventions for common emergencies seen in homes and community settings. Some emergency conditions that require further medical attention are covered in greater detail elsewhere in this book.

GENERAL PRINCIPLES OF EMERGENCY CARE

When accidents or emergencies occur, the victim and any observers are often anxious and frightened. Knowing that a nurse is present can be very reassuring to them but you must remember the cardinal rule: Remain calm! Victims react to emergencies in various ways, from stunned silence to hysteria. Your priority is to preserve life and minimize the effects of injuries but the manner in which you conduct yourself can also soothe and reassure the victim.

The nursing process is used in emergencies just as it is in other nursing situations. The important difference is that assessment and intervention must be accomplished very quickly and efficiently to identify and treat priority needs immediately.

The first step in initiating first aid is to survey the scene. You must determine if the area is safe for you, the victim(s), and any bystander(s) before you proceed. Once you have determined safety, the next steps are to determine how many are injured, how are they injured, and who is around that can help. Identify yourself as a nurse and obtain their consent to provide them with care; then activate, or have a bystander activate, medical assistance.

The focused assessment begins when approaching the victim so that he or she does not have to move his or her head to see you. Ask the victim's name to determine whether the victim can speak, which would reveal airway or neurologic problems. Determine the nature of the emergency; that is, was the injury caused by a motor vehicle accident, a fall, a diving accident, or an electrocution? In addition, look for any hazards to the victim and the rescuer. For example, is the victim in a burning vehicle or lying in the middle of the highway? Failure to recognize such dangers may result in injuries to the rescuer and additional injuries to the victim.

During the primary survey, assess for life-threatening injuries and intervene immediately if indicated in the following sequence:

1. Evaluate the ABCs: airway, breathing, circulation.
2. Initiate cardiopulmonary resuscitation or rescue breathing as needed.
3. Look for uncontrolled bleeding, identify the source, and apply pressure to the source.
4. Systematically examine for injuries from the head to the feet and immobilize the spine, limbs, or both as indicated.
5. Look for a medical alert tag, usually a necklace or a bracelet.

After the primary survey, once again conduct a systematic head-to-toe inspection (called the *secondary survey*) to detect significant changes and other findings that might have been missed initially.

GUIDELINES FOR FIRST-AID TREATMENT

General guidelines for first-aid treatment of emergency patients are as follows:

1. Protect the airway.
2. Splint injured parts in the position they are found.
3. Prevent chilling but do not add excessive heat.
4. Do not remove penetrating objects.
5. Do not give anything by mouth to an unconscious person or to one with potentially serious injuries.
6. Stay with the injured person until medical care or transportation arrives.

NURSING ASSESSMENT IN EMERGENCIES

Patient emergencies can occur in every setting. In some situations, nurses observe the events and know what has happened but at other times evidence at the scene is needed to determine the circumstances. Intervening appropriately in emergencies whose cause cannot be immediately determined can be difficult. Be prepared to make a quick appraisal and then act promptly to provide appropriate care that may save a life. The health history and physical examination are presented separately here but, in fact, may be conducted almost simultaneously in emergencies. Depending on the nature of the injury outside the health care setting, the assessment focuses on the specific injury. The more complete assessment described next would be conducted in the health care setting where the licensed vocational nurse/licensed practical nurse (LVN/LPN) may assist with data collection.

HEALTH HISTORY

If the victim is able to speak or a witness is available, obtain a brief health history of the victim. Data collection is limited in emergency situations and should include the chief complaint, any treatment given, and the relevant medical history. The acronym SAMPLE may help you to remember to inquire about Symptoms, Allergies, current Medications, Past illness/Pregnancy, Last oral intake, and Events related to injury.

Chief Complaint

Determine the nature of the problem, the signs and symptoms, and the circumstances under which the injury or illness occurred. If the victim is or has been unconscious, note the length of time that the person has been unconscious if possible.

Medical Treatment

Determine whether any treatment has been given and, if so, the effect of the treatment. In the presence of an injury, note whether the victim has been moved.

Past Medical History

If possible, determine known health problems, including diabetes and cardiac or pulmonary disease, which may provide important clues to the immediate problem or influence the care provided. Check for a medical alert tag, which may provide essential information if the patient cannot. If possible, identify current medications and known allergies. Note any evidence of alcohol or other drugs.

Pharmacology Capsule

The medical alert tag can provide clues about medical emergencies and alert rescuers to known allergies and chronic conditions.

PHYSICAL EXAMINATION

Begin collecting objective data as soon as the victim is seen, and quickly determine whether the patient is responsive. The first assessment priorities must be the ABCs: Airway, Breathing, and Circulation—followed by D (Disability) and E (Exposure). Watch the victim's chest for rhythmic breathing and listen near the patient's mouth and nose for air movement. Palpate the carotid and peripheral pulses. Once the adequacy of respiration and circulation has been established, assess for uncontrolled bleeding and shock. Note the level of consciousness, pupil response, and gross sensory and motor function to determine disability. Exposure refers to the removal of clothing to permit a more complete inspection for injuries. If no evidence of uncontrolled bleeding or shock is noted, the next step is a systematic head-to-toe examination. At each step, look for obvious injury, bleeding, swelling, bruising, and drainage. Note circulation, mobility, sensation, symmetry, and alignment of the entire body. Also note skin color, warmth, and temperature at each step of the head to toe assessment.

The systematic assessment, or secondary survey, will be a more thorough assessment of the injured person. It begins with inspection of the head. Speak to the victim and evaluate the response to determine level of consciousness (alert, disoriented, unresponsive). Evaluate comprehension by asking the patient to follow simple commands such as opening and closing the eyes. Inspect the eyes for pupil size, equality, and reaction to light. Ask the alert victim about neck pain or stiffness and the ability to swallow. Inspect the chest for symmetry of the chest wall movement. Next, assess respiratory effort, dyspnea, and abnormal sounds associated with respirations. Examine the contour of the abdomen to detect distention. Use light palpation to detect areas of pain or tenderness. Inspect the extremities for deformity or injury and evaluate movement. Then assess peripheral pulses and warmth and sensation in the extremities. Box 16-1 summarizes the focused assessment of the patient who requires first aid or emergency care.

SPECIFIC EMERGENCIES

CARDIOPULMONARY ARREST

When the heart stops beating, a person is in cardiac arrest. When respirations cease, the person is in **respiratory**, or pulmonary, **arrest**. **Cardiopulmonary arrest** is the absence of a heartbeat and respirations. The cardiac and respiratory systems are so dependent on each other that when one fails, the other quickly fails as well.

Nerve tissue is so susceptible to hypoxia (low levels of oxygen) that, in most circumstances, the brain cells begin to die after 4 minutes without oxygen. Unless circulation and oxygenation are restored very quickly after cardiopulmonary arrest, permanent brain damage results. Prompt recognition and treatment of cardiopulmonary arrest can maintain the oxygen supply to the brain until circulation and respiration are restored.

Cardiopulmonary resuscitation (CPR) can be part of basic life support or advanced life support. Basic life support is the immediate care given to maintain oxygenation of the brain until advanced life support is available. Only nursing diagnoses and goals are listed below. Literature published by the American Heart Association (AHA) and the American Red Cross provide specific information. All nurses should be familiar with the automated external defibrillator (AED), which is now available in many public places. Advanced life support is discussed in Chapter 36.

Causes. Among the causes of cardiopulmonary arrest are myocardial infarction, heart failure, electrocution, drowning, drug overdose, anaphylaxis, and asphyxiation.

Signs and Symptoms. Victims of cardiopulmonary arrest collapse and quickly lose consciousness. They have no pulse or respiration.

Nursing Assessment. In cardiopulmonary arrest, assessment and interventions are quickly interwoven. To obtain the most current recommendations for CPR, refer to AHA references.

Box 16-1 Assessment of the Patient Who Requires First Aid or Emergency Care

HEALTH HISTORY

Chief Complaint
Nature of illness or injury, signs and symptoms, circumstances of illness or injury, how long unconscious

Treatment
Efforts that have been made, effects, whether moved after injury

Past Medical History
Current health problems, current medications, allergies

PHYSICAL EXAMINATION

ABCs
Airway, breathing, circulation

Skin
Color, temperature, obvious injury

Head
Level of consciousness

Eyes
Opening, pupil size, equality, response to light

Neck
Stiffness, pain, ability to swallow

Chest
Symmetry of movement, dyspnea, respiratory rate and effort

Abdomen
Contour, rigidity, distention, pain, tenderness

Extremities
Deformity, movement, sensation, peripheral pulses

Nursing Diagnoses, Goals, and Outcome Criteria: Cardiopulmonary Arrest

Nursing Diagnoses	Goals and Outcome Criteria
Ineffective Peripheral Tissue Perfusion related to cessation of heartbeat **and Decreased Cardiac Output** related to cessation of heartbeat	Adequate oxygenation until heartbeat and respirations are restored: improving skin color, palpable pulse, spontaneous respirations
Ineffective Breathing Pattern related to inadequate or absent respirations	Effective ventilation: spontaneous respirations, improving skin color

Interventions. Refer to the latest AHA guidelines for CPR because the guidelines are revised at intervals.

CHOKING OR AIRWAY OBSTRUCTION

Choking is airway obstruction caused by a foreign body that enters the airway.

Assessment. The initial response when a person appears to be choking depends on the severity of the airway obstruction.

Mild Airway Obstruction. If the victim has good air exchange, is responsive, and can cough forcefully, do not interfere.

1. Encourage the victim's efforts to breathe and cough.
2. If symptoms persist, activate the emergency response system.

Severe Airway Obstruction. Signs of severe airway obstruction are poor or no air exchange, poor or no cough, high-pitched noise or no noise on inhalation, respiratory distress, cyanosis, inability to speak, inability to move air, and clutching the neck (the universal choking sign, depicted in Fig. 16-1).

Nursing Diagnoses, Goals, and Outcome Criteria: Choking

Nursing Diagnoses	Goals and Outcome Criteria
Ineffective Airway Clearance related to inability to expel an aspirated foreign object **and Risk for Suffocation** related to aspirated foreign object	Patent airway with normal respirations: expulsion of foreign object, audible respirations, improving skin color, decreased coughing, reduced anxiety, normal pulse

Interventions. Perform abdominal thrusts for the conscious or unconscious choking victim per the latest AHA guidelines for choking (Fig. 16-2). Adaptive measures should be taken for obese or pregnant individuals.

Complications from Abdominal Thrusts. Because of the risk for damage to internal organs, a person who has received abdominal thrusts should subsequently be examined by a health care provider.

Prevention. Most choking deaths could be prevented if people would do the following:

1. Cut food into small pieces, eat slowly, and chew food thoroughly before swallowing.
2. Not laugh and talk while chewing and swallowing.
3. Perform abdominal thrusts promptly when a person is in distress because of an obstructed airway.

SHOCK

Shock results from acute circulatory failure caused by inadequate blood volume, heart failure, overwhelming infection, severe allergic reactions, or extreme pain or fright. Because of the complexity of the topic, shock is covered in detail in Chapter 19.

HEMORRHAGE

Hemorrhage is the loss of a large amount of blood. The loss of more than 1 liter of blood in an adult may lead to hypovolemic shock. Continued uncontrolled bleeding results in death. Bleeding may be external or internal. Internal bleeding is suspected if a trauma victim shows signs of shock but no external bleeding is evident.

Assessment. Assess for signs and symptoms of hemorrhage, which may include obvious bleeding; cool, sweaty, pale skin; thready pulse; rapid respirations; and decreasing alertness. The victim who is bleeding

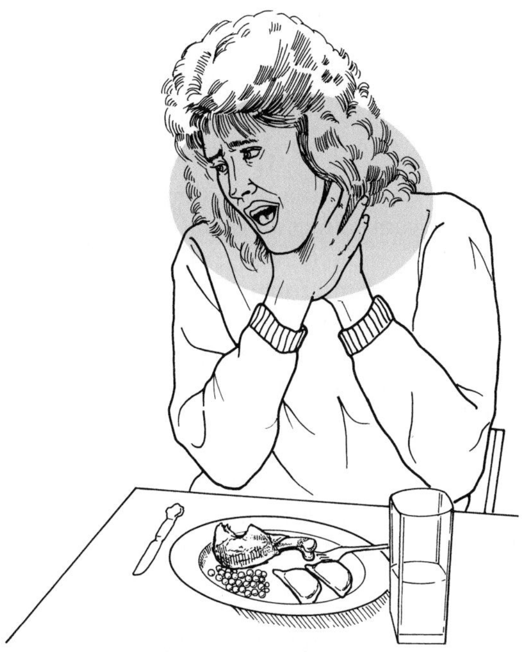

FIGURE 16-1 The universal choking sign.

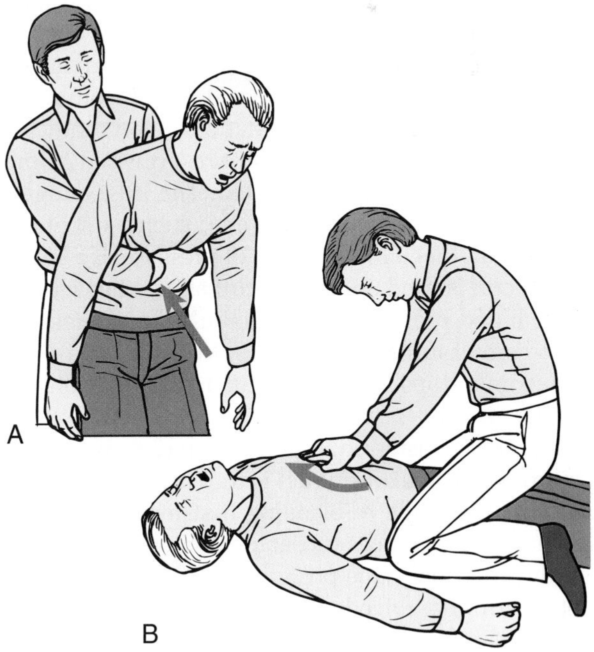

FIGURE 16-2 **A,** Abdominal thrusts for the conscious choking victim. **B,** Abdominal thrusts for the unconscious choking victim. (A, From Lewis SM, Heitkemper MM, Dirksen SR, et al: *Medical-surgical nursing: assessment and management of clinical problems*, ed 7, St. Louis, 2007, Mosby. B, From Lewis SM, Heitkemper MM, Dirksen SR: *Medical-surgical nursing: assessment and management of clinical problems*, ed 5, St. Louis, 2000, Mosby.)

internally may also have abdominal distention, pain, hematemesis, or dyspnea, depending on the site of the bleeding. Ask if the patient has a bleeding disorder or takes any drugs that affect blood coagulation.

Nursing Diagnoses, Goals, and Outcome Criteria: Hemorrhage

Nursing Diagnoses	Goals and Outcome Criteria
Decreased Cardiac Output related to hypovolemia	Increased cardiac output: pulse and blood pressure within normal range, skin warm and dry, no visible bleeding
Fear related to possible impending death	Decreased fear: patient appears more relaxed, states is less fearful

Interventions. The immediate treatment for external bleeding is direct, continuous pressure. Ideally, a sterile dressing is placed over the wound. If sterile supplies are unavailable, use a clean cloth. Elevate and immobilize the injured part (unless fracture is suspected). Elevation decreases blood flow to the area; immobilization prevents dislodging of clots that have formed. After bleeding stops, secure a large dressing, if available, over the wound. Reinforce the dressing but do not change it.

If direct wound pressure and elevation fail to control bleeding, apply indirect pressure, that is, pressure to the main artery that supplies the area (Fig. 16-3).

The use of a tourniquet to control severe bleeding in an extremity is controversial. Tourniquets that are inappropriately placed or left in place too long may result in unnecessary amputations. Therefore tourniquets should be applied only by people with advanced training in first aid. Some sources do not recommend a tourniquet under any circumstances; others indicate that it should be used only as a last resort when a limb is mangled, crushed, or amputated. The least dangerous tourniquet is a pneumatic one, such as a blood pressure cuff, that allows control of pressure. If a blood pressure cuff is used, inflate the cuff above the victim's systolic blood pressure. If the victim's blood pressure cannot be measured, the cuff should be inflated until the bleeding stops. Once the cuff is inflated, only a physician should remove it. When a victim with a tourniquet is transferred, the receiving caregiver must be informed that a tourniquet is in place.

Epistaxis. One type of bleeding that requires special intervention is **epistaxis** (nosebleed). Blood may come from the anterior or the posterior portion of the nose. Most anterior nosebleeds respond to pressure. Instruct the patient to sit down and lean the head *forward* in order to prevent aspiration of blood. Pinch the nostrils of the patient shut for at least 10 minutes (Fig. 16-4). In most cases, this action stops the bleeding. Afterward, advise the patient not to blow or pick at the nose for several hours. Continued bleeding or bleeding from the posterior area of the nose requires medical treatment (see Chapter 30).

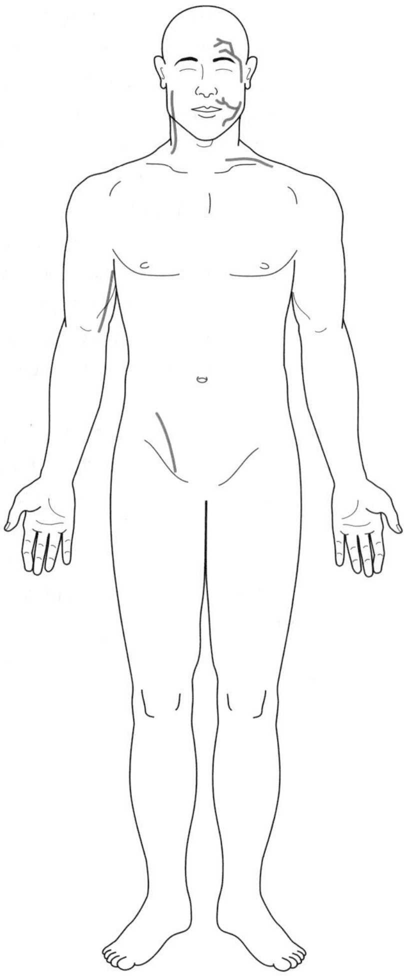

FIGURE 16-3 Major arterial pressure points.

TRAUMATIC INJURY

Traumatic injuries result from a variety of events. Sports injuries, motor vehicle accidents, falls, and acts of violence often require emergency treatment at the scene of the injury.

Fractures

A fracture is a break in a bone that may be described as simple or compound, open or closed, complete or incomplete. A simple (closed) fracture does not break the skin. A compound (open) fracture is one in which the ends of the broken bone protrude through the skin. In a complete fracture, the broken ends are separated. The bone ends in an incomplete fracture are not separated. (See Chapter 44 for a discussion of other types of fractures.)

Assessment. Check the victim of traumatic injury for signs and symptoms of fractures. The primary symptom is pain, although some people, especially older adults, do not always have severe pain with fractures. Numbness and tingling may be present as a result of injury to nerves and blood vessels. Objective

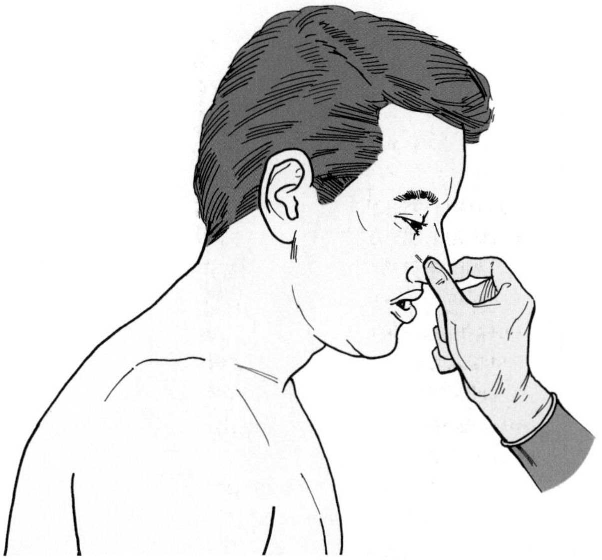

FIGURE 16-4 Epistaxis may be controlled by having the patient sit up and lean forward slightly. Then pinch the patient's nostrils closed.

signs of fracture include deformity, swelling, discoloration, decreased function, and bone fragments protruding through the skin. Suspected fractures should be treated as such until they are ruled out by the physician.

Nursing Diagnosis, Goal, and Outcome Criterion: Fractures. The primary nursing diagnosis for the emergency treatment of the person with a suspected fracture is **Risk for Trauma** related to movement of unstable fractures. The goal is reduced risk for trauma and the outcome criterion is stabilization of the fractured bone with minimal tissue damage.

Interventions. The key to emergency management of fractures is immobilization. Immobilize the injured part, including the joints above and below the injury, to prevent further trauma to the bone and surrounding soft tissue. Do not attempt to straighten a broken bone. Instead, splint the bone in the position in which it was found, with as little movement as possible. Boards, sticks, magazines, and strips of cloth can all be used to immobilize an injured limb. A cool pack may be applied to reduce swelling.

Severe bleeding may be present with compound fractures. In such cases, apply direct pressure to the artery above the injury. Give the victim nothing by mouth and seek transportation to a medical care facility as soon as possible.

Strains and Sprains

Strains are injuries to muscles or to the tendons that attach muscles to bones, or to both. **Sprains** are injuries to ligaments. Ligaments are bands of tissue that hold bones in position in the joints. These injuries are painful and swelling may be present. Emergency treatment for both of these injuries is immobilization, elevation, and application of a cool pack. The victim should see a physician for further evaluation.

Head Injury

Head injury is not always apparent immediately after an accident. It should be suspected with any type of blow to the head or any unexplained loss of consciousness. A critical complication of head injury is increased intracranial pressure caused by bleeding or swelling associated with trauma. Increased intracranial pressure progressively impairs brain function and may lead to cessation of breathing.

Older adults are at special risk for head injuries because they are more likely than younger people to have sensory deficits, unstable gait, or circulatory disorders. Head injury in an older person may be overlooked if a state of confusion is attributed to age without determining the person's usual level of mental function.

Assessment. When head injury is suspected, assessment includes inspection and palpation of the head and evaluation for signs and symptoms of increased intracranial pressure. Signs of increased intracranial pressure are as follows:

- Change in behavior, agitation, confusion
- Decreasing level of consciousness
- Pupil dilation or constriction, pupillary inequality, slow or no pupillary response to light
- Impaired sensory or motor function
- Increasing blood pressure with widening pulse pressure
- Decreasing pulse and respiratory rates
- Projectile vomiting

Be alert for the leakage of cerebrospinal fluid (CSF) that occurs with basilar skull fractures. CSF leakage is usually seen as clear, colorless fluid draining from the nose or ear. If the fluid drains onto a white cloth, it appears as a yellowish stain. If blood is in the fluid, a yellow "halo" is produced around the pink (bloody) center. While other fluids also can produce the "halo" sign, it is one piece of data in assessing for CSF leakage.

Nursing Diagnoses, Goals, and Outcome Criteria: Head Injury

Nursing Diagnoses	Goals and Outcome Criteria
Ineffective Breathing Pattern related to neurologic trauma	Effective breathing pattern: normal respiratory rate and depth, normal pulse
Risk for Injury related to increasing intracranial pressure, improper movement after spinal fracture	Decreased risk for injury: prompt recognition of rising intracranial pressure (altered mental function, unequal pupils, abnormal response of pupils to light), secure immobilization of spine

Interventions. The victim of a head injury must be assessed by a physician as soon as possible. Because head injuries often accompany spinal injuries, always treat the victim as if a spinal injury has occurred until it is ruled out. This precaution is especially important when the victim is unconscious or when no history can be obtained. Immobilize the neck and keep the victim flat with proper alignment of the neck and head. A backboard should be used to transport the victim.

Even if the head injury seems to be minor, the physician may admit the victim to the hospital for observation as a precaution. This safety measure is initiated because bleeding and swelling are sometimes so slow that signs and symptoms of increased intracranial pressure may not appear until hours or even weeks after the initial injury. (See Chapter 27 for detailed neurologic assessment and care of the hospitalized patient with a head injury.)

Neck and Spinal Injuries

Suspect neck and spinal injuries in any patient with a head injury, especially if the victim has had a diving or motor vehicle accident. Do not move the victim during the initial assessment unless absolutely necessary. Improper movement of the patient with a spinal injury may increase the damage to the spinal cord, causing permanent paralysis. After a diving injury, the neck and back should be immobilized while removing the victim from the water.

Assessment. When a victim has a neck or spinal injury, first evaluate the victim's breathing and circulation and then begin resuscitation if needed. Use the jaw thrust method to open the airway. DO NOT use the head tilt–chin lift technique until the spine has been cleared by a physician! Then determine the victim's movement and sensation in all extremities.

Nursing Diagnosis, Goal, and Outcome Criteria: Neck and Spinal Injuries. The priority nursing diagnosis for the person with a neck or spinal injury is **Risk for Trauma** related to improper movement of the fractured spine. The goal is decreased risk of additional injury. Outcome criteria include continuous immobilization of the spine and transport for medical care.

Interventions. Immediately summon an expert emergency team when neck or spinal injury is suspected. A professional team has the equipment and the expertise to immobilize and transport the victim properly. In remote or life-threatening settings, the victim may have to be moved. If so, a rolled towel or article of clothing can be used as a collar to support the neck. The victim can then be moved by logrolling to one side and then rolling back onto a board, keeping the spine as straight as possible. Throughout the movement, one rescuer supports the head while two others support the shoulders, hips, and legs.

Eye Injury

Eye conditions that warrant immediate attention include presence of foreign bodies, chemical contact, perforation of the globe, and eyelid trauma.

Assessment. After an injury of the eye, inspect the patient's eyelid for trauma and the eye itself for redness, foreign bodies, or penetrating objects. To inspect for foreign bodies, evert the eyelids (Fig. 16-5). If the eye has been exposed to a chemical irritant, attempt to determine what the substance is.

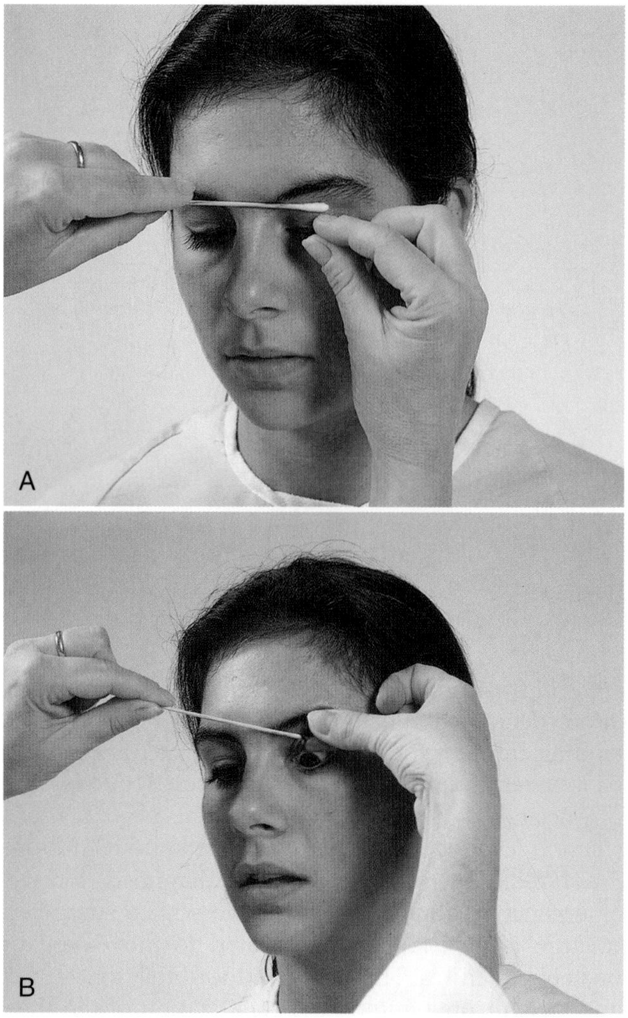

FIGURE 16-5 Eversion of the upper eyelid for inspection. **A,** Gently hold a cotton-tipped applicator against the closed lid and lift the lashes up. **B,** Use your thumb to evert the lid over the applicator and hold the lashes against the bony orbit. (From Jarvis C: *Physical examination and health assessment*, ed 5, Philadelphia, 2008, Saunders.)

Nursing Diagnosis, Goal, and Outcome Criteria: Eye Injury. The primary nursing diagnosis is **Risk for Injury** related to foreign body, direct trauma, or exposure to harmful substances. The goal is to minimize injury to the eye. Outcome criteria, depending on the nature of the injury, may be removal of a foreign body or chemical or protection of the eye from further damage while medical attention is being obtained.

Interventions. Interventions are summarized in Table 16-1.

Ear Trauma

The position and structure of the external ear make it vulnerable to traumatic injury. The most serious injury to the external ear is avulsion. **Avulsion** means that all or part of the auricle is torn loose.

Table 16-1 Interventions for Specific Eye Injuries

TYPE OF INJURY	EMERGENCY INTERVENTION
Foreign bodies	If not embedded: Remove by irrigation or by gently touching the object with the corner of a clean cloth or gauze pad or a moistened cotton-tipped applicator. Embedded foreign bodies should be removed only by a physician.
Chemical contact	Immediately flush the eye for at least 20 minutes. Sterile normal saline or water is ideal but tap water may be used. Direct the irrigating fluid to flow from the inner canthus to the outer canthus of the eye. Even if the flushing seems to relieve all symptoms, the patient should be examined by a physician to assess the eye for injury.
Perforation of the globe	Do not attempt to remove an object that has perforated the eye! You could cause additional harm. Instead, limit movement of the object and the eye and transport the victim for immediate medical care. Protect the injured eye by covering it with a shield that does not touch the object. An inverted paper cup can be taped over the eye. Patch the unaffected eye as well because the eyes move together. This precaution limits movement in both eyes. Tell the patient why both eyes need to be covered.
Eyelid trauma	Seek medical evaluation because injury of the globe, as well as the lid, is always possible. Do not apply direct pressure to a bleeding eyelid. If the globe has been injured, pressure could cause additional harm. Apply a loose dressing and transport the victim for medical care.

Assessment. Determine the extent of the injury; note whether any tissue is fully separated and the severity of bleeding. If necessary, apply direct pressure to the site of the injury to control bleeding.

Nursing Diagnosis, Goal, and Outcome Criteria: Ear Trauma. If bleeding is under control, the priority nursing diagnosis for a traumatic injury to the auricle is **Impaired Tissue Integrity** related to trauma. The goal is to preserve the tissue to maximize successful repair. Outcome criteria for successful interventions are recovery and protection of avulsed tissue.

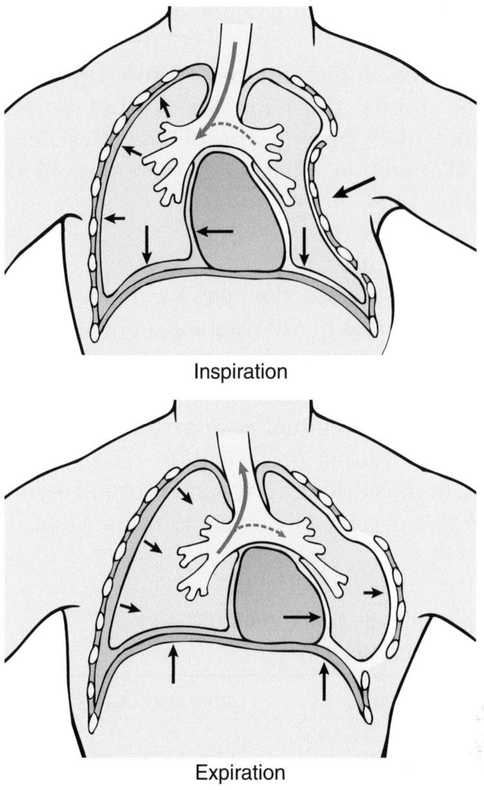

FIGURE 16-6 Paradoxical motion caused by loss of chest wall support. (From Lewis SM, Dirksen SR, et al: *Medical-surgical nursing*, ed 8, St. Louis, 2011, Mosby.)

Interventions. If the injured part is actually separated, reattachment may be possible. Retrieve the tissue, wrap it in plastic, keep it cool, and transport it with the victim.

Chest Injury

Injuries to the chest can result in serious impairment of respiratory function. Chest injuries are described as open or closed. The most critical injuries are open **pneumothorax**, **flail chest**, massive **hemothorax**, and **cardiac tamponade**. Any injury at or below the nipple line may cause both chest and abdominal injuries.

Assessment. Assessment of respiratory status always takes first priority when the victim has sustained a chest injury. Note the rate and character of the victim's respirations, skin color, pulse rate and rhythm, symmetry of the chest wall movement, and the presence of any apparent injuries to the chest. Signs and symptoms of chest injuries that impair respirations are dyspnea, tachycardia, restlessness, cyanosis, asymmetric or other abnormal chest wall movement, and abnormal sounds associated with breathing (Fig. 16-6). Note the patient's mental state and level of consciousness.

Nursing Diagnosis, Goal, and Outcome Criteria: Chest Injury. For the patient with a chest injury, the priority nursing diagnosis is **Impaired Gas Exchange** related to altered anatomic structure. The goal is adequate oxygenation and the outcome criteria are absence of dyspnea, normal pulse and respiratory rates, and normal skin color.

Interventions. Interventions for emergency management of specific chest injuries are briefly described in Table 16-2. (See "Care of the Patient with a Chest Wound" in Chapter 31 for a more detailed discussion.)

Abdominal Injury

Assessment. Assess the abdomen for evidence of injury. In addition to asking the patient about abdominal symptoms, inspect the abdomen for abnormalities. Suspect internal abdominal injuries when the patient complains of abdominal pain or the abdomen shows evidence of trauma or distention. The protrusion of internal organs through a wound is called **evisceration**. Eviscerated organs are subject to trauma and drying.

Nursing Diagnoses, Goals, and Outcome Criteria: Abdominal Injury

Nursing Diagnoses	Goals and Outcome Criteria
Impaired Tissue Integrity related to traumatic injury or exposed internal organs	Protection of eviscerated tissue: proper covering of wound to maintain moisture and warmth
Risk for Infection related to break in skin, possible injury to intestinal tract	Decreased risk of infection: wound protected from contamination

Interventions. Possible internal injuries require medical evaluation. Do not give the patient anything by mouth while preparing for transport. Do not attempt to replace eviscerated organs in the abdomen because additional harm may result. Cover eviscerated organs with some material such as plastic wrap or foil to conserve moisture and warmth. A saline-soaked sterile dressing is ideal but is not likely to be available at the scene of an accident. Cover the wound with a clean cloth and seek transportation to a hospital.

Traumatic Amputation

If body tissue has been partially or completely detached, reattachment may be possible. If supplies are available, clean the wound surfaces with sterile water or saline and place the tissue in its normal position. Ideally, a body part that is completely detached should be wrapped in sterile gauze moistened with sterile saline, placed in a watertight container such as a resealable plastic bag, and placed in an iced saline bath. The tissue should not be frozen or placed in contact with ice. Amputated extremities may be healthy enough for reattachment for 4 to 6 hours whereas digits (fingers and toes) may be viable for as long as 8 hours.

BURNS

Care of the burn patient is discussed in detail in Chapter 52. This chapter addresses only emergency measures for burn care. When a burn accident occurs, the immediate concern is to stop the burning process. A victim whose clothing is burning should be told to

Table 16-2 Emergency Interventions for Chest Injuries

TYPE OF INJURY	EMERGENCY INTERVENTION
Pneumothorax: An open chest wound penetrates the pleural cavity, allowing air to enter, which collapses lung on affected side. *Signs and symptoms:* Dyspnea, asymmetric chest wall movement, "sucking" sound as air moves in and out of wound with respirations.	• Apply vented dressing: sealed on three sides so air can escape but not enter the wound, *OR* • Apply airtight dressing. *IF* patient's condition worsens, suspect tension pneumothorax and loosen the dressing.
Flail chest: Several adjacent ribs are broken in more than one place, causing a loss of support in the affected section of the chest wall. *Signs and symptoms:* The affected section moves inward on inspiration and outward on expiration. This abnormal chest wall movement, called *paradoxical motion*, impairs gas exchange (see Fig. 16-6).	Provide support for the injured area. Hold or tape a small pad or pillow over the injury to splint the ribs.
Hemothorax: Accumulation of blood in the pleural cavity; causes the lung or lungs to collapse. *Signs and symptoms:* Increasing respiratory or circulatory failure.	Cannot be diagnosed directly or treated by the first-aid care provider. The victim requires prompt treatment in a medical facility.
Cardiac tamponade: Presence of blood in the pericardial sac. *Signs and symptoms:* Increasing respiratory or circulatory failure.	Cannot be diagnosed directly or treated by first-aid care. Causes decreased cardiac output. The victim requires prompt treatment in a medical facility.

drop to the ground and roll to extinguish the flames. Smother the flames with coats or blankets or extinguish the flames with water if no chemicals or flammable liquids are present on the clothing. Remove burning or smoldering materials from the victim. Protection of the airway is of primary importance in a burn patient.

Assessment. First determine the type of burn that has occurred. If the victim has had a flame burn or has been in a closed, smoke-filled area, begin with assessment of respirations. Assess airway patency. The patient who has singed areas around the mouth or nose, or any areas of blackness around the mouth and nose or the eyes, must be treated as having an inhalation injury. Then determine the extent and depth of the burns. Inspect the skin for color, blisters, and tissue destruction. Superficial burns are typically pink or red and painful. Deeper burns may be red, white, or black and may destroy not only the skin, but also the underlying tissues. The deepest burns are not painful because nerves have been destroyed. However, because the depth of a burn is often not uniform, patients with deep burns can still have pain. Determining the extent of the body surface area injured is very important. (See guidelines for assessing the extent of burn injury in Chapter 52.)

Electrical burns are difficult to assess initially because the full extent of tissue damage may not be apparent for several days. In the event of chemical burns, note and immediately remove any remaining chemical.

Interventions. Ensuring a patent airway and respirations for burn victims is critical. If the burns have been caused by flames, fumes, or chemicals, the victim may have inhaled substances that cause respiratory impairment. Immediately apply oxygen and anticipate an order for arterial blood gas analysis. Rescue breathing, if needed, is described in AHA publications under Cardiopulmonary Arrest. Other interventions are addressed in Table 16-3 for each of the major types of burns.

Nursing Diagnoses, Goals, and Outcome Criteria: Burns

Depending on the severity and type of the burn, nursing diagnoses and goals for the burn victim immediately after the injury may include the following.

Nursing Diagnoses	Goals and Outcome Criteria
Impaired Gas Exchange related to inhalation or thermal injury, edema of airway tissues	Improved gas exchange: normal pulse and respiratory rates; no dyspnea, confusion, or cyanosis; normal arterial blood gases
Impaired Skin or **Tissue Integrity** (or both) related to thermal destruction, chemical injury	Limited extent of injury: no additional damage after initial burn, skin surfaces protected and free of burning materials
Acute Pain related to thermal injury	Reduced pain: victim calmer, states pain is lessened

HEAT AND COLD EXPOSURE

Extreme heat or cold may have local or systemic effects. Several mechanisms work to maintain body temperature within a fairly narrow range. If the body temperature rises or falls excessively, vital functions begin to fail. Infants and older adults are less able to adapt to temperature extremes than other people. This tendency places them at increased risk for excessive alterations in body temperature.

Hyperthermia

Excessive heat exposure may cause **hyperthermia**, a condition in which body temperature rises above 37.2°C (99°F). Heat edema and heat cramps are mild

Table 16-3 Emergency Interventions for Burns

TYPE OF BURN	EMERGENCY INTERVENTION
Minor or superficial	Immerse the injured body part in cool water for 2 to 5 minutes. Applying butter to the burn is contraindicated. Medical care usually is not required.
Sunburn	Topical preparations with benzocaine may be soothing. Many people believe that aloe vera is very effective in treating minor burns but this treatment is still being studied. Children and older adults with extensive sunburn may require hospitalization for dehydration.
Extensive burns	Apply cool water only until the burned area is cool. Do not apply butter, lotions, ice, medications, or absorbent materials. Call the nearest burn center for instructions before applying any dressing. You may be advised to cover burns with a clean, dry dressing or cloth. Wrap burned fingers and toes separately to prevent sticking together. Have the victim transported for medical care immediately.
Chemical burns	Remove contaminated clothing. Thoroughly dust powdered chemicals from the skin and then flush with water for 30 minutes. If the dry chemical is not removed before flushing, the water may cause the chemical to become caustic, resulting in additional injury. Flush liquid chemicals from the skin with running water for at least 30 minutes. Apply a dressing or covering and have the victim transported for medical care.

degrees of hyperthermia. These mild forms of hyperthermia usually can be treated by moving the individual into a cool place and providing fluids with electrolytes such as sports drinks. Salt tablets are not generally recommended. Heat exhaustion and heat stroke are more serious. Treatment details are presented in Table 16-4. (See also the *Patient Teaching* box.)

Patient Teaching

Prevention of Heat Exhaustion

- Avoid strenuous activities outdoors when the temperature or humidity is very high.
- Increase fluid intake to replace excessive fluid loss.
- Take frequent rest breaks when working in hot, humid weather.

Pharmacology Capsule

Diuretics and anticholinergics increase the risk of heat stroke by affecting the body's heat-reducing defenses.

Hypothermia

Hypothermia is a decrease in body core temperature below 35°C (95°F). It may be caused by prolonged exposure to cold, extremely cold temperatures, or immersion in cold water. Hypothermia causes depression of vital functions and, if it is not corrected, death results from cardiac dysrhythmias. Hypothermia is classified based on core body temperature as mild (32°C to 35°C), moderate (28°C to 32°C), or severe (<28°C). In the mild stage, the patient shivers in an effort to generate body heat. Blood vessels in the extremities are constricted and performance of complex motor tasks is impaired. Persons in moderate hypothermia appear dazed and have poor motor coordination, slurred speech, and violent shivering; they also may behave irrationally. Severe hypothermia is characterized by waves of shivering, rigid muscles, and pale skin. The pulse rate is slow and the pupils are dilated.

Older adults are susceptible to hypothermia because of loss of subcutaneous fat, diminished circulation, and reduced neural control over circulation; they are also unable to conserve heat effectively. Research shows that confusion in some older people is the result of hypothermia. (See Table 16-4 for treatment of systemic responses to heat and cold exposure and local cold injuries. Local thermal injuries were discussed earlier under "Burns.")

POISONING

A **poison** is any substance that, in small quantities, is capable of causing illness or harm after ingestion, inhalation, injection, or contact with the skin. Large quantities of most chemicals, including all medications, can act as poisons. Even common drugs such as aspirin, acetaminophen, and vitamins can be poisonous if taken in excessive amounts.

Carbon Monoxide Poisoning

Carbon monoxide is an odorless, invisible gas emitted by internal combustion engines, gas stoves and furnaces, and burning charcoal and other combustible materials. When carbon monoxide is inhaled, it enters the bloodstream and promptly binds with hemoglobin. Carbon monoxide binds to hemoglobin much more readily than oxygen. Therefore it soon occupies many of the sites on the hemoglobin needed to transport oxygen to the cells. The victim becomes hypoxemic and can die.

Assessment. Evaluate for early signs and symptoms of carbon monoxide poisoning, which include headache and shortness of breath with mild exertion. Dizziness, nausea, vomiting, and mental changes appear next. As the amount of carbon monoxide in the bloodstream rises, the victim loses consciousness and develops cardiac and respiratory irregularities. A victim usually dies when the carbon monoxide bound with hemoglobin exceeds 70%. Although a cherry-red skin color is a clear indicator of carbon monoxide poisoning, skin color is often found to be pale or bluish with reddish mucous membranes.

Nursing Diagnosis, Goal, and Outcome Criteria: Carbon Monoxide Poisoning. The primary nursing diagnosis for the victim of carbon monoxide poisoning is **Impaired Gas Exchange** related to carbon monoxide poisoning. The goal of nursing care for the emergency treatment of the victim of carbon monoxide poisoning is normal oxygenation. Criteria for evaluating the effects of nursing interventions are regular pulse with a rate of 60 to 100 beats per minute (bpm), oxygen saturation of 95% or higher, regular respirations with a rate of 12 to 20 breaths per minute, and alert mental state.

Interventions. Immediately move the victim of carbon monoxide poisoning to fresh air. If the person is not breathing, start rescue breathing. Seek emergency medical assistance immediately. Give the victim oxygen as soon as it is available. At the hospital, the patient may be placed in a hyperbaric oxygen chamber. A hyperbaric chamber uses pressure to force oxygen into the blood and tissues. See the *Patient Teaching* box for ways to prevent carbon monoxide poisoning.

Patient Teaching

Prevention of Carbon Monoxide Poisoning

- Keep gas furnaces and stoves in proper repair.
- Burners that use gas must be vented to the outside.
- Do not use charcoal or wood-burning devices in a closed area without ventilation.
- Never let an engine run in a closed garage.
- Use a carbon monoxide detection alarm device.

Pharmacology Capsule

Common drugs such as aspirin, acetaminophen, and vitamins can be poisonous if taken in excessive amounts.

Table 16-4 Emergency Interventions for Heat and Cold Exposure

TYPE OF EXPOSURE OR INJURY	EMERGENCY INTERVENTION
Heat Exhaustion	
Caused by excessive fluid loss when exposed to high environmental temperature and humidity. Rising body temperature and metabolic rate increase oxygen demand. Cardiac output and heart rate first increase then fall. Loss of fluids causes hypovolemia (low blood volume) and electrolyte imbalances. *Signs and symptoms:* Dizziness, headache, muscle cramps, nausea and vomiting, and collapse. Skin is usually pale and damp. Elevated rectal temperature; may be as high as 41.1°C (106°F).	Move the person to cooler environment, preferably one that is air-conditioned, and loosen clothing. Splash cool water on the skin. If the victim is alert, offer fluids such as commercially prepared electrolyte drinks, if available.
Heat Stroke	
Body core temperature of 41.1°C (106°F) or greater. Temperature-regulating mechanisms in the brain fail. Heart, kidneys, and central nervous system functions are depressed. The victim is unable to sweat and will die if the temperature is not lowered. Usually associated with strenuous activity in hot, humid weather. *Signs and symptoms:* Similar to heat exhaustion at first: dizziness, weakness, nausea. As the condition worsens, the skin becomes red, hot, and dry. *Perspiration is noticeably absent*. If the condition is not reversed, the victim may collapse and have seizures. The body temperature may reach as high as 43.3°C (110°F).	Cooling the person quickly is critical. Immediate transport for medical care is recommended. Anyone who cannot be transported immediately should be moved into the shade or to an air-conditioned area if possible. Apply wet, cool towels to the trunk and the extremities and place ice packs on the forehead and axillae. If a tub is available, the victim can be placed in a cool bath. Continue cooling measures until the body temperature falls below 38.3°C (101°F).
Frostnip and Frostbite	
Frostnip: Mild tissue damage caused by cold.	Immediate treatment of mild cold injury: Rapid rewarming. For example, have the patient place cold hands in his or her axillae or between the thighs.
Frostbite: More serious cold injury. Blood vessels in the skin and the extremities constrict when exposed to extreme cold. Blood clots form and circulation to the affected areas decreases. Cells die because of lack of oxygen and nutrients and because of formation of crystals that cause them to swell and rupture. Nose, cheeks, fingers, and toes are affected most often. *Signs and symptoms:* Pain is noted at first, then tingling followed by numbness.	Patient should be transported for medical treatment as soon as possible. If transport is delayed, seek a setting where warm water is available. *Do not attempt to thaw the tissue unless warmth can be maintained*. Frostbitten extremities are best rewarmed by immersion in a warm water bath of 37.7°C to 40.5°C (100°F to 105°F). Handle affected areas very gently to prevent additional tissue trauma. Do not rub, massage, or apply cold to the tissue. As tissue warms, the skin turns bright pink and blisters. Rewarming is very painful. If the procedure is performed in a medical facility, analgesics will be ordered before rewarming. After warming the extremities, pat dry and wrap in sterile dressings. Wrap each finger or toe separately to prevent injured tissues from sticking together. Immobilize and elevate affected parts. With severe or deep frostbite, thawed tissue dies and eventually has to be surgically debrided (removed).
Hypothermia	
Rectal temperature lower than 35°C (95°F). *Signs and symptoms:* Mild hypothermia: shivering and impaired performance. Progressive chilling: decreasing heart and respiratory rates and blood pressure. Irregular heart and breathing patterns; cardiopulmonary arrest if not treated.	Mild hypothermia: Wrap victim in warm, dry clothing and blankets. Severe hypothermia: Transport immediately for treatment. Victim must be rewarmed aggressively but gradually, because excessive rewarming sends lactic acid and cold blood from the extremities to the heart, possibly triggering cardiac dysrhythmias. Warm the torso first. It may be wrapped in blankets or immersed in tepid water. Once the rectal temperature reaches 35°C (95°F), turn attention to warming the extremities also. Internal rewarming (warmed oxygen and intravenous fluids, peritoneal lavage, and extracorporeal blood warming) may be ordered in a medical facility.

Drug or Chemical Poisoning

Poisoning by drugs or chemicals can result from accumulation, excessive dose level, drug interactions, or ingestion of inappropriate substances.

Assessment. In situations that suggest poisoning, collect data about relevant signs and symptoms. The signs and symptoms vary with the type of poison. The history is an important part of the assessment of a poisoning victim and should include the following:

1. Name of the drug or chemical involved (If the victim cannot provide the information, look for clues and save the container.)
2. Amount of substance consumed
3. Length of time since the substance was taken
4. Last food consumed: amount, time
5. Signs and symptoms that may be caused by poisons
6. Victim's age and approximate weight
7. Other medications, drugs, or alcohol ingested

Nursing Diagnosis, Goal, and Outcome Criterion: Drug or Chemical Poisoning. The primary nursing diagnosis for the victim of drug or chemical poisoning is **Risk for Injury** related to poison. The general goal of nursing intervention for a poisoning victim is decreased or minimized risk for injury caused by the poisoning agent. The criterion for evaluating successful intervention for drug or chemical poisoning is the absence of ill effects from the substance.

Interventions. In the event of poisoning, immediately call the American Association of Poison Control Centers (2013) at 1-800-222-1222 to be put in contact with your local poison control center. Having the product container with you is helpful because specific interventions depend on knowing exactly what poison was consumed. The poison control center staff person will ask about the condition, age, and weight of the individual; exactly when the poisoning occurred; and your name and telephone number. While some poisonings can be treated at home, others require treatment by a physician or in a hospital.

In years past, syrup of ipecac was commonly used to induce vomiting after ingestion of poisons. However, the benefits of this drug are questionable and it has significant contraindications and adverse effects. Under limited circumstances, the poison control center or an emergency department physician may recommend its use. Vomiting is specifically contraindicated if the victim is already vomiting, is unconscious, or is having seizures, or if the substance ingested was a caustic substance or a petroleum product. Treatment of poisoning in an emergency facility may involve activated charcoal, total bowel lavage, cathartics, or any combination. Activated charcoal is useful because it binds to many poisons, thus preventing their absorption. Bowel lavage and cathartics cause rapid transit of the poison through the intestinal track for elimination.

Food Poisoning

Food poisoning is caused by ingesting contaminated food. Contaminants can be bacteria, chemicals, or natural toxins. Bacteria most often associated with food poisoning are *Clostridium botulinum, Staphylococcus aureus, Clostridium perfringens,* and *Salmonella* (Table 16-5).

Assessment. Victims of food poisoning often recognize the relationship between their symptoms and the ingestion of food. The most common symptoms of food poisoning are nausea, vomiting, abdominal cramps, and diarrhea. Botulism caused by *C. botulinum* produces neurotoxic effects, including difficulty breathing, seeing, and swallowing. An important clue that food poisoning is causing the victim's symptoms is that all who consumed a certain food become ill. To assist in identifying poisons, the nurse should collect samples of stool or vomited materials for possible laboratory analysis.

Nursing Diagnosis, Goal, and Outcome Criterion: Food Poisoning. The primary nursing diagnosis for the victim of food poisoning is **Risk for Injury** related to poisoning. The specific type of injury depends on the action of the contaminant. In general, the treatment of food poisoning involves identifying the poison and decreasing the symptoms. The goal of nursing care for the victim of food poisoning is the absence or reduction of ill effects from the poison. The criterion for evaluating the effects of intervention for food poisoning is diminished symptoms (e.g., decreased pain, respiratory rate of 12 to 20 breaths per minute, depending on the poison).

Interventions. Medical care is necessary if symptoms are severe or persistent, especially in children and older adults. Although the physician may order antiemetics and antidiarrheals, vomiting and diarrhea are sometimes allowed to continue within limits to eliminate the offending substances. Intravenous fluids may be prescribed with severe vomiting and diarrhea. Patients with botulism may require ventilatory support.

Prevention. Most cases of food poisoning can be attributed to improper cooling, storage, or preparation of perishable foods. People need to be taught the importance of cleanliness when handling and cooking food and the correct way to cool and prepare food for storage.

Bites and Stings

Snakes, ticks, bees, wasps, household pets, and even humans are capable of causing serious harm with their bites or stings. The most serious effects of bites are anaphylactic shock, infection, and tissue destruction.

Assessment. Try to determine the type of bite the patient has received. Inspect the bite wound to identify the characteristics of the actual bite site and any changes in surrounding tissue. Ask the patient about

Table 16-5 Food Poisoning

ORGANISM	SOURCE	SIGNS AND SYMPTOMS	TREATMENT	PREVENTION
Clostridium botulinum	Improper home canning; food left out	Onset 18–36 hours after ingestion: nausea and vomiting, headache, dry throat and mouth, dysphagia, diplopia 4–5 days after ingestion: descending paralysis affecting speech, breathing, and swallowing Can be fatal	Gastric lavage, intravenous (IV) fluids, trivalent botulism antitoxin (ABE), mechanical ventilation if needed	Discard food containers that are swollen or have broken seals Spores are not destroyed by boiling Do not depend on taste or odor to detect *C. botulinum* Do not allow hot foods to cool below 145°F outside the refrigerator
Staphylococcus aureus	Poor hygiene of food handlers; inadequate refrigeration of food, especially milk products and mayonnaise	Onset within 6 hours: weakness, nausea and vomiting, diarrhea, abdominal cramps Rarely fatal	IV fluids, antiemetics, sedation	Proper refrigeration of food Good hygiene
Clostridium perfringens	Improper canning; inadequately cooked meat or poultry	Onset 6–12 hours after ingestion: abdominal cramps, diarrhea	Antidiarrheals	Thorough cooking
Salmonella	Contaminated food; undercooked meat, eggs	Abdominal cramps, diarrhea, nausea and vomiting	Antidiarrheals, antiemetics, IV fluids	Thorough washing and cooking

any symptoms that developed after the bite, such as pain, edema, numbness, tingling, nausea, fever, dizziness, and dyspnea.

Nursing Diagnoses, Goals, and Outcome Criteria: Bites and Stings

Nursing Diagnoses	Goals and Outcome Criteria
Risk for Infection related to break in skin by bite of human, animal, or insect	Reduced risk for infection: clean wound
Risk for Injury related to exposure to allergens or toxins	Reduced risk for injury: antihistamine, epinephrine, or antitoxin drugs prevent dyspnea or other specific toxic effects

Interventions. See Table 16-6 for interventions related to bites. The *Patient Teaching* boxes discuss insect bite allergy and Lyme disease.

Pharmacology Capsule

Many drugs and chemicals have antidotes. Antidotes are substances that block or reverse the effects of other substances. If the poisonous substance is known, an antidote may be ordered.

ACTS OF BIOTERRORISM

In the past 20 years, numerous events, including the terrorist attacks on the World Trade Center and Pentagon, have made us aware that we are vulnerable to attacks using various means. Bioterrorism is the deliberate release of pathogens to kill and injure people. The biologic agents most likely to be used in terrorism attacks are anthrax, botulism, plague, smallpox, and tularemia. Because these agents are easily spread, they have the potential to cause many deaths. Imagine the public panic that might follow an outbreak of smallpox! A major problem in the United States is lack of experience in recognizing and treating these infections. Basic information about the biologic agents most likely to be used as bioterrorism weapons is provided in Table 16-7.

In the event of an outbreak of disease related to bioterrorism, health care providers must know how to protect themselves and others. Health care facilities should have readily available information on resources, including the local health department and the Centers for Disease Control and Prevention (CDC). Staff should know where to obtain personal protective equipment and what types of precautions (e.g., patient isolation) should be taken. Staff members who are exposed should obtain prophylactic therapy if appropriate. Persons with weakened immune systems should not provide direct care for affected individuals.

Table 16-6 Interventions for Specific Bites

TYPE OF BITE	EFFECTS	INTERVENTIONS
Snake bite	Venom that is injected through the fangs into the victim may affect the nervous system or the blood and blood vessels. Venom that affects the nervous system is *neurotoxic* and can cause nausea, vomiting, dizziness, tachycardia, muscle twitching, and respiratory distress. *Local effects:* Discoloration, pain, mild to severe edema. Bites of poisonous snakes usually leave two distinct fang marks, although a finger or a toe may be pierced by only one fang.	Seek medical care immediately. A description of the snake (shape of head, color) assists in identification, which may affect treatment. To limit absorption of venom, immobilize the part where the bite is located and keep it at or below the level of the heart. Try to keep the patient still. Wipe the wound. If available, a suction cup can be applied to aspirate the wound. Antivenin, which may be given to counteract the effects of the venom, is most effective if given within 6 hours of the bite. Some tissue around the bite often becomes necrotic and must be removed surgically. *No longer recommended* (risks outweigh benefits): Tourniquet, ice, incision and suction.
Insect bite or sting	*Common reactions:* Local itching, edema, and erythema. People who have serious allergies react with systemic symptoms of urticaria (hives), edema, and possibly fatal anaphylaxis. Characteristics of anaphylaxis are difficulty breathing and a drop in blood volume and blood pressure. If the process is not reversed, the victim quickly loses consciousness and dies (see Chapter 34).	Especially anticipate anaphylaxis in victims who develop systemic symptoms rapidly. *Mild reactions:* Calamine lotion or a paste of baking soda or meat tenderizer is soothing. *Severe allergic responses:* The patient with severe allergies should be taken to a medical facility. Epinephrine (intramuscular), diphenhydramine chloride (Benadryl), aminophylline, and hydrocortisone may be administered after a bite or sting to prevent anaphylaxis. *Prevention:* People who are severely allergic to insect venom should carry emergency epinephrine that can be given intramuscularly after a bite or sting to prevent anaphylaxis. Only the honeybee leaves its stinger, which continues to inject venom into the victim. Immediately remove the stinger with a scraping motion rather than by grasping and pulling on it. Pinching the stinger to grasp it injects additional venom.
Animal bite	All animal bites should be taken seriously because of the risk of wound infections and rabies. Rabies is an infection of the central nervous system that is almost always fatal.	Clean the wound thoroughly; apply a bulky dressing. Advise the patient to have a tetanus booster if immunizations are not current. Patient should see a physician for antibiotic therapy. Follow local protocol to assess whether the animal has rabies. If the animal shows signs of rabies or cannot be located, *previously unvaccinated people* should receive the vaccine intramuscularly at 0, 3, 7, and 14 days. In addition, these people should also receive rabies immune globulin (HRIG) at the same time as the first dose of the vaccine to provide rapid protection that persists until the vaccine works. If the victim was bitten on the face or head, the virus may reach the central nervous system more quickly. Therefore treatment may be started before the disease is confirmed in the animal.
Human bite	Human bites are potentially very dangerous because of the risk of infection. The most common site is the hand or fingers, caused by hitting a person in the mouth.	Clean thoroughly and apply a dressing. Advise the victim to seek medical attention for antibiotic therapy.

Table 16-6 Interventions for Specific Bites—cont'd

TYPE OF BITE	EFFECTS	INTERVENTIONS
Tick bite	Tick bites require attention because ticks carry organisms that cause Lyme disease and Rocky Mountain spotted fever. *Lyme disease:* *Early localized stage:* Influenza-like symptoms with or without a ring-shaped reddened area around the bite ("bull's-eye lesion"). *Early disseminated stage:* Fatigue, anorexia, vomiting, neurologic symptoms. *Late disseminated stage:* Joint (Lyme "arthritis") and muscle involvement, progressive neurologic symptoms ("arthritis"). *Rocky Mountain spotted fever*: *Symptoms*: Appear 3 to 10 days after the bite: chills, fever, headache, pain behind the eyes, joint and muscle pain, and a rash that begins on the wrists and ankles and spreads to the extremities, the trunk, and sometimes the face. Can be fatal if not treated.	When a tick is discovered, remove it promptly. *CDC recommendation*: Grasp the tick near the skin with tweezers and use a firm, steady motion to remove the tick. After tick removal, inspect to see if it is intact (no part remaining in the victim's skin). Wash the site with soap and water; apply antiseptic. *Lyme disease:* Tell the patient to notify the physician if influenza-like symptoms or a "bull's-eye lesion" develops in next 7 to 10 days. *Diagnosis:* Skin biopsy to detect the causative organism, *Borrelia burgdorferi*. A blood test can detect antibodies about 2 months after onset of the infection. *Treatment:* Early localized or disseminated stages: doxycycline or amoxicillin. *Lyme "arthritis" and neurologic symptoms:* Penicillin, cephalosporin, or chloramphenicol. *Rocky Mountain spotted fever treatment:* Tetracycline and chloramphenicol.
Spider bite	Most spider bites cause only local irritation.	For any bite, wash the site and apply a cool compress. Transport the victim for medical care if bite was by black widow or brown recluse.
	Black widow: Venom is neurotoxic; causes pain, nausea and vomiting, fever, weakness, muscle cramps, headache. *More serious effects:* Respiratory distress, hypertension, seizures, and shock.	*Black widow* is shiny black with red hourglass on abdomen. *Treatment:* Antivenin is available for black widow spider bites. *Not recommended:* Constricting bands.
	Brown recluse: Bite not especially painful; area usually swells within a few hours. Initially, a bluish ring appears around the bite. Later it is surrounded by a white ring with a red "halo." Some people experience nausea and vomiting, fever, and joint pain. Severe cardiac, renal, and neurologic reactions are uncommon. In 3–4 days after a bite, the affected tissue becomes necrotic.	*Brown recluse* is light brown with a fiddle-shaped mark on the thorax. Medical attention should be sought for these bites. *Treatment:* No specific antivenin is available to counteract the venom of the brown recluse. Eventually the tissue sloughs off or needs to be debrided. The injury can be so extensive that reconstructive surgery is needed.

CDC, Centers for Disease Control and Prevention.

Table 16-7 **Biologic Agents Most Likely to Be Used as Bioterrorism Weapons**

BIOLOGIC AGENT	CHARACTERISTICS	TREATMENTS AND OUTCOMES
Anthrax	After exposure, symptoms may appear in 7–42 days. Three types: 1. Skin (cutaneous): painless lesion begins as small sore and then blisters, ulcerates, and blackens. 2. Lungs (inhalation): sore throat, mild fever, muscle aches, cough, shortness of breath. 3. Digestive tract (gastrointestinal): nausea, anorexia, bloody diarrhea, severe stomach pain.	Antibiotic treatment with fluoroquinolones used for prevention following exposure (along with vaccine); antibiotics alone for infection Cutaneous: usually responds to antibiotics Gastrointestinal: fatal in 25% to 50% of cases Inhalation: fatal in about one half of all cases
Botulism	Toxins are ingested in foods. Onset of symptoms 6 hours to 2 weeks after ingestion. Causes progressive paralysis with double vision, drooping eyelids, slurred speech, and dry mouth. Progresses downward to arms, chest, and legs. Can paralyze muscles of respiration.	Centers for Disease Control and Prevention stocks antitoxin, which can reduce severity of symptoms if given early. Most people recover after weeks to months of supportive care.
Pneumonic plague	Normally spread by rodents but can be spread in an aerosol form and then transmitted from one person to another. Causes fever, weakness, rapidly developing pneumonia, shortness of breath, and cough.	Prompt antibiotic therapy (within 24 hours after onset of symptoms) may be effective in prevention after exposure. Antibiotics include tetracyclines, chloramphenicol, streptomycin, and gentamicin.
Smallpox	Caused by a virus transmitted from person to person. Onset of symptoms 10–12 days after exposure includes high fever and pain. Rash with small papules progresses to pustules and then to scabs.	Can be prevented with vaccine but this is not routinely given now in the United States. No specific treatment is available. Among infected persons who have not been vaccinated, 25% to 30% die.
Tularemia	In nature, is carried by rodents and rabbits. As a weapon, can be made into an aerosol or dispersed in food or water. Onset of symptoms usually 3–5 days after exposure. Manifestations: sudden fever, chills, headache, diarrhea, muscle aches, joint pain, dry cough, progressive weakness.	Antibiotics usually are effective. Efforts to have a vaccine approved are underway.

Data from Henderson DA: *Bioterrorism as a public threat* (1998; updated 2010): http://www.cdc.gov/ncidod/eid/vol4no3/hendrsn.htm. Accessed September 24, 2013; Centers for Disease Control and Prevention: *Emergency preparedness and response* (2012): http://emergency.cdc.gov/bioterrorism/prep.asp. Accessed September 24, 2013.

Patient Teaching

Insect Bite Allergy

People who are very sensitive to venom should be taught how to avoid and treat bites. The teaching plan should include the following:

- Always wear a medical alert tag stating "Allergic to insect bites."
- Obtain an emergency allergy treatment kit. Learn to use it. Teach a family member to use it. Carry it with you at all times.
- Avoid perfumes, hair spray, and bright colors when working outside. Insects are drawn to strong scents and bright colors.
- Wear long pants and sleeves, shoes and socks, and gloves when gardening.
- Keep the car windows closed when driving.
- Consider desensitizing injections if recommended by a physician. These injections gradually reduce sensitivity to venom.
- Use an insect repellant containing DEET.

Patient Teaching

Lyme Disease

Untreated Lyme disease, transmitted by the deer tick, can have serious chronic effects on the brain, eyes, joints, muscles, heart, blood vessels, lungs, skin, liver, spleen, stomach, and intestines. Adherence to the following guidelines can reduce the risk of contracting Lyme disease:

- After engaging in outdoor activities, inspect body folds and hairy areas for ticks. If ticks are removed within 36 hours, the odds of getting Lyme disease are greatly reduced.
- If you have a tick bite and develop influenza-like symptoms within 7 to 10 days, seek medical care. Antibiotic therapy can arrest Lyme disease at this early stage.

DISASTER PLANNING

A challenge for the health care system is to be ready for natural disasters that often occur with short warning. Organizations such as the American Red Cross and the Salvation Army, which are experienced in handling these situations, quickly move in to help. However, a call for nurse volunteers usually follows. Regardless of the area of clinical expertise, each nurse can certainly contribute. The American Red Cross offers courses in disaster training for nurses and nursing students. With appropriate supervision, nursing students can assist with many services in disaster situations. When Hurricanes Katrina, Ike, and Sandy struck the United States, local nurses, nursing faculty, and nursing students were indispensable in providing care to persons affected and displaced by the storm. The competencies for nurses related to emergency and disaster preparedness are listed in Box 16-2. See the *Health Promotion* box for a review of how the Health Insurance Portability and Accountability Act (HIPAA) applies during disaster response situations.

Box 16-2 Emergency and Disaster Preparedness: Core Competencies for Nurses

- Describe the agency's role in responding to a range of emergencies that might arise.
- Describe the chain of command in emergency response.
- Identify and locate the agency's emergency response plan (or the pertinent portion of it).
- Describe emergency response functions or roles, and demonstrate them in regularly performed drills.
- Demonstrate the use of equipment (including personal protective equipment) and the skills required in emergency response during regular drills.
- Demonstrate the correct operation of all equipment used for emergency communication.
- Describe communication roles in emergency response.
- Identify the limits of your own knowledge, skills, and authority, and identify key system resources for referring matters that exceed these limits.
- Apply creative problem-solving skills and flexible thinking to the situation, within the confines of your role, and evaluate the effectiveness of all actions taken.
- Recognize deviations from the norm that might indicate an emergency, and describe appropriate action.
- Participate in continuing education to maintain up-to-date knowledge in relevant areas.
- Participate in evaluating every drill or response, and identify necessary changes to the plan.

Additional competencies specific to nurses with managerial or leadership responsibilities are:

- Ensure that a written plan for major categories of emergencies is available.
- Ensure that all parts of the emergency plan are practiced regularly.
- Ensure that identified gaps in knowledge or skills are filled.

From Gebbie KM, Qureshi K: Emergency and disaster preparedness: core competencies for nurses. Copyright 2002. *Am J Nurs* 102(1):46–51, 2002. Used with permission. All rights reserved.

Internet resources for emergency preparedness information include the following:

- U.S. Department of Health and Human Services, Office of the Assistant Secretary for Preparedness and Response: www.phe.gov/about/oem/Pages/default.aspx.
- Federal Emergency Management Agency (FEMA): www.fema.gov
- Centers for Disease Control and Prevention: www.cdc.gov

Health Promotion

HIPAA Privacy and Disclosures in Emergency Situations

The HIPAA Privacy Rule allows patient information to be shared to assist in disaster relief efforts, such as those that occurred after Hurricane Katrina. Providers and health plans covered by the HIPAA Privacy Rule can share patient information in all of the following ways.

TREATMENT

Health care providers can share patient information as necessary to provide treatment. Treatment includes:

- Sharing information with other providers (including hospitals and clinics)
- Referring patients for treatment (including linking patients with available providers in areas where the patients have relocated)
- Coordinating patient care with others (e.g., emergency relief workers or others that can help in finding patients appropriate health services)

NOTIFICATION

Health care providers can share patient information as necessary to identify, locate, and notify family members, guardians, or other persons responsible for the individual's care or the individual's location, general condition, or death. Thus, when necessary, the hospital may notify the police, the media, or the public at large to the extent necessary to help locate, identify, or otherwise notify family members and others as to the location and general condition of their loved ones.

IMMINENT DANGER

Providers can share patient information with anyone as necessary to prevent or lessen a serious and imminent threat to the health and safety of a person or the public, consistent with applicable law and the provider's standards of ethical conduct.

FACILITY DIRECTORY

Health care facilities that maintain a directory of patients can tell people who call or ask about individuals whether the individual is at the facility, the individual's location in the facility, and the individual's general condition.

Of course, the HIPAA Privacy Rule does not apply to disclosures if they are not made by entities covered by the Privacy Rule. Thus, for instance, the HIPAA Privacy Rule does not restrict the American Red Cross from sharing patient information.

From www.hhs.gov/ocr/hipaa.

LEGAL ASPECTS OF EMERGENCY CARE

Although we do not ordinarily treat people without their permission, in emergencies patients may be unable to consent to care. In such cases, treatment can be provided under the assumption (called the *emergency doctrine*) that the patient would have consented if able.

In the first-aid treatment of emergencies outside the hospital, the nurse is expected to demonstrate the same skill, knowledge, and care that would be provided by other nurses in the same community with the same credentials. The Good Samaritan doctrine in most states is intended to limit liability and provide protection against malpractice claims when health care providers render first aid at the scene of an emergency. Although many Good Samaritan laws cover nurses, not all do. An important point to remember is that these laws do not protect the nurse in the event of gross negligence or willful misconduct. In addition, recent court cases have challenged the Good Samaritan doctrine.

Be aware that situations involving legal matters may depend on evidence at the scene of the injury. Remember that clothing and other materials may provide important information and should not be discarded. Victims who require first aid have the same rights to privacy and confidentiality as those treated in health care facilities. Do not disclose to the public any information about the victim's condition or treatment. In cases involving possible criminal activity, preserving all evidence, such as soiled or damaged clothing and body fluids, may be critical.

Put on Your Thinking Cap!

You are traveling with your spouse when a van in front of you swerves, runs off the road, and rolls over. You summon help on your cellphone and then stop to help. You find the following: Mr. A., in the driver's seat, complains of severe chest pain from striking the steering wheel; Mrs. B., lying on the ground, has an open compound fracture that is bleeding heavily; Teenager C., in the back seat, complains of severe neck pain; Teenager D., beside the van, has blood streaming from her nose and a cut on her forehead; and Grandmother E. is wandering around in a dazed state with her hands to her head. Fill in the table below to show the type of injury you think each person may have sustained, the priority of each injury, the assessment (relevant data), and interventions for each injury, and the sequence of your interventions. Compare your completed table with that of your classmates and reach agreement on the best answers.

VICTIM	TYPE OF INJURY	PRIORITY	ASSESSMENT	INTERVENTIONS
Mr. A.	______	______	______	______
Mrs. B.	______	______	______	______
Teen C.	______	______	______	______
Teen D.	______	______	______	______
Grandmother E.	______	______	______	______

Get Ready for the NCLEX® Examination!

Key Points

- Knowledge of first aid can make the difference between life and death in many situations.
- The cardinal rule in emergency situations: Remain calm!
- The primary survey includes evaluation of airway, breathing, and circulation.
- Look for medical alert tags, which may give some clues about the patient's health status.
- Critical interventions that may be needed are CPR or rescue breathing, application of pressure to control bleeding, head-to-toe inspection, and immobilization of injured spine or limbs.
- Because brain cells begin to die after 4 minutes without oxygen, treatment of cardiopulmonary arrest must begin immediately.
- The universal sign of choking is grabbing the throat with one or both hands.
- Abdominal thrusts use pressure on the diaphragm to force air and obstructions out of the airway.
- Shock results from acute circulatory failure caused by inadequate blood volume, heart failure, overwhelming infection, severe allergic reactions, and extreme pain or fright.
- The immediate treatment for external bleeding is direct, continuous pressure.
- Tourniquets are controversial but may be used to control bleeding as a last resort.
- For epistaxis, the patient should be told to sit down and lean forward; then pinch the nostrils shut for at least 10 minutes.
- The key to emergency management of fractures is immobilization.
- Sprains and strains are treated initially with immobilization, elevation, and cool packs.
- Assess for increased intracranial pressure with any head injury.
- Improper movement of the patient with a spinal injury may damage the spinal cord, causing permanent paralysis.

- Only a physician removes foreign bodies embedded in the eye.
- When tissue is actually torn from the body, it should be retrieved, wrapped in saline-moistened gauze, placed in a plastic bag, kept cool, and transported with the patient for possible reattachment.
- When a chest injury occurs, assessment of respiratory status always takes first priority.
- Open chest wounds that penetrate the pleural cavity allow air to enter (pneumothorax), causing the lung on the affected side to collapse.
- Cover eviscerated organs with some material such as plastic or foil to conserve moisture and warmth; do not attempt to replace the organs in the abdomen.
- The first concern with burns is to stop the burning process and then to ensure a patent airway and respirations.
- Cover large burns with clean, dry dressings and transport the victim to a care facility immediately.
- Extreme heat or cold can have serious local or potentially fatal systemic effects.
- People with heat stroke will die if the body temperature is not lowered quickly.
- Perspiration is noticeably absent with heat stroke.
- Victims of severe hypothermia must be rewarmed gradually to prevent triggering cardiac dysrhythmias.
- A hyperbaric oxygen chamber may be used to treat carbon monoxide poisoning.
- Instructions about treatment of poisoning can be obtained from the poison control center; instructions also may be found on product labels.
- In the event of poisoning, the first action is to call the local poison control center for expert guidance.
- The most serious effects of bites and stings are anaphylactic shock, infection, and tissue destruction.
- Lyme disease, transmitted by tick bites, can lead to chronic cardiac, neuromuscular, and musculoskeletal disorders.
- Among the agents used as bioterrorism weapons are anthrax, botulism, pneumonic plague, smallpox, and tularemia.
- HIPAA privacy rules allow patient information to be shared to assist in disaster relief efforts.
- The emergency doctrine assumes that people would give consent for treatment of life-threatening conditions if they were able.
- Good Samaritan laws do not protect nurses against gross negligence or willful misconduct.

Additional Learning Resources

SG Go to your Study Guide for additional learning activities to help you master this chapter content.

evolve Go to your Evolve website (http://evolve.elsevier.com/Linton/medsurg) for the following learning resources and much more:

- Interactive Prioritization Exercises
- Fluid & Electrolyte Tutorial
- Pharmacology Tutorial
- Review Questions for the NCLEX® Examination

Review Questions for the NCLEX® Examination

1. After determining that an accident victim is breathing and has a pulse, you should next assess for ______________.
   NCLEX Client Need: Physiological Integrity: Physiological Adaptation
2. Circulation must be restored within 4 minutes of cardiopulmonary arrest because:
   1. Irreversible kidney failure develops
   2. The blood begins to coagulate
   3. The lungs fill with fluid
   4. Brain cells begin to die

   NCLEX Client Need: Physiological Integrity: Physiological Adaptation
3. A person with dementia living at home is found with an empty bottle of aspirin. The caregiver suspects that the patient has consumed an unknown quantity of the drug. What should the caregiver's *first* action be?
   1. Have the victim drink a large glass of water
   2. Administer syrup of ipecac
   3. Call the poison control center for guidance
   4. Drive the victim to the emergency department

   NCLEX Client Need: Physiological Integrity: Physiological Adaptation
4. ______________ ____________ are used to dislodge a foreign body from the airway.
   NCLEX Client Need: Physiological Integrity: Physiological Adaptation
5. During a hike, a participant fell and injured his leg. Suspecting a fracture, the first-aid care provider should take what action?
   1. Immobilize the leg in the position in which it was found
   2. Gently straighten the leg and immobilize it
   3. Apply a tourniquet above the fracture if bleeding is present
   4. Elevate the injured part above the level of the victim's heart

   NCLEX Client Need: Physiological Integrity: Reduction of Risk Potential
6. Your assessment of a person who has sustained a head injury reveals the following: headache, decreasing blood pressure, increasing respiratory rate, unequal pupils, and confusion. Which of these findings would cause you to suspect increased intracranial pressure? (Select all that apply.)
   1. Headache
   2. Decreasing blood pressure
   3. Increasing respiratory rate
   4. Unequal pupils
   5. Confusion

   NCLEX Client Need: Physiological Integrity: Physiological Adaptation
7. While at a picnic at the lake, a person catches his clothing on fire while trying to start a charcoal fire. What should bystanders do *first*?
   1. Tell him to run and jump in the lake
   2. Try to extinguish the flames with their hands
   3. Tell him to drop to the ground and roll
   4. Run to a telephone to call for help

   NCLEX Client Need: Physiological Integrity: Reduction of Risk Potential

8. A high school football player collapses during practice on a hot, humid day. He is breathing but not responding verbally. His skin is hot, red, and dry. Which of the following actions should be taken? (Select all that apply.)
   1. Move him to a cool location
   2. Activate the emergency medical services system
   3. Notify his parents to take him to the hospital
   4. Encourage him to take sips of ice cold liquids
   5. Apply cool, wet towels

   NCLEX Client Need: Physiological Integrity: Physiological Adaptation
9. The patient with hypothermia must be *gradually* rewarmed to prevent ____________________.

   NCLEX Client Need: Physiological Integrity: Reduction of Risk Potential
10. The nurse in an immunization clinic notices a peculiar ring-shaped, reddened area on the leg of a child. When asked about it, the mother states that she removed a tick from that area last week. What should the nurse do?
    1. Suspect early Lyme disease and refer the child for medical treatment
    2. Advise the mother to apply antibiotic ointment to the lesion daily
    3. Recognize the bite of a black widow spider and apply a constrictive band
    4. Contact the physician for an order for brown recluse spider antivenin

    NCLEX Client Need: Physiological Integrity: Physiological Adaptation

chapter 17

Surgical Care

http://evolve.elsevier.com/Linton/medsurg

Objectives

1. State the purpose of each type of surgery: diagnostic, ablative, palliative, reconstructive or restorative, procurement for transplant, constructive, and cosmetic.
2. List data to be included in the nursing assessment of the preoperative patient.
3. Identify the nursing diagnoses, goals and outcome criteria, and interventions during the preoperative phase of the surgical experience.
4. Outline a preoperative teaching plan.
5. List the responsibilities of each member of the surgical team.
6. Explain the nursing implications of each type of anesthesia.
7. Explain how the nurse can help to prevent postoperative complications.
8. List data to be included in the nursing assessment of the postoperative patient.
9. Identify nursing diagnoses, goals and outcome criteria, and interventions for the postoperative patient.
10. Explain patient needs that should be considered in discharge planning.

Key Terms

Ablative surgery
Anesthesiologist (ăn-ĕs-thē-zē-Ŏ-lō-jĭst)
Anesthetic (ăn-ĕs-THĔ-tĭk)
Constructive surgery
Cosmetic surgery
Dehiscence (dē-HĬS-ĕns)
Diagnostic surgery
Evisceration (ē-vĭs-ĕr-Ā-shŭn)
Nurse anesthetist
Palliative surgery
Paralytic ileus
Procurement for transplant
Reconstructive or restorative surgery
Sanguineous (săn-GWĬN-ē-ŭs)
Serosanguineous (sĕ-rō-săn-GWĬN-ē-ŭs)
Serous (SĔ-rŭs)

Surgical treatments have been attempted since early times. However, until fairly recently surgery was considered the last resort, to be used only when more conservative measures had failed. However, twentieth-century advances brought antibiotics, safe anesthesia, refined surgical techniques, and improved diagnosis and treatment of illness and injury. Through these advances, surgery became safer than ever before and it is now almost commonplace (Fig. 17-1).

Surgical procedures are performed in physicians' offices, clinics, ambulatory surgery centers, and full-service hospitals. Over recent years, cost control measures resulted in a tremendous shift toward ambulatory surgery centers for many procedures. In all of these settings, nurses play important roles. Nurses who care for patients before, during, and after surgery are called *perioperative nurses.* They admit surgical patients, perform initial assessments and prepare them for surgery, assist in the procedures, and provide post-operative care. Because hospital stays for surgical procedures have shortened dramatically and many procedures are performed in ambulatory settings, nurses are challenged to provide adequate postoperative teaching. Verbal instructions should be supplemented with written materials. Follow-up phone calls provide a chance to answer questions, reinforce instructions, and assess postoperative status (pain, nausea, wound healing, etc).

PURPOSES OF SURGERY

Surgery may be performed for a variety of reasons. Surgical procedures classified by purpose include diagnostic, ablative, palliative, reconstructive or restorative, procurement for transplant, constructive, and cosmetic.

Diagnostic surgery is done to make an accurate diagnosis. It often involves the removal and study of tissue, as with a biopsy of a skin lesion or the removal of a lump in breast tissue. More extensive procedures require opening a body cavity to diagnose and to find out the extent of a disease process. A common example is an exploratory laparotomy, in which the abdomen is opened to find the cause of unexplained pain. Some

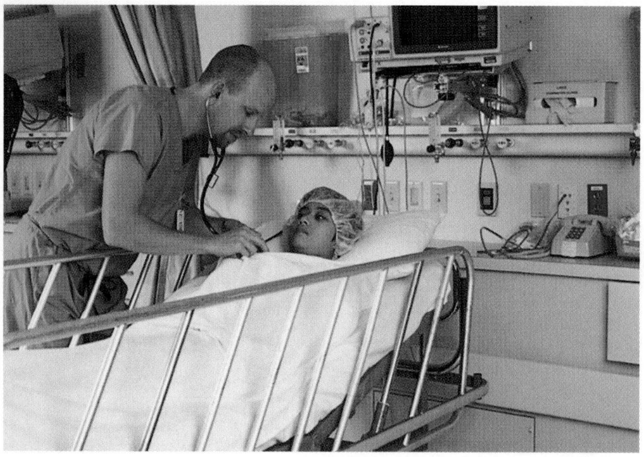

FIGURE 17-1 The nurse provides continuity of care for the surgical patient. (From Harkreader H, Hogan MA: *Fundamentals of nursing: caring and clinical judgment*, ed 3, St. Louis, 2007, Saunders.)

exploratory surgery can be performed using specialized scopes inserted into the body through small incisions.

Ablative surgery is performed to remove diseased tissue such as an inflamed gallbladder.

Palliative surgery relieves symptoms or improves function without correcting the basic problem. For example, palliative surgery may be performed just to remove a malignant tumor obstructing the intestine even though the cancer is widespread elsewhere in the body.

Reconstructive or restorative surgery restores function or structure to damaged or malfunctioning tissue. Breast reconstruction after mastectomy is an example.

Procurement for transplant refers to the removal of organs (e.g., heart, lungs, liver) for transplantation into another person.

Constructive surgery restores function lost because of congenital defects such as a cleft palate.

Cosmetic surgery is performed to improve a person's appearance. It is often chosen simply because the patient wants to change a physical feature. Common cosmetic procedures are performed to change the shape of facial features, remove wrinkles, flatten the abdomen, and change the size or shape of the breasts.

VARIABLES AFFECTING SURGICAL OUTCOMES

Among the variables that must be considered when caring for surgical patients are age, nutritional status, fluid and electrolyte balance, medical diagnoses, drugs, and habits.

AGE

Health care providers and older adults themselves often believe that surgery is dangerous for older people. This belief is unfortunate because modern surgical techniques can restore many lost functions and often can greatly improve the patient's quality of life. Improved monitoring, less invasive procedures, and better drugs have made surgery safer for everyone. People over age 70 who are frail or have cardiovascular disease, renal disease, or diabetes are at increased risk for surgical complications. Hospitalization and surgery may disrupt control of chronic conditions, leading to impaired healing and recovery. However, older adults who are in good health are likely to do just as well in surgery as younger people.

As a general rule, inactivity is not good for anyone; it is especially bad for the older person, who takes longer to regain strength. One other important consideration is that older people may respond differently to drugs because of age-related changes in liver and kidney function and drug interactions.

Surgical risks for the older adult can be greatly reduced if chronic conditions are well controlled, drug therapy is carefully evaluated, and the patient is well hydrated and nourished before surgery. For this reason, emergency procedures carry greater risks for older patients than scheduled procedures.

NUTRITIONAL STATUS

Patients who are overweight or underweight require special care when surgery is indicated. The patient who is malnourished is at risk for poor wound healing and infection. Obese patients are generally in surgery longer and are more likely to have postoperative respiratory and wound complications than patients of normal weight. Effective deep-breathing exercises are limited by the excess weight. Because adipose tissue has poor blood supply, the healing process is slower than normal. The obese patient may also need additional time to recover from anesthesia because the drug tends to remain longer in adipose tissue than in other tissue.

FLUID AND ELECTROLYTE BALANCE

Fluid and electrolyte status can have a significant bearing on the outcome of surgery. Adequate fluids are necessary to maintain blood volume and urine output. However, excess body fluid can overload the heart, aggravating the stress of surgery. Sudden changes in fluid volume are especially dangerous for the older patient who cannot adapt as efficiently as a younger person. Electrolyte imbalances also may predispose the patient to dangerous cardiac dysrhythmias. Diuretics (e.g., Lasix) can play a part in balancing fluid overload; they can also play a part in creating electrolyte imbalances, including potassium deficit. Many older patients are taking diuretics on a regular basis. Physicians usually order laboratory tests to measure serum electrolytes before surgery. Fluid and electrolyte imbalances can then be corrected preoperatively.

MEDICAL DIAGNOSES

A significant number of medical conditions increase surgical risks or require special attention in the perioperative period. Patients with bleeding disorders or those who are taking anticoagulants are at risk for excessive bleeding and must be monitored closely. People with heart disease are at risk for cardiac complications related to anesthesia and the stress of surgery. Chronic respiratory disease increases the risk of pulmonary complications as a result of anesthesia or hypoventilation. Obstructive sleep apnea increases the risk for postoperative airway obstruction, especially if opioids are given. A patient who has liver disease may have impaired wound healing and impaired blood clotting and may experience drug toxicity arising from the inability to metabolize drugs effectively. Disorders of the immune system and chemotherapy or immune-suppressing drugs place the patient at risk for infection and delayed wound healing. Patients with diabetes mellitus also heal more slowly and are at greater risk for infection than nondiabetics. In addition, the control of chronic conditions may be disrupted by surgery, which may mandate adjustments in therapy. In addition, patients who undergo surgery in life-threatening situations are at increased risk of complications.

DRUGS

Many drugs, especially those that depress the central nervous system (CNS), have the potential to interact with anesthetics. Serious adverse effects may result. The effects of surgery or additional drugs may require dosage adjustments in drugs that the patient had been taking routinely. Therefore it is important to document all drugs that the patient has been taking.

Pharmacology Capsule

Drugs that should be held or modified before surgery include anticoagulants, nonsteroidal antiinflammatory drugs (NSAIDs), aspirin, and herbal products, including ginger, ginkgo, and ginseng.

HABITS

Habits that alert the nurse to the possibility of specific perioperative complications are smoking and the use of recreational drugs, herbal medications, and alcohol. Smoking increases the risk of pulmonary complications because smokers have more copious and tenacious secretions and their ciliary activity is less effective compared to nonsmokers. Recreational drugs, such as cocaine and methamphetamine, can increase the heart rate, alter cardiac function, and increase the need for higher-than-usual doses of anesthesia. Herbal medication is thought to interact with certain medications and experts recommend that they be discontinued 1 to 2 weeks before surgery (Table 17-1). Alcohol interacts with many drugs. In addition, patients who use alcohol excessively may need a higher-than-normal dose of anesthetic agent because of increased drug tolerance. If liver damage has occurred, the metabolism of drugs, including anesthetics, can be impaired. In addition, patients with liver disease are at increased risk for bleeding. Individuals who habitually use alcohol may experience withdrawal after 24 hours.

PREOPERATIVE PHASE

Preoperative Nursing Care

The preoperative phase begins when a decision is made to perform a surgical procedure and ends when the patient enters the operating room. During the preoperative phase, the goals of nursing care are for the patient to know what to expect in the surgical experience and to have minimal anxiety.

Assessment

When nonemergency surgery is scheduled, a thorough assessment is made that starts with the patient's health history and physical examination. Although not responsible for total patient assessment as described here, the licensed vocational nurse/licensed practical nurse (LVN/LPN) often assists by collecting specific, relevant data. This assessment is usually performed before admission to the nursing care unit. If not done before admission, laboratory studies of blood and urine, blood grouping and crossmatching,

Table 17-1 Herbs That May Pose Risks in Patients Undergoing Surgery

HERB	EFFECT
Black cohosh	Can cause blood pressure decrease and may increase bleeding
Echinacea	Can cause immune suppression and liver inflammation
Garlic	Can cause blood pressure changes and risk of prolonged bleeding
Ginger	Has sedative effects and can cause risk of bleeding especially if taken with aspirin and ginkgo
Ginkgo	May increase bleeding
Ginseng	Has risk of cardiac effects
Hoodia	Can cause changes in blood sugar and possible arrhythmia
Kava	Has potential liver toxicity and increases risk of additive effect to medications
St. John's wort	Can cause sedation, blood pressure, changes, and has risk of interaction with other medications that prolong effects of anesthesia
Valerian	Can cause increased sedative effects

From Wong A, Townley SA: Herbal medicines and anaesthesia, *Contin Educ Anaesth Crit Care Pain* 11(1):14–17, 2010. Cited in Prieto-Garcia JM: Common herbal-drug and food-drug interactions, *Nurse Prescribing* 11(5):240–244, 2013.

chest radiography and other imaging procedures, pulmonary function tests, and electrocardiography (ECG) may be ordered. A nasal swab test may be done to rule out methicillin-resistant *Staphylococcus aureus* (MRSA).

Most surgical facilities have standardized forms for assessing the newly admitted patient. The nursing assessment should obtain important data needed to plan preoperative, intraoperative, and postoperative care; it also provides baseline data for monitoring the patient's status. Box 17-1 shows the elements of the preoperative assessment. For outpatient surgery, obtaining some information in advance is especially important because the time available for a comprehensive assessment will be limited.

Health History

Identifying Data. Record identifying data, including the patient's age.

History of Present Illness. Describe the problem that is being treated surgically.

Box 17-1 Assessment of the Preoperative Patient

HEALTH HISTORY

Identifying Data
Age, marital status

History of Present Illness
Problem being treated surgically

Past Medical History
Acute and chronic conditions, previous hospitalizations and surgeries, allergies, recent and current medications (to include recreational and herbal medications)

Review of Systems
Disabilities and limitations: hearing or vision loss, paralysis, stiffness, weakness, cognitive impairment; any current health deviations

Functional Assessment
Occupation, roles, responsibilities, diet and fluid intake, exercise, tobacco and alcohol use, sources of stress and support, coping strategies, expectations of surgery

PHYSICAL EXAMINATION

General Survey
Emotional state, ability to communicate, response to directions

Height and Weight

Vital Signs

Skin
Color, lesions, bruises, warmth, turgor, moisture

Thorax
Respiratory pattern and effort, breath sounds, apical pulse

Abdomen
Distention, scars, bowel sounds

Extremities
Color, hair distribution, lesions, deformities, range of motion, crepitus, pain, weakness

Prostheses
Hearing aids, eyeglasses, contact lenses, dentures, artificial limbs, other devices

Past Medical History. Include acute and chronic conditions, hospitalizations, surgeries, allergies, and drug history. Record all chronic health problems such as diabetes, heart failure, pulmonary disease, sleep apnea, or liver or kidney disease. Note if any family member has had complications with anesthesia.

Document any known allergies (food, drug, tape, latex, chemical) according to agency policy. Place an allergy alert bracelet on the patient's wrist if any allergies are found. A large number of drugs are routinely given to surgical patients. During and immediately after surgery, the patient is unable to report allergies; therefore if an emergency should arise, any allergies can be determined promptly by checking the patient's allergy alert bracelet.

Compile a complete list of medications and complementary and alternative therapies that the patient is taking or has recently taken. Knowledge of the patient's drug history enables the health care team to anticipate possible effects of drug interactions.

Pharmacology Capsule

Long-term drug therapy with agents such as anticoagulants and hypoglycemics may require dosage adjustments before and after surgery.

Review of Systems

Collect data about each body system, noting any abnormalities. Record any disabilities or limitations. Include the presence of acute problems (e.g., a cold, a urinary tract infection, a bout of diarrhea) that could necessitate delay of a surgical procedure. In addition to the conditions identified in the past medical history, document problems that may be significant during the surgical experience, such as vision or hearing loss, partial paralysis or joint stiffness, weakness, or cognitive impairment. Strategies such as bracelets may be used to alert staff to these issues.

Functional Assessment

Describe the patient's usual activity pattern, including occupation, roles, and responsibilities. Determine the usual diet and fluid intake, as well as the use of tobacco, recreational drugs, herbal medications, over-the-counter drugs, and alcohol. Note exercise and rest patterns. Ask about sources of stress and support, usual ways of coping, and specific fears or concerns about this surgery. Although some anxiety is normal, be alert for indications of excessive anxiety (e.g., tearfulness, trembling, tachycardia).

Physical Examination

Throughout the physical examination, be alert to the patient's emotional state, ability to communicate, and ability to understand directions.

Height and Weight. Measure height and weight. Unless the patient is very ill or malnourished, the admission weight provides a goal weight to be maintained after surgery.

Vital Signs. Vital signs assessed shortly after admission provide a baseline for evaluating readings during and after surgery. If the patient's pulse and blood pressure are slightly higher than expected on admission, the cause may be anxiety. After allowing the patient to rest, reassess the vital signs. If they remain abnormal, notify the physician.

Skin. Inspect the skin for color, lesions, and bruises. Palpate to determine texture, warmth, turgor, and moisture.

Thorax. Observe the patient's respiratory rate, pattern, and effort. Auscultate the lungs to assess breath sounds. Assess the apical heartbeat for rate and rhythm.

Abdomen. Inspect the abdomen for distention and scars and auscultate bowel sounds.

Extremities. Inspect the extremities for skin color, hair distribution, lesions, edema, and deformities. Assess range of motion while listening for crepitus and noting pain or weakness.

Prostheses. Note the presence of any prosthetic devices, including hearing aids, contact lenses, eyeglasses, dentures, artificial limbs, or other devices used to maintain appearance or function.

Nursing Diagnoses, Goals, and Outcome Criteria: Preoperative Nursing Goals

Some of the nursing diagnoses and goals that might be made during the preoperative phase are as follows.

Nursing Diagnoses	Goals and Outcome Criteria
Anxiety related to uncertain outcome of surgery, anticipated pain, potential disfigurement, or loss of function	Patient's anxiety is reduced: patient is calm, states that anxiety is reduced
Deficient Knowledge of the surgical experience related to lack of exposure to information	Patient understands the surgical experience: patient describes preoperative and postoperative routines, what to expect

More specific diagnoses and goals are made based on individual patient data and specific surgical procedures.

Interventions

Anxiety

Most patients are somewhat anxious about surgery. Determine the presence and the level of anxiety, the contributing factors, and the need for intervention. The patient's previous experiences, if any, with hospitalization and surgery can be especially important. If a patient admitted for heart surgery had an acquaintance who died after similar surgery, the patient might be understandably frightened. However, a person whose previous experiences have been positive is more likely to expect this procedure to go well. If the patient seems excessively nervous or fearful about the surgery, report this behavior to the surgeon or to the anesthesia personnel. Extreme fear is associated with surgical complications; thus it should be controlled with preoperative medication and other therapeutic interventions. In some cases, surgery is postponed until anxiety is reduced.

Deficient Knowledge

Patient teaching may be performed in the physician's office, in the clinic, during the preadmission workup, or after admission to the hospital. Ideally, patient teaching is not left until shortly before surgery, when many activities are scheduled and the patient may be distracted. A cost-saving trend is to admit patients very early in the morning on the day of surgery. In this case, the burden of preoperative teaching rests heavily on the physician, the office nurse, the admission nurse, or the clinic nurse.

Preoperative teaching should include the patient and those who will be with the patient during the recovery period. An attentive family member or companion can reinforce instructions and help to reassure the patient. Telling the patient and family or friends what to expect in the immediate postoperative phase can prevent unnecessary stress. An appropriate teaching plan is based on an assessment of what the patient already knows, wants to know, and needs to know (Fig. 17-2). Verbal instructions should be supplemented with written material or media.

Teaching Methods. The teaching methods selected depend on the situation. Direct patient teaching that the nurse provides is probably used most often. This method has advantages in that the teaching plan can

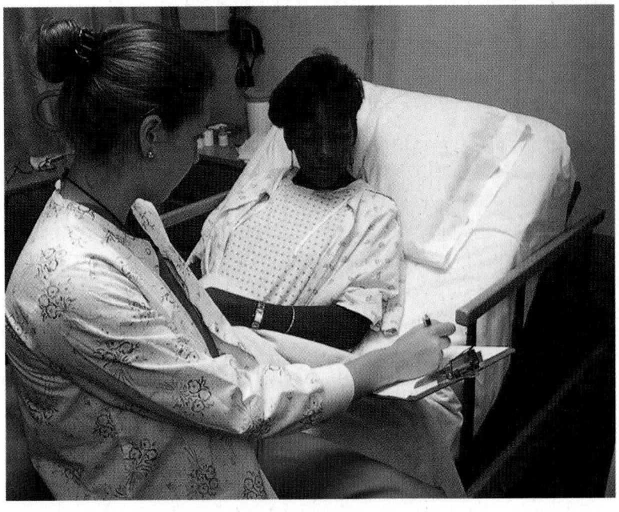

FIGURE 17-2 Preoperative teaching prepares the patient for the surgical experience. (From Harkreader H, Hogan MA: *Fundamentals of nursing: caring and clinical judgment*, ed 3, St. Louis, 2007, Saunders.)

be individualized and the patient can ask questions freely. The main disadvantage of one-to-one instruction is that it is time consuming.

Some hospitals have group classes for all preoperative patients. The main advantage of group classes is economy of time. In addition, some people like talking to others who are having similar procedures. Group classes have several disadvantages. Scheduling times that are accessible to multiple patients before admission may be difficult. Some patients are less likely to ask questions or express fears in a group setting. In addition, information presented to mixed groups of patients is necessarily rather generalized.

Written material, media, and computer-based products are available for patient use. Unfortunately, many patient teaching materials are appropriate only for a limited audience. The reading level may be above the patient's ability or too many technical terms may be used. Many people in the United States do not speak or read English well enough to learn from these materials. If foreign language materials are not available, the services of a professional translator should be obtained. While media can be very helpful, do not depend on them completely for patient teaching. Personal follow-up allows the nurse to assess the patient's understanding of the material and to answer questions (see the *Patient Teaching* box).

Patient Teaching

Preoperative Patient

Most people need basic information and simple explanations without technical details. The family members will probably want to know the expected time of surgery, where to wait for the patient, and how they will be informed when the procedure is over. The teaching plan should include an orientation to the unit and the following:

- In preparation for surgery, you will have specific treatments based on the specific surgical procedure, agency protocols, and physician's orders.
- In the postanesthesia care unit (PACU; sometimes called the *recovery* room):
  - You may have tubes, dressings, or equipment in place.
  - Nurses will check your pulse and blood pressure often and perform other procedures specific to your surgery.
  - You will be coached to deep breathe, cough, turn, and exercise your legs to help you eliminate the anesthetic and to prevent complications.
  - You may be asked to respond to various commands, depending on your surgery.
  - You need to report pain so that measures can be taken to provide pain relief. You will be asked to rate your pain on a scale of 1 to 10, with 1 being "no pain" and 10 being "the worst pain imaginable."

Preparation for Surgery

Preparation of the patient for surgery starts before or shortly after admission. Patients admitted for emergency surgery may not have the benefit of preoperative teaching.

Informed Consent

Before surgery, a patient must sign a legal document called a *consent form* (Fig. 17-3). It states that the patient has been informed about the procedure to be performed, the alternative treatments, and the risks involved and that the patient agrees to the procedure. Written consent is also required for blood or blood products to be used. The purpose of written consent is to protect the patient from unwanted procedures; it also protects the health care facility and caregivers. Explaining the procedure and risks to the patient is the physician's responsibility but the nurse may obtain and witness the patient's signature on the form if agency policy allows. If the patient has questions or seems to be in doubt, contact the physician.

Because the consent form is a legal document, the patient must be fully alert and aware of what it contains when signing it. If the patient is a minor, a parent or guardian must sign the form. The age at which a person is considered an adult varies from state to state. Know the law in the state in which you practice.

A patient who is confused, mentally incompetent, or under the influence of drugs cannot give informed consent. For this reason, the consent form is always signed before the patient is given preoperative medications.

The patient should sign the consent form in the presence of a witness who also signs the form. The nurse who witnesses the consent is confirming that the signature is authentic, consent was given voluntarily, and the patient appeared to be competent at the time. Nursing students should not serve as witnesses. The consent form becomes part of the patient's record.

Preparation of the Digestive Tract

The extent of bowel preparation, if any, depends on the type of anesthesia and the type of surgery planned. For surgery on the lower abdomen or the digestive tract, laxatives and enemas may be given to empty the bowel. In some instances, patients are instructed to take a cathartic to empty the bowel at home before being admitted to the hospital.

Bowel cleansing serves three purposes. First, it reduces the risk of contamination from fecal matter during the operation. Second, it helps to prevent postoperative distention until normal bowel function returns. Third, it prevents constipation and straining in the postoperative period. Straining can create pressure on the surgical wound. Surgery may be canceled if bowel preparation is inadequate.

Food and Fluid Restriction

Even if bowel cleansing is not ordered, ingestion by mouth of fluids and foods is restricted for a specific period. The evening meal before the day of surgery

Consent to Medical/Surgical Procedure
Office/Practice Name
Address
Telephone

I, ____________________, request and consent to the medical/surgical procedure(s) ____________________ to be performed by____________________ and whomever he or she may delegate to assist with the procedure and any additional operations that may be deemed necessary based on conditions that may be revealed during the planned procedure.

This procedure has been explained to me in terms that I understand. The potential risks and benefits, possible complications, and potential alternatives have been explained to me.

I authorize and consent to the administration of such anesthetics and/or other medications deemed necessary. The risks and benefits of sedation or analgesia have been explained to me.

The disposition of any tissues or parts surgically removed should be handled as is the customary practice of the facility.

I am aware that the practice of medicine and surgery is not an exact science, and I acknowledge that no guarantees have been made to me concerning the results of this procedure.

I certify that I have read and understand the above consent statements. Additionally, I have been given the opportunity to ask my provider questions regarding the procedure(s) to be performed and all have been answered to my satisfaction.

Signature of Patient/Decision Maker	Date	Time
Signature of Provider	Date	Time
Signature of Witness	Date	Time

____

Relationship to the Patient/Decision Maker

FIGURE 17-3 Surgical consent form.

may be restricted to fluids. This precaution is employed to reduce the risk of vomiting and aspiration during or after anesthesia. The American Society of Anesthesiologists recommends minimal fasting times, depending on the type of food and liquid taken (Table 17-2). If a patient routinely takes an oral medication that is considered essential (e.g., antihypertensive drugs, asthma inhalers), it may be ordered early on the morning of surgery with a few sips of water or given parenterally.

Skin Preparation

When an incision is made in the skin, microorganisms can enter the wound. Skin preparation is intended to reduce the number of organisms near the incision site. The process usually includes scrubbing and sometimes removing hair from a wide margin around the planned surgical site. The exact skin preparation is ordered by the physician or outlined in a procedure manual.

A typical procedure requires the patient (if able) to shower and wash with an antiseptic soap the evening before the surgery and again the next morning. The perioperative nurse or operating room technician scrubs the operative site shortly before surgery. If the patient's skin is very hairy or if the hair might interfere with the surgical procedure or dressing, it can be removed by clipping with electrical surgical clippers or by shaving the area. Shaving is no longer routine because it causes tiny nicks in the skin that can shelter organisms and cause infection. Therefore if shaving is done at all, it is best delayed until shortly before surgery to allow less time for organisms to multiply.

Dress and Grooming

On the morning of surgery, provide a clean gown and instruct the patient to remove all undergarments unless agency policy dictates otherwise. All jewelry should be removed, which includes body piercings. If a ring

INTRAOPERATIVE PHASE

Operating room personnel transfer the patient from the nursing unit to the surgical suite. They assist the patient onto a gurney (wheeled stretcher) and take the patient and the medical record to the surgical area.

The patient may be taken directly to an operating room or to a holding room first. In the holding room, skin preparation may be performed and intravenous fluids started, if these procedures were not performed earlier. The patient who knows what to expect will feel more secure in the surgical area. When moved into the operating room, the patient will see many pieces of equipment, bright lights, and various people. The patient is helped to move to the operating room table and positioned in a specific way for the type of surgery being performed. Safety straps are applied carefully because of the risk of impaired circulation or nerve damage caused by pressure. Comfort and alignment are confirmed while the patient is awake (Fig. 17-5). The anesthetic agent is then administered and is maintained throughout the procedure.

SURGICAL TEAM

On arrival in the surgical suite, the patient is greeted by the nurse, the physician, the anesthesiologist, or the nurse anesthetist. A large number of people participate in the intraoperative period. Depending on the procedure, they may include the following:

- The surgeon who actually performs the procedure.
- An assistant surgeon, a nurse first assistant, or a physician assistant, who assists the surgeon in the procedure.
- The registered nurse (RN) in the circulating role. This nurse is responsible for assessing the patient, planning intraoperative nursing care, functioning as patient advocate, and maintaining patient safety. This person oversees the operating room. Responsibilities include setting up the room, monitoring aseptic technique, assisting in positioning and monitoring the patient, preparing the skin, providing needed supplies and equipment, and documenting nursing care (Fig. 17-6).
- A registered nurse first assistant (RNFA) works collaboratively with the surgeon and has advanced training for specific duties such as suturing and handling tissue with instruments.
- An RN, LVN/LPN, or surgical technician who scrubs and handles instruments within the sterile field and monitors the sterility of the surgical field.
- The anesthesia care provider (ACP) can be a nurse anesthetist or anesthesiologist. The ACP administers anesthetics and monitors the patient's status throughout the procedure. A **nurse anesthetist** is an advanced practice registered nurse (APRN) with special training in anesthesia and a graduate degree. An **anesthesiologist** is a physician who specializes in anesthesia.
- Other technical personnel with specialized jobs. For example, a perfusionist operates the heart bypass machine during open heart surgery.

ANESTHESIA

Although surgery has been performed since prehistoric times, anesthesia has been used only for approximately 150 years. **Anesthetics** are used to alter sensation so that surgical procedures can be performed painlessly and safely. Agents used for anesthesia include local and general anesthetics.

Local and Regional Anesthesia

Regional anesthesia is achieved by using local anesthetics that block the conduction of nerve impulses in

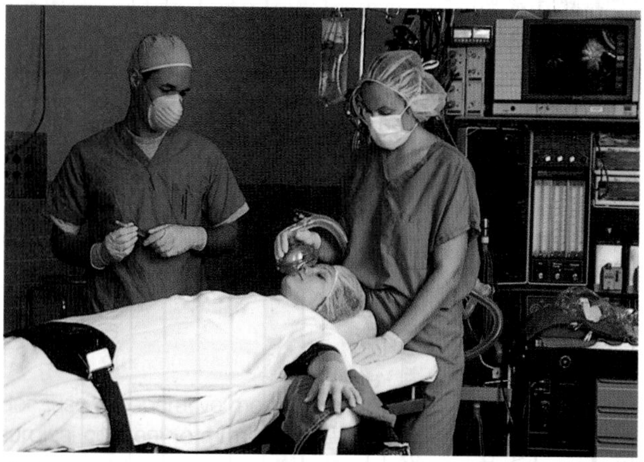

FIGURE 17-5 The nurse ensures the patient's safety on the operating table. (From Harkreader H, Hogan MA: *Fundamentals of nursing: caring and clinical judgment*, ed 3, St. Louis, 2007, Saunders.)

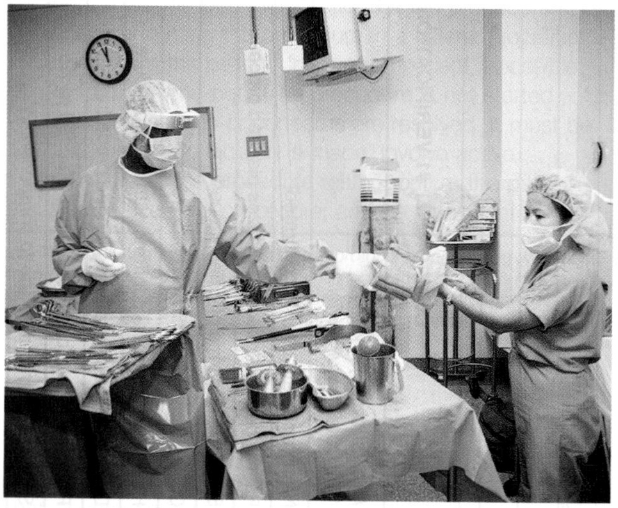

FIGURE 17-6 The nurse sets up the operating room. (From Ignatavicius DD, Workman ML: *Medical-surgical nursing: patient-centered collaborative care*, ed 6, St. Louis, 2010, Saunders.)

a specific area. These anesthetics do not cause the patient to lose consciousness. For some procedures, intravenous sedatives are given in addition to the local anesthetic.

Examples of local anesthetics are lidocaine hydrochloride (Xylocaine), bupivacaine hydrochloride (Marcaine HCl), tetracaine (Pontocaine), and ropivacaine (Naropin). These agents are commonly used for dental procedures, eye surgery, cosmetic surgery on the face, repair of lacerations, childbirth, and other procedures in which general anesthesia is not needed or desired by the patient. Local anesthetics are often the agents of choice for older adult patients because of other medical conditions.

Local anesthetics may be administered topically, by local infiltration, and by nerve-blocking techniques. Topical anesthetics are applied directly to the area to be anesthetized. For local infiltration, the anesthetic agent is injected into and under the skin around the area of treatment. A nerve block is administered by injecting an anesthetic agent around a nerve to block the transmission of impulses. Epidural anesthesia and subarachnoid anesthesia are examples of regional nerve blocks. Both methods are achieved by injecting the anesthetic agent into the area around the spinal nerves. Motor and sensory functions are blocked below the level of the anesthetic administration. This anesthesia is especially useful for surgical procedures on the lower abdomen and legs. The level of anesthesia is controlled by the amount of the drug injected and the position of the patient on the operating table. Regional nerve blocks may be done to control postoperative pain in some procedures.

As a rule, spinal and epidural anesthesia pose less risk for respiratory, cardiac, and gastrointestinal (GI) complications than general anesthesia. However, if the level of spinal or epidural anesthesia rises higher in the spinal cord than intended, a risk of respiratory and cardiovascular depression increases.

One complication of spinal anesthesia is postspinal headache, which is caused by the leaking of cerebrospinal fluid at the puncture site. Postspinal headache can be severe and may last for several weeks. It is relieved by lying flat. Postspinal headache is more common in women, especially postpartum women, than in men. Keeping the patient flat for a specified period after spinal anesthesia may reduce the risk of headache. Always check the postoperative orders, however, for any positioning or activity restrictions. Forcing fluids in the postoperative period, if allowed, may help.

Severe spinal headache is sometimes treated by injecting a small amount of the patient's blood into the epidural space at the site of the previous subarachnoid puncture. The blood clot forms a "blood patch" that prevents further leaking. The procedure can be repeated if it is unsuccessful the first time. A successful patch relieves the headache immediately. Postanesthesia headache should not occur with epidural anesthesia.

As the effect of a regional anesthetic wears off, the patient often reports that the affected limbs feel numb and heavy. You should assure the patient that this feeling is normal and that movement and sensation gradually return to normal. Passive range-of-motion exercises, compression hose, and sequential compression devices (SCDs) help to prevent thrombus (clot) formation until mobility returns. Typically, motor function returns before sensory function. At this time, the patient is susceptible to injury resulting from trauma or pressure because movement is possible but pain is not perceived. !

Complications of local anesthesia include toxic effects caused by overdose, local tissue damage, and allergic responses. Initial signs and symptoms of toxic effects are excitement and CNS stimulation followed by depression of the CNS and the cardiovascular system. Local tissue effects may be inflammation and edema. Abscesses and necrosis sometimes develop at the injection site. This circumstance is thought to be caused by poor technique rather than by the anesthetic agent.

General Anesthesia

General anesthesia acts on the CNS, causing loss of consciousness, sensation, reflexes, pain perception, and memory. Combinations of drugs are used to achieve these effects without excessive CNS depression. This use of multiple drugs, known as *balanced anesthesia*, allows lower dose levels of each drug, which reduces the risks of adverse effects. General anesthetics are most often given by inhalation or intravenous infusion. Although the intramuscular and rectal routes can be used to administer anesthetics, the use of these routes is uncommon.

Near the end of procedures performed under general anesthesia, the anesthetist or anesthesiologist administers drugs to reverse the effects of the anesthetic. When the procedure is completed, a member of the surgical team escorts the patient to the PACU, where careful monitoring can be maintained until the patient recovers from the anesthesia.

Inhalation Agents. Inhalation agents include isoflurane (Forane), sevoflurane (Ultane), enflurane (Ethrane), desflurane (Suprane), and nitrous oxide. For most procedures using inhalation agents, the patient is first induced with a short-acting intravenous agent that causes rapid loss of consciousness. An endotracheal tube is then inserted into the patient's trachea to permit administration of the maintenance inhalation anesthesia and to control mechanical ventilation. A cuff on the endotracheal tube is inflated to prevent leakage during mechanical ventilation and aspiration of gastric contents while the patient is unconscious (Fig. 17-7). The laryngeal mask airway (LMA) is an alternative to the endotracheal tube.

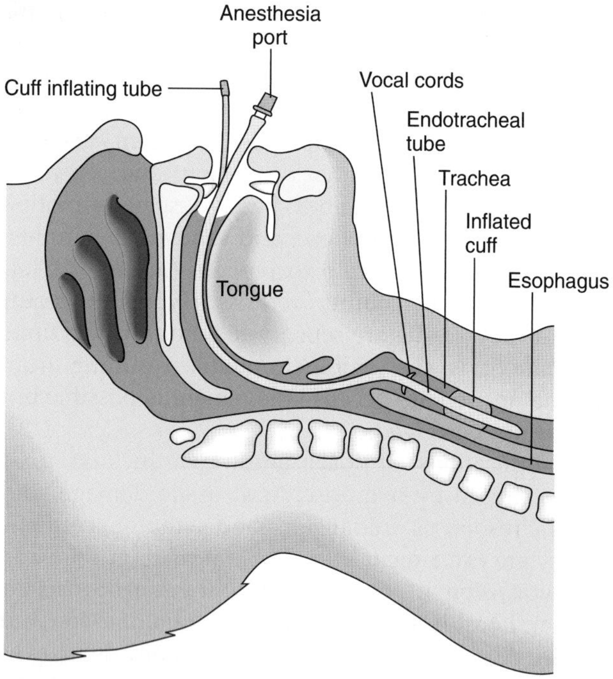

FIGURE 17-7 Inhalation anesthetic is given through an endotracheal tube. (From Ignatavicius DD, Workman ML, Mishler MA: *Medical-surgical nursing across the health care continuum*, ed 3, Philadelphia, 1999, Saunders.)

Intravenous Agents. Intravenous agents include thiopental sodium (Pentothal), methohexital sodium (Brevital Sodium), diazepam (Valium), propofol (Diprivan), midazolam (Versed), etomidate (Amidate), sufentanil (Sufenta), alfentanil (Alfenta), fentanyl (Duragesic), and ketamine hydrochloride (Ketalar).

Other Agents. Muscle relaxants, opioids, benzodiazepines, and antiemetics are often given with the anesthetics. Muscle relaxants such as succinylcholine (Anectine, Quelicin), vecuronium (Norcuron), rocuronium (Zemuron), atracurium (Tracrium), and cisatracurium (Nimbex) prevent movement of muscles during the surgical procedure. Opioids supplement anesthetics and support postoperative pain management. Benzodiazepines are used to induce and maintain anesthesia, for moderate sedation, and to sedate patients during local or regional anesthesia. Antiemetics help to prevent vomiting during surgery.

Complications. Inhalation anesthetics and the endotracheal tube itself can cause irritation of the respiratory tract and the larynx. Individual agents may have the potential to cause serious adverse effects such as cardiac dysrhythmias, seizures, liver damage, nausea and vomiting, and death.

Malignant Hyperthermia

Malignant hyperthermia is a rare but life-threatening complication that occurs in response to certain drugs. Susceptibility to this response is inherited. It is characterized by increasing body temperature and metabolic rate, tachycardia, hypotension, cyanosis, and muscle rigidity. Immediate measures must be taken to cool the patient. Oxygen is administered and the patient is given dantrolene sodium (Dantrium), furosemide (Lasix), mannitol, and sodium bicarbonate.

Moderate Sedation

Moderate (or procedural) sedation was previously called conscious sedation. It refers to the use of intravenous drugs to reduce pain intensity or awareness without loss of reflexes. It is used with some diagnostic and therapeutic procedures, including cardiac catheterization and endoscopy. Only patients who meet specific psychologic and physiologic criteria are candidates for moderate sedation. Registered nurses with specialized training may administer the drugs used for moderate sedation. During the procedure, the patient's vital signs, oxygen saturation, airway, level of consciousness, and ECG readings must be closely monitored. Documentation must include assessment data; interventions such as oxygen therapy; and the time, dose level, route, and effects of all drugs administered. Complications include respiratory depression and apnea, hypotension, excessive sedation approaching that of general anesthesia, and agitation and combativeness. !

After procedures using moderate sedation, the patient may be discharged home with a responsible person when the following conditions are met: stable vital signs, patent airway, intact motor function and reflexes, satisfactory surgical site, no nausea or vomiting, and the patient is alert and able to void.

❖ Intraoperative Nursing Care

Intraoperative nursing care is a specialty and is beyond the scope of this chapter. Only potential nursing diagnoses and goals are listed here.

Nursing Diagnoses, Goals, and Outcome Criteria: Intraoperative Nursing Care

Nursing Diagnoses	Goals and Outcome Criteria
Risk for Injury related to the effects of anesthesia, positioning, use of restraints, wrong surgery or site error, hypothermia	Absence of physical injury: complete recovery from anesthesia, no pressure or traumatic tissue damage associated with positioning or restraints. The Joint Commission guidelines to confirm site, procedure, and patient verified and documented. Body temperature of 36°C (96.8°F) (normothermia).
Impaired Gas Exchange related to the effect of anesthesia and immobility	Adequate gas exchange: normal arterial blood gases

Nursing Diagnoses, Goals, and Outcome Criteria: Intraoperative Nursing Care—cont'd

Nursing Diagnoses	Goals and Outcome Criteria
Decreased Cardiac Output related to drug effects or blood loss	Adequate cardiac output: heart rate and blood pressure consistent with patient norms
Risk for Deficient Fluid Volume related to blood loss, insensible loss of water, NPO status	Normal fluid volume: balanced intake and output, pulse and blood pressure consistent with patient norms

NPO, Nothing by mouth.

POSTOPERATIVE PHASE

When the surgical procedure is completed, the patient is usually transferred to the PACU (also known as the recovery room) or the critical care unit before returning to the nursing unit. Exceptions are patients who have undergone minor procedures with only local anesthesia. The information communicated from the perioperative nurse to the PACU nurse should include patient diagnosis, surgical procedure performed, any relevant medical history, how the procedure was tolerated by the patient, medication given and times, blood loss, any blood given, latest vital signs, drains present and outputs, and any peripheral or central infusion lines. This information is known as the "hand off."

SURGICAL COMPLICATIONS

The postoperative patient is at risk for a significant number of complications. These complications may be related to the surgical procedure itself, to the drugs used before and during the procedure, or to immobility during and after the procedure. The types of postoperative complications vary depending on the length of time that has elapsed since the surgical procedure. For example, shock and hypoxia are most likely to occur in the immediate recovery period. Wound infection, however, does not appear until several days after surgery. Complications in the immediate and later postoperative periods are described in Table 17-4. Prevention, recognition, and nursing implications are discussed in the section on nursing care.

Pharmacology Capsule

Opioid analgesics given before the effects of general anesthesia wear off may cause a drop in blood pressure and slow respirations.

Shock

Shock is inadequate tissue perfusion, which is most likely to occur as an effect of anesthesia or loss of blood. If opioid analgesics are given before the anesthesia wears off, they may contribute to a drop in blood pressure.

Shock may also result from low blood volume (hypovolemic shock). Bleeding is an obvious cause of low blood volume but other factors may contribute as well. Dehydration without adequate fluid replacement or fluid losses through wounds and suction can explain low blood volume.

Interest in "bloodless" surgical procedures is growing. These procedures employ a variety of strategies to reduce the need for blood replacement necessitated by excessive blood loss. Such strategies include drug therapy to stimulate production of red blood cells; the use of Gamma Knife radiosurgery, electrocautery, and laser beam coagulation; and the collection and reinfusion of the patient's own blood during the procedure.

Hypoxia

Hypoxia refers to inadequate oxygenation of body tissues. The patient is at risk for hypoxia in the immediate postoperative phase for several reasons. First, general anesthetics depress respirations such that the patient's breathing efforts may be inadequate initially. Second, when the patient is unconscious, the tongue may fall back and block the airway. Third, anesthesia depresses the cough and swallowing reflexes. Until these reflexes return, vomitus and saliva can enter the airway. A fourth reason that hypoxia may occur in the immediate postoperative period is the risk of laryngospasm or bronchospasm. Spasm of the larynx or bronchi narrows the airway and obstructs airflow. Because they are at increased risk for hypoxia, patients with sleep apnea may be treated with continuous positive airway pressure (CPAP) in the PACU.

Pharmacology Capsule

Regional anesthesia blocks sensation and movement; as a result, the affected body part is at risk for injury.

Injury

Immediately after surgery, the patient is at risk for injury because of the decreased level of consciousness associated with general anesthesia or other sedatives. If regional anesthesia was used, the affected body part may be injured because it lacks sensation.

Pharmacology Capsule

General anesthetics and opioid analgesics depress respirations.

Pneumonia and Atelectasis

Drug effects and immobility place the surgical patient at risk for pneumonia and atelectasis. Patients who are most prone to these complications are older adults, the obese, those with chronic pulmonary disease, and those who have undergone chest or abdominal surgery.

Table 17-4 Surgical Complications

COMPLICATIONS	PREVENTION	TREATMENT
Shock related to deficient fluid volume	Inspect wound dressing Report excessive drainage or bleeding Monitor vital signs every 15 min until stable Note early changes in vital signs Report tachycardia, tachypnea, hypotension Monitor input and output Keep intravenous fluid rate on schedule Evaluate respirations before giving opioids	Fluid or blood replacement Vasopressors (drugs to raise blood pressure) as ordered Additional surgery may be needed to control bleeding
Hypoxia related to ineffective airway clearance, ineffective breathing pattern	Keep airway in place until patient awakens Position unconscious patient on side, if not contraindicated Suction as necessary Monitor vital signs every 15 min until stable Encourage deep breathing	Position to promote effective ventilation Suction as necessary Administer oxygen Encourage deep breathing and coughing
Wound complications related to impaired wound healing and/or infection Dehiscence Evisceration Infection	Provide adequate fluids and nutrition Splint incision during activity, coughing, and deep breathing Good hand washing; sterile or clean technique or wound care as appropriate	Cover open wound with sterile dressing If organs protrude, saturate dressing with normal saline and cover wet dressing with dry, sterile dressing; notify physician Keep patient still and quiet with knees flexed Anticipate return to surgery; withhold opioids until consent form signed
Impaired gas exchange related to pneumonia Atelectasis	Change position at least every 2 hours Assist to cough and deep breathe hourly Incentive spirometry	Rest Administer oxygen and antibiotics as ordered
Digestive disturbances Nausea and vomiting	Withhold oral fluids until nausea subsides Give antiemetics to prevent vomiting as soon as nausea is reported	Administer antiemetic drugs as ordered
Altered elimination Urine retention Kidney failure Abdominal distention "Gas" pains Constipation	Provide privacy; offer warm bedpan; position comfortably; take to bathroom or bedside commode chair if allowed; pour warm water over the perineum; let tap water run Promptly report urine output of less 30 mL/h Nothing by mouth until bowel sounds return Encourage ambulation as allowed Encourage fluids, food, and ambulation as ordered; use stool softeners as ordered	Catheterize catheterization as ordered Use heat to abdomen, bisacodyl suppositories as ordered Position on right side Initiate nasogastric intubation with suction as ordered Ambulate frequently when permitted Administer laxatives or enemas, or both, as ordered
Thrombophlebitis	Avoid pressure on blood vessels Encourage leg exercises every 1–2 hours Early, frequent ambulation as ordered Elastic or automatic compression stockings	Bed rest Administer anticoagulant therapy as ordered
Fluid and electrolyte imbalances	Monitor intravenous fluid rate Provide a variety of oral fluids when permitted; treat vomiting promptly Recognize signs of imbalances (see Chapter 14)	Give intravenous fluids as ordered Encourage oral intake when allowed

General anesthetics and opioid analgesics depress respiratory function. Anticholinergics cause pulmonary secretions to be drier and thicker than normal.

Immobility limits lung expansion and allows fluids to pool in the lungs. Fluid provides a medium for infectious organisms to grow. An infection of the lungs associated with immobility is called *hypostatic pneumonia*.

As secretions accumulate, they begin to block off branches of the respiratory tree. When gases can no longer enter or leave the affected alveoli, they collapse. *Atelectasis* is the term used to describe collapse of alveoli, which may affect a portion or an entire lobe of the lung. Because atelectasis impairs the exchange of gases, it can be very serious.

WOUND COMPLICATIONS

Complications in wound healing include dehiscence, evisceration, and infection. All of these complications are, to some extent, preventable.

Dehiscence and Evisceration

Dehiscence is the reopening of the surgical wound. It involves one or more layers of tissue. Dehiscence is most likely to happen when strain on the suture line is excessive. Factors that increase the risk of dehiscence include wound infection, malnutrition, obesity, dehydration, and extensive abdominal wounds or injuries. Dehiscence is most likely to occur between the fifth and twelfth postoperative days. **Evisceration** is the term used when body organs protrude through the open wound. Dehiscence and evisceration are illustrated in Figure 17-8.

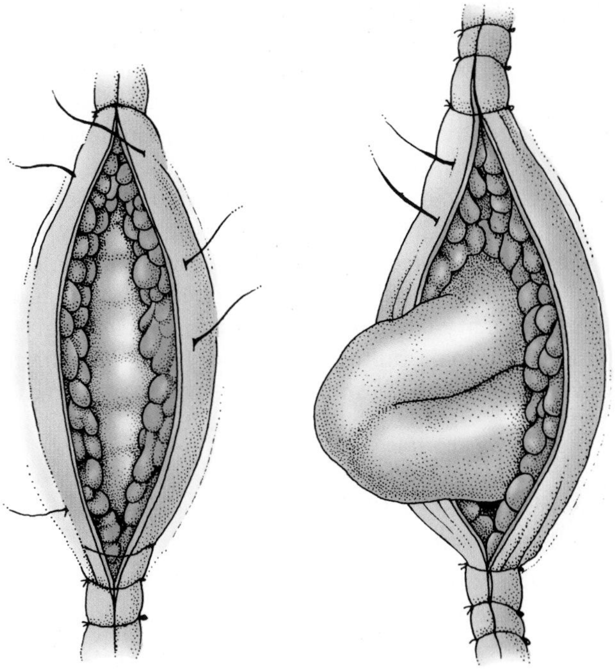

FIGURE 17-8 Complications of wound healing. **A,** Dehiscence. **B,** Evisceration. (From Ignatavicius DD, Workman ML, Mishler MA: *Medical-surgical nursing across the health care continuum*, ed 3, Philadelphia, 1999, Saunders.)

Infection

The risk of wound infection is greatest in cases of traumatic injuries, wounds that were not treated promptly, and wounds that were infected before surgery. Obese patients and those with diabetes mellitus or immune suppression are also at increased risk.

GASTROINTESTINAL DISTURBANCES

The primary GI problems that follow surgery are nausea, vomiting, impaired peristalsis, and constipation. Nausea and vomiting are most common in the early postoperative period. Causative factors include anesthesia, pain, opioids, decreased peristalsis, and resuming oral intake too soon.

Factors that cause peristalsis to be impaired after surgery include anesthesia, immobility, opioid analgesics, and handling of the bowel during surgery. Patients who develop metabolic imbalances, respiratory problems, or shock are also at risk for GI disturbances.

The effects of slowed peristalsis can be mild or severe. Gas normally forms in the digestive tract. When peristalsis is slow, the gas builds up and causes cramping pain and distention. Mild effects are generally experienced as gas pains that typically occur on the second or third postoperative day. Constipation is also related to slow peristalsis.

If peristalsis stops completely, the patient is said to have a **paralytic ileus**. The patient with a paralytic ileus has abdominal distention that may be severe enough to impair lung expansion and decrease blood return from the legs, causing cardiac output to fall. Distention also causes strain on an abdominal incision.

URINARY RETENTION AND RENAL FAILURE

With urinary retention, the kidneys produce urine but the patient is unable to empty the bladder. Urinary retention can be caused by the effects of anesthesia or opioids, trauma to the urinary tract, or anxiety about voiding. Urine volume may also be decreased because of dehydration or blood loss.

With kidney failure, the kidneys are unable to produce enough urine to remove wastes from the body. Urine production falls dangerously low.

Put on Your Thinking Cap!

Use the stress response (discussed in Chapter 8) to explain the signs and symptoms of deficient fluid volume during the immediate postoperative period.

THROMBOPHLEBITIS

The risk of hemorrhage and shock decreases after the immediate postoperative period. A more common circulatory problem in the later period is thrombophlebitis. Thrombophlebitis is the inflammation of veins with the formation of blood clots. It occurs most often in the legs after a period of immobility. Patients who have very lengthy surgical procedures or who must be immobilized are at greatest risk for thrombophlebitis and frequently will come to PACUs or nursing units with an SCD in place as a preventive measure.

Clots that cling to the walls of blood vessels are called *thrombi.* Thrombi that break loose and flow with the blood are called *emboli.* Emboli formed in the legs are most likely to pass through the heart and lodge in the pulmonary circulation. If they are large enough to seriously impair pulmonary blood flow, the patient develops severe respiratory distress and may even die.

IMMEDIATE POSTOPERATIVE NURSING CARE in the Postanesthesia Care Unit

Assessment

When the patient is admitted to the PACU, determine the medical diagnosis and the surgical procedure and other assessment data listed earlier. Promptly assess the patient's status (level of consciousness, vital signs, pain) and inspect the wound or dressing. Check and set up equipment, such as suction devices, wound drains, oxygen, urinary drainage, and intravenous lines, as needed. When the patient returns to the nursing unit, a more complete assessment will be performed.

Interventions

Decreased Cardiac Output

Be alert to the possibility of shock. To detect impending shock, the patient's vital signs are monitored every 5 to 15 minutes in the PACU. Signs and symptoms of impending shock include a rapid, thready pulse; restlessness; decreasing blood pressure; and decreasing urine output. Use the patient's preoperative vital signs to evaluate whether postoperative vital signs are normal. An increasing pulse usually precedes a fall in blood pressure. Monitor intravenous fluid intake and urinary output. When blood volume is low (hypovolemia), the kidneys reduce urine production. Continuous cardiac monitoring is often performed to identify early signs of hypovolemia or potentially dangerous changes in cardiac rhythm.

Measures to reduce the risk of shock include prompt recognition and treatment of bleeding, replacement of lost fluids, and the cautious use of opioid analgesics. Frequently inspect wound dressings and drains for the color and amount of drainage. The amount of bleeding expected varies with different surgical procedures.

An open intravenous route must be maintained during the early postoperative period. This access permits the infusion of fluids, blood, and emergency medications if needed. Therefore check the venipuncture site to ensure that the fluid is infusing properly. The intravenous fluid infusion rate is ordered by the physician but the nurse regulates the rate. If the rate falls behind, the patient may not receive adequate fluids to replace losses during surgery. If given too rapidly, intravenous fluids can overload the circulatory system, causing heart failure. !

Nursing Diagnoses, Goals, and Outcome Criteria: Immediate Postoperative Care

Depending on the specific surgical procedure, nursing diagnoses and goals for the patient immediately after surgery may include the following.

Nursing Diagnoses	Goals and Outcome Criteria
Decreased Cardiac Output related to excessive loss of blood and other body fluids or the effects of drugs	Normal cardiac output: pulse and blood pressure consistent with patient norms, normal skin color
Ineffective Breathing Pattern and/or **Ineffective Airway Clearance** related to effects of anesthetics or pain	Adequate oxygenation: respiratory rate, effort, and pattern consistent with patient norms; normal arterial blood gases; breath sounds clear; SpO_2 of 95% to 100%
Acute Pain related to tissue trauma or to positioning during surgical procedures	Decreased pain: relaxed expression, patient statement of pain relief
Acute Confusion related to the effects of anesthetics	Absence of confusion; orientation to person and place
Risk for Injury related to decreased level of consciousness or loss of sensation and movement as effect of anesthesia	Patient remains safe during recovery period: no falls, bruises, trauma when under effects of anesthesia

SpO_2, Oxygen saturation.

Ineffective Breathing Pattern

To detect early signs of hypoxia in the PACU, monitor the patient's respiratory status. Assess respiratory depth, rate, and effort. Listen for abnormal breath sounds that suggest breathing difficulty. In addition, be alert for changes in the pulse rate because an increasing pulse rate is often an early indicator of poor oxygenation. The oximeter is a device with a wire that clips to a finger or an earlobe and provides a continuous reading of blood oxygenation as SpO_2.

The patient's color, especially in the nail beds and lips, provides a clue to oxygenation. Because cyanosis is a late sign of hypoxia, however, you should detect problems long before color changes develop.

Take measures to reduce the risk of hypoxia during the immediate postoperative period. An airway is inserted to keep the air passages open until the patient begins to awaken. Position the unconscious patient (if permitted) on one side to reduce the risk of aspiration. Suction if necessary to remove secretions or vomitus. When the gag reflex returns, the airway can be removed.

Acute Pain

Decisions to medicate for pain in the early postoperative phase are based on physician's orders and nursing judgment. If opioid analgesics are given too early, their effects when combined with the effects of the anesthesia may lead to shock. However, severe pain also may cause shock.

Acute Confusion

As patients begin to regain consciousness, they may move around and touch dressings and drains. Tell patients where they are, that the surgery is over, and what is happening. Simple explanations and gentle reminders are often sufficient to calm and reassure them. The amnesic effects of drugs used in surgery may cause the patient to forget what was said, making it necessary to repeat information.

Risk for Injury

Patients who have had local anesthesia may be sent to the PACU postoperatively or they may be returned directly to the nursing unit or the ambulatory surgery unit. In the immediate postoperative period, patients are usually drowsy because preoperative and intraoperative sedatives typically have been given.

When regional block anesthesia is used, remember that sensation in that area is impaired. Take care therefore to prevent injury to the anesthetized body region. !

After spinal anesthesia, the patient regains the ability to move the legs before sensation returns. Chart the times that the patient regains both movement and sensation. Assess the bladder for distention because the patient is unable to feel pressure. Patients may be kept flat for a specific time period in the belief that it may help to prevent spinal headache.

Patient's Family

The time between the patient leaving the nursing unit and returning can be 3 or 4 hours, even with relatively simple procedures. This period may seem like a very long time for family and friends who are waiting. Most hospitals have some system for communicating the patient's status to those who wait. These visitors are usually relieved to know when the patient is in the recovery room. Many surgeons take time to speak with the family shortly after the surgery is completed. When problems arise, offer visitors privacy and the services of a patient representative or a spiritual counselor.

Discharge from the Postanesthesia Care Unit

Most patients remain in the PACU for 1 to 2 hours, although the time varies considerably. The patient's progress in the PACU is carefully monitored. Patients who are unstable or who need very close observation may be transferred to a critical care unit. Several systems of scoring have been used to determine when recovery is adequate and the patient can be transferred. The modified Aldrete score is used to assess patients at intervals while in the PACU (Box 17-3). For inpatients, only the first five criteria are included and a total score of 8 or more is required for the patient to be discharged from the PACU. Patients in ambulatory care settings are assessed on all 10 criteria and indices and must have a score of 18 to be discharged.

POSTOPERATIVE NURSING CARE on the Nursing Unit

When the patient is transferred to the nursing unit, the PACU nurse reports on the patient to the nurse who will be caring for that patient, again using the "hand-off" procedure of SBAR. Several people are usually necessary to move the patient safely from the gurney to the bed. Be careful to prevent pulling or dislodging tubes and to prevent a shearing force on the skin. Hang intravenous fluids and set infusion at the ordered rate. Connect nasogastric suction tubes to suction equipment. Identify and arrange drains to avoid obstruction. For safety, raise the side rails, lower the bed, place the call bell within reach, and instruct the patient not to get up without assistance (see Nursing Care Plan: Postoperative Patient).

Assessment

Health History

Review the patient's preoperative assessment (as outlined in Box 17-1), noting long-term conditions, disabilities, prostheses, drugs, and allergies. When the patient is able to respond, ask about significant symptoms, including pain, nausea, and altered sensations (as explained in Box 17-4).

Physical Examination

Vital Signs. Take vital signs and compare the results with the preoperative readings. Note the respiratory rate, depth, and effort. Take the pulse, noting rate, rhythm, and quality. Record the blood pressure. Document patient's rating of pain. Measurements are usually repeated every 15 minutes until the vital signs stabilize.

Neurologic Status. The assessment of neurologic status includes level of consciousness and pupil size, equality, and reaction to light. Evaluate sensation in affected body areas. Note spontaneous movements and the patient's ability to move affected parts on command. For example, when a cast has been applied

Box 17-3 Modified Aldrete Score

Criteria	Score
Activity	
Able to move four extremities voluntarily or on command	2
Able to move two extremities voluntarily or on command	1
Unable to move extremities voluntarily or on command	0
Respiratory	
Able to breathe deeply and cough freely	2
Dyspnea or limited breathing	1
Apneic	0
Circulation	
BP 20% of preanesthetic level	2
BP 20% to 49% of preanesthetic level	1
BP 50% of preanesthetic level	0
Consciousness	
Fully awake	2
Arousable on calling	1
Not responding	0
Oxygen (O_2) Saturation	
Able to maintain O_2 saturation > 92% on room air	2
Needs O_2 inhalation to maintain O_2 saturation > 92%	1
O_2 saturation < 90% even with O_2 supplement	0
TOTALS: Possible score range of 0–10	
For patients in ambulatory surgical settings, the Aldrete score is derived by assessing the criteria above plus these indices:	
Dressing	
Dry and clean	2
Wet but marked and not increasing	1
Growing area of wetness	0
Pain	
Pain free	2
Mild pain handled by oral medication	1
Severe pain requiring parenteral medication	0
Ambulation	
Able to stand up and walk straight*	2
Vertigo when erect	1
Dizziness when supine	0
Fasting-feeding	
Able to drink fluids	2
Nauseated	1
Nausea and vomiting	0
Urine output	
Has voided	2
Unable to void but comfortable	1
Unable to void and uncomfortable	0
TOTALS: Possible score range of 0–20	

Modified from Aldrete JA: Modifications to the post anesthesia score for use in ambulatory surgery, *J Perianesth Nurs* 13(3):148, 1998; Aldrete JA, Kroulik D: A post-anesthesia recovery score, *Anesth Analg* 49:924, 1970.
BP, Blood pressure.
*May be substituted by Romberg test, or by picking up 12 paper clips in one hand.
Note: Total score must be at least 18 for the patient to be discharged to the home; a lower score is allowed if the patient was unable to walk or move the extremities before surgery.

Box 17-4 Assessment of the Postoperative Patient

HEALTH HISTORY
Reason for surgery, name of procedure, medical diagnosis, disabilities, prostheses, drugs, allergies, intravenous (IV) fluids, dressings, drains, tubes

Presence of pain, nausea, altered sensations

PHYSICAL EXAMINATION
Vital Signs
Neurologic Status
Level of consciousness; pupil size, equality, response to light; sensation; spontaneous movement, response to commands
Integument
Color, temperature, incision or dressing appearance, amount and appearance of drainage on dressing and in closed drainage systems. Appearance of IV insertion site
Thorax
Chest expansion, symmetry, breath sounds
Heart
Apical pulse
Abdomen
Contour, bowel sounds, bladder distention, tenderness
Extremities
Color, capillary refill, pulses, edema, warmth, redness

to a fractured arm, test the patient's ability to move the fingers.

Integument. Inspect the skin color and palpate for temperature. Inspect the surgical area. If the wound is visible, assess the incision for intactness of the wound margins, drainage, and excessive redness or swelling. If a dressing covers the incision, inspect the dressing for bleeding or other drainage. If closed drains are in place, observe the amount and appearance of the drainage (Table 17-5).

Thorax. Observe chest expansion with respirations. Chest movement should be symmetric. Auscultate for breath sounds to detect atelectasis, crackles, and wheezes.

Heart. Auscultate the apical pulse if the peripheral pulse is weak or irregular or if the patient has heart disease.

Abdomen. Inspect the abdomen for distention and auscultate for bowel sounds. Light palpation also may be performed to assess bowel and bladder distention and tenderness. Check the patency of GI tubes and note the characteristics of any output.

Extremities. Assess the color and capillary refill of nail beds and the presence and quality of peripheral pulses in affected extremities. Note the presence of edema or excessive warmth or redness. Simultaneously compare the color and temperature of both arms and then both legs to detect differences.

Interventions

Acute Pain

Pain is expected in the early postoperative phase. Pain receptors are stimulated because tissues are cut and

Nursing Care Plan: Postoperative Patient

HEALTH HISTORY Ms. M, 37 years old, was admitted for an abdominal hysterectomy and surgical excision of endometriosis implants. She is a secretary, married, and the mother of a 3-year-old child. On day 1 after the surgery: Complains of moderate abdominal and incisional pain (7 on a scale of 1–10); has been out of bed three times since surgery; ambulated well with assistance; has not voided since Foley catheter removed 3 hours ago; intravenous fluids infusing at 100 mL/h; no nausea but NPO until noon, when 550 mL of clear liquids were taken and retained.

PHYSICAL EXAMINATION Patient is alert and oriented. Vital signs: temperature 99.4°F orally; pulse 90 bpm, respirations 16 breaths/min, blood pressure 130/86 mm Hg. (Admission vital signs were temperature 98°F orally; pulse 84 bpm, respirations 20 breaths/min, blood pressure 126/82 mm Hg.) Breath sounds diminished in lower lobes; abdomen soft; no bladder distention; wound covered with dry dressing; bowel sounds present but hypoactive.

Nursing Diagnosis	Goals and Outcome Criteria	Interventions
Acute Pain related to tissue trauma	Patient will report pain relief and appear more relaxed.	Assess nature, location, and severity of pain. Evaluate effectiveness of analgesia. Assure patient that opioids can be taken safely for acute pain for a limited time. Assist to change positions at least every 2 hours. Give back rub. Coach in relaxation exercises and mental imagery. Assess anxiety and explore causes. Be available. Reassure.
Impaired Tissue Integrity related to surgical incision	Patient's wound edges will remain clean and closed until discharge.	Check dressing hourly for bleeding first 24 hours then twice each shift. Report bleeding to physician. Protect wound by supporting during respiratory exercises. Treat nausea promptly.
Risk for Infection related to break in skin, invasive devices, and procedures	Patient will remain free of infection, as evidenced by oral temperature less than 100°F, decreasing redness of incision; no purulent drainage; clear breath sounds; no dysuria; no phlebitis.	Monitor vital signs every 4 hours. Report increasing temperature. Assess wound for increasing redness, edema, or drainage each shift. Inspect for purulent drainage. Exercise good hand washing. Use aseptic technique for wound care. Monitor and encourage fluid intake. Collect specimens for culture if ordered. Teach patient how to care for wound after discharge.
Impaired Gas Exchange related to stasis of pulmonary secretions	Patient's breath sounds will remain clear and respiratory rate will be between 12 and 20 breaths/min without dyspnea.	Help patient to support incision and turn, cough, and deep breathe or use incentive spirometry at least every 2 hours. Teach to take 10 deep breaths each hour. Auscultate breath sounds for crackles or atelectasis every 2 hours. Encourage fluid intake. Assist out of bed to walk as tolerated.
Urinary Retention related to effects of anesthesia	Patient's urine output will be approximately equal to fluid intake; no bladder distention.	Measure all fluid intake and output. Palpate for distended bladder every 2 hours. Provide privacy and try to stimulate voiding. Catheterize using sterile technique as ordered if patient is unable to void.
Constipation related to effects of drugs, immobility, bowel manipulation during surgery	Patient will have bowel sounds and pass flatus before discharge.	Assess bowel sounds and ask patient to report passage of flatus ("gas"). Count and document gurgles per minute in each quadrant of abdomen. Encourage frequent ambulation as allowed. Position the patient on the right side. Report distention.
Risk for Deficient Fluid Volume related to blood loss, wound drainage, NPO status	Patient's fluid intake and output will be approximately equal; serum electrolytes will remain within normal limits.	Measure fluid intake and output. Assess fluid status: tissue turgor, mucous membranes, pulse quality. Administer antiemetics promptly for nausea or vomiting. Offer fluids as prescribed.
Impaired Physical Mobility related to weakness, tissue trauma	Patient will gradually increase activity and assume more self-care.	Assist out of bed until patient can do so alone. Teach patient importance of ambulation to promote healing and prevent complications.
Disturbed Body Image related to abdominal wound	Patient will state any concerns about appearance of wound.	Observe patient's reaction to the incision. Elicit any patient questions or concerns. Answer questions honestly or refer to surgeon. Tell the patient the incision will fade and the edema will diminish.
Deficient Knowledge of postoperative routines related to lack of exposure.	Patient will correctly describe postoperative routines and self-care during hospitalization and after discharge. Patient will identify complications that should be reported to the physician.	Reinforce physician's instructions for wound care and activity limitations. Encourage consideration of adaptations needed in work or home roles and responsibilities. Stress need for good nutrition. Explain any drugs being prescribed: dose level, schedule, side effects, and adverse effects that should be reported to the physician. Include husband in teaching.

Continued

Nursing Care Plan — Postoperative Patient—cont'd

CRITICAL THINKING QUESTIONS

1. In addition to your desire to ensure that the patient is comfortable, why is collecting data about postoperative pain necessary?
2. Members of the health care team often repeat and reinforce one another's instructions when talking to the patient. List at least three reasons to explain the importance of doing so.

bpm, Beats per minute; *NPO*, nothing by mouth.

Table 17-5 Expected Drainage from Tubes and Catheters

SUBSTANCE	DAILY AMOUNT	COLOR	ODOR	CONSISTENCY
Indwelling catheter: urine	800–1500 ml first 24 hrs; minimal expected output: 0.5 mL/kg/hr	Clear, yellow	Ammonia	Watery
Nasogastric tube/ Gastrostomy tube: gastric contents	Up to 1500 ml/day	Pale, yellow-green Bloody after gastrointestinal surgery	Sour	Watery
Hemovac: wound drainage	Variable with procedure; may decrease over hours or days	Variable with procedure; initially, may be sanguineous or serosanguineous, changing to serous	Same as wound dressing	Variable
T-tube: bile	500 ml	Bright yellow to dark green	Acid	Thick

From Lewis SM, Dirksen SR, Heitkemper MM, Bucher L, Camera IAM: *Medical-surgical nursing: assessment and management of clinical problems*, ed 8, St. Louis, 2011, Mosby.

Nursing Diagnoses, Goals, and Outcome Criteria: Postoperative Nursing Care

Once the immediate postoperative phase has passed, the types of potential complications change somewhat. The risks of shock and hypoxia lessen. The nurse's attention turns toward other nursing diagnoses and goals, which are detailed in this chart.

Nursing Diagnoses	Goals and Outcome Criteria
Acute Pain related to tissue trauma	Reduced pain: relaxed expression, patient statement of pain reduction or relief
Impaired Tissue Integrity related to poor wound healing	Normal wound healing: intact wound margins
Risk for Infection related to break in skin or invasive devices and procedures	Absence of infection: minimal redness, clear drainage, no purulence; no fever
Impaired Gas Exchange related to stasis of pulmonary secretions, thrombosis, or emboli	Adequate oxygenation: respiratory rate and effort consistent with patient norms, normal arterial blood gases Absence of thrombophlebitis: no redness or swelling in legs
Urinary Retention related to the effects of anesthesia or restricted position	Normal bladder emptying: urine output approximately equal to fluid intake, no bladder distention

Nursing Diagnoses, Goals, and Outcome Criteria: Postoperative Nursing Care—cont'd

Nursing Diagnoses	Goals and Outcome Criteria
Constipation related to the effects of drugs, immobility, or bowel manipulation during surgery	Normal bowel function: bowel sounds present, passage of flatus
Risk for Deficient Fluid Volume related to wound drainage, inadequate intake, vomiting, or gastrointestinal decompression	Normal hydration: approximately equal fluid intake and output, normal serum electrolytes, pulse and blood pressure consistent with patient norms
Imbalanced Nutrition: Less Than Body Requirements related to nausea and vomiting or medical restriction of intake	Adequate nutrition for metabolic demands: retention of oral food and fluids, stable body weight
Impaired Physical Mobility related to weakness, tissue trauma, or medical activity restrictions	Improved physical mobility: gradual increase in mobility to preoperative level
Disturbed Body Image related to change in body appearance and function	Adaptation to changes in body image: patient looks at and touches affected area, patient verbalizes acceptance of physical changes

stretched during surgery. Muscle spasms in the area around the incision add to the patient's discomfort. The pain is usually most severe during the first 48 hours after surgery. During this time, an intravenous opioid analgesic such as morphine is most appropriate. Patient-controlled analgesia (PCA) may be used to provide prompt relief of pain and to maintain a more stable blood level of the drug. PCA is discussed in Chapter 15. By the third postoperative day, most patients require less medication for pain relief. The dose level or frequency may be reduced or the order may be changed to an oral analgesic such as acetaminophen with codeine on an as-needed basis.

When postoperative patients complain of pain, determine the exact nature of the complaint. Where is the pain located? An easy assumption would be that the pain is incisional when, in fact, the patient may have a headache or a backache. Chest pain, leg pain, or gas pain requires additional assessment and interventions. How severe is the pain? Ask the patient to rate the severity of the pain on a scale of 1 to 10, with 1 being no pain and 10 being the worst pain imaginable. This system provides a means for evaluating response to comfort measures.

During the first few days after surgery, promptly medicate the patient for pain. Pain is controlled better if it is treated before it becomes severe. Some physicians will order routine (rather than as-needed) analgesics for the first 24 to 36 hours, which maintains consistent therapeutic blood levels of the analgesic and reduces episodes of acute pain. Pain medication can also be given before activities that normally cause pain. Some patients are afraid that they will become addicted to opioids. Assure them that the short-term use of opioids for acute pain relief generally has not been associated with addiction.

A patient whose pain is controlled adequately is better able to participate in the exercises necessary to prevent postoperative complications. Schedule turning, coughing, deep breathing, and even walking to take advantage of periods when the patient is most comfortable. Of course, a medicated patient must be closely supervised when out of bed.

Although drugs are the mainstay of pain management in the early postoperative phase, other nursing measures can be used to help reduce pain. Position changes and back rubs can be very soothing. Relaxation exercises and mental imagery are often very effective alone or in combination with other nursing measures.

One source of discomfort in the postoperative patient is singultus, commonly known as *hiccups*. Hiccups are caused by intermittent spasms of the diaphragm. They are uncomfortable and may put stress on the incision, disrupt rest, and interfere with the intake of food and fluids. If hiccups persist, notify the physician.

Anxiety seems to intensify discomfort. Measures to decrease anxiety may therefore enhance the effects of pain relief measures. Recognize when the patient is tense and try to discover the source of the anxiety. Patients need to feel safe and need reassurance about what is happening to them.

Pain management in older adults can pose special challenges. The older patient may be stoic, reluctant to request analgesics, and fearful of addiction and overdose. Nurses who are concerned about the increased risk of adverse drug effects or who believe that the older person experiences less pain than younger patients may fail to treat the older person adequately. Good management of postoperative pain in the older person can often be attained with NSAIDs or acetaminophen in combination with opioids at somewhat reduced dose levels. The rule of thumb with opioids is to start with a low dose and gradually increase it. Drugs that are likely to have increased adverse effects in the older person are meperidine (Demerol) and long-acting benzodiazepines such as diazepam (Valium). Regardless of age, well-prepared patients can participate in pain management by describing and rating their pain, informing the nurse of the effects of treatment, and using PCA when appropriate.

The management of pain in cognitively impaired older adults is especially difficult. You may have to rely on your observations of patient behavior or family perceptions to recognize pain. Inappropriate behaviors such as pulling at tubes, striking out, and yelling may be manifestations of pain. Some impaired older adults can use pediatric pain rating scales, which provide you with some measure of pain intensity. After procedures that are known to be painful, it is reasonable to assume that the patient has pain. Provide analgesics in combination with other comfort measures.

Impaired Tissue Integrity

Various techniques are used to close the wound after surgery. The patient's incision may be closed with sutures, staples, surgical skin glue, or tape, as shown in Figure 17-9. When the patient returns to the nursing unit, a dressing probably covers the wound. After some procedures such as rectal, vaginal, nasal, or ear surgery, the operative site may be packed with gauze. In some situations, wounds are left open and covered with a dressing.

In healthy people, surgical wounds begin to heal immediately. By the third or fourth day, the healing process is increased. Although the wound appears to be healed after approximately 10 days, complete healing may take as long as a year.

Clean sutured incisions heal by first *(primary)* intention. Because the wound edges are closed, tissue bonds with little scarring. An infected wound is left open to heal from the bottom up. This method is called *healing*

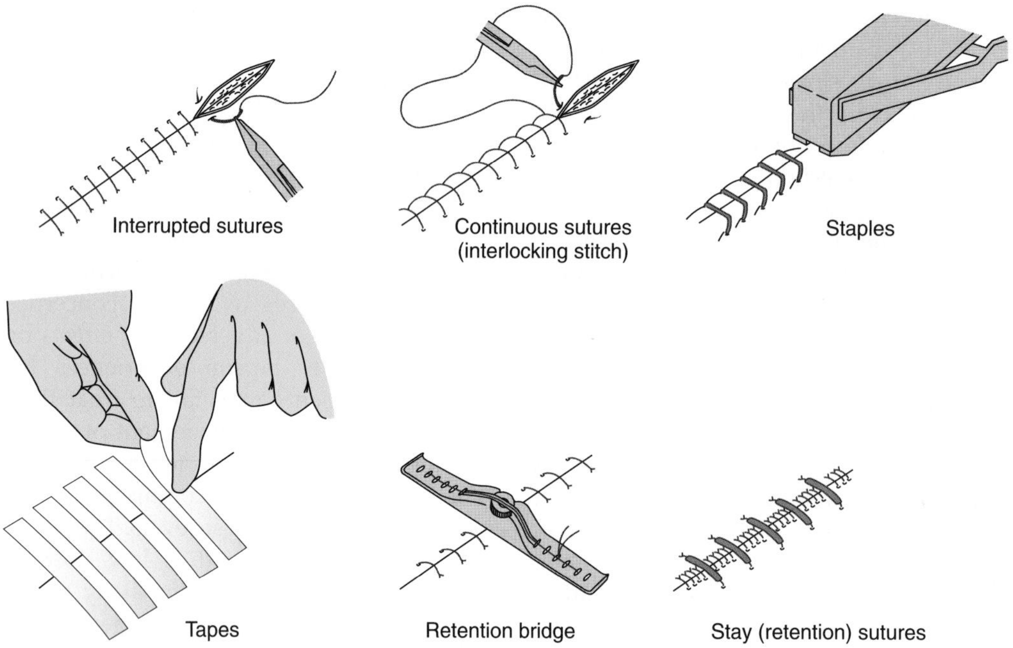

FIGURE 17-9 Methods of wound closure. (From Ignatavicius DD, Workman ML, Mishler MA: *Medical-surgical nursing across the health care continuum*, ed 3, Philadelphia, 1999, Saunders.)

by secondary intention. Some sources refer to healing by *tertiary intention* when the wound is initially left open and later closed. Figure 17-10 illustrates these three types of healing.

The physician usually performs the first dressing change, inspects the wound, and orders specific wound care. For the first 24 hours, check the dressing hourly for bleeding or drainage. If dressings become saturated, reinforce them using aseptic technique. Depending on physician preference and agency policy, reinforcement may be accomplished several ways. One method is simply to place dry dressings over the wet ones. Another method is to remove bulky outer layers of the wet dressing and replace them with dry dressings. After the first 24 hours, check the dressing once or twice each shift. Bleeding should be minimal and should stop within a few hours after the wound is closed. Report continued or excessive bleeding to the physician.

Some wounds have drains in a "stab" wound close to the incision (Fig. 17-11). Drains remove fluids from the operative site. Fluid accumulation in a wound interferes with healing. A Penrose drain is a soft tube that permits passive movement of fluids from the wound. The drainage is absorbed by the wound dressing.

Other types of drains are attached to collection devices that create suction to draw fluid from the wound. This type of drain is called an *active drain.* Examples of low-suction active drains are the Hemovac and the Jackson-Pratt drain. Both create negative pressure when they are compressed. As they fill with fluid, the collection devices expand. They must be emptied and recompressed ("recharged") using aseptic technique to maintain their effectiveness. The frequency of emptying depends on the amount of drainage and the physician's orders. Wound drains may also be connected to a suction device. Record drainage as output. Vacuum-assisted closure devices are used to apply negative pressure to certain open wounds.

In the immediate postoperative phase, wound drainage is often bright red (**sanguineous**). As the amount of blood in the drainage decreases, the fluid becomes pinkish (**serosanguineous**). It should become progressively lighter in color and thinner until it is straw colored and clear (**serous**). At the same time that the color is changing, the amount of drainage should steadily decrease.

Take care to reduce the risk of wound complications: dehiscence (separation of wound margins), evisceration (protrusion of abdominal organs thorough an open wound), and infection. Although dehiscence is not expected in a clean wound, always avoid strain on the suture line. Teach the patient to support the incision during coughing and when getting in and out of bed (Fig. 17-12). Patients who have had abdominal surgery should not use trapeze bars to move themselves. Promptly treat nausea to avoid the stress of retching and vomiting. Because many surgical patients go home within a few days, they need verbal and written instructions about safe activities. The exact type of surgery that was performed determines the restrictions. Consult with the physician about correct instructions.

Wounds that are healing normally are unlikely to undergo dehiscence. If infection develops under surgical sutures, the sutures dissolve too soon. Fluid accumulates in the wound and the wound dehisces. A sudden increase in wound drainage may precede

▶ Healing by First Intention

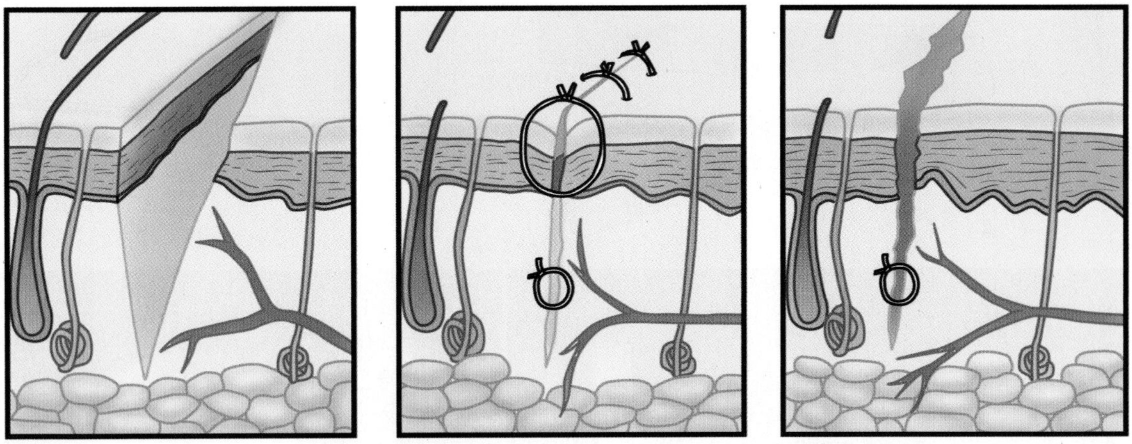

Clean incision | Early suture | "Hairline" scar

An aseptically made wound with minimal tissue destruction and minimal tissue reaction begins to heal as the edges are approximated by close sutures or staples. No open areas or dead spaces are left to serve as potential sites of infection.

▶ Healing by Second Intention (Granulation) and Contraction

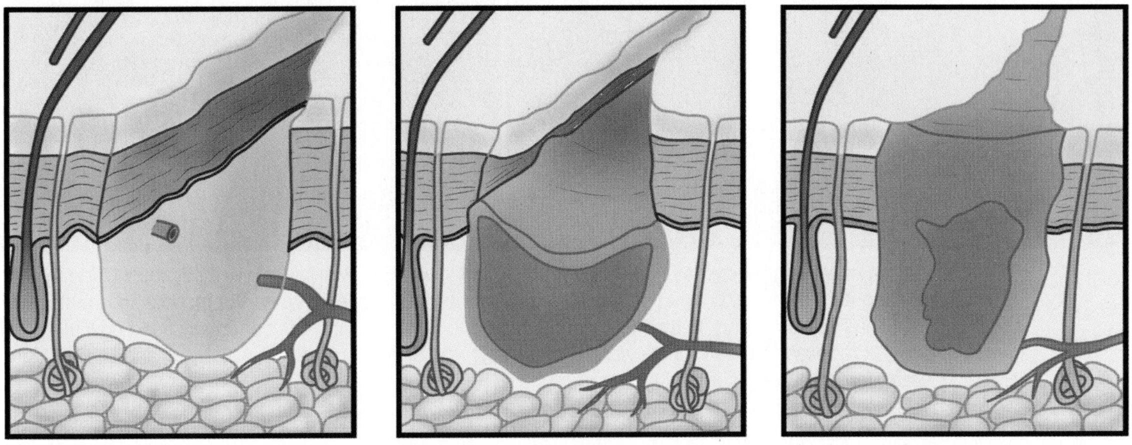

Gaping, irregular wound | Granulation and contraction | Growth of epithelium over scar

An infected or chronic wound or one with tissue damage so extensive that the edges cannot be smoothly approximated is usually left open and allowed to heal from the inside out. The nurse periodically cleans and assesses the wound for healthy tissue production. Scar tissue is extensive, and healing is prolonged.

▶ Healing by Third Intention (Delayed Closure)

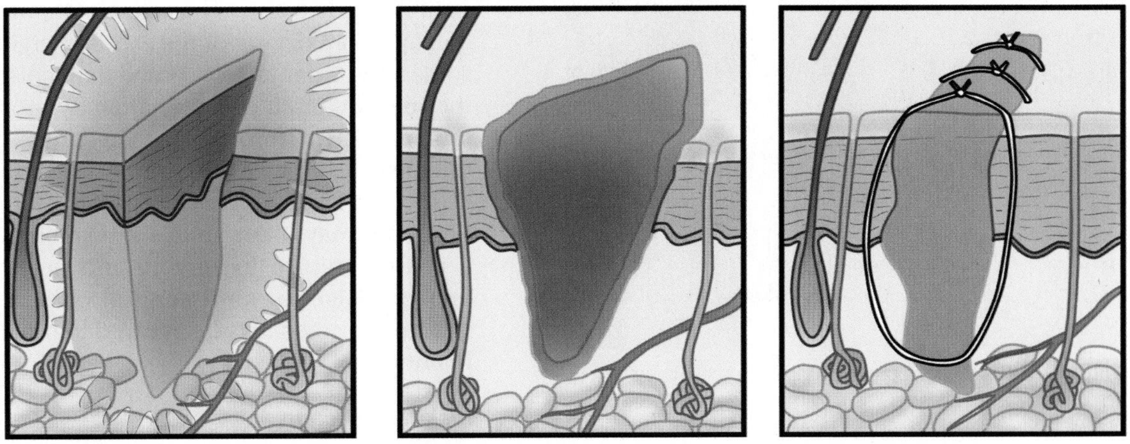

Infected wound | Granulation | Closure with wide scar

A potentially infected surgical wound may be left open for several days. If no clinical signs of infection occur, the wound is then closed surgically.

FIGURE 17-10 Wound healing. (From Rothrock, JC: *Alexander's care of the patient in surgery*, ed 15, St. Louis, 2015, Mosby.)

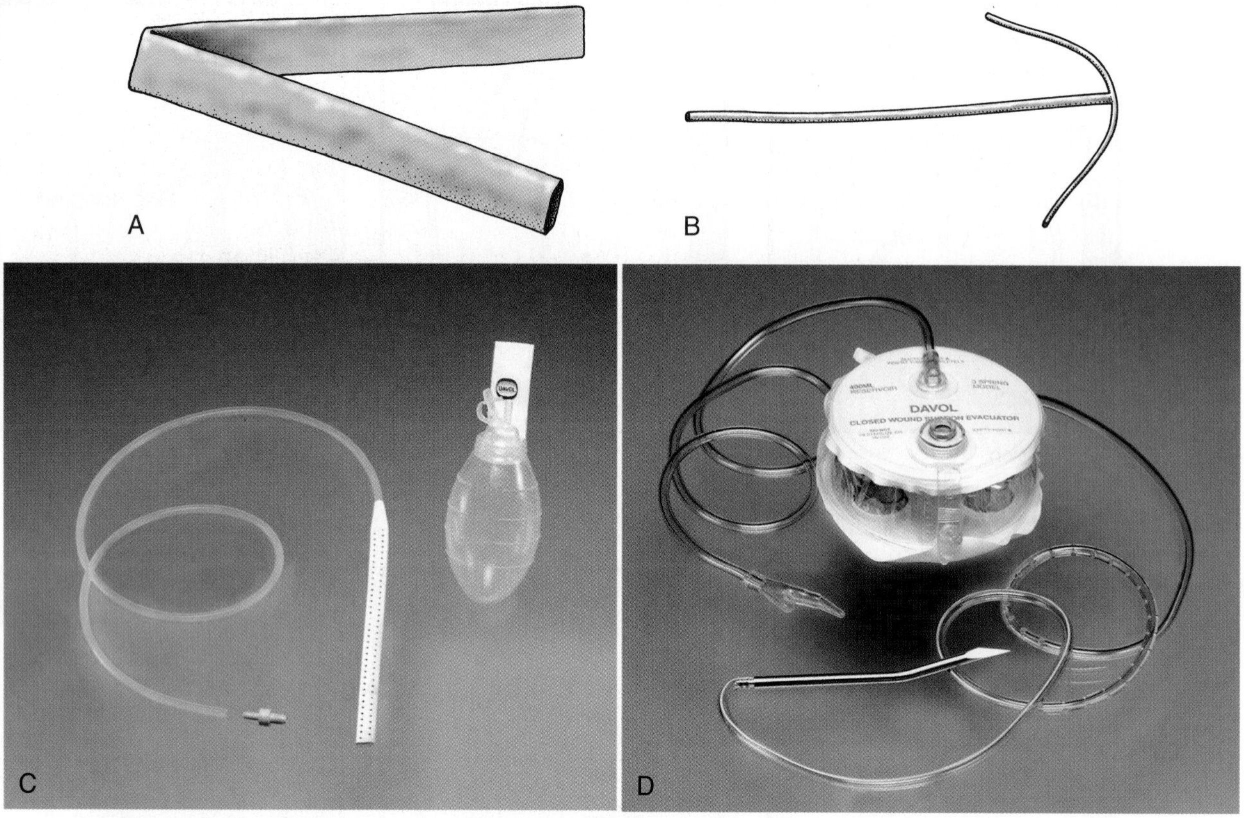

FIGURE 17-11 Types of surgical drains used to remove fluid from wounds. Passive or gravity drains include (**A**) the Penrose drain and (**B**) the T-tube. Drains that work by creating negative pressure when the receptacle is compressed are (**C**) the Jackson-Pratt drain and (**D**) the Hemovac. (T-tube and Hemovac are less commonly used now.) (A and B, From Rothrock, JC: *Alexander's care of the patient in surgery*, ed 15, St. Louis, 2015, Mosby. C and D, Copyright 2014 C.R. Bard, Inc. Used with permission.)

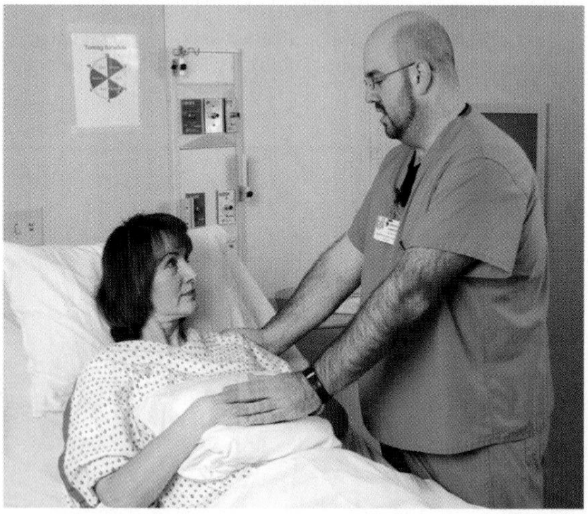

FIGURE 17-12 Splinting supports the incision during coughing. (From Potter P, Perry A, et al: *Fundamentals of nursing*, ed 8, St. Louis, 2013, Mosby.)

wound dehiscence. When the suture line ruptures, the patient may feel as though the wound is "pulling apart."

If dehiscence occurs, keep the patient in bed and in a position to decrease strain on the wound and decrease the risk of evisceration. For example, the patient with an abdominal wound should be in semi-Fowler position with the knees flexed. If dehiscence or evisceration occurs, the usual practice is to cover the wound with sterile dressings saturated with normal saline and to notify the physician. The saline is thought to prevent damage from drying of the exposed organs. However, some authorities are concerned that moisture increases the risk of wound contamination by promoting bacterial movement through the dressings. Covering the saline-soaked gauze with a dry dressing may prevent this complication. After inspecting the wound, the physician may order an abdominal binder. Anticipate a possible return to surgery and do not administer opioid analgesics until surgical consent is obtained. Infected wounds may be allowed to heal by secondary intention.

Risk for Infection

Continuously assess the patient for indications of infection. Signs and symptoms of wound infection usually do not develop until the third to fifth day after the operation; they may appear as late as a week after surgery. The classic signs and symptoms of wound infection include pain, fever, redness, swelling, and purulent drainage. Surgical pain should decrease as the days go by. Continued or increasing pain suggests the possibility of infection. A low-grade fever is common during the first 2 postoperative days because of the normal inflammation stage of healing. However, if the temperature is higher than 38°C (100.4°F) or lasts more than 2 days, infection may be present. Early signs of infection are sometimes hard to detect in older surgical patients because these patients typically do not develop high fevers even with serious infections. Some redness is expected at the wound suture line and around the sutures or staples. Increasing redness or redness that spreads to surrounding tissue is not normal.

Prevention of wound infection requires decreasing the exposure to microorganisms and maintaining the patient's resistance to infection. Good hand washing, the use of sterile or clean gloves (as appropriate), aseptic dressing changes, and diligent wound care prevent the introduction of infectious organisms. Good hydration and nutrition support the patient's healing and resistance to infection.

If infection is suspected, a culture of any drainage may identify the infectious organism or organisms. The antibiotics that are most likely to be effective can then be prescribed. While awaiting results of the culture and sensitivity tests, the physician often orders a broad-spectrum antibiotic. Collect the culture specimen before antibiotic therapy begins. Various wound care procedures may also be ordered. The patient may need to be isolated from other patients to prevent transfer of the organisms. The presence of highly contagious organisms such as MRSA requires patient isolation.

Because infection may develop after the patient is discharged, patient teaching should include signs and symptoms of infection that should be reported to the physician. The patient also should know whether the wound requires any special treatment. If wound care is needed at home, ensure that the patient or a family member is able to perform wound care before the patient leaves the hospital.

Impaired Gas Exchange

Document the patient's respiratory status every hour for the first 24 hours and once or twice per shift after that. Signs and symptoms of pneumonia include dyspnea, fatigue, fever, cough, purulent or bloody sputum, and "wet" breath sounds. When gas exchange is impaired, as with pneumonia or atelectasis, the pulse rate generally increases and the arterial blood oxygen saturation (SaO_2) falls. Breath sounds are absent in areas of atelectasis.

The most important nursing measures to prevent pneumonia and atelectasis are frequent position changes and coughing and deep-breathing exercises. Initially, assist the patient to turn at least every 2 hours. Patients are often assisted out of bed on the day of surgery. They are usually ambulated several times daily, beginning on the second day. Early ambulation has been found to greatly reduce the respiratory complications of surgery.

Deep breathing inflates the lungs fully and coughing removes secretions. Help the patient to cough and deep breathe every hour. Instruct the patient to take in a deep breath through the nose and gradually blow out through the mouth. After taking several deep breaths, a cough should be attempted to bring up secretions.

The incentive spirometer is a device used to promote lung expansion (Fig. 17-13). It consists of a tube through which air is inhaled and a cylinder containing a ball. The ball rises in the cylinder as the patient inhales through the tube. The more air that is taken in, the higher the ball moves. Markings on the cylinder indicate the volume of air taken in, which gives the patient a measurable goal toward which to work while using the spirometer.

Deep breathing and coughing are painful for the patient who has had abdominal or chest surgery. To reduce discomfort, coordinate the exercises with

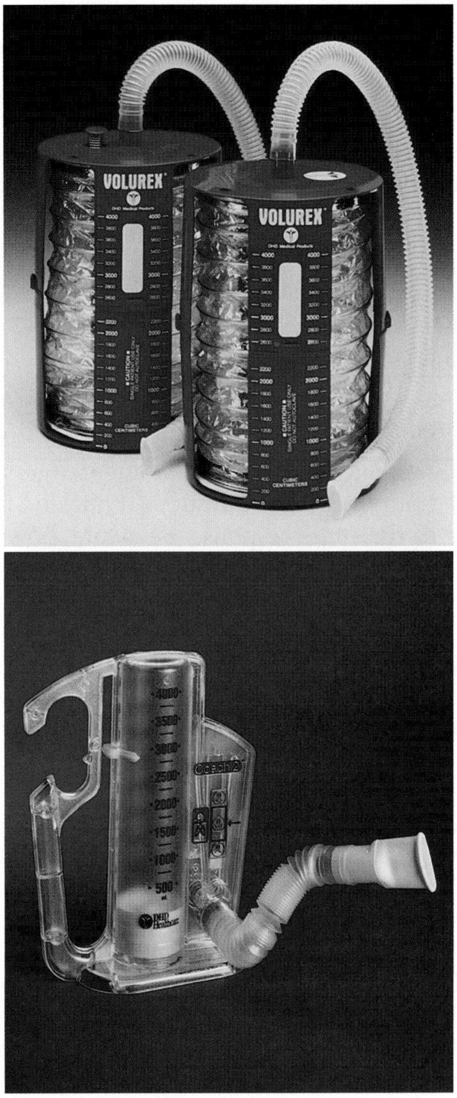

FIGURE 17-13 The incentive spirometer is used to promote lung expansion. (Courtesy Smiths Medical, Dublin, OH. All rights reserved.)

analgesics and splint the incision. The patient can splint by holding a pillow firmly over the surgical area while coughing.

The best course of action is to teach the patient about turning, deep breathing, coughing, and using the incentive spirometer before surgery. A patient who is in pain or drowsy from anesthesia is not in the best condition for learning. Instances in which coughing is contraindicated are few. They include surgeries for hernias and cataracts as well as brain surgery.

If the patient develops pneumonia, treatment includes rest, oxygen, and antibiotics. Care of the patient with pneumonia is discussed in Chapter 31.

Another factor that may cause severe, sometimes fatal, respiratory complications is pulmonary embolism. Pulmonary emboli usually arise from thrombi that develop in veins, especially the veins of the legs and pelvis. Measures to prevent thrombophlebitis and related pulmonary emboli include leg exercises, early ambulation, drug therapy as described earlier in the chapter, and frequent position changes within the limits of any restrictions imposed by the physician (Fig. 17-14). Antiembolic stockings such as thromboembolic disorder (TED) hose or an SCD may be ordered. Signs and symptoms that alert the nurse to possible pulmonary embolism are dyspnea, tachypnea, chest pain, and hemoptysis. If the embolus is very large, the patient may become cyanotic and go into shock. Emboli may be treated with heparin, thrombolytics, or both.

Pharmacology Capsule

Anesthesia, anticholinergics, and opioid analgesics can contribute to urinary retention.

Urinary Retention

Carefully monitor urinary output after surgery. In the first 24 hours, urinary output is typically reduced because of the stress response. Be aware, however, of the possibilities of urine retention or kidney failure in the early postoperative phase. Monitor urinary function by measuring intake and output. Bladder distention can be detected by palpation and by use of a bladder scanner. If the patient does not void within 6 to 8 hours, catheterization is usually performed to empty the bladder.

Patients who have had perineal or abdominal surgery are most likely to have difficulty voiding. They often have indwelling catheters inserted before or during surgery. The patient with a urine retention problem usually reports feelings of fullness and pressure over the lower abdomen. Some patients are unable to void at all. When a patient passes small amounts of urine frequently without feeling relief of fullness, suspect urine retention with overflow. The bladder releases just enough urine to reduce the pressure but does not empty completely. Gentle palpation of the lower abdomen usually reveals the smooth, rounded, full bladder. Distention can be confirmed with the scanner. If the patient is unable to void, catheterization is necessary. Because catheterization can cause urinary infection, it should be performed only if other interventions fail. Interventions must take the physician's activity orders into consideration. The patient should be provided with privacy while attempting to void. The toilet is preferred if the patient can go to the bathroom. If a bedpan must be used, raise the head of the bed, if permitted, to create a normal position for voiding. Men who need to stand to void should be assisted to do so if not contraindicated.

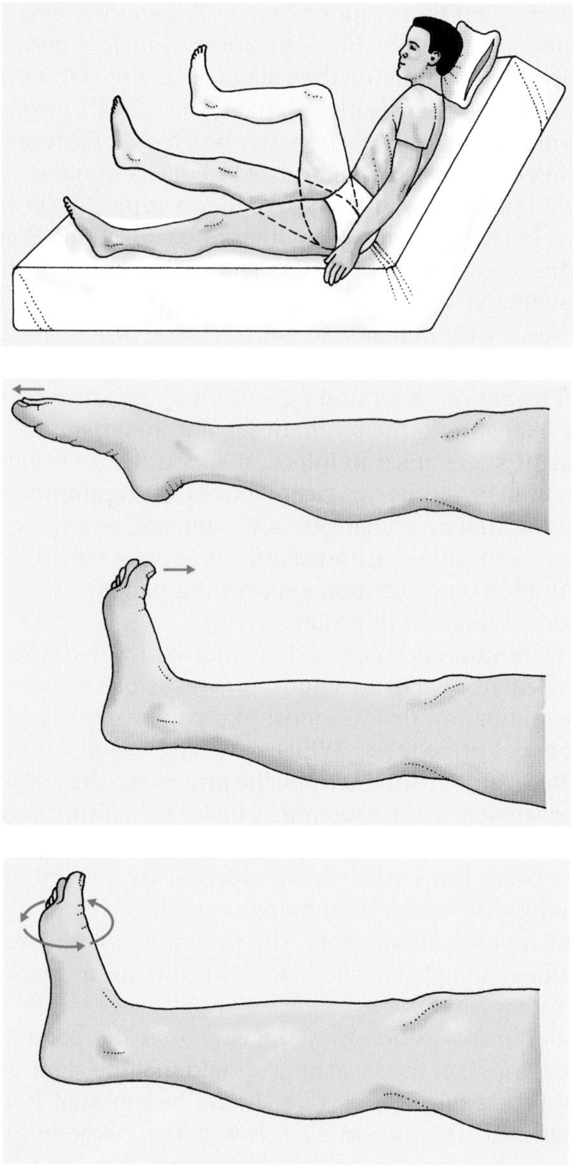

FIGURE 17-14 Postoperative leg exercises promote venous return. (From Ignatavicius DD, Workman ML, Mishler MA: *Medical-surgical nursing across the health care continuum*, ed 3, Philadelphia, 1999, Saunders.)

Sensory stimuli help some people to overcome difficulty voiding. The sound of running water or the sensation of warm water poured over the perineum or hands may encourage voiding. Use a measured amount of the water so it can be subtracted from the urine output.

If all independent measures fail, a physician's order is required for catheterization. In most instances, an "as necessary" order is given to empty the bladder with a catheter if the patient does not void within 6 to 8 hours after surgery.

If the patient has to be catheterized several times, the physician may order the insertion of an indwelling catheter. Catheterization and the care of the patient with a catheter are discussed in Chapter 42.

If the bladder is not distended but little or no urine output occurs, the patient may be in kidney failure. The minimal urine output is considered to be 30 mL/h. Failure to produce at least 30 mL/h should be reported promptly to the physician. The diagnosis and treatment of kidney failure are discussed in Chapter 42.

Constipation

Gastrointestinal function is disrupted by surgery, especially surgery on GI structures. Postoperatively, inspect and palpate for abdominal distention and auscultate for bowel sounds. Document the passage of flatus and the first bowel movement. The patient may not realize the significance of passing flatus and may wonder why it should be reported. Explain that passing flatus means that the digestive tract is beginning to function again. Most patients pass flatus approximately 48 hours postoperatively. After GI surgery, a normal diet usually can be resumed once the patient passes flatus.

Early, frequent ambulation is the best way to prevent GI discomfort. The intake of oral fluids and ingestion of a normal diet also help to stimulate peristalsis. Oral intake is usually withheld, however, until bowel sounds return (normally 24 to 48 hours after surgery).

Measures to promote the passage of flatus may be ordered, including early ambulation, application of heat to the abdomen, positioning the patient prone or on the right side, and insertion of bisacodyl suppositories.

If the patient develops a paralytic ileus, a nasogastric tube may be ordered to permit decompression of the intestines. If the surgical procedure is one that often causes GI problems, the nasogastric tube may be inserted during surgery to prevent problems.

The patient should have a bowel movement within a few days after resuming the intake of solid foods. In some instances, a suppository or an enema is necessary to stimulate emptying of the bowel.

Pharmacology Capsule

Antiemetic drugs control postoperative nausea and vomiting.

Deficient Fluid Volume and Imbalanced Nutrition: Less Than Body Requirements

Depending on the type of surgery performed, fluid and nutrition needs are met in a variety of ways. Some patients are given regular diets on the evening of surgery; others receive nothing by mouth for several days. Most patients return from the PACU with intravenous infusions. Patients are traditionally given clear liquids at first and then full liquids. If liquids are retained, the diet is advanced to include soft foods and then regular foods. Physiologically, no reason has been found to delay the introduction of solids once GI function has returned and a few oral liquids are retained, but this practice persists in many settings.

When the patient is able to tolerate liquids well, the intravenous infusion is usually discontinued unless it is needed for the administration of medication. Monitor the flow rate and the patient response. Nursing care of the patient receiving intravenous fluids is discussed in Chapter 18.

To promote healing, the patient's diet must provide adequate carbohydrates, protein, zinc, iron, folate, and vitamins C, B_6, and B_{12}. Alternative methods of feeding may be ordered if the patient is unable to resume oral intake for a long time. These methods are discussed in Chapter 39.

Fluid intake and output are usually measured for several days after surgery. In addition, laboratory studies of serum electrolytes often are ordered.

Nausea and vomiting interfere with the intake of food and fluids and can cause considerable fluid loss. Antiemetics (drugs used to control nausea and vomiting) are usually ordered as necessary (see the *Patient Teaching* box). General nursing measures for the patient with nausea and vomiting are discussed in Chapter 39.

Patient Teaching

Postoperative Patient

Patient teaching in the postoperative phase emphasizes recovery from the surgical experience and preparation for return to maximal possible function. Discharge planning should be started when the patient is admitted for surgery and revised as needed during the course of hospitalization. Topics to include in the discharge teaching plan are the following:

- Take your prescribed drugs as directed but notify the physician if you have adverse effects (specify drug, dose level, schedule, side effects, and adverse effects).
- Wound care: You will need to continue your wound care as I have demonstrated. Notify your physician if you have symptoms of infection (fever, increasing redness, swelling, pain, drainage at the incision site).
- When regular activities can be resumed, do not lift anything heavier than specified by your physician.
- If you need assistance, community services are available. (Specify services for patient needs.)
- If the physician advises specific fluids and nutritional requirements, you need to follow this special diet or take the prescribed amounts of fluids.
- You will need some specialized equipment and supplies. (Tell the patient how to obtain and use assistive devices, special equipment, and supplies.)

Continued

Patient Teaching—cont'd

- Can you identify any adaptations that will be needed in your home environment before you are discharged?
- You need to keep medical appointments to ensure that you are healing properly.

Pharmacology Capsule

Discharge teaching includes information about drug therapy.

Put on Your Thinking Cap!

Observe the room of a recent postoperative patient and identify four ways in which the environment can be modified to promote safety.

Impaired Physical Mobility

After general anesthesia and invasive surgical procedures, patients are usually weak and tire quickly. The physician prescribes measures to increase the patient's activity level (progressive ambulation in most cases). Assist the patient out of bed the first few times until the patient can safely get up alone. Help the patient to sit on the bedside, press the feet on the floor, stand, and then walk increasingly greater distances. Monitor for weakness and dizziness associated with orthostatic hypotension. Emphasize the physical benefits of early ambulation to the patient.

Disturbed Body Image

The effects of surgery (scars, loss of body organs, altered physical functions) can be very traumatic. A sense of loss can be demonstrated by anger, depression, or even denial. Understand and accept these responses. Nursing care of the grieving patient is discussed in detail in Chapter 24. Surgery can also produce positive changes in body image when it improves appearance or function or relieves symptoms.

Get Ready for the NCLEX® Examination!

Key Points

- Surgical procedures classified by purpose are diagnostic, ablative, palliative, reconstructive or restorative, procurement for transplant, constructive, or cosmetic.
- Variables that affect surgical outcomes are age, nutritional status including weight, fluid and electrolyte balance, medical diagnoses, drugs, and habits such as use of tobacco and alcohol.
- The phases of the surgical experience are preoperative, intraoperative, and postoperative.
- Nursing measures to reduce patient anxiety and increase knowledge about the surgical experience may actually decrease complications.
- Preoperative teaching should include surgical preparation; what to expect in the surgical suite and the PACU; what tubes, dressings, or equipment may be in place after surgery; and how patient participation can promote recovery.
- Before surgery, the patient or legal guardian must sign a legal consent form. Consent from the patient must be obtained *before* preoperative medications are given.
- Preparation for surgery may involve bowel cleansing, food and fluid restriction, skin scrubbing and hair removal, securing and covering hair, and administering preoperative medications as ordered. Clothing, jewelry, nail polish, and prostheses are usually removed.
- After preoperative medications are given, the patient should remain in bed with the call bell in reach and the side rails up.
- The surgical team consists of nurses who circulate, nurses who scrub, a RNFA, one or more surgeons, an anesthesiologist or a nurse anesthetist, and other technical personnel.
- Several types of drugs are used for general anesthesia; combined drug effects induce unconsciousness, alter sensation, and prevent movement so that surgical procedures can be performed painlessly and safely.
- The nursing diagnoses in the intraoperative phase may include Risk for Injury, Impaired Gas Exchange, Decreased Cardiac Output, and Risk for Deficient Fluid Volume.
- Postoperative surgical complications may include shock, hypoxia, wound infection, wound dehiscence and evisceration, injury, pneumonia, atelectasis, nausea and vomiting, impaired peristalsis, urinary retention, renal failure, and thrombophlebitis.
- Nursing diagnoses in the immediate postoperative period are Decreased Cardiac Output, Ineffective Breathing Pattern, Acute Pain, Acute Confusion, and Risk for Injury.
- Confirm the person or persons who the patient has approved to be given information about the patient and inform visitors where to wait and how they will be notified of the patient's status.
- Nursing diagnoses after recovery from anesthesia may include Acute Pain, Impaired Tissue Integrity, Risk for Infection, Impaired Gas Exchange, Urinary Retention, Constipation, Risk for Deficient Fluid Volume, Imbalanced Nutrition: Less Than Body Requirements, Impaired Physical Mobility, and Disturbed Body Image.
- Patient teaching for discharge emphasizes drug therapy, wound care, activity limitations, fluid and nutrition needs, equipment and supplies needed, adaptation of the home environment, and the importance of follow-up care.

Additional Learning Resources

SG Go to your Study Guide for additional learning activities to help you master this chapter content.

Online Resource

- Herbal Medications and Safety: www.sgna.org/Issues/SedationFactsorg/PatientCare_Safety/HerbalSupplements.aspx

evolve Go to your Evolve website (http://evolve.elsevier.com/Linton/medsurg) for the following learning resources and much more:

- Interactive Prioritization Exercises
- Fluid & Electrolyte Tutorial
- Pharmacology Tutorial
- Review Questions for the NCLEX® Examination

Review Questions for the NCLEX® Examination

1. An older adult who is scheduled for a surgical procedure expresses fear that he is too old for surgery and asks what you think. Your response should be based on the knowledge that:
   1. Older adults are twice as likely to have surgical complications as younger people
   2. An older adult in good health is likely to do just as well in surgery as a younger person
   3. For most older adults, the risks of surgery are too great to justify any possible benefits
   4. Older adults who have chronic health problems are poor candidates for surgery

   NCLEX Client Need: Physiological Integrity: Physiologic Adaptation
2. New LVNs/LPNs are being oriented to an ambulatory surgical center. The educator should explain that the nurse's responsibility when obtaining a patient's signature on a surgical consent form includes:
   1. Explaining the surgical procedure to the patient
   2. Obtaining the signature before the patient is given sedatives
   3. Informing the patient of possible risks associated with the procedure
   4. Assessing which alternative options the patient has explored

   NCLEX Client Need: Safe and Effective Care Environment: Coordinated Care
3. A patient is recovering from a surgical procedure that was done using spinal anesthesia. The PACU nurse assesses whether the patient has sensation and movement in his legs. Why is this data especially important?
   1. Regional anesthesia can impair blood flow to the extremities, causing gangrene.
   2. The patient cannot move the extremities despite feelings of pain or pressure.
   3. The extremities are susceptible to injury because movement returns before sensation.
   4. The effects of regional anesthesia may persist for several weeks.

   NCLEX Client Need: Physiological Integrity: Pharmacologic Therapies
4. Complications that are most likely to occur during the immediate postoperative period include which of the following? (Select all that apply.)
   1. Wound infection
   2. Pneumonia
   3. Shock
   4. Hypoxia
   5. Thrombophlebitis

   NCLEX Client Need: Physiological Integrity: Physiological Adaptation
5. In the PACU, a patient's vital signs are as follows: temperature 98°F, pulse 66 bpm and regular, respirations 14 breaths/min, blood pressure 100/56 mm Hg. Which other piece of information is *most important* to allow the nurse to evaluate these vital signs?
   1. Medications given during surgery
   2. Length of time under general anesthesia
   3. Whether the patient is having pain
   4. Patient's preoperative vital signs

   NCLEX Client Need: Physiological Integrity: Physiologic Adaptation
6. A patient with an abdominal incision reports that his dressing is soaked with drainage and that he felt a pulling sensation when getting out of bed. On inspection, the nurse observes that a loop of intestine is protruding from the open wound. The appropriate action is to:
   1. Have the patient lie flat in bed
   2. Gently reapply the surgical dressing and call the physician
   3. Administer a dose of prescribed opioid analgesic for pain
   4. Apply saline-soaked gauze and cover with a sterile, dry dressing

   NCLEX Client Need: Physiological Integrity: Reduction of Risk Potential
7. After surgery, a patient voids 20 to 30 mL of urine at frequent intervals. You should suspect:
   1. Urinary retention with overflow
   2. Damage to the bladder during surgery
   3. Fluid volume excess
   4. Kidney failure

   NCLEX Client Need: Physiological Integrity: Reduction of Risk Potential
8. During the shift "hand off," a postoperative patient reportedly has a paralytic ileus. The nurse should anticipate which of the following? (Select all that apply.)
   1. The patient will be unable to walk.
   2. A nasogastric tube and suction may be in place.
   3. Bowel sounds should be auscultated.
   4. The patient will be limited to a liquid diet.
   5. Blood transfusions will probably be needed.

   NCLEX Client Need: Physiological Integrity: Reduction of Risk Potential

9. Preoperative medications typically include: (Select all that apply.)
1. Sedative-hypnotic agent
2. Opioid analgesic
3. Antiemetic agent
4. Anticholinergic drug
5. Nonsteroidal antiinflammatory drug
NCLEX Client Need: Physiological Integrity: Pharmacologic Therapies

10. Guidelines to prevent wrong-site surgery include: (Select all that apply.)
1. Confirm that the operative site is marked before giving any sedating drugs
2. Verify that the appropriate equipment is available for the procedure
3. Confirm that the surgical consent form has been signed and witnessed
4. Verify with the patient the procedure that is expected to be performed
5. Conduct a time out before the first incision to resolve any concerns
NCLEX Client Need: Safe and Effective Care Environment: Coordinated Care

chapter 18

Intravenous Therapy

Carl Flagg

http://evolve.elsevier.com/Linton/medsurg

Objectives

1. List the indications for intravenous fluid therapy.
2. Describe the types of fluids used for intravenous fluid therapy.
3. Describe the types of venous access devices and other equipment used for intravenous therapy.
4. Given the prescribed hourly flow rate, calculate the correct drop rate for an intravenous fluid.
5. Explain the causes, signs and symptoms, and nursing implications of the complications of intravenous fluid or drug therapy.
6. Explain the nursing responsibilities when a patient is receiving intravenous therapy.
7. Identify intravenous medications that require dilution because they are vesicants or irritants.

Key Terms

Cannula (KĂN-yū-lă)
Embolism (ĔM-bō-lĭzm)
Embolus (*pl.* Emboli) (ĔM-bō-lŭs, ĔM-bō-lī)
Extravasation (ĕks-tră-vā-SĀ-shŭn)
Hypertonic (hī-pĕr-TŎN-ĭk)
Hypotonic (hī-pō-TŎN-ĭk)
Infiltration (ĭn-fĭl-TRĀ-shŭn)
Isotonic (ī-sō-TŎN-ĭk)
Phlebitis (flĕ-BĪ-tĭs)
Solution
Thrombus (pl. *Thrombi*) (THRŎM-bŭs)
Tonicity (tō-NĬS-ĭ-tē)
Vesicant (VĔS-ĭ-kănt)

Intravenous therapy is the administration of fluids directly into a vein. Most hospitalized patients receive some form of intravenous therapy. Home infusion of intravenous products has become common as well.

INDICATIONS FOR INTRAVENOUS THERAPY

Intravenous therapy is used to administer drugs, fluids (including nutrients), and blood or blood components. Intravenous administration of drugs may be ordered when a rapid drug effect is needed, when the drug is not available in an oral form, or when the patient is unable to take drugs by mouth. The intravenous route is also recommended when a drug must be maintained at a certain level in the blood.

In addition to drugs, intravenous fluids can provide water, normal saline, electrolytes, amino acids, lipids, vitamins, and glucose. Intravenous lines also may be used to provide continuous venous access for intermittent drug administration and emergency drug administration.

Whole blood and blood components are also given intravenously. Blood components include packed red blood cells, frozen red blood cells, platelets, and plasma proteins. Blood transfusions are discussed in Chapter 33.

TYPES OF INTRAVENOUS FLUIDS

By definition, a fluid is any liquid or gas. A **solution** is a liquid containing one or more dissolved substances. The terms *fluid* and *solution* are often used interchangeably in relation to intravenous therapy. Fluids that contain water and electrolytes and that can diffuse through a semipermeable membrane are called *crystalloids*. Fluids in which substances are suspended, such as blood plasma, are *colloids*.

TONICITY

Fluids can be classified by **tonicity**, a measure of the concentration of electrolytes in the fluid. The normal concentration of electrolytes in body fluids is approximately 285 milliequivalents per liter (mEq/L). Solutions that have the same concentration as body fluids are called **isotonic**. When the concentration of a solution is greater than 300 mEq/L, the solution is said to be **hypertonic**. **Hypotonic** solutions have a concentration of less than 280 mEq/L. The tonicity of fluids is important because it affects blood volume. Fluid that is hypertonic draws and retains water in the circulation, increasing the blood volume. Hypotonic fluid allows water to shift out of the capillaries into body tissues, resulting in decreased blood volume.

COMPONENTS

Many types of fluids are available for intravenous use. The physician selects the appropriate fluid to meet the patient's needs. The most commonly used intravenous solutions are specific combinations of water, sugar (in the form of dextrose), sodium chloride, and other electrolytes.

In most intravenous solutions, dextrose is the only source of calories. The patient receives 34 calories for each 1% of dextrose in a liter of fluid; thus 1 liter of 5% dextrose provides 170 calories (34 × 5 = 170). Dextrose fluids given in a peripheral vein are 2.5%, 5.0%, or 10.0% dextrose. Fluids infused into a larger (central) vein may have a much higher percentage of dextrose.

Sodium chloride solutions also are commonly used. An isotonic solution is 0.9% sodium chloride and is called *normal saline.* It is used to supply balanced amounts of water and sodium chloride. A hypotonic solution of 0.45% sodium chloride may be ordered if the patient's body fluids are concentrated owing to excessive water loss. More concentrated hypertonic solutions are needed when the patient has had excessive losses of both sodium and chloride.

Dextrose, sodium chloride, and other electrolytes are available in numerous combinations. Some commonly used electrolyte solutions are Plasma-Lyte and lactated Ringer solution. Dextrose 5% in Ringer solution is a combined dextrose and electrolyte solution.

When a patient needs long-term or aggressive intravenous therapy for nutrition, total parenteral nutrition (TPN) may be indicated. A catheter is placed in the distal superior vena cava for administering TPN. TPN fluids provide dextrose, water, amino acids, electrolytes, vitamins, and minerals. Fat emulsions can also be given intravenously. TPN is discussed in greater detail in Chapter 9.

Pharmacology Capsule

Always check the "six rights" when administering intravenous fluids.

VENOUS ACCESS DEVICES

Intravenous fluid is delivered by various types of venous access devices (Fig. 18-1). These devices include needles, over-the-needle catheters, inside-needle catheters (rarely used), subcutaneous infusion ports, and subcutaneously implanted pumps. The term **cannula** can be used to describe both a needle and a catheter. Cannula size is based on the inside diameter and is expressed as a *gauge.* The smaller the gauge is, the larger the inside diameter of the cannula is. Therefore a 14-gauge cannula is larger than a 22-gauge cannula.

The intravenous administration of fluids requires placement of the venous access device into a peripheral or central vein. Peripheral veins are located in the extremities (and in the scalp of an infant). They are used for short-term therapy, when a patient has healthy veins, and when relatively nonirritating fluids are given.

Central veins, large vessels located nearer the heart, are used when long-term therapy is required, when the patient has poor peripheral veins, and when **vesicant** fluids are administered. Central lines are inserted into the left or right subclavian or jugular or femoral veins with the tip of the catheter resting in the superior vena cava. The line may be placed in the subclavian vein through venipuncture, inserted into a peripheral vein and advanced to the desired location, or inserted through a skin incision and tunneled under the skin and into the large vessel. Devices placed through a cutdown incision are called *percutaneous catheters.* The central line threaded through a peripheral vein is called a *peripherally inserted central catheter* (PICC).

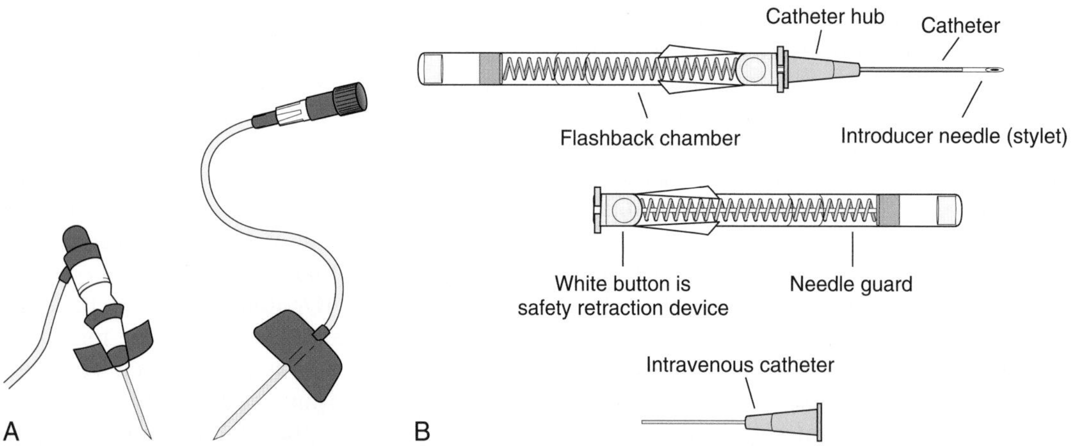

FIGURE 18-1 Venous access devices. **A,** Winged infusion needles. **B,** Catheter. (From Potter PA, Perry AG, editors: *Fundamentals of nursing*, ed 8, St. Louis, 2013, Mosby.)

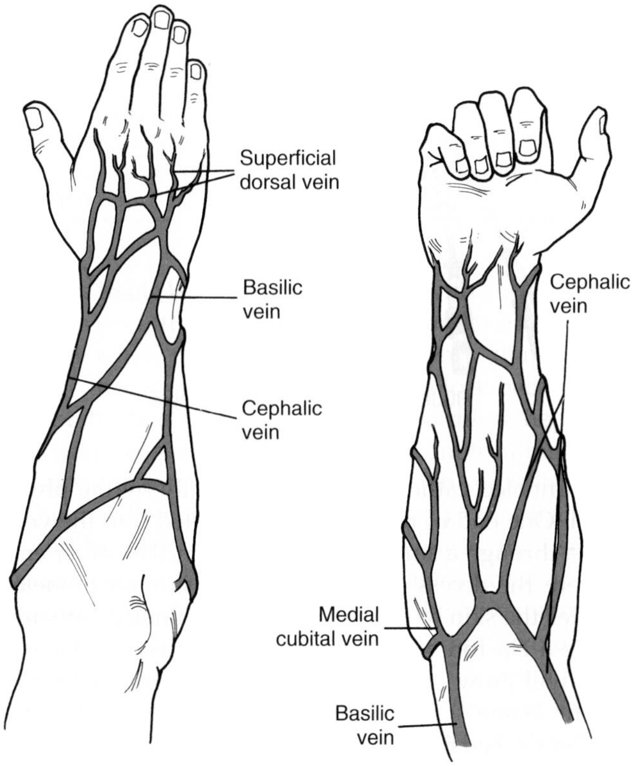

FIGURE 18-2 Common peripheral intravenous infusion sites.

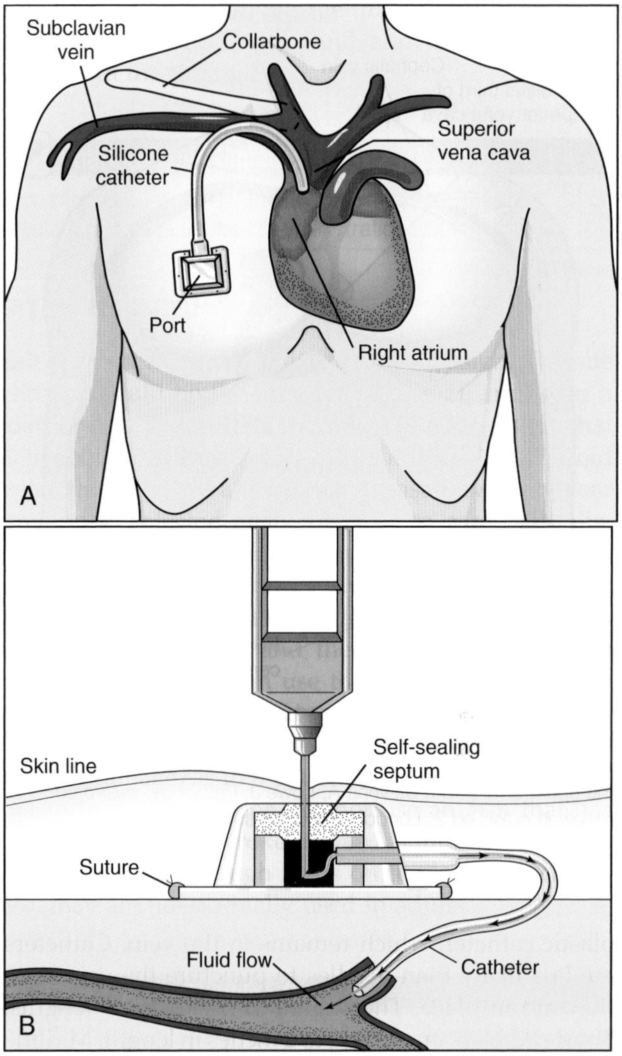

FIGURE 18-3 **A,** An implantable port in place. The entire unit is under the skin. **B,** Injection of medication into the port. (Adapted with permission from "Implantable Vascular Access Devices" by V. Winters, 1984, *Oncology Nursing Forum, 11*[6], p. 26. Copyright 1984 by ONS. All rights reserved.)

Examples of central venous tunneled catheters are the Hickman, Broviac, Groshong, Hickman-Broviac, and Raaf, and the implanted venous access ports. Figure 18-2 shows common peripheral infusion sites for intravenous fluids.

A port is a device with a central catheter that is surgically implanted in the subcutaneous tissue. It consists of a venous catheter and a port through which fluids can be injected but it has no external parts (Fig. 18-3, A). The catheter is inserted into a central vein and the port, which has a rubber septum, can be felt under the skin. A noncoring needle catheter that does not damage the septum is used to puncture the skin and access the port to deliver fluid and medications (Fig. 18-3, B). A port requires less care and is less restrictive than other access devices but it does require a needle puncture for each infusion.

For therapy over a period of days to weeks, the percutaneous catheter or PICC is preferred. Sometimes midline catheters are also used. Tunneled catheters and implanted ports are more appropriate for long-term use.

NEEDLES

One type of needle used is a winged ("butterfly") infusion needle, a short needle with two plastic wings that are held during insertion. A winged infusion needle is useful in infants when a scalp vein is used for intravenous therapy. It is also used at times in adults who have very poor or small veins, for one-time therapy, to draw blood samples, and for therapy of short duration (less than 24 hours).

To reduce the risk of bloodborne injuries acquired through needlesticks, various devices have been developed. One style has a self-sheathing stylet that retracts into a rigid chamber at the catheter hub after insertion; others use Luer-Lok connections rather than diaphragms that must be punctured with a needle. Concern about bloodborne pathogens has led to the development of various devices to reduce the risk of needlesticks. Among the products that make venipunctures safer for the nurse are safety needles that cover the needle after it has been used.

CATHETERS

A catheter is a small plastic tube that fits over or inside a needle. After insertion into the vein, the needle is withdrawn, leaving the catheter in the vein. The tubing that will deliver the fluid is then connected to the

Box 18-1 Sample Flow Rate Calculation

PHYSICIAN'S ORDER

1000 mL 5% dextrose in 0.45% normal saline every 8 hours. Delivery set: 20 drops = 1 mL.

Step 1: Calculate how many milliliters should be given in 1 hour. Divide the total number of milliliters to be given by the prescribed number of hours.

1000 mL ÷ 8 hr = 125mL/h

Step 2: Calculate how many drops should be given in 1 hour. Multiply the number of milliliters to be given each hour by the number of drops in 1 mL using the specific delivery set.

125 mL × 20 = 2500 drops/h

Step 3: Calculate how many drops should be given in 1 minute. Divide the number of drops per hour by 60 to find out how many drops should be given in 1 minute.

2500 drops ÷ 60 min = 41.6, or 42 drops/ min

Some people prefer to use a formula to calculate the drop rate. The formula is:

(Fluid volume to be infused) × (Number of drops per mL with selected infusion set) ÷ Time (min) = Drops per minute

fluid. However, they do not excuse you from monitoring the flow rate at intervals and assessing the catheter or needle insertion site. Box 18-1 gives step-by-step instructions for calculating the flow rate.

INTRAVENOUS INFUSION OF MEDICATIONS

Agency policies usually dictate what medications the nurse may give by piggyback or by direct injection through a cannula into the vein (intravenous push). Many states do not permit LVNs/LPNs to administer medications by intravenous push. When giving such medications, you must know how to dilute the medication and the correct rate of infusion. Improper administration of intravenous medications can be extremely dangerous. For example, potassium is *never* given by direct injection because of the risk of potentially fatal cardiac dysrhythmias. !

You also must be aware that some medications and intravenous solutions are incompatible; that is, they cannot be given together.

CHANGING VENOUS ACCESS DEVICES AND ADMINISTRATION SETS

The Infusion Nurses Society recommends that administration sets be changed no more frequently than every 96 hours for continuous infusions and every 24 hours for intermittent infusions. Exceptions are for lipids and blood and blood components. Blood administration sets should be changed every 4 hours. Administration sets for intravenous fat emulsion should be changed every 24 hours. Continuous parenteral nutrition *without* fat emulsions should be changed every 96 hours. An intravenous fluid container should not be used for more than 24 hours.

PICC lines have been in place for up to 3 years. Even though many factors influence the length of time that PICC lines are maintained, as long as adequate care and maintenance has taken place, a hard-and-fast rule no longer exists about how long they can remain in place and be used. Tunneled catheters and ports can be left in place for years. Agency policies are generally quite specific about the schedule.

TERMINATION OF INTRAVENOUS THERAPY

To discontinue intravenous therapy with needles or short catheters, put on gloves, stop the flow of fluid, loosen or remove the tape and dressing, gently press a dry gauze pad over the site, and remove the cannula, keeping the hub parallel to the skin. Dispose of the needle or catheter according to standard precautions guidelines. Elevate the extremity, apply pressure to the puncture site with a sterile gauze pad for 2 or 3 minutes to prevent bleeding, and then secure the gauze with tape. Record the appearance of the site, the condition of the catheter, and how the patient tolerated the procedure. Removal of midlength and long catheters requires special training. Document the length of these devices upon removal and compare it with the insertion length. Also report any signs and symptoms of infection.

PRECAUTIONS

When performing a venipuncture or handling used needles or catheters, always be aware of the risk of exposure to bloodborne pathogens. The most serious pathogens that can be transmitted by this route are the human immunodeficiency virus (HIV) and hepatitis B virus.

Several products for venipuncture and intravenous therapy that reduce the risk of needle punctures or other exposure to blood are available. Every nurse should be familiar with the agency needle puncture and body fluid exposure guidelines. In the event of an accidental needlestick, most policies require blood specimens to be drawn from the nurse and the patient to test for bloodborne infections. Drug therapy may be advised if the patient has an infectious disease. Documentation of the incident and the health status of the nurse at the time of the exposure may be very important if the nurse becomes ill as a result of the exposure. !

COMPLICATIONS OF INTRAVENOUS THERAPY

Intravenous therapy is so widely used that safety is often taken for granted. Several potential complications of intravenous therapy can be very serious, however. Complications include tissue trauma, infiltration, inflammation, infection, fluid volume excess, bleeding, and embolism. Each of these complications is discussed in detail in the Nursing Care During Intravenous Therapy section.

THE OLDER PATIENT AND INTRAVENOUS THERAPY

The older patient requires special consideration during intravenous therapy. Key points include the following:

- Anchor the vein with the thumb of your nondominant hand to maintain traction until the catheter is inserted to the hub.
- When performing the venipuncture, you may be able to distend the vessel by simply pressing on or touching the vein. If a tourniquet is needed, protect fragile skin by using the sleeve of the patient's gown or wrapping a washcloth under the tourniquet or use a blood pressure cuff inflated just above the patient's diastolic pressure. In some cases, a tourniquet is not used at all because it may cause the vein to rupture when punctured.
- Special adhesives or dressings may be needed to prevent damage to the skin. A skin polymer solution can be applied to protect the skin from adhesives.
- If the hand or arm is secured to an armboard, the armboard must be padded; apply another piece of tape or gauze to the back of the tape to prevent direct contact of the adhesive with the skin.
- Because older people have less subcutaneous tissue than younger patients, infiltrated fluid may drain away from the cannula insertion site. For example, if the hand is elevated, fluid may collect in the elbow area.
- If the patient is confused or restless, protect the infusion site and tubing with a commercial securement device or conceal the site under long sleeves or an ACE wrap.
- If a soft wrist immobilizer is justified, secure the immobilizer to the armboard and then secure the arm with the infusion to the armboard.
- Never apply an immobilizer *over* an infusion site; the immobilizer must be *below* the site.
- Confusion during acute illness is common. Reassure the confused patient, use a calm and gentle approach, and frequently reinforce instructions.
- With dementia patients, distraction may take their attention away from the intravenous apparatus. Keeping the infusion equipment out of sight may reduce attempts to handle it.
- Monitoring for fluid volume excess is especially important because older people often have less efficient cardiac and renal function.

❖ NURSING CARE During Intravenous Therapy

Assessment

When a patient is receiving intravenous therapy, frequent assessment is needed to ensure that the correct fluid is infusing at the correct rate and that the patient is not suffering any complications from this therapy (see Nursing Care Plan: Patient Receiving Intravenous Therapy).

Check the physician's order to ensure that the correct intravenous solution is infusing. Determine the prescribed rate of flow and assess the actual flow rate. Inspect the infusion site for edema, pallor or redness, bleeding, and drainage. Palpate the infusion site for edema and warmth or coolness. Ask the patient if the infusion site is painful.

Nursing Diagnoses, Goals, and Outcome Criteria: Intravenous Therapy

When a patient is receiving intravenous therapy, nursing diagnoses address the risk for complications, the need for assistance with activities of daily living, and the need for patient teaching. Specific nursing diagnoses and related goals are as follows.

Nursing Diagnoses	Goals and Outcome Criteria
Risk for Injury related to trauma, infiltration, inflammation	Absence of trauma, inflammation, infiltration: no bruising, bleeding, edema, pallor, redness, or drainage at infusion site
Risk for Infection related to disruption of skin integrity or presence of a cannula in a vein	Absence of infection: normal body temperature, no purulent drainage or redness at venipuncture site
Excess Fluid Volume related to rapid fluid infusion	Normal fluid volume: fluid output approximately equal to intake, no dyspnea or edema
Decreased Cardiac Output related to blood loss through disrupted intravenous line	Normal cardiac output: pulse and blood pressure within normal limits, skin warm and dry, tubing connection intact
Ineffective Peripheral Tissue Perfusion related to obstruction of blood flow by an embolus	Unobstructed blood flow: normal skin color and warmth in extremities
Self-Care Deficit (bathing, dressing, feeding, toileting) related to restricted movement of infusion site and connection to fluid delivery system	Patient's performance of self-care activities: activities completed without disruption of intravenous therapy

Nursing Care Plan — Patient Receiving Intravenous Therapy

ASSESSMENT

HEALTH HISTORY A 77-year-old patient was admitted for nausea and vomiting of 3 days' duration. He reported fluid intake of only water and cola in the previous 2 days and complained of dizziness and fatigue. Intravenous fluids were begun at 150 mL/h via a 21-gauge cannula.

PHYSICAL EXAMINATION Lethargic but oriented. Vital signs: blood pressure 96/58 mm Hg, pulse 102 bpm, respirations 22 breaths/min, temperature 101.6°F orally. Mucous membranes dry and sticky; urine dark yellow; intravenous infusion site: no swelling or redness.

Nursing Diagnosis	Goals and Outcome Criteria	Interventions
Risk for Injury related to trauma, infiltration	The patient will experience minimal trauma, as evidenced by absence of bruising, bleeding, swelling.	Use gentle technique to start the infusion. Inspect the infusion site for swelling and bleeding. Palpate for warmth or coolness. Anchor the tubing securely. Exercise caution to prevent movement of the cannula. Stop the infusion if signs of infiltration (swelling near infusion site, pain, slow infusion rate) and restart.
Risk for Infection related to disruption of skin integrity, presence of cannula in vein	The patient will remain free of infection at infusion site, as evidenced by absence of redness, swelling, edema, or drainage.	Use strict aseptic technique when starting the infusion and handling the site. Assess for signs of inflammation and infection: redness, swelling, warmth, purulent drainage, fever. Report signs to physician. Administer antibiotics and apply warm compress to inflamed site as ordered.
Excess Fluid Volume related to rapid fluid infusion	The patient's fluid status will be normal, as evidenced by normal vital signs and fluid intake approximately equal to output.	Monitor rate of fluid infusion and maintain correct rate of flow. Measure all fluid intake and output. Assess for signs and symptoms of fluid volume excess (hypervolemia): increasing blood pressure, bounding pulse, dyspnea. If patient is hypervolemic, slow infusion rate, elevate patient's head, and notify physician.
Decreased Cardiac Output related to blood loss	The patient will have no bleeding at infusion or tubing connections.	Check connections to be sure they are secure. Tape tubing to prevent accidental disconnection.
Ineffective Peripheral Tissue Perfusion related to obstruction of blood flow by embolus	The patient will maintain normal circulation, as evidenced by usual skin color and absence of respiratory distress.	Do not irrigate obstructed cannula. Aspirate gently or administer thrombolytic if permitted per agency protocol. Assess and report any signs of respiratory distress.
Self-Care Deficit (bathing, dressing, feeding, toileting) related to restricted movement of infusion site and connection to fluid delivery system	The patient will accomplish self-care activities without disruption of intravenous therapy.	Provide assistance with meals, hygiene, dressing, and toileting as needed. Provide gown that unfastens at the shoulder. Assure the patient that he/she can move with the infusion.
Deficient Knowledge of intravenous therapy management related to lack of exposure to information	The patient will demonstrate ability to protect and manage the infusion.	Tell the patient the purpose of the infusion and what symptoms should be reported: pain, bleeding, swelling. Assure the patient that movement is possible with the infusion as long as it is protected and the tubing is not disconnected.

Critical Thinking Questions

1. What is the importance of telling the patient the purpose of the infusion and possible symptoms?
2. What type of aseptic technique should be used in this situation in the initiation, maintenance, and discontinuance of intravenous infusion? Explain your answer.

Many people believe that the infusion is not infiltrating if blood flows into the tubing when the fluid container is lowered. This test is not accurate because blood may return even when fluid is escaping into the tissue. Notably, the lack of blood return does not necessarily mean that the needle is out of the vein. Therefore this time-honored test for needle placement is not reliable. Inspection and palpation of the infusion site remain the best means of evaluating for infiltration.

Assess the patient's vital signs and compare the readings with previous findings to detect increased pulse and blood pressure. Measure and record the fluid intake and output and auscultate the patient's lungs for crackles.

Interventions

Risk for Injury

Trauma. The insertion of a cannula is traumatic to the skin and underlying tissues. Tape may irritate or tear the skin. If a dressing such as Tegaderm is in place, excess tape will prevent loss of moisture under the dressing and it will loosen. Use gentle technique when performing the venipuncture and anchor the cannula to reduce tissue trauma. Apply a commercial site protector, if available, to shield the intravenous site.

Infiltration. Infiltration is the collection of infused fluid in the tissue surrounding the cannula. The term **extravasation** is often used interchangeably with **infiltration** but extravasation specifically refers to leakage of fluid from a blood vessel. Infiltration can be caused by leakage at the point where the cannula enters the vein or by puncture of a second site in the vein by the cannula. Drugs that are especially toxic to subcutaneous tissues are called *vesicants.* Common vesicants are vasopressors, potassium chloride, and antineoplastic agents.

Frequently inspect the site for signs and symptoms of infiltration. When the infusion is infiltrated, the patient may report pain or a burning sensation in the area. On inspection, the site may be pale and puffy. If an excessive amount of fluid is in the tissue, it may feel hard and cool. When evidence of infiltration is noted, stop the infusion and restart it in a different vein; otherwise the patient may not be receiving the drug or fluid as intended. Tissue that is edematous with infiltrated fluid is fragile, so handle it gently. Elevate the affected arm on a pillow to promote reabsorption of excess fluid.

Because many medications harm subcutaneous tissue, the physician should be notified if a solution containing a vesicant infiltrates. When administering vesicants, selecting a large, soft vein is especially important. Use the smallest appropriate cannula, ensure cannula placement before giving the vesicant, and flush the cannula after the vesicant is given. Examples of medications that are irritants or vesicants or that have a pH less than 5 or more than 9 or osmolarity above 500 mOs are presented in Box 18-2.

Put on Your Thinking Cap!

A patient complains of pain at an intravenous insertion site. The site feels cool and is slightly swollen. When the intravenous fluid container is lowered, blood flows back into the tubing. Do you think the infusion is infiltrated? What should you do?

Box 18-2 Partial List of Intravenous Drugs and Solutions That Require Proper Dilution to Prevent Harm to Blood Vessels

10% dextrose ($D_{10}W$)
3% sodium chloride
Acyclovir (Zovirax)
Amiodarone hydrochloride (Cordarone)
Amphotericin B (Fungizone/Abelcet)
Ampicillin (Unasyn)
Calcium chloride
Calcium gluconate
Ciprofloxacin (Cipro)
Dobutamine (Dobutrex)
Dopamine (Intropin)
Doxycycline (Vibramycin)
Epinephrine
Erythromycin
Ganciclovir (Cytovene)
Gentamicin (Garamycin)
Nafcillin
Norepinephrine (Levophed)
Penicillin G
Piperacillin/tazobactam (Zosyn)
Potassium chloride (minibags)
Sodium bicarbonate
Sulfamethoxazole/trimethoprim (Bactrim)
Tobramycin (Nebcin)
Total or peripheral parenteral nutrition
Vancomycin (Vancocin)

Data from Motley LC: *Target drug list for central line access*, 2007: www.iv-therapy.net/node/901. Accessed January 28, 2009.

Risk for Infection

Inflammation of the vein is called **phlebitis**. With intravenous fluid therapy, phlebitis may be caused by irritation by the cannula or by medications. Redness, swelling, warmth, and tenderness near the insertion site suggest phlebitis. The inflammation may be mild or severe and carries the possibility of the formation of blood clots in the vein (thrombophlebitis). If a venipuncture site is infected, there may be purulent drainage in addition to redness and swelling and the patient may have a fever.

To reduce the risk of inflammation and infection, use strict aseptic technique when starting and handling intravenous infusions. Agency policy describes specific site care, including the frequency of dressing changes.

If the infusion site appears to be inflamed or infected, stop the infusion and restart it in another site. If agency policy permits, a warm compress can be applied to the inflamed site. If evidence of infection is noted, notify the physician. Antibiotic therapy may be ordered.

Pharmacology Capsule

Drugs that are toxic to body tissues are called *vesicants.* They can cause phlebitis or tissue necrosis.

Excess Fluid Volume

The patient's blood volume may increase excessively when fluid is delivered directly into the bloodstream. This situation is most likely to happen when large volumes of fluid are infused, especially in patients who have impaired renal or cardiac function.

Signs and symptoms of fluid volume excess include rising blood pressure, bounding pulse, and edema. Severe fluid volume excess produces congestive heart failure and pulmonary edema (discussed in Chapter 36).

The risk of fluid volume excess is reduced by controlling the rate of fluid infusion. If the infusion falls behind schedule, correct the rate as noted previously but do not increase it to make up for the slow infusion. Normally, fluid intake and output are approximately equal. When the heart or kidneys are unable to handle excess blood volume, heart failure may develop. Young children and older adults must be monitored closely for fluid volume excess because they do not adapt to fluid changes as readily as a young adult. If indications of fluid volume excess (increasing blood pressure, bounding pulse, dyspnea) appear, slow the infusion rate, elevate the patient's head, and notify the physician.

Pharmacology Capsule

Rapid intravenous administration of drugs or fluids may cause fluid volume excess, leading to heart failure.

Decreased Cardiac Output

Bleeding may occur if the cannula is moved excessively after insertion. Even more serious bleeding is possible if the tubing becomes disconnected from the cannula, allowing blood to flow freely from the vein.

To prevent bleeding, make sure that all connections in the infusion set are secure. Tape tubing so that it cannot be pulled loose easily. Protect the infusion site and tubing when the patient moves. If a large amount of blood is lost, assess the patient's vital signs and notify the physician. Institute emergency measures if the patient is in shock.

Ineffective Peripheral Tissue Perfusion

An **embolus** (*pl.* **emboli**) is an unattached blood clot or other substance in the circulatory system. An embolus can have serious, even life-threatening, effects if it lodges and obstructs blood flow in a critical blood vessel. The obstruction created by a trapped embolus is called an **embolism**.

Intravenous therapy presents risks of emboli from blood clots, air, and broken catheters. A blood clot, or **thrombus** (*pl.* **thrombi**), can develop in intravenous needles or catheters. Air can enter the bloodstream if the infusion system is opened. As little as 10 mL of air can cause serious complications. The risk of air embolism with peripheral lines has been greatly reduced by the use of plastic rather than glass fluid containers. The danger is greatest with central venous lines such as the subclavian, Hickman-Broviac, and triple-lumen catheters. If a port is disconnected, air may be drawn into the bloodstream. The patient experiences shortness of breath, hypotension, and possibly shock and cardiac arrest.

A rare occurrence is a catheter embolus. This event occurs when a piece of the catheter breaks off in the vein. Broken catheters may be caused by defects in the catheter, reintroduction of the needle into the catheter, accidental cutting with scissors, forceful flushing of a PICC line, and pulling catheters through needles.

Chest discomfort may be caused by a catheter embolism and should be reported to the physician immediately. If a catheter breaks in a peripheral vein, keep the patient calm with the head elevated, and notify the physician. A radiograph will be ordered to locate the broken catheter, usually in the right ventricle or pulmonary artery. The fragment may be removed with a snare that is passed through the femoral vein.

When the cannula seems to be obstructed, blood clots may have formed in it. Irrigation of the cannula is not recommended because it may force clots into the bloodstream. Depending on agency policy, gentle aspiration may be attempted to remove the obstruction. Alteplase (tPA) may be ordered to dissolve clots that are obstructing the cannula.

Exercise extra caution to prevent an air embolism when a patient has a central line. The chance of this event happening with PICC lines that have valves is greatly reduced. The infusion set must remain closed. When hanging new bags of fluid, clamp the catheter port to prevent air entering the bloodstream. When a central catheter is inserted or removed, instruct the patient to take a deep breath and bear down. This action helps to prevent air entering the bloodstream. If air accidentally enters the line, close the leak immediately. Turn the patient on the left side with the head lowered. This position traps the air in the right atrium, where it can be absorbed gradually. Air in the bloodstream is an emergency situation in which cardiac arrest is possible; thus close monitoring is vital. Notify the physician immediately and keep the emergency supply cart close at hand. One-hundred percent oxygen with a nonrebreather mask may be ordered.

Self-Care Deficit (Bathing, Feeding, Dressing, Toileting)

Provide assistance as needed with eating, dressing, toileting, and hygiene. Dressing may be easier if the patient is provided with a gown or shirt that unfastens at the shoulder. These garments are simpler to remove than garments that must be removed over the arm. Some patients are fearful of moving with an intravenous infusion. Explain what restrictions, if any, are needed to protect the infusion (see the *Patient Teaching* box). If a commercial intravenous shield is available, consider using one to reduce the risk of trauma at the insertion site.

Patient Teaching

Intravenous Therapy in the Home

When intravenous therapy is ordered outside the acute care setting, explain what will be performed and why. Teaching should begin well before discharge so that the patient's ability to perform the care can be assessed. With long-term therapy, teaching the patient (and family, if appropriate) the following is especially important:

- Infusion site care
- Proper administration of fluids or drugs
- Signs that should be reported to the physician or home health nurse
- How to flush infusion ports if appropriate
- Care of central lines or implanted infusion ports

Details depend on the situation.

Get Ready for the NCLEX® Examination!

Key Points

- Intravenous therapy is used to administer drugs, fluids including nutrients, and blood or blood products.
- The terms *fluid* and *solution* are used interchangeably in relation to intravenous therapy.
- Tonicity is a measure of the concentration of electrolytes in a fluid.
- Hypertonic intravenous solutions tend to increase blood volume whereas hypotonic intravenous solutions tend to decrease blood volume.
- A patient receives 34 calories for each 1% of dextrose in a liter of fluid.
- Devices used to deliver intravenous fluids include needles, over-the-needle catheters, inside-needle catheters, subcutaneous infusion ports, and subcutaneously implanted pumps.
- Central veins are large veins located nearer the heart that are used for long-term therapy, when the patient has poor peripheral veins, and when irritating or vesicant medications or fluids are administered.
- Peripheral veins in the extremities and scalp are used for short-term therapy, when a patient has healthy veins, and when relatively nonirritating fluids are given.
- Nurse practice acts and agency policies govern who can perform venipuncture and who can administer intravenous fluids and intravenous medications.
- Cannula size is selected based on the patient's vein size and general condition and the type of fluid to be administered.
- Use the "six rights" when administering intravenous fluids as well as drugs.
- Administration sets are changed every 24 hours for intermittent infusions, parenteral nutrition, and fat emulsion; for continuous infusions other than blood or blood products or lipids, sets are changed every 96 hours.
- On the site dressing, record the date and time that the cannula was inserted, the length and gauge of the cannula, and your initials.
- When an infusion flows by gravity, the rate is influenced by the height of the fluid container, fluid volume in the container, fluid viscosity, cannula diameter, venting of the fluid container, and position of the extremity.
- If your state permits you to administer drugs per intravenous push, you must know how to dilute the medication, the correct rate of infusion, and whether the drug is compatible with the infusing fluid.
- Use standard precautions when starting infusions, providing site care, discontinuing infusions, and making dressing changes.
- Complications of intravenous therapy are tissue trauma, infiltration, inflammation, infection, fluid volume excess, bleeding, and embolism.
- Monitor for fluid volume excess in the older person who is receiving intravenous fluids.
- When a cannula appears to be obstructed, irrigation is not recommended because you may force blood clots into the bloodstream.
- With central lines, take precautions to prevent air entering the line, which can cause an air embolism—a potentially fatal complication.

Additional Learning Resources

SG Go to your Study Guide for additional learning activities to help you master this chapter content.

evolve Go to your Evolve website (http://evolve.elsevier.com/Linton/medsurg) for the following learning resources and much more:

- Interactive Prioritization Exercises
- Fluid & Electrolyte Tutorial
- Pharmacology Tutorial
- Review Questions for the NCLEX® Examination

Review Questions for the NCLEX® Examination

1. Which intravenous cannula is largest?
   1. 12 gauge
   2. 14 gauge
   3. 18 gauge
   4. 22 gauge

   NCLEX Client Need: Physiological Integrity: Pharmacological Therapies

2. A patient is receiving an intravenous infusion of 0.45% sodium chloride. The nurse knows that this solution is:
   1. Isotonic
   2. Hypotonic
   3. Hypertonic
   4. Concentrated

   NCLEX Client Need: Physiological Integrity: Pharmacological Therapies
3. Solutions that have the same concentration of electrolytes as body fluids are called _______________ solutions.

   NCLEX Client Need: Physiological Integrity: Pharmacological Therapies
4. When intravenous fluid is given to increase blood volume, the tonicity of the solution should be _______________.

   NCLEX Client Need: Physiological Integrity: Pharmacological Therapies
5. A central line is preferred over a peripheral line under which of the following conditions? (Select all that apply.)
   1. Irritating intravenous fluids are to be administered.
   2. The patient is an infant.
   3. Short-term therapy is required.
   4. The patient has poor peripheral veins.
   5. Antibiotics will be infused.

   NCLEX Client Need: Physiological Integrity: Pharmacological Therapies
6. A patient is to receive 1000 mL of intravenous fluid every 8 hours at a rate of 34 drops/min. If the infusion has slowed so that he has received only 700 mL near the end of one 8-hour shift, the correct action is to:
   1. Quickly infuse an additional 300 mL before the end of the shift
   2. Increase the infusion rate to deliver an additional 300 mL over the next shift
   3. Notify the physician to determine what action should be taken
   4. Reset the infusion rate at 34 drops/min to continue the infusion

   NCLEX Client Need: Physiological Integrity: Pharmacological Therapies; Reduction of Risk Potential
7. An older patient is receiving intravenous fluids to treat dehydration. When she complains of shortness of breath, your assessment reveals a 20-point increase in her systolic blood pressure and a heart rate of 100 beats per minute (bpm). The most likely cause of these findings is:
   1. Shock caused by deficient fluid volume
   2. Anxiety associated with hospitalization
   3. Fluid volume excess related to fluid overload
   4. Renal failure caused by circulatory collapse

   NCLEX Client Need: Physiological Integrity: Reduction of Risk Potential
8. Which of the following interventions is/are recommended when an older adult requires peripheral intravenous therapy? (Select all that apply.)
   1. Pad the armboard, if used
   2. Protect the skin from adhesive tape
   3. Place an immobilizer over the infusion site
   4. Use a blood pressure cuff rather than a tourniquet
   5. Release traction on the vein after the needle pierces the skin

   NCLEX Client Need: Physiological Integrity: Reduction of Risk Potential
9. A PICC line is inserted into a vein and advanced into the ____________________.

   NCLEX Client Need: Physiological Integrity: Pharmacological Therapies; Therapeutic Procedures
10. The *greatest* danger of irrigating an obstructed intravenous line is:
    1. Embolism
    2. Trauma to the blood vessel
    3. Rupture of the cannula
    4. Infusion site irritation

    NCLEX Client Need: Physiological Integrity: Reduction of Risk Potential

chapter 19

Shock

Catherine Robichaux

Objectives

1. List the types of shock.
2. Describe the pathophysiologic features of each type of shock.
3. List the signs and symptoms of each stage of shock.
4. Explain the first-aid emergency treatment of shock outside the medical facility.
5. Identify general medical and nursing interventions for shock.
6. Explain the rationale for medical-surgical treatment of shock.
7. Assist in developing care plans for patients in each type of shock.

Key Terms

Ischemia (ĭs-KĒ-mē-ă)
Metabolic acidosis (mĕt-ă-BŎL-ĭk ă-sĭ-DŌ-sĭs)
Multiple organ dysfunction syndrome (MODS)
Sepsis (SĔP-sĭs)
Shock
Systemic inflammatory response syndrome (SIRS)

DEFINITION OF SHOCK

Shock is a syndrome characterized by inadequate tissue perfusion resulting in impaired cellular metabolism. Inadequate tissue perfusion deprives cells of essential oxygen and nutrients, forcing cells to rely on anaerobic (without oxygen) metabolism. As a result, a reduced amount of energy is produced and lactic acid, a by-product of anaerobic metabolism, causes tissue acidosis and subsequent organ dysfunction. Several types of shock have been identified, each with a different cause that requires specific interventions. Although some aspects of treatment may be appropriate for treating the effects of all types of shock, patient responses will vary; therefore continual and astute nursing assessments and prompt interventions are required.

TYPES OF SHOCK

Historically, shock has been classified into one of four types based on the etiology or cause: hypovolemic (inadequate circulating volume), cardiogenic (decreased myocardial contractility), obstructive (inadequate circulatory blood flow caused by a physical impairment or obstruction), and vasogenic or distributive shock (widespread vasodilation). Distributive shock further encompasses anaphylactic, septic, and neurogenic shock (Anderson & Watson, 2013; Kleinpell, 2012).

HYPOVOLEMIC SHOCK

Hypovolemic shock is the most common type of shock and occurs when the circulating blood volume is inadequate to maintain the supply of oxygen and nutrients to body tissues. It can result from loss of blood, plasma volume loss of more than 20% of circulating volume, or extreme dehydration. Intravascular or circulating volume deficits can occur from external or internal losses. Rapid blood loss is the most frequent cause of hypovolemic shock. Additional causes include severe diarrhea or vomiting and excessive perspiration. Excessive shift of plasma can result in hypovolemic shock and is associated with conditions such as burns, pancreatitis, and intestinal obstruction (Kolecki, 2012; Strickler, 2013).

CARDIOGENIC SHOCK

Cardiogenic shock occurs when the heart fails as a pump. A decrease in myocardial contractility results in decreased cardiac output and impaired tissue perfusion. This type of shock is one of the most difficult to treat and usually results when diseased coronary arteries cannot meet the demand of the working myocardial cells, such as occurs in acute myocardial infarction (MI). Although only about 7% of patients with an MI develop cardiogenic shock, mortality rates are 70% to 90% in the absence of aggressive, experienced care (Ren, 2013). Other causes of cardiogenic shock are conditions that result in ineffective myocardial cell function, such as dysrhythmias, cardiomyopathy, myocarditis, valvular disease, and structural disorders.

OBSTRUCTIVE SHOCK

In obstructive shock, blood flow is reduced and prevented from entering or leaving the heart by a

Table 19-1 Obstructive Shock

TYPE	DEFINITION AND SYMPTOMS	CAUSES
Tension pneumothorax	Complete collapse of a lung, causing increase in intrathoracic pressure and compression of the vena cava and resulting in decreased preload and cardiac output	Blunt or penetrating trauma, barotraumas, central venous catheter placement, chest compressions during cardiopulmonary resuscitation
Cardiac tamponade	Fluid collects within the pericardial sac, causing compression of the myocardium and resulting in reduced cardiac output and myocardial ischemia	Malignancies, uremia, idiopathic pericarditis, infectious diseases
Pulmonary embolism	A blockage of the pulmonary artery or one or more of its branches, resulting in shortness of breath and hemodynamic compromise	Deep vein thrombosis; air, fat, or tissue emboli resulting from surgery or trauma
Abdominal compartment syndrome	Increase in pressure within the confined anatomic space of the abdominal cavity, resulting in vascular or organ compression and decreased blood flow	Abdominal surgery, fluid resuscitation, ileus, intraperitoneal bleeding, ascites, peritonitis
Superior vena cava syndrome	Obstruction of the superior vena cava, resulting in facial or chest edema, shortness of breath, tachycardia, and hypotension	Malignancies, tuberculosis, indwelling central venous catheters, pacemaker wires

mechanical obstruction. The lack of blood flow results in circulatory arrest, causing the heart to stop pumping blood through the body. Causes of obstructive shock include tension pneumothorax, pericardial tamponade, pulmonary embolus, superior vena cava syndrome, and abdominal compartment syndrome (Gallagher, 2009; Table 19-1).

DISTRIBUTIVE SHOCK

In distributive shock, the problem is not loss of blood but rather excessive dilation of blood vessels or decreased vascular resistance, causing the blood to be improperly distributed. To demonstrate this point, imagine pouring 5 mL of water into a test tube and another 5 mL into a mixing bowl. The water would nearly fill the test tube, exerting even pressure against the walls of the tube. The water in the mixing bowl, however, might just barely cover the bottom of the bowl. The diameter of the mixing bowl is so large that the water exerts pressure primarily against the container bottom. This example is similar to what happens in the vascular system when the diameter enlarges due to dilation. Fluid pools in the dependent areas of the body and is not returned to the arterial circulation to supply critical cellular metabolic needs. Distributive shock can be complicated by increased capillary permeability, which permits plasma to leak into the interstitial compartment, thereby decreasing intravascular blood volume. The three types of distributive shock are (1) anaphylactic, (2) septic, and (3) neurogenic.

Anaphylactic Shock

Anaphylactic shock occurs when a person has a severe allergic reaction that results in the release of chemicals that dilate blood vessels and increase capillary permeability. Fluid leaks out of the capillaries into the tissues. Pooling of blood in peripheral tissues and the shift of fluid out of the capillaries cause venous return and cardiac output to fall. In addition, the allergic reaction causes constriction of the bronchi and airway obstruction. People can be allergic to many substances, including drugs, vaccines, contrast media, insect bites and stings, foods and food additives, pet dander, molds, and pollens. Insect stings present the greatest number of cases of anaphylaxis. The onset of anaphylaxis is typically sudden and dramatic after exposure to a substance to which the patient has developed antibodies. If untreated, anaphylaxis can result in a shock state with cardiac, renal, pulmonary, and multisystem organ failure.

Septic Shock

Sepsis is a systemic inflammatory response to a documented or suspected infection. Sepsis can progress to septic shock, which is hypotension unresponsive to fluid resuscitation along with signs of inadequate tissue perfusion such as metabolic acidosis, acute encephalopathy, oliguria, or coagulation disorders. Septic shock develops when pathogenic organisms (e.g., bacteria, fungi, viruses, rickettsiae) release toxic substances that cause blood vessels to dilate, thereby decreasing vascular resistance and increasing capillary permeability. The increased permeability results in leakage of plasma proteins and reduced intravascular volume, preload, and cardiac output that contributes to inadequate tissue perfusion and oxygenation as in other shock states. This process is more complex in sepsis, however, as microcirculatory clot formation further compromises perfusion to tissues and cells (Kleinpell, 2012).

The incidence, hospitalization, and mortality rates of patients diagnosed with sepsis makes sepsis one of the leading causes of morbidity and mortality worldwide. Although these statistics are alarming, proof that evidence-based interventions decrease sepsis-related mortality is growing. Initiatives such as the Surviving Sepsis Campaign (SSC), which involves adherence to guidelines and implementing "sepsis bundle" components, can improve patient outcomes (Dellinger et al., 2013). The committee of the SSC is composed of international experts from 30 organizations who published updated guidelines in 2013 designed to increase the early recognition and treatment of sepsis. Additional information on these guidelines and sepsis bundles can be found at www.survivingsepsis.org/.

Neurogenic Shock

Neurogenic shock occurs when a disruption in the nervous system affects the vasomotor center in the medulla. Normally, the vasomotor center initiates sympathetic stimulation of nerve fibers that travel down the spinal cord and out to the periphery where they cause the smooth muscles of the blood vessels to constrict. In neurogenic shock, disruption of sympathetic nerve impulses results in vasodilation or loss of vascular resistance. The patient will have signs and symptoms similar to those just described in the distributive shock syndromes, including pooling of blood in peripheral tissues with subsequent decreased venous return and cardiac output. The classic signs of shock may be absent in neurogenic shock because of the alteration in sympathetic tone resulting in bradycardia and skin that is warm, dry, and pink below the level of spinal cord injury (Chinn, 2013). The most common cause of neurogenic shock is spinal cord injury from trauma or regional anesthesia (Kleinpell, 2012). Other causes of neurogenic shock are disease of the upper spinal cord and depression of the vasomotor center from certain drugs.

EFFECTS OF SHOCK ON BODY SYSTEMS AND FUNCTIONS

- **Respiratory system:** tissue hypoxia and anoxia, respiratory failure, acute respiratory distress syndrome
- **Acid-base balance:** metabolic acidosis
- **Cardiovascular system:** myocardial depression, disseminated intravascular coagulation (widespread clotting caused by sluggish flow of acidic blood combined with bacterial endotoxins or clotting factors released by destruction of red blood cells)
- **Neuroendocrine system:** release of catecholamines (epinephrine and norepinephrine), mineralocorticoids (aldosterone and desoxycorticosterone), glucocorticoids (hydrocortisone), and antidiuretic hormone; decreased level of consciousness when cerebral blood flow falls
- **Hematologic system:** inflammation and coagulation increases clotting and coagulopathy, resulting in peripheral ischemia and necrosis of digits and extremities
- **Integumentary system:** cyanosis may be present but it is a late, unreliable sign; central cyanosis of mucous membranes, nose; cyanosis of nails and earlobes
- **Immune system:** depressed immune response
- **Gastrointestinal system:** decreased peristalsis, ischemia of intestinal submucosa, impaired liver function
- **Renal system:** reduced glomerular filtration, inadequate renal perfusion, tubular necrosis, renal ischemia

STAGES OF SHOCK

Although patient response to shock is individualized, a continuum consisting of four stages has been identified: (1) initiation (2) compensatory (3) progressive, and (4) refractory. Although no clear-cut division between the stages has been found, they appear to occur regardless of the type of shock experienced.

INITIATION STAGE

Shock is initiated by a decrease in the delivery of oxygen, inadequate extraction of oxygen, or both, resulting from one of the types of shock discussed above. There may be no obvious clinical symptoms in this stage other than a decrease in cardiac output if the patient is being monitored invasively.

COMPENSATORY STAGE

The compensatory stage of shock begins when the continued reduction in cardiac output triggers a set of neural, endocrine, and chemical compensatory mechanisms in an effort to overcome the consequences of anaerobic metabolism and maintain blood flow to vital organs. During this stage the following symptoms may become apparent but can be reversed if interventions are begun:

1. Activation of baroreceptors in the carotid arteries and the aorta stimulates the sympathetic nervous system.
2. Sympathetic stimulation causes increased heart rate, constriction of peripheral blood vessels, and reduced blood flow to the kidneys, lungs, muscles, skin, and gastrointestinal tract.
3. Decreasing renal blood flow triggers the release of renin and a sequence of events that produces angiotensin II, a potent vasoconstrictor.
4. The adrenal cortex secretes aldosterone, which promotes sodium retention by the kidneys.
5. Antidiuretic hormone is released by the posterior pituitary, resulting in additional retention of water by the kidneys.
6. Falling blood pH and increasing arterial carbon dioxide are detected by chemoreceptors in the

carotid arteries that stimulate the respiratory center. Increased respiratory rate and depth help to eliminate excess carbon dioxide and normalize the blood pH.

During this stage, the following symptoms may be found on assessment, although shock may be reversed with minimal morbidity if appropriate interventions are initiated (Gallagher, 2009).

- **Mental status:** anxiety, restlessness
- **Blood pressure:** possibly normal initially, decreasing pulse pressure later
- **Pulse:** slight increase in rate progressing to tachycardia; decreased rate (bradycardia) that may be present in neurogenic shock as a result of loss of sympathetic stimulation
- **Respirations:** increased rate and depth
- **Urine output:** decreased to less than 0.5 to 1.0 mL/kg
- **Skin:** cool and pale; *exception:* warm and dry with septic shock
- **Abdomen:** decreased bowel sounds; hypoperfusion and ischemic injury, which can result in translocation of bacteria from the intestine to the circulation with subsequent development of sepsis
- **Blood glucose:** increased
- **Other:** thirst

Table 19-2 summarizes the compensatory mechanisms activated in the first stage of shock.

PROGRESSIVE STAGE

If the cause of shock is not corrected or if compensatory mechanisms continue without reversing the shock, the patient enters the decompensated or progressive stage. Even though the neural, endocrine, and chemical compensatory mechanisms worked together in the early stage, they now begin to function independently and in opposition. In the decompensated or progressive stage of shock, the systemic circulation continues to constrict in the attempt to maintain blood flow to vital organs. The decrease in peripheral blood flow, however, leads to weak or absent pulses and **ischemia** of the extremities. As intravascular blood volume decreases, the blood becomes increasingly viscous (or thick), causing clumping of red blood cells, platelets, and proteins. Deprived of adequate oxygen, cells resort to anaerobic metabolism, which produces lactic acid and results in **metabolic acidosis**, which has a depressant effect on myocardial cells. In septic shock, progression from the hyperdynamic or "warm phase" to the hypodynamic or "cold phase" indicates progression from compensation to decompensation (Gallagher, 2009). Typical assessment findings are as follows:

- **Mental status:** listlessness, confusion
- **Blood pressure:** hypotension, which is the hallmark finding indicating the transition from compensated to decompensated stage
- **Pulse:** weak and thready, tachycardia, dysrhythmias
- **Respirations:** increased, deep, crackles on auscultation
- **Temperature:** subnormal, except with septic shock
- **Urine output:** decreased, possible renal failure
- **Skin:** cold, pale, clammy, slow capillary refill, cyanosis
- **Other:** dry mouth, thirst, sluggish pupillary response, peripheral edema, muscle weakness

Aggressive interventions are necessary in this stage of shock to prevent the development of widespread organ dysfunction.

REFRACTORY STAGE

The final stage of shock is marked by irreversible changes in vital organs as compensatory mechanisms

Table 19-2 Compensatory Mechanisms in Shock

MECHANISM	RESPONSE	BENEFITS
Baroreceptors activate the SNS	Increased heart rate	Speeds delivery of oxygen and nutrients to tissues
	Peripheral vasoconstriction	Shunts blood to vital organs, helps maintain BP
	Constriction of renal arteries	Activates renin-angiotensin-aldosterone system
	Renin-angiotensin-aldosterone system activation (angiotensin is a potent vasoconstrictor)	Vasoconstriction shunts blood to vital organs and helps maintain BP
	Aldosterone causes the kidneys to retain sodium, which induces ADH secretion and water retention	Fluid retention increases blood volume by decreasing urine output
Chemoreceptors in the carotid arteries respond to acidic blood pH and increased arterial carbon dioxide by stimulating the respiratory center	Increased respiratory rate and depth	Helps eliminate the excess carbon dioxide and normalize the blood pH; takes in additional oxygen

ADH, Antidiuretic hormone; *BP,* blood pressure; *SNS,* sympathetic nervous system.

fail. Tissue perfusion deteriorates, as blood remains pooled in the capillary bed, where clumping and the formation of clots further compromise sluggish flow. Coronary artery perfusion is reduced, causing ischemia and dysrhythmias. Cerebral ischemia occurs as a result of the decrease in cerebral blood flow. Death is imminent. Even patients who are resuscitated during this stage often die within a week or two from widespread organ dysfunction. Assessment findings in the irreversible stage include the following:

- **Mental status:** loss of consciousness
- **Blood pressure:** systolic continuing to fall, diastolic approaching zero
- **Pulse:** progressive slowing, irregular
- **Respirations:** slow, shallow, irregular
- **Urine output:** minimal
- **Skin:** cold, clammy, cyanosis

DIAGNOSIS

A diagnosis of shock is based on the health history and physical examination. Tests and procedures that help to establish the type of shock, the stage, and the cause include blood and urine studies, measurement of hemodynamic pressures, chest radiograph, electrocardiographic and continuous cardiac monitoring, pulse oximetry and arterial blood gases, and urine output.

FIRST AID FOR SHOCK OUTSIDE THE MEDICAL FACILITY

Treatment that is provided to patients in shock before medical care is available can have a significant impact on the chances of survival. The overall goal of treatment is restoration and maintenance of oxygen delivery to the tissues. Essential to this process is a systematic approach to patient assessment to determine life-threatening issues with initial interventions based on these findings. Employing a modified application of the ABC—airway, breathing, circulation—approach is recommended (Gallagher, 2009). The *Healthy People 2020* objectives identify the necessity for both increasing public awareness of how and whom to call for emergency assistance and providing education on initial life-saving procedures to be followed until emergency responders arrive. Box 19-1 describes emergency first-aid care.

Box 19-1 Assessment in First Aid for the Patient in Shock

DATA COLLECTION

Pulse
Rapid and weak, "thready"

Respirations
Air hunger initially, then increased rate; shallow

Blood Pressure
Stable initially, then decreased

Skin
Cool and moist at first; diaphoresis; later, cyanosis of lips and nail beds

Mental Status
Restless, then listless; confused; unconscious

Thirst
Increased

INTERVENTIONS

- Summon medical assistance.
- Establish or maintain patent airway.
- Control external bleeding with direct pressure or pressure dressing.
- Maintain blood flow to the brain.
- Keep still and quiet.
- Position flat; legs may be elevated unless the shock is caused by heart failure, the head or neck is bleeding, injury is possible, intracranial pressure is increased, or the patient has dyspnea.
- Protect the patient from cold but do not overheat (patient should not shiver or perspire).
- Even if the patient complains of thirst, withhold oral fluids in case surgical intervention is needed.
- Tell the patient what actions are being taken, that someone will stay with him or her, and that help is coming.

GENERAL MEDICAL TREATMENT

General medical interventions for the patient in shock are directed toward maintaining perfusion of vital organs until the cause is found and treated. Care is directed toward correcting or reversing the altered circulatory component or components, including blood volume, myocardial contractility, blood flow, and vascular resistance, in addition to improving oxygen delivery to the cells. Interventions to increase oxygen delivery and a combination of fluid, pharmacologic, and mechanical therapies are implemented to maintain tissue perfusion.

OXYGENATION

Maintaining a patent airway and improving tissue oxygenation are priorities. Proper head position is maintained and use of appropriate airways or intubation may be indicated, depending on the patient's condition. Oxygen is administered by methods ranging from nasal cannula to mechanical ventilation. In addition to standard assessment of respiratory rate, pattern, and quality of breath sounds, adjuncts such as pulse oximetry, end-tidal carbon dioxide monitoring, and positive end expiratory pressure may be used to determine and enhance adequate oxygenation (Kleinpell, 2012). Prompt treatment of pain, agitation, fever, or other underlying causes of unnecessary oxygen consumption is essential. Paralytics, sedatives, and analgesics may be ordered to decrease oxygen requirements.

FLUID REPLACEMENT

Shock results in major alterations in fluid balance. Patients experiencing hypovolemic or distributive shock require administration of intravenous (IV) fluids to restore intravascular volume and adequate tissue perfusion. In general, aggressive fluid administration is not routinely indicated for patients in cardiogenic shock, as large volumes of fluid may further compromise a failing heart.

After IV access is established, a fluid challenge consisting of rapid administration of 250 mL of a crystalloid solution may be administered to assess the patient's hemodynamic response to fluid administration. Nursing responsibilities at this time may include obtaining hemodynamic measurements, administering the fluid challenge, and assessing the patient's response.

The administration of additional fluids depends on the cause of volume deficit, the patient's status, and the physician's preference. Normal saline may be administered initially. Subsequent fluids may include various crystalloids and colloids depending on the situation. The optimal choice of resuscitation fluid in the critically ill is constantly debated. Crystalloids provide replacement water and electrolytes for all fluid compartments. Colloids, such as albumin, remain in the vascular system and draw fluid into the bloodstream, thereby increasing circulatory volume, but are more expensive. A recent systematic review found no evidence to support the use of colloids over crystalloids in critically ill patients (Perel et al., 2013).

Patient response must be monitored closely during fluid replacement to ensure adequate but not excessive replacement. Fluid replacement is best determined by monitoring pulmonary artery wedge pressure, cardiac output, and urine output. Generally, volume replacement continues until a mean arterial pressure of 60 mm Hg or greater is attained and evidence of adequate tissue perfusion is noted. Once sufficient fluids have been administered, an inotropic agent may be ordered to increase myocardial contractility.

PHARMACOLOGIC THERAPY

Pharmacologic interventions for the patient in shock are based on management of the cardiac dynamics: contractility, preload, afterload, and heart rate. Although no single drug will provide nutrients and oxygen to the cells, several agents have been developed that assist in manipulation of the four circulatory components, thus improving the availability of these vital components (Table 19-3).

MECHANICAL MANAGEMENT

The management of shock may also include the use of mechanical devices that assist in the restoration of cellular perfusion (Fig. 19-1). These devices are listed in Table 19-4.

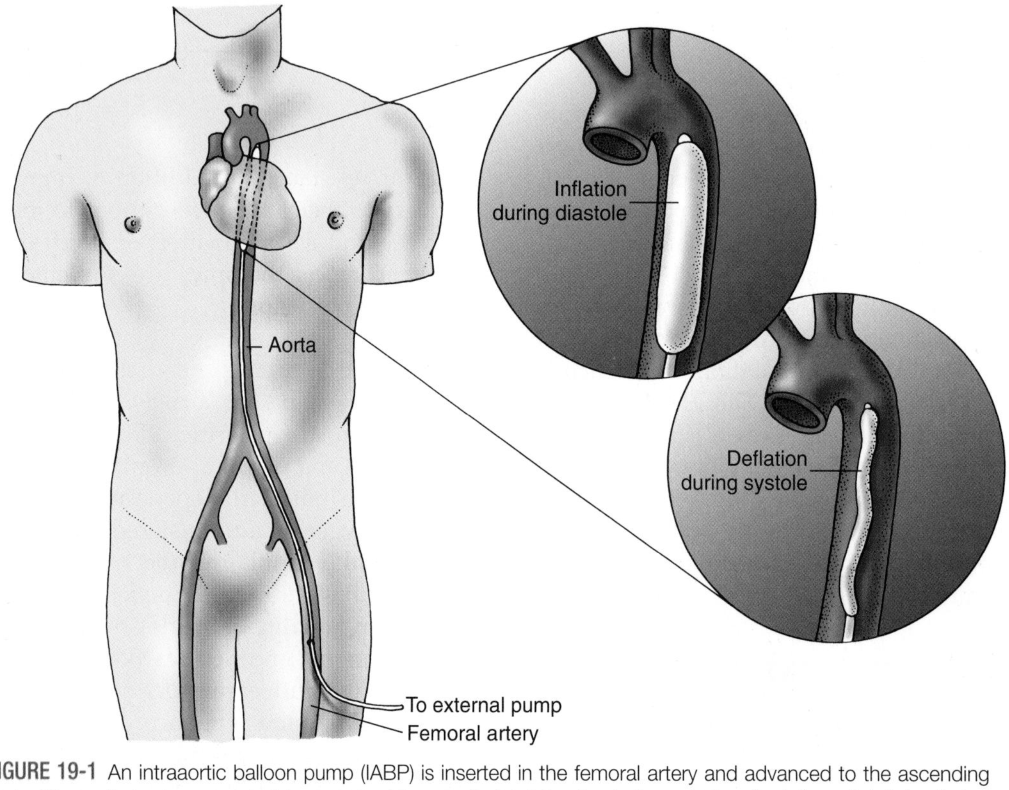

FIGURE 19-1 An intraaortic balloon pump (IABP) is inserted in the femoral artery and advanced to the ascending aorta. The catheter is connected to an external pump that inflates the balloon during diastole and deflates it during systole. (From Black JM, Hawks JH, Keene AM: *Medical-surgical nursing: clinical management for continuity of care*, ed 6, Philadelphia, 2001, Saunders.)

Table 19-3 Drug Therapy: Medications Commonly Used in Shock

DRUG	ACTION	TYPE OF SHOCK	INDICATIONS	SIDE EFFECTS	NURSING IMPLICATIONS
Dopamine (action is dose dependent)	Renal vasodilation Positive inotropic at low to moderate dosage Vasopressor at high dosage	Cardiogenic	↑ Myocardial contractility ↑ Afterload ↑ BP when not caused by hypovolemia	↑ HR, dysrhythmias ↑ MVO_2 Nausea, vomiting	Monitor BP at least every 15 min Administer with IV pump Should be tapered gradually If IV infiltrates, may cause sloughing
Dobutamine	Positive inotropic	Cardiogenic with severe systolic dysfunction Septic with normal CO_2 that is not meeting metabolic demands	↑ BP in low CO_2 states	↑ HR, dysrhythmias ↑ MVO_2 Headache, tremors, nausea	Monitor BP at least every 15 min Administer with IV pump Should be tapered gradually
Norepinephrine	Vasopressor; some inotropic effects	Cardiogenic after myocardial infarction Septic (increases vascular resistance)	↑ Afterload ↑ BP refractory to other drugs	↑ MVO_2 Dysrhythmias Severe nausea	Monitor BP at least every 15 min Administer with IV pump Should be tapered gradually If IV infiltrates, may cause sloughing
Epinephrine	Vasopressor Bronchodilator	Cardiogenic combined with afterload reduction Anaphylactic	↑ HR, BP Bronchodilation	Chest pain Dysrhythmias Tremors Headache	Monitor BP at least every 15 min Monitor for HR >110 bpm Monitor for dyspnea, pulmonary edema
Nitroglycerin	Vasodilator	Cardiogenic	↓ Preload Pump failure	Headache Hypotension Bradycardia	Monitor BP at least every 15 min Administer with IV pump Should be tapered gradually Use glass or nonabsorbable container and special IV tubing
Nitroprusside	Vasodilator	Cardiogenic with ↑ SVR	↓ Preload and afterload	Myocardial ischemia Hypotension Nausea	Monitor BP at least every 15 min Administer with IV pump Should be tapered gradually Protect from light Monitor patient for cyanide toxicity (tinnitus, hyperreflexia, seizures)
Vasopressin	Vasoconstrictor	Cardiogenic Septic	↑ BP ↑ SVR ↑ Myocardial contractility BP unresponsive to catecholamines	Diaphoresis Tremors Nausea, vomiting ↓ CO_2 Bradycardia	Monitor BP at least every 15 min Administer with IV pump

Adapted from Sole M, Klein D, Moseley, M: *Introduction to critical care nursing*, ed 6, St. Louis, 2013, Saunders Elsevier; and Dellinger RP, Levy MM, Rhodes A, et al: Surviving sepsis campaign: international guidelines for management of severe sepsis and septic shock: 2012. *Crit Care Med* 2013; 41:580-637.

BP, Blood pressure; *bpm,* beats per minute; *CO_2,* carbon dioxide; *HR,* heart rate; *IV,* intravenous; *MVO_2,* myocardial oxygen consumption; *SVR,* systemic vascular resistance.

Table 19-4 Mechanical Devices Used in the Treatment of Shock

DEVICE	DESCRIPTION	PURPOSE
Hypothermic devices—Thermo Suit	Maintains body temperature at 33°C; circulates ice water in direct contact with patient's skin.	May improve neurologic recovery after cardiac arrest of cardiac origin.
Intraaortic balloon pump (IABP)	A balloon-tipped catheter is inserted into the descending thoracic aorta. The balloon inflates during diastole and deflates just before systole.	Reduces preload with cardiogenic shock. Heart pumps more efficiently; increases cardiac output.
Ventricular assist devices (VADs)	Various devices include pulsatile and nonpulsatile pumps, external and implantable devices.	Decreases myocardial workload and oxygen demand. Supports circulation until the heart recovers or is replaced.
Extracorporeal membrane oxygenation (ECMO)	Blood is removed from the inferior vena cava, oxygenated, and returned via the femoral artery.	Used for short-term stabilization.

Put on Your Thinking Cap!

Three patients are in the emergency department. All of them are in the compensatory stage of shock. Patient A is in hypovolemic shock. Patient B is in cardiogenic shock. Patient C is in septic shock.

1. What assessment finding would you expect in Patient C but not in Patient A or B?
2. For which patient or patients would colloid intravenous fluids be contraindicated? Why?
3. Which patient would you expect to have a history of:
   a. Coronary artery disease
   b. Severe vomiting and diarrhea
   c. Urinary tract infection

NURSING CARE of the Patient in Shock

Assessment

Assessment of the patient who is at risk for shock should include continuous monitoring of cardiac rate and rhythm; blood pressure; body temperature; hemodynamic values; respiratory rate, rhythm, and depth; and arterial blood gases. In the routine nursing assessment, observe the color of the skin and palpate for skin warmth and moisture. Note pupil size, equality, and response to light. Describe the patient's level of consciousness and response to commands and assess reflexes. Auscultate heart, lung, and bowel sounds. Observe the movement of the chest wall with respirations. Inspect and palpate the abdomen for distention. Palpate for bladder distention and note the appearance of urine and the hourly output. Inspect the extremities for color and palpate for peripheral pulses and edema. Inspect intravenous infusion sites for pallor, swelling, or coolness that suggests extravasation.

Nursing Diagnosis

The primary nursing diagnosis for all patients in shock is Ineffective Peripheral Tissue Perfusion. This diagnosis may be related to one or more alterations in circulating blood volume, myocardial contractility, blood flow, or vascular resistance.

Interventions

Ineffective Peripheral Tissue Perfusion

Your continuous assessment must include all body systems because shock, if not corrected, eventually results in failure of all major organs. Specific organ failures are addressed here under other nursing diagnoses.

Decreased Cardiac Output

Administer intravenous fluids as ordered and assess for both fluid volume deficit and fluid volume excess. With cardiogenic shock, monitoring hemodynamic parameters is especially important. Administer inotropic and antidysrhythmic agents as ordered. Continuous cardiac monitoring enables you to assess the effectiveness of these drugs. You can reduce oxygen requirements by handling the patient gently and coordinating care to allow for rest. Maintain adequate body heat to prevent shivering, which also increases metabolic (and circulatory) demands. Fever may be treated with acetaminophen or nonsteroidal antiinflammatory drugs. In some situations, a tepid sponge bath or a cooling blanket is ordered.

Acute Confusion and Anxiety

As patients progress through the stages of shock, they may be anxious, then confused and disoriented, and finally unconscious. For the anxious patient, you must remain calm and give simple explanations of what actions are being taken. Remember that the intensive care environment is foreign and frightening to most people. As much as possible, protect the patient from constant, excessive noise and light.

Protect confused patients from harm. Repeat orientation, instructions, and reassurance often. In the

Nursing Diagnoses, Goals, and Outcome Criteria: Shock (General)

Goals and Nursing Diagnoses	Outcome Criteria
Ineffective Peripheral Tissue Perfusion related to decreased blood volume (hypovolemic shock); decreased myocardial contractility (cardiogenic shock); impaired circulatory blood flow (obstructive shock); widespread vasodilation (distributive shock)	Normal tissue perfusion: urine output at least 0.5 mL/kg/h, patient alert and oriented, normal heart rate and rhythm, normal blood pressure, active bowel sounds, extremities warm with palpable pulses
Decreased Cardiac Output related to hypovolemia, peripheral vasodilation, myocardial disorders	Normal cardiac output: normal hemodynamic values, vital signs consistent with patient norms, mental alertness
Acute Confusion related to inadequate cerebral perfusion, metabolic acidosis	Improved orientation: patient alert and oriented, responds to commands appropriately, behaves appropriately
Deficient Fluid Volume related to hemorrhage, inadequate fluid intake, excessive fluid loss	Normal fluid balance: vital signs consistent with patient norms, capillary refill in 3 to 5 seconds
Anxiety related to hypoxia, life-threatening situation	Reduced anxiety: patient calm, states is less anxious
Risk for Injury related to confusion, adverse effects of drugs, invasive treatments	Absence of injury: no trauma
Risk for Infection related to trauma, invasive therapeutic procedures	Absence of infection: body temperature within normal range, normal white blood cell count
Disabled or Compromised Family Coping related to anxiety, uncertainty of patient's outcome	Effective coping: family members are supportive of the patient and each other and indicate that they have adequate resources to cope with present situation

presence of unconscious patients, remember that they may hear even when they cannot respond. Continue to speak to the patient and beware of negative comments made in the patient's presence.

Deficient Fluid Volume

Monitor for hypovolemia (tachycardia, hypotension, tachypnea, decreased urine output, decreased central venous pressure and pulmonary artery pressure). Administer intravenous fluids cautiously while assessing output of urine. Notify the physician if urine output falls below 0.5 mL/kg/h because low urine output may signal inadequate fluid replacement or renal failure, or both. Assess for fluid overload, especially with renal impairment and with intravenous colloids. Signs and symptoms of overload include full, bounding pulse; dilute urine; increased respiratory rate; abnormal lung sounds; dyspnea; and edema.

Risk for Injury

In addition to the risk for injury related to changes in consciousness, the patient in shock can be harmed by the therapeutic measures being used. For example, antidysrhythmics can depress cardiac activity, anticoagulants can permit excessive bleeding, and extravasation of vasopressors (drugs that raise blood pressure by vasoconstriction) can cause local tissue necrosis. Therefore you must closely monitor the patient for both therapeutic and adverse effects of drugs used to treat the patient in shock.

Because of poor peripheral tissue perfusion and the need to minimize activity, the patient in shock is at high risk for complications of immobility. Institute measures to prevent prolonged pressure on susceptible sites. Pressure ulcers can develop very rapidly. In addition, personal hygiene may be limited by the patient's tolerance of such activity. A partial bath and gentle range-of-motion activities may be provided if the patient is stable enough. Mouth care provides some comfort and helps to prevent cracking of the lips and dryness of the oral mucosa. Apply water-soluble lubricant to the lips and moisten the mouth with normal saline. Brushing teeth with a soft toothbrush is recommended.

> **Put on Your Thinking Cap!**
>
> Why would a vasopressor be harmful to surrounding tissues if it leaked out of the vein?

Risk for Infection

Intravenous lines, indwelling urinary catheters, chest tubes, airways, ventricular assist devices, and other equipment provide avenues for infection in the patient in shock. The risk of infection is greatest in very young, very old, and immunocompromised patients. To reduce the risk of infection, wash your hands thoroughly between patients. Follow agency guidelines for care of intravenous and urinary catheters. Use aseptic technique when inserting these devices, caring for insertion sites, and providing wound care. Monitor for signs of infection (elevated body temperature and white blood cell count; redness, swelling, and warmth of wounds and tube insertion sites; purulent drainage; abnormal breath sounds; and yellow or green sputum). When antibiotics are ordered, administer them on schedule to maintain a therapeutic blood level. Oral care, including tooth brushing, is essential to reduce the accumulation and colonization of dental plaque that can result in health care–associated infection risk (Kleinpell, 2012).

Disabled or Compromised Family Coping

The patient in shock often may have one or more family members present. Members of the health care team should be sensitive to the family's needs for information and support (see *Cultural Considerations* box). You can explain the nursing care and encourage family members to ask questions. Offer the services of a counselor or patient representative.

Table 19-5 summarizes the interventions for each type of shock.

> **Cultural Considerations**
>
> **What Does Culture Have to Do with Shock?**
>
> A Japanese or Vietnamese family would expect to participate in patient care or to remain at the bedside. Extended families may gather to be near the patient and to support one another. In Mexico, important decisions may be deferred to male relatives in traditional families. In Italy, patients and families would not discuss a fatal prognosis before death. In many cultures, rituals related to illness and death are very important to the patient and the family.

SYSTEMIC INFLAMMATORY RESPONSE SYNDROME

Inflammation is a normal response to tissue injury. However, in certain clinical situations, generalized inflammation that threatens vital organs occurs. This

Table 19-5 Interventions for Each Type of Shock

CAUSE	CLINICAL SITUATION	INTERVENTION*
Blood loss	Massive trauma Gastrointestinal bleeding Ruptured aortic aneurysm Surgery Erosion of vessel from lesion, tubes, or other devices DIC	Stop external bleeding with direct pressure, pressure dressing, tourniquet (as last resort) Reduce intraabdominal or retroperitoneal bleeding or prepare for emergency surgery Administer lactated Ringer solution or normal saline Transfuse with fresh whole blood, packed cells, fresh-frozen plasma, platelets, or other clotting factors, if significant improvement does not occur with crystalloid administration Conduct autotransfusion if appropriate Use of non–blood plasma expanders or colloids remains controversial
Plasma loss	Burns Accumulation of intraabdominal fluid Malnutrition Severe dermatitis DIC	Administer low-dose cardiotonics (dopamine, dobutamine) Administer lactated Ringer solution or Plasma-Lyte Use of 5% albumin, fresh-frozen plasma, and dextran are possible
Crystalloid loss	Dehydration (e.g., diabetic ketoacidosis, heat exhaustion)	Administer isotonic or hypotonic saline with electrolytes as needed to maintain normal circulating volume and electrolyte balance
Myocardial disease or injury	Acute myocardial infarction Myocardial contusion Cardiomyopathies	Fluid challenge with up to 300 mL of normal saline solution or lactated Ringer solution to rule out hypovolemia, unless heart failure or pulmonary edema is present Vasodilators (e.g., sodium nitroprusside, nitroglycerin, calcium channel blockers, morphine) Diuretics (e.g., mannitol or furosemide) Cardiotonics (e.g., digitalis) Beta-blockers (e.g., propranolol) Intraaortic balloon pump, ventricular assist device, or extracorporeal life support may be used Reperfusion interventions, including percutaneous transluminal angioplasty or coronary artery bypass graft Thrombolysis for treatment of myocardial infarction depends on timely drug delivery to the clot
Valvular disease or injury	Ruptured aortic cusp Ruptured papillary muscle Ball thrombus	Same as above: if rapid response does not occur, prepare for prompt cardiac surgery

Table 19-5 **Interventions for Each Type of Shock—cont'd**

CAUSE	CLINICAL SITUATION	INTERVENTION*
External pressure on heart interferes with heart filling or emptying	Pericardial tamponade caused by trauma, aneurysm, cardiac surgery, pericarditis Massive pulmonary embolus Tension pneumothorax Hemoperitoneum Mechanical ventilation	Relieve tamponade with ECG-assisted pericardiocentesis; surgical repair if it recurs Thrombolytic (streptokinase) or anticoagulant (heparin) therapy; surgery for removal of clot Relieve air accumulation with needle thoracostomy or chest tube insertion Relieve fluid accumulation with paracentesis Reduce inspiratory pressure
Cardiac dysrhythmias	Tachydysrhythmias Bradydysrhythmias Pulseless electrical activity	Treat dysrhythmias; be prepared to initiate CPR, cardiac pacing
Anaphylactic shock	Allergy to food, medicines, dyes, insect bites, stings, or latex	Prepare for surgical management of airway Decrease further absorption of antigen (e.g., stop IV fluid, place tourniquet between injection or sting site and heart if feasible) Epinephrine (1 : 100) per inhalation *or* Epinephrine (1 : 1000) subcutaneously, *or* Epinephrine (1 : 10,000) intravenous infusion IV fluid resuscitation with isotonic solution Diphenhydramine HCl or H_1-receptor antagonist IV Theophylline IV drip for bronchospasm Steroids IV Vasopressors (e.g., norepinephrine, metaraminol bitartrate, high-dose dopamine) Gastric lavage for ingested antigen Ice pack to injection or sting site Meat tenderizer paste to sting site
Septic shock	Often gram-negative septicemia but also caused by other organisms in debilitated, immunodeficient, or chronically ill clients	Identify origin of sepsis; culture all suspected sources Vigorous IV fluid resuscitation with normal saline Empirical antibiotic therapy until sensitivities are reported Administer vasopressors (e.g., norepinephrine, epinephrine, vasopressin, dopamine [only in selected patients as alternative to norepinephrine]) Dobutamine may be used in selected patients Corticosteroid use in selected patients IV insulin to maintain serum glucose at or less than 180 mg/dL DVT prophylaxis with low-molecular-weight heparin in severe sepsis Temperature control (both hypothermia and hyperthermia are noted) Platelet administration considered in severe sepsis when counts $<10{,}000/mm^3$
Neurogenic (spinal) shock	Spinal anesthesia Spinal cord injury	Normal saline to restore volume Treat bradycardia with atropine Vasopressors (e.g., norepinephrine, metaraminol bitartrate, high-dose dopamine, and phenylephrine) may be given Place client in modified Trendelenburg position Place client in a head-down or recumbent position
Vasovagal reaction	Severe pain Severe emotional stress	Place client in a head-down or recumbent position Atropine if bradycardia and profound hypotension; eliminate pain

CPR, Cardiopulmonary resuscitation; *DIC,* disseminated intravascular coagulation; *DVT,* deep vein thrombosis; *ECG,* electrocardiography; *IV,* intravenous.
*Assumes that airway management and cardiac monitoring are ongoing.

state is called **systemic inflammatory response syndrome (SIRS)**. In addition to shock, some of the conditions that can lead to SIRS are multiple transfusions, massive tissue injury, burns, and pancreatitis.

The effects of SIRS include damage to the endothelium of blood vessels and a hypermetabolic state. Damaged endothelium increases capillary permeability, allowing fluid to leak into body tissues. Hypotension, microemboli, and shunting of blood flow compromise organ perfusion. The hypermetabolic state is characterized by increased serum glucose, which eventually depletes carbohydrate, fat, and protein stores.

A diagnosis of SIRS is made when a patient exhibits two or more of the following symptoms:

- Temperature less than 97°F (36°C) or more than 100.4°F (38°C)
- Heart rate more than 90 beats per minute (bpm)
- Respiratory rate more than 20 breaths/min or arterial pressure of carbon dioxide less than 32 mm Hg
- White blood cell count less than 4000 cells/μl or more than 12,000 cells/μl or more than 10% immature (band) neutrophils

Manifestations of SIRS range from mild to severe. The term **sepsis** is used when a patient has two or more of the symptoms mentioned above and a known or suspected infection. With advanced SIRS and failure of more than one organ, deterioration of the cardiac, pulmonary, renal, and central nervous systems; liver; pancreas; and gastrointestinal tract occurs. Thrombocytopenia may develop and progress to disseminated intravascular coagulation.

When more than one organ begins to fail as a result of SIRS, the patient is said to have **multiple organ dysfunction syndrome (MODS)**. A recent review indicated that there was a 71% increase in the number of hospitalizations for severe sepsis between 2003 and 2007 and, among these, an increased number of patients diagnosed with three or more organ dysfunctions (Lagu et al., 2012).

MEDICAL TREATMENT AND NURSING INTERVENTIONS

A discussion of detailed care of the patient with SIRS and MODS is beyond the scope of this text but early detection or prevention is important, given that no specific treatment exists once SIRS or MODS occurs. Again, adherence to the guidelines and interventions developed by the SSC and the Institute for Healthcare Improvement are recommended for treatment of SIRS and MODS. They include initial resuscitation, management of infection, hemodynamic support, and other selective and supportive interventions, including mechanical ventilation, sedation, deep vein thrombosis and stress ulcer prophylaxis, glucose control, and renal replacement therapy (Kleinpell, 2012).

Prevent and Treat Infection

Prevention and early identification of sepsis may enable prompt treatment and prevention of SIRS or MODS. The following have been identified as priority prevention measures: monitor potential infection sites and assess for signs and symptoms of infection; maintain strict asepsis with invasive procedures and equipment; exercise scrupulous hand washing; provide frequent oral care including tooth brushing (decontamination with oral chlorhexidine gluconate is suggested to reduce the risk of ventilator-associated pneumonia in patients with severe sepsis); position the patient in the semirecumbent position, if tolerated, as this may reduce ventilator-associated pneumonia; administer antimicrobials as ordered; and administer enteral feedings as ordered to enhance perfusion of the gastrointestinal tract (Kleinpell et al., 2013).

Maintain Tissue Oxygenation

Administer sedatives and analgesics as ordered to reduce oxygen requirements. Monitor the patient on mechanical ventilation. Administer drugs to improve cardiac output and tissue perfusion as ordered. Plan care to minimize physical demands on the patient.

Provide Nutritional and Metabolic Support

Provide enteral or parenteral nutrition as ordered (see the *Nutrition Considerations* box). Monitor blood glucose and weight.

Nutrition Considerations

1. Hypermetabolism in shock causes protein-calorie malnutrition.
2. Early enteral feedings for all patients who are unable to consume adequate calories orally is thought to (1) prevent and treat shock, (2) improve perfusion of the gastrointestinal tract, and (3) reduce the movement of bacteria through the intestinal walls into the bloodstream.
3. Nutritional status of the patient in shock is assessed by monitoring serum protein, nitrogen balance, blood urea nitrogen, serum glucose, and serum electrolytes.

Support Failing Organs

Examples of measures to support failing organs include mechanical ventilation for respiratory distress syndrome and replacement therapy for renal failure.

Get Ready for the NCLEX® Examination!

Key Points

- Shock is a state of acute circulatory failure and impaired tissue perfusion.
- Untreated shock progresses to SIRS and then to MODS or death.
- The types of shock are hypovolemic, cardiogenic, obstructive, and distributive.
- Hypovolemic shock results from inadequate circulating blood volume.
- Cardiogenic shock occurs when the heart fails as a pump.
- Obstructive shock occurs when physical impairment of adequate circulating blood flow occurs.
- Distributive shock results from the excessive dilation of blood vessels or decreased vascular resistance that causes blood to be improperly distributed.
- The three types of distributive shock are anaphylactic, septic, and neurogenic.
- Compensatory responses to shock represent neurologic, endocrine, and chemical stimulation intended to maintain blood flow to vital organs.
- In the progressive stage of shock, continued vasoconstriction deprives the extremities of blood, blood thickens, and cells must resort to anaerobic metabolism, which leads to acidosis.
- The final stage of shock is marked by irreversible changes in vital organs; death is imminent.
- Because brain cells begin to die within 4 minutes without oxygen, a priority in the first-aid treatment of shock is to maintain blood flow to the brain.
- Positioning of the patient is dependent on the type of shock identified and is somewhat controversial.
- Except for cardiogenic shock, all types of shock may require significant fluid volume replacement.
- Normal saline is usually administered first followed by various crystalloids. Administration of colloids remains controversial but they may be used.
- The physician should be notified if urine output falls below 0.5 mL/kg/h.
- Assessment of the patient in shock includes monitoring of vital signs, hemodynamic values, respiratory status, and arterial blood gases.
- General nursing diagnoses for the patient in shock include Ineffective Peripheral Tissue Perfusion, Decreased Cardiac Output, Acute Confusion, Anxiety, Deficient Fluid Volume, Risk for Injury, Risk for Infection, and Disabled or Compromised Family Coping.
- SIRS is generalized inflammation that damages the lining of blood vessels and creates a hypermetabolic state.
- Failure of more than one organ as a result of SIRS is called MODS; failure of three or more organs presents a very poor prognosis.
- The goals of care with SIRS and MODS are to prevent and treat infection, maintain tissue oxygenation, provide nutritional and metabolic support, and support individual failing organs.

Additional Learning Resources

SG Go to your Study Guide for additional learning activities to help you master this chapter content.

evolve Go to your Evolve website (http://evolve.elsevier.com/Linton/medsurg) for the following learning resources and much more:

- Interactive Prioritization Exercises
- Fluid & Electrolyte Tutorial
- Pharmacology Tutorial
- Review Questions for the NCLEX® Examination

Review Questions for the NCLEX® Examination

1. A patient has developed peritonitis after a traumatic injury to the abdomen. The nurse knows that this patient is at greatest risk for which type of shock?
   1. Cardiogenic
   2. Anaphylactic
   3. Neurogenic
   4. Hypovolemic

   NCLEX Client Need: Physiological Integrity: Reduction of Risk Potential
2. A patient is admitted to the emergency department in distributive shock. Which of the following factors can lead to distributive shock? (Select all that apply.)
   1. Bacterial infection
   2. Blood or fluid loss
   3. Dilation of blood vessels
   4. An antigen-antibody reaction
   5. Failure of the heart as a pump

   NCLEX Client Need: Physiological Integrity: Physiological Adaptation
3. A patient in anaphylactic shock has massive edema. What would explain this condition?
   1. Increased capillary permeability
   2. Pooling of blood in dependent parts of the body
   3. Retention of excess water by the kidneys
   4. Overproduction of antidiuretic hormone

   NCLEX Client Need: Physiological Integrity: Physiological Adaptation
4. What do anaphylactic shock, septic shock, and neurogenic shock have in common?
   1. Infection
   2. Allergic reactions
   3. Vasodilation
   4. Heart failure

   NCLEX Client Need: Physiological Integrity: Physiological Adaptation
5. Which acid-base disturbance should the nurse anticipate with the intermediate or progressive stage of shock?
   1. Metabolic alkalosis
   2. Respiratory alkalosis
   3. Metabolic acidosis
   4. Respiratory acidosis

   NCLEX Client Need: Physiological Integrity: Reduction of Risk Potential

6. The nurse is concerned about cerebral perfusion in a patient who is in shock. Which assessment provides the best indicator of cerebral perfusion?
   1. Presence of reflexes
   2. Level of consciousness
   3. Emotional state
   4. Mean arterial pressure

   NCLEX Client Need: Physiological Integrity: Physiological Adaptation
7. When patients have lost large amounts of plasma proteins, which fluid is most appropriate for restoring blood volume?
   1. Packed red blood cells
   2. Crystalloid fluids
   3. Normal saline
   4. Colloids

   NCLEX Client Need: Physiological Integrity: Pharmacological Therapies
8. What is the most common cause of cardiogenic shock?
   1. Pancreatitis
   2. Anaphylaxis
   3. Acute myocardial infarction
   4. Gastrointestinal bleed

   NCLEX Client Need: Physiological Integrity: Physiological Adaptation
9. A patient in shock has been given blood, crystalloids, and osmotic fluids. The nurse's assessment reveals: pulse rate 80 bpm, bounding, regular; respiratory rate 30 breaths/min; blood pressure 140/86 mm Hg; dyspnea and crackles throughout lung fields. Which complication should the nurse suspect?
   1. Sepsis
   2. Multiple organ failure
   3. Pneumonia
   4. Circulatory overload

   NCLEX Client Need: Physiological Integrity: Physiological Adaptation
10. Which interventions reduce the risk of SIRS and MOD in a patient with pancreatitis? (Select all that apply.)
    1. Maintain strict asepsis with invasive procedures
    2. Provide frequent oral care with chlorhexidine gluconate
    3. Position the patient in high Fowler position
    4. Practice scrupulous hand washing
    5. Administer enteral feedings as ordered

    NCLEX Client Need: Physiological Integrity: Basic Care and Comfort

chapter 20

Falls

http://evolve.elsevier.com/Linton/medsurg

Objectives

1. Define *falls*.
2. State the incidence of falls.
3. Describe factors that increase the risk of falls.
4. Discuss the relationship between restraint use and falls, types of restraints, and regulations for restraint use.
5. Describe fall prevention techniques in acute care and long-term care and the home.
6. Describe nursing interventions to use when a fall occurs.
7. Explain what is meant by *least restrictive* interventions for fall prevention.

Key Terms

Chemical restraint
Extrinsic factors
Fall
Intrinsic factors
Omnibus Budget Reconciliation Act (OBRA)
Physical restraint

If you were to ask several people whether they had fallen in the past 6 months, the chances are that many would say "yes." The chances are even greater that those who have fallen, particularly the young and healthy adults, have not sustained a significant injury. Although falls do not necessarily result in serious physical injuries or death, many older people who have fallen become less confident in their ability to function independently. Those who fear falling tend to restrict their physical and social activities, become more dependent, and have an increased need for long-term care (LTC). In addition, caregivers tend to restrict older persons' activities out of the concern that ill or frail people who have been weakened from sickness, hospitalization, or inactivity may fall and be injured.

DEFINITION OF FALLS

The Hartford Institute for Geriatric Nursing (2008) defines an actual **fall** as "an unexpected event in which the participant comes to rest on the ground, floor, or lower level."

INCIDENCE AND RISK FACTORS

Although falls and fall-related injuries occur at every age, the greater severity of injuries in old age, combined with longer recovery periods, makes a fall a particularly serious threat to the health and functioning of older people.

The risk of injury from falls is highest in people over 75 years of age and falls are the most frequent cause of accidental injury and death among older adults. It is estimated that one in three community-dwelling older adults fall each year, with less than half of those incidents reported to health care providers. Twenty percent to 30% of falls result in serious injury, including traumatic brain injury and fractures. Whereas older adults constitute only 12% to 13% of the total U.S. population, they account for 72% of deaths as a result of falls. More than 20,000 older Americans died as a result of falls in 2009.

The U.S. Public Health Service (USPHS) has estimated that two thirds of the deaths as a result of falls are preventable. Potentially avoidable environmental factors cause about half of fatal falls. According to the USPHS, adequate medical evaluation and treatment for underlying medical conditions probably could prevent most of the remaining fatal falls.

Falling is not a normal part of aging. However, older adults are at particular risk for accidents because of predisposing and precipitating factors that are more common in older adults. Falls occur because of two major factors: (1) **intrinsic factors**, or factors related to the functioning of the individual; and (2) **extrinsic factors**, or environmental factors. Intrinsic factors enhance the possibility of falling whereas extrinsic factors enhance the opportunity to fall.

Intrinsic factors related to falls include sensory impairments such as reduced vision and hearing, changes in posture and gait, confusion, depression, lack of exercise leading to weakness, urge or stress urinary incontinence, acute infections, neurologic conditions that affect balance, and overestimation of abilities. In addition, the medications that many older adults take for various chronic illnesses may cause dizziness or drowsiness.

Extrinsic factors may differ according to the setting. For example, potential hazards in the home environment include low-lying and poorly visible tables, trailing electrical wires, pets, steep and unlit stairs, loose carpeting, throw rugs, unsafe walking aids, and inconvenient bathroom or kitchen arrangements. Falls occurring in the institutional setting as a result of various environmental factors are often related to changes in position, such as transferring to and from a bed or chair, toileting procedures, and unstable and defective equipment (e.g., nonfunctioning brake locks on wheelchairs); wet or excessively waxed floors; use of assistive devices, and obstructions in hallways. In addition, falls may result from imposed immobility. Patients who spend much of their time in a bed or chair weaken and develop problems with balance. Falls often occur during periods of high activity when staff members are busy.

Injury-causing falls are more likely to occur in LTC facilities than in the community. Among community-dwelling older persons, approximately 30% fall every year, compared with 50% to 75% of those living in residential care facilities. However, in most incidents no injuries occur. Contusions, cuts, or lacerations occur in 25% to 30% of all reported falls and deep tissue damage or concussion occurs in approximately 5%. Fractures occur in 1% to 5% of all reported falls.

The cost of falls is greater than simply the billions of dollars spent in required treatments; the loss of independence and confidence, as well as the loss of life, must be considered. To address this important problem, the National Patient Safety Goals (The Joint Commission, 2008) recommend that each patient care organization or setting design a fall reduction program that is appropriate for the population it serves (Nursing Care Plan).

Put on Your Thinking Cap!

Assess one of your patients in the clinical setting to identify intrinsic and extrinsic risk factors for falling. Develop nursing interventions to prevent falls in this specific situation.

RESTRAINTS

Restraints restrict an individual's movement and are classified as either *physical* or *chemical.* A **physical restraint** can be anything that restricts movement and that cannot be removed by the patient. Examples of physical restraints are side rails; chairs with trays; and vest, waist, wrist, or ankle ties. Physical restraints are sometimes classified as safety restraint devices (SRDs). A **chemical restraint** is a drug that is given to subdue agitated or confused patients.

SAFETY RESTRAINT DEVICE (SRD)

Older patients, particularly those who are confused, are more likely to be physically restrained than younger patients, probably because they are at greater risk of falling. The most common reasons given for using SRDs with older patients in hospitals or LTC facilities are to (1) protect the patient or others from harm or prevent tampering with medical devices (e.g., feeding tube, catheter), (2) prevent falls from the bed or chair, and (3) prevent wandering. The most common incidents precipitating the use of restraints involve attempts to get out of bed or resistance to treatment while confused or disoriented.

It is difficult to justify the use of restraints to prevent injuries because research has shown that restraints actually cause injuries. Physical restraints can tear the skin and impair circulation and joint mobility. Accidental strangulation has occurred when patients slide down while secured to a chair or bed by a vest or strap restraint. Nurses have long been taught to raise side rails so that vulnerable patients will either stay in bed or call for help. The wisdom of using side rails to keep a person in bed is now in question. Although properly installed modern bed rails should be safe, patients have been injured, sometimes fatally, after crawling over side rails or becoming trapped between side rail bars or between the side rails and the mattress. It has been found that many patients who had fallen out of bed had raised side rails. Half rails may be safer than full rails.

Restraints likely have damaging psychologic effects on older patients. Patients may experience anger, discomfort, resistance, and fear in response to physical restraint. Other possible outcomes include poor self-image, growing dependency, increased confusion and disorientation, regressive behavior, and withdrawal.

The many negative effects of physical restraints prompted passage of the **Omnibus Budget Reconciliation Act (OBRA)** of 1987, which included policies to protect patients from unnecessary restraint in LTC facilities. The law specified that patients have the right to be free from restraint used for purposes of discipline or convenience and that is not required to treat patients' medical symptoms. Restraint use requires a physician's order that specifies the duration and circumstances under which the restraint may be used. Although the number of falls rose as restraint use declined, most of those incidents did not result in serious injury. In fact, the most serious injuries occurred among patients who were restrained.

According to OBRA regulations, the only people who are candidates for restraints are those who:

Nursing Care Plan — Patient with a History of Falling

ASSESSMENT

HEALTH HISTORY A 75-year-old woman resides in an LTC facility because of chronic health problems that include hypertension, emphysema, and mild dementia. She has a history of several falls at home, including one that resulted in a wrist fracture that led to her admission to the LTC facility. She is able to walk but requires assistance because her balance is poor, she becomes short of breath, and she experiences dizziness with position changes. The nursing staff frequently reminds her to call for help and often checks on her but she continues to get up unassisted when unsupervised. In the past she enjoyed daily walks but gave them up when she began to have trouble breathing and sometimes had dizzy spells. Her only activity since admission has been attendance at religious services and bingo games. She enjoys reading large-print romance novels.

PHYSICAL EXAMINATION Vital signs: blood pressure 144/76 mm Hg, pulse 90 bpm; respiration 22 breaths per minute; oral temperature 97°F (35°C). Height 5′1″, weight 98 lb. Skin is warm and dry. Wheezing is noted on expiration. The patient is oriented to person, time, and place.

Nursing Diagnosis	Goals and Outcome Criteria	Interventions
Risk for Falls related to weakness, dizziness, and poor balance	Patient will remain free from fall-related injury.	Ask the patient whether she is concerned about falling. Explain the fall risk and need to call for assistance. Provide the nurse call button and respond quickly to her calls. Discuss possible physical therapy consultation to evaluate the use of cane or walker and to recommend appropriate strengthening and balance exercises. Advise her to wear supportive, nonslip shoes. Provide the patient's glasses or hearing aid.
Risk for Falls related to environmental hazards		Assess the patient and environment for possible hazards. Discuss possible environmental hazards and measures to reduce risks. Consider rearranging furniture to provide clear pathways. Keep her bed at its lowest level. Consult with the patient about providing a bedside commode if she has difficulty getting to the toilet.
Risk for Falls related to postural hypotension		Consult with a registered nurse about drugs that may be causing postural hypotension; a change may be indicated. Suggest elastic stockings to improve venous return. Teach the patient to change positions slowly and to exercise her legs before rising. Determine usual fluid intake and encourage adequate fluids to prevent dehydration.

Critical Thinking Questions

1. How could glasses and a hearing aid reduce the risk of falls?
2. When in a clinical site, examine the patient's room to identify possible hazards in the patient's environment that might contribute to falls.

- Have a history of severe falls or are at extremely high risk of taking a fall that is *life threatening*;
- Are neurologically, orthopedically, or muscularly impaired and need postural support for safety or comfort, or both;
- Experience any number of mental dysfunctions that may cause them to be a *serious hazard* to themselves, objects, or others; or
- Have medical symptoms that are life threatening and require the *temporary* use of a restraint to provide necessary treatment.

When restraints are employed, data indicating the need for restraints *must* be documented in the patient record. If a physical restraint is used, the least restrictive device is best. For example, use a mitt rather than a wrist restraint that limits movement. Check the patient frequently, at least every 15 to 30 minutes. A patient who is agitated or combative must be monitored continuously. Ensure that the restraint is used properly and is providing adequate protection and comfort without impeding circulation or breathing. Remove and release physical restraints *every 2 hours* for 10 minutes to provide for range of motion, toileting, nourishment, and comfort measures. Document ongoing assessments while the patient is restrained. !

Identify patients at risk for restraint so that you can try alternatives. Several alternatives to physical restraint are physical therapy, engaging the patient in group activities, sitting and talking with patients for short periods of time, recruiting family members or volunteers to spend time with the patient, and assigning staff to be responsible for high-risk patients in small blocks of time. Box 20-1 lists more alternatives to physical restraint. In addition, patients, family members, or both should be involved in the decision to use or not to use physical restraint. Special units for the care of persons with dementia typically are designed so that wanderers can move about freely without fear of leaving the premises.

Box 20-1 Alternatives to Physical Restraint

1. Anticipate needs.
2. Provide companionship and supervision by involving family, friends, or volunteers, especially at night.
3. Distract attention with television, radio, CD player, or other activities that interest patient.
4. Arrange environment for easy access to equipment and personal items (e.g., call bell, water, bedside commode)
5. Change forms of treatment contributing to restraint use (e.g., substitute oral feedings for intravenous or nasogastric tubes, remove catheters).
6. Redesign furniture (e.g., lower beds, place mattress on floor, remove wheels from furniture).
7. Use bed and chair alarms to alert caregiver that patient is up.
8. Use exit alarms on exterior doors. Disguise exit doors or doorknobs to discourage exiting (e.g. shower curtain or drape over door). Install slide lock near bottom of door.
9. Enroll patient in Safe Return program that includes identification device with contact information.

Put on Your Thinking Cap!

When in the clinical setting, observe the methods used as alternatives to physical restraint. Could other steps be taken?

CHEMICAL RESTRAINTS

The same guidelines that apply to the use of physical restraints apply to chemical restraints. Never use psychotropic drugs for the purposes of discipline or convenience. They should be used only when the danger of self-injury or injury to others exists. The administration of a psychotropic drug requires a physician's written order that specifies the duration and circumstance under which the medication is to be used. Always document the patient assessment prior to giving a psychotropic drug and after administering the drug.

Psychotropic drugs, including antidepressants, sedatives/hypnotics (e.g., benzodiazepines), and antipsychotic drugs, are the most commonly prescribed chemical restraints. All can have serious adverse effects, such as greater confusion, agitation, postural hypotension, and an increased number of falls in older persons. Other drugs that increase the risk of falls because of postural hypotension are some of the antihypertensives and diuretics, both commonly used by older persons. Avoid the use of psychotropic drugs if at all possible. The same alternatives to physical restraints apply to chemical restraints (see Box 20-1).

NURSING ASSESSMENT AND INTERVENTION

FALL PREVENTION

The most important intervention for falls is prevention. The best prevention is education of patients, families, and caregivers about the ways to prevent falls.

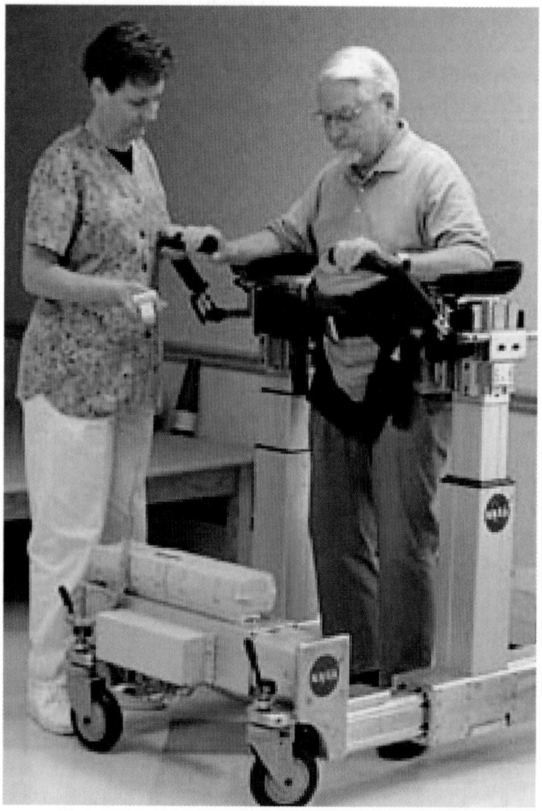

FIGURE 20-1 The National Aeronautics and Space Administration (NASA) has developed a secure ambulation mode (SAM) that allows patients to ambulate safely and securely as they regain the ability to walk after a traumatic injury or receive physical therapy for a degenerative disease. A unique harness supports the patient's body weight without restricting hip movement. (Courtesy National Aeronautics and Space Administration.)

Prevention is aimed toward minimizing both the intrinsic and the extrinsic factors that cause falls and increase the potential for injury.

The first step in preventing falls and injury is to determine who is at risk. People who are at greatest risk for falls and injury are those who have fallen before and those who have multiple intrinsic risk factors. Table 20-1 lists intrinsic risk factors for falling and possible interventions. The more risk factors a person has, the greater the risk of falling. Several tools for the assessment of fall risk exist, including the Hendrich II Fall Risk Model for use in acute care settings. A simple screening tool for fall risk is to have the patient sit in an armless chair, rise, walk, return, and sit back down in the chair. Patients who have difficulty with this task should be assessed in greater detail. Be ready to assist if the patient is unsteady. Other related tools assess gait, balance, and fear of falling (Box 20-2). One strategy that can be used to alert staff to patients at risk for falling is the use of a yellow wristband. It is important for staff to include information about fall risk and known effective interventions when patients are transferred to other units or settings.

Fall prevention strategies are carried out in the home and in institutional environments (Fig. 20-1).

Table 20-1 Intrinsic Risk Factors for Falling and Possible Interventions

RISK FACTORS	INTERVENTIONS
Impaired Vision	
Reduced visual acuity	Ensure that the individual wears glasses, if appropriate. Keep glasses clean. Encourage regular eye examinations. Paint last step a lighter color.
Impaired dark adaptation	Maintain adequate lighting, reduce glare from shiny floors, and allow time to adjust to light levels (e.g., as patient moves from a dark room to the outside). Wear sunglasses in sunlight. Use a night-light in the bedroom and bathroom.
Impaired Hearing	
Impacted cerumen (earwax)	Remove earwax.
Presbycusis	Speak slowly, use a low voice, and decrease background noise. Encourage the use of a hearing aid. Advise to scan environment while walking.
Balance and Gait Problems	
Musculoskeletal disorders	Encourage balance and gait training and muscle-strengthening exercises.
Balance disorders	Encourage balance exercises. Provide and educate the patient on the use of assistive devices. Avoid alcohol.
Peripheral neuropathy	Encourage the patient to use correctly sized footwear with firm soles.
Foot disorders	Trim toenails. Encourage patient to wear appropriate footwear. Advise podiatry for foot care.
Cardiovascular Disease	
Postural hypotension	Encourage dorsiflexion exercises. Use pressure-graded stockings. Elevate the head of the bed before rising. Teach the patient to get up from a chair or bed slowly. Advise patient not to tip the head backward.
Neurologic Disease	
Stroke	Place the call bell in the visual field and within reach of an unaffected arm. Anticipate needs for toileting, dressing, eating, and bathing. Assist with transfer. Provide active and/or passive range-of-motion exercises to improve functional ability.
Slowed reaction time	Encourage patient to avoid rushing and to assess pathway ahead for uneven surfaces and barriers.

Box 20-2 Hendrich II Fall Risk Model™

Risk Factor	Risk Points	Score
Confusion/Disorientation/Impulsivity	4	
Symptomatic Depression	2	
Altered Elimination	1	
Dizziness/Vertigo	1	
Gender (Male)	1	
Any Administered Antiepileptics (anticonvulsants): (Carbamazepine, Divalproex Sodium, Ethotoin, Ethosuximide, Felbamate, Fosphenytoin, Gabapentin, Lamotrigine, Mephenytoin, Methsuximide, Phenobarbital, Phenytoin, Primidone, Topiramate, Trimethadione, Valproic Acid)[1]	2	
Any Administered Benzodiazepines:[2] (Alprazolam, Chloridiazepoxide, Clonazepam, Clorazepate Dipotassium, Diazepam, Flurazepam, Halazepam[3], Lorazepam, Midazolam, Oxazepam, Temazepam, Triazolam)	1	
GET-UP-AND-GO TEST: "RISING FROM A CHAIR"		
If unable to assess, monitor for change in activity level, assess other risk factors, document both on patient chart with date and time.		
Ability to rise in single movement—No loss of balance with steps	0	
Pushes up, successful in one attempt	1	
Multiple attempts but successful	3	
Unable to rise without assistance during test	4	
If unable to assess, document this on the patient chart with the date and time.		
(A score of 5 or greater = High Risk)	**TOTAL SCORE**	

[1]Levetiracetam (Keppra) was not assessed during the original research conducted to create the Hendrich Fall Risk Model. As an antieptileptic, levetiracetam does have a side effect of somnolence and dizziness which contributes to its fall risk and should be scored (effective June 2010).

[2]The study did not include the effect of benzodiazepine-like drugs since they were not on the market at the time. However, due to their similarity in drug structure, mechanism of action and drug effects, they should also be scored (effective January 2010).

[3]Halazepam was included in the study but is no longer available in the United States (effective June 2010).

Patient Teaching

Fall Prevention Guidelines for the Home: Instructions for the Patient

LIGHTS AND LIGHTING

1. Eyes tire quickly in improper lighting. Illuminate reading material or the object worked on. Illuminate steps, entranceways, and rooms before entering. Use 70- or 100-watt bulbs, not 60-watt bulbs.
2. Avoid glaring light caused by highly polished floors or large expanses of uncovered glass. Use sunglasses to avoid the glare of highway driving but use light tints or photo-ray lenses.
3. Allow more time to adjust to changes in light levels. When entering a light room from a dark area or vice versa, allow 1 to 2 minutes for the eyes to accommodate to the change in light before proceeding.
4. Dirty glasses or outgrown prescription lenses inhibit vision. Schedule regular eye examinations to identify changes in vision and to get new glasses when needed. If possible, do not use bifocals when walking because the ground cannot be seen clearly. Keep glasses clean.
5. Ability to see up, down, and sideways decreases with age. Observe the "lay of the land"; learn to look ahead at the ground to spot and avoid hazards such as cracks in the sidewalks. Use canes, walking sticks, and walkers that are prescribed.
6. At night, keep a night-light on in the bedroom and bathroom. When getting out of bed at night, turn the light on and wait 1 to 2 minutes for the eyes to adjust before getting up. Have a telephone in the bedroom so you do not have to get out of bed to answer the telephone. Before leaving in the evening or late afternoon, turn on a light for your return.

ACTIVITY

1. Get up from a chair slowly.
2. When getting out of bed, sit up and then wait 1 to 2 minutes. Move to the side of the bed, exercise the legs, and wait another minute. Stand after sitting for a few minutes.
3. If you are dizzy, sit down immediately. Sit on a step or a chair, or ease yourself to the sidewalk if you are outdoors.
4. Avoid tipping the head backward (extending the neck). Activities to avoid (because they extend the neck) include washing windows, hanging clothes, and getting things from high shelves.
5. Use shelves at eye level. Avoid rapid turning of the head.
6. If weather is rainy and windy, avoid going out.
7. Use alcohol and tranquilizers with caution.
8. Exercise programs help your flexibility, balance, and strength. Enroll in a senior exercise program if your physician approves.
9. Shoes and slippers should be low-heeled with rubber soles. Avoid clothing such as long robes and loose-fitting garments that may catch on furniture or doorknobs.

AROUND THE HOUSE

1. Avoid scatter rugs and small bathroom mats that can slide. Repair loose, torn, wrinkled, or worn carpet.
2. Avoid slick, glossy polish on floors.
3. Put things in easy reach and avoid reaching to high shelves.
4. Use nonskid treads on stairs and nonskid mats in the bathtub.
5. Install grab rails in the bath, in the shower, and also by the toilet.
6. Install handrails on both sides of the stairs. Paint stair edges in a bright contrasting color.
7. Remove door thresholds.
8. Remove low-lying objects, such as coffee tables and extension cords.
9. Wipe up spills immediately.
10. Watch for pets underfoot and scattered pet food.
11. Check for even, nonglare lighting in every room with easily accessible light switches.
12. Avoid floor coverings with complex patterns.
13. Avoid clutter in living areas.
14. Select furniture that provides stability and support, such as chairs with arms.
15. Check walking aids routinely, such as rubber tips on canes and screws on walkers.

Adapted from Chenitz WC, Stone JT, Salisbury SA, editors: *Clinical gerontological nursing*, Philadelphia, 1991, Saunders.

Evidence-based interventions that are likely to be effective include muscle strengthening and balance training, Tai Chi, modification of the home environment, withdrawal of psychotropic medications and drugs that cause hypotension, and cardiac pacing for selected patients. Effective interventions need to be individualized based on the specific factors that create a fall risk for the individual patient. Fall prevention guidelines for the home are listed in the *Patient Teaching* box; those for use in institutional settings are listed in Box 20-3. Finally, the *Health Promotion* box offers general tips for preventing falls.

REDUCING FEAR

Even if all recommended measures are taken, the older adult may restrict activity out of fear of falling. Part of

Health Promotion

Strategies for Preventing Falls

In summary, basic strategies for reducing all types of falls include the following:

- Increase physical activities that enhance and maintain muscular strength, endurance, balance, and flexibility.
- Increase regular, moderate physical exercise.
- Reduce visual impairments.
- Teach and encourage proper use of aids (e.g., cane, walker) for ambulation.
- Increase health care provider review of prescribed and over-the-counter medications.
- Increase health care provider screening and referral for alcohol and drug problems.
- Modify the environment to reduce or eliminate factors that can cause falls or to minimize injury if a fall occurs.

Box 20-3 Fall Prevention Techniques Used in Hospitals and Long-Term Care Facilities

PATIENT-ORIENTED TECHNIQUES

1. Encourage exercise to strengthen muscles and improve balance. Use electronic alarm devices such as Bed-Check or Ambularm.

MEDICATIONS

1. Monitor effects of drugs that cause sedation or orthostatic hypotension.
2. Inform physician of adverse drug effects so that alternatives might be considered.
3. Administer diuretics and laxatives in the morning to reduce nighttime toileting.

ACTIVITIES OF DAILY LIVING

1. Assist the patient to the toilet at regular intervals.
2. Check for proper footwear (e.g., nonskid footwear).
3. Keep the patient's belongings close to the bed; consider on which side of the bed to place items based on patient's abilities.
4. Request referrals for rehabilitation training by Physical Therapy and/or Occupational Therapy to improve function.

ENVIRONMENT-ORIENTED TECHNIQUES

1. Relocate the patient at high risk for falling to rooms close to the nurses' station. Place the nurse call light system within reach (e.g., pinned to pillow); assess ability to use.
2. Use the bed rails judiciously; half rails are best.
3. Keep the bed in the low position (ideally, 14 to 20 inches above the floor, including the mattress).
4. Keep the room light on during waking hours; illumination should be bright and even without glare.
5. Keep the rooms and hallways free of clutter.
6. Carpet all hard surfaces.
7. Clean up spills.
8. Lock all equipment with wheels.
9. Keep equipment on one side of hallway.
10. Use night-lights in rooms during sleeping hours.
11. Place safety (grab) bars in the bathroom and hall.
12. Install high-seated toilets or use bedside commodes. Remove wheels from bedside commodes.

PATIENT EDUCATION

1. Hand out safety brochure to patient and family on admission.
2. Teach the patient about proper use of room equipment and assistive devices.
3. Encourage the patient to request help.
4. Encourage the use of the bathroom and corridor handrails.
5. Teach the patient how to transfer from the bed to the chair.
6. Teach the patient to rise slowly and pump ankles before standing.

NURSING ASSESSMENT

1. Perform assessment at admission and throughout the hospital stay.
2. Apply agency protocol for "Fall Risk" based on assessment.
3. Check hourly and offer fluids, assistance to toilet, etc.

OTHER

1. Monitor falls, watch for trends, and conduct in-service training when a trend emerges.
2. Have staff move slowly around ambulatory, unsteady patients.

patient education is helping the patient to view fall risks as controllable. Just as a good driver practices defensive driving, a safe walker recognizes risks and makes adaptations to reduce their risks. When people have the facts about falling and proactive measures, they are empowered to remain active.

REDUCING FALL-RELATED INJURIES

Some falls will occur no matter what precautions are taken. In some societies, falls are viewed as indicators of greater activity and independence. Health care providers generally accept an increased number of falls as an inevitable risk that is outweighed by the benefits of physical activity and rehabilitation. Evidence is growing to support exercise interventions to improve balance, thereby reducing the risk of falls. Recommended exercises include walking; balance, coordination, and functional exercises; muscle strengthening; and multiple exercise types. Individuals at risk for falling can also be taught how to fall in a way that reduces the risk for hip injury. The patient is less likely to sustain a fracture if he or she can rotate forward or backward to avoid falling sideways. Measures to prevent osteoporosis may reduce the risk of fractures associated with falls. These measures are discussed in Chapter 44. Because persons with low vitamin D levels have been found at greater risk for fractures, some physicians recommend calcium and vitamin D supplementation for susceptible patients. The use of hip protectors is one strategy that accepts the risk of falling but aims to decrease the severity of fall-related injuries. Overall, research has not found a significant reduction in hip fractures when the protectors are worn in institutional settings or by persons living in the community. Many patients who have been offered hip protectors decline to wear them, citing discomfort and not liking the way they look.

Put on Your Thinking Cap!

A patient who fell near the bathroom door was found to be wet with urine. What intervention might reduce future falls for this patient?

WHEN A FALL OCCURS

When a fall occurs in a hospital or LTC facility, determine the circumstances of the fall and any injuries sustained. Document the fall according to the agency protocol. Note what the patient was doing at the time of the fall, the patient's mental and emotional status,

Patient Teaching

Methods for Getting Up After a Fall: Instructions for the Patient

ROLL
1. Roll onto your right side.
2. Bend the right knee.
3. Lever upward to the kneeling position by pressing down on the right forearm.
4. Reach out with the left arm to a nearby chair or bed.
5. With a twist of the trunk, pull yourself into a sitting position.
6. Sit on the chair or bed to recover.

CRAWL
1. Roll to a prone position.
2. Get up on all fours.
3. Crawl to a sturdy couch, chair, or bed and place your hands on it.
4. Bring one foot forward, putting the foot flat on the floor.
5. Pull yourself up to a standing position.
6. Sit on the chair or bed to recover.

SHUFFLE
1. Pull yourself to a sitting position on the floor.
2. Shuffle on the buttocks to a nearby piece of furniture.
3. Pull yourself up onto your knees directly in front of the item of furniture.
4. Stand up.

STAIR SHUFFLE
1. Pull yourself to a sitting position on the floor.
2. Shuffle on the buttocks to the stairs.
3. Gradually move up and backward to a stair height suitable for standing.
4. Grab on to the handrail and pull up.

Data from Chenitz WC, Kussman HL, Stone JT: Preventing falls. In Chenitz WC, Stone JT, Salisbury SA, editors: *Clinical gerontological nursing*, Philadelphia, 1991, Saunders.

and environmental factors that may have contributed to the fall. When the cause of the fall is determined, take steps to remove or correct the cause. After a fall, the patient should be examined for injury. Inspect the extremities for deformity or trauma. Inspect and palpate the head for bleeding or swelling and collect data for a mental status assessment. Describe the nature and severity of any pain that the patient reports. Have the patient begin ambulating as soon after the fall as possible and at least several times a day to prevent the hazards of bed rest and to restore confidence.

Dealing with falls in the home requires the cooperation of the person who is at risk, the family, and possibly neighbors. A plan of action for when a fall occurs should include information about getting up and seeking help.

Several ways to get up after a fall in the home are described in the *Patient Teaching* box. These techniques should be practiced by the potential faller to ensure confidence in managing the problem. If none of the methods is possible, the person at risk for falling would be wise to have a call system to obtain help from others. Devices worn around the neck that can send signals to a control center are effective and provide a feeling of well-being for the potential faller. A cellphone attached to the waist also provides a means of calling for help. In addition, having a person or agency call every day can provide reassurance.

Put on Your Thinking Cap!

Practice the methods for getting up after a fall described in the *Patient Teaching* box. Consider the limitations on patients with restricted movements. Which methods would work best for patients you have seen?

Get Ready for the NCLEX® Examination!

Key Points

- The risk of injury from falls is highest in people over age 75 and falls are the most frequent cause of accidental injury and death among older adults.
- The USPHS estimates that two thirds of the deaths as a result of falls are preventable.
- Falls occur in older adults because of intrinsic factors (i.e., factors related to the functioning of the individual, such as weakness, drug side effects, or physical illness) and extrinsic factors (i.e., environmental factors).
- In an institutional setting, falls often occur during periods of high activity when the staff is busy.
- Serious fall injuries occur in 20% to 30% of all falls; fractures occur in approximately 1% to 5% of all reported falls.
- People who are at greatest risk for falls and injury are those who have fallen before and those who have multiple intrinsic risk factors.
- Older patients, particularly those who are confused, are more likely to be physically restrained than younger patients.
- Safety restraint devices (physical restraints) seldom eliminate the risk for injury and may actually cause or worsen problems.
- The OBRA of 1987 was enacted to protect patients from unnecessary restraint in LTC facilities.
- A physician's order is required for restraint use and the order must specify the duration of use and the circumstances under which the restraint may be used.
- Remove restraints for at least 10 minutes every 2 hours, assess the skin and mental status, and reapply, if indicated. Document.

- Alternatives to using physical restraint include physical therapy, sitting and talking with patients for short periods, and asking staff to be responsible for wanderers in small blocks of time.
- Special care units for persons with dementia allow patients to wander in a safe environment.
- The most important intervention for falls is prevention and the first step in preventing falls and injury is to determine who is at greatest risk.
- When a fall occurs in a hospital or LTC facility, nurses should assess the circumstances of the fall and any injuries sustained and report the fall according to the protocol of the institution.
- When the cause of a fall is determined, steps should be taken to remove or correct the cause.
- Because most people who fall have multiple risk factors, fall prevention usually requires individualized care plans.

Additional Learning Resources

SG Go to your Study Guide for additional learning activities to help you master this chapter content.

evolve Go to your Evolve website (http://evolve.elsevier.com/Linton/medsurg) for the following learning resources and much more:

- Interactive Prioritization Exercises
- Fluid & Electrolyte Tutorial
- Pharmacology Tutorial
- Review Questions for the NCLEX® Examination

Review Questions for the NCLEX® Examination

1. The nurse in a retirement center is conducting a fall prevention program. She explains to the residents that fractures occur in what percentage of falls among older adults?
   1. Less than 10%
   2. 15%
   3. 40%
   4. 65%

   NCLEX Client Need: Safe and Effective Care Environment: Safety and Infection Control
2. The health history of a resident of an assisted living facility includes the data below. Which is the strongest predictor of falling for this resident?
   1. History of falling
   2. Diagnosis of heart disease
   3. Recent weight loss
   4. Urinary incontinence

   NCLEX Client Need: Safe and Effective Care Environment: Safety and Infection Control
3. Part of the orientation for new nurses in a long-term care facility includes information about restraint devices. Which statement should be included in the orientation?
   1. Anything that restricts movement and cannot be released by the patient is a restraint.
   2. Physical restraints greatly reduce the risk of injury.
   3. Side rails have been found to be the safest means of preventing falls.
   4. Restraints must be removed once each shift for exercise and to assess skin and circulation.

   NCLEX Client Need: Safe and Effective Care Environment: Safety and Infection Control
4. A patient who has fallen twice is being given a psychotropic drug to control agitation. The nurse recognizes that psychotropic drugs may contribute to falls because they often cause which of the following?
   1. Hallucinations and delusions
   2. Constipation
   3. Postural hypotension
   4. Insomnia

   NCLEX Client Need: Physiological Integrity: Pharmacological Therapies
5. The home health nurse is conducting a fall risk assessment. Which of these are *intrinsic* risk factors for falling? (Select all that apply.)
   1. Confusion
   2. Inadequate lighting
   3. Weakness
   4. Poor vision
   5. Broken wheelchair brakes

   NCLEX Client Need: Safe and Effective Care Environment: Safety and Infection Control
6. A newly admitted patient has an order for restraints. Under OBRA, the physician's order for the use of restraints should include which of the following? (Select all that apply.)
   1. Duration that restraints may be used
   2. Circumstances under which restraints may be used
   3. Nursing assessment data to be recorded
   4. Measures to be taken to prevent injury
   5. Patient consent to be restrained for safety reasons.

   NCLEX Client Need: Safe and Effective Care Environment: Coordinated Care
7. A restraint device is applied to a confused postoperative patient who is pulling on her intravenous tubing and surgical dressing. How often must the restraint be released?

   NCLEX Client Need: Safe and Effective Care Environment: Safety and Infection Control

8. Classes of drugs that may be used as chemical restraints include which of the following? (Select all that apply.)
   1. Antipsychotic drugs
   2. Sedatives and hypnotic drugs
   3. Antidepressants
   4. Analgesics
   5. Skeletal muscle relaxants

   NCLEX Client Need: Physiological Integrity: Pharmacological Therapies
9. Which of the following nutritional supplements may reduce the risk of fall-related fractures? (Select all that apply.)
   1. Vitamin C
   2. Iron
   3. Vitamin D
   4. Calcium
   5. Vitamin B_{12}

   NCLEX Client Need: Health Promotion and Maintenance
10. The nurse is encouraging regular exercise for residents of a retirement center. The nurse should explain that physical training can help to prevent falls by improving which of the following? (Select all that apply.)
    1. Muscle strength
    2. Balance
    3. Flexibility
    4. Alertness
    5. Bone mass

    NCLEX Client Need: Health Promotion and Maintenance

chapter 21

Immobility

http://evolve.elsevier.com/Linton/medsurg

Objectives

1. Describe common problems associated with immobility.
2. Discuss the impact of exercise and positioning on preventing complications related to immobility.
3. Identify the risk factors for pressure ulcers.
4. Describe the stages of pressure ulcers.
5. Describe methods of preventing and treating pressure ulcers.
6. Discuss measures to manage the effects of immobility on respiratory status, nutrition, elimination, and circulation.

Key Terms

Active exercise
Contracture (kŏn-TRĂK-shŭr)
Erythema (ĕr-ĭ-THĒ-mă)
Immobility
Isometric exercise (ī-sō-MĔT-rĭk)
Passive exercise
Pressure ulcer (ŬL-sĕr)
Range-of-motion exercises
Shearing forces

Immobility (the inability to move) is a restriction imposed on all or part of the body. People become immobilized by physical factors such as joint disease, paralysis, or pain or psychologic factors such as depression or fear. Sometimes immobilization is prescribed for beneficial purposes. Therapeutic outcomes of immobility include (1) pain relief and prevention of further injury of a part, as in a fractured bone; (2) reduced workload of the heart in a cardiac condition; (3) healing and repair; and (4) reversal of the effects of gravity, as in abdominal hernias and prolapsed organs.

Immobility can have a profound impact on both the mind and the body. Psychosocial effects may include depression, fear, anxiety, social withdrawal, apathy, loss of independence, and a feeling that life has no meaning. Almost every body system can be affected by immobility, depending on the extent and duration of the immobilization. The physiologic effects of immobility are summarized in Table 21-1.

Common aging changes, combined with common medical conditions, place the older adult at risk for immobility and its consequences. Examples of age-related physical changes that affect mobility are decreased flexibility and strength and changes in posture and gait. Chronic medical conditions such as arthritis, stroke, Parkinson disease, cardiovascular disease, anemia, pulmonary disease, and foot deformities can lead to decreased mobility. Pain also may be a factor that leads to immobility in older adults. Drugs that cause drowsiness, hypotension, or dizziness can affect mobility as well.

Psychosocial factors that can impair mobility include depression, dementia, bereavement, lack of motivation, fear of falling, isolation, and loss of friends. The older person's environment also can promote or hinder mobility. An unsafe home setting, hospitalization, or institutionalization, for example, may be associated with reduced activity. The older person who is hospitalized may quickly become debilitated and dependent as a result of the combined effects of inactivity, pain, drugs, various therapies such as bed rest or traction, and an unfamiliar environment.

The impact of immobilization depends on the duration, degree, and type of mobility limitation. Temporary immobilization can begin a vicious cycle that leads to an ever-increasing loss of independence for patients. As patients become less able to move, they become more dependent. As they become more dependent, they are less able to care for themselves, which in turn leads to an increasing number of adverse effects from immobility.

Whatever the reason for resting a part or all of the body, measures must be taken to manage the adverse effects of immobility. You can prevent the vicious cycle of events from the beginning by helping patients to maintain normal functioning as much as possible and for as long as possible (see Nursing Care Plan: Preventing Hazards of Immobility). Before patients begin to suffer the ill effects of immobilization, therapeutic

Table 21-1 Consequences of Immobility of Body Systems

BODY SYSTEM	CONSEQUENCES
Musculoskeletal	Thickening of joint capsule; loss of smoothness of cartilage surface; decreased flexibility of connective tissues; changes similar to osteoarthritis—joint contractures, demineralization of bone, bone loss; atrophy and shortening of muscle; decreased muscle strength; decreased muscle oxidative capacity; decline in aerobic capacity
Pulmonary	Arterial oxygen desaturation; increased hypostatic pooling; increased risk of atelectasis and infection
Cardiovascular	Decreased cardiac output and stroke volume; increased peripheral resistance; net loss of total body water and total blood volume; stasis of blood in veins of legs may allow blood clots to form (deep vein thrombosis, or DVT)
Integumentary	Pressure ulcers
Gastrointestinal	General weakening of muscles, causing altered colonic motility; constipation
Urinary	Increased levels of nitrogen, phosphorus, total sulfur, sodium, potassium, and calcium excretion; renal insufficiency; decreased glomerular filtration rate; loss of ability to concentrate urine; low creatinine clearance
Metabolic	Decreased basal metabolic rate; increased storage of fat or carbohydrates; negative nitrogen and calcium metabolic balance as a result of decreased protein and calcium intake; decreased glucose tolerance; metabolic alkalosis
Sensory	Decreased sensory stimulation (kinesthetic, visual, auditory, tactile); decreased social interaction; changes in affect, cognition, and perception

Modified from Chenitz WC, Stone JT, Salisbury SA: *Clinical gerontological nursing*, Philadelphia, 1991, Saunders.

Nursing Care Plan Preventing Hazards of Immobility

ASSESSMENT

HEALTH HISTORY A 90-year-old retired general lives alone in the assisted living section of a senior retirement community. He has multiple medical conditions and has become increasingly frail. He has fallen three times, with the last fall resulting in a serious knee injury. While recovering from this injury, he has been instructed to use a walker or wheelchair and to avoid full weight-bearing activities. Therefore he was moved to the nursing home area until he can again care for himself. In the nursing home, he has been irritable and insists on caring for himself. He attempts to transfer himself without assistance by bearing weight on one leg. On several occasions he has been unable to delay urination until he could get help. He eats very little other than toast at breakfast and he is drinking little fluid.

PHYSICAL EXAMINATION Vital signs: blood pressure 94/52 mm Hg, pulse 88 bpm; respirations 18 breaths per minute, temperature 97°F orally. Height 5′10″, weight 140 lb. All extremities exhibit muscle atrophy and weakness. Reddened areas are noted on the elbows and sacrum. Urine is dark with a strong odor.

Nursing Diagnosis	Goals and Outcome Criteria	Interventions
Risk for Falls related to weakness	Patient will remain safe from falls during his recovery.	Ask the patient to request help with transferring. Arrange his room for easy movement in a wheelchair. Assist with active range-of-motion exercises for unaffected limbs. Suggest physical therapy referral to strengthen upper body and his weight-bearing leg.
Risk for Infection (Urinary) related to stasis of body fluids associated with low fluid intake	Patient's daily fluid intake will be at least 1200 mL. The patient's urine will be clear and light in color.	Explain the need to increase fluid intake to prevent urinary tract infections. Determine preferred liquids and make them available. Instruct the CNA to offer 3 ounces of fluids hourly while the patient is awake, for a total of 1600 mL/day, and to record intake. Report foul urine odor. Provide urinal. Assure easy access to toilet.
Risk for Impaired Skin Integrity related to prolonged pressure while sitting.	Patient's skin will remain intact throughout the recovery period.	Obtain pressure-reducing pad for wheelchair. Teach patient to shift weight every 15 minutes. Plan periods of bed rest to prevent constant pressure on sacrum. Keep sacral area clean and dry.
Ineffective Coping related to loss of independence, situational crisis, uncertainty.	The patient will adapt to temporary dependence by participating in rehabilitation efforts. The patient will resume self-care activities by discharge to his home.	Explain the benefits of rehabilitation activities in relation to regaining independence. Stress goal of returning to his former residence and need to avoid further injuries. Encourage self-care within limitations. Compliment efforts. Arrange for him to attend social function in previous living section. Request consult for occupational therapist to improve self-care abilities.

Critical Thinking Questions

1. How do age-related changes increase the risk of complications of immobility for this patient?
2. Why is it important to consider both physical and emotional needs of the patient with reduced mobility?

bpm, Beats per minute; *CNA*, certified nursing assistant.

interventions must be implemented. The health care team must work together to develop a plan of care that includes preventive and therapeutic measures that address the individual's needs. The patient and family, as central members of the health care team, should participate in care planning if able. The *Health Promotion* box discusses how the family and health care team can collaborate to support the patient's self-care as he or she regains independence.

Health Promotion

Promoting Independence in Self-Care Activities

Regaining independence in self-care activities requires the collaboration of all members of the health care team. Following a thorough assessment, the team designs a rehabilitation plan. Each discipline then develops the parts of the plan for that discipline. The overall goal is for the patient to reach the highest level of wellness possible to achieve an acceptable quality of life. Rehabilitation seeks to help patients relearn lost skills and compensate for temporary or permanent losses. Family members need to be included in all teaching so that they understand how to support independence rather than dependence. Given adequate time, most motivated patients with moderate impairments can relearn the skills needed for basic activities of daily living.

Assistive devices can play a major role in regaining independence immobility, eating, and dressing. Nurses or therapists should instruct patients and families in the proper use and care of these devices. Any measures that simplify tasks can improve independence. For example, slip-on shoes, Velcro closures, loose pullover shirts, and elastic-waist pants can promote independence in dressing and toileting. Encourage patients to dress in simple workout-type clothes, rather than in pajamas and gowns, as soon as active rehabilitation is started.

Pharmacology Capsule

Drugs that cause drowsiness, hypotension, or dizziness can impair mobility.

NURSING ASSESSMENT AND INTERVENTION

A thorough assessment of the patient's abilities and limitations is essential to planning interventions. Data collected by the licensed vocational nurse/licensed practical nurse (LVN/LPN) make an important contribution to the assessment. While the physician may order specific activities or therapies related to immobility, there are many measures the nurse can implement independently to prevent the adverse effects of immobility. Nursing interventions focus on promoting exercise and maintaining adequate respiratory status, food and fluid intake, normal elimination, skin integrity, joint mobility, and circulation (Box 21-1).

EXERCISE

Regardless of the severity of their condition, most people can engage in some form of exercise. For example, patients with fractures can tighten and relax muscles in an immobilized extremity; debilitated patients can gradually increase their range of movement, number of movements, or resistance against movement; and patients in pain can coordinate activity with pain medication and adapt their pace or intensity for comfort.

Exercises may be **active** (performed by the patients themselves) or **passive** (movement of the patient's body by another person). Active and passive exercises may be performed in bed, in a chair, or standing. The

Box 21-1 Case Study: Immobility

Mrs. Smith is an 84-year-old woman who has resided in an intermediate care facility for 2 years. She was admitted to the facility because she had been living at home alone and had become unable to shop and cook for herself or to dress herself after sustaining a broken wrist as a result of a fall. She was incontinent of urine and mildly confused.

Mrs. Smith had previously been quite active in the community but in the residential home she remained confined to her room and was not interested in interacting with other people. Her daughter visited her two or three times a week.

Because Mrs. Smith preferred to stay in bed or in a chair most of the time, the nurses and other members of the interdisciplinary team were concerned about the consequences of her immobility. She had fallen many times, usually on the way to the dining room to eat. She had reached the point where she stayed in a wheelchair most of the time because she had become too weak to walk.

The team held a case conference and identified problems associated with her immobility: (1) continued falling, (2) incontinence, and (3) isolation and perhaps depression. They formulated a plan to get her up and moving while at the same time avoiding falls. The nurse walked with Mrs. Smith three times daily. The first week they walked around the bed. The second week they walked to the door and back. The third week they walked a few feet outside the door to her room. As the weeks progressed, Mrs. Smith was able to walk to the dining room at the end of the hall without falling. The nurses encouraged in-bed and in-chair exercises to further build up her strength.

Eventually, Mrs. Smith was able to walk to the bathroom independently. The nurses worked with her to develop a regular schedule of toileting so that the number of "accidents" decreased. Because she was slightly confused and disoriented, the nurses provided gentle reminders for her to go to the bathroom. After a meal, they would guide her back to her room to use the bathroom. At other times they would stop by her room, look in, and suggest that she go to the bathroom.

With all of the increased activity, Mrs. Smith became more outgoing and involved in activities. She sat with the same group at meals and developed friendships with others around her. The nurses found that taking small steps with a walking program can have many benefits for a person of any age in any condition.

exercises can be performed while giving other care, such as during a bed bath or while grooming. Examples of bed and chair exercises are listed in the *Health Promotion* box.

Health Promotion

Sample Bed and Chair Exercises

IN-BED EXERCISES	IN-CHAIR EXERCISES
Deep breathing (slow inhalation and full exhalation)	Deep breathing
Neck rolls (neck forward flex, backward extend, lateral flex, rotate)	Head rolls (neck forward flex, backward extend, lateral flex, rotate)
Knee to chest (on back or side, bring one knee to chest, wrap arms around, hold and breathe, straighten leg slowly)	Knee to chest
Pelvic tilts (on back, knees bent, feet flat, tuck in tummy, relax)	Head to knees
Bridging (on back, feet flat on bed, raise hips, lower slowly)	Shoulder rolls (forward and back)
Head raising in prone and supine positions	Weight shifts (hip to hip)
Unilateral leg lifts	Hands on head, elbows out and in, lateral trunk flex-extension, trunk rotation
Foot dorsiflexion	Leg lifts
Rolling	Ankle rotation and dorsiflexion
Prone lying	Ankle on knee (external hip rotation, place ankle on opposite knee and lower the bent leg)
Arms straight over head of bed in supine position	Push down on legs as if to stand, lean forward, bear weight
Arms out to sides, palms up, in supine position	
Hands behind head, elbows bent	
Hands at lower back	

From Giduz BH, Snow TL, Wildman DL, McConnell ES: *Geriatric first aid kit*, Chapel Hill, NC, 1986, Program on Aging–University of North Carolina.

Range-of-Motion Exercises

Range-of-motion exercises are effective in preventing some disabilities of the musculoskeletal system. Each of the joints of the body has a range of motion, meaning the limits to which it may be safely moved. Muscular activity maintains range of motion by allowing the joint to remain flexible and functional. When little or no movement of a joint occurs, its structures change. Normal muscle tissue is replaced by fibrous tissue. Muscles shorten and lose their elasticity. Shortening of muscles and tendons creates a **contracture** that is defined as "a lack of full active or passive range of motion due to joint, muscle, or soft tissue limitations" (Wagner et al., 2008). A contracture can severely and permanently limit joint movement.

The purpose of range-of-motion exercises is to put each joint that is at risk for loss of motion through its full range of motion to the highest degree possible. These exercises may be active or passive. Range-of-motion exercises should be initiated early in immobile patients to prevent contractures.

Isometric Exercises

Isometric exercises maintain muscle tone without moving the joint. The muscle is contracted and held in that position for several seconds. The muscle is then relaxed briefly and contracted again. This type of exercise is especially helpful in maintaining muscle strength after a fracture.

POSITIONING

Proper positioning in a bed or chair is extremely important for preventing many of the side effects of immobility (see *Coordinated Care* box). The patient's position should be changed *at least every 2 hours* to prevent prolonged pressure on the skin. If redness from pressure persists after 2 hours, the interval between repositioning needs to be shortened. Maintain joints in their functional positions so that they are not abnormally flexed or extended. Use pillows, trochanter rolls, footboards or positioning boots, and splints to maintain proper positioning for patients lying in bed. Footboards and positioning boots keep the feet at right angles to the legs so that foot drop is avoided. Splinting the limbs keeps them straight. For example, a firm splint in the hands prevents the fingers from curling up into a tight fist. Avoid positioning the patient with the knees and hips flexed. Imagining how a person looks while standing helps to achieve that position while the patient is lying down. Patients who are seated in chairs should be encouraged to shift their weight every 15 minutes.

Coordinated Care

Preventing Complications of Immobility

Educate certified nursing assistants (CNAs) about the importance of turning, positioning, exercise, and hydration to prevent complications of immobility. Explain how turning and proper positioning relieve pressure on sensitive or painful areas.

Monitor care to ensure that patients are being repositioned on schedule and that fluids are being provided. Show CNAs what the early signs of pressure ulcers look like and stress the importance of promptly reporting such observations. Ask CNAs to report constipation, incontinence, or diarrhea if it occurs so that corrective measures can be taken.

SKIN INTEGRITY

Pressure ulcers are localized areas of tissue necrosis (tissue death) that develop when soft tissue is compressed between a bony prominence and an external surface or when pressure occurs in combination with shearing force or friction or both. Pressure points are

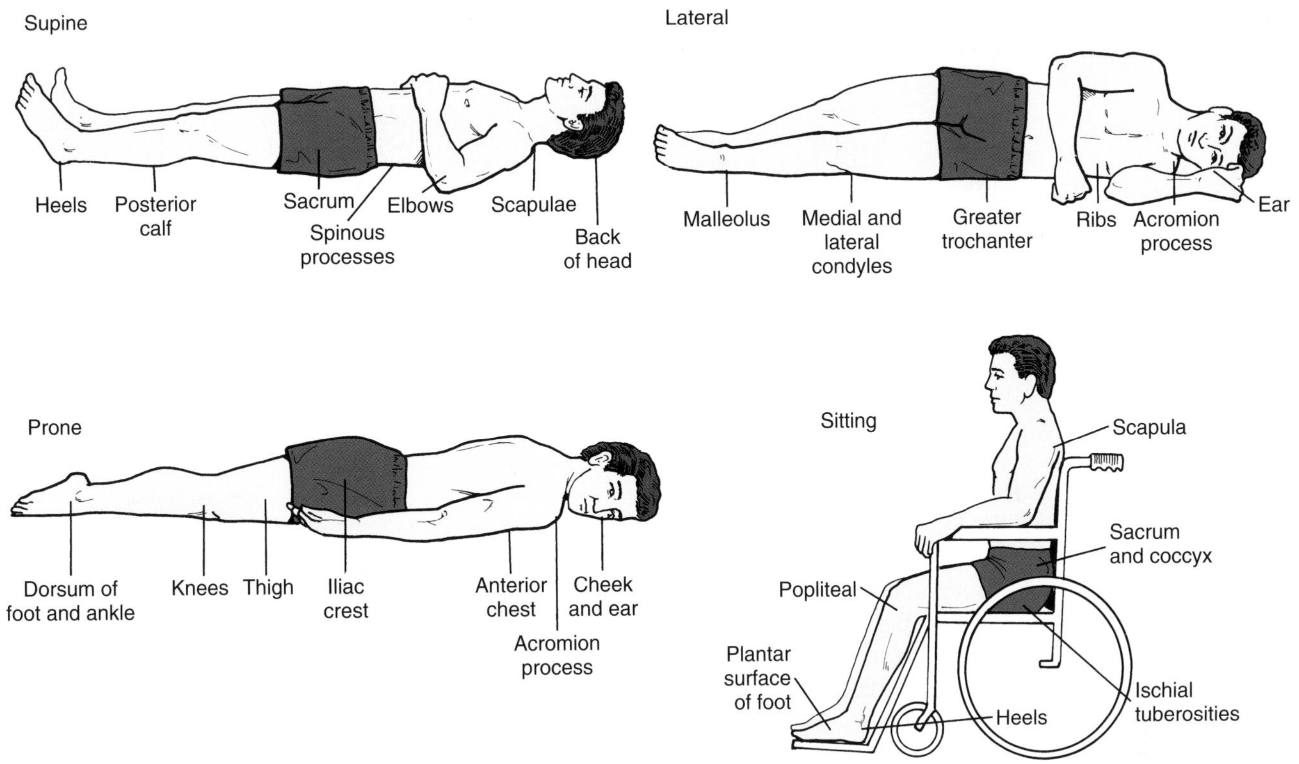

FIGURE 21-1 Possible locations of pressure ulcers.

areas over bony prominences such as the elbows, hips, shoulders, and sacrum (Fig. 21-1). The most frequent sites of skin breakdown are the sacrum (35%), ischial tuberosities (16%), heels (11%), trochanters (7%), ankles (3%), and scapulae (2%). The term *pressure ulcers* is preferred for what are commonly called "bedsores," "decubitus ulcers," or "decubiti." The word *decubitus* means "lying down" and an ulcer is a lesion produced by the sloughing of necrotic, inflammatory tissue (Fig. 21-2). Thus a decubitus ulcer is an open wound that is associated with lying in bed. However, skin breakdown can just as easily develop in patients who are sitting for a long period, because of pressure against blood vessels.

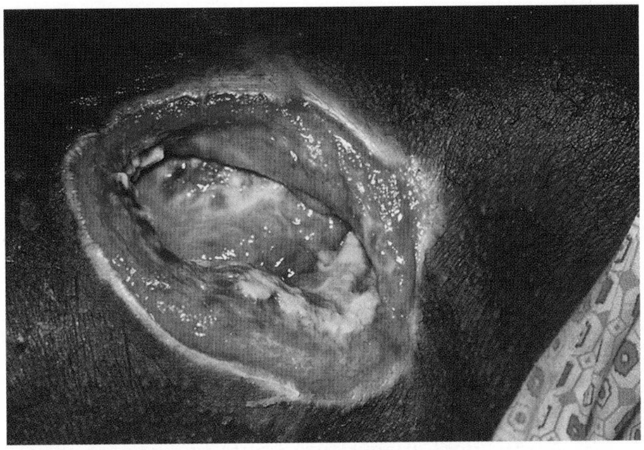

FIGURE 21-2 Stage IV pressure ulcer with full-thickness involvement of all soft tissue. (From Ignatavicius DD, Workman ML: *Medical-surgical nursing: patient-centered collaborative care*, ed 6, St. Louis, 2010, Saunders.)

Development of Pressure Ulcers

An area of **erythema** (redness) is the beginning of a pressure ulcer and a sign that capillaries in the area have become congested because of impaired blood flow. Erythema can occur within 1 to 2 hours in a person with healthy skin and adequate circulation. Persons who are malnourished, obese, aged, or suffering from circulatory disease are even more likely to develop erythematous areas that progress rapidly to an ulcerated stage.

In addition to immobility, factors that contribute to the development of pressure ulcers are shearing forces, chemical irritants such as urine, sedation, and poor nutrition. **Shearing forces** exert a downward and forward pressure on tissues underlying the skin. Shearing action occurs when a patient slumps down while sitting in bed or in a chair; it also can occur when boosting a patient up in bed.

Pressure ulcers are expensive to treat, result in longer hospital stays, increase the likelihood of placement in a long-term care facility, and increase mortality. Therefore prevention is vital. *Nursing care is a major factor in pressure ulcer prevention.*

Preventing Pressure Ulcers

The first step in the prevention of pressure ulcers is to identify patients who are at risk for developing them. The Norton scale is a useful instrument for identifying

NORTON SCALE

		PHYSICAL CONDITION	MENTAL CONDITION	ACTIVITY	MOBILITY	INCONTINENT	
		Good 4 Fair 3 Poor 2 Very bad 1	Alert 4 Apathetic 3 Confused 2 Stupor 1	Ambulant 4 Walk/help 3 Chairbound 2 Bedrest 1	Full 4 Slightly limited 3 Very limited 2 Immobile 1	Not 4 Occasional 3 Usually/urine 2 Doubly 1	TOTAL SCORE
Name	Date						

FIGURE 21-3 Norton scale for the identification of those at risk for the development of pressure ulcers. (From Norton D, McLaren R, Exton-Smith AN: *An investigation of geriatric nursing problems in the hospital*, London, 1962, Centre for Policy on Ageing. Reproduced with permission from the Centre for Policy on Ageing [formerly NCCOP], London, UK.)

those at risk (Fig. 21-3). The scores in all five categories of the scale are added. If the total score is greater than 14, little risk exists for developing pressure ulcers. If the score is less than 14, a significant risk exists for developing pressure ulcers. Any patient with a score of less than 14 needs a formal pressure ulcer prevention program started as soon as the risk is recognized. The skin of patients "at risk" should be assessed and documented every day.

A pressure ulcer prevention protocol consists of the following:

1. Use a special mattress or bed designed to reduce pressure, such as an egg crate–type foam (minimum 2 inches thick), static air, alternating air, gel, fluidized air, or water mattress (Fig. 21-4).
2. Keep bed linens dry, smooth, and free of wrinkles.
3. Post a *written* schedule for repositioning the bed patient *at least every 2 hours* (more often if redness persists).
4. Position patients so that they are not resting on pressure points of the skin.
5. When the patient is in bed, keep the head lowered 30 degrees or less to reduce shearing force caused by sliding down in bed.
6. Apply heel suspension boots to prevent shearing forces to the feet, or use pillows or wedges to prevent heel pressure.
7. For the side-lying position, avoid pressure on the trochanter by tilting at a 30-degree angle.
8. Use pillows or foam wedges to separate knees and ankles.
9. Use a draw sheet or transfer device to avoid friction when moving patients to prevent damage to the uppermost layers of the skin.
10. Teach patients in wheelchairs to shift their weight every 15 minutes. Patients who cannot do this should be repositioned at least hourly.
11. Protect the skin from urine and stool (e.g., absorbent pads or briefs for incontinence). Gently cleanse the skin when soiled and at regular intervals, using warm water and a mild cleansing agent.

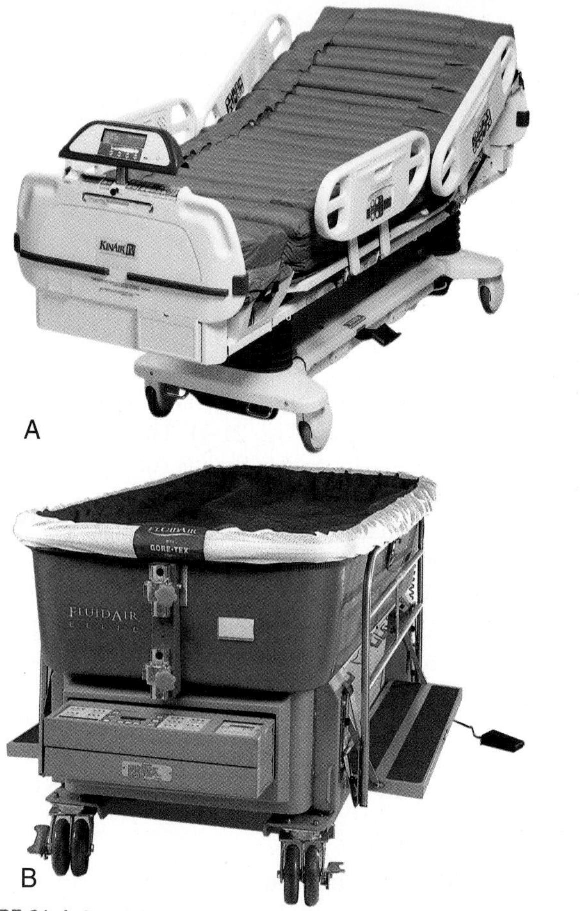

FIGURE 21-4 Specialty beds prevent pressure on bony prominences. **A,** KinAir IV beds provide controlled air suspension. **B,** FluidAir Elite beds use airflow and bead fluidization. Both are covered with tough GORE-TEX fabric that is waterproof and serves as a barrier to bacteria. (Courtesy ArjoHuntleigh.)

12. Use moisturizers, lubricants, protective films, barriers, and dressings to reduce friction and shearing.
13. Institute measures that enhance patient mobility, such as installing trapeze bars.
14. Instruct the patient and family about risk factors and strategies for preventing pressure ulcers.
15. Request an evaluation by the dietitian regarding nutritional needs.

16. Offer a glass of water each time the patient is repositioned to maintain hydration.

The best preventive measure is frequent position change. Do *not* massage pressure points. Any kind of massage around or on a reddened area of skin can damage fragile capillaries. In addition, rubber rings should *not* be used to elevate heels or sacral areas. Rings cause a concentrated area of pressure that places patients at a higher risk for developing pressure ulcers. *Remember: No massage on reddened skin and no rings!* Another important factor that must be considered is the patient's nutritional status. Adequate nutrients are essential to maintain or restore skin integrity.

If pressure ulcers develop despite all preventive measures, assess and precisely describe the stage. Proper documentation helps to evaluate the effectiveness of treatment and progress toward healing and repair. Documenting the skin condition and presence of pressure ulcers on admission to a health care facility is especially important.

Stages of Pressure Ulcers

Pressure ulcers are classified into six stages (Fig. 21-5).

Stage I: Nonblanchable Erythema. The major characteristic of stage I pressure ulcers is erythema (redness) that does not blanch (turn white at the point of pressure) when pressed. Before stage I begins, a finger pressed on a reddened area causes temporary blanching, followed by a return of the erythema when the finger is removed. In stage I, the redness does not fade when the finger is removed. The color ranges from red to the dusky blue called *cyanosis.* The area of pressure reflects the shape of the object creating the pressure or the bony prominence underlying the skin. Pain and tenderness may be present, with warmth, swelling, and hardening of the tissue. In individuals with dark skin, congestion is apparent in increased warmth or coolness, induration (hardening caused by edema), and tenderness. Although not white, the affected skin may appear a different color from surrounding tissue. At this stage, little destruction of tissue has occurred, and the condition is reversible.

Stage II: Partial Thickness. In stage II, some skin loss has occurred in the epidermis and dermis. A blister or shallow ulcer develops. The ulcer bed is pink without dead tissue or bruising. The ulcer is surrounded by a broad, irregular, and painful reddened area that is warmer than normal.

Stage III: Full-Thickness Skin Loss. Stage III is characterized by full-thickness skin loss involving damage or necrosis of the dermis and subcutaneous tissue. Subcutaneous fat may be visible but not bone, tendon, or muscle. A craterlike sore with a distinct outer margin has formed as the epidermis thickens and rolls over the edge toward the ulcer base. The wound may be infected and is usually open and draining with a loss

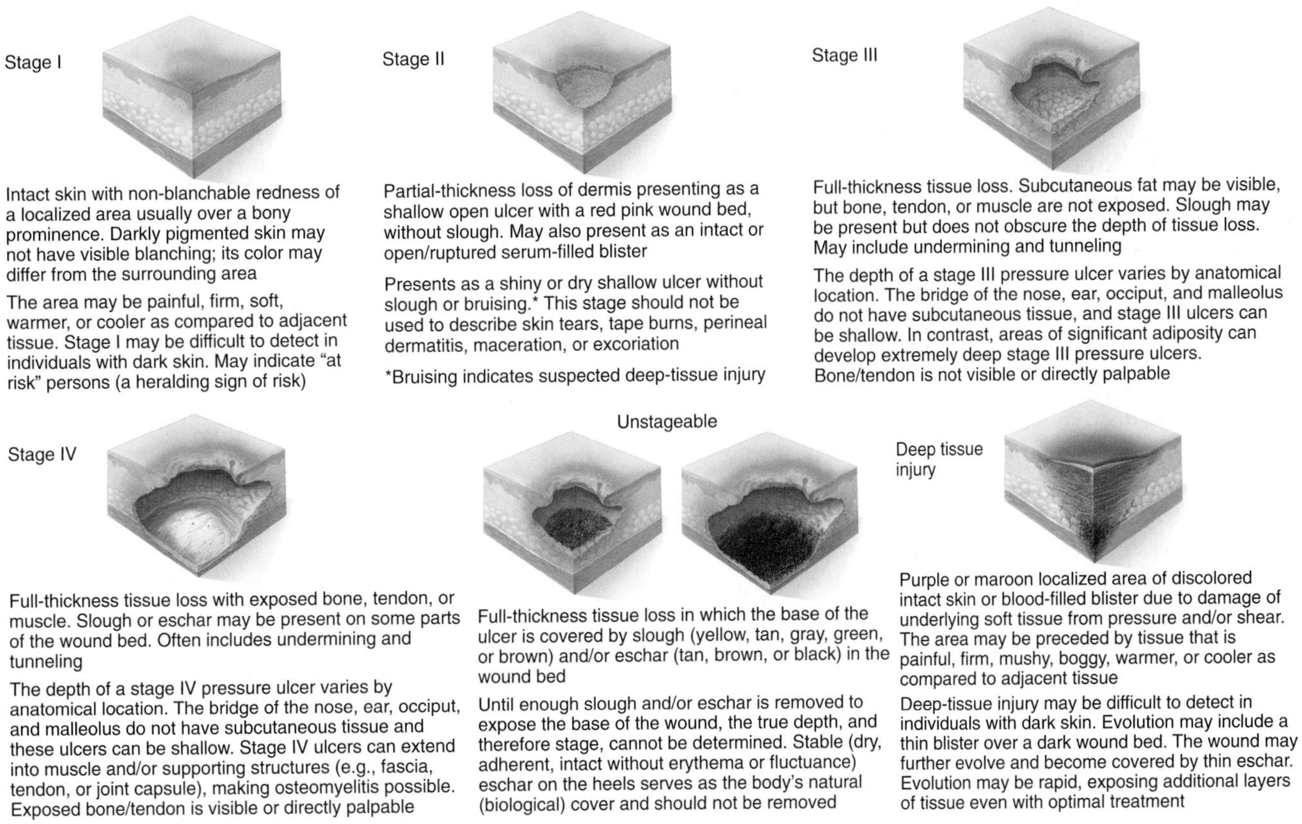
Stage I
Intact skin with non-blanchable redness of a localized area usually over a bony prominence. Darkly pigmented skin may not have visible blanching; its color may differ from the surrounding area
The area may be painful, firm, soft, warmer, or cooler as compared to adjacent tissue. Stage I may be difficult to detect in individuals with dark skin. May indicate "at risk" persons (a heralding sign of risk)
Stage II
Partial-thickness loss of dermis presenting as a shallow open ulcer with a red pink wound bed, without slough. May also present as an intact or open/ruptured serum-filled blister
Presents as a shiny or dry shallow ulcer without slough or bruising.* This stage should not be used to describe skin tears, tape burns, perineal dermatitis, maceration, or excoriation
*Bruising indicates suspected deep-tissue injury
Stage III
Full-thickness tissue loss. Subcutaneous fat may be visible, but bone, tendon, or muscle are not exposed. Slough may be present but does not obscure the depth of tissue loss. May include undermining and tunneling
The depth of a stage III pressure ulcer varies by anatomical location. The bridge of the nose, ear, occiput, and malleolus do not have subcutaneous tissue, and stage III ulcers can be shallow. In contrast, areas of significant adiposity can develop extremely deep stage III pressure ulcers. Bone/tendon is not visible or directly palpable
Stage IV
Full-thickness tissue loss with exposed bone, tendon, or muscle. Slough or eschar may be present on some parts of the wound bed. Often includes undermining and tunneling
The depth of a stage IV pressure ulcer varies by anatomical location. The bridge of the nose, ear, occiput, and malleolus do not have subcutaneous tissue and these ulcers can be shallow. Stage IV ulcers can extend into muscle and/or supporting structures (e.g., fascia, tendon, or joint capsule), making osteomyelitis possible. Exposed bone/tendon is visible or directly palpable
Unstageable
Full-thickness tissue loss in which the base of the ulcer is covered by slough (yellow, tan, gray, green, or brown) and/or eschar (tan, brown, or black) in the wound bed
Until enough slough and/or eschar is removed to expose the base of the wound, the true depth, and therefore stage, cannot be determined. Stable (dry, adherent, intact without erythema or fluctuance) eschar on the heels serves as the body's natural (biological) cover and should not be removed
Deep tissue injury
Purple or maroon localized area of discolored intact skin or blood-filled blister due to damage of underlying soft tissue from pressure and/or shear. The area may be preceded by tissue that is painful, firm, mushy, boggy, warmer, or cooler as compared to adjacent tissue
Deep-tissue injury may be difficult to detect in individuals with dark skin. Evolution may include a thin blister over a dark wound bed. The wound may further evolve and become covered by thin eschar. Evolution may be rapid, exposing additional layers of tissue even with optimal treatment

FIGURE 21-5 Classification of pressure ulcers. (From Black JM, Hawks JH: *Medical-surgical nursing: clinical management for positive outcomes*, ed 8, St. Louis, 2009, Saunders.)

of fluid and protein. The patient may have fever, dehydration, anemia, and leukocytosis (increased white blood cells in the blood).

Stage IV: Full-Thickness Tissue Loss. In stage IV, full-thickness skin loss has occurred with extensive destruction and exposure of bone, tendons, or muscles. The ulcer is usually extensively infected and may appear black with exudation, foul odor, and purulent drainage.

Additional Stages. In the United States, two additional stages are used. The first is labeled *Unstageable/Unclassified: Full-thickness skin or tissue loss—depth unknown*. In this stage, slough (yellow, green, tan, gray, or brown) or eschar (tan, brown, or black) covers the base of a full-thickness ulcer. The true stage cannot be determined until at least part of the wound base can be examined. The second additional stage is *Suspected Deep Tissue Injury—depth unknown*. This stage is characterized by purple or maroon color to intact skin or blood-filled blisters. The actual depth of tissue injury cannot be determined at this point.

Treatment

The first step in treating pressure ulcers is to continue all preventive measures. A pressure ulcer cannot heal unless measures are taken to relieve the pressure that initially caused it. Numerous treatments are used to promote wound healing. The National Pressure Ulcer Advisory Panel provides an excellent summary of research-based recommendations for prevention and treatment. These materials are available under Educational and Clinical Resources at www.npuap.org. In general, stages I and II pressure ulcers should be cleaned with water or normal saline. Avoid pastes, creams, ointments, and powder because they may interfere with healing. In addition, alcohol, antiseptics, and disinfectants are not used because their effectiveness has not been proved; they may actually cause harm. Stages I and II ulcers are not usually infected, therefore topical and oral antibiotics are not appropriate. Heat is not used because a rise in temperature increases the metabolic demands of the tissue and places additional stress on the affected area.

The most effective dressing for a stage I or II pressure ulcer is one that provides a moist environment and maintains a temperature close to body temperature. All wound covers should allow oxygen to pass through. Wound healing is enhanced when the ulcer and surrounding tissues can freely take up oxygen and eliminate carbon dioxide.

Stages III and IV pressure ulcers require more extensive treatment and supportive care. Mechanical devices used for irrigation include spray bottles, bulb and piston syringes, and other specialized irrigating devices such as a Waterpik. Excess pressure can cause trauma and may force bacteria into the wound, therefore the Waterpik should be used only on the lowest setting. Cleansing solutions and antimicrobials may be needed if the wound is infected or has debris. Debridement of necrotic tissue is necessary to promote granulation of new, healthy tissue. Methods of debridement include surgical techniques; autolysis; and enzymatic, mechanical, and biosurgical (maggot therapy) debridement. Debridement is sufficient when the ulcer bed appears pink, indicating healthy granulation tissue. Negative pressure wound care, described in Chapter 52, can significantly decrease the healing time for pressure ulcers. Supportive care consists of measures to treat anemia, dehydration, and protein depletion. Nutritional intervention consists of oral supplements high in protein and vitamins, nasogastric feedings, or parenteral nutrition to provide the additional nutrients necessary for healing.

Stages II, III, and IV pressure ulcers are normally colonized with bacteria. Good wound care usually prevents the bacteria from causing a clinical infection. Topical broad-spectrum antibiotics may be ordered if the wound fails to heal despite good care. If evidence of widespread infection exists, systemic antibiotics are indicated.

Patients may have pain associated with pressure ulcers. Administer an analgesic before dressing changes and debridement procedures. Topical opioids are sometimes applied to the ulcer surface. Allow time for the drug to take effect before the procedure. Patients with chronic ulcer pain may be treated with a local anesthetic and an antidepressant or antiepileptic agent. Transcutaneous electrical nerve stimulation (TENS) may be helpful.

RESPIRATORY STATUS

Oxygen and carbon dioxide are exchanged in the thin, moist mucous membrane that lines the airway passages and the alveoli. Most healthy people take between six and eight deep, sighing breaths every hour. Sighs help to keep the lungs expanded and move secretions upward along the air passages. When a person remains immobile or does not take deep breaths, thick secretions can accumulate and pool in the lower respiratory structures. These secretions interfere with the normal exchange of gases, can cause areas of the lung to collapse (atelectasis), and can provide an environment for growth of pathogens. A lung infection associated with immobility is called *hypostatic pneumonia*.

Individuals who are at risk for impaired gas exchange related to immobility include those who:

- Are given drugs that depress respirations, such as general anesthetic agents, opioids, or sedatives
- Have tight binders or bandages that limit chest expansion
- Have abdominal distention from gas, fluid, or feces
- Lie in one position for extended periods

Older adults are also at risk for respiratory problems related to immobility because age-related changes reduce lung expansion and breathing capacity (see *Patient Teaching* box).

Patient Teaching

Coughing and Deep Breathing

- Coughing and deep breathing are most effective in a sitting position.
- If you have a chest or abdominal surgical incision, support the area with a pillow to minimize discomfort.
- Use the abdominal muscles and diaphragm to expand the lower chest. Inhale deeply through the nose, hold the breath for 1 to 3 seconds, and exhale slowly while pursing your lips. Focus on how much air you can exhale rather than on the force with which you exhale it.
- After 4 to 6 deep breaths, cough deeply. Some sources recommend taking a single deep breath followed by three consecutive coughs, trying to clear all air from the lungs with each cough.

Nursing interventions for patients at risk for respiratory complications include frequent turning and position changes and coughing and deep-breathing exercises. These interventions must be performed every 2 hours to be effective. Coughing and deep-breathing exercises are done at the same time to allow for periods of rest and to obtain the best results.

Effective coughing may be difficult for patients, especially for those who are in pain from a surgical incision or for those who have chronic coughs and are worried that the coughing may trigger a long, exhausting coughing experience. The objective of coughing is to move the secretions gradually upward and to cough them out a little at a time. Teach patients how to cough and to deep breathe effectively (see *Patient Teaching* box). Incentive spirometry (IS) is widely used; however, by itself, it is not adequate to prevent complications. The patient must use the spirometer correctly and practice coughing and deep breathing as well.

To evaluate the effectiveness of nursing interventions, monitor the patient's respiratory status. Count the respiratory rate, observe the respiratory effort and chest movement, check the oxygen saturation if oximetry is used, and listen for crackles in the lung fields.

FOOD AND FLUID INTAKE

In relation to food and fluid intake, the most common problem associated with immobility is *anorexia* (loss of appetite). Factors that contribute to anorexia are worry, depression, anxiety about dependence on others, and decreased metabolic needs resulting from inactivity. *Hypoproteinemia* (protein deficiency) can develop in patients who are immobilized.

Immobilized patients also may have inadequate fluid intake. Getting up for a drink of water may be too difficult and time consuming for inactive individuals or they may not think to drink liquids regularly. Older people are particularly prone to becoming dehydrated from an inadequate fluid intake, resulting in complications such as confusion, constipation, or urinary tract infection.

Maintain accurate records of patients' dietary and fluid intakes. Small, frequent meals may be more acceptable than three large meals for patients with anorexia. Dietary supplements that are high in protein content also may be encouraged. Offer fluids, even small sips of water, juice, or other liquids, at least every hour while awake. Fluids need to be within reach so that patients may have easy access to them if they are able to drink without help. Encourage family members to offer fluids while they are visiting.

ELIMINATION

Constipation

Constipation is one of the most common problems associated with immobility. Contributing factors in the immobile patient include changes in the usual routine and environment, inability to defecate on a bedpan because of embarrassment or discomfort, and weakened muscle tone. In addition, many medications cause constipation by slowing intestinal motility. Constipated individuals may strain to defecate, causing an increase in intraabdominal pressure. This pressure is called the *Valsalva maneuver* or vasovagal reflex and it can lead to cardiovascular alterations and even to lightheadedness and fainting. The vasovagal reflex can be especially problematic in the older person whose circulation may be somewhat impaired.

Confused patients may ignore the normal urge to have a bowel movement. If the impulse is ignored for a considerable time, the natural urge to defecate can diminish and eventually disappear.

Long-standing constipation can result in a fecal impaction. *Fecal impaction* is the presence of hardened or puttylike feces in the rectum and sigmoid colon. If the condition is not relieved, intestinal obstruction can occur. Symptoms of a fecal impaction include painful defecation, a feeling of fullness in the rectum, abdominal distention, and sometimes cramps and watery stool. The presence of diarrhea does not mean that a fecal impaction has been removed, because the liquid fecal material may flow around the hardened mass.

When an impaction develops, the mass of feces must be broken up with a gloved finger (a physician's order is usually needed). Before digital removal of the mass, giving an oil retention enema to soften the mass may be helpful. In addition, an analgesic may be given 1 hour before digital removal of an impaction.

Inactivity, medications, decreased fluid intake, and lack of adequate fiber in the diet all contribute to constipation. A vicious cycle may begin when immobility promotes inactivity, decreased fluid intake, and poor appetite. Patients become weaker, more immobile, and less likely to eat and drink adequately. Encouraging proper foods with adequate roughage, fluids, and as much activity as possible can help to prevent or relieve constipation. Whenever possible, patients should use a bedside commode or be taken to the bathroom to defecate rather than try to use a bedpan. Laxatives should be used sparingly; however, stool softeners may be helpful if the stools are hard and difficult to pass. Patients with long-established laxative dependence may require continued laxative therapy during the period of immobility.

Put on Your Thinking Cap!

With pencil and paper in hand, note the time. Now, sit perfectly still for 10 minutes. At the end of that time, note what sensations and thoughts you experienced. When the time was up, what was the first thing you did? Discuss what a nurse could have done to make you more comfortable. Compare your experience with that of a patient who is immobilized.

Urinary Incontinence

The urinary system functions best when the body is upright. Urine flows downward from the kidney by gravity. When the body is in a reclining position, the kidney must force urine into the ureters against the pull of gravity. Urine is continually being formed in the kidney but the peristaltic action of the ureters is not strong enough to maintain a constant flow of urine. If the body remains in a supine (lying down) position for even a few days, the flow becomes sluggish and the urine pools, which sets the stage for the development of a urinary tract infection.

Lying in bed also can cause a loss of control of the urinary sphincter muscles and result in incontinence. Without the downward pressure of the full bladder against the sphincter muscles, awareness of the need to void is less. The result can be bladder distention with an overflow or a dribbling of urine that the patient cannot control.

Older persons who have problems with mobility may have functional incontinence because they are unable to respond to the urge to void in time. The bladder is usually fuller when the urge to void occurs; consequently, less time is available to get to the bathroom. In addition, they may not be able to move quickly enough because of the slowed reaction time associated with older age or chronic illness.

The most effective way to prevent urinary incontinence associated with immobility is to set up a toileting program. Patients should have scheduled toiletings with adjustments in schedule based on the patients' voiding patterns. If voiding patterns cannot be assessed, patients should, at the very least, be taken to the bathroom or commode or offered a bedpan every 2 hours during waking hours. Some individuals restrict fluids at certain times of the day, especially after dinner and through the night to avoid nighttime incontinence. However, studies have been inconclusive regarding the effectiveness of limiting fluids. Incontinence is covered in greater detail in Chapter 23.

CIRCULATORY EFFECTS

Immobility is a key risk factor for the formation of blood clots in the deep veins of the pelvis and legs. Deep vein thrombosis (DVT) may be manifested by edema, warmth, and tenderness in the affected area. However, about half of patients with DVT have no symptoms. The most serious complication of DVT is pulmonary embolism (PE). Patients considered to be at risk for DVT may be treated with preventive anticoagulants. Other preventive measures include positioning to maintain circulation, range-of-motion exercises, and good hydration. Treatment of DVT is discussed in Chapter 37, and treatment of PE is covered in Chapter 31.

Put on Your Thinking Cap!

Observe a person during class, church, a movie, or other situation where people are expected to stay seated. Note the number of movements by that person in a 5-minute period. Identify the therapeutic value of those motions.

Get Ready for the NCLEX® Examination!

Key Points

- The psychologic effects of immobility may include depression, fear, anxiety, social withdrawal, apathy, loss of financial and personal independence, and lack of meaningful existence.
- Among the complications of immobility are pressure ulcers, respiratory problems, impaired nutrition, constipation, and urinary tract infection and incontinence.
- Exercise is the best medicine for immobility.
- Exercises may be active (performed by the patient) or passive (movement of the patient's body performed by another person without assistance from the patient).
- Pressure ulcers are expensive to treat, extend hospital stays, increase the likelihood of placement in a long-term care facility, and increase mortality.
- The best preventive measure for pressure ulcers is frequent position changes.
- The major principles of pressure ulcer wound management are: (1) clean the area, (2) promote the formation of granulation tissue, and (3) ensure adequate nutritional intake for wound healing.
- Especially in older adults, immobility can contribute to respiratory problems, including impaired gas exchange, atelectasis, and hypostatic pneumonia.
- Factors that contribute to respiratory complications of immobility include drugs that depress respirations and

dry secretions; tight binders or bandages that limit chest expansion; abdominal distention from gas, fluid, or feces; and lying in one position for extended periods.
- Frequent turning and position changes and encouraging coughing and deep-breathing exercises help to prevent respiratory complications of immobility.
- Anorexia (loss of appetite) is the most common nutritional problem associated with immobility.
- Immobility contributes to constipation by causing a change in the usual routine and environment, an inability to defecate on a bedpan because of embarrassment or discomfort, and a weakening of muscle tone.
- Immobility can promote a loss of control of the urinary sphincter muscles, resulting in incontinence.
- The most effective way to prevent urinary incontinence associated with immobility is to set up a toileting program.
- Urinary stasis increases the risk of urinary tract infections.
- Anticoagulants may be prescribed to prevent deep vein thrombosis (DVT) in the immobilized patient.

Additional Learning Resources

SG Go to your Study Guide for additional learning activities to help you master this chapter content.

evolve Go to your Evolve website (http://evolve.elsevier.com/Linton/medsurg) for the following learning resources and much more:
- Interactive Prioritization Exercises
- Fluid & Electrolyte Tutorial
- Pharmacology Tutorial
- Review Questions for the NCLEX® Examination

Review Questions for the NCLEX® Examination

1. A patient who sustained a head injury has not regained consciousness. The nurse moves the patient's joints through their normal movements twice a day. This exercise intervention is called:
   1. Isometric
   2. Active
   3. Passive
   4. Isotonic

   NCLEX Client Need: Physiological Integrity: Basic Care and Comfort
2. The home health nurse is teaching family members how to move a patient up in bed by using a draw sheet to prevent which of the following?
   1. Tissue trauma from shearing force
   2. Strain on the caregiver
   3. Disturbing the bed linens
   4. Extension contractures of the spine

   NCLEX Client Need: Physiological Integrity: Basic Care and Comfort
3. The nursing care plan for an immobilized patient includes the following interventions. Which one is specifically intended to maintain skin integrity?
   1. Keep joints in functional positions
   2. Reposition the patient at least every 2 hours
   3. Perform range-of-motion exercises twice daily
   4. Give at least eight 8-ounce glasses of fluids each day

   NCLEX Client Need: Physiological Integrity: Basic Care and Comfort and Reduction of Risk Potential
4. During a bed bath, you observe a reddened area over the sacrum. You should:
   1. Document erythema and instruct nursing assistants to keep the patient off his back
   2. Gently massage the reddened area with skin lotion to provide protective moisture
   3. Place a round inflatable cushion under the patient's buttocks to relieve pressure on the sacrum
   4. Position the patient on one side and use a heat lamp to stimulate circulation to the area

   NCLEX Client Need: Physiological Integrity: Basic Care and Comfort
5. Instructions in effective coughing for the patient after abdominal surgery should include which of the following?
   1. Try not to use the abdominal muscles during coughing and deep-breathing exercises
   2. Assume a comfortable position on your side to reduce strain on the incision
   3. Exhale as forcefully and for as long as you can
   4. Take one deep breath and then cough three times, trying to clear all air from the lungs

   NCLEX Client Need: Physiological Integrity: Reduction of Risk Potential
6. A postoperative patient reports that she was straining to have a bowel movement when she became lightheaded. You should suspect which of the following?
   1. Valsalva maneuver
   2. Internal hemorrhage
   3. Dehydration
   4. Wound dehiscence

   NCLEX Client Need: Physiological Integrity: Physiological Adaptation
7. What is the effect of immobility on the urinary tract?
   1. Decreased urine production by the kidneys
   2. Pooling of urine in the urinary system
   3. Increased blood flow to kidneys
   4. Increased bladder sensitivity to fullness

NCLEX Client Need: Physiological Integrity: Reduction of Risk Potential

chapter

22 Delirium and Dementia

http://evolve.elsevier.com/Linton/medsurg

Objectives

1. Describe the neurocognitive disorders (NCDs): delirium, mild NCD, and major NCD.
2. Describe the subtypes of mild and major NCDs.
3. Identify the common causes of delirium.
4. Explain the differences between delirium and dementia.
5. Identify drugs used to treat delirium and dementia.
6. Discuss nursing assessment and interventions related to delirium and dementia.

Key Terms

Delirium (dĕ-LĒ-rē-ŭm)

Dementia (dĕ-MĔN-shēă)

The thing that the majority of people fear most about aging is the prospect of losing independence. When significant disturbances in cognition occur, the ability to care for oneself declines as well. Fortunately a decline in cognitive ability is not a part of normal aging, despite some changes in information processing described in Chapter 11. Nevertheless, older age is a risk factor for various states that cause cognitive impairment.

Altered mental function may develop suddenly or gradually depending on the underlying pathology. Some causes can be treated, resulting in a return to usual cognition, whereas other causes are not reversible. Altered cognitive states are commonly diagnosed as delirium or dementia depending on the onset, duration, contributing factors, response to intervention, and progression. It is possible to have both conditions at the same time. In general, the term *delirium* is used to describe a state of impaired cognition that occurs rather suddenly and usually resolves when the underlying problem is corrected. Examples of factors that may cause delirium in the older adult are infection, fever, and drug effects.

The *Diagnostic and Statistical Manual of Mental Disorders*, 5th edition (DSM-5) is published by the American Psychiatric Association. The DSM-5 provides guidelines for the diagnosis and classification of mental disorders. Neurocognitive disorders (NCDs) include delirium, mild NCD, major NCD, and numerous subtypes based on cause. NCDs exist along a continuum from mild to moderate depending on the severity of impairment. The term *dementia* is commonly used to refer to major NCDs.

Each of the neurocognitive disorders affects one or more domains of cognitive function. These domains are complex attention, executive function, learning and memory, language, perceptual-motor function, and social cognition. Disorders of complex attention result in difficulty staying on task and sorting through multiple stimuli. Executive function allows us to plan, make decisions, carry out plans, and evaluate our activities. Therefore a person with impaired executive function has difficulty with multitasking and carrying out multiple steps. Disorders of learning and memory may affect short-term and long-term memory, which can affect all aspects of function. A person might forget appointments, leave food on a hot stove, be unable to dress or shop, or become lost. Language disorders can affect the ability to understand or use words. Perceptual-motor disorders can affect the ability to perform usual activities, such as driving a car. Various defects in vision may be present. Social cognition is concerned with recognizing emotions. When social cognition is disturbed, people may say or do socially inappropriate things. They may have personality changes and become insensitive to the feelings of others. These disturbances can be mild or major.

DELIRIUM

Delirium is a decline from a person's usual attention and awareness (orientation to the environment). People with delirium may have difficulty focusing or paying attention; consequently they are easily distracted. Engaging them in a conversation may be difficult and often questions must be repeated. Delirium develops over a short period of time and tends to vary in severity throughout the day. In addition to altered attention and awareness, the patient has an additional disturbance such as memory deficit, disorientation, or a language or perceptual problem. Speech may be slurred and disjointed with aimless repetitions. Individuals may misinterpret what is happening in the environment and may develop delusional thinking and experience hallucinations. For example, they may think that the banging of a door is a gunshot. A common delusion is that someone is trying to steal from them. Sleep-wake disturbances are common. A delirious person may be hyperactive, hypoactive, or alternate between the two. The level of consciousness may fluctuate from drowsiness to stupor or coma. At the other extreme, the individual may be extremely alert and agitated.

For a diagnosis of delirium, evidence must exist that the symptoms can be explained by a medical condition, substance intoxication or withdrawal, exposure to a toxin, or multiple causes. Examples of medical conditions that can cause delirium are infections, liver or kidney failure, fluid and electrolyte imbalances, and hypoxia. Among the many drugs that can cause delirium are alcohol, opioids, cannabis, hallucinogens, sedatives, antianxiety drugs, amphetamines, and cocaine. Withdrawal after regular use of these and other drugs can cause substance withdrawal delirium. Anticholinergics have been found to contribute to delirium among older persons. In addition to drugs and some medical conditions, immobility and boredom also are risk factors for delirium. Although delirium can occur at any age, it is more prevalent in older adults. Examples of factors that can contribute to delirium are listed in Box 22-1.

Delirium typically responds to treatment, with the patient returning to the previous level of cognitive function. The medical management of delirium includes managing the symptoms and treating or removing the cause. For example, if delirium is the result of a drug or drug interaction, medication orders will need to be changed. If delirium occurs with an infection, antimicrobial medications are ordered. If the patient is so severely agitated that essential care cannot be given or the patient poses a danger to self or others, an antipsychotic drug may be ordered. Examples of

Box 22-1 Systemic and Central Nervous System Causes of Delirium

SYSTEMIC CAUSES

Cardiovascular Disease
Congestive heart failure
Dysrhythmias
Cardiac infarction
Hypovolemia (deficient fluid volume)
Aortic stenosis

Infections
Pneumonia
Urinary tract infections
Bacteremia
Septicemia

Medications
Alcohol
Amphetamines
Analgesics
Anticholinergics
Antidepressants
Antihistamines
Antiparkinsonian agents
First-generation H2-receptor blockers (e.g., cimetidine [Tagamet])
Diuretics
Neuroleptics (e.g., haloperidol [Haldol])
Sedatives or hypnotic agents (benzodiazepines [e.g., diazepam {Valium}, barbiturates])

Metabolic Conditions
Electrolyte and fluid imbalance
Hepatic, renal, or pulmonary failure
Diabetes, hyperthyroidism, hypothyroidism, or other endocrine disorders
Nutritional deficiencies
Hypothermia and heat stroke

Neoplasm

Postoperative State

Poisons
Heavy metals
Solvents
Pesticides
Carbon monoxide

Trauma
Head injury
Burns
Hip fracture

CENTRAL NERVOUS SYSTEM CAUSES

Infections
Meningitis
Encephalitis
Septic emboli
Neurosyphilis
Brain abscess
HIV

Neoplasm
Primary intracranial
Metastatic

Trauma
Subdural hematoma
Extradural hematoma
Contusion

Vascular Incidents
Transient ischemic attack
Stroke
Chronic subdural hematoma
Vasculitis
Arteriosclerosis
Hypertensive encephalopathy
Subarachnoid hemorrhage

Seizures
Ictal and postictal states

From Zisook S, Braff DL: Delirium: recognition and management in the older patient, *Geriatrics* 41(6):67–78, 1986.
HIV, Human immunodeficiency virus.

antipsychotic drugs are haloperidol (Haldol), risperidone (Risperdal), aripiprazole (Abilify), quetiapine (Seroquel), and olanzapine (Zyprexa). However, because antipsychotic drugs increase the risk of death in elderly patients, they should be used with great caution. There is some evidence of benefit from the following nonneuroleptics: carbamazepine, sodium valproate, trazodone, and citalopram. Some antipsychotics can cause serious reactions in patients with Lewy body dementia or Parkinson disease dementia. Benzodiazepines should be avoided in older persons because they are more likely to cause oversedation or worsen confusion.

MILD NEUROCOGNITIVE DISORDER

Mild NCD is a modest decline from one's usual function in one or more cognitive domains. The individual functions well enough to live independently. The disorder can be due to various types of dementia described below in the section on major NCD as well as to other medical conditions. Patients may or may not exhibit behavioral symptoms such as agitation, apathy, sleep disturbances, depression, anxiety, hallucinations, and delusions.

Nursing care with mild NCD focuses on compensating for the functions that are declining. For example, numerous strategies can be used to cope with impaired memory. A medication container with daily dividers can help the person to take the correct drugs each day and avoid double dosing. Written "to do" lists can provide reminders of activities or chores. If executive function is impaired, the person can be helped to focus on a single task at a time and to break tasks into smaller steps that can be readily done.

MAJOR NEUROCOGNITIVE DISORDER (DEMENTIA)

Major NCDs (dementias) are characterized by a "significant cognitive decline from a previous level of performance in one or more of the cognitive domains" (DSM-5, p. 602). **Dementia** is not a disease in itself; it is a clinical syndrome, a collection of symptoms that can occur with many types of diseases. The onset and progression vary with the subtype. Features of the major subtypes are described in Table 22-1. (Also, see *Cultural Considerations* box.) The most prevalent types of dementia are due to Alzheimer disease (AD), vascular disease, frontotemporal dementia (FTD), Lewy body disease, and Parkinson disease. Other conditions that are associated with dementia include traumatic brain injury, substance use and medication effect, human immunodeficiency virus (HIV) infection, prion disease, Huntington disease, and specific or multiple medical

Table 22-1 Major Neurocognitive Disorder (Dementia) Subtypes

DEMENTIA ETIOLOGIC SUBTYPE	USUAL FEATURES
Alzheimer disease	Insidious onset. Gradual, steady progression in cognitive and behavioral symptoms. Decline in memory and learning and at least one other cognitive domain. Depression and apathy common in early stage. Irritability, agitation, combativeness, delusions, hallucinations, and wandering may occur in later stages. Final stage marked by gait disturbance, dysphagia, incontinence, muscle spasms, and possible seizures. Patient becomes mute and totally dependent for care.
Frontotemporal lobar degeneration	Insidious onset. Progression is gradual but faster than AD. Two variants (forms) exist: behavioral and language. Behavioral symptoms: disinhibition, apathy, loss of sympathy or empathy, repeated or compulsive behavior, excessive eating. Persons with behavioral form also decline in social cognition and executive function. Individuals with language form decline in speech production, word finding, object naming, grammar, or word comprehension.
Lewy body disease	Insidious onset and gradual progression. Often seen with AD or vascular disease. Attention and awareness fluctuates. May have auditory hallucinations, orthostatic hypotension, and incontinence. Repeated falls and syncope (fainting) are common, as are Parkinson symptoms (tremor, slow movement, shuffling gait). Cognitive symptoms appear about the same time as motor symptoms. Patients are very sensitive to antipsychotic drugs.
Vascular disease	Onset is related to a cerebrovascular event. Primary decline is in complex attention and executive function. Personality and mood changes, depression, emotional lability, and psychomotor slowing are common.
Parkinson disease	Insidious onset and gradual progression. Established diagnosis of Parkinson disease. May have apathy, depression, anxiety, hallucinations, delusions, personality changes, REM sleep behavior disorder, and excessive daytime sleepiness.

Data from Mayo Clinic: *Alzheimer's disease.* Accessed June 5, 2014 from http://www.mayoclinic.org/diseases-conditions/alzheimers-disease/indepth/alzheimers-stages/art-20048448?pg=2&p=1; Mayo Clinic: *Frontotemporal dementia.* Accessed June 5, 2014 from http://www.mayoclinic.org/diseases-conditions/frontotemporal-dementia/basics/definition/con-20023876?p=1; Mayo Clinic: *Lewy body dementia.* Accessed June 5, 2014 from http://www.mayoclinic.org/diseases-conditions/lewy-body-dementia/basics/definition/con-20025038?p=1; Mayo Clinic: *Parkinson's disease.* Retrieved June 5, 2014 from http://www.mayoclinic.org/diseases-conditions/parkinsons-disease/basics/definition/con-20028488?p=1; Mayo Clinic: *Vascular dementia.* Accessed June 5, 2014 from http://www.mayoclinic.org/diseases-conditions/vascular-dementia/basics/definition/con-20029330?p=1.
AD, Alzheimer disease; *NCD*, neurocognitive disorder; *REM*, rapid eye movement.

conditions. People can have more than one type of dementia at the same time and also can have delirium in addition to dementia.

The cause of AD is unknown but characteristic changes in the brain include deposits of amyloid (a protein), neurofibrillary tangles (i.e., tangled microtubules in neurons) associated with altered tau protein, and a deficiency of neurotransmitters, especially acetylcholine. Neurotransmitters are chemicals that transmit signals in the brain. These changes affect the structure and function of the neurons in the brain. Vascular dementia results from damage to brain cells caused by inadequate blood supply. Patients with vascular dementia often have had a series of small strokes that cause progressive damage. Lewy body disease is characterized by the presence of a protein called synuclein, first seen in the substantia nigra and later in the cerebral cortex. Parkinson disease is associated with a deficiency of dopamine. Frontotemporal dementia is manifested by behavioral symptoms and/or language disorders, depending on the areas of the brain affected. Atrophy of the frontal lobes are associated with behavioral changes, while problems with language are the result of temporal lobe changes.

Cultural Considerations

What Does Culture Have to Do with Dementia?

Caregivers from lower socioeconomic families are more likely to be caring for older parents at an earlier age, when the caregiver is employed or still has children at home.

At this time there is no "cure" for dementia; it is generally considered irreversible. The medical treatment offered depends on the type of dementia. Several drugs are available for patients with AD. The response to these drugs is highly variable; a small percentage of individuals have significantly improved function whereas most others do not. Most AD drugs act to increase the amount of acetylcholine in the brain. They are most effective in the early to middle stages of AD. These include donepezil (Aricept), rivastigmine (Exelon), and galantamine (Razadyne). Memantine (Namenda) is used in mid- to late-stage dementia. It prevents the effects of galantamine, a harmful substance released by AD-damaged cells, and prevents excess calcium entry into the neurons. None of the AD drugs is curative and eventually the patient will decline despite drug therapy. All of these drugs have significant side effects that some patients may not be able to tolerate. Antidepressant and antipsychotic medications are sometimes prescribed as well; however, antipsychotic drugs increase the risk of death, so their use requires careful consideration. If antidepressants are used, selective serotonin reuptake inhibitors (SSRIs) such as citalopram or sertraline are recommended. If sleep is disturbed, mirtazapine or trazodone is recommended. Treatment of cerebrovascular disease and Parkinson disease is discussed in other chapters of this book.

Cultural Considerations

What Does Culture Have to Do with Dementia?

Tests used in the diagnosis of dementia may not be appropriate for individuals with less than high school education or those whose primary language is not English.

NURSING CARE of the Patient with a Neurocognitive Disorder

Assessment

The first step in collecting data about a person with an NCD is to observe the behavior and to collect data about mental status. Licensed vocational nurses/licensed practical nurses (LVNs/LPNs) may use standardized tools for a focused assessment of orientation and memory. Orientation is commonly based on the patient's ability to state his or her name, location, and date and time. The person who cannot accurately report his or her name, location, and time is said to be disoriented or confused. However, for patients in long-term care, uncertainty about days of the week and dates is not unusual. Note the patient's response to questions and instructions to determine use of language. If a change in cognitive status is recent, note any events surrounding the change (i.e., infection, relocation, major loss). Also record other symptoms such as depression, apathy, agitation, restlessness, and wandering. If the patient has exhibited aggression or agitation, ask what factors trigger these behaviors. In the community, the patient or family may be able to supply information about acute or chronic illnesses and current medications. In long-term care settings, the physician's health history should provide this information. Be alert for medications that most often cause confusion in older adults. These include anticholinergic drugs, digoxin, H2 receptor blockers, benzodiazepines, nonsteroidal antiinflammatory drugs (NSAIDs), and many antidysrhythmic and antihypertensive drugs (see Box 22-1). Also ask about any drugs prescribed for neurocognitive symptoms.

Of greatest importance for nursing care is a description of the patient's usual routine, preferences, use of assistive devices, and ability to carry out activities of daily living. Note patterns of activity and rest, dietary needs, mobility, and elimination. If the patient lives independently, it is important to assess the ability to prepare meals, shop, use the telephone, manage finances, and maintain the living environment. With delirium, self-care should improve as confusion diminishes. The person with dementia will need increasingly more assistance as the condition progresses.

Determining when confusion started and whether it has been constant or intermittent can help

Table 22-2 Clinical Features in Delirium and Dementia

FEATURE	DELIRIUM	DEMENTIA
Onset	Sudden onset	Months to years
Duration	Hours to days	Long term or lifetime
Mood	Labile, suspicious, mood swings	Fluctuating, depressed, apathetic, uninterested
Behavior	Variable; hyperactive or hypoactive	Variable; psychomotor retardation or agitation
Cognition		
Orientation	Impaired; variable severity	Slow decline over time
Alertness	Lethargic or hypervigilant	Generally normal
Memory	Impaired recent memory	Initially, impaired recent memory; later, remote memory also impaired
Thought processes	Poor concentration; disorganized, fragmented thinking	Impaired abstract thinking; difficulty finding words; impaired judgment
Perception	Possible visual, auditory, and tactile hallucinations or delusions	Hallucinations and delusions may occur
Speech and language	Slurred, forced, or rambling	Disordered

Adapted from Kazer, MW: Cognitive and neurologic function. In Meiner SE, editor: *Gerontological nursing*, ed 4, St. Louis, 2011, Elsevier-Mosby.

to differentiate delirium and dementia. Some major differences between the clinical features of delirium and dementia are described in Table 22-2. Nursing care of delirium and dementia is addressed separately, although there are some common interventions. The *Coordinated Care* box offers tips on helping certified nursing assistants (CNAs) to provide nursing care for patients with delirium and dementia.

Nursing Diagnoses, Goals, and Outcome Criteria: Delirium

Nursing Diagnoses	Goals and Outcome Criteria
Acute Confusion related to drugs, infection, dehydration, unfamiliar setting, sensory overload or deprivation	Improved thought processes: orientation to person, place, and time; calm behavior, no combative actions
Disturbed Sleep Pattern related to agitation, mood alterations, drug effects	Restoration of patient's usual sleep pattern: fewer nighttime awakenings, patient reports feeling rested
Risk for Injury related to agitation, disorientation, unfamiliar setting	Safety maintained: absence of injury

Interventions: Delirium

When managing the patient with delirium, the physician focuses on identifying and treating the cause of the problem. The nurse focuses on supporting the patient to maintain safety and comfort and to reduce anxiety. Nursing care can be more effective than drugs in managing confusion.

Acute Confusion

Delirium may develop during hospitalization or may be a reason for hospitalization. If possible, the patient should be in a private room with continual supervision. Keep the room quiet and uncluttered to avoid agitation caused by extraneous stimuli. Lighting should be soft and diffuse to avoid shadows that may be misinterpreted and add to the patient's fears. Familiar objects such as photographs, a clock, and a large calendar placed in the room may help orient the patient to time and person. Encourage patients who normally wear hearing aids and glasses to use them.

Communication with a confused patient should be simple and direct. Anyone dealing with a delirious patient should be calm, warm, and reassuring. Speak before touching the patient and always explain what you are doing. It is helpful if the same personnel are assigned to care for the patient from day to day. Handle the patient gently when providing care.

Patients with delirium may have frightening hallucinations that cause them to strike out, cry, or scream. The best response is to orient the patient to the reality of being sick and hospitalized and to explain that the hallucinations are not real even though they seem to be. You might say, "You are sick in the hospital and what you are seeing is part of the illness." Hallucinating patients in a delirious state need one-to-one nursing observation and repeated verbal reorientation. They need to be assured that the medical and nursing staff are helping them and keeping them safe.

Frequent orientation to the surroundings and the situation is important for patients with delirium. Orienting phrases such as "here in the hospital" or "now that it is evening" can be woven into conversation. Keep choices to a minimum. Simple, direct statements ("Now it is time to take your bath") are better than

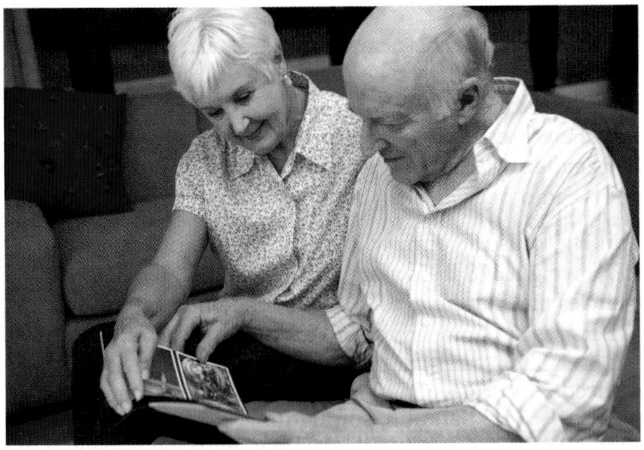

FIGURE 22-1 Presence of a family member may help to calm a confused patient. (Copyright ThinkStockPhotos.com. All rights reserved.)

questions ("When would you like to take a bath?"). All communication and nursing care should be carried out in a way that conveys respect and preserves the patient's dignity.

Disturbed Sleep Pattern

Sleep deprivation can cause or contribute to disorientation and confusion. Nursing measures such as giving a back rub, providing a glass of warm milk, and having a soothing conversation may help the patient to relax and fall asleep. Encourage the patient to void before bedtime. Schedule medications or treatments at times that do not interrupt nighttime sleep. The presence of a family member may help to calm an agitated and confused patient (Fig. 22-1).

Risk for Injury

The patient with delirium may pull on tubes, try to get out of bed unassisted, or attempt to leave the setting. Protecting the patient from harm without imposing excessive restrictions can be challenging. Avoid physical restraints, which tend to increase anxiety and agitation in confused patients and often result in injuries, Instead, ask a family member to remain with the patient or assign a staff member to do so. Use common sense. Position tubes out of sight. Place the bed in the low position. Postpone activities that are flexible. If the confused patient does not need to stay in bed, allow him or her to sit in a chair or even to "visit" the nurses' station in a wheelchair. Avoid arguing with delirious patients. Give a gentle explanation of what is being done and the reason why it is being done.

These nursing diagnoses are only a few that might apply to the patient with delirium. Depending on the situation, different priorities will present themselves (see Nursing Care Plan 22-1: Patient with Delirium).

Interventions: Dementia

Most people with dementia suffer from chronic, debilitating, progressive illness. The goal for individuals with dementia is to maintain the highest level of functioning possible as their abilities gradually diminish (see Nursing Care Plan 22-2: Patient with Dementia).

Nursing Diagnoses, Goals, and Outcome Criteria: Dementia

Nursing Diagnoses	Goals and Outcome Criteria
(Bathing, Dressing, Feeding, Toileting) Self-Care Deficit related to impaired thinking, sensory and motor dysfunction	Maximum possible independence in activities of daily living: patient participates in bathing, grooming, feeding, and toileting with assistance as needed.
Imbalanced Nutrition: Less Than Body Requirements related to difficulty with self-feeding, inattention	Adequate nutrition: weight is stable (within 5 pounds of the ideal weight).
Disturbed Sleep Pattern related to neurologic changes, altered perceptions	Adequate sleep: patient rests at night and remains physically active and awake during the day.
Risk for Injury related to poor judgment, physical decline, sensorimotor changes	Absence of injuries: patient has no falls, suffers no bruises, cuts, or fractures.
Chronic Confusion/ Impaired Verbal Communication related to memory loss, altered perception, impaired judgment, anxiety	Cooperative behavior: patient is calm; no combative or dangerous behavior is demonstrated. Effective communication: patient needs are recognized by caregivers.

Coordinated Care

Working with Patients with Dementia

Working with patients with dementia can be frustrating for CNAs. The best thing the LVN/LPN can do is to model good interactions with patients. In addition, give the following explanations to CNAs:

- Rudeness and uncooperative behavior are symptoms of dementia and are best managed with kindness and patience.
- Because patients with dementia have memory impairments, information and instructions may have to be repeated at intervals.
- When patients resist care, let the LVN/LPN know and try a different approach later.

Self-Care Deficit

As with patients with delirium, the first priority for patients with dementia is to meet their basic needs. Adequate nutrition, fluid and electrolyte balance, sleep, elimination, and hygiene must be maintained. Patients with dementia have varying levels of competence when it comes to carrying out these functions. Determine the patient's level of functioning and then

Disturbed Sleep Pattern

Sleep and awakening hours are often reversed in patients with dementia. Providing stimulation to keep them awake during the day may help them to sleep at night. Schedule tests and treatments during the morning and early afternoon to allow the patient time to wind down by bedtime. Some caregivers have found that a quiet hour in the evening with soft music playing promotes sleep at night. However, sometimes the patient persists in nighttime awakening. When that occurs, assist the patient to the toilet, offer fluids and/or a snack, and provide comfort measures. Offer reassurance in a soft, soothing manner. The patient may go back to sleep afterward. Avoid regular use of sedatives; however, prolonged periods of wakefulness can lead to delirium. If a sleeping aid is needed, trazodone (Oleptro) is preferred.

Risk for Injury

A safe, structured environment is essential for the person with dementia. Nothing harmful should be left around. Falls and injuries may be prevented with environmental modifications, careful observation, muscle strengthening, and a fall prevention program (see Chapter 20). Avoid restraints, if possible; they may aggravate agitation and have been associated with injuries such as skin tears, obstructed circulation, and even strangulation. Arrange furniture for easy access to toilets from the patient's bed or chair. Use nightlights to illuminate the path to the bathroom. Lights that turn on in response to detected motion may be used as well.

Chronic Confusion and Impaired Verbal Communication

Communication usually becomes increasingly difficult. Patients with dementia are disoriented and their thinking ability is impaired. They are confused by what is going on around them. Communication should be simple and direct. Approach them gently, calmly, and quietly. They tend to copy the behavior of people around them; consequently a caregiver who is anxious or upset can easily convey these feelings to a patient. Nonverbal communication is extremely important. Cues from the patient's actions and facial expressions are important because patients are frequently unable to express their needs verbally. When patients resist activities such as bathing or dressing, avoid confrontations, which only provoke agitation and possible violence. Instead, come back at another time. A consistent schedule of care given by the same caregivers provides security for the patient with dementia.

Whereas frequent reality orientation is helpful for the patient with delirium, such orientation is not effective for the patient with dementia. Clocks, calendars, constant mention of the date and time, and other such orientation reminders used to be a staple of care for patients with dementia. However, reality orientation may agitate people with dementia. Furthermore, patients may not be able to use clocks and calendars. Assisting them in a nonconfrontational manner and redirecting activities without constantly reminding them of their deficits is a better approach.

> **Put on Your Thinking Cap!**
>
> A patient's daughter is distressed because her mother does not seem to recognize her at times. What could you say to help the daughter? What suggestions could you give her to promote communication with her mother?

GUIDELINES FOR WORKING WITH PATIENTS WITH DEMENTIA

Two important concepts are helpful to keep in mind when taking care of patients with dementia: (1) they usually forget things relatively quickly and (2) they are usually unable to learn new things. For example, if persons with dementia start to become agitated, it may be effective to divert their attention somewhere else. They may be gently guided to another activity; usually within a relatively short period they will forget what was bothering them and focus on the new activity (Fig. 22-2). Sometimes agitation indicates pain, hunger, stress, fear, or the need for toileting. Investigate whether any of these problems are present. Take advantage of the fact that patients with dementia are usually slow or unable to learn new things. For example, putting new locks on the doors in new places may prevent wandering patients from opening exit doors. Using these two concepts as a basis for care allows the caregiver to be creative in the care of patients with dementia.

The cognitive developmental approach (CDA) can also guide care for patients with dementia. The CDA

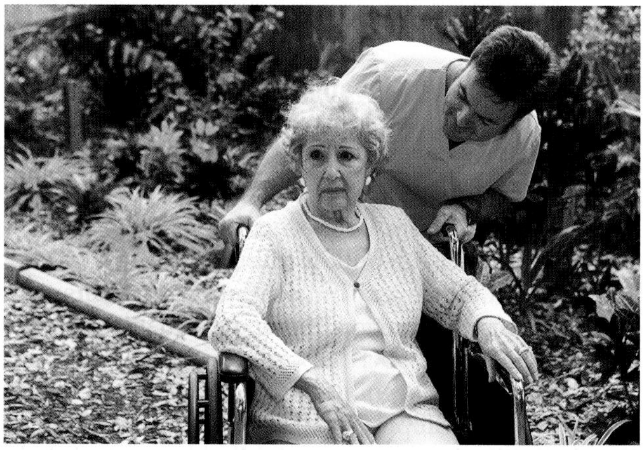

FIGURE 22-2 Calmly diverting the attention of confused, agitated patients somewhere else by gently guiding them to another activity is best. (Copyright ThinkStockPhotos.com. All rights reserved.)

adapts interventions based on the patient's cognitive abilities. Eliminating unrealistic expectations and allowing the patient to do as much as he or she is able is believed to reduce patient stress and frustration. Some principles derived from the CDA that can be applied are as follows:

- Accept that the patient with dementia may no longer be able to make adult decisions and behave as a healthy adult would. Offer limited choices to simplify decision making.
- Adapt the environment to the patient rather than the patient to the environment. For example, create a safe environment for wandering instead of trying to keep the patient from wandering.
- Encourage self-care at whatever level the patient can function. If the patient can eat independently with his or her hands but not with utensils, provide finger foods.
- Recognize irrational fears such as a fear of the bathtub; arrange for alternative ways to give personal care.
- Accept that, in advanced dementia, patient behaviors and thinking are not typical of a healthy adult. Some strategies that work with children often work with dementia patients.
- Recognize that the patient deserves to be treated with dignity, regardless of abilities or behaviors. Even the most impaired patient can probably sense compassion in a caregiver.

Get Ready for the NCLEX® Examination!

Key Points

- Neurocognitive disorders (NCDs) include delirium, mild NCD, and major NCD.
- The domains of cognitive function that may be affected by NCDs are complex attention, executive function, learning and memory, language, perceptual-motor function, and social cognition.
- Patients who are not oriented to person, place, and time are said to be disoriented or confused.
- Delirium is a rather sudden decline from a person's usual attention and awareness (orientation to the environment) that is usually reversible.
- Symptoms of delirium may include memory deficit, disorientation, delusions, hallucinations, and a language or perceptual problem.
- Delirium is usually caused by some underlying medical condition such as infection, liver or kidney failure, fluid and electrolyte imbalances, hypoxia, substance intoxication or withdrawal, exposure to a toxin, or multiple causes.
- Dementia is chronic, progressive, and generally considered irreversible.
- Dementia exists on a spectrum from mild to major neurocognitive dysfunction.
- Dementia is characterized by a "significant cognitive decline from a previous level of performance in one or more of the cognitive domains" (DSM-5, p. 602). Dementia is not a disease entity in itself; it is a clinical syndrome, a collection of symptoms that may be cause by a variety of conditions.
- The most common types of dementia are Alzheimer disease (AD), vascular dementia, frontotemporal dementia (FTD), Lewy body dementia, and Parkinson disease dementia.
- The first step in the focused assessment of a cognitively impaired person is to observe the patient's behavior and to evaluate mental status.
- Determine how long the symptoms have been present and how and when they started.
- In caring for a patient with delirium, provide safety and comfort measures, as well as frequent orientation to the surroundings and situation.
- The goal for patients with dementia is to maintain the highest level of functioning possible as their abilities gradually diminish.
- A safe, structured environment is essential for patients with dementia and tasks should be broken down into steps that can be performed one at a time.
- When patients with dementia resist activities such as bathing or dressing, avoid confrontations and divert their attention elsewhere.
- The cognitive developmental approach (CDA) adapts interventions to the patient's cognitive level.

Additional Learning Resources

SG Go to your Study Guide for additional learning activities to help master this chapter content.

evolve Go to your Evolve website (http://evolve.elsevier.com/Linton/medsurg) for the following learning resources and much more:

- Interactive Prioritization Exercises
- Fluid & Electrolyte Tutorial
- Pharmacology Tutorial
- Review Questions for the NCLEX® Examination

Review Questions for the NCLEX® Examination

1. What is the primary difference between delirium and dementia?
   1. Delirium is typically reversible; dementia is usually irreversible.
   2. Agitation is constant with delirium but intermittent with dementia.
   3. The onset of delirium is gradual; the onset of dementia is typically rapid.
   4. Delirium usually lasts only a few minutes; dementia lasts weeks to months.

   NCLEX Client Need: Physiological Integrity: Physiological Adaptation

2. A delirious patient repeatedly cries out for her daughter in the middle of the night. What is the best intervention?
    1. Check to see whether she has an order for a sedative
    2. Call the daughter and ask her to come see the patient
    3. Calmly tell her where she is and that her daughter is not there
    4. Tell her she needs to be quiet because she is disturbing other patients

    NCLEX Client Need: Physiological Integrity: Basic Care and Comfort
3. A patient with AD wanders away from the table during meals, leaving most of his food uneaten. What should you do?
    1. Consult with the dietitian about providing finger foods
    2. Restrain the patient in his seat during meals
    3. Tell him he must sit down and finish his meal
    4. Ask another patient to try to keep him at the table

    NCLEX Client Need: Physiological Integrity: Basic Care and Comfort
4. When addressing a person who has dementia, which message is *most* appropriate?
    1. "You need to be dressed for church in 30 minutes."
    2. "Put your arm in the sleeve of your shirt."
    3. "Put your shirt on."
    4. "What would you like to wear today?"

    NCLEX Client Need: Physiological Integrity: Basic Care and Comfort
5. A new nurse on the special care unit for patients with AD repeatedly asks patients what time it is and if they know where they are. What information should you share with her?
    1. If a patient cannot answer the questions correctly, wait 5 minutes and ask again.
    2. Consistently tell patients the time, date, and place to keep them oriented.
    3. Frequent attempts at orientation tend to agitate patients with AD.
    4. Ask the patient to repeat the date, time, and place after you say them.

    NCLEX Client Need: Psychosocial Integrity
6. If you applied the principles of the CDA to the care of a patient with dementia, you would:
    1. Consistently use the same interventions for all patients with dementia
    2. Have patients confront irrational fears so they can be overcome
    3. Insist that the patient behave as a mature adult at all times
    4. Adapt expectations and interventions to the patient's abilities

    NCLEX Client Need: Psychosocial Integrity
7. Which type of dementia is most common?

    ________________.

    NCLEX Client Need: Physiological Integrity: Physiological Adaptation
8. Most drugs used to treat AD work by increasing the amount of which neurotransmitter in the brain?

    ____

    NCLEX Client Need: Physiological Integrity: Pharmacological Therapies
9. When a patient and her family are informed that the patient probably has early Alzheimer disease, the patient says, "Don't they have drugs to cure this disease?" To explain drug therapy for AD, the health care provider should include which statements? (Select all that apply.)
    1. Drugs are curative only if started early in the course of the disease.
    2. Drugs currently used for the treatment of AD have no side or adverse effects.
    3. There are no drugs for moderate dementia.
    4. Benefits gained from taking AD drugs vary greatly among individuals.
    5. A combination of drugs usually arrests the progression of AD.

    NCLEX Client Need: Physiological Integrity: Pharmacological Therapies
10. Your home health patient has become confused over the past week. He is taking all of the drugs listed below. Which of these can cause confusion? (Select all that apply.)
    1. Digoxin for heart failure
    2. Antacid for heartburn
    3. First generation H2 receptor blocker for peptic ulcer disease
    4. Anticholinergic for seasonal allergies
    5. Nonsteroidal antiinflammatory drug for arthritis

    NCLEX Client Need: Physiological Integrity: Pharmacological Therapies

chapter 23

Incontinence

http://evolve.elsevier.com/Linton/medsurg

Objectives

1. Identify common therapeutic measures used for the patient with incontinence.
2. Identify the types of urinary and fecal incontinence.
3. Explain the pathophysiology and treatment of specific types of incontinence.
4. List nursing assessment data needed to assist in the evaluation and treatment of incontinence.
5. Assist in developing a nursing care plan for the patient with incontinence.

Key Terms

Anorectal incontinence (ā-nō-RĔK-tăl ĭn-KŎN-tĭ-nĕns)
Credé technique (kră-DĀ)
Detrusor overactivity
Bowel incontinence
Fecal overflow incontinence
Functional incontinence
Micturition (mĭk-tŭ-RĬSH-ŭn)
Neurogenic bladder (nū-rō-JĔN-ĭk)
Neurogenic incontinence
Overflow urinary incontinence
Stress incontinence
Symptomatic incontinence
Transient incontinence (TRĂN-zē-ĕnt)
Urge incontinence
Urinary incontinence
Void

Incontinence is the term used to describe the involuntary passage of urine (**urinary incontinence**) or feces (**fecal or bowel incontinence**). Many conditions and situations can cause either temporary or permanent incontinence. Incontinence deserves special attention because of the toll it takes on the individual. The person who is troubled by incontinence faces physical, psychosocial, and financial burdens. The management of incontinence in patient care settings also requires many hours of nursing care.

The goals of treatment for the incontinent person include the restoration or improvement of control for treatable incontinence, the management of irreversible incontinence, and the prevention of complications.

URINARY INCONTINENCE: PREVALENCE AND COSTS

Statistics on urinary incontinence vary greatly depending on the gender, age, type of incontinence, and place of residence (community versus institution) of the individuals studied. Exact figures are difficult to obtain because people often do not report the problem to health care providers. General surveys of adults have found that 5% to 25% note leakage at least once a week and 5% to 15% experience it daily or most of the time. Among U.S. women who live in the community, 15% to 50% are affected by urinary incontinence, with 7% to 10% having severe leakage. Although urinary incontinence is twice as common among women as among men, 17% of men older than 60 years of age also have this condition. Among men who have had a radical prostatectomy, as many as 30% have some degree of incontinence.

The cost of medical care related to incontinence in the United States is estimated to be more than $400 million per year. This figure is compounded by the cost of supplies and management of complications such as skin breakdown and urinary tract infections. Health care providers need to recognize the economic and personal value of aggressively treating incontinence. Nurses play an important role in educating people about the need for evaluation and treatment. Although urinary incontinence is more common in older people, it should not be considered a normal age-related change. It often can be improved or cured, regardless of the patient's age.

PHYSIOLOGY OF URINATION

Terms used to describe the passage of urine are *urination*, **micturition**, and *voiding*. The terms **void** and *voiding* are used in this chapter because they are common in medical settings.

Normal controlled voiding requires a healthy bladder muscle (detrusor muscle), a patent (open) urethra, normal transmission of nerve impulses, and mental alertness. Alterations in any of these factors may result in incontinence.

Urine continually drains from the kidneys to the urinary bladder, where it is stored until it can be eliminated. When 200 to 250 mL of urine collects in the bladder, stretch and tension receptors in the muscular bladder wall are stimulated. The bladder contracts and the internal sphincter relaxes. A message is sent to the brain, making the person aware of the need to void. Because the act of voiding is normally voluntary, it can be delayed until an appropriate time. Then the external sphincter can be relaxed, permitting urine to flow out through the urethra (Fig. 23-1).

Of course, a limit exists to the amount of urine the bladder can hold. When the limit is exceeded, pressure causes the bladder to contract and force urine out involuntarily. If the bladder cannot be emptied, then urine backs up into the kidneys (a condition called *hydronephrosis*) and can cause kidney damage.

DIAGNOSTIC TESTS AND PROCEDURES

The presence and specific type of urinary incontinence are diagnosed based on the patient's history, physical examination, and various diagnostic tests and procedures. A diary of fluid intake and voiding kept over several days can reveal patterns characteristic of specific types of incontinence. Also, a record may be kept of the number or weight of wet incontinence pads. If additional assessment is needed, diagnostic studies may include laboratory tests, measurement of residual urine volume, stress tests, imaging procedures (computed tomography [CT] or magnetic resonance imaging [MRI]), cystoscopy, renal ultrasound, and urodynamic studies. Urodynamic procedures assess the neuromuscular function of the lower urinary tract. These procedures include uroflowmetry, which measures voiding duration and the amount and rate of urine voided. Cystometry is used to evaluate the neuromuscular function of the bladder. Cystoscopy involves the insertion of a scope through the urethra to visualize the urethra and bladder. The results help to define the type of incontinence, which in turn guides treatment decisions. Details of these and other urological tests are presented in Chapter 42.

LABORATORY TESTS

A clean-catch urinalysis with culture and sensitivity testing is usually ordered to assess for infection. If the patient cannot cooperate with the clean-catch procedure, catheterization may be necessary. Collection devices similar to those used for pediatric patients can be used for frail persons. The specimen is studied for bacteria, red blood cells (RBCs), white blood cells (WBCs), and glucose. Sometimes bacteria are found in

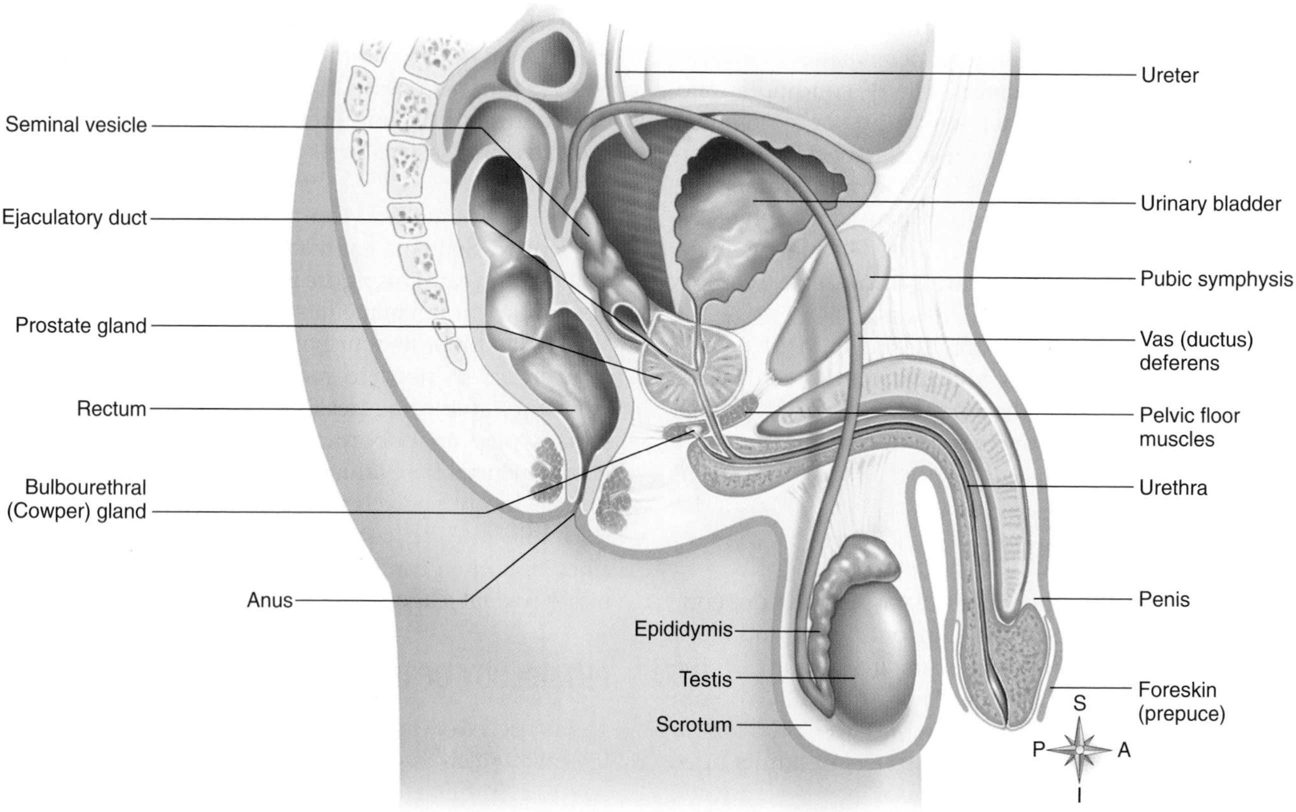

FIGURE 23-1 The bladder, urethra, and adjacent structures. **A,** Female patient. **B,** Male patient. (From Patton K, Thibodeau G: *Anatomy & physiology*, ed 8, St. Louis, 2013, Mosby.)

the urine when there are no symptoms of infection. Such asymptomatic bacteriuria does not require treatment and treatment will not improve bladder control. A blood sample may be analyzed for blood urea nitrogen (BUN), creatinine, glucose, and calcium.

POSTVOID RESIDUAL VOLUME

Knowing whether the patient is emptying the bladder completely is useful. Postvoid residual (PVR) volume is the amount of urine remaining in the bladder after voiding. Several methods are used to determine the PVR volume. The preferred method uses an ultrasound device to estimate the amount of urine remaining in the bladder after voiding. A second method involves catheterizing the patient immediately after voiding and measuring the amount of urine obtained by catheterization. Normally less than 50 mL of urine remains after voiding. However, because of common aging changes a PVR volume up to 100 mL may be acceptable in older adults.

Put On Your Thinking Cap!

Why is it better to use ultrasound to assess postvoid residual (PVR) volume instead of catheterizing the patient?

PROVOCATIVE STRESS TESTING

Provocative stress testing is performed to detect involuntary passage of urine when abdominal pressure increases. The patient may be positioned in a standing or lithotomy position. The physician encourages the patient to relax and then to cough vigorously. The examiner observes for urine loss during coughing.

COMMON THERAPEUTIC MEASURES

Depending on the type of urinary incontinence, a number of therapeutic measures may be prescribed. These are generally classified as *behavioral, pharmacologic,* or *surgical* treatments. Despite the variety of treatments available, many people do not seek medical care for urinary incontinence. Some individuals manage the condition with commonsense practices such as limiting activities outside the home, emptying the bladder frequently, restricting fluids, wearing pads, and avoiding activities that induce leakage. Unfortunately, some of these strategies can have negative consequences, such as inadequate fluid intake and giving up social and recreational activities.

BEHAVIORAL INTERVENTIONS

Behavioral interventions include bladder training or retraining, habit training, prompted voiding, and pelvic muscle rehabilitation. These techniques are low risk and are often effective in decreasing the frequency of incontinent episodes. Also, toileting can be simplified by providing a urinal or bedside commode at night. In general, these interventions require patient cooperation.

Bladder Training

Bladder retraining uses patient education, scheduled toileting, and positive reinforcement. The teaching plan includes information about normal urinary function and the bladder retraining program. With scheduled toileting, the patient is encouraged to delay voiding and void only at scheduled times. Initially voiding is usually scheduled every 2 to 3 hours while the patient is awake. The length of time between voidings is then gradually increased. If the patient voids ahead of schedule, the next voiding may be rescheduled at the prescribed interval. Another approach is to ignore the unscheduled voiding and have the patient void again at the previously scheduled time. The patient's efforts and improvement are positively reinforced throughout the treatment period, which usually lasts several months.

Habit Training

Habit training is also called *timed voiding* and is similar to bladder training in that the patient is encouraged to void at scheduled intervals. The difference is that the patient is not advised to resist the urge and delay voiding. The voiding schedule is based on the patient's usual pattern.

Prompted Voiding

Prompted voiding is often used with habit training for people who are dependent or cognitively impaired. The caregiver checks the patient for wetness at regular intervals and asks the patient to state whether he or she is wet or dry. The caregiver then encourages the patient to try to use the toilet. The caregiver praises the patient for trying to use the toilet and for remaining dry. This process is intended to help the patient recognize incontinence and to ask caregivers for help with toileting.

Pelvic Muscle Rehabilitation

Pelvic muscle rehabilitation aims to strengthen the pelvic floor and includes pelvic muscle exercises, with or without biofeedback; pelvic floor electrical stimulation; and vaginal weight training. Pelvic muscle exercises, commonly called *Kegel exercises,* are described in the *Patient Teaching* box. They actively exercise the pubococcygeus muscle, which helps to close the urethra and strengthen muscles of the pelvic floor.

Biofeedback may be used in conjunction with other pelvic muscle exercises. Electronic or mechanical sensors are used to help the patient isolate the appropriate pelvic muscles to contract while keeping the abdominal muscles relaxed. Electrical stimulation of the muscles of the pelvic floor can also be used along with Kegel exercises to cause muscle contraction.

Patient Teaching

Pelvic Muscle (Kegel) Exercises

- Uncontrolled loss of urine is commonly caused by a weakness in the perineal muscles that normally control urination.
- Strengthening perineal muscles, which are located around the vagina and rectum, can improve urinary control.
- To identify the correct muscles you need to exercise, practice tightening the perineal muscles as if you were trying to control the passage of intestinal gas.
- To improve muscle strength and endurance, two types of exercises should be done:
  - Short (2 to 4 seconds), firm contractions, followed by a brief period of relaxation, improves strength.
  - Long (6 to 12 seconds) contractions, followed by relaxation for 6 to 12 seconds, improves endurance.
- Perform both exercises several times a day starting with just three to five repetitions or as recommended by your physician.
- Gradually work up to 40 to 50 of each contraction each day.
- You may notice improvement in urinary control after 3 weeks; however, it may take 6 to 8 weeks before improvement is noticed.
- Continue the exercises indefinitely to maintain control.
- You can perform these exercises anywhere: at your desk, while driving, or while standing in line at the grocery store. No one can tell!

Sometimes vaginal weights (cones) are used with pelvic muscle training in women. The cones are ceramic devices of various weights that are inserted into the vagina. The patient begins with the lightest cone, inserts it, and tries to retain it for up to 15 minutes twice daily. When the lightest cone is successfully retained, the heavier cones are then used in succession.

Urge Suppression. Patients with urge incontinence may find the following strategy helpful (Miller, 2000):

- If you have the urge to void, then stop what you are doing. Sit down or stand quietly.
- Quickly squeeze the pelvic floor muscles several times without resting between squeezes.
- Take a few deep breaths and try to relax except for the pelvic floor muscles.
- Try to suppress the urge to void.
- Wait until the urge passes.
- While continuing to squeeze the pelvic floor muscles, walk to the bathroom at a normal pace.

REFLEX TRAINING

Reflex training is sometimes used by people with a spinal cord injury. This technique uses the Valsalva maneuver with rectal stretching to force urine from the bladder. The Valsalva maneuver is performed by taking a deep breath, holding it, and bearing down. At the same time, the rectum is stretched by inserting a gloved finger into the rectum and pulling toward the back. This creates pressure on the urinary sphincter and relaxes the pelvic floor, allowing urine to flow. Patients who use this method of emptying the bladder should be checked for PVR volume at times. Ideally the PVR volume will be less than 100 mL. Patients who learn to use this method successfully may no longer need catheterization.

DRUG THERAPY

Drug therapy is most effective in the management of urge and reflex incontinence. Classification of drugs most commonly used are anticholinergic and muscarinic receptor antagonist (antispasmodic) medications. Alpha-adrenergic agonists, tricyclic antidepressants, and serotonin-norepinephrine reuptake inhibitors may be helpful for stress incontinence. However, side effects of alpha-adrenergic agonists include tachycardia and hypertension. Older adults should be started on a low dose with gradual increases. It may take up to 2 months to achieve the full benefit. Postmenopausal women with urge or stress incontinence may obtain improvement using intravaginal estrogen cream or tablets. Examples of these and other types of drugs, their side effects, and nursing considerations are presented in Table 23-1. Suburethral bulking agents such as glutaraldehyde cross-linked (GAX) collagen (Contigen), silicone microimplants in gel (Macroplastique), or zirconium oxide beads (Durasphere) may be injected into the tissues around the urethra. The substance adds bulk to the bladder neck, thereby increasing resistance to urine outflow. This procedure, called *periurethral bulking*, is helpful in certain situations for both men and women. The effects typically last only 2 to 3 years; the procedure can then be repeated.

In addition to drugs used to control incontinence, a variety of creams and sprays are available to coat and protect the skin of the perineum and buttocks of the incontinent patient. A light dusting powder can be used to absorb moisture. Cornstarch is not recommended because it promotes the development of yeast infections. Do not use talc and lotion together on the same area because the combination creates an abrasive paste.

URINE COLLECTION DEVICES

External Devices

External urine collection devices are useful for men who do not have retention or bladder outlet obstruction. These latex sheaths, sometimes called *condom catheters*, drain urine into a bag that is usually secured to the leg. These devices are quite effective in maintaining dryness but the adhesive may cause skin irritation on the penis. The directions for applying a condom catheter must be followed carefully. *The patient and all caregivers should know NOT to encircle the penis with tape.* To do so can restrict circulation. Elastic tape should be used and wrapped in a spiral pattern. No external device is in common use at this time for women. !

Table 23-1 **Medications for Treating Urinary Incontinence**

DRUG	USE	ACTION	NURSING INTERVENTIONS
Cholinergic Medications			
bethanechol chloride (Urecholine)	Overflow incontinence (atonic bladder)	Bladder contraction	Common side effects: sweating, flushing, GI distress, headache, visual disturbances. Toxicity: nausea, dyspnea, irregular pulse, headache Antidote: atropine Contraindications: bladder or intestinal obstruction, asthma, hyperthyroidism, ulcer, cardiac disease, parkinsonism Works within 1 hour; ensure bedpan or toilet is accessible
Anticholinergic Medications/Muscarinic Receptor Antagonists (Blockers)			
oxybutynin chloride (Ditropan) darifenacin (Enablex) solifenacin (VESIcare)	Urge incontinence	Bladder relaxation	Side effects: dry mouth, constipation, tachycardia, drowsiness, urinary retention, insomnia, blurred vision (less with tolterodine)
tolterodine (Detrol)		Increased bladder capacity Delayed urge to void	Administer 1 hour before meals; provide oral care; potentiates other CNS depressants
trospium (Sanctura)		Bladder relaxation	Administer 1 hour before meals on empty stomach; no CNS side effects.
Alpha-Adrenergic Medications			
duloxetine (Cymbalta)	Stress incontinence (off-label use)	Sphincter contraction	Common side effects: dry mouth, constipation, drowsiness, dizziness, trouble sleeping, low energy, excessive sweating, loss of appetite, nausea, diarrhea
Alpha-Adrenergic Antagonists (Blockers)			
doxazosin (Cardura) terazosin (Hytrin) tamsulosin (Flomax)	Overflow incontinence	Relaxation of internal sphincter	Side effects: postural hypotension (especially in older adults), tachycardia, headache, dizziness, nasal congestion
phenoxybenzamine hydrochloride (Dibenzyline)			After the first dose, patient should lie down for 2 hours to prevent fainting; elastic stockings may help During dose adjustments, monitor blood pressure; most side effects decrease over time
Bulking Agents			
glutaraldehyde cross-linked (GAX) collagen (Contigen)	Stress incontinence	Adds bulk to sphincter to increase resistance to urine	Injected around urethra by physician Monitor voiding and assess bladder for distention

Continued

Table 23-1 Medications for Treating Urinary Incontinence—cont'd

DRUG	USE	ACTION	NURSING INTERVENTIONS
5-Alpha Reductase Inhibitors			
finasteride (Proscar)	Used to treat overflow incontinence associated with prostate enlargement	Inhibit a male hormone that is thought to cause prostate enlargement	Adverse effects include impotence, decreased libido, decreased volume of ejaculate
dutasteride (Avodart)		Shrinking the enlarged prostate allows urine to flow through the urethra more easily	Inform patients that pregnant women and women who may become pregnant should not come in contact with this drug or the semen of a man taking the drug
Tricyclic Antidepressants			
imipramine (Tofranil) amitriptyline (Elavil)	Used to treat urge incontinence (overactive bladder)	Reduces overactive bladder contractions	Common side effects: constipation, dry mouth, blurred vision (pupil dilation), fatigue, tachycardia

CNS, Central nervous system; *GI*, gastrointestinal.

Indwelling Catheters

An indwelling catheter may be ordered to control urinary incontinence when all other measures have failed and skin integrity is endangered. A catheter also may be needed temporarily if urine is coming in contact with a wound. Use of indwelling catheters for the management of incontinence in nursing home residents is *not* considered appropriate. Care of the patient with an indwelling catheter is discussed in Chapter 42.

Intermittent Self-Catheterization

Some patients are quite successful at using intermittent self-catheterization but its use requires dexterity, adequate vision, and the ability and motivation to learn. A clean technique rather than a sterile technique is usually taught for use in the home setting. Initially the bladder is drained every 4 hours. If more than 500 mL of urine is obtained, the time interval is shortened. If less than 200 mL is obtained, the time interval is extended. Most people produce more urine at certain times of the day. Individual schedules can be adjusted to accommodate this variation.

GARMENTS AND PADS FOR INCONTINENCE

A variety of incontinence products are available that help to maintain dryness. Disposable briefs and pads are found in most pharmacies and grocery stores. Some women wear perineal pads to absorb urine. Some nursing homes use washable waterproof briefs with absorbent cotton liners. Another style has a stretchy brief with a perineal pouch through which absorbent pads can be changed. The best product is one that draws urine away from the skin through a liner that remains dry. However, these products do not protect the skin against feces.

Those who discourage the use of incontinence briefs and pads believe that their use encourages patients to void in their clothing. Although this may be true at times, these items have their place. They may give a person the confidence to be socially active without the risk of having an embarrassing accident. When trying to restore control, use briefs that can be removed easily for toileting. For patients who are unlikely to ever be continent, these products are an acceptable management tool.

For the immobile patient, an absorbent pad with a waterproof backing may be used instead of briefs. These pads can also be placed under the buttocks of a bedridden patient who wears briefs in case leakage occurs. One factor to remember is that multiple layers of padding interfere with special beds or mattresses designed to prevent decubitus ulcers. Some paper pads stick to the skin and become lumpy when wet; therefore they should be checked frequently for wetness. Never place the patient directly on a plastic surface; doing so keeps the skin wet from perspiration and urine.

PENILE COMPRESSION DEVICE

The penile compression (penile clamp) is a device that is applied to the penis. It compresses the urethra, preventing the passage of urine. Patients typically continue to have a small amount of leakage, requiring a pad to protect the clothing. To prevent circulatory impairment and pressure sores, the clamp must be removed and repositioned frequently. Use of the penile clamp is controversial because it can cause injury if not used correctly. The patient must be mentally and physically capable of managing the device.

PELVIC ORGAN SUPPORT DEVICES

A *pessary* is a device that is inserted into the vagina to hold the pelvic organs in place. It is sometimes used as a tool to treat incontinence in women with relaxation of the pelvic structures. A doughnut-shaped pessary exerts pressure on the vaginal wall, lifting the uterus and holding it in the pelvis. When incontinence occurs as a result of the bladder prolapsing into the vagina, other types of pessaries may be used to support the urethra as well. Pessaries are generally recommended for patients who are awaiting surgical treatment or those for whom surgery is contraindicated. The patient must be reexamined within 24 hours after pessary placement to ensure proper placement and to rule out urinary obstruction. The device must then be removed periodically for cleansing and replacement. ! *Document that the patient has a pessary to ensure that it will not be forgotten.*

For women with stress incontinence, a bladder neck support prosthesis may be helpful. When the silastic device is fitted into the vagina, it supports the area where the urethra connects to the bladder, thereby reducing the incidence of involuntary urine loss. Another device used to prevent leakage is the urethral insert, a small plastic device that creates a mechanical barrier to urine loss.

SURGICAL TREATMENT

Surgical intervention may be recommended for some conditions that cause urinary incontinence. Specific surgical procedures may be performed to remove obstructions, treat severe detrusor overactivity, implant an artificial sphincter, reposition the sphincter unit, improve perineal support, and inject substances that increase urethral compression (suburethral bulking agents). Electrostimulation is the use of electrodes that stimulate the pelvic floor muscles. Electrodes can be surgically implanted in the vagina or rectum. Retropubic urethropexies and pubovaginal slings are surgical procedures most often used for stress urinary incontinence in women. A sling procedure for men creates a support system for the urethra so that it does not open inappropriately. Nursing care of the patient undergoing surgery on the urinary tract is described in Chapter 42.

The artificial sphincter (Fig. 23-2) consists of an inflatable cuff, a reservoir of fluid that fills the cuff, and a pump. The cuff is positioned around the urethra or bladder neck. The reservoir is placed in the abdomen and the pump is positioned in the scrotum or labia. Fluid fills the cuff, applying pressure to the urethra to prevent urine passage. To void, the patient compresses the pump, which deflates the cuff by transferring fluid from the cuff to the reservoir and allowing urine to pass through the urethra.

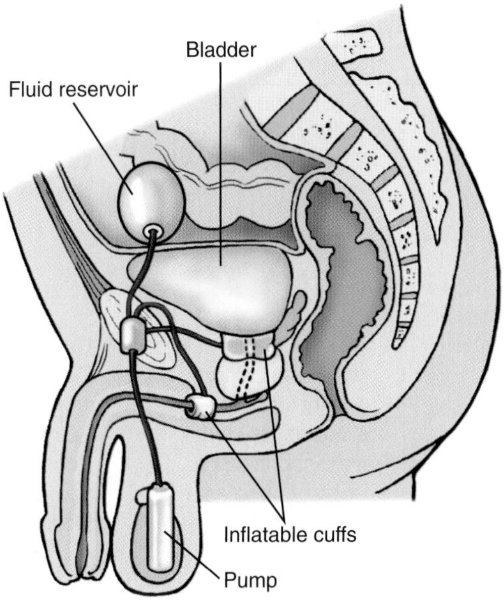

FIGURE 23-2 An artificial urinary sphincter in place. (From Monahan FD, Drake DT, Neighbors M, editors: *Medical-surgical nursing: foundations for clinical practice*, ed 2, Philadelphia, 1998, Saunders-Elsevier.)

TYPES OF URINARY INCONTINENCE

Urinary incontinence is classified into four basic types: (1) urge, (2) overflow, (3) stress, and (4) functional (Table 23-2). A patient may have more than one type of incontinence at the same time (mixed incontinence). Urinary incontinence may be transient or persistent. **Transient incontinence** is caused by reversible conditions and is often corrected by treatment of the underlying problem.

URGE INCONTINENCE

Description

Urge incontinence is the involuntary loss of urine shortly after a strong, abrupt urge to urinate. It most often results from an overactive detrusor (bladder) muscle. Urge incontinence is associated with neurologic disorders such as stroke, multiple sclerosis, and spinal cord lesions; however, the cause cannot always be identified. **Detrusor overactivity** is the most common cause of incontinence in older adults. Some patients with urge incontinence have involuntary urethral

Table 23-2 Types of Urinary Incontinence

TYPE	DESCRIPTION	CAUSES	NURSING CARE	TREATMENTS
Urge	Loss of urine that usually follows a strong desire to void	Nervous system disorder Urinary tract infection Bladder obstruction	Schedule toileting. Limit fluids 2 hours before bedtime. Administer drugs as ordered to control bladder contractions (see Table 23-1). Keep incontinence record.	Behavior modification Drug therapy: anticholinergics Surgical procedures to increase bladder capacity or to decrease bladder contractions
Overflow	Loss of urine associated with a full bladder Frequent voiding Volume usually small Reflex incontinence: loss of urine as a result of reflexive contraction	Urethral obstruction Disorders of bladder, nerves, or muscles Spinal cord injury Postanesthesia Spinal cord injury Radiation cystitis	Catheterize as ordered; teach self-catheterization as appropriate. Administer drugs as ordered to stimulate the bladder and to relax the internal sphincter (see Table 23-1). Cutaneous triggers; teach stimulation techniques.	Surgery to relieve obstruction Drug therapy to stimulate the bladder and to relax the sphincter Catheterize as necessary
Stress	Loss of urine during physical exertion	Relaxation of pelvic floor muscles Urethral trauma Sphincter injury	Teach Kegel exercises. Advise patient to void frequently. Administer drugs as ordered to stimulate the sphincter (see Table 23-1).	Surgical correction Bladder suspension Artificial sphincter Drug therapy to improve sphincter contraction
Functional	Bladder functions normally but patient voids inappropriately	Dementia Head injury Cerebrovascular accident (stroke)	Schedule toileting. Reinforce appropriate behavior. Remove environmental barriers.	

relaxation in addition to abnormal detrusor activity. Urinary tract infection and fecal impaction sometimes cause temporary urge incontinence.

Management

Treatment of urge incontinence is aimed at correcting the cause, if possible, and includes antibiotics for infection and the removal of impaction. When the problem is not related to reversible conditions, behavioral techniques, drug therapy, or surgical intervention may be used. A simple measure is to consume 6 to 8 glasses of water each day instead of caffeine-rich drinks. Bladder training with scheduled voiding and positive reinforcement may be effective. Pelvic muscle exercises may be prescribed to supplement bladder training. Anticholinergic and muscarinic antagonists (antispasmodics) are the drugs most commonly used for urge incontinence. Anticholinergic drugs may cause confusion and agitation that might be mistaken for dementia in the older patient. Tolterodine (Detrol) is an antispasmodic that is effective in many people, particularly those with an overactive bladder. It generally has fewer side effects than anticholinergic medications. Botulinum toxin injected into the detrusor may improve symptoms for as long as 9 months. If behavioral techniques, drugs, or both do not work, some surgical procedures may be recommended. Clam ileocystoplasty is a very effective procedure but it leaves the patient unable to empty the bladder except with intermittent self-catheterization. Some older adults can do this but others cannot. Sacral neuromodulation involves the implantation of a stimulator that improves nerve function in the pelvic floor.

OVERFLOW INCONTINENCE

Description

Overflow urinary incontinence is the involuntary loss of urine associated with an overdistended bladder. Small amounts of urine are lost either continually or at frequent intervals. In addition to passing through the urethra, urine may flow from the bladder back into the ureters and kidneys and cause hydronephrosis—a condition that can damage the kidneys. Patients who have normal sensation usually feel uncomfortable because of bladder distention. Factors that contribute to overflow incontinence are obstruction to urine flow, an underactive detrusor muscle, or impaired transmission of nerve impulses. In addition, some women have overflow incontinence after surgery to treat other types of incontinence.

These patients are not aware of bladder fullness and the bladder becomes overdistended. Urinary retention with overflow is also fairly common after general anesthesia or childbirth or after the removal of an indwelling catheter. Medications that may cause urinary retention include antihistamines, epinephrine, anticholinergics, and theophylline (Table 23-3). **Neurogenic bladder** is any type of bladder dysfunction caused by neurologic dysfunction associated with a spinal cord injury, radical pelvic surgery, or radiation cystitis. The pattern of bladder emptying varies with the specific cause of dysfunction. It may be classified as reflex, areflexic, or sensory incontinence.

Management

The medical treatment of overflow incontinence depends on the cause. The physician may prescribe drugs to stimulate the bladder (e.g., bethanechol chloride [Urecholine]) and relax the internal sphincter (e.g., prazosin hydrochloride [Minipress]). A common reason for obstruction in men is prostate enlargement. Surgical removal of all or part of the prostate gland often restores normal emptying of the bladder. Sphincterotomy, in which an incision is made in the sphincter, is another surgical procedure that may be indicated when the sphincter is obstructing the outflow of urine. Sacral neuromodulation is another option that may be helpful.

In some cases, intermittent or indwelling catheterization is necessary. Postoperative and postpartum patients may require intermittent catheterization once or twice before normal bladder function returns. The indwelling catheter is considered the measure of last resort in the management of overflow incontinence. Self-catheterization using clean technique may be taught to patients who are able to perform it in the home setting. This technique works very well for many patients.

Other techniques that may be used to empty the bladder are the Credé method, the Valsalva maneuver, and the anal stretch maneuver. The **Credé technique** involves using the open hand to gently press the abdomen over the bladder and promote urine passage. Ask the physician about the safety of this procedure for individual patients. These techniques and others are described more fully in rehabilitation texts.

For patients who have reflex incontinence, bladder drainage *must* be maintained! Overdistention of the bladder may trigger a serious reaction called *autonomic dysreflexia,* in which the blood pressure rises to life-threatening levels. This can be prevented by emptying the bladder often enough to prevent overdistention. Among the techniques that may be used to stimulate bladder emptying in patients with reflex incontinence are cutaneous triggering methods, which include tapping the suprapubic area and stroking the inner thigh. These techniques and others are more fully described in texts on rehabilitation. The Credé method is *not* used for patients with reflex incontinence. Chapter 29 discusses in detail the care of the patient with spinal cord injury.

Table 23-3 Medications That Cause Urinary Retention or Incontinence

CLASS	EXAMPLE
Urinary Retention	
Anticholinergics	atropine sulfate
Antihistamines	diphenhydramine hydrochloride (Benadryl)
Alpha-adrenergic agonists	epinephrine hydrochloride (Adrenalin)
Xanthine	theophylline (Theo-Dur)
Incontinence	
Alpha-adrenergic blockers	prazosin hydrochloride (Minipress)
Anticholinergics	atropine sulfate
Antihistamines	diphenhydramine hydrochloride (Benadryl)
Antiparkinsonian drugs	levodopa (Dopa), trihexyphenidyl hydrochloride (Artane)
Antipsychotics	chlorpromazine (Thorazine)
High ceiling diuretics	furosemide (Lasix)
Opiate agonists	morphine sulfate (Epimorph)
Sedatives or hypnotics	phenobarbital sodium (Luminal Sodium), diazepam (Valium)
Sympathomimetics	phenylephrine hydrochloride (Neo-Synephrine), isoproterenol hydrochloride (Isuprel)

STRESS INCONTINENCE

Description

Stress incontinence is the involuntary loss of small amounts of urine during physical activity that increases abdominal pressure. Coughing, laughing, sneezing, and lifting are examples of activities that often result in urine loss. In women, stress incontinence is usually caused by a relaxation of the pelvic floor muscles and the ureterovesical junction as a result of pregnancy, childbirth, obesity, and aging. Urethral trauma, sphincter injury, congenital sphincter weakness, urinary infection, neurologic disorders, and stress can cause stress incontinence in men and women. It may occur after prostatectomy or radiation therapy.

Management

Sometimes stress incontinence is successfully treated with behavioral methods such as scheduled voiding and pelvic muscle exercises (see Nursing Care Plan: Patient with Stress Urinary Incontinence). In addition, the patient is advised to maintain a fluid intake of at least 2000 mL/day. If the patient has hypertension, heart failure, or renal disease, consult a registered nurse (RN) about the appropriate recommended fluid intake. Remember that older adults whose fluid intake has been low will need to increase fluid intake gradually to prevent fluid volume overload. Fluids that have a diuretic effect (e.g., tea, coffee, cola) should be avoided. Alpha-adrenergic drugs such as pseudoephedrine hydrochloride (Sudafed) may be prescribed to increase bladder outlet resistance. Oral or topical estrogen may be given to strengthen the bladder outlet in postmenopausal women. The most common surgical interventions now are retropubic urethropexies,

Nursing Care Plan — Patient with Stress Urinary Incontinence

ASSESSMENT

HEALTH HISTORY Mrs. Seigel is an 85-year-old resident in a long-term care facility. She complains of having trouble "holding my urine." She is unable to control urination if she strains, coughs, or laughs. She is the mother of five children, all born at home. She reports no other physical complaints except for arthritis in her hips and knees, and hypertension. Her medications are acetaminophen, 325 mg, three times daily, and hydrochlorothiazide, 25 mg daily. Fear of losing control of her urine has caused her to avoid leaving her room except for meals. She is wearing perineal pads to keep her clothing dry.

PHYSICAL EXAMINATION Vital signs: blood pressure 130/86 mm Hg, pulse 72 bpm, respiration 16 breaths per minute, temperature 98°F (36.67°C) orally. Height 5′3″, weight 179 lb. Heart and breath sounds are normal. Abdomen is rounded and soft. No bladder distention is noted. Faint urine odor is present. Rises with some difficulty. Walks slowly with walker. Has limited range of motion in the knees and hips.

Nursing Diagnosis	Goals and Outcome Criteria	Interventions
Stress Urinary Incontinence related to weak pelvic muscles and high intraabdominal pressure	Improved urinary control: Patient will report fewer incidents of stress incontinence.	Explain to the patient how weak perineal muscles cause stress incontinence. Instruct her how to do Kegel perineal exercises (see *Patient Teaching* box). Advise the patient to empty her bladder every 2 hours while awake. Encourage the intake of normal amounts of fluid but discourage liquids with diuretic effects (e.g., coffee, tea, alcohol). Explain that obesity increases intraabdominal pressure and contributes to stress incontinence. Explore her interest in weight loss and refer her to a dietitian.
Risk for Impaired Skin Integrity related to prolonged contact of urine with skin	Reduced risk of skin breakdown: Skin is kept clean and dry; remains intact and free of excessive redness.	Inspect the perineal area and buttocks and report signs of irritation (e.g., redness, breaks in the skin). Apply skin protectants as ordered or per agency protocol. Teach the patient the importance of good perineal care to remove urine from the skin. Encourage her to cleanse the area with mild soap, rinse, and gently dry twice daily. Perineal pads or other incontinence pads should be changed promptly if they are wet.
Social Isolation related to fear of embarrassment as a result of incontinence	Decreased social isolation: Patient resumes usual social activities.	Identify activities that the patient would like to resume. Discuss strategies to decrease embarrassment about incontinent episodes: (1) empty bladder before leaving room; (2) wear perineal pads or special incontinence pads to absorb urine and protect clothing and furniture. Avoid any comments that could humiliate the patient, such as references to "diapers." Avoid discussing her problem in front of others.

Critical Thinking Questions

1. What are the possible contributing factors to stress incontinence in this resident?
2. How would you teach the resident the importance of perineal care?

pubovaginal slings, and collagen injections. These procedures have largely replaced anterior colporrhaphy and needle suspension.

FUNCTIONAL INCONTINENCE

Description

Functional incontinence is the term used when a person voids inappropriately because of an inability to get to the toilet or to manage the mechanics of toileting. The problem can be related to confusion, immobility, or barriers in the environment.

Management

The treatment of functional incontinence depends on the cause. Arrange the environment to permit independent toileting and provide assistive devices that enable the immobile patient to void appropriately. The confused patient may respond well to scheduled or timed voiding and periodic orientation to toilet facilities. In long-term care facilities, promoting the attitude that incontinence usually can be improved even in physically and cognitively impaired patients is important.

❖ NURSING CARE of the Patient with Urinary Incontinence

■ Assessment

Health History

Data collection helps to determine the type of incontinence, the possible causes, and the patient's response to treatment.

Chief Complaint. A thorough description of the chief complaint is essential. Ask whether the patient is aware of the need to void and is able to hold the urine once the need is felt. Determine the pattern of incontinent voiding, urine volume, and related symptoms.

Pattern. Ask the patient how often incontinent episodes occur and whether they are associated with any particular activities, such as sneezing or laughing. A voiding diary is a helpful tool in identifying the pattern of urinary incontinence. Many patients are able to keep their own diaries. If the patient is unable to maintain an accurate record, a caregiver must do so for the patient.

Volume. If a patient is incontinent, measurements of urine can only be estimated but the patient can probably describe the amount voided as being *large, moderate,* or *small.* If pads or briefs are used, record the number used and the degree of saturation. Weighing wet pads and subtracting the dry weight of the pad is more precise but not very practical in the home setting. When the patient resides in a long-term care facility or hospital, measure and record the amount of urine passed with continent voiding as well.

Related Symptoms. Ask whether the patient has had dysuria (painful voiding), pain in the suprapubic area (the lower abdomen where the bladder is located), or polyuria (large urine volume).

Medical History. Past problems that might be related to incontinence include urologic, gynecologic, neurologic, and endocrine conditions. Specifically ask whether the patient has diabetes mellitus. People who have diabetes may develop neurologic problems that affect the bladder. In addition, a person with poorly controlled diabetes may produce large volumes of urine that quickly fill the bladder.

Document all abdominal disorders, surgeries, and trauma. Record the number of pregnancies and types of deliveries. Inquire about current and recent medications because many drugs can affect kidney or bladder function. Drugs that might contribute to urinary incontinence are high ceiling (loop) diuretics, major tranquilizers, antihistamines, decongestants, some sedatives or hypnotics, and antiparkinsonian drugs. Anticholinergics, which are used to treat some types of incontinence, could actually cause overflow incontinence. Other drugs that can disrupt normal voiding are epinephrine, theophylline, isoproterenol, and prazosin.

Pharmacology Capsule

When urinary incontinence develops suddenly, check the patient's drug profile for drugs known to contribute to incontinence.

Review of Systems. The review of systems may offer clues to conditions that contribute to incontinence. For example, the patient with severe arthritis in the hands or severely impaired vision may have difficulty managing toileting independently. Constipation is a common problem that can contribute to incontinence.

Functional Assessment. A description of the patient's usual activities and habits provides clues about possible contributing factors and about the effect of incontinence on the individual. Of special interest in relation to incontinence are usual fluid intake (amount, type, timing) and the consumption of alcohol.

Physical Examination

The physical examination begins with the measurement of vital signs and height and weight. Be alert for fever, tachycardia, and weight gain. Note the patient's level of awareness and appropriateness of responses. Inspect and palpate the skin for edema.

Sometimes incontinence is first recognized when an odor of urine is detected during the examination or when providing care. When examining the incontinent patient, palpate the abdomen for masses, tenderness, fullness, or distention. A distended bladder or abdominal distention associated with constipation is an important finding. Examination of the male genitalia includes inspection for abnormalities and for skin irritation. Inspect the female perineum for redness or irritation. The physician or nurse practitioner (NP) performs a pelvic examination on the female patient to assess for

Box 23-1 Focused Assessment of Patients with Urinary Incontinence

HEALTH HISTORY

Chief Complaint

The pattern of continent and incontinent voiding, behaviors or activities associated with incontinent voiding, amount of urine passed with continent and incontinent voiding, awareness of the need to void, ability to hold urine once aware of the need to void, dysuria

Medical History

Urologic, gynecologic, neurologic, and endocrine problems; abdominal operations, trauma, disorders; mental confusion; current and recent medications

Review of Systems

Disorders that might contribute to incontinence: diabetes mellitus, cerebrovascular accident, paralysis

Functional Assessment

Usual activities, fluid intake, alcohol consumption

PHYSICAL EXAMINATION

Vital Signs

Fever, tachycardia

Height and Weight

Weight gain

Level of Consciousness

Orientation

Odor of urine

Abdomen

Masses, tenderness, fullness, distention

Male Genitalia

Abnormalities of foreskin, glans penis, perineal skin

Female Genitalia

Redness, irritation

Rectal Examination

Sensation, sphincter tone, fecal impaction

prolapse of abdominal organs and to evaluate perineal muscle tone. A rectal examination is performed to determine sensation, sphincter tone, and presence of fecal impaction. In male patients, the prostate is palpated for contour and consistency.

Assessment of the patient with urinary incontinence is outlined in Box 23-1. In addition, the environment must be assessed, including toilet accessibility, grab bars, lighting, and availability of toileting options (e.g., urinals, commode chairs).

Nursing Diagnoses, Goals, and Outcome Criteria: Urinary Incontinence

Nursing diagnoses and goals for the patient with urinary incontinence may include the following:

Nursing Diagnoses	Goals and Outcome Criteria
Deficient Knowledge of causes of incontinence and corrective measures	Patient understands condition and management: accurately describes and participates in the treatment plan
Functional Urinary Incontinence related to physical, cognitive, or environmental barriers	Continent voiding with appropriate support: decreased episodes of incontinent voiding
Overflow Urinary Incontinence related to obstruction or neurologic impairment accomplished with minimal involuntary leakage	Adequate management of incontinence: bladder emptying
Stress Urinary Incontinence related to weak pelvic structures, increased intraabdominal pressure	Improved control of urine flow: decreased episodes of involuntary voiding when under stress
Urge Urinary Incontinence related to decreased bladder capacity or bladder spasms	Ability to hold increasing volume of urine: time between voiding increases without leakage
Social Isolation related to fear of embarrassment	Decreased social isolation: patient participates in usual social activities
Situational Low Self-Esteem related to loss of control of voiding	Improved self-esteem: patient demonstrates positive self-image (confidence, pride in appearance)
Risk for Impaired Skin Integrity related to the presence of urine on the skin	Reduced risk of skin breakdown: skin kept clean, dry, and free of urine or feces
Risk for Infection related to chronic bladder distention or catheterization	Absence of urinary tract infection: normal body temperature and WBC count

Interventions

Deficient Knowledge

Patient and caregiver education are key elements in the management of urinary incontinence. Do not assume that improvement is not possible, especially in frail older adults. In fact, improvement or correction is possible for most people. Sometimes the incontinent patient is very discouraged and reluctant to try retraining techniques. Therefore remain positive and encouraging and praise the patient's attempts and successes. Many people believe that patients will be more motivated if they are dressed in street clothes and are not wearing incontinence garments. However, when the best outcome includes some continued leaking, pads or briefs may always be needed.

The teaching plan should explain normal urination, the type of incontinence the patient is experiencing, and the prescribed treatment. Supplement verbal information with written material and inform the patient that improvement takes time and to not expect immediate results. Praise the patient's participation in the treatment plan and interest in working toward continence. The appropriate methods for managing various types of incontinence are emphasized in the next section (see previous sections for a discussion of the specific methods for improving continence).

Incontinence

Nursing interventions for various types of incontinence overlap. Therefore interventions are discussed in general terms here. Table 23-2 summarizes the treatments for each type of incontinence.

Bladder Training or Retraining

Bladder training or retraining may be recommended for stress and urge incontinence. Teach the patient (and caregiver, if appropriate) the basic principles of bladder training. Establish a schedule for voiding every 2 to 3 hours while awake; pads or an external collection device may be needed during sleep hours. Emphasize the importance of trying to delay voiding until the scheduled time. In addition, praise the patient's efforts.

Habit Training

If habit training is prescribed, initiate an incontinence record to help establish the schedule for timed voiding (Fig. 23-3). Remind the patient to try to void at the scheduled times.

If the patient has difficulty voiding at the scheduled time, attempt to stimulate voiding. To promote voiding, establish a comfortable position for the patient and provide privacy. Stimuli that may encourage voiding include stroking the inner thigh, pouring warm water over the perineum, running water in the lavatory or tub, and having the patient drink water while on the toilet.

Fluid intake may be spaced at 2-hour intervals to provide regular filling of the bladder. Nighttime wetness can be reduced by limiting fluids after 7 PM. Patients or their caregivers sometimes decrease fluid intake excessively to reduce urinary incontinence. This makes it harder to schedule toileting and can lead to other problems (e.g., urinary tract infection, urinary calculi). Most references recommend 1500 to 3000 mL of fluid daily unless contraindicated. If a patient has cardiovascular or renal disease, consult the RN or physician about the ideal fluid intake. Gradually increase fluid intake for older patients because they often do not adapt well to rapid changes in blood volume.

Social Isolation

The person with urinary incontinence may curtail social activities out of fear of having embarrassing accidents. In addition, access to toilets in public places is often limited, so patients who cannot delay voiding may be afraid to venture far from home. If continence is unlikely or not yet established, a variety of incontinence products are available that may permit the patient to venture out without fear of wetness or odor. Specially designed pads and undergarments as well as some external urine collection devices may be used. As mentioned earlier, effective external collection devices for men are readily available. The patient also can be encouraged to maintain the voiding schedule during the social outing. If the patient has an incontinent episode, those responsible for his or her care should be careful not to show disapproval.

Situational Low Self-Esteem

The ability to control elimination is an important childhood accomplishment. Adults who become incontinent may be so embarrassed that they are reluctant to tell anyone about it. Nurses often discover that a newly admitted patient has concealed incontinence from family and physicians. Some older people do not seek help for incontinence because they think it is caused by old age and cannot be corrected.

You can help patients learn to manage incontinence and see that it is not a barrier to achieving a full life. Your attitude toward the patient and toward incontinence influences how the patient deals with the change in body function. Caregivers must be committed to efforts to help patients avoid incontinence. The following situation should not be allowed to happen:

A stroke patient in a long-term care facility calls out, "I need to go to the bathroom!"

A busy nursing staff member rushes by, pats the patient on the hand, and says, "That's all right. You have a diaper on. Go ahead and pee."

Encourage patients to attend to dress and grooming to promote a more positive self-image. The patient who takes an active role in carrying out the treatment plan may feel less helpless and better able to cope with incontinence. Advise caregivers not to refer to incontinence pads and undergarments as *diapers* because of that term's association with infants.

Risk for Impaired Skin Integrity

A major problem for the incontinent patient is the risk of skin breakdown. Urine and feces, if left in contact with the skin, cause a rash. Continuous moisture causes the skin to lose its oily protective barrier. Skin breakdown may follow. The key to preventing breakdown is to keep the skin clean, dry, and free of urine or feces. If a patient is incontinent and unable to report voiding, check hourly for wetness. Remove wet garments and linens immediately and wash the patient's

INCONTINENCE MONITORING RECORD

INSTRUCTIONS: EACH TIME THE PATIENT IS CHECKED:
1) Mark *one* of the circles in the BLADDER section at the hour closest to the time the patient is checked.
2) Make an X in the BOWEL section if the patient has had an incontinent or normal bowel movement.

● = Incontinent, small amount ⊘ = Dry X = Incontinent BOWEL
● = Incontinent, large amount △ = Voided correctly X = Normal BOWEL

PATIENT NAME________ ROOM #______ DATE______

	BLADDER			BOWEL			
	INCONTINENT OF URINE	DRY	VOIDED CORRECTLY	INCONTINENT X	NORMAL X	INITIALS	COMMENTS
12 am	● ●	○	△ cc ___				
1	● ●	○	△ cc ___				
2	● ●	○	△ cc ___				
3	● ●	○	△ cc ___				
4	● ●	○	△ cc ___				
5	● ●	○	△ cc ___				
6	● ●	○	△ cc ___				
7	● ●	○	△ cc ___				
8	● ●	○	△ cc ___				
9	● ●	○	△ cc ___				
10	● ●	○	△ cc ___				
11	● ●	○	△ cc ___				
12 pm	● ●	○	△ cc ___				
1	● ●	○	△ cc ___				
2	● ●	○	△ cc ___				
3	● ●	○	△ cc ___				
4	● ●	○	△ cc ___				
5	● ●	○	△ cc ___				
6	● ●	○	△ cc ___				
7	● ●	○	△ cc ___				
8	● ●	○	△ cc ___				
9	● ●	○	△ cc ___				
10	● ●	○	△ cc ___				
11	● ●	○	△ cc ___				
TOTALS:							

C 1984

FIGURE 23-3 An incontinence record. (From Williamson M: Reducing post-catheterization bladder dysfunction by reconditioning, *Nurs Res* 31:28-30, 1982.)

skin with mild soap and warm water, rinse, and gently pat dry. Inspect the genitals, perineum, thighs, and buttocks for redness and skin breakdown. In addition, apply a protective cream as ordered or according to agency policy. If skin breakdown does occur, notify the RN or physician and provide treatment as ordered or according to agency policy.

Risk for Infection

The patient who is incontinent of urine is at risk for urinary tract infection and urinary calculi (stones). These complications are most likely to occur in patients who retain urine and in those who restrict their fluids. Retained urine is a good medium for bacterial growth and the overstretched bladder wall is susceptible to infection. Patients may restrict fluid intake to try to reduce the frequency of incontinence. However, concentrated urine is a risk factor for infections and calculi. Patients with indwelling catheters are at increased risk for urinary tract infections.

To reduce the risk of urinary tract infection, encourage the patient to empty the bladder as scheduled, provide adequate fluids, and use strict aseptic technique during catheterization. Keep the perineal area clean and encourage an intake of 1500 to 3000 mL of fluid per day unless contraindicated. Details of catheter care are covered in Chapter 42.

BOWEL (FECAL) INCONTINENCE

Bowel incontinence is less common than urinary incontinence but it can be very distressing for patients who are affected by it. It is believed to affect 20% of community dwelling older persons and 50% of long-term care residents. Bowel incontinence is usually related to anal sphincter dysfunction caused by anal surgery, trauma during childbirth, Crohn disease affecting the anus, or diabetic neuropathy. Some patients experience temporary incontinence with severe diarrhea because they do not have time to reach the toilet. Incontinent diarrhea may also be present with fecal impaction. Diminished muscle strength associated with aging also may be a factor.

PHYSIOLOGIC PROCESS OF DEFECATION

The structures that maintain bowel control are the internal and external sphincters and the puborectal muscle. The muscles of the pelvic floor and the external sphincter are under voluntary control (Fig. 23-4). The bowel has its own nerve network that stimulates peristalsis when distended. Therefore disorders of the central nervous system (CNS) and spinal cord do not impair bowel control as much as they do bladder control.

The fecal mass enters the rectum by mass movement. The presence of feces in the rectum creates a desire to defecate. Defecation occurs when the anal sphincter relaxes and the rectum contracts. Tightening of the diaphragm and abdominal muscles promotes defecation by increasing pressure in the abdomen. If defecation does not occur soon after this pressure is felt, the sensation of needing to defecate soon fades. People who often ignore or delay defecation tend to become constipated.

DIAGNOSTIC TESTS AND PROCEDURES

Evaluation of fecal incontinence may include assessment of rectal sphincter tone, laboratory examination of a stool specimen for blood or pathogens, and endoscopic or radiologic procedures to detect underlying problems. Diagnostic tests and procedures for the lower gastrointestinal (GI) system are presented in detail in Chapter 40.

COMMON THERAPEUTIC MEASURES

ENEMAS

Enemas may be necessary to stimulate emptying of the bowel in the patient who is prone to impaction. In general, frequent use of large-volume enemas is not advised because it overstretches the bowel and may contribute to loss of muscle tone. Sometimes, however, enemas are necessary. The patient with poor rectal

Put on Your Thinking Cap!

Four of the patients you have cared for in the past week have had diagnoses of "urinary incontinence." Mrs. A., age 55, was admitted for treatment of her asthma. She has five adult children and often babysits for two toddlers. She says that she loses a small amount of urine when she coughs or picks up a toddler.

Mr. B., age 72, had a prostatectomy 2 weeks ago. His catheter has been removed but he was readmitted with a severe urinary tract infection. He complains of constant dribbling of urine that requires him to wear incontinence pads. His bladder is not palpable.

Mrs. C., age 25, had an appendectomy. On the afternoon of the procedure, she voided 25 to 60 mL of urine at frequent intervals. Her bladder was distended and she complained of a constant urge to void.

Mr. D., age 85, was admitted with pneumonia. He has a diagnosis of moderate dementia. On two occasions he was found out of bed and urine was found on the floor. On another occasion he urinated in the wastebasket.

Decide which type of incontinence each patient probably had and fill in the chart below with the probable cause or causes for the specific patient, the recommended treatment, and the appropriate nursing interventions for each patient related to incontinence.

PATIENT	TYPE OF INCONTINENCE	PROBABLE CAUSE	TREATMENT	NURSING CARE
Mrs. A.				
Mr. B.				
Mrs. C.				
Mr. D.				

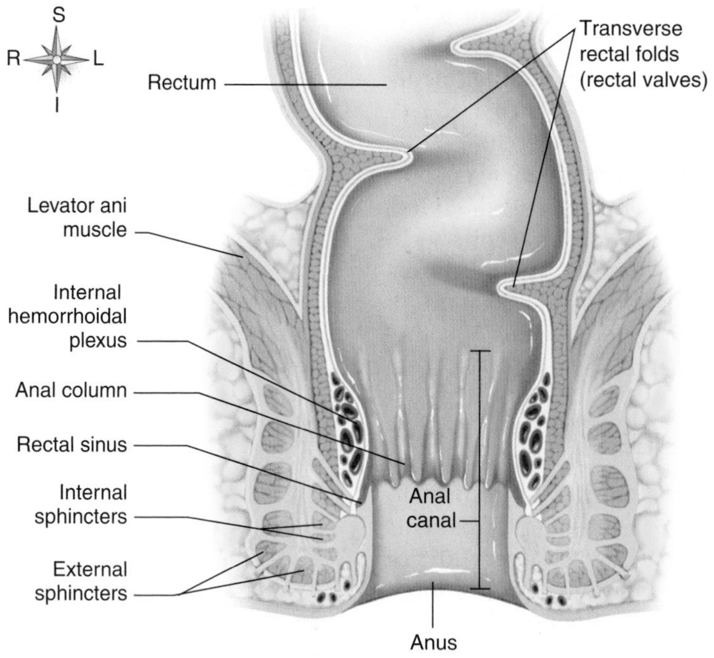

FIGURE 23-4 The anal sphincters and musculature. (From Patton K, Thibodeau G: *Anatomy & physiology*, ed 8, St. Louis, 2013, Mosby.)

sphincter tone may have difficulty retaining enema solutions. An adapter can be placed on the enema tubing and inserted into the anus. The nipplelike adapter helps the patient to retain the solution.

POUCHES

Plastic pouches, much like ostomy bags, may be applied to the perianal area and held in place with adhesive. They are helpful for patients who have frequent stools. Because they are bulky and uncomfortable, they are not practical for ambulatory patients. Another disadvantage is the skin irritation caused by the adhesive. When the pouch is changed, provide meticulous skin care. An alternative to the pouch is an adult incontinent brief or (for bed patients) linen protectors.

DRUG THERAPY

Types of drugs used to prevent or treat fecal incontinence include laxatives, stool softeners, and antidiarrheal drugs, depending on the cause of the incontinence. If the patient has had fecal impactions, laxatives or stool softeners are appropriate. Antidiarrheal drugs are appropriate if diarrhea is causing the problem. These drugs are discussed in Chapter 39.

Put on Your Thinking Cap!

When would a patient with fecal incontinence need laxatives?

SURGICAL TREATMENT

Surgical options include repair of anal muscles, implanting electrodes to stimulate and strengthen the perineal muscles, and placement of an artificial sphincter. The artificial sphincter functions like the urinary artificial sphincter described earlier. A fluid-filled chamber around the anus maintains continence. The patient deflates the chamber by pressing a reservoir in the scrotum or labia to allow bowel movements. Although the idea is appealing, infection and other complications often require removal of the device. Therefore some experts believe that sacral modulation is more effective and less costly.

BIOFEEDBACK

Patients who are motivated and able to follow directions and whose external anal sphincter is capable of responding to rectal distention may achieve bowel control with biofeedback. A balloon is inserted into the rectum and inflated. A manometer creates a tracing of the normal response of the sphincter to rectal pressure. The patient tries to consciously reproduce the pattern by contracting the muscles that delay defecation. The size of the balloon is progressively decreased to help the patient recognize and respond to the amount of rectal distention expected with normal stool volume. Biofeedback has been effective for many patients but has not proven useful for patients with fecal incontinence associated with diabetes, spinal cord injury, rectal trauma, or radiation injury. Pelvic muscle strengthening exercises, as described with urinary incontinence, may be helpful.

DIETARY CHANGES

The patient can be advised to avoid foods that stimulate the anal sphincters to relax. These include chocolate, coffee, tea, and other caffeinated beverages. Raw fruits, fruit juices (especially prune and grape juice), raw vegetables, cabbage, sweets, alcohol, and highly spicy foods stimulate stool production. Conversely, foods that thicken the stool include bananas, rice, bread, potatoes, cheese, yogurt, oatmeal, oat bran, boiled milk, and pasta. Until fecal incontinence is corrected, the patient may also wish to avoid foods that cause odor and gas. Odor-causing foods include cabbage family vegetables, beans, garlic, eggs, fish, and turnips. Beans, beer, carbonated beverages, cucumbers, cabbage, broccoli, dairy products, and corn produce gas.

TYPES OF BOWEL (FECAL) INCONTINENCE

The four types of bowel incontinence are overflow, neurogenic, symptomatic, and anorectal. Table 23-4 summarizes the features of each type.

OVERFLOW INCONTINENCE

Description

Overflow incontinence is caused by constipation in which the rectum is constantly distended. The fecal mass backs up until the entire colon is full. A fecal impaction may or may not be present. The patient passes semisolid stools frequently. This condition may be related to a long-standing dependence on laxatives or enemas.

Medical Treatment

Medical management of bowel overflow incontinence is concerned with immediate relief of the constipation and long-term control of the problem. The first step is to cleanse the colon. Phosphate enemas and suppositories may be ordered to empty the rectum. Daily enemas for 7 to 10 days are then needed to empty the entire colon. Instead of the enemas, the physician may order oral laxatives such as bisacodyl, polyethylene glycol, or mannitol. If hard masses of stool are present, they can be softened with oil retention enemas and then removed digitally.

Once the colon has been cleansed, regular evacuation is essential. Increased fluids and fiber may be helpful but some patients need regular aids to elimination. The physician may order enemas or suppositories twice a week or daily laxatives. For older patients, senna or lactulose is preferred by many geriatric specialists. Mineral oil should be avoided because it interferes with absorption of fat-soluble vitamins and because it may be aspirated, causing lipid pneumonia.

NEUROGENIC INCONTINENCE

Description

Many people report having a bowel movement shortly after the first meal of the day. This is caused by the gastrocolic reflex. When food enters the stomach, it stimulates activity throughout the digestive tract and causes the movement of the fecal mass into the rectum. Patients who do not voluntarily delay defecation are said to have bowel **neurogenic incontinence**. This occurs most often in patients with dementia. These patients usually have one or two formed stools daily after meals.

Medical Treatment

Neurogenic incontinence is usually treated with scheduled toileting based on the patient's usual time of defecation. If this is not successful, some physicians order a constipating drug (e.g., codeine) each morning and a laxative (e.g., senna, milk of magnesia) each night. This routine results in a controlled bowel movement each morning and avoids later accidents. However, it does not correct the underlying problem.

Table 23-4 Types of Bowel Incontinence

TYPE	DESCRIPTION	CAUSES	NURSING CARE
Overflow	Uncontrolled, frequent passage of small, semisoft stools Fecal impaction may be present	Constipation in which entire colon is full of fecal matter	Administer laxatives and enemas as ordered. Increase fluids and fiber as appropriate.
Anorectal	Uncontrolled passage of stool several times a day	Weak pelvic muscles Loss of anal reflexes Poor rectal sphincter tone Rectal prolapse	Teach Kegel exercises. Prepare for surgery, if planned.
Neurogenic	Formed stools passed after meals Usually seen in dementia patients	Gastrocolic reflex stimulates defecation Patient does not delay until appropriate time	Ensure scheduled toileting.
Symptomatic	Incontinent stools, usually diarrhea Not related to other types of fecal incontinence	Colon or rectal disease	Provide comfort measures and proper skin care. Prepare for diagnostic tests and procedures.

SYMPTOMATIC INCONTINENCE

Description

Symptomatic incontinence is the result of colorectal disease. These patients usually have incontinence with diarrhea. Blood or mucus may be seen in the stool.

Medical Treatment

When a patient has symptomatic incontinence, medical care should be sought to identify and treat the cause. Reducing intake of caffeine, alcohol, sorbitol, dairy products, and fiber may be helpful.

ANORECTAL INCONTINENCE

Description

Anorectal incontinence is associated with nerve damage that causes the muscles of the pelvic floor to be weak. Rectal abnormalities may be present, including loss of anal reflex and loss of anal sphincter tone. Patients typically have several incontinent stools a day.

Medical Treatment

Anorectal incontinence is treated with pelvic muscle exercises and sometimes biofeedback. If these techniques are ineffective, surgical repair of the anal sphincter may be advised.

NURSING CARE of the Patient with Bowel Incontinence

Assessment

The data the licensed vocational nurse/licensed practical nurse (LVN/LPN) collects can contribute to a thorough nursing assessment that can help to diagnose the type and cause of bowel incontinence and guide the selection of treatment.

Health History

Chief Complaint. When a patient has bowel incontinence, determine the usual bowel pattern, changes, stool characteristics, and related symptoms such as pain or cramping.

Bowel Pattern. Bowel patterns are usually well established in the adult. Document the patient's usual frequency of bowel movements. Regarding incontinent episodes, ask if the patient is aware of the need to defecate. For dementia patients, a caregiver may be able to detect clues that the patient is about to have a bowel movement (e.g., restlessness, trying to remove clothing). If the patient is confused, initiate a record of times and circumstances when defecation occurs.

Characteristics of Stools. Describe the consistency, color, and constituents of the patient's stools. Terms used to describe consistency include *liquid, watery, pasty, tarry, semiformed, formed,* and *hard.* Most of these terms are self-explanatory. Tarry is used to describe stools that are shiny, sticky, and black. Stool is normally brown in color. Abnormal colors are black, red, green, and white. Abnormal stool constituents might include blood, mucus, or undigested food.

Past Medical History. Document chronic illnesses, past acute illnesses, and surgeries or trauma to the abdomen or rectum. Neurologic conditions, including stroke, spinal cord injury, and dementia, are significant. List recent and current medications and all allergies. It is especially important to determine the use of laxatives, enemas, or suppositories. Because these are often purchased without a prescription, the patient may not mention them when reporting medications. Record the obstetric history of female patients, including the number of pregnancies, types of deliveries, and complications of childbirth.

Review of Systems. The review of systems identifies problems that may be related to bowel incontinence, such as motor, sensory, or cognitive impairments.

Functional Assessment. The functional assessment focuses on habits that may be related to bowel function, including diet, fluid intake, and exercise or activity pattern. Determine whether the patient has the mobility and dexterity needed to manage toileting independently. Recent travel to other countries may be significant because travelers sometimes acquire uncommon intestinal infections.

Physical Examination

Inspect and palpate the abdomen for distention and auscultate for bowel sounds. In addition, inspect the perianal area for irritation or breakdown. The physician or NP may perform a rectal examination and test the strength of the rectal sphincter.

Assessment of the patient with bowel incontinence is outlined in Box 23-2.

Box 23-2 Focused Assessment of Patients with Bowel Incontinence

HEALTH HISTORY

Chief Complaint
Bowel pattern changes, stool characteristics (consistency, color, constituents), awareness of need to defecate, symptoms associated with passage of incontinent stool

Past Medical History
Chronic illnesses, past acute illnesses, abdominal or rectal trauma or surgery, abdominal radiotherapy, recent and current medications, dementia, allergies

Review of Systems
Motor, sensory, or cognitive dysfunction that could affect continence

Functional Assessment
Diet, fluid intake, exercise or activity pattern, foreign travel

PHYSICAL EXAMINATION

Abdomen
Distention, bowel sounds

Perianal Area
Irritation, breakdown

Nursing Diagnoses, Goals, and Outcome Criteria: Fecal Incontinence

Nursing diagnoses and goals for the patient with fecal incontinence may include the following:

Nursing Diagnoses	Goals and Outcome Criteria
Bowel Incontinence related to impaction, cognitive impairment, neurologic impairment, environmental barriers, or impaired mobility	Controlled bowel elimination: regular voluntary bowel evacuation of soft, formed stool
Impaired Skin Integrity related to contact of feces with skin	Normal skin integrity: no redness or skin breakdown
Situational Low Self-Esteem related to loss of control of elimination	Improved self-esteem: patient's comments and behavior reflect positive view of self (e.g., confidence, takes pride in appearance)

Interventions

Bowel Incontinence

Continued monitoring is an essential part of the nurse's role in caring for the patient with bowel incontinence. Documentation of the patient's usual bowel pattern provides a guideline for scheduled elimination and for setting realistic goals. To establish a bowel program, take the patient to the toilet at the usual time of defecation, commonly 30 minutes after eating. If suppositories or enemas are ordered, administer them and document the results.

When enemas or laxatives are prescribed on a routine basis for overflow incontinence, caregivers often fear creating laxative or enema dependency. For these patients, however, normal bowel function may not be a realistic goal. They may do better with a program that promotes regular bowel evacuation. Such a program is far better than the miserable process of emptying a full colon every few weeks.

Explain normal bowel physiology and interventions for incontinence to the patient. Advise the patient to consume adequate fluids and fiber to prevent constipation and impaction. A fluid intake of at least 1500 mL/day is recommended if not contraindicated. Increase fluids gradually in older patients because fluid overload can lead to heart failure. Work with the dietitian to teach the patient that fresh fruits and vegetables provide bulk and fiber that keep the stool moist and soft. Encourage ambulation if the patient is able to walk. If perineal exercises are prescribed, advise the patient to practice contracting the muscles that control defecation. The contraction should be held for at least 10 seconds and repeated several times each day.

Impaired Skin Integrity

After each incontinent stool, cleanse the patient's perianal area thoroughly and apply protective creams or ointments as ordered or per agency policy. Incontinence undergarments may be needed to prevent soiling and embarrassment but they must be checked frequently so that stool does not remain in contact with the skin. Fecal pouches may be used but the adhesive and plastic can irritate the skin, so good skin care is still a priority.

Situational Low Self-Esteem

Loss of bowel control can be devastating for the patient. Express understanding of the patient's distress and encourage the patient to strive for as much improvement as possible. In addition, praise the patient for participation in the treatment program and for decreased frequency of incontinent stools. Encourage the patient to practice good grooming and to resume social activities. It is important to help patients to coordinate their social schedule with their bowel programs.

Get Ready for the NCLEX® Examination!

Key Points

- Incontinence is the inability to control the passage of urine or feces.
- Normal controlled voiding requires healthy bladder muscle, a patent urethra, normal transmission of nerve impulses, and mental alertness.
- Data collection relevant to urinary incontinence includes recording the voiding pattern, urine volume, associated signs and symptoms, medications, medical history, and physical findings.
- The types of urinary incontinence are urge, stress, overflow (including reflex), and functional.
- Transient incontinence is caused by reversible conditions and is often corrected by treatment of the underlying problem.
- Urge urinary incontinence—involuntary loss of urine after a strong urge to void—may be corrected by treating the cause with behavior modification and drug therapy.
- Overflow urinary incontinence—involuntary loss of urine associated with a full bladder—may be corrected by treating the cause (e.g., enlarged prostate) or by using drugs that stimulate the bladder and relax the internal sphincter.

- Reflex urinary incontinence is a type of overflow incontinence.
- Stress urinary incontinence—the involuntary loss of urine during physical exertion—may be improved by strengthening the perineal muscles, surgical intervention, or placement of an artificial sphincter.
- Functional urinary incontinence is inappropriate voiding despite normal urinary function.
- Assessment of bowel incontinence includes recording the usual bowel pattern, stool characteristics, related symptoms, activity, diet, fluid intake, medications, and use of aids to help elimination, as well as performing an abdominal assessment.
- Types of bowel incontinence include overflow, anorectal, neurogenic, and symptomatic.
- Fecal overflow incontinence is caused by constipation in which the rectum is constantly distended and is treated by relieving the constipation and preventing future episodes.
- Anorectal incontinence is caused by abnormalities in the pelvic muscle, anus, or rectum and may require pelvic floor muscle exercises or surgery.
- Neurogenic bowel incontinence is automatic defecation seen in people (e.g., patients with dementia) who do not voluntarily delay defecation; it may be corrected by scheduled toileting.
- Symptomatic bowel incontinence results from colorectal disease and requires correction of the basic problem.
- Nursing care of the patient who is incontinent may address measures to correct the specific type of incontinence, to maintain skin integrity, to improve situational low self-esteem, and to improve knowledge of management.
- Techniques to restore bladder control include bladder retraining using scheduled toileting, Credé technique for emptying the bladder, Kegel exercises to strengthen pelvic floor muscles, and reflex training.
- Bowel training may be accomplished by scheduled toileting, stimulation techniques, or both.

Additional Learning Resources

SG Go to your Study Guide for additional learning activities to help you master this chapter content.

evolve Go to your Evolve website (http://evolve.elsevier.com/Linton/medsurg) for the following learning resources and much more:

- Interactive Prioritization Exercises
- Fluid & Electrolyte Tutorial
- Pharmacology Tutorial
- Review Questions for the NCLEX® Examination

Review Questions for the NCLEX® Examination

1. Habit training is being used to treat a patient with urinary incontinence. What should the nurse instruct the nursing assistant to do?
   1. Check the patient for wetness every 2 hours and ask the patient to state whether he or she is wet or dry
   2. Encourage the patient to void every 2 hours on a schedule based on the patient's usual pattern
   3. Encourage the patient to delay voiding and to void only at scheduled times
   4. Have the patient practice interrupting urine flow by contracting perineal muscles

   NCLEX Client Need: Safe and Effective Care Environment: Coordinated Care
2. The nurse is teaching a patient to perform pelvic muscle exercises. Instructions should include which of the following? (Select all that apply.)
   1. You should contract perineal muscles for 30 seconds, then relax for 30 seconds.
   2. You will notice improvement within 1 week after starting exercises.
   3. Strengthening perineal muscles can improve urinary control.
   4. To do these exercises correctly, you must be in a sitting position.
   5. You will need to continue the exercises indefinitely to maintain control.

   NCLEX Client Need: Health Promotion and Maintenance
3. The nurse is preparing to discharge a patient who will be doing self-catheterization at home. How does intermittent self-catheterization in the home setting differ from that in an institution?
   1. Clean technique may be used at home but not in a hospital.
   2. Sterile technique must be used regardless of the setting.
   3. Clean technique may be used anywhere as long as the patient performs the procedure.
   4. Clean technique can be used in long-term care facilities because patients live there.

   NCLEX Client Need: Safe and Effective Care Environment: Safety and Infection Control
4. A clinic patient has had a pessary inserted because of urinary incontinence. Care of this patient includes:
   1. Evaluation of placement position within 1 week after insertion
   2. Documentation of pessary placement so it will not be forgotten
   3. Monitoring for signs of bowel obstruction
   4. Removal for cleansing each time perineal care is done

   NCLEX Client Need: Safe and Effective Care Environment: Safety and Infection Control

5. An older adult patient has been diagnosed with urge urinary incontinence. Her husband asks what this means. Which statements accurately describe this diagnosis? (Select all that apply.)
   1. A strong, abrupt urge to urinate occurs shortly before involuntary urine loss.
   2. Urge incontinence is often caused by anticholinergic drugs.
   3. Urge incontinence commonly is the result of an overactive bladder muscle.
   4. In urge incontinence the bladder overfills so that small amounts of urine are passed to relieve pressure.
   5. Medications are often effective in reducing bladder overactivity.

   NCLEX Client Need: Physiological Integrity: Physiological Adaptation
6. Autonomic dysreflexia is a very serious complication of which type of incontinence?

   NCLEX Client Need: Physiological Integrity: Physiological Adaptation
7. Which statement should be included when teaching a woman about stress urinary incontinence?
   1. It is usually caused by relaxation of the pelvic floor muscles.
   2. You should limit fluid intake to 1000 mL/day.
   3. Fluids containing caffeine stimulate contraction of perineal muscles.
   4. The only effective treatment for stress incontinence is surgical repair.

   NCLEX Client: Physiological Integrity: Physiological Adaptation
8. A patient in the independent living unit of a retirement home reports that she has had several incidents of bowel incontinence. The nurse's assessment reveals that the patient consumes all of the items listed below. Which one might be related to the patient's fecal incontinence?
   1. Bananas
   2. Alcohol
   3. Pasta
   4. Cheese

   NCLEX Client Need: Physiological Integrity: Physiological Adaptation
9. A bedridden patient with no history of bowel incontinence has been involuntarily passing liquid stools for 2 days. What additional data should the nurse collect?
   1. Last formed bowel movement
   2. Urine output
   3. Temperature
   4. Usual mental status

   NCLEX Client Need: Physiological Integrity: Basic Care and Comfort

chapter 24

Loss, Death, and End-of-Life Care

http://evolve.elsevier.com/Linton/medsurg

Objectives

1. Describe beliefs and practices related to death and dying.
2. Describe responses of patients and their families to terminal illness and death.
3. Identify data required in assessing the terminally ill or dying patient.
4. Assist in the development of a care plan for the terminally ill patient.
5. Discuss the ways in which nurses can intervene to meet the needs of the terminally ill patient's significant others.
6. Explore the needs of the nurse who works with terminally ill patients.
7. Identify issues related to caring for the dying patient, including advance directives, artificial feeding and hydration, do not resuscitate decisions, brain death, organ donations, and pronouncement of death.

Key Terms

Advance directives
Algor mortis (ĂL-gōr MŌR-tĭs)
Autopsy (ĂW-tŏp-sē)
Bereavement (bĕ-RĒV-mĕnt)
Cerebral death (sĕ-RĒ-brăl)
Denial
Grief
Livor mortis (LĪ-vōr MŌR-tĭs)
Loss
Mourning
Palliative care (PĂL-ē-ă-tĭv)
Rigor mortis (RĬ-gōr MŌR-tĭs)
Shroud

Aging and death are topics often avoided in a society that admires youth and beauty. However, for health care providers caring for people of all ages as they near death, it is an important and moving experience. It was not until the 1960s that we began to look at death as a holistic process and began to study it systematically. Scientists, health care professionals, theologians, and laypersons have examined the processes associated with dying and death. Information concerning death and dying can be found in popular and professional literature and is openly discussed. The result has been better understanding of the needs and wishes of patients and those who love them. The public has become better informed about death and patients often are able to express their fears and hopes. Communication between health care providers, patients, and families is more transparent. Palliative care and hospice care, which provide specialized care before and after the end of life, have flourished. Nowhere is the art and science of nursing needed more that when caring for patients through the dying process.

This chapter presents information concerning the dying process in persons near the end of life. The grieving process for the dying person experienced by the person's friends and family is presented, with a special emphasis on nursing care.

A **palliative care** movement is aimed at providing care rather than achieving a cure. Palliative care refocuses health care on allowing natural death in a pain- and symptom-controlled environment with psychosocial support. Palliative care can be provided in any setting. When a cure is no longer expected and the person's life expectancy is limited, hospice care may be chosen. Hospice care embraces palliative care with a focus on quality of life, comfort, and dignity near the end of life. It also includes bereavement care for survivors after the death of the patient. Hospice care, discussed in Chapter 1, can be provided in any setting. It involves a multidisciplinary team and has a strong nursing component.

CONCEPT OF LOSS

Loss may be defined as a real or potential absence of someone or something that is valued. Real losses occur when something actually happens so that valued people or possessions are no longer available. Potential losses relate to an individual's perceptions of what *might* occur if a valued person or object were lost permanently. For example, families of soldiers who are deployed to combat zones must face the potential loss of the soldier. Death may be thought of as the ultimate loss. Whatever the loss, people experience similar feelings and thoughts when it happens. Anxiety, fear, and grief are common with both real and potential losses. The intensity of feelings varies with the importance of the specific loss to each person.

TYPES OF LOSSES

Loss is experienced in many ways. Changes in self-image, developmental changes, loss of possessions, and loss of significant others are common types of loss.

Change in Self-Image

Each of us has a self-image, which is our perception of our own identity, worth, abilities, and limitations. These components of our self-image are subject to change. While some change is planned, other change is beyond our control. Various normal life events such as pregnancy, hair loss, and aging as well as health deviations that require surgery or result in disability can alter a person's self-image.

Developmental Changes

Across the life cycle, numerous changes or milestones take place. Despite the feelings of pride associated with gaining skills and achieving goals, we also experience insecurities, fears, and feelings of loss as we change and grow. New parents have a loss of freedom and a change in lifestyle along with increased financial demands. During the child-rearing stage, parents experience a loss of control of their children as they gain independence and self-control. Young adults may feel a sense of loss related to changes in routines that were previously secure and dependable. These changes include moving away from parents, getting a job, finding a partner, and a general loss of dependence and innocence.

Parents may experience a sense of loss once all of their children have left the home. Retirement represents a huge change in roles, functions, and place in the community. In general, changes associated with old age occur gradually. However, health crises can bring rapid changes and possible sudden loss of independence. The older person's social network shrinks as friends die, relocate, or become disabled. Facing one's own dying and death is the final change that all humans face.

Loss of Possessions

Possessions have a perceived value to the owner that may not be readily apparent to others. An object may be irreplaceable because of the memories associated with it or it may be valuable in monetary terms. For example, the loss of an appointment calendar may be as distressing as the loss of a family heirloom. The loss of a pet can affect the owner as significantly as the loss of a family member. For older persons, the loss of a lifetime's accumulation of possessions through placement in housing for older adults can be devastating.

Loss of Significant Others

Loss of significant others occurs through death but also may occur through separation, growth of children, relocation, divorce, or lack of communication.

Separation from significant others may be related to actual distance or it may be emotional in nature. Children leaving their parents to go to school or to start their own families can produce feelings of loss in all concerned. Relocation to a long-term care residence can lead to prolonged separation and feelings of loss.

Emotional aspects of loss may be related to a lack of fulfillment of expected roles. Persons who have remained unmarried or who have not had children may feel a loss because their expectations were not fulfilled. Communication breakdowns or barriers can divide significant others as completely as a physical separation would. The loss of a loved one through death is a permanent loss. In American society, death is frequently seen as a tragic event to be delayed for as long as possible. Americans expect to live into old age, even if old age is not considered as attractive as youth.

Loss that occurs during normal development can be anticipated and possibly prepared for, depending on an individual's ability to do so. When death occurs suddenly and unexpectedly, survivors must deal with the shock as well as the loss. Regardless of who or what is lost, those left behind react to the event. Not all people react in the same way to similar situations.

GRIEF

Grief is the normal personal response to a loss. It is an emotional reaction that serves to maintain emotional and physical well-being. The grieving process is a complex and intense experience that affects a person's thoughts, feelings, and behaviors. The grief process is usually most profound when the loss experienced is death. **Mourning** is the outward part of coping with grief. It represents a period of grieving marked by social customs. Most societies have expectations for appropriate behavior during the period of mourning. The concept of **bereavement** is broader in that it includes the total grief and mourning experience.

Working through the grief process helps the dying person and significant others to adapt to the loss. Grief that assists the person in accepting the reality of death may be called *uncomplicated grief.* Various terms are used to describe grief that does not progress in the "normal" fashion. Grief that is prolonged, unresolved, or disruptive to the person who experiences it may be termed *complicated grief.* Complicated grief may relate to a real loss or a perceived loss. It may occur when grief is not resolved from a prior experience or when the expression of grief is blocked in some way. Feelings and behaviors may become exaggerated and disruptive to a person's typical lifestyle. Specific behaviors are associated with complicated grief. Many times distress at the loss is expressed. Unresolved issues may be identified and past experiences reviewed. Complicated grief is sometimes described as dysfunctional.

When a person's relationship to the person or lost object is not socially recognized, the survivor may experience *disenfranchised grief*. For example, when a same-sex partner dies, others may not be aware of or may not accept the relationship and fail to provide the same level of support offered to others.

Uncomplicated grief is a healthy response. When it begins before a death actually occurs or when the reality that death is inevitable is known, it is referred to as *anticipatory grief*. Anticipatory grief is usually related to an impending loss or death. Both the patient and the family members can experience anticipatory grieving.

Emotions such as anger, sadness, guilt, and denial may be present in all types of grief. Some people have difficulty expressing these feelings. The person experiencing grief may demonstrate changes in eating, sleeping, and other activities of daily living. Difficulty concentrating and making decisions may occur.

GRIEVING PROCESS

People who are facing the inevitability of death need caregivers who understand how personal attitudes affect the experience. The attitudes of the dying person, those of the significant others, and the nurse's own attitudes affect the death experience.

Understanding how culture, spirituality, family, and stage of development influence the dying person will help you to appreciate the person's needs, wants, and fears. Culture, religious beliefs, and age affect a person's understanding of and reaction to death or loss. Frequently, beliefs and attitudes are interrelated between culture and religion. The American work ethic is closely related to the Protestant ethic, which emphasizes independence, self-reliance, hard work, and rugged individualism. Death and dying tend to be private matters shared only with significant others. Often feelings are repressed or internalized. People who believe in "toughing it out" or "being strong" may not express themselves when they face a tragic loss.

Members of African-American and Latin cultures commonly express their feelings more easily than do European Americans. Kinship tends to be very strong within the Latino culture. Family members, both immediate and extended, provide support for one another. Expressing feelings of loss is encouraged and accepted.

Religious teachings usually include beliefs about death and life after death. These beliefs can have a powerful influence on the way a person reacts to loss and death. Most religious groups have common practices related to care of the dying person, care of the body after death, and final rites. Specific information about religious preferences should be obtained from the family.

Family members' past experiences and stages of development influence their responses to death and dying. Through experience with other losses, a generalized acceptance of dying can take place. Past experience with death of a loved one provides a frame of reference for some members of the family. Adaptive skills that have worked in the past may help individuals to cope with the loss of a loved one.

The age or stage of development also affects a person's reactions to death and dying. Children have a different understanding of loss and death than adults do. Some adults believe that children should be protected from the pain associated with the death of a loved one. Often, however, children who are "protected" feel abandoned, frightened, and alone with their feelings. A child who loses a loved one to death may regress or be delayed in emotional development until the grief can be resolved.

Maturity contributes to understanding and accepting death. During adulthood people must come to terms with the death of their parents and other older family members. Coping with the death of one's parents is often identified as a developmental crisis. During adulthood people also have to confront their own mortality. The death of a spouse has a profound impact on older adults. Widowed persons reportedly have an increase in health problems during the first year after the death of the spouse. Loss of one's child at any age is an especially traumatic event. Table 24-1 identifies some common age-related attitudes associated with death.

STAGES OF GRIEVING

Various scholars have studied grief as a process that has stages. Among these scholars of grief are Kübler-Ross, Martocchio, and Rando.

Kübler-Ross

In 1969 Dr. Elisabeth Kübler-Ross shattered the taboo against talking about death and dying when she published a book that identified five stages of grieving that occur in response to impending death. The five stages are (1) denial, (2) anger, (3) bargaining, (4) depression, and (5) acceptance. The stages represent categories of responses to a diagnosis of a fatal illness. The term *stages* is not intended to imply sequence or mutually exclusive categories. Indeed, stages can overlap and multiple stages can exist at the same time. Kübler-Ross identified behaviors common to each stage. Not all people experience all stages and there is no predictable timetable on which the stages occur. This model is often applied to other individuals who experience significant losses, such as loss of a loved one, an amputation, loss of vision, or paralysis.

Denial. The person refuses to acknowledge the terminal diagnosis and may put forth a cheerful appearance to prolong the denial of the loss. **Denial** is a defense

Table 24-1 Age-Related Beliefs about Death

AGE RANGE	BELIEFS
Infancy to 5 years (preschool)	Child has little or no understanding of death. Child believes death is temporary and reversible, like sleep.
6 to 9 years (school age)	Child believes death is final. Child believes one's own death can be avoided. Child believes death is related to violence. Child believes that wishing or hoping for death can make it happen.
10 to 12 years (preadolescent)	Preadolescent believes death is an inevitable end to life. Preadolescent grasps his or her own mortality by discussing fear of death or life after death. Preadolescent expresses feelings of death based on adult attitudes.
13 to 18 years (adolescent)	Adolescent is afraid of prolonged death. Adolescent may act out defiance for death through dangerous or self-destructive acts. Adolescent has a philosophical or religious approach to death. Adolescent seldom thinks about death.
19 to 45 years (young adulthood)	Young adult's cultural and religious beliefs influence his or her attitudes about death. Young adult sees death as a future event.
45 to 65 years (middle adulthood)	Middle-aged adult accepts his or her own mortality as inevitable. Middle-aged adult faces the death of parents and peers. Middle-aged adult may experience death anxiety.
65 years and older (older adulthood)	Older adult is afraid of prolonged health problems. Older adult faces the death of family members and peers. Older adult sees death as inevitable. Older adult examines death as it relates to various meanings, such as freedom from discomfort.

mechanism that helps the patient and others to manage anxiety evoked by the threat.

Anger. The patient expresses anger toward themselves or others. The anger may be directed at the health care providers, the institution, or even significant others.

Bargaining. In the bargaining stage, the person recognizes the terminal nature of his or her illness and seeks to "buy" more time. The individual may express feelings that the loss is a punishment for past actions and try to negotiate with a higher power to gain time. For example, the patient may pray to live through some important event, such as a child's wedding or a landmark birthday.

Depression. The depressed patient may experience many emotions, including sadness, regret, and fear. The patient needs to review his or her life. In this stage the person has begun to accept the reality of impending death.

Acceptance. The individual may become somewhat emotionally detached and objective. The patient identifies the loss as inevitable and may want to make plans.

Martocchio

B.C. Martocchio has described five clusters of grief: (1) shock and disbelief; (2) yearning and protest; (3) anguish, disorganization, and despair; (4) identification in bereavement; and (5) reorganization and restoration.

Shock and Disbelief. The individual may feel numb and may express feelings of anger, sadness, or guilt. Denial may be present.

Yearning and Protest. Anger may be directed toward God, health care providers, survivors, and even the deceased for dying. Surviving loved ones may withdraw into themselves and not wish to share their feelings.

Anguish, Disorganization, and Despair. A decreased interest in the future may be felt. Decision making is difficult. Survivors may express a general lack of purpose for living. Crying is common in this stage.

Identification in Bereavement. Survivors may imitate the deceased's habits, traits, or goals.

Reorganization and Restoration. Grieving does not stop all at once. Typical patterns of life gradually return. No timetable can be set for the process of grieving. Some people seem to recover from grief quickly whereas others may experience recurrent grief throughout their lives.

Rando

T. A. Rando described grief in terms of a series of processes that occur in one of three phases of mourning. The three phases are (1) avoidance, (2) confrontation, and (3) accommodation. Specific processes occur in each phase (Table 24-2)

Avoidance. Individuals respond to grief with denial, shock, and disbelief regarding the loss.

Confrontation. Feelings are intense and charged with great emotion. Individuals face the loss and experience emotional upheaval.

Accommodation. Emotional healing begins. The intensity of grief gradually subsides. Individuals learn to deal with the loss.

Table 24-2 Rando's Phases of Mourning and Related Processes

PHASE	PROCESS
Avoidance	**Recognize the loss** by acknowledging and understanding the death
Confrontation	**React to the separation**; experience the pain; react to the loss **Recollect and re-experience feelings**; review and remember the deceased **Relinquish old attachments** to the deceased
Accommodation	**Readjust** by moving forward, establishing a new identity **Reinvest** emotional energy in new people, goals, activities

Despite differences in terminology, Kübler-Ross stages of grief, Martocchio's clusters of grief, and Rando's phases of grieving are more alike than they are different. Each provides a framework for anticipating and understanding the experience of the dying and their survivors.

COMMON SIGNS AND SYMPTOMS OF GRIEF

Common signs and symptoms of grief are shared by the terminally ill person and those who lose a significant other. Knowledge of the signs and symptoms allows the nurse to better communicate with everyone involved.

Physical symptoms are experienced during the grief process. Physical symptoms might include tightness in the chest, sensations of shortness of breath or suffocation, generalized weakness, intense tightening in the abdomen, and emptiness or churning in the stomach. These symptoms may fluctuate throughout the grief process. Generally they occur with the initial acknowledgment of death as the outcome. The patient and the family members may experience symptoms of a stress reaction (see *Cultural Considerations* box). You should be aware that the stress reaction is a very real experience. Nursing intervention may be needed to assist a person in regaining a sense of physical function.

Cultural Considerations

What Does Culture Have to Do with Grief?

Culture strongly influences the way people handle grief. For example, traditional Vietnamese value stoicism, traditional Mexicans express grief openly, and traditional Swedes accept quiet or open grief. Traditional widows in Greece wear black for the rest of their lives.

Awareness of Terminal Illness

Awareness of terminal illness and impending death affects the dying person and the family both emotionally and physiologically. Strauss and Glaser (1970) have identified three states of awareness: (1) closed awareness, (2) mutual pretense, and (3) open awareness.

Closed Awareness. When closed awareness occurs, the family and the patient recognize that the patient is ill. They may not understand the severity of the illness and impending death.

Mutual Pretense. With mutual pretense, the patient, the loved ones, and the care providers know of the terminal prognosis. However, no one discusses the issue openly and they may make every effort to avoid the subject. Frequently the patient avoids the subject to protect the family and the caregivers from discomfort.

Open Awareness. With open awareness, the patient and others involved freely discuss the impending death. The discussions may be difficult but they allow the patient and the family to become comfortable with the topic. Patients who wish to do so can participate in making final arrangements and wrapping up personal business. Even though health care providers should respect the individual's right to know, some people let it be known that they do not want some information. That wish should be respected. The law requires that patients identify who, if anyone, else can be informed about their condition. Nurses must be careful not to share information with anyone without the patient's permission.

FEARS ASSOCIATED WITH TERMINAL ILLNESS AND DEATH

Fear is a typical feeling associated with dying. The nurse is frequently called on to deal with the dying person's fears. Three specific fears associated with dying are (1) fear of pain, (2) fear of loneliness, and (3) fear of meaninglessness.

Fear of Pain

People tend to associate death with pain. Common sayings such as "on pain of death" or "a violent death" have colored the way we perceive death. A dying person who has lost a loved one to a painful death may expect the same type of experience. Therefore many people assume that pain always accompanies death.

Physiologically, no absolute indication exists that death is always painful. Psychologically, pain may occur based on the anxieties and separations related to dying.

Terminally ill patients who experience physical pain should have medication available. The patient and family members need assurance that medication will be given promptly when it is needed. Patients can participate in their own pain relief by discussing pain relief measures and their effects. Most patients want their pain relieved without excessive grogginess or sleepiness (see *Cultural Considerations* box). Pain relief measures such as medication need not deprive the patient of the ability to interact with others.

Cultural Considerations

What Does Culture Have to Do with Pain?

Culture influences how patients respond to pain. Some readily report pain whereas others try to be stoic. Assess all patients for pain and explain how it can be reduced or relieved to improve quality of life.

Prevention of pain and relief from discomfort should be handled with compassion. Pain control will be better if analgesics are given on a regular schedule rather than waiting until the pain is unbearable and then trying to relieve it. Addiction to opioid drugs should not be a concern when dealing with the terminally ill patient. When death is inevitable, nursing interventions are aimed at maintaining comfort rather than promoting wellness. Pain management is discussed in Chapter 15.

Pharmacology Capsule

The terminally ill patient should not be denied pain relief measures. Pain relief is best achieved by scheduled administration of analgesic agents rather than administration only when pain returns.

Fear of Loneliness

Most terminally ill and dying people do not want to be alone. Many are afraid that they will be abandoned by loved ones who cannot cope with imminent death. Dying patients typically want someone they know and trust to stay with them. It may be a loved one or a caregiver. The simple presence of another person provides support and comfort. Neither words nor actions are necessary unless the patient requires something. Holding hands, touching, and listening are meaningful nursing responses. Simply being there can provide a sense of security.

Fear of Meaninglessness

During the dying process most people review their lives. They review their intentions during life, examining actions and expressing regrets about what might have been. Patients need to look at the positive aspects of their lives. Relatives, as well as nurses, can help patients to review their lives. This process helps to confirm the worth of the dying person.

You can assist patients and their families by focusing on the positive qualities of the patient's life. Prayers and shared thoughts and feelings may provide comfort for the patient. Respect the patient's practices and rituals even if they are different from your own.

CLINICAL SIGNS OF IMPENDING DEATH

Death occurs when all vital organs and systems cease to function. During the death process, systems and organs slow and lose their ability to maintain life. All systems are involved. Table 24-3 summarizes the clinical signs of impending death.

Loss of Muscle Tone

The muscular system weakens gradually. Body movements are slowed. Facial muscles lose tone, and the jaw may sag. Speech may be difficult because of decreased muscle coordination. Swallowing becomes increasingly difficult and the gag reflex is eventually lost. The functions of the gastrointestinal (GI) and genitourinary systems slow down. Peristalsis diminishes, which can lead to constipation, gas accumulation, distention, and nausea. Pain medications may enhance the GI slowing. Loss of sphincter control may result in fecal and urinary incontinence.

Circulatory and Respiratory Changes

Vital signs reflect cardiovascular and respiratory changes that precede death. The pulse slows and weakens. Blood pressure drops. Temperature may be elevated. Respirations may be rapid, shallow, and irregular, or they may be very slow. Noisy, wet-sounding respirations, termed the *death rattle,* are caused by mouth breathing and the accumulation of mucus in the upper airways. Cheyne-Stokes respirations are irregular with periods of apnea and develop as a person nears death.

Decreased circulation causes the skin to become fragile. The extremities become mottled and cyanotic. The skin feels cool to the touch, first in the feet and legs, then progressing to the hands and arms. However, the patient may feel warm because of an elevated temperature.

Sensory Changes

Sensory changes include decreasing pain and touch perception, blurred vision, and decreasing sense of taste and smell. The sense of touch decreases first in the lower extremities as a result of circulatory changes. The blink reflex is lost eventually and the patient appears to stare. Liquid tears may be ordered to lubricate the eyes.

Hearing is commonly believed to be the last sense lost during the death process. You should assume that the patient can hear and understand. Speaking slowly and clearly may increase the patient's understanding. Inform the patient's family and visitors that the patient may still be able to hear. Encourage family members to talk to the patient in a comforting way.

During the death process the body gradually relaxes until all function ends. Generally the respirations cease first. The heart stops beating within a few minutes. The

Table 24-3 Physical Manifestations of Approaching Death

FUNCTION AND SYSTEM	MANIFESTATION
Hearing	Usually last sense to disappear *Remember that comatose patients may still be able to hear.*
Touch	Decrease of sensation Decrease of pain and touch perception
Taste	Decreases as illness progresses
Smell	Decreases with disease progression Related to loss of taste
Sight	Blurring of vision Sinking and glazing of eyes Blinking stops; eyelids remain halfway open
Skin	Mottling on hands and feet Cold, clammy skin High fever because of improper functioning of thermoregulator in the brain or dehydration "Waxlike" skin appearance very near death
Respiration	Becomes rapid and deep with periods of apnea (Cheyne-Stokes respiration) Becomes irregular, gradually slowing down to terminal gasps (may be described as "guppy breathing") Grunting and noisy tachypnea (death rattle) common *Families need to be reassured that these symptoms do not signal emotional or physical distress.*
Urinary tract	Becomes incontinent of urine or unable to excrete or pass urine
Bowel	Slowing of digestive tract and possible cessation of function (may be enhanced by pain medications) Accumulation of gas, distention, and nausea because of diminished peristalsis Loss of sphincter control (may produce incontinence) May have a bowel movement when death is imminent
Muscle tone	Sagging of jaw because of loss of tone of the facial muscles Possible speaking difficulty because of decreased muscle coordination Possible swallowing difficulty (taking food, fluids, and medications by mouth becomes increasingly difficult) Loss of gag reflex Jerking movements (myoclonic jerking) seen in patients on large amounts of opioid agents
Circulation	Slowing and weakening of pulse Drop in blood pressure

physician is responsible for ordering discontinuation of life support if it is in use. The physician is also responsible for pronouncement of death in most situations. In some states, under specific circumstances, registered nurses (RNs) are legally permitted to pronounce death. A death certificate must be completed and signed. State laws designate who can sign a death certificate. This person is usually a physician, medical examiner, or nurse practitioner. Licensed vocational nurses/licensed practical nurses (LVNs/LPNs) should know the policies and procedures in their state and their employing institution.

The Harvard criteria were developed in 1968 to standardize the criteria used to determine death. According to the Harvard criteria, the following must occur in order to pronounce death:

1. Unresponsiveness to external stimulation that would normally be painful
2. A complete absence of spontaneous movement and breathing
3. A total lack of reflexes that are normally found on a neurologic examination, particularly the reaction of the pupils to light
4. A flat electroencephalogram (EEG) for 24 hours, which indicates that no electrical activity exists in the brain
5. The lack of circulation to the brain for 24 hours as identified by technology

Usually the first three criteria are enough for a pronouncement of death. The EEG and other technology are generally used when life support equipment is in use. The Harvard Committee recommended that if the final two criteria are used, the tests be repeated 24 hours later to confirm results.

Another definition associated with the diagnosis of death is cerebral or brain death. **Cerebral death** occurs when the cerebral cortex stops functioning or is irreversibly destroyed. The cerebral cortex, or the higher brain, is responsible for voluntary movement, actions, and thought. Some believe that cerebral cortex function *is* the individual.

Life-sustaining technology has raised many issues. Scientists ask whether cerebral or brain death occurs when the whole brain (cortex and brainstem) ceases activity or when cortical function alone stops. In 1995 the Quality Standards Subcommittee of the American Academy of Neurology recommended diagnostic criteria guidelines for clinical diagnosis of brain death in adults. The criteria include coma or unresponsiveness, absence of brainstem reflexes, and apnea as three findings in brain death. Specific assessments by a physician are required to validate each of the criteria.

Currently, legal and medical standards require that all brain function must cease for brain death to be pronounced and life support to be disconnected. Diagnosis of brain death is of particular importance when organ donation is an option.

PHYSICAL CHANGES AFTER DEATH

After death, many changes occur in the body as decomposition takes place. Three specific changes are (1) rigor mortis, (2) algor mortis, and (3) livor mortis.

Immediately after death, some involuntary jerking movements may take place. Within 2 to 4 hours, the body stiffens, a condition referred to as **rigor mortis**. Rigor mortis is caused by chemical changes within the body's cells that prevent muscle relaxation. It is usually fully developed in 6 to 12 hours and resolves within 36 hours.

After death, the body begins to cool. This is known as **algor mortis**. Body temperature falls until it reaches the environmental temperature in approximately 24 hours. As the body cools, the skin tends to lose elasticity and can be broken easily.

The breakdown of red blood cells (RBCs) after death causes a discoloration in the skin, which is called **livor mortis**. The skin may appear bruised with reddish-purple discoloration, usually in the dependent parts of the body. Livor mortis usually occurs within 30 minutes to 2 hours.

Decomposition happens faster in warmer temperatures because of bacterial growth. To slow decomposition, the body must be kept cool. Embalming reverses the process of decomposition by replacing the body's fluids with chemicals that prevent further growth of the bacteria that cause decomposition.

NURSING CARE of Terminally Ill and Dying Patients

Nursing care of patients who are terminally ill or dying must address their psychologic and physical needs. Respect, dignity, and comfort are important for the patient and the family. In addition, nurses and other care providers must recognize their own responses and needs when dealing with grief and dying.

Assessment

Assessment of the terminally ill or dying patient varies with the patient's condition. In general, the assessment is limited to essential data.

If the patient is admitted to an in-patient facility, document the specific event or change that brought the patient to the health care facility. Record the patient's medical diagnoses, medication profile, and allergies. If the patient is alert, briefly review the body systems to detect important signs and symptoms. In addition, document discomfort such as pain or nausea for prompt intervention. Depending on the specific terminal condition, other relevant information should be recorded. For example, if the patient has colon cancer, you would assess elimination in more detail.

The functional assessment of activities of daily living (ADL) elicits information about the patient's abilities, food and fluid intake, patterns of sleep and rest, and response to the stress of terminal illness. It is important to determine how the patient (if able to communicate) and family are coping. You can draw inferences about the stage of grief and the coping mechanisms based on statements reflecting sorrow, anger, guilt, or denial.

The physical assessment is abbreviated and detects changes that accompany terminal illness. The frequency of assessment depends on the patient's stability but is performed at least every 8 hours. As changes occur, documentation is performed more frequently.

Neurologic assessment is especially important and includes level of consciousness, reflexes, and pupil responses. Evaluation of vital signs, skin color, and temperature detects changes in circulation. Monitor the patient's respiratory status and describe the character and pattern of respirations and breath sounds. Renal and GI functions are assessed by monitoring nutritional and fluid intake, urinary output, and bowel sounds. Skin condition also must be monitored because skin becomes very fragile and may break down. To reemphasize, it is important to be sensitive and not to impose repeated, unnecessary assessments on the dying patient. If health history data are available in the chart, you can use that resource rather than tiring the patient with an interview. However, it is important to check on the patient frequently so that he or she does not feel abandoned.

Nursing Diagnoses, Goals, and Outcome Criteria: Terminally Ill and Dying Patients

The nursing care plan for the grieving patient must be individualized depending on individual patient data. The following is an example of nursing diagnoses, goals, and outcome criteria frequently used during the process of grieving. Discussion of other diagnoses follows.

Nursing Diagnoses	Goals and Outcome Criteria
Grieving related to an actual or perceived loss	Resolution of grief: patient expresses feelings related to grief, progresses through stages of grief resolution
Grieving related to an anticipated loss	Resolution of grief: patient acknowledges impending loss, demonstrates behaviors that reflect progress in grief resolution
Complicated Grieving related to the inability to adapt to the loss	Resolution of grief: patient verbalizes feelings related to grief process, begins to move toward resolution of grief

Additional diagnoses for the dying patient and the family include acute or chronic pain, fear, impaired skin integrity, imbalanced nutrition (less than body requirements), ineffective airway clearance, spiritual distress, hopelessness, powerlessness, ineffective coping, and compromised or disabled family coping. Refer to Chapter 21 for specific nursing diagnoses and interventions for the immobile patient and to Chapter 15 for pain management.

Interventions

Priority interventions for anticipatory grieving and complicated grieving focus on providing an environment that allows the patient to express feelings. Open discussion of feelings helps the patient and family to work toward resolution of the grief process. Accept expressions of anger, fear, or guilt without judgment. Assure the patient and family that these feelings are a normal part of grieving. Demonstrate respect for the patient's privacy and need or desire to talk (or to not talk). Be honest in answering questions and giving information.

Encourage families and patients to continue their usual activities as much as possible. They need to discuss their activities and maintain some control of their lives. You might help them to identify what they can and cannot change.

Grieving relatives, friends, and significant others can provide emotional support for one another. Be sensitive to the importance of significant others who are not necessarily relatives. Provide information about resources such as community counseling and support groups that may assist some people in working through their grief. Support groups share experiences and coping strategies that can help individuals to deal with their grief.

It is useful to identify the stage of grief (denial, anger, bargaining, depression, acceptance) that the person is experiencing. Awareness of the stage permits you to react according to the individual's needs. Respect the person's right to privacy, right to have a wide range of emotions, and right to talk when he or she chooses. Suggest a referral to a social worker if the family needs assistance with planning for the future or for the funeral. Anger is a common and normal response to grief. Recognize that the grieving person cannot be forced to accept the loss. Acknowledge and encourage the expression of feelings but at the same time realize how difficult it is to come to terms with grief. If you find yourself the target of the patient's anger, try to understand what is happening and to not react on a personal level.

Feelings of hopelessness and powerlessness are common in terminal illness and during grief. Encourage realistic hope within the limits of the situation. Allow the patient and the family to identify and deal with what is within their control and to recognize what is beyond their control. Encourage patient-identified goals to restore some sense of power.

During terminal illness and impending death, meeting the patient's safety and physiologic needs is the priority. Physical requirements for oxygen, nutrition, pain relief, mobility, elimination, and skin care remain throughout the life cycle. Physical care, including comfort measures and skin care, should be continued. People who are dying deserve and require the same physical care as people who are expected to recover. However, intrusive monitoring need not be continued.

CARE OF THE BODY AFTER DEATH

After death, the body must be prepared for transfer to the morgue or funeral home. Nurses are responsible for the care and preparation of the body. Dignity and privacy for the deceased and the family must be maintained. Table 24-4 identifies nursing management for preparation of the body for family viewing after death.

Table 24-4 Preparation of the Body for Family Viewing After Death

TOPIC	NURSING MANAGEMENT
Autopsy	Identification band remains on the body. Contact medical examiner/coroner if required. Consent form signed by next of kin if autopsy is requested. Follow legal requirements and agency policy.
Positioning	Place body in supine position with arms at sides or hands folded across the abdomen. Place small pillow under the head and shoulders. Close eyelids gently and hold for a few minutes or apply moist cotton balls as needed. Close mouth. Place a rolled towel under the chin as needed. Follow agency policy.
Hygiene	Wash soiled areas of the body. Apply a clean gown. Place linen savers under the buttocks. Comb hair. Apply clean top linens and cover body to shoulder level. Follow agency policy.
Personal effects	Insert dentures gently. Do not force. If dentures cannot be inserted, place them in denture container marked with appropriate identification. Secure jewelry that cannot be removed easily with tape. Inventory all valuables and possessions with the family, the funeral director, or the medical examiner/coroner staff. Clearly document the disposition of possessions. Follow agency policy.

Legal and religious issues may affect the care required for the disposition of the body. In certain instances an autopsy may be required. An **autopsy** is a postmortem examination of the deceased. It may be requested by the next of kin, suggested by the physician, or required by law. Consent for an autopsy must be given before the procedure can be performed, unless the law requires that the procedure be performed.

Each state has its own laws regarding autopsy. Under the law in most states, an autopsy is required if a person expires by suicide, by homicide, within 24 hours of admission to a health care facility, or from unknown causes. In such cases the coroner or the medical examiner must be notified.

During an autopsy, organ specimens and samples may be removed for examination. Body parts that are removed are either disposed of or preserved for burial, depending on the situation and the family's wishes. An autopsy is no more disfiguring than a surgical procedure. When the body is dressed, signs of an autopsy are not visible.

The family may wish to view the body before it is transported to the mortuary or morgue. It is important to make the environment as comfortable as possible for the family. It is your responsibility to prepare the body for viewing before the transfer (see *Cultural Considerations* box).

Cultural Considerations

What Does Culture Have to Do with Care After Death?

Cultural practices related to care of the body after death must be respected. Examples of traditional practices include the following:

- Greece: Body is washed by a relative or older woman.
- Roman Catholics: Body should not be shrouded until sacraments have been performed.
- Orthodox Jews: Dying person is not left. Body is not left alone between death and burial, which must occur within 24 hours. Body must not be touched for up to 30 minutes after death. Only designated Orthodox persons or Jewish Burial Service care for the body.

Normally, after death you will place the body in the supine position with the arms at the sides or with the hands across the abdomen. Identification bands should remain in place. A single pillow is placed under the head and shoulders to prevent discoloration of the face from pooling of the blood. Avoid use of large, overstuffed pillows.

Gently holding the eyelids closed for a few seconds helps them to remain closed. If the eyelids do not remain closed after a few seconds, the application of moist cotton balls for a few minutes may help.

Dentures may be inserted gently to maintain the normal facial appearance. If the dentures cannot be inserted easily, they should not be forced. Dentures that are not in place should be stored in a denture container, marked with identification, and sent with the body to the mortuary. The mouth should be closed. A rolled towel placed under the chin helps to hold the mouth closed.

Areas of the body that are soiled should be washed. Linen savers are placed under the buttocks to absorb urine or feces that may be released as the sphincters relax. A clean gown is applied and the hair is combed.

Tubes that are present in the body may be removed unless an autopsy is required. Some agencies require that tubes remain in place or that they be trimmed to approximately 1 inch and taped in place. It is important to review state and agency requirements.

Jewelry is generally removed, except for wedding bands, which may be taped to the patients' fingers. If other rings cannot be removed easily, they should be taped in place.

An inventory of possessions and valuables is done with the family. Each valuable is listed and signed for by the family. If no family is available, the inventory of valuables is listed and signed for by the funeral home director. The disposition of possessions is documented in the medical record.

After the positioning and preparation of the body, top linens should be straightened and pulled up to the deceased's shoulder level. The family may view the body after preparation is complete.

Often the family needs the nurse's emotional support while viewing the body. If only one family member is present, it is wise to accompany the person who is viewing the body. Close the door to allow for privacy and allow the family as much time as desired.

When the family leaves, apply additional identification tags to the wrist and ankle or toe of the deceased. The gown is removed and the body may be wrapped in a shroud. The **shroud** may be a large square or rectangle of cloth or plastic material. An identification tag is placed on the outside of the shroud. Additional identification markings may be required if the deceased had a communicable disease. The body is then transported to the morgue or removed by the mortician. Agency policy regarding the transport of a body from the room may vary. Some agencies require that all patient doors be closed before transport and that service elevators be used. Table 24-5 lists the nursing management for preparation of the body for transfer.

THE EFFECT OF PATIENT DEATH ON NURSES

The nurse-patient relationship often extends over weeks or even months. Throughout the terminal illness, nurses may experience feelings of helplessness, sorrow, guilt, and frustration. Nurses who are in touch with their own feelings are better able to help patients and families deal with their feelings. When the patient finally dies, the caring nurse will experience a personal sense of loss. Grieving is the normal response. The nurse must work through the stages of grief even if his or her grief is less intense than that of the patient or

Table 24-5 Preparation of the Body for Transfer

TOPIC	NURSING MANAGEMENT
Body identification	Identification band remains on the body. Apply additional identification tags to the wrist, ankle, or toe per agency policy. Place additional identification on the outside of the shroud. Communicable disease identification should be listed on the body and outside the shroud. Follow agency policy.
Autopsy	Tubes and medical appliances frequently are left as originally placed in accordance with agency policy and legal requirements. Follow agency policy.
Positioning	Place body in supine position with arms at sides or hands folded across the abdomen. Wrists and ankles may be bound based on agency policy. Remove gown. Apply shroud. Follow agency policy.
Personal effects	Inventory all valuables and possessions with the family, the funeral director, or the medical examiner/coroner staff. Clearly package and document the disposition of possessions. Follow agency policy.
Transport	Transport via stretcher to the morgue based on agency policy. Assist with transfer of the body to the mortician's stretcher for transport.

family. It is acceptable to cry with the patient or family during the grief process. If possible, nurses or a representative member of the nursing staff may attend the patient's viewing or funeral. Nursing staff also need to be supportive of one another when dealing with the death of a patient. Failure to deal with the grief experience can lead to nurse burnout and a loss of sensitivity to patient needs. Some agencies have formal grief support groups for nurses. Another helpful activity is a periodic memorial service in which patients who have died recently are remembered.

ISSUES RELATED TO TERMINAL ILLNESS AND DEATH

Patients and families struggle with many emotional decisions during the terminal illness and dying experience. These decisions often focus on physical and emotional comfort, such as whether to initiate artificial feeding. The decisions may involve the choice of advance directives, medical power of attorney, living wills, organ donations, and resuscitation (Fig. 24-1). Advance directives are especially helpful because they specify the patient's wishes.

ORGAN DONATION

Organ donation may be made by any person who is legally competent. Any body part or the entire body may be donated. The decision to donate organs or to provide anatomic gifts may be made by a person before death. The decision to donate organs after death may be made by immediate family members.

Some people carry donor cards. Some states allow for organ donation to be marked on drivers' licenses. The names of agencies that handle organ donation vary by locale. Some common names for such an agency are *organ bank, organ-sharing network, tissue bank*, or *organ-sharing alliance.* Legal requirements and facility policy for organ donation must be followed. The physician should be notified immediately when organ donation is intended because some tissues must be used within hours after death.

CARDIOPULMONARY RESUSCITATION

In the past 40 years cardiopulmonary resuscitation (CPR) has become common practice in health care. CPR is initiated when patients suffer respiratory or cardiac arrest unless a physician has given a do not resuscitate (DNR) order. A DNR order is usually written when a patient or his or her representative has made it clear that CPR should not be initiated. Several different types of CPR decisions can be made. Complete and total heroic measures, which may include CPR, medications, and mechanical ventilation, can be referred to as a *full code.* Some states offer DNR protocols that enable the patient to specify exactly which actions may be carried out during CPR.

The Patient Self-Determination Act was an important part of the Omnibus Budget Reconciliation Act (OBRA) of 1990. This Act requires all institutions that participate with Medicare to provide written information to patients concerning their right to accept or refuse treatment. The information must explain the patient's right to initiate advance directives. **Advance directives** are written statements of a person's wishes regarding medical care. The first advance directive document, developed in 1974, was called the *Living Will.*

Most states have replaced the idea of living wills with Natural Death Acts. Within many of these Acts are specific aspects related to the individual's wishes and durable powers of attorney for health care. Directives to physicians may be included. Under the Natural Death Acts, an individual can tell the physician exactly what is desired. Each state will have its own unique

FLORIDA LIVING WILL

Declaration made this _______ day of _______________, _______________,
(day) (month) (year)

I, ___________________________, willfully and voluntarily make known my desire that my dying not be artificially prolonged under the circumstances set forth below, and I do hereby declare that:

If at any time I am incapacitated and
__ I have a terminal condition, or
__ I have an end-stage condition, or
__ I am in a persistent vegetative state

and if my attending or treating physician and another consulting physician have determined that there is no reasonable medical probability of my recovery from such condition, I direct that life-prolonging procedures be withheld or withdrawn when the application of such procedures would serve only to prolong artificially the process of dying, and that I be permitted to die naturally with only the administration of medication or the performance of any medical procedure deemed necessary to provide me with comfort care or to alleviate pain.

It is my intention that this declaration be honored by my family and physician as the final expression of my legal right to refuse medical or surgical treatment and to accept the consequences for such refusal.

In the event that I have been determined to be unable to provide express and informed consent regarding the withholding, withdrawal, or continuation of life-prolonging procedures, I wish to designate, as my surrogate to carry out the provisions of this declaration:

Name: ______________________________
Address: ______________________________
______________________________ Zip code: __________
Phone: ______________________________

I wish to designate the following person as my alternate surrogate, to carry out the provisions of this declaration should my surrogate be unwilling or unable to act on my behalf:

Name: ______________________________
Address: ______________________________
______________________________ Zip code: __________
Phone: ______________________________

Additional instructions (optional):

I understand the full import of this declaration, and I am emotionally and mentally competent to make this declaration.

Signed: ______________________________

Witness 1:
Signed: ______________________________
Address: ______________________________

Witness 2:
Signed: ______________________________
Address: ______________________________

A

FIGURE 24-1 Sample advance directive. **A,** Health care treatment instructions in the event of end-stage medical condition or permanent unconsciousness (Living Will).

Continued

FLORIDA DESIGNATION OF HEALTH CARE SURROGATE

Name: ____
(Last) (First) (Middle initial)

In the event that I have been determined to be incapacitated to provide informed consent for medical treatment and surgical and diagnostic procedures, I wish to designate as my surrogate for health care decisions:

Name: ____
Address: ____
______________________________ Zip code: ____________
Phone: ____

If my surrogate is unwilling or unable to perform his or her duties, I wish to designate as my alternate surrogate:

Name: ____
Address: ____
______________________________ Zip code: ____________
Phone: ____

I fully understand that this designation will permit my designee to make health care decisions and to provide, withhold, or withdraw consent on my behalf; to apply for public benefits to defray the cost of health care; and to authorize my admission to or transfer from a health care facility.

Additional instructions (optional):

I further affirm that this designation is not being made as a condition of treatment or admission to a health care facility. I will notify and send a copy of this document to the following persons other than my surrogate so they may know who my surrogate is:

Name: ____
Address: ____
Name: ____
Address: ____

Signed: ____
Date: ____

Witness 1:
Signed: ____
Address: ____

Witness 2:
Signed: ____
Address: ____

B

FIGURE 24-1, cont'd B, Durable health care power of attorney. (Copyright 2008 National Hospice and Palliative Care Organization. All rights reserved. Reproduction and distribution by an organization or organized group without the written permission of the National Hospice and Palliative Care Organization is expressly forbidden. Visit caringinfo.org for more information.)

requirements and rules for the use of advance directives. Special forms for durable power of attorney, medical power of attorney, and directives for physicians, family members, or surrogates can be obtained from local medical associations and the internet. Specific details as to withholding or withdrawing treatments must be included. What is to be done and what is not to be done must be included in very clear terms.

A person may write a durable power of attorney or directive to physicians without special forms. Verbal directives with specific instructions may be given to physicians in the presence of two witnesses. Attorneys and notaries are not necessarily required.

In the event that the person is not capable of communicating his or her wishes, the family and the physician can agree on what measures will or will not be taken. The physician should document the family's decision.

Another option is the durable power of attorney for health care or medical power of attorney. This document allows individuals to select someone to make health care decisions for them if they are unable to do so for themselves. This power of attorney can be used only if the physician certifies in writing that the person is incapable of making decisions. Until the physician does this, the individual remains in control of his or her own decisions.

In addition to advance directives, another initiative called *Five Wishes* has been put in place. Figure 24-2 shows the first page of this document. The organization Aging with Dignity (www.agingwithdignity.org) developed *Five Wishes*™ to promote better care for individuals and families facing the end of life. This document focuses on a patient's needs and includes personal, medical, spiritual, and emotional needs. Currently, 42 states and the District of Columbia legally recognize the *Five Wishes* document as an advance directive; the remaining states accept it as an attachment to another legal form.

The *Five Wishes* document specifies how the family and the health care team are expected to treat the patient. It includes the following:

- The name of the person who will make decisions for health care if the patient cannot do it
- The type of medical care the patient wants or does not want
- The amount of comfort the patient wants
- How the patient wants to be treated
- What information the patient wants the loved ones to know

You must be aware of legal issues and the wishes of the patient. Advance directives and organ donor information should be located in the medical record and identified on the nursing care plan. All caregivers responsible for the patient need to know the patient's wishes.

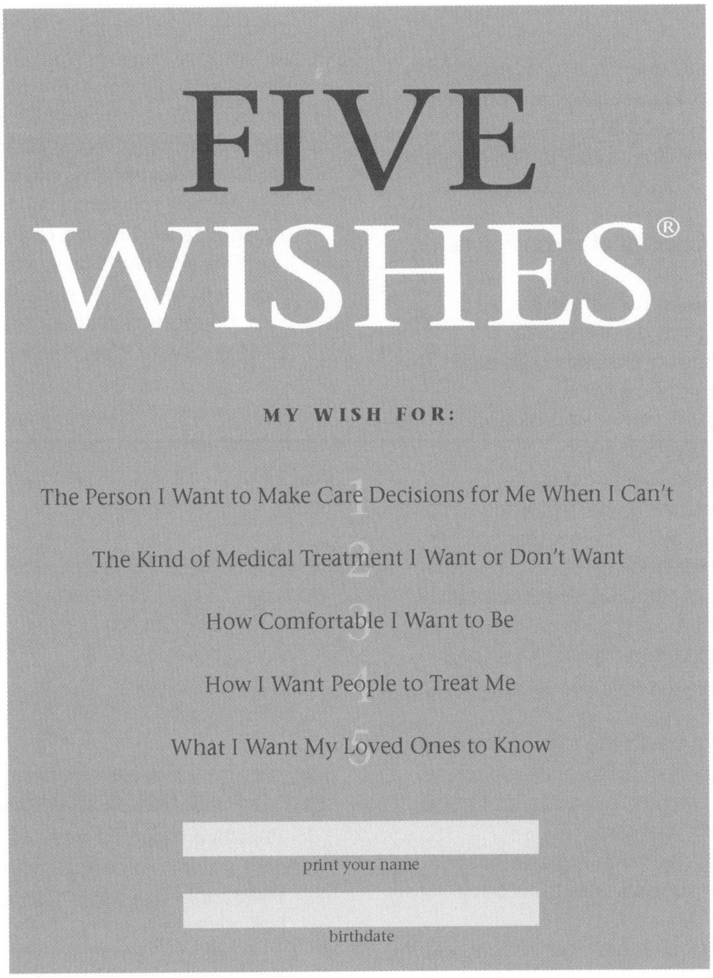
FIVE WISHES®

MY WISH FOR:

1 The Person I Want to Make Care Decisions for Me When I Can't

2 The Kind of Medical Treatment I Want or Don't Want

3 How Comfortable I Want to Be

4 How I Want People to Treat Me

5 What I Want My Loved Ones to Know

print your name

birthdate

FIGURE 24-2 The *Five Wishes* document (www.agingwithdignity.org) helps patients to communicate their wishes to their families and to members of the health care team. Written in language that is easily understood by those outside the medical and legal professions, the document helps people to discuss and make reasoned decisions about issues that are often difficult to face. This is the first page of the 12-page document that allows individuals to express their wishes on various issues. (Copyright AGING WITH DIGNITY, www.agingwithdignity.org.)

Put on Your Thinking Cap!

1. Write down the customs and rituals that are followed in your family in relation to deaths: care of the body, viewing, wake, spiritual counselors, services, burial or cremation, types of memorials, support for survivors.
2. Discuss your answers with others in your clinical group.
3. Consider how you reacted to others' customs and rituals. Recognize the importance of your customs and rituals to you and appreciate the need to be accepting of different practices. Do not assume that your patients will handle death in the same way you do.

SUMMARY

Terminal illness and dying are very personal events that affect the patient, the family, and the caregivers. Grief is experienced by everyone differently but with similar patterns of behavior. The dying process and death require specific physical, emotional, spiritual, and legal nursing interventions. Caring for the terminally ill and dying is a challenging and rewarding experience.

Get Ready for the NCLEX® Examination!

Key Points

- Loss is the real or potential absence of someone or something that is valued.
- People experience loss when faced with changes in self-image, developmental changes, loss of possessions, and loss of significant others through death or other means.
- The response to loss, called grief, is similar regardless of the nature of the loss but is usually most profound when the loss experienced is death.
- Uncomplicated (adaptive) grief is a healthy response to loss; complicated grief is a delayed or exaggerated response.
- Grieving can occur in anticipation of a loss before it happens.
- Culture, religion, and age affect a person's understanding and reaction to death or loss.
- Kübler-Ross stages of grieving are denial, anger, bargaining, depression, and acceptance.
- Martocchio's five clusters of grief are shock and disbelief; yearning and protest; anguish, disorganization, and despair; identification in bereavement; and reorganization and restoration.
- Rando's three phases of grieving are avoidance, confrontation, and accommodation.
- The stages of awareness of terminal illness are closed awareness, mutual pretense, and open awareness.
- Common fears associated with terminal illness and dying are fear of pain, fear of loneliness, and fear of meaninglessness.
- Clinical signs of impending death are loss of muscle tone, bradycardia, hypotension, abnormal respiratory pattern, abnormal breath sounds, cyanosis, cool skin, blurred vision, and sensory changes.
- Current legal and medical standards require that all brain function must cease for brain death to be pronounced.
- Changes in the body after death are rigor mortis, algor mortis, and livor mortis.
- Assessment of the terminally ill or dying person varies with the person's condition but is often limited to essential data.
- Nursing diagnoses for the patient who is terminally ill or dying may include grieving, complicated grieving, acute pain, fear, impaired skin integrity, imbalanced nutrition (less than body requirements), ineffective airway clearance, spiritual distress, hopelessness, powerlessness, and ineffective coping.
- The nurse is responsible for the care and preparation of the body after death.
- An autopsy (postmortem examination of the body) requires family consent unless it is required by law.
- Decisions that terminally ill patients and their families may record in advance directives include desired medical interventions and organ donations.
- Cultural and religious beliefs strongly influence the grief experience and rituals related to death.
- The *Five Wishes*™ document records the patient's desires in relation to decision-making authority, medical care, comfort measures, treatments, and information to be shared with loved ones.

Additional Learning Resources

SG Go to your Study Guide for additional learning activities to help you master this chapter content.

evolve Go to your Evolve website (http://evolve.elsevier.com/Linton/medsurg) for the following learning resources and much more:
- Interactive Prioritization Exercises
- Fluid & Electrolyte Tutorial
- Pharmacology Tutorial
- Review Questions for the NCLEX® Examination

Review Questions for the NCLEX® Examination

1. Palliative care has been recommended to a patient with advanced cancer who has decided to discontinue treatment. The patient should be told that the focus of palliative care is:
1. Finding alternative methods of treatment of disease
2. Providing supportive care while allowing natural death
3. Delaying death for as long as possible by any means
4. Hastening death when no hope exists for a cure
NCLEX Client Need: Psychosocial Integrity

2. Which of the following represent a loss related to a change in self-image? (Select all that apply.)
   1. A worker is required to retire after 30 years.
   2. Family records are destroyed in a house fire.
   3. An adult child accepts a job in another country.
   4. A patient's hair falls out because of chemotherapy.
   5. An electrician has an arm amputated after an injury.

   NCLEX Client Need: Psychosocial Integrity
3. When a patient was diagnosed with a terminal illness, his wife began to grieve. Which nursing diagnosis describes the wife's response?
   1. Dysfunctional grief related to unresolved issues
   2. Grieving related to anticipated loss
   3. Normal grief related to uncertain future
   4. Complicated grieving related to failure to accept prognosis

   NCLEX Client Need: Psychosocial Integrity
4. Ms. A. has been diagnosed with terminal lung cancer. She tells the nurse: "If God will just let me live to see my children finish school, I will never smoke another cigarette." This illustrates which stage of grief according to Kübler-Ross?

   NCLEX Client Need: Psychosocial Integrity
5. A year after her husband's death, Mrs. B. has her wedding rings made into a dinner ring. She also begins attending the singles group at her church. According to Martocchio's model, this demonstrates which cluster of grief?
   1. Yearning and protest
   2. Anguish, disorganization, and despair
   3. Confrontation and avoidance
   4. Reorganization and restoration

   NCLEX Client Need: Psychosocial Integrity
6. The hospice nurse is visiting Miss C., whose mother died the previous year. Miss C. says, "I am finally feeling normal again." According to Rando, Miss C. is in which stage of grieving?
   1. Acceptance
   2. Avoidance
   3. Confrontation
   4. Accommodation

   NCLEX Client Need: Psychosocial Integrity
7. A new hospice patient reports that her pain has been getting worse. The nurse should explain that the hospice approach to pain management is guided by which of the following principles?
   1. Make relief of pain a priority
   2. Use caution to prevent addiction
   3. Keep the patient heavily sedated
   4. Medicate only when pain is severe

   NCLEX Client Need: Psychosocial Integrity
8. During the last few days of Ms. B.'s life, family members visited her and talked about shared happy memories and how much Ms. B. meant to them. How might this be helpful to Ms. B.? (Select all that apply.)
   1. This would probably benefit the visitors more than Ms. B.
   2. Reviewing her life can help Ms. B. to find meaning in her life.
   3. Visitors will prevent Ms. B. from focusing on her impending death.
   4. This sharing experience helps to confirm Ms. B's worth.
   5. Both the visitors and the patient are in denial about Ms. B's illness.

   NCLEX Client Need: Psychosocial Integrity
9. As Mrs. C. nears death, her husband says, "I wish I could do something for her." What could the nurse tell her?
   1. "It may be comforting if you will talk to her slowly and clearly."
   2. "Unfortunately, nothing can be done at this point."
   3. "She probably cannot hear you but she may be able to feel your touch."
   4. "It's just a matter of time now. Why don't you take a break?"

   NCLEX Client Need: Psychosocial Integrity
10. A new nursing assistant leaves the room in tears the first time one of her patients dies. What is the most appropriate comment by the nurse?
    1. "Get back in there and take care of your patient."
    2. "It hurts to lose a patient but you will get used to it."
    3. "You really can't get so emotionally involved with patients."
    4. "It is normal for you to feel upset. How can I help you?"

    NCLEX Client Need: Psychosocial Integrity

chapter 25

The Patient with Cancer

http://evolve.elsevier.com/Linton/medsurg

Barbara Owens

Objectives

1. List the most common sites of cancer in men and women.
2. Explain the differences between benign and malignant tumors.
3. Define terms used to name and classify cancer.
4. Describe measures to reduce the risk of cancer.
5. List nursing responsibilities in the care of patients having diagnostic tests to detect possible cancer.
6. Explain the nursing care of patients undergoing each type of cancer therapy: surgery, radiation, chemotherapy, and biotherapy.
7. Assist in developing a nursing care plan for the terminally ill patient with cancer and the patient's family.

Key Terms

Adjuvant (ĂJ-ă-vănt)
Alopecia (ă-lō-PĒ-shă)
Alternative therapy
Antineoplastic (ăn-tī-nē-ō-PLĂS-tĭk)
Benign (bĕ-NĪN)
Biotherapy
Carcinogens (kăr-SĬN-ō-jĕn)
Chemotherapy (kē-mō-THĔR-ă-pē)
Complementary therapy
Extravasation (ĕks-tră-vă-SĀ-shŭn)
Gray (Gy)
Malignant (mă-LĬG-nănt)
Metastasis (mĕ-TĂS-tă-sĭs)
Neoadjuvant (nē-ō-ĂJ-ă-vănt)
Neoplasms (NĒ-ō-plăsm)
Neutropenia (nū-trō-PĒ-nē-ă)
Radiotherapy
Xerostomia (zē-rō-STŌ-mē-ă)

WHY STUDY CANCER?

Specific cancers are discussed with every body system in this text. Why, then, is a separate chapter devoted to the subject? The American Cancer Society defines cancer as a large group of diseases characterized by uncontrolled growth and spread of abnormal cells. More than 200 diseases are classified as *cancer.* They share some common characteristics, progress in similar ways, and respond to similar types of treatments. To reduce repetition throughout the text, this chapter addresses the common features of those diseases known as *cancer.*

Health statistics often group all types of cancer together. Not surprisingly, cancer is listed as the second most common cause of death in the United States. Almost everyone has been touched by cancer. It is estimated that 1 in 3 Americans will have cancer at some time. The most common sites of cancer in men and in women are shown in Figure 25-1. Because so many die of cancer, many people assume that a diagnosis of cancer is a death sentence. In reality, more than 9 million Americans with a history of cancer are alive today.

Some cancers can be prevented by avoidance of causative agents (see *Nutrition Considerations* box). Early diagnosis has been found to make a significant difference in survival with many types of cancer and advances in treatment have prolonged the lives of many cancer patients.

Nutrition Considerations

1. Thirty-five percent of all cancers are believed to be related to diet.
   - Diets high in salt-cured, smoked, and nitrate-cured foods are associated with esophageal and stomach cancers.
   - Obesity is associated with cancers of the colon, breast, prostate, gallbladder, ovary, and uterus.
   - Cancers of the breast, colon, and prostate may be associated with high-fat diets.

Continued

Leading New Cancer Cases and Deaths – 2014 Estimates

Estimated New Cases*		Estimated Deaths	
Male	**Female**	**Male**	**Female**
Prostate 233,000 (27%)	Breast 232,670 (29%)	Lung & bronchus 86,930 (28%)	Lung & bronchus 72,330 (26%)
Lung & bronchus 116,000 (14%)	Lung & bronchus 108,210 (13%)	Prostate 29,480 (10%)	Breast 40,000 (15%)
Colon & rectum 71,830 (8%)	Colon & rectum 65,000 (8%)	Colon & rectum 26,270 (8%)	Colon & rectum 24,040 (9%)
Urinary bladder 56,390 (7%)	Uterine corpus 52,630 (6%)	Pancreas 20,170 (7%)	Pancreas 19,420 (7%)
Melanoma of the skin 43,890 (5%)	Thyroid 47,790 (6%)	Liver & intrahepatic bile duct 15,870 (5%)	Ovary 14,270 (5%)
Kidney & renal pelvis 39,140 (5%)	Non-Hodgkin lymphoma 32,530 (4%)	Leukemia 14,040 (5%)	Leukemia 10,050 (4%)
Non-Hodgkin lymphoma 38,270 (4%)	Melanoma of the skin 32,210 (4%)	Esophagus 12,450 (4%)	Uterine corpus 8,590 (3%)
Oral cavity & pharynx 30,220 (4%)	Kidney & renal pelvis 24,780 (3%)	Urinary bladder 11,170 (4%)	Non-Hodgkin lymphoma 8,520 (3%)
Leukemia 30,100 (4%)	Pancreas 22,890 (3%)	Non-Hodgkin lymphoma 10,470 (3%)	Liver & intrahepatic bile duct 7,130 (3%)
Liver & intrahepatic bile duct 24,600 (3%)	Leukemia 22,280 (3%)	Kidney & renal pelvis 8,900 (3%)	Brain & other nervous system 6,230 (2%)
All sites 855,220 (100%)	All sites 810,320 (100%)	All sites 310,010 (100%)	All sites 275,710 (100%)

*Excludes basal and squamous cell skin cancers and in situ carcinoma except urinary bladder.

©2014, American Cancer Society, Inc., Surveillance Research

FIGURE 25-1 American Cancer Society estimates, 2014: Leading site of new cancer cases and deaths. (Copyright 2014, American Cancer Society, Inc., Surveillance Research.)

Nutrition Considerations—cont'd

- High alcohol intake is associated with cancers of the oral cavity, larynx, esophagus, liver, colon, and breast.

2. To *reduce the risk* of cancer, the American Cancer Society recommends the following:
   - Consume adequate fruits and vegetables (five or more servings each day).
   - Consume adequate grains, rice, pasta, and beans (several servings each day).
   - Limit consumption of fats.
   - Engage in moderate physical activity of at least 30 minutes or more on most days and maintain a healthy weight.
   - Limit alcohol consumption (or do not drink any alcohol).

Nurses use their teaching and assessment skills in the prevention and detection of cancer. They also care for patients undergoing diagnostic procedures and treatments for cancer. In almost any specialty, nurses work with patients who are being treated for cancer.

WHAT IS CANCER?

NORMAL BODY CELLS

A normal cell has the following characteristics:

- A distinct, recognizable appearance typical of all cells from a particular tissue ("tissue of origin"); has a single small nucleus
- The ability to perform a specific function when mature
- The production of substances that hold cells from the same type of tissue closely together
- The ability to recognize other cells and identify the other cells' tissue of origin
- The ability to reproduce in a controlled manner to produce additional identical cells only as needed for growth and replacement
- The ability for cell division to be inhibited by inadequate space or insufficient nutrients
- The ability to remain in their tissue of origin (except for blood cells, which migrate)

Cells that reproduce abnormally and in an uncontrolled manner form **neoplasms** or tumors. Such cells may be benign or malignant.

BENIGN TUMORS

Benign tumors are relatively harmless, primarily because they do not spread to other parts of the body. However, benign tumors present problems if they create pressure on or obstruct body organs. Because of this, surgical removal of benign tumors is often recommended.

MALIGNANT TUMORS

The presence of **malignant** cells is the basis for a diagnosis of cancer. Characteristics of cancer cells are the following:

- Change in appearance from normal cells of tissue of origin (said to be *undifferentiated* if tissue of origin cannot be determined); large nucleus or multiple nuclei
- Inability to properly perform the function of the tissue of origin; may assume functions of other cells
- Cells not readily recognized by other cells
- May have abnormal proteins (called *tumor markers*) on cell surface
- Random, disorganized, uncontrolled growth pattern
- Continue dividing even when no need exists for additional cells, inadequate space, or inadequate nutrients
- Ability to migrate from one tissue or organ to another

As they grow, malignant tumors cause some of the same problems as benign tumors. They press on normal tissues and compete with normal cells for nutrients. Malignant growths are more threatening, however, because they can invade nearby tissues or disperse cells to colonize distant parts of the body. *Regional invasion* is the term used to describe the movement of cancer cells into adjoining tissue. The process by which cancer spreads to distant sites is called **metastasis**. Tumors found away from the original site of malignant cells are called *metastatic growths*. The most common sites of metastasis are liver, brain, bone, and lungs. Once metastasis has occurred, cancer treatment is more difficult and less likely to be curative.

A comparison of the features of benign and malignant cells is presented in Table 25-1.

MALIGNANT TRANSFORMATION

Examples of factors that promote the transformation of normal cells to malignant cells are increasing age, diet, hormones, and chronic irritation. A person's general emotional and physical health also may be factors in promoting or slowing the growth of cancer cells. Malignant transformation occurs when normal cells are exposed to substances (called **carcinogens**) that damage cell deoxyribonucleic acid (DNA). The transformation occurs in four steps as outlined in Table 25-2. It seems that carcinogens stimulate the initial change of normal cells, making them susceptible to malignant changes.

CLASSIFICATION OF TUMORS

Tumors are classified by anatomic site, stage, and cell appearance and differentiation. The term *differentiation* refers to how cells are different from their parent cells ("tissue of origin"). When it is difficult to recognize the original type of tissue from which tumor cells came, they are described as *poorly differentiated cells*. When cells are well differentiated, the tissue of origin is recognizable.

Anatomic Site

The suffix *-oma* means "tumor." Technically, a tumor is a swelling. However, the word is most commonly used to refer to a malignant or benign neoplasm. Tumors are named according to the type of tissue from which they developed originally. These names are summarized in Table 25-3.

Additional prefixes may be used to designate the exact type of malignant tissue. For example, a sarcoma could be an osteosarcoma or a chondrosarcoma. An osteosarcoma is a tumor of the bone whereas a chondrosarcoma is a cartilage tumor. Many other combinations of terms are used to describe tumors precisely by origin and location.

Staging System for Cancer

Because cancers tend to grow and spread in predictable ways, their progress can be described in stages. Specific stages exist for all types of cancer. Staging is done at the time of diagnosis and at intervals during and after treatment. Such staging is helpful in planning treatments and in predicting long-term survival.

One method of describing the extent of cancer is shown in Table 25-4. A second, more specific system is the TNM staging system (Table 25-5), which specifies the status of the primary tumor, regional lymph nodes, and distant metastases. In the TNM system, *T* refers to the tumor, *N* to regional lymph nodes, and *M* to distant

Table 25-1 A Comparison of Benign and Malignant Tumors

CHARACTERISTIC	BENIGN	MALIGNANT
Growth rate	Usually slow and encapsulated	Usually rapid but may be slow
Growth mode	Enlarges and expands	Invades surrounding tissue
Cell structure and differentiation	Cells closely resemble those of tissue of origin	Tissue of origin not readily identifiable
Recurrence after removal	Unlikely	Common
Metastasis	No	Yes
Tissue destruction	Usually none unless compression or obstruction occurs	Can cause necrosis, ulceration, perforation, tissue sloughing; effects can be fatal

Table 25-2 Steps in Transformation of Normal Cells to Malignant Cells

STEP	PROCESS	EFFECTS ON CELLS AND TISSUE
Initiation	Deoxyribonucleic acid (DNA) exposed to a carcinogen	Cell appears somewhat abnormal
	Irreversible changes occur in DNA	Continues to function normally
Promotion	Sufficient exposure to an agent (a *promoter*) to encourage or enhance cell growth	Latent period before increased growth forms tumors (early detection period)
Progression	Accelerated growth rate Enhanced invasiveness Altered appearance and biochemical activity	Tumor development Cells mutate so that they are not all identical and have differing sensitivities to treatment
Metastasis	Tumor develops internal blood vessels Tumor cells produce enzymes that dissolve substances that hold normal cells together Tumor penetrates capillaries, other body structures, and cavities Tumor cells transported throughout the body; most destroyed by body's defenses Tumor cells trapped in capillary bed and form a fibrin meshwork that prevents detection by immune system Enzymes dissolve lining of blood vessels; cells invade surrounding tissue Cells attempt to establish blood supply to support development of metastatic colony	Transformed cells relocate by direct extension, invasion, establishment of remote sites

Table 25-3 Tumor Names by Anatomic Site

TYPE OF TUMOR BY ANATOMIC SITE	TISSUE OF ORIGIN
Benign Tumor	
Fibroma	Fibrous connective tissue
Lipoma	Fat tissue
Leiomyomas	Smooth muscle tissue
Malignant Tumor	
Carcinoma	Skin; glands; linings of digestive, urinary, and respiratory tracts
Sarcoma	Bone, muscle, other connective tissue
Melanoma	Pigment cells in the skin
Leukemia and lymphoma	Blood-forming tissues: lymphoid tissue, plasma cells, and bone marrow

metastases. To illustrate, a patient whose primary tumor has grown and spread to regional lymph nodes but not to distant sites would be staged *T2, N1, M0.*

Put on Your Thinking Cap!

You are assigned to care for a patient who has cancer. The cancer has been staged T4, N3, M1. How would you interpret this information?

Table 25-4 Staging Classification for Cancer

STAGE	DESCRIPTION
Stage I	The malignant cells are confined to the tissue of origin. No invasion of other tissues takes place.
Stage II	Limited spread of the cancer occurs in the local area, usually to nearby lymph nodes.
Stage III	The tumor is larger or has spread from the site of origin to nearby tissues (or both). Regional lymph nodes are likely to be involved.
Stage IV	The cancer has metastasized to distant parts of the body. The term *advanced* is also used to describe Stage IV.

RISK FACTORS

A single, specific cause of cancer has not been identified. Genetic and environmental factors appear to increase the risk for development of cancer. Changes in genetic information of a normal cell can cause alterations that lead to malignancies. Cancer-causing agents, called *carcinogens,* include a variety of chemicals, radiation, and viruses. Box 25-1 shows a partial list of carcinogens. Carcinogens such as cigarette smoke, asbestos, and nitrites are commonly found in the environment. Drugs that may act as carcinogens include diethylstilbestrol, androgenic steroids, and high-dose unopposed synthetic estrogens.

Table 25-5 TNM Staging System for Cancer

T (PRIMARY TUMOR)	N (REGIONAL LYMPH NODES)	M (DISTANT METASTASIS)
T0—no sign of tumor after treatment	N0—no regional lymph nodes involved	M0—no distant metastasis
Tis—malignancy in epithelial tissue but not basement membrane	N1—minimal regional lymph node involvement	M1—distant metastasis present
T1—minimal size and extension	N2—increased involvement of regional lymph nodes	
T2, T3—progressively increasing size and extension	N3—extensive involvement of regional lymph nodes	
T4—large size and extension		

Box 25-1 Common Carcinogens

VIRUSES AND CHEMICALS
Tar
Soot
Asphalt
Aniline dyes
Hydrocarbons
Crude paraffin oils
Nickel
Arsenic
Benzene
Cadmium

PHYSICAL AGENTS
Radiation
Asbestos
Tobacco smoke

HORMONAL AGENTS
Synthetic estrogens
Androgenic anabolic steroids

IMMUNOSUPPRESSANT AGENTS
Antimetabolites
Corticosteroids
Alkylating agents
Antilymphocyte serum

CYTOTOXIC DRUGS
Phenylalanine mustard
Cyclophosphamide

Other factors thought to be associated with cancer development are increasing age, heredity, and hormones. Cancers that appear at a higher rate than expected in one family are called *familial cancers.* In these situations, no single genes have been identified to explain the frequency. Hereditary cancers, on the other hand, have clearly predictable patterns of inheritance based on a single gene. For people with family histories of familial or hereditary cancers, genetic counseling can direct the person to appropriate screening and lifestyle changes and serve as a basis for making decisions about reproductive options.

Pharmacology Capsule

Some drugs are carcinogenic, meaning they can cause cancer. Examples are diethylstilbestrol, androgenic steroids, high-dose unopposed synthetic estrogens, and some antineoplastic drugs used to treat cancer.

SEVEN WARNING SIGNS

The signs and symptoms of cancer vary with the location and severity of the disease. The American Cancer Society has identified seven warning signs that are associated with many common types of cancer. They can serve to guide the nurse and the public in identifying signs and symptoms that require medical evaluation. The first letters of the warning signs spell out *CAUTION,* making it easier to remember them (see *Health Promotion* box).

Health Promotion

Warning Signs of Cancer

Change in bowel or bladder habits
A sore that does not heal
Unusual bleeding or discharge
Thickening or lump in a breast or elsewhere
Indigestion or difficulty swallowing
Obvious change in a wart or a mole
Nagging cough or hoarseness

PREVENTION AND EARLY DETECTION

A number of things can be done to reduce the risk of development of cancer or to detect it in the early stages. They include (1) general measures to promote health, (2) avoidance of known carcinogens, (3) identification of high-risk people, and (4) cancer screening.

Health Promotion

Many behaviors associated with good health may reduce the risk of some cancers. The recommended diet is low in fat, calories, and preservatives and high in fiber, with at least five servings of various fruits and vegetables daily. Alcoholic beverages and foods that are salt cured, smoked, or nitrite preserved should be consumed in limited quantities. Appropriate calorie intake to maintain or attain normal body weight is also important because obesity is a risk factor for some cancers. A balanced program of activity and rest with stress management may enable the body to resist diseases, including cancer.

Avoidance of Carcinogens

Some specific carcinogens were mentioned earlier. They include cigarette smoke, alcohol, intercourse with multiple partners, a variety of chemicals and drugs, and even excessive sun exposure. Public education has focused attention on carcinogens and people are becoming more aware of the need to avoid them.

For example, smoking tobacco has long been considered a risk factor for cancers of the lung, bladder, head and neck, mouth, and stomach. Only in the past few years, however, have antismoking programs had a real effect on tobacco use. The fact that 1 million people quit smoking each year demonstrates that public education is making a difference. On a broader scale, legal restrictions on public smoking are reducing the exposure of nonsmokers to so-called second-hand smoke.

A harmful effect associated with use of smokeless tobacco is the increased risk of oral cancers. Alcohol consumption also increases the risk of cancers of the mouth, head and neck, and stomach. Many industrial products are recognized as carcinogens as well. Their use is regulated by the Occupational Safety and Health Administration's guidelines for the safety of workers and consumers. Unprotected sun exposure is a risk factor for skin cancers, including the most deadly type—melanoma. Increased awareness of the dangers of excessive sun exposure has boosted the use of sunscreens.

Identification of High-Risk People

Identifying people at risk for development of specific cancers serves several purposes. It helps researchers and health care providers to recognize factors that may contribute to the development of various cancers. In addition, people who are known to fall into high-risk categories can be monitored closely to detect cancer early (see *Cultural Considerations* box). Examples of people at risk for specific cancers are those with familial rectal polyposis, those with family histories of breast cancer, and those with Down syndrome, who are at increased risk for leukemia. In addition, people with high-risk behaviors and certain racial and ethnic groups have increased risk of specific cancers.

Cultural Considerations

What Does Culture Have to Do with Cancer?

Of all racial and ethnic groups, African-American men have the highest rates of cancers of the prostate, colon and rectum, and lung and bronchus and are most likely to die of those cancers. Although Caucasian women have the highest rates of breast cancer, African-American women are more likely to die from breast cancer. Nurses should encourage African Americans to participate in screenings and to seek early treatment for warning signs of cancer.

Put on Your Thinking Cap!

1. What are possible reasons that minorities in the United States have higher rates of several types of cancer and are more likely to die from cancer?
2. How can you use your knowledge of culture to intervene?

Screening for Cancer

When cancer does occur, early diagnosis and treatment often increase the chances of a cure. Public education should emphasize the following:

- The value of early detection and treatment
- The seven warning signs of cancer
- How to do self-examinations (breast, skin, testicular)
- The importance of periodic examinations for common cancers

The American Cancer Society recommends specific examinations or procedures to detect cancers of the colon, prostate, cervix, endometrium, and breast. The recommendations are summarized in Table 25-6.

DIAGNOSIS OF CANCER

The health history and physical examination often provide the first clues to the presence of cancer. Diagnostic procedures may be used when cancer is suspected, when high-risk people are screened, or when determining the extent of known disease. Diagnostic procedures rely on tissue examinations, imaging studies, endoscopic procedures, and laboratory tests. Combinations of procedures may be indicated for cancers that are difficult to locate or to determine whether more than one site exists. It is important to note that many laboratory tests are nonspecific for cancer. Abnormal laboratory results can have many causes but, combined with other data, they assist in the diagnostic process. In addition, the same diagnostic tests and procedures may be used during and after cancer treatment to assess treatment effectiveness. Table 25-7 presents examples of tests and procedures that might be used in the diagnostic process.

MEDICAL TREATMENT OF CANCER

Methods of treating cancer include surgery, radiotherapy, chemotherapy, biotherapy, transplantation of bone marrow and hematopoietic stem cells, and hormone therapy. Various complementary therapies may be used as well. One treatment or a combination may be recommended, depending on the type and location of the cancer.

SURGERY

Surgery is performed in the majority of patients to diagnose and stage the cancer, relieve symptoms, maintain function, effect a cure, or reconstruct affected structures. Although not common, surgery is sometimes done prophylactically in people who are at very high risk for development of specific cancers. For example, those with familial polyposis may have a portion of the colon removed to prevent colon cancer. Surgery is commonly used in the treatment of cancer, often in combination with other therapies. Surgery for cancer may be extensive or simple. A thorough preoperative diagnostic evaluation enables the surgeon to plan the most appropriate procedure.

Surgery is most likely to be curative when tumors are detected early, are slow growing, are confined to

Table 25-6 Screening Guidelines for the Early Detection of Cancer in People With No Symptoms and Average Risk

CANCER SITE	POPULATION	TEST OR PROCEDURE	FREQUENCY
Breast	Women, age 20+	Breast self-examination (BSE)	It is acceptable for women to choose not to do BSE or to do BSE regularly (monthly) or irregularly. Beginning in their early 20s, women should be told about the benefits and limitations of BSE. Whether or not a woman ever performs BSE, the importance of prompt reporting of any new breast symptoms to a health professional should be emphasized. Women who choose to do BSE should receive instruction and have their technique reviewed on the occasion of a periodic health examination.
		Clinical breast examination (CBE)	For women in their 20s and 30s, it is recommended that CBE be part of a periodic health examination, preferably at least every three years. Asymptomatic women aged 40 and over should continue to receive a CBE as part of a periodic health examination, preferably annually.
		Mammography	Begin annual mammography at age 40.*
Cervix	Women, ages 21–65	Pap test; human papillomavirus (HPV) DNA test	Cervical cancer screening should begin at age 21. For women ages 21–29, screening should be done every 3 years with conventional or liquid-based Pap tests. For women ages 30–65, screening should be done every 5 years with both the HPV test and the Pap test (preferred), or every 3 years with the Pap test alone (acceptable). Women aged 65+ who have had ≥ 3 consecutive negative Pap tests or ≥ 2 consecutive negative HPV and Pap tests within the last 10 years, with the most recent test occurring within 5 years, and women who have had a total hysterectomy should stop cervical cancer screening. Women should not be screened annually by any method at any age.
Colorectal	Men and women, age 50+	Fecal occult blood test (FOBT) with at least 50% test sensitivity for cancer, or fecal immunochemical test (FIT) with at least 50% test sensitivity for cancer, or	Annual, starting at age 50. Testing at home with adherence to manufacturer's recommendation for collection techniques and number of samples is recommended. FOBT with the single stool sample collected on the clinician's fingertip during a digital rectal examination is not recommended. Guaiac-based toilet bowl FOBTs also are not recommended. In comparison with guaiac-based tests for the detection of occult blood, immunochemical tests are more patient-friendly, and are likely to be equal or better in sensitivity and specificity. There is no justification for repeating FOBT in response to an initial positive finding.
		Stool DNA test,† or	Interval uncertain; starting at age 50.
		Flexible sigmoidoscopy (FSIG), or	Every 5 years, starting at age 50. FSIG can be performed alone, or consideration can be given to combining FSIG performed every 5 years with a highly sensitive gFOBT or FIT performed annually.
		Double contrast barium enema (DCBE), or	Every 5 years, starting at age 50.
		Colonoscopy	Every 10 years, starting at age 50.
		CT colonography	Every 5 years, starting at age 50.
Endometrial	Women, at menopause	At the time of menopause, women at average risk should be informed about risks and symptoms of endometrial cancer and strongly encouraged to report any unexpected bleeding or spotting to their physician.	

Table 25-6 Screening Guidelines for the Early Detection of Cancer in People With No Symptoms and Average Risk—cont'd

CANCER SITE	POPULATION	TEST OR PROCEDURE	FREQUENCY
Lung	Current or former smokers ages 55–74 in good health with at least a 30 pack-year history	Low-dose helical CT (LDCT)	Clinicians with access to high-volume, high-quality lung cancer screening and treatment centers should initiate a discussion about lung cancer screening with apparently healthy patients ages 55–74 who have at least a 30 pack-year smoking history, and who currently smoke or have quit within the past 15 years. A process of informed and shared decision making with a clinician related to the potential benefits, limitations and harms associated with screening for lung cancer with LDCT should occur before any decision is made to initiate lung cancer screening. Smoking cessation counseling remains a high priority for clinical attention in discussions with current smokers, who should be informed of their continuing risk of lung cancer. Screening should not be viewed as an alternative to smoking cessation.
Prostate	Men, ages 50+	Digital rectal examination (DRE) and prostate-specific antigen test (PSA)	Men who have at least a ten-year life expectancy should have an opportunity to make an informed decision with their health care provider about whether to be screened for prostate cancer, after receiving information about the potential benefits, risks, and uncertainties associated with prostate cancer screening. Prostate cancer screening should not occur without an informed decision-making process.
Cancer-related checkup	Men and women, ages 20+	On the occasion of a periodic health examination, the cancer-related checkup should include examination for cancers of the thyroid, testicles, ovaries, lymph nodes, oral cavity, and skin, as well as health counseling about tobacco, sun exposure, diet and nutrition, risk factors, sexual practices, and environmental and occupational exposures.	

From American Cancer Society (ACS): *Cancer facts and figures 2014,* Atlanta, 2014, American Cancer Society.
*Beginning at age 40, annual clinical breast examination should be performed prior to mammography.
†The stool DNA test approved for colorectal cancer screening in 2008 is no longer commercially available. New stool DNA tests are presently undergoing evaluation and may become available at some future time.

Table 25-7 Diagnostic Tests and Procedures: Cancer

TEST OR PROCEDURE	EXAMPLES OF USES
Tissue Examination	
Specimens of body fluids, secretions, or tissues are obtained and examined microscopically to detect the presence of malignant cells.	Papanicolaou (Pap) test detects cancer cells in cervical smear. Body fluids from digestive and respiratory tracts are examined for presence of cancer cells.
Fluids and secretions can be obtained by swabs or smears, by venipuncture, or by withdrawal of fluids from body structures.	Blood cells are examined to diagnose leukemias and lymphomas.
Tissue samples are obtained by biopsy. Specimen may be entire growth, sample cut from the growth, or cells drawn from the growth with a needle.	Samples can be taken from any accessible growth. Tissue is examined for cancer cells.
Imaging Studies	
Plain Radiographs Images produced result from the different absorption rates of different tissues. Calcium in bones absorbs x-rays the most; therefore bones look white on the radiograph. Fat and other soft tissues absorb less and look gray. Air absorbs the least and therefore lungs look black.	Chest radiographs detect changes in lung tissue and bones. Can reveal organ size, position, abnormal structures and shapes. Mammography detects potentially malignant breast calcifications before they can be felt.

Continued

Table 25-7 Diagnostic Tests and Procedures: Cancer—cont'd

TEST OR PROCEDURE	EXAMPLES OF USES
Contrast Radiographs Contrast media given orally or intravenously to outline hollow organs. Shadows of abnormal structures can be visualized.	Used primarily to detect cancers of the digestive and urinary tracts.
Computed Tomography (CT) Provides cross-sectional, three-dimensional views of body tissue (Fig. 25-2). Details are much clearer than radiographs. Can be done plain or with contrast media.	Used to detect cancers of the head and trunk, spine, joints, and soft tissue. Also useful in staging bronchogenic and gastrointestinal (GI) tumors.
Positron Emission Tomography (PET) PET is a nuclear scan that reveals patterns of tissue metabolism.	Used to detect solid tumors in the brain and breast and to assess the effects of cancer treatment.
Magnetic Resonance Imaging (MRI) Radiofrequency waves are used in the presence of a strong magnetic field. Energy changes are measured and converted to computer images. Does not expose patient to radiation.	Used to detect cancers of the central nervous system (CNS), spinal column, neck, bones, joints, lungs, kidneys, and others.
Radionuclide Scans Radionuclides are radioactive substances that are taken up by specific body tissues. The patient is given a radionuclide, usually intravenously, and is then scanned to study the pattern of uptake of the radionuclide in target tissues. The radionuclide accumulates in target tissue, with greater uptake in abnormal tissue.	Used to detect tissue abnormalities. For example, technetium tagged with phosphorus is used for bone scans because technetium is absorbed in increased amounts in bone tissue where abnormal activity or increased metabolism is evident. Other radionuclides are used to detect cancers of the thyroid, liver, lung, and breast as well as lymphoma and melanoma.
Endoscopic Procedures Lighted tubes are inserted into hollow organs or body cavities to visualize and take specimens of suspicious tissue for examination.	Examples of endoscopic procedures and the areas they examine include: bronchoscopy (bronchi), colonoscopy (colon), cytoscopy (urinary bladder), and laparoscopy (abdominal cavity).
Laboratory Tests	
Oncofetal Antigens Oncofetal antigens are substances found on fetal cells and the surface of cancer cells. They are called *tumor markers* because elevations are associated with certain cancers. Can be elevated by nonmalignant conditions also, yielding a false-positive result for cancer. Often used to monitor response to cancer treatments. If treatment is successfully destroying the cancer, the antigen level goes down.	The following are examples of oncofetal antigens and the types of cancers with which they are associated: Carcinoembryonic antigen (CEA): digestive tract, breast; also elevated in heavy smokers Alpha-fetoprotein (AFP): liver, testicle Cancer antigen (CA)-50: GI tract, biliary tract, pancreas, transitional cell carcinoma, non–small cell lung cancer
NOTE: Elevated oncofetal antigens can have causes other than cancer. For example, oncofetal antigens may be elevated with cirrhosis of the liver and ulcerative colitis.	CA-125: ovary, breast, cervix, colon, endometrium, fallopian tube, GI tract, liver, lung, lymphoma, non-Hodgkin lymphoma, pancreas Prostate-specific antigen (PSA): prostate CA-19-9: pancreas, liver, lung, colon, rectum Pancreatic oncofetal antigen: pancreas and lung CA 15-3: breast, liver, lung, prostate Bladder tumor antigen (BTA): urinary bladder Human chorionic gonadotropin (HCG): testicle
Other Studies	
Other laboratory studies of body fluids do not specifically diagnose cancer but may suggest possible malignancies.	The following are examples of other useful laboratory tests: Serum alkaline phosphatase: elevated with metastatic bone cancer, hyperparathyroidism Serum acid phosphatase: elevated with metastatic bone cancer, hairy cell leukemia, prostate cancer Serum and urine calcium: elevated with bladder, breast, kidney, lung, endocrine cancer, leukemia, lymphoma Thyroid antithyroglobulin antibody: elevated with thyroid cancer ***NOTE:*** Elevations can be caused by numerous other, nonmalignant conditions.

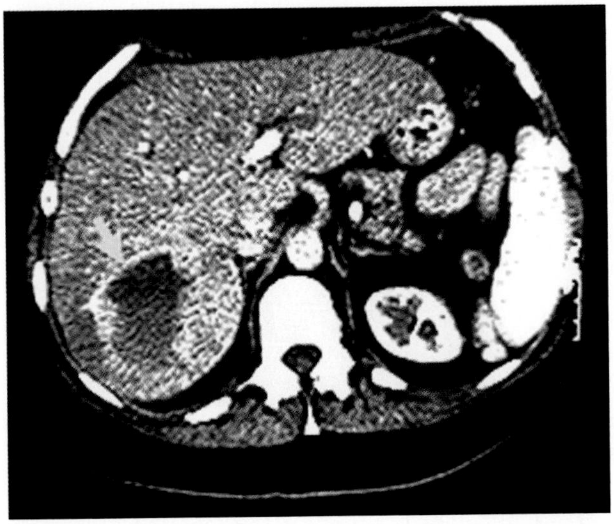

FIGURE 25-2 Computed tomography (CT) provides cross-sectional, three-dimensional views of body tissue. This upper abdominal CT scan shows a blood vessel tumor (hemangioma) in the liver. (Courtesy National Institutes of Health.)

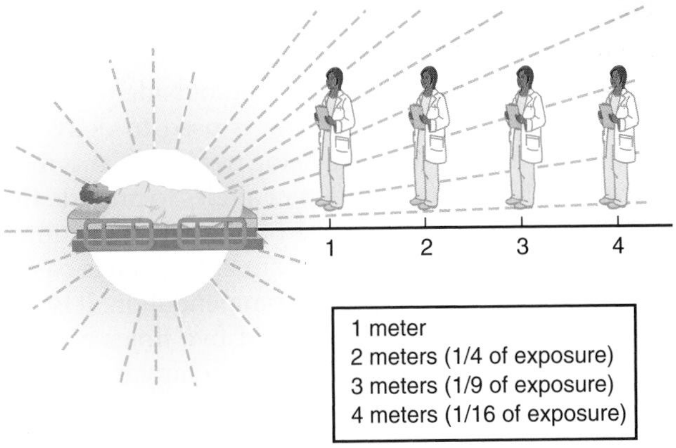

FIGURE 25-3 Radiation exposure decreases as distance from the source increases. (From Black JM, Hawks JH: *Medical-surgical nursing: clinical management for positive outcomes*, ed 8, St. Louis, 2009, Saunders.)

one area, and do not invade vital body structures. Surrounding tissues, including lymph glands, are often removed to eliminate malignant cells that have escaped the tumor mass. When surgery is extensive, it is often referred to as a *radical procedure.*

The preoperative and postoperative care of the surgical cancer patient varies with the specific surgery. General care of the surgical patient is detailed in Chapter 17. Specific surgeries are discussed in individual chapters. After surgery, other therapies may be recommended. The recommended treatment is based on the type of cancer, its location, the staging, and the extent of metastasis. The surgeon often consults with a radiologist and an oncologist (a physician who specializes in treating patients who have cancer) to determine the best therapy.

Adjuvant and **neoadjuvant** therapies are relatively recent approaches to cancer treatment. Adjuvant therapy may be used when a patient has had surgery or radiotherapy and is free of signs of disease but has a high likelihood of recurrence. Such patients may be given chemotherapy to eradicate any remaining undetected cells. Adjuvant therapy is often used in the treatment of breast cancer. Neoadjuvant therapy uses chemotherapy to reduce the extent of the tumor before surgery or radiotherapy.

RADIOTHERAPY

Radiotherapy is the use of ionizing radiation in the treatment of disease. The unit of measure for radiation doses is now the **gray (Gy)**. Formerly, the *rad* was the unit of measure (1 Gy equals 100 rad). Radiation is used to treat cancer because malignant cells are more sensitive than normal cells to radiation. Radiation has immediate and delayed effects on cells. The immediate effect is cell death because of damage to the cell membrane. The delayed effect is alteration of DNA, which impairs the cell's ability to reproduce. Types of cancer cells vary in their sensitivity to radiation. A tumor is considered *radiosensitive* if it can be destroyed by radiation at a dose that is tolerated by surrounding normal tissue.

Radiotherapy may be given internally or externally. Internal radiation requires the introduction of the radioactive substance into the body. External radiation is given by way of a beam directed at the tumor.

Caregiver Safety

To work with radiation safely, the medical professional must understand it. The amount of radiation received by those who come in contact with the patient depends on the time of exposure, the distance from the radiation source, and the amount of shielding between the caregiver and the source. The less time spent near the patient with a radiation implant, the less exposure is incurred. Doubling the distance from the source decreases the exposure to one fourth. When the distance from the source is tripled, the exposure is reduced to one ninth (Fig. 25-3). Unless direct care is being given, nurses and caregivers should remain at least 6 feet from the source. There should be limits on visitors when a radiation implant is in place. As a precaution, most hospitals do not allow pregnant women or children younger than 18 years to visit patients who have a radiation implant. Visitors need to check with the staff before they enter the room. They may be asked to stay at least 6 feet from the patient and visit for less than 30 minutes each day (American Cancer Society, 2012). Effective shielding depends on the type of rays being emitted. In general, the denser the material composing the shield, the better protection it provides. Therefore lead is more protective than concrete or wood. Because shielding is awkward and cannot provide complete protection during patient care, many agencies rely more on time and distance to limit exposure.

External Radiation

Procedure. With external radiation therapy, the source of the radioactivity is located outside the body. A special type of x-ray machine is used to deliver a beam of radiation to the area being treated. Beams may be directed from several different angles to provide the greatest dose to the tumor and minimal exposure of other tissues. The number of treatments given is based on the radiation oncologist's recommendation. It is not unusual for a patient to be treated five times a week for 2 to 8 weeks. A variation of this therapy is intraoperative radiation therapy (IORT), a technique in which the tumor or tumor bed is radiated directly during surgery.

Patient Preparation. Before the first radiation treatment, the patient goes through a treatment *simulation*, which includes computed tomography (CT) scanning, to determine the exact location to be treated. The patient is positioned in various ways while radiographs are taken. The radiation therapist then marks the skin over the area to be treated. The markings are usually made with waterproof ink; however, tiny permanent markings are sometimes made. The markings must remain visible throughout the course of radiation. Instruct the patient not to remove the markings until given permission to do so by the physician. For the actual treatments, various devices are used to shield healthy tissue.

Internal Radiation

Internal radiation involves the introduction of a radiation source into the body. Sources of radiation used for therapy include radioactive forms of iodine, phosphorus, radium, iridium, radon, and cesium. The source may be either sealed or unsealed. In general, patients being treated with internal radiation emit radiation and *do* pose a threat to others until the source is removed or excreted. An exception is the patient who has small radioactive beads permanently implanted to treat localized prostate cancer or inoperable lung cancer.

Sealed-Source Radiation. Sealed-source radiation is inserted in the body in a sealed container. One example of sealed-source radiation is cesium, which is contained in a sealed applicator that is inserted into body cavities to treat cancer of the prostate, mouth, tongue, vagina, and cervix. Sealed-source radiation also may be placed in threads, beads, needles, or seeds and implanted in body tissues or may be enclosed in a mold and applied externally. The radiologist determines how long the source is left in place. The patient's body fluids, as well as objects the patient touches, are not radioactive because the radiation source is closed. However, because radiation is emitted from the source while it is in the patient, the following safety measures are necessary in most cases to protect all visitors and nurses from excessive exposure to radiation:

1. The patient is placed in a private room, preferably one that is lined with lead.

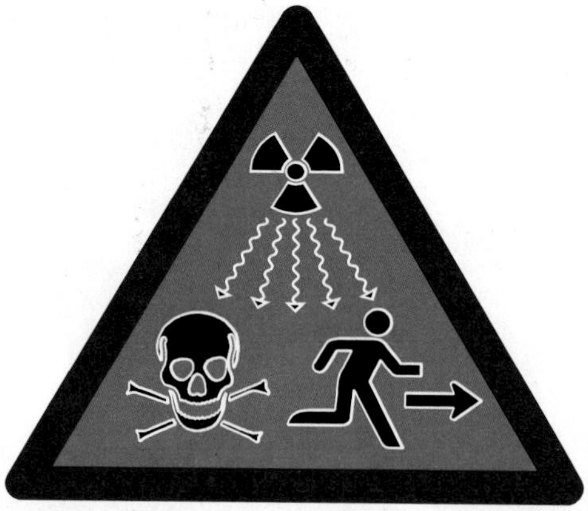

FIGURE 25-4 The radiation sign alerts others to the dangers of radiation.

2. A sign is placed on the door to the patient's room indicating that the room is a radiation area. A standard sign is usually available for this purpose (Fig. 25-4).
3. Anyone who might enter the room for any reason is informed of the proper precautions to take. People younger than 18 years old and pregnant women should not enter the room. This restriction applies to staff as well as to others. Exposure to radiation is potentially harmful to a fetus.
4. The amount of radiation exposure is reduced by limiting time spent in the room and by working as far as possible from the radiation source. Institutional policies prescribe the time restrictions for implants. Nursing personnel who spend the most time with the patient should wear film badges to monitor their radiation exposure. As noted above, nurses and visitors who are pregnant should not enter the room.
5. Work must be organized efficiently. For most patients, care can be provided in a total of 30 minutes per shift. Portable lead shields can be used to provide some protection. Lead aprons do not provide adequate protection in this situation.
6. Recognize that sealed sources can be dislodged accidentally. The placement of the source is selected to exert the direct effects of radiation on the area being treated. Specific positions may be ordered for the patient to decrease the risk of displacing the source. Check bedpans and linens for any dislodged source before disposal. If the source moves out of position, immediately notify the physician and the radiation safety personnel. If the source comes out of the patient's body, *do not touch it with bare hands.* Forceps and a lead container (called a *pig*) that are routinely placed in the room are used to retrieve and contain the source.

Unsealed-Source Radiation. When unsealed sources are used, additional considerations exist. Because body fluids may be contaminated, you must wear gloves when working with the patient. Contaminated fluids, dressings, and the like may require special care, as outlined in the agency policy. Disposable utensils are recommended. Equipment used in the room may need to be checked for radioactivity before it can be removed from the room. The radiologist can advise the staff on specific precautions and how long they are necessary. Nurses and visitors who are pregnant should not enter the room.

Side Effects

The ideal radiation treatment destroys the tumor with the least harm to surrounding cells. Because cells that regenerate rapidly are more susceptible to radiation, cancer cells and some normal cells may be harmed. Normal cells that are most sensitive to radiation include those of the hair follicle, bone marrow, lining of the digestive and urinary tracts, ovaries, testes, and lymph tissue. Radiation damage to these cells explains many of the side effects of the therapy. Depending on the area being irradiated, the following side effects may occur: bone marrow suppression; alopecia (hair loss); anorexia; dry mouth; nausea and vomiting; diarrhea; and inflammation of the skin, esophagus (esophagitis), lungs (pneumonitis), and bladder (cystitis). Regardless of the site treated, radiation therapy commonly causes skin changes and fatigue. Side effects are usually not evident until at least 1 week after treatments are started. These side effects are slow to start and slow to subside. Some people tolerate therapy well whereas others become very ill. Factors that influence the severity of side effects include the area being treated, total and daily radiation doses, volume of tissue treated, method of treatment, and individual factors.

Bone Marrow Suppression. In healthy people, the bone marrow produces red blood cells (RBCs), white blood cells (WBCs), and platelets. Depending on the treatment site, total area irradiated, and daily radiation dose, radiation treatment can suppress the production of these cells. Anemia results from a deficiency of RBCs. Without adequate WBCs, the patient's ability to resist infection is reduced. Without adequate platelets, the patient is at risk for bruising and bleeding. Bone marrow suppression is most common among patients whose treatment area involves a large area of bone.

Blood counts are usually ordered every other week during radiation therapy, depending on the treatment area, to detect excessive bone marrow suppression. If blood counts are too low, transfusions may be required. The radiation treatments may have to be temporarily stopped until the bone marrow recovers. WBC and platelet counts usually recover in 2 to 6 weeks. When radiation treatments are used in combination with chemotherapy treatments, an increased chance of bone marrow suppression exists. Growth factors for WBCs and RBCs can be used to help the blood cell counts recover sooner.

Alopecia. Because the cells in the hair follicles are very sensitive to radiation, radiation of the head often produces partial or complete **alopecia** (loss of hair). Whether the hair grows back depends on the radiation dosage. If the hair does grow back, it may be different in color or texture than it was before treatment.

Anorexia. Anorexia is a loss of appetite. Factors that may cause the patient undergoing radiation therapy to have anorexia include inflammation of the mouth and tongue, altered taste perception, and nausea. Anorexia is a significant problem because it can lead to inadequate nutrition and weight loss. It is especially problematic for patients being treated for cancer of the esophagus, stomach, neck, or head. Depression may contribute to anorexia in the patient undergoing radiation therapy.

Dry Mouth. Dry mouth, called **xerostomia**, is a special problem with radiation of the head and neck. The production of saliva decreases, putting the patient at risk for infections of the teeth and gums. Diseased teeth are often extracted before radiation of the head or neck because the risk of osteoradionecrosis is so great. Osteoradionecrosis is destruction of bone caused by radiation. It is a debilitating complication of head and neck radiation. Medication is available that can help to protect the salivary glands as well as any mucus-producing tissue. These medications are called *radioprotectors* and are given before radiation treatment on a daily basis or as ordered by the physician.

Effects on Reproduction. Radiation is potentially harmful to reproductive cells as well as to the developing fetus and embryo. Therefore radiotherapy is not recommended during pregnancy and patients are advised to avoid becoming pregnant during the therapy. The major side effects of radiation are summarized in Table 25-8.

CHEMOTHERAPY

Chemotherapy is the use of chemical agents in the treatment of disease. Chemical agents specifically used to treat cancer are called **antineoplastic** or *anticancer drugs*. The terms *chemotherapy, anticancer,* and *antineoplastic drugs* are used interchangeably in this chapter, just as they are in common practice. These drugs act in a variety of ways and may be used alone or in combination with other forms of treatment. In some cases chemotherapy is curative. In other circumstances it may reduce the number of cancer cells, causing symptoms to decrease and often prolonging life.

Types of Antineoplastic Drugs

Types of antineoplastic drugs now commonly used in chemotherapy include cytotoxic agents, hormones and hormone antagonists, agents classified as biotherapy, and others listed in Box 25-2. The term *targeted drugs* applies to those that promote cell death by binding with specific targets on cancer cells. Kinase inhibitors, proteasome inhibitors, and angiogenesis inhibitors are examples of targeted anticancer drugs.

Table 25-8 Side Effects of Radiation Therapy and Nursing Implications

SITE	SIDE EFFECTS	NURSING IMPLICATIONS
Skin	Erythema (redness), desquamation (peeling), permanent darkening	Skin is easily injured. Avoid exposure to sun, trauma, harsh chemicals, or soaps. Until therapy is completed, no lotions or topical medications should be applied. Do not remove markings.
Scalp	Partial or complete alopecia (hair loss); may be permanent	New hair may be different color and texture. Cover scalp with wig, cap, or scarf if patient desires. Refer to American Cancer Society for free hairpieces and help with styling and care.
Digestive tract	Anorexia, inflammation and dryness of the mouth, decreased or altered sense of taste	Schedule small, frequent feedings. Respect patient preferences. Promote frequent oral hygiene. Suggest artificial saliva and ice chips. Monitor weight to assess nutritional state.
	Dental caries	Encourage good dental care. Conduct mouth care per protocol.
	Painful swallowing	Provide antacids and viscous lidocaine as ordered.
	Nausea, vomiting	Provide antiemetics as ordered. Monitor intake.
	Diarrhea	Provide antidiarrheals as ordered. Encourage good perianal care.
Urinary tract	Cystitis	Increase fluid intake.
	Contracted bladder	Have patient empty bladder often.
	Crystalluria	Keep intake and output records.
Bone marrow	Suppressed production of red blood cells (RBCs), white blood cells (WBCs), and platelets	Schedule activities to prevent overtiring. Protect patient from infection and injury. Watch for excessive bruising or bleeding. Check results of blood tests. Report fever. Encourage use of soft toothbrush and electric razor.
Lungs	Pneumonitis	Encourage coughing and deep breathing to prevent pneumonia. Use humidifier if ordered. Protect patient from respiratory infections. No one with an elevated temperature or children should visit.
Reproductive organs	Harm to embryo or fetus; sterility, impotence	Advise patient not to become pregnant during therapy or for specified time afterward. Physician may counsel male patient about banking sperm.

Box 25-2 Examples of Drugs Used to Treat Cancer

CYTOTOXIC DRUGS

Mitotic Inhibitors (Plant Alkaloids)
docetaxel (Taxotere)
paclitaxel (Taxol)
vinblastine (Velban)
vincristine (Oncovin)
vinorelbine (Navelbine)

Alkylating Agents
busulfan (Myleran)
carboplatin (Paraplatin)
carmustine (BiCNU)
chlorambucil (Leukeran)
cisplatin (Platinol)
cyclophosphamide (Cytoxan)
ifosfamide (Ifex)
lomustine (CCNU)
mechlorethamine hydrochloride (Mustargen)
melphalan (Alkeran)
streptozocin (Zanosar)
temozolomide (Temodar)

Antitumor Antibiotics
bleomycin (Blenoxane)
dactinomycin (Cosmegen)
daunorubicin (Cerubidine, and others)
doxorubicin (Adriamycin)
epirubicin (Ellence)
idarubicin hydrochloride (Idamycin)
mitomycin (Mutamycin)
mitoxantrone (Novantrone)
plicamycin (Mithramycin)
valrubicin (Valstar)

Antimetabolites

Folic Acid Analog
methotrexate (Folex)

Pyrimidine Analogs
capecitabine (Xeloda)
cytarabine (Cytosar-U)
fluorouracil (Adrucil)
floxuridine (FUDR)
gemcitabine (Gemzar)

Purine Analogs
fludarabine (Fludara)
mercaptopurine (Purinethol)
pentostatin (Nipent)
thioguanine (Tabloid)

Topoisomerase Inhibitors
etoposide (Etopophos, VePesid, and others)
irinotecan (Camptosar)

Box 25-2 Examples of Drugs Used to Treat Cancer—cont'd

teniposide (Vumon)
topotecan (Hycamtin)

Miscellaneous Cytotoxic Medications
altretamine (Hexalen)
asparaginase (Elspar)
dacarbazine (DTIC-Dome)
hydroxyurea (Hydrea)
pegaspargase (Oncaspar)
mitotane (Lysodren)
procarbazine (Matulane)

HORMONES AND HORMONE ANTAGONIST DRUGS

Androgens
fluoxymesterone (Halotestin)
testosterone (generic only)
testolactone (Teslac)

Gonadotropic-Releasing Hormone Analogs
leuprolide (Lupron)
goserelin (Zoladex)

Androgen Receptor Blockers
flutamide (Eulexin)
bicalutamide (Casodex)
nilutamide (Nilandron)

Estrogens
diethylstilbestrol diphosphate (Stilphostrol)
ethinyl estradiol (Estinyl)

Estrogen Mustard
estramustine (Emcyt)

Antiestrogens
tamoxifen (Nolvadex)
raloxifene (Evista)
toremifene (Fareston)

Progestins
medroxyprogesterone acetate (Depo-Provera)
megestrol acetate (Megace)

Aromatase Inhibitors
anastrozole (Arimidex)
letrozole (Femara)
exemestane (Aromasin)

Glucocorticoid
prednisone (Deltasone, and others)

BIOLOGIC RESPONSE MODIFIERS (IMMUNOSTIMULANTS)

Monoclonal Antibodies
alemtuzumab (Campath)
gemtuzumab (Mylotarg)
rituximab (Rituxan)

Radioimmunoconjugates
tositumomab (Bexxar)
ibritumomab (Zevalin)

Epidermal Growth Factor Receptors
trastuzumab (Herceptin)
cetuximab (Erbitux)
panitumumab (Vectibix)
trastuzumab (Herceptin)
bevacizumab (Avastin)

Tyrosine Kinase Inhibitors
imatinib (Gleevec)
erlotinib (Tarceva)
lapatinib (Tykerb)
sorafenib (Nexavar)
sunitinib (Sutent)
temsirolimus (Torisel)

Proteasome Inhibitors
bortezomib (Velcade)

Interferons
interferon alfa-2a (Roferon-A)
interferon alfa-2b (Intron A)
interferon alfa-n3 (Alferon N)
interferon beta-1a (Avonex)
interferon beta-1b (Betaseron)
interferon gamma-1b (Actimmune)

Interleukins
aldesleukin/interleukin-2 (Proleukin)
oprelvekin/interleukin-11 (Neumega)

Vaccines
bacillus Calmette-Guérin (BCG) vaccine (TheraCys, and others)

Colony-Stimulating Factors
erythropoietin (Procrit, Epogen)
darbepoetin alfa/erythrocytes (Aranesp)
filgrastim (G-CSF, Neupogen)
sargramostim (GM-CSF, Leukine)
interleukin-3
macrophage CSF
pegfilgrastim (Neulasta)

Other Medications
levamisole (Ergamisol)

Various types of cancer are sensitive to different drugs or drug combinations. Combinations are sometimes used to attack cells at different stages of development. Drugs that are effective only during a particular phase of cell development are said to be *cell cycle phase specific*. Drugs that are effective during any phase of cell development are said to be *cell cycle phase nonspecific*.

A physician or a nurse who has had specialized education administers chemotherapy. Some drugs may be given in an outpatient setting; others must be given in an inpatient setting. The route may be oral, intramuscular, intravenous, intracavity, or intrathecal. *Intracavity* means that the drug is instilled in a body cavity such as the bladder. *Intrathecal* chemotherapy is given in the subarachnoid space.

Chemoembolization is a technique in which the drug is injected directly into an artery supplying the tumor. Chemoembolization has been used in the treatment of metastatic liver cancer. The goal of this approach is to stop liver tumors from growing or cause them to shrink; shrinkage occurs in about two thirds of cases treated. This benefit lasts 10 to 14 months on average (NCCN, 2010).

Pharmacology Capsule

The most dangerous adverse effect of antineoplastic drugs used in chemotherapy is bone marrow suppression.

Side Effects

Like radiotherapy, antineoplastic drugs act on normal cells and malignant cells. The major systemic side effects of antineoplastic drugs are the same as those of radiation: bone marrow suppression, nausea and vomiting, and alopecia. Depending on the specific antineoplastic agent, the patient is also at risk for toxic effects to the heart, lungs, nerve tissue, kidneys, and bladder. These problems and related nursing interventions are discussed in "Nursing Care of the Patient Who Has Cancer" and are summarized in Table 25-9.

Although bone marrow suppression is the most *dangerous* side effect, nausea and vomiting are likely to be the most distressing. Antineoplastic drugs simultaneously irritate the lining of the digestive tract and stimulate the vomiting center in the brain. Some agents have toxic effects on the heart that may lead to heart failure. Others are neurotoxic, with effects manifested most often by numbness and tingling of extremities, paralytic ileus, and loss of deep tendon reflexes. Hypersensitivity reactions can occur with many chemotherapeutic agents that require vigilant assessment, especially during the initial stage of infusion. Like

Table 25-9 Side Effects of Antineoplastic Therapy and Nursing Implications

SITE	SIDE EFFECTS	IMPLICATIONS
Bone marrow	Suppressed production of red blood cells (RBCs), white blood cells (WBCs), and platelets	Monitor blood test results. Balance activity and rest. Prevent overtiring and stress. Protect from infection. Report fever. Watch for excessive bruising or bleeding. Apply pressure to injection sites. Avoid rectal temperatures if WBC count is low. Use soft toothbrush and electric razor.
Digestive tract	Nausea and vomiting	Give antiemetics as ordered. Assess for dehydration. No fluids with meals. Pleasant environment. Respect food preferences.
	Anorexia	Schedule small, frequent feedings and frequent oral hygiene. Monitor weight. Give supplements as ordered.
	Xerostomia	Increase fluid intake. Recommend artificial saliva, sugarless gum or hard candy, and ice chips. Moisten dry food.
	Stomatitis	Encourage dental care and mouth care as ordered or per protocol. Assess for lesions.
	Diarrhea	Provide antidiarrheals as ordered. Promote correct perianal care.
	Constipation	Encourage fluids and high-fiber foods and exercise as tolerated. Give laxatives, stool softeners, enemas as ordered.
Heart	Cardiomyopathy Heart failure	Monitor for dyspnea, edema, increasing pulse pressure. Request electrocardiograms (ECGs) as ordered.
Lungs	Inflammation, fibrosis	Encourage turning, coughing, and deep breathing to prevent pneumonia. Use humidifier as ordered. Elevate head if dyspneic. Protect from respiratory infections. Monitor activity tolerance.
Nerve tissue	Numbness, tingling, loss of deep tendon reflexes	Assess sensation. Protect affected areas from injury.
Scalp	Alopecia	Cover scalp with hairpiece, scarf, or turban if patient wishes. Refer to American Cancer Society for free hairpieces and help with grooming.
Veins	Phlebitis at infusion site	Watch for possible necrosis of surrounding tissue with extravasation. Monitor infusion carefully. Protect infusion site. Report signs of extravasation immediately.
Reproductive cells	Harm to developing embryo or fetus Sterility, impotence with some agents	Discourage pregnancy while on therapy and for specified period thereafter. (Physician may discuss banking sperm with male patients.)

radiation, antineoplastic drugs are hazardous to reproductive cells and some cause erectile dysfunction and sterility.

Antineoplastic drugs also can cause very serious tissue injury to the vein during administration. If the agent leaks out of the vein, surrounding tissue destruction may occur. When **extravasation** is suspected, stop the infusion immediately and notify the physician or clinical nurse specialist. The physician or clinical nurse specialist may use various interventions to limit potential harm done by a particular agent (Schulmeister, 2010).

Pharmacology Capsule

Tissue destruction can result from a group of intravenous antineoplastic drugs classified as *vesicants.* Extravasation is leakage of these intravenous drugs into surrounding tissues.

BIOTHERAPY

Agents that work by affecting biologic processes (referred to as **biotherapy**) include hematopoietic growth factors, BRMs, and monoclonal antibodies (MAbs). Hematopoietic growth factors (see Box 25-2) are colony-stimulating factors (CSFs). Because antineoplastic drugs suppress the bone marrow, CSFs may be used to stimulate the bone marrow to produce platelets, RBCs, and WBCs in patients receiving chemotherapy. This reduces the risk of infection by shortening the period of **neutropenia**, which occurs when WBCs are low and is associated with chemotherapy as well as with anemia and thrombocytopenia. Chapters 33 and 34 provide additional information about CSFs. With CSFs, higher doses of chemotherapy can be given for longer periods of time.

Surgery, radiotherapy, and chemotherapy work by destroying malignant cells and thereby reduce the size of the tumor. It is hoped that the body's natural defenses will then destroy the remaining malignant cells. Therapy using BRMs is intended to boost the body's existing defenses. BRMs act directly on malignant cells or stimulate the immune system to act against them. Such therapy is most effective if the immune system is functioning adequately. A skin test may be performed to evaluate the immune response before therapy is started. Examples of BRMs are interferons and interleukins.

MAb therapy uses antibodies made in large numbers in a laboratory rather than by a person's own immune system. Scientists can now produce MAbs designed to recognize very specific targets, or antigens, that are present on certain kinds of cancer cells. This type of treatment is considered a form of *passive* immunotherapy. These treatments often do not require the person's immune system to take an "active" role in fighting the cancer. The first MAbs were made entirely from mouse cells. One problem with this is that the human immune system can see these antibodies as foreign (because they are from a different species) and can mount a response against them. In the short term, this can sometimes cause allergic-type reactions. Over time, researchers have learned how to replace some parts of these mouse antibody proteins with human parts. Depending on how much of the MAb is human, these are called *chimeric* or *humanized* antibodies. Some MAbs are now fully human, which means that they are likely to be safer and may be more effective than older MAbs. The most common side effects are extreme fatigue, headache, muscle aches, chills, and fever. Side effects are more common in older people and in people who are dehydrated, anemic, and malnourished. Previous cardiac, neurologic, gastrointestinal (GI), hepatic, or renal disease also increases the risk of side effects. Table 25-10 outlines side effects of BRM therapy. The patient should be told to report a rash, a blister, or pain at the injection site or a fever. Since 1997 the U.S. Food

Table 25-10 Common Side Effects of Biologic Response Modifiers and Nursing Implications

SITE	SIDE EFFECTS	NURSING IMPLICATIONS
Generalized	Flulike symptoms: fever, chills, muscle aches, severe fatigue, malaise, headaches, tachycardia	Side effects may mask signs and symptoms of infection, so assess carefully. Give acetaminophen as ordered (meperidine is sometimes ordered for severe chills). Help patient plan for adequate rest.
Heart	Serious dysrhythmias, myocardial infarction	Monitor heart rate and rhythm. Report abnormal findings.
Capillaries	Increased permeability, pulmonary and dependent edema, hypotension	Assess for edema. Monitor blood pressure. Have patient change positions slowly; avoid prolonged standing, hot baths, and showers. For hypotension, give colloids or vasopressors as ordered.
Bronchi and lungs	Anaphylaxis with bronchial constriction Pulmonary edema	Note signs of allergy: rash, wheezing, itching. For anaphylaxis, give epinephrine or diphenhydramine as ordered. Maintain airway. Assess lungs for crackles. Position for comfort (head elevated).

NOTE: Many other side effects occur with individual biologic response modifiers (BRMs). These include nausea, diarrhea, anorexia, weight loss, skin redness or rash, pruritus, desquamation, bone pain, renal toxicity, anemia, thrombocytopenia, leukopenia, leukocytosis, altered mental status, and liver toxicity. The nurse should identify the specific effects and implications for the specific agents the patient is receiving.

and Drug Administration (FDA) has approved several MAbs for the treatment of certain cancers.

Clinical trials of MAb therapy are also in progress for people with almost every type of cancer. As researchers have found more cancer-associated antigens, they have been able to make MAbs against more and more cancers.

Pharmacology Capsule

Biologic response modifiers (BRMs) boost the body's natural defenses to combat malignant cells.

BONE MARROW AND STEM CELL TRANSPLANTATION

Bone marrow transplantation is most often used after treatment of leukemia and lymphoma with chemotherapy, radiation, or both that destroys the patient's bone marrow. Stem cell transplantation can be used to treat the destruction of the bone marrow caused by the chemotherapy and radiotherapy. Transplantation of bone marrow or peripheral blood stem cells is done to restore the blood manufacturing cells. If a patient donates his or her own stem cells or bone marrow before therapy, it is classified as an *autologous transplant.* If a patient receives cells from a sibling or other relative, it is classified as an *allogeneic transplant;* if the cells are donated from an unrelated donor, it is classified as a *matched unrelated donor* (*MUD*) *transplant.* See Chapter 34 for additional discussion of CSFs and bone marrow and stem cell transplants.

HORMONE THERAPY

Because some tumors are affected by hormones, various treatments may be used to suppress natural hormone secretion, block hormone actions, or provide supplemental hormones. For example, hormones may be used to block the male sex hormones in the treatment of prostate cancer and female hormones in the treatment of breast cancer.

COMPLEMENTARY AND ALTERNATIVE THERAPIES

Some patients choose to use nontraditional treatments such as relaxation techniques, guided imagery, music, meditation, herbal remedies, and acupuncture (see *Complementary and Alternative Therapies* box). If a nontraditional therapy is used with conventional treatment, it is called **complementary therapy**. The term **alternative therapy** is used if the patient uses nontraditional therapy in place of traditional treatment. The National Center for Complementary and Alternative Medicine, part of the National Institutes of Health, is conducting research to determine the therapeutic value of nontraditional therapies.

Many patients with cancer or other chronic conditions use alternative therapies, including herbal remedies, and many are "secretive" about their use. It is important for patients to report all herbal products used to their physician and to consider their use carefully. Generally, very few clinical trials take place evaluating the true safety and efficacy of these products. In addition, some affect the action of prescribed medications.

Complementary and Alternative Therapies

The American Cancer Society identifies some complementary therapies that can help to relieve symptoms or side effects, ease pain, and increase enjoyment of life. These include the following:

- Aromatherapy
- Art therapy
- Biofeedback
- Massage therapy
- Music therapy
- Prayer, spiritual practices
- Tai chi
- Yoga

UNPROVEN METHODS OF CANCER TREATMENT

It is important for health care providers to incorporate clear assessment strategies to ascertain the type of complementary and alternative medicine (CAM) the patient is using or plans to use. The American Cancer Society discourages the use of treatments that have not been studied and found to be safe and effective. Alternative therapies can be harmful and may delay treatment with potentially effective conventional therapies (see *Patient Teaching* box and *Complementary and Alternative Therapies* box). Barns et al. (2008) found in their study that almost 12% of children are involved in some sort of CAM therapies. The safety and efficacy of CAM in children requires further research. The nurse can direct patients to the American Cancer Society for further information about questionable therapies. Special considerations about the use of herbs as therapy can be found in Box 25-3.

Patient Teaching

Herbal Therapy

- "Natural" does not always mean safe.
- Discuss herbal products with your physician before use.
- Try to research the product thoroughly.
- Use products with a single component or ingredient (additional ingredients add to the potential toxicity).
- Use products from a reputable manufacturer. The label should have the manufacturer's address and expiration date.
- Look for products that have a drug identification number (DIN). The DIN guarantees that the specified medicinal components will be present. For example, Tanacet 125 guarantees that an exact amount of tanacet, the medicinal component of feverfew, is present and that the product is quality controlled.

Box 25-3 Herbs: A Few Things to Think About

The following are common problems with herb use:

- The quantity and quality of any medicinal components in an herbal product can vary considerably. Herbal products are not regulated by FDA. Safety and effectiveness do not have to be demonstrated before these products are marketed.
- No legal standards are applied to herbs' growing conditions, harvesting, processing, or packaging. The possibilities of poor quality, adulteration, contamination, and varying strengths must be kept in mind when evaluating them (e.g., sprayed with pesticides, grown in contaminated soil). The country of origin in which the herb is grown is often not known.
- If the product label has *whole plant* listed, the amount of active medicine or chemical in the product is not known and can vary considerably. This can make dosing difficult or inaccurate. If the label indicates the chemical in *total weight,* this can be considered a specific amount of that product. See information about drug identification number (DIN) in *Patient Teaching* box.
- Finding herbs in the wild can be dangerous. For example, wild parsley looks very similar to poison water hemlock; poisonous mushrooms are (virtually) indistinguishable from edible ones.
- Many herbs interfere with prescription medications.
- Some natural products such as thymus are derived from animal sources and could be contaminated by prions, which can cause Creutzfeldt-Jakob disease (the human equivalent of mad cow disease). Another example: products that contain thyroid can alter the body's natural balance of thyroid hormone.
- Some herbal products *decrease* the risk of cancer; others may *increase* the risk of cancer or increase cancer growth.
- The American Cancer Society has published *Complete Guide to Complementary & Alternative Cancer Therapies* (2009).
- Internet resources concerning herbs are as follows:
  - FDA and Center for Food Safety and Applied Nutrition (CFSAN)
  - FamilyDoctor.org—Herbal Products and Supplements (www.familydoctor.org)

Complementary and Alternative Therapies

Myth: Herbs are natural products and therefore are safe.
Truth: Many herbs have serious side effects, including liver toxicity and even death.
Plants are composed of many different chemicals; some are medicinal and others are poisonous.

NURSING CARE of the Patient Who Has Cancer

When working with someone who has cancer, it is easy to focus on the cancer and forget the person. However, medical professionals can do many things that can significantly affect the patient's quality of life. (See Nursing Care Plan: Patient with Cancer. Assessment of the patient who has cancer is discussed, along with nursing care for each phase of illness: diagnostic phase, treatment phase, rehabilitation, and recurrence of terminal illness.)

Diagnostic Phase

People who develop one of the common signs of cancer are often unaware of the seriousness of the condition. Out of fear, some ignore the signs until the disease is advanced. When people seek evaluation of the signs, they are likely to be very worried. Patients often say that "not knowing" is the hardest part. They go through tests and procedures, some uncomfortable, and then wait for the final word. Cancer is often what they fear most.

Assessment

When a patient is having diagnostic procedures related to an actual or potential diagnosis of cancer, collect data needed for the planning and provision of care. A complete list of data follows. The data collected by the licensed vocational nurse/licensed practical nurse (LVN/LPN) depend on agency policy and individual training.

Health History

Chief Complaint. Begin with the chief complaint. The patient may complain of pain, lesions, lumps, or changes in some body function. Elicit a complete description of the problem and the related signs and symptoms.

Past Medical History. Document chronic illnesses, serious injuries, surgeries, and hospitalizations.

Family History. Inquire about the incidence of cancer and other serious diseases in the patient's immediate family.

Review of Systems. In the review of systems, record any of the following signs and symptoms, if present: pain, lumps, fatigue, activity intolerance, lesions of the skin or mucous membranes, easy bruising or bleeding, headache, vision or hearing disturbances, hoarseness, cough, dyspnea, hemoptysis, loss of appetite, difficulty swallowing, digestive disturbances, blood in the urine or stool, and change in bowel pattern.

Functional Assessment. Describe the patient's diet, use of alcohol and tobacco, safe sex practices, activity, and sleep routines. Document the patient's occupation and describe a usual day. Document health practices, including frequency of breast self-examination, testicular examination, and medical checkups. Identify the patient's concerns about living conditions and location. Ask about sources of stress and of support and usual coping strategies.

Nursing Care Plan: Patient with Cancer

ASSESSMENT

HEALTH HISTORY Mr. Silas Wilson is a 63-year-old African-American man who was recently diagnosed with lung cancer that is being treated with radiotherapy and chemotherapy. He reports a chronic, nonproductive cough but denies dyspnea or hemoptysis. He states that he has been fatigued and weak since starting his therapy. He has had mild nausea, anorexia, and occasional diarrhea. He complains of dry mouth and is having some dysphagia. The skin over the area being radiated is tender. He is married, is the father of three grown children, and is an insurance salesperson. He smoked one pack of cigarettes a day for 30 years until he quit smoking in 1996. He continues to work part time and expresses concern about his financial situation. He states that he has excellent insurance coverage.

PHYSICAL EXAMINATION Vital signs: blood pressure 176/92 mm Hg, pulse 72 bpm, respiration 18 breaths per minute, temperature 98°F (37°C) measured orally. Height 5′9″, weight 175 lb. Patient is alert and oriented but does not initiate conversation. Mucous membranes are dry and lips are cracked. Skin on the upper chest and neck is more darkly pigmented. A central venous catheter is in place; the insertion site is free of swelling and drainage. Respirations are not labored and breath sounds are clear throughout lung fields. Abdomen is soft and bowel sounds are present. Extremities are warm, with strong peripheral pulses. No edema is seen. Patient is unable to distinguish warm and cold or sharp and dull sensations in lower legs.

Nursing Diagnosis	Goals and Outcome Criteria	Interventions
Anxiety related to effects of treatment of uncertain outcomes	Patient will experience reduced anxiety as evidenced by patient statements and by objective observation of decreased anxiety.	Encourage the patient to talk about his illness and his feelings about it. Listen attentively and use touch to convey concern. Help the patient identify sources of anxiety and strategies to deal with it, such as teaching, counseling, spiritual guidance, and support groups.
Ineffective coping related to multiple stressors	Patient will identify stressors and strategies to deal with them to improve coping.	Help the patient to set priorities during therapy. Provide information about management of therapy side effects. Encourage self-care as much as possible. Emphasize his strength. Teach relaxation techniques. Refer the patient to the American Cancer Society for information about support services in the community.
Deficient knowledge of the prescribed therapy, effects, and precautions	Patient will correctly describe his disease, treatment, the effects of therapy, and the precautions needed.	Determine what the patient already knows and what additional information he wants. Reinforce pretreatment teaching. Remind him not to wash off skin markings until the radiologist gives permission to do so and not to apply lotion to irritated skin. Recommend cotton clothing over irritated skin. Provide information about specific drugs used in his chemotherapy. Refer the patient to the Cancer Information Service (CIS) (1-800-4CANCER) if he is interested (available in English and Spanish).
Risk for injury related to side effects of therapy	Patient will have no injuries related to therapy, as evidenced by absence of bleeding, dyspnea, skin lesions, or bruises.	Monitor for excessive bruising or prolonged bleeding, edema, dyspnea, and impaired sensation. Report blood in stool, urine, or sputum. Handle gently. Apply pressure for 5 minutes after venipunctures or injections. Instruct the patient to use a soft toothbrush and an electric razor and to protect his feet and legs from trauma. Inspect daily for injury. Advise the patient to wear shoes whenever out of bed.
Risk for infection related to decreased white blood cells, venous access devices	Patient will remain free of infection, as evidenced by normal body temperature and absence of swelling or warmth at central line insertion site.	Teach basic infection preventions such as hand washing, avoiding raw foods that have high bacteria possibility, and avoiding crowds and people with infections. Report fever, foul wound drainage, or confusion to physician promptly. Teach the patient proper care of central venous catheter and have him return demonstration.
Imbalanced nutrition: less than body requirements related to anorexia and nausea	Patient will maintain adequate nutrition, as evidenced by body weight within 10 lb of usual (180 lb).	Emphasize the importance of good nutrition. Request a dietary consult. Consider frequent feedings. Respect preferences and aversions. Suggest soft diet eaten slowly for dysphagia. Tell the patient not to drink alcohol while receiving chemotherapy. Advise him not to drink fluids with meals and to decrease intake of sweets and fatty foods. Create a pleasant environment without offensive odors. Suggest mild exercise before meals and rest afterward. Give ordered antiemetics as necessary. Additional protein in the form of shakes is often well tolerated.

Nursing Care Plan Patient with Cancer—cont'd

Nursing Diagnosis	Goals and Outcome Criteria	Interventions
Impaired oral mucous membrane related to decreased salivation, inflammation	Patient will report successful management of dry mouth and oral mucous membranes will be intact.	Tell the patient to do frequent, gentle mouth care. Recommend artificial saliva for dryness. Encourage increased fluids, sugarless gum or candies, and ice chips. Suggest moistening food before eating. When the mouth is inflamed, avoid acidic, salty, or spicy foods.
Fatigue related to anemia, effects of cancer	Patient will report adaptations in lifestyle that reduce fatigue.	Determine the patient's need for assistance and schedule activities to conserve energy.
Interrupted family processes related to illness and therapy	Patient and family will discuss need to alter roles and relationships during treatment.	Include the family in patient teaching. Encourage them to plan with the patient for accomplishment of family tasks and responsibilities. Acknowledge family stress and fears. Refer to American Cancer Society, National Cancer Institute, and Oncology Nursing Society resources for help as needed. Ask the social worker to assist with financial arrangements.

Critical Thinking Questions

1. How could you find out what the patient already knows about his disease and what he wants to know?
2. How might the patient's emotional reaction to the diagnosis of cancer affect his prognosis or treatment?
3. Identify safety threats and specific nursing interventions to maintain safety for this patient.

Physical Examination

The physical examination begins with measurement of vital signs, height, and weight. Note whether there has been a change in weight. Inspect the face, scalp, and oral mucosa for lesions. Palpate the neck for enlarged lymph nodes. Throughout the examination, inspect the skin for color, lesions, edema, and bruising. Auscultate breath sounds and observe respiratory effort. Inspect the breasts for symmetry, dimpling, and abnormal skin color and palpate for lumps or thickened areas. Inspect the abdomen for distention, auscultate for bowel sounds, and palpate for masses. Inspect the genitalia for lesions. The scrotum should be palpated for descended testicles and, if present, for testicular lumps.

Nursing Diagnoses, Goals, and Outcome Criteria: Diagnostic Phase

Nursing Diagnoses	Goals and Outcome Criteria
Ineffective Denial related to fear of diagnosis of cancer, medical evaluation, and treatment	Acceptance and seeking out of medical evaluation and treatment by patient
Anxiety related to threat of or change in health status	Reduced anxiety: patient states anxiety reduced, demonstrates calm manner
Deficient Knowledge of diagnostic tests and procedures to tests related to lack of exposure to information	Knowledge of tests and procedures: patient correctly describes tests and follows directions related to them

Interventions

Ineffective Denial

When people detect possible signs or symptoms of cancer, they may be so anxious that they cannot cope with their fears. Instead, they deny the seriousness of the situation and do not seek medical care. Such delays may allow the disease to progress, making treatment more difficult and less likely to be successful. Encourage people to learn the warning signs of cancer and to report them promptly. Emphasize that these signs may be caused by conditions other than cancer but medical evaluation is needed for a correct diagnosis. Stress the fact that many cancers are curable, especially in the early stages.

Anxiety

During the diagnostic phase, the patient needs encouragement, support, and honest information. Be careful to remain hopeful yet not give false reassurance ("I'm sure it will not be cancer."). Clichés are not helpful either ("Everything has a purpose."). It *is* helpful to recognize what the patient seems to be feeling (e.g., "You seem to be very worried."). Information about tests and procedures allows the patient to prepare mentally.

Remember that patients who are being evaluated for cancer are under stress. They may show this stress through anger, irritability, fear, or depression. All of these reactions are normal under the circumstances and should be accepted with understanding (Fig. 25-5).

The physician reports findings to the patient and informs the patient of the diagnosis. In the past, it was not uncommon for the diagnosis of cancer to be kept from the patient. Now most patients are told of their diagnoses. This change has come about because

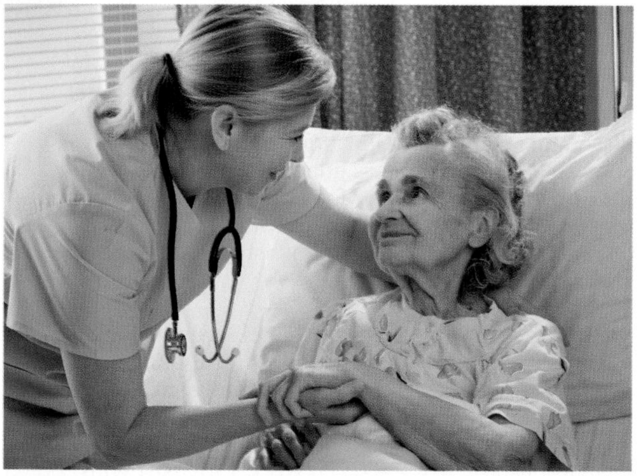

FIGURE 25-5 Listening and touching convey acceptance and caring. (Courtesy ThinkStockPhotos. Used with permission. All rights reserved.)

patients are better informed, cancer treatment has improved the odds of survival, and the patient's right to know is recognized. Nevertheless, you should know what the patient has been told, to avoid giving the patient conflicting messages. At times, you may need to help patients to communicate their needs and questions to the physician.

Once a diagnosis of cancer has been made, the patient needs support to adapt to the situation. Even at this phase of the illness, the patient may show various responses related to grief. Responses could include denial, shock and disbelief, anger, depression, bargaining, and acceptance. It is useful to understand and recognize how to help the grieving patient. Chapter 24 discusses nursing care of the grieving patient.

Patients struggle to adjust to the knowledge that they have cancer. For many, this is the first time they have seriously considered the possibility of their own deaths. They are typically preoccupied with what will happen to them. Researchers (Sigal et al., 2008) discovered that avoidant coping correlated positively with fear of the unknown and social diversion correlated positively with fear of pain and suffering.

People have different ways of coping with a diagnosis of cancer. Poor coping is sometimes related to lack of information about the disease and its treatment. In that case the oncology clinical nurse specialist may be consulted to provide patient education. Some coping styles are more effective than others. Recent research by Franks and Roesch (2007) found that individuals with cancer who appraise their illness as a *threat* are likely to use more problem-focused coping strategies, those who appraise their cancer as *harm* or *loss* are likely to use more avoidance coping strategies, and those who appraise their cancer as a *challenge* are likely to use approach coping strategies. Factors found to modify the relationship between appraisals and coping included age of the participant, time since diagnosis, and type of cancer (Franks & Roesch, 2007).

In the diagnostic phase of cancer care, patients typically use their usual methods of dealing with stress. When coping is not effective, a referral to a psychiatric clinical nurse specialist or a mental health counselor may be in order.

Deficient Knowledge

Tell the patient about diagnostic procedures, including preparation, what the procedure is like, and any specific postprocedure care.

Treatment Phase

Assessment

During the treatment phase, specific assessments depend on the type and site of cancer and the prescribed treatment. Information obtained in the initial assessment provides baseline data. Frequently and systematically collect data to determine changes related to the disease process and for effects and side effects of therapy. Areas of ongoing data collection are presented here.

Health History

Note the patient's diagnosis and treatment plan. Take the past medical history to reveal other acute and chronic conditions that require attention during cancer therapy. Obtain a complete drug profile and record allergies prominently. Review the systems to detect significant symptoms related to cancer or the treatment, including fatigue, weakness, headache, sore or dry mouth, dyspnea, palpitations, altered taste sensations, nausea, diarrhea, constipation, blood in stools, change in urinary frequency, hematuria or dysuria, sexual dysfunction, numbness, and tingling sensations. In the functional assessment, determine the effects of the illness and therapy on the patient's daily functioning. Explore the patient's knowledge, fears, concerns, and coping strategies. Also explore adaptations made by the patient and family during this phase.

Physical Examination

Note the patient's general appearance, level of consciousness, posture, and gait. Be alert for clues to the patient's mental and emotional state (e.g., eye contact, mannerisms, tone of voice). Measure weight and vital signs and compare with previous measurements. Assess the skin for lesions and bruises. Inspect the scalp for hair loss. Inspect the oral mucous membranes for lesions and inflammation. Observe the patient's respiratory effort and auscultate the lung fields for atelectasis or abnormal breath sounds. Inspect the abdomen for distention and auscultate bowel sounds. Inspect and palpate the extremities for color, edema, and peripheral pulses. Test reflexes and sensation in the extremities.

Assessment of the patient with cancer during the treatment phase is summarized in Box 25-4.

Box 25-4 Assessment of the Patient with Cancer in the Treatment Phase

HEALTH HISTORY

Chief Complaint
Diagnosis, prominent symptoms related to disease or treatment

Past Medical History
Acute and chronic conditions, previous surgeries and hospitalizations, drug profile, allergies

Review of Systems
Fatigue, weakness, headache, sore mouth, dyspnea, palpitations, altered taste sensations, nausea and vomiting, diarrhea, constipation, blood in stools or urine, urinary frequency, dysuria, numbness or tingling sensations, sexual dysfunction

Functional Assessment
Effects of illness and treatment on functioning, patient knowledge and concerns, stresses and coping strategies, family adaptation

PHYSICAL EXAMINATION

General Survey
Level of consciousness, posture and gait, eye contact, mannerisms, tone of voice

Height and Weight
Present and previous weight

Vital Signs
Present and previous readings, fever, tachypnea, tachycardia, hypotension, hypertension

Skin
Lesions, bruises, darkened or irritated areas

Scalp
Hair loss

Mouth
Condition of mucous membranes, dryness

Thorax
Respiratory effort, breath sounds

Abdomen
Distention, bowel sounds

Extremities
Color, edema, peripheral pulses, reflexes, sensation

Nursing Diagnoses, Goals, and Outcome Criteria

Nursing Diagnoses	Goals and Outcome Criteria
Anxiety related to effects and outcomes of treatment	Reduced anxiety: patient states less anxiety, demonstrates relaxed manner
Ineffective Coping related to multiple stressors or overwhelming threat to self	Effective coping: patient identifies and uses strategies that decrease distress
Risk for Injury related to adverse effects of therapy	Absence of serious adverse effects: patient has no signs/symptoms of injuries associated with therapy
Risk for Infection related to decreased white blood cell count and invasive procedures/devices	Decreased risk/presence of infection: precautions in place to avoid exposure to infectious agents; patient has normal body temperature; absence of redness, drainage from wounds, or venous access sites
Imbalanced Nutrition: Less Than Body Requirements related to anorexia, nausea, vomiting	Adequate nutrition: patient's body weight remains stable
Impaired Oral Mucous Membranes related to decreased salivation and/or inflammation	Decreased oral discomfort: patient states is more comfortable, moist mucous membranes
Constipation related to decreased activity, drug side effects	Normal bowel elimination: soft, formed stool passed at least every 3 days
Fatigue related to anemia or effects of cancer	Adaptation to decreased energy level: patient completes essential activities without exhaustion
Disturbed Body Image related to alopecia, surgical scars, loss of function, stoma	Adaptation to change in body: patient demonstrates acceptance of hair loss and scars or conceals them; adapts to functional changes; adjusts to stoma and learns self-care
Grieving related to loss of body part or altered appearance or function	Patient recognizes losses and moves toward resolving grief:—patient discusses feelings of loss, touches affected body parts
Interrupted Family Processes related to illness and therapy	Adjustment of family roles and relationships: reassignment within family
Ineffective Self-Health Management related to lack of knowledge, inadequate resources, denial, hopelessness	Effective management of treatment program: patient describes and carries out plan and self-care measures

Interventions

Anxiety

The thought of having surgery or of receiving cancer therapy may be very frightening to the patient. Suspect anxiety when a patient seems tense, apprehensive, or helpless. The patient may have poor eye contact, increased pulse and respirations, perspiration, and trembling. Tactfully share your observations and offer the patient an opportunity to talk. Encourage the patient to express feelings and identify the source of the anxiety. Listening and touch can be very effective in reducing anxiety. Recognize the need for patient teaching or for referrals.

Ineffective Coping

The patient may need help in setting priorities and in coping with the side effects of therapy. Strategies to promote coping include teaching, encouraging self-care within the patient's limitations, treating physical signs and symptoms, emphasizing abilities, coaching in relaxation strategies, and encouraging the use of coping strategies that have been effective in the past.

Support groups may be most effective at this phase. People who have been through the same treatments as the patient can be especially informative and supportive. The local chapter of the American Cancer Society can provide information about services in the patient's community. Some agencies can arrange transportation for therapy and medical care. The Reach for Recovery program trains women who have had mastectomies to counsel others in adapting to their losses. Groups are also available to help patients with ostomies resulting from cancer of the colon, bladder, or larynx.

When a patient must be isolated physically (as when receiving internal radiotherapy), it is difficult to provide emotional support. Remember to check on the patient frequently. Intercom conversations let the patient know that he or she has not been forgotten.

Risk for Injury

The patient may exhibit various signs and symptoms of tissue injury associated with cancer therapy. Specific nursing measures are described as follows for some of the injurious effects of cancer therapy.

Pneumonitis and Pulmonary Fibrosis. Encourage patients with pneumonitis to do coughing and deep-breathing exercises to reduce the risk of pneumonia. Protect the patient from exposure to people who have upper respiratory infections. If the patient has dyspnea, elevate the head and schedule care to allow adequate rest and avoid exhaustion.

Cardiac Toxicity. Patients receiving doxorubicin (Adriamycin) and BRMs (interferon, interleukin-2, and Trastuzumab) may show signs of heart failure, so monitor for dyspnea, increasing pulse pressure, and edema. Notify the registered nurse (RN) promptly if these signs occur. Care of the patient with heart failure is covered in Chapter 36.

Neurotoxicity. The patient who has neurotoxic effects of chemotherapy has special needs as well. Extremities that lack normal sensation (neuropathy) are prone to injury and must be protected.

Cystitis and Diarrhea. If the abdomen or lower back is irradiated, encourage the patient to increase fluid intake and empty the bladder often because of the risk of cystitis. Assessments of tissue turgor and mucous membrane moisture help to detect dehydration. Diarrhea may require the administration of antidiarrheal drugs and special perianal care.

Thrombocytopenia. Radiation and chemotherapy can suppress the production of platelets. When a patient has a low platelet count (thrombocytopenia), the blood does not clot promptly. Gentle handling is necessary to avoid trauma and bruising. Minimize invasive procedures, including rectal temperatures. After venipunctures or injections, apply pressure for 5 minutes to control oozing. Instruct the patient to use a soft toothbrush and an electric razor to prevent trauma to the oral tissues or the skin.

Immediately report any blood in the stool, urine, or sputum to the physician. Signs and symptoms of internal bleeding include increased pulse and respirations, restlessness, pallor, decreased urine output, and falling blood pressure (a late sign).

Anemia. Anemia is common after repeated cycles of chemotherapy, so patients should have hemoglobin and hematocrit testing done. Anemia is treated with packed RBCs and erythropoietin (epoetin alfa). A diet high in iron is recommended. Tell the patient to report palpitations, pallor, and excessive fatigue to the physician.

Reproductive Cells. Because of the potential for harm to the developing embryo or fetus, women are usually advised not to become pregnant within 2 years of chemotherapy or while receiving radiotherapy. Female patients of childbearing age should discuss specific guidelines with their physicians. Because sperm production is reduced, male patients are counseled about the advisability of banking sperm before beginning therapy with certain drugs.

Risk for Infection

Patients with low WBC counts because of radiation or chemotherapy must be protected from infection. They should avoid crowds and close contact with others who have infectious diseases. Promptly report any signs of infection (elevated temperature, foul wound drainage, confusion).

If the WBC count is very low, compromised host precautions (or neutropenic precautions) may be needed to protect the patient. Such precautions include a private room and strict hand washing by all who enter the room. Fresh flowers, fruits, and vegetables are not allowed in the room because they harbor organisms. Additional details on compromised host precautions are presented in Chapters 13 and 34.

Patients who receive chemotherapy may have a venous access device implanted to permit frequent intravenous access without repeated venipunctures. An access device also delivers the antineoplastic drug into a large vein with turbulent blood flow. This decreases the local tissue injury caused by the drug. The venous access device presents a potential portal for infection. Most agencies have standard procedures for care of the device. Because the device usually remains in place for the entire treatment period, the patient or a helper must know how to care for it at home. Care of venous access devices is discussed in Chapter 18.

Imbalanced Nutrition: Less Than Body Requirements

Anorexia is common with cancer therapy but maintaining good nutrition is essential. The patient is advised to eat a high-protein, high-calorie diet. Small, frequent feedings are sometimes easier to take than three large meals a day. Light exercise before meals may stimulate the appetite. If patients have specific food preferences and aversions, these should be respected. Many patients find that red meat and some other foods taste bitter when on chemotherapy. Use of plastic utensils may decrease the bitter taste. Nutritional supplements (e.g., Carnation Instant Breakfast, Ensure, Boost), enteral feedings, or both may be ordered if the patient has excessive weight loss (see *Nutrition Considerations* box).

Nutrition Considerations

1. Impaired nutrition in patients with cancer can result from the disease itself or from the various treatment modalities, such as chemotherapy and radiation.
2. Cancer cachexia is a complex metabolic problem characterized by weight loss, anemia, and abnormalities in fat, protein, and carbohydrate metabolism.
3. The goals of nutritional care for patients with cancer are to prevent or correct nutritional deficiencies and to minimize weight loss.
4. Interventions for common problems associated with cancer therapy (nausea and vomiting, food aversions, anorexia, dry mouth, diarrhea, constipation) should be geared toward individual needs.
5. Immunotherapy indirectly affects nutrition by causing fatigue, chills, fever, and flulike symptoms, which may affect appetite.
6. Diets for cancer patients must be individualized depending on their baseline nutritional status, symptoms, and therapy side effects.
7. If oral intake is inadequate, enteral tube feedings or parenteral nutrition is considered.

Nurses should be familiar with the specific antineoplastic drugs so that the patient can be advised of any specific food restrictions. For example, patients taking procarbazine (Matulane) may have severe hypertensive reactions if they consume foods containing tyramine while on this drug. Foods rich in tyramine are produced by fermentation or decay. Foods that are spoiled, pickled, aged, smoked, fermented, or marinated, such as aged beef or cheeses and alcoholic beverages, have a higher tyramine level. Other foods that contain tyramine are avocados, bananas, beverages containing caffeine, eggplants, figs, pineapple, red plums, raspberries, yogurt, Brazil nuts, coconuts, peanuts, and liver. Patients taking procarbazine should not consume alcohol.

Persistent nausea and vomiting can lead to dehydration and malnutrition. Various combinations of antiemetics and sedatives can be tried as ordered to obtain relief, as outlined in Table 25-11. Newer antiemetic drugs such as palonosetron (Aloxi), dolasetron (Anzemet), ondansetron (Zofran), and granisetron (Kytril) have greatly improved the management of nausea and vomiting associated with chemotherapy and have fewer side effects.

Contrary to common belief, not all patients with cancer have problems with weight loss. Patients with breast cancer and Hodgkin disease often are nauseated but actually gain weight during therapy, possibly because they eat often to settle their stomachs. The important point for the nurse is to assess and treat each patient individually.

While antineoplastic drugs are being administered, sedatives are sometimes ordered so that the patient can sleep. Nursing measures to manage nausea and vomiting are detailed in Chapter 39. The following are additional suggestions for patients from the American Cancer Society (2013):

1. Take your antinausea medicine. Call your doctor or nurse if the medicine is not working.
2. Stay away from some foods. Eat less greasy, fried, salty, sweet, or spicy foods if you feel sick after eating them. If the smell of food bothers you, ask others to cook for you. Eat food at room temperature.
3. Have enough to eat and drink. Take small sips of water during the day.
4. On days you get treatment, talk with your nurse to learn about ways to relax if you feel sick before treatment.
5. Learn the best time for you to eat and drink. Some people feel better when they eat a little before treatment and others feel better when they do not eat before treatment.
6. After treatment wait at least 1 hour before eating or drinking.

Food and beverages that are helpful for patients with nausea and vomiting are listed in Box 25-5.

Pharmacology Capsule

Many newer drugs are in oral formulation. Patients may feel that taking pills will produce fewer side effects than intravenous medications. However, the actual emetic potential of a drug, not necessarily the route of administration, determines the degree of chemotherapy-induced nausea and vomiting. Patients who are receiving oral medicines need as much education as those receiving intravenous drugs. It is vital that they receive the appropriate antiemetics to take at home.

Impaired Oral Mucous Membranes

A number of measures are helpful when the patient has xerostomia (dry mouth). Patients should try frequent, gentle mouth care and artificial saliva to increase comfort. Several commercial products on the market

Table 25-11 Medication Therapy: Antiemetics Used with Cancer Therapy

CLASSIFICATION	SPECIFIC DRUGS	SIDE EFFECTS
Phenothiazines	prochlorperazine maleate (Compazine) chlorpromazine hydrochloride (Thorazine) thiethylperazine maleate (Torecan) promethazine hydrochloride (Phenergan) perphenazine hydrochloride (Trilafon) fluphenazine hydrochloride (Prolixin)	Sedation, hypotension, extrapyramidal symptoms
Antihistamines	diphenhydramine (Benadryl) hydroxyzine hydrochloride (Vistaril) cyclizine hydrochloride (Marezine) meclizine hydrochloride (Bonine, Antivert) dimenhydrinate (Dramamine)	Sedation, dry mouth, constipation
Butyrophenones	droperidol (Inapsine) haloperidol lactate (Haldol)	Extrapyramidal symptoms (such as akathisia, dystonia, pseudoparkinsonism, and dyskinesia) Sedation, hypotension
Corticosteroids	dexamethasone (Decadron)	Fluid retention
Hypnotics or sedatives	diazepam (Valium)	Sedation, ataxia
	lorazepam (Ativan)	Amnesia, sedation, dizziness
Cannabinoid	dronabinol (Marinol)	Visual hallucinations, somnolence, ataxia, hypotension
5-HT_3 Receptor Blockers	ondansetron hydrochloride (Zofran) granisetron (Kytril) dolasetron (Anzemet) palonosetron (Aloxi)	Constipation, diarrhea, headache Headache, constipation, somnolence, diarrhea, asthenia, fever, taste disorders Headache, bradycardia Headache, constipation, diarrhea, dizziness
Miscellaneous agents	metoclopramide hydrochloride (Reglan) aprepitant (Emend)	Sedation, diarrhea, dizziness, extrapyramidal symptoms Abdominal pain, fatigue, dehydration, dizziness

Box 25-5 Recommended Food and Beverages for the Patient with Nausea and Vomiting

SOUPS
- Clear broth, such as chicken, beef, and vegetable

BEVERAGES
- Clear soda such as ginger ale
- Cranberry or grape juice
- Oral rehydration solution drinks, such as Pedialyte
- Tea
- Water

MEALS AND SNACKS
- Chicken—broiled or baked, without the skin
- Cream of Wheat or Cream of Rice cereal
- Crackers or pretzels
- Oatmeal
- Pasta or noodles
- Potatoes—boiled, without the skin
- White rice
- White toast

FRUITS AND SWEETS
- Bananas
- Canned fruit such as applesauce, peaches, and pears
- Gelatin (Jell-O)
- Popsicles and sherbet
- Yogurt (plain or vanilla)

moisten the mouth. Various protocols for mouth care can be used. For example, the patient can rinse the mouth with normal saline, a solution of 1 tablespoon of hydrogen peroxide in a glass of water, or a solution of ½ teaspoon of bicarbonate of soda in a glass of water. Encourage the patient to increase fluid intake, chew sugarless gum or candies, suck on ice chips, and moisten dry food before eating. Lemon and glycerin swabs are no longer recommended because lemon juice dehydrates oral tissues and glycerin provides a medium for bacterial growth.

Mucositis is inflammation of the mucosa and it may extend from the mouth and affect the entire intestinal tract. It is a painful condition that can interfere with adequate food intake. The patient who has stomatitis should continue mouth care as prescribed, eat soft foods, and avoid foods that are acidic, salty, or spicy. A soft-bristled or foam toothbrush should be used. Normal saline alone or with sodium bicarbonate makes a soothing mouthwash and should be used at least four times a day.

Constipation

Some patients are constipated while on cancer therapy because of reduced activity, opioid analgesics, and the effects of some antineoplastic drugs. Monitor the patient's bowel movements to detect constipation. The physician may prescribe a high-fiber diet, stool softeners, laxatives, and phosphate or biphosphate enemas to prevent or treat constipation.

Fatigue

Fatigue is a common symptom in the patient with cancer. In addition, side effects of therapy may cause the patient to tire easily. Determine the patient's need for assistance and schedule activities to conserve energy. In addition, encourage the patient to prioritize activities and ask others to assume less important ones. Daily naps and mild exercise may be helpful.

Disturbed Body Image

The effects of cancer and cancer treatments can alter physical appearance and function. For example, patients receiving chemotherapy may have hair loss. Surgical interventions may result in visible scars, altered functioning, loss of body structures, and ostomies.

Be sensitive to the patient's concern about hair loss. At first, the patient may just note extra hair in the brush or comb. Later, hair often comes out in clumps. Hair loss may be partial or complete. Typically, hair begins to grow back soon after the completion of chemotherapy and 4 to 6 months after the completion of radiotherapy. It is not unusual for the new hair to be a different color or texture. After large doses of radiation to the head, hair in the treated area may not return. Although some patients take this in stride, others may wish to use wigs, scarves, or hats to cover the head. Some insurance companies cover the price of wigs; others do not. The American Cancer Society gives wigs to patients free of charge. The society also sponsors the "Look Good … Feel Better" program to assist patients in looking their best during therapy.

Whereas hair usually grows back, other effects of cancer treatment are often permanent. Patients need time and support to incorporate those changes into their body images and to regain a healthy self-concept.

Grieving

Treatment of cancer often results in temporary or permanent changes in body appearance or function. Changes or losses often trigger a grief response. The patient may be sad or tearful or verbalize feelings about the loss. Listen in an accepting way that lets the patient know that the feelings are understood. Behaviors that suggest that the patient is beginning to accept the loss or change include talking about the loss and looking at or touching the affected part. Support the patient as needed and provide practical information about adapting to the loss. Participation in a support group may help the patient to learn new coping strategies and begin to resolve the grief process.

Interrupted Family Processes

While undergoing treatment for cancer, the patient may be concerned with meeting responsibilities at home and at work. Some treatments extend over many months and make it difficult to maintain one's usual activities. Side effects of the treatment may make the patient feel tired and discouraged. Family and friends need to understand what the patient is going through and what they can do to help. Encourage them to remain involved with the patient. Family members may need help in handling their own responses to the patient's illness.

Financial concerns may be very serious for the patient and family. Obtain a social work consultation if necessary to assist them with insurance and disability claims and financial assistance referrals.

Ineffective Self-Health Management

A pretreatment teaching plan informs the patient of what the prescribed therapy involves and what the experience will be like. Know what the physician has told the patient and reinforce that teaching. One source of information is the National Cancer Institute's Cancer Information Service (CIS). Booklets on cancer, cancer therapy, and coping can be obtained by calling CIS at 1-800-4CANCER. A variety of materials is available from the American Cancer Society that can be accessed by calling 1-800-227-2345 (or at www.cancer.org).

Chemotherapy. If chemotherapy is prescribed, the teaching plan includes a description of the drugs to be administered, the potential side effects, and related precautions. Provide written information to supplement the verbal teaching. Explore what the patient has heard about chemotherapy and correct any misconceptions. Many patients have heard horror stories about drug side effects, especially nausea and vomiting. Inform the patient of measures that can be taken that usually make the side effects more tolerable. Key teaching points for the patient who is receiving chemotherapy or radiation therapy are summarized in the *Patient Teaching* boxes.

Patient Teaching

External Radiation Therapy

- Having the treatment is much like having a radiograph (x-ray). You are positioned on a table and the machine is adjusted to direct the beam appropriately. During the treatment, you are alone in the room but closed-circuit television permits the staff to see you. In addition, a two-way intercom allows you and the therapist to talk as needed during the procedure.
- The treatment is not painful. In fact, no sensations at all are felt related to the radiation. The machine that houses the radiation is controlled by a radiotherapist. You will hear whirring or clicking sounds as the machine operates.

Continued

Patient Teaching—cont'd

- These treatments do not cause you to be radioactive. The radioactive material remains in the machine. Only the rays emitted by the material come in contact with you. When the machine is turned off, no radiation exposure occurs.
- The skin markings made by the therapist are used to direct the radiation to the treatment site. Do not wash the marks off until the physician gives you permission to do so.
- Skin over the area being treated may become irritated. Keep irritated skin clean and dry but do not apply lotions. Cotton clothing may feel more comfortable over irritated skin. Antiperspirants should not be applied to a treatment site but cornstarch can be used to absorb moisture. Special lotions are available from your radiation nurse or physician, who will instruct you on how and when to use them.

Patient Teaching

Internal Radiation Therapy

- The radioactive material is given orally, injected into a vein, or a physician implants it.
- You are placed in a private room for a specified period of time for the treatment.
- Visitors and staff are restricted in the amount of time they can spend in your room, to limit their exposure to radiation. They also will maintain some distance from you when they are in the room.
- If a sealed source is to be placed in a body cavity, you may be required to maintain a certain position to keep the source positioned correctly.

Recovery and Rehabilitation

If the outcome of treatment appears to be a cure, the patient and family are usually overjoyed. However, some patients become excessively concerned with their bodies, constantly monitoring for new evidence of cancer. Periodic checkups are essential but may be dreaded because the patient realizes that complete or permanent recovery cannot be guaranteed. If any signs of a possible recurrence appear, patients are understandably concerned.

As patients recover from the effects of cancer and cancer therapy, rehabilitation may be needed to restore them to the highest possible level of functioning.

Put on Your Thinking Cap!

You are assigned to two patients who are being treated for cancer. One is receiving external radiation; the other is receiving chemotherapy.

1. Identify nursing diagnoses that might appear in the care plans of *both* of these patients.
2. Identify one adverse effect that occurs with radiation but not with chemotherapy.
3. Identify one adverse effect that occurs with chemotherapy but not with radiation.

Terminal Illness

Although increasing numbers of people are surviving cancer, it is still the second leading cause of death. If treatment is unsuccessful, the patient eventually begins to decline. Patients need to know what resources are available to them and to their families. The oncology clinical nurse specialist is an excellent resource person for the patient. Provide information about home health care, hospice, and voluntary and charitable organizations whose services might be needed. For patients who wish to die at home, hospice provides the support and teaching needed for this to be honored. The focus of hospice is to keep the patient's symptoms, especially pain, under control during the final period of the illness. In addition, hospice staff provides bereavement care after the patient's death.

To work effectively with these patients, you must be aware of your own feelings about dying. You can help the terminal patient in many ways. Continue to be attentive and accepting. New nurses often fear that patients will ask them questions they cannot answer. It is all right to admit that you do not know but acknowledge the patient's concerns. Listening carefully is more important than talking. Guide patients to claim their accomplishments and find peace with their failures. Terminally ill patients should remember that although they are going to die eventually, they are living now and can still have some pleasure. Chapter 24 discusses care of the dying patient in more detail.

People with terminal cancer often express fear of having great pain as the disease progresses. Although cancer is usually painless in the early stages, advanced disease often causes pain. Cancer pain can be caused by pressure on nerves, interference with circulation, obstruction of hollow structures (e.g., ureter, bowel, bronchi), and local tissue destruction.

General medical and nursing measures for the management of pain are discussed in Chapter 15. An especially good resource is the Agency for Healthcare Research and Quality (AHRQ—formerly AHCPR) publication on management of cancer pain. A variety of approaches should be tried to keep the patient as comfortable as possible. With severe, chronic pain, it is appropriate to medicate the patient at fixed intervals rather than on request. The patient may have pain at specific times or during certain activities despite the routine analgesic. This is referred to as *breakthrough pain.* If that happens, there may be an order for the additional as-needed (PRN) use of a short-acting drug with a rapid onset of action. Do not withhold ordered opioids out of concern about causing addiction. Analgesics that may be ordered include long-acting opioids (morphine sulfate [MS-Contin, Roxanol], fentanyl patches) that may be supplemented with short-acting opioids for breakthrough pain. Combinations of drugs, including opioids, a stimulant, and an antiemetic, may be effective for the patient with cancer. These "cocktails," although not used as much as they once were, often control pain when given regularly without causing excessive sedation. Advise the RN or physician if pain control is not achieved.

ONCOLOGIC EMERGENCIES

In the patient with cancer, conditions sometimes develop that require emergency intervention as a result of the disease process or the therapy. Some of the conditions requiring prompt recognition and action are hypercalcemia, syndrome of inappropriate antidiuretic hormone (ADH), disseminated intravascular coagulation, superior vena cava syndrome, and spinal cord compression. Characteristics of these conditions and related interventions are outlined in Table 25-12.

Put on Your Thinking Cap!

A patient who is receiving outpatient chemotherapy for cancer tells you that he is using natural vitamins and herbal products to help combat his cancer. He says, "They are all natural products, so they can't be harmful, right?"

1. How should you answer him?
2. What should you advise him to do?

Table 25-12 Oncologic Emergencies

EMERGENCY	RISK FACTORS	SIGNS AND SYMPTOMS	TREATMENT	NURSING CARE
Hypercalcemia	Multiple myeloma, metastatic bone cancer; cancer of lung, breast, or kidney; prolonged immobility	Fatigue, confusion, weakness, constipation, polyuria, hypertension, tachycardia, poor muscle tone If untreated, possible renal failure, coma, cardiac dysrhythmias, or death	IV normal saline and furosemide (Lasix) Drugs to promote excretion of calcium: plicamycin, calcitonin, etidronate disodium	Monitor fluid status. Give IV fluids and drugs as ordered. Record intake and output.
Syndrome of inappropriate antidiuretic hormone (ADH)	Thoracic or mediastinal tumors, thymoma, lymphomas, pancreatic cancer, cyclophosphamide (Cytoxan) or vincristine (Oncovin) therapy	Water intoxication and dilutional hyponatremia because of water retention: nausea and vomiting, anorexia, weakness Lethargy at first, followed by confusion, psychosis, loss of deep tendon reflexes, seizures, coma, and death	Fluids restricted to 500 mL/day; demeclocycline (Declomycin); IV fluids and diuretic agents administered only in late stage	Explain and enforce fluid restriction. Monitor vital signs. Keep intake and output records. Do not give demeclocycline with food or dairy products.
Disseminated intravascular coagulation	Septicemia, transfusion reaction Some drugs: vincristine, methotrexate, mercaptopurine, prednisone, asparaginase	Normal clotting process exaggerated, which depletes clotting factors Early signs: petechiae, ecchymoses, prolonged bleeding from venipuncture Late signs: signs of vascular obstruction, tachycardia, dyspnea, gastrointestinal (GI) bleeding, heart failure, and shock	Platelets, fresh frozen plasma, other blood components; heparin may be prescribed	Avoid trauma. Handle gently. Give blood products and heparin as ordered. Monitor vital signs. Look for bleeding.

Continued

Table 25-12 Oncologic Emergencies—cont'd

EMERGENCY	RISK FACTORS	SIGNS AND SYMPTOMS	TREATMENT	NURSING CARE
Superior vena cava syndrome	Breast or lung cancer, lymphoma, Kaposi's sarcoma, or metastatic testicular cancer that puts pressure on the superior vena cava	Redness and edema of face, conjunctiva; distended neck and thoracic veins; dyspnea, cough, tachypnea, tachycardia, cyanosis progressing to increased intracranial pressure	Radiation therapy, diuretic agents, steroidal agents	Give medications as ordered. Elevate head and arms but not legs. Tell patient not to bend forward. Reassure patient that symptoms usually subside in 2–3 days.
Spinal cord compression	Lung and breast cancers, lymphomas	Tumor in epidural space presses on spinal cord, causing intense pain, weakness, altered sensation in arms or legs, impaired bowel and bladder function	High-dose radiation, corticosteroid agents, surgery to relieve pressure	Give analgesic agents as ordered. Assess for full bladder, constipation. Do neurologic checks on affected extremities.

From Lewis MA, Hendrickson AW, Moynihan TJ: Oncologic emergencies: pathophysiology, presentation, diagnosis, and treatment, *CA Cancer J Clin* 61(5): 287–314, 2011.
IV, intravenous.

Get Ready for the NCLEX® Examination!

Key Points

- Cancer is the second most common cause of death in the United States.
- Early diagnosis and treatment increase the chances of survival with many types of cancer.
- The risk of developing certain types of cancers, and dying from some cancers, varies with race and ethnicity.
- Cells that reproduce abnormally and in an uncontrolled manner form neoplasms that can be benign or malignant.
- Benign neoplasms do not spread to other parts of the body whereas malignant neoplasms invade nearby tissues and can form metastases in distant parts of the body.
- Tumors are classified by anatomic site, cell appearance and differentiation, and staging.
- Carcinogens are factors that appear to increase the risk for development of cancer.
- The seven warning signs of cancer are change in bowel or bladder habits, a sore that does not heal, unusual bleeding or discharge, thickening or a lump, indigestion or difficulty swallowing, obvious change in a mole or wart, and a nagging cough or hoarseness.
- A diagnosis of cancer is based on tissue studies, laboratory tests, endoscopic examinations, and radiologic and imaging procedures.
- Surgery is a common treatment for malignant tumors.
- Internal or external radiotherapy is used to treat cancer because malignant cells are more sensitive than normal cells to radiation.
- Chemotherapy is the use of chemical agents in the treatment of disease.
- Radiotherapy and chemotherapy have serious side effects and adverse effects, including bone marrow suppression, anorexia, alopecia, nausea and vomiting, and local inflammation.
- Patients who receive internal radiation emit rays that can be harmful to others.
- BRMs act directly on malignant cells and promote the body's natural defenses against cancer.
- Patients who have suspected or confirmed cancer are under great stress and may respond with anger, irritability, fear, denial, or depression.
- In addition to helping with specific physical problems, nursing care of the patient with cancer addresses anxiety, risk for injury, deficient knowledge, ineffective coping, imbalanced nutrition: less than body requirements, risk for infection, and ineffective self-health management.

Additional Learning Resources

SG Go to your Study Guide for additional learning activities to help you master this chapter content.

evolve Go to your Evolve website (http://evolve.elsevier.com/Linton/medsurg) for the following learning resources and much more:
- Interactive Prioritization Exercises
- Fluid & Electrolyte Tutorial
- Pharmacology Tutorial
- Review Questions for the NCLEX® Examination

Review Questions for the NCLEX® Examination

1. Benign and malignant tumors are alike in that *both:*
   1. Press on normal tissues and compete with normal cells for nutrients
   2. Usually grow very rapidly
   3. Invade nearby tissues or disperse cells to colonize distant parts of the body
   4. Contain cells that closely resemble the tissue of origin

   NCLEX Client Need: Physiological Integrity: Physiological Adaptation
2. A chemical, viral, or radioactive substance that can cause cancer is called a(n) ____________________.

   NCLEX Client Need: Health Promotion and Maintenance: Disease Prevention
3. The nurse is teaching a class on healthy living. Select the dietary recommendation(s) believed to reduce the risk of some cancers that should be included in the lesson plan. (Select all that apply.)
   1. Limited alcohol consumption
   2. No dairy products or red meat
   3. High fiber, low fat, and low calories
   4. A variety of fruits and vegetables
   5. Limited smoked and nitrate-preserved foods

   NCLEX Client Need: Health Promotion and Maintenance: Disease Prevention
4. A patient's blood level of the oncofetal antigen CA-125 has continued to rise during 6 months of chemotherapy for ovarian cancer. What is the most likely explanation?
   1. The chemotherapy is effectively destroying the cancer cells.
   2. The patient is having an adverse response to the chemotherapy.
   3. The cancer is continuing to grow despite chemotherapy.
   4. The patient's immune system has been strengthened.

   NCLEX Client Need: Physiological Integrity: Reduction of Risk Potential
5. When working with a patient who has an internal radiation source, safety precautions include which of the following? (Select all that apply.)
   1. Always wear a lead apron when providing direct care to the patient with internal radiation.
   2. If the radiation source comes out of the patient's body, gloves should be worn to pick it up.
   3. When not providing direct care, stay at least 3 feet from the source.
   4. No pregnant visitors or staff should enter the patient's room.
   5. The patient must be in a private room

   NCLEX Client Need: Safety and Infection Control: Handling Hazardous and Infectious Materials
6. Adverse effects of radiation therapy commonly affect the bone marrow, hair follicles, and GI tract. What makes these tissues especially sensitive to the effects of radiation?
   1. They have inadequate defenses against harmful substances.
   2. These tissues attract radioactive substances.
   3. These tissues have very poor circulation.
   4. These tissues regenerate rapidly.

   NCLEX Client Need: Pharmacological Therapies: Adverse Effects
7. A patient asks why she is receiving a CSF as part of her cancer treatment. Which replies by the nurse are accurate? (Select all that apply.)
   1. CSFs stimulate the production of white blood cells by the bone marrow.
   2. With CSFs, the dosage of chemotherapy drugs can be reduced.
   3. CSFs reduce the risk of anemia that commonly occurs with chemotherapy.
   4. CSFs eliminate the need for bone marrow or stem cell transplantation.
   5. CSFs reduce the nausea and vomiting associated with chemotherapy.

   NCLEX Client Need: Pharmacological Therapies: Expected Effects
8. To monitor patients who are taking antineoplastic drugs, the nurse must be aware that the *most dangerous* adverse effect is:
   1. GI bleeding
   2. Increased intracranial pressure
   3. Bone marrow suppression
   4. Nausea and vomiting

   NCLEX Client Need: Pharmacological Therapies: Adverse Effects
9. Which of the following describes the action of BRMs?
   1. Treat mental depression that is common during cancer treatment
   2. Promote the body's natural defenses against cancer cells
   3. Immunize patients against some types of cancer
   4. Prevent the spread of cancer cells before metastasis occurs

   NCLEX Client Need: Pharmacological Therapies: Pharmacological Actions
10. Three patients at a urology clinic received diagnoses of prostate cancer. All were in an early stage and had similar expectations of cure. Mr. A. asked many questions and started to plan his work schedule around his treatments. Mr. B. stalked out of the office and slammed the door, saying that he would rather die than give up sex. Mr. C. was stunned and seemed unable to take in any more information at that time. Which of these patients' responses would be considered "normal" in this situation?
    1. Mr. A.'s
    2. Mr. B.'s
    3. Mr. C.'s
    4. They are all normal reactions to grief.

    NCLEX Client Need: Psychosocial Integrity: Grief and Loss

chapter

26 The Patient with an Ostomy

http://evolve.elsevier.com/Linton/medsurg

Objectives

1. List the indications for ostomy surgery to divert urine or feces.
2. Describe nursing interventions to prepare the patient for ostomy surgery.
3. Explain the types of procedures used for fecal diversion.
4. Assist in developing a nursing process to plan care for the patient with each of the following types of fecal diversion: ileostomy, continent ileostomy, ileoanal reservoir, and colostomy.
5. Explain the types of procedures done for urinary diversion.
6. Assist in developing a nursing care plan for the patient with each of the following types of urinary diversion: ureterostomy, ileal conduit, and continent internal reservoir.
7. Discuss content to be included in teaching patients to learn to live with ostomies.

Key Terms

Anastomosis (ă-năs-tŏ-MŌ-sĭs)
Colostomy (kŏ-LŎS-tō-mē)
Continent (KŎN-tĭ-nĕnt)
Ileostomy (ĭ-lē-ŎS-tō-mē)
Nephrostomy (nĕ-FRŎS-tō-mē)
Ostomy (ŎS-tō-mē)
Prolapse (PRŌ-lăps)
Stoma (STŌ-mă)
Ureterostomy (yŭ-rē-tĕr-ŎS-tō-mē)
Vesicostomy (vĕ-sĭ-KŎS-tō-mē)

Ostomy is the term used to describe an artificial opening into a body cavity. The site of the opening on the skin is called a **stoma**. An **ostomy** in the digestive tract may be a gastrostomy, jejunostomy, duodenostomy, ileostomy, or colostomy. The gastrostomy is an opening through the abdominal wall into the stomach that is used for long-term feedings. Jejunostomies, duodenostomies, ileostomies, and colostomies are created to drain fecal matter from the intestines. Examples of stomas in the urinary tract are the ureterostomy, ileal or colonic conduit, cystostomy, vesicostomy, and continent internal reservoir. Ostomies of the urinary tract drain urine from the kidney, ureters, or bladder. Ostomies are sometimes described as a means of urinary or fecal diversion. The term *ostomate* refers to a person who has an ostomy. However, many people prefer to be thought of as *individuals with ostomies* rather than as *ostomates*. This chapter describes the care of patients with ostomies created to pass urine or feces.

INDICATIONS AND PREPARATION FOR OSTOMY SURGERY

Ostomy surgery is done for a number of reasons. A temporary ostomy may be indicated after surgery or trauma or when severe inflammation or infection exists. The ostomy bypasses the affected portion of the bowel or urinary tract, giving it time to heal. Permanent ostomies are usually necessitated by cancer of the bladder or colon or severe inflammatory bowel disease (see *Cultural Considerations* box). Pouches are external appliances that are used with most ostomies to collect drainage. Whether ostomies are temporary or permanent, patients require considerable assistance as well as educational and psychologic support to learn to manage them.

Cultural Considerations

What Does Culture Have to Do with Colon Cancer?

In the United States, African Americans have the highest rates of colon and rectal cancers, which often are treated with ostomies. Therefore nurses should counsel African-American patients about the importance of periodic screening, emphasizing that early detection and treatment improve the chances of a cure.

Ideally the patient is prepared for the ostomy before surgery. The physician informs the patient of the need for the ostomy, what it is, and whether it will be temporary or permanent. Sometimes the procedure is done in emergency situations, as when treating acute bowel obstruction or trauma. In these situations, the ostomy may come as a great shock to the patient.

An important resource for the nurse and the patient is the wound, ostomy, continence nurse (WOC nurse). The WOC nurse is a registered nurse (RN) who has special training in stoma care. The WOC nurse may be a certified ostomy care nurse (COCN) or a certified wound, ostomy, continence nurse (CWOC nurse). The WOC nurse is often an appropriate person to assess and teach the ostomy patient. However, this does not relieve the staff nurse of all teaching responsibility. The staff nurse follows up and reinforces the instructions of the WOC nurse. In settings in which specialists are not available, the responsibility for teaching may fall primarily on the staff nurse.

The exact placement of the stoma is very important. The WOC nurse often consults with the surgeon regarding the ideal site. Two factors must be considered: (1) secure pouch placement and (2) ease of self-care. To provide a good seal, the site must not be too close to the umbilicus, bony prominences, scars, folds, or creases. If the pouch does not fit smoothly around the stoma, liquid stool or urine may leak around it. The stoma is placed below the waistline if possible. If it can be placed within the margins of the rectus muscle, the muscle will help to prevent peristomal hernias. The stoma also must be placed where it can be seen and touched by the patient. A patient cannot learn to care for a stoma that is located where it cannot be seen.

NURSING CARE of the Patient Having Ostomy Surgery

General preoperative nursing care is discussed in detail in Chapter 17. This section emphasizes only those aspects that are unique to the patient with an ostomy.

Assessment

Before ostomy surgery, you should be especially concerned with determining the patient's expectations, understanding of the procedure, information desired, and fears. The health history reveals the reason for the procedure. The medical history documents other acute and chronic conditions that will require management before and after surgery. Note drug therapy and allergies. During the physical examination, expect to see a mark on the abdominal skin where the stoma will be created. See Chapter 17 for other details of the preoperative assessment.

Nursing Diagnoses, Goals, and Outcome Criteria: Ostomy Surgery: Preoperative Phase

The nursing diagnoses and goals that require particular attention are as follows:

Nursing Diagnoses	Goals and Outcome Criteria
Anxiety and **Grieving** related to perceived threat to self-image, anticipated changes in body appearance and function	Reduced anxiety: patient states anxiety is reduced; relaxed manner Grieving: verbalizes reality of impending loss
Deficient Knowledge of what to expect after surgery in relation to the stoma related to lack of exposure to information	Patient understanding of postoperative routines and procedures in relation to ostomy care: patient describes routines correctly and participates in postoperative care

Interventions

Anxiety and Grieving

Be accepting of the patient's anxiety and try to help the patient identify exactly what his or her concerns are. Some patients may be concerned about appearance and others about how their jobs or family lives might be disrupted. The anticipated loss of normal function and change in self-image triggers the grief response. Encourage patients to talk and to use coping strategies that have been effective in the past. In addition, inform them about support groups and psychologic counseling that may be helpful at this time. Because moderate or severe anxiety interferes with learning, try to reduce anxiety before teaching.

Deficient Knowledge

Basic aspects of ostomy care should be taught before surgery. The patient's responses and questions guide you as to how much detail is appropriate. However, preoperative teaching usually requires repetition and reinforcement after surgery.

In addition to the WOC nurse, an important resource is a volunteer from an organization such as the American Cancer Society or the United Ostomy Associations of America (UOAA). Volunteers are people with ostomies who have been trained to counsel other patients about adjustment to their ostomies. Their personal experiences in everyday ostomy management can make them very effective role models. Another good reason for using these volunteers is that the patient has a chance to meet a person who is living fully with an ostomy. When a patient is referred to an ostomy group (with the patient's permission, of course), the organization tries to send a volunteer who is similar in age, gender, and occupation.

FECAL DIVERSION

Intestinal ostomies divert fecal matter through a surgically created opening in the abdomen. Although the various types of ostomies (e.g., ileostomy, colostomy) have much in common, differences exist and should be noted. The characteristics of the fecal material vary with the location of the ostomy and influence the type of care needed. Normally the colon absorbs water from the fecal mass as it moves toward the rectum so that it becomes progressively more solid. When the mass is diverted from the colon, it may be liquid, semisolid, or formed depending on the section of the colon where the ostomy is created. Fecal matter in the ileum is liquid. The closer the ostomy is to the rectum, the more formed the fecal matter will be.

Depending on the way an ostomy is constructed, it is described as an end (single-barreled) stoma, a double-barreled stoma, or a loop stoma (Fig. 26-1). An end stoma is constructed from the proximal end of the resected portion of bowel. The distal bowel may be removed or closed and left in place. If left in place, it is possible for the ends of the bowel to be reconnected, a procedure called *reanastomosis*. A double-barreled stoma has two stomas but they are no longer attached (i.e., the bowel is completely divided). The proximal stoma, which is continuous with the upper intestinal tract, drains fecal matter. The distal stoma is nonfunctional; it is referred to as a *mucus fistula.* A loop stoma is created by bringing a loop of bowel to the abdominal surface and opening it so that fecal matter can drain. The posterior wall of the bowel remains connected so that the loop stoma has two openings: one to the proximal bowel and one to the distal bowel. Both loop and double-barreled ostomies are usually temporary.

Before fecal diversion, a low-fiber diet may be prescribed for several days. This would require the patient to avoid consuming whole grains and most fruits and vegetables. Antibiotics that are not absorbed but pass through the intestinal tract may be given to reduce the bacterial flora in the intestines. Cathartics and laxatives are usually ordered to empty the digestive tract. Clearing feces and reducing the bacteria in the bowel aims to lower the risk of bacterial contamination of the abdominal cavity when the bowel is opened surgically.

ILEOSTOMY

An **ileostomy** is an opening in the ileum. The ileum is the distal portion of the small intestine that empties into the large intestine. An ileostomy is necessary when the entire colon must be bypassed or removed. Conditions that require colon bypass include congenital defects, cancer, inflammatory bowel disease, bowel trauma, and familial conditions such as multiple polyposis. Multiple polyposis is characterized by the presence of many polyps in the colon. Because these polyps often become malignant, removal of the colon may be recommended.

Procedure

A surgical incision is made in the abdomen and a loop or the end of the ileum is brought out through a second abdominal incision. The edges of the loop or the end of the ileal segment are everted and sutured to the abdominal skin to create a stoma. Loops may be supported with a device such as a rod or bridge instead of being sutured to the skin.

The physician applies a temporary plastic pouch or a fluffy dressing to absorb drainage in the operating room. The pouch collects fecal drainage to keep it from contaminating the surgical incision and to protect surrounding skin. The plain ileostomy frequently or intermittently drains liquid to pasty stool, so the patient will always have to wear a pouch. The stool output may be as high as 2000 mL per day initially. The small bowel gradually adapts and the output falls to about 500 mL per day.

Alternatives to the plain ileostomy are the Kock pouch (Fig. 26-2) and the ileal J-pouch anal anastomosis (Fig. 26-3). The Kock pouch creates a reservoir for the liquid stool so that it can be drained at intervals. The Barnett continent intestinal reservoir is a modification of the Kock procedure. The ileal J-pouch anal **anastomosis** essentially creates a new rectum from the terminal ileum. This procedure allows for nearly normal bowel evacuation. The letter *J* describes the

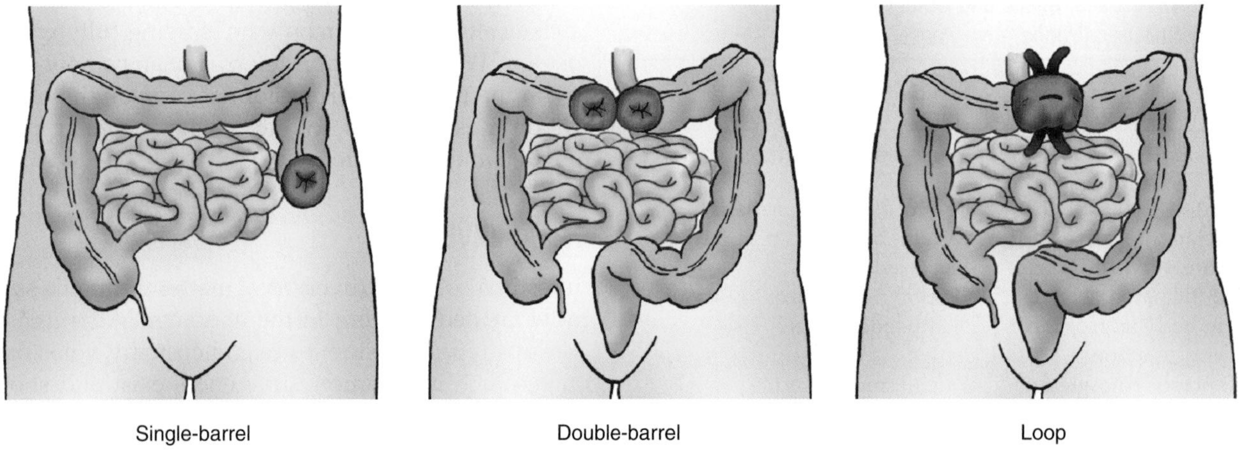

FIGURE 26-1 Types of colostomies. Single-barreled (end) colostomies are usually permanent. Double-barreled colostomies are usually temporary and stomas may be adjacent or several inches apart. Loop colostomies are temporary and are formed by bringing a loop of colon through the abdominal wall and supporting it with a plastic brace. (From Black JM, Hawks JH: *Medical-surgical nursing: clinical management for positive outcomes*, ed 8, St. Louis, 2009, Saunders-Elsevier.)

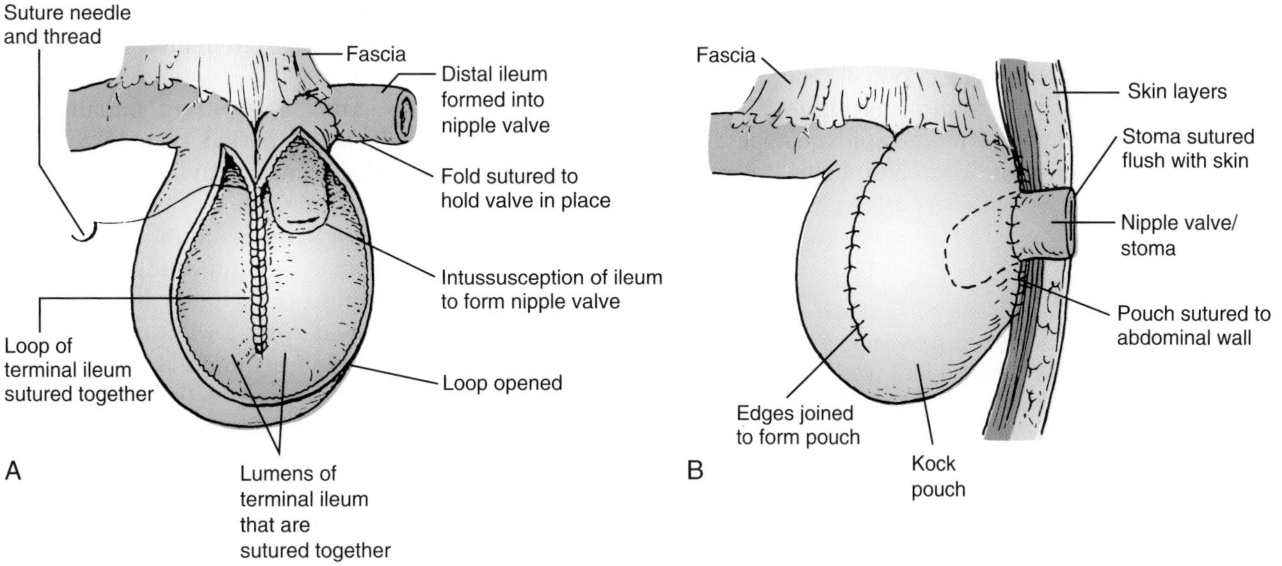

FIGURE 26-2 Continent ileostomy (Kock pouch). The pouch to hold fecal matter is created from a loop of ileum folded back on itself. (From Black JM, Hawks JH: *Medical-surgical nursing: clinical management for positive outcomes*, ed 8, St. Louis, 2009, Saunders-Elsevier.)

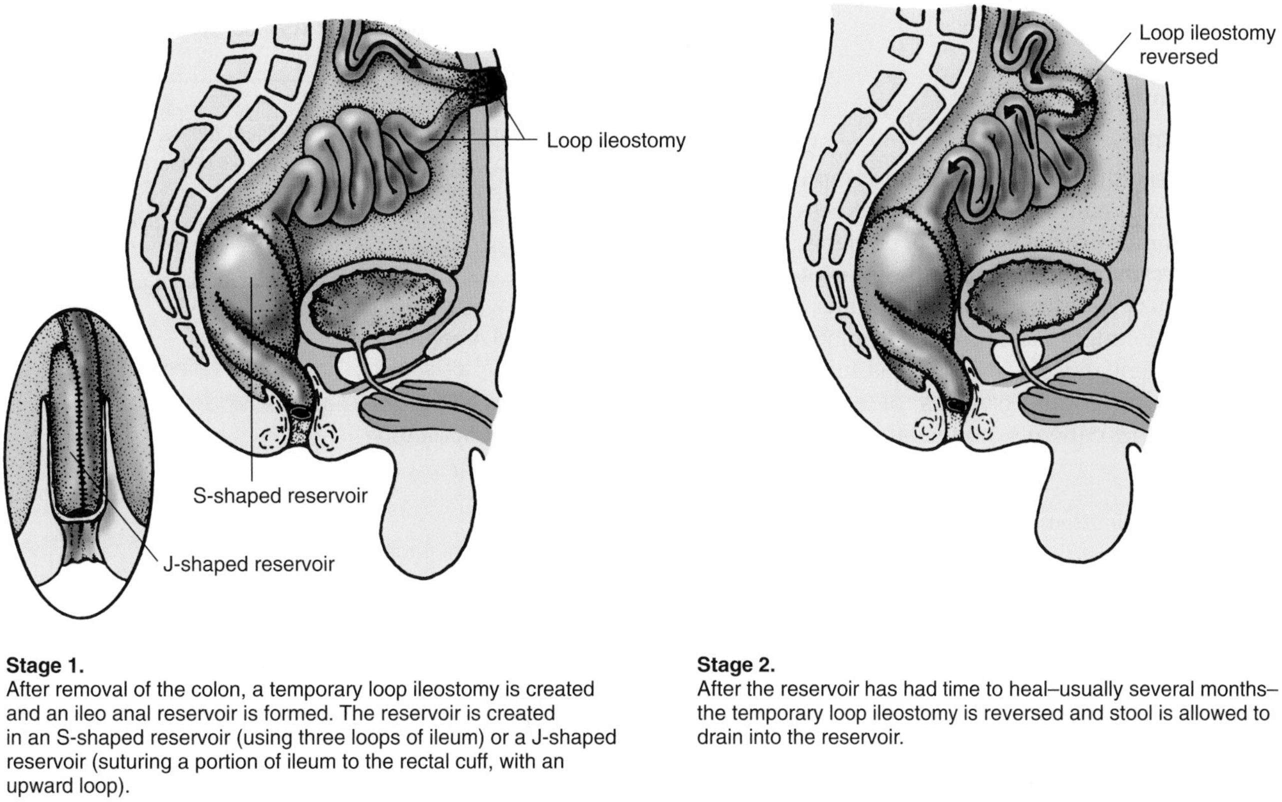

Loop ileostomy
S-shaped reservoir
J-shaped reservoir
Loop ileostomy reversed
Stage 1.
After removal of the colon, a temporary loop ileostomy is created and an ileo anal reservoir is formed. The reservoir is created in an S-shaped reservoir (using three loops of ileum) or a J-shaped reservoir (suturing a portion of ileum to the rectal cuff, with an upward loop).
Stage 2.
After the reservoir has had time to heal–usually several months–the temporary loop ileostomy is reversed and stool is allowed to drain into the reservoir.

FIGURE 26-3 Creation of an ileoanal reservoir. **A,** Stage 1: The colon is removed, a temporary loop ileostomy is created, and an ileoanal reservoir is formed. The reservoir may be J-shaped or S-shaped, depending on the technique used. **B,** Stage 2: After the reservoir heals (usually several months), the temporary loop ileostomy is reversed and stool drains into the reservoir for storage until it is eliminated through the rectum. (From Ignatavicius DD, Workman ML: *Medical-surgical nursing: patient-centered collaborative care*, ed 7, St. Louis, 2013, Saunders.)

shape of the reconstructed bowel; in addition, *S*, *W*, or *H* pouches exist that are shaped accordingly. The patient may have a temporary loop ileostomy while the pouch heals. Laparoscopic procedures are relatively new but promise a more rapid postoperative recovery, lower infection risk, and better cosmetic outcome.

Pharmacology Capsule

Ileostomy patients are usually not given timed-release capsules or enteric-coated tablets because they are likely to be eliminated before they can dissolve and be absorbed.

POSTOPERATIVE NURSING CARE of the Patient with an Ileostomy

The immediate postoperative care of the patient with an ileostomy is like that of most other patients having abdominal surgery. The patient has a nasogastric tube attached to low intermittent suction. Intravenous fluids are ordered for several days, after which oral intake is gradually increased.

General care of the surgical patient is discussed in Chapter 17. This section emphasizes only the special needs of the ileostomy patient beyond the immediate recovery period.

Assessment

Health History

After surgery, document significant symptoms such as pain, anorexia, nausea, vomiting, weakness, thirst, and muscle cramps in the review of systems. The functional assessment reveals how the patient is reacting to the surgery and how he or she thinks it will affect usual functioning. In addition, determine what stressors the patient perceives as well as his or her usual coping strategies and sources of support. Finally, determine the patient's understanding of ileostomy care.

Physical Examination

Begin the physical examination with observation of the patient's general status: level of consciousness, orientation, posture, and expression. Take vital signs and weight and compare them with preoperative findings. Inspect and palpate the skin color, warmth, and turgor and inspect oral tissues for moisture. Observe respiratory effort and auscultate breath sounds. In addition, examine the abdomen for distention and bowel sounds.

Inspect the stoma for color and bleeding. A new intestinal stoma should be beefy red. When healed it should be rose red, somewhat darker than the color of the oral mucosa. A very pale, bluish, or black stoma has impaired circulation and *must* be reported to the RN or physician immediately. Prompt surgical intervention is needed to restore circulation and prevent tissue necrosis. !

Swelling of the stoma is expected initially, after which it shrinks during a period of 6 to 8 weeks. Inspect the base of the stoma for redness, skin breakdown, and purulent drainage. A small amount of bleeding around the base of a new stoma is not unusual. In fact, it may be a positive sign indicating an adequate blood supply. If edema occurs later, it is probably caused by pressure created by an improperly fitting collection device. The device should be removed and replaced with one that has a correctly sized opening. Note the characteristics of draining fluid or fecal matter. The presence of some blood and mucus in the drainage is normal at first.

Record urine appearance and volume. Palpate extremities for warmth and peripheral pulses. It is important to observe for neuromuscular symptoms such as trembling, twitching, or cramping, which may indicate electrolyte imbalances.

General postoperative assessment of the patient with an ostomy is summarized in Box 26-1.

Box 26-1 Postoperative Assessment of the Patient with an Ostomy

HEALTH HISTORY

Chief Complaint and History of Present Illness
Type of ostomy procedure done and reason

Past Medical History
Acute and chronic conditions, prescribed drugs, allergies

Review of Systems
Pain, anorexia, nausea, vomiting, abdominal cramping or pain, weakness, thirst, muscle cramps

Functional Assessment
Response to surgery, anticipated effects on lifestyle, sources of stress and support, usual coping strategies

PHYSICAL EXAMINATION

General Survey
Level of consciousness, orientation, posture, expression

Skin
Color, warmth, turgor

Mouth
Moisture

Thorax
Respiratory effort, breath sounds

Abdomen
Distention, bowel sounds

Stoma
Color, bleeding, edema; condition of skin at base of stoma

Characteristics of Drainage
Amount, color, odor, blood, mucus

Extremities
Warmth, peripheral pulses

Neuromuscular Status
Trembling, twitching, cramping, change in mental status

Nursing Diagnoses, Goals, and Outcome Criteria: Ileostomy

Nursing diagnoses and goals common to most postoperative patients (acute pain, ineffective airway clearance, risk for infection, ineffective peripheral tissue perfusion, and urinary retention) are discussed in Chapter 17. Additional diagnoses specific to the ileostomy patient in the immediate postoperative phase are as follows:

Nursing Diagnoses	Goals and Outcome Criteria
Risk for Deficient Fluid Volume related to nothing by mouth (NPO) status, nasogastric suction, passage of liquid stool	Normal fluid balance: pulse and blood pressure consistent with patient norms, moist mucous membranes, urine output approximately equal to fluid intake, absence of neuromuscular symptoms
Risk for Ineffective Peripheral Tissue Perfusion (of Stoma)	Effective gastrointestinal perfusion (of stoma): stoma is beefy red
Impaired Skin Integrity related to adhesive, fecal drainage	Normal skin integrity: skin intact with minimal redness around stoma
Disturbed Body Image related to presence of stoma, altered body function	Adjustment to change in body image: patient makes positive statements about ability to adapt, learns and takes over ostomy care
Sexual Dysfunction and/or Ineffective Sexuality Pattern related to altered body structure and function or reactions to those changes	Fulfilling sexual expression: patient reports satisfying sexual expression, makes adaptations as necessary
Ineffective Self-Health Management related to lack of understanding of self-care with ostomy, failure to accept ostomy, lack of resources for proper care	Patient effectively manages ostomy: patient accepts responsibility for self-care, demonstrates proper care of ostomy, obtains necessary supplies
Risk for Injury related to obstruction of the ileum	Absence of injury: ostomy remains patent, drainage is continuous or frequent

Interventions

Risk for Deficient Fluid Volume

The loss of fluids and electrolytes through nasogastric suction and the passage of liquid stool can lead to deficient fluid volume and electrolyte imbalances. Administer intravenous fluids as ordered, with careful monitoring of hydration status. Maintain accurate intake and output records including urine, gastric contents, and fecal drainage. Monitor serum electrolytes closely and watch for signs and symptoms of imbalances: changes in mental status (confusion, anxiety), changes in neuromuscular status (twitching, trembling, weakness), poor tissue turgor, edema, and dry mucous membranes.

When the patient resumes oral intake, advise a daily fluid intake of 2 to 3 L. During hot weather or illness, additional fluids may be required. It is best to consume a variety of fluids, rather than plain water, to obtain electrolytes. The loss of bicarbonate in ileostomy drainage can result in metabolic acidosis. To prevent this, the physician may order bicarbonate replacement.

Risk for Ineffective Tissue Perfusion (of Stoma)

As noted above, a healthy stoma is beefy red during the postoperative period. As it heals, the color becomes more rose red. If blood flow to the stoma is impaired, the stoma may appear pale, bluish, or even black. Unless adequate circulation is restored quickly, the tissue will become necrotic. The surgeon must be informed immediately because surgical intervention will be needed to restore blood flow.

Impaired Skin Integrity

Check the pouch hourly at first to detect leakage. When the pouch is emptied or changed, try to keep fecal matter from contaminating the primary incision. Cleanse the skin around the stoma gently but thoroughly. Maintaining skin integrity is an ongoing problem for the patient with an intestinal ostomy. The presence of fecal matter on the skin provides a medium for bacterial, fungal, and yeast infections. In addition, the materials used to hold the pouch securely can cause traumatic injuries and allergic responses.

A protective barrier must be maintained to prevent skin breakdown. A plastic pouch is used to collect fecal drainage. A good pouch is one that protects the skin, contains wastes and gas, is odor proof, permits freedom of movement, provides security for the patient, and is not noticeable. Many kinds of pouches are available, as seen in Figure 26-4, but their features are basically the same. Some type of adhesive is needed to secure the pouch around the stoma. The pouch has an opening at the bottom that allows for emptying and rinsing. Some have gas filters that allow gas to escape while minimizing odor. Reusable and disposable pouches exist, including one that is flushable for easy disposal. The WOC nurse is a good resource person to help the patient find the right appliance.

Periodically (about every 3 to 7 days) remove the appliance for thorough cleansing of the skin surrounding the stoma. Gently peel the adhesive off the skin. Rough handling and frequent changes contribute to skin breakdown. Commercial adhesive removers are available if needed. After removing the adhesive, wash the stoma and the area around it with water. If soap is used, it should be nonoily and must be rinsed off thoroughly. Then pat the skin dry. The patient may be

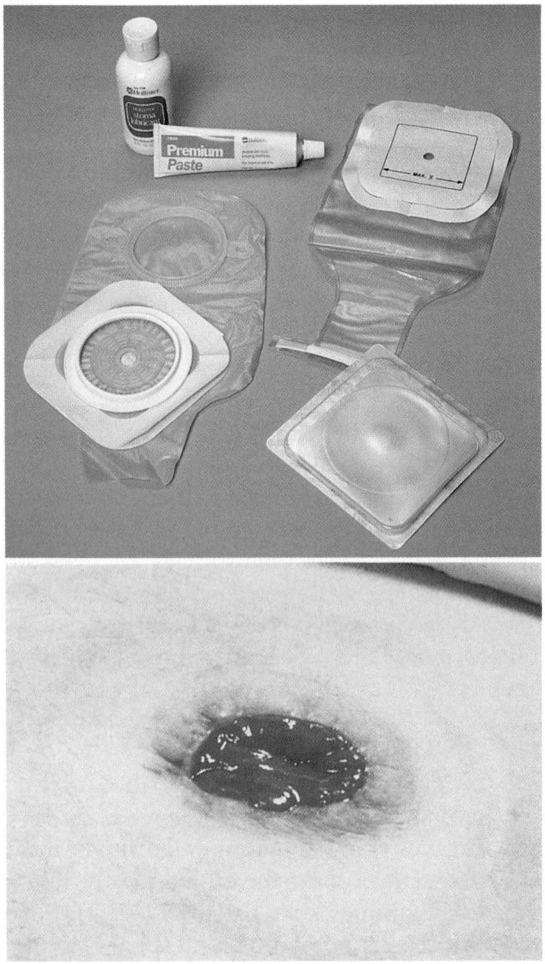

FIGURE 26-4 Supplies needed for an ostomy may include a pouch with an attached or separate skin barrier, a pouch closure device, skin barrier, paste, and adhesive remover. (**A,** From Potter PA, Perry AG, editors: *Fundamentals of nursing*, ed 5, St. Louis, 2001, Mosby-Elsevier. **B,** Permission to use and/or reproduce this copyrighted material has been granted by the owner, Hollister, Inc., Libertyville, Ill.)

surprised to find that although the stoma itself has no sensation, the surrounding skin may be tender.

A protective barrier must be applied before the pouch can be replaced. Skin sealants that come in the form of gels, wipes, sprays, liquids, and roll-ons may be applied to the skin. Sealants protect the skin; they do not hold the pouch in place. Next, apply a skin barrier. Commonly used skin barriers include powders, pastes, wafers, and washers. If the skin around the stoma is broken, ostomy powder may be applied followed by a special coating material or hydrocolloid dressing. Dust away excess powder before the wafer is applied. Wafers and washers may be precut or may have to be cut to fit around the stoma. The opening should be no more than ⅛ inch larger than the stoma because a larger opening permits more fecal matter to come in contact with the skin. If a paste is used, apply it around the stoma or on the cut edge of the wafer. Place the wafer over the stoma and press down. Some pouching systems have the pouch attached to the wafer; other systems consist of a wafer that is placed around the stoma and a pouch that adheres to the wafer. Some patients have an uneven skin surface around the stoma, making it difficult to create a seal. In that case a caulking material such as Nu-Hope Barrier Strips can be applied around the stoma to create a smooth surface. Clamp the pouch after it is securely placed. Initially, the pouch opening will probably need to be custom cut. As the stoma heals and shrinks, precut appliances may work well. Custom-cut pouches can be ordered for stomas of unusual size or shape. Patients whose barriers quickly erode and those with very convex stomas can obtain special barriers to maintain good fit. Once the stoma heals, some patients will prefer to cleanse the peristomal skin in the shower.

Disturbed Body Image

Establishment of bowel control is an important developmental task of childhood. The patient who has an ileostomy is no longer able to control the passage of fecal matter and must learn to manage bowel elimination in a new way. This can be very distressing to the adult who fears spillage and exposure.

Inability to control odor associated with passage of gas through the stoma is another concern for the patient with an intestinal ostomy. The characteristic odor of stool is generally considered unpleasant. Because the ostomy patient may have fecal matter draining intermittently, the source of odor is almost always present.

Assure the patient that odor is normal when the pouch is being changed or emptied but that it can be controlled at other times. Causes of odor include certain foods and poor hygiene. Foods that produce gas or stimulate bowel activity are most likely to contribute to odor problems. These generally include spicy foods, onions, garlic, some vegetables such as cabbage and beans, and high-fiber foods such as whole grains and fresh fruits and vegetables. Reactions to specific foods depend on the individual. Therefore advise the patient to delete and reintroduce various foods to find those that are most troublesome. Because flatus is usually evident several hours after eating gas-forming foods, the patient can eat those foods selectively at times when flatus would not be embarrassing.

Good hygiene also helps to control odor. Reusable collection pouches should be washed with soap and water. Rinsing with a vinegar solution neutralizes odors that cling to the pouch. Odor-proof pouches and commercial pouch deodorizers are available as well.

Sexual Dysfunction and/or Ineffective Sexuality Pattern

One area that often worries patients with an ostomy is sexuality. Encourage patients to ask questions about how the ostomy might affect sexual function or behavior. Patients may feel unattractive or fear rejection by their partner. Some men have erectile dysfunction or disruption of emission, especially if they have had nerve damage associated with perineal surgery. The surgeon and the WOC nurse counsel these men about options, which may include penile implants. Other patients have problems because of psychologic factors, which may improve with counseling.

Some practical suggestions may help the patient to resume sexual activity. The pouch should be emptied and taped down before sexual intercourse. Pouch covers are available to conceal the appliance and its contents. The partner wearing the pouch should experiment with positions that are most comfortable. Female patients should know that ostomy surgery does not interfere with pregnancy or delivery.

Ineffective Self-Health Management

After surgery, some teaching should be included every time stoma care is done. At first you may simply tell the patient what is being done and why. Then encourage the patient to take over more and more of the procedure. Ask the patient to demonstrate and practice as much as possible before discharge.

Some patients adjust more easily than others to an ostomy. A first step in accepting the stoma is looking at it. Note when the patient begins to watch stoma care. Patients should be encouraged but not forced to participate in the care. If a patient does not begin to show some interest in learning self-care after a few days, consider seeking help from supportive resources such as the WOC nurse or an ostomy club volunteer. You may feel frustrated if patients seem unwilling to learn self-care (see *Patient Teaching* box). You must be sensitive to the patient's feelings. An ostomy requires adjustments in body image and self-concept. Patients also have a grief response to this type of surgery. Chapter 24 explores nursing interventions to help the patient cope with feelings of loss.

Patient Teaching

Ostomy Surgery

The staff nurse, WOC nurse, or both must help the patient to plan for discharge. General topics to include in the teaching plan after ostomy surgery are outlined below. Specifics must be individualized to the patient and the surgical procedure.

- Stoma and skin care: Recommended procedures and supplies (and provide written care instructions and some temporary supplies when the patient is discharged).
- Appliances: Provide a list of the supplies needed and where they can be purchased.
- Irrigation (if appropriate) or drainage: Explain about the frequency, procedure, and supplies needed.

Other helpful points include the following:

- You can bathe or shower with your appliance in place because the pouch and the seal are waterproof.
- You can wear regular clothing but avoid direct pressure over the stoma.

Patient Teaching—cont'd

- You will learn to recognize foods that cause excess gas or odor, so that these can be avoided.
- Maintain a fluid intake of at least 2000 mL daily.
- Avoid heavy lifting and strenuous activities at first; usually no restrictions are made after approximately 3 months; ask your physician about specific activities and contact sports.
- Adaptations for sexual activity can include concealing the pouch and experimenting with positions.
- Contact your physician or the WOC nurse if you observe skin breakdown, prolapse (bulging out) of the stoma, or obstruction (output absent or markedly decreased).
- Resources for information about living with an ostomy include the American Cancer Society (www.cancer.org), United Ostomy Associations of America (www.uoaa.org), Crohn's and Colitis Foundation of America (www.ccfa.org), Wound Ostomy and Continence Nurses Society (www.wocn.org), and home health agencies.
- If you enjoy traveling, you can continue doing that. Tips on traveling include the following:
- Take adequate supplies.
- If flying, keep the supplies in a hand-carried bag. This could prevent problems if luggage is lost or delayed.
- Include sealable plastic bags to dispose of used supplies.
- Exercise caution with new foods that may cause diarrhea or gas.
- If visiting a country where drinking the water is not advised, do not irrigate a colostomy with the water. Use only water that is safe for drinking.

Risk for Injury

The lumen (interior diameter) of an ileostomy is less than 1 inch; therefore it can easily become obstructed. To reduce the risk of obstruction, the patient is initially given a low-fiber diet. High-fiber foods are then added gradually. Certain foods such as dried fruit, mushrooms, olives, popcorn, and foods with skins must be chewed very thoroughly so that they do not create an obstruction in the ileum.

Put on Your Thinking Cap!

Locate a resource in the area where you live that provides information for people with an ostomy. Share this with classmates.

CONTINENT (POUCH) ILEOSTOMY

The **continent** ileostomy has an internal pouch created from a loop of ileum for storing fecal matter. The advantage of this type of ileostomy is that the patient does not have continuous drainage and so does not have to wear a pouch.

Not all patients are candidates for the continent ileostomy. The patient must be capable of draining the pouch and the ileum must be sufficient for the valve to be constructed. People with ulcerative colitis are candidates for the continent ileostomy but patients with Crohn disease usually are not eligible.

Procedure

To create a continent ileostomy, a loop of the ileum is sutured together and then opened. A portion of the distal end of the ileum is inverted within itself to create a nipple valve. The valve prevents the leakage of fluid from the pouch. The looped section of the ileum is then closed, leaving a pouch capable of expanding and storing fecal matter. The distal end of the ileum is brought through the abdominal wall and sutured into place to create a stoma (see Fig. 26-2). During surgery, a catheter is placed through the stoma into the pouch and sutured in place. The catheter is connected to low intermittent suction to keep the pouch empty. This prevents stress on the suture lines while the pouch heals.

❖ POSTOPERATIVE NURSING CARE of the Patient with a Continent Ileostomy

In general, postoperative nursing care is like that described for the patient with an ileostomy. This section provides information on additional nursing measures that are specific to the patient with a continent ileostomy.

Assessment

Postoperative assessment of the patient who has a continent ileostomy is essentially the same as that of the patient with an ileostomy. When the patient has a continent ileostomy, it is especially important to assess for continuous drainage because obstruction of the catheter may occur. Absence of drainage or patient complaints of a feeling of fullness in the pouch suggests obstruction. The drainage from the catheter is bloody at first and then brownish.

Nursing Diagnoses, Goals, and Outcome Criteria: Continent Ileostomy

Nursing diagnoses and goals in addition to those previously listed are as follows:

Nursing Diagnoses	Goals and Outcome Criteria
Risk for Injury related to obstruction of the pouch drainage	Absence of injury: patient's pouch drains readily
Deficient Knowledge of technique for draining pouch and caring for stoma and pouch related to lack of exposure to information	Patient understands pouch and stoma care: patient demonstrates proper pouch drainage and stoma care

Interventions

Risk for Injury

In the initial postoperative period the patient is given only intravenous fluids. This allows the bowel to heal and peristalsis to resume. The catheter is removed after several days and the pouch is drained at intervals. At first the pouch can hold only 70 to 100 mL of fluid. Later it can hold as much as 600 mL. For the first 2 weeks the pouch is drained every 3 to 4 hours. During the next 2 weeks the interval is lengthened to every 5 hours. Eventually the patient will need to drain the pouch only two to four times a day. As the patient's body adapts to the ileostomy, the drainage gradually becomes thicker and the color of normal stool.

Deficient Knowledge

Key points in draining the continent ileostomy are as follows:

1. Have the patient sit or lie down for the procedure.
2. Gather supplies: lubricant, No. 28 catheter, drape, basin, irrigating syringe, irrigating solution, gauze dressing.
3. Lubricate the catheter and insert it gently into the stoma.
4. Resistance will be felt when the catheter reaches the nipple valve (approximately 2 inches past the stoma). Instruct the patient to bear down and then roll the catheter between your fingers and advance it into the pouch.
5. As soon as the catheter is in the pouch, gas and fecal matter begin to be expelled. Drainage usually continues for approximately 10 minutes and produces a total volume of 50 to 200 mL.
6. If the drainage is too thick, instill 30 mL of normal saline as ordered. Gently aspirate. Do not do this unless it is necessary because it may cause dislocation of the nipple.
7. When drainage stops, quickly remove the catheter.
8. Place a gauze dressing over the stoma to absorb any secretions.
9. Measure, describe, and discard the drainage.
10. Instruct the patient on how to perform this procedure as soon as possible.
11. Advise the patient to wear a medical alert bracelet at all times that states he or she has a continent diversion that must be drained.

See the *Health Promotion* box and the *Nutrition Considerations* box for a review of dietary considerations for the patient with a continent ileostomy.

ILEOANAL RESERVOIR (ILEOANAL ANASTOMOSIS)

An ileoanal reservoir is somewhat like the pouch ileostomy except that fecal matter is stored and then eliminated through the rectum. It is an alternative to an

Health Promotion

Dietary Considerations for the Patient with a Continent Ileostomy

Patients with a continent ileostomy will have some dietary restrictions and it is helpful to request a postoperative dietary consultation. The diet is intended to avoid excess gas, maintain a soft stool, and avoid obstruction of the catheter. Be sure that patients know they should avoid the following foods:

- Coffee, alcohol, and gas-forming foods (initially)
- Skins, seeds, and nuts (including corn, olives, and peas)
- Pineapple, berries, and fresh fruit (initially)
- Milk products, if they cause excessive gas

Nutrition Considerations

1. The patient with an ileostomy or colostomy may eat a normal diet and simply omit foods that seem to cause problems.
2. The main concern of the patient with an ileostomy or colostomy is odor, which is caused by flatulence.
3. Patients should be encouraged to avoid foods tending to cause bad odor, especially corn, dried beans, onions, cabbage, spicy foods, and fish.
4. Fibrous vegetables should be avoided and all food should be chewed well.

ostomy and information about it is included in this chapter because the patient has a temporary ileostomy and the nursing care is similar to that of the ostomy patient.

Procedure

The ileoanal reservoir requires a complex set of surgical procedures that are done in two stages. In the first stage, the colon is removed and an internal pouch that is created from the ileum is attached to the anorectal canal. A temporary ileostomy diverts stool while healing occurs. Approximately 2 to 3 months later, the ileostomy is closed if the reservoir does not leak and stool is then eliminated through the anus (see Fig. 26-3). The procedure is not recommended for patients with Crohn disease or poor rectal sphincter control.

Complications

The major complications of the ileoanal reservoir are (1) small bowel obstruction, (2) leaking of suture lines leading to peritonitis, and (3) inflammation of the reservoir.

Obstruction. Scar tissue or strictures may cause obstruction. Signs and symptoms of small bowel obstruction are abdominal distention, nausea and vomiting, decreased bowel sounds, and a change in bowel pattern.

Peritonitis. If fecal matter leaks through the suture lines of the reservoir into the abdominal cavity, abscesses or peritonitis can develop. Signs and symptoms are increased pulse, respirations, and temperature; rigid abdomen and abdominal pain; and elevated white blood cell count.

Inflammation. Inflammation of the reservoir may be manifested by bloody diarrhea, anorexia, and pain.

POSTOPERATIVE NURSING CARE of the Patient with an Ileoanal Reservoir

Assessment

The nursing assessment after surgery to create an ileoanal reservoir is the same as for the patient with an ileostomy. In addition, assess for rectal drainage and condition of the perianal skin.

Nursing Diagnoses, Goals, and Outcome Criteria: Ileoanal Reservoir

In addition to the nursing diagnoses and goals for the patient with an ileostomy, the following diagnoses may be appropriate for the patient with an ileoanal reservoir:

Nursing Diagnoses	Goals and Outcome Criteria
Risk for Impaired Skin Integrity related to frequent passage of liquid stool through the rectum	Healthy skin: intact skin without excessive redness around the rectum and the perianal area
Bowel Incontinence related to inability to control passage of frequent liquid stools	Control of bowel elimination: decreasing number of incontinent episodes
Risk for Injury related to possible small bowel obstruction, leaking of reservoir suture line, inflammation of reservoir	Absence of signs and symptoms of obstruction, suture leakage, or reservoir inflammation: no fever, abdominal pain or distention, bloody stools

Interventions

Risk for Impaired Skin Integrity

After the first surgical procedure, the patient's skin around the ileostomy stoma and in the perianal area needs special care (see *Cultural Considerations* box). Ileostomy care is discussed earlier in this chapter. Until the reservoir is well healed, liquid discharge may be expelled without warning. Thorough, gentle cleansing and protective creams help to prevent skin breakdown.

Cultural Considerations

What Does Culture Have to Do with Stoma Care?

The Muslim patient is expected to perform a washing ritual and pray five times each day. Because the patient will need to have a clean appliance for each prayer, a two-piece appliance should be used that will allow frequent pouch changes without skin trauma.

Bowel Incontinence

Initially the patient may have as many as 20 stools a day. After 1 week the number decreases to 8 to 10 daily. By 6 months the frequency is usually only approximately 4 to 6 a day. Nighttime control may continue to be a problem. Perineal pads or incontinence briefs may be needed to prevent soiling of clothing.

The patient must learn to strengthen the perineal muscles to restore control of fecal elimination. A recommended exercise is to tighten the anus, count to 10, and relax. This should be repeated five to six times, four times daily. In addition, drugs can be prescribed to decrease the frequency of stools and to make them less watery.

No absolute dietary restrictions exist. Advise patients to avoid fatty foods at first. The patient learns through trial and error how his or her body handles specific foods. Caffeine and fresh fruits and vegetables tend to cause loose, frequent stools. Pasta, boiled rice, and low-fat cheese tend to produce thicker stools.

Risk for Injury

Be alert for signs and symptoms of bowel obstruction (abdominal distention, pain, no stool passage), peritonitis (pain, fever), and inflammation (pain, bloody stools), which should be reported to the physician. If obstruction occurs, the patient is given intravenous fluids and kept NPO. A nasogastric tube is inserted to decompress the bowel. If the obstruction is caused by adhesions (scar tissue), surgery may be necessary to release the restriction.

Sometimes a stricture or narrowing develops at the site where the ileum is joined to the rectum. This is most likely to happen in the fourth week after surgery. The physician may be able to stretch the tissue manually and relieve the obstruction. If an abscess or peritonitis develops, the infection is treated with antibiotic drugs. Intravenous fluids are ordered and a nasogastric tube is inserted for decompression of the bowel. Surgery may be necessary to drain abscesses and repair the leaking suture line.

If the inner lining of the reservoir becomes inflamed or infected, the physician may do a proctoscopic examination to identify the cause. The condition may be treated with metronidazole (Flagyl) and steroids given orally.

COLOSTOMY

A **colostomy** is an opening in the colon through which fecal matter is eliminated. The location of the colostomy affects the characteristics of the fecal drainage; the closer to the rectum it is, the more formed the stool.

Procedure

A colostomy is performed by bringing a loop or an end of the intestine through the abdominal wall and creating a stoma for the passage of fecal matter. The location of the stoma depends on the portion of the intestine removed. Colostomies are classified by location in the colon. Therefore ascending, transverse, descending, and sigmoid colostomies exist (Fig. 26-5). An ascending colostomy passes relatively liquid material. The drainage from a transverse colostomy is liquid to semisolid. A descending or sigmoid colostomy passes softly formed stool. The colostomy begins to function on the third to fifth postoperative day.

A colostomy may be temporary or permanent. A temporary colostomy is done to allow healing of the intestine after surgery, trauma, or in certain disease states. Because the intestine below the colostomy is intact, the temporary colostomy may have two stomas. The stoma that drains fecal matter from the intestine is the proximal stoma. The distal stoma opens into the portion of the colon connected to the rectum. This is called a *double-barreled colostomy*. Sometimes the opening of the distal portion is brought through another location on the abdominal wall, creating a fistula through which mucus drains. If there is more than one stoma, the patient record should clarify which is the functional stoma that drains feces. An end colostomy with a Hartmann pouch for the distal segment is now more common than the double-barreled colostomy. A Hartmann pouch is created by closing the distal bowel and leaving it in place. The patient with a Hartmann pouch passes mucus through the rectum.

When it is necessary to remove a large part of the colon or the rectum, a permanent colostomy is made. If the colostomy is created in two stages, the patient returns from the first procedure with a loop of intestine protruding from an abdominal wound. The loop is held in place by a rod or a bridge. Later, the surgeon cuts the loop to create the stoma.

The main long-term complications of colostomy are **prolapse** and stenosis. A prolapsed stoma protrudes farther out than usual. It is caused by increased abdominal pressure, as can occur with coughing or sneezing. Other contributing factors might include an abdominal opening that is too large or a poorly attached stoma. Stenosis is the narrowing of the abdominal opening around the base of the stoma. If severe, stenosis blocks the passage of feces. Additional complications are associated with poor blood supply to the stoma, leading to necrosis and peristomal hernia. Peristomal hernia can limit bowel function, causing constipation, strangulation of the bowel, and poor results from colostomy irrigation.

❖ POSTOPERATIVE NURSING CARE of the Patient with a Colostomy

■ Assessment

The postoperative care of the patient with a colostomy is essentially the same as that for the patient with an ileostomy.

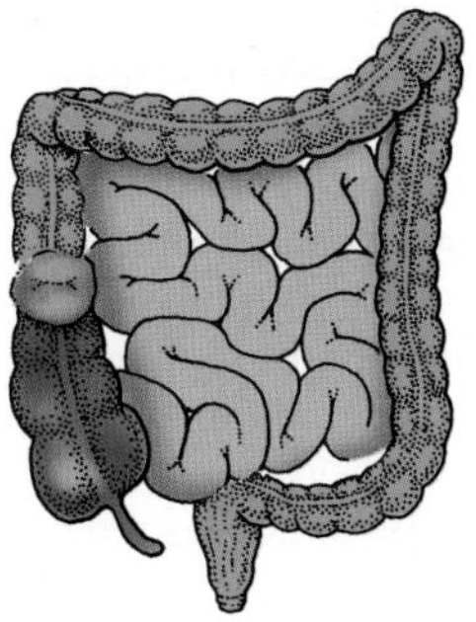

The **ascending colostomy** is done for right-sided tumors. This is an example of an end stoma.

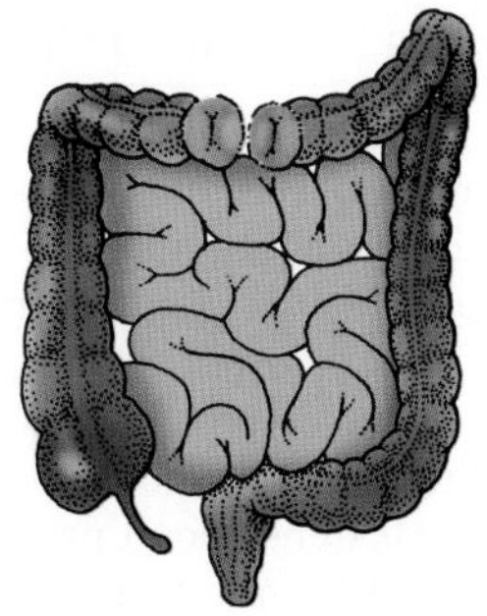

The **transverse (double-barreled) colostomy** is often used in such emergencies as intestinal obstruction or perforation because it can be created quickly. There are two stomas. The proximal one, closest to the small intestine, drains feces. The distal stoma drains mucus.

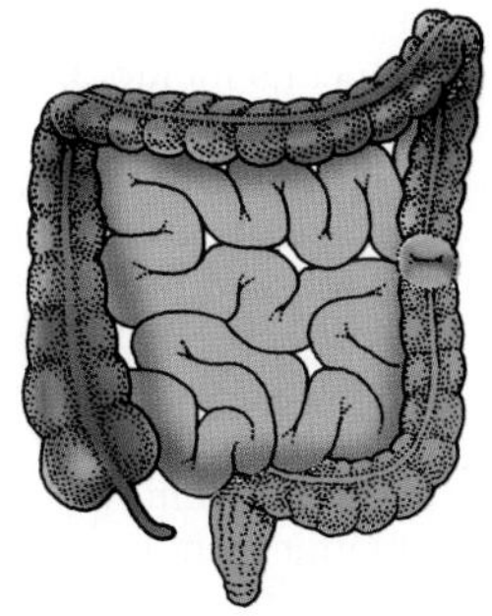

The **descending colostomy** is done for left-sided tumors.

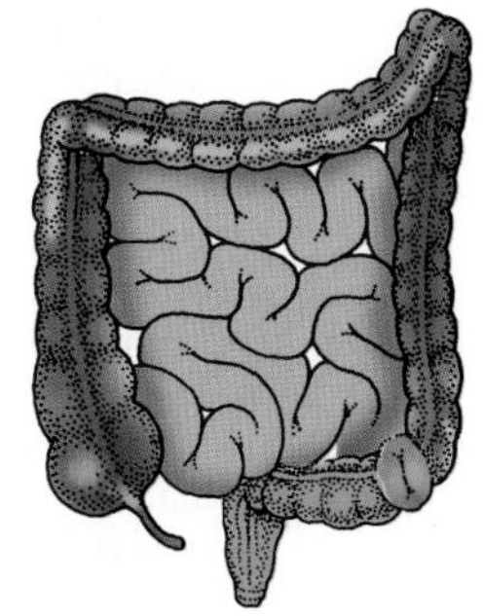

The **sigmoid colostomy** is done for rectal tumors.

FIGURE 26-5 Colostomy location depends on the reason for the surgery and, in the case of cancer, the location of tissue that must be removed. (From Ignatavicius DD, Workman ML: *Medical-surgical nursing: patient-centered collaborative care*, ed 7, Philadelphia, 2013, Saunders.)

Nursing Diagnoses, Goals, and Outcome Criteria: Colostomy

In addition to the nursing diagnoses and goals already identified, the following may also apply to the patient with a colostomy:

Nursing Diagnoses	Goals and Outcome Criteria
Ineffective Self-Health Management related to lack of knowledge of care and irrigation procedure (if ordered), lack of confidence, colostomy, lack of resources, failure to accept ostomy	Patient manages colostomy effectively: patient demonstrates irrigation (if ordered) and other ostomy care correctly; uses resources as needed
Risk for Injury related to prolapse or stenosis	Absence of injury: no signs of prolapse, no protrusion of stoma; patent stoma with lumen of adequate diameter: regular elimination of feces through stoma

Interventions

Most aspects of care are the same as those discussed for the patient with an ileostomy. A few points specific to the patient with a colostomy are presented here (see also Nursing Care Plan: Patient with a Colostomy).

Ineffective Self-Health Management

People with a sigmoid or descending colostomy may be taught to irrigate it every day or two to maintain regular, controlled elimination. Many patients have regular bowel movements without irrigation. Others are unlikely to establish controlled elimination and may find the procedure not worth the trouble. Patients who have liquid stools do not benefit from irrigation because they drain fecal matter continuously. Irrigation is unlikely to establish control if the patient has diarrhea when under stress, has had radiotherapy, has a poor prognosis, or has a history of inflammatory bowel disease. The surgeon and WOC nurse will decide whether irrigation is appropriate in individual cases.

Nursing Care Plan — Patient with a Colostomy

ASSESSMENT

HEALTH HISTORY Mr. Chin is a 47-year-old Asian American who had a bowel resection and permanent colostomy in the descending colon to remove a malignant tumor. He is 3 days postsurgery. He has been receiving intravenous morphine by patient-controlled analgesia and reports adequate pain control. He has had no nausea or vomiting but has a nasogastric tube attached to low suction. He is allowed nothing by mouth (NPO) and is receiving intravenous fluids at 150 mL/h. He participates in turning, coughing, deep breathing, and using incentive spirometry every 2 hours. He has discussed his fear of cancer with the nurse, stating that his mother died of stomach cancer.

PHYSICAL EXAMINATION Vital signs: blood pressure 118/64 mm Hg, pulse 92 bpm, respiration 20 breaths per minute, temperature 100°F (38°C) measured orally. Height 5′5″, weight 140 lbs. The patient is alert and oriented. His skin is warm and dry with good turgor. Oral mucous membranes are moist. Breath sounds are clear to auscultation. The abdomen is soft and bowel sounds are present in all four quadrants. The stoma is beefy red and edematous. A temporary drainage device is in place and the collection pouch has approximately 100 mL of greenish-brown liquid stool. Extremities are warm with palpable peripheral pulses. No muscle twitching or cramps are noted.

Nursing Diagnosis	Goals and Outcome Criteria	Interventions
Risk for Deficient Fluid Volume related to NPO status, nasogastric suction, passage of liquid stool	Patient will maintain normal fluid balance, as evidenced by pulse and blood pressure consistent with patient's baseline, moist mucous membranes, and approximately equal fluid intake and output.	Monitor for signs of hypovolemia: tachycardia, hypotension, decreasing urine output, and dry mucous membranes. Keep accurate intake and output (i.e., urine, liquid stool, gastric fluid) records. Monitor for signs of electrolyte imbalances: confusion, anxiety, twitching, trembling, muscle weakness, and cardiac dysrhythmias. Give intravenous fluids as ordered, monitoring rate of flow carefully.
Impaired Skin Integrity related to stoma adhesive, fecal drainage	Skin at the base of the stoma will be healed by time of discharge.	Check pouch hourly to detect leakage. When pouch is removed for emptying, prevent fecal matter from contaminating the incision. When changing the appliance, gently remove adhesive. Cleanse skin around stoma with soap and water, rinse, and pat dry. Apply a protective skin barrier before replacing the pouch. If washers or wafers are used, make the opening not more than ⅛ inch larger than the stoma. Report rash or skin breakdown.
Disturbed Body Image related to presence of stoma, altered body function	Patient will adapt to colostomy as evidenced by self-care and ability to resume normal activities.	Provide an opportunity for the patient to share his thoughts about colostomy. Identify specific concerns such as activity limitations, stoma care, odor control, and effect on sexuality. Provide information. Be accepting of the patient's feelings. Encourage him to attend to grooming and appearance. Offer to have a volunteer from the American Cancer Society or United Ostomy Associations of America visit him. Advise the patient that services are available from a WOC nurse, a mental health counselor, and a spiritual counselor if he desires.
Ineffective Self-Health Management related to complexity of ostomy care, lack of understanding of self-care with ostomy, lack of resources, failure to accept ostomy	Patient will manage ostomy care effectively: patient demonstrates proper ostomy care, uses available resources, and resumes valued activities with adaptations as needed.	During stoma care in early postoperative period, tell the patient what is being done and why. When the patient begins to watch the procedure, gradually encourage him to participate and then to take over care. Recognize the patient's need to grieve and that the patient may use denial as a coping mechanism. Develop a teaching plan that includes skin care, pouches, diet fluids, irrigation if appropriate, activity, sexuality, complications, tips on traveling, and resources.

Critical Thinking Questions

1. What would be some behaviors that indicate the patient is beginning to accept the permanent colostomy?
2. Why might a patient with a new colostomy experience grief?

Irrigation can cause complications. The tube used to introduce irrigating fluid can perforate the bowel. A perforated bowel permits fecal matter to flow into the abdominal cavity, causing peritonitis, a very serious infection. The risk of perforation can be reduced greatly by using a cone-tipped catheter. Other complications are caused by the type, amount, or temperature of the solution used. Plain tap water may cause fluid and electrolyte imbalances if used repeatedly or in large amounts. If too much solution is used or if it is too cold, the patient may experience cramping, nausea, and dizziness. Inform the physician if weakness occurs after irrigation even after the amount and temperature of the solution are adjusted.

If irrigations are indicated, you or the WOC nurse may perform them initially. However, the goal is for the patient or significant other to learn to do the procedure, so an explanation of the process must be provided (see *Cultural Considerations* box).

Cultural Considerations

What Does Culture Have to Do with Ostomies?

The involuntary passage of feces and gases, which is common with a colostomy, invalidates ablution, a ritual cleansing performed by Muslims. Refer the Muslim patient to the WOC nurse to see if colostomy irrigations are appropriate. Irrigations typically reduce the spontaneous output of stool and gas.

The following are key points to remember when irrigating a colostomy:

1. Have the patient select the time of day that is most convenient. The procedure should be done at approximately the same time every day. The entire process takes 45 minutes to 1 hour.
2. Have the patient sit on or in front of the toilet if possible. If the patient cannot get out of bed, the procedure can be done while the patient is in bed.
3. Remove the old pouch and apply an irrigating sleeve. This device opens at the top so that the tubing can be inserted into the stoma and it opens at the bottom so that fecal matter can drain into the toilet.
4. Pour 500 to 1000 mL of lukewarm irrigating solution into an enema fluid container and hold it at the level of the patient's shoulder. Initially, 500 mL is used but adults eventually increase the fluid to 1000 mL.
5. Clear the air from the tubing, lubricate the tubing, and insert it gently 2 to 4 inches into the stoma. The direction to insert the tubing can be assessed by first inserting a gloved, lubricated finger into the stoma. Do not use force! If a cone-tipped catheter is used, the catheter can be inserted only approximately 1 inch. This reduces the risk of perforation.
6. Allow the solution to flow slowly into the stoma. If the patient has cramping, slow down or stop the flow for a few minutes. Remove the catheter after the solution has been administered.
7. If the solution does not drain promptly, close the bottom of the sleeve so that the patient can carry out other activities. Complete emptying may take 20 to 30 minutes.
8. When elimination is complete, remove, wash, and dry the sleeve.
9. Measure the stoma before applying a new pouch, especially in the first 4 to 6 weeks, because the stoma size will change as healing occurs. The opening in the skin barrier should be just slightly larger than the stoma.
10. Apply a clean pouch if additional drainage usually occurs during the day. Some patients need only a small dressing or a stoma cap.
11. Rectal suppositories can be inserted into a colostomy stoma to stimulate evacuation.
12. Patients who have double-barreled colostomies can be given rectal medications through the distal stoma. Be sure you identify which stoma is the distal one.

Risk for Injury

Be alert for indications of colostomy complications. Although a prolapsed stoma may look frightening, it is not usually serious. No reason exists for immediate action if it continues to drain feces. It can usually be gently put back in place by the surgeon or WOC nurse. If the prolapse is severe or causes fecal obstruction, surgical repair is indicated.

Inform the physician if the ostomy is not draining properly. The surgeon may be able to dilate the stoma and enlarge the opening. If dilation is not successful, surgery may be needed.

URINARY DIVERSION

When the normal route for urine elimination is disrupted, it may be necessary to divert urine out of the body in a different way. The most common type of incontinent urinary diversion is the ileal conduit. Other incontinent diversions include cutaneous ureterostomy, colonic (sigmoid) conduit, cystostomy, vesicostomy, and nephrostomy (Fig. 26-6). Continent urinary diversions use a segment of bowel to create an internal reservoir that is drained via an abdominal stoma at intervals. The orthotopic bladder construction, or "neobladder," is a new bladder constructed from a segment of bowel. The orthotopic bladder is placed in the normal bladder location. It is attached to the urethra so that the patient voids normally. Not all patients are good candidates for the neobladder. Ureterosigmoidostomy and ureteroileosigmoidostomy are not performed as commonly now as in the past;

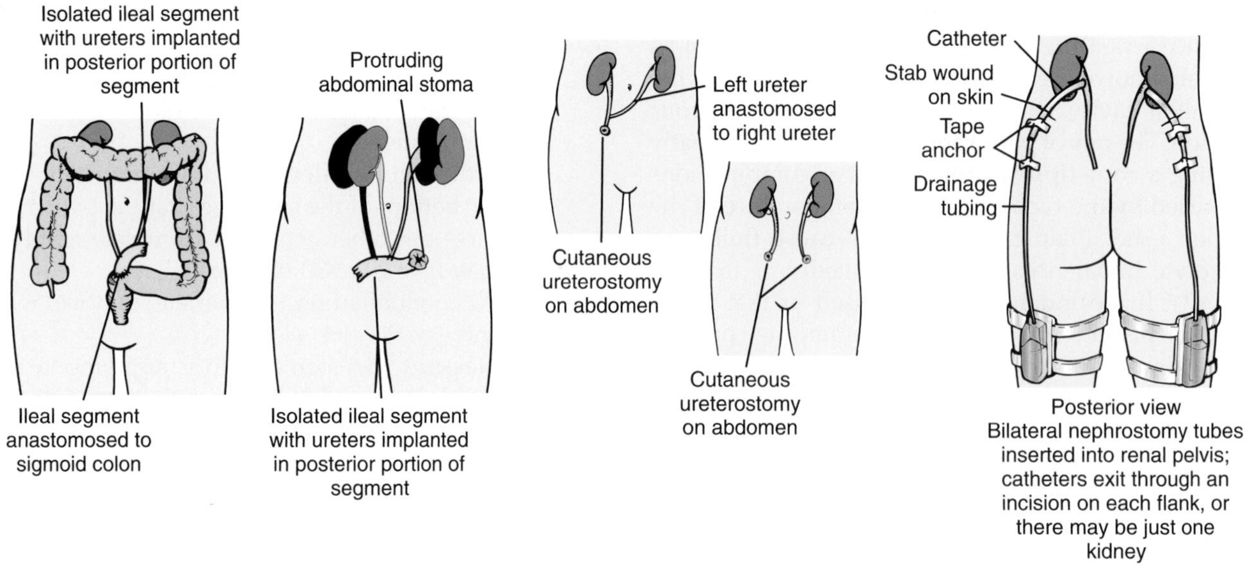

FIGURE 26-6 Types of urinary diversion. (From Lewis SM, Heitkemper MM, Dirksen SR, Bucher L, Camera I: *Medical-surgical nursing: assessment and management of clinical problems*, ed 8, St. Louis, 2011, Mosby-Elsevier.)

however, patients who have had them are still encountered. Decisions about which procedure to use are based on the patient's ability to tolerate surgery, life expectancy, and ability to carry out the care required for the various options.

Urinary diversion may be temporary or permanent. Permanent urinary diversion is necessary when the bladder is congenitally absent or removed because of malignancy or trauma or when extensive pelvic malignancy obstructs urine flow. Temporary diversion may be used when obstruction to urine flow occurs, as might be caused by a urinary calculus, or to permit healing of the ureters or bladder.

Preparation of the patient for ostomy surgery is discussed at the beginning of this chapter. Postoperative care after each type of diversion is discussed separately.

ILEAL CONDUIT

The ileal conduit is the most common type of urinary diversion. Other names for the ileal conduit are *ureteroileostomy, ureteroileocutaneous anastomosis, ileal loop,* and *Bricker procedure.*

Procedure

The ileal conduit is a urinary drainage system made out of a portion of small intestine. A 6- to 8-inch segment of ileum is first removed. The remaining ends of the ileum are then anastomosed (stitched) to restore bowel function. The ureters are cut from the bladder and attached to the ileal segment at an angle to prevent reflux. One end of the ileal segment is sutured closed. The other end of the ileal segment is brought through an abdominal incision and sutured to create a stoma for urine drainage. A similar procedure that uses a segment of large intestine is called a *colonic* or *sigmoid conduit.* The stoma of an ileal or colonic conduit is bright red because it is intestinal mucosa.

Complications

During the postoperative period, the patient is at risk for a number of complications. Complications related to the surgical procedure include leakage of the anastomosed ureters and intestinal segments, ureteral obstruction, and separation of the stoma from surrounding skin.

Other problems include wound infection, necrosis of the stoma, and paralytic ileus. The stoma may become necrotic if the blood supply in the resected segment is inadequate. If the stoma turns gray or black, circulation is impaired; the physician should be notified at once.

Complications that may occur in the later postoperative period are infection, crystal formation, and calculi (stones). The patient may also have problems with the stoma, including retraction, prolapse, or hernia.

❖ POSTOPERATIVE NURSING CARE of the Patient with an Ileal Conduit

Nursing care of the patient who has an ileal conduit is essentially the same as that for the patient with an ileostomy. A few special points should be made about the ileal conduit. This patient will have a nasogastric tube attached to suction to prevent abdominal distention and stress on the resected portion of the ileum while it heals. The patient is allowed NPO and is given intravenous fluids until bowel sounds return. A temporary ileus (absence of bowel activity) is expected after bowel resection. A ureteral catheter or stent may be in place to drain urine. If one is present, output is monitored because obstruction can occur. Mucus is normally present in drainage from a conduit because it is produced by the lining of the bowel segment. The pouch should be emptied when it is one-third to one-half full. The pouch should be attached to a Foley collection device during the night because the output may exceed the pouch capacity.

CONTINENT INTERNAL RESERVOIRS

All of the methods of urinary diversion already discussed permit urine to flow steadily through a stoma. Newer procedures allow for the storage and controlled drainage of urine. Examples of these, called *continent internal reservoirs*, are the Kock, Mainz, Indiana, and Florida pouches. The orthotopic neobladder (also called *ileum neobladder*) eliminates the need for a stoma. The neobladder is an internal urinary reservoir constructed using a resected segment of the ileum that is attached to the urethra and the ureters. Urine drains into the reservoir and is eliminated through the urethra instead of a stoma. The neobladder is used more often in men than in women. Continence varies with the neobladder, so an artificial urinary sphincter is sometimes implanted. Another option for patients who cannot achieve continence with the neobladder is intermittent self-catheterization. Even though the procedure is well received by patients, some surgeons are reluctant to spare the urethra with bladder cancer, fearing the urethra could be a site for recurrent cancer.

The Kock pouch is constructed with a segment of ileum. The ureters are implanted in one side of the ileum segment. A nipple valve is constructed from the other side and attached to the skin, where a stoma is created. The valve prevents urine from flowing from the reservoir. A catheter is used to drain the reservoir at 4- to 6-hour intervals. Other types of pouches are constructed from different parts of the bowel. The Indiana pouch is similar to the Kock pouch, except that it is made of a portion of the terminal ileum and the ascending colon. This reservoir is larger than that of the Kock pouch. The Indiana pouch is also drained with a catheter every 4 to 6 hours.

Complications

Complications of the continent pouches are incontinence, difficult catheterization, and urinary reflux leading to pyelonephritis, obstruction, and bacteriuria.

❖ POSTOPERATIVE NURSING CARE of the Patient with a Kock or Indiana Pouch

Immediately after surgery, the patient may have a drain to remove fluid from the operative site and a clear tube in place for continuous urine drainage. Irrigations may be ordered to remove clots and mucus. When the tube is removed, the pouch may be drained every 2 to 3 hours at first. Later the patient may need to drain the pouch only every 4 to 6 hours during the day and once during the night. If the pouch functions properly, the patient does not have to wear an external appliance. A small gauze dressing may be placed over the stoma to absorb mucus drainage. Advise the patient to wear a medical alert bracelet that identifies the presence of a continent device that needs intubation to drain.

CUTANEOUS URETEROSTOMY

A cutaneous **ureterostomy** is created when one or both ureters are brought out through an opening in the abdomen or flank. Often the two ureters are joined surgically so that only one stoma is needed. In some situations, a stoma is created from each ureter.

A ureterostomy stoma is much smaller than an intestinal stoma. Immediately after surgery the urinary stoma is pink but it quickly fades to a lighter color. Because no reservoir exists to hold it, urine drains from the stoma continuously. A pouch is needed to collect the urine and protect the skin.

Complications

Complications experienced by patients with a cutaneous ureterostomy include stenosis and urinary tract infections. Stenosis is a narrowing of the opening that interferes with the flow of urine. If the obstruction is not relieved, urine backs up in the kidney. The kidney may become swollen with urine, a condition called *hydronephrosis*, which leads to serious kidney damage. The kidneys can also be damaged by urinary tract infections.

❖ POSTOPERATIVE NURSING CARE of the Patient with a Cutaneous Ureterostomy

■ Assessment

Health History

The preoperative health history may be used to determine the reason for the ureterostomy as well as pertinent past medical history, drug profile, and allergies. In the postoperative period, the review of systems should include questions about the presence of flank or abdominal pain, fatigue, malaise, and chills. Also determine the patient's response to the ostomy, knowledge about it, and readiness to learn.

Physical Examination

Begin the physical examination with a survey of the patient's general state. Take vital signs and compare them with preoperative readings. Observe respiratory effort and auscultate for breath sounds. In addition, examine the abdomen for distention and bowel sounds and inspect the stoma. It is usually much smaller than an intestinal stoma and lighter in color. Document the amount, appearance, and odor of the urine. Some blood in the urine is normal at first but it should clear gradually. Ureterostomy drainage should not contain mucus.

Nursing Diagnoses, Goals, and Outcome Criteria: Cutaneous Ureterostomy

In addition to the common diagnoses and goals for postoperative patients (see Chapter 17), the following diagnoses may apply to the patient who has a cutaneous ureterostomy:

Nursing Diagnoses	Goals and Outcome Criteria
Impaired Skin Integrity related to contact of urine with skin	Normal skin around stoma: healed stoma base without redness or edema
Risk for Infection related to contamination of stoma	Absence of infection: no fever or foul urine odor
Risk for Injury related to obstruction of urine flow	Unobstructed urine flow: urine output approximately equal to fluid intake
Disturbed Body Image related to presence of stoma, altered body function	Adjustment in body image: patient acknowledges stoma, shows increasing interest in self-care, resumes previous sexual activity
Ineffective Self-Health Management of ostomy related to complexity of therapeutic regimen	Patient assumes self-care of ostomy: patient demonstrates proper techniques of ostomy care and describes self-care with an ostomy

Interventions

Impaired Skin Integrity

After a ureterostomy, the patient has a ureteral catheter for 1 or 2 weeks. The catheter is attached to a collection device. Once the catheter is removed, an appliance is needed to collect urine drainage. A variety of pouches are available (see Fig. 26-4). Some have antireflux valves to prevent the flow of urine back into the stoma. A skin barrier product can be used around the stoma for protection. Karaya products are used for intestinal ostomies but not for urinary drainage because urine breaks down the product. Belts can be worn with some appliances to hold them in place. Some pouches can be connected to a leg bag for urine collection.

The pouch is usually cleaned once or twice daily. It is changed every 4 to 6 days or when it leaks, because frequent changes are irritating to the surrounding skin. When it is changed, gently remove any adhesive. A gauze pad, tampon, or tissue may be placed at the opening of the stoma to absorb urine. Pouch changes are usually done in the morning when urine production is lowest. Steps in the application of a urinary pouch are illustrated in Figure 26-7. Wash the peristomal area with water and pat dry. If soap is used, it should be nonoily and rinsed off thoroughly. If crystals are present, a gauze pad saturated in a dilute vinegar solution can be used to dissolve them. Urinary stoma problems are summarized in Table 26-1.

Risk for Infection

The stoma serves as a portal for pathogens to enter the urinary tract, causing infection. Urinary tract infections can have serious consequences, including kidney damage and septicemia. Pouch care is treated as a clean rather than sterile procedure because the stoma is not sterile. However, you still must take care to avoid introducing organisms to the area.

Yeast infections that sometimes develop around the stoma are characterized by a skin rash surrounding the stoma. These are usually treated with nystatin powder applied under the skin barrier.

Risk for Injury

If urine does not flow readily, an obstruction is possible; notify the RN or surgeon immediately.

Disturbed Body Image

Adjustment to a stoma can be very difficult. The patient may be afraid of leakage and odor and may feel disfigured. Demonstrate acceptance of the patient and care for the stoma in a matter-of-fact manner. In addition, express understanding of the patient's feelings and encourage the patient to groom and dress normally. If odor is a problem, the pouch can be soaked in vinegar water for 20 to 30 minutes. Odor-proof pouches also should be recommended. Learning to care for the ureterostomy boosts the patient's self-confidence and may help to restore a more positive body image.

Patients with ostomies commonly experience grief in response to the loss of normal function and perceived disfigurement. This may be exhibited as denial, shock, anger, bargaining, or depression. Chapter 24 offers guidance for dealing with the patient who is grieving.

The change in body image may affect the patient's sexuality. Provide opportunities for patients with an ostomy to ask questions or discuss how the ostomy might affect sexual function or behavior. Patients may feel unattractive or fear rejection by their partners. People who have had radical perineal surgeries may have physical barriers to sexual performance; other patients have problems because of psychologic factors.

The same practical suggestions identified for the patient with an intestinal ostomy may be useful to the patient with a urinary ostomy. The pouch should be emptied before sexual intercourse. Pouch covers are available to conceal the appliance and its contents. The partner wearing the pouch should experiment with positions that are most comfortable. Female patients should know that ostomy surgery does not interfere with pregnancy or delivery.

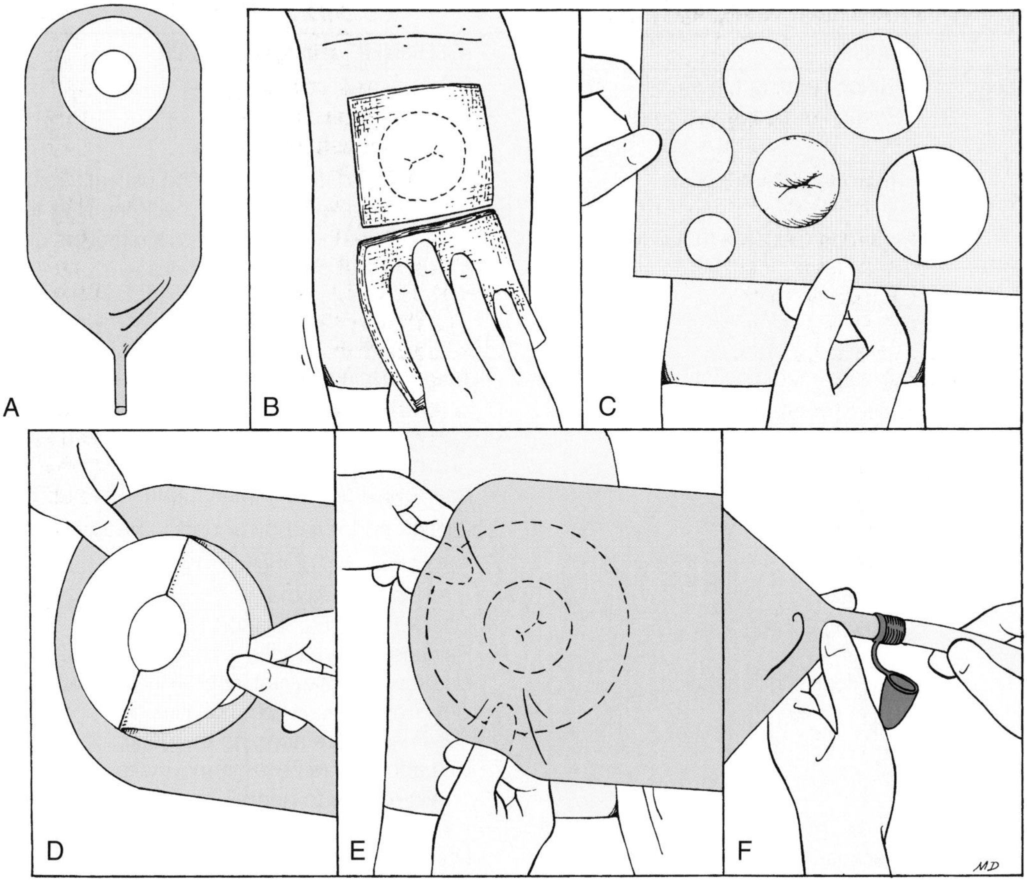

FIGURE 26-7 Procedure for applying pouch. **A,** Gather supplies: pouch, ostomy belt, skin barrier, stoma template, gauze pads, pouch clamp or rubber band, safety pin, and clean gloves. Wash hands and put on gloves. **B,** After removing the old pouch and cleaning the area around the stoma, place a gauze square over the stoma to absorb the drainage. **C,** Use a stoma template to measure the size of the stoma and then cut an opening the same size as the stoma into the skin barrier and adhesive. **D,** Remove the backing from the adhesive of the new pouch. **E,** Place the opening in the new pouch over the stoma and gently press into place with the pouch drain pointed toward the floor. **F,** Connect the drain to the tubing or close the drain if appropriate. Secure the tubing to sheets or according to agency policy. (From Black JM, Hawks JH: *Medical-surgical nursing: clinical management for positive outcomes*, ed 8, St. Louis, 2009, Saunders-Elsevier.)

Ineffective Self-Health Management

Many aspects of teaching the patient with a ureterostomy are the same as those identified for the patient with an ileostomy. The topics to include in the teaching plan are ostomy care, pouches, diet, fluids, activity, sexuality, complications, and resources. See the teaching plan in the section on Ileostomy.

From the early postoperative period, try to help the patient learn independent ostomy care. At first, patient teaching may take place each time stoma care is done by simply telling the patient what is being done and why. Encourage the patient to participate and gradually assume more responsibility for the care. Practice builds confidence and provides the patient with the opportunity to identify problems while help is available.

Some people adapt more readily to the stoma than others. You must be sensitive to the patient's feelings and encourage the patient in a kind way. A volunteer from the American Cancer Society or the UOAA can be especially helpful as a role model for the patient with a new ostomy. With the patient's and the physician's approval, the agency can be contacted about sending a volunteer to visit the patient.

The nurse, WOC nurse, or both must help the patient to plan for discharge. Provide written care instructions. The patient needs a list of supplies and places where they can be purchased. In addition, send some temporary supplies home with the patient. Finally, give the patient information (and referrals as needed) regarding resources such as home health care and community organizations.

In general, normal activities can be resumed within 3 months but specific directions should be obtained from the physician or WOC nurse. Because the pouch and seal are waterproof, the patient can bathe or shower with the appliance in place. Regular clothing

Table 26-1 Problems Associated with Urinary Stomas

PROBLEM	CAUSE	ASSESSMENT AND INTERVENTION
Stomal laceration	Pouch opening too small Pouch not positioned correctly	Enlarge pouch opening. Reposition pouch. Monitor healing.
Peristomal laceration	Improperly fitting pouch Improper pouch removal technique	Evaluate the pouch fit with the patient in sitting, lying, and standing positions. Check the fit of the belt. Consider the need for adhesive removers and/or specialized pouching systems.
Bleeding	Trauma	Apply a cool cloth. Cleanse gently.
Crystal formation	Urinary tract infection, stasis	Treat the infection and acidify the urine. Apply a vinegar compress to the stoma during dressing change. Put 1 to 2 oz of vinegar solution in the pouch for 20 minutes twice a day, then rinse. Use a vinyl or plastic pouch rather than a rubber one.
Stenosis	Scar formation	Dilation performed by or under direction of physician.
Skin irritation	Skin barrier or wafer too small Leaking appliance Hair follicle inflammation Perspiration under pouch Allergy to pouching products *Candida* ("yeast") infection	Adjust the size of the skin barrier or wafer to cover skin around the stoma. Check the belt. If it is too tight, the seal can break. Replace the appliance as needed (PRN). Use topical antimicrobial powder and skin barrier powder. Cover any lesions with nonstick dressing and with a barrier before applying the pouching system. Use adhesive remover; remove sealants gently. After the skin returns to normal, shave or cut any hair around the stoma. Dry the skin well. Apply a protective barrier. Apply powder to skin under pouch. Use a soft pouch cover. Spot test other brands to find one that does not cause irritation. Dry well. Apply nystatin powder as ordered.
Hernia/prolapse	Muscle weakness Increased intraabdominal pressure	Condition requires surgical repair.
Wartlike lesions	Excessive peristomal wetness	Reduce pouch opening size or acquire custom-cut system to reduce moisture on the skin. Condition may require debridement by a physician.
Odor	Urinary tract infection Appliance soiled or leaking	Treat infection. Check the seal; change the appliance. Provide deodorant tablets PRN.

can be worn but should not apply pressure to the stoma. Pouches can be attached to a collection device at night to permit continuous drainage.

Patients with an ostomy who enjoy traveling are encouraged to continue to do so. When traveling, patients are advised to take adequate supplies, including sealable plastic bags to dispose of used materials. If the patient is flying, his or her supplies should be kept in a hand-carried bag to avoid problems if luggage is lost or delayed. On a long flight, a leg bag attached to the pouch may be beneficial in case the patient must remain seated because of turbulence.

URETEROSIGMOIDOSTOMY AND URETEROILEOSIGMOIDOSTOMY

Ureterosigmoidostomy and ureteroileosigmoidostomy are not done as often now as in the past. However, you may care for patients who have had these diversions for some time and have adapted well to them. In a ureterosigmoidostomy, the ureters are implanted into the sigmoid colon. Urine drains into the colon and is eliminated through the rectum. In a ureteroileosigmoidostomy, a segment of the ileum is anastomosed to the sigmoid and the ureters are implanted into that part of the ileum. Neither procedure provides continence and both procedures present problems with kidney infections and urinary calculi (stones). Additional complications are caused by the colon's absorption of electrolytes from the urine. Patients are at risk for deficits in potassium and bicarbonate and for excesses in sodium, chloride, and hydrogen. These imbalances may lead to metabolic acidosis.

VESICOSTOMY

Vesicostomy or cystostomy is an opening into the urinary bladder. Several types exist. Some are drained continuously through a catheter; others have a nipple valve and are drained at intervals.

NEPHROSTOMY

A **nephrostomy** tube diverts urine directly from the kidney through a tube that exits through the skin. This device may be used as a temporary or permanent method of urinary diversion. Conditions that may be treated with these tubes are discussed in Chapter 42.

Get Ready for the NCLEX® Examination!

Key Points

- An ostomy is an artificial opening into a body cavity; a stoma is the site of the opening on the skin.
- Ostomy surgery may be done to bypass a section of the digestive or urinary tract, either temporarily or permanently.
- Nurses who have specialized training in ostomy management are an important resource for staff nurses and ostomy patients. They include the wound, ostomy, continence nurse (WOC), certified ostomy care nurse (COCN), and the certified wound, ostomy, continence nurse (CWOC).
- Before ostomy surgery it is important to determine the patient's expectations, understanding of the procedure, information desired, and fears.
- Intestinal ostomies include the ileostomy, the continent ileostomy, the ileoanal reservoir, and the colostomy.
- The characteristics of fecal material depend on the location of the ostomy; liquid stool drains from the ileum and softly formed stool drains from the descending colon.
- The new intestinal stoma should be beefy red and a small amount of bleeding around the base is not unusual.
- Postoperative nursing care after intestinal ostomy surgery addresses risk for deficient fluid volume, impaired skin integrity, disturbed body image, sexual dysfunction, and ineffective self-health management.
- Protective barriers are applied around the stoma to fill creases and create a seal, and a pouch is secured over the stoma with adhesive to collect fecal drainage.
- Elimination of gas-forming foods and good hygiene can help to control odor associated with an intestinal ostomy.
- The continent pouch ileostomy and the ileoanal reservoir both store fecal matter but the continent ileostomy is drained periodically with a catheter whereas the ileoanal reservoir allows fecal elimination through the rectum.
- Routine colostomy irrigations are no longer recommended.
- The most common types of urinary diversion are ileal conduit and continent internal reservoirs; other urinary diversions are cutaneous ureterostomy and colonic conduit.
- A urinary stoma is pink immediately after surgery but quickly fades to a light color.
- Ureterostomies and ileal conduits drain urine continuously, so collection pouches are needed and meticulous skin care must be provided.
- A continent internal reservoir allows for storage and controlled drainage of urine.
- Complications of urinary stomas include urinary infections, obstruction of urine flow, and skin breakdown.

Additional Learning Resources

SG Go to your Study Guide for additional learning activities to help you master this chapter content.

evolve Go to your Evolve website (http://evolve.elsevier.com/Linton/medsurg) for the following learning resources and much more:

- Interactive Prioritization Exercises
- Fluid & Electrolyte Tutorial
- Pharmacology Tutorial
- Review Questions for the NCLEX® Examination

Review Questions for the NCLEX® Examination

1. Which of the following is/are created surgically to drain fecal matter from the intestines? (Select all that apply.)
   1. Colostomy
   2. Ileostomy
   3. Ileal conduit
   4. Vesicostomy
   5. Ureterosigmoidostomy

   NCLEX Client Need: Physiological Integrity: Physiological Adaptation
2. Which of the intestinal stoma sites will produce the most formed stool?
   1. Jejunostomy
   2. Duodenostomy
   3. Ileostomy
   4. Colostomy

   NCLEX Client Need: Physiological Integrity: Physiological Adaptation

3. What color should a new intestinal stoma be on the first postoperative day?
   NCLEX Client Need: Physiological Integrity: Physiological Adaptation
4. The nursing team is reviewing the care plan for a patient having ileostomy surgery that day. One of the postoperative nursing diagnoses is Risk for Deficient Fluid Volume. What does the licensed vocational nurse/licensed practical nurse (LVN/LPN) know is the reason for this risk?
   1. A significant loss of blood occurs during the surgical procedure.
   2. Patients with ileostomies often have anorexia, nausea, and vomiting.
   3. Fluid normally reabsorbed in the colon is lost through the ileostomy.
   4. Fluid intake will be restricted until the stoma heals completely.

   NCLEX Client Need: Physiological Integrity: Physiological Adaptation
5. The LVN/LPN is reviewing stoma care with a patient before discharge. What teaching point should the nurse reinforce?
   1. Remove the drainage appliance daily to cleanse skin around the stoma
   2. Wash the stoma and surrounding skin with a moisturizing soap
   3. Vigorously rub the skin surrounding the stoma to stimulate circulation and healing
   4. Cut the opening on the wafer no more than ⅛ inch larger than the stoma.

   NCLEX Client Need: Physiological Integrity: Physiological Adaptation
6. When teaching a new colostomy patient how to control odor, the nurse provides a list of foods that commonly cause gas. The patient says, "You mean I can't eat any of these foods?" Which of the following is the most appropriate reply?
   1. "Gradually try them one at a time to see how you tolerate them."
   2. "That is correct. You can never eat any of these foods again."
   3. "Because flatus production is unpredictable, you never know what will happen if you eat these foods."
   4. "It would be better if you took vitamins instead of eating fresh fruits and vegetables."

   NCLEX Client Need: Physiological Integrity: Physiological Adaptation
7. Mr. Y. had ostomy surgery 3 days ago. Which of the following is most likely to help Mr. Y. adjust to his stoma and learn how to perform self-care?
   1. Shield the stoma from Mr. Y's sight until he asks to see it
   2. Tell Mr. Y.: "If you don't do your stoma care, then no one will do it for you."
   3. Encourage Mr. Y. to participate in care once he begins looking at the stoma
   4. Teach a family member how to do the care

   NCLEX Client Need: Psychosocial Integrity: Coping Mechanisms; Unexpected Body Image Changes
8. A patient with a new continent ileostomy has abdominal distention and hypoactive bowel sounds. These observations suggest which complication?
   NCLEX Client Need: Physiological Integrity: Reduction of Risk Potential
9. The nurse on a urology unit has patients with each of the types of urinary diversion listed below. The nurse should anticipate needing to changes pouches on three of the patients. The patient with which type of urinary diversion will not need to wear a pouch?
   1. Cutaneous ureterostomy
   2. Ileal conduit
   3. Indiana pouch
   4. Ureteroileostomy

   NCLEX Client Need: Physiological Integrity: Basic Care and Comfort
10. The surgeon has explained the advantages and disadvantages of various types of procedures that might be done for a patient who has bladder cancer. Which of the following is the main advantage of the ileum neobladder?
    1. The patient does not have a stoma for urine drainage.
    2. Urinary continence is always maintained.
    3. Urine is eliminated through the rectum.
    4. The neobladder has to be drained only once a day.

    NCLEX Client Need: Physiological Integrity: Physiological Adaptation

chapter 27

Neurologic Disorders

Sherry Dawn Weaver

http://evolve.elsevier.com/Linton/medsurg

Objectives

1. Identify common neurologic changes in the older person and the implication of these for nursing care.
2. List the components of the nursing assessment of the patient with a neurologic disorder.
3. Describe the diagnostic tests and procedures used to evaluate neurologic function and the nursing responsibilities associated with each.
4. Identify the uses, side effects, and nursing interventions associated with common drug therapies used in patients with neurologic disorders.
5. Describe the signs and symptoms associated with increased intracranial pressure and the medical therapies used in treatment.
6. Describe the pathophysiologic condition, signs and symptoms, complications, and medical or surgical treatment for patients with selected neurologic disorders.
7. Assist in developing a nursing care plan for the patient with a neurologic disorder.

Key Terms

Aura (ĂW-ră)
Contralateral (kŏn-tră-LĂT-ĕr-ăl)
Decerebrate (dē-SĔR-ă-brāt)
Decorticate (dē-KŎR-tĭ-kāt)
Encephalitis (ĕn-sĕf-ă-LĪ-tĭs)
Hemiparesis (hĕm-ē-pă-RĒ-sĭs)
Hemiplegia (hĕ-mē-PLĒ-jă)
Intracranial pressure (ĭn-tră-KRĀ-nē-ăl PRĔ-shŭr)
Ipsilateral (ĭp-sĭ-LĂT-ĕr-ăl)
Neuralgia (nū-RĂL-jă)
Neurotransmitter (nū-rō-TRĂNS-mĭ-tĕr)
Paresthesia (pā-rĕs-THĒ-zhă)
Postictal (pōs-TĬK-tĕl)
Seizure (SĒ-zhŭr)

Neurologic disease and injury present some of the greatest challenges in health care today. Nurses face the challenge of caring for people with neurologic disorders during the acute and rehabilitation phases of recovery from injuries and diseases. The long-term effects of many neurologic disorders are frequently devastating to the patient and the family. An important aspect of care is assisting the patient and family to adjust physically and emotionally to the alterations that often result from neurologic dysfunction.

ANATOMY AND PHYSIOLOGY OF THE NERVOUS SYSTEM

In this age of computers, it may be helpful to think of the nervous system as an elaborate control system. The system coordinates and regulates all bodily functions. It receives and interprets information from the external environment and initiates responses to the received information.

The functional unit of the nervous system is the neuron (nerve cell), which conducts electrical impulses within the nervous system. The main cell body has branches called *axons* and *dendrites* (Fig. 27-1). Axons conduct impulses away from the cell body and dendrites convey impulses toward the cell body. Many axons and dendrites are covered with a material called *myelin*, which enhances conduction along nerve fibers. Myelin gives the axons a white appearance (white matter) whereas cell bodies without myelin are gray (gray matter).

Neurons are classified according to their particular functions. Those that transmit information from distal parts of the body or environment toward the central nervous system (CNS) are sensory neurons, also known as *afferent* ("bearing toward") *neurons*. Motor information is carried from the CNS to the periphery by motor neurons, also known as *efferent* ("bearing away from") *neurons*. Interneurons also exist and are like relay stations between sensory and motor neurons.

Coordinated, organized function is a result of a well-integrated system of impulse transmission. When the end of a dendrite is stimulated, a series of electrochemical events are initiated. At the point of

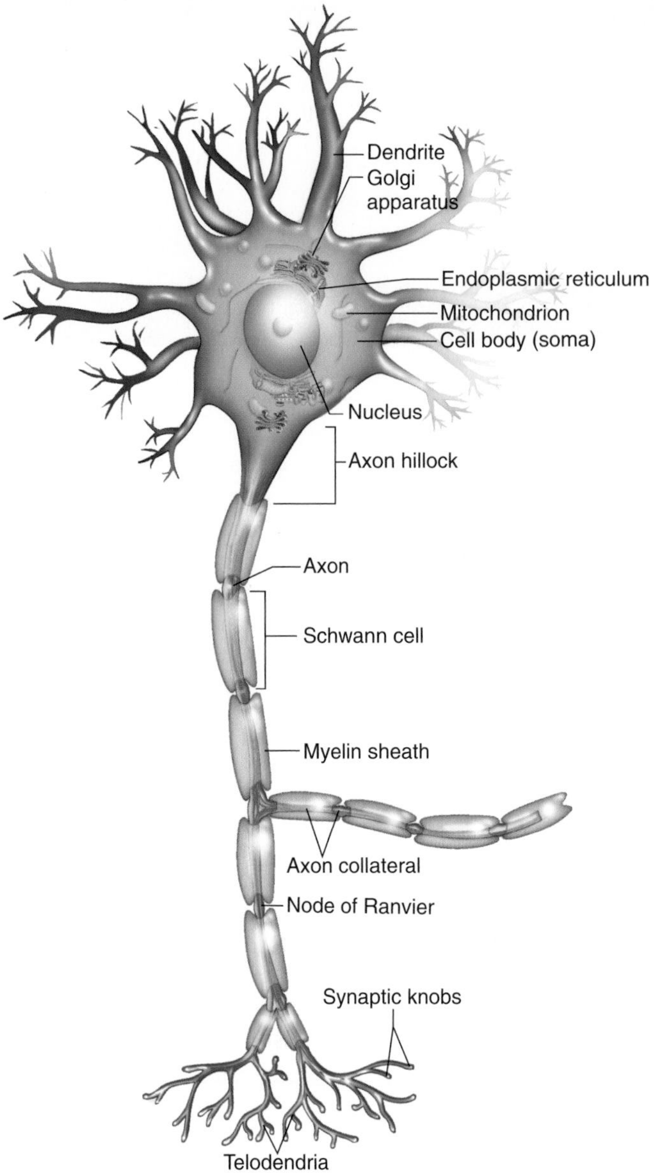

FIGURE 27-1 A neuron (nerve cell). The dendrites receive incoming messages. The axons convey outgoing signals. (From Patton K, Thibodeau G: *Anatomy & physiology*, ed 8, St. Louis, 2013, Mosby.)

stimulation, sodium and potassium ions are exchanged, resulting in a process called *depolarization*. This process continues down the dendrite to the axon, until the ions return to their resting state. This return to the resting state is known as *repolarization*.

Impulses must be able to pass from one neuron to another across the neural synapse—the space between the axons of one neuron and the dendrites of the next neuron. When an impulse reaches the end of its axon, a biochemical messenger called a **neurotransmitter** is released. Among the best understood neurotransmitters are acetylcholine, norepinephrine, epinephrine, and dopamine. The neurotransmitter crosses the synapse to the neighboring dendrite, where it stimulates an electrical impulse. The process of depolarization then continues down the length of the nerve cells.

Structurally, the nervous system is divided into two main parts: (1) the CNS, made up of the brain and spinal cord, and (2) the peripheral nervous system, which comprises all nerves of the peripheral parts of the body, including both spinal and cranial nerves. The brain is divided into the cerebrum, cerebellum, and brainstem (Fig. 27-2). The cerebrum is composed of left and right hemispheres, which are subdivided into specific lobes. The thalamus, hypothalamus, and basal ganglia are other important structures identified in the cerebrum. Box 27-1 lists the functions of the major parts of the brain.

Cerebrospinal fluid (CSF) is composed primarily of water, glucose, sodium chloride, and protein. It is produced in the ventricles of the brain in the arachnoid granulations. CSF circulates within the subarachnoid

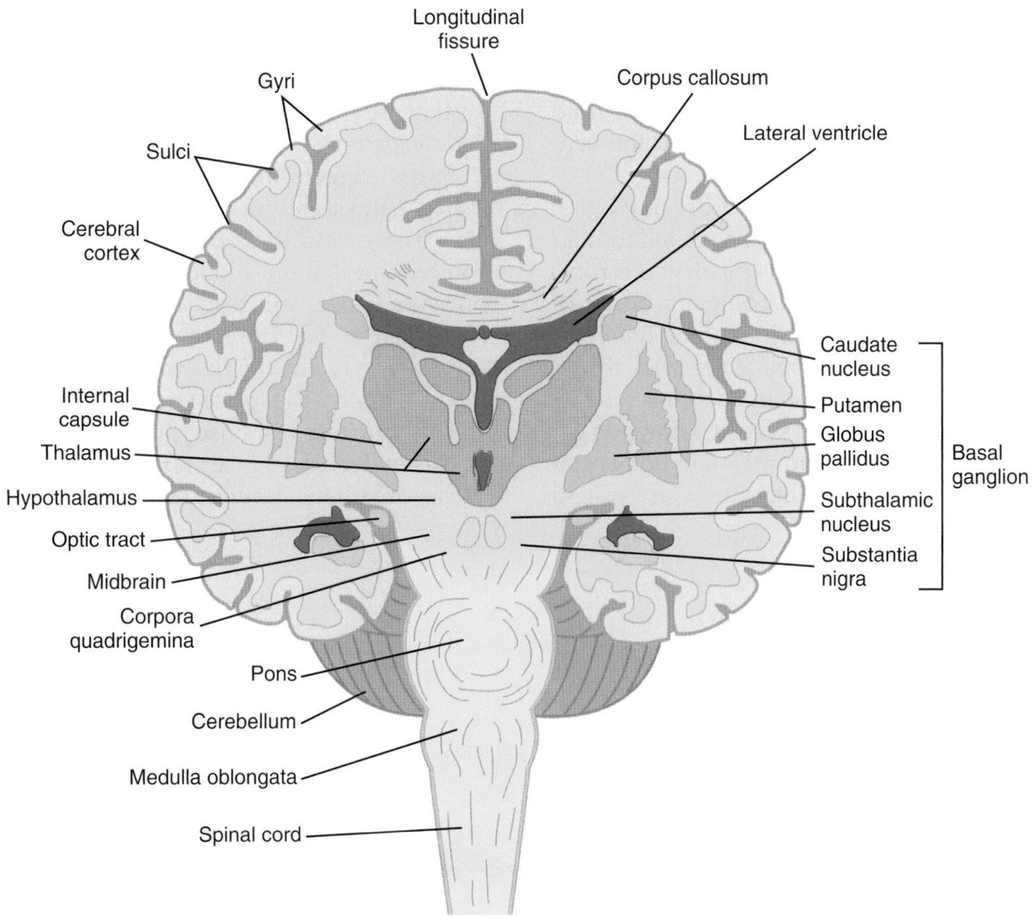

FIGURE 27-2 Structures of the brain (coronal section). (From Black JM, Hawks JH: *Medical-surgical nursing: clinical management for positive outcomes*, ed 8, St. Louis, 2009, Saunders-Elsevier.)

Box 27-1 Functions of the Major Parts of the Brain

BRAINSTEM AND DIENCEPHALON
Control awareness or alertness through the reticular activating system, composed of fibers scattered throughout the midbrain, pons, and medulla.

MEDULLA
Links the higher brain centers to other parts of the body through the spinal cord. Controls muscles of respiration through the respiratory reflex center. Controls the heartbeat (to some extent) through the cardiac reflex center. Constricts blood vessels to raise blood pressure through the vasomotor reflex center. Is the point of origin for some cranial nerves.

PONS
Relays messages from the medulla to the higher centers in the brain. Is a reflex center for some cranial nerves.

CEREBELLUM
Coordinates movement, balance, posture, and spatial orientation.

HYPOTHALAMUS
Controls the pituitary. Controls appetite, sleep, and some emotions. Controls much activity of the autonomic nervous system.

FOREBRAIN (CEREBRUM)
Controls the higher functions and activities: conscious mental processes, sensations, emotions, and voluntary movements.

FRONTAL LOBE
Controls the voluntary muscle movements, verbal and written speech.

PARIETAL LOBE
Contains the sensory reception areas to interpret pain, touch, temperature, distances, sizes, and shapes.

TEMPORAL LOBE
Contains the auditory center for hearing and understanding spoken language. Contains the olfactory center for smell.

OCCIPITAL LOBE
Contains the visual center for seeing and reading.

Data from Jacob SW, Francone CA: *Elements of anatomy and physiology*, ed 2, Philadelphia, 1989, Saunders.

space, the ventricles, and the central canal of the spinal cord (Fig. 27-3). The fluid is reabsorbed in the arachnoid villi. The CSF acts as a shock absorber for the brain and spinal cord. If excess fluid forms or if fluid is not normally reabsorbed, pressure within the ventricular system increases.

The spinal cord extends from the border of the first cervical vertebra (C1) to the level of the second lumbar vertebra (L2). Thirty-one pairs of spinal nerve roots exit from the spinal cord, each consisting of a posterior sensory (afferent) root and anterior motor (efferent) root (Fig. 27-4). These nerve roots, along with the 12 cranial nerves, make up the peripheral nervous system.

Part of the peripheral nervous system, known as the *autonomic nervous system*, helps to maintain homeostasis for the body. The autonomic nervous system controls the involuntary activities of the viscera, including smooth muscles, cardiac muscle, and glands. The two major subdivisions of the autonomic nervous system are (1) the *sympathetic nervous system* and (2) the *parasympathetic nervous system.*

Stress triggers the sympathetic nervous system to increase the secretion of epinephrine and norepinephrine. These neurotransmitters increase heart rate and constrict peripheral blood vessels, causing the blood pressure to rise. This reaction to stress is called the *fight or flight response.* The sympathetic nervous system is also referred to as the *thoracolumbar system.*

Conversely, the parasympathetic nervous system mediates a rest response. Stimulation of this system results in decreased heart rate and blood pressure. The parasympathetic nervous system is also known as the

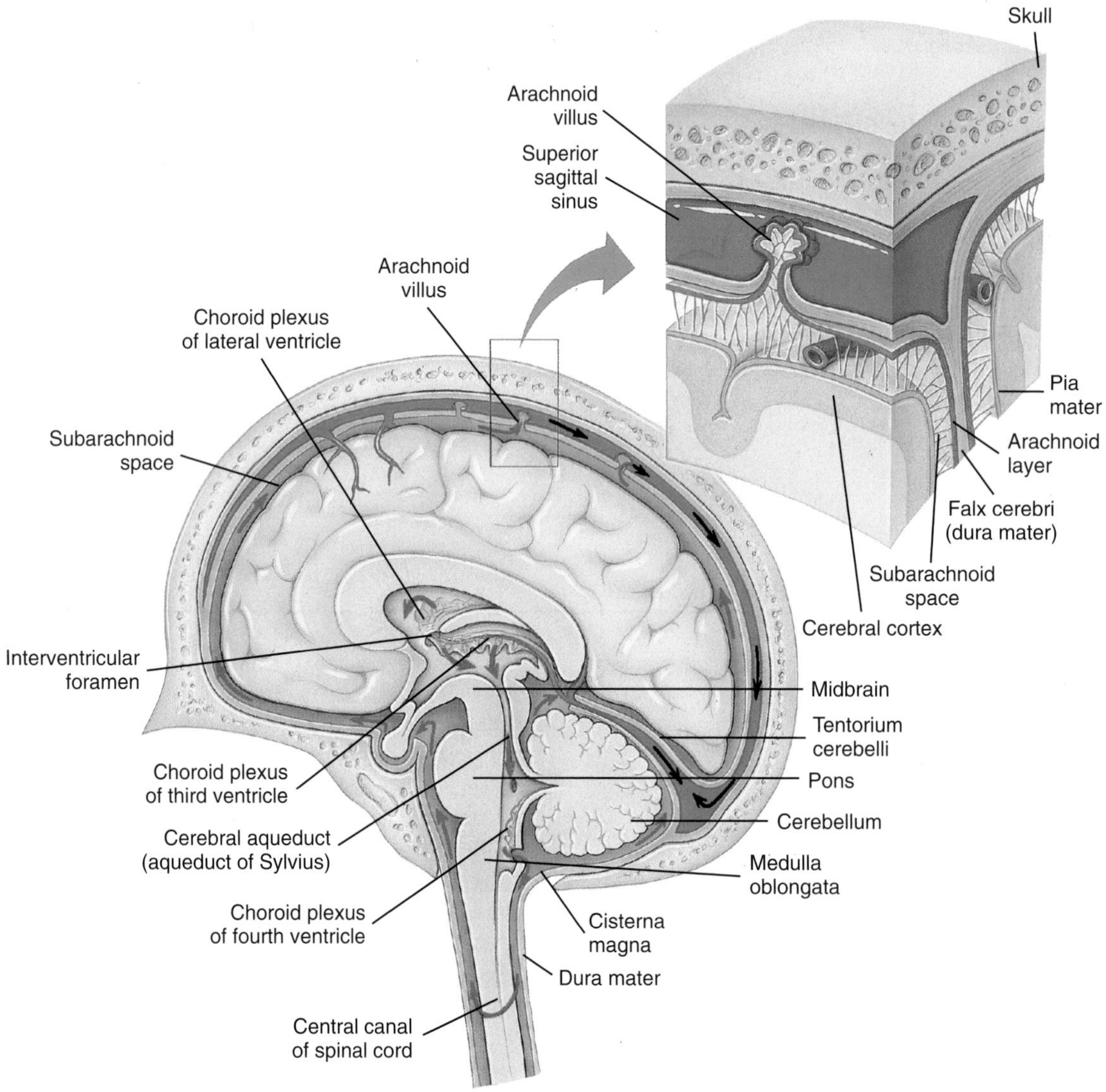

FIGURE 27-3 Structures of the brainstem and cerebrospinal fluid (CSF) circulation. Red arrows represent the route of the CSF. Black arrows represent the route of blood flow. CSF is produced in the ventricles, exits the fourth ventricle, and returns to the venous circulation in the superior sagittal sinus. The inset depicts the arachnoid granulations in the superior sagittal sinus, where the CSF enters the circulation. (From Wilson SF, Giddens JF: *Health assessment for nursing practice*, ed 5, St. Louis, 2013, Mosby.)

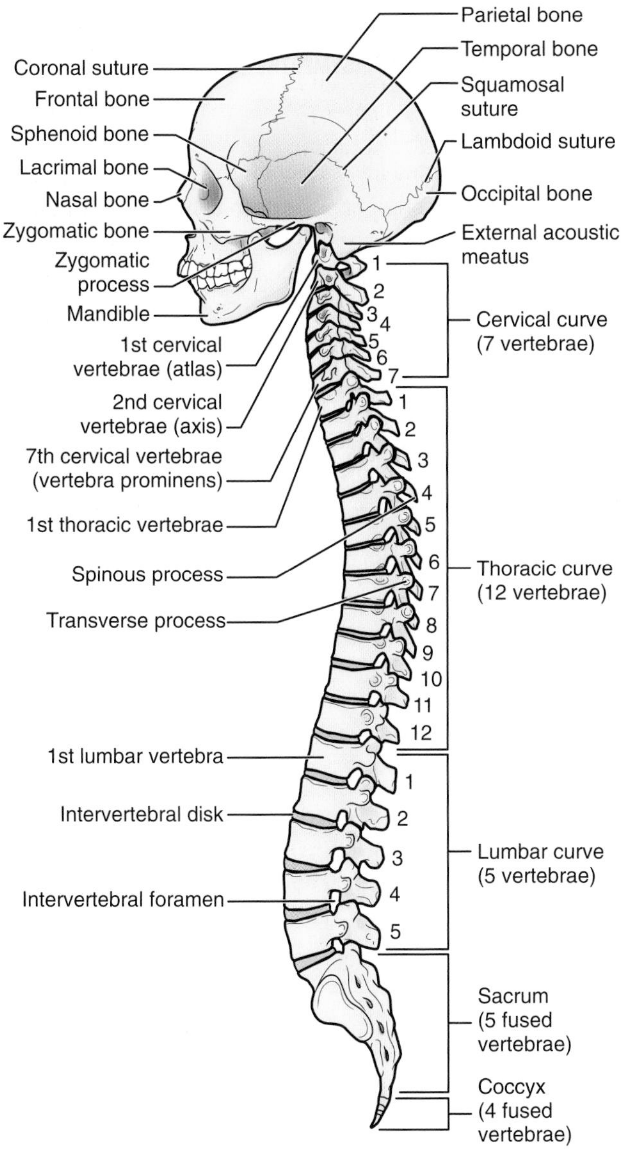

FIGURE 27-4 Bony structure of the skull and vertebral column.

craniosacral system. Specific effects of the stimulation of the sympathetic and parasympathetic nervous systems are outlined in Table 27-1.

AGE-RELATED CHANGES

With normal aging, the number of nerve cells decreases. Brain weight is reduced and the ventricles increase in size. An aging pigment called *lipofuscin* is deposited in nerve cells, along with *amyloid*, a type of protein. Increased plaques and tangled fibers are found in nerve tissue. These changes are associated with Alzheimer disease but also are seen in the brains of people who have no symptoms of dementia. Fortunately, many more nerve cells are present than are needed for normal function. Therefore most older people retain normal cognition and function despite the decreasing number of nerve cells.

The physical examination reveals some neurologic changes typical of aging. The pupil of the eye is often smaller and may respond to light more slowly. When asked to track (follow with the eyes) a moving object, the older person's eye movements may be jerky rather than smooth. Reflexes are usually intact except for the Achilles tendon jerk, which is often absent.

Older people often demonstrate some changes in functional abilities as well. Reaction time increases with aging, especially for complex reactions. Tremors in the head, face, and hands are common. Some older people develop dizziness and problems with balance. These are not considered normal age-related changes.

Put on Your Thinking Cap!

Identify three implications for nursing care related to normal neurologic changes that occur with age.

PATHOPHYSIOLOGY OF NEUROLOGIC DISEASES

Potential causes of neurologic disorders include developmental and genetic disorders, trauma, infections and inflammation, neoplasms, degenerative processes, vascular disorders, and metabolic and endocrine disorders.

- **Developmental and genetic disorders.** Developmental disorders include structural problems such as hydrocephalus. An example of a genetic disorder is Huntington disease.
- **Trauma.** CNS injuries resulting from trauma can be life threatening or severely disabling. Physical trauma to the nervous system may follow accidental injury, violent crime, or chemical injury caused by drugs, alcohol, or other harmful substances.
- **Infections and inflammation.** Meningitis and encephalitis are examples of disease states that cause inflammation of meningeal tissue and brain tissue, respectively. Causative agents may be viruses or bacteria and may be transmitted by a variety of vectors and routes.
- **Neoplasms.** CNS tumors may be primary or metastatic in origin. Although considerable progress has been made in treating these tumors, definitive therapy is often difficult to achieve, depending on the cell type involved in the tumor and the degree of invasion of surrounding tissue.
- **Degenerative processes.** The primary degenerative disease of the brain is Alzheimer disease, a progressive condition that begins with memory loss and eventually results in severe mental and physical deterioration. Alzheimer disease is discussed in Chapter 22. Other degenerative disorders are multiple sclerosis (MS), Parkinson disease, amyotrophic lateral sclerosis (ALS, also known as *Lou Gehrig's disease*), and Huntington disease.

Table 27-1 Effects of Sympathetic and Parasympathetic Stimulation

ORGAN	EFFECT OF SYMPATHETIC STIMULATION	EFFECT OF PARASYMPATHETIC STIMULATION
Eye		
Pupil	Dilated	Constricted
Ciliary muscle	Slight relaxation (far vision)	Constricted (near vision)
Glands: nasal, lacrimal, parotid	Vasoconstriction and slight secretion	Stimulation of copious secretions
Sweat glands	Copious sweating (cholinergic)	Sweating on palms of hands
Apocrine glands	Thick, odoriferous secretion	None
Blood vessels	Mostly constricted	Most often little or no effect
Heart		
Muscle	Increased rate	Slowed rate
	Increased force of contractions	Decreased force of contractions (especially atria)
Coronary arteries	Dilated ($beta_2$), constricted (alpha)	Dilated
Lungs		
Bronchi	Dilated	Constricted
Blood vessels	Mildly constricted	Dilated
Gut		
Lumen	Decreased peristalsis and tone	Increased peristalsis and tone
Sphincter	Increased tone (most times)	Relaxed (most times)
Liver	Glucose released	Slight glycogen synthesis
Gallbladder and bile ducts	Relaxed	Contracted
Kidney	Decreased output; increased renin secretion	None
Bladder		
Detrusor	Relaxed (slight)	Contracted
Trigone	Contracted	Relaxed
Penis	Ejaculation	Erection
Systemic Arterioles		
Abdominal viscera	Constricted	None
Muscle	Constricted (alpha adrenergic) Dilated ($beta_2$ adrenergic) Dilated (cholinergic)	None
Skin	Constricted	None
Blood		
Coagulation	Increased	None
Glucose	Increased	None
Lipids	Increased	None
Basal metabolism	Increased up to 100%	None
Adrenal medullary secretions	Increased	None
Mental activity	Increased	None
Piloerector muscles	Contracted	None
Skeletal muscle	Increased glycogenolysis	None
	Increased strength	
Fat cells	Lipolysis	None

Adapted from Hall JE: *Guyton and Hall textbook of medical physiology*, ed 12, Philadelphia, 2011, Saunders.

- **Vascular disorders.** Any factor that interferes with blood flow to nervous tissue can lead to cell death, with resulting loss of function. Nerve tissue is so sensitive to hypoxia that cells begin to die after being deprived of oxygen for 4 minutes. Neurologic disorders associated with impaired blood flow include cerebrovascular accident (see Chapter 28) and multiinfarct dementia. Vascular abnormalities, including aneurysms and arteriovenous malformations, can rupture or prevent the delivery of adequate oxygen to affected tissue.
- **Metabolic and endocrine disorders.** The brain depends on constant supplies of glucose and other nutrients. Disturbances in glucose metabolism and electrolyte imbalances can lead to deterioration in thought processes and level of consciousness. Neurologic dysfunction can also result from accumulation of toxins, as in poisoning, renal failure, and liver failure.

NURSING ASSESSMENT OF NEUROLOGIC FUNCTION

A number of diagnostic tests may be done to evaluate and diagnose neurologic problems. However, any evaluation begins with an accurate assessment, which may be initiated by the nurse. The licensed vocational nurse/licensed practical nurse (LVN/LPN) assists with the assessment by collecting relevant data. Much of the assessment requires simply observing the patient and then recording the findings.

Health History

The general nursing assessment of the patient with a neurologic disorder is described here. Throughout the assessment, the patient's speech, behavior, coordination, alertness, and comprehension should be noted. More sophisticated assessments are described in Table 27-2.

Chief Complaint and History of Present Illness. An initial portion of the neurologic assessment includes an investigation of the patient's health history, particularly as it relates to the chief complaint. Document the event that prompted the patient to seek medical attention and describe any injuries. If the patient has pain, note the onset, severity, location, and duration.

Past Medical History. Past neurologic disorders and pertinent signs and symptoms are vital pieces of information. Ask about a history of head injury, seizures, diabetes mellitus, hypertension, heart disease, and cancer. Record dates and types of immunizations, including influenza, and list current medications. In addition, record current drugs and highlight allergies according to agency policy.

Table 27-2 Diagnostic Tests and Procedures: Neurologic Disorders

TEST AND PURPOSE	PATIENT PREPARATION	POSTPROCEDURE NURSING CARE
Lumbar Puncture		
Lumbar puncture is used to diagnose infections and other CNS disorders. CSF pressure is measured. A CSF sample is taken for analysis.	Informed consent is required. Tell the patient a fluid sample will be taken from the spinal column. Have the patient void to reduce the discomfort of a full bladder. Support the patient on one side in a knee-to-chest position during the procedure (see Fig. 27-8).	The risk of headache may be reduced by lying flat for a specific period after the procedure. Encourage oral fluids. Assess for numbness, tingling, or pain in the extremities; CSF or bleeding from the puncture site; and changes in vital signs. Promptly deliver labeled specimens to the lab. The puncture site is covered with a small bandage.
Electroencephalography		
EEG is used to detect seizure activity by monitoring electrical activity in the brain.	Explain that electrodes will be applied to the scalp; patient will not feel any electrical shocks. Shampoo hair before EEG. Withhold medications (anticonvulsants, sedatives, stimulants, and tranquilizers) and caffeine for up to 48 hours before EEG as ordered.	Help patient shampoo hair to remove electrode paste.
Electromyography		
EMG is useful in diagnosing neuromuscular abnormalities such as ALS, peripheral neuropathy, myasthenia gravis, and carpal tunnel syndrome	Signed consent is required. Tell patient procedure takes 1–2 hours. No caffeine or smoking for 3 hours before EMG.	Inspect the sites of needle electrode placement. Patient may be instructed to return within 5 days to have blood drawn for enzyme tests (AST, CK, LD).

Continued

Table 27-2 Diagnostic Tests and Procedures: Neurologic Disorders—cont'd

TEST AND PURPOSE	PATIENT PREPARATION	POSTPROCEDURE NURSING CARE
Imaging Studies		
A **brain scan** depicts the pattern of distribution of a radioactive isotope that has been injected intravenously. Used to diagnose brain abscesses, tumors, contusions, vascular occlusions or hemorrhage, and hematomas.	Informed consent is required. Contraindicated during pregnancy. KCl is given several hours before the procedure. Tell patient that scan is painless and radiation exposure is minimal. An isotope will be injected and the patient will lie on a stretcher while the scanner moves over the head. The scan will be repeated 1 hour later.	Encourage oral fluids to promote elimination of the isotope.
Cerebral angioplasty uses computer-based images taken after injection of contrast medium to assess abnormalities in cerebral, carotid, and vertebral blood vessels.	Informed consent is required. Inform radiologist if patient is allergic to contrast media, shellfish, or iodine. Remove any metal from head area. Tell patient a "dye" will be injected and radiographs taken as the patient lies on a stretcher. When medium is injected, patient may feel flushed, warm, and nauseated and report a salty taste.	Apply pressure to puncture site and monitor for bleeding. Bed rest may be ordered for specified period. Extremity used to inject contrast medium may be immobilized for a specified period of time; assess circulation and neurologic function. Allergic response to contrast medium causes hives, nausea, swollen salivary glands. Treat with antihistamines as ordered.
Computed tomography (CT) shows intracranial structures. Used to diagnose tumors, inflammation, edema, hematomas, and infarctions. Distinguishes normal from clotted blood. CT may be done along with angiography.	Patient may be NPO 4–8 hours before scan if contrast medium is planned; can take prescribed medications and diabetic diet. Patient must lie still on a stretcher that fits into a donut-shaped frame that moves around the head. A mechanical sound can be heard. Procedure is painless and takes 15–20 minutes. Give sedatives as ordered for patients who cannot stay still.	No special aftercare needed. Observe patient who receives contrast medium for a delayed allergic reaction.
Magnetic resonance imaging/ magnetic resonance angiogram (MRI/MRA) creates images of intracranial structures without radiation.	Tell patient he or she will lie on a stretcher that passes into a tubular structure. Loud drumming noises will be heard while imager is in use. No special preparation is required. Sedation may be ordered for confused patients or those who are claustrophobic. Open MRI may be available for claustrophobic patients. Patients with some metal implants cannot be exposed to MRI because magnet can cause metal to move in the body. Special oxygen equipment, ventilators, and infusion pumps must be used.	No special aftercare needed.
Pneumoencephalography uses injected gas by lumbar puncture and radiography to provide an outline of the cerebral ventricles and cisterns. Used to diagnose masses, congenital abnormalities, cysts, and atrophy of cerebral and cerebellar cortex.	Informed consent is required. Remove metal objects from head area. Support patient during lumbar puncture.	Perform neurologic checks per agency protocol. Keep patient flat and logroll for up to 48 hours as ordered. Inspect puncture site for CSF leakage or bleeding. Encourage oral fluids if permitted.
Blood Flow Studies		
Doppler flow uses ultrasound to assess carotid blood flow. Can be used with a duplex scanner to detect plaques in blood vessels.	Signed consent is required. Inform patient that test is painless and not to smoke for 30 minutes before test. Patient will need to lie supine while instrument is moved over the neck area.	No special aftercare needed unless activity restrictions are ordered.

ALS, Amyotrophic lateral sclerosis; *AST*, aspartate aminotransferase; *CK*, creatine kinase; *CNS*, central nervous system; *CSF*, cerebrospinal fluid; *EEG*, electroencephalography; *EMG*, electromyography; *KCl*, potassium chloride; *LD*, lactic dehydrogenase; *NPO*, nothing by mouth.

Family History. Questions about the presence of neurologic disease or other diseases in the immediate family may elicit valuable information about risk factors, such as those for stroke or neuromuscular diseases. Therefore ask whether any immediate family members have had heart disease, stroke, diabetes mellitus, cancer, seizure disorders, muscular dystrophy, or Huntington disease.

Review of Systems. Important signs and symptoms to be documented in reviewing the system are fatigue or weakness, headache, dizziness, vertigo, changes in vision or hearing, tinnitus, drainage from the ears or nose, dysphagia, neck pain or stiffness, vomiting, problems with bladder or bowel function, sexual dysfunction, fainting, blackouts, tremors, paralysis, incoordination, numbness or tingling, memory problems, and mood changes.

Functional Assessment. Document whether present symptoms interfere with the patient's usual activities and occupation. Explore sources of stress, usual coping strategies, and sources of support.

Physical Examination

A complete physical examination, including the neurologic examination, should be done when the patient is stable. A neurologic assessment provides baseline data to compare with ongoing assessments and serves as the basis for developing the nursing care plan. Four major components of a routine neurologic examination that provide valuable information regarding the overall integrity of the CNS are (1) level of consciousness, (2) pupillary evaluation, (3) neuromuscular response, and (4) vital signs. You must look at the trends in the patient's neurologic status. A single finding considered in isolation may not provide a true picture of the patient's status. For example, one elevated blood pressure reading may not be significant but continuing increases may be associated with increased **intracranial pressure** (ICP).

Basic Neurologic Examination

Level of Consciousness. The most accurate and reliable indicator of neurologic status is level of consciousness. Evaluate patients for orientation to person, place, and time by asking them to state their names, where they are, and what time it is. It is important to consider the degree of stimulation required to evoke a response from the patient. If the patient responds only to vigorous physical stimulation, consciousness is more impaired than if the patient responds immediately to a verbal greeting. Consider patient behavior in response to stimulation. Does the patient respond pleasantly or is he or she combative, agitated, or lethargic? All of these observations provide additional information regarding mental status.

Some of the common terms used to describe altered levels of consciousness are *somnolence, lethargy, stupor, semicoma,* and *coma*. Somnolence is unnatural drowsiness or sleepiness. Lethargy also is used to describe excessive drowsiness. Stupor suggests decreased responsiveness accompanied by lack of spontaneous motor activity. If a patient is in a stupor (stuporous) but can be aroused, the term *semicomatose* is used. A patient who cannot be aroused even by powerful stimuli is said to be in a coma, or comatose.

Because the terms related to altered levels of consciousness are open to interpretation, it is clearer to describe the patient's response to specific stimuli. The description should always begin with the mildest stimuli and stop when a response is elicited. The mildest stimulus is simply approaching the patient. This can be followed in order with verbal stimuli, with tactile stimuli (shaking the shoulder gently), and finally with painful stimuli. Appropriate methods of applying painful stimuli include applying pressure on the nail bed using an object such as a pen or pinching the trapezius muscle firmly between the thumb and forefinger and twisting.

Pupillary Evaluation. The second major component of the neurologic assessment is the pupillary evaluation. To evaluate the pupils, assess and compare their size, shape, and reactivity. Pupils are normally about 3 mm in size, round, and react briskly to light. Changes in equality or reactivity from one assessment to the next may indicate neurologic deterioration.

Neuromuscular Response. Assessment of neuromuscular response provides a means of evaluating cerebral and spinal cord function. All electrical impulses responsible for eliciting motor responses are initiated in the frontal lobe of the cerebral cortex. The impulses travel down the brainstem into the spinal cord. Motor spinal nerve roots then stimulate muscle movement. Additional techniques for assessing specific neuromuscular responses are found in Table 29-5.

Vital Signs. Monitoring pulse, respirations, and blood pressure provides highly reliable information regarding neurologic well-being. However, changes in vital signs are late indicators of deterioration. The significance of these values is discussed in detail in the section titled "Increased Intracranial Pressure". Elevated temperature may be associated with infection or with impaired thermoregulation. Figure 27-5 is a sample assessment tool that includes the Glasgow Coma Scale. This scale is commonly used to rate the patient's eye-opening response, motor response, and verbal response. The numeric ratings are totaled for a summary score. A normal, alert person would score 15; a person in a coma would score 7 or less.

General Physical Examination. Once the neurologic assessment is done, complete the remaining physical examination. If possible, measure the patient's height and weight. Throughout the examination, inspect the skin for lesions and color change and palpate for temperature. Assess hydration status by evaluating tissue turgor and moisture of mucous membranes. Inspect

MISSION HOSPITAL
REGIONAL MEDICAL CENTER

ADULT NEURO FLOW SHEET

TIME

			0700	0800	0900	1000	1100	1200	1300	1400	1500	1600	1700	1800	1900	2000	2100	2200	2300	2400	0100	0200	0300	0400	0500	0600
GLASGOW COMA SCALE		Eyes open																								
		Best motor																								
		Best verbal																								
		TOTAL																								
VOLUNTARY MOTOR	Right	Upper extremity																								
		Lower extremity																								
	Left	Upper extremity																								
		Lower extremity																								
CRANIAL NERVES	PUPILS Right	Size																								
		Reaction																								
	PUPILS Left	Size																								
		Reaction																								
	EOMS	Conjugate																								
		Disconjugate																								
		Tracking Right																								
		Left																								
		Blink reflex																								
		Gag reflex																								
		Facial symmetry																								
			0700	0800	0900	1000	1100	1200	1300	1400	1500	1600	1700	1800	1900	2000	2100	2200	2300	2400	0100	0200	0300	0400	0500	0600

TIME

Date

KEY

MOTOR
5+ Normal power
4+ Weakness
3+ Anti-gravity
2+ Not anti-gravity
1+ Trace
0 No movement

Pupil Size
B = Brisk
S = Sluggish
A = Absent

2 mm 3 mm 4 mm 5 mm
6 mm 7 mm 8 mm

✓ = Present
O = Absent
S = Symmetrical
A = Asymmetrical

Speech patterns: ____________________

Comments: ____________________

GLASGOW COMA SCALE			
	Eyes Open	4	Spontaneously
		3	To verbal command
		2	To pain
		1	No response
	Best Motor Response	6	Obeys command
		5	Localize pain
		4	Flexion to pain withdraw
		3	Flexion decorticate
		2	Extension to pain (decerebrate)
		1	No response to pain
	Best Verbal Response	5	Oriented
		4	Confused
		3	Inappropriate words
		2	Incomprehensible sounds
		1	No response

Unit ____________________

R.N. signature ____________________ Shift: __________

R.N. signature ____________________ Shift: __________

R.N. signature ____________________ Shift: __________

ADDRESSOGRAPH

Form: 408 5/92 **Adult Neuro Flow Sheet**

FIGURE 27-5 A neurologic flow sheet is used to record the assessment of neurologic function. (Courtesy Linda R. Littlehohn, RN, BSN, CCRN, Neuro Clinician, and Mission Hospital Regional Medical Center, Mission Viejo, Calif.)

the head for lesions and palpate for masses or swelling. Observe the patient's respiratory effort and auscultate breath sounds. In addition, examine the abdomen, palpate for bowel and bladder distention, and auscultate bowel sounds. Finally, inspect the extremities for injuries or abnormal positions. Assessment of motor and sensory function is detailed in Chapter 29.

Assessment of the patient with a neurologic disorder is summarized in Box 27-2.

Box 27-2 Assessment of the Patient with a Neurologic Disorder

HEALTH HISTORY

Chief Complaint and History of Present Illness
Event requiring medical attention

Past Medical History
Head injury, seizures, other neurologic disorders, other diseases (diabetes mellitus, hypertension, heart disease, cancer), dates of immunizations, current medications, allergies

Family History
Stroke, neuromuscular diseases, heart disease, diabetes mellitus, cancer, seizures

Review of Systems
Fatigue, weakness, headache, dizziness, vertigo, changes in vision or hearing, tinnitus, drainage from nose or ears, dysphagia, neck pain or stiffness, vomiting, bladder or bowel dysfunction, fainting, blackouts, tremors, paralysis, incoordination, numbness or tingling, memory problems, mood changes

Functional Assessment
Usual occupation and activities, effect on life, changes in sexuality, changes in activities of daily living (ADL), sources of stress, usual coping strategies, sources of support

PHYSICAL EXAMINATION

Initial Level of Consciousness
Response to stimulation

Pupils
Size, shape, response to light, equality

Neuromuscular Status
Voluntary movement, reflexes

Vital Signs
Blood pressure, pulse, respirations, temperature

If/When Stable

Height and Weight

Skin
Lesions, injuries, turgor

Head
Lesions, injuries, masses, swelling

Oral Cavity
Moisture

Thorax
Respiratory effort, breath sounds

Abdomen
Distention, bowel sounds

Extremities
Injuries, abnormal positions

DIAGNOSTIC TESTS AND PROCEDURES

Once an initial evaluation and history have been obtained, more detailed diagnostic tests and procedures are often indicated (see Table 27-2).

Advanced Neurologic Examination

Baseline and serial examinations are critical in the evaluation of the patient with a neurologic disorder. Cranial nerve function, coordination and balance, neuromuscular function, sensory function, and reflexes are the components that can assist the practitioner in localizing the area of injury or disease and in developing a plan of care relevant to the individual patient. (See Figure 27-5 for an example of a flow sheet used to record the findings on periodic neurologic assessments.)

Cranial Nerves. The cranial nerves mediate various motor, sensory, and autonomic functions. The cranial nerves enter and exit the brain rather than the spinal cord. The primary function of the cranial nerve is to control sensory, motor, and autonomic activities of the head and neck. The vagus nerve affects autonomic cardiac, respiratory, gastric, and gallbladder function. The examiner with advanced assessment skills may assess each nerve individually (Table 27-3).

Coordination and Balance. Both the cerebellum and the cerebral cortex influence coordination and balance. Cerebellar dysfunction creates loss of steady, balanced posture and gait on the **ipsilateral** side (same side) as the brain lesion. Lesions of the cortex, however, cause motor dysfunction on the **contralateral** side (opposite side) of the lesion.

Observation of routine activity, such as ambulation, feeding, or performing activities of daily living (ADL), can provide valuable information about coordination and balance. In the assessment of balance, ask the patient to walk 10 to 20 feet away, turn, and walk back toward you. Observe the patient's gait and arm swing, then ask the patient to walk a straight line in a heel-to-toe fashion.

To perform the Romberg test, have the patient stand with feet together and arms at his or her sides. Instruct the patient to close their eyes and maintain that position (while you stay close by in case the patient starts to fall). Normally the patient will display only slight swaying. To evaluate coordination of movements:

1. Ask the patient to pat his or her knees with the palms of the hands and then with the backs of the hands in a rapid, alternating pattern.
2. Hold up one of your fingers and instruct the patient to touch it with his or her index finger.
3. Ask the patient to touch his or her nose with the index finger, first with the eyes open and then with the eyes closed.
4. Ask the patient to run the heel of one foot down the shin of the other leg and then repeat with the opposite heel.

Table 27-3 Cranial Nerves

NUMBER/NAME		FUNCTION	TEST
I	Olfactory	Smell	Common odors to one nostril at a time
II	Optic	Vision	Visual acuity Visual fields Optic disc
III	Oculomotor	Movement of eye (medially, upward and inward, downward and outward, upward and outward), pupillary accommodation and constriction, raises upper eyelid	EOMs Doll's eyes (when head is moved, eyes move in opposite direction) Light examination direct and consensual; accommodation
IV	Trochlear	Movement of eye (down and inward)	EOMs Doll's eyes
V	Trigeminal	Facial sensation to hot/cold; light touch Chewing Branches: ophthalmic, maxillary, mandibular	Respective testing of three divisions. Clench jaw and check masseter and temporalis muscles; jaw and corneal reflex
VI	Abducens	Movement of eye (laterally)	EOMs Doll's eyes
VII	Facial	Facial expression; salivation; lacrimation, taste	Smile, frown, show teeth, puff out checks. Taste (anterior ⅔ of tongue), close eyes
VIII	Acoustic	Hearing (cochlear) Equilibrium (vestibular)	 Vestibular usually not tested
IX	Glossopharyngeal	Motor response limited; sensory on posterior tongue Innervates carotid body and sinus	Swallow on command, gag reflex Taste (posterior ⅓ of tongue)
X	Vagus	Movements of pharynx and larynx (raises the palate) Innervates organs of thorax abdomen	Gag reflex, midline elevation of uvula
XI	Spinal accessory	Movements of shoulders and neck	Shrug shoulders and turn head against resistance
XII	Hypoglossal	Movement of tongue for speech and swallowing	Protrude tongue (deviates to affected side)

EOMs, Extraocular movements.

5. Alternate tapping with the heel and then the toes of one foot and then the other foot.

Normally these responses are done smoothly and rapidly.

Neuromuscular Function. Evaluate individual muscle groups by assessing their size, tone, and strength. Upper arm strength is evaluated by having the patient provide resistance to a movement. For example, you can ask the patient to extend the arms and bend the elbows, while alternately trying to push the examiner away or pull the examiner forward. Strength of the intrinsic muscles of the hand is tested by having the patient spread the fingers apart and then resist having them pushed together. Strength of hand grasp is tested by putting one finger on top of another so that a firm squeeze will not painfully press the knuckles together. You also instruct the patient to lift each hand or to raise a finger on each hand. A subtle weakness in upper arm strength is assessed by having the patient extend both arms forward with the palms up. Ask the patient to close his or her eyes and maintain the position for 10 to 20 seconds. With normal strength, the arms remain steady. In the presence of a slight weakness, the weak arm will rotate internally and drift slightly downward. This is referred to as *ulnar* or *motor drift.*

To evaluate strength of the legs, position the patient supine and ask him or her to raise one leg at a time. The patient with normal strength can lift the leg 90 degrees. Test the strength of other muscles as indicated.

Sensory Function. Many tests of sensory function exist, including evaluation of the patient's perception of pain, temperature, light touch, vibration, position, and tactile discrimination. All sensory testing is done with the eyes closed. Apply various stimuli to the skin and ask the patient to identify the type of stimulus perceived.

Pain. Pain can be evaluated by using a wooden applicator that is broken to create a sharp point. This broken applicator is used as the "sharp" stimulus whereas the cotton end is used as a "dull" control stimulus. Ask the patient to state whether sharp or dull sensations are felt. Recognition of sharp pricks indicates ability to perceive painful stimuli.

Temperature. Temperature perception can be tested by touching test tubes containing hot or cold water to the patient's skin and asking the patient to distinguish hot from cold.

Light Touch. A wisp of cotton brushed against the skin is used to assess perception of light touch. Ask the patient to state when the sensation is felt.

Vibration. To test vibration, strike a tuning fork and touch the base to a joint in the great toe or a finger. Then ask the patient to report when the vibration is felt and when it stops. The examiner actually stops the tuning fork from vibrating. If the sensation is not perceived, repeat the test on a more proximal joint until the patient perceives it.

Position. To test direction, lightly hold the patient's great toe or a finger on the sides and move it up and down. Then ask the patient to identify the direction of the movement.

Tactile Discrimination. Tests for tactile discrimination include stereognosis, graphesthesia, and point localization. To test stereognosis, place a familiar object (e.g., paper clip, cotton ball) in the patient's hand and request identification using only one hand. Graphesthesia tests the patient's ability to recognize a number or letter "written" on the palm with a dull object. To test point localization, briefly touch the skin and ask the patient to touch the place where the sensation was felt.

Reflexes. A reflex is an unconscious, involuntary response that is entirely mediated at the level of the spinal cord, without input from higher brain centers. The knee jerk represents a simple reflex. When a stimulus is applied to the patella, the sensory root of the spinal nerve transmits the impulse to the spinal cord. At the cord, the impulse is relayed to the motor nerve root, which then elicits the knee jerk (Fig. 27-6). Other commonly tested reflexes are listed in Table 27-4.

Although these common reflexes are normal, others appear only with pathologic states. The Babinski reflex accompanies abnormalities in the motor pathways originating in the cerebral cortex. Assess for it by stroking the lateral side of the bottom of the foot and across the ball of the foot with a blunt object and observing the resulting movement of the toes. Normally the toes curl downward. However, in the presence of cortical

Table 27-4 Commonly Tested Reflexes

REFLEX	EXPECTED RESPONSE
Biceps	Flexion of forearm
Triceps	Extension of forearm
Brachioradialis	Flexion and supination of forearm
Quadriceps	Extension of lower leg
Achilles (ankle jerk)	Plantar flexion of foot
Clonus	Repetitive movement after brisk dorsiflexion of foot

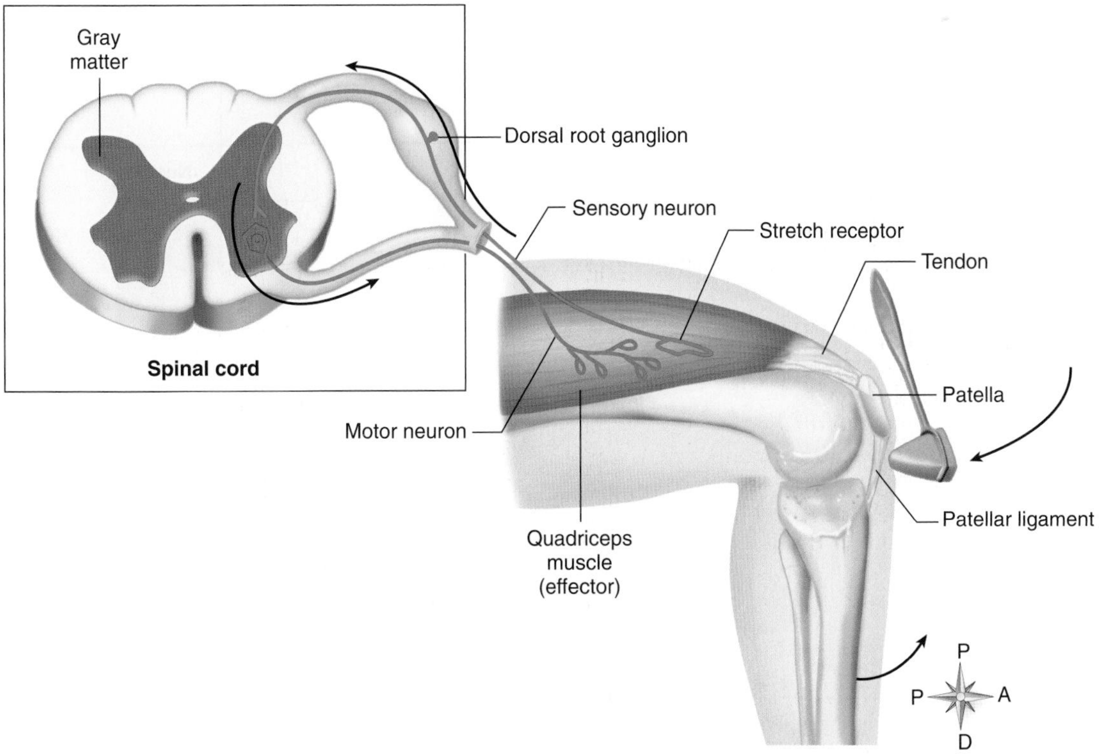

FIGURE 27-6 Reflexes are elicited by stimulating a sensory nerve, which conveys an impulse to the spinal cord. An impulse is then conveyed by a motor nerve to cause the muscle to contract. (From Patton K, Thibodeau G: *Anatomy & physiology*, ed 8, St. Louis, 2013, Mosby.)

dysfunction, the big toe bends upward and the other toes fan out. Figure 27-7 illustrates the response.

Lumbar Puncture

A lumbar puncture is an invasive procedure that is used most often to detect infections and other disorders of the CNS, tumors, and hydrocephalus. A local anesthetic is used to anesthetize the puncture site. Then a cannula is inserted into the subarachnoid space at the level of the fourth or fifth lumbar vertebra (Fig. 27-8). Entering at this level allows the physician to avoid traumatizing the spinal cord, which ends at the level of the second lumbar vertebra. Once the needle is in place, a sample of CSF is collected for laboratory analysis. CSF specimens are placed in test tubes and labeled, with the first specimen usually being discarded because it may contain blood from the puncture. Normal CSF has the following characteristics: pressure 50 to 175 mm H_2O; pH 7.30 to 7.40; clear, colorless appearance; fasting glucose 40 to 80 mg/dL; white blood cells 0 to 5 small lymphocytes/mm^3.

Injuries resulting from lumbar puncture are rare. However, some patients experience severe headaches resulting from a CSF leak. Leaks are sometimes treated with a blood patch, which is created by injecting a small amount of the patient's blood into the lumbar puncture site. The blood clots and seals the puncture site, preventing further loss of CSF.

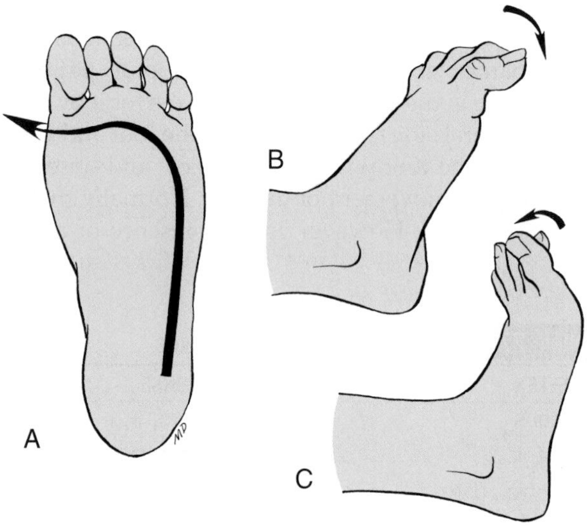

FIGURE 27-7 Babinski reflex. **A,** The examiner scrapes the foot as shown, using a blunt point. **B,** The normal response (absence of Babinski response) is plantar flexion of the toes. **C,** An abnormal response (presence of Babinski response) is characterized by dorsiflexion of the big toe and often fanning of the other toes. (From Black JM, Hawks JH: *Medical-surgical nursing: clinical management for positive outcomes*, ed 8, St. Louis, 2009, Saunders-Elsevier.)

Electroencephalography

The electroencephalogram (EEG) is a graphic representation of electrical activity in brain cells. Small electrodes are placed at various positions on the head to detect electrical signals generated from neurons located near the surface of the cerebral cortex. It is an excellent tool in the diagnosis of seizure activity (Fig. 27-9).

Some people have misconceptions about EEG. Assure the patient that no electrical shock will be experienced, that the examiner is not able to "read the

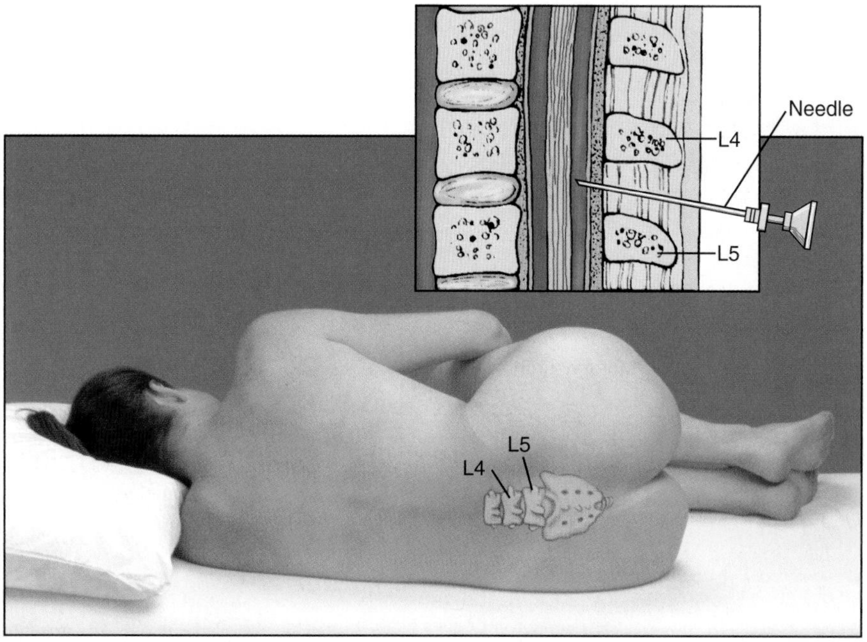

FIGURE 27-8 Lumbar puncture. With the patient in a flexed position to maximize the space between vertebrae, the lumbar puncture needle is inserted between L4 and L5 or L3 and L4 to gain entry to the subarachnoid space. During the actual procedure, the patient would be gowned and draped to protect privacy. (From Monahan FD, Drake DT, Neighbors M, editors: *Medical-surgical nursing: foundations for clinical practice*, ed 2, Philadelphia, 1998, Saunders.)

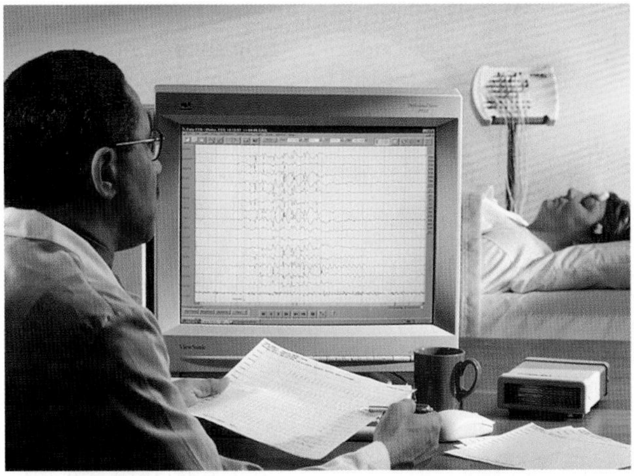

FIGURE 27-9 Client undergoing an electroencephalogram (EEG). (From Black JM, Hawks JH, Keene AM: *Medical-surgical nursing: clinical management for continuity of care*, ed 6, Philadelphia, 2001, Saunders.)

patient's mind," and that the test is not done to detect mental illness. Fatigue stresses the brain and may evoke abnormal activity not usually seen on the EEG. Therefore patients may be evaluated with a sleep-deprived EEG, in which they are awakened after a short sleep period in an effort to elicit such activity during the test.

Electromyography

Electromyography (EMG) studies the response of peripheral motor and sensory nerves to electrical stimuli. Needle electrodes are placed on several points over a nerve and over the muscles supplied by the nerve. Stimuli are administered and the effects are recorded on an oscilloscope.

Radiologic Studies

Brain Scan. The brain scan shows the pattern of distribution of a radioactive isotope injected intravenously. It is useful in detecting brain abscesses, tumors, contusions, vascular occlusion or hemorrhage, and hematomas. The patient is given potassium chloride (KCl) 2 hours before the isotope is injected to prevent excessive isotope uptake. The isotope is given immediately before the scan is done. While the patient lies still on a stretcher, the scanner, which is somewhat like a radiograph machine, moves back and forth over the head. No sensation is associated with the scanning process. The scan is repeated 1 hour later.

Cerebral Angiography and Digital Subtraction Angiography. Cerebral angiography provides images of the cerebral, carotid, and vertebral blood vessels. A catheter is inserted into an artery (usually femoral) and advanced to the carotid or vertebral arteries. A contrast dye is injected and a series of radiographs are taken. Angiography is the most definitive diagnostic test in the diagnosis of cerebral aneurysm or congenital vascular disorders, such as arteriovenous malformation. Risks include severe allergy to contrast media, embolus, hematoma, hemorrhage, renal toxicity, transient ischemic attack, infection, and loss of consciousness. Digital subtraction angiography (DSA) is a complementary, computer-assisted radiographic procedure for visualization of cerebral vessels.

Computed Tomography. The evolution of computed tomography (CT) represents one of the most significant developments in neurologic diagnostic procedures. CT is an excellent tool in the evaluation of trauma, tumors, and hemorrhage (Fig. 27-10). Enhancement of an area may be achieved by injecting contrast medium; therefore any allergy to such media must be reported to the radiologist in advance. The entire scanning procedure lasts 15 to 20 minutes and generally requires no advance preparation or postprocedure care.

Magnetic Resonance Imaging. One of the latest tools in neuroradiology is magnetic resonance imaging (MRI). Unlike CT, MRI does not expose the patient to radiation. It is a noninvasive examination that involves placing the patient in a strong magnetic field and then applying bursts of radiofrequency waves. Sophisticated technology converts information about the movement of molecules in the tissue into precise, clear images (Fig. 27-11). Magnetic resonance angiography (MRA) is a special technique that allows the measurement of flow through blood vessels. Depending on the type of equipment available, metal prostheses, pacemakers, and various implants may contraindicate MRI. This noninvasive diagnostic procedure is painless, has no known risks, and requires no preparation.

COMMON THERAPEUTIC MEASURES

DRUG THERAPY

A number of drugs are used to treat neurologic disorders. They include antimicrobials, analgesics, antiinflammatory agents, corticosteroids, anticonvulsants, diuretics, chemotherapeutic agents, and dopaminergic, anticholinergic, cholinergic, and antihistamine medications. Because of the great variety of drugs used for neurologic conditions, specific drugs are discussed with individual conditions.

Pharmacology Capsule

Many drugs stimulate or depress the central nervous system (CNS). For example, caffeine is a stimulant whereas morphine is a depressant.

SURGERY

A craniotomy (surgical opening of the skull) may be done to treat tumors, correct defects, evacuate hematomas, and relieve pressure associated with trauma. A craniectomy is the excision of a segment of the skull and a cranioplasty is any procedure done to repair a

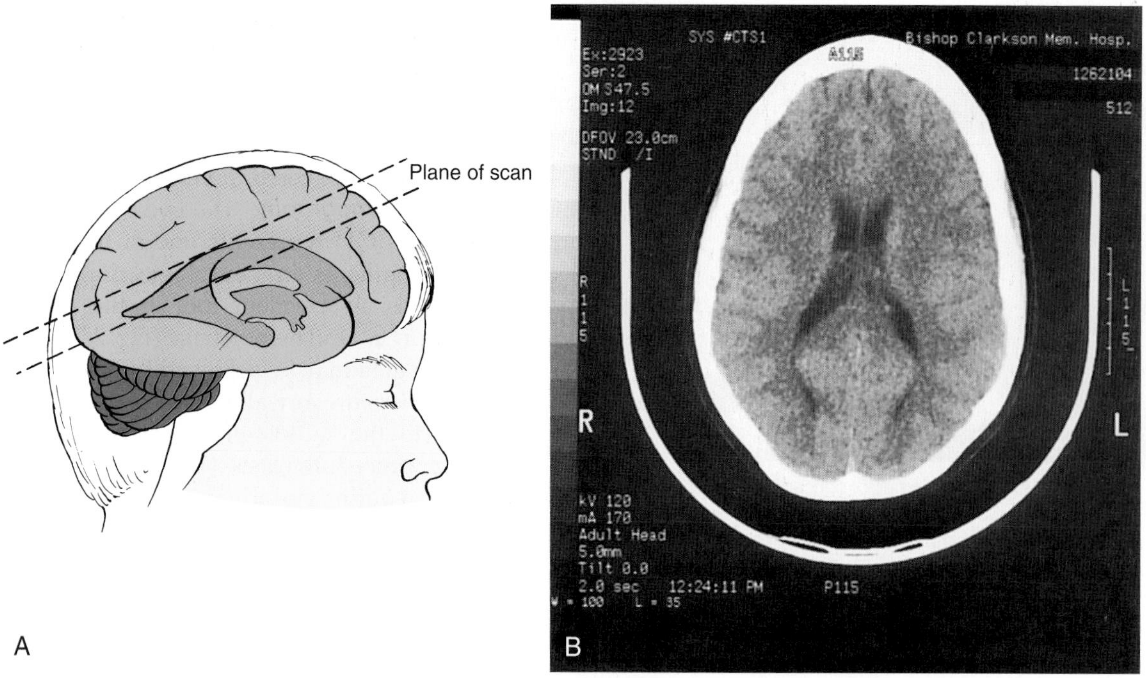

FIGURE 27-10 Computed tomography (CT) scans are taken at various cross-sections of the brain. The image in **A** illustrates the cross-section used for the scan shown in **B.** (From Black JM, Hawks JH, Keene AM: *Medical-surgical nursing: clinical management for continuity of care*, ed 6, Philadelphia, 2001, Saunders.)

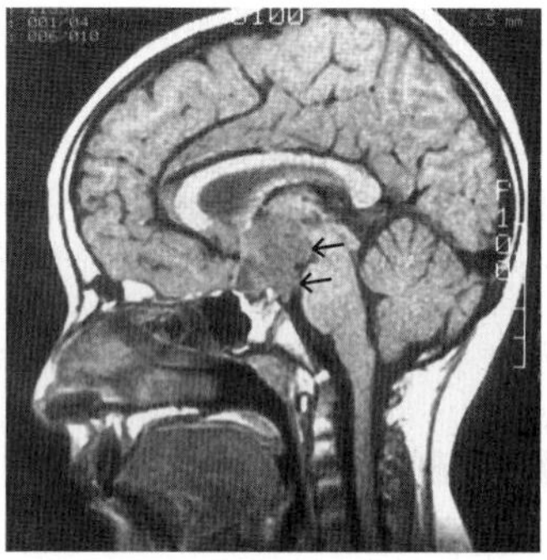

FIGURE 27-11 Magnetic resonance imaging (MRI) uses magnetic fields to create cross-sectional views of the brain. This sagittal section shows the cerebrum, ventricles, cerebellum, and medulla. (From Bontrager K, Lampignano J: *Textbook of radiographic positioning and related anatomy*, ed 8, St. Louis, Mosby, 2014.)

skull defect. General care of the surgical patient is discussed in Chapter 17 but interventions specific to neurologic surgery are emphasized here.

Preoperative Nursing Care

Preoperatively, document the patient's neurologic status to provide a baseline for evaluating postoperative progress. Encourage the patient to ask questions and to express fears. If the patient has cerebral edema, parenteral corticosteroids may be ordered to help reduce cerebral swelling. Hair on part of the scalp is usually clipped. Because shaving the head can be very stressful for patients, they should be assured that the hair will grow back. Sometimes clipping is done after the patient is anesthetized to reduce the trauma. Advise the patient's family that a craniotomy can take as long as 12 hours and that they will get progress reports during the procedure.

Postoperative Nursing Care

Postoperative craniotomy care includes monitoring level of consciousness, vital signs, movement and strength, pupil size and response to light, and speech. Signs and symptoms that may be related to complications are headache, visual disturbances, vomiting, seizures, and respiratory depression. Vital signs are recorded and neurologic checks are done hourly until the patient is stable. Maintain intake and output records and inspect any dressings for evidence of bleeding or CSF drainage. Note drainage from the ears or nose (if this occurs, a dressing may be placed loosely to absorb the drainage). Replace the dressing if it becomes wet because the moisture can harbor bacteria. On dressings, CSF appears as a pink stain surrounded by a lighter ring described as a *halo*. However, other fluids may produce halos as well. It is no longer recommended to check CSF with a dipstick for glucose because dipsticks are calibrated only for the specific fluids they were designed to test. Report any signs of deteriorating neurologic status to the physician immediately. The physician prescribes the patient's position and usually specifies that the head of the bed be elevated about 30 degrees.

If the patient has an external ventricular drainage system, use strict aseptic technique when changing the insertion site dressing and the drainage bag. Keep the zero reference point of the drip chamber of the drainage bag at the level of the external auditory canal (or at the level the physician prescribes) to prevent drainage of excessive CSF. When the patient is being repositioned, clamp and then restore the drainage tube to the correct level and unclamp it.

In addition to the usual surgical complications, the patient having a craniotomy is at risk for increased ICP, CSF leak, meningitis, and seizures. Other complications depend on the area of the brain affected and could include paralysis; memory loss; confusion; and impaired speech, vision, or hearing. Because increased ICP is a concern with cranial surgery, as well as with many neurologic disorders, it is described here.

INCREASED INTRACRANIAL PRESSURE

Increased ICP poses an extremely serious threat to the neurologic patient. Understanding the physiology as well as the signs and symptoms will enable you to recognize the problem and respond appropriately to prevent life-threatening consequences.

Pathophysiology

Anatomically, the skull is an empty cavity with rigid sides and an opening at the bottom. This cavity contains the brain, blood, and CSF, which are the components that exert pressure in the cranium. This pressure, or ICP, is normally 0 to 15 mm Hg.

In the course of a day, ICP fluctuates minimally because alterations are usually corrected rapidly. The Monro-Kellie hypothesis describes the adaptations that must occur in the three components (brain, blood, and CSF) for ICP to remain normal. If the volume of one component increases, ICP will rise unless a subsequent decrease occurs in the other two components. For example, if a brain tumor increases the volume of brain tissue, ICP will rise unless the volume of both blood and CSF decreases.

As ICP increases, the perfusion (delivery of blood and oxygen) to brain tissue decreases. This can be measured by calculating cerebral perfusion pressure (CPP), which is obtained by subtracting the ICP from the mean arterial pressure (MAP):

$$CPP = MAP - ICP$$

A minimum perfusion pressure of 70 mm Hg is necessary to ensure adequate cerebral functioning. If perfusion pressure falls to 40 mm Hg, ischemia occurs. A perfusion pressure of 30 mm Hg or less is incompatible with life. Perfusion pressure can be increased by decreasing ICP.

Signs and Symptoms

You can detect increases in ICP and assess the adequacy of perfusion based on the presence of specific signs and symptoms. Assess the patient's level of consciousness, pupillary characteristics, motor function, sensory function, and vital signs to detect signs of increasing ICP and initiate prompt treatment, if necessary.

Level of consciousness is the most reliable indicator of mental status because of its extreme sensitivity to oxygen levels in the cerebral blood. As ICP increases and perfusion is reduced, oxygen delivery to cerebral tissue also is reduced. Changes in level of consciousness are the earliest changes seen in ICP. These changes may be very subtle, with minimal agitation or drowsiness, or quite extreme, with profound unresponsiveness. Patients who are restless and agitated or suddenly quiet must be closely monitored and significant changes must be reported.

Classic pupillary changes are seen with increasing ICP. As pressure rises, the pupil progresses from its normal size to a dilated state described as a *blown pupil*. The pupil becomes dilated and fixed and no longer reacts to light. These changes occur because of pressure on the oculomotor nerve (third cranial nerve). This is a late sign of increased ICP.

Another major indicator of increased ICP is altered motor function. As the motor areas of the frontal lobe are compressed by rising pressure, deficits develop on the side opposite the expanding mass. When deficits are on the opposite side from brain injury, they are said to be *contralateral to the injury*. For example, if a tumor exists in the right side of the brain, motor deficits will appear in the left side of the body. The deficits may involve a single extremity or an entire side. **Hemiparesis** (weakness on one side) or **hemiplegia** (paralysis on one side) may be seen. The earliest sign of a change in motor function is a motor drift.

As increased pressure becomes more extensive, abnormal posturing may be evident. As increasing pressure is exerted on the cerebral tissue above the midbrain, a pattern known as *abnormal flexion* (**decorticate**) *posturing* can be observed. The patient exhibits abnormal flexion in the upper extremities, with extension of the lower extremities. Increasing pressure affecting the midbrain or upper pons causes *extension* (**decerebrate**) *posturing*. The lower extremities remain extended and the upper extremities are abnormally extended as well. These motor changes may occur spontaneously or may be seen only with painful stimuli (Fig. 27-12).

Hypothalamic impairment results in the loss of temperature control. As ICP compresses the tissue around the hypothalamus, it becomes ischemic and unable to regulate body temperature.

ICP elevations evoke an increase in systolic blood pressure with little or no associated increase in diastolic blood pressure. This results in a widening pulse pressure, defined as an increasing difference between systolic and diastolic blood pressure values. Initially the heart rate may be slightly accelerated. However, as ICP compresses the center for cardiac control in the brainstem, the heart rate becomes slow and irregular. Alterations in respiratory pattern are directly related

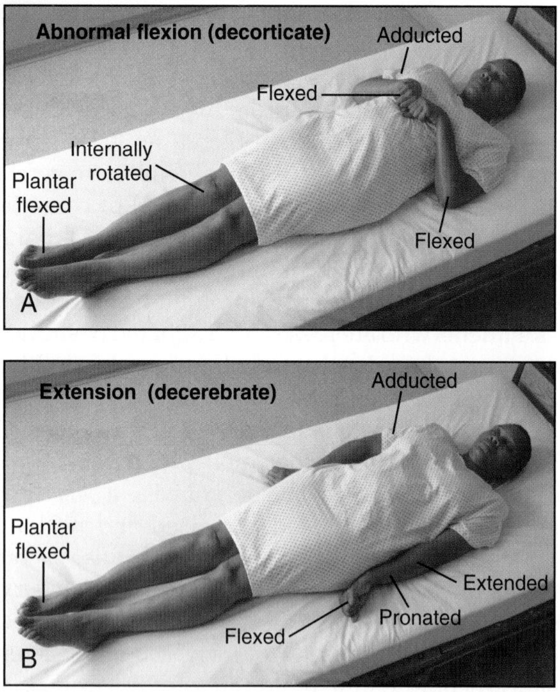

FIGURE 27-12 Abnormal postures may be seen in the patient with neurologic impairment. **A,** Abnormal flexion posturing (decorticate rigidity). **B,** Abnormal extension posturing (decerebrate rigidity). (From Monahan FD, Neighbors M, Sands JK, et al.: *Phipps' medical surgical nursing: Health and illness perspectives*, ed 8, St. Louis, 2008, Mosby.)

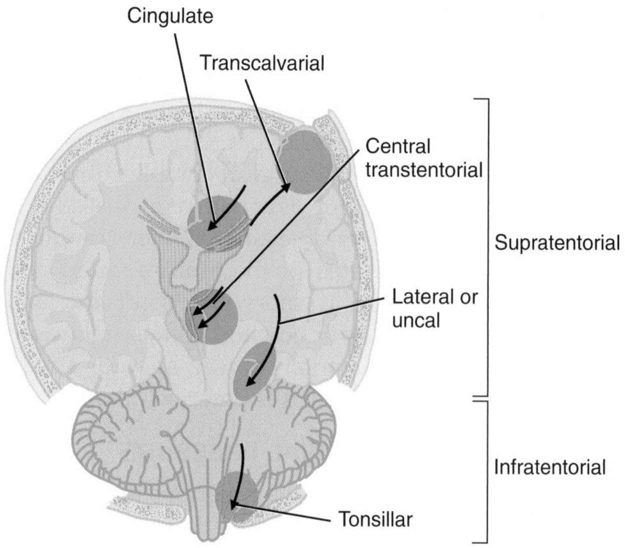

FIGURE 27-13 Types of intracranial herniation. In transcalvarial herniation, edematous brain tissue is extruded through a fracture in the skull. In central transtentorial herniation, the lesion is located centrally or superior in the cranium and compression of central and midbrain structures may result. In lateral or uncal herniation, the lesion is located laterally within the cranium and can cause pressure on the midbrain. Cingulate herniation occurs between the two frontal lobes; the brain is pressed under the falx cerebri. In tonsillar herniation, the cerebellar tonsils are driven between the posterior arch of the atlas and the medulla and may be compressed. (From Black JM, Hawks JH: *Medical-surgical nursing: clinical management for positive outcomes*, ed 8, St. Louis, 2009, Saunders.)

to the extent of tissue compression. Figure 27-13 illustrates areas of tissue compression (types of "herniation" syndromes).

Although it is extremely important to monitor vital signs in the neurologic patient, remember that changes in pulse, respiratory pattern, and blood pressure are late signs of increasing ICP. The combination of hypertension, bradycardia, and a widening pulse pressure is known as *Cushing's triad.* Cushing's triad is generally associated with increased ICP but it is unreliable in determining the severity of neurologic compromise.

Medical Treatment

Prompt treatment of increased ICP is vital for survival. Measures to lower ICP include positioning, hyperventilation, fluid management, mechanical drainage, and drug therapy.

The jugular vein is the primary route for venous outflow from the brain. It has long been thought that raising the head of the bed 30 to 45 degrees improves the flow of venous blood from the brain, thereby decreasing cerebral blood volume and ICP. However, recent research indicates that perfusion pressure may be better preserved if the head of the bed is elevated no more than 30 degrees. Further investigations may lead to some changes in current practice.

As oxygen delivery to cerebral tissue becomes more impaired, the level of carbon dioxide in the tissue increases. Increased carbon dioxide leads to dilation of cerebral blood vessels, thereby increasing the cerebral blood volume and ICP. With controlled hyperventilation, the excess carbon dioxide is eliminated, causing blood vessels to constrict and ICP to fall. Controlled hyperventilation is best achieved by mechanical ventilation. It decreases ICP within 1 to 2 minutes but its effectiveness is diminished after 36 to 48 hours. Hyperventilation does have risks. Excessive vasoconstriction reduces cerebral oxygenation and worsens ischemia. Hyperventilation may be reserved for situations in which other treatments fail to reduce ICP. The goal is to achieve normocapnia.

The patient must have adequate fluids to maintain CPP. Fluid volumes are often increased in an effort to boost perfusion. Patients with questionable cardiac function must be monitored closely for fluid volume excess. A specialized catheter, called a *ventriculostomy catheter*, can be placed in the brain to drain excess CSF. After placement, the catheter is connected to tubing and a collection bag for gravity drainage. Drainage of CSF lowers ICP. Absolute sterility must be maintained in managing this system, because it presents an open avenue for contamination.

Intravenous mannitol administration is one of the mainstays in the treatment of increased ICP. Mannitol is a hyperosmolar diuretic that draws edema fluid from the tissue spaces into the bloodstream. The mannitol and excess fluid are then eliminated through the kidneys. A rebound phenomenon may occur after administration. During administration some of the mediation crosses the blood-brain barrier. As mannitol is eliminated from the bloodstream, fluid is pulled into the brain. Other diuretics, such as furosemide, also may be used in an effort to reduce edema.

Corticosteroids, although controversial, may be used to help decrease cerebral edema and ICP. They decrease the edema, thereby lowering the elevated ICP associated with CNS tumors. Dexamethasone (Decadron) is a major agent used for patients with neurologic disorders.

Pharmacology Capsule

Diuretics used to treat increased intracranial pressure (ICP) can cause fluid and electrolyte imbalances.

DISORDERS OF THE NERVOUS SYSTEM

HEADACHE

Headache is the most common type of pain. It is a symptom, rather than a disease, that has many causes. Four common types of headaches are (1) migraine headache; (2) cluster headache; (3) tension headache; and (4) headache related to disorders of the eyes, teeth, or sinuses. For headaches associated with these and other conditions, treatment depends on the underlying cause (see *Complementary and Alternative Therapies* box).

Complementary and Alternative Therapies

Complementary and alternative therapies are excellent adjuncts in the management of headache. Progressive muscle relaxation techniques, imagery, acupuncture, and electromyography (EMG) biofeedback may reduce the frequency and intensity of headaches.

Migraine Headache

Migraine headache is thought to be caused by intracranial vasoconstriction followed by vasodilation. Although no single cause is known, it may be triggered by menstruation, ovulation, alcohol, some foods, and stress.

Patients may experience depression, irritability, vision disturbances, nausea, and paresthesias before the onset of pain. The pain is usually unilateral, often begins in the temple or eye area, and is often very intense. Tearing and nausea and vomiting may occur. The patient is hypersensitive to light and sound and prefers a dark, quiet environment.

Mild migraines may be treated with acetaminophen or aspirin but more severe ones may be treated with ergotamine (Cafergot) or sumatriptan (Imitrex), administered as a tablet or by autoinjector for self-injection. However, prevention should be emphasized. Medications such as beta-blockers or calcium channel blockers may help to control the vascular influences. Identification and avoidance of triggering agents, such as particular foods (e.g., chocolate, yogurt, aged meats, cheeses), beverages (e.g., alcohol, red wine), or emotional stress, may also prove helpful.

Cluster Headache

Cluster headaches occur in a series of episodes followed by a long period with no symptoms. They are intensely painful and seem to be related to stress or anxiety. Unlike migraines, cluster headaches usually have no warning symptoms. They are also shorter in duration than migraines. Treatment may include cold application, indomethacin (Indocin), and tricyclic antidepressants.

Tension Headache

Tension headaches result from prolonged muscle contraction associated with anxiety, stress, or stimuli from other sources such as a brain tumor or an abscessed tooth. The location of the pain may vary and the patient may have nausea and vomiting, dizziness, tinnitus, or tearing. Tension headaches may persist for days or even years. Treatment measures include correction of known causes, psychotherapy, massage, heat application, and relaxation techniques. Analgesics, usually nonopioid drugs, may be prescribed along with other medications to reduce anxiety.

SEIZURE DISORDER

The electrical impulses generated in the brain normally spread in a very organized fashion. However, in the patient with a seizure disorder, electrical impulses are conducted in a highly chaotic pattern that yields abnormal activity and behavior. **Seizure** activity involves a large number of hyperactive neurons that use excessive oxygen and glucose. Therefore oxygen and glucose stores may be depleted, leading to permanent neurologic damage.

Seizure activity may be related to trauma, reduced cerebral perfusion, infection, electrolyte disturbances, poisoning, or tumors. A genetic tendency for such activity may also exist.

Medical Diagnosis

Diagnostic testing for seizure activity is often directed toward ruling out specific problems. An accurate history of the seizure disorder can provide clues to the type of seizure disorder, possible triggering events, and the origin of activity. Because unexpected seizure activity is often very frightening to the family, the nurse or other health care provider may be the first reliable eyewitness. If you observe a seizure, note the patient's behavior before, during, and after the seizure, as well as the duration of the seizure.

The patient's EEG tracing, which records the electrical activity of the brain, is used to detect abnormal brain activity.

Seizure Classification

The two broad classifications of seizures, based on the patterns of activity, are (1) partial seizures and (2) generalized seizures. Abnormal electrical activity may be generated in a specific area of the brain, remain localized and stop, or the activity may spread to adjacent neurons but remain fairly localized. These patterns of activity are termed *partial* (or focal) *seizures* because they involve only a part of the brain. The observed activity corresponds to the area of the brain affected.

In addition, partial seizures may recruit a sufficient number of adjacent cells and the activity can spread throughout the cerebral hemispheres. This is known as a *partial seizure with secondary generalization. Generalized seizures* involve the entire brain from the onset and are associated with loss of consciousness.

Some sources use the term *unclassified seizures* for those that are not readily classified as *partial* or *generalized.*

Partial Seizures. Partial seizures are described as *simple* or *complex.* Simple seizures affect part of one cerebral hemisphere and consciousness is not impaired. A simple partial seizure may include motor, somatosensory, autonomic, or psychic symptoms. Focal motor seizures are a subtype of simple seizures in which the abnormal brain activity remains localized to a specific motor area. This may occur with or without *jacksonian march,* the term used when the abnormal activity begins in one area and then "marches" (spreads) to adjacent motor areas. For example, the simple focal motor seizure may begin with the eyelid, then spread to the same side of the face, and continue on to involve the arm and leg on that side.

In a complex partial seizure (previously called a *psychomotor* or *temporal lobe seizure*), the patient's consciousness is impaired and the patient may exhibit bizarre, repetitive behavior. Simple partial and complex partial seizures can progress to involve the entire brain. These are referred to as *partial seizures with secondary generalization.*

Generalized Seizures. Generalized seizures involve the entire brain from the onset. Consciousness is lost during the *ictal* (seizure) period. One type of generalized seizure is the tonic-clonic seizure, previously referred to as a *grand mal seizure.* The *tonic phase* of the seizure is characterized by stiffening of the muscles or extremities with loss of consciousness. After the tonic phase, a rhythmic movement of the extremities occurs, called the *clonic phase* of the seizure. When seizure activity ceases (the *postictal* phase), the patient is sleepy and has no memory of the seizure. These phases are illustrated in Figure 27-14. The patient may be incontinent of urine during a generalized seizure.

Other types of generalized seizures are absence, myoclonic, and atonic seizures. Absence seizures (previously called *petit mal*) are brief periods of loss of consciousness in which the person may appear to be daydreaming. Absence seizures may be associated with automatisms such as eye blinking and lip smacking. These seizures are generally identified during childhood. During a myoclonic seizure, the person has only brief jerking or stiffening of the extremities. Atonic seizures were formerly called *drop attacks* because a sudden loss of muscle tone causes the patient to collapse.

Status Epilepticus. Status epilepticus is a medical emergency in which the patient has continuous seizures or repeated seizures in rapid succession for 30 minutes or more. The prolonged seizure activity depletes the brain of oxygen and glucose, which can lead to permanent brain damage.

Aura. Some people experience an aura preceding a seizure. The **aura** is a sensation such as dizziness, numbness, visual or hearing disturbance, perception of an offensive odor, or pain. It occurs before loss of consciousness. The individual retains the memory of the aura and so is able to recognize the oncoming seizure.

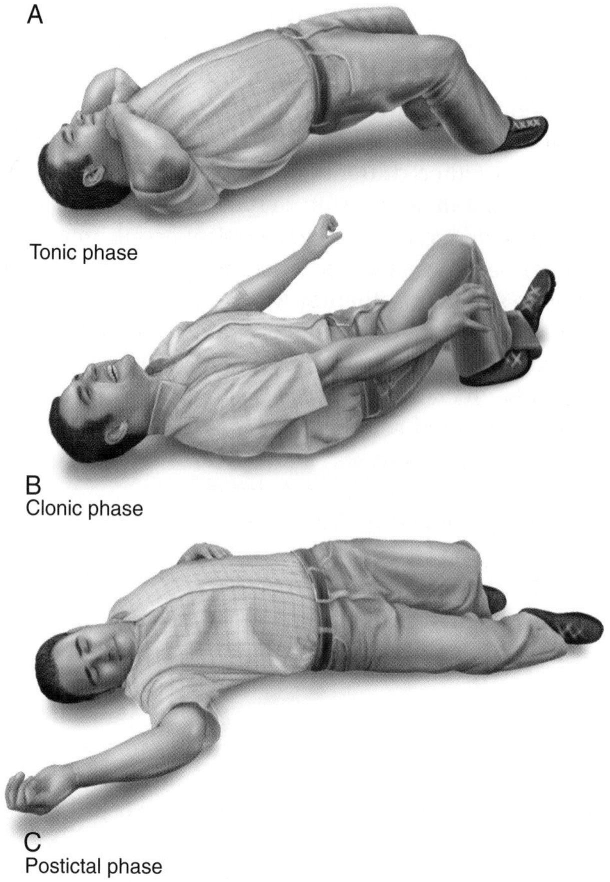

FIGURE 27-14 Phases of a generalized tonic-clonic seizure. **A,** Tonic phase is marked by loss of consciousness, falling, crying, and generalized stiffness. Incontinence may occur. **B,** During the clonic phase, jerking of the limbs and salivary frothing occurs. **C,** During the postictal phase, seizure activity has ceased. The patient is drowsy and has no memory of the seizure. (From Black JM, Hawks JH: *Medical-surgical nursing: clinical management for positive outcomes*, ed 8, St. Louis, 2009, Saunders.)

Medical Treatment

The most desirable treatment of a seizure disorder is the resolution of the underlying condition. For example, if a tumor is causing seizure activity, surgical excision of the tumor would be the most desirable therapy. However, if a cause is not readily identifiable or correctable, medical management is implemented.

Anticonvulsant drug therapy provides satisfactory chemical control of seizure activity in about 75% of patients. A variety of drugs are available, some being more effective in particular seizure disorders than others. The selected drug is introduced and the dose is gradually increased until a therapeutic level is achieved. If good seizure control is not accomplished with one drug, combinations of drugs may be prescribed. Examples of specific drugs used to treat epilepsy are presented in Table 27-5.

Status epilepticus is treated with intravenous anticonvulsant drugs. If the patient does not respond to anticonvulsants, general anesthetics and neuromuscular blockers may be used (see *Health Promotion* box).

Health Promotion

Seizures

Patients with seizure disorders should receive the following interventions as necessary.

PREVENTION OF SEIZURE DISORDER

- Promote general safety behaviors such as use of helmets and seat belts.
- Obtain perinatal care (for pregnant women and those planning to become pregnant).

PATIENTS WITH SEIZURE DISORDER SHOULD

- Avoid alcohol use.
- Get adequate rest.
- Engage in stress-reducing activities such as meditation and visualization.
- Maintain general health through proper diet and exercise.

Surgical Treatment

Patients whose seizures are poorly controlled with medication may be candidates for surgical procedures to decrease or control seizures. Procedures include removal of seizure foci in the temporal lobe and pallidotomy or implantation of a vagal nerve stimulator.

Pharmacology Capsule

Sudden discontinuance of anticonvulsant drugs can trigger seizure activity.

NURSING CARE of the Patient with a Seizure Disorder

Assessment

Assessment of the neurologic patient is summarized in Box 27-2. With a seizure disorder, it is especially important to describe the seizure episode, including the **postictal** period and to document drug therapy.

Nursing Diagnoses, Goals, and Outcome Criteria: Seizure Disorder

Nursing Diagnoses	Goals and Outcome Criteria
Risk for Injury related to seizure activity	Absence of injury: no bruises, breaks in skin, or fractures
Ineffective Coping related to social stigma of seizure disorder or chronicity	Effective coping: patient makes positive statements about life with seizure disorder, patient adheres to prescribed therapy
Deficient Knowledge of seizure disorders, treatment, and self-care	Patient understands self-care: patient and family accurately describe condition, drug therapy, and care; demonstrate appropriate care

Interventions

Risk for Injury

You must protect the patient from injury during and after a seizure. Most agencies require that the side rails of the bed be up and padded, a suction machine be readily available, and the bed be maintained in the low position. Some experts believe that padding the side rails is unnecessary, is cumbersome, and may have a negative emotional effect on the patient and visitors. However, it is a common practice used in an effort to protect the patient in case he or she strikes the rails during a seizure.

If the patient has a seizure, quickly move objects away from the patient. If the patient falls to the floor, the head may be cradled in your lap to prevent injury. Do not attempt to restrain the patient. In the past it was common practice to attempt to insert a tongue blade or oral airway between the teeth to prevent biting of the tongue. However, this is no longer recommended. Attempts to force an object between clenched teeth may result in injury to the mouth and do not help if the tongue has already been bitten. The patient will not "swallow the tongue" but it may fall back and occlude the airway. Turning the patient to one side can help to maintain a patent airway. Measures to prevent injury are described in Box 27-3. !

When seizure activity ceases, the patient is typically drowsy and needs to rest. During this postictal period, the nurse should provide for quiet and privacy. Afterward, he or she should document the conditions and any unusual behaviors that preceded the seizure, the length of the seizure, associated patient activity, deviation of the eyes, and any incontinence. In addition, document any lingering effects and the time before recovery.

Box 27-3 Management of Seizures

"DOS"

DO remove any objects that could cause harm.
DO turn the person to one side if possible.
DO note the time the seizure began and how it progressed.
DO assess and document postictal (postseizure) status.
DO allow the person to rest quietly.
DO call a medical emergency if a generalized tonic-clonic seizure lasts more than 4 minutes or if seizures occur in rapid succession.

"DO NOTS"

DO NOT restrain the person unless he or she is in grave danger of severe injury.
DO NOT attempt to force anything between the person's teeth.

Ineffective Coping and Deficient Knowledge

Ineffective coping can be related to lack of information or misconceptions and may be reflected in noncompliance with prescribed therapy, anxiety, or social isolation. Important aspects of nursing management include not only the care of the patient during hospitalization but also teaching the family and patient about the seizure disorder and the therapy. For guidelines on teaching, see the *Patient Teaching* box.

Patient Teaching

Seizures

- Factors that may trigger a seizure are fatigue, stress, fever, visual disturbances, alcohol, failure to take medication, and large caffeine intake.
- When an impending seizure is perceived, immediately seek a safe place.
- Know your prescribed drug names, dosages, schedules, and side effects to be reported to the physician.
- Consult your physician regarding the use of generic substitutions for your drugs.
- Never stop taking your seizure medication without direction from your physician.
- Psychologic counseling may help you to deal with stress associated with this disorder.
- Always wear a medical alert tag, which states that you have a seizure disorder, and carry a card that specifies drug therapy, physician, and individuals to be contacted in an emergency.
- The local chapter of the Epilepsy Foundation is an excellent resource (1-800-332-1000; www.EFA.org).
- A sensation that warns of an impending seizure is called an *aura;* common sensations include dizziness, numbness, visual or hearing disturbance, pain, and perception of an offensive odor.

Because a seizure disorder is often a lifelong problem, patient teaching must be directed toward helping the patient and family adjust to a chronic condition. Patients must adjust physically, psychologically, and vocationally to the changes brought on by the disorder itself as well as to the side effects of the medications. The nurse should encourage the patient to ask questions and to express concerns.

HEAD INJURY

Traumatic brain injury is a leading cause of death caused by trauma in the United States. The most common causes of head injury are motor vehicle accidents, assaults, and falls, with drug and alcohol abuse being major contributing factors. Several different types of injuries can be identified.

Types of Head Injuries

Scalp Injuries. Scalp injuries include lacerations, contusions, abrasions, and hematomas. They may bleed profusely and may or may not be associated with skull or brain injuries.

Concussion. A concussion is head trauma in which no visible injury exists to the skull or brain. The patient has a loss of consciousness lasting less than 5 minutes and may have a headache, amnesia about the event, nausea, and vomiting.

Contusion. A contusion is more serious than a concussion because actual bruising and bleeding exist in the brain tissue. Contusions can be very serious, especially if the brainstem is affected.

Hematomas. A hematoma is a collection of blood, usually clotted, that may be classified as *subdural* or *epidural.*

Subdural Hematoma. A subdural hematoma is usually the result of tearing of the veins that drain the brain, allowing blood to accumulate in the space beneath the dura (Fig. 27-15, A). The three types of subdural hematomas are (1) acute, (2) subacute, and (3) chronic. Acute subdural hematomas develop within 24 hours of the injury. Subacute subdural hematomas are seen more than 24 hours and less than 1 week after the initial injury. Chronic subdural hematomas occur within weeks or even months of the original injury and are associated with low-impact injuries that cause very slow, diffuse bleeding. Because the bleeding associated with any hematoma can cause potentially serious consequences, astute assessment is needed to determine patient status. Surgical intervention is usually indicated for these types of injuries.

Epidural Hematoma. An epidural hematoma forms in the space between the inner surface of the skull and the outermost meningeal covering of the brain, known as the *dura* (see Fig. 27-15, A). Generally, epidural hematomas result from arterial bleeding secondary to a laceration and tearing of the middle meningeal artery. The patient typically has a momentary lapse of consciousness, then a period of alertness, followed by rapid deterioration. Therefore you must be alert for any indication of increasing ICP, especially drowsiness progressing to coma. Surgical intervention may be necessary to relieve pressure, remove the clot, and stop the bleeding.

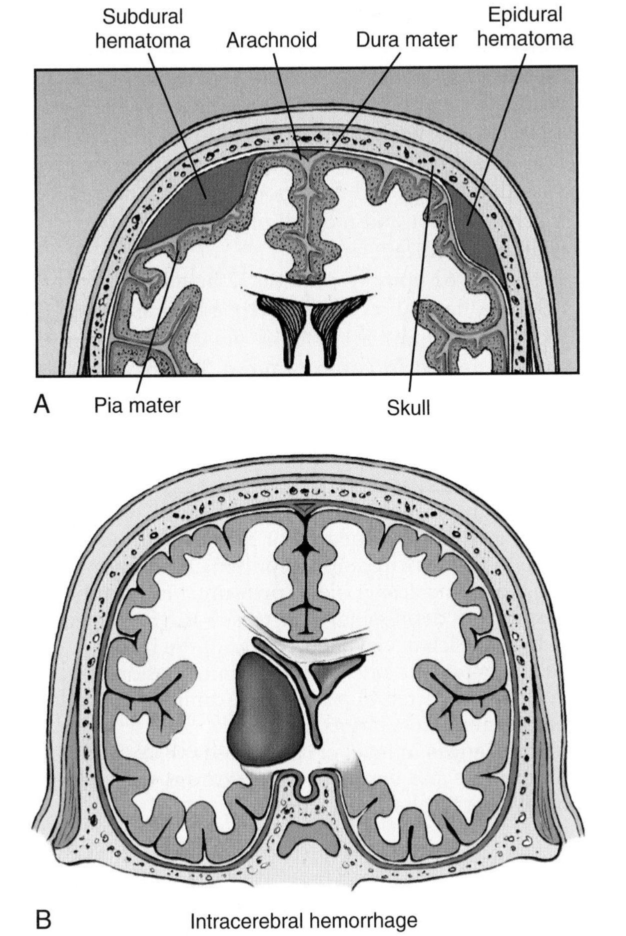

FIGURE 27-15 **A,** Epidural hematoma and subdural hematoma. **B,** Intracerebral hemorrhage. (From Black JM, Hawks JH, Keene AM: *Medical-surgical nursing: clinical management for continuity of care*, ed 6, Philadelphia, 2001, Saunders.)

Intracerebral Hemorrhage. Intracerebral hemorrhages result from lesions within the tissue of the brain itself (Fig. 27-15, B). These injuries may be small or large and may be accompanied by massive neurologic deficits.

Penetrating Injuries. Penetrating injuries result from sharp objects that penetrate the skull and brain tissue. In addition to the obvious brain injury, a scalp laceration exists along with a skull fracture. All penetrating injuries require prompt surgical intervention and pose an extremely high risk of infection for the patient because of the wound contamination that occurs.

Surgical Treatment

Surgical intervention for each of these types of trauma is directed at evacuating (removing) hematomas and debriding damaged tissue.

❖ NURSING CARE of the Patient with a Head Injury

■ Assessment

Nursing assessment of the patient with a neurologic disorder is outlined in Box 27-2. (See also Nursing Care Plan: Patient with a Head Injury and the *Health Promotion* box.

Health Promotion

Preventing Head Injury

Everyone should practice general safety by using the following:

- Helmets for sports activities such as football, baseball, skydiving, snowboarding, and skateboarding
- Helmets for riding bikes and motorcycles
- Seat belts while in automobiles
- Helmets on job sites for high-risk jobs such as construction and mining

Nursing Diagnoses, Goals, and Outcome Criteria: Head Injury

Nursing Diagnoses	Goals and Outcome Criteria
Risk for Ineffective Cerebral Tissue Perfusion related to increased intracranial pressure (ICP)	Adequate cerebral tissue perfusion: patient alert and oriented
Ineffective Breathing Pattern related to increased ICP	Normal oxygenation: respiratory rate of 12 to 20 breaths/min with normal arterial blood gas values
Risk for Injury related to seizures, decreased level of consciousness, disorientation, vision disturbances	Absence of injury: no abrasions, fractures, or severe bruising incurred during seizures or falls
Risk for Infection related to traumatic wounds or invasive procedures	Absence of infection: normal body temperature without signs of wound infection (redness, edema, purulent drainage), urinary infection (cloudiness, foul odor), or phlebitis (redness, tenderness)
Impaired Physical Mobility related to neuromuscular impairment, decreased mental alertness	Absence of complications of immobility (contractures, pressure ulcers, pneumonia, atelectasis, constipation, urinary retention): intact skin, mobile joints, regular bowel movements, no bladder distention, breath sounds clear on auscultation
Disturbed Body Image related to loss of function	Adaptation to altered body function: patient verbalizes way to compensate for changes in body function
Ineffective Role Performance related to neurologic impairment	Adjustment of roles and responsibilities consistent with abilities: patient assumes new roles within abilities

Nursing Care Plan Patient with a Head Injury

ASSESSMENT

HEALTH HISTORY Austin Mandrel is a 17-year-old male who was injured in a motorcycle accident 2 days ago. He reportedly struck his head on the pavement and was unconscious on admission. He is now alert and oriented to person and place but not to time. He asks if he has any permanent injuries. He had a seizure the evening of admission but is now being given anticonvulsant drugs and has had no seizures since. His mother reports that he has had no serious illnesses, hospitalizations, or operations and that he has no known allergies. He is a high school junior and football player. He has two close friends who visit frequently. He is receiving intravenous fluids and antibiotic medications.

PHYSICAL EXAMINATION Vital signs: blood pressure 150/84 mm Hg, pulse 62 bpm, respiration 12 breaths per minute, temperature 98°F (37°C) measured orally. Height 6′1″, weight 145 lbs. Sutured laceration on the forehead; abrasions on the forehead and right cheek. Edematous. Serosanguineous drainage. Pupils equal and react to light. No drainage from the ears. No stiffness of the neck. Reflexes normal in right extremities but decreased in left extremities. Patient moves left extremities on command but they are weaker (4/5) than the right.

Nursing Diagnosis	Goals and Outcome Criteria	Interventions
Risk for Ineffective Cerebral Tissue Perfusion related to increased intracranial pressure (ICP)	Patient will have adequate cerebral tissue perfusion, as evidenced by alertness and orientation to person, place, and time.	Monitor for signs of increased ICP: decreasing level of consciousness, pupil inequality or dilation without response to light, increasing motor deficits, abnormal posture, fever, increasing blood pressure, bradycardia, and respiratory depression. If increased ICP is suspected, notify the physician; elevate the head of the bed as ordered. Monitor the rate of fluid administration to ensure adequate cerebral perfusion. Administer diuretic and antiinflammatory drugs as ordered.
Ineffective Breathing Pattern related to increased ICP	Patient will have adequate oxygenation, as evidenced by respiratory rate of 12 to 20 breaths per minute with normal arterial blood gas values.	Monitor for changes in level of consciousness, decreasing respiratory rate and depth, and tachycardia. Check the results of arterial blood gas studies.
Risk for Injury related to lethargy, possible seizures	Patient will remain free of injury during hospitalization.	Use seizure precautions per agency policy. Place the bed in low position. Have a call bell available and within reach of patient's right hand. Provide assistance with transferring.
Risk for Infection related to traumatic wounds	Patient will remain free of infection, as evidenced by normal temperature and white blood cell count.	Assess temperature for elevation. Assess wounds for increasing redness, edema, and foul drainage. Use Standard Precautions for wound care and when handling invasive equipment. Administer antibiotic drugs as ordered.
Impaired Physical Mobility related to neuromuscular impairment, lethargy	Patient will retain normal range of motion in all extremities and will participate in activities to restore strength to left extremities.	Explain the importance of frequent position changes (at least every 2 hours) and assist the patient to do so. Position the affected extremities in functional alignment. Assist in active range-of-motion exercises at least three times a day. Apply antiembolism stockings as ordered. Assess skin, especially bony prominences, for signs of pressure or breakdown. Monitor elimination to detect urinary retention or constipation. Encourage fluids and high-fiber diet as needed.
Disturbed Body Image related to loss of function	Patient will adapt to altered body function, as reflected in positive statements about self.	Encourage the patient to ask questions and to express thoughts and feelings about injuries. Include him in planning sessions. Show acceptance through touch and genuine interest. Encourage his friends to continue visits. Explain helping process and how rehabilitation measures can help. Emphasize abilities rather than disabilities. Promote independence in light of abilities. Refer the patient to a support group.
Ineffective Role Performance related to neurologic impairment	Patient will participate in rehabilitation efforts and explore potential new roles and activities.	Explain the healing process and how rehabilitation measures can help. As the patient improves, help him learn to perform activities of daily living (ADL) with limitations.

Critical Thinking Questions

1. How does increased ICP affect respirations?
2. Why would the patient lose consciousness when the ICP is elevated?

Interventions

Risk for Ineffective Cerebral Tissue Perfusion

Monitor the patient closely for signs of increased ICP and impaired cerebral blood flow: decreasing level of consciousness, pupillary dilation with no response to light, motor deficits, abnormal posture, fever, increased blood pressure, bradycardia, and respiratory depression. Particularly note early signs of deterioration, including restlessness, agitation, or lethargy, and promptly report changes to the physician or the registered nurse (RN). Nursing care that can decrease ICP includes positioning to prevent neck and hip flexion, limiting suctioning, spacing nursing care, and preventing isometric muscle contraction. Elevate the head of the bed as ordered. Carefully regulate the rate of administration of intravenous fluids to prevent fluid volume excess. Also monitor urine output to assess fluid balance. If a ventriculostomy catheter is in place, inspect and measure the drainage fluid as ordered using strict aseptic technique. Administer diuretic and antiinflammatory drugs as ordered.

Ineffective Breathing Pattern

Closely monitor the patient's respiratory status using pulse oximetry or measurement of arterial blood gases. Immediately advise the physician of signs of respiratory depression or changes in the patient's respiratory pattern.

Risk for Injury

Nursing measures to prevent injuries associated with seizures are discussed in previous sections of this chapter and are summarized in Box 27-3.

Risk for Infection

The patient who has suffered a head injury may have serious lacerations or abrasions that can admit pathogenic organisms. Intravenous lines and urinary catheters also place the patient at risk for infection. Use Standard Precautions when handling all invasive lines and when dressing wounds. In addition, monitor the patient's temperature and inspect wounds for increasing redness, swelling, or foul drainage. Administer antibiotic drugs as ordered.

Impaired Physical Mobility

After a head injury, the patient may have temporary or permanent motor impairment. While confined to bed, the patient should be turned and positioned and encouraged to deep breathe at least every 2 hours. Routinely inspect the patient's skin for signs of pressure or breakdown and use antiembolism stockings if ordered. Encourage the patient to perform range-of-motion exercises and position joints in functional alignment. Assess urine and bowel elimination frequently to detect retention or constipation. As soon as permitted, help the patient out of bed and encourage as much activity as possible. Unfortunately, some head-injured patients have permanent impairments that necessitate lifelong care. Care of the immobile patient is discussed in detail in Chapter 21.

Disturbed Body Image and Ineffective Role Performance

The losses associated with a serious head injury can render the patient unable to resume usual activities. The injury also may leave disfiguring scars or distorted features. Demonstrate acceptance of the patient through touch and genuine interest. Encourage the patient to ask questions, express concerns, and anticipate problems and solutions. Be realistic about the patient's disabilities while emphasizing abilities.

Patients with serious deficits are usually treated by a team that includes rehabilitation specialists. These experts help the patient to regain physical mobility, learn to carry out ADL, learn new job skills, and deal with the emotional trauma of the injury and its effects.

Include the patient's family in the rehabilitation process. In many cases, family members serve as the caregivers after head injury. Activities provided by families include providing personal care, obtaining rehabilitation services, providing a safe environment, seeking reminders of the preinjury person, exploring what abilities might be regained, encouraging return to preinjury activities, encouraging active decision making, becoming active members of the rehabilitation team, and staying open to potential gains.

Put on Your Thinking Cap!

You are caring for a patient with a head injury. The patient has been lethargic for most of the day but now seems more difficult to arouse. His vital signs and pupils are the same as they have been. What do you think is your best course of action in this situation?

BRAIN TUMORS

Brain tumors account for a relatively small percentage of cancer deaths annually. Brain tumors develop in some cancer patients as a result of metastasis from other primary sites. Tumor cells can spread to the CNS through the blood and CSF.

Not all brain tumors are malignant. Some tumor types, such as the meningioma, a tumorous growth of the meningeal tissue, are often benign. One might assume that benign tumor cells would suggest an excellent chance of complete recovery. However, the invasion of any kind of tumor into normal brain tissue is never insignificant. This invasion can cause significant damage that may prove fatal because of increasing ICP or surgical inaccessibility of the tumor.

Causes and Risk Factors

The causes of brain tumors are generally unknown but some appear to be congenital in origin whereas others may be related to heredity. In addition, drug influences and environmental factors may play a role in the development of some brain tumors.

Signs and Symptoms

The signs and symptoms of brain tumors are directly related to the area of the brain that is invaded by the tumor. Motor and sensory symptoms, visual disturbances, and headache all may be early manifestations of tumor growth. New-onset seizure activity in an adult patient often indicates the presence of a tumor. Cerebellar tumors may cause difficulties with balance and coordination. Other tumors, depending on their location, may involve cranial nerves.

Medical Treatment

Management of the patient with a brain tumor depends on the type of cells present in the tumor. Surgery can be done to remove as much of the tumor tissue as possible. If the tumor is malignant, surgery is often followed by radiation therapy with or without chemotherapy.

NURSING CARE of the Patient with a Brain Tumor

Nursing care of the patient with a brain tumor depends on the specific deficits, treatment, and prognosis and may be similar to the care of the patient with a head injury. Care of the patient with cancer is discussed in Chapter 25.

Assessment

The complete neurologic assessment is summarized in Box 27-2. The assessment is especially important before brain surgery to provide a baseline for comparing postoperative findings.

Nursing Diagnoses, Goals, and Outcome Criteria: Brain Tumor

Nursing diagnoses vary with the patient's specific symptoms and disabilities and the type of treatment used. Common nursing diagnoses and goals include the following.

Nursing Diagnoses	Goals and Outcome Criteria
Acute Pain related to pressure of expanding tumor mass	Pain relief: patient states pain is relieved, has relaxed manner
Risk for Acute Confusion and Impaired Memory related to effects of tumor on brain tissue	Adaptation to altered thinking: improved mental orientation
Risk for Injury related to impaired conduction of sensory information	Safety maintained: absence of injury associated with sensory or perceptual impairment
Impaired Physical Mobility and **Self-Care Deficit (Bathing, Dressing, Feeding, Toileting)** related to motor disturbances, impaired cognition	Accomplishment of activities of daily living (ADL): maximum possible patient mobility level and absence of complications of immobility (contractures, pneumonia, constipation, urinary retention)
Ineffective Coping related to life-threatening disease, changes in behavior function	Effective coping: patient and family make positive statements about ability to deal with the illness

Interventions

Acute Pain

Document pain and administer analgesics as ordered. Codeine or acetaminophen is often used. Small doses of morphine also may be used for pain relief. If pain relief is not achieved, inform the physician and assess for signs of increased ICP.

Risk for Acute Confusion and Impaired Memory

Monitor the patient for changes in cognitive function by assessing orientation and response to instructions. Patients may demonstrate cognitive dysfunction, including impaired short-term memory, poor judgment, poor decision making, and impaired problem solving. Investigate sudden changes in mental status that may be caused by the tumor or by correctable factors such as drugs, hypoxia, and fluid and electrolyte imbalances. Listen carefully to the patient and present reality in a straightforward manner. Devices to help the patient maintain orientation include clocks, calendars, and seasonal decorations.

Risk for Injury

Explain to the patient that the effects of the brain tumor may cause unusual sensations and perceptual disturbances. Implement safety measures as needed to prevent injury because of impaired vision, spatial perceptual problems, or sensation.

Impaired Physical Mobility and Self-Care Deficits (Bathing, Dressing, Feeding, Toileting)

Patients with brain tumors may have varying degrees of physical impairment. Assess the patient's ability to perform ADL and provide assistance as needed. Encourage the patient to remain as active as possible. If the patient's mobility is severely impaired, a high risk exists for disuse syndrome and the associated complications. Care of the immobilized patient is described in Chapter 21.

Ineffective Coping

The patient and family need assistance in dealing with a difficult diagnosis in addition to the obvious residual physical effects. A diagnosis of a malignant brain tumor is devastating for the family and emotional support is vital to help family members understand the nature of the disease and the anticipated problems and outcomes. Nursing care depends on the specific deficits, treatment, and prognosis and may be similar to the care of the patient with a head injury. Care of the patient with cancer is discussed in Chapter 25.

INFECTIOUS AND INFLAMMATORY CONDITIONS: MENINGITIS

Meningitis is inflammation of the meningeal coverings of the brain and spinal cord caused by either viruses or bacteria. Organisms may reach the meninges through the blood, through head wounds, or from other cranial structures such as the sinuses or inner ear. A number of organisms may be responsible for bacterial infection, including *Neisseria meningitidis, Streptococcus pneumoniae,* and *Haemophilus influenzae.*

Complications of meningitis include seizures, septicemia, vasomotor collapse, and increased ICP. *N. meningitidis* is particularly problematic because septicemia develops in approximately 10% of patients.

Signs and Symptoms

The common signs and symptoms of meningitis are related to meningeal irritation. These include headache, nuchal rigidity (stiffness of the back of the neck), irritability, diminished level of consciousness, photophobia (sensitivity to light), hypersensitivity, and seizure activity. The presence of Kernig sign and Brudzinski sign also is indicative of meningeal irritation. To assess for Kernig sign (Fig. 27-16, A), flex the patient's hip to a 90-degree angle and then extend the knee. In the presence of a meningeal infection, this movement produces pain in the hamstring area. Brudzinski sign (Fig. 27-16, B) is flexion of both hips when the examiner flexes the patient's neck.

Medical Diagnosis

A lumbar puncture is done to obtain a CSF sample for laboratory analysis. The sample is examined to detect the presence of microorganisms in the CSF and to identify the infecting organism. With bacterial meningitis, the CSF appears milky and purulent because of white blood cells suspended in the fluid. CT or MRI scans are used to assess for complications.

Medical Treatment

Management of bacterial meningitis requires prompt recognition and treatment with antimicrobial agents. In severe infections, broad-spectrum antimicrobials are used after a CSF specimen is obtained. Changes in therapy may be made when the results of culture and sensitivity tests are reported. Bacterial infections usually respond to antimicrobial therapy but no specific drugs are effective against most viral infections of the CNS. Anticonvulsants are used to control seizure activity if necessary.

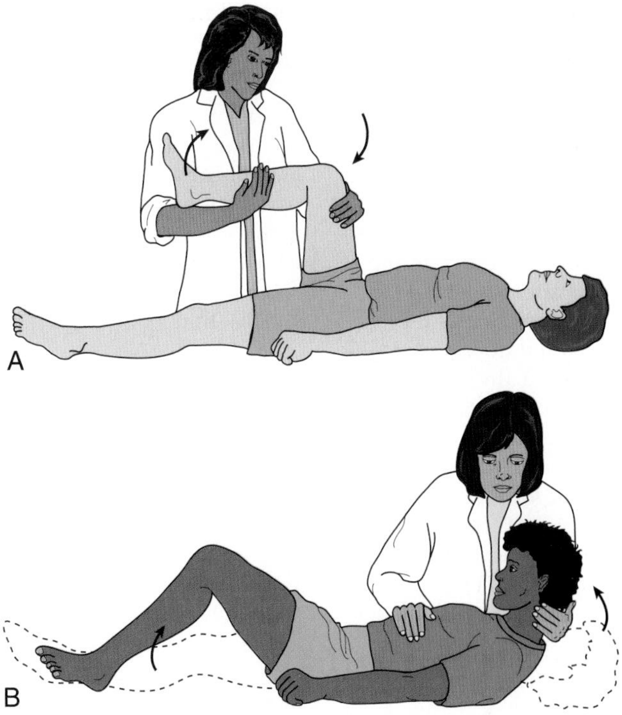

FIGURE 27-16 A, Positive Kernig sign: When the patient's leg is flexed as shown, the patient is unable to completely extend the leg. **B,** Brudzinski sign: When the nurse flexes the patient's neck, hip flexion occurs. (From Lewis S et al: *Medical-surgical nursing*, ed 7, St. Louis, 2007, Mosby.)

If needed, Isolation Precautions should be initiated. Organisms responsible for meningococcal meningitis are spread by the respiratory route and appropriate safeguards must be used to protect other patients, family, and staff until the organism is no longer in the nares (see Chapter 13).

❖ NURSING CARE of the Patient with Meningitis

■ Assessment

The routine neurologic assessment is summarized in Box 27-2. When a patient has meningitis, assess vital signs and neurologic status frequently to determine further deterioration or the onset of complications (see *Health Promotion* box).

Health Promotion

Meningitis

Patients with meningitis and those who interact with them should receive the following interventions as necessary:

- Vaccination to prevent pneumococcal pneumonia and influenza
- Treatment of respiratory and ear infections
- Prophylactic antibiotics for anyone in close contact with bacterial meningitis

Nursing Diagnoses, Goals, and Outcome Criteria: Meningitis

Nursing Diagnoses	Goals and Outcome Criteria
Risk for Ineffective Cerebral Tissue Perfusion related to increased intracranial pressure (ICP)	Adequate cerebral tissue perfusion: vital signs and level of consciousness consistent with patient norms
Ineffective Breathing Pattern related to depression of the respiratory center	Adequate oxygenation: respiratory rate of 12 to 20 breaths/min
Acute Pain related to irritation of meninges and increased ICP	Pain relief: patient states pain has been relieved, relaxed manner
Risk for Injury related to confusion, seizures, restlessness	Absence of injury: no falls or other trauma
Deficient Fluid Volume related to vomiting and fever	Normal fluid balance without vomiting or fever: fluid intake and output approximately equal, moist mucous membranes, blood pressure within patient norms
Risk for Disuse Syndrome related to bed rest	Absence of complications of immobility: clear breath sounds, intact skin, normal muscle strength and joint mobility, regular bowel movements without straining

Interventions

Risk for Ineffective Cerebral Tissue Perfusion

Elevate the head of the patient's bed as ordered. Instruct the patient to avoid coughing and not to hold his or her breath during turning because these behaviors increase ICP. Do not use restraints unless they are absolutely necessary. Monitor for signs of increasing ICP: decreased level of consciousness, headache, nausea, vomiting, abnormal pupillary responses, and respiratory depression. If ICP does increase, administer prescribed treatments (e.g., diuretics, barbiturates, and opioids). Measures to lower the body temperature may be ordered to reduce the metabolic rate.

Ineffective Breathing Pattern

Monitor the patient's respiratory status and gag and swallowing reflexes. Position the patient to maintain a patent airway (and use suction if necessary). Arterial blood samples should be drawn and analyzed for gas values as ordered. If the respiratory rate is decreasing, the physician should be notified immediately.

Acute Pain

Assess the location and severity of any patient discomfort. Nursing measures to decrease pain include position changes, massage, and a quiet environment. Give analgesics as ordered and document their effect. Chapter 15 provides additional information about the nursing management of pain.

Risk for Injury

Because of the prevailing risk of seizures, take appropriate precautions to ensure patient safety. A subdued environment should be maintained to reduce irritability and contribute to patient comfort. Keep the bed in a low position, with the side rails padded and raised. Reorient the patient to the setting as needed and keep the call bell within easy reach. Remind patients who are dizzy not to get up without assistance.

Deficient Fluid Volume

Monitor the patient's vital signs, tissue turgor and moisture, and fluid intake and output. Weight may be measured daily to assess fluid status. Encourage oral fluid intake if permitted and if the patient is alert. Administer intravenous fluid therapy as ordered and monitor to ensure the correct flow rate. Antipyretics may be ordered for fever and antiemetics for vomiting.

Risk for Disuse Syndrome

The patient who is confined to bed is at risk for all complications of immobility, especially stasis of pulmonary secretions, pressure sores, muscle weakness, joint stiffness, and constipation. Measures to prevent these complications are discussed in detail in Chapter 21.

INFECTIOUS AND INFLAMMATORY CONDITIONS: ENCEPHALITIS

Encephalitis is inflammation of brain tissue that is usually caused by one of several viruses. These viruses may be prevalent during certain times of the year or in a specific geographic area. For example, certain types of mosquitos found in the United States are carriers of a virus commonly associated with encephalitis. In addition, toxic substances or other types of viral infections, such as herpes simplex, may precipitate encephalitis. Complications of encephalitis include changes in level of consciousness, increased ICP, cranial nerve palsies, motor and sensory changes, and speech function. Therefore ongoing assessments should monitor for these changes. The complications are not specific to the agent causing the inflammation.

Signs and Symptoms

The patient with encephalitis has symptoms directly related to the area of the brain that is involved. Fever, nuchal rigidity (stiff neck), headache, confusion, delirium, agitation, and restlessness are commonly seen. However, the patient also may become comatose or exhibit aphasia, hemiparesis, facial weakness, and other alterations in motor activity.

Medical Treatment

Care for the patient with encephalitis is focused on enhancing patient comfort and increasing strength. Because seizure activity is a potential problem, you must take appropriate safety precautions.

❖ NURSING CARE of the Patient with Encephalitis

The nursing plan of care parallels that of the patient with meningitis.

GUILLAIN-BARRÉ SYNDROME

Although its specific cause is unknown, Guillain-Barré syndrome (GBS), also known as *acute inflammatory polyneuropathy*, is believed to be an autoimmune response to a viral infection. It is a rapidly progressing disease that affects the motor and sensory component of the peripheral nervous system. Although the spinal nerves are usually affected, the cranial nerves also may be involved.

Patients with GBS often report some recent viral infection or vaccination. This apparently triggers an autoimmune response that destroys the myelin sheath around the peripheral nerves, slowing the conduction of impulses across the involved nerves. The four recognized types of GBS are (1) ascending GBS, (2) descending GBS, (3) Miller Fisher syndrome, and (4) pure motor GBS.

Signs and Symptoms

GBS has three phases: (1) initial, (2) plateau, and (3) recovery, as described in Table 27-6. The initial phase is characterized by symmetric muscle weakness that typically begins in the lower extremities and ascends to the trunk and upper extremities. The disease process may affect cranial nerves, resulting in visual and hearing disturbances, difficulty chewing, and lack of facial expression. The muscles of respiration also may be affected, resulting in the need for mechanical ventilation. Respiratory dysfunction is the greatest threat to patients with GBS. They require close monitoring for incipient respiratory failure requiring intubation.

Mild **paresthesia** (abnormal sensations) or anesthesia (numbness) in the feet and hands may be present in a glove or stocking distribution pattern. In addition, some patients experience pain associated with the sensory changes. Despite all the motor and sensory changes, level of consciousness and intellectual functioning remain unchanged.

Effects on the autonomic nervous system may include hypertension, orthostatic hypotension, cardiac dysrhythmias, profuse sweating, paralytic ileus, and urinary retention. Dysautonomia, characterized by the effects just mentioned, occurs most frequently in patients with respiratory involvement and is potentially life threatening.

In the plateau phase, the patient with GBS remains essentially unchanged. Although no further neurologic deterioration exists, no improvement is seen.

As recovery begins and progresses, remyelinization occurs and muscle strength returns in a proximal to distal pattern (head to toes). Because the underlying axon generally remains undamaged, approximately 95% of patients with GBS have a nearly complete recovery. Others have residual numbness, stiffness, or paresis.

Table 27-6 Phases of Guillain-Barré Syndrome

PHASE	CHARACTERISTICS	DURATION
Initial	Begins with onset of symptoms	Usually 1–3 weeks Ends when disease ceases to progress
Plateau	No further changes; neither deterioration nor improvement	Several days to 2 weeks
Recovery	Gradual improvement	May be as long as 2 years; some residual effects may be permanent

Medical Diagnosis

The characteristic onset and pattern of ascending motor involvement provide the basis for the diagnosis of GBS. An elevated protein level in the CSF obtained by lumbar puncture provides additional evidence for the diagnosis. Nerve conduction velocity studies reveal slowed conduction speed in the involved nerves.

Medical Treatment

Management during the acute phase of the illness is directed at preserving vital function, particularly respiration. Respiratory status is closely monitored and mechanical ventilation initiated if the vital capacity falls to 15 mL/kg of body weight. In the presence of pharyngeal paresis and difficulty handling secretions, intubation and ventilation can be done earlier.

Massive doses of corticosteroids may be prescribed to suppress the inflammatory process.

Because GBS is believed to be an autoimmune disease, plasmapheresis has emerged as a major treatment intervention. Plasmapheresis is a process in which blood is removed, centrifuged, and returned to the patient. In the process, antibodies that trigger the autoimmune disease are removed from the blood by a machine equipped with a special filtration system. The patient with GBS generally undergoes a series of treatments, ideally delivered within 7 to 14 days after the onset of the disease. Those patients benefiting from plasmapheresis often recover faster.

NURSING CARE of the Patient with Guillain-Barré Syndrome

Assessment

Assessment of the patient with a neurologic disorder is summarized in Box 27-2. When GBS is suspected, the health history describes the progression of symptoms. Note the patient's fears, coping strategies, and sources of support. Record information about important social data such as occupation and family roles and responsibilities. The physical examination focuses on cranial nerve, motor, sensory, respiratory, and cardiovascular function.

Nursing Diagnoses, Goals, and Outcome Criteria: Guillain-Barré Syndrome

Nursing Diagnoses	Goals and Outcome Criteria
Ineffective Breathing Pattern related to neurologic impairment	Adequate oxygenation: normal arterial blood gases and skin color
Decreased Cardiac Output related to labile blood pressure, cardiac dysrhythmias	Normal cardiac output: regular pulse with rate of 60 to 100 beats/min and blood pressure consistent with patient norms
Risk for Disuse Syndrome related to motor impairment	Absence of complications of immobility: intact skin, no contractures, clear breath sounds, regular bowel movements
Imbalanced Nutrition: Less Than Body Requirements related to dysphagia, endotracheal tube	Adequate nutrition: stable body weight
Risk for Injury related to loss of sensation in hands and feet, motor impairment, inability to speak	Absence of injury in affected body areas: no falls, bruises, corneal damage, or other injuries
Anxiety related to paralysis, doubts about recovery, loss of verbal communication	Decreased anxiety: patient states anxiety is reduced, calm manner
Deficient Knowledge of Guillain-Barré syndrome (GBS) and its treatment	Knowledge of GBS and its treatment: patient confirms understanding and (if possible) demonstrates self-care

Interventions

Ineffective Breathing Pattern

Some patients with GBS need mechanical ventilation because of neuromuscular failure. Closely monitor the patient for signs of respiratory mechanical failure. Assess the patient's oxygenation status frequently. A respiratory rate greater than 30 breaths per minute, abnormal chest and abdominal movements, and decreasing vital capacity signal increasingly ineffective breathing. Turn the patient at least every 2 hours and suction when indicated by increased pulse or adventitious breath sounds.

Decreased Cardiac Output

Be alert to rapid or slow cardiac dysrhythmias and administer antidysrhythmic drugs as ordered.

Risk for Disuse Syndrome

Immobility is a major issue to address in the patient with GBS. If mobility is severely impaired, the patient is at high risk for disuse syndrome. These patients generally benefit from the use of rotational bed therapy to help promote pulmonary hygiene, peristalsis, and urinary bladder emptying. Careful positioning is crucial, with emphasis on maintaining joint function, muscle tone, and range of motion. Active and passive exercises, splints, and continuous passive motion machines may be used to prevent contractures.

Imbalanced Nutrition: Less Than Body Requirements

Impaired swallowing or the presence of an endotracheal tube mandates an alternative means of feeding. Enteral feedings are usually provided by way of a gastrostomy or nasoduodenal tube. Feedings may be given continuously or intermittently. Elevate the head of the bed 30 degrees during feedings to reduce the risk of aspiration. Aspirate and measure the residual (amount of feeding remaining in the stomach) at intervals to assess emptying of the stomach and prevent overfilling. In some cases, total parenteral nutrition may be used.

Risk for Injury

Progressive weakness makes the patient susceptible to falls. When the patient is in bed, raise the side rails, place the call bell within reach, and put the bed in low position. If the eyes do not close completely, ophthalmic drops or ointments should be applied as ordered. A moisture chamber for the eye is used to prevent eye injury from excessive drying. Carefully inspect the skin, especially areas without sensation, to detect pressure or injury. !

Anxiety

Anxiety is understandable with progressive paralysis and increasing dependence on others for basic needs. You must work to develop trust and establish a therapeutic relationship with the patient. If the patient is able to speak, encourage him or her to discuss thoughts, fears, and feelings and explore previously used coping strategies. To promote some sense of control, give the patient some choices about aspects of care. Explain equipment and procedures to the patient. Other strategies to reduce anxiety include the use of imagery, music, and deep breathing (if possible) and controlling anxiety-producing thoughts. Boredom is a problem that must be considered for the patient with GBS. Orienting devices such as clocks, calendars, and daily schedules are helpful. The patient may enjoy television, radio, CDs, and visits from friends and family (see *Complementary and Alternative Therapies* box).

Complementary and Alternative Therapies

Strategies to reduce anxiety include music therapy and massage. The herb *valerian* is used by some people as a sedative; its safety is under study.

One source of anxiety for many patients is impaired communication. While the patient is able to speak, establish an alternative system of communication, such as blinking (one blink means *yes*, two blinks mean *no*) or a communication board. If the condition does affect speech or if mechanical ventilation is required, the patient will have a simple, alternative means of expression.

Deficient Knowledge

From admission through rehabilitation, the patient with GBS needs education about the condition and its usual course. Patients can deal with the condition better if they know how the symptoms progress and that reversal and improvement are expected.

Rehabilitation

As function is restored, emphasis is placed on both respiratory and physical rehabilitation. Total recovery of respiratory function determines how quickly physical rehabilitation can begin. Once rehabilitation is initiated, attention must be devoted to maximizing motor function through exercises and occupational therapy. Because complete recovery may take several years, a prolonged rehabilitation period is sometimes necessary. Before the patient is discharged from the hospital, referrals may be made to rehabilitation or home health agencies as appropriate. The patient and family may benefit from a support group for people with long-term or chronic illnesses. The Guillain-Barré Foundation is a source of information (610-667-0131; www.gbs-cidp.org).

PARKINSON DISEASE

Parkinson disease is a progressive degenerative disorder of the basal ganglia that results in an eventual loss of coordination and control of involuntary motor movement. It is generally recognized as a disease of older adults, first appearing in individuals in their 50s, with men affected more often than women. Idiopathic Parkinson disease has no known cause but is related to decreased levels of dopamine in the basal ganglia. A deficiency of dopamine, a neurotransmitter, contributes to the loss of motor function. Other types of parkinsonism are caused by atherosclerosis, the long-term use of phenothiazines, and some toxins.

Signs and Symptoms

Several symptoms are characteristic of Parkinson syndrome. The major triad of symptoms is tremor, rigidity, and bradykinesia. Tremor is a trembling or shaking type of movement most often seen in the upper extremities of the patient with Parkinson syndrome. Tremors are more pronounced during resting postures and often relieved by movement. Typically they disappear during sleep. A movement associated with the tremor is pill rolling, in which the tremor repetitively moves the individual's thumb against the fingertips as if rolling a small object. Rigidity is stiffness and *bradykinesia* refers to extremely slow movements. Other signs and symptoms are loss of dexterity and power in affected limbs, aching, monotone voice, handwriting changes, drooling, lack of facial expression, rhythmic head nodding, reduced blinking, and slumped posture. Those with advanced disease demonstrate cogwheel rigidity (jerky movements with passive muscle stretching) and gait disturbances. The individual may appear to freeze and may have difficulty initiating the action of walking. Depression is common and dementia develops in some patients. Figure 27-17 illustrates the typical facial appearance, posture, and gait of individuals with Parkinson syndrome.

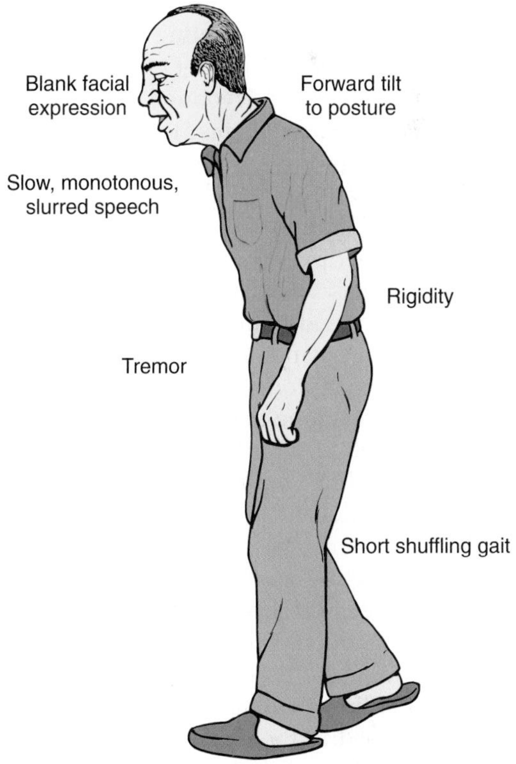

FIGURE 27-17 Clinical manifestations of Parkinson syndrome. (From Monahan F, Sands J, Neighbors M, et al: *Phipps' medical-surgical nursing: health and illness perspectives*, ed 8, St. Louis, 2006, Mosby.)

Medical Diagnosis

Parkinson syndrome is diagnosed from the health history and the physical examination results. MRI may be done to rule out other causes of the symptoms.

Medical Treatment

Management of the patient with Parkinson syndrome is directed toward controlling the symptoms with physical therapy and drug therapy. The most beneficial physical therapy programs incorporate massage, heat, exercise, and gait retraining. Speech therapy has been used with swallowing issues as well as difficulty with speech, with variable results.

Drug therapy relieves many of the symptoms of the disease. Early in the course of the disease, dopamine receptor agonists pramipexole (Mirapex) or ropinirole (Requip) are used to maximize the intrinsic dopamine. The cornerstone of therapy is the use of L-dopa (L-dihydroxyphenylalanine). L-dopa can cross the blood-brain barrier and is converted to dopamine in the basal ganglia, thereby supplementing levels of the neurotransmitter and reducing the symptoms of the disease. The conversion of L-dopa to dopamine must occur in the basal ganglia and not in the peripheral tissue. To ensure this, inhibitors are administered to prevent the breakdown of L-dopa by decarboxylase enzymes. The decarboxylase inhibitor most commonly used is carbidopa. It is frequently given in combination as carbidopa/levodopa (Sinemet). When the two drugs are used in combination, therapeutic levels may be achieved with lower doses. Carbidopa/levodopa also comes in orally disintegrating tablets (Parcopa, Carbilev). The enzyme catechol-*O*-methyltransferase (COMT) also breaks down levodopa in the peripheral circulation. Entacapone (Comtan) blocks this breakdown and prolongs the effectiveness of carbidopa/levodopa (Sinemet). Carbidopa/levodopa/entacapone (Stalevo), a combination drug, provides maximum blocking in the peripheral circulation and decreases the number of pills taken at one time. Because the benefits of L-dopa tend to decline after about 2 years, various other drug combinations may be used in an effort to control symptoms. Selegiline hydrochloride (Eldepryl), a monoamine oxidase (MAO) inhibitor, is used with Sinemet. MAO is the enzyme that degrades dopamine. Selegiline hydrochloride increases the available dopamine.

Anticholinergic drugs such as trihexyphenidyl (Artane) and benztropine (Cogentin) may be used in patients who have less severe symptoms or who are unresponsive to L-dopa. These are useful in managing tremors. Although the exact mechanism of action is unclear, amantadine (Symmetrel), an antiviral compound, also is used in the management of Parkinson syndrome. Amantadine is thought to release dopamine from storage sites in the neurons. Amantadine is effective for tremor as well as akinesia. It is often used in combination with L-dopa.

Treatment for depression may include antidepressant drug therapy, psychotherapy, and electroconvulsive therapy.

Several surgical procedures, among them thalamotomy, thalamic stimulation, and pallidotomy, may be used to treat parkinsonism, although the benefits are variable. Surgical implantation of fetal dopamine-producing cells continues to be done experimentally. Adrenal medullary transplant entails implantation of the patient's own adrenal cells in the brain. It has produced limited improvement in some patients and is not widely accepted. All of these surgical procedures are considered palliative rather than curative.

Put on Your Thinking Cap!

Write a short teaching plan for a home health patient who has started taking selegiline (Eldepryl) for Parkinson syndrome.

NURSING CARE of the Patient with Parkinson Syndrome

Nursing management for the patient with Parkinson syndrome is primarily related to maintaining mobility and preventing injury.

Assessment

The complete neurologic assessment is summarized in Box 27-2. The health history of a patient with Parkinson syndrome should specifically include assessment for weakness, fatigue, muscle cramps, sweating, dysphagia, constipation, difficulty voiding, and unusual movements. Describe the effects of the disease on the patient's life. During the physical examination, be alert for lack of facial expression, eyes fixed in one direction, drooling, slurred speech, tearing, tremors, muscle stiffness, and poor balance and coordination.

As the disease progresses, the patient becomes more immobilized, requiring additional nursing diagnoses, as addressed in Chapter 21.

Nursing Diagnoses, Goals, and Outcome Criteria: Parkinson Syndrome

Nursing Diagnoses	Goals and Outcome Criteria
Impaired Physical Mobility related to neuromuscular disease	Maximum possible mobility: patient participates in prescribed exercise program and performs self-care within abilities
Risk for Injury related to poor balance and coordination	Absence of injury: no bruises, lacerations, or fractures because of trauma
Imbalanced Nutrition: Less Than Body Requirements related to dysphagia, difficulty with self-feeding	Adequate nutritional intake: stable body weight

Nursing Diagnoses, Goals, and Outcome Criteria: Parkinson Syndrome—cont'd

Nursing Diagnoses	Goals and Outcome Criteria
Ineffective Coping related to physical changes and effects of disease on lifestyle	Effective coping with disease effects: patient makes statements confirming ability to deal with condition, adheres to plan of care
Deficient Knowledge of disease, management, and self-care	Compliance with the prescribed plan of care: patient correctly describes and adheres to drug therapy, demonstrates exercise routine, uses resources, adapts to continue self-care

Interventions

Impaired Physical Mobility

Assess the patient's mobility and ability to perform self-care. Provide assistance as needed but encourage the patient to remain as independent in self-care as possible. Assistive devices, including walkers and wheelchairs, may enable the patient to be mobile despite some deterioration in coordination and balance. Stress the value of exercise in maintaining strength and mobility. Active and passive range-of-motion exercises may be done. Both the physical therapist and the occupational therapist may participate in designing programs to maintain or improve function.

Suggestions to improve mobility with Parkinson syndrome include the following:

- Scoot to the edge of a chair before trying to stand.
- Use satin sheets to make it easier to move in and out of bed.
- March in place before starting to walk.
- Practice lifting the foot as if to step over an object on the floor to initiate walking.

Risk for Injury

The patient with Parkinson syndrome is at special risk for injury-related falls. Place the call bell within easy reach and instruct the patient to call for assistance when rising. If the patient is ambulatory, remove obstacles on the floor. Recommend firm shoes, which provide better support than soft slippers. Provide assistive devices (e.g., canes, walkers, wheelchairs) as needed. Allow the patient to move at his or her own speed to decrease the risk of injury. Because this is a chronic condition, the patient's home setting should be evaluated and adapted for safe ambulation.

Imbalanced Nutrition: Less Than Body Requirements

To promote ease of swallowing, position the patient comfortably for meals, with the head elevated and food conveniently arranged. Provide assistance as needed (this may involve simply cutting meat and opening containers or may entail actually feeding the patient). Patients must never be rushed while they are eating. If the patient chokes on liquids, the dietitian should be consulted about the need for semisolids and thick liquids, which are often easier to swallow. Thickening agents can be added to thin fluids to facilitate swallowing. Small, frequent meals may be better tolerated than three large ones. Monitor the patient's weight to assess the adequacy of nutritional intake. Some researchers believe that patients with Parkinson syndrome benefit from a low-protein diet during the day and an evening meal high in protein but this is still experimental.

Ineffective Coping

Patients with Parkinson syndrome must deal with loss of mobility that may affect their jobs, home and family responsibilities, social relationships, and leisure activities. Voice changes may severely impair verbal communication. Explore how the patient is dealing with these changes. Nurses and other members of the health care team help the patient to identify strategies to adapt to changing abilities. These professionals should be alert to expressions of depression and inform the physician of such findings. A referral may be made to a mental health counselor, clinical nurse specialist, or support group. Administer antidepressant drugs as ordered and monitor their effects (see *Complementary and Alternative Therapies* box).

Complementary and Alternative Therapies

St. John's wort is used widely as an antidepressant. It is a monoamine oxidase (MAO) inhibitor and can interact with prescribed drugs. Ask the patient to report use of herbal remedies to the physician. Other measures to treat depression are physical exercise, massage, and light therapy.

Caution patients with Parkinson syndrome not to use herbal supplements without physician approval. Kava can worsen symptoms of Parkinson syndrome. Chaste tree fruit interferes with the drug selegiline. Indian snakeroot interferes with the actions of levodopa and carbidopa.

Deficient Knowledge

Management of this progressive condition requires the patient or a caregiver to understand Parkinson syndrome and how it is treated (see *Patient Teaching* box). Supplement verbal information with written material (see *Health Promotion* box).

Patient Teaching

Parkinson Disease

- Drugs relieve symptoms but do not cure Parkinson syndrome. You must continue therapy as prescribed to control symptoms.
- Know your drug names, dosages, schedule, and adverse effects that should be reported to your physician.

Continued

Patient Teaching—cont'd

- Exercise is essential to maintain mobility.
- Resources include the American Parkinson Disease Association (1-800-223-2732; www.apdaparkinson.org), the Parkinson Foundation (222-923-4700; www.parkinsonfoundation.org), and the National Parkinson Foundation (1-800-327-4545; www.parkinson.org).

Health Promotion

Patients with Parkinson Syndrome

Patients with Parkinson syndrome and those who interact with them should receive the following interventions as necessary:

- Maintain general health and have regular checkups.
- Follow a regular routine of stretching and exercise to maintain mobility and balance.
- Prevent falls through environmental control.

MULTIPLE SCLEROSIS

A chronic, progressive degenerative disease, MS attacks the protective myelin sheath around axons and disrupts the conduction of impulses through the CNS (Fig. 27-18). It may affect motor, sensory, cerebellar, and other pathways. The course of the disease is variable. Several patterns have been identified. The disease may progress steadily (chronic, progressive MS), may be characterized by exacerbations and remissions (exacerbating-remitting MS), may have less stable periods than exacerbating-remitting MS (relapsing-progressive MS), or may become stable with no active disease for at least 1 year (stable MS). MS is the second most common neurologic cause of disability. The incidence is highest in persons between 20 and 40 years of age and MS affects women more often than men.

Cause

Although the exact cause of MS is unknown, viral infections and autoimmune processes have been implicated. Some studies have implicated a retrovirus in the disease process but more research is needed to determine whether this is indeed the cause of MS. The myelin sheath surrounding the axons is destroyed, eventually leaving areas of sclerotic tissues (see Fig. 27-18). As the sclerotic tissue develops, the patient may have a period of remission. The involved fibers eventually degenerate, resulting in permanent damage. Nerve impulses then are no longer able to travel down the affected axon.

Signs and Symptoms

Because the exact pattern of damage varies from patient to patient, the signs and symptoms vary as well. The most common symptoms of MS are fatigue, weakness and tingling in one or more extremities, visual disturbances, problems with coordination, bowel and bladder dysfunction, spasticity, and depression.

For patients who have exacerbating-remitting MS, the progression is variable. As the disease progresses, the periods of remission become shorter and the neurologic deficits present during exacerbations become more severe and permanent.

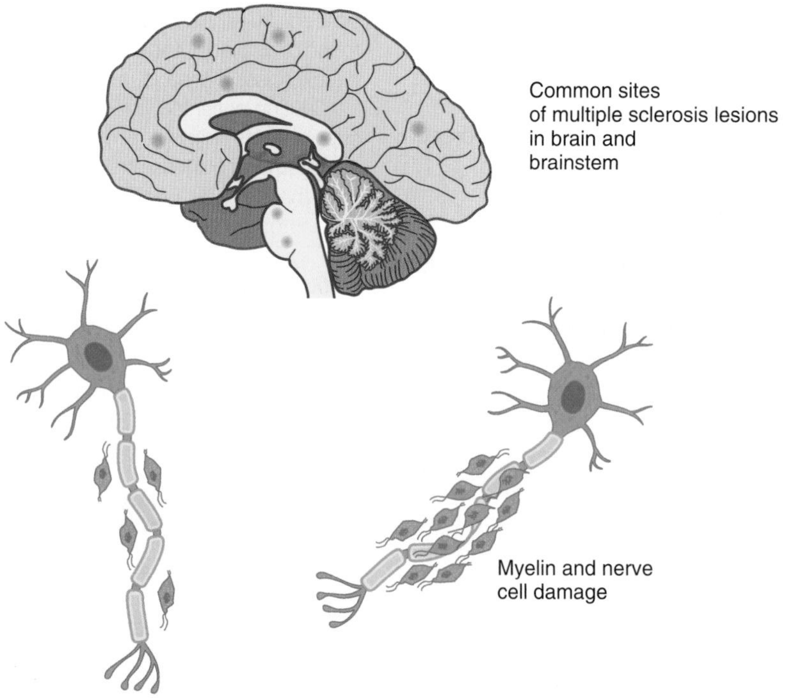

FIGURE 27-18 The lesions in multiple sclerosis (MS): location and effects. (From Hopper T: *Mosby's pharmacy technician*, ed 3, St. Louis, 2012, Saunders.)

Medical Diagnosis

The diagnosis of MS is based primarily on the physical examination and history of cyclic remission-exacerbation periods. A familial history of the disease is significant, as is worsening of symptoms when the patient is exposed to warm weather. MRI of the brain and spinal cord may reveal plaques characteristic of MS. Currently, specific MRI requirements support a diagnosis of MS. Slow, absent, or abnormal visual-evoked responses are seen with MS.

Medical Treatment

Because of its chronic, progressive nature, the treatment of MS is symptomatic and supportive. Drug therapy during periods of exacerbation may involve administration of adrenocorticotropic hormone (ACTH). Corticosteroids (ACTH, prednisone, methylprednisolone) may be used to control exacerbations but they do not slow the progression of the disease. Treatment often includes drugs that modulate the immune response and thus the course of the disease. The specific drug will depend on the type of MS. Drugs in this category include interferon beta-1b (Betaseron) and interferon beta-1a (Avonex). Glatiramer acetate (Copaxone) is an immune modulator that is unrelated to interferon. Immunosuppressant drugs such as mitoxantrone (Novantrone) and natalizumab (Tysabri) also are used for exacerbations. When immunosuppressive agents are used, patients must be carefully monitored for bone marrow suppression. Glucocorticosteroids are used for acute exacerbation and relapses. The spasticity experienced by MS patients may respond to treatment with baclofen (Lioresal) or tizanidine (Zanaflex). Carbamazepine (Tegretol) and gabapentin (Neurontin) are used to relieve neuropathic pain. Amantadine (Symmetrel) is used to relieve fatigue associated with the disease. Electrical neuromuscular stimulation is being used to decrease spasticity and improve active movement and function but studies of its effectiveness have not found consistent evidence of improvement. Urinary retention is treated with cholinergic drugs such as bethanechol (Urecholine) or neostigmine (Prostigmine). Urinary frequency and urgency resulting from spasticity of the bladder can be treated with anticholinergics such as propantheline bromide (Pro-Banthine) or oxybutynin (Ditropan). Tolterodine (Detrol) is a competitive muscarinic receptor antagonist and is more specific for the bladder than oxybutynin. Tamsulosin (Flomax) is also useful for urinary issues related to failure to store and empty urine.

❖ NURSING CARE of the Patient with Multiple Sclerosis

■ Assessment

Complete assessment of the patient with a neurologic disorder is summarized in Box 27-2. When a patient has MS, the health history specifically includes the onset and progression of symptoms, especially those that affect mobility, vision, eating, and elimination. Explore the effects of the disease on the person's lifestyle (see *Health Promotion* box). In addition, identify the patient's usual coping strategies. Important aspects of the physical examination are evaluation of range of motion and strength and observation for gait abnormalities, tremors, and muscle spasms.

Health Promotion

Patients with Multiple Sclerosis

Patients with multiple sclerosis (MS) should receive the following interventions as necessary:

- Maintain general health through diet and exercise.
- Avoid or minimize effects of triggers for MS such as infections, trauma, climate changes, and immunizations.
- Seek regular medical checkups for disease prevention.

Nursing Diagnoses, Goals, and Outcome Criteria: Multiple Sclerosis

Nursing Diagnoses	Goals and Outcome Criteria
Impaired Physical Mobility related to weakness or spasticity	Maximal possible mobility: patient continues physical activity within capabilities
Risk for Injury related to neurologic impairment	Absence of injury associated with impaired sensation: intact skin without redness related to pressure, no falls
Self-Care Deficit (Dressing, Bathing, Feeding, Toileting) related to impaired voluntary movements and poor coordination	Achievement of self-care: activities of daily living (ADL) completed independently or with assistance as needed
Impaired Urinary Elimination related to impaired conduction of bladder nerve impulses	Normal bladder filling and emptying: bladder not palpable, no uncontrolled passage of urine
Risk for Infection related to inadequate resistance	Absence of infection: normal body temperature and white blood cell count
Ineffective Coping related to chronic illness, uncertain course of disease	Adaptation to changes in physical functioning: behavior and statements reflect intent to maximize abilities
Deficient Knowledge of disease, treatment, and self-care	Patient understands disease, treatment, and self-care: patient accurately describes MS, its treatment, and self-care measures to reduce risk of complications

Interventions

Impaired Physical Mobility

Encourage the patient to be as independent as possible. Provide assistance with ambulation as needed; a cane or walker may enable the patient to walk safely. If the patient has muscle spasms, administer muscle relaxants as ordered. To prevent contractures, the patient should perform range-of-motion exercise. If the patient cannot do the exercises independently, teach a caregiver how to do the exercises. Physical therapy may be ordered. The patient who is not able to move independently is at risk for disuse syndrome. If the patient becomes disabled to this extent, decisions must be made about home nursing services or care in a long-term facility.

Risk for Injury

If the patient has impaired sensation, give special attention to the skin. Inspect extremities and pressure points for signs of pressure or trauma and encourage the patient to wear shoes when out of bed to prevent injury. Other measures instituted to prevent injury include using caution with sources of heat and cold.

Self-Care Deficit (Bathing, Feeding, Dressing, Toileting)

Encourage patients to do as much as they can for themselves. Provide assistance as needed to carry out ADL. Difficulty with feedings, especially if the patient is dysphagic, may result in inadequate food intake. Alternative means of feeding may be necessary. Discuss with the patient and family their needs for assistance with caregiving. Home nursing care can support the patient who wishes to remain in a home setting.

Impaired Urinary Elimination

Palpate the patient's lower abdomen for bladder distention and carry out intermittent catheterization as ordered. If urine retention is a problem, assess the patient for signs and symptoms of urinary tract infection: fever, burning on urination, foul odor, sediment. If the patient has urinary incontinence, take steps to reduce the incontinent episodes as described in Chapter 23. Incontinence briefs may be needed and meticulous skin care is a must. Loss of bladder control is very distressing and you must be sensitive in helping the patient to deal with it.

Risk for Infection

The MS patient who is being treated with immunosuppressive drugs has decreased resistance to infection. Take steps to reduce the risk of infection, including protecting the patient from people with infections (e.g., avoiding crowds during seasons with increased respiratory infections). Encourage intake of fluids to maintain adequate hydration and emphasize good hygiene practices. In addition, teach the patient and family the signs of infection that should be reported promptly to the physician.

Ineffective Coping

MS is a chronic, progressive disease. Most patients have increasing disability, which requires considerable adaptation. Because the initial symptoms typically occur in young adults, patients often must learn to balance work, home, and family responsibilities. Provide the patient with opportunities to talk about the illness and its effects. Be accepting of the patient's concerns and guide the patient to identify strengths, abilities, and usual coping strategies (see *Complementary and Alternative Therapies* box). With the patient's permission, a referral may be made to the clinical nurse specialist, mental health counselor, or spiritual counselor. Support groups can be helpful to many patients and their families.

Complementary and Alternative Therapies

Imagery, breathing exercises, and progressive relaxation can help the MS patient to reduce stress. Various special diets and nutritional supplements (commonly fatty acids, niacin, zinc, magnesium, selenium, beta-carotene, and vitamins C, B_6, and B_{12}) have been proposed but research has not consistently shown benefits to the MS patient.

Deficient Knowledge

Assess what the patient knows about MS and what he or she would like to know. The teaching plan is individualized to the patient's needs and may include problems associated with immobility and measures to prevent complications.

AMYOTROPHIC LATERAL SCLEROSIS

Cause

ALS, also known as *Lou Gehrig's disease,* is a degenerative neurologic disease. It affects males two to four times as often as females and most often strikes those between 40 and 70 years of age. The disease generally progresses rapidly and death ensues approximately 3 years after the onset of symptoms. Although a viral cause has been suspected, the exact cause is unknown.

Pathophysiology

In ALS, degeneration of the anterior horn cells and the corticospinal tracts occurs, so the patient exhibits both upper and lower motor neuron symptoms. Evidence of upper motor neuron disease includes spasticity and hyperreflexia. Lower motor neuron disease is demonstrated by weakness, atrophy, cramps, and muscle twitching. Some patients have difficulty swallowing and slurred speech. Despite involvement of the motor nuclei of the brainstem, intellectual ability, sensory perception, vision, and hearing are all unaffected.

Signs and Symptoms

Initially the patient exhibits weakness of voluntary muscles of the upper extremities, particularly the hands. In addition, some patients may experience difficulty swallowing and speaking because of progressive weakness of the oropharyngeal muscles. Spasticity of the involved muscle groups may be evident. The disease progresses steadily until the patient is completely incapacitated. Eventually, respirations become shallow and the patient has difficulty clearing the airway of pulmonary secretions. Death results from aspiration, respiratory infection, or respiratory failure.

Medical Diagnosis

The patient's history and physical examination findings lead to the diagnosis of ALS. EMG provides supporting evidence of impaired impulse conduction in the muscles. More sophisticated tests are used to rule out other degenerative motor diseases such as MS or myasthenia gravis.

Medical Treatment

Because no known cure or treatment for ALS exists, therapy is supportive, focusing on the prevention of complications and the maintenance of maximum function.

NURSING CARE of the Patient with Amyotrophic Lateral Sclerosis

Assessment

The complete neurologic assessment is outlined in Box 27-2. When a patient has ALS, the nurse's history assessment of the patient determines the presence of dyspnea, dysphagia, muscle cramps, weakness, twitching, and joint stiffness. Describe the effects of the disease on the patient's lifestyle. During the physical examination, anticipate finding weakness, muscle atrophy, abnormal reflexes and gait, and paralysis.

Nursing Diagnoses, Goals, and Outcome Criteria: Amyotrophic Lateral Sclerosis

Nursing Diagnoses	Goals and Outcome Criteria
Ineffective Airway Clearance related to paralysis of respiratory muscles	Patent airway: respiratory rate of 12 to 20 breaths/min without crackles or wheezes
Impaired Physical Mobility related to progressive weakness and atrophy	Maximal possible mobility: patient participates in activities to maintain joint mobility
Imbalanced Nutrition: Less Than Body Requirements related to dysphagia	Adequate nutritional intake: stable body weight

Nursing Diagnoses, Goals, and Outcome Criteria: Amyotrophic Lateral Sclerosis—cont'd

Nursing Diagnoses	Goals and Outcome Criteria
Impaired Verbal Communication related to oropharyngeal muscle weakness	Effective communication: patient conveys needs without excessive frustration
Impaired Skin Integrity related to immobility	Normal skin integrity: intact skin without signs of pressure (redness, blanching)
Grieving related to progressive, fatal disease	Adaptation to losses: patient verbalizes losses, their importance, and acceptance of losses; makes realistic plans
Situational Low Self-Esteem related to loss of independence	Stable or improved self-esteem: patient makes positive statements about self
Interrupted Family Processes related to progressive illness of patient	Family adapts to patient condition: positive family communication and interactions, patient's role shifted

Interventions

Ineffective Airway Clearance

Monitor the patient's respiratory rate and effort, breath sounds, and pulse rate to detect inadequate oxygenation. Instruct or assist the immobile patient in turning, coughing, and deep breathing at least every 2 hours. Chest physiotherapy may be ordered to mobilize secretions to prevent atelectasis and pneumonia. If the patient has difficulty removing secretions, gentle suction may be needed. Oxygen therapy is indicated if evidence of hypoxia (restlessness, tachycardia) is noted.

Impaired Physical Mobility

Progressive muscle wasting, spasticity, and paralysis cause increasing immobility. Perform active or passive range-of-motion exercises to prevent contractures and give antispasmodic drugs as ordered. Maintain extremities in functional positions and encourage use of assistive devices (e.g., cane, walker, wheelchair) as needed to maintain mobility as long as possible. Monitor the patient's ability to perform ADL and provide assistance as needed. The patient who is immobile is at high risk for complications of immobility. Nursing care of the immobile patient is discussed in Chapter 21.

Imbalanced Nutrition: Less Than Body Requirements

Muscle weakness and cranial nerve involvement eventually make it difficult for the patient to consume adequate food for good nutrition. Monitor the patient's weight to assess adequacy of the diet. Meals may be supplemented with high-protein snacks. Recommend high-fiber foods if the patient can eat them, because constipation is a common problem. Adequate fluids are needed but may be difficult to swallow. The patient may be able to increase fluid intake by eating semisolids such as ice cream, milkshakes, or gelatin desserts.

The patient with ALS is at risk for aspiration because of impaired swallowing. While the patient is eating, the head of the bed must be elevated or the patient must be seated in a chair. Consult the dietitian about providing a diet of the appropriate texture for the patient and arrange dietary instruction for any caregivers who might be involved in preparing food for the patient. A speech therapist can recommend techniques to facilitate swallowing. Eventually, oral intake becomes inadequate. The decision to insert a feeding tube should be based on the desires of the patient and family. If a feeding tube is in place, administer feedings and monitor for tube placement and residual. Teach the family or other caregivers how to do the feedings.

Impaired Verbal Communication

Speech becomes impaired by muscle weakness and dyspnea. Establish alternatives to verbal communication. These might include the use of blinks or gestures or the use of boards with pictures, words, or letters that the patient can select. Use questions that can be answered with "yes" or "no" and give the patient time to respond. Electronic communication devices can prolong the patient's ability to communicate.

Impaired Skin Integrity

Muscle wasting, incontinence, and immobility put these patients at risk for skin breakdown. Reposition them at least every 2 hours and inspect bony prominences for redness. Special beds that alternate or distribute pressure may be used. Promptly change wet or soiled clothing to avoid skin irritation. Meticulous skin care is essential. Once again, if the patient will be cared for at home, caregivers must be able to care for the skin.

Anticipatory Grieving

Once the implications of a diagnosis of ALS are understood, patients and their families may begin the grieving process. Encourage patients to talk; listen compassionately and help them to make realistic plans. Remember the stages of grief and be understanding when patients and families show anger, denial, and depression (see *Cultural Considerations* box). Referrals to visiting nurse agencies and hospice services can provide needed emotional and physical support at various times in the progress of the disease.

> **Cultural Considerations**
>
> **What Does Culture Have to Do with Incurable Illness?**
>
> Patients facing progressive, incurable illness may find comfort in religious symbols, charms, incense, candles, and native healers.

Situational Low Self-Esteem

Explore the patient's thoughts, feelings, and concerns about living with this progressive, terminal disease. Although it is difficult not to offer false reassurance, let the patient cry or otherwise express grief and anger. Stress the patient's strengths, abilities, and contributions and identify and enlist sources of support (e.g., family, friends, support groups, spiritual counselors, therapists). Stress-reducing techniques include imagery, breathing exercises, and progressive relaxation. To preserve the patient's dignity, it is important to provide privacy during personal care and to help the patient attend to grooming and appearance.

Interrupted Family Processes

The disease is painful for both the patient and the family as it steadily takes its toll. Patients with ALS are often middle-aged, with family responsibilities, jobs, and places in the community. The family must plan for transfer of responsibilities and care of the patient when he or she becomes disabled. Issues that need to be discussed are patient feelings about advance directives, insurance, and wills. These topics may be difficult to address but are best handled while the patient can participate. Care of the dying patient is discussed in Chapter 24.

HUNTINGTON DISEASE

Huntington disease is an inherited degenerative neurologic disorder. It usually begins in middle adulthood with abnormal movements, emotional disturbance, and intellectual decline. Symptoms progress steadily, with increasing disability and death in 15 to 20 years. Medical and nursing care are supportive; no cure exists.

MYASTHENIA GRAVIS

Myasthenia gravis is a chronic, progressive disease in which a defect exists at the neuromuscular junction, where electrical impulses are transmitted to muscle tissue.

Cause

Evidence indicates that myasthenia gravis has an autoimmune basis. Some patients display an increase in the titer of acetylcholine receptor antibody. The presence of these antibodies interferes with the normal activity at the acetylcholine receptor sites and reduces muscle strength. Some patients have antibodies to muscle-specific receptor tyrosine kinase (MuSK). This

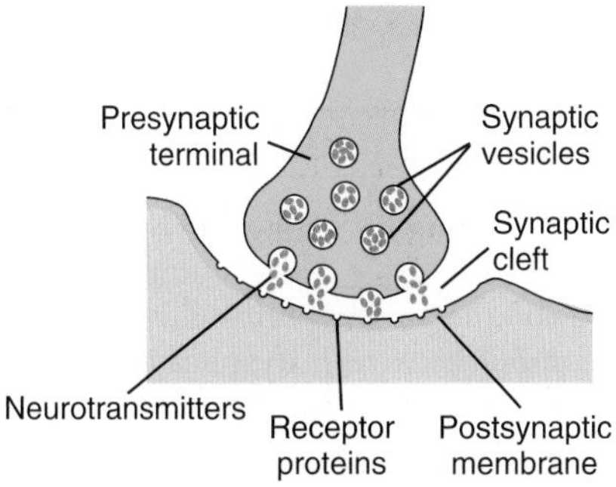

FIGURE 27-19 Neurotransmitters (norepinephrine, acetylcholine, dopamine) are released from the axon, travel across the synaptic cleft, and produce some response in the receptors of target cells. (From Black JM, Hawks JH, Keene AM: *Medical-surgical nursing: clinical management for continuity of care*, ed 6, Philadelphia, 2001, Saunders.)

polypeptide is found on the muscle side of the myoneural junction.

Pathophysiology

Normally, as a nerve impulse travels down a peripheral nerve, the neurotransmitter acetylcholine is released at the presynaptic membrane (Fig. 27-19). The impulse is then transmitted across the synaptic junction to postsynaptic receptor sites on the effector muscle. This causes contraction of the involved muscle.

In myasthenia gravis, insufficient receptor sites exist at the junction of the motor nerve with the muscle. With repeated stimulation, the muscle becomes exhausted and is eventually unable to contract at all. If respiratory muscles become involved, death from respiratory insufficiency or arrest is a possibility.

Signs and Symptoms

Myasthenia gravis is characterized by the following features: weakness of voluntary muscles, particularly those of chewing, swallowing, and speaking; partial improvements of strength with rest; and dramatic improvement with the use of anticholinesterase drugs.

The onset of symptoms is gradual and early weakness may be so subtle that it goes unnoticed. Muscles responsible for fine movements, such as eye, facial, or hand muscles, are often affected early in the disease process. Ptosis and diplopia are commonly seen. The patient becomes unable to perform any activity that demands sustained muscular contractions, such as brushing the hair, walking upstairs, or holding the hands over the head. The fatigue may abate with rest but rapidly returns when the activity is tried again. If the diaphragm or intercostal muscles are involved, breathing is compromised.

Medical Diagnosis

The diagnosis is made by administering edrophonium (Tensilon). This is an anticholinesterase drug that increases the relative amount of acetylcholine in the neuromuscular junction by destroying acetylcholinesterase. In the patient with myasthenia gravis, muscle tone is markedly improved within 1 minute of injection and this improvement persists for 4 to 5 minutes. The serum is tested for antiacetylcholine receptor antibodies. CT and MRI are performed to screen for thymoma (a tumor of the thymus gland).

Medical Treatment

Anticholinesterase Drugs. Therapy is directed primarily toward pharmacologic management with anticholinesterase drugs and corticosteroids. Neostigmine and pyridostigmine (Mestinon) are anticholinesterase drugs that increase the availability of acetylcholine at the neuromuscular junction. Both drugs inhibit the action of cholinesterase, the enzyme that destroys acetylcholine. The availability of acetylcholine is improved, thereby enhancing muscle strength. Dosages are individualized for each patient, based on response and needs rather than a standardized dosing schedule. Stress or sustained levels of activity can alter the need for these agents. The patient must be monitored for pyridostigmine overdose, which is characterized by gastrointestinal (GI) discomfort, diarrhea, nausea, and vomiting. The adverse events of increased bronchial and oral secretions are particularly risky for patients with dysphagia and respiratory involvement. Other common adverse events are cramping and muscle fasciculation.

Neuromuscular blockers must be used very cautiously in the patient with myasthenia gravis.

Corticosteroids. Corticosteroids may be useful in those patients who do not respond well to the anticholinesterase drugs. ACTH or prednisone is administered concurrently with the anticholinesterase drug in an effort to induce remission. During the first 7 to 10 days of therapy symptoms may worsen, requiring hospitalization to monitor for respiratory depression. With improvement, corticosteroids may be tapered and maintained at the lowest effective dose.

Cytotoxic Therapies. Cytotoxic therapies are useful in patients who are unable to significantly taper corticosteroid drugs. Azathioprine and cyclosporine have been used in these cases.

Thymectomy. Because a large number of patients with myasthenia gravis have hyperplasia of the thymus gland, thymectomy is performed early after the initial diagnosis. Close monitoring is essential postoperatively because a risk of respiratory compromise exists as a result of possible pneumothorax. About 40% of patients enjoy some degree of remission after thymectomy.

Plasmapheresis. Plasmapheresis is an adjunctive therapy based on the autoimmune theory of myasthenia. It is a process of plasma exchange in which the acetylcholine receptor antibodies are washed from the plasma. A temporary catheter, similar to a renal dialysis access catheter, is used for venous access. Blood is then routed through a pheresis field, where the antibodies are separated from the plasma. The washed blood is then returned to the patient. The procedure takes 3 to 4 hours and is repeated over several days to ensure adequate treatment. Improvement in muscle strength may be noted within 24 to 48 hours after treatment. As progress is made with plasmapheresis, drug doses may be decreased.

Myasthenic and Cholinergic Crises

Emergency respiratory support requiring mechanical ventilation may be necessary in the event of myasthenic or cholinergic crises. Myasthenic crisis is marked by a sudden exacerbation of myasthenic symptoms, including difficulty swallowing and breathing, with possible respiratory arrest. Infection often precipitates the event and symptoms do not decrease even with increased doses of medications.

Cholinergic crisis presents with sudden, extreme weakness and respiratory impairment. It is precipitated by overmedication with anticholinesterase drugs, which literally bombard the receptor sites with excess amounts of acetylcholine. Intubation and mechanical ventilation are required to manage the respiratory compromise.

Because the two crises present similarly, differentiation is critical. Once again, edrophonium is used to distinguish the two entities. Rapid improvement in muscle strength after administration of edrophonium indicates an underlying myasthenic crisis. If no improvement is observed, the patient is experiencing a cholinergic crisis.

Because myasthenia gravis is a chronic neurologic disease, the patient is generally managed at home. However, hospitalization is likely on the initial diagnosis and during periods of crisis and respiratory compromise.

Pharmacology Capsule

Edrophonium (Tensilon) rapidly reverses a myasthenic crisis but has no effect on a cholinergic crisis.

NURSING CARE of the Patient with Myasthenia Gravis

Assessment

The complete neurologic assessment is outlined in Box 27-2. When the patient has myasthenia gravis, the health history describes the onset of symptoms, particularly muscle weakness, diplopia, dysphagia, slurred speech, breathing difficulties, and loss of balance. Record the effects of the condition on the patient's lifestyle. In the physical examination, evaluate muscle strength, balance, respiratory effort, and oxygenation status.

Nursing Diagnoses, Goals, and Outcome Criteria: Myasthenia Gravis

Nursing Diagnoses	Goals and Outcome Criteria
Ineffective Breathing Pattern related to impaired conduction of nerve impulses	Adequate oxygenation: respiratory rate of 12 to 20 breaths/min without dyspnea
Impaired Physical Mobility and **Self-Care Deficit (Bathing, Feeding, Dressing, Toileting)** related to muscle weakness, fatigue	Improved mobility and self-care: performance of activities of daily living (ADL) without excessive fatigue
Impaired Verbal Communication related to weakness of the muscles involved in speech	Effective communication: patient makes needs known
Impaired Swallowing related to muscle weakness	Adequate intake of fluids and food: stable body weight and absence of respiratory distress associated with aspiration
Deficient Knowledge of disease and treatment	Patient understands disease and treatment: patient accurately describes condition and treatment, follows plan of care

Interventions

Ineffective Breathing Pattern

You must monitor the patient for early signs and symptoms of ineffective breathing and hypoxia (tachycardia, restlessness). Progressive symptoms that do not respond to prescribed drug therapy may require mechanical ventilation. Management of the patient on a ventilator is discussed in Chapter 31.

Impaired Physical Mobility and Self-Care Deficit (Bathing, Feeding, Dressing, Toileting)

Because of weakness, the patient may be relatively inactive and unable to provide self-care. Monitor the patient's capabilities and assist as needed (see *Patient Teaching* box). Measures to prevent complications, discussed in Chapter 21, include turning and repositioning at least every 2 hours.

Patient Teaching

Myasthenia Gravis

- Myasthenia gravis is a chronic disease that can be treated but not cured.
- You must know your drug names, dosages, schedule, side effects, and adverse effects that should be reported to the physician. It is very important to take the prescribed drugs on time.
- Myasthenic crisis indicates too little acetylcholine.

Patient Teaching—cont'd

- Cholinergic crisis occurs when too much acetylcholine is present.
- Difficulty swallowing and breathing are symptoms of both types of crises and each requires immediate medical treatment.
- You will need to adjust your routine based on your symptoms.
- A good source of information is the Myasthenia Gravis Foundation of America (1-800-541-5454; www.myasthenia.org), which may have a local chapter where you live.

Impaired Verbal Communication

Patients may have weakness of the muscles used in speech, especially when drug effects are wearing off, and after a long conversation. Therefore, delay questioning when the patient's voice is fading.

Impaired Swallowing

Patients may have difficulty chewing and swallowing. Anticholinesterase drugs may be ordered 30 minutes before meals to improve muscle strength. The patient should be seated upright for meals and allowed (or assisted) to eat in an unhurried manner. Teach the patient to lower the chin toward the chest when swallowing to help prevent aspiration. Small, frequent meals may be tolerated better than three large ones. A soft diet is usually ordered so that minimal chewing is required. If swallowing is severely impaired, a feeding tube may be inserted and liquid feedings given as ordered. Adequate fluid intake is important to maintain hydration and prevent constipation.

Deficient Knowledge

Patient teaching with myasthenia gravis is essential because this chronic condition requires lifelong treatment (see *Health Promotion* box).

Health Promotion

Patients with Myasthenia Gravis

Patients with myasthenia gravis should receive the following interventions as necessary:

- Maintain general health through diet.
- Seek regular medical checkups for disease prevention.
- Plan rest periods.
- Tailor activities to conserve energy.

TRIGEMINAL NEURALGIA (TIC DOULOUREUX)

Trigeminal **neuralgia** is characterized by intense pain along the distribution of one of the three branches of the trigeminal nerve (fifth cranial nerve): (1) ophthalmic, (2) mandibular, or (3) maxillary (Fig. 27-20). The pain has an abrupt onset and is usually unilateral in nature, lasting from seconds to a few minutes. Despite the intense pain, no associated motor or sensory deficit exists. The pain may be crippling,

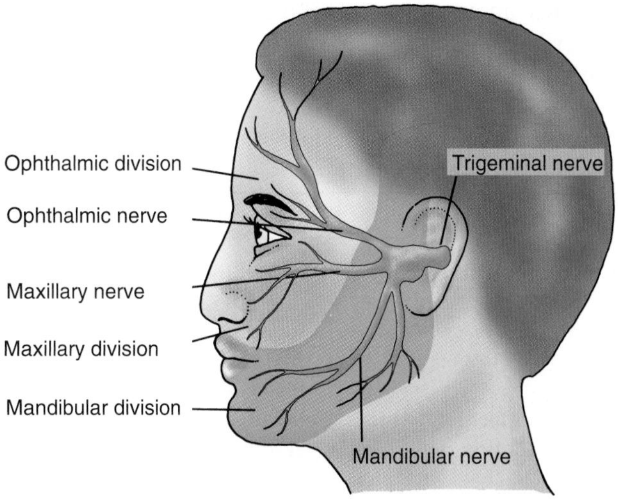

FIGURE 27-20 Distribution of the trigeminal nerve and its three divisions: (1) ophthalmic, (2) maxillary, and (3) mandibular. (From Ignatavicius DD, Workman ML: *Medical-surgical nursing: patient-centered collaborative care*, 6 ed, St. Louis, 2010, Saunders.)

restricting the patient's daily routine. Attacks may be triggered by ingestion of hot or cold liquids, chewing, shaving, or washing the face. Between episodes the patient may experience a dull ache or be pain free.

Cause

Although the exact cause of trigeminal neuralgia is undetermined, various contributing factors can be identified. Trauma or infection may precipitate the characteristic pain, as may compression of the nerve by an aneurysm, artery, or tumor.

Medical Diagnosis

Because no specific test exists, the diagnosis is based on the history. Stimulation of certain trigger points may precipitate the pain.

Medical Treatment

Pharmacologic management is the preferable course of therapy. Phenytoin (Dilantin) and carbamazepine (Tegretol) are most commonly used to suppress the pain episodes. During the acute attack, alcohol or phenol may be injected into the affected branch of the trigeminal nerve, with pain relief lasting from 8 to 16 months.

Patients with the most severe, debilitating pain may undergo surgical intervention. Electrocoagulation, a procedure in which heated electrodes are used to destroy the sensory fibers of the nerve, is effective in providing lasting pain relief without compromising motor or tactile function.

NURSING CARE of the Patient with Trigeminal Neuralgia

Assessment

Assessment of the patient with trigeminal neuralgia focuses on describing the pain, factors that trigger it, and treatments found to be effective or ineffective. Describe the effects of the condition on the patient's life.

Nursing Diagnoses, Goals, and Outcome Criteria: Trigeminal Neuralgia

Nursing Diagnoses	Goals and Outcome Criteria
Chronic Pain related to disease process	Reduced frequency and severity of attacks: patient reports attacks are less frequent and pain is lessened
Self-Neglect related to debilitating pain	Self-care activities accomplished: activities of daily living (ADL) completed independently
Imbalanced Nutrition: Less Than Body Requirements related to pain associated with chewing	Adequate nutrition: stable body weight
Fear related to anticipated painful episodes	Lessened fear: patient expresses less fear and increased confidence in ability to manage condition
Deficient Knowledge of trigeminal neuralgia and its treatment	Patient understands condition and treatment: patient accurately describes condition, prevention of episodes, and treatment

Interventions

The focus of nursing care for the patient with trigeminal neuralgia is pain assessment and management. It may be beneficial to assist the patient in developing alternative strategies for pain relief, such as guided imagery or relaxation therapy. Because of the debilitating nature of the pain, the patient may need encouragement and assistance in performing self-care activities. Nutrition may be affected because chewing may trigger pain. Psychologic effects are also a consideration in management because the fear of engaging in some activity that may trigger pain can lead to social isolation. Chapter 15 provides additional information about care of the patient in pain. Patient teaching emphasizes the nature of the condition and avoidance of factors that trigger episodes.

NEUROFIBROMATOSIS, TYPES 1 AND 2

Neurofibromatosis type 1, also known as *von Recklinghausen disease,* is characterized by multiple subcutaneous nerve tumors. The tumors are benign but may be removed to relieve compression of the nerves or for cosmetic reasons. Neurofibromatosis type 2 is characterized by tumors affecting the inner ear, cranial and peripheral nerves, and brain tissue. The primary treatment is surgical intervention.

BELL'S PALSY

Bell's palsy is acute paralysis of the seventh cranial nerve, which serves the face. The condition usually begins with pain behind the ear or on the face. The patient then has a drawing sensation followed by paralysis of the muscles on the affected side. The affected eyelids do not close, taste is impaired, and eating may be difficult. Most patients recover during a period of weeks or months but some have residual weakness.

Bell's palsy is treated on an outpatient basis with prednisone and analgesic drugs. Artificial tears are needed if the eyelids do not close and the affected eye should be closed and an eye shield used on the affected eye at night to prevent drying of the cornea. When function begins to return, the patient can do simple exercises to improve muscle tone: grimacing, opening and closing the eye, whistling, and puffing out the cheeks. Be sensitive to the patient's concerns about the condition and his or her appearance.

CEREBRAL PALSY

Cerebral palsy is a paralysis associated with a loss in motor coordination caused by cerebral damage. Although the cause is uncertain, the damage is generally believed to occur at birth and to be related to hypoxia, premature birth, or birth trauma.

Individuals with cerebral palsy are often frustrated by people who equate the disorder with mental retardation. Although the staggering gait and unclear speech may resemble a stereotype of a person with mental retardation, the individual with cerebral palsy is fully capable of comprehending his or her situation and is willing to strive for as much independence as possible.

Types of Cerebral Palsy

The three types of cerebral palsy are: (1) spastic paralysis, (2) athetoid, and (3) ataxic. Spastic paralysis is characterized by overall exaggerated reflexes and muscle spasms. Random, purposeless movement with extreme muscle tone is indicative of the athetoid type whereas the ataxic variety is characterized by poor balance; an uncoordinated, staggering gait; and speech or vision defects.

Medical Treatment

Although no cure exists for cerebral palsy, early muscle training and exercises can be beneficial in an effort to prevent complications and promote optimal function. Orthopedic surgery, braces, and casts may be useful in limiting deformities and disabilities.

❖ NURSING CARE of the Patient with Cerebral Palsy

Nursing care of the patient with cerebral palsy is covered in depth in pediatric nursing texts because it is typically a lifelong condition diagnosed in infancy. Therefore although many adults have cerebral palsy, it is not discussed in detail here.

POSTPOLIO SYNDROME

Before the advent of the polio vaccine, many people suffered varying degrees of motor impairment caused by the polio virus. Many years after having had the initial infection, some patients once again experience progressive muscle weakness, fatigue, pain, and respiratory problems typical of polio infections. The reason for the recurrence of symptoms is not known. Medical and nursing care are primarily supportive, aimed at helping the patient to adapt to the symptoms and maintain maximum possible function.

SUMMARY

Management of the patient with a neurologic disorder can be demanding and challenging. Astute observation and assessment are vital to any treatment plan and other therapies are often based on the nursing assessment. As is apparent from this chapter, many nursing diagnoses and modes of management are common to almost any patient with a neurologic disorder. Because of the complicated nature of many of these disorders, the management of other body systems also must be considered in a comprehensive care plan.

Get Ready for the NCLEX® Examination!

Key Points

- The functional unit of the nervous system is the neuron (nerve cell), which conducts electrical impulses throughout the nervous system.
- The brain and the spinal cord compose the CNS whereas the nerves in the peripheral parts of the body compose the peripheral nervous system.
- CSF circulates through the CNS.
- The neurologic assessment includes evaluation of the level of consciousness, pupillary size and response, coordination and balance, sensory function, reflexes, and vital signs.
- Increased ICP may impair cerebral tissue perfusion, resulting in ischemia and possibly respiratory arrest.
- Signs and symptoms of increased ICP and impaired cerebral blood flow are decreasing level of consciousness, pupil dilation with no response to light, motor deficits, abnormal posture, fever, increased blood pressure, bradycardia, and respiratory depression.
- Measures to decrease ICP include positioning, hyperventilation, fluid restriction, mechanical drainage, and drug therapy.
- Seizures are abnormal activity and behavior caused by abnormal electrical impulses in the brain that may be treated with anticonvulsant therapy and, when possible, measures to correct the cause.
- Nursing care of the patient with a seizure disorder addresses risk for injury, ineffective coping, and deficient knowledge.
- Nursing care of the patient with a head injury may focus on risk for ineffective cerebral tissue perfusion, ineffective breathing pattern, risk for injury, risk for infection, impaired physical mobility, disturbed body image, and ineffective role performance.
- Meningitis and encephalitis are infections of the nervous system.
- GBS, thought to be an autoimmune response to a viral infection, is characterized by progressive ascending neurologic deficits that, in most cases, eventually resolve.
- Nursing care of the patient with GBS addresses ineffective breathing pattern; decreased cardiac output; risk for disuse syndrome; imbalanced nutrition: less than body requirements; risk for injury; anxiety; and deficient knowledge.
- Parkinson syndrome, a progressive disorder that results in loss of coordination and control over involuntary movement, is treated with physical therapy and drugs that increase dopamine levels in the brain.
- The focus of nursing care for the patient with Parkinson syndrome is impaired physical mobility; risk for injury; imbalanced nutrition: less than body requirements; ineffective coping; and deficient knowledge.
- MS is a progressive degenerative disease that disrupts the motor pathways of the CNS and may lead to severe neurologic disabilities.
- ALS is a rapidly progressive degenerative disease that usually results in death from respiratory complications within 3 years.
- The patient with ALS has increasing needs for nursing care, eventually becoming completely dependent for all aspects of care.
- Myasthenia gravis is caused by a defect in impulse conduction that is manifested as weakness of voluntary muscles and is treated with anticholinesterase drugs and corticosteroids.
- Trigeminal neuralgia is intense pain along a branch of the trigeminal nerve that may be treated with drug therapy or surgical intervention.
- Cerebral palsy is associated with a loss in motor coordination caused by cerebral damage.

Additional Learning Resources

SG Go to your Study Guide for additional learning activities to help you master this chapter content.

evolve Go to your Evolve website (http://evolve.elsevier.com/Linton/medsurg) for the following learning resources and much more:
- Interactive Prioritization Exercises
- Fluid & Electrolyte Tutorial

- Pharmacology Tutorial
- Review Questions for the NCLEX® Examination

Review Questions for the NCLEX® Examination

1. Neurotransmitters include which of the following? (Select all that apply.)
   1. Acetylcholine
   2. Norepinephrine
   3. Epinephrine
   4. Dopamine
   5. Monoamine oxidase

   NCLEX Client Need: Physiological Integrity: Physiological Adaptation
2. Which of the following statements about normal aging of the neurologic system are true? (Select all that apply.)
   1. The number of neurons decreases.
   2. Lipofuscin and amyloid are deposited in nerve cells.
   3. Despite loss of neurons, most older people retain normal cognition.
   4. By age 80 the only intact reflex is the Achilles tendon jerk reflex.
   5. Brain size decreases and ventricles enlarge.

   NCLEX Client Need: Health Promotion and Maintenance
3. A male patient who is being treated for a closed head injury is lying still and appears to be sleeping even in the noisy emergency department. When you shake his shoulder and call his name, he opens his eyes and says, "Huh?" Then he closes his eyes again. Which of the following is a term that describes his level of consciousness?
   1. Somnolent
   2. Lethargic
   3. Stuporous
   4. Semicomatose

   NCLEX Client Need: Physiological Integrity: Physiological Adaptation
4. To evaluate neuromuscular function, the patient is instructed to raise one leg at a time while lying supine. How many degrees (at a minimum) would a patient with normal strength be able to lift each leg?

   NCLEX Client Need: Physiological Integrity: Reduction of Risk Potential
5. A postoperative craniotomy patient has an external ventricular drainage system. Proper management of the system includes which of the following instructions?
   1. Do not clamp the drainage tube under any circumstances.
   2. Use strict aseptic technique to cleanse the insertion site.
   3. Keep the zero point of the drip chamber at the level of the external auditory canal.
   4. Irrigate the tube with sterile normal saline at least every 8 hours.

   NCLEX Client Need: Physiological Integrity: Reduction of Risk Potential
6. A patient with a head injury is being monitored for increased ICP. The earliest sign of increased ICP is a change in which of the following?
   1. Pupil response to light
   2. Level of consciousness
   3. Blood pressure
   4. Motor and sensory function

   NCLEX Client Need: Physiological Integrity: Reduction of Risk Potential
7. Factors that may trigger migraine headaches include which of the following? (Select all that apply.)
   1. Alcohol
   2. Menstruation
   3. Exposure to bright light
   4. Changes in environmental temperature
   5. Certain foods

   NCLEX Client Need: Physiological Integrity: Physiological Adaptation
8. Nursing measures when a patient has a generalized seizure include which of the following? (Select all that apply.)
   1. Apply soft arm restraints to prevent injury.
   2. Insert a tongue blade between the teeth to prevent biting of the tongue.
   3. Turn the patient to one side to maintain a patent airway.
   4. Move objects away from the patient to prevent injury.
   5. Note the time the seizure began.

   NCLEX Client Need: Physiological Integrity: Reduction of Risk Potential
9. Which one of the following is a nursing measure used to decrease ICP?
   1. Suction the patient frequently.
   2. Encourage isometric exercises.
   3. Avoid flexing the neck and hips.
   4. Provide continuous stimulation.

   NCLEX Client Need: Physiological Integrity: Reduction of Risk Potential
10. Parkinson syndrome is associated with a deficit of which neurotransmitter?

    NCLEX Client Need: Physiological Integrity: Physiological Adaptation

chapter 28

Cerebrovascular Accident

Cheryl Ann Lehman

http://evolve.elsevier.com/Linton/medsurg

Objectives

1. Discuss the risk factors for cerebrovascular accident (CVA).
2. Identify the two major types of CVA.
3. Describe the pathophysiology, signs and symptoms, and medical treatment for each type of CVA.
4. Describe the neurologic deficits that may result from CVA.
5. Explain the tests and procedures used to diagnose CVA and nursing responsibilities for patients undergoing those tests and procedures.
6. Discuss criteria used to identify patients eligible for treatment with recombinant tissue plasminogen activator (rt-PA).
7. List data to be included in the nursing assessment of the CVA patient.
8. Assist in developing a nursing care plan for a CVA patient during the acute and rehabilitation phases.
9. Specify criteria used to evaluate the outcomes of nursing care for the CVA patient.
10. Identify resources for the CVA patient and family.

Key Terms

Aphasia (ă-FĀ-zhă)
Diplopia (dĭ-PLŌ-pē-ă)
Dysarthria (dĭs-ĂR-thrē-ă)
Dysphagia (dĭs-FĀ-zhă)
Dyspraxia (dĭs-PRĂK-sē-ă)
Expressive aphasia
Global aphasia
Hemiplegia (hĕm-ē-PLĒ-zhă)
Homonymous hemianopsia (hō-MŎN-ĭ-mŭs hĕm-ē-ă-NŎP-sē-ă)
Intracerebral (ĭn-tră-sĕ-RĒ-brăl)
Nonfluent aphasia
Ptosis (TŌ-sĭs)
Receptive aphasia
Subarachnoid (sŭb-ă-RĂK-nōyd)
Transient ischemic attack (TRĂN-zē-ĕnt ĭs-KĒ-mĭk ă-TĂK)

The brain is the body's center of thinking, feeling, and physical function. A continuous blood supply is essential to maintain function in the brain. A cerebrovascular accident (CVA) is an interruption of blood flow to part of the brain. Without normal blood flow, the affected area is deprived of oxygen and cell death begins to occur in as little as 4 minutes. The effects of oxygen deprivation vary depending on the area of the brain involved and the length of time the brain is deprived of oxygen. If blood flow is restored to the deprived area in time, recovery of the brain tissue may occur.

ANATOMY AND PHYSIOLOGY

The central structures of the brain include the cerebrum, the brainstem, and the cerebellum. A brief review of the anatomy and physiology of the brain is presented here. Refer to Chapter 27 for a more detailed review.

CEREBRUM

The cerebrum is the largest and most highly developed part of the brain. It has many complex functions, including initiation of movements, recognition of sensory input, higher-order thinking, regulation of emotional behavior, and regulation of endocrine and autonomic functions.

The cerebrum is divided into two halves, called *hemispheres*, connected by the corpus callosum. Each hemisphere controls the opposite side of the body; that is, the right hemisphere controls the left side of the body and the left hemisphere controls the right side of the body. For most people, the left hemisphere is dominant. This hemisphere controls the more analytic mental processes such as language acquisition and use, mathematics, and reasoning powers. The right hemisphere encompasses emotional and artistic tendencies.

The outer layer of the cerebrum is called the cortex. Each hemisphere of the brain is divided into the parietal, frontal, temporal, and occipital lobes. Each lobe has a different area of function (Fig. 28-1).

BRAINSTEM

The brainstem includes the midbrain, pons, medulla, and part of the reticular activating system. The brainstem controls vital basic functions, including respiration, heart rate, and consciousness.

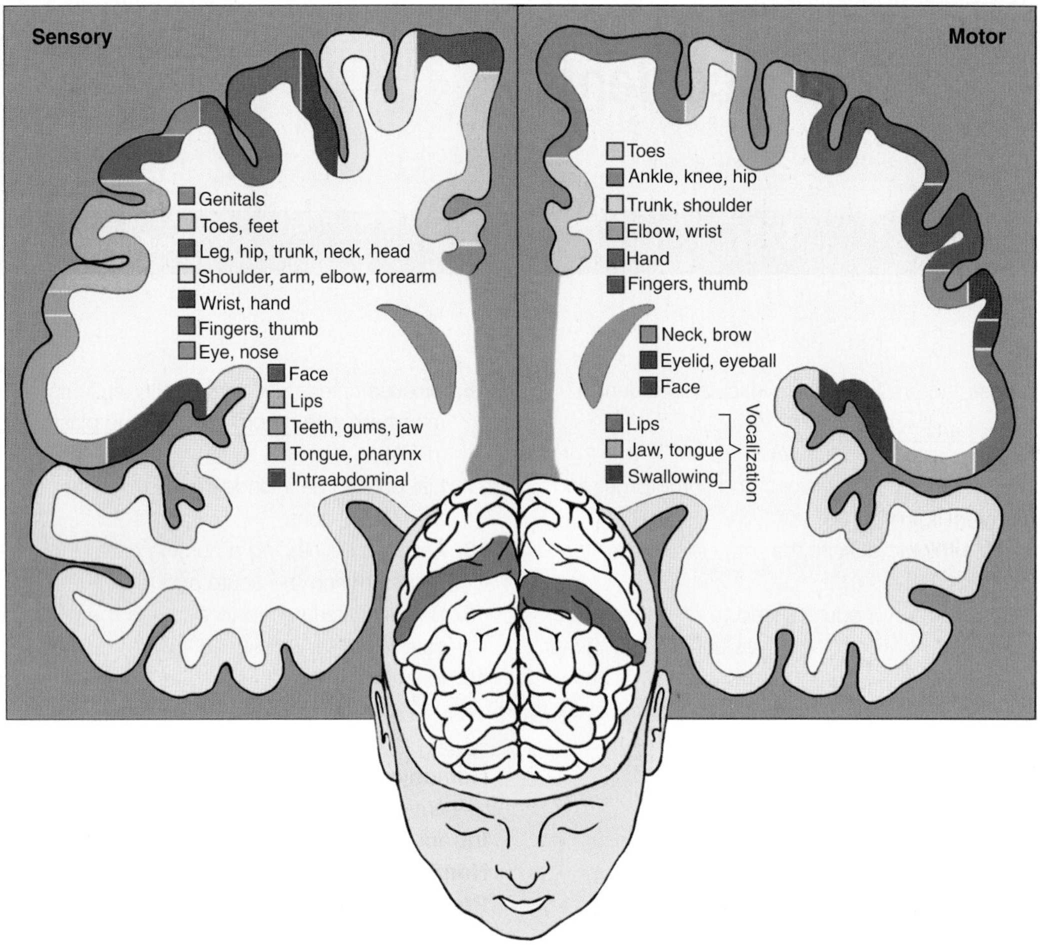

FIGURE 28-1 Control zones of the brain. This drawing represents a slice of each side of the brain. The diagram on the left shows the areas of the cerebral cortex that receive sensory information for specific body areas. The diagram on the right shows where motor activity is initiated for various areas of the body. (From Monahan FD, Drake DT, Neighbors M, editors: *Medical-surgical nursing: foundations for clinical practice*, ed 2, Philadelphia, 1998, Saunders.)

CEREBELLUM

The cerebellum uses information received from the cerebrum, muscles, joints, and inner ear to coordinate movement, balance, and posture. Unlike the cerebrum, the right side of the cerebellum controls the right side of the body and the left side of the cerebellum controls the left side of the body.

CIRCULATION

The brain is rich with arterial circulation to satisfy its high need for oxygen. Figure 28-2 shows the major cerebral arteries. Although the brain comprises only 2% of the body's weight, it consumes 20% of the oxygen supply and cardiac circulation each minute. The two major arterial systems that supply the brain are (1) the carotid and (2) the vertebral arteries. The carotid system begins as one common artery that later divides into the external and internal carotid arteries. The external carotid arteries divide to supply blood to the face. The internal arteries further divide into the middle cerebral artery and the anterior cerebral artery to supply blood to the brain. The vertebral arteries originate from the subclavian artery and travel up the anterior neck to merge and form the basilar artery at the brainstem. A second division forms the posterior cerebral artery. The internal carotid arteries and vertebral-basilar arteries unite to form the circle of Willis. Some people have anatomic differences in blood vessels that can increase the likelihood that they will sustain a CVA.

CEREBROVASCULAR ACCIDENT

A CVA is commonly referred to as a *stroke* or "brain attack." Stroke is the third leading cause of death and the leading cause of adult disability in the United States. Nearly 795,000 Americans experience a new or recurrent stroke each year, resulting in the deaths of approximately 130,000 people annually. (An additional 200,000 to 500,000 individuals experience a **transient ischemic attack** [TIA]). The economic effect of stroke is estimated to be more than $60 billion each year, with monies spent on treatment, medications, and missed

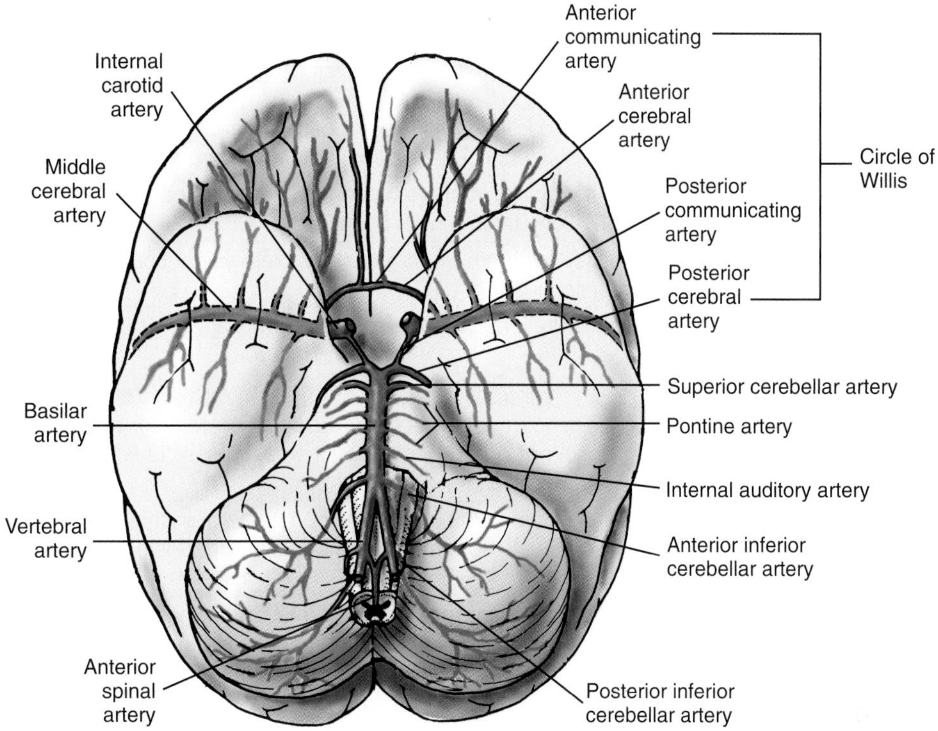

FIGURE 28-2 Cerebral circulation. (From Ignatavicius DD, Workman ML: *Medical-surgical nursing: patient-centered collaborative care*, ed 7, St. Louis, 2013, Saunders.)

Box 28-1 Signs of a Stroke

- Sudden numbness or weakness of the face, arm, or leg, especially on one side of the body
- Sudden confusion, trouble speaking or understanding
- Sudden trouble seeing in one or both eyes
- Sudden trouble walking, dizziness, loss of balance or coordination
- Sudden, severe headache with no known cause

work. Despite these statistics, a reason for hope exists. Approximately 7 million Americans are stroke survivors. Stroke is considered one of the most preventable of catastrophic events in the United States. With risk factor modification and new treatments emerging, the outlook for patients and families continues to improve. Box 28-1 lists the common signs of a stroke.

RISK FACTORS FOR STROKE

Stroke experts believe that the majority of strokes could be prevented. Unfortunately, the public has limited knowledge about stroke in relation to signs and symptoms of impending stroke or TIA, prevention of stroke, or medical treatment available. Nurses are becoming more involved in community education through outreach programs directed at assisting the public to learn more about stroke, identify risk factors, and teach individuals methods to adopt a healthy lifestyle so as to reduce their risk of suffering a stroke. The national Know Stroke campaign aims to educate the public to recognize the signs and symptoms of stroke and to take immediate action. To learn more, visit the Know Stroke website at http://stroke.nih.gov/.

Risk factors for stroke are classified as *modifiable* and *nonmodifiable.* Nonmodifiable factors are risk factors that cannot be changed: age, race, gender, heredity, having had a previous TIA or CVA, fibromuscular disease, and patent foramen ovale. CVAs are more common in men, African Americans, people aged 51 to 74 years, and those with a family history of CVA. Stroke has been considered mostly a disease of older individuals but at least 5% of strokes occur in individuals younger than 45 years. Causes of strokes among the young include drug abuse, use of birth control pills in combination with smoking, congenital heart conditions, mitral valve prolapse, atrial fibrillation, infectious endocarditis, sickle cell anemia, rheumatic fever, and leukemia. For more information on risk factors, visit www.stroke.org/site/PageServer?pagename=Risk. Modifiable risk factors are those that can be eliminated or controlled, thereby dramatically reducing the risk for CVA. The modifiable risk factors are listed in Table 28-1 along with the interventions used for each factor. (For a discussion of the nation's goals for stroke prevention, see *Health Promotion* box.)

A common denominator of many of the risk factors (hypertension, cardiac disease, diabetes mellitus) is atherosclerosis. Therefore many interventions include measures to slow the progression of atherosclerosis (see Chapter 36 for more complete coverage).

Table 28-1 Modifiable Cerebrovascular Accident Risk Factors and Related Interventions

MODIFIABLE RISK FACTOR	INTERVENTIONS TO MODIFY EFFECTS OF RISK FACTOR
Pathologic Disorders	
Hypertension	Antihypertensive drugs, weight control, stress management, smoking cessation, limited alcohol consumption, low-fat diet, reduced sodium intake.
Cardiac disease	Drug therapy to improve blood flow and prevent clots. Treatment of atrial fibrillation. Treatment of hyperlipidemia.
Diabetes mellitus	Balanced program of drug therapy, diet, weight control, exercise. Blood glucose monitoring.
Conditions that increase risk of blood clotting (e.g., sickle cell anemia)	Good hydration. Drug therapy as appropriate.
Lifestyle Factors	
Excessive alcohol consumption	Limit alcohol to 1 ounce of pure alcohol or less (not more than 1 ounce of pure alcohol per day: 2 cans beer, 2 small glasses of wine, 2 average cocktails). Avoid binge drinking.
Cigarette smoking	Advise patients of risks of tobacco use. Explain that risk falls with smoking cessation. Recommend self-help programs. Refer to physician for drug therapy.
Obesity	Encourage patient to maintain normal body weight. Instruction in proper diet. Weight control programs that help patients modify eating behaviors and establish healthy nutritional practices. Exercise programs as specified by the physician.
High-fat diet	Instruction in meal planning and preparation. Reduce saturated fats in diet.
Drug abuse	Drug abuse treatment programs.
Sedentary lifestyle	Education, structured exercise program.

Health Promotion

***Healthy People 2020*: Implications for Nurses**

Healthy People 2020 presents a comprehensive set of disease prevention and health promotion objectives developed to improve the health of all people in the United States during the second decade of the twenty-first century. Nurses are in a unique position within the community to promote and participate in this initiative.

ROLE OF THE NURSE IN STROKE PREVENTION AND TREATMENT

- Spread the word about risk factors for and warning signs of stroke.
- Assist patients in addressing and lowering their risks for stroke.
- Participate in community education programs for cardiovascular health.
- Get involved in Operation Stroke in your community.
- Participate in stroke and blood pressure screenings.
- Promote evidence-based care and best practices for a healthy lifestyle.
- Engage in and promote physical activity.
- Participate in antismoking campaigns and assist patients to locate such programs.
- Recognize depression after stroke and help patients to obtain adequate treatment.

TRANSIENT ISCHEMIC ATTACK

TIA is a "transient episode of neurologic dysfunction caused by focal brain, spinal cord, or retinal ischemia, without acute infarction" (Easton et al., 2009). Blood vessels may be occluded by spasms, fragments of plaque, or blood clots. It is believed that at least 85% of blood flow to an area must be blocked before signs and symptoms of a TIA appear. These episodes of temporary neurologic changes were previously thought to be "benign." It is now known that TIAs are important warning signs for the individual who could potentially experience a full stroke in the future. Previously, TIA was defined as lasting less than 24 hours but it is now defined as a temporary onset of stroke symptoms without permanent damage. It is recommended that a patient experiencing a TIA receive a full medical evaluation within 24 hours. This may be completed in an inpatient or outpatient setting.

Approximately 30% of individuals who experience a TIA have a stroke within 5 years. One tool used to assess the risk of stroke after TIA is the $ABCD^2$ score. Points are assigned based on age, blood pressure on first evaluation, clinical symptoms, and duration of symptoms and diagnosis of diabetes. The score can range from 0 to 7; the greater the score is, the more increased the risk of stroke is within 2 days. Try out the $ABCD^2$ score at www.mdcalc.com/abcd2-score-for-tia/.

Signs and Symptoms

With TIA, neurologic signs and symptoms resolve with no permanent effects. Some common signs and symptoms of TIA are dizziness, momentary confusion, loss of speech, loss of balance, tinnitus, visual disturbances, ptosis, dysarthria, dysphagia, drooping mouth, weakness, and tingling or numbness on one side of the body. The nature and severity of the symptoms depend on the area of the brain involved and the extent of tissue deprived of adequate oxygen.

Medical Diagnosis

TIA is generally suspected based on the health history and physical examination findings. Confirmation requires brain imaging studies, preferably with magnetic resonance imaging (MRI). In addition, noninvasive imaging of blood vessels, laboratory studies, and cardiac evaluation may be ordered to detect risk factors for TIA and stroke. Noninvasive vascular studies can show narrowing of cervical and cerebral blood vessels. Doppler studies may also be done to assess cerebral blood flow. Ultrasonic duplex scanning is useful in detecting carotid artery disease. Computed tomography (CT) and electroencephalogram (EEG) may be used to rule out intracranial lesions such as tumors, aneurysms, and abscesses. Key features of diagnostic tests are presented in Table 27-2.

On auscultation, a swooshing noise may be heard over a carotid artery. Its sound is similar to that of a rush of water through a narrow or dammed-up area. This sound, called a *bruit*, reveals that the artery is partially obstructed as with an atherosclerotic plaque.

Treatment

Treatment of TIA depends on the cause. The common causes of TIA are thought to be carotid artery disease, large or small artery disease from atherosclerosis, and atrial fibrillation. The treatment of atherosclerotic disease depends on the location of the narrowed vessel and the degree of narrowing. Based on research evidence, the American Stroke Association recommends initial treatment with acetylsalicylic acid (aspirin) alone or in combination with extended-release dipyridamole (Aggrenox), or clopidogrel bisulfate (Plavix) alone to decrease platelet clumping. In atrial fibrillation, microscopic emboli are believed to form, which later are released from the heart and travel to the arteries of the brain to cause TIA or stroke. Warfarin (Coumadin) and heparin are anticoagulants that may be given alone or in combination in patients exhibiting a cardioembolic TIA. The dosage for warfarin therapy is based on the prothrombin time (PT) and the international normalized ratio (INR). For therapeutic anticoagulation, the PT is usually kept in a therapeutic range of 1.5 to 2.0 times normal and the INR at 2.0 to 3.0. The effect of unfractionated heparin therapy is monitored with the activated partial thromboplastin time (aPTT). If low molecular weight heparin (enoxaparin and others) is used, laboratory values for Heparin anti-Xa may be monitored. Statin drugs are recommended for patients with elevated lipids or coronary artery disease, or when evidence exists that the TIA is related to atherosclerosis. Treatment of hypertension is recommended as well. Additional information about drug therapy is provided in Table 28-2.

Because of the operative risks and controversy about the value of surgical intervention in terms of stroke prevention, surgery is often reserved for the most serious stenosis. The most common surgical procedures are carotid endarterectomy (Fig. 28-3) and transluminal angioplasty. Carotid endarterectomy is the surgical removal of plaques in the artery to permit improved blood flow. Patients who are at high risk for surgical intervention because of other health problems may benefit from angioplasty. A stent may be placed in the artery to keep it open. Transluminal angioplasty improves blood flow by dilating the narrowed artery with a balloon that is inserted into the artery. A patent foramen ovale is sometimes identified in the patient with TIA. Closure of this defect in the heart can be accomplished through an open surgical approach or a transcatheter closure.

Pharmacology Capsule

When patients are taking antiplatelet or anticoagulant medications, take care to prevent injuries and bleeding.

STROKE

A stroke is an abrupt impairment of brain function resulting in a set of neurologic signs and symptoms that are caused by impaired blood flow to the brain and that last more than 24 hours. When symptoms progress over hours or days, the condition is described as *stroke in evolution*. When the neurologic deficits do not change for 2 to 3 days, the stroke is said to be *completed*. Unlike TIA, a completed stroke causes lingering motor, sensory, or cognitive damage with varying disabilities. As noted earlier, stroke is the third leading cause of death and the leading cause of adult disability in the United States. Approximately 795,000 Americans experience strokes each year, resulting in the deaths of approximately 130,000 people annually (see *Cultural Considerations* box). When the occurrence of TIAs is added to these numbers, the total may reach 2 million CVAs each year in the United States alone. Acute care and rehabilitation of stroke patients is a long and expensive process. Advances in care have improved the outlook for many individuals who experience a stroke. More than half of stroke victims acquire independence in activities of daily living (ADL) within 1 year after the stroke. Thirty percent of stroke survivors return to work or productive lives within 1 year. These are important figures to remember when caring for the stroke patient.

Cultural Considerations

What Does Culture Have to Do with Stroke?

For unknown reasons, people in the Southeastern United States have the highest stroke mortality rates in the country.

Table 28-2 **Medications for Cerebrovascular Accident**

DRUG	USE/ACTION	SIDE EFFECTS	NURSING INTERVENTIONS
Corticosteroids			
Dexamethasone (Decadron)	Reduces ICP by reducing inflammation in brain after stroke.	Fluid retention, hypertension, hypokalemia, hyperglycemia, suppressed response to infection, fat deposits in cheeks and upper back, gastric ulcers, insomnia, easy bruising, mood swings. Dose usually tapered over 7–10 days to prevent acute withdrawal and adrenal insufficiency.	Monitor I&O, BP, blood glucose in people with diabetes. Protect from infection. Report even minor signs of infection. Protect from bumps and other minor injuries.
Hyperosmotic Agents			
Mannitol (Osmitrol) Glycerin (Osmoglyn)	Induces diuresis, which reduces ICP. Mannitol is first-choice drug.	Circulatory overload, heart failure, hypertension, renal failure.	15% to 25% mannitol solutions should be filtered. Monitor infusion site; stop flow and restart if infiltrated to avoid tissue damage. Monitor for signs of fluid volume excess: hypertension, bounding pulse, edema, urine output less than fluid intake.
Anticoagulants			
Unfractionated heparin sodium (Liquaemin sodium)	Prevents formation of new blood clots; does not dissolve existing clots.	Bleeding or hemorrhage due to excessive anticoagulation, hyperkalemia, alopecia allergy period.	Effect is monitored by partial thromboplastin time (PTT) or activated partial thromboplastin time (aPTT). Therapeutic goal is 1.5–2.0 times the control of 30–40 sec. If patient's aPTT is greater, withhold drug and contact physician. Assess for bruises, bleeding from GI and urinary tracts, mouth, or nose. Contraindicated with active bleeding. Heparin antidote is protamine sulfate. Caution with venipuncture—apply pressure to site.
Low molecular weight heparin: enoxaparin, dalteparin, and others	Prevents formation of new blood clots; does not dissolve existing clots.	Bleeding or hemorrhage, allergic reactions, injection site reactions, increases in liver enzyme tests.	Lab values not routinely followed. If monitored, the anti-Xa assay will be used. Protamine as an antidote will be only partially effective. Assess for bruises, bleeding from GI and urinary tracts, mouth, or nose. Contraindicated with active bleeding.
Warfarin sodium (Coumadin, Panwarfin)	Prevents formation of new blood clots; does not dissolve existing clots.	Bleeding or hemorrhage due to excessive anticoagulation.	Effect is monitored by prothrombin time (PT) and international normalized ratio (INR). Therapeutic goal is a PT of 1.5–2.0 times control and INR of 2.0–3.0. Check PT/INR before initiating medication and daily until maintenance dose is reached. Assess for bruising, bleeding from GI and urinary tracts, mouth, or nose. Apply pressure after venipuncture. Antidote for warfarin overdose is vitamin K_1 (AquaMEPHYTON).

Table 28-2 Medications for Cerebrovascular Accident—cont'd

DRUG	USE/ACTION	SIDE EFFECTS	NURSING INTERVENTIONS
Dabigatran (Pradaxa)	A direct thrombin inhibitor indicated to reduce the risk of stroke for patients with nonvalvular atrial fibrillation.	Can cause serious and sometimes fatal bleeding. Promptly evaluate signs and symptoms of blood loss.	Do not break, chew, or empty the contents of the capsule. Discontinuing abruptly may increase risk of new stroke. Antidote not available.
Thrombolytics			
Recombinant tissue plasminogen activator (rt-PA)	Initiates dissolution of clots by breaking down fibrin.	Hemorrhage, especially within the first 24 h after administration.	Minimize venipunctures; protect arterial line sites; assess for bleeding; monitor coagulation studies.
Platelet Aggregation Inhibitors			
Aspirin	Reduces risk of stroke in male patients with recurrent ischemic attacks. May be given in combination with other antiplatelets.	Excessive bruising, bleeding; bronchoconstriction; nausea, vomiting, gastric bleeding, urticaria, confusion, drowsiness, tinnitus. May be given in combination with other antiplatelets.	Tinnitus and confusion suggest overdosage. Teach patients that aspirin can be harmful if not taken properly.
Dipyridamole (Persantine)	Prevents thromboembolism with heart valve prostheses. Used with coumarin anticoagulants.	Hypotension, dizziness. Caution with hypotensive patients. MI, dysrhythmias with IV use. Constipation, dry mouth.	Teach patient to manage orthostatic hypotension. Monitor pulse and blood pressure.
Aspirin/extended-release dipyridamole (Aggrenox)	Prolongs bleeding time, decreasing the risk of stroke.	Rash, diarrhea, itching, bruising. Not associated with neutropenic purpura as with Ticlid.	May be given with or without food; assess for bruising.
Clopidogrel (Plavix)	Reduces risk of stroke by inhibition of clotting.	GI bleeding, epistaxis, neutropenia, intracranial hemorrhage, hypertension, dyspnea. Risk of hemorrhage increases if given with aspirin.	Give with food. Advise patients of need for periodic lab studies, including liver function tests with long-term therapy.
Calcium Channel Blockers			
Nimodipine (Nimotop)	Prevents spasms in cerebral blood vessels after a hemorrhagic stroke.	Headache, fatigue, depression, confusion, dysrhythmias, hypotension, MI, renal failure.	Monitor pulse and blood pressure. Assess for edema. Monitor urine output. Count pulse before each dose; withhold if less than 60 beats/min.

BP, Blood pressure; *GI*, gastrointestinal; *I&O,* intake and output; *ICP,* intracranial pressure; *IV,* intravenous; *MI,* myocardial infarction.

Pathophysiology

The two main classifications of stroke are (1) hemorrhagic and (2) ischemic.

Hemorrhagic Stroke. Hemorrhagic stroke accounts for only about 20% of all strokes. In hemorrhagic stroke, a blood vessel in the brain ruptures and bleeding into the brain occurs. As a result, intracranial pressure (ICP) may increase, disrupting normal cerebral function. Hemorrhagic strokes are further classified by location. An **intracerebral** (within the cerebrum) hemorrhage is associated with trauma, uncontrolled hypertension, and aneurysms. When a hemorrhage occurs within the spaces of the brain, the terms *subdural, subarachnoid,* or *ventricular* are used to describe the location. Hemorrhagic strokes are often sudden in onset and require emergent, life-sustaining treatment.

Box 28-3 Assessment of the Cerebrovascular Accident Patient

HEALTH HISTORY

Source of Data
Reliability and ability of patient to provide information

Present Illness
Description of onset and progression

Past Medical History
Cardiovascular conditions, liver disorder, diabetes mellitus, gout, previous cerebrovascular accidents (CVAs), head injury, previous disability, current medications

Family History
Neurologic or vascular conditions

Review of Systems
Visual disturbances, motor or sensory impairments, pain, dysphagia, incontinence, mental and emotional changes

Functional Assessment
Usual activities, help required from others to complete usual activities, use of adaptive equipment, diet, occupation, use of alcohol and tobacco, interpersonal relationships, stressors

PHYSICAL ASSESSMENT

General Appearance
Level of consciousness, behavior, gait, posture

Height and Weight

Vital Signs
Blood pressure, temperature, pulse, respiration

Face
Symmetry

Eyes
Pupil size, equality, alignment, reaction to light; gross visual acuity, eyelid closure, ptosis

Skin
Moisture, turgor, color

Abdomen
Bowel or bladder distention

Genitalia and Anus
Presence or odor of urine or stool

Extremities
Muscle tone, strength, voluntary movement, sensation

Nursing Care Plan — Patient with a Stroke

ASSESSMENT

HEALTH HISTORY An obese 78-year-old male was admitted with weakness on the right side and slurred speech. His daughter assisted with the history because the patient had some difficulty responding verbally. He has had type 2 diabetes mellitus for 10 years, which he treats with an oral hypoglycemic, and had a myocardial infarction at age 75. He has no recent changes in vision but does wear reading glasses. He has good hearing and no headaches. He is right-handed. He was unable to stand when he awoke this morning. He tried to drink some water but had difficulty swallowing. He has had no loss of bowel or bladder control. He is divorced. An adult daughter and her two teenagers live with him. He is a retired construction worker; his hobbies are carpentry and watching television.

PHYSICAL EXAMINATION Vital signs: blood pressure 210/104 mm Hg, pulse 96 bpm, respiration 22 breaths per minute, temperature 97°F (36°C) measured orally. Height 6′1″, weight 285 lb. Acknowledges he is in the hospital but is uncertain about day or date and time. Uses gestures to respond to some questions when he seems unable to find the right words. Pupils are equal and react to light. Ptosis of right eyelid is noted. Hand grips; voluntary movements; and reflexes of leg, arm, and hand are normal on left side but diminished on right side. Leans toward right side when not supported.

Nursing Diagnosis	Goals and Outcome Criteria	Interventions
Deficient Fluid Volume related to inadequate intake, dysphagia	The patient will maintain adequate hydration, as evidenced by moist mucous membranes, dilute urine, and pulse and blood pressure within usual range.	Record fluid intake and output. Administer intravenous fluid as ordered. After assessment by the speech-language pathologist (SLP), monitor oral fluid intake and assess swallowing. Assist the patient to sit up while eating and drinking. If thin fluids are difficult to swallow, try semisolids such as ice cream, pudding, and Popsicles. Have an oral suction device available in case of choking or aspiration. Detect and report signs and symptoms of fluid volume deficit: tachycardia, concentrated urine, and dry mucous membranes.
Imbalanced Nutrition: Less Than Body Requirements related to dysphagia, inability to feed self	The patient will maintain adequate nutrition, as evidenced by stable weight.	Document food intake. Assist with meals as needed. Use positioning and food consistency guidelines as provided by the SLP. Seat the patient upright for meals. Do not make him feel rushed. Provide alternative means of feeding (nasogastric or gastrostomy tube, total parenteral nutrition [TPN]) as ordered. Weigh weekly to assess adequacy of food intake.

Nursing Care Plan Stroke Patient—cont'd

Nursing Diagnosis	Goals and Outcome Criteria	Interventions
Impaired Verbal Communication related to aphasia	The patient will use nonverbal means to supplement verbal communication and will participate in speech therapy exercises.	Establish a code system of blinks or nods for nonverbal communication; use pictures or cards that the patient can select to express his needs. Encourage verbalization but recognize his frustration and provide words if he cannot retrieve them. Discuss referral to SLP with the physician. Tell the patient that improvement is usually possible with therapy.
Impaired Physical Mobility related to weakness, paralysis, poor balance	The patient will maintain intact skin, joint mobility, regular bowel and bladder elimination, good peripheral circulation, and normal breath sounds.	While on bed rest, assist the patient to change positions at least every 2 hours. He should not lie on his right side for more than 30 minutes at a time. Use positioning techniques and devices to reduce pressure points. Inspect the skin for redness and edema associated with pressure. Position the limbs in functional alignment and perform range-of-motion exercises three times a day. Do not pull on the affected side. Monitor bowel and bladder function. Administer stool softeners and laxatives as ordered. Encourage fluids and fiber when able to take orally. Palpate the lower abdomen for bladder distention and catheterize as ordered as necessary. Use bladder scanner if available to assess need for urinary catheterization. Report any tenderness, pain, or swelling in calves. Exercise the legs with each position change. Apply graduated compression stockings or sequential compression devices (SCDs) as ordered. Ambulate using gait belt when able. Discuss consults for physical therapy (PT) and occupational therapy (OT) with physician. Encourage coughing and deep breathing with each position change. Auscultate lung fields for breath sounds, wheezes, or rales. Report temperature elevation.
Risk for Injury related to paralysis	The patient will have no falls or injuries associated with motor impairment or altered sensory perception.	Keep the bed in low position with the side rails raised according to hospital policy. Put the call bell within reach on nonparalyzed side and instruct the patient to call for help getting out of bed. A bed check device may be implemented when patient has difficulty understanding directions or is in a confused state. Check on him frequently. Monitor the position of affected extremities to prevent trauma that might not be detected because of poor sensation. Use a sling or brace if ordered to support affected limbs. Assess the effects of ptosis on vision. If vision is impaired, approach the patient from the unaffected side and arrange personal articles on that side. When the patient is out of bed, be sure he is seated safely. Use pillows to prevent excessive leaning to one side. When ambulatory, use a gait belt if needed and assist the patient as appropriate.
Anxiety related to loss of function or fear of disability	The patient will have a reduction in anxiety, as evidenced by calm manner and patient statement.	Acknowledge signs of anxiety and attempt to identify sources. Provide information about what is happening, what you are doing, and what the patient can expect. Check on him often. Encourage his family to visit.
Interrupted Family Processes related to anticipated need of patient for assistance after discharge	The patient and family will plan for altered roles and responsibilities to support the patient during and after discharge.	Give family members an opportunity to ask questions and share their concerns. Provide information and facilitate communication with the physician as needed. Refer them to sources of support and resources, including a social worker and community agencies. Start planning for discharge. Assess family strengths and resources and willingness to help care for the patient after discharge. Identify new responsibilities they might need to assume and discuss how these can be fulfilled.

Critical Thinking Questions

1. What effect might this patient's stroke have on his daughter and her family?
2. Describe three examples of signs of anxiety that the patient may exhibit.
3. What data in this assessment are consistent with stroke?

Family History. The health history includes a family history of neurologic or cardiovascular disease as well as strokes.

Review of Systems. Ask the patient about significant problems in the review of systems. Important items to assess include weakness, impaired movement, pain (especially headache), dysphagia, bowel or bladder incontinence, visual disturbances, mental or emotional changes, and altered sensation.

Functional Assessment. The last component of the health history, the functional assessment, addresses the patient's usual activities and health practices. It is important to inquire about activity level, use of adaptive equipment at home, prior disability, dietary pattern, occupation, use of alcohol and tobacco, drug use, interpersonal relationships, and current stressors. These are important elements that will be used to identify risk factors for stroke and cardiovascular disease.

Physical Examination

During the physical examination, observe the patient's general appearance, responsiveness, and behavior and record any displays of restlessness or agitation. The patient's level of consciousness is important because subtle changes in level of consciousness such as confusion, irritability, or a decrease in level of consciousness may suggest a stroke in evolution or increasing ICP. Measure vital signs. A description of the patient's breathing pattern and effort are especially important. If possible, obtain the patient's weight and height.

Inspect the face for symmetry and assess the mouth for moisture and drooling. Then evaluate the alert patient's ability to swallow and inspect the patient's pupils for size, equality, and reaction to light. Conduct a gross vision assessment by asking the patient to read something. Inspect the patient's skin for color and palpate for moisture and turgor. Assess extremities for muscle tone and strength, sensation, and voluntary movement. Instruct the patient to move each extremity individually and observe the responses. Impaired movement or inappropriate response may be caused by aphasia or dyspraxia as well as by neuromuscular damage. The patient who has aphasia has difficulty interpreting messages and may not perform the requested movement for that reason. The patient with dyspraxia may comprehend instructions but be unable to direct the body part to move. Also record any evidence of incontinence or bladder distention.

Neurologic checks consisting of evaluating level of consciousness, pupil appearance and response to light, the patient's ability to follow commands, and the movement and sensation of extremities should be conducted frequently. These checks, along with vital signs, are essential to detect increasing ICP if ICP is not being monitored. For additional neurologic assessment, see Chapter 27.

The NIH Stroke Scale (Table 28-4) is a tool often used to assess patients who have experienced a stroke. This tool provides a method to guide systematic assessment of neurologic deficits often associated with an acute stroke. The examination addresses motor function, visual fields, ataxia, speech, language, cognition, and motor and sensory abnormalities. A point system is used to rate function; then points are combined to offer a "score." A research neurologist designed it to standardize and document neurologic assessments of stroke patients. Most facilities that use this assessment tool require those administering the examination to go through a certification process to ensure accuracy and consistency among examiners.

Nursing assessment of the stroke patient is summarized in Box 28-3.

Nursing Diagnoses, Goals, and Outcome Criteria: Acute Phase of Stroke

Depending on location and extent of brain damage, appropriate diagnoses and goals may include the following.

Nursing Diagnoses	Goals and Outcome Criteria
Ineffective Airway Clearance related to impaired cough reflex, altered consciousness, impaired swallowing	Patent airway: breath sounds clear to auscultation
Ineffective Breathing Pattern related to impaired cerebral circulation, increased intracranial pressure (ICP)	Effective breathing pattern: normal respiratory rate and depth, arterial blood gases within normal limits
Risk for Injury related to seizure activity, confusion, motor and sensory impairment, increased ICP, hemorrhage after recombinant tissue plasminogen activator (rt-PA) administration	Absence of injury: no bruising, skin breaks, falls, or fractures; stable neurologic status (level of consciousness, pupil equality and reaction to light)
Risk for Deficient Fluid Volume related to inadequate intake or excessive diuresis	Adequate hydration: balanced fluid intake and output
Excess Fluid Volume related to overhydration	Normal extracellular fluid volume: pulse and blood pressure consistent with patient norms, no edema, breath sounds clear
Imbalanced Nutrition: Less Than Body Requirements related to dysphagia, inability to feed self, inability to chew	Adequate intake of nutrients: maintenance of body weight

Nursing Diagnoses, Goals, and Outcome Criteria: Acute Phase of Stroke—cont'd

Nursing Diagnoses	Goals and Outcome Criteria
Ineffective Thermoregulation related to effects of neurologic impairment and/or metabolic processes	Effective thermoregulation: temperature within patient's normal range
Risk for Acute Confusion related to impaired cerebral circulation	Improved mental function: patient is oriented to self and environment
Impaired Verbal Communication related to aphasia	Effective communication: patient successfully communicates needs
Impaired Physical Mobility related to weakness, paralysis, spasticity, impaired balance	Absence of complications of immobility: joints have full range of motion, skin intact
Functional Urinary Incontinence related to inability to manage toileting process, impaired cognition. **Impaired Urinary Elimination** related to initial effects of stroke.	Improved control of urine elimination: episodes of uncontrolled voiding decrease; patient voids, voluntarily
Constipation related to immobility, dehydration, drug side effects	Normal bowel elimination: regular passage of soft, formed stool without straining
Bowel Incontinence related to impaired conduction of impulses	Controlled bowel elimination: no involuntary bowel evacuation
Ineffective Coping related to adapting to neurologic deficits	Effective coping strategies: patient verbalizes acceptance of stroke and strives for maximum recovery
Interrupted Family Processes related to disruption of family roles and functions	Adaptation of the family to the patient's condition: family demonstrates willingness and ability to adapt to patient's condition

Interventions

Ineffective Airway Clearance and Ineffective Breathing Pattern

To ensure effective airway clearance and breathing, maintain the patient's body alignment and elevate the head of the bed 25 to 30 degrees. Closely monitor the patient's respiratory status. Maintaining a patent airway is a priority for patients who have suffered strokes. Neurologic deficits may cause altered breathing patterns and impaired swallowing, gag, and cough reflexes. Increasing ICP may affect the respiratory center in the brain, causing respiratory depression. If the patient exhibits signs of increased ICP (e.g., rising blood pressure, bradycardia, abnormal pupil response, decreasing level of consciousness), elevate the head of the bed 30 degrees and notify the physician.

After a stroke the patient is at risk for airway obstruction for a number of reasons. If the patient is unconscious, the tongue may fall back and block the airway. A side-lying position helps to prevent such obstruction. An oral or nasal airway is sometimes used to keep the airway open.

Immobility and dehydration cause thick secretions to be retained in the respiratory tract, possibly leading to pneumonia and atelectasis. Good hydration helps to thin respiratory secretions for easier expectoration. Dysphagia may cause the patient to aspirate fluids or food, causing airway obstruction and contributing to the development of pneumonia. Pneumonia is, in fact, the most frequent cause of death after stroke. Feeding the patient with dysphagia is discussed in Chapter 39.

Suctioning and frequent position changes can help to prevent aspiration and promote removal of secretions. Respiratory treatments for the patient, with regular reminders to do deep-breathing exercises, can be helpful. Forceful coughing may be discouraged in the acute phase after a hemorrhagic stroke because it tends to increase ICP. Ask the physician if and when coughing is permitted. Administer oxygen therapy as ordered.

Risk for Injury

Many factors place the stroke patient at risk for injury. Seizures may occur, causing the patient to lose consciousness and to have abnormal motor activity. Therefore it is important to raise bed side rails and pad them according to agency protocol to reduce trauma if the patient strikes the rails. During a seizure, turn the patient to one side and move hard objects away from the patient. Never force anything between the patient's clenched teeth. To do so may injure the teeth and gums. ! Additional information about seizures is presented in Chapter 27.

Safety precautions are also essential for confused patients and patients with motor impairments. Orient patients to their surroundings and explain why they should not get up unassisted. The staff must respond promptly to the patient's calls for help. Although restraints are needed at times, they should only be used as a last resort because they often agitate the patient and can actually cause injuries. A bed check system may be of more benefit when the patient is having difficulty understanding directions. Get sufficient help or use mechanical devices to assist the patient in and out of the bed.

Sensory perceptual problems in the stroke patient may include visual disturbances, sensory deprivation or overload, and impaired tactile sensation. Among

Table 28-4 National Institutes of Health Stroke Scale

1a. Level of Consciousness	0 Alert 1 Not alert, but arousable with minimal stimulation 2 Not alert, requires repeated stimulation to attend 3 Coma
1b. Ask patient the month and his or her age	0 Answers both correctly 1 Answers one correctly 2 Both incorrect
1c. Ask patient to open and close eyes and grip and release hand	0 Obeys both correctly 1 Obeys one correctly 2 Both incorrect
2. Best Gaze (only horizontal eye movement)	0 Normal 1 Partial gaze palsy 2 Forced deviation
3. Visual Field Testing	0 No visual field loss 1 Partial hemianopia 2 Complete hemianopia 3 Bilateral hemianopia (blind including cortical blindness)
4. Facial Paresis (ask patient to show teeth or raise eyebrows and close eyes tightly)	0 Normal symmetric movement 1 Minor paralysis (flattened nasolabial fold, asymmetry on smiling) 2 Partial paralysis (total or near total paralysis of lower face) 3 Complete paralysis of one or both sides (absence of facial movement in the upper and lower face)
5. Motor Function—Arm (right and left) Right arm — Left arm —	0 Normal (extends arms 90 [or 45] degrees for 10 seconds without drift) 1 Drift 2 Some effort against gravity 3 No effort against gravity 4 No movement
6. Motor Function—Leg (right and left) Right leg — Left leg —	0 Normal (holds leg at 30 degrees for 5 seconds) 1 Drift 2 Some effort against gravity 3 No effort against gravity 4 No movement 9 Untestable (joint fused or limb amputated)
7. Limb Ataxia	0 No ataxia 1 Present in one limb 2 Present in two limbs
8. Sensory (use pinprick to test arms, legs, trunk, and face—compare side to side)	0 Normal trunk and face 1 Mild-to-moderate decrease in sensation 2 Severe-to-total sensory loss
9. Best Language (describe picture, read items, read sentences)	0 No aphasia 1 Mild-to-moderate aphasia 2 Severe aphasia 3 Mute
10. Dysarthria (read several words)	0 Normal articulation 1 Mild-to-moderate slurring of words 2 Near unintelligible or unable to speak 9 Intubated or other physical barriers
11. Extinction and Inattention	0 Normal 1 Inattention or extinction to bilateral simultaneous stimulation in one of the sensory modalities 2 Profound hemiinattention or extinction to more than one sensory modality (e.g., does not recognize own hand)

the visual disturbances are **diplopia** (double vision), loss of the corneal (blink) reflex, **ptosis** (drooping of the upper eyelid), homonymous hemianopsia, and inability to close the eyelids on the affected side. All of these pose threats to safety and self-care. They may also contribute to confusion. The cornea is susceptible to injury when not protected and, in healthy patients, kept moist by the closed eyelid and the blink reflex. Artificial tears may be used to provide moisture in patients with disturbed corneal reflex.

Patients who have homonymous hemianopsia see only half of the field of vision. Some patients have unilateral neglect, a condition in which visual fields are intact but the patient does not attend to certain parts of the fields. Unilateral neglect is most common in patients with right-brain damage. These patients may not attend to one side of the body and may overlook objects on one side of the visual field.

It is helpful to encourage patients to scan the affected side. Differences in the nursing approaches during the acute and rehabilitative phases are well contrasted here. In the acute phase, position patients with homonymous hemianopsia so that their unimpaired side is approached by the staff, to reduce stress to the patients. In rehabilitation, the patient should be positioned so that deliberate scanning by and use of the affected side are required. This is designed to stimulate return of function. Balanced sensory input is essential to reduce the risk of sensory deprivation or overload. The environment should be pleasant but not overly stimulating.

Another type of sensory disturbance after stroke is diminished sensation in affected body parts. The patient who does not feel pressure or pain is susceptible to injury. For example, a paralyzed foot can easily slip between the bed frame and side rails. Catheter tubing under the leg may create pressure that the patient cannot feel. Protect susceptible areas and remind the patient of the need for extra caution. In addition, check positioning of affected extremities to ensure that they are free of pressure and reposition them as needed.

! If rt-PA is administered for ischemic stroke, the patient must be monitored closely for hemorrhage for 24 to 36 hours. Intracranial bleeding is the most common location of hemorrhage associated with rt-PA therapy. Signs of intracerebral hemorrhage include change in level of consciousness, elevation in blood pressure, deterioration in motor function, new headache, and nausea and vomiting. Treatment of the bleeding requires administration of factor VIII and platelets.

Cerebral edema is common after large cerebral infarctions, especially in younger patients. It is most common 3 to 5 days after an ischemic stroke. Early signs of increased ICP include deterioration in level of consciousness and motor function, headache, visual disturbances, change in respiratory pattern, and changes in blood pressure and heart rate. Keep the head of the bed elevated at 30 degrees and maintain the alignment of the head with the rest of the body. Medical interventions include diuretic and barbiturate drugs, hyperventilation, and in some cases surgical intervention.

Risk for Deficient Fluid Volume or Excess Fluid Volume

Close monitoring of fluid status is especially important in the acute phase of stroke. Accurate intake and output records are essential. Measure vital signs, compare for trends suggesting excess or deficient fluid volume, and assess the mouth for moisture. In a well-hydrated person, the mucous membranes of the mouth are moist. Evaluate tissue turgor, remembering that it is not a very reliable indicator of fluid status in the older person. Age-related changes in the skin and subcutaneous structures cause a loss of tissue elasticity that may be mistaken for dehydration. Laboratory studies, including urine specific gravity, serum electrolytes, and hematocrit, are also useful indicators of fluid balance.

The patient is at risk for excess fluid volume if excessive intravenous fluids are administered or if the patient's kidneys are unable to eliminate excess fluid rapidly enough. Excess fluid volume may lead to edema and heart failure. Signs of excess fluid volume are fluid intake greater than output, bounding pulse, venous distention, increased blood pressure, crackles in the lungs, and edema. Report evidence of excess fluid to the registered nurse (RN) or physician. The rate of intravenous fluid may be decreased and diuretics may be ordered. Explain to the patient and family the need to temporarily restrict fluids. If the patient is thirsty, frequently provide small amounts of fluids in small containers and record all intake.

Factors that place the stroke patient at risk for deficient fluid volume include age, dysphagia, drug therapy with diuretics, and immobility. The stroke patient is likely to be older and older people are less able to conserve water through the kidneys. The patient with dysphagia may be unable to take in adequate oral fluids. If diuretics are given for excess fluid volume or increased ICP, they can precipitate excess loss of water and electrolytes. The patient with motor deficits may not be able to obtain fluids independently.

Deficient fluid volume contributes to constipation, skin dryness, urinary tract infections, and renal calculi (stones). Signs of deficient fluid volume are a thready pulse, tachycardia, low blood pressure, low urine output, concentrated urine, dry mucous membranes, and sometimes confusion. Report evidence of deficient fluid volume to the RN or physician. If intravenous fluids are being administered, the physician may order an increase in the hourly flow rate. Fluids may also be given through enteral feeding tubes.

To reduce the risk of deficient fluid volume, monitor the fluid intake record to ensure that the patient is getting at least eight 8-oz glasses of fluids each day (unless contraindicated). All staff and family members should know to offer fluids and record the amounts taken.

Place fluids within sight and easy reach of the patient and explain the need for adequate hydration. If the patient has hemiplegia, the fluids must be placed on the nonparalyzed side. Spill-proof containers that are easily held with one hand can facilitate independent drinking. If the patient is able to take oral fluids but has difficulty swallowing, it is important to proceed slowly. Have suction equipment on hand in case of aspiration. Thin liquids are more readily aspirated. Jell-O, ice cream, Popsicles, and frozen juice may be substituted to provide adequate fluids. Thickening agents can be added to other liquids as needed, as prescribed by the SLP.

Imbalanced Nutrition: Less Than Body Requirements

The patient's nutritional status is of concern throughout stroke treatment. Factors that may lead to inadequate nutrition include dysphagia, paralysis, difficulty chewing, and depression. The patient who is malnourished is at risk for skin breakdown and infection. Obesity hampers mobility and can interfere with rehabilitation.

The patient who has dysphagia may not be able to consume adequate nutrients orally. Sometimes a nasogastric tube is inserted for feeding purposes. The physician may order TPN for the malnourished patient. Aggressive treatment of dysphagia is delayed until the rehabilitative phase. Dysphagia often resolves spontaneously during the first few months of recovery. Feeding the dysphagic patient is discussed in Chapter 39.

If the patient has a nasogastric or nasointestinal feeding tube in place, check its placement and residual according to agency policy. Be certain to provide the correct formula and to ensure that it flows at the prescribed rate. Bolus feedings may be ordered at intervals or pumps may be used to dispense continuous feedings. Keep the head of the patient's bed slightly elevated to reduce the risk of fluid flowing back into the esophagus and being aspirated. The nasogastric tube irritates the naris and the nasal passages. Gently cleanse the naris several times a day. Concentrated formulas may cause diarrhea. If that happens, the physician should be consulted about diluting the formula or changing to another type of formula.

TPN is given through an intravenous line inserted in a large vein (a central line). Unlike enteral feedings, the flow of TPN fluids is always controlled with a mechanical infusion pump. The nurse hangs new bottles of prescribed fluids. ! Take special care to prevent air from entering the tubing. The insertion site also requires special care to prevent infection. Change dressings according to agency protocol, using strict aseptic technique. Patients on TPN may develop hyperglycemia; therefore it is important to monitor blood glucose levels at regular intervals. Care of the patient receiving TPN is explained in Chapter 9.

Ineffective Thermoregulation

After a stroke the body's temperature-regulating mechanism may be impaired, causing the temperature to rise. Metabolic processes that are also in play may increase the body temperature. It is important to monitor the patient's temperature and treat elevations promptly. Fever is treated aggressively, most often with antipyretic drugs. Some studies even suggest a decrease in infarction size in those patients aggressively treated for hyperthermia. Always assess the patient for an underlying infection as a potential cause for any temperature elevation.

Risk for Acute Confusion

After a stroke, patients may suffer functional losses, alterations in sensation and perception, and impaired communication. In addition, they find themselves in the hospital, where they are poked, monitored, and prodded by strangers and where days and nights all seem the same. All of these factors combined can cause the patient to become disoriented or confused. Neglect associated with right-brain strokes may also be manifested as denial. In extreme cases, patients deny that they have even had a stroke.

To orient patients, introduce yourself as often as necessary, remind patients where they are, and tell them what is being done and why. Be sure that eyeglasses and hearing aids are worn if the patient normally uses them. In addition, place clocks and marked calendars in view and tell the patient what time it is and what to expect next. Confused patients require frequent reassurance and reinforcement. Instructions and information should be concise and repeated as needed. Sometimes a familiar person can be helpful with a confused patient. If the visitor is disturbed by the patient's behavior, provide guidance on how to deal with the patient.

Impaired Verbal Communication

The alert patient who has aphasia is understandably anxious about his or her inability to speak, to understand words, or both. Use brief, clear statements accompanied by gestures, pictures, and facial expressions. Questions that can be answered with "yes" or "no" may allow the patient to respond more easily. Pause attentively when the patient struggles to respond (excessive chatter can be distressing to the aphasic patient). Explain the communication problem and approaches to the family. Speech therapy may be initiated once the patient's medical condition is stable. Speech rehabilitation is discussed further in the section titled "Nursing Care in the Rehabilitation Phase."

Impaired Physical Mobility

Impaired motor function is common after stroke and places the patient at risk for complications of immobility. Care of the immobilized patient is discussed in detail in Chapter 21 and is summarized here.

Skin Integrity. The potential for skin breakdown in this patient population is great because of motor impairment, altered consciousness or sensation, poor nutritional status, and incontinence. Measures to maintain skin integrity include cleanliness, pressure relief, and good hydration and nutrition. When skin is dry, as it often is in older patients, it is important to reduce bathing frequency, use soap sparingly, and apply lotions to retain skin moisture.

It is essential to turn and reposition the acute stroke patient at least every 2 hours. Skin breakdown can occur at vulnerable pressure points after just 30 minutes in one position. If reddened pressure areas remain when it is time to turn the patient, shorten the intervals between turnings. Do not allow the patient to lie on the affected side for more than 30 minutes. Because of impaired sensation, the risk of excessive pressure and trauma is much greater on the affected side. Pressure must be alternated on main pressure points such as hips, knees, heels, and lower back. An air floatation mattress or fluidized bed may be used for the high-risk patient. Some of the newer therapeutic beds automatically turn patients. These beds do not stress the usual pressure points of the patient but regular skin assessments and breathing exercises are still required. As soon as possible, position the patient comfortably in a chair for brief periods. Remember to monitor for a drop in blood pressure when getting the patient out of bed.

Good nursing care is time consuming, so take advantage of this time to stimulate the patient with conversation and explanations of care. This is helpful even if the patient is unresponsive.

Joint Mobility. The immobilized patient is at risk for muscle atrophy and joint contractures. In the stroke patient, the affected side is especially vulnerable when loss of voluntary movement occurs. During the acute phase, be concerned with maintaining joint mobility. This can be done with frequent, gentle range-of-motion exercises and proper positioning. Determine whether the patient had any preexisting limitations of joint mobility. Older patients may have arthritic changes that reduce the range of motion. Never force resistant joints. Once the acute phase has passed, the patient is usually referred for vigorous physical therapy.

Affected extremities must be supported. Never grab or pull the extremities on the patient's affected side. Dislocation or further injury can easily occur because the patient may not be able to accurately perceive the pressure or pain that is normally felt.

Circulation. DVT is a major complication of immobility, especially in this patient population. Regular passive and active range-of-motion exercises encourage venous blood return, thereby reducing the risk of thrombus formation. The physician may order elastic stockings or alternating pressure wraps to promote venous return. Low-dose anticoagulation therapy should be initiated to help prevent thrombus formation. Ambulation is generally encouraged (if the patient is able) as soon as possible after the medical condition stabilizes.

Functional Urinary Incontinence and Impaired Urinary Elimination

It is not unusual for urinary incontinence to occur after stroke. This may be caused by a temporarily flaccid bladder or an inability of the brain to coordinate information to be able to store urine in the bladder or wait once the urge to void is felt. Check the patient hourly for wetness and remove wet clothing and linens promptly. Wash the skin, rinse, and pat dry. A variety of incontinence products are available to minimize the contact of urine with the skin (see Chapter 23). Sometimes an indwelling catheter is ordered to prevent incontinence. The catheter protects the skin and allows for more accurate measurement of output. The disadvantage is that an indwelling catheter is frequently the cause of urinary tract infections. A regular toileting schedule with bladder scanning and intermittent catheterization is a better alternative to indwelling catheterization. External condom catheters are options for male patients. Bladder retraining, discussed in Chapter 23, is actively pursued in the rehabilitation phase.

Many older men have prostatic hypertrophy, which can cause dribbling of urine or urine retention. Scheduled toileting may be helpful but catheterization may be required. The enlarged prostate makes catheterization more difficult. If the catheter cannot be inserted easily, *never* force it; instead notify the RN or physician. Sometimes a special type of catheter is needed for the patient with prostate enlargement.

Constipation and Bowel Incontinence

As with urinary incontinence, the ability of the brain to coordinate the information to wait once the urge to move the bowels is felt may be damaged. During the acute phase of stroke, it is especially important to monitor bowel elimination, because the patient may develop constipation or incontinence. It is helpful to know the patient's usual patterns of elimination, although they cannot always be determined.

Constipation may develop as a result of immobility, dehydration, and drug therapy. A bowel program, consisting of a mild laxative or stool softener and a high-fiber diet, can help to prompt regular fecal elimination. Explain to patients and family members the importance of sufficient fluids to prevent dry stools. Some older people are laxative dependent. It is unrealistic to try to reverse the effects of years of laxative use during the acute phase of stroke. Inform the RN or physician of the pattern and document bowel movements. Laxatives and enemas may be needed to maintain bowel elimination in these patients.

Bowel incontinence may be related to the inability to toilet independently or to confusion and can often be prevented in the alert patient by taking the patient to the toilet at the usual time of defecation. A raised toilet seat with armrests is easier and safer for the patient with hemiplegia. If incontinence occurs, take special care to clean the skin thoroughly. Be careful not to make comments that embarrass the patient. Remember that incontinence, especially with liquid stools, may indicate a fecal impaction. Removal of an impaction usually requires repeated enemas and manual removal of hard stool. Restoration of bowel control receives more attention in the rehabilitation phase and is detailed in Chapter 23.

Ineffective Coping

The effects of stroke may be temporary or permanent. It is difficult to predict how much function will be lost permanently or returned during recovery. Patients typically exhibit responses that reflect the grief process: shock, denial, depression, withdrawal, and bargaining. Determine how the patient is coping and whether the coping strategies are constructive and effective.

An example of unhealthy coping is the patient who denies having problems with vision or balance and refuses to call for help when getting out of bed. Another example is the depressed and withdrawn patient who resists doing therapeutic exercises that would minimize complications. In this type of situation, the nurse can point out the behavior to the patient, explain its consequences, and encourage the patient to take an active role in rehabilitation activities. Depression is a major problem associated with stroke and can occur in up to 70% of stroke patients. The depression seen after a stroke may be the result of a loss of brain chemicals associated with the injury or a reaction to the loss of one's functional abilities. Antidepressant medications may be ordered for patients experiencing depression after a stroke and have been associated with improved outcomes in those patients treated. Sometimes a mental health counselor or support group is beneficial to help the patient learn to deal with the effects of stroke more constructively.

Interrupted Family Processes

In the acute phase of stroke, family members are often frightened and confused. They may fear the patient's death or severe disability. They also may experience emotional and financial strain during the long rehabilitation process. Family members have to assume roles and responsibilities normally carried by the patient. It is important to recognize that the family, as well as the patient, experiences a sense of loss when a loved one has a stroke. Provide support by telling family members what is happening, what is being done, and how they can help the patient. If necessary, a referral may be made to a social worker, mental health specialist, or spiritual counselor.

NURSING CARE in the Rehabilitation Phase

A patient's transition from the acute phase to the rehabilitation phase of stroke is an important one. Early and attentive care for the stroke patient shortens the recovery time and hastens the return of function. The general goals of treatment in the rehabilitation phase are to maximize functional abilities and to teach new ways to compensate for losses. Stabilization of vital signs with no further neurologic deficits indicates that the patient has entered the rehabilitation phase of stroke. At this time the patient's functional and cognitive problems can vary widely, depending on the location and extent of brain damage. The patient may regain complete independent functioning, partially recover previous abilities, or lose functional abilities completely.

The rehabilitation phase is usually managed by an interdisciplinary team that includes nurses, physicians, physical therapists, occupational therapists, SLPs, social workers, psychologists, recreational therapists, vocational rehabilitation counselors, and dietitians.

During the rehabilitation phase of a stroke, vast changes can occur in the brain. The extent to which collateral blood circulation and alternative neuronal pathways develop affects the ultimate outcome for the patient. The goals of rehabilitation to enhance the ultimate recovery of functional abilities are reached through a program of stimulation and practice. It has been said that rehabilitation is the respectful challenging of the patient facing a chronic health problem. With this in mind, this section describes nursing care in the management of long-term problems that can follow a stroke.

Assessment

Nursing assessment of the stroke patient was described earlier in this chapter and is summarized in Box 28-3. In the rehabilitation phase, reassess the patient's abilities as well as his or her expectations, knowledge, motivation, and resources.

Nursing Diagnoses, Goals, and Outcome Criteria: Rehabilitation Phase of Stroke

Nursing Diagnoses	Goals and Outcome Criteria
Self-Care Deficit (Bathing, Dressing, Feeding, Toileting) related to sensory and motor impairments	Self-care needs met: care accomplished with assistance as needed
Risk for Injury related to sensory and motor impairments	Absence of injury: no falls, bruises, skin tears, pressure sores
Ineffective Coping related to cognitive impairments	Effective coping: patient uses adaptive strategies to cope with disability
Impaired Verbal Communication related to aphasia, dysarthria	Effective communication: meaningful verbalizations or effective use of nonverbal communication to make needs known

Nursing Diagnoses, Goals, and Outcome Criteria: Rehabilitation Phase of Stroke—cont'd

Nursing Diagnoses	Goals and Outcome Criteria
Imbalanced Nutrition: Less Than Body Requirements related to dysphagia, anorexia	Adequate nutrition: achievement and maintenance of ideal body weight
Impaired Physical Mobility related to residual motor impairment	Improved physical mobility: increasing independent physical activity
Constipation related to inactivity	Normal bowel elimination: regular, formed stools without straining
Impaired Urinary Elimination and/or **Functional Urinary Incontinence** related to neurologic and motor impairment	Normal urine elimination: voluntary urination, decreasing incontinent episodes

Interventions

Self-Care Deficit (Bathing, Dressing, Feeding, Toileting)

The main focus of the rehabilitation phase is to return the stroke patient to the highest level of functioning possible. One of the most frustrating problems after a stroke for many patients and caregivers is the patient's inability to complete ADL. To improve, patients need to use affected parts as much as they are able. It is important for the nurse to demonstrate patience and a supportive attitude. Allow time for patients to try to do things for themselves. Discouragement is a major factor in unsuccessful rehabilitation and demands prompt attention by the rehabilitation team.

A variety of personal devices and environmental adaptations can foster a return to independence. Prosthetic devices that assist patients with dressing, bathing, and eating are available. Simple measures such as replacing buttons with Velcro fasteners and replacing complicated trousers with elastic-waist pants can make a big difference. Collaboration between the nurse and the occupational therapist will help to identify equipment and environmental adaptations that will support the patient's progress in rehabilitation.

A referral for follow-up at home should be initiated so that the safety and accessibility of the home environment can be assessed before discharge. The trend toward shorter hospital stays means that this must be addressed very early. Many patients are discharged to rehabilitation or skilled nursing facilities until they are ready to return home. A home visit by the patient, home health nurse, physical therapist, and occupational therapist can be made to identify problems and make plans for adaptations. Adaptations should promote access in and out of the home and enable patients to be as independent as possible. The addition of a raised commode seat, bathtub handrails, shower seat, or other devices can facilitate toileting and bathing. Cooking may be assisted by adjusting the height of counters, creating shelves that roll out, and rearranging cabinet contents to improve access. Patients need to practice daily tasks under conditions similar to those at home. Rehabilitation centers usually have activity centers that allow patients to practice self-care skills with their disabilities (Fig. 28-6).

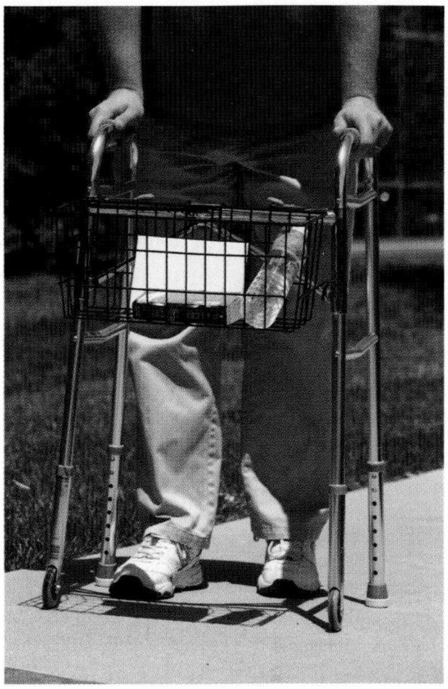

FIGURE 28-6 Assistive devices can enable a person with mobility impairment to be active at home and in the community. (From Birchenall J, Streight E: *Mosby's textbook for the home care aide*, ed 3, St. Louis, 2012, Mosby.)

Risk for Injury

Alterations in motor function, sensation, and vision are distressing changes that affect the patient's ability to carry out self-care and pose a threat to safety.

Motor Function. Alterations in motor functioning may leave the patient at risk for injury. Safety precautions are a vital part of nursing care of the patient. Teaching should include calling for assistance as needed, using assistive devices for mobilization, and adaptation of the environment to promote safety. Physical and occupational therapists are invaluable in assisting with providing a safe environment.

Sensation. As noted previously, patients may have altered sensation in the affected body parts after a stroke. This may appear as loss of sensation or as exaggerated response in which every sensation is perceived as painful. The patient may be injured without even knowing it because of impaired sensation. Teach the patient and family to assess the affected area frequently for signs of pressure and to protect it from injury. In addition to teaching the patient how to avoid pressure, advise the patient not to apply heat or cold to that area because of the risk of injury. Remind the patient and family not to pull on the affected side or use that side to move or support the patient in ambulation.

Patients with abnormal pain perception may benefit from regular physical therapy, using a kind of desensitization. During therapy, the patient is reminded and encouraged that the pain is not real and is only misinterpreted by the brain.

Vision. Homonymous hemianopsia, in which half of the field of vision is lost, also presents problems with self-care and safety. In the acute phase, the patient's environment is arranged so that people approach and important items are available on the unaffected side. In the rehabilitation phase, the patient is challenged more to promote adaptation to the disability. Place objects in the field of the visual deficit. Remind the patient to scan the affected visual field, especially when walking, wheeling, and eating. The patient forms new habits of observation through constant practice.

Ineffective Coping

Intellectual and emotional changes after stroke are distressing to patients and their families. Explain these changes and demonstrate how to help patients adapt. Cognitive processes may continue to be slow for quite some time after the stroke. It is important to avoid rushing the patient. The patient may become frustrated and give up trying. Emotional lability is manifested as sudden laughing, crying, or outbursts of anger without apparent reason. Caregivers and families may attribute this emotional unpredictability to depression. It is generally believed that depression is frequently associated with brain trauma of any kind. The patient can often be easily distracted from crying or from anger with simple redirection to the task at hand. This is an indication that the depression, if it exists, may be of a different type than the usual emotional state and require specific interventions. Treatment of depression, whatever the cause, is an important part of the rehabilitation process. Research clearly demonstrates a positive relationship to outcomes when patients are identified and treated aggressively for depression after a stroke. Adaptation and rehabilitation efforts may be impeded by disabling CPSP. This pain may respond to amitriptyline or lamotrigine therapy.

Impaired Verbal Communication

Helping the patient to improve or regain effective communication is an extremely important goal of the rehabilitation phase. Aphasia may affect the ability to understand spoken words or to use words to express oneself. Types of aphasia were explained with the signs and symptoms of stroke (see Table 28-3).

Patients with aphasia need encouragement as they struggle to communicate. Be patient because the aphasic person requires more time to plan and deliver a response. Take time to allow the patient to respond while providing verbal cues or picture boards to avoid frustrating the patient. The physician often refers patients with severe communication impairments to SLPs.

Imbalanced Nutrition: Less Than Body Requirements

The patient with dysphagia must be reevaluated at intervals for the ability to swallow. If the patient is able to swallow saliva, the physician may allow liquids to be introduced. Initially, ¼ teaspoon of ice chips might be given with a spoon. The amount is increased and water may be added until the patient is able to swallow a teaspoon of water. If problems with this simple assessment occur, a video fluoroscopic test of swallowing may be ordered. This test, conducted by the SLP and the radiologist, traces the route of swallowed fluid to detect swallowing abnormalities. Because water is thin, some patients find it difficult to swallow. It may be helpful to add a thicker substance to liquids to facilitate swallowing.

The patient who has some difficulty swallowing may be placed on a supervised feeding program. SLPs are trained to help patients relearn swallowing but everyday feeding falls to the nursing staff. Through use of radiologic procedures, the SLP will determine the patient's best position to ensure safe swallowing and eating. Often this will be sitting with the head tilted forward and toward the unaffected side. Fluid intake must still be encouraged for the dysphagic person, despite the increased work for patient and staff. Special utensils can greatly facilitate self-feeding (Fig. 28-7). Acknowledge even small improvements as the patient struggles in rehabilitation.

Impaired Physical Mobility

Mobility can continue to be a problem for patients in the rehabilitation phase. Hemiplegia, dyspraxia, and visual field disturbances all create unique problems. Hemiplegia is rarely a motor problem alone. It is often accompanied by disturbances in balance and spatial perception (Fig. 28-8).

Regular physical therapy and occupational therapy promote optimal return of motor function. Regular exercise can facilitate a dramatic return of function for some patients. Therefore affected arms and legs need to be used to maintain muscular function and circulation if and until neurologic ability is recovered. In the meantime, assistance is needed with motor activities. When the patient is moving, assess gait (if applicable), strength in arms and legs, and balance. Correct body mechanics and transfer techniques are essential when working with the patient. A gait belt helps the patient in transfers and in ambulation and may protect the patient and staff members from injury. This is a fabric belt with a toothed buckle that is applied between the nipple line and the waist and is used to support and assist the patient. Assistive devices such as the quad cane and walkers may improve safety with ambulation (Fig. 28-9).

Patients who have dyspraxia are unable to initiate voluntary motor acts. It is interesting to note that they

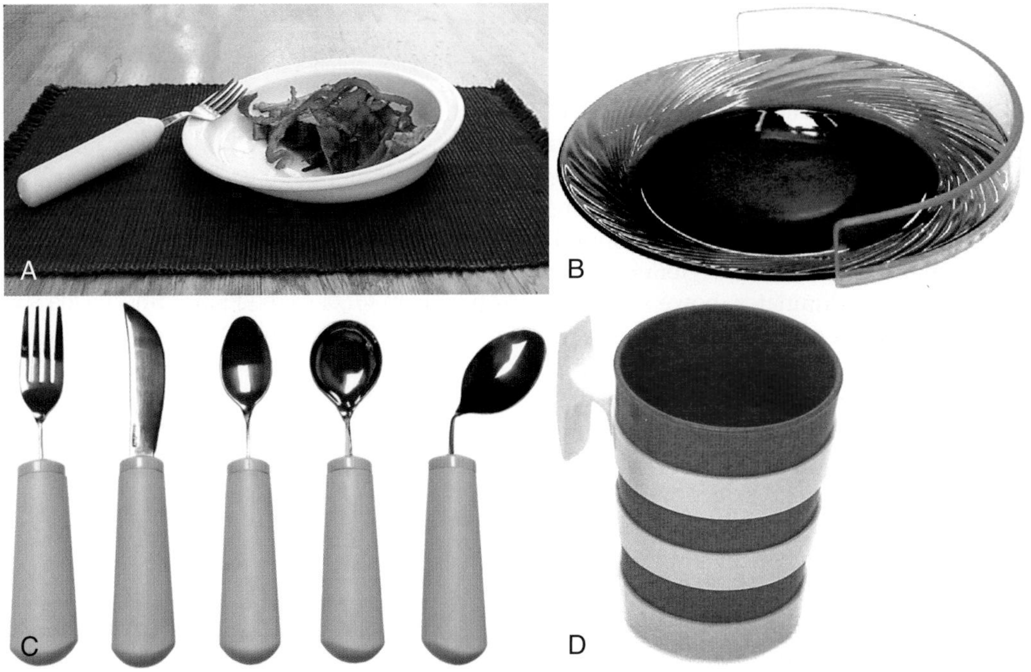

FIGURE 28-7 Assistive devices for eating. **A,** A scoop plate keeps food from being pushed off the edge. **B,** Plate guards keep food on the plate. **C,** Utensils adapted to special needs. The rocker blade knife allows a person to cut with only one hand. **D,** The special handle is easier to grasp and hold. (Courtesy Kinsman Enterprises Inc.)

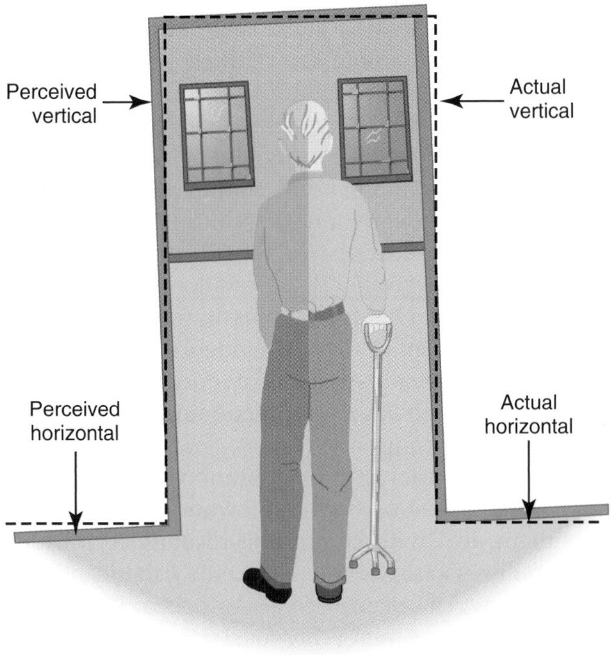

FIGURE 28-8 Perceptual disturbances in hemiplegia may affect the patient's ability to maneuver safely in the environment. (From Black JM, Hawks JH: *Medical-surgical nursing: clinical management for positive outcomes*, ed 8, St. Louis, 2009, Saunders.)

sometimes exhibit those actions spontaneously. To help the patient remember to initiate voluntary responses, provide verbal cues. Teach family members about dyspraxia and advise them to be patient and to use cues to induce the desired motor performance.

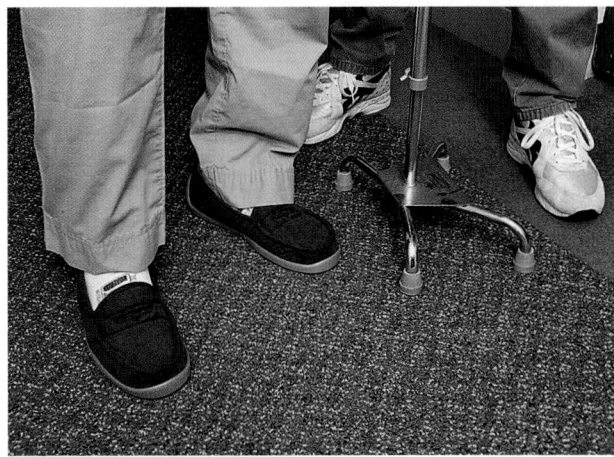

FIGURE 28-9 A quad cane provides good support for a patient with hemiplegia. (From Potter PA, Perry AG, Stockert PA, Hall AM: *Fundamentals of nursing*, ed 8, St. Louis, 2013, Mosby.)

Remind the patient who has unilateral neglect to use and support the affected side.

Put on Your Thinking Cap!

Use a towel or other material to make an arm sling. Place your dominant arm in the sling while you prepare a meal, eat, and clean up. Immediately after this exercise, write down: (1) what adaptations you had to make, (2) what things you were unable to do unassisted, (3) how you felt during the exercise, and (4) how you behaved during the exercise. Compare responses with your classmates. Discuss implications for patient care.

Constipation

Bowel elimination problems may continue into the rehabilitation phase. Incontinence is not usually a problem for the alert patient except when it is caused by inability to access toileting devices or manage clothing. Document the timing of incidents of bowel incontinence so that a toileting schedule can be developed. Often simply taking the patient to the toilet at the usual time of defecation eliminates bowel incontinence. Additional discussion of bowel incontinence is found in Chapter 23.

Constipation is a common challenge in the rehabilitation phase. A regular bowel program with toileting, orientation, and reminders is needed. Provide sufficient fluids to promote bowel regularity. Many stroke patients do not receive adequate fluid intake because of dysphagia or fear of incontinence. In addition, caregivers may not take the extra time needed to provide fluids for the patient who responds slowly. Stool softeners, laxatives, and suppositories may be used to reestablish regular bowel elimination and then gradually be discontinued. Some patients continue to need stool softeners. As noted earlier, some patients with long-standing laxative dependency may not respond to more conservative measures to promote bowel elimination.

Impaired Urinary Elimination and Functional Urinary Incontinence

If an indwelling catheter was inserted in the acute phase of stroke treatment, it will probably be removed and efforts made to restore bladder control. Immediately after the catheter is removed, the patient may have poor sphincter control or may retain urine. Therefore it is important to monitor urine output and check for bladder distention until normal voiding is established. Perineal muscle exercises (see Chapter 23) may be prescribed to improve sphincter control.

Intermittent catheterization may continue to be necessary in the rehabilitation phase. The urine volume obtained is measured and intermittent catheterization is done every 4 to 6 hours, depending on the volume obtained. Bedside ultrasound scanners may be used by the nurse, as ordered and available, to assess the amount of urine in the bladder and to determine the need for intermittent catheterization.

Incontinence of urine is more difficult to correct than bowel incontinence. A bladder program should be initiated promptly. Document the patient's fluid intake and frequency of voiding. Scheduled toileting based on the patient's usual pattern often helps to control incontinence.

Discharge

Patients may be discharged to their homes or may go to specialized rehabilitation centers for continued therapy. Outpatient therapy is an option for some patients. The rehabilitation phase is defined in various ways. In acute rehabilitation settings, patients will be evaluated by all disciplines and goals will be set. Continuous assessments and goal setting occur throughout the rehabilitation process. When able, patients are transitioned back to the home setting. It is essential to include family, friends, and significant others in this process. Medicare defines the rehabilitation phase as 3 months after the stroke. Rehabilitation specialists say that rehabilitation continues indefinitely but progress slows down. A great deal of evidence indicates that rehabilitation helps patients recovering from a stroke to achieve a high level of functioning and improve safety after returning home.

During and after the rehabilitation phase, patients and families need to be made aware of resources to help them deal with continuing disabilities. Patients and families should be referred to the American Heart Association, American Stroke Association, National Stroke Association, and other local agencies within the community. Support groups are available in many communities to offer assistance and generally have a positive effect on the stroke survivor.

Although stroke remains a major health problem, the risk can be reduced. The acute phase of stroke, from diagnosis to stabilization of blood pressure, requires support and careful evaluation of the patient's remaining abilities. In rehabilitation the patient is respectfully challenged to return to the highest level of function possible.

Nutrition Considerations

1. A major nutritional concern for the stroke patient is dysphagia (difficulty swallowing), which may lead to malnutrition and dehydration because of inadequate intake.
2. Swallowing thin liquids is frequently a problem. Thin liquids can be thickened with dry milk powder, cornstarch, fruit and vegetable flakes, or commercial thickening agents.
3. Very warm or chilled foods stimulate the swallowing reflex better than bland, lukewarm foods.
4. In addition to thickened liquids, foods that are better for chewing and swallowing are soft bread, cooked cereal, ice cream, yogurt, cooked eggs, moist ground beef, canned fruits and vegetables, thick soups, and puddings.

Put on Your Thinking Cap!

List all of the factors you can think of that might cause a patient recovering from a stroke to be incontinent of urine *besides* the physiologic effects of the stroke on the bladder.

Get Ready for the NCLEX® Examination!

Key Points

- CVA, commonly called a *stroke* or *brain attack*, is an interruption of blood flow to part of the brain.
- The risk factors for CVA are atherosclerosis, atrial fibrillation, hypertension, diabetes mellitus, cardiac disease, excessive alcohol consumption, and, for women, smoking while taking oral contraceptives.
- CVA can be classified as a *TIA, a stroke in evolution,* or a *completed stroke.*
- TIA is an episode of temporary neurologic dysfunction caused by focal brain, spinal cord, or retinal ischemia that occurs without acute infarction.
- TIA, sometimes considered a warning sign of impending stroke, is treated with diet modification, exercise, drug therapy to prevent clot formation, surgery to clear or bypass obstructed blood vessels, or a combination of these therapies.
- A stroke is a set of neurologic signs and symptoms caused by impaired blood flow to the brain that persists for more than 24 hours.
- A hemorrhagic stroke is caused by rupture of a blood vessel in the brain and an ischemic stroke is caused by obstruction of a blood vessel by an embolus or a thrombus.
- Signs and symptoms of stroke depend on the type, location, and extent of brain injury but may include one-sided weakness, numbness, visual problems, confusion and memory lapses, headache, dysphagia, and speech problems.
- Aphasia is the inability to understand words or respond with appropriate messages.
- Dysarthria is the inability to speak clearly because of neurologic damage that affects the muscles of speech.
- Dysphagia is difficulty swallowing.
- Dyspraxia is the partial inability to initiate coordinated voluntary motor acts in an unparalyzed extremity.
- Paralysis of one side of the body (the side opposite the brain injury) is called *hemiplegia.*
- Medical treatment of CVA may use oxygen therapy, diuretics, corticosteroids, anticoagulants, thrombolytics, intravenous fluids, dietary modifications, and catheterization, as well as treatment of risk factors.
- The focus of nursing care after stroke is on ineffective airway clearance; ineffective breathing pattern; risk for injury; risk for deficient fluid volume; excess fluid volume; imbalanced nutrition: less than body requirements; ineffective thermoregulation; risk for acute confusion; impaired verbal communication; impaired physical mobility; impaired urinary elimination and/or functional urinary incontinence; constipation; bowel incontinence; ineffective coping; and interrupted family processes.
- After experiencing a stroke, the patient may regain complete independent functioning, partially recover previous abilities, or lose functional abilities completely.
- The goal of rehabilitation after stroke is to enhance the recovery of functional abilities through a program of stimulation and practice.

Additional Learning Resources

SG Go to your Study Guide for additional learning activities to help you master this chapter content.

evolve Go to your Evolve website (http://evolve.elsevier.com/Linton/medsurg) for the following learning resources and much more:
- Interactive Prioritization Exercises
- Fluid & Electrolyte Tutorial
- Pharmacology Tutorial
- Review Questions for the NCLEX® Examination

Review Questions for the NCLEX® Examination

1. In which part of the brain are the structures that control respirations and heart rate located?
   NCLEX Client Need: Physiological Integrity: Physiological Adaptation
2. The licensed vocational nurse/licensed practical nurse (LVN/LPN) recognizes symptoms of a TIA in a homebound patient. Why is it important for the nurse to recognize a TIA?
   1. Because TIA is a symptom of a brain tumor
   2. Because TIA can cause permanent disability
   3. Because TIA is a warning sign of future stroke
   4. Because TIA occurs shortly before a hemorrhage

   NCLEX Client Need: Physiological Integrity: Physiological Adaptation
3. Which of the following may be present in both TIA and stroke? (Select all that apply.)
   1. Visual disturbances
   2. Dysphagia
   3. Drooping mouth
   4. Confusion
   5. Weakness

   NCLEX Client Need: Physiological Integrity: Physiological Adaptation
4. How are TIAs and strokes different?
   1. Weakness and loss of balance are symptoms of TIA but not stroke.
   2. Imaging studies show circulatory changes with stroke but not with TIA.
   3. Anticoagulants are used with some strokes but not with TIAs.
   4. An infarction occurs with stroke but not with TIA.

   NCLEX Client Need: Physiological Integrity: Physiological Adaptation
5. A clinic patient who is taking an anticoagulant to reduce the risk of stroke has regular blood tests to measure INR. The LVN/LPN knows that the physician should be notified if the INR exceeds which of the following measurements?
   1. 1.5
   2. 2.0
   3. 2.5
   4. 3.0

   NCLEX Client Need: Physiological Integrity: Pharmacological Therapies

6. Which of the following is the most common type of stroke?
   1. Ischemic
   2. Incomplete
   3. Hemorrhagic
   4. Subarachnoid

   NCLEX Client Need: Physiological Integrity: Physiological Adaptation
7. Ms. Y. is recovering from a stroke. She is able to follow directions and communicate nonverbally. However, she struggles to speak and her words are slurred. When you can understand her, her message is appropriately expressed. What is the correct term to describe this pattern?

   NCLEX Client Need: Physiological Integrity: Physiological Adaptation
8. Which of the following are modifiable risk factors for stroke? (Select all that apply.)
   1. Age
   2. Obesity
   3. Gender
   4. Hypertension
   5. Cigarette smoking

   NCLEX Client Need: Physiological Integrity: Reduction of Risk Potential
9. Which of the following are necessary for the most successful use of rt-PA in the stroke patient? (Select all that apply.)
   1. Patient not currently taking warfarin (Coumadin)
   2. Administration only after an ischemic stroke
   3. Intravenous administration within 3 hours of the onset of symptoms
   4. Concurrent use with heparin to prevent additional clots from forming
   5. Deep intramuscular administration into a large muscle mass

   NCLEX Client Need: Physiological Integrity: Pharmacological Therapies
10. A patient with aphasia is admitted to a long-term care facility. The care plan should include which nursing interventions? (Select all that apply.)
    1. Insist that patients try to express needs verbally
    2. Help them to find the right word if they become frustrated
    3. Give praise when patients attempt to verbalize
    4. Encourage families to speak for patients rather than expecting patients to speak
    5. Establish a system such as blinks for the nonverbal patient to communicate

    NCLEX Client Need: Psychosocial Integrity and Physiological Integrity: Physiological Adaptation

chapter 29

Spinal Cord Injury

Sherry Dawn Weaver

http://evolve.elsevier.com/Linton/medsurg

Objectives

1. Explain the effects of spinal cord injury.
2. Describe the diagnostic tests used to evaluate spinal cord injuries and related nursing responsibilities.
3. Explain the physical effects of spinal cord injury.
4. Describe the medical and surgical treatment during the acute phase of spinal cord injury.
5. List the data to be included in the nursing assessment of the patient with a spinal cord injury.
6. Identify nursing diagnoses, goals, interventions, and outcome criteria for the patient with a spinal cord injury.
7. State the goals of rehabilitation for the patient with spinal cord injury.
8. Describe the nursing care for the patient undergoing a laminectomy.

Key Terms

Autonomic dysreflexia (ăw-tō-NŌ-mĭk dĭs-rē-flĕk-sē-ă)
Dermatome (DĔR-mă-tōm)
Flaccid (FLĂ-sĭd)
Myelinated (MĪ-ĕ-lĭ-nā-tĕd)
Paraplegia (păr-ă-PLĒ-jă)
Spasticity (spas-TĬ-sĭ-tē)
Tetraplegia (tĕ-tră-PLĒ-jă)

Few injuries are as physically and emotionally distressing to a person as a permanent spinal cord injury (SCI). The Spinal Cord Injury Information Network estimates that 12,000 new cases of SCI occur each year in the United States. Average cost for the first year varies from $775,567 for high tetraplegia (paralysis of all four extremities) to $283,388 for paraplegia (paralysis of lower extremities). When the spinal cord is injured but not completely severed, the patient is said to have an *incomplete motor lesion.* The costs associated with incomplete motor lesions average $228,566 in the first year. Subsequent year averages are lower, ranging from $138,923 to $16,018.

Since 2005, the average age at injury has increased to 39.5 years. Additionally, the percentage of individuals older than age 60 at the time or injury has increased from 4.7% before 1980 to 11.5% since 2000. Since 2000, 77.8% of SCI have occurred among male subjects. This is down slightly from numbers reported before 1980. The leading cause of SCI since 2005 is trauma sustained in motor vehicle crashes (42%), falls, assaults, and recreational sports–related mishaps. The cord also can be damaged by degenerative conditions and tumors.

Medical advances and more rapid transport of accident victims to trauma centers have increased the life expectancy of individuals with SCI. Life expectancy is still somewhat below those without SCI. However, the effects of the injury may lead to other health problems that require long-term care and potentially affect quality of life. Quality nursing care during the acute and rehabilitative phases of injury can minimize the effect of lifelong problems that plague the person with an SCI. Consequently, the potential for rehabilitation and full quality of life can be enhanced.

ANATOMY AND PHYSIOLOGY OF THE SPINAL CORD

To understand the effects of SCI fully, it is important to know the anatomy and physiology of the spinal cord. Normal spinal cord function requires an intact cord with a good blood supply and bony support. Disruption of any one of these components can result in neurologic dysfunction.

VERTEBRAL COLUMN

The bony vertebral column consists of 33 vertebrae: 7 cervical (C1 through C7), 12 thoracic (T1 through T12), 5 lumbar (L1 through L5), 5 sacral (S1 through S5), and 4 coccygeal, which are fused (Fig. 29-1). The individual vertebra consists of a body and an arch, as shown in Figure 29-2. The body is the round structure that forms the anterior portion of the vertebra. The arch is the posterior portion of the vertebra. The spinal cord passes through an opening in the center of each arch. The structures that form the posterior section of the arch are called *laminae.* Each arch has articulating surfaces against which adjacent vertebrae smoothly glide

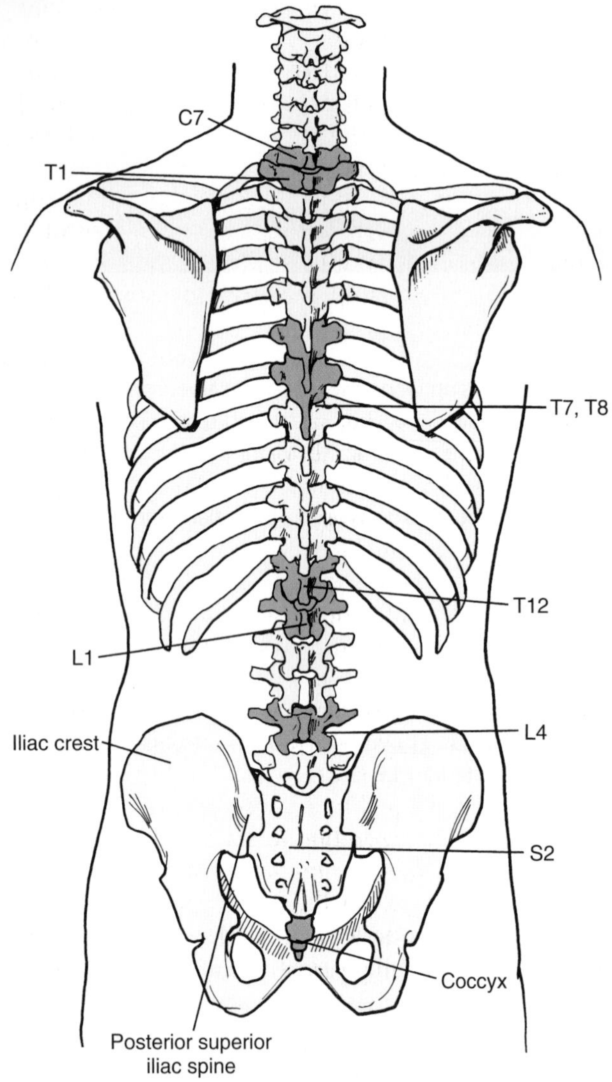

FIGURE 29-1 The bony vertebral column consists of 33 vertebrae. (From Jarvis C: *Physical examination and health assessment*, ed 6, St. Louis, 2012, Saunders.)

with movement. In addition, each arch has locations for the attachment of ribs and muscles. Muscles and ligaments, which permit mobility and flexibility, support the bony column.

DISKS

Vertebrae are separated by intervertebral disks, which serve as shock absorbers for the vertebral column (see Fig. 29-2). Disks are composed of the annulus fibrosus and the nucleus pulposus. The annulus fibrosus is the fibrous ring of tissue that encircles the nucleus pulposus. The nucleus pulposus is the central saclike structure with a gelatinous filling that has a high water content. As a person ages, the nucleus pulposus loses a great deal of its water, so it becomes less effective as a shock absorber. Therefore older people are at increased risk for back injuries and herniated disks.

SPINAL CORD

The spinal cord extends from the brainstem to the level of L2 in the pelvic cavity (Fig. 29-3). It has a central canal, which is continuous with the fourth ventricle of the brain. The cord is surrounded by three protective meningeal layers: (1) the dura mater, (2) the arachnoid, and (3) the pia mater. The dura mater is the outermost layer. The arachnoid, the middle layer, is a network of spaces containing cerebrospinal fluid (CSF). The pia mater is the innermost layer; it directly covers the spinal cord. The CSF circulates through the brain and spinal column, bathing and protecting the entire central nervous system (CNS).

A cross-section of the spinal cord reveals an inner area of H-shaped gray matter surrounded by white matter. The gray matter consists of the bodies of nerve cells that control motor and sensory activities. The white matter, which is **myelinated** (surrounded by a sheath), consists of bundles of fibers. These fibers,

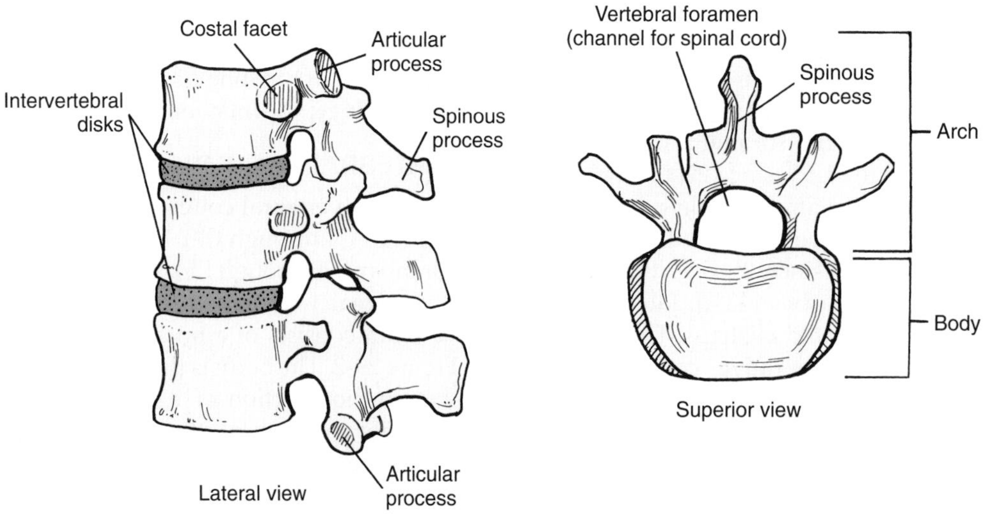

FIGURE 29-2 Intervertebral disks separate the vertebrae, each of which consists of a body and an arch. (From Jarvis C: *Physical examination and health assessment*, ed 6, St. Louis, 2012, Saunders.)

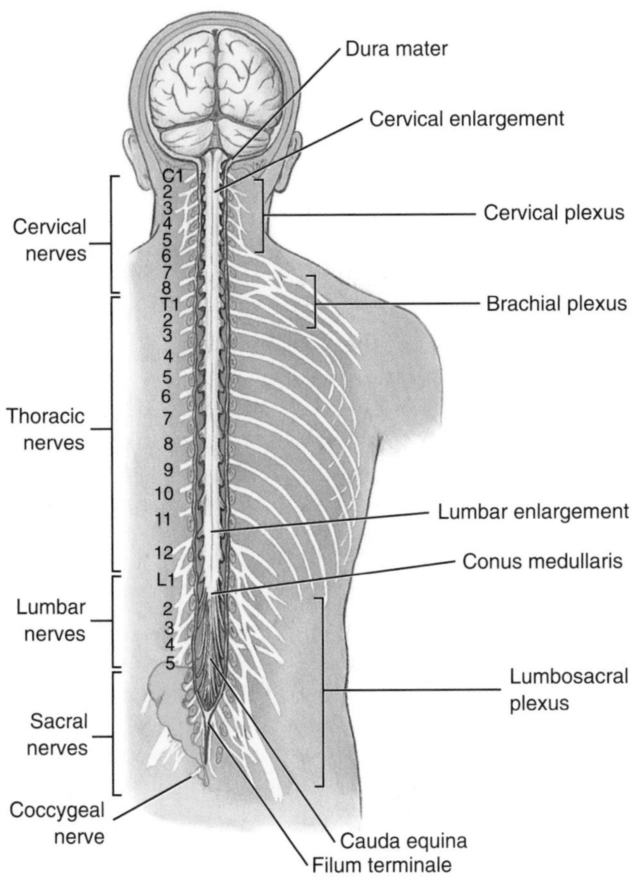

FIGURE 29-3 The spinal cord extends from the medulla of the brainstem to the level of the second lumbar vertebra. (From Applegate E: *The anatomy and physiology learning system*, ed 4, St. Louis, Saunders, 2011.)

known as *columns* or *tracts*, convey information between the brain and the spinal cord. The tracts may be either ascending or descending. Ascending tracts carry sensory information from the spinal cord to the brain. Descending tracts carry motor information from the brain to the spinal cord (Fig. 29-4).

Blood supply to the spinal cord is vital. Any disruption in blood flow can lead ultimately to neurologic damage. The major arterial supply to the spinal cord consists of the vertebral arteries posteriorly and the anterior spinal artery.

Spinal cord function may be classified as either *reflexive* or *relay* in nature. With reflexive activity, the sensory stimulus is received and a response is initiated at the level of the spinal cord. The knee jerk is an example of reflexive activity. When the knee is tapped, impulses travel by sensory neurons to the spinal cord, where they are relayed to motor neurons. The impulse travels back to the muscles at the front of the thigh, causing muscle contraction and jerking of the leg. This circuit of impulse transmission is called a *reflex arc.*

With relay activity, the stimulus enters the spinal cord and travels up the ascending tracts to relay sensory signals from the external environment to the brain. Information is processed in the brain and responses are initiated by impulses transmitted to the body by way of descending tracts.

The descending white matter tracts also participate in the relay function of the spinal cord. These tracts relay motor information, with messages being sent from the brain, down the cord, to muscles, which affect

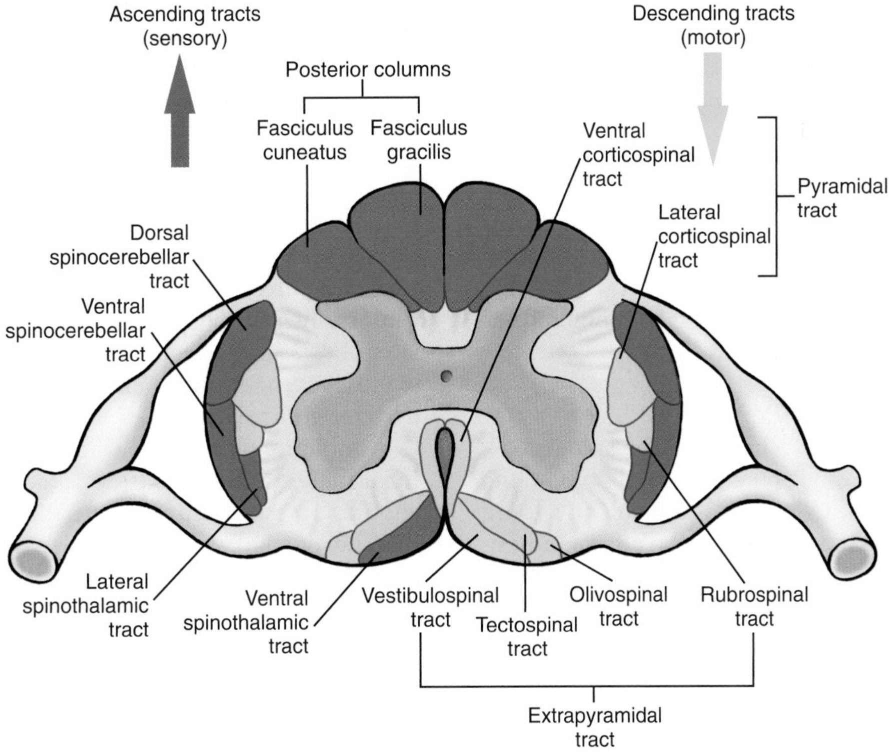

FIGURE 29-4 Cross-section of spinal cord. Sensory tracts convey sensory information to the brain; motor tracts convey information from the brain.

Table 29-1 Summary of the Four Major Spinal Cord Tracts

TRACT	TYPE	FEATURES	FUNCTION
Spinothalamic	Ascending (sensory: pain and temperature)	Originates in spinal cord and ascends to thalamus in brain; on entering cord, impulses cross over to opposite side (contralateral)	Carries pain and temperature lateral sensation from opposite side
Corticospinal, lateral	Descending (motor)	Initiates in motor tract of brain, crosses over to opposite side at level of medulla, proceeds down to appropriate spinal cord level	Controls voluntary motor action
Spinocerebellar	Ascending (sensory)	Initiates in spinal cord and terminates in cerebellum	Assists in coordination of muscle contraction
Posterior columns	Ascending (sensory: touch, vibration, position sense)	Made up of several tracts that relay messages from body to brain; initiates in sensory fibers of spinal nerves, crosses over in medulla, and terminates in sensory cortex of opposite hemisphere	Carries touch, deep pressure, vibration, and position sense

various kinds of responses. Four of the most important spinal cord tracts are summarized in Table 29-1.

Information is conveyed by the senses to the brain and spinal cord via the peripheral nervous system. This system consists of 31 pairs of spinal nerves (8 cervical, 12 thoracic, 5 lumbar, 5 sacral, and 1 coccygeal), which branch from the cord and pass between the vertebrae to muscles and visceral organs. Each spinal nerve has a dorsal root, which transmits sensory information, and a ventral root, which transmits motor information. The 12 cranial nerves, arising from the brainstem, also are part of the peripheral nervous system.

DIAGNOSTIC TESTS AND PROCEDURES

Emergency care of the patient with SCI is discussed in Chapter 16. When the victim of SCI arrives at the hospital, the extent of injury must be determined. Specific tests are performed to determine the type of injury and to provide direction for treatment. Throughout the diagnostic process, the spine must be immobilized continuously.

NEUROLOGIC EXAMINATION

In the initial neurologic evaluation of the spinal cord, the injured patient provides the nurse with a baseline assessment of both function and problems. Ongoing assessment is necessary to monitor the effects of neurologic injury, detect related complications, and determine the patient's need for assistance in activities of daily living (ADL).

In the patient with SCI, neurologic evaluation focuses on the motor and sensory systems. Movement, muscle strength, and reflex activity are evaluated on an ongoing basis as described in the Assessment section. Basic neurologic assessment is discussed in Chapter 27. Refer to a textbook on physical assessment for the detailed steps of the neurologic evaluation.

IMAGING STUDIES

Radiography

Standard radiographs are obtained to detect vertebral compression, fractures, or problems with alignment. The entire spine may be radiographed because patients sometimes have multiple fractures separated by sections of normal spine. The physician also may order special radiographs, called *coned-down views,* which reveal fractures more clearly. Radiography is repeated at intervals to evaluate the achievement of proper alignment with treatment.

Computed Tomography

Computed tomography (CT) provides a noninvasive examination of the specific levels of the spinal cord to be visualized as well as the bony vertebrae and the spinal nerves. The physician can readily identify bony fractures, floating bone fragments, dislocations, tumors, hemorrhage, and cord and nerve compressions. In some injuries, soft tissue swelling may obscure some structures and make visualization of the cord and vertebrae difficult.

Although no special physical preparation is needed for a patient undergoing CT, this imaging procedure should be explained to the patient. Tell the patient that he or she will be asked to lie very still for a period of time while on a small table that slowly moves through the scanner. Enhanced scanning also may be done, in which a radiopaque dye is infused intravenously into the patient. This testing is contraindicated in the patient who is allergic to the dye. Encourage patients who receive the dye to take plenty of fluids after the procedure to promote renal excretion.

Magnetic Resonance Imaging

Magnetic resonance imaging (MRI), unlike CT, does not expose the patient to radiation. The patient is slowly moved through a strong magnetic field and then subjected to short bursts of radio waves. Sophisticated technology translates information about body tissue to produce precise, clear images of internal structures.

This noninvasive diagnostic imaging study is painless, has no known risks, and requires no preparation. Tell the patient to expect to hear a hammering sound as the radio waves are turned on and off. Metal materials or equipment (including prostheses) are not permitted in the scanning suite. Because the magnetic field in the scanner is very strong, any metal object may be attracted into the field. Patients with pacemakers cannot undergo MRI because the magnetic field would inactivate the pacer. This is also true of patients with aneurysm clips that are not made of inert metal. A quartz watch would be disrupted because the magnetic field has a detrimental effect on the battery. If an intravenous pump is being used, the site must first be converted to a heparin lock or changed over to a specialized pump because the metal in most pumps cannot be placed in the scanning room. If oxygen (O_2) is required, adequate tubing is needed to allow the O_2 tank to be placed a safe distance outside the suite.

Myelography

A myelogram is obtained to visualize the spinal cord and vertebrae. A puncture is made in the lumbar area between L3 and L4. Radiopaque dye is then injected into the subarachnoid space of the spinal canal. Any obstruction that impedes the flow of the dye can be seen on radiography. Because of the invasive nature of the procedure, informed consent must be obtained. Nursing care before and after myelography is summarized in Box 29-1.

Box 29-1 Nursing Care of the Patient Having Myelography

PREPARATION

- Ensure that signed consent has been obtained.
- Inquire about any allergies to dye, iodine, and shellfish; inform the radiologist if the patient is allergic.
- Allow nothing by mouth (NPO) for 4 to 6 hours before the procedure, according to agency protocol.
- Administer the prescribed premedications.
- Have the patient empty the bladder if he or she is able to do so.
- Determine whether any medications should be withheld.

POSTPROCEDURE CARE

- Frequently assess the patient's vital signs and neurologic status.
- Encourage increased fluid intake to promote elimination of dye, if not contraindicated.
- Measure and record fluid intake and output.
- Position the patient as ordered: flat or head of bed elevated 30 to 45 degrees, depending on type of contrast medium used.
- Administer analgesics as ordered for headache.
- Assess the patient for back pain, increased temperature, difficulty voiding, neck stiffness, and nausea and vomiting.

PATHOPHYSIOLOGY OF SPINAL CORD INJURY

Traumatic injury creates abnormal forces on the neck and structural components of the spinal cord. The cervical vertebrae support the head and neck and permit movement in various directions. The thoracic vertebrae, on the other hand, permit little movement because of the restrictions of the ribs. Because the thoracic spine has limited flexibility, the neck and cervical spine are extremely vulnerable to injury.

TYPES OF INJURIES

Spinal cord injuries may be classified (1) by location, (2) as *open* or *closed*, and (3) by extent of damage to the cord. Injuries classified by location are described as *cervical, thoracic,* or *lumbar,* depending on the level of the cord affected.

Closed injuries involve trauma in which the skin and meningeal covering that surrounds the spinal cord remain intact. However, it is important to keep in mind that stretching or twisting the spinal cord can lead to injury as extensive as partial or complete transection (i.e., cutting all the way through). Common causes of closed injuries include compression, flexion, hyperextension, rotation, and blunt trauma (Fig. 29-5). Degeneration of the vertebrae or intervertebral disks, hematomas, or spinal cord tumors also may compress the cord or one of the spinal nerves. Fractures of the vertebral bodies may cause a subluxation (partial dislocation) of bone fragments, which may further damage the cord. Open injuries with damage to protective skin and meninges are most commonly caused by bullets or stabbing.

The injury may be classified as *complete* or *incomplete,* depending on the extent to which the cord is transected (i.e., cut across). A complete SCI occurs when the cord has been completely severed whereas an incomplete injury results from partial cutting of the cord. Open injuries often result in either complete or partial transection of the cord.

EFFECTS OF SPINAL CORD INJURY

Early recognition of the effects of SCI is vital to maintain maximum possible function. Factors that determine the effects of SCI include the extent of the damage and the level of the injury. Sometimes the extent of injury cannot be fully determined because the symptoms of spinal cord edema may mimic partial or complete transection. A complete injury cuts all descending and ascending tracts. The result is disruption of all voluntary motor and sensory activity below the level

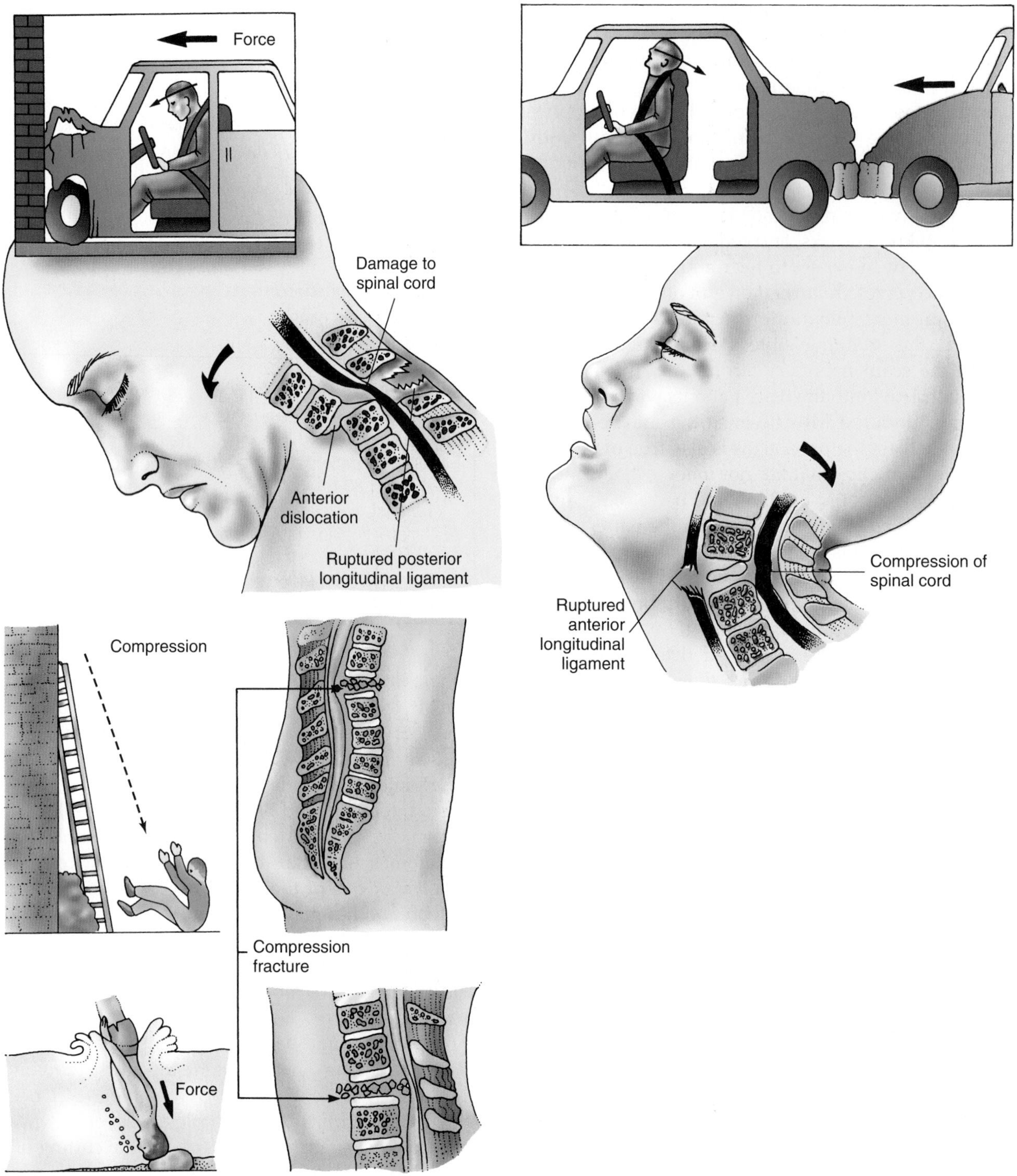

FIGURE 29-5 Mechanisms of spinal cord injury (SCI). (From Ignatavicius DD, Workman ML: *Medical-surgical nursing: patient-centered collaborative care*, ed 7, St. Louis, 2013, Saunders.)

of the injury. However, reflex activity continues below the level of injury because it occurs by completing the reflex arc without the transmission of impulses to and from the brain.

Trauma also may produce a variety of incomplete spinal cord injuries. These are injuries in which some function remains below the level of the injury. Specific tracts may be involved, causing particular patterns of neurologic dysfunction. Table 29-2 describes the major types of incomplete injuries and the resulting neurologic losses.

The higher the level of the injury is, the more encompassing is the neurologic dysfunction (because increasingly more of the body is affected). High cervical spine injuries may result in the loss of motor and sensory function in all four extremities. This condition,

Table 29-2 **Incomplete Injuries and Related Neurologic Deficits**

INJURY	MECHANISM OF INJURY	ACCOMPANYING DEFICIT
Anterior cord syndrome	Herniation of disk occurring with flexion injury or dislocation of vertebrae	Loss of bilateral pain and temperature perception and motor function below level of lesion without loss of position sense
Central cord syndrome	Hyperextension injury	Motor and sensory loss in upper extremities
Brown-Séquard syndrome	Transverse hemisection of cord	Ipsilateral loss of motor function with contralateral loss of pain and temperature perception

Table 29-3 **Degree of Loss and Functional Capability with Injury to Each Level of the Spinal Cord**

CORD LEVEL	DEGREE OF LOSS	FUNCTIONAL CAPABILITY
C1 to C4	Motor and sensory function from neck down Respiratory function Bowel and bladder control	Mechanical ventilation with home care
C5	Motor and sensory function below shoulders Intercostal function in ventilation Bowel and bladder control	Has remaining head control, which facilitates use of "joystick" for writing, typing, and control of mechanical wheelchair
C6	Motor and sensory function below shoulders but increased degree of sensation in arm and thumb Intercostal function in ventilation Bowel and bladder control	Requires some assistive devices for upper extremity use but may be able to help feed and dress self Requires mechanical wheelchair but may be capable of using hand control
C7	Motor control of portion of upper extremities Sensation below clavicle Intercostal function Bowel and bladder control	Remaining intact muscles enhance ability to carry out activities of daily living (ADL) Increased ability to manage specially equipped wheelchair and automobile
C8	Motor control of portions of upper extremities Sensation below chest Intercostal function Bowel and bladder control	Improved upper extremity mobility enhances hand grasp, independence in ADL, and use of wheelchair Capable of self-catheterization
T1 to T6	Trunk muscles below midchest Sensation from midchest Some intercostal function Bowel and bladder control	Complete control of upper extremities makes independence in wheelchair and ADL possible Employment possible
T6 to T12	Motor control below waist Sensation below waist Bowel and bladder control	Capable of unassisted respiratory function Good upper back and abdominal strength, making increased wheelchair activities and athletics possible
L1 to L3	Motor and sensory function to lower extremities Sensation to lower abdomen Bowel and bladder function	Full control of upper extremities allows independence in wheelchair and appropriate athletic activity
L3 to L4	Motor and sensory function to distal portions of lower extremities Bowel and bladder control	Control of hip extensors remains, making ambulation possible with leg braces
L4 to S5	Variable motor and sensory function to knee, ankle, and foot Sensation to perineum Variable bowel and bladder control	Ambulation with braces possible Considerable independence in ADL can be expected

previously known as **quadriplegia**, is now referred to as **tetraplegia**. Injuries at or below T2 may cause **paraplegia**, which is paralysis of the lower part of the body. Table 29-3 describes the activities that are possible with SCI at various levels.

Respiratory Impairment

The phrenic nerve, which is formed by the nerve roots of C1 to C4, innervates the diaphragm. Therefore injuries at or above the level of C5 (called *high cervical injuries*) may result in instant death because the nerves that control respiration are interrupted. Many patients with high cervical injuries die before reaching the hospital. If these patients receive immediate attention and rapid transport to an acute care facility, mechanical ventilation may be possible. However, they remain dependent on ventilators and face challenges for rehabilitation.

Modern technology affords the ventilator-dependent patient a variety of options for pulmonary rehabilitation. A small portable ventilator can be mounted on the back of a mechanized wheelchair, enabling the patient to be mobile. Phrenic nerve stimulators also may be implanted in the patient to help stimulate diaphragmatic movement and enhance respiratory function. Even with a ventilator or phrenic nerve stimulator, pulmonary hygiene is an issue because these patients may have difficulty clearing the airway.

Cervical injuries below the level of C4 spare the diaphragm but can involve impairment of intercostal and abdominal muscles. Patients with these injuries usually can breathe independently but often experience some degree of respiratory compromise related to weakened exhalation and cough.

Spinal Shock

Spinal shock is an immediate, transient response to injury in which reflex activity below the level of the injury temporarily ceases. It may appear as early as 30 to 60 minutes after the injury and may persist for days, weeks, or months. During the period of spinal shock, paralysis is described as **flaccid**, meaning that the involved extremity or muscle group has no tone. The involved neurons in the spinal cord gradually regain their excitability. Resolution of spinal shock is marked by the appearance of spastic, involuntary movements of the extremities.

Autonomic Dysreflexia

One of the most serious and potentially dangerous problems for the patient with SCI is **autonomic dysreflexia**, an exaggerated response of the autonomic nervous system to some noxious (painful) stimuli. It occurs in patients whose injury is at or above the level of T6. As spinal shock begins to subside and reflex activity returns, the risk of autonomic dysreflexia increases. It may occur even in patients with long-standing injuries.

Excessive stimulation of sensory receptors below the level of the injury precipitates autonomic dysreflexia. The sympathetic nervous system is stimulated but an appropriate parasympathetic modulation response cannot be elicited because of the SCI that separates the two divisions of the autonomic nervous system. Arterioles constrict, causing severe hypertension, which may lead to seizures or a stroke if not corrected. In an attempt to reduce the excessively increased blood pressure, regulatory mechanisms cause the blood vessels to dilate. The vasodilating response is effective only above the level of the injury, where superficial vasodilation, flushing, and profuse sweating occur. The patient experiences nasal congestion, facial flushing, and a pounding headache.

Increased blood pressure also stimulates the vagus nerve, causing bradycardia. Normally, vagal stimulation also would serve to dilate the constricted vessels. However, because the cord has been severed, these impulses never reach the affected blood vessels below the level of the lesion.

Autonomic dysreflexia is triggered by a variety of stimuli, including a distended bladder, constipation, renal calculi, ejaculation, or uterine contractions, but it also may be caused by pressure sores, a skin rash, enemas, or even sudden position changes. In the event of autonomic dysreflexia, indwelling catheters must be inspected for possible occlusions or kinks. If no indwelling catheter exists and the bladder is distended, intermittent catheterization may be done. If constipation is the triggering event, disimpaction may be necessary. Pressure ulcers need to be treated with a topical anesthetic to decrease the stimuli and skin rashes can be treated with appropriate topical ointments to decrease itching.

Autonomic dysreflexia is an emergent situation. It is important to obtain a history related to autonomic dysreflexia on any quadriplegic being cared for in a health care setting. This will allow the provider to be on the alert for symptoms and respond in a timely manner.

Spasticity

Most patients with SCI display some degree of **spasticity** (increased muscle tone) after the resolution of spinal shock. Muscle spasms may prove to be quite incapacitating for these patients, hampering efforts at rehabilitation. Generally, after 1 or 2 years, a gradual reduction in spastic episodes occurs.

Muscle tone is evaluated by assessing the amount of resistance to passive movement. The spastic muscle displays a brief period of increased resistance, which is followed by a sudden relaxation. Reflexes also are assessed because hyperactive reflexes accompany spasticity. Spastic activity may be elicited by passive movement, positioning, or even the slight stimulation of a sheet moving over the lower extremities. A number of drugs are available to treat spasticity.

Impaired Sensory and Motor Function

As stated earlier, the higher the level of the lesion is, the more extensive is the neurologic dysfunction. Any complete cord injury results in the loss of motor and sensory function below the level of the lesion. The effects of incomplete lesions on sensation and motor function are variable. Impaired motor function can significantly affect the patient's mobility and self-care and thus result in complications from immobility. Loss of sensation puts the patient at risk for skin breakdown and other injuries because pressure and pain are not perceived.

Put on Your Thinking Cap!

1. In the community, observe (without being noticed) a person who is using a wheelchair to determine any difficulties he or she may have with access to public facilities, including buildings, transportation, water fountains, and restrooms.
2. Describe any insights this experience provided that could help you to take care of a patient with SCI who uses a wheelchair.

Impaired Bladder Function

During the period of spinal shock, all bladder and bowel function ceases. An indwelling catheter is inserted to empty the bladder and permit close monitoring of urinary output. As soon as the patient's fluid status is stabilized, the indwelling catheter often is removed and the bladder drained by intermittent catheterization. Once spinal shock resolves, reflex activity returns. The bladder becomes spastic and may spontaneously empty. Bladder retraining protocols can be specifically designed for individual patients.

Medications may be used to aid in the prevention of urinary tract infections. Methenamine mandelate (Mandelamine) is a urinary antiseptic that may be used in the regimen. Because the action of methenamine requires an acidic environment, vitamin C (ascorbic acid) often is prescribed to lower urine pH.

Impaired Bowel Function

The absence of bowel activity in the first day or two after injury may require insertion of a nasogastric tube for decompression. Peristalsis usually returns by the third day postinjury. Most patients with SCI can maintain bowel function because the large bowel musculature has its own neural center that responds to distention by the fecal mass. To assist in evacuation of the bowel, the patient must take advantage of the abdominal muscles as well as have an appropriate diet. Bowel retraining programs are initiated to aid in the regular evacuation of the bowel.

Impaired Temperature Regulations

Depending on the level of the injury, the patient may have difficulty maintaining body temperature within a normal range. If a person becomes too cold, the body normally responds with vasoconstriction and shivering to increase the temperature. If a person becomes too hot, sweating helps to dissipate heat. The patient with SCI may lose these regulatory mechanisms and be unable to adapt to temperature extremes. The quadriplegic person is especially vulnerable to environmental temperature changes because such a large part of the body is affected.

Impaired Sexual Function

Spinal levels S2, S3, and S4 control sexual function, so injury at or above these levels results in sexual dysfunction. The ability of the male patient to achieve erection and ejaculation is variable, depending on the level of injury. In women, menses resumes normally after injury. Women with SCI can have sexual intercourse but lack vaginal sensation. Some women with SCI do experience orgasm, although it is not vaginally triggered. They also can bear children, regardless of the level of the lesion. In the event of pregnancy, vaginal delivery is possible if pelvic proportions are adequate. If the lesion is high, however, the woman will not be aware of labor contractions.

Impaired Skin Integrity

Immobility and loss of sensation put the patient at risk for skin problems. One of the most common complications in the patient with SCI is pressure ulcers. Because the immobile patient is unable to change positions, skin in the sacral area and across the bony prominences may break down. This presents a portal for infection in the patient. In addition, the presence of a pressure sore in the sacral area impedes early rehabilitation efforts because the patient is unable to begin wheelchair training until the ulcer heals.

The complete SCI also interrupts the vasomotor tone of the vascular system. This loss of tone results in vasodilation and pooling of blood in the periphery, impeding perfusion of the skin and encouraging the development of pressure sores.

Disturbed Body Image

The effect of SCI on the patient's self-concept and body image is tremendous. Depending on the extent of the injury, every aspect of the patient's life (e.g., occupation, family roles and responsibilities, socialization, hobbies) may be affected. Timing of information is essential to prevent overwhelming the patient and family after injury. For some patients, psychologic counseling may be helpful. Psychologic adaptation occurs over time. Because patients are in the acute care setting for shorter periods, they do not have time to fully process the meaning of the injury to their personhood. The sudden nature of SCI precipitates a crisis. As with many crisis situations, it is met with shock, disbelief, and denial. These stages are incompatible with acceptance of the situation.

The patient moves into a period of reaction, which may last a long time. The reaction can include anger, rage, depression, bargaining, inappropriate sexual behavior, verbal abuse, and suicidal ideation. Any mention of suicide should be taken seriously. Appropriate referrals should be made while protecting the patient from harm. As the period of reaction resolves, the patient begins to seek information about the injury and the future. Patient independence and control should be facilitated at this time.

MEDICAL TREATMENT IN THE ACUTE PHASE

The goals of medical treatment guide the plans for the patient with SCI through all phases of the injury. Three major medical goals exist for the patient with spinal injury: (1) to save the patient's life, (2) to prevent further injury to the cord, and (3) to preserve as much cord function as possible. Each medical goal has specific implications for nursing care and is directed at maximizing the patient's potential for recovery and rehabilitation.

SAVING THE PATIENT'S LIFE

The patient with SCI may have additional life-threatening injuries. As mentioned earlier, patients with high cervical cord injuries (C1 to C4) often die from impaired respiratory function before arriving at the hospital.

The first priority is to establish a patent airway. The conventional head-tilt–chin-lift method of opening the airway is inappropriate in patients with SCI because of the risk of increasing cord damage. The risk of additional damage is especially high with cervical injury. Avoid flexion of the neck, even that caused by a pillow or other support. The jaw-thrust method of opening the airway is preferred for these patients. Once the airway has been opened, 100% O_2 may be administered by mask and manual resuscitator (e.g., an Ambu bag).

An endotracheal or tracheostomy tube may be placed to allow direct access to the airway and to facilitate optimal oxygenation. Any injury that compromises ventilation must be treated immediately.

PREVENTING FURTHER CORD INJURY

Immobilization is essential to prevent further damage to the spinal cord after the initial injury. At the scene of an accident, emergency personnel will apply a hard cervical collar, also known as a *Philadelphia collar*, around the patient's neck to immobilize the spinal column. Various types of devices and traction may be used once the patient arrives at an acute care facility.

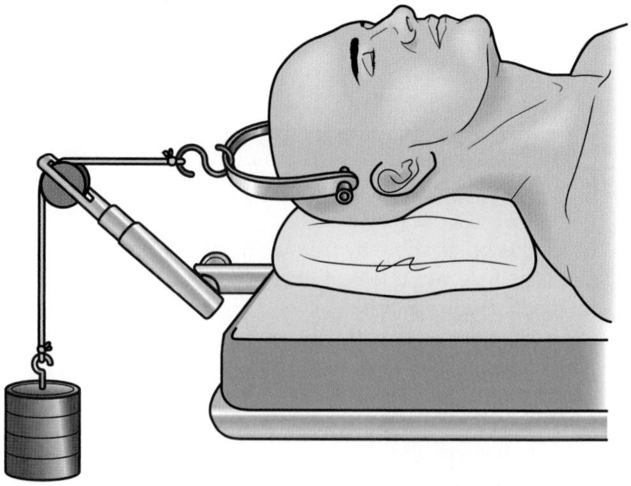

FIGURE 29-6 Gardner-Wells tongs are used to immobilize the cervical spine.

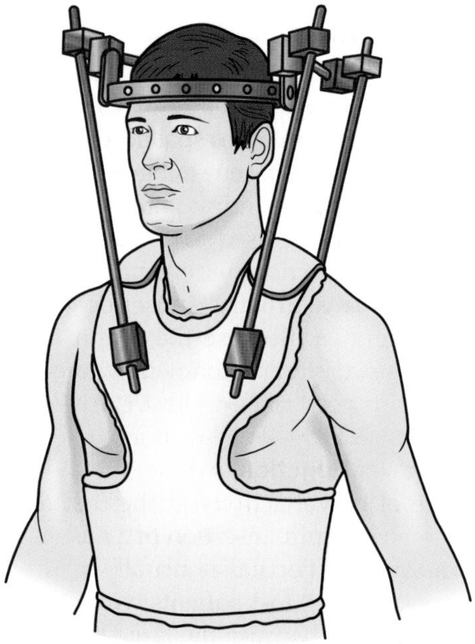

FIGURE 29-7 The halo device immobilizes and aligns the cervical vertebrae.

Traction

Initially, immobilization with skeletal traction often is used to manage cervical SCI. A variety of skull traction devices may be used, including Gardner-Wells and Crutchfield tongs. Gardner-Wells tongs are secured just above the ears but do not actually penetrate the skull. Crutchfield tongs, which are less commonly used now than in the past, are applied directly to the skull, just behind the hairline. The tongs allow traction to be applied, which separates and aligns the vertebrae to prevent further cord damage and reduces painful muscle spasms (Fig. 29-6). After the tongs are applied, radiographs are ordered to confirm alignment of the spine. Ongoing neurologic assessment is done to monitor for further deficits.

The halo vest is used to immobilize and align the cervical vertebrae and usually is placed at the time of surgery that is done to internally stabilize fractures and relieve the compression of nerve roots (Fig. 29-7). A ring is applied to the skull using four pins and then attached to a fiberglass vest by adjustable rods. The vest allows the paralyzed patient to be moved out of bed and allows the patient who is not paralyzed to be ambulatory. Because good immobilization of the spine is achieved, attention can be turned to other aspects of treatment and rehabilitation can be initiated.

Special Beds and Cushions

A number of special beds are available to help prevent complications of immobility while maintaining spinal

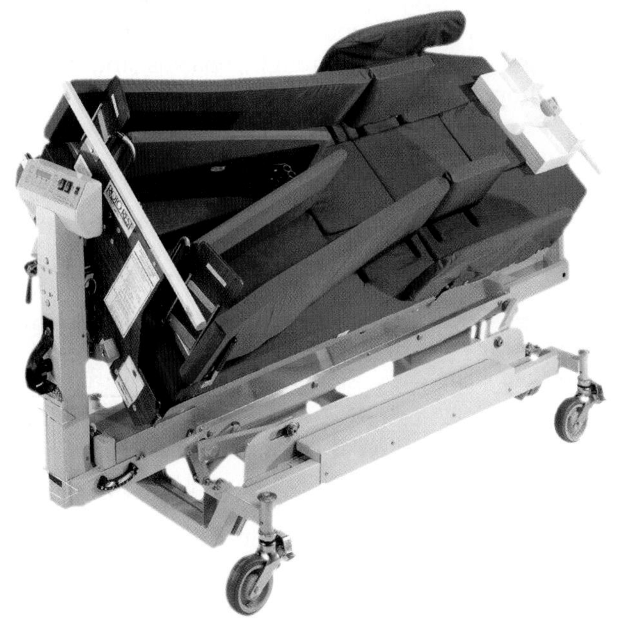

FIGURE 29-8 The RotoRest bed slowly turns the patient from side to side. (Courtesy ArjoHuntleigh.)

immobilization. A kinetic bed, such as the RotoRest bed, slowly but continually rotates the patient from side to side (Fig. 29-8). This rotation is especially helpful in preventing pulmonary complications by mobilizing secretions. Overlay air mattresses are flotation devices that are placed on standard hospital beds. Air-fluidized and flotation beds may be used *after* the spine has been stabilized but they are *never* used when a patient is in tongs because of the potential damage that could occur if the bed should unexpectedly deflate.

The Stryker wedge frame is a canvas and metal frame bed that may be used to help turn the patient. It is not used as often as it was in the past. The patient lies supine on the posterior frame for approximately 2 hours at a time; then the anterior frame is secured on top of the patient and the device is turned over so that the patient is prone on the anterior frame. Two people are needed each time to turn the patient and the patient must be tightly secured to the frame. Every 2 hours the patient is turned from the supine to the prone position or vice versa. Many patients have a difficult time adjusting to such a bed because the prone position leaves the patient feeling as though suspended in midair. Because of this, most patients are managed on a conventional or other specialty bed.

Once the patient is able to be up in a chair, cushioning is needed to prevent excessive pressure and pressure ulcers. Types of cushions include those inflated with air, flotation devices, and gel pads. Examples of pressure-reducing cushions are the ROHO cushion, Bye Bye Decubiti (BBD) cushion, Jay cushion, AKRO cushion, and VARILITE cushion. The cushion that best meets the needs of the individual patient is selected. The physical therapist is a good resource person to consult for this recommendation.

Drug Therapy

Until the early 1990s, management of the patient with SCI relied almost exclusively on surgical and immobilization techniques. However, the use of methylprednisolone to reduce the damage to the cellular membrane has become standard practice in the acute management of SCI. The optimal time of administration is within the first 8 hours of injury. Completely paralyzed patients have been found to regain about 20% of function whereas those partially paralyzed have regained up to 75% of function. This treatment modality is controversial.

Pharmacology Capsule

The administration of high doses of methylprednisolone sodium succinate during the first 8 hours after spinal cord injury (SCI) may help to limit the neurologic effects of injury.

PRESERVING CORD FUNCTION

Early surgical intervention may be necessary to repair cord damage. Situations in which surgery is required include cord compression by bony fragments, compound vertebral fractures, and gunshot and stab wounds. In these cases, surgery within the first 24 hours is most desirable.

A laminectomy involves removing all or part of the posterior arch of the vertebra. This may be done to alleviate compression on the cord or spinal nerves. If multiple vertebrae are involved, spinal fusion also may be done to stabilize the area. A spinal fusion entails placing a piece of donor bone, commonly taken from the hip, into the area between the involved vertebrae. After healing, the fusion immobilizes the affected section of the spine. Postoperative immobilization of the area is necessary to allow for adequate healing, permanent fusion, and correct alignment. If the cervical area is involved, a halo jacket will be used. If the thoracic or lumbar area is involved, other brace-like devices may be fitted to the patient. Neither laminectomy nor spinal fusion can be attempted until the patient has been fully stabilized during the acute phase of the injury.

NURSING CARE in the Acute Phase

Assessment

A complete assessment as described here may be delayed until the patient is stabilized. Until then, monitor the patient's level of consciousness, vital signs, respiratory status, motor and sensory function, and intake and output.

Health History

Present Illness. Record the event that brought the patient to the hospital, noting any specific injuries incurred in the incident. This may be the initial hospitalization after the injury or the patient may be admitted at a later time for other reasons. Describe pain and other symptoms in detail.

Past Medical History. It is important not to overlook other medical problems when the patient has SCI. Inquire about other accidents or injuries and chronic illnesses such as diabetes, hypertension, heart disease, cancer, or seizure disorder. Record previous hospitalizations and operations and obtain an obstetric history if the patient is female. Identify and record any current medications and allergies.

Family History. A routine family history is taken but is not considered specifically relevant to a diagnosis of SCI resulting from trauma.

Review of Systems. Inquire about signs and symptoms that may be related to neurologic dysfunction or its consequences. Data to be collected include skin condition, headache or dizziness, vision disturbances, hearing impairment or tinnitus, nasal or ear drainage (especially if a head injury occurred), dyspnea, nausea and vomiting, constipation or diarrhea, fecal incontinence, bladder dysfunction, sexual dysfunction, and impaired motor and sensory function.

Functional Assessment. Investigate the patient's self-care abilities and explore the patient's roles and responsibilities as a family member. It is also important to record the patient's occupation, hobbies, usual activity pattern, habits (including use of tobacco and alcohol), and diet. Identify the patient's significant others and whether those relationships are supportive. In addition, determine the patient's emotional response to the spinal injury and ask about usual coping strategies, Explore spiritual beliefs and other sources of support (see the *Health Promotion* box).

Physical Examination

Record the patient's reported height and weight (an actual weight measurement may have to be deferred until the patient can tolerate the procedure). Take vital signs. Be alert for hypotension and bradycardia that may accompany spinal shock (discussed earlier in Effects of Spinal Cord Injury). Take the patient's temperature to detect alterations that may reflect failure of regulatory mechanisms or infection. In the general survey, observe the patient's level of responsiveness, posture, and spontaneous movements.

It is important to inspect the patient's skin for lesions (i.e., lacerations, bruises) that may have occurred at the same time as the SCI as well as for signs of pressure that may have resulted from immobility. Inspect and palpate the skin to evaluate tissue turgor, examine the head for lesions, and palpate the head for masses and swelling. Ask the patient to read available print to assess visual acuity and examine the pupils of the eyes for size, equality, and reaction to light.

Observe the patient's respiratory effort and auscultate breath sounds. Inspect the abdomen for distention and auscultate for bowel sounds. In addition, inspect the extremities for open fractures or abnormal positions. Assess range of motion, voluntary and involuntary movement, muscle strength, spasms, and sensory perception in all extremities. If the patient is conscious, ask him or her to move the extremities through the various ranges of motion. This simply indicates whether the patient is capable of such movement and gives some early indication as to the involvement of particular spinal cord levels.

Health Promotion

Spinal Cord Injury

PREVENTION

- Identify high-risk activities and provide safety counseling and education.
- Support safety-focused legislation such as laws related to seat belts, child safety seats, helmets, and driving under the influence of drugs.

AFTER SPINAL CORD INJURY

- Conduct a general health screening appropriate to age and gender.
- Promote positive health behaviors (e.g., smoking cessation, healthy diet, exercise programs).
- Provide spinal cord injury (SCI) preventive care (e.g., bowel and bladder program, skin care, pressure relief, euthermia).

Muscle strength is assessed by using passive range-of-motion exercises and by testing strength against gravity and against resistance applied by the examiner. Instruct the patient to try to move the extremity against the examiner's hand. Evaluate both upper and lower extremities and compare one side to the other. Function is graded on a scale of 0 (complete paralysis) to 5 (normal strength) (Table 29-4). If the patient is unconscious, some noxious stimulus, such as pressure on the nail bed, must be applied to determine whether movement is possible. In the event of cranial involvement, such movement in response to noxious stimuli may be described as *decorticate* or *decerebrate* posturing. Both of these are described in Chapter 27.

Table 29-4 Grading Scale for Muscle Strength

SCORE	FINDINGS
0	No movement, total paralysis
1	Weak contraction palpated or observed
2	Muscle moves when supported against gravity
3	Active muscle movement against gravity
4	Full active range of motion against gravity but with some weakness when resistance is tested
5	Full active range of motion against gravity and resistance

Involuntary movement also may be observed in the injured patient. This type of movement is evidenced by the appearance of muscle spasms. Record the location and severity of such spasms. Techniques for assessing the movement of the major muscle groups in the upper and lower extremities are described in Table 29-5.

To evaluate sensory function, determine the patient's ability to perceive sharp and dull sensations and touch with the eyes closed. As with the motor evaluation, compare one side of the body to the other to assess equality. Include the hands, forearms, upper arms, trunk, thighs, lower legs, feet, and perineal area in the assessment. Sensory loss is best described with the aid of a dermatome chart (Fig. 29-9). A **dermatome** defines an area of the skin that is innervated by a particular subcutaneous nerve root. In the initial postinjury period, frequently reassess sensation because the injury may ascend (rise) and affect vital functions.

Table 29-5 Assessment Techniques for Major Muscle Groups

NERVE ROOT	MUSCLE ACTION	ASSESSMENT TECHNIQUE
C4 to C5	Abduction of shoulder	Shrug shoulder against downward pressure
C5 to C6	Elbow flexion (biceps)	Arm flexed toward body against resistance
C7	Elbow extension (triceps)	Arm extended away from body against resistance
C8	Hand grasp (finger flexors)	Hands grasped around examiner's fingers with attempts to withdraw fingers from grasp
L2 to L4	Hip flexion	Leg raised against resistance
L2 to L4	Knee extension	Knee extended away from body against resistance
L5	Foot dorsiflexion	Foot pulled upward against resistance
L5 to S1	Knee flexion	Knee flexed toward body against resistance
S1	Plantar flexion	Foot and toes pointed downward against resistance

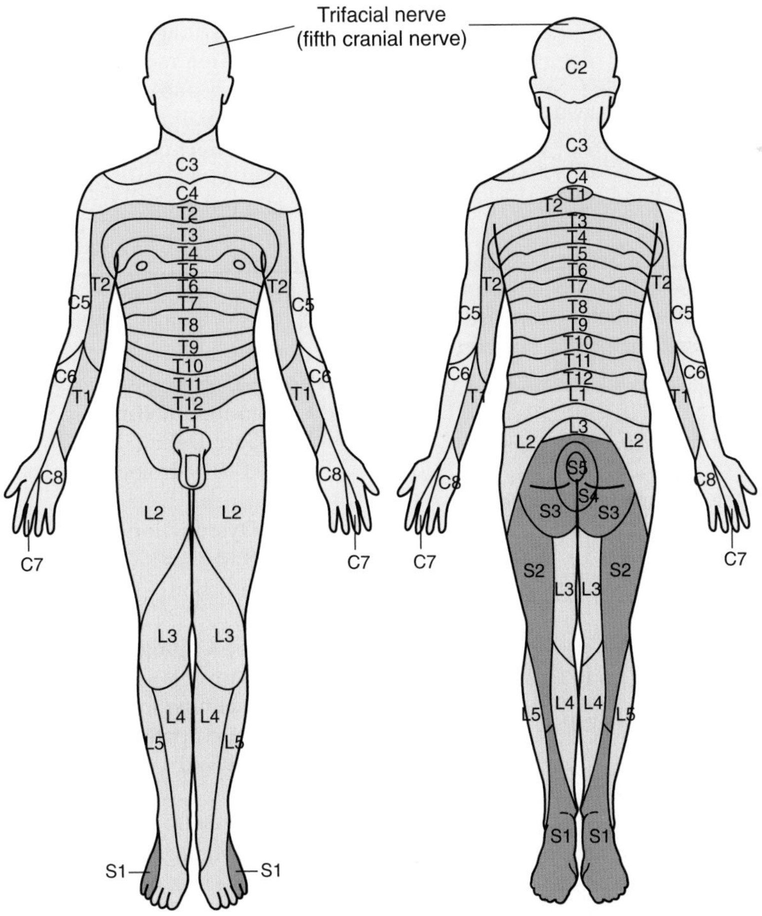

FIGURE 29-9 A dermatome chart. A dermatome is an area of the skin that a particular nerve root innervates. (From Phillips NM: *Berry & Kohn's operating room technique*, ed 12, St. Louis, 2013, Mosby.)

To test proprioception (position sense), ask the patient to close his or her eyes and identify the position of a toe or finger as you move it up or down.

Nursing assessment of the patient with SCI is summarized in Box 29-2.

Interventions

Ineffective Breathing Pattern

Respiratory problems may result from neurologic damage or may be associated with immobility. The patient with an injury at or above C5 has complete loss of spontaneous respirations and requires mechanical ventilation. When a person has an injury to the lower

Box 29-2 Assessment of the Patient with a Spinal Cord Injury

HEALTH HISTORY

Present Illness
Specific event that caused injury, other apparent injuries, pain location, and severity

Past Medical History
Past accidents, injuries, hospitalizations, and operations; history of diabetes mellitus, hypertension, heart disease, cancer, seizure disorder; obstetric history; current medications; allergies

Family History
Routine family history

Review of Systems
Skin condition, headache, dizziness, vision disturbances, hearing impairment, tinnitus, nasal drainage, dyspnea, nausea, vomiting, constipation, diarrhea, fecal incontinence, bladder dysfunction, sexual dysfunction, impaired motor or sensory function

Functional Assessment
Self-care abilities, roles and responsibilities, occupation, hobbies, usual activity pattern, use of tobacco and alcohol, diet, interpersonal relationships, emotional response to injury, usual coping strategies, spiritual beliefs, sources of support

PHYSICAL EXAMINATION

Height and Weight

Vital Signs

Level of Consciousness, Posture, Spontaneous Movements

Skin
Lesions, bruises, redness, tissue turgor

Head
Lesions, masses, swelling

Eyes
Visual acuity; pupil size, equality, reaction to light

Thorax
Respiratory effort, breath sounds

Abdomen
Distention, bowel sounds

Extremities
Range of motion, voluntary and involuntary movements, muscle strength, spasms, sensory perception, abnormal posturing, ability to recognize position of digits without looking

Nursing Diagnoses, Goals, and Outcome Criteria: Acute Phase of Spinal Cord Injury

Nursing Diagnoses	Goals and Outcome Criteria
Ineffective Breathing Pattern related to neurologic impairment	Adequate oxygenation: normal respiratory rate and measures of oxygenation (blood gases, oximeter)
Risk for Injury related to involuntary muscle spasms, lack of motor and sensory function, orthostatic hypotension	Reduced risk for injury: protective measures are taken to prevent injury associated with uncontrollable movement or sensory loss
Risk for Autonomic Dysreflexia related to bladder or bowel distention, renal calculi, pressure sores	No signs of autonomic dysreflexia: pulse and blood pressure consistent with patient norms
Risk for Disuse Syndrome related to pathologic or prescribed immobility (or both)	Absence of complications of immobility: no pressure sores, maximal possible range of motion, clear breath sounds
Bowel Incontinence related to impaired conduction of impulses	Controlled bowel elimination: regular bowel movements under controlled circumstances
Impaired Urinary Elimination related to sensory and motor impairment	Absence of urinary retention and urinary infection: no bladder distention, urine clear with normal odor
Risk for Infection related to skeletal traction pins	Pin sites free of infection: minimal redness and swelling around pins, no purulent drainage
Ineffective Thermoregulation related to spinal cord trauma	Maintenance of normal body temperature: temperature within normal range
Feeding-Dressing-Grooming-Toileting Self-Care Deficit related to neurologic impairment	Adaptation to self-care deficits: patient participates in self-care as much as possible, accepts help as needed
Sexual Dysfunction related to altered body function	Adaptation to altered sexual function: patient verbalizes sexual capabilities and adaptive techniques
Ineffective Coping related to overwhelming losses and limited potential for recovered function	Effective coping: patient expresses feelings about losses, makes realistic plans for future
Ineffective Self-Health Management related to lack of knowledge, physical impairment, denial, depression	Patient effectively manages self-care within capabilities: follows plan of care, plans realistically, uses resources

thoracic cord, abdominal and intercostal muscles are affected, resulting in weakened exhalation and cough. Nursing care is individualized for these patients depending on the extent of respiratory impairment. Ventilator-dependent patients may be taught techniques to allow independent breathing for limited periods of time. The ventilator-dependent patient needs special care, as described in Chapter 31.

A variety of techniques may be used to help patients with spontaneous but impaired breathing to clear the airway more effectively. These include breathing exercises, assisted coughing, and vibration and percussion with postural drainage. For assisted coughing, apply firm pressure to the diaphragm just below the rib cage as the patient exhales or coughs. Because timing is important, it is vital to establish some form of communication with the patient (e.g., a blink) to identify when inspiration is completed. You should be properly trained in this technique before using it.

Turn and reposition the immobile patient as permitted to decrease pooling of secretions in the lungs. If the patient is breathing independently, coach the patient in deep-breathing exercises and use of the incentive spirometer. Adequate hydration helps to thin secretions so that they can be removed more readily.

Risk for Injury

Safety is of prime consideration during the period of spastic paralysis. Involuntary muscle spasms can be so violent that the patient may be thrown from the wheelchair or bedside chair. Therefore it is imperative that the patient be adequately secured with a protective strap across the chest. Even while in bed, the patient requires protection. It is important to avoid undue stimulation of the spastic extremity or muscle group. When performing range-of-motion exercises or positioning the patient, avoid grasping the muscle. Instead, support the joints above and below the affected muscle groups with the palms of the hands.

For the patient maintained in cervical traction on a conventional bed, position changes must be done by "logrolling." A minimum of three nurses is needed to correctly logroll a patient. Some prior planning must be done so that the movement is coordinated. It is helpful to identify the desired position and place pillows and equipment in the proper locations before turning the patient. One nurse stands at the head of the bed and stabilizes the traction by placing his or her hands firmly on the patient's head and neck without flexing the neck. The second nurse prepares to move the patient's shoulders while the third nurse prepares to move the patient's hips and legs. After explaining the procedure to the patient, turn the patient as a unit ("logroll") to the desired position while maintaining proper alignment. Then place pillows against the patient's back and shoulders and between the legs (to protect any pressure spots and to promote comfort). The nurse holding the head and neck should not release the patient until all movement has been completed to ensure that traction does not slip out of place.

Venous thromboembolism prevention is essential. Sequential compression devices are important to promote venous return. Use these when the patient is in bed. Pressure stockings can decrease venous stasis and edema.

If injections are necessary, administer them above the level of paralysis. Two reasons for this exist. First, circulation is impaired below the level of injury, causing drug absorption to be poor. Second, the patient is at increased risk for infection when the skin integrity is broken in affected parts of the body.

Sensory loss presents definite implications for nursing care. The patient with a complete SCI is unable to detect any temperature or pain sensation below the level of the injury. The individual is not able to determine if a painful stimulus, such as a burn, is present. Therefore you must provide meticulous skin care and take all necessary measures to protect the patient from harm.

Risk for Autonomic Dysreflexia

The focus of nursing management for the patient at risk for autonomic dysreflexia is directed primarily toward the prevention of the triggering stimulus. Teach the patient and family members the causes, signs and symptoms, and management of autonomic dysreflexia.

When autonomic dysreflexia occurs, it is a medical emergency. Once it is recognized, immediate action is required to raise the patient's head to a 45-degree angle or to place the patient in a sitting position to help decrease the pressure. If the cause can be identified, make every effort to eliminate it. Check the indwelling catheter for occlusion. If the bladder is distended and no indwelling catheter is present, straight catheterization may be indicated. Fecal impactions, if present, need to be digitally removed after the application of a local anesthetic as ordered. Monitor the patient with severe hypertension for seizures or signs of a stroke. Immediately notify the physician so that appropriate medications or other interventions can be initiated. Administer antihypertensive drugs as ordered. Features of autonomic dysreflexia are summarized in Box 29-3.

Risk for Disuse Syndrome

To avoid the development of pressure ulcers, turn the patient at least every 2 hours. Massaging the bony prominences may be harmful and is not recommended. As the patient is turned, inspect the back and sacral area for skin breakdown or signs of pressure and provide back care using a gentle lotion or other agent designed specifically to prevent skin breakdown. It is vital to relieve pressure on any reddened or broken areas. When the patient is resting in the lateral supine position, place a pillow between the legs to keep the

Box 29-3 Autonomic Dysreflexia

CAUSES
Distended bladder or plugged catheter
Fecal impaction
Urinary calculi
Pressure ulcer
Ejaculation
Uterine contractions

SIGNS AND SYMPTOMS
Sudden hypertension
Pounding headache
Anxiety
Flushed face
Diaphoresis
Nasal congestion
Bradycardia
Vasoconstriction below lesion with cold skin and "goose flesh"
Vasodilation above lesion with warm, moist skin

POTENTIAL EFFECTS
Seizures
Stroke

MANAGEMENT
Assessment to identify cause
Elevation of head of bed
Irrigation or replacement of urinary catheter
Intermittent catheterization
Application of topical anesthetic and digital disimpaction
Removal of pressure from irritated skin
Administration of antihypertensives as ordered

heels free of pressure and to prevent pressure between the knees. Keep bed linens clean, dry, and free of wrinkles. Teach the patient and caregiver how to inspect the skin and recognize signs of pressure.

Specialty beds and cushions also may be used to help alleviate pressure and enhance circulation. Even if special padding is used, patients in wheelchairs should still be instructed or assisted to reposition at least every 15 minutes. Some wheelchairs designed for quadriplegic patients can be tilted backward to allow shifting of body weight.

Patients with tongs are maintained on strict bed rest. Therefore it is imperative that meticulous skin care be provided. With the vertebral column stabilized, the patient may be turned for position changes and skin assessment.

When the patient has spasticity, nursing management is directed toward preventing contractures and muscle atrophy. Pharmacologic agents, such as diazepam (Valium), baclofen (Lioresal), and dantrolene sodium (Dantrium), may be effective muscle relaxants. Electrical stimulators, used with heat and physiotherapy, also may help to relieve spasms. Nursing management of the patient with muscle spasms is summarized in Box 29-4.

During the time of flaccid paralysis, you must diligently perform passive range-of-motion exercises and position and align the patient's extremities to reduce the risk of subluxation or contractures. A more complete discussion of the nursing care of the immobilized person is given in Chapter 21.

Box 29-4 Management of Spasticity in the Patient with Spinal Cord Injury

Perform passive range-of-motion exercises at least four times a day.
Properly position and splint extremities to prevent contractures.
Limit tactile stimuli.
Avoid incidence of noxious stimuli, such as anxiety, pain, bladder or bowel distention, and pressure ulcers.
Turn and reposition at least every 2 hours.
Properly administer medications to reduce spasms.

Pharmacology Capsule

Muscle relaxants may be ordered to control muscle spasticity.

Bowel Incontinence

In the early postinjury period, an ileus may develop, meaning that peristalsis ceases. The abdomen becomes distended and bowel sounds are absent. If this happens, fluids are administered intravenously and nothing is given by mouth. A nasogastric tube may be inserted and connected to suction for decompression. Peristalsis usually returns by the third day postinjury.

Once peristalsis resumes, the patient is given oral fluids and food. Encourage adequate fluids and high-fiber foods to promote soft stools and administer bulk laxatives, stool softeners, suppositories, and lubricants as ordered. It is important to document bowel movements and institute measures to prevent constipation and impaction. Work with the patient to determine the best schedule for bowel elimination and to help the patient carry out the program. A bowel retraining program must be a cooperative effort between the caregiver and the patient. The program can succeed only when the patient is prepared physically and emotionally. Bowel retraining is discussed in detail in Chapter 23.

Impaired Urinary Elimination

While the patient has an indwelling catheter, meticulous catheter care is essential. Because catheterization increases the risk of urinary tract infections, monitor the patient's temperature and assess the urine for cloudiness and foul odor. Administer prescribed urinary acidifiers, antiseptics, and antimicrobials as ordered. In addition, encourage the oral intake of fluids, when permitted, to maintain dilute urine. Discourage the ingestion of dairy products because they contain calcium, which may promote formation of urinary calculi.

In the rehabilitation phase, bladder retraining is addressed. As bladder retraining is instituted, work with the patient to carry out the retraining program. To help improve tone and relieve bladder spasms, the catheter may be periodically clamped and then released in an effort to increase bladder capacity. When the bladder can hold 300 to 400 mL of urine, the catheter may be removed for a trial period. Details of bladder retraining are provided in Chapter 23.

Put on Your Thinking Cap!

D.J. is a 22-year-old who has a spinal cord injury (SCI) at T5. His physician has indicated that he no longer is experiencing spinal shock. How would you know that spinal shock has resolved? Why is management of the bowel and bladder very important at this time?

Risk for Infection

The risks of pulmonary and urinary infections have already been discussed. If the patient has skeletal traction (Gardner-Wells tongs, halo ring), a risk of infection exists at the pin insertion sites. It is important to provide specific skin care as ordered or per agency policy. Risk of infection is minimized by cleaning the pin site twice daily with sterile saline and keeping it dry. After the initial healing, the area can be cleaned with soap and water. Report increasing redness or purulent drainage at the pin sites to the physician.

Ineffective Thermoregulation

Maintain the environmental temperature at a level that avoids chilling or overheating the patient. A room temperature of 70°F (21°C) will keep the quadriplegic's body temperature stable at 95°F. To prevent hypothermia, provide adequate clothing and blankets and promptly change wet clothing and linens.

To prevent excessive warming (hyperthermia), the patient should avoid the outdoors during very hot, humid weather. Some patients carry a water spray bottle when outdoors in the heat or during intense activity. The water can be sprayed on the skin, where it evaporates and cools the body. Fans also can help to cool the patient. An increase in temperature after exercise is normal.

Self-Care Deficit (Feeding, Dressing, Grooming, Toileting)

It is important to continually reassess the patient's abilities and need for assistance with self-care activities. The patient may need total care initially. As soon as the patient is able, begin preparing him or her for self-care consistent with the patient's expected abilities. During rehabilitation, the patient learns to use specialized equipment and strategies to be as independent as possible in self-care.

Sexual Dysfunction

Sexuality and sexual function in the patient with SCI must be addressed when the patient first brings up the subject. Sexual function is controlled by spinal levels S2 to S4. Because sexual gratification is an important aspect of emotional and psychologic well-being, it is an issue that requires thoughtful discussion and counseling. Patients must be apprised of their physical abilities to achieve erection or to bear children. Information about the possibility of pregnancy and about birth control should be provided, if the patient expresses a desire to know.

Advise the patient of resources available in the agency and in the community. The expertise of a trained counselor often is needed and the counselor is usually a member of the rehabilitation team. Honest discussion must occur between the patient and the counselor. Both parties must be willing to explore the physical and emotional aspects of the injury. Additional information on management of impaired sexual function is presented in Chapters 49 and 50.

Ineffective Coping

Ineffective coping may occur at any phase but is particularly evident during rehabilitation as the patient begins to deal with the realities of his or her situation. Ineffective coping may present as hopelessness. Hopelessness may manifest as withdrawal, passive behavior, and decreased affect. A person who feels hopeless sees few or no personal choices available and cannot mobilize the energy needed to move forward. Offer opportunities for the patient to discuss feelings about his or her situation and future. Listen actively and accept the patient's feelings. When the patient is withdrawn, encourage (but do not force) participation in self-care. As the patient begins to acknowledge the injury and assess its effect, encourage him or her to identify strengths and coping strategies. Refocus attention on things other than the injury and losses. Begin rehabilitation efforts in earnest and give generous praise for effort.

The health care team also works with the patient's significant others to create a supportive atmosphere that conveys hope, acceptance, and confidence. Patients and families often continue to hope for physical improvement that is unlikely. For example, they may interpret the movement associated with spastic paralysis as a return of voluntary motor function. You can avoid this misconception by explaining this phenomenon in advance and emphasizing that it is expected and does not signify improved function.

Ineffective Self-Health Management

During the acute phase of SCI, explain routines and procedures. The physician or clinical nurse specialist usually informs the patient of the extent of the injury and probable effects. The nurse reinforces that information and helps the patient and family to obtain any additional information requested. An important resource is the National Spinal Cord Injury Association (www.spinalcord.org; 1-800-962-9629), which has a 24-hour service to provide information about rehabilitation, research, organizations, and local contacts. Many communities have local chapters of the Spinal Cord Society, Paralyzed Veterans of America, and National Spinal Cord Injury Association that can provide information and resources.

The following are the essential components of the teaching plan. The details will vary with the level of the injury:

- Effects of SCI
- Types of treatments and their purposes
- Breathing exercises and adaptive techniques
- Range-of-motion exercises and positioning
- Management of orthostatic hypotension
- Skin care and assessment (see the *Health Promotion* box)
- Management of bowel and bladder elimination
- Recognition of signs and symptoms of infection
- Changes in sexual function and resources for information about adaptation
- Protection of body areas that lack sensation
- Adaptive techniques and devices to maximize self-care
- Emotional responses to SCI and coping strategies
- Community resources

See Case Study (Box 29-5).

Health Promotion

Skin Care: Key Points for the Patient with Spinal Cord Injury

- Avoid excessive pressure, shearing force, and trauma.
- Bathe in tepid water with mild soap; dry thoroughly.
- Soak the feet for 20 minutes once a week; keep toenails trimmed and smooth.
- Keep the skin dry and free of contact with urine or stool.
- Avoid tight clothing with heavy seams.
- Wear cotton undergarments and avoid clothing made of fabrics that do not absorb moisture.
- Eat a balanced diet with adequate vitamins A and C and protein.
- Drink 2000 to 3000 mL of fluid (8 to 12 8-oz glasses) each day unless directed otherwise.
- When in bed, turn at least every 2 hours.
- When in a chair, shift your weight at least every 15 minutes.
- Inspect the skin every morning and every evening for redness, bruising, blisters, and dryness and feel for swelling and hardness.
- If redness is present, try to determine the cause. Are you are turning or shifting your weight often enough? Are you transferring correctly? Are your cushions in good condition?

Box 29-5 Case Study: Spinal Cord Injury

Todd is a 16-year-old Caucasian teenager who was injured while playing football in the park. His friends called emergency medical services and kept him motionless until their arrival. After his arrival at the hospital, his radiographs revealed a C5 fracture dislocation. The fracture was immobilized using tongs and he received methylprednisolone before admission to the intensive care unit. His condition has stabilized and he now has a halo brace in place for stabilization of the fracture. He is being transferred to your floor before future admission to rehabilitation.

CRITICAL THINKING QUESTIONS

1. What strategies would you use to ease the patient's transition to your unit?
2. Identify key components of the nursing care plan to consider based on the level of the patient's injury.
3. Does the patient have a potential risk for autonomic dysreflexia? If it occurs, what assessment data would you gather and what would you do during this crisis?

REHABILITATION

The saying "rehabilitation begins at admission" may sound trite but for the patient with SCI its truth is astounding. The newly paralyzed person is faced with many sobering physical and psychologic challenges. The acute care staff and the rehabilitation staff strive to ensure that the patient is fully equipped to face the challenge.

Nursing care during the acute phase of the injury focuses on preventing further disability and avoiding complications that could prolong hospitalization and hamper rehabilitation. Rehabilitation is best described as those activities that assist the individual to achieve the highest possible level of self-care and independence.

The rehabilitation process involves a well-organized interdisciplinary team that can address all aspects of function. Members of the team include the physician, nurse, physical therapist, occupational therapist, speech therapist, dietitian, social worker, psychologist, and counselor. Each plays a vital role in helping the patient to achieve the highest level of independence. What was once regarded by the patient as a normal lifestyle or occupation may no longer be possible. Rather, modifications and adjustments must be made. The patient and family must be emotionally and physically prepared to make those adjustments. The team not only helps the patient to accomplish ADL and self-care but also addresses successful adjustment to social integration and gainful employment in the workplace. Although this phase of treatment may take more than 1 year to accomplish, the patient, family, and rehabilitation team can take pride in the realization that the patient's life can once again be productive and happy.

Put on Your Thinking Cap!

You are assigned to a 19-year-old man who sustained a C8 spinal cord injury (SCI) 2 weeks ago. His condition is stable at this time and he is alert and oriented. When the nursing assistant brings his breakfast tray, he closes his eyes, says he is not hungry, and asks her to turn off the lights and close the drapes.

1. What phase of adjustment do you think the patient's behavior represents?
2. With adequate support, education, and encouragement, the patient will move into the next phase of adjustment. Describe expected behaviors at that time.

NURSING CARE of the Laminectomy Patient

Laminectomy is the removal of part of a vertebra. It usually is done to relieve pressure on spinal nerves. In addition to traumatic cord injury, it may be used to treat herniated disks or spinal tumors. See Chapter 17 for general surgical care.

Preoperatively, record the patient's vital signs and neurologic status to establish baselines. Determine the patient's understanding of surgical routines and tell the patient what to expect in the immediate postoperative period.

For the patient who has undergone a laminectomy, postoperative care focuses on ongoing assessment of neurologic status and on promoting healing at the operative site. Specific nursing responsibilities are summarized in Box 29-6.

Assessment

After a laminectomy, monitor the patient's vital signs, neurologic status, and breath sounds. Frequently assess movement, strength, range of motion, and ability to localize sensory stimulus. Measure fluid intake and output. In addition, auscultate the abdomen for bowel sounds and palpate for bladder distention. Inspect the surgical dressing for bleeding, clear CSF drainage, and foul drainage. If the patient has pain, obtain a complete description of it for the record.

Nursing Diagnoses, Goals, and Outcome Criteria: After Laminectomy

Nursing Diagnoses	Goals and Outcome Criteria
Risk for Injury related to immobility, neurologic trauma, spinal fluid leakage	Freedom from injury: stable or improving neurologic and vital signs, absence of bleeding or cerebrospinal fluid (CSF) drainage, absence of fever, normal white blood cell count
Ineffective Peripheral Tissue Perfusion related to hypovolemia, obstruction to blood flow	Adequate tissue perfusion: normal pulse, blood pressure, respirations, skin color, and tissue turgor
Acute Pain related to tissue trauma, muscle spasms	Pain relief: patient states pain relieved, relaxed expression

Continued

Box 29-6 Nursing Care After Laminectomy

NEUROLOGIC ASSESSMENT AND VITAL SIGNS
- Frequently assess movement, strength, and range of motion.
- Assess the patient's ability to localize sensory stimulus.
- Frequently measure vital signs to determine any postoperative complications, such as hemorrhage or infection.

CIRCULATION AND RESPIRATION
- Maintain elastic stockings on lower extremities to prevent deep vein thrombosis (DVT).
- Encourage range-of-motion exercises four times a day.
- Encourage deep-breathing exercises every 2 hours.
- Auscultate breath sounds every 2 to 4 hours.
- Have the patient perform incentive spirometry every 2 hours while awake.

PROGRESSIVE AMBULATION AS APPROPRIATE
- Help the patient to progress from sitting at the edge of the bed to ambulating with assistance.
- Encourage increasing distances and independence while ambulating.
- Ensure that the patient uses a back brace or other apparatus as ordered.

BED OR POSITIONING
- Maintain the bed flat or only slightly elevated to reduce strain on the operative site.
- Maintain a soft collar for cervical laminectomy.
- Encourage position changes every 2 hours.

BOWEL AND BLADDER FUNCTION
- Measure urinary output.
- Assess the patient for urinary distention and complete emptying of the bladder after spontaneous void.
- Encourage fluid intake.
- Perform intermittent catheterization (as needed) if the patient is unable to void.
- Auscultate bowel sounds.
- Initiate a bowel program as appropriate.

SURGICAL INCISION
- Change the dressing aseptically.
- Check the dressing for blood or cerebrospinal fluid (CSF) drainage.

PAIN OR DISCOMFORT
- Medicate the patient for pain and spasms as needed.
- Encourage ambulation if possible to reduce spasms.

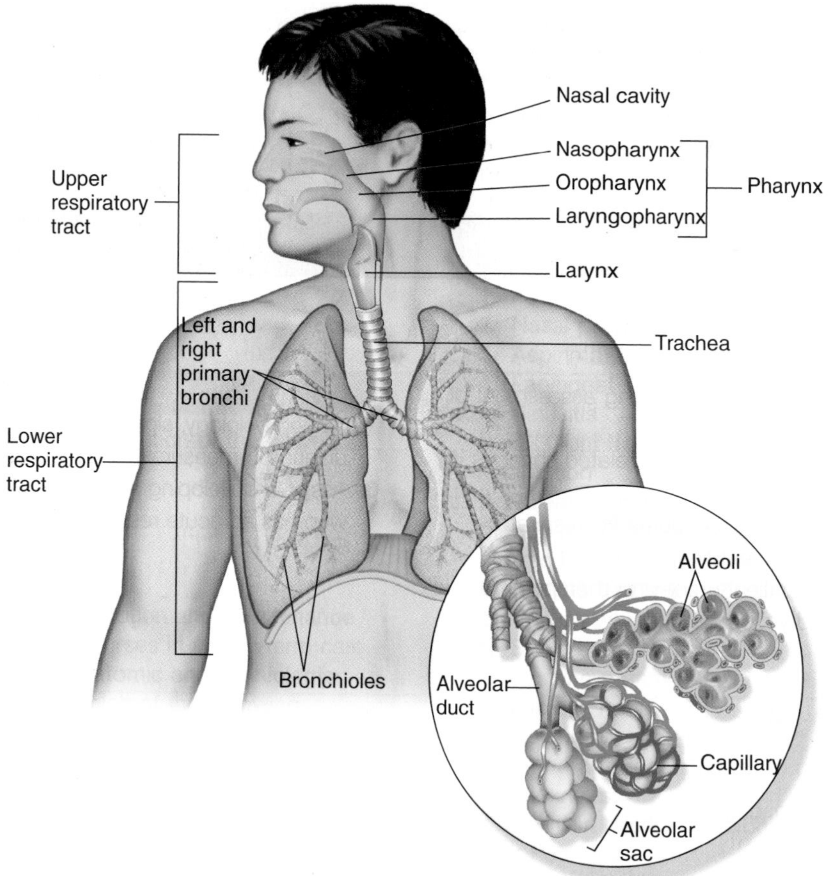

FIGURE 31-1 Structure of the respiratory system: the alveoli and capillaries. (From McCance KL, Huether SE: *Understanding pathophysiology*, ed 5, St. Louis, 2013, Mosby.)

pleura. The pleura are a sac containing a small amount of fluid that acts as a lubricant for the lungs when they expand and contract.

RESPIRATORY PHYSIOLOGY

Mechanism of Breathing

The process of air entering the lungs is called *inspiration* and the process of air leaving the lungs is called *expiration.* The terms *inhalation* and *exhalation* are used interchangeably with inspiration and expiration. The movement of the diaphragm and the muscles in the chest accomplish both of these processes. Inspiration involves an active contraction of the muscles and diaphragm and can be noted by an enlargement of the chest cavity. Expiration is a passive process during which the muscles relax and the chest returns to its normal size (Fig. 31-2).

During normal, quiet breathing, approximately 500 mL of air is inhaled and exhaled. Most of the air movement occurs because of the contraction and relaxation of the diaphragm. A temporary interruption in the normal breathing pattern in which no air movement occurs is called *apnea.* Shortness of breath is called **dyspnea**. Difficulty with breathing in a lying position is called **orthopnea**. Different types of breathing patterns are described in Table 31-1.

Respiratory Center

Breathing is controlled by the respiratory center, which is located in the medulla. The medulla is part of the brainstem immediately above the spinal cord. The respiratory center is stimulated by changing levels of CO_2 and O_2 in arterial blood. Chemoreceptors in the aorta and carotid artery monitor the pH and the amount of CO_2 and O_2 in the bloodstream. Changes in the pH, increased levels of CO_2, or decreased levels of O_2 cause signals to be sent to the phrenic nerves, which in turn send signals to the respiratory muscles to carry out the major work of breathing.

AGE-RELATED CHANGES

Older people may experience difficulty with respiration because they may have loss of lung elasticity, enlargement of the bronchioles, and a decreased number of functioning alveoli. The trachea may deviate from midline in individuals who have scoliosis of the upper spine. Older adults are also more susceptible to lung infections because of less effective respiratory defense mechanisms. In addition, the respiratory muscles atrophy, the rib cage becomes more rigid, and the diaphragm flattens. The consequences of these changes include reduced chest movement and ability

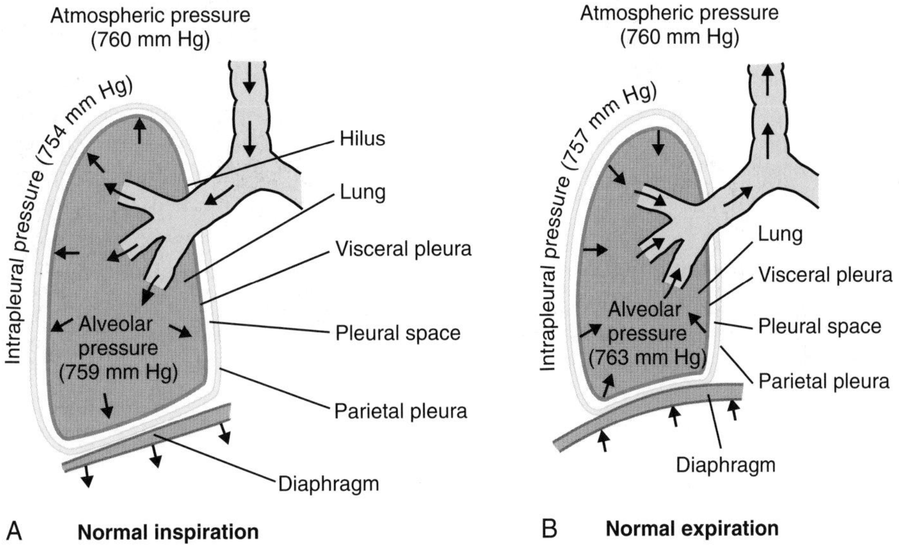

FIGURE 31-2 **A,** Normal inspiration and **(B)** normal expiration. Note the visceral pleura, pleural space, and parietal pleura as well as the changes in pressure in the alveoli and pleural space on inspiration and expiration. (From Black JM, Hawks JH: *Medical-surgical nursing: clinical management for positive outcomes*, ed 8, St. Louis, 2009, Saunders.)

Table 31-1 Types of Breathing Patterns

PATTERN	CHARACTERISTICS	CAUSES
Normal	Pattern: regular Depth: even Rate: 12–20 breaths/min	Normal respiratory drive
Tachypnea	Pattern: regular Depth: even Rate: faster than 20 breaths/min	Fever, pain, anxiety
Bradypnea	Pattern: regular Depth: even Rate: slower than 12 breaths/min	Sedatives, opioids, and alcohol; brain, metabolic, and respiratory disorders
Sighing respirations	Pattern: regular Depth: uneven: periodic deep breaths (more than 3 sighs/min) Rate: 12–20 breaths/min	Severe anxiety
Cheyne-Stokes respirations, apnea	Breaths progressively deeper, then becoming more shallow, followed by period of apnea	Severe brain pathology
Kussmaul respirations (with hyperventilation)	Pattern: regular Depth: deep Rate: faster than 20 breaths/min	Metabolic acidosis; diabetic ketoacidosis, renal failure
Biot's respirations; apnea	Pattern: irregular Depth: varies, sudden periods of apnea	Neurologic disorders
Obstructive breathing, rising end-expiratory level with forced rapid breathing	Gradual rise in end-expiratory level with each successive breath	Emphysema

Adapted from Kersten LD: *Comprehensive respiratory nursing,* Philadelphia, 1989, Saunders.

to inhale and exhale, less effective cough, increased work of breathing, and less tolerance for exercise and stress.

NURSING ASSESSMENT OF THE RESPIRATORY SYSTEM

HEALTH HISTORY

The health history encompasses the chief complaint, history of the present illness, the past medical history, family history, the review of systems, and the functional assessment. If the patient is in respiratory distress, the nurse focuses on the immediate problem, any conditions that might affect treatment, and allergies. Detailed assessment may be deferred until the patient's respiratory status improves. The components of a complete assessment of the patient with a respiratory disorder are discussed here.

Chief Complaint and History of Present Illness

Common complaints associated with respiratory disorders are cough, dyspnea, and pain. To describe a cough, include the onset, duration, frequency, type (wet or dry), severity, and related symptoms such as sputum production and pain. The frequency of expectoration and the sputum characteristics (i.e., color, consistency, odor, amount) should be documented. The patient's efforts to self-treat the cough with measures such as medication, vaporizers, and humidifiers, as well as the response to the treatments, should also be recorded.

If the patient complains of dyspnea, determine the onset, duration, severity, and precipitating events. Note whether the dyspnea becomes worse with activity or certain positions and whether it is more frequent during certain seasons. Identify associated symptoms such as fatigue or palpitations. Describe the effectiveness of methods used to manage dyspnea, which might include medications, O_2, and positioning.

When the patient has chest pain, the location, severity, onset, duration, and precipitating events (trauma, coughing, inspiration) should be recorded. Determine whether the pain causes shallow breathing and whether it radiates up to the jaw or down the arms. Record the presence of fever, sweating, or nausea and document measures that bring relief, such as splinting, heat, analgesics, and antitussive medications.

Past Medical History and Family History

The patient's past medical history determines previous respiratory disorders, allergies, trauma, and surgery. Conditions that are important to document when a patient has a respiratory disorder include allergies, colds, pneumonia, tuberculosis, chronic bronchitis, emphysema, asthma, cancer of the respiratory tract, cystic fibrosis, sinus infections, ear infections, diabetes mellitus, and heart disease. It is especially important to note conditions that suppress the immune response, making the patient more susceptible to infection. Record all recent and current medications, including the use of over-the-counter (OTC) drugs, and the dates of the most recent chest radiograph and tuberculin skin test. Inquire about immunizations against pneumonia and influenza and include questions regarding family history. In addition, ask the patient to describe any major respiratory conditions and smoking history of members of the household.

Review of Systems

The review of systems assesses signs and symptoms that may be directly or indirectly related to the respiratory disorder. Ask about fatigue, weakness, fever, chills, and night sweats. Other data that may be significant are earaches, nasal obstructions, sinus pain, sore throat, hoarseness, edema, dyspnea, and orthopnea.

Functional Assessment

Describe the patient's occupational history, including any exposure to pathogens or to substances that might irritate or harm the respiratory tract. Note exposure to any fumes, toxins, coal dust, silica, or sawdust. Ask the patient to describe a typical day, and to give particular attention to any limitations imposed by the respiratory disorder. Ask about the usual diet and fluid intake. In addition, a smoking history is important; for the cigarette smoker, this is usually reported in pack-years (see *Cultural Considerations* box). Pack-years are calculated by multiplying the number of years the patient smoked cigarettes by the number of packs smoked each day. To illustrate, a person who smoked 2 packs a day for 30 years would have a 60 pack-year smoking history (see *Health Promotion* box). The functional assessment also includes the patient's role in the family, sources of stress, and coping strategies.

Cultural Considerations

What Does Culture Have to Do with Smoking?

Among adolescents, smoking is most prevalent among Caucasians, followed by Latinos and then African Americans. However, programs aimed at smoking prevention and cessation need to target all segments of the population because smoking, which is a health threat to everyone, typically begins before high school.

Health Promotion

How to Calculate Pack-Years

Number of years the patient has smoked × Number of packets smoked each day

Put on Your Thinking Cap!

A patient has smoked 1 pack of cigarettes each day for 15 years. Calculate the pack-years of the patient's smoking history.

PHYSICAL EXAMINATION

The physical examination begins with observing the patient's general appearance. Note facial expression, posture, alertness, speech pattern, and any obvious signs of distress. Take the vital signs and measure height and weight. Be alert to unusually rapid or slow breathing and to tachycardia, which may be a sign of **hypoxia**. The normal respiratory rate for adults is 12 to 20 breaths per minute.

Head and Neck

Examine the head and neck. Inspect the nose for symmetry and deformity and gently palpate for tenderness. The patency of each naris can be assessed by closing one at a time and asking the patient to breathe in through the nose. Note flaring of the nares, because it is a common sign of air hunger. Use a nasal speculum to inspect the nasal cavity for swelling, discharge, bleeding, or foreign bodies. The nasal mucosa is normally light red in color. Tilt back the patient's head to inspect for deviation of the nasal septum, the structure that separates the nares. A deviation may be seen as a hump in the nasal cavity. Palpate the sinuses for tenderness by using the thumbs to apply pressure over the frontal and maxillary sinuses (see Chapter 30).

Inspect the lips, the tip of the nose, the top of the auricles, the gums, and the area under the tongue for cyanosis—a bluish color related to inadequate tissue oxygenation. Document the presence of pursed-lip breathing, a common technique for decreasing dyspnea with chronic respiratory disease. Inspect the pharynx for redness and tonsil exudate or enlargement, which are signs of infection.

Inspect the trachea to see if it is midline; if not midline, it is said to be *deviated*. A deviated trachea can be indicative of a large **atelectasis**, pleural effusion, aortic aneurysm, enlargement of part of the thyroid gland, or tension **pneumothorax**. Place the thumbs on either side of the trachea just above the clavicles and gently move the trachea from side to side. Compare the spaces between the sternocleidomastoid muscles on either shoulder and the trachea. An experienced examiner palpates for enlargement and tenderness of the lymph glands in the neck.

Thorax

Inspect the chest for deformities and lesions and observe the breathing pattern and effort. The rise and fall of the chest should be regular and symmetric. See Table 31-1 for the different types of breathing patterns. Palpate the thorax for tenderness and lumps. Additional, more sophisticated aspects of the examination that require special training include palpating for symmetric chest expansion and tactile fremitus. The skilled examiner also may percuss (tap) the thorax in a systematic manner to elicit sounds that give clues about the density of underlying tissues.

Using the diaphragm of the stethoscope, auscultate the lungs bilaterally in a systematic manner (Fig. 31-3), usually the posterior, the sides, and then the anterior chest. Listen for the normal movement of air in and out of the lungs and for abnormal breath sounds: wheezes, rhonchi, and **crackles**. A wheeze is a high-pitched sound caused by air passing through narrowed passageways that may be present with asthma or chronic obstructive pulmonary disease (COPD). A **rhonchus** is a dry, rattling sound caused by partial bronchial obstruction. Crackles are abnormal sounds associated with many cardiac and pulmonary disorders. Fine crackles are the result of fluid accumulation in the alveoli and do not clear with coughing. To demonstrate the sound of fine crackles, rub a few strands of hair between the thumb and forefinger next to the ear. Coarse crackles are described as sounding like a Velcro fastener opening. Course crackles are due to secretions accumulating in the larger airways and usually clear with coughing. One other abnormal sound that may be heard on auscultation is a pleural friction rub, which is indicative of pleurisy. A pleural friction rub is a grating, scratchy noise similar to a creaking shoe.

In addition to the examination of the thorax and the auscultation of lung sounds, assess for signs of circulatory disorders that could affect respirations. Inspect the abdomen for distention that might interfere with full expansion of the lungs. Inspect the extremities for color and palpate for edema. Examine the fingers for clubbing, which is associated with chronic respiratory problems (Fig. 31-4). Deep veins in the legs and pelvis are the source of most pulmonary emboli, so it is important to assess for any circulatory changes in the lower extremities. Assess for unilateral leg or calf swelling, pitting edema confined to one leg, and localized redness and tenderness along the distribution of the deep venous system. Patients with a history of previous pulmonary emboli or deep vein thrombosis, recent surgery or immobilization, or a diagnosis of cancer are at an increased risk for developing a deep vein thrombosis. If a deep vein thrombosis is suspected, it is important to avoid moving the leg vigorously and to immediately notify the health care provider. The nursing assessment of the patient with a respiratory disorder is summarized in Box 31-1.

Put on Your Thinking Cap!

A patient in respiratory distress usually has tachycardia. Explain why this happens and what purpose the increased heart rate serves.

DIAGNOSTIC TESTS AND PROCEDURES

A variety of tests and procedures may be performed to diagnose disorders of the respiratory system. These tests and procedures are described briefly here. Details

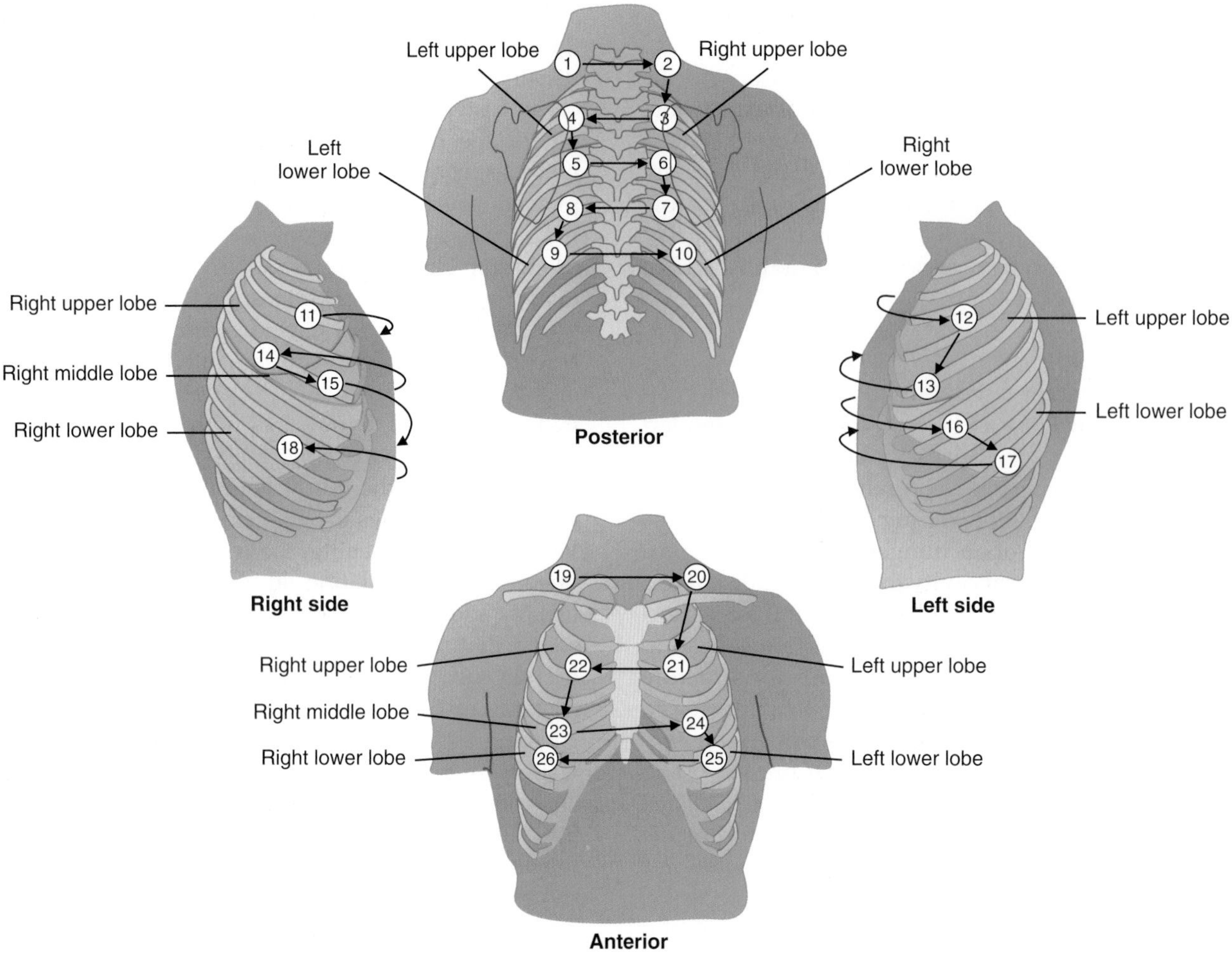

FIGURE 31-3 Sequence for percussion and auscultation of the lungs. (From Black JM, Hawks JH: *Medical-surgical nursing: clinical management for positive outcomes*, ed 8, St. Louis, 2009, Saunders.)

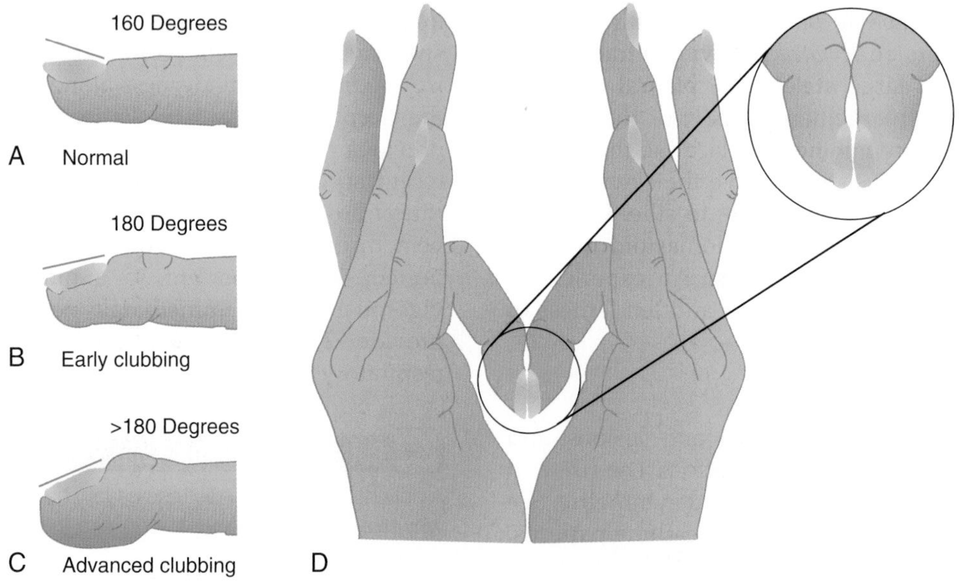

FIGURE 31-4 Clubbing is a flattening of the angle between the nail and the skin. **A,** Normal angle of 160 degrees. **B,** Early clubbing: The angle is flattened to 180 degrees. **C,** Advanced clubbing: The angle is greater than 180 degrees. **D,** The Schamroth technique: The patient puts the nails of the ring fingers of each hand together and holds the other fingers straight up. The examiner then looks at the space between the touching nails. If no clubbing exists, the space is diamond shaped. (From Black JM, Hawks JH: *Medical-surgical nursing: clinical management for positive outcomes*, ed 8, St. Louis, 2009, Saunders.)

Box 31-1 Assessment of the Patient with a Respiratory Disorder

HEALTH HISTORY

Present Illness
Cough: onset, duration, frequency, type, severity, sputum production and characteristics, pain

Dyspnea
Onset, duration, severity, precipitating events, associated symptoms

Pain
Location, onset, duration, precipitating events, effects on breathing, measures that reduce or relieve, associated symptoms

Past Medical History
Colds, pneumonia, tuberculosis, chronic bronchitis, emphysema, asthma, cancer of the respiratory tract, cystic fibrosis, sinus infections, ear infections, diabetes mellitus, heart disease, allergies, trauma, surgeries, hospitalizations, conditions that suppress the immune response, immunizations against pneumonia and influenza, last chest radiograph, last tuberculin skin test, recent and current medications

Family History
Major respiratory conditions, smoking history

Review of Symptoms
Fatigue, weakness, fever, chills, night sweats, earaches, nasal obstruction, sinus pain, sore throat, hoarseness, edema, dyspnea, orthopnea

Functional Assessment
Occupation, exposure to pathogens or respiratory irritants, typical day, usual diet and fluid intake, smoking history, role in family, stressors, coping strategies

PHYSICAL EXAMINATION

General Survey
Appearance, facial expression, posture, alertness, speech pattern, obvious distress

Height and Weight

Vital Signs
Blood pressure, temperature, pulse, respiration

Nose
Nasal shape, tenderness, patency, flaring; swelling, discharge, bleeding, foreign bodies in nasal cavity, septal deviation

Sinuses
Tenderness

Lips
Pursed-lip breathing, color

Pharynx
Redness, tonsil exudate or enlargement

Trachea
Midline

Lymph Nodes
Enlargement, tenderness

Thorax
Breathing pattern and effort, accessory muscles, lung sounds

Abdomen
Distention

Extremities
Color, clubbing, edema

of patient preparation and postprocedure care are presented in Table 31-2.

RADIOLOGIC STUDIES

Chest Radiography

Radiographic examination of the chest is one of the most frequently used methods for respiratory screening and diagnosis. It also is used to assess progression of a disease and response to treatment. The radiograph (x-ray) produces a picture in which the bony structures (e.g., ribs, sternum, clavicle), heart shadow, trachea, bronchi, and blood vessels are visible. Bone appears white on the film because it is very dense and does not absorb much energy. In contrast, the lungs appear black because they are filled with air and absorb the x-ray energy. Chest films usually are taken posteroanterior (back to front), anteroposterior (front to back), and lateral (side) to view the chest cavity from different angles.

Fluoroscopy

Fluoroscopy is a radiograph of the chest taken to observe deep structures in motion. It is possible to observe both lungs at the same time during inspiration and expiration. Instead of producing a single, still image, the screen registers a constant image of the chest. The fluoroscopic examination can give information about the speed and degree of lung expansion and structural defects in the bronchial tree.

Ventilation-Perfusion Scan

When the lungs are working efficiently, a balance exists in the ventilation-perfusion ratio, which means that areas receiving ventilation are well perfused with blood and areas perfused with blood are well ventilated. When the alveolus and pulmonary blood flow are normal, ventilation and perfusion are said to match. A mismatch occurs when there is ventilation without perfusion or perfusion without ventilation, as illustrated in Figure 31-5.

A lung scan or ventilation-perfusion scan is used to assess lung ventilation and lung perfusion. Its chief purpose is to detect pulmonary embolism (PE) or some other obstruction. The patient is given a radioactive substance either by inhalation (to evaluate ventilation) or intravenously (to evaluate perfusion). Ventilation images are compared with the pictures taken during the perfusion scan to determine whether an equal amount of radioactivity exists on both the ventilation and the perfusion pictures. Any areas indicating good ventilation but poor perfusion suggest the presence of a pulmonary embolus or obstruction.

IMAGING PROCEDURES

Computed Tomography

Tomography or tomograms allow visualization of slices or layers of the chest. A computed tomography (CT) scan is a computerized method of tomography in

Table 31-2 Diagnostic Tests and Procedures: Respiratory System

General nursing implications: Always tell the patient what to expect before, during, and after the procedure. When a venous blood sample is required, tell the patient to expect a venipuncture. Following venipuncture, apply pressure and a Band-Aid. Check for oozing.

TEST AND PURPOSE	PATIENT PREPARATION	POSTPROCEDURE CARE
Pulmonary Function Tests		
Used to evaluate lung function, gas exchanges, pulmonary blood flow, and acid-base balance.	Advise the patient not to smoke or eat a heavy meal for 4–6 hours before the test. Patient should rest comfortably in bed and should void before the tests. Determine whether any medications or treatments should be withheld.	Resume medications. No special care is required.
Fiberoptic Bronchoscopy		
Used to visualize abnormalities, take biopsy samples of lesions, or remove foreign bodies.	Obtain signed consent. Patient status should be NPO for 6–8 hours or as specified. Have the patient remove any dentures and provide oral hygiene. Document any loose teeth. Ask the patient not to smoke. Administer sedative and anticholinergics as ordered.	Patient status should be NPO until gag reflex returns and placed in semi-Fowler position. Monitor the patient's vital signs as well as for gross hemoptysis, swelling of face and neck, stridor, decreased or asymmetric chest movement, diminished lung sounds, and dyspnea. Report any abnormal findings to the physician.
Thoracentesis		
Pleural fluid is aspirated and examined for pathogens and other abnormal components. Cells are studied for malignancy.	Obtain signed consent. Stress the importance of not moving or coughing during the procedure. Support the patient during the thoracentesis and monitor his or her skin color, respiratory rate, and general response. Label any specimens and send them to the laboratory.	Monitor the patient's vital signs, lung sounds, and chest movement. If noted, report dyspnea and asymmetric chest movement. Assess the patient for bleeding. Document the amount and color of fluid removed. Check the dressing for bleeding.
Tuberculin Skin Test		
Used to determine past or present exposure to tuberculosis.	Inform the patient that the procedure causes brief pain. Cleanse the skin and inject it intradermally into the lower anterior forearm. Mark and record the site. Tell the patient that a skin reaction may persist for 1 week and not to scratch it. Stress the need to return to the clinic in 48–72 hours so that the reaction can be read. A reaction (swelling, redness) of 5 mm or more is positive for tuberculosis exposure. A patient who has ever been vaccinated with BCG will test positive regardless of actual exposure.	Follow-up depends on the response to the test. If it is positive, the patient will be evaluated for active tuberculosis.
Radiographic and Imaging Studies		
General interventions: Confirm that signed consent has been obtained, if required. Inform the patient what to expect during the procedure. Inform patient if fasting is required. *Dye precautions: If contrast dye is to be used, assess for allergy to iodine or shellfish; notify radiologist if patient reports allergy.		
Chest Radiography		
Used to screen and diagnose some respiratory disorders.	Patient will be asked to remove jewelry on the neck and chest and clothing above waist and to put on hospital gown.	No special care is required.
Fluoroscopy		
Used to provide motion radiographs of lungs.	Preparation is the same as for chest radiography.	No special care is required.

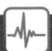

Table 31-2 Diagnostic Tests and Procedures: Respiratory System—cont'd

TEST AND PURPOSE	PATIENT PREPARATION	POSTPROCEDURE CARE
Ventilation-Perfusion Scan (Lung Scan)		
Used to demonstrate lung ventilation and perfusion. Detects pulmonary embolism (PE) and other obstructive conditions.	Assure the patient that the radiation dose is small, that the isotope is quickly eliminated, and that the procedure is painless except for venipuncture. If sedation is needed for agitated patients or small children, the patient is usually maintained NPO for 4 hours. The procedure takes approximately 2 hours. Monitor the patient for 1 hour after the procedure for anaphylaxis.	Check the venipuncture site. Apply a small dressing and pressure if needed. Radioactive material is excreted in the urine. Tell the patient to wash his or her hands after voiding. Anyone who handles the patient's urine should wear rubber gloves. Gloves and hands should be washed after urine is discarded.
Computed Tomography		
Used to visualize lesions and tumors.	Inform the patient that the procedure is painless. Stress the importance of remaining still during the scanning. *Dye precautions. NPO status may be required.	Assess the patient for side effects of contrast: headache, nausea, vomiting.
Magnetic Resonance Imaging		
Produces images of multiple body planes without radiation. Used to detect abnormalities, lesions, and tumors.	Obtain signed consent. Inform the patient that he or she will lie on a stretcher that slides into a tubelike device; mechanical clanging noises are heard as the machine operates. Aneurysm clips, intraocular metal, heart valves made before 1964, and middle-ear prostheses generally contraindicate MRI. MRI may also affect metal implants such as cardiac pacemakers and orthopedic implants but they are not absolute contraindications. Assess the patient for claustrophobia; if found, report it to the physician. Patients who are anxious or restless may require sedation. Special equipment must be used for oxygen (O_2) therapy or mechanical ventilation. Have the patient remove metal watches and other jewelry.	Use safety precautions if the patient is sedated; otherwise, no special care is needed.
Laboratory Studies		
General interventions: Inform the patient that a blood sample or urine sample will be required and whether fasting is necessary. After venipuncture, apply pressure and a Band-Aid; check for oozing.		
Arterial Blood Gas Analysis		
Used to detect alkalosis or acidosis and alterations in oxygenation status.	Tell the patient that a blood sample will be drawn from an artery (usually the radial artery). An Allen test *must* be done before an arterial puncture to ensure that the arteries to the hand are patent. (Arterial punctures require specialized training.)	Apply pressure to the puncture site for 5–10 minutes. Note on the laboratory slip the concentration of any O_2 therapy. Transport the blood gas syringe containing the specimen to the laboratory in an ice bath within 15 minutes.
Sputum Analysis Volume, consistency, odor, color provide clues to clinical disorders. Sputum Culture and Sensitivity (C&S) Reveals pathogens and effective antimicrobials. Sputum for Cytology Detects malignant cells and inflammatory changes.	Collect the specimen early in the morning before breakfast. Provide a sterile container. Instruct the patient to (1) brush the teeth and rinse the mouth, (2) cough deeply and expectorate directly into the container, (3) immediately cap the container, and (4) inform the nurse that the specimen is ready. *For cytology*, a special container and solution must be used for specimens. Send the specimen to the laboratory promptly. Refrigerate if it will be more than 1 hour before delivery to the laboratory.	No special care is required.

BCG, Bacillus Calmette-Guérin; *MRI*, magnetic resonance imaging; *NPO*, nothing by mouth.

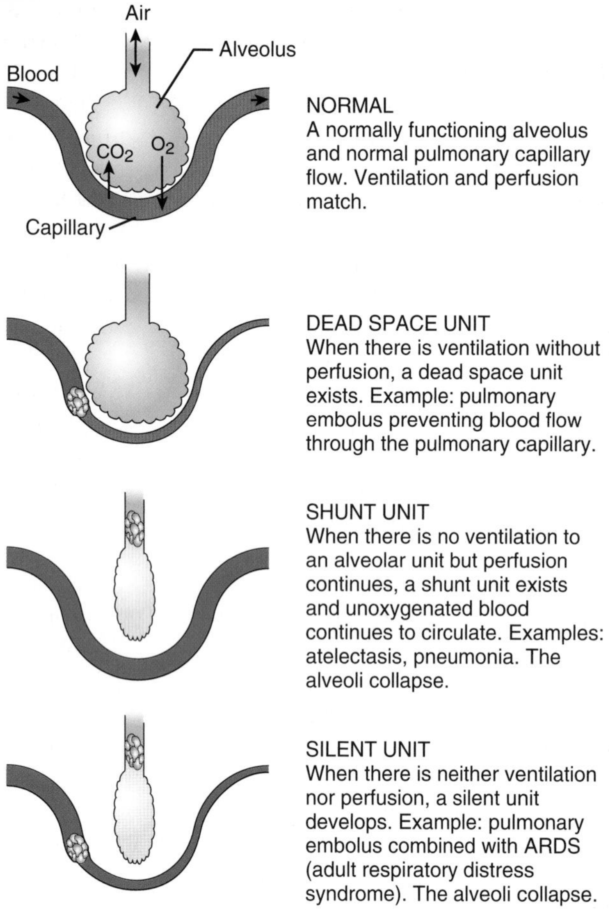
Air
Alveolus
Blood
CO2
O2
Capillary
NORMAL
A normally functioning alveolus and normal pulmonary capillary flow. Ventilation and perfusion match.
DEAD SPACE UNIT
When there is ventilation without perfusion, a dead space unit exists. Example: pulmonary embolus preventing blood flow through the pulmonary capillary.
SHUNT UNIT
When there is no ventilation to an alveolar unit but perfusion continues, a shunt unit exists and unoxygenated blood continues to circulate. Examples: atelectasis, pneumonia. The alveoli collapse.
SILENT UNIT
When there is neither ventilation nor perfusion, a silent unit develops. Example: pulmonary embolus combined with ARDS (adult respiratory distress syndrome). The alveoli collapse.

FIGURE 31-5 Normal functioning alveolus and pulmonary capillary blood flow. When both are normal, the ventilation and perfusion match. Blockage of the bronchiole or the pulmonary capillary creates a ventilation-perfusion mismatch. CO_2, Carbon dioxide; O_2, oxygen. (From Black JM, Hawks JH: *Medical-surgical nursing: clinical management for positive outcomes*, ed 8, St. Louis, 2009, Saunders.)

which a camera rotates in a circular pattern around the body to provide a three-dimensional assessment of the thorax. The test usually is used to look for the presence of lesions or tumors.

Radioactive dye containing iodine may be injected intravenously. Each layer of the chest is photographed before and after the injection of the dye. It is extremely important to find out whether the patient is allergic to iodine before the procedure is performed. Make sure to ask the patient about allergies to shellfish, which contain iodine. Failure to determine sensitivity to iodine could result in an allergic reaction, anaphylaxis, and death.

Pharmacology Capsule

Dyes used in computed tomography (CT) contain iodine, which can produce fatal reactions in people with iodine allergies.

Magnetic Resonance Imaging

A magnetic resonance imaging (MRI) scan is similar to a CT scan but without the harmful radiation. The MRI scanner encloses the patient in a donut-shaped magnet and picks up signals from the body to make electronic images. The patient must remain as quiet and as motionless as possible during the procedure. No preparation is necessary but patients should be warned that no metal may be worn inside the unit (with the exception of dental fillings). Patients with implanted devices such as pacemakers and orthopedic plates, pins, or screws may be ineligible for MRI scanning.

Positron Emission Tomography

Positron emission tomography (PET) scans of the lungs are used most often to distinguish malignant from benign cells and to evaluate the effectiveness of cancer treatment. PET scans use special radionuclides attached to a natural body compound, usually glucose. This substance is administered to the patient intravenously and the radioactivity localizes in the appropriate areas of the body and is detected by the PET scanner. Cancerous tissue, which uses more glucose than normal tissue, will accumulate more of the substance and appear brighter than normal tissue on the PET images. The patient must remain quiet, avoiding movement or talking during the test. Because glucose is the substance most often tagged with the radionuclides, it is important to ensure that the patient has not eaten for at least 4 hours before the test.

PULMONARY FUNCTION TESTS

Pulmonary function tests are used to diagnose pulmonary disease, monitor disease progression, evaluate the extent of disability, and assess the effects of medication. The tests measure lung volumes and capacities including total lung capacity (TLC), forced expiratory volume (FEV), functional residual capacity (FRC), inspiratory capacity (IC), vital capacity (VC), forced vital capacity (FVC), minute volume (MV), and thoracic gas volume (TGV).

A clip is applied to the nose and the patient breathes through a mouthpiece as directed while various measurements are taken to assess the mechanics of breathing (flow rates of gas in and out of the lungs) and to measure diffusion (the movement of the gas across the alveolar-capillary membrane).

Spirometry

A spirometer is an instrument that measures the ventilatory function of the lung. It measures the volume of air that the lung can hold, the rate of flow of air in and out of the lung, and the compliance (elasticity) of lung tissue. The test enables the physician to detect impaired pulmonary function, classify the pulmonary impairment, estimate the severity of the impairment, monitor the cause of pulmonary disease, evaluate treatment, give information helpful in planning care, and provide preoperative assessment.

The test involves inserting a mouthpiece; taking as deep a breath as possible; and blowing as hard, as fast, and for as long as possible. Patients should be encouraged to continue blowing out until exhalation is complete.

Spirometry measures FVC and FEV. These and other lung volumes and capacities are defined in Table 31-3.

People who are to undergo spirometry should be taught what to expect during the test and how to prepare. They may be anxious about taking a breathing test if they have respiratory problems, because they may fear increased dyspnea or exhaustion. They should be advised not to smoke or use bronchodilator medications for 4 to 6 hours before testing.

Pharmacology Capsule

Bronchodilators should not be given before pulmonary function testing because they can alter the results.

Arterial Blood Gas Analysis

Ventilation and diffusion also are measured by testing for concentrations of O_2 and CO_2 in the arterial blood to determine whether the exchange is adequate across the alveolar membrane. Blood gas analysis is useful in the care of patients with respiratory disorders, problems of circulation and distribution of blood, body fluid imbalances, and acid-base imbalances. *Drawing an arterial blood sample requires special training.* Samples are often obtained from the radial artery after first performing the Allen test to ensure adequate circulation to the hand from other arteries (Fig. 31-6). After the arterial puncture, pressure must be applied for 5 to 10 minutes to ensure no bleeding. In the critical care setting, the physician may place an arterial line, commonly called an *ART line.* This line allows for frequent monitoring of arterial blood gases without repeated arterial punctures.

The arterial blood sample is analyzed for pH, $PaCO_2$ (partial pressure of carbon dioxide in arterial blood), PaO_2 (partial pressure of oxygen in arterial blood), HCO_3^- (bicarbonate), and O_2 saturation to detect alkalosis or acidosis and alterations in oxygenation status. Normal values for adults are pH 7.35 to 7.45, $PaCO_2$ 35 to 45 mm Hg, PaO_2 80 to 100 mm Hg (some references give a lower limit of 75 mm Hg), HCO_3^- 22 to 26 mEq/L, and O_2 saturation 96% to 100%.

PULSE OXIMETRY

Pulse oximetry permits the noninvasive measurement of O_2 saturation. A sensor is clipped to an earlobe or fingertip. A beam of light passes through the tissue and the amount of light absorbed by O_2-saturated hemoglobin is measured. The O_2 saturation is presented as a percentage and registered on a digital readout. Factors that interfere with accurate measurement of the oximeter are hypotension, hypothermia, vasoconstriction, and finger movement. Normal pulse oximetry is 95% or higher. Notify your supervisor or the physician of readings <90%.

Table 31-3 Lung Volumes and Capacities

VOLUME	DEFINITION	SIGNIFICANCE OF INCREASE	SIGNIFICANCE OF DECREASE
Total lung capacity (TLC)	Total lung volume when fully inflated	Overdistention of lung caused by obstructive lung disease	Restrictive lung disease
Forced expiratory volume (FEV)	Volume of air expired during specified time intervals (0.5, 1.0, 2.0, 3.0 sec)	Not significant	Restrictive or obstructive lung disease depending on measurements at time intervals
Functional residual capacity (FRC)	Volume of air remaining in the lungs after normal exhalation	Chronic obstructive pulmonary disease (COPD)	Acute respiratory distress syndrome (ARDS)
Inspiratory capacity (IC)	Maximum volume of air that can be inhaled after a normal exhalation	Excessive use of positive end-expiratory pressure	Restrictive lung disease
Vital capacity (VC)	Total volume of air that can be exhaled after maximum inspiration	Not significant; increased or normal VC with normal flow rates: pulmonary edema	Decreased VC with normal or increased flow rates: impaired respiratory effort
Forced vital capacity (FVC)	Total volume of air exhaled rapidly and forcefully after maximum inhalation	Not significant	Obstructive or restrictive lung disease
Minute volume (MV)	Total amount of air breathed in 1 min	Not significant	Restrictive parenchymal lung disease; fatigue
Thoracic gas volume (TGV)	Total volume of air in the lungs, including ventilated and nonventilated areas	Obstructive lung disease with air trapping	Not significant

Data from Chernecky CC, Berger BJ: *Laboratory tests and diagnostic procedures*, ed 3, Philadelphia, 2001, Saunders; Jaffe MS, McVan BF: *Davis's laboratory and diagnostic test handbook*, Philadelphia, 1997, Saunders.

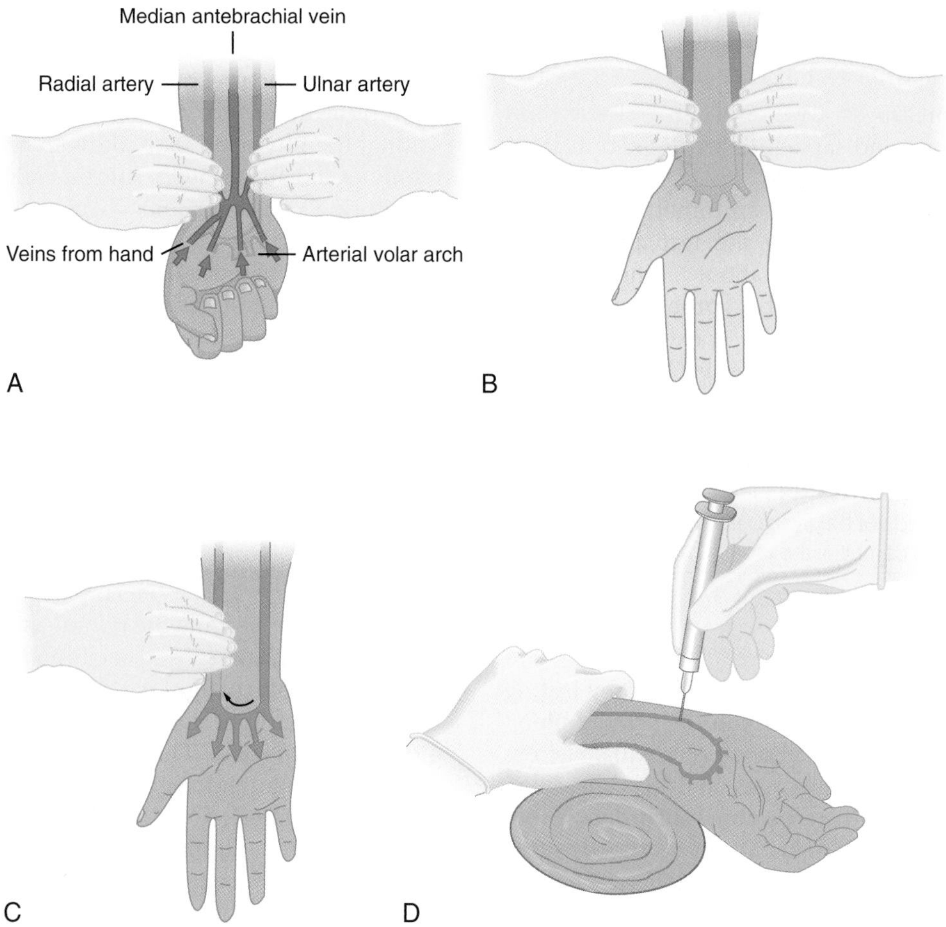

FIGURE 31-6 The Allen test should be done before each radial arterial puncture to ensure adequate collateral circulation. Because an arterial puncture may injure the radial artery, the adequacy of blood supply to the area by other arteries must be determined. A puncture is not done on an artery if the other blood supply is not adequate. **A,** To perform the Allen test, occlude the radial and ulnar arteries and have the patient make a fist. **B,** While maintaining pressure on the arteries, have the patient open the hand. The hand is pale if the arteries are occluded. **C,** Release the pressure on the ulnar artery. If collateral circulation is adequate, color will return to the hand. This is a positive Allen test result; the puncture can proceed on the radial artery. If color does not return, the Allen test result is negative and the radial artery should not be punctured. **D,** A blood sample is drawn from the radial artery after a positive Allen test result. (From Black JM, Hawks JH: *Medical-surgical nursing: clinical management for positive outcomes*, ed 8, St. Louis, 2009, Saunders.)

SPUTUM ANALYSIS

Sputum is material that originates in the bronchi. Sputum analysis may be performed when respiratory disease is suspected. The mucous membrane lining of the lower respiratory tract responds to acute inflammation by increasing the production of secretions, which may contain bacterial or malignant cells. These cells may be detected by examination of sputum. Sputum specimens are examined also for volume, consistency, color, and odor. Sputum that is thick; foul smelling; and yellow, green, or rust colored may indicate a bacterial infection. Instruct the patient to expectorate the specimen directly into a sterile container after coughing deeply. If the patient is unable to expectorate a specimen, sputum production may be induced with aerosol therapy or obtained by suctioning.

Culture and Sensitivity

Sputum culture and sensitivity tests are ordered to determine the presence of bacteria, identify the specific organisms, and identify appropriate antimicrobials. Collect specimens before antimicrobial therapy begins to ensure that sufficient bacterial growth is present.

Acid-Fast Test

An acid-fast test on a sputum specimen is performed to determine the presence of acid-fast bacilli, which include the bacteria that cause tuberculosis. Specimens are usually collected on 3 consecutive days. Keep each sputum specimen covered and refrigerated or delivered to the laboratory within 1 hour. Use a new sterile container for each collection.

Cytologic Specimens

Sputum specimens are obtained for cytologic examination to determine the presence of lung carcinoma or infectious conditions. Because sputum contains cells from the tracheobronchial tree, malignant cells may be detected in the specimen. A special container with fixative solution may be used for this type of specimen collection. Consult the agency laboratory manual for directions.

FIBEROPTIC BRONCHOSCOPY

A bronchoscopic examination is performed by inserting a flexible fiberoptic scope through the nose or mouth into the bronchial tree after local anesthesia of the patient's throat. The scope allows for direct visualization of the bronchial tree structures for assessment, diagnosis, or removal of foreign bodies or mucus plugs. Lesions suggestive of malignancy may be located and a biopsy performed as well. Before the procedure, signed consent should be obtained. Have the patient remove dentures. Give sedatives as ordered. Afterward, monitor the patient's respiratory status and level of consciousness. The patient should take nothing by mouth (NPO) until the gag reflex returns. Complications of bronchoscopy include bronchospasm, bacteremia, bronchial perforation, pneumonia, laryngospasm, hemorrhage, and pneumothorax.

Additional details about diagnostic tests and procedures are presented in Table 31-2.

COMMON THERAPEUTIC MEASURES

THORACENTESIS

A thoracentesis is the insertion of a large-bore needle through the chest wall into the pleural space. Usually the physician performs the procedure at the patient's bedside. Thoracentesis is done to remove pleural fluid, blood, or air or to instill medication. Pleural fluid may be removed to reduce respiratory distress caused by fluid accumulation in the pleural space. In addition, fluid obtained in the procedure may be studied to obtain blood cell counts or to measure protein, glucose, lactic dehydrogenase, fibrinogen, or amylase levels. The study of pleural fluids may aid in the diagnosis of infectious diseases and cancer.

The patient sits on the side of the bed and leans the upper torso over the bedside table with the head resting on folded arms or pillows (Fig. 31-7). If the patient is unable to sit up, a side-lying position with the head of the bed elevated 30 degrees may be used. The skin is cleansed thoroughly and a local anesthetic is injected. The physician inserts a 20-gauge or larger needle between the ribs and through the parietal membrane. Fluid or air is then aspirated, the thoracentesis needle is removed, and a sterile dressing is applied to the puncture site. The patient is positioned on the unaffected side. A chest radiograph may be ordered after the procedure to detect any pulmonary complications caused by accidental injury to the lung. Complications of thoracentesis include air embolism, hemothorax, pneumothorax, and pulmonary edema. Immediately report uneven chest movements, respiratory distress, or hemorrhage to the supervisor and the physician. Details of nursing responsibilities are included in Box 31-1.

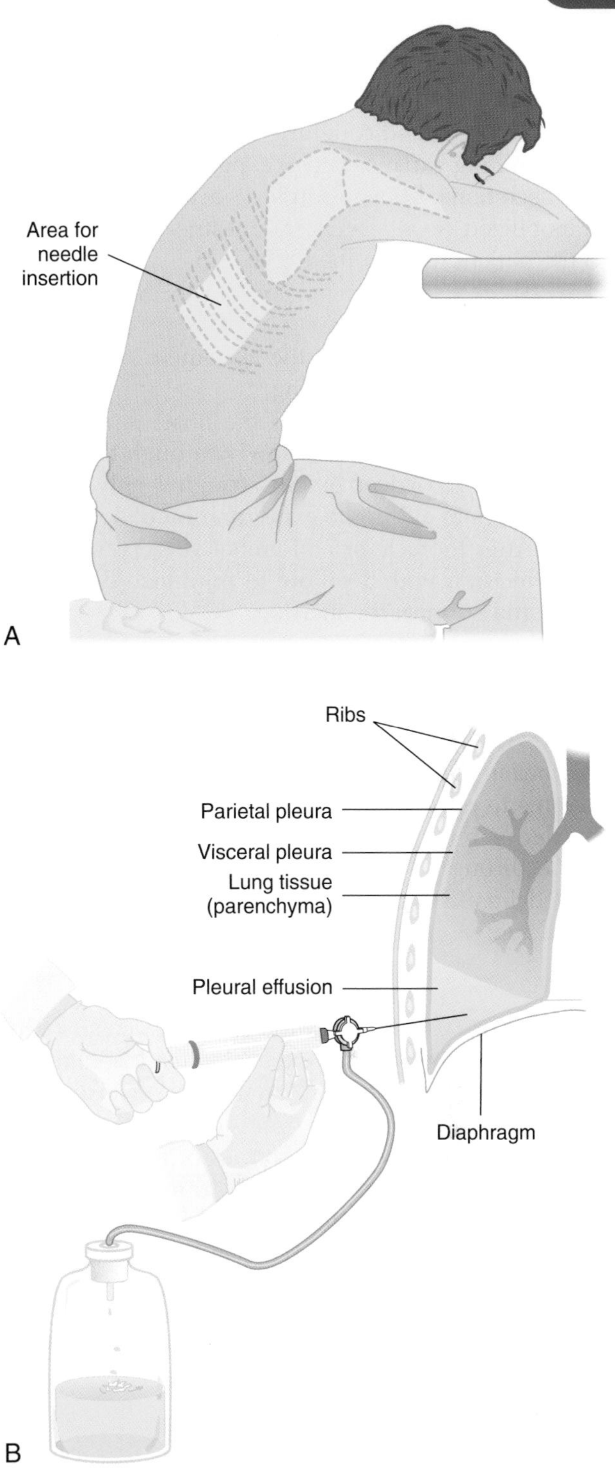

FIGURE 31-7 **A,** The patient is positioned for a thoracentesis. **B,** The needle is inserted into the pleural space, avoiding lung tissue and the diaphragm. The exact location of the puncture varies. (From Black JM, Hawks JH: *Medical-surgical nursing: clinical management for positive outcomes*, ed 8, St. Louis, 2009, Saunders.)

BREATHING EXERCISES

Deep-Breathing and Coughing Exercises

Deep-breathing and coughing exercises are performed to aid in lung expansion and expectoration of respiratory secretions. They are indicated when patients are immobilized or after general anesthesia. Instructions to the patient include the following:

1. Sit in a semi-Fowler position for maximal lung expansion.
2. Place one hand on the abdomen to feel it rise and fall with breathing.
3. Inhale deeply through the nose, pause 1 to 3 seconds, and exhale slowly through the mouth.
4. After 4 to 6 deep breaths, cough deeply from the lungs to aid in the expectoration of sputum.
5. After thoracic or abdominal surgery, splint the incision with a pillow to minimize discomfort and support the incision.

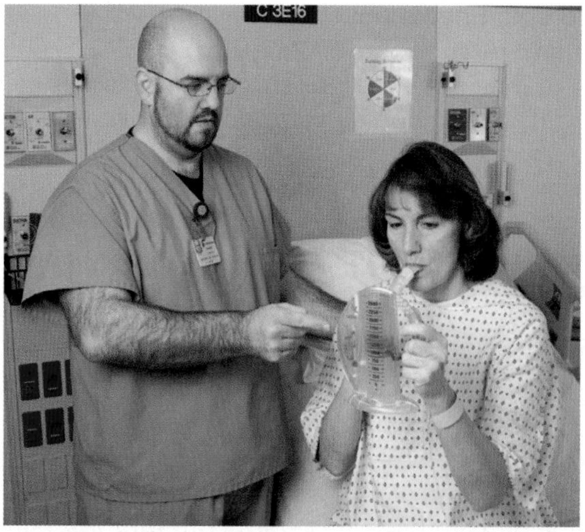

FIGURE 31-8 Incentive spirometry encourages deep breathing by providing a visual cue to the patient about the efficiency of deep breathing. (From Potter PA, Perry AG, Stockert P, Hall A, editors: *Fundamentals of nursing*, ed 8, St. Louis, 2013, Mosby-Elsevier.)

Pursed-Lip Breathing

Another type of breathing exercise is pursed-lip breathing. It is used to inhibit airway collapse and to decrease dyspnea in patients with chronic lung disease. Instruct patients to pucker the lips as if to whistle, blow out a candle, or blow through a straw. They should then inhale through the nose and slowly exhale through pursed lips. Exhalation should last twice as long as inhalation.

Sustained Maximal Inspiration

Sustained maximal inspiration is used to ensure deep inspiration for maximal expansion and aeration of the lungs. An incentive spirometer is an instrument that frequently is used to encourage maximal inspiration. Spirometers basically consist of a cylinder that contains balls or disks and a tube through which the patient inhales. As the patient inhales through the tube, the balls or disks rise (Fig. 31-8). Instruct the patient to inhale deeply and slowly to move the balls or disks in the cylinder upward. For maximum effect, the spirometer is kept upright because tilting the device reduces respiratory effort. Some spirometers provide a digital readout of the volume of air displaced. If the patient's maximal inspiration can be measured before surgery, that reading can be used as a target after surgery.

CHEST PHYSIOTHERAPY

Chest physiotherapy consists of percussion, vibration, and postural drainage. These mechanical techniques are used to facilitate the mobilization and expectoration of secretions in patients with large mucus-producing or chronic mucus-retaining respiratory disorders such as chronic bronchitis and cystic fibrosis. Although this therapy is usually performed in the acute care setting by a respiratory therapist, the nurse often does this in long-term and home care settings. Therefore you should be familiar with the procedures and be able to evaluate the patient's response. In an outpatient setting, you also may monitor the caregiver's technique in administering the treatment. Chest physiotherapy should be performed before meals to reduce the risk of regurgitation and aspiration of stomach contents. Chest physiotherapy can also cause a decrease in appetite, so the timing of the treatment should allow adequate time for the patient to regain his or her appetite.

Chest Percussion and Vibration

Chest percussion and vibration are performed to facilitate the movement of respiratory secretions so that sputum can be expectorated. Percussion is clapping of the cupped palms against the chest wall to dislodge and mobilize respiratory secretions (Fig. 31-9, A). The procedure is performed with the hands cupped to create a pocket of air when striking the patient's chest—first with one hand and then with the other. Percussion is confined to areas protected by the rib cage and is never done over the sternum, kidney, liver, spleen, stomach, or spine. In general, percussion is done for 20 to 30 seconds, followed by vibration.

Vibration is performed by the therapist placing one hand on the top of the other, keeping the arms straight, and pressing the hands flat against the patient's chest (Fig. 31-9, B). As the patient exhales, the therapist creates a shaking (vibrating) movement with the palms. The therapist pauses during inhalation. The vibration is repeated during three or four breathing cycles. Devices designed to loosen and mobilize secretions include various mechanical vibrators, ultra-low frequency airway oscillation devices, and manual percussor cups. Contraindications to percussion and vibration include lung cancer, bronchospasm, pain in the area being treated, hemorrhage, hemoptysis,

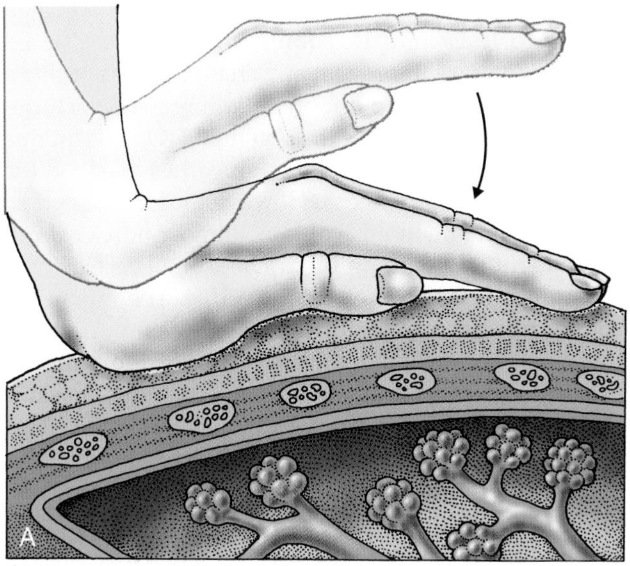

Chest percussion (with cupped hand)

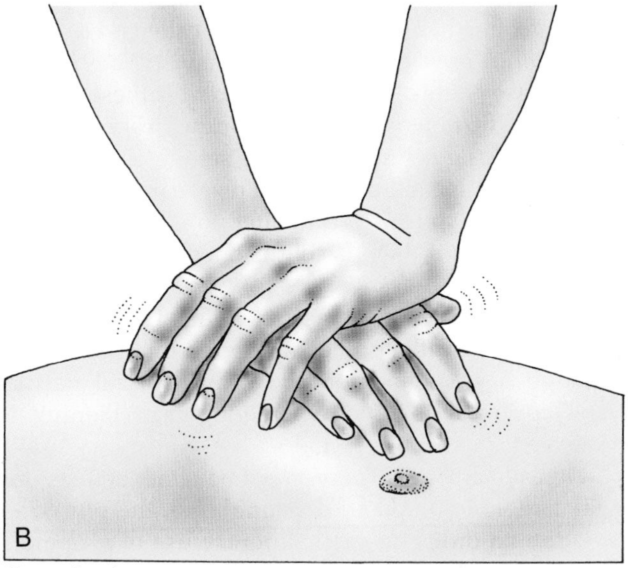

Chest vibration

FIGURE 31-9 Chest physiotherapy. **A,** Percussion. **B,** Vibration. (Modified from Ignatavicius DD, Workman ML: *Medical-surgical nursing: patient-centered collaborative care*, ed 6, St. Louis, 2010, Saunders.)

increased intracranial pressure, chest trauma, pulmonary embolism, pulmonary edema, gastric reflux, pneumonectomy with open pericardium, extreme agitation or anxiety, and high risk for rib fractures.

Postural Drainage

Postural drainage is the technique of positioning the patient to facilitate gravitational movement of respiratory secretions toward the bronchi and trachea for expectoration. Various positions are used to drain all 18 segments of the lungs. If a patient cannot tolerate a specific position, it should be omitted or modified. Instruct the patient to breathe slowly and deeply throughout the procedure. Drain the upper lobes first and the posterior basal segments of the lower lobes last. The patient should not sit up between position changes. Provide tissues and a disposal receptacle. Maintain each position for 5 to 15 minutes. Perform postural drainage before meals or tube feedings. It may be ordered after respiratory treatments with bronchodilators. The frequency is ordered by the physician. Discontinue the procedure and inform the physician if the patient experiences a heart rate over 120 beats per minute, dysrhythmias, hypertension, hypotension, dizziness, or signs of **hypoxemia**.

HUMIDIFICATION AND AEROSOL THERAPY

The upper respiratory system is designed to moisturize and warm the air that is inspired through the nose. Humidity is necessary in the respiratory tract to prevent secretions from becoming inspissated (thickened and dried). Inspissated secretions irritate the mucosa, making it more susceptible to bacterial infection.

Humidifiers

A humidifier creates water vapor to raise the relative humidity of inspired gas to 100%. Several types of humidifying devices are available for use. Room humidifiers deliver water vapor directly into the air. Medical O_2 is humidified as it bubbles through a container of water. Humidifiers that require heat to create water vapor pose a risk of heat injury. The fluid reservoir can become contaminated, making it a source of airborne infection. To prevent the spread of bacteria, sterile water should be used to fill the reservoir and the equipment must be cleaned between each use. Finally, the equipment can present an electrical hazard.

Aerosol Therapy

Aerosol therapy is used to liquefy and mobilize respiratory secretions and to deliver medications. Aerosols are suspended liquid particles of bronchodilators or inactive fluids such as water or saline that are delivered by devices called *nebulizers*. Nebulizers deliver a humidified aerosol through large tubing, which may be connected to an O_2 mask or a handheld device. When handheld nebulizers are used, the patient should sit upright and slowly inhale the nebulizer aerosol deeply, hold the breath briefly, and exhale slowly. Once secretions are mobilized, the patient may require deep-breathing and coughing techniques, postural drainage, suctioning, or a combination of these techniques to clear the secretions. Because aerosols can cause bronchospasm, bronchodilators may be ordered before administering some types of aerosol therapy. A risk of fluid retention, infection, and drug toxicity also exists.

Pharmacology Capsule

Oxygen (O_2) should be thought of as a pharmacologic agent with risks of adverse effects.

OXYGEN THERAPY

Air in the atmosphere contains approximately 21% O_2. Usually this is sufficient for oxygenation to maintain the tissue's ability to function normally. In the presence of cardiopulmonary disease or injury, it may be necessary to provide a patient with supplemental O_2, in order to enrich the atmospheric air with increased concentrations than the patient normally breathes. O_2 should be treated as a pharmacologic agent, as serious side effects (as well as benefits) may occur from its use.

O_2 therapy requires a medical order that should be carried out like any other drug order. If a patient is observed becoming lethargic or bradypneic (abnormally slow breathing), the nurse should immediately notify a supervisor or physician because these are symptoms of adverse effects of O_2 therapy.

To administer O_2 to the patient, it is necessary to alter the gas from a compressed form such as a bulk O_2 supply or cylinder to a form with a usable, safe flow rate. Modern hospitals have bulk O_2 systems with wall adapters to which flowmeters are attached. When patients with O_2 must be transported, a cylinder on wheels is necessary. A regulator with a flowmeter must be used. After a flowmeter has been attached to the O_2 source, it may be necessary to humidify the gas before delivering it to the patient. Humidification is usually unnecessary when using a low-flow cannula at a flow setting of 2 L (or less) per minute or when using an air entrainment (Venturi mask) O_2 delivery system.

A tube is needed to connect the flowmeter to the specific O_2 delivery device being used. In some devices the tube is incorporated as an integral component but in others it is not. It is possible to use extension tubes for some devices but increasing the length of the tube increases the resistance to gas flow, thus causing pressure to back up in the system so that the patient may not receive the desired O_2 flow.

O_2 therapy is ordered in liters per minute—or fraction of inspired O_2 (FiO_2). This measurement is written, for example, as 0.30 FiO_2, which means 30% O_2 concentration. Various devices can deliver different amounts of O_2 (Fig. 31-10).

The most commonly used device is the nasal cannula, which fits around the face and directly into the nares by way of two prongs. It is designed to deliver a low flow of O_2 from 1 to 6 L/min with an approximate FiO_2 of 0.24 to 0.40 (24% to 40% O_2). The nasal catheter is also a low-flow device that is inserted into one naris and then into the pharyngeal space approximately at the uvula. The FiO_2 and flow rates are the same as those for the cannula. This catheter is rarely used, except during short-term procedures.

Four types of masks are available: (1) the simple oxygen mask, (2) the partial rebreathing mask, (3) the nonrebreathing mask, and (4) the air entrainment (Venturi) mask. The simple O_2 mask is designed to deliver an FiO_2 ranging from 0.35 to 0.55 (35% to 55% O_2). Flow rates from the flowmeter may be adjusted from 6 to 10 L/min. The minimum flow rate of 6 L/min is necessary to prevent any chance of CO_2 buildup from occurring. The partial rebreathing mask includes a reservoir bag to elevate the potential FiO_2. It is unique because the patient actually rebreathes part of the exhaled gas in the system. However, it is designed so that the rebreathed gas contains almost no CO_2 from the patient's lungs—only enriched O_2. The expected FiO_2 range is 0.35 to 0.60 (35% to 60%). The flowmeter setting must be from 6 to 10 L/min. The nonrebreathing mask is so named because none of the patient's exhaled gas is rebreathed. Like the previous mask, it also includes a reservoir bag to enhance the FiO_2 but it has a series of valves to direct the flow of O_2 in such a way that the patient receives a fresh supply of gas with each breath. The expected FiO_2 should be near 1.0 (100%). However, experimental research has shown that the highest FiO_2 obtained is approximately 0.7 (70%). The air entrainment mask is designed to provide a specific FiO_2. This device has been called a *Ventimask* or a *Venturi mask* in the past and may still be referred to by these names. The manufacturers of these devices list a specific flowmeter setting for the desired FiO_2. It is also necessary either to adjust a setting on the device or to place a specific attachment on the mask to obtain the desired results. Read the literature accompanying the mask and, if there is confusion, consult a respiratory therapist.

Transtracheal O_2 therapy delivers O_2 through a small, flexible catheter that is inserted into the trachea through a small incision or with a special needle. This approach is used when long-term therapy is indicated.

Occasionally an O_2 mask must be removed (e.g., for oral care, for eating and drinking). Ask the physician to write an order for the temporary use of a cannula during these times.

Advances in outpatient O_2 therapy have the potential to improve greatly the quality of life for patients with chronic pulmonary or cardiac conditions. Whereas patients used to have to rent large cylinders for home use, they can now rent O_2 concentrators that process room air and deliver air with an increased percentage of O_2. The concentrator is about the size of a canister vacuum cleaner and has a 50-foot tubing connected to a nasal cannula. This allows the patient considerable freedom of mobility in the home setting.

To leave the home, patients can use small tanks of compressed O_2. The tanks weigh approximately 3 pounds and can deliver 2 L/min of O_2 for approximately 3 hours. A device that can be used with the canister delivers O_2 only "on demand," when the patient inhales. This conserves the O_2, making the canister last longer. Portable liquid O_2 canisters that can deliver a very high flow of O_2 are also available. These canisters can be refilled from a larger tank that can be kept in the patient's home. A weekend version of the

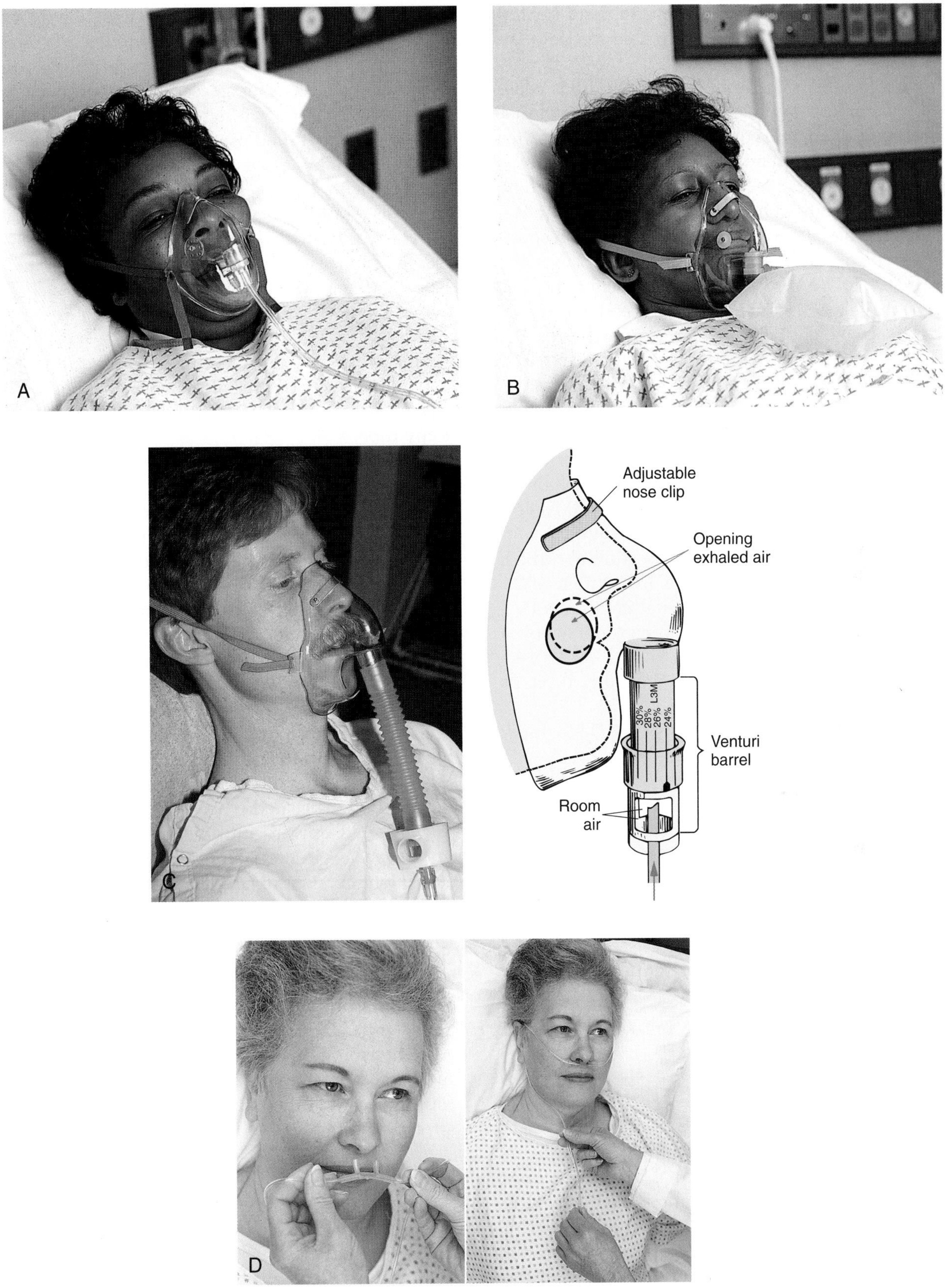

FIGURE 31-10 Oxygen (O_2) delivery systems. **A,** Standard O_2 mask. **B,** Partial rebreathing O_2 mask. **C,** Venturi O_2 mask. **D,** Nasal cannula (From Potter PA, Perry AG, Stockert P, Hall A, editors: *Fundamentals of nursing*, ed 8, St. Louis, 2013, Mosby-Elsevier.)

tank fits in the backseat of a car and lasts several days. These devices allow considerable freedom for the patient.

The nurse must recognize the complications of O_2 therapy, including hypoventilation, toxicity, atelectasis, and ocular damage. Patients at the greatest risk for O_2-induced hypoventilation are those with chronic respiratory disorders. Because they may have become insensitive to high CO_2 levels in the blood, low O_2 levels in the blood serve as the stimulus for respirations ("hypoxic drive"). O_2 administration raises the level of O_2 in the blood and the patient who has hypoxic drive may hypoventilate or even have apnea. The primary goal of supplemental oxygen for the patient with a chronic respiratory disorder is to maintain the pulse oxygen saturation (SpO_2) at 90% to 93% and the arterial oxygen tension (PaO_2) at 60 to 70 mm Hg. O_2 toxicity can result from exposure to a high concentration of O_2 for a prolonged period of time. Toxicity progresses from tracheobronchitis to lung fibrosis and atelectasis and may be fatal. Atelectasis can result from the replacement of nitrogen normally in the alveoli with O_2. O_2 is readily absorbed, predisposing the alveoli to collapse. Exposure to 100% O_2 can cause retinal injury and visual impairment.

The following are key points to consider when a patient is receiving O_2 therapy:

1. Monitor the liter flow to be sure it is as prescribed.
2. Assess the patient's response to O_2 therapy; monitor reports of blood gas analyses.
3. Inspect the tubing for kinks, obstructions, and loose connections; listen for a hissing sound in the O_2 mask; feel for adequate O_2 flow.
4. Maintain sterile water in the humidifier reservoir.
5. Clean and replace O_2 therapy equipment according to agency policy.
6. Post a NO SMOKING sign and advise the patient and visitors that smoking is not allowed because O_2 supports combustion.
7. Monitor for potential skin breakdown around the oxygen delivery device.

INTERMITTENT POSITIVE PRESSURE BREATHING TREATMENTS

Intermittent positive pressure breathing (IPPB) treatments are used to achieve maximal lung expansion. The IPPB equipment delivers humidified gas with positive pressure, which forces air into the lungs with inhalation and allows passive exhalation. This facilitates maximal exchange of O_2 and CO_2 gases in the alveoli and promotes a productive cough. Aerosol medications, including mucolytics (which liquefy secretions) and bronchodilators, can be administered through IPPB treatments with a nebulizer device. Although respiratory therapists administer most IPPB treatments, in some settings nurses administer them.

In the past, IPPB was used for a wide range of conditions. The American Association for Respiratory Care now recommends it only for specific conditions, including atelectasis, decreased lung compliance with kyphoscoliosis, and cardiogenic pulmonary edema. In addition to its limited usefulness, IPPB is losing favor because it may cause a tension pneumothorax in patients with COPD. It also may cause respiratory alkalosis because of hyperventilation. The desired effects of IPPB usually can be achieved by other, less expensive measures such as incentive spirometry and handheld nebulizers.

ARTIFICIAL AIRWAYS

Artificial airways are sometimes required to maintain a patent airway. Artificial airways include the oral airway, nasal airway, endotracheal tube, and tracheostomy tube.

Oral Airway

The oral airway is a curved tube used to maintain an airway temporarily. The oropharyngeal airway is inserted by tilting the head back, opening the mouth, and inserting the airway into the patient's mouth with the tip pointed toward the roof of the mouth. The tube is turned over while being advanced so that the end of the tube rests on the base of the patient's tongue.

Nasal Airway

A nasopharyngeal airway is a soft rubber tube that is inserted through the nose and extended to the base of the tongue. After ruling out a deviated septum, the nasal airway is coated with a water-soluble lubricant and inserted upward into the nose so that the distal end is located in the pharynx at the level of the base of the tongue. A nasal airway should be changed from one naris to the other every 8 hours.

Endotracheal Tube

An endotracheal tube is a long tube inserted through the mouth or nose into the trachea. These tubes have cuffs—inflatable balloons that seal the trachea to prevent aspiration of foreign material and to facilitate mechanical ventilation. Insertion of an endotracheal tube and care of the patient who is intubated require specialized training.

Tracheostomy Tube

A tracheostomy is a surgically created opening through the neck into the trachea. A variety of tracheostomy tubes exist and they may be used with or without cuffs. Care of the patient with a tracheostomy is discussed in Chapter 30.

MECHANICAL VENTILATION

Mechanical ventilation is the process of providing respiratory support by means of a mechanical device called a *ventilator.* Ventilators are required most commonly for patients with acute respiratory failure who are unable to maintain adequate gas exchange in the lungs. This may be evidenced by **tachypnea** or bradypnea with an elevated or a stable $PaCO_2$, low PaO_2, or low pH. To ventilate a patient mechanically, a cuffed endotracheal or tracheostomy tube must be used to deliver the air. Once the tube is in place, the cuff must be inflated to create a closed system in the patient's airway. Otherwise, air being forced into the lungs could simply flow back out through the trachea.

A volume-limited ventilator is used most commonly for patients with acute respiratory failure. It inflates the lungs with a preset volume of oxygenated air that is delivered under pressure during the inspiratory cycle. The expiratory cycle may be conducted passively or with pressure as indicated.

Three types of positive pressure ventilators exist: (1) volume cycled, (2) pressure cycled, and (3) time cycled. A volume-cycled ventilator, which delivers a constant preset amount of oxygenated air to the patient, is the most commonly used type. A pressure-cycled ventilator, which pushes air into the lungs until a preset pressure is reached, is not widely used for continuous mechanical ventilation. Time-cycled ventilators deliver oxygenated air during a preset length of time. This type is used most frequently in infants and children.

Depending on the patient's needs, ventilators may be programmed to control or assist the rate of ventilation. The most frequently used modes are intermittent mandatory ventilation and synchronized intermittent mandatory ventilation. These modes provide assistance with ventilation by allowing the patient to breathe spontaneously between a preset number of ventilator breaths. Ventilators deliver O_2 ranging in concentration from 21% O_2 (atmospheric air) to 100% O_2. The O_2 concentration, or FiO_2, is adjusted for individual patient needs.

Tidal volume is the preset amount of oxygenated air delivered during each ventilator breath. This is usually 10 to 15 mL/kg of the patient's body weight.

The respiratory rate setting is the total number of breaths delivered per minute. The ventilator alone may govern the respiratory rate, or the ventilator and the patient's spontaneous respirations may determine it.

Positive end-expiratory pressure may be prescribed to keep the pressure in the lungs greater than the atmospheric pressure at the end of expiration. This reduces collapse of small airways and alveoli, thereby increasing the FRC and improving ventilation.

Other mechanical ventilation modalities include options such as pressure support ventilation, flow-by ventilation, continuous positive airway pressure (CPAP) ventilation, and high-frequency ventilation. These are mentioned only for completeness and not for discussion. If the nurse encounters any of these modalities, specific training is needed that is beyond the scope of this text.

Like much other health care technology, mechanical ventilation can now be managed in the home. With proper training, a family member can manage these devices. Individuals with sleep apnea use a CPAP unit. CPAP maintains positive pressure in the airway during sleep, thereby preventing periods of apnea. CPAP units are small and have a face mask that is worn during sleep.

Nursing care of patients on mechanical ventilation requires special training but key aspects of care include the following:

1. Monitor settings to ensure that they are set as prescribed.
2. Ensure that high- and low-pressure alarm settings are activated.
3. Have a manual resuscitator and O_2 source readily available.
4. Do not allow water to accumulate in the tubing.
5. Monitor the patient's vital signs and breath sounds; suction as necessary.
6. Establish an alternate method of communication because the patient cannot speak while intubated.

CHEST TUBES

Chest tubes are inserted to drain air or fluid from the pleural space of the lungs. This permits reexpansion of a collapsed lung in the patient with a hemothorax, pneumothorax, or pleural effusion. The physician inserts chest tubes under sterile conditions in the operating room or at the patient's bedside. Multiple tubes may be inserted. A small incision is made to insert one chest tube in the second to fourth intercostal space to remove air. A tube placed in the eighth or ninth intercostal space is for fluid removal. The tubes are sutured in place and an airtight sterile dressing is applied. The distal ends of the plastic chest tubes are connected to sterile rubber tubing that leads to a pleural drainage device composed of three compartments: (1) the collection chamber, (2) the water seal chamber, and (3) the suction control chamber (Fig. 31-11). Chest fluid and air drain into the collection chamber. Air is diverted to the water seal chamber, where it can be seen bubbling up through the water. Suction pressure is controlled in the suction control chamber. The tubing in the suction chamber is partially submerged in water; the depth of the tube in the water regulates the amount of suction. After the tubes have been inserted, a chest radiograph is obtained to confirm placement.

Monitor the patient's vital signs, breath sounds, and oxygen status frequently. Assess the dressing to ensure that a tight seal is maintained. Tape tubing connections and inspect the connections frequently to detect air leaks. Coil extra tubing on the bed to avoid kinks and keep the drainage system on the floor. Monitor the drainage for blood clots or lung tissue, which may

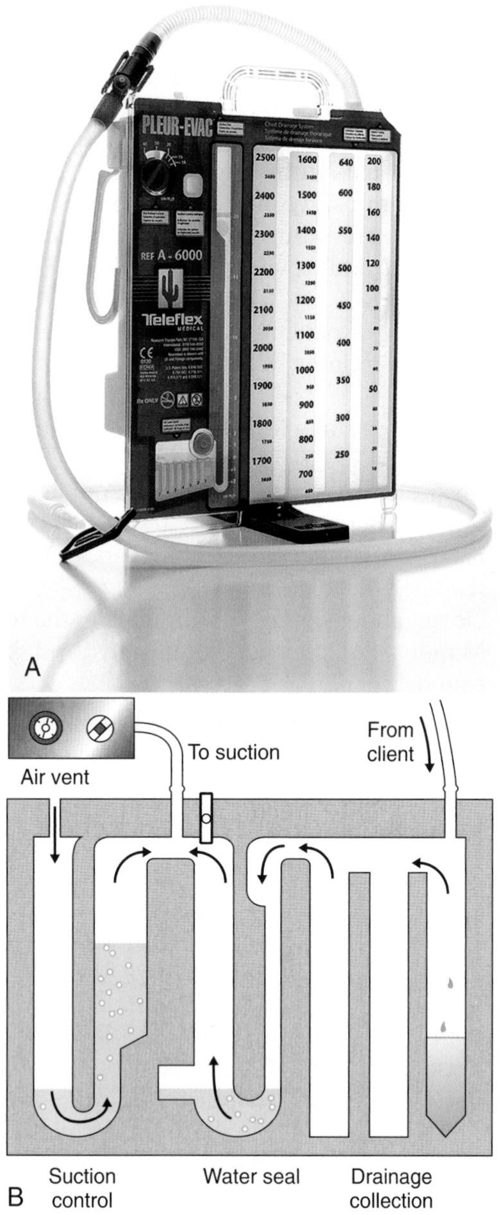

FIGURE 31-11 A, A commonly used disposable chest drainage system. **B,** Diagram of chambers of water seal chest drainage. (A, Courtesy Teleflex Medical Incorporated. B, From Ignatavicius DD, Workman ML, Mishler MA: *Medical-surgical nursing across the health care continuum*, ed 3, Philadelphia, 1999, Saunders.)

have to be gently kneaded downward to keep the tube patent. Agency and physician preferences dictate whether chest tubes are stripped or milked (Fig. 31-12). Observe the chambers for bubbling. When the system is initially connected to the patient, bubbles are usually seen in the water seal chamber. After a short time, bubbling in this chamber will stop until the lung has reexpanded or the tubing is occluded. If suction is prescribed, you will also see bubbling in the suction control chamber.

The rate of drainage is monitored by marking the drainage level on the drainage receptacle. The middle water seal chamber is observed for the expected rise in the fluid level with inspiration and the expected

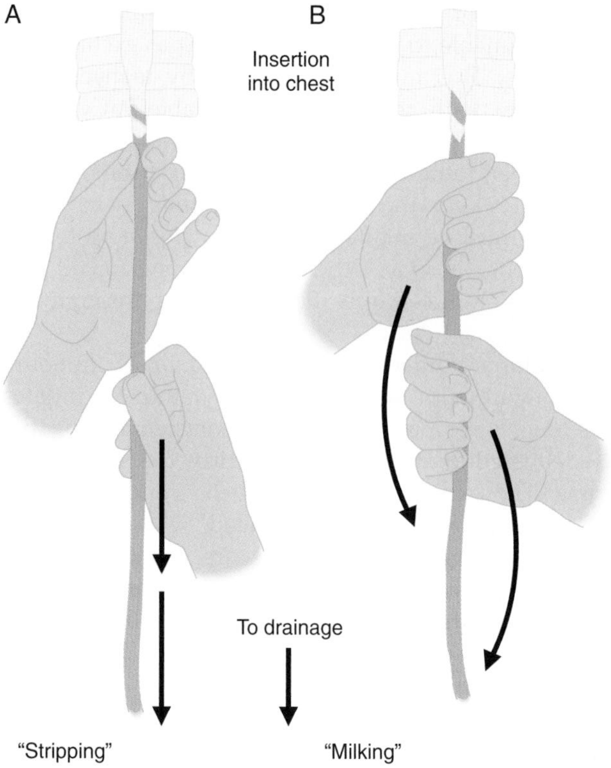

FIGURE 31-12 Two techniques for removing blood clots from chest tubes. **A,** Stripping. **B,** Milking. Both can create excessive negative pressure in the pleural space but milking is safer than stripping. Follow agency policies and physician orders in relation to these procedures. (From Black JM, Hawks JH, Keene AM: *Medical-surgical nursing: clinical management for continuity of care*, ed 6, Philadelphia, 2001, Saunders.)

fall with expiration. This is called *tidaling*. Continuous bubbling in the water seal chamber suggests an air leak. If an air leak is suspected, agency policy may permit the tubing to be clamped for a maximum of 10 seconds while locating the leak. Wet or dry drainage systems may be used. Wet chambers are regulated by maintaining the water level that is ordered by the physician. Gentle bubbling is expected in the wet suction chamber. Dry chambers are regulated by adjusting the dry suction until the float appears. The drainage receptacle is not usually changed unless the drainage chamber is full. Use sterile technique to change the receptacle. Know the agency policies and procedures for managing chest tubes.

An alternative to the large chest drainage systems is the Heimlich flutter valve. The valve is a disposable unit that is attached to the chest tube and to a sterile drainage receptacle. Air and fluid can flow into the receptacle but cannot flow backward into the chest. The patient who has a flutter valve can assume any position and can ambulate easily. A system with a flutter valve can be attached to chest suction if necessary.

THORACIC SURGERY

A thoracotomy is the surgical opening of the chest wall. Surgical procedures on the lung include pneumonectomy, lobectomy, segmental resection, and wedge resection. *Pneumonectomy* is the removal of an entire lung whereas a *lobectomy* is removal of one lobe of a lung. The extensive dissection and removal of a section of the lung is called a *segmental resection.* A *wedge resection* is the removal of a small, triangular section of lung tissue. Other procedures that require a thoracotomy are *decortication* and *thoracoplasty.* Decortication is stripping of the membrane that covers the visceral pleura and thoracoplasty is the removal of ribs. Among the most common purposes for thoracic surgery are evaluation of chest trauma, removal of tumors and cysts, and treatment of empyema.

PREOPERATIVE NURSING CARE of the Patient with a Thoracotomy

Preoperative nursing care is described in Chapter 17. Before thoracotomy, the nurse should emphasize postoperative breathing exercises. If the insertion of a chest tube is anticipated, the nurse should explain the procedure to the patient.

Assessment

After surgery, the nurse should monitor vital signs, lung sounds, mental status, dressings, and chest tube function and drainage.

Nursing Diagnoses, Goals, and Outcome Criteria: Thoracotomy

General postoperative nursing diagnoses are presented in Chapter 17. Diagnoses and goals specific to the patient who has had a thoracotomy may also include the following.

Nursing Diagnoses	Goals and Outcome Criteria
Impaired Gas Exchange related to ventilation-perfusion mismatch	Improved gas exchange: vital signs consistent with patient's norms, arterial blood gases within normal limits
Ineffective Breathing Pattern related to preexisting respiratory disease or pain	Effective breathing pattern: regular respirations without cyanosis or dyspnea
Ineffective Airway Clearance related to dry secretions or ineffective cough	Effective airway clearance: breath sounds clear to auscultation

Interventions

Impaired Gas Exchange

After a thoracotomy, the patient is at risk for pneumonia and atelectasis because of the effects of anesthesia (which impairs ciliary motion), drugs that dry secretions, and immobility. To improve gas exchange, position the patient with the head of the bed elevated 20 to 40 degrees. In the immediate postoperative period, the patient is usually placed on the unaffected side. Thereafter, various positions are permitted depending on the specific surgical procedure. Avoid the operative side after wedge resection or segmentectomy to encourage expansion of remaining lung tissue on the affected side. After pneumonectomy, also avoid the complete side-lying position on the affected side because this may encourage mediastinal shift. Administer oxygen as ordered.

Ineffective Breathing Pattern

Splint the thoracic incision while assisting the patient to breathe deeply and cough. An incentive spirometer may be used to encourage full expansion of the lungs. Adequate pain control enables the patient to breathe more effectively. Chest physiotherapy and bronchodilators are indicated for some patients. When permitted, assist the patient to sit on the edge of the bed with the feet flat on the floor. An overbed table can be placed in front of the patient, who can lean on it with folded arms. This position fosters movement of the diaphragm and chest expansion.

Ineffective Airway Clearance

Adequate oral fluid intake reduces the viscosity of mucus; therefore encourage fluids if not contraindicated. If the patient cannot tolerate adequate oral fluids, intravenous fluids may be ordered. For management of chronic respiratory conditions, see Chapter 32.

VIDEO THORACOSCOPY

Many procedures that formerly required thoracic surgery now can be done with video thoracoscopy. Thoracoscopy is performed by inserting an endoscope through a small thoracic incision. Procedures that can be done with this instrument include resection of pulmonary and mediastinal lesions, biopsy, drainage of effusions, sympathectomy, vagotomy, and thymectomy. Potential complications of thoracoscopy include atelectasis, pneumonia, air leaks, and injury to thoracic organs. A chest tube is usually needed to promote full reexpansion of the lung on the operative side. Otherwise, patient care is much less complicated than it is after thoracotomy. Monitor the patient's respiratory status, including lung sounds. Immediately report sudden dyspnea or other signs of respiratory distress to the surgeon. Document the amount and appearance of chest tube drainage. Inspect the closed drainage system for proper functioning. Incentive spirometry may be used to encourage lung expansion. Administer analgesics as ordered. Patients are usually permitted out of bed 4 to 6 hours after surgery and can return to work in 1 week. Before discharge, instruct the patient to notify the physician of dyspnea or a temperature greater than 101°F (38.3°C).

Pharmacology Capsule

People with hypertension, heart disease, and hyperthyroidism should not take over-the-counter (OTC) cold remedies without consulting a pharmacist or a physician. Many cold remedies stimulate the heart and raise the blood pressure.

DRUG THERAPY

Drugs used to treat respiratory disorders include decongestants, antitussives, antihistamines, expectorants, antimicrobials, bronchodilators, corticosteroids, mast cell stabilizers, leukotriene inhibitors, mucolytics, and thrombolytics, as described in Table 31-4.

Decongestants

Decongestants are adrenergics. They mimic the action of epinephrine and norepinephrine, causing constriction of nasal blood vessels and reducing the swelling of mucous membranes. OTC decongestants such as pseudoephedrine (Sudafed) are commonly used to treat the common cold. With oral decongestants, constriction of the blood vessels is not limited to the nasal passages, so systemic vasoconstriction and elevated blood pressure may result. Systemic effects are less severe with topical drops and sprays. Nevertheless, people with hypertension, heart disease, diabetes mellitus, and hyperthyroidism are usually advised to avoid decongestant drugs except under medical supervision.

Antitussives

Antitussives suppress the cough reflex. Antitussive action is not always desirable because coughing removes secretions from the airways. However, when a cough is nonproductive, creates pain, interferes with sleep, or impairs wound healing, temporary cough suppression may be indicated. Codeine is an effective antitussive; however, as an opioid drug, it can produce many unwanted side effects and has the potential for abuse. Therefore dextromethorphan, which is not an opioid, is more commonly used.

Table 31-4 Drug Therapy: Drugs Used to Treat Respiratory Disorders

DRUG	USE AND ACTION	SIDE EFFECTS	NURSING INTERVENTIONS
Decongestants			
pseudoephedrine (Sudafed)	Vasoconstriction. Reduce swelling of mucous membranes. Used to treat nasal discharge, common cold.	Occasional mild CNS stimulation, especially in older adults. Toxicity can cause lightheadedness, tachycardia, palpitations, nausea, vomiting, hallucinations, and seizures.	Monitor the patient's pulse, blood pressure, and mental and emotional state. Contraindicated in those with severe hypertension and coronary artery disease as well as those who are breastfeeding. Tell patients to swallow extended-release tablets whole.
Antitussives			
codeine, hydrocodone bitartrate (Hycodan), dextromethorphan	Suppression of cough reflex. Appropriate uses: control nonproductive cough or cough that interferes with rest or wound healing.	Codeine is an opioid and therefore has abuse potential and can cause sedation. Dextromethorphan does not have these effects.	Encourage fluids unless contraindicated to facilitate expectoration of secretions. Take safety measures with codeine.
Antihistamines			
diphenhydramine (Benadryl)	Block allergic response. Dry respiratory secretions. Also antiemetic and sedative effects.	Drowsiness, dry mouth, blurred vision, photophobia, thickening of mucus secretions, decreased sweating, constipation, urinary retention, and increased heart rate.	Take safety precautions if the patient is drowsy and monitor the patient's respiratory status (not recommended for patients with asthma). Encourage fluids if not contraindicated. Monitor elimination and oral hygiene.
Expectorants			
guaifenesin (Robitussin)	Thin respiratory secretions for easier expectoration.	Nausea and vomiting with large doses.	Assess the patient's cough productivity. Do not crush sustained-release capsules.

Table 31-4 **Drug Therapy: Drugs Used to Treat Respiratory Disorders—cont'd**

DRUG	USE AND ACTION	SIDE EFFECTS	NURSING INTERVENTIONS
Antimicrobials			
	Kill or inhibit the growth of bacteria, viruses, or fungi.	Side and adverse effects are specific to each antimicrobial classification. Common side effects are nausea, vomiting, and diarrhea. A risk of superinfections exists, such as yeast infections of the mouth and genitourinary tract. A risk of severe allergic response also exists.	Assess the patient's allergies before administration. Be alert for an allergic response: rash, dyspnea, loss of consciousness. Withhold the drug if an allergy is suspected. Instruct the patient to complete the entire course of therapy. Monitor the patient for improvement and for superinfections. Report continued symptoms to the physician.
Bronchodilators			
	Relax smooth muscle in the bronchial tree to relieve bronchial constriction.		
1. Methylxanthine drugs: theophylline, aminophylline	Methylxanthine drugs also cause increased heart rate and force of cardiac contraction, CNS stimulation, and increased gastric acid secretion.	Anxiety, restlessness, tachypnea, tachycardia, dysrhythmias, and GI distress. Rapid intravenous administration can cause hypotension and fatal dysrhythmias.	Monitor the patient's vital signs, mental state, and serum drug levels. Measure the patient's intake and output. Give the medication with milk or food to decrease GI distress. Do not administer the drug before bedtime because it may keep the patient awake.
2. Adrenergic drugs: sympathomimetics, epinephrine, isoproterenol hydrochloride (Isuprel), ephedrine	Adrenergic drugs also decrease mucus secretion, increase mucociliary clearance, and stabilize mast cells.	Restlessness, anxiety, tachycardia, headache, hypertension, disorientation, nausea, vomiting, and diarrhea.	Do not exceed the prescribed dosage. Teach the patient to use an inhaler and to rinse the mouth after inhalation to decrease dryness and irritation. Avoid excessive caffeine. Monitor the patient's respiratory and cardiovascular status.
Selective beta$_2$ agonists: albuterol sulfate (Proventil), terbutaline sulfate (Brethine), isoetharine hydrochloride (Bronkosol)		Less cardiac stimulation occurs with beta$_2$ agonists than with nonselective adrenergics.	
3. Inhaled muscarinics: ipratropium bromide (Atrovent)	Inhaled muscarinic drugs act directly on the respiratory passages to cause bronchodilation. Not effective for acute asthma attacks.	Increased intraocular pressure with narrow-angle glaucoma. Rare: hypotension.	Monitor the patient's respiratory status. Evaluate the patient for improvement. Tell the patient not to use more than two inhalations at a time and to rinse the mouth after inhaling to reduce dry mouth and throat. Avoid excessive caffeine intake.

Continued

these droplets through breathing, sneezing, or coughing or by direct hand contact. Touching contaminated surfaces and then carrying the virus to the nasal membranes and eyes is the most common means of spreading a cold. Therefore careful attention to hand washing is one of the best preventive measures for avoiding this illness.

Signs and Symptoms

Colds occur most frequently during the winter months when people tend to stay indoors and can more easily contaminate one another. A cold lasts 2 to 14 days and people are most contagious during the first 3 days. Symptoms include a feeling of nasal dryness and stuffiness, sneezing, runny nose, headache, sore throat, lethargy, and fatigue. In severe cases, chills, fever, and marked prostration may be present.

Complications

Although most people with colds recover without incident, viral or bacterial pneumonitis develops in some patients.

Medical Diagnosis

The common cold is diagnosed on the basis of patient history and clinical presentation.

Medical Treatment

The most common treatment for a cold is a combination of rest, fluids, proper diet, antipyretics, and analgesic medications. Antibiotics and currently available antivirals are usually not indicated because they are not effective against cold viruses. Studies have been inconclusive about the value of using large doses of vitamin C for treating and preventing a cold. Other drugs that may be used to relieve the symptoms of the common cold by drying secretions are antihistamines and decongestants. Herbal products commonly used to treat the common cold include echinacea and goldenseal. However, limited research exists to support the efficacy of these products. Thorough hand washing can help to prevent colds (see *Health Promotion* box).

Health Promotion

Meeting *Healthy People 2020* Objectives for Inappropriate Use of Antibiotics

The *Healthy People 2020* objective for immunizations and infectious diseases is to increase immunization rates and reduce preventable infectious diseases. Inappropriate use of antibiotics multiplies the potential for worldwide epidemics of all types of infectious diseases. Nurses caring for patients suffering from the common cold can help to advance this objective through the following actions:

- Teach patients the difference between bacterial and viral infections.
- Teach patients that the common cold from a viral cause does not require antimicrobial therapy.

Health Promotion—cont'd

- Reinforce health promotion considerations such as frequent hand washing using soap and warm water for at least 20 seconds. Instruct the patient to cover his or her mouth and nose when coughing or sneezing.
- Teach patients the importance of adequate nutrition to reduce their susceptibility to infectious organisms.

NURSING CARE of the Patient with Acute Viral Rhinitis

Assessment

The complete assessment of the patient with a respiratory disorder is summarized in Box 31-1. The health history may be limited in scope and include a complete description of symptoms, past medical history, and drug history. The physical examination focuses on the nose, throat, ears, neck, and chest.

Nursing Diagnosis, Goal, and Outcome Criteria: Common Cold

The primary diagnosis for the patient with a common cold is *ineffective self-health management* related to lack of understanding of treatment, prevention, and signs and symptoms of complications. The goal of nursing care is effective patient management of the cold with full recovery and no complications. If the patient is at risk for secondary infection, the goal is absence of signs of worsening infection.

Criteria for assessing the effective patient management of the plan of care are the patient's verbalization of understanding the content presented and a statement of intent to follow the plan of care. Absence of infection is evidenced by normal vital signs, clear breath sounds, and clear sputum.

Interventions

The common cold is unlikely to require inpatient care unless a patient is immunocompromised. Therefore the primary nursing intervention is usually patient teaching. Advise the patient to rest and to maintain a daily fluid intake of 2 to 3 liters, if not contraindicated. Hydration is essential for keeping secretions thin for ease of expectoration. A room humidifier may provide comfort by moistening mucous membranes. Fever can be treated with antipyretics. If the physician has prescribed or recommended drugs, inform the patient of the proper use, dosage, and side effects. Many drugs used to treat symptoms of the common cold cause drowsiness, so advise the patient to avoid activities that require mental alertness.

Infection control measures are needed to prevent the spread of the cold and to protect the patient who has a cold from secondary bacterial infections. During the first 3 days, the patient is most contagious. The patient should avoid contact with others, especially those who are at increased risk for infection (i.e., young children, older adults, and people who are immunosuppressed), to prevent the spread of the cold (see *Patient Teaching* box).

Patient Teaching

Common Cold

To reduce the risk of spreading the cold or of acquiring secondary bacterial infection:

- Avoid close contact with other people who have bacterial infections.
- Avoid crowded places.
- Avoid sharing drinking glasses or eating utensils.
- Practice good hand washing with antibacterial soap.
- Cover the mouth when coughing or sneezing.
- Use disposable tissues for expectorated secretions; dispose of them promptly.
- If you develop purulent (greenish) sputum; chest pain; a temperature higher than 100°F (37.8°C); a red, sore throat; or lung congestion, contact the physician, because these signs and symptoms suggest a more severe respiratory condition that may require additional treatment.

Pharmacology Capsule

Explain to patients that antibacterials are not usually prescribed for the common cold, because they are effective only against bacteria (and the common cold is caused by a virus).

ACUTE BRONCHITIS

Cause and Risk Factors

Acute bronchitis is a common condition that may follow a viral infection such as a cold or influenza. Bronchitis is usually viral in origin but bacterial causes (*Streptococcus pneumoniae* or *Haemophilus influenzae*) also are common. Irritation and inflammation may occur throughout the upper respiratory tract, resulting in an increased production of mucus. Excess production of mucus leads to coughing and sputum production.

Signs and Symptoms

Symptoms of acute bronchitis include fever, cough, yellow or green sputum, rapid breathing, and chest pain.

Medical Diagnosis

Acute bronchitis is usually diagnosed on the basis of the health history and clinical presentation.

Medical Treatment

Treatment consists of a broad-spectrum antibiotic (e.g., ampicillin, tetracycline, erythromycin) for 7 to 10 days; hospitalization is usually not necessary.

❖ NURSING CARE of the Patient with Acute Bronchitis

Nursing care for acute bronchitis is similar to that for the common cold. In addition, the nurse should encourage patients who are taking antibiotics to take the full course of the medication.

INFLUENZA

The term *flu* is commonly used to describe a number of ailments involving various body systems. However, influenza is actually an acute viral respiratory infection that is accompanied by a fever. Several strains of the influenza virus exist (i.e., influenzas A, B, and C). A strain is further subtyped according to the place and year it was isolated. Influenza usually occurs in epidemics during the winter months, with approximately 10% to 15% of people worldwide contracting the virus annually. Acute respiratory infections, including influenza, are the 8th leading cause of death in the United States, accounting for 56,000 deaths annually. On average, influenza leads to more than 200,000 hospitalizations and 36,000 deaths each year. The 2009 H1N1 influenza pandemic caused an estimated 270,000 hospitalizations and 12,270 deaths (1270 of which were children) in North America between April 2009 and March 2010. Global pandemics of viral infections can be devastating because of their wide geographic spread. Those most susceptible to the influenza virus are very young children, older adults, people living in institutional settings, people with chronic diseases, and health care personnel.

Complications

The most common complications of influenza are bronchitis and viral or bacterial pneumonia. Other, less common complications are myocarditis, pericarditis, Reye syndrome, confusion, seizures, Guillain-Barré syndrome (GBS), toxic shock syndrome, myositis, and renal failure.

Signs and Symptoms

Influenza is similar to the common cold in the way it is spread (i.e., through droplet infection); however, its symptoms differ from those of the common cold. People with colds experience nasal symptoms and malaise and usually are afebrile (without fever) whereas those with influenza typically experience an abrupt onset of symptoms. These symptoms include headache, fever, general aches, weakness, and myalgia, accompanied by respiratory tract symptoms, particularly cough and sore throat. However, a wide spectrum of clinical presentations may occur, ranging from a mild, afebrile upper respiratory illness to prostration and severe systemic signs and symptoms. The most common complication that occurs during outbreaks of influenza is pneumonia (both viral and bacterial).

Medical Diagnosis

A diagnosis of influenza is usually based on the patient's history and physical findings. Laboratory tests for confirming infections caused by the influenza virus are improving dramatically and can provide results in less than 48 hours. However, viral tests in general are expensive and may not be available in all facilities.

Medical Treatment

Treatment of influenza is similar to the treatment of the common cold: rest, fluids, proper diet, antipyretics, and analgesics. First-generation antiviral agents such as amantadine hydrochloride (Symmetrel) or rimantadine (Flumadine) can be used to treat type A influenza. Second-generation antiviral medications such as oseltamivir (Tamiflu) and zanamivir (Relenza) treat influenza types A and B. With either generation, therapy must be started within 24 to 48 hours after the onset of symptoms and continued for 10 days. For the latest information on the use of antivirals to treat influenza, visit www.cdc.gov/flu/professionals/antivirals.

The best treatment for influenza is prevention through immunization, especially for older adults, people with chronic illnesses, health care personnel, and people living in crowded environments. The *Department of Health and Human Services Centers for Disease Control and Prevention National Immunization Guidelines* recommends an annual influenza vaccine. Two types of vaccine are available: (1) an inactivated vaccine and (2) a live vaccine. The live attenuated influenza vaccine (LAIV) FluMist is indicated for healthy, nonpregnant persons aged 2 through 49 years. FluMist is given intranasally. The inactivated influenza vaccine is recommended for all others, including health care workers. These immunizations are usually given in the fall of each year. "Flu shots," the inactivated vaccines, are given with a needle via the intramuscular or intradermal route. The three types of influenza injections being produced for the United States market now include the regular vaccine approved for use in people 6 months of age and older, given intramuscularly; a high-dose vaccine for people ages 65 and older, also give intramuscularly; and an intradermal vaccine for people ages 18 to 64 years.

The protection rate for influenza vaccines is approximately 70% in the general population but may be lower among older adults. Although the incidence of adverse reactions to influenza immunizations is low, some people report having a sore arm, headache, fever, muscle aches, nausea, and diarrhea. Reported intranasal vaccine reactions include runny nose, nasal congestion, or cough. Acetaminophen, 325 mg taken every 4 hours for the first 12 hours, may reduce these symptoms. Other measures to reduce the risk of influenza are good nutrition and hygiene (see *Complementary and Alternative Therapies* box). An antiviral also may be prescribed for people who are at increased risk of acquiring viral infections.

Complementary and Alternative Therapies

Echinacea is an herb taken orally to stimulate immune function, suppress inflammation, and treat viral infections such as the common cold and influenza. Scientific studies have found no effect on the incidence, severity, or duration of colds.

Pharmacology Capsule

Antiviral drugs must be administered soon after the onset of influenza symptoms to be effective.

❖ NURSING CARE of the Patient with Influenza

Nursing care of the patient with influenza is similar to care of the patient with the common cold. Ongoing monitoring is particularly important with influenza because of the risk of serious complications, especially in older adults. Routine annual influenza vaccination is now recommended for all persons 6 months of age and older but most importantly for those individuals at high risk: those with serious chronic cardiopulmonary disorders, residents of long-term care facilities, health care providers who have contact with high-risk patients, people older than 65 years, and those who have chronic metabolic disorders such as diabetes mellitus.

PNEUMONIA

Cause and Risk Factors

The term *pneumonia* describes inflammation of certain parts of the lung such as the alveoli and bronchioles. Pneumonia may be caused by either infectious or noninfectious agents. Examples of infectious agents are bacteria, fungi, and nonspecific viruses. Noninfectious agents may include irritating fumes, dust, or chemicals that are inhaled or foreign matter that is aspirated. Nosocomial pneumonia is a health care–associated infection that may be attributed to inadequate hand washing, poor sterile technique with suctioning, contaminated equipment, and exposure to others who have infectious respiratory conditions.

People who are most likely to contract pneumonia are smokers; those with altered consciousness from alcohol, seizures, anesthesia, drug overdose, or other neurologic disorders; those who are immunosuppressed; chronically ill people who are malnourished or debilitated; and people on bed rest with prolonged immobility.

Patients at increased risk for aspiration pneumonia are those with impaired swallowing or cough reflexes, decreased gastrointestinal (GI) motility, esophageal abnormalities, tube feedings, tracheostomies, and endotracheal tubes.

Pathophysiology

Pneumonia may be classified according to the causative organism—usually bacteria or viruses.

Gram-positive bacteria cause pneumococcal, staphylococcal, and streptococcal pneumonias and gram-negative bacteria cause pseudomonal and influenza pneumonias and legionnaires' disease. Pneumococcal pneumonia *(Streptococcus pneumoniae)* is the most common cause of bacterial pneumonia. Several different viruses, including the influenza virus, cause viral pneumonias.

The pathophysiology of pneumonia follows a predictable course. When pathogens invade the lungs, the inflammatory process causes fluid to accumulate in the affected alveoli. In a process called *hepatization*, capillaries dilate and neutrophils, red blood cells (RBCs), and fibrin fill the alveoli, causing the lung to appear red and granular. Next, blood flow decreases and leukocytes (white blood cells) and fibrin infiltrate the area and consolidate (solidify). As the infection resolves, the consolidated material dissolves and is ingested and removed by macrophages.

Complications

Although most people recover from pneumonia, it remains one of the leading causes of death, especially in older adults (Centers for Disease Control and Prevention, 2013). Relatively common pulmonary complications of pneumonia include pleurisy, pleural effusion, and atelectasis. Pleurisy is inflammation of the pleura that causes pain with breathing. Pleural effusion is the accumulation of fluid between the pleura that encases the lungs and the pleura that lines the thoracic cavity. A large amount of fluid can lead to collapse of the lung. Atelectasis refers to collapsed alveoli. Other less common pulmonary complications of pneumonia are lung abscesses, delayed resolution, and empyema. Empyema is the presence of purulent exudate in the pleural cavity. Potential systemic complications include pericarditis, arthritis, meningitis, and endocarditis.

Signs and Symptoms

Usual symptoms of pneumonia are fever, chills, sweats, chest pain, cough, sputum production, hemoptysis (coughing up blood), dyspnea (difficulty breathing), headache, and fatigue. Older adults, however, may experience confusion, anorexia, and weakness but no fever or cough. People with bacterial pneumonia may experience an abrupt explosive onset: severe, shaking chills; sharp, stabbing lateral chest pain, especially with coughing and breathing; and intermittent cough with rusty sputum. Viral pneumonia is characterized by burning or searing chest pain in the sternal area; a continuous, hacking, barking cough producing small amounts of sputum; and headache.

Medical Diagnosis

Diagnosis of pneumonia is based on the findings of the history and clinical presentation, sputum culture and Gram stain, chest radiograph, complete blood count, and blood culture.

Medical Treatment

Treatment usually consists of increased fluid intake (at least 3 L every 24 hours), limited activity or bed rest, antipyretics and analgesics, and in some cases O_2 and aerosol IPPB therapy. Bacterial pneumonias are treated with appropriate antibacterial agents; however, antibacterials are not used with viral pneumonias because they do not kill viruses.

The pneumococcal conjugate vaccine (PCV13) is recommended for all children under 24 months of age; children ages 24 to 59 months who have sickle cell disease, human immunodeficiency virus (HIV) infection, chronic disease, or immunosuppression; and children ages 24 to 59 months who are African American, Alaska Native, or American Indian. PCV13 is also recommended to help prevent pneumococcal disease in adults with certain medical conditions. The unconjugated pneumococcal vaccine (PPSV23) is recommended for all adults 65 years and older and for anyone who is 2 years and older and at high risk. PPSV23 is also recommended for adults 19 through 64 years of age who smoke cigarettes; have chronic diseases, particularly cardiovascular and respiratory diseases; have diabetes mellitus; are recovering from severe illness; or are living in nursing homes or other community living facilities. Vaccination with the unconjugated vaccine is not recommended for children younger than 2 years. A booster may be given to select patients after 6 years.

NURSING CARE of the Patient with Pneumonia

Assessment

Assessment of the patient with a respiratory disorder is summarized in Box 31-1 (see also Nursing Care Plan: Patient with Pneumonia).

Interventions

Ineffective Airway Clearance

Accumulated secretions in the respiratory tract impair gas exchange and may result in alveolar collapse. Therapeutic measures are taken to decrease the production and promote the expectoration of secretions. Administer antimicrobials, decongestants, and expectorants as ordered. A good cough is essential for removal of secretions but antitussive medications may be given as ordered if the patient becomes exhausted because of constant coughing. Encourage or assist the patient to change positions at least every 2 hours to help mobilize secretions. Other measures used to mobilize secretions are deep-breathing and coughing exercises, chest physiotherapy, and aerosol therapy. The patient who has a very weak cough may require suctioning. Provide tissues and a receptacle for disposal of secretions. Note the amount, color, and consistency of secretions. Auscultate lung sounds frequently to assess the effects of interventions to clear the airways.

Nursing Care Plan Patient with Pneumonia

ASSESSMENT

HEALTH HISTORY A 77-year-old retired schoolteacher comes to the clinic complaining of chills and fever, cough, sore throat, and chest pain. The physician diagnosed viral pneumonia and recommended hospitalization. She states that she had a cold for about 1 week and seemed to get progressively worse. She states that she has "a little" shortness of breath and tires very easily. Her chest pain is aggravated by coughing. She has been taking over-the-counter (OTC) cold remedies. She has a history of hypertension and congestive heart failure (CHF), for which she takes an angiotensin-converting enzyme (ACE) inhibitor and a diuretic. She lives alone in a one-story apartment. She has a close friend next door who visits frequently.

PHYSICAL EXAMINATION Vital signs: blood pressure 160/94 mm Hg, pulse 92 bpm, respiration 24 breaths per minute, temperature 100.6°F (38.1°C) measured orally. Height 5′9″, weight 175 lb. Alert, slightly dyspneic. Skin color pale. Nail beds slightly dusky. Lung sounds clear to auscultation over right lung fields. Wheezes and crackles auscultated in left lung. Frequent cough producing greenish sputum. No retractions or use of accessory muscles of respiration. Abdomen soft.

Nursing Diagnosis	Goals and Outcome Criteria	Interventions
Ineffective Airway Clearance related to increased sputum production and thick secretions	The patient will have a patent airway, as evidenced by clear breath sounds without wheezes or crackles.	Administer decongestants and expectorants as ordered. Administer antitussive medications as ordered if the cough interferes with rest. Suction only if necessary. Have the patient turn, deep breathe, and cough at least every 2 hours. Perform chest physiotherapy and provide aerosol therapy as ordered. Assess response. Monitor lung sounds, respiratory rate, and characteristics of secretions. Dispose of tissues in a sanitary manner.
Impaired Gas Exchange related to obstruction of airways by edema and secretions or atelectasis	The patient will have adequate oxygenation, as evidenced by normal arterial blood gases and vital signs.	Monitor vital signs, lung sounds, skin color, blood gas reports, and level of consciousness. Be alert for signs of hypoxemia: restlessness, tachycardia, and tachypnea. Report abnormal findings to the physician. Elevate the head of the bed. Administer oxygen (O_2) therapy as ordered.
Activity Intolerance related to fatigue or hypoxia	The patient will perform activities of daily living (ADL) as ordered without excessive fatigue or dyspnea.	Instruct the patient in activity restrictions. Plan care to allow periods of uninterrupted rest. Assist the patient with ADL as needed. Gradually encourage increased activity while monitoring for dyspnea and fatigue. Keep interactions short and limit visitors.
Imbalanced Nutrition: Less Than Body Requirements related to anorexia, dyspnea, or fatigue	The patient will maintain optimal nutritional status, as evidenced by stable body weight.	Monitor food intake and weight. If intake is poor, consult with the dietitian about patient preferences. Suggest small, frequent meals. Provide a pleasant environment for meals. Position the patient for comfort. Use an O_2 cannula during meals if permitted. Weigh the patient daily.
Risk for Deficient Fluid Volume related to inadequate fluid intake, fever, or mouth breathing	The patient's hydration will remain normal, as evidenced by fluid intake equal to output, moist mucous membranes, and blood pressure consistent with patient's norms.	Monitor the patient's fluid status for signs of fluid volume deficit: decreased skin turgor, concentrated urine, decreased urine output, dry mucous membranes, and elevated hemoglobin and hematocrit levels. Administer intravenous fluids as ordered. Encourage fluids by mouth up to 3 L/day as permitted. Record intake and output. Monitor the patient's temperature and treat fever as ordered. Keep the patient dry and lightly covered. Administer tepid sponge baths as ordered for fever but do not induce shivering. Use hypothermia blanket as ordered.
Acute Pain related to inflammation, cough, or muscle aches	The patient will report pain relief, as measured with a pain scale.	Use a pain scale to assess the patient's pain. Administer analgesics as ordered. Reposition the patient for comfort. Splint painful areas during coughing and deep breathing. Use massage and relaxation techniques. Document the effects of interventions.

Critical Thinking Questions

1. Identify the factors that make fluid balance a challenge for this patient.
2. What are the risks that occur when patients self-medicate?
3. How is body temperature related to fluid balance?

Nursing Diagnoses, Goals, and Outcome Criteria: Pneumonia

Nursing Diagnoses	Goals and Outcome Criteria
Ineffective Airway Clearance related to increased sputum production, thick secretions, ineffective cough	Effective airway clearance: clear breath sounds without wheezes or crackles
Impaired Gas Exchange related to obstruction of airways by edema and secretions or atelectasis	Adequate oxygenation: normal arterial blood gases, heart rate, and respiratory rate
Activity Intolerance related to obstruction of airways by edema and secretions or atelectasis	Improved activity tolerance: performance of daily activities without fatigue or dyspnea
Imbalanced Nutrition: Less Than Body Requirements related to anorexia, dyspnea, fatigue	Optimal nutritional status: stable body weight
Risk for Deficient Fluid Volume related to inadequate fluid intake, fever, mouth breathing	Normal hydration: fluid intake approximately equal to fluid output, moist mucous membranes, blood pressure consistent with patient norms
Acute Pain related to inflammation, cough, muscle aches	Pain relief: patient statement of pain relief, relaxed appearance

Impaired Gas Exchange

The edema and secretions that occur with pneumonia interfere with the exchange of gases in the lungs. The patient may have hypoxemia, meaning that the level of O_2 in the blood is low. At the same time, excess CO_2 may accumulate in the blood, a condition called **hypercapnia**. Because normal oxygenation is essential for all body tissues, efforts must be made to improve the patient's gas exchange.

To assess gas exchange, monitor vital signs, lung sounds, and skin color. Be alert for signs of hypoxemia: restlessness, tachycardia, and tachypnea. If arterial blood gases are being measured, report abnormal results to the physician. Hemoglobin may also be measured. Low hemoglobin is significant because it indicates the reduced O_2-carrying capacity of RBCs.

Measures that mobilize secretions, discussed earlier, are important in improving gas exchange. In addition, elevate the head of the bed. Some patients are more comfortable in a reclining chair that permits alterations in position. A semi-Fowler position decreases the pressure of the abdominal organs on the diaphragm so that the patient breathes more easily. Maintain oxygen therapy as ordered.

Activity Intolerance

Activity is usually restricted for the patient with pneumonia and may range from complete bed rest to limited activities. Schedule nursing care to prevent overtiring and allow periods of uninterrupted rest. Provide assistance as needed until the patient is able to resume self-care. Keep conversations short and encourage visitors not to tire the patient with long visits. When the patient begins to resume activities of daily living (ADL), evaluate the ability to tolerate daily activities.

Imbalanced Nutrition: Less Than Body Requirements

Good nutrition is essential to combat the infection and to promote healing (see *Nutrition Considerations* box). Assess the patient's usual dietary habits to provide baseline information so that the diet may be individualized. Monitor weight to determine the adequacy of nutrition. Weigh the patient before breakfast using the same scale each time. Monitor albumin and lymphocyte blood counts to detect low levels that are common with inadequate protein.

A typical diet for the patient with pneumonia is a high-protein, soft diet. Unfortunately, fatigue, dyspnea, and anorexia may interfere with adequate food intake. Provide the diet as ordered, assist the patient with the meal if needed, and document intake. To enhance the appetite, provide oral care before and after meals, elevate the head of the bed, and arrange the tray in an attractive and convenient manner. The diet should conform to the patient's preferences as much as possible. If oxygen is needed, a nasal cannula is recommended during meals. If the patient tires quickly, more frequent meals with smaller servings may be better received.

Nutrition Considerations

1. Adequate fluids may help to mobilize pulmonary secretions for expectoration.
2. Approximately 40% of patients admitted to intensive care units with acute respiratory failure are undernourished.
3. Nutritional support for patients with respiratory failure should begin within the first 3 to 4 days of hospitalization.
4. Patients who receive nutritional support are more easily weaned from ventilators than those who receive only intravenous glucose support.
5. A diet for patients who have been in acute respiratory failure should be high in nutrients.
6. Lung disease can substantially increase energy needs.
7. The patient who is malnourished is at increased risk for respiratory infections because of impaired immunity and possible impairment of defense mechanisms.
8. When a patient has a fever, each degree Celsius of elevation increases the metabolic rate 10% to 13%. For each degree Fahrenheit, the metabolic rate rises 7.2%.
9. Excessive intake of vitamin K–rich foods (e.g., cabbage, broccoli, cauliflower, asparagus, onions, spinach, fish, liver) can interfere with anticoagulation therapy.

Risk for Deficient Fluid Volume

The patient with pneumonia may lose excess fluid because of fever and mouth breathing and fluid intake may be inadequate because of fatigue and dyspnea. Dehydration causes respiratory secretions to be thicker and more difficult to mobilize. Signs and symptoms of deficient fluid volume include decreased skin turgor, concentrated urine, dry mucous membranes, and elevated hemoglobin and hematocrit levels. Therefore the patient should consume 3 L of fluid a day unless contraindicated. If the patient's oral intake is low, intravenous fluids may be ordered. Hard candy, if permitted, stimulates thirst and fluid intake. Intake and output records may be kept (see *Patient Teaching* box).

Patient Teaching

Pneumonia

The teaching plan for the patient with pneumonia should include the following points:

- Gradually increase your activities as you recover because fatigue may persist for several weeks.
- Avoid people with colds or other infections.
- You need plenty of rest, good nutrition, and 3 L of fluids each day (unless contraindicated).
- Complete any prescribed drugs after discharge.

Monitor the patient's temperature every 2 to 4 hours to detect fever. Administer antipyretics as ordered. Keep the patient dry and lightly covered. Keep the room at a comfortable temperature that avoids chilling. Tepid sponge baths may be given for high fevers as ordered but do not induce shivering. A hypothermia blanket may be needed to reduce body temperature.

Acute Pain

Treat pain with ordered analgesics. Also use positioning, splinting painful areas during deep breathing and coughing, and massage to promote comfort. Document the effects of comfort measures and notify the physician if the patient's pain is unrelieved or worsens. Other measures to manage pain are detailed in Chapter 15.

Prevention of Aspiration Pneumonia

Aspiration pneumonia may be prevented by using measures to avoid aspiration or to treat aspiration promptly should it occur. If a patient is at risk for aspiration, keep suction equipment on hand. Position patients with dysphagia (difficulty swallowing) upright with the neck in a neutral position or slightly bent forward during meals. Because semisolids are swallowed more easily than thin liquids, thickening agents may be added to liquids.

If a patient is receiving enteral feedings, elevate the head of the bed while the feeding is being delivered and for 30 minutes afterward. Check tube position per agency policy before each bolus feeding or at specified intervals. Measure residual before each bolus feeding and withhold the feeding according to physician orders or agency policy.

Stop continuous feedings for 20 to 30 minutes before lowering the patient's head. If a patient must be kept flat, the best position is on the right side. Check residual every 4 hours. If the residual is 20% more than the hourly rate, consult the physician about reducing the rate of feeding.

To reduce the risk of aspiration, position the unconscious patient on alternating sides with the head of the bed elevated unless contraindicated. Do not put fluids in the patient's mouth until the presence of a gag reflex has been established.

If aspiration is suspected, use suction to try to remove the foreign material. A side-lying position, if not contraindicated, may promote drainage from the airway. Stop the enteral feeding until it is ruled out as the source of the aspirated material. Monitor the patient closely and notify the physician. Administer oxygen as ordered.

PLEURISY (PLEURITIS)

Pleurisy is inflammation of the pleura. The most common causes are pneumonia, tuberculosis, injury to the chest wall, pulmonary infarction, and tumors. The most characteristic symptom of pleurisy is abrupt and severe pain. The pain almost always occurs on one side of the chest and patients usually can point to the exact spot where the pain is occurring. Breathing and coughing aggravate the pain.

Treatment of pleurisy is aimed at the underlying disease and at pain relief. Analgesics, antiinflammatory agents, antitussives, antimicrobials, and local heat therapy may be ordered.

❖ NURSING CARE of the Patient with Pleurisy

■ Assessment

Assessment of the patient with a respiratory disorder is summarized in Box 31-1.

Nursing Diagnoses, Goals, and Outcome Criteria: Pleurisy

The primary nursing diagnoses when a patient has pleurisy are listed here. Other diagnoses related to the underlying cause of pleurisy are possible.

Nursing Diagnoses	Goals and Outcome Criteria
Acute Pain related to inflammation	Pain relief: patient statement of pain relief, relaxed expression
Ineffective Breathing Pattern related to splinting, pleural effusion	Effective breathing pattern: vital signs within patient norms, normal breath sounds

Interventions

Acute Pain

When the patient reports pain, obtain a complete description including location, severity, precipitating factors, and alleviating factors. Use analgesics and splinting of the affected side to relieve pain. It is also helpful to splint the rib cage when coughing. If ordered, apply heat to the painful area and give antitussives to decrease painful coughing. If bed rest is prescribed, assist the patient with regular position changes. Administer nonsteroidal antiinflammatory drugs (NSAIDs) as ordered to reduce pain and inflammation (see *Patient Teaching* box). Monitor patients on NSAIDs for GI distress and bleeding.

Patient Teaching

Pleurisy

- Take deep breaths every 1 to 2 hours while awake.
- Sitting upright will make breathing more comfortable.
- If being discharged on nonsteroidal antiinflammatory drugs (NSAIDs):
  - Avoid aspirin because it increases the risk of bleeding.
  - Take NSAIDs with food, milk, or antacids if gastrointestinal (GI) distress occurs.

Ineffective Breathing Pattern

Monitor the patient's breathing pattern with attention to the symmetry of chest movement. Encourage the patient to turn, take deep breaths and cough, and ambulate if permitted to mobilize secretions and maximize ventilation. Elevate the head of the bed to improve lung expansion. If pleural effusion develops, the patient experiences progressive dyspnea, decreased or absent breath sounds in the affected area, and decreased chest wall movement on the affected side. A thoracentesis may be done to remove the accumulated fluid. If the procedure is done at the bedside, the nurse assists as described in the section titled "Common Therapeutic Measures."

CHEST TRAUMA

Traumatic chest injuries fall into two major categories: (1) nonpenetrating injuries and (2) penetrating injuries. Nonpenetrating or blunt injuries most commonly result from automobile accidents, falls, or blast injuries. In automobile accidents, 40% of the people killed have sustained blunt injuries from the steering wheel. The extent of the injury depends on the force and effect of the trauma. Common nonpenetrating injuries include rib fractures, pneumothorax, pulmonary contusion, and cardiac contusion. Penetrating injuries most commonly result from gunshot or stab wounds to the chest. Common penetrating injuries include pneumothorax and life-threatening tears of the aorta, vena cava, or other major vessels.

Chest trauma can result in changes in normal pressure relationships between air inside and outside the body, interference with normal breathing patterns and protective mechanisms such as cough, disturbances in blood flow to the lungs, swelling, and pain. Patients are therefore at risk for air entering the pleural space, infection and increased secretions in the tracheobronchial tree, hemorrhage, and abnormal fluid collection in the lung.

Signs and Symptoms

Signs and symptoms of chest injury may include obvious trauma to the chest wall (e.g., bruising); chest pain; dyspnea; cough; asymmetric movement of the chest wall; marked cyanosis of the mouth, face, nail beds, and mucous membranes; rapid, weak pulse; decreased blood pressure; deviation of the trachea; distended neck veins; and bloodshot or bulging eyes.

Medical Treatment

Immediate care of a person with a chest injury is directed at stabilization and prevention of further injury. Remove clothing to assess injury sites and to observe for other injuries such as bleeding. Immediately treat bleeding. Cover any open chest wound with an airtight dressing taped on three sides. This is called a *vented dressing*; it permits air to escape through the chest wound but prevents additional air from entering the chest through the wound. If you were to completely seal an open chest wound, air could continue to leak from the lung into the pleural space. With no exit, the leaking air could accumulate in the pleural space and create a tension pneumothorax (discussed under "Pneumothorax" below).

If an airtight dressing has been applied, be alert for worsening respiratory status (increasing dyspnea, cyanosis, distended neck veins, trachea deviated from midline, decreased breath sounds on the affected side), which requires removal of the airtight dressing. Do not remove impaled objects but stabilize them with bulky dressings. Monitor vital signs and level of consciousness, keeping in mind the potential for shock. Oxygen may be administered by nasal cannula. To facilitate breathing, put the client in a semi-Fowler position or on the injured side.

PNEUMOTHORAX

Chest injuries often cause pneumothorax, which is an accumulation of air in the pleural cavity that results in complete or partial collapse of a lung. Pneumothorax occurs in nearly half of the people who have chest injuries. Air enters the space between the chest wall and the lung, either through a hole in the chest wall or through a tear in the bronchus, bronchioles, or alveoli.

Two types of pneumothorax exist: (1) open and (2) tension. An open pneumothorax results from a chest wound that allows air to move in and out freely with inspiration and expiration. The lung on the affected

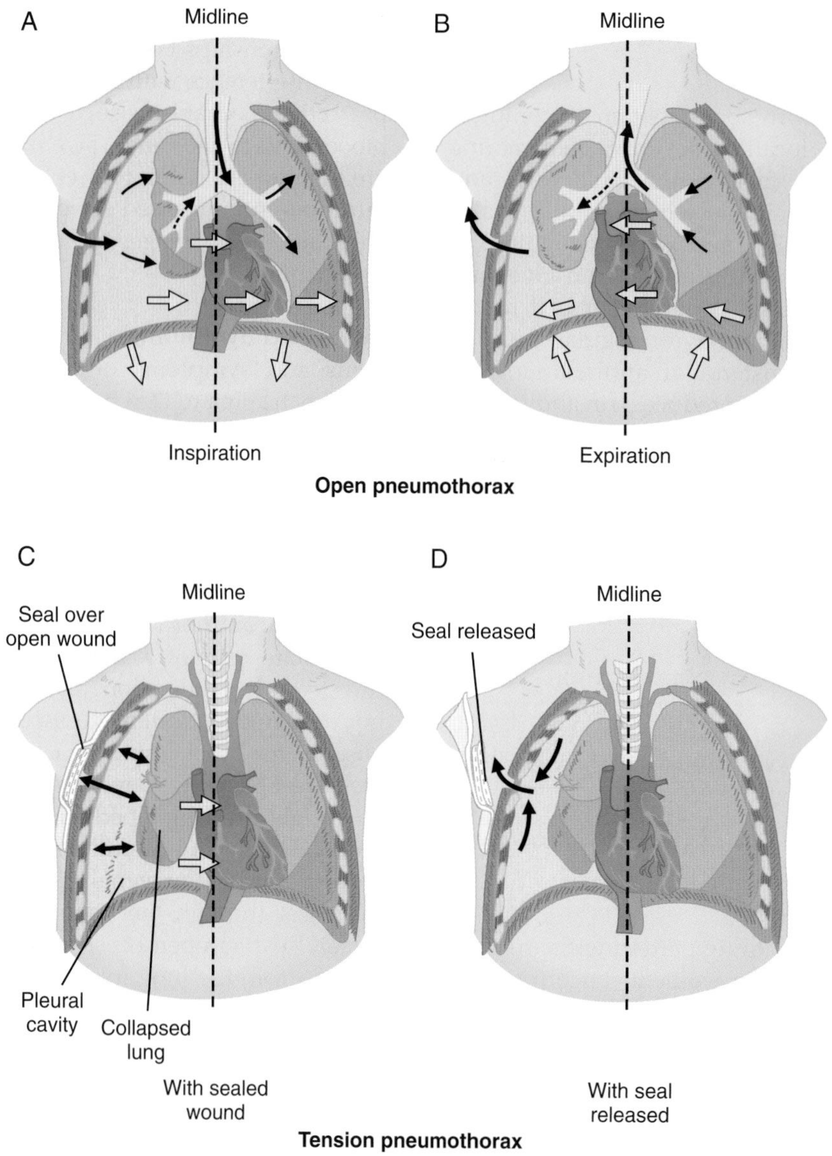

FIGURE 31-13 **A,** Open pneumothorax. Air movement (*solid and dashed arrows*); structural movement (*open arrows*). On inspiration, air is sucked into the pleural space through the open chest wound and the lung on the affected side collapses. The mediastinal contents shift toward the unaffected side. On expiration, air exits through the open wound and the mediastinal contents swing back toward the affected side (mediastinal flutter). **B,** An airtight dressing can cause a tension pneumothorax when air accumulates in the pleural space through a tear in the lung tissue. The air cannot exit if no open chest wound exists and pressure builds, shifting the contents of the mediastinum toward the unaffected side and impairing circulatory and respiratory function (mediastinal shift). (Modified from Black JM, Hawks JH: *Medical-surgical nursing: clinical management for positive outcomes*, ed 8, St. Louis, 2009, Saunders.)

side collapses. The heart, trachea, esophagus, and great blood vessels may shift back and forth toward the unaffected side with inspiration, and then toward the affected side with expiration. This condition is called *mediastinal flutter.* Like mediastinal shift, it is potentially fatal (Fig. 31-13, A and B).

With a tension pneumothorax, air repeatedly enters the pleural space with inspiration, causing the pressure to rise. Because air is not escaping from the wound, the accumulating pressure causes the affected lung to collapse. The heart, trachea, esophagus, and great blood vessels shift toward the unaffected side. This is called a *mediastinal shift*, a condition that interferes with blood return to the heart. This is a medical emergency because both the respiratory and the circulatory systems are affected. If not corrected, cardiac output falls and the patient dies (Fig. 31-13, C and D).

Signs and Symptoms

Symptoms of pneumothorax are dyspnea, tachypnea, tachycardia, restlessness, pain, anxiety, decreased movement of the involved chest wall, asymmetric chest wall movement, diminished breath sounds on the injured side, and progressive cyanosis. In trauma cases, a chest wound may be present. If air can be heard or felt moving in and out of the wound, it is called a *sucking* chest wound.

Medical Treatment

The physician may insert an 18-gauge needle through the chest wall into the pleural space, aspirate accumulated air or fluid, and insert a chest tube. An alternative is to omit the needle aspiration and immediately insert the chest tube. If air is entering the pleural space from a tear in the lung or bronchus, surgery may be needed to repair the tear. A variety of materials are being studied for use in sealing persistent air leaks, including intrapleural tetracycline, autologous "blood patches," and fibrin glue.

NURSING CARE of the Patient with Pneumothorax

Assessment

The complete assessment of the patient with a respiratory disorder is outlined in Box 31-1. In addition, if the patient has a chest tube, the nurse should monitor the insertion site as well as the amount and characteristics of any drainage from the tube. Care of patients with chest tubes is covered in the "Chest Tubes" section.

Nursing Diagnoses, Goals, and Outcome Criteria: Pneumothorax

Nursing Diagnoses	Goals and Outcome Criteria
Ineffective Breathing Pattern related to decreased lung expansion	Effective breathing pattern: regular respirations at a rate of 12 to 20 breaths/min, normal arterial blood gases, no dyspnea, normal skin color
Fear related to difficulty breathing	Decreased fear: calm demeanor, patient statement that fear is reduced
Decreased Cardiac Output related to mediastinal shift	Adequate cardiac output: pulse and blood pressure consistent with patient norms
Acute Pain related to trauma, altered pressure in chest cavity, chest tube	Pain relief: patient statement that pain is reduced or relieved, relaxed manner
Risk for Infection related to traumatic injury, chest tube insertion	Absence of infection: normal body temperature, normal white blood cell count

Interventions

Ineffective Breathing Pattern

Monitor the patient closely for increasing respiratory distress as indicated by tachycardia, dyspnea, cyanosis, restlessness, and anxiety. Inspect the trachea for deviation that may be caused by mediastinal shift. Check arterial blood gas results for hypoxemia (low blood oxygen) and hypercapnia (high blood carbon dioxide). Immediately report signs and symptoms of deteriorating respiratory status to the physician. After the chest tube has been inserted, protect the tube and monitor its function.

Position the patient for comfort in Fowler or semi-Fowler position. Avoid the side-lying position until the affected lung has reexpanded because this position could foster mediastinal shift. Support and encourage the patient to do deep-breathing and coughing exercises at least every 2 hours while awake. Administer oxygen as ordered.

Fear

A pneumothorax is frightening. Patients feel like they are suffocating and may fear that they are dying. Speak to the patient calmly and explain what is happening. Tell the patient that the chest tube will allow the lung to reexpand and relieve the dyspnea. Also, tell the patient how to prevent dislodging the tube. Give the patient the opportunity to ask questions and express fears.

Decreased Cardiac Output

Monitor the patient's pulse and blood pressure. If cardiac output decreases because of mediastinal shift, the blood pressure falls and the pulse rate increases. Immediately notify the physician of signs of this potentially life-threatening change.

Acute Pain

Be alert for signs of pain and document the characteristics of the patient's pain. Administer analgesics as ordered and document the effects. In addition to drug therapy, use positioning, massage, distraction, and other measures described in Chapter 15. Notify the physician if pain is not relieved.

Risk for Infection

Monitor the patient for signs and symptoms of infection: fever, increased pulse and respirations, foul drainage from the tube insertion site, and elevated white blood cell count. Various possible sites of infection must be considered: traumatic wounds, chest tube insertion site, intravenous infusion sites, indwelling catheter, and lungs. Use sterile technique for invasive procedures and dressing changes and administer prescribed antimicrobials. Encourage increased activity when permitted. Monitor hydration status and promote fluid intake of 2 to 3 L per day unless contraindicated. Before discharge, instruct the patient to keep the chest tube insertion site clean and dry and to notify the physician of signs of infection: fever or increasing redness, swelling, or drainage from the insertion site.

chapter 33

Hematologic Disorders

http://evolve.elsevier.com/Linton/medsurg

Stacey Young-McCaughan

Objectives

1. List the components of the hematologic system and describe their role in oxygenation and hemostasis.
2. Identify data to be collected when assessing a patient with a disorder of the hematologic system.
3. Describe tests and procedures used to diagnose disorders of the hematologic system and nursing considerations for each.
4. Describe nursing care for patients undergoing common therapeutic measures for disorders of the hematologic system.
5. Describe the pathophysiology, signs and symptoms, medical diagnosis, and medical treatment for selected disorders of the hematologic system.
6. Assist in planning nursing care for a patient with a disorder of the hematologic system.

Key Terms

Anemia (ă-NĒ-mē-ă)
Ecchymosis (ĕk-ĭ-MŌ-sĭs)
Hemostasis (hē-mō-STĀ-sĭs)
Orthostatic vital sign changes (ŏr-thō-STĂ-tĭk)
Oxygenation (ŏk-sĭ-jĕ-NĀ-shŭn)
Petechiae (pĕ-TĒ-kē-ă)
Purpura (PŬR-pūr-ă)
Universal donor
Universal recipient

The primary functions of the hematologic system are **oxygenation** and **hemostasis** (control of bleeding). Disorders of the hematologic system can be either a primary disease or a complication of another disease. The diagnosis and treatment of these disorders can be very complex. The nurse plays an important role in helping to assess, plan, and manage the care of these patients.

ANATOMY AND PHYSIOLOGY OF THE HEMATOLOGIC SYSTEM

ANATOMIC STRUCTURES AND COMPONENTS OF THE HEMATOLOGIC SYSTEM

Important structures and components of the hematologic system are the bone marrow, the kidneys, the liver, the spleen, and the blood.

Bone Marrow

The bone marrow is the spongy center of the bones where the red blood cells (RBCs) and platelets are made. The marrow of all bones produces these cells; however, the majority of RBCs and platelets are produced in the vertebrae, ribs, sternum, skull, pelvis, and long bones of the legs.

Kidneys

The kidneys are located in the back of the abdominal cavity to the right and left of the aorta and inferior vena cava. The kidneys perform many functions for different body systems. As part of the hematologic system, the kidneys manufacture hematopoetin, a hormone that is released by the kidneys in response to hypoxia. Hematopoetin stimulates the production of RBCs in the bone marrow.

Liver

The liver is located in the upper right quadrant of the abdomen, under the rib cage and below the diaphragm. The liver performs many functions for different body systems. As part of the hematologic system, the liver manufactures clotting factors. In addition, the liver clears old and damaged RBCs from circulation.

Spleen

The spleen is located in the upper left quadrant of the abdomen. Like the liver, the spleen performs many functions for different body systems. As part of the hematologic system, the spleen removes old RBCs from circulation.

Blood

Blood is a generic term referring to a mixture of RBCs, platelets, clotting factors, and plasma, as well as white blood cells (WBCs), proteins, electrolytes, hormones, and enzymes that travel through vessels in the body (Fig. 33-1). Blood serves many functions but as part of the hematologic system it transports oxygen (O_2) from the lungs to tissues and maintains hemostasis. A healthy adult has about 6 L of blood circulating through the body pumped by the heart.

Red Blood Cells (RBCs or Erythrocytes). RBCs, also known as erythrocytes, are made in the bone marrow. Once released from the marrow, they circulate in the body, transporting O_2 from the lungs to the tissues and carbon dioxide (CO_2) from the tissues back to the lungs. Hemoglobin (Hgb) in the RBCs makes the transport of O_2 and CO_2 possible. The tough, flexible membrane of the RBCs allows these disk-shaped, biconcaved cells to maneuver through the smallest capillaries. After about 120 days, the old RBCs are filtered out of circulation by the liver and spleen. The iron and heme in the old RBCs are recycled to make new RBCs.

RBCs normally have various proteins, called *antigens*, as part of their cell membranes. The two major antigens are named *A* and *B*. Based on the presence or absence of the A and B antigens, a person's blood type is determined. People with type A blood have the A antigen, those with type B blood have the B antigen, those with type AB blood have both the A and B antigens, and those with type O blood have neither the A nor the B antigen. Rhesus (Rh) is another type of RBC antigen that is either present or absent. People with the Rh antigen are designated Rh positive (Rh^+) while those without the Rh antigen are designated Rh negative (Rh^-). Both blood type and Rh factor are genetically determined.

Platelets (Thrombocytes). Platelets also are produced in the bone marrow. Platelets activate the blood-clotting system by going to a break in a blood vessel and forming a platelet plug. At the same time, other clotting mechanisms are activated and the body begins repairing itself. Once released into circulation from the bone marrow, the normal life span of a platelet is 10 days.

Clotting Factors. Once platelets activate the blood-clotting system, several clotting factors are activated. The clotting factors are numbered I through XIII and include fibrinogen (factor I) and thrombin (factor II).

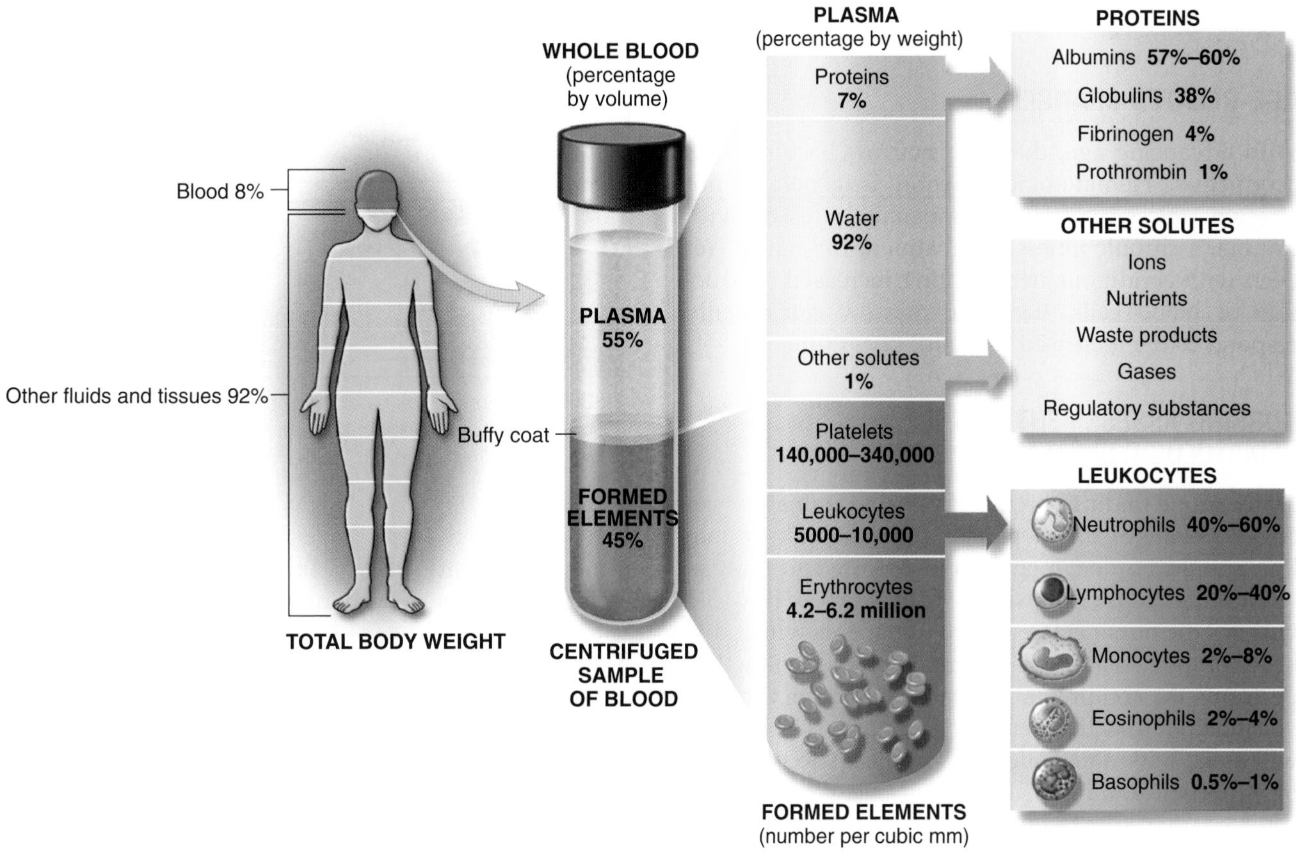

FIGURE 33-1 Blood is composed of plasma (about 55%) and cellular elements (about 45%). Cellular elements include leukocytes (white blood cells [WBCs]), thrombocytes (platelets), and erythrocytes (red blood cells [RBCs]). There are 600 times as many erythrocytes as leukocytes. (From McCance KL, Huether SE: *Understanding pathophysiology*, ed 5, St. Louis, 2013, Mosby.)

The clotting factors form a stable fibrin matrix over the wounded area, protecting the injured site while the healing process is completed.

Plasma. Plasma is the clear, straw-colored fluid that carries the RBCs, platelets, and clotting factors through the circulatory system. Plasma is primarily water. The other major components of plasma are the plasma proteins, albumin, and globulins.

PHYSIOLOGIC FUNCTIONS OF THE HEMATOLOGIC SYSTEM

Oxygenation

RBCs transport O_2 from the lungs to the tissues and carry CO_2 from the tissues back to the lungs for excretion. The Hgb in the RBCs combines easily with O_2 and CO_2 to accomplish oxygenation.

Hemostasis

Hemostasis means *control of bleeding*. It is how the body maintains the integrity of the circulatory system. If a blood vessel is injured, three things occur: (1) the blood vessel constricts, reducing the amount of bleeding; (2) platelets adhere to the injured blood vessel, forming an unstable platelet plug; and (3) the coagulation cascade is initiated, forming a stable fibrin matrix, which is commonly recognized as a scab. The *coagulation cascade* is a term used to describe the series of events that occur in the process of blood clotting (Fig. 33-2).

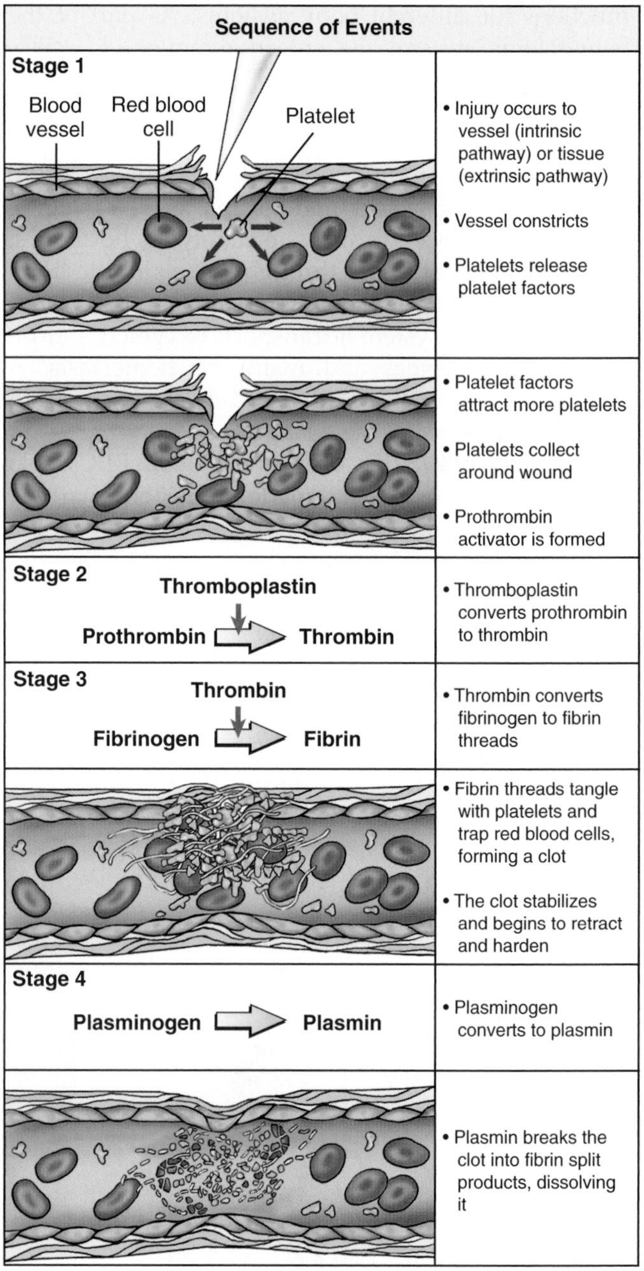

FIGURE 33-2 Formation of a blood clot. (From Monahan F, Sands J, Neighbors M, et al: *Phipps' medical-surgical nursing: health and illness perspectives*, ed 8, St. Louis, 2006, Mosby.)

AGE-RELATED CHANGES

With advancing age, the bone marrow becomes less productive. Hematologic function is generally not affected unless a person is unusually stressed with trauma, a chronic illness, or treatment for cancer. Yet even with conditions necessitating increased production of blood cells, the bone marrow can usually respond to the increased demand, given time.

NURSING ASSESSMENT OF THE HEMATOLOGIC SYSTEM

Many subtle findings on the physical examination can suggest changes in the patient's hematologic system that should be documented and reported to a registered nurse (RN) or physician for evaluation. Box 33-1 outlines the nursing assessment of patients with a disorder of the hematologic system. Even though the RN performs the comprehensive assessment, the licensed vocational nurse/licensed practical nurse (LVN/LPN) will assist with data collection and needs to be aware of important findings.

HEALTH HISTORY

Chief Complaint and History of Present Illness

Pay special attention to the patient who remarks that he or she bruises easily, bleeds for an unusually long time, or is chronically fatigued. These may be the symptoms of an underlying hematologic disorder.

Past Medical History

A patient could have an underlying hematologic problem if he or she reports any of the following: cancer or prior treatment for cancer, human immunodeficiency virus (HIV) infection, liver disease, kidney disease, malabsorption disease, prolonged bleeding or delayed healing with surgery or dental extractions, a history of blood transfusion, placement of prosthetic heart valves, or placement of an indwelling venous access device (indicating that the patient needed

Box 33-1 Assessment of Patients with Disorders of the Hematologic System

HEALTH HISTORY

History of Present Illness
Easy bruising, prolonged bleeding, chronic fatigue

Past Medical History
Cancer or prior treatment for cancer, human immunodeficiency virus (HIV) infection, liver disease, kidney disease, malabsorption disorder; prolonged bleeding or delayed healing with surgery or dental extractions; history of having blood transfused; placement of prosthetic heart valves or placement of an indwelling venous access device, indicating that the patient needed long-term venous access; current medications, including over-the-counter (OTC) medications and any recent changes in medication

Family History
Blood disorders, death of a family member at a young age for reasons other than trauma

REVIEW OF SYSTEMS

Integumentary
Change in skin color, dryness, pruritus, brittle fingernails or toenails

Neurologic
Dizziness, vertigo, confusion, pain, headache, mental status changes, change in vision

Respiratory
Epistaxis, hemoptysis, dyspnea

Cardiovascular
Palpitations, chest pain, dizziness or fainting with position changes

Gastrointestinal
Change in eating habits, nausea, vomiting, bleeding, abdominal pain, change in bowel habits, blood in stool

Genitourinary
Blood in urine, heavy menses in women

Musculoskeletal
Numbness or pain in bones or joints

Endocrine
Fatigue, cold intolerance

Functional Assessment
Occupation and hobbies, self-concept, activities and exercise, sleep and rest, nutrition, interpersonal relationships, coping and stress, perception of health

PHYSICAL EXAMINATION

Vital Signs
Tachycardia, tachypnea, hypotension, orthostatic vital sign changes

Height and Weight

General Survey
Responsiveness, mood, expression, posture

Skin
Color, dryness, brittle fingernails and toenails, bruising, petechiae, purpura, ecchymoses

Head and Neck
Bleeding, cracking at the corners of the mouth

Thorax
Respiratory rate, breath sounds, heart rate

Abdomen
Liver enlargement, stool guaiac test, dipstick urine sample for blood

long-term venous access). Also note any history of blood transfusions.

Medications the patient is currently using or a recent change in medication may suggest an underlying hematologic problem. It is important to find out what over-the-counter (OTC) medications the patient uses because many of these contain aspirin or nonsteroidal antiinflammatory drugs (NSAIDs) that may prolong bleeding.

Family History

Note any family history of blood disorders such as sickle cell disease or hemophilia. Death of a family member at a young age for reasons other than trauma may indicate a genetic hematologic disorder.

Review of Systems

The review of systems is aimed at finding out what symptoms the patient has been experiencing over the past weeks or months that might provide clues as to what specific medical disorder the patient may now have.

In relation to the integumentary system, ask the patient about changes in skin (color, dryness, pruritus [itching]) and brittle fingernails or toenails. Data relevant to the assessment of the neurologic system include dizziness, vertigo, confusion, and pain. Patients with low RBC counts may have headaches. If the patient has had headaches, record the location, duration, and intensity of the pain, as well as what, if anything, relieves the pain. Patients with intracranial bleeding from low platelet counts may report sudden mental status changes or severe headaches. Note changes in vision, which may indicate bleeding behind the eye. While collecting data about the respiratory and cardiovascular systems, ask the patient about epistaxis (nosebleeds), hemoptysis (coughing up blood), dyspnea (shortness of breath), heart palpitations, and chest pain, which may be symptoms of a low RBC count. Heart palpitations accompanied by dizziness may occur with position changes as the heart beats faster in an attempt to move what little blood exists quickly from the lungs to the body tissues to deliver O_2. Significant data for assessment of the gastrointestinal (GI) system include any changes in eating habits, including changes in appetite or episodes of nausea or vomiting. Inquire about bleeding or pain in the mouth, gums, or tongue. In addition, record the patient's normal bowel function and any recent changes in frequency of bowel movements or consistency of the stool. Also note any report of blood in the stool as well as any report of blood in the urine as an abnormality of the genitourinary system. Ask female patients about unusually heavy menses, which may indicate a bleeding disorder. Any musculoskeletal numbness or pain should also be noted; joint pain can occur if bleeding has taken place in the joint (hemarthrosis). Finally, to collect data about the endocrine system, ask the patient about fatigue or cold intolerance, which may be a symptom of a low RBC count.

Functional Assessment

Patients newly diagnosed with blood disorders may not experience dramatic changes in their functional abilities. However, many blood disorders are chronic conditions that the patient has lived with for many years.

Occupation and Hobbies. Knowing a patient's job and hobbies can alert the nurse to unusual chemical exposures. Because the bone marrow and blood can be affected by various chemicals, it is important to document any recent chemical exposure. For example, someone who builds models for a hobby may be exposed to unusual glues or paints, which may affect the blood count.

Self-Concept. Assess the patient's self-concept by exploring the patient's feelings about himself or herself. For many people, their self-concept is related to their job. If the patient is unable to work, his or her self-concept can be adversely affected. In addition, medical insurance is often contingent on employment. Loss of medical insurance and the need to receive state or federal assistance can further erode a patient's self-concept. Another factor that can adversely affect the patient's self-concept is a change in appearance because of the disease.

Activity and Exercise. Describe the patient's current activity level and the effects of the disease and treatment on the patient's usual pattern of activity and exercise. Ask about the layout of the patient's home, specifically the location of bathrooms in relation to living areas and bedrooms. Determine if the patient must climb stairs to enter the home or get to a second floor. Having to climb stairs can quickly tire a patient with a hematologic disorder. Inquire about what the patient does for recreation and whether these activities can still be done during times of decreased energy.

Sleep and Rest. Note the number of continuous hours the patient sleeps every night, whether any sleeping aids are used, what interrupts the patient's sleep, and whether the patient naps during the day.

Nutrition. Ask the patient to describe his or her usual diet and any recent changes in appetite or weight (see *Nutrition Considerations* box). Identify factors that might be interfering with eating, such as nausea, vomiting, and taste changes. Depression and loneliness can adversely affect a patient's nutritional status. Limited financial resources can also limit a patient's ability to maintain a nutritious diet.

Nutrition Considerations

A balanced diet should include foods rich in iron, which is required for hemoglobin (Hgb) production. Foods rich in iron include red meats, fish, dried fruits, beans, and dark-green vegetables.

Interpersonal Relationships. Explore the patient's view of himself or herself as a husband or wife, father or mother, son or daughter, friend, and co-worker. Discuss the effects of the disease on these relationships and on the patient's roles in the home. In addition, ask what household chores the patient is responsible for and who does the shopping, cooking, and cleaning. If the patient has children who need to be cared for, note whether the patient is able to perform the usual child care.

Coping and Stress. Ask what worries the patient has and how he or she usually deals with stress. In addition, explore sources of support, which might include family, support groups, and spiritual beliefs and practices.

Perception of Health. Ask the patient to discuss feelings about his or her own health and health practices. This might include measures taken to prevent complications from the disease and keeping regular medical appointments.

PHYSICAL EXAMINATION

Begin the physical examination by measuring the patient's vital signs, height, and weight. Be alert for tachycardia (pulse >100/min), tachypnea (respiratory rate >20/min), and hypotension (systolic blood pressure <90 mm Hg).

Patients with low RBC counts may experience **orthostatic vital sign changes** in pulse and blood pressure when they rise. The body tries to maintain the blood pressure when the patient changes position from lying to standing. If the patient's blood volume is inadequate, the heart rate increases and the blood pressure decreases as the patient stands. This can be why patients complain of feeling dizzy or lightheaded when they stand up quickly. Box 33-2 describes how to assess for orthostatic changes in vital signs. Patients who have orthostatic changes in their vital signs

Box 33-2 Assessing for Orthostatic Changes in Vital Signs

1. Have the patient lie down on a bed or in a reclining chair for at least 1 minute.
2. Record the patient's heart rate and blood pressure.
3. Have the patient sit up.
4. After the patient has been sitting for no more than 30 seconds, record the heart rate and blood pressure again.
5. Have the patient stand up. Stay near the patient to ensure the safety of the individual.
6. After the patient has been standing no more than 30 seconds, record the heart rate and blood pressure again.
7. If the blood pressure decreases 10 to 15 points with the change from the lying to the standing position and the heart rate increases 10 to 15 points from lying to standing, the patient is described as having orthostatic or tilt-positive changes.

usually need some type of hydration. Often the patient is simply dehydrated and needs extra fluids. However, a patient with a low RBC count who needs a blood transfusion can also be orthostatic.

General Survey

Note the patient's responsiveness, mood, expression, and posture. Throughout the examination, carefully inspect and describe any reddened, swollen, or painful areas the patient identifies.

Skin

Note the general color of the skin. A patient with a low RBC count may appear pale. In dark-skinned people, this may be difficult to assess. Look at the conjunctiva of the eyes, the nail beds, and around the mouth to detect any paleness. Patients also may appear jaundiced, or yellow, if many RBCs have been destroyed or if the body is having trouble clearing the blood of old RBCs. Indications of a vitamin deficiency that might cause a blood disorder include dry, itchy skin and scalp or brittle fingernails and toenails (see *Complementary and Alternative Therapies* box).

> **Complementary and Alternative Therapies**
>
> Be sure to note any herbal products that the patient uses. Herbs that can affect blood clotting include black cohosh, feverfew, garlic, ginkgo, and ginseng.

Describe any bruising. **Petechiae** are small (1 to 3 mm), red or reddish-purple pinpoint spots on the skin resulting from blood capillaries breaking and leaking small amounts of blood into the tissues. Petechiae are often confused with a skin rash. Petechiae almost always signal that the patient has a very low platelet count. Severe coughing can cause petechiae on the chest, neck, and face of a patient. A blood pressure cuff pumped up to greater than 250 mm Hg on a patient with a low platelet count can cause petechiae on the arm below the blood pressure cuff as the small capillaries break with the high cuff pressure. This is not dangerous but can be frightening to the patient and the nurse if it happens. Red or reddish-purple spots denote **purpura** and are the result of larger blood vessels breaking. Purpura are larger than petechiae, usually 3 mm or more. Purpura can suggest a low platelet count or a problem with clotting factors in the blood. Ecchymoses are larger purplish areas of skin resulting from a larger amount of blood leaking outside the blood vessels. The common name for **ecchymosis** is a bruise. Ecchymoses do not necessarily indicate a bleeding disorder but if the patient has a number of ecchymotic areas or notes that he or she bruises easily, it may be a symptom of a blood disorder.

Head and Neck

When evaluating the eyes, ears, nose, mouth, and throat, note any signs of bleeding. Look for cracking at the corners of the mouth, which may be a symptom of iron or B vitamin deficiency.

Thorax

Lungs. Assess the patient's respiratory rate and effort and auscultate breath sounds. Patients with low RBC counts often are dyspneic, or short of breath, because they do not have enough RBCs to carry O_2 to all their tissues, yet the lungs will sound clear to auscultation without wheezing, crackles, or rhonchi. As a result, they are tachypneic, with a respiratory rate greater than 20 breaths per minute, in an attempt to oxygenate what little blood they have. Any strenuous activity may exacerbate the shortness of breath.

Heart and Vascular System. Assess the patient's heart rate, resting blood pressure, and adaptation of blood pressure to position changes. Patients with low RBC counts can be tachycardic, with a heart rate greater than 100 beats per minute. Again, because not enough RBCs exist to carry O_2 to all the tissues, the heart beats faster in an attempt to move what little blood exists quickly from the lungs to the body tissues to deliver O_2.

Abdomen

Inspect and palpate the patient's abdomen for distention and tenderness. The examiner with advanced skills may also palpate for organ enlargement. The liver and spleen can become enlarged with blood cell disorders, causing abdominal fullness and tenderness. If a stool specimen is available, a guaiac test may be done to detect microscopic blood. If the patient can provide a urine sample, it also can be tested for blood.

DIAGNOSTIC TESTS AND PROCEDURES

Primarily, blood studies determine the function of the patient's hematologic system. Diagnostic tests and procedures done to diagnose disorders of the hematologic system are described in Tables 33-1 and 33-2. The laboratory performing the test should provide normal values for the various blood tests. Ranges of normal values can be found in various textbooks of laboratory and diagnostic tests.

BLOOD TESTS

The RBC count, the Hgb, and the hematocrit (Hct) are the three main blood tests used to monitor RBCs. The RBC count is the total number of RBCs found in a cubic millimeter (mm^3) of blood. The Hgb indicates the O_2-carrying capacity in the blood. The Hct is the percentage of RBCs in whole blood. Normally, the Hct is approximately three times the Hgb value. Iron is an essential part of RBCs; therefore serum iron, total iron-binding capacity (TIBC), and ferritin are measured to assess the patient's resources for producing RBCs.

Normal platelet counts range from 140,000 to 440,000 platelets/mm^3 of blood. Many times the

Table 33-1 Diagnostic Tests and Procedures **Laboratory Tests**

General Interventions: Check your agency procedure manual for diagnostic tests and procedures. Always tell the patient what to expect when tests are ordered. Explain if fasting prior to the test is necessary. Document the care provided and relevant assessment data. If venipuncture is to be done, tell the patient to expect a sharp pain as the needle goes through the skin. Apply pressure for 1 minute and elevate the arm if the patient's blood clotting is impaired. Apply dressing for at least 1 hour.

Different blood tests are collected in different laboratory tubes containing specific reagents or no reagents at all. Usually the tubes have color-coded tops. Be sure to collect the blood in the blood tube specific for the blood test ordered. Usually each institution's laboratory publishes a manual identifying what colored tube to use for each blood test.

TEST/STUDY	PURPOSE AND PROCEDURE	PATIENT PREPARATION	POSTPROCEDURE NURSING CARE
Blood tests (CBC, RBC count, Hgb, Hct, serum iron, TIBC, ferritin, platelet count, PT, PTT, fibrinogen, TT, FSP or FDP, D-dimers, INR, HbS, serum bilirubin, Coombs tests)	Blood tests measure various blood components.	Choose the correct blood tubes in which to collect the blood. See General Interventions.	See General Interventions.
Bleeding time	The bleeding time measures the time it takes for the platelet plug to form.	Tell the patient that a blood pressure cuff is placed above the elbow and inflated to 40 mm Hg. The forearm is cleaned and a puncture is made. A stopwatch is started. The wound is blotted with filter paper every 30 seconds until all bleeding has stopped. The time is noted.	Apply a bandage.

Data from Fischbach FT, Dunning MB: *A manual of laboratory and diagnostic tests*, ed 8, Philadelphia, 2009, Lippincott-Williams & Wilkins.
CBC, Complete blood count; *FDP,* fibrinogen degradation products; *FSP,* fibrin split products; *HbS,* sickle cell hemoglobin; *Hct,* hematocrit; *Hgb,* hemoglobin; *INR,* international normalized ratio; *PT,* prothrombin time; *PTT,* partial thromboplastin time; *RBC,* red blood cell; *TIBC,* total iron-binding capacity; *TT,* thrombin time.

Table 33-2 Diagnostic Tests and Procedures **Bone Marrow Biopsy**

TEST/STUDY	PURPOSE AND PROCEDURE	PATIENT PREPARATION	POSTPROCEDURE NURSING CARE
Bone marrow biopsy	A bone marrow biopsy is used to evaluate how well the bone marrow is making white blood cells (WBCs), red blood cells (RBCs), and platelets. The patient is positioned on an examining table according to the location of where the bone marrow biopsy will be collected. The most common site is the posterior iliac crest, requiring the patient to be in the prone position, although the anterior crest, sternum, and tibia can also be biopsy sites, allowing for alternative positioning. The selected site is prepared and draped as for a minor surgical procedure. A local anesthetic is injected. A Jamshidi needle is forced into the bone marrow. Bone marrow fluid is aspirated and a core biopsy is taken through and with the Jamshidi needle. The needle is removed and a pressure dressing is applied to the site. A laboratory technician must be present during the procedure to immediately fix and stain the specimens. Sometimes a short-acting benzodiazepine, such as midazolam (Versed), is used to sedate the patient during the procedure.	Explain the purpose and procedure to the patient. A permit must be signed. No fasting is necessary. Some local discomfort may be experienced as the local anesthetic is injected. The patient usually feels pressure as the Jamshidi needle is inserted into the bone and a momentary sharp pain down the leg as the bone marrow fluid is aspirated. The procedure takes approximately 30 minutes.	If intravenous sedation is used, monitor the patient's pulse, blood pressure, respirations, and pulse oximetry until the patient is fully recovered. The pressure dressing can be removed in 2 hours.

Data from Fischbach FT, Dunning MB: *A manual of laboratory and diagnostic tests*, ed 8, Philadelphia, 2009, Lippincott-Williams & Wilkins.

platelet count is abbreviated as a multiple of 1000. For example, a platelet count of 200,000 is abbreviated 200K.

The function of the clotting factors is measured with the prothrombin time (PT), the partial thromboplastin time (PTT), and the bleeding time. If the results of these tests are abnormal, other blood tests that may be done to determine the specific abnormality include measurements of fibrinogen; thrombin time (TT); fibrinogen degradation products (FDP), also known as fibrin split products (FSP); and D-dimers. If the patient is taking heparin to anticoagulate the blood, the PTT is used to monitor therapy. If the patient is taking warfarin (Coumadin) to anticoagulate the blood, the PT, the international normalized ratio (INR), or both are used to monitor therapy.

BONE MARROW BIOPSY

If blood tests show abnormalities, the physician may perform a bone marrow biopsy to see how well the blood cells are being made in the bone marrow (Fig. 33-3). Table 33-2 describes the bone marrow biopsy procedure.

COMMON THERAPEUTIC MEASURES

Treatment of disorders of the hematologic system is aimed at correcting the underlying problem. Blood product transfusions and colony-stimulating factors are used to symptomatically manage the patient.

NURSING ACTIONS FOR THE PATIENT AT RISK FOR INJURY FROM LOW RED BLOOD CELL COUNTS

Box 33-3 outlines typical nursing actions for the patient at risk for injury from low RBC counts.

NURSING ACTIONS FOR THE PATIENT AT RISK FOR INJURY FROM BLEEDING

Box 33-4 outlines typical nursing actions for the patient at risk for injury from bleeding.

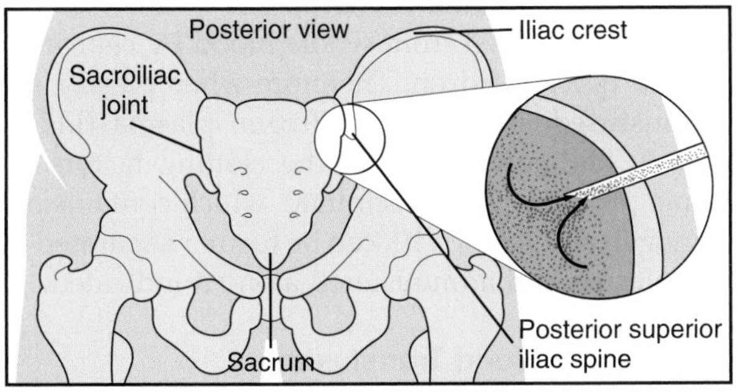

FIGURE 33-3 Most common site of bone marrow biopsy. (From Pagana KD, Pagana TJ: *Mosby's manual of diagnostic and laboratory tests*, ed 4, St. Louis, 2010, Mosby.)

BLOOD PRODUCT TRANSFUSIONS

Because of the risk for infections, such as with hepatitis or HIV, blood product transfusions are no longer automatically given when the patient's laboratory values fall below a certain value. Instead the patient is evaluated clinically and a decision is made with the patient whether or not to administer a blood transfusion. Symptoms of a low RBC count that would prompt an RBC transfusion include shortness of breath, tachycardia, decreased blood pressure, chest pain, lightheadedness, or extreme fatigue. For each unit of packed red blood cells (PRBCs) transfused, the patient's Hgb should increase approximately 1 g/dL and the Hct approximately 3%. Table 33-3 provides an overview of commonly transfused blood components.

Typing for Transfusions

Before a blood transfusion, a sample of the patient's blood is sent to the blood bank for typing and crossmatching. As discussed previously, depending on which antigens are present in the RBC membrane, a person has either type A, B, AB, or O blood. In addition, depending on the presence or absence of the Rh antigen, a person is either Rh^+ or Rh^-. People with any of these antigens cannot be given blood containing a different antigen. Therefore persons with type O^- blood are considered **universal donors** because their blood does not contain any of the A, B, or Rh antigens and can safely be given to anyone. Those with AB^+ blood are considered **universal recipients** because their blood contains the A, B, and Rh antigens. They can safely receive any type of blood. Unless it is a medical emergency, blood banks exactly match the blood to be transfused with the blood of a patient needing a transfusion.

Box 33-3 Nursing Actions for the Patient at Risk for Injury from Insufficient Oxygenation Related to Low Red Blood Cell Counts (Anemia)

1. Administer oxygen (O_2) as prescribed.
2. Administer blood products as prescribed (see Tables 33-3 and 33-4 and Box 33-5).
3. Administer the hematopoietic growth factor erythropoietin as prescribed (see Table 33-5).
4. Monitor position changes from bed or chair to standing to ensure safety.
5. Allow for rest between periods of activity because the patient with anemia can tire easily.
6. Elevate the patient's head on pillows for shortness of breath.
7. Provide extra blankets if the patient feels too cool.
8. Teach the patient and family about the underlying pathophysiology and how to manage the symptoms of anemia.

From Young-McCaughan S, Jennings BM: Hematologic and immunologic systems. In Alspach JG, editor: *Core curriculum for critical care nursing*, ed 5, Philadelphia, 1998, Saunders.

Box 33-4 Nursing Actions for the Patient at Risk for Injury from Bleeding

1. Administer blood product transfusions as prescribed. If a platelet transfusion is to be given in preparation for a procedure, then it is best to give the transfusion immediately before the procedure so the greatest number of platelets will be available to stop bleeding caused by the procedure (see Tables 33-3 and 33-4 and Box 33-6).
2. Minimize the number of invasive procedures done to the patient that might result in prolonged bleeding by taking the following measures:
   a. Draw blood for as much laboratory work as possible with one venipuncture.
   b. Avoid prolonged tourniquet use.
   c. Apply direct pressure for 5 to 10 minutes after all invasive procedures such as venipuncture or bone marrow biopsies.
   d. Avoid intramuscular injections.
3. Avoid damage to the rectal mucosa that might cause bleeding by taking the following measures:
   a. Avoid taking rectal temperatures.
   b. Avoid use of suppositories.
   c. Avoid use of enemas.
   d. Prevent constipation by increasing fiber in the diet or administering stool softeners as ordered.
4. When measuring blood pressure, inflate the cuff only until the pulse is obliterated to prevent petechiae along the arm. Set automated sphygmomanometers to the lowest appropriate pressure.
5. Instruct the patient to use a soft-bristled toothbrush. If oral bleeding occurs, then toothettes or mouth rinses can be used to maintain oral hygiene.
6. Instruct the patient to use an electric razor to shave, not a straight-edged razor.
7. As much as possible and as prescribed by the physician, avoid the use of drugs that interfere with platelet function such as aspirin, aspirin-containing drugs (e.g., Pepto-Bismol, Percodan), and the nonsteroidal antiinflammatory drugs (NSAIDs).
8. Teach the patient and family about the underlying pathophysiology that puts the patient at risk for hemorrhage and precautions to minimize the risk of bleeding.

From Young-McCaughan S, Jennings BM: Hematologic and immunologic systems. In Alspach JG, editor: *Core curriculum for critical care nursing,* ed 5, Philadelphia, 1998, Saunders.

Transfusions of Packed Red Blood Cells

The physician should counsel and get the signed consent of the patient before any blood transfusion. A blood sample is drawn from the patient and sent to the blood bank for type and crossmatch. One procedure for administering a PRBC transfusion is outlined in Box 33-5. The policies for administering blood products vary from hospital to hospital, so the LVN/LPN must be familiar with his or her institution's policies.

One way to prevent the risks of infection and reactions with blood transfusions is to collect the patient's own blood before a planned procedure and then transfuse the patient's own blood back into the patient if needed as an autologous RBC transfusion. The patient donates his or her own blood several times before the planned procedure. The blood is stored by the blood bank and reinfused into the patient if needed intraoperatively or postoperatively. Autologous transfusion—using the patient's own blood—is recommended if significant blood loss is expected during the procedure, especially if the patient has a rare blood type or religious beliefs against receiving donated blood.

Platelet Transfusions

Like RBC transfusions, platelet transfusions are not automatically administered when the patient's platelet count falls below a certain value. However, the lower a patient's platelet count goes, the greater is the chance of bleeding. Generally, when the platelet count falls below 20,000 cells/mm^3, platelets are administered. If the platelet count is greater than 20,000 cells/mm^3, platelets usually are not given unless the patient is actively bleeding. For each multidonor (from multiple donors) pack of platelets, the patient's platelet count should increase by 5000 to 10,000 cells/mm^3.

As with blood transfusions, the physician should counsel and get the signed consent of the patient for the platelet transfusion. A blood sample is drawn from the patient and sent to the blood bank for typing. If the patient has been previously typed and crossmatched for either a RBC transfusion or a platelet transfusion, the blood bank can usually use this information to provide platelets. Platelets are commonly ordered in four-packs or six-packs. Each pack contains approximately 60 mL. One procedure for administering a platelet transfusion is outlined in Box 33-6. Because the policies for administering blood products vary from hospital to hospital, the LVN/LPN must be familiar with his or her institution's policies.

If platelets are ordered before an invasive procedure that might cause bleeding, such as a lumbar puncture or endoscopy, the platelets should be administered just before the procedure is started. No indication exists to "get the platelets in early" for a procedure scheduled for later in the day. Instead, with the physician, the nurse should plan to administer the platelets just before the procedure begins.

Fresh Frozen Plasma Transfusions

Plasma is separated from whole blood by centrifugation and quickly frozen. Therefore when plasma is to be transfused, usually fresh frozen plasma (FFP) is ordered. FFP contains all of the clotting factors and plasma proteins. Cryoprecipitate, which contains only fibrinogen and factor VIII, can be further separated out from plasma and administered alone if indicated.

Reactions to Blood Transfusions

Four main types of transfusion reactions can occur with transfusions of blood or any of the blood components: (1) hemolytic, (2) anaphylactic, (3) febrile, and

Table 33-3 Commonly Transfused Blood Products

BLOOD COMPONENT	INDICATIONS	USUAL AMOUNT IN ONE UNIT	RECOMMENDED INFUSION RATE	SPECIAL CONSIDERATIONS
Packed red blood cells (PRBCs)	Anemia; symptoms caused by low hematocrit (Hct) or hemoglobin (Hgb), such as shortness of breath, tachycardia, decreased blood pressure, chest pain, lightheadedness, or fatigue	250–300 mL	2–4 h/unit	An 18 or 20 gauge needle must be used to prevent damage to RBCs. The transfusion should be started within 30" of leaving the blood bank.
Platelets	Bleeding from thrombocytopenia	30–60 mL/pack; usually four to six packs are pooled for platelet transfusion	Run infusion slowly the first 15 minutes, watching for any transfusion reaction, and then increase rate as patient can tolerate	Platelets should be stored on an agitator prior to administration to maximize oxygenation of the cells and prolong their effectiveness.
Fresh frozen plasma (FFP)	Clotting deficiencies, hemophilia B, rapid reversal of warfarin (Coumadin), massive red blood cell (RBC) transfusions	100–300 mL/U	Run infusion slowly the first 15 minutes, watching for any transfusion reaction, and then increase rate as patient can tolerate	FFP contains all clotting factors except platelets
Cryoprecipitate	Hemophilia A	10 mL/bag; usually 10 bags are pooled for transfusion	Run infusion slowly the first 15 minutes, watching for any transfusion reaction, and then increase rate as patient can tolerate	Cryoprecipitate contains factors I (fibrinogen) and VIII

Data from American Association of Blood Banks, America's Blood Centers, & American Red Cross: *Circular of information for the use of human blood and blood components* (website): www.aabb.org. Accessed September 8, 2013.

Box 33-5 Administration of a Red Blood Cell Transfusion

1. After the patient has been counseled and has given signed consent for the transfusion, draw a sample of blood and send it to the blood bank with a request for a type and crossmatch. Start a peripheral intravenous line of normal saline using an 18- or 20-gauge needle. Blood should not be infused through a cannula smaller than 20 gauge because of the chance of lysing (destroying) the individual blood cells as they go through the cannula. Similarly, normal saline is used in the administration of blood products rather than 5% dextrose solution or lactated Ringer solution to avoid the possibility of agglutination and/or hemolysis of the transfused blood in the intravenous (IV) line.
2. When the blood arrives, two licensed people should check them at the patient's bedside. Be certain to check the expiration date of the blood. Once the blood has arrived from the blood bank, the transfusion should be started within 30 minutes. In many states licensed vocational nurses/licensed practical nurses (LVNs/LPNs) cannot initiate a blood transfusion. However, the LVN/LPN is responsible for monitoring the patient while the transfusion is in progress. Check the practice laws in your state and your institution's policies.
3. Take and record the patient's vital signs.
4. To administer blood, use a special blood transfusion tubing that has a built-in filter to screen for clots. Piggyback the blood into the normal saline line. Each unit of blood is usually between 250 and 300 mL. Generally blood is infused over 2 to 4 hours.
5. Stay with the patient for 5 to 10 minutes after the blood is started to observe for any immediate untoward reactions that might signal a reaction to the transfusion, such as back pain, fever, chills, or a decreased blood pressure.
6. Continue to monitor vital signs during the transfusion per your institution's policy.
7. When the transfusion is complete, document the procedure, the patient's vital signs, and how the patient tolerated the procedure.
8. Subsequent units of blood can be hung immediately as just described. Sometimes the same blood tubing can be used for administering several units of blood.

Box 33-6 Administration of a Platelet Transfusion

1. After the patient has been counseled and has given signed consent for the transfusion, draw a sample of blood and send it to the blood bank with a request for typing and crossmatch. Start an intravenous line of normal saline using at least a 24-gauge needle. Platelets are smaller than red blood cells (RBCs); therefore a smaller intravenous needle can be used to administer the platelets without risk of lysing the cells.
2. When the platelets arrive, two licensed people should check them at the patient's bedside. Once the platelets have arrived from the blood bank, the transfusion should be started immediately. In many states licensed vocational nurses/licensed practical nurses (LVNs/LPNs) cannot initiate a blood transfusion. However, the LVN/LPN is responsible for monitoring the patient while the transfusion is in progress. Check the practice laws in your state and your institution's policies.
3. Take and record the patient's vital signs.
4. Run the platelets through blood transfusion tubing that has a built-in filter in the system. Piggyback the platelets into the normal saline line. Platelets can be infused as fast as the patient can tolerate them.
5. Stay with the patient for 5 to 10 minutes after the platelets are started to observe for any immediate untoward reactions that might signal a reaction to the transfusion, such as back pain, fever, chills, or decreased blood pressure.
6. Continue to monitor the patient's vital signs during the infusion per your institution's policy.
7. When the transfusion is complete, document the procedure, the patient's vital signs, and how the patient tolerated the procedure.

(4) circulatory overload. If the patient experiences back or chest pain, fever, chills, a decreased blood pressure, urticaria, wheezing, dyspnea, coughing, or blood in the urine during the transfusion, stop the transfusion immediately and keep the intravenous line open with normal saline. Notify the physician, nursing supervisor, and blood bank immediately; be prepared to administer O_2, epinephrine, Solu-Cortef, furosemide (Lasix), and antipyretics as prescribed by the physician. Save the unused portion of the blood bag for the blood bank. Also be prepared to collect blood and urine samples from the patient for evaluation. Documentation of the event is important; usually each institution has a blood transfusion reaction form that needs to be completed. A delayed hemolytic reaction can also occur 2 to 14 days after the transfusion in patients previously treated with RBC transfusions and alloimmunized so that the patient's own immune system attacks the transfused RBCs. Usually delayed hemolytic reactions do not require treatment. Table 33-4 outlines the types, symptoms, and treatments for the different blood transfusion reactions.

COLONY-STIMULATING FACTORS

Colony-stimulating factors are naturally occurring hormones that stimulate the bone marrow to produce more blood cells. Certain of the colony-stimulating factors have been isolated and are available for therapeutic use. Erythropoietin (Epogen) and darbepoetin (Aranesp) stimulate the bone marrow to produce more RBCs whereas oprelvekin (Neumega) stimulates the bone marrow to produce more platelets. The effects of these drugs on the Hct and platelet count are not apparent for several days; therefore they are not an option for patients who need to elevate their blood cell counts immediately. These patients need a transfusion of the appropriate blood component. Erythropoietin and darbepoetin are predominantly used by hemodialysis patients who are chronically anemic as a result of dialysis; these medications have also been used to prevent the complications and relieve the symptoms of anemia in patients with cancer or HIV infection. Table 33-5 describes the nursing care of patients receiving these drugs.

DISORDERS OF THE HEMATOLOGIC SYSTEM

RED BLOOD CELL DISORDERS

Patients with RBC disorders may have either too many RBCs (i.e., polycythemia vera) or too few RBCs (i.e., anemia). Having too few RBCs is more common. Because the main function of RBCs is oxygenation, anemia results in tissue hypoxia. Anemia can result from a major blood loss over a short period of time, too few RBCs being made, or increased RBC destruction. Acute blood loss, such as with an arterial rupture, dramatically changes the patient's hemodynamic status, requiring emergency intervention. Chronic blood loss, such as with sickle cell disease, allows the body to compensate. Depending on whether the **anemia** is acute or chronic, the body compensates in three ways: (1) by increasing heart rate and respiratory rate to circulate the existing RBCs as quickly as possible with as much O_2 as possible; (2) by redistributing the blood away from the skin, GI tract, and kidneys to the brain and heart; and (3) by increasing the production of erythropoietin, the hormone that stimulates the bone marrow to produce more RBCs. Anemia can be a primary disease or a symptom of another disease. Descriptions of the different types of RBC disorders follow.

Polycythemia Vera

Polycythemia vera is a condition in which too many RBCs are produced. The increased number of RBCs makes the blood more viscous, or thicker, so that it does not circulate freely through the body. Symptoms of polycythemia vera include headache, dizziness, ringing in the ears, and blurred vision. Patients

Table 33-4 **Blood Transfusion Reactions**

REACTION	MECHANISM	SYMPTOMS	OCCURRENCE	TREATMENT
Hemolytic	Antigen-antibody reaction to transfusion of ABO-incompatible blood	Fever, chills, nausea, dyspnea, chest pain, back pain, hypotension, hematuria (blood in urine)	Shortly after starting transfusion	Stop the transfusion. Notify the physician immediately. Be prepared to provide supportive therapy to maintain heart rate and blood pressure.
Anaphylactic	Type I hypersensitivity reaction to plasma proteins	Urticaria, wheezing, dyspnea, hypotension	Within 30 minutes of starting transfusion	Stop the transfusion. Notify the physician immediately. Be prepared to administer epinephrine and steroids.
Febrile	Recipient's antibodies react to donor leukocytes	Fever, chills	Within 30–90 minutes of starting transfusion	Stop the transfusion. Notify the physician immediately.
Circulatory overload	Patient's cardiovascular system is unable to manage the additional fluid load	Cough, frothy sputum, cyanosis, decreased blood pressure	Any time during transfusion and up to several hours afterward	Stop the transfusion. Call for help. Be prepared to administer oxygen (O_2) and/or furosemide (Lasix).
Delayed hemolytic reactions	Reaction occurs in patients previously treated with red blood cell (RBC) transfusions and alloimmunized so that patient's own immune system attacks transfused RBCs	Unexplained fever, unexplained decrease in hemoglobin (Hgb) and hematocrit (Hct)	2–14 days after transfusion	Most delayed reactions require no treatment.

with this disorder may have a ruddy (reddish) complexion.

Treatment for polycythemia vera is to have 1 U of blood (250 to 500 cc) phlebotomized, or taken off, to keep the patient's Hct normal. This procedure is usually done in the blood bank. A large-bore intravenous needle is inserted in the patient's antecubital vein and 1 U of blood is drawn (taken off). This is the same procedure used when a person goes to the blood bank to donate blood; however, the blood taken from the patient with polycythemia vera cannot be used as donor blood.

Aplastic Anemia

Aplastic anemia results from the complete failure of the bone marrow. The term *aplastic anemia* is misleading because patients with this condition have more than an extremely low RBC count; they also have extremely low WBC counts and low platelet counts because their bone marrow is not making any of these cells. Certain drugs such as streptomycin and chloramphenicol, as well as exposure to toxic chemicals or radiation, can cause bone marrow failure. Yet in many cases the cause of a patient's bone marrow failure is never identified.

Signs and symptoms of aplastic anemia can include pallor, extreme fatigue, tachycardia, shortness of breath, hypotension, unusually prolonged or spontaneous bleeding, and frequent infections that do not resolve. In addition to abnormally low RBC, WBC, and platelet counts on blood tests, patients with aplastic anemia have abnormally low numbers of blood-making cells in their bone marrow.

Medical treatment for aplastic anemia focuses on identifying and treating the cause. Transfusions are given to replace RBCs and platelets. Antibiotics are given to prevent or treat infections. Corticosteroid drugs also may be given. If the patient's bone marrow does not recover on its own, a bone marrow transplant may be considered if a donor can be found. The patient with aplastic anemia is critically ill and requires intensive nursing support similar to the care provided to a patient who is undergoing a bone marrow transplant, as described in Chapter 34.

Table 33-5 Drug Therapy: Drugs Used to Treat Disorders of the Hematologic System

DRUG	USE AND ACTION	SIDE EFFECTS	NURSING INTERVENTIONS
epoetin alfa (Epogen)	Stimulates bone marrow to produce red blood cells (RBCs)	Hypertension, headache, arthralgia	Usually administered by subcutaneous injection; may also be administered intravenously. Patient is usually treated three times per week until the hematocrit (Hct) is 30–33.
darbepoetin alfa (Aranesp)	Stimulates bone marrow to produce RBCs	Hypertension, headache, arthralgia	Usually administered by subcutaneous injection; may also be administered intravenously. Patient is usually treated only once per week until the Hct is 30–33.
oprelvekin (Neumega)	Stimulates bone marrow to produce platelets	Fluid and electrolyte abnormalities, dysrhythmias, visual disturbances, dizziness, insomnia, dyspnea, oral candidiasis	Given by subcutaneous injection once a day for up to 21 days. Most patients receiving this drug experience side effects.
ferrous sulfate (Feosol, Fer-In-Sol)	Iron replacement	Constipation, black stools, mild nausea	Have the patient take the drug with food but not with milk, eggs, or caffeinated drinks because milk, eggs, and caffeine inhibit drug absorption. If the patient is taking liquid iron, dilute the drug and administer it through a straw to prevent the drug from staining the teeth.
iron dextran	Iron replacement	Hypersensitivity reactions, brown skin discoloration at the injection site	Test dose the patient before starting treatment. Give intramuscular injections only in the upper, outer quadrant of the buttock using the Z-track technique. To give an injection using the Z-track technique, firmly pull the skin over the upper, outer quadrant of the buttock laterally. Insert the needle. Slowly inject the medication. Remove the needle and let go of the skin.
vitamin B_{12} (cyanocobalamin)	Vitamin B_{12} replacement	Diarrhea, hypokalemia; itching, rash at injection site; RARELY heart failure, anaphylaxis	Given via intramuscular or deep SubQ injection. For patients with pernicious anemia, vitamin B_{12} injections must be given every month for the rest of the person's life.
hydroxyurea	Prevention of sickle cell crisis	Nausea, vomiting	Reinforce to the patient that this drug must be taken regularly to prevent sickle cell crises and that it is of no use once a crisis occurs.

Autoimmune Hemolytic Anemia

With aplastic anemia, the bone marrow does not make adequate amounts of the blood cells; with autoimmune hemolytic anemia, the bone marrow makes adequate amounts of the blood cells but they are destroyed once they are released into the circulation. Causes of autoimmune hemolytic anemia can include certain infections, drug reactions, and certain cancers. Hemolytic anemia of the newborn can occur after delivery if the mother has Rh^- blood and the baby has Rh^+ blood. Blood transfusions can cause hemolytic anemia if lymphocytes in the transfused blood make antibodies against the person receiving the blood. As with aplastic anemia, many times the cause of the hemolytic anemia is never identified.

Signs and symptoms of hemolytic anemia include pallor, extreme fatigue, tachycardia, shortness of breath, and hypotension. Patients may appear jaundiced. Patients with hemolytic anemia usually have high bilirubin levels in their blood from all the RBCs being lysed (broken down). Patients with hemolytic anemia have a positive result on a direct Coombs antiglobulin blood test.

Medical treatment of this type of anemia focuses on identifying and treating the cause. Blood transfusions may be needed to replace RBCs. Corticosteroids may be administered to the patient. The patient usually recovers in a few days to weeks.

Iron Deficiency Anemia

Iron deficiency anemia results from a diet too low in iron or from the body not absorbing enough iron from the GI tract. As a result, the body does not have enough iron to make adequate amounts of Hgb. Older adults with poor eating habits frequently suffer from anemia. Symptoms of this anemia include fatigue and pallor. In severe cases, patients may have orthostatic changes in their heart rate and blood pressure. In addition to a low RBC count, a low Hgb value, and a low Hct, patients with iron deficiency anemia have a low serum iron level, a low ferritin level, and a high TIBC.

Physicians treat iron deficiency anemia by prescribing iron supplements such as ferrous sulfate and iron dextran. Table 33-5 describes the nursing care of the patient taking iron supplements. Nurses caring for patients with iron deficiency anemia can suggest incorporating foods high in iron in the diet. Foods that are rich in iron include liver, oysters, red meats, fish, dried fruits, legumes (e.g., dried beans, peas), dark-green vegetables, and iron-enriched whole-grain breads and cereals (see *Nutrition Considerations* box).

Nutrition Considerations

1. Inadequate dietary intake of iron or inadequate absorption of dietary iron causes iron deficiency anemia.
2. The lack of intrinsic factor, which is normally manufactured in the stomach, prevents the absorption of vitamin B_{12} and leads to pernicious anemia.

Pharmacology Capsule

Large doses of supplemental iron can be toxic to the gastrointestinal tract and eventually to the brain and liver if not recognized and treated. Caution patients not to exceed recommended dose and to keep the drug out of the reach of children.

Pernicious Anemia (Vitamin B_{12} Anemia)

Pernicious anemia occurs when a person does not absorb vitamin B_{12} from the stomach. The person may lack intrinsic factor, a substance made in the stomach that is essential for B_{12} absorption. The individual may have had a gastrectomy, in which part or all of the stomach was surgically removed, and so cannot make intrinsic factor and therefore cannot absorb vitamin B_{12}. In addition to the fatigue and pallor commonly seen with all anemias, symptoms of pernicious anemia characteristically include weakness, a sore tongue, and numbness of the hands or feet. Physicians treat pernicious anemia by prescribing a monthly intramuscular injection of vitamin B_{12} (cyanocobalamin). Table 33-5 describes the nursing care of patients receiving vitamin B_{12}.

Sickle Cell Anemia

Sickle cell anemia is a disease in which the normally disk-shaped RBCs become sickle shaped (Fig. 33-4). These misshapen blood cells are much more fragile than normal RBCs and as a result the sickled cells easily rupture as they pass through small capillaries, resulting in chronic anemia. In addition, these abnormally shaped, sickled cells become stuck in the small capillaries of the body, obstructing blood flow.

Sickle cell anemia is a genetic disease that occurs almost exclusively in African Americans (see *Cultural*

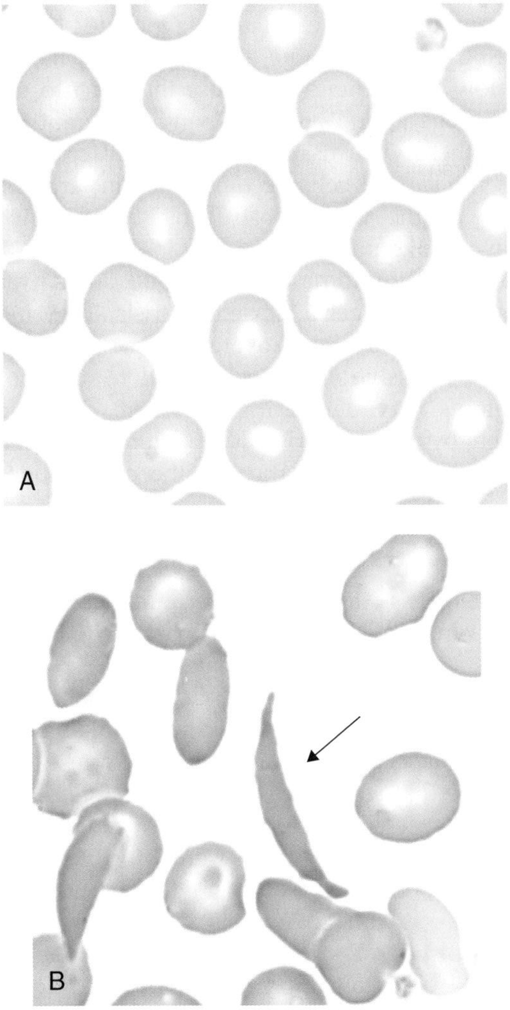

FIGURE 33-4 Comparison of **(A)** normal red blood cells (RBCs) and **(B)** sickled cells (*arrow*). (From Carr JH, Rodak BF: *Clinical hematology atlas*, ed 3, St. Louis, 2009, Saunders.)

Considerations box). Eight percent of African Americans carry the genetic trait for sickle cell anemia. Because sickle cell anemia is carried on a recessive gene, a person must inherit the gene from the mother and father to actually have the disease. A person with the trait for sickle cell on only one gene does not experience any symptoms. Newborn screening for sickle cell hemoglobin (HbS) can be done to identify infants with sickle cell disease and to educate parents about the disease and prevention of crises. Unfortunately, this screening is not required in every state.

Cultural Considerations

What Does Culture Have to Do with Recruitment for Clinical Trials?

Diseases like sickle cell occur predominantly in African Americans. This population may be reluctant to join research studies because of unethical studies such as the Tuskegee syphilis experiment, which started in the 1930s. In the Tuskegee study, African-American men enrolled but were not treated when effective treatment, penicillin, became available in the 1940s.

Symptoms of sickle cell anemia include persistently low RBC counts, fatigue, and jaundice. The chronically low RBC counts can cause the heart to enlarge (cardiomegaly) and beat faster in an attempt to oxygenate the body's tissues. A sickle cell crisis occurs when the sickled cells become stuck in larger blood vessels of the body, obstructing blood flow and causing severe pain.

Signs and Symptoms of Sickle Cell Crisis. Various stressors can trigger a sickle cell crisis. They include dehydration, infection, overexertion, cold weather changes, excessive alcohol consumption, and smoking. Symptoms vary depending on where circulation is blocked by the sickled RBCs. Commonly during a sickle cell crisis, circulation to the chest, abdomen, bones, joints, bone marrow, brain, or penis may be compromised. With circulation obstructed, tissue hypoxia occurs, causing severe pain. Patients in a sickle cell crisis often have a fever, either because infection precipitated the crisis or as part of the inflammatory response to tissue hypoxia.

Medical Diagnosis of Sickle Cell Disease. Patients with known sickle cell disease who complain of severe pain are suspected of being in crisis. No test exists to determine that a patient is in sickle cell crisis. Rather, physicians use clinical judgment to make the diagnosis. Crises can last anywhere from 1 to 10 days. Some patients experience crises every few weeks whereas other patients can go months without experiencing painful episodes. Radiographs and scans of the painful area are usually taken to evaluate for bleeding.

Medical Treatment of the Patient in Sickle Cell Crisis. No cure exists for sickle cell disease. Medical treatment for patients experiencing a sickle cell crisis is symptomatic. The physician usually prescribes intravenous fluids and pain medication. Aggressive intravenous hydration helps the kidneys to clear the metabolic wastes from ruptured RBCs. The pain can be very severe and the patient needs adequate pain relief during these episodes, even if they last for several days. Intravenous morphine commonly is prescribed for pain relief. Patients with sickle cell disease can become addicted to opioids. Therefore physicians try to transition the patient quickly from intravenous opioids to oral opioids to nonopioid pain relievers as the crisis resolves. RBC transfusions may be prescribed to correct the anemia and help the body to oxygenate tissues. Although O_2 therapy is often prescribed, it is of little benefit in reversing the crisis.

For patients who experience frequent crises, the drug hydroxyurea can be prescribed. Hydroxyurea has been used for many years as a treatment for leukemia. The drug also stimulates the production of a certain type of Hgb that is resistant to sickling. Patients with sickle cell disease who regularly take hydroxyurea experience fewer crises. However, once a patient is in crisis, hydroxyurea does not work quickly enough to reduce either the severity or the duration of the crisis. Table 33-5 describes the nursing care of patients receiving hydroxyurea.

NURSING CARE of the Patient in Sickle Cell Crisis

Patients in sickle cell crisis have specialized needs beyond treatment of the simple anemia (see Nursing Care Plan: Patient in Sickle Cell Crisis).

Assessment

Obtain a complete description of the pain that the patient in sickle cell crisis is experiencing. Note the location, intensity, duration, and precipitating events. Measure vital signs every 4 hours. Be especially alert for a fever, which may indicate an infection that precipitated the crisis. Investigate any symptoms of an infection, such as sore throat, cough, abnormal breath sounds, dysuria, or diarrhea. In addition, monitor the patient for signs and symptoms of dehydration, such as concentrated urine, low blood pressure, or poor skin turgor, which may have precipitated the crisis.

Interventions

Acute Pain

Give pain medications as prescribed. Usually intravenous morphine is prescribed. Initially it is not unusual for patients to need large amounts of medication to control their pain. One option for medication delivery is patient-controlled analgesia. Closely monitor the patient's pain level and medication use. Good documentation can contribute to effective pain management. Keeping a flow sheet of patient reports of pain on a 10-point scale can be helpful, especially if different nurses care for the patient throughout the day. A

Nursing Care Plan Patient in Sickle Cell Crisis

ASSESSMENT

HEALTH HISTORY A 19-year-old African-American woman was diagnosed with sickle cell anemia at age 12 years. She has been in stable health until 3 days ago, when she complained of nausea and began to have diarrhea and vomiting. She has taken only soup and cola beverages since that time. When she began to complain of severe pain in her abdomen, she was brought to the emergency department by her mother, who suspected sickle cell crisis.

PHYSICAL EXAMINATION Vital signs: blood pressure 110/56 mm Hg, pulse 106 bpm, respiration 24 breaths per minute, temperature 102°F (38.9°C) measured orally. Oral mucosa dry. Skin dry and warm to touch. Breath sounds clear to auscultation. Abdomen soft but tender to light palpation. Bowel sounds hyperactive in all four quadrants. No bladder distention. Mild joint enlargement noted in both knees.

Nursing Diagnosis	Goals and Outcome Criteria	Interventions
Acute Pain related to sickle cell crisis	The patient states that pain has been relieved and appears relaxed.	Administer analgesics as prescribed. Assess the effects and notify the physician if pain is not relieved. Have the patient rate her pain (0 = no pain, 10 = worst pain) before and after medication administration. Use the distraction technique. Respond to calls quickly. Reassure the patent.
Anxiety related to pain and hospitalization	The patient states that anxiety is reduced and appears calm.	Respond quickly to the patient's needs. Check on her often. Assign a consistent caregiver. Listen and use attention and touch to convey concern.
Risk for Injury related to orthostatic hypotension	The patient experiences no injuries or falls caused by dizziness.	Assist the patient to get out of bed when permitted. Have her sit on the side of the bed and exercise her legs before rising. Check the patient's blood pressure in lying, sitting, and standing positions to detect orthostatic hypotension. Advise her to sit and lower her head if she feels dizzy.
Risk for Deficient Fluid Volume related to inadequate intake and excess loss of fluids	The patient is adequately hydrated and has a consistent intake of 4 to 6 L of fluid daily. In addition, she has moist oral tissues and normal urine specific gravity.	Administer intravenous fluids as ordered. Teach the patient the importance of fluid intake. Weigh the patient daily to assess any change in fluid status. Monitor her fluid intake and output and note urine characteristics.
Ineffective Self-Health Management related to lack of knowledge of disease process and self-care	The patient accurately describes the disease process and implications of self-care measures.	Assess what the patient knows about sickle cell disease. Initiate teaching when the crisis has resolved. Make sure she knows to avoid smoking, alcohol, and high altitudes. Emphasize the need to maintain good hydration (4 to 6 L of fluids each day) and to keep regular medical appointments.

Critical Thinking Questions

1. Why would genetic counseling be recommended for a young woman with sickle cell disease?
2. Describe the order in which you should implement the listed interventions for this patient.

0 represents no pain and a *10* represents the worst pain that a patient has ever experienced. The patient report of pain, coupled with the amount of pain medication he or she is receiving, can guide you and the physician in determining the appropriate type and amount of pain medication for the patient. A detailed discussion of pain management strategies is presented in Chapter 15.

Anxiety

Sickle cell crises can be extremely frightening to a patient, especially because of the severe pain that accompanies these crises. Patients fear not obtaining adequate pain relief. The unpredictability of the timing and severity of the crises can be especially frustrating to patients. Provide consistent care to the patient in sickle cell crisis to establish a trusting relationship. In addition, listening closely to the patient can reduce anxiety. Once the patient is discharged from the hospital, he or she can contact one of the many support groups available for patients with sickle cell disease and their families. Patients should be encouraged to attend meetings of these groups so that they can better cope with this chronic disease.

Risk for Injury

The primary treatment for anemia is RBC transfusions. Nursing considerations in administering blood transfusions are outlined earlier in the chapter. Nursing actions that should be taken when patients are anemic are outlined in Box 33-3. Procedures for administering a RBC transfusion are outlined in Box 33-5.

Nursing Diagnoses, Goals, and Outcome Criteria: Sickle Cell Crisis

Nursing Diagnoses	Goals and Outcome Criteria
Acute Pain related to sickle cell crisis	Pain relief: patient states pain has been relieved, relaxed manner
Anxiety related to pain and hospitalization	Reduced anxiety: patient states anxiety is reduced, calm manner
Risk for Injury related to orthostatic hypotension	Absence of injury: no falls caused by dizziness
Risk for Deficient Fluid Volume related to inadequate intake or excess loss of fluids	Adequate hydration: consistent intake of 4 to 6 L of fluid daily
Ineffective Self-Health Management related to lack of knowledge of the disease process and self-care	Effective management of condition: patient accurately describes disease process and implications for self-care measures

Risk for Deficient Fluid Volume

Administer intravenous fluids as prescribed and keep records of fluid intake and output. Measure weight daily to assess gross fluid status and encourage the patient to drink 4 to 6 L of fluids each day to maintain adequate hydration.

Ineffective Self-Health Management

When the patient is not in crisis, he or she should be taught about the disease (see *Patient Teaching* box). Help the patient to identify stressors that bring on a crisis and strategies to avoid these stressors. Encourage the patient not to smoke or drink large amounts of alcoholic beverages, because these are two common stressors that can bring on a crisis. Traveling to high altitudes where less O_2 exists can bring on an attack, so caution the patient about vacationing at high altitudes. Drinking 4 to 6 L of nonalcoholic fluids a day helps to maintain adequate hydration. Regular medical follow-up is extremely important in keeping the patient with sickle cell disease out of a crisis. Genetic counseling can be done with people who have the sickle cell gene to inform them of the risk of passing on the trait or disease to their children. With this information, some people choose not to have their own children and risk passing on this painful, life-threatening disease. Several resources are available for patients, families, and health care providers. An example is the Sickle Cell Disease Association of America (scdaa@sicklecelldisease.org). This and other such organizations provide excellent free literature on sickle cell disease and can help to locate groups in specific regions of the country.

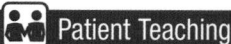

Patient Teaching

Sickle Cell Anemia

- To prevent crises, maintain good hydration and avoid smoking, alcoholic beverages, and high altitudes.
- Drink 4 to 6 L of fluid each day to maintain adequate hydration.
- Genetic counseling can help you with decisions about having children by exploring the risk of passing on sickle cell trait or disease.
- You can get additional information from the Sickle Cell Disease Association of America.

Put on Your Thinking Cap!

How would a high fluid intake decrease the risk of sickle cell crisis?

Put on Your Thinking Cap!

Why would immunizations be particularly important for people with sickle cell disease?

COAGULATION DISORDERS

Coagulation disorders can result from a platelet abnormality or from a clotting factor deficiency.

Thrombocytopenia

Thrombocytopenia is a condition in which a person has too few platelets circulating in the blood. This may be because not enough platelets are being made in the bone marrow or because too many platelets are being destroyed in circulation.

The major cause of thrombocytopenia related to inadequate production of platelets is treatment of cancer with chemotherapy or radiation therapy. Chemotherapy and radiation therapy kill rapidly dividing cells. Unfortunately, the therapy cannot tell the difference between rapidly dividing cancer cells and rapidly dividing normal cells like those that produce platelets. In patients treated with chemotherapy or radiation therapy, thrombocytopenia can be expected 10 to 14 days after treatment and lasts until the bone marrow is able to make more platelets, which is usually 1 week.

Two examples of thrombocytopenia resulting from too many platelets being either destroyed or consumed are idiopathic thrombocytopenic purpura (ITP) and thrombotic thrombocytopenic purpura (TTP). Both of these disorders are abnormal immunologic processes that result in thrombocytopenia. ITP and TTP are discussed in more detail in Chapter 34.

Symptoms of thrombocytopenia include petechiae and purpura, gingival bleeding, epistaxis (nosebleeds), or any other unusual or prolonged bleeding. The diagnosis is made with blood tests and a bone marrow biopsy. Treatment for thrombocytopenia is to treat or stop the causative factor. If the cause is cancer chemotherapy or radiation therapy, platelet transfusions may be prescribed. Nursing actions for the patient who is at risk for injury from bleeding are outlined in Box 33-4. Procedures for administration of a platelet transfusion are outlined in Box 33-6.

Disseminated Intravascular Coagulation

Disseminated intravascular coagulation (DIC) is a hypercoagulable state, meaning that blood clotting is abnormally increased. DIC occurs when overstimulation of the normal coagulation cascade results in simultaneous thrombosis and hemorrhage. DIC is always secondary to another pathologic process, such as overwhelming sepsis, shock, major trauma, crush injuries, burns, cancer, acute tumor lysis syndrome, or obstetric complications such as abruptio placentae or fetal demise (death). Coagulation occurs at so many sites in the body that eventually all available platelets and clotting factors are depleted and uncontrolled hemorrhage results.

Blood tests that help to diagnose DIC include the PT and PTT, FDPs, and D-dimers. A patient with DIC has an increased PT/PTT, FDPs, and increased D-dimers. In combination, these three test results are diagnostic for DIC.

Blood component replacement therapy may be prescribed. However, some physicians believe that additional platelets and clotting factors perpetuate the abnormal DIC feedback loop and so do not prescribe blood component replacement. Heparin may be prescribed to interrupt the DIC cycle and allow the body to replenish platelets and clotting factors. However, heparin therapy is also controversial, because some physicians believe that it only makes the bleeding worse. Nursing actions for the patient who is at risk for injury from bleeding are outlined in Box 33-4.

Put on Your Thinking Cap!

Explain how heparin could be helpful for a patient with DIC.

Hemophilia

Hemophilia is a genetic disease in which the affected person lacks some of the blood-clotting factors normally found in plasma. The incidence of hemophilia is 1 case per 5000 to 30,000 persons, depending on the type of hemophilia. In hemophilia A, factor VIII is missing whereas in hemophilia B, factor IX is missing. Hemophilia is sometimes called *Christmas disease* after Stephen Christmas, the first patient described with the disease. Hemophilia A has a much higher incidence than hemophilia B. Because the trait is carried on the X chromosome, women carry the trait and can pass it on to their sons, who manifest the disease. However, approximately 30% of cases arise from a spontaneous mutation in patients without any family history of hemophilia. Whether the trait is inherited or spontaneous, it is rare for women to have this disease.

Signs and Symptoms. Uncontrollable bleeding is the hallmark of hemophilia. Bleeding generally occurs after some sort of trauma; however, bleeding can also occur spontaneously for no clear reason. Most commonly, bleeding occurs into the joints, causing swelling and severe pain. Bleeding also can occur into the skin; from the mouth, gums, and lips; and from the GI tract. Because any surgical procedure puts the patient at great risk for bleeding, a complete preoperative evaluation must be done. In addition, the availability of replacement factors for transfusion must be confirmed (see *Cultural Considerations* box).

Cultural Considerations

What Does Culture Have to Do with Blood Transfusions?

Members of some religious groups do not accept blood transfusions from other people. Autotransfusion may be an acceptable alternative.

Medical Diagnosis. The diagnosis of hemophilia is made by measuring factors VIII and IX in the blood. In addition, the PTT is prolonged in people with hemophilia.

Medical Treatment. No cure exists for hemophilia. Medical treatment for patients experiencing a bleeding episode is symptomatic. The physician usually prescribes transfusions of FFP or cryoprecipitate, or both. Patients with hemophilia A need factor VIII, which is found in FFP and cryoprecipitate. Patients with hemophilia B need factor IX, which is found in FFP. RBC transfusions are frequently used to replace blood lost from the profuse bleeding to which hemophiliacs are prone. The pain can be very severe. The patient needs adequate pain relief during these episodes, even if they last several days. Intravenous morphine is commonly prescribed for pain relief. Because patients with hemophilia can become addicted to opioids, pain must be assessed carefully. Usually physicians try to transition the patient quickly from intravenous opioids to oral opioids to nonopioid pain relievers as the crisis resolves.

NURSING CARE of the Patient with Hemophilia

Assessment

Assess the patient for bleeding and pain, noting what measures have stopped the bleeding and relieved the pain in the past. In addition, monitor vital signs and urine output.

Interventions

Risk for Injury

The primary treatment to control bleeding in hemophilia is to transfuse FFP, cryoprecipitate, or both (see *Coordinated Care* box). Nursing considerations in

Nursing Diagnoses, Goals, and Outcome Criteria: Hemophilia

Nursing Diagnoses	Goals and Outcome Criteria
Risk for Injury related to bleeding	Cessation of bleeding: no visible bleeding, stable vital signs
Acute Pain related to bleeding into closed spaces, creating pressure on nerves	Pain relief: patient states pain is relieved, relaxed manner
Ineffective Self-Health Management related to lack of knowledge about the disease process and self-care	Effective management of condition: patient accurately describes condition and demonstrates self-care measures

administering these products are outlined in Table 33-1. Bleeding precautions that should be taken when patients have hemophilia are similar to bleeding precautions taken when patients are thrombocytopenic (see Box 33-4 for these bleeding precautions).

Coordinated Care

Helping the Certified Nursing Assistant to Care for Patients with Blood Disorders

- Instruct the certified nursing assistant (CNA) to allow periods of rest for patients with anemia (low red blood cell counts).
- Show the CNA how to handle patients with thrombocytopenia (low platelet counts) gently to prevent trauma and bleeding.
- Stress the importance of maintaining accurate records of oral fluid intake of patients in sickle cell crisis.

Acute Pain

Administer pain medications as prescribed. If the patient is experiencing a great deal of pain, patient-controlled analgesia may be appropriate. Closely monitor the patient's pain level on a scale of 0 to 10. Keeping a flow sheet of patient reports of pain on a 10-point scale can be helpful, especially if different nurses care for the patient throughout the day. The patient's report of pain, coupled with the amount of pain medication he or she is receiving, can guide the nurse and physician in selecting the appropriate type and amount of pain medication. A detailed discussion of pain management is presented in Chapter 15.

Ineffective Self-Health Management

Hemophiliacs bleed with even the smallest blow or abrasion (see *Patient Teaching* box). Patients and their families should be taught to prevent injury and to safeguard their environment against accidents as much as possible. Some patients and families are taught to administer the replacement concentrate at home so that, should an injury occur, prompt treatment can be initiated and blood loss minimized. Genetic counseling can be done with people with the hemophilia gene to inform them of the risk of passing on the disease to their children. With this information, some people choose not to have their own children and risk passing on this painful, life-threatening disease. The National Hemophilia Foundation (116 West 32nd Street, 11th floor, New York, NY 10001; www.hemophilia.org; telephone: 1-800-42-HANDI or 1-212-328-3700; email: handi@hemophilia.org) provides information and support to patients with hemophilia and their families.

Patient Teaching

Hemophilia

- Protect yourself from injuries by avoiding activities that could result in trauma.
- Know the emergency treatment of bleeding episodes: first-aid measures (apply pressure, immobilize and elevate affected part if possible), seek medical attention, administer replacement concentrate (if prescribed).
- Remember that the National Hemophilia Foundation is a resource for additional information.

Get Ready for the NCLEX® Examination!

Key Points

- The hematologic system includes the bone marrow, kidneys, liver, spleen, and blood.
- A healthy adult has about 6 L of blood circulating through the body.
- Components of the blood are RBCs (erythrocytes), platelets (thrombocytes), clotting factors, and plasma, as well as WBCs (leukocytes), proteins, electrolytes, hormones, and enzymes.
- Signs of hematologic abnormalities can include petechiae, purpura, and ecchymoses.
- The four major blood groups are A, B, AB, and O; each group may be Rh^- or Rh^+.
- People with type O^- blood are universal blood donors and people with type AB^+ blood are universal blood recipients.
- Types of reaction that can occur when blood or blood components are transfused include hemolytic, anaphylactic, febrile, and circulatory overload.
- Anemia is a deficiency of RBCs or Hgb that may be caused by blood loss, an iron deficient diet, vitamin B_{12} deficiency, bone marrow failure, or genetic abnormalities.
- Sickle cell anemia is an incurable genetic condition in which RBCs can become abnormally sickle shaped so that they rupture easily and can obstruct capillaries.

- Sickle cell crisis occurs when blood flow is obstructed. Patients in crisis can experience severe pain.
- Nursing diagnoses during sickle cell crisis focus on the patient's acute pain, anxiety, risk for injury, risk for deficient fluid volume, and ineffective self-health management.
- Thrombocytopenia is a deficiency of platelets that can lead to excessive or prolonged bleeding.
- Hemophilia is an incurable genetic disease in which some of the factors needed for blood clotting are absent.
- Nursing diagnoses for the patient with hemophilia include the patient's risk for injury, acute pain, and ineffective self-health management.

Additional Learning Resources

SG Go to your Study Guide for additional learning activities to help you master this chapter content.

evolve Go to your Evolve website (http://evolve.elsevier.com/Linton/medsurg) for the following learning resources and much more:
- Interactive Prioritization Exercises
- Fluid & Electrolyte Tutorial
- Pharmacology Tutorial
- Review Questions for the NCLEX® Examination

Review Questions for the NCLEX® Examination

1. If a person has no A or B antigens, what is his or her blood type?
   NCLEX Client Need: Health Promotion and Maintenance
2. When inspecting a patient's skin, you notice multiple ecchymoses and petechiae. This should lead you to suspect a deficiency of which blood component?
   NCLEX Client Need: Physiological Integrity: Physiological Adaptation
3. A patient says that he is a "universal donor." This means his blood type is ______________?
   NCLEX Client Need: Health Maintenance and Promotion
4. While receiving a blood transfusion, a patient complains of chest and back pain and chills. Which of the following should be your *initial* action?
   1. Notify the blood bank
   2. Take vital signs
   3. Administer acetaminophen
   4. Stop the transfusion

   NCLEX Client Need: Physiological Integrity: Reduction of Risk Potential
5. Which of the following nursing interventions are appropriate for a patient with a low RBC count? (Select all that apply.)
   1. Avoid taking rectal temperatures and using suppositories
   2. Allow for rest between periods of activity
   3. Encourage increased fluids and dietary fiber
   4. Do not allow fresh flowers in the room
   5. Provide extra blankets as needed to maintain warmth

   NCLEX Client Need: Physiological Integrity: Physiological Adaptation
6. A patient's laboratory report reflects a deficiency of RBCs, WBCs, *and* platelets. The nurse recognizes that these findings are characteristic of which condition?
   1. Aplastic anemia
   2. Hemolytic anemia
   3. Sickle cell anemia
   4. Iron deficiency anemia

   NCLEX Client Need: Physiological Integrity: Physiological Adaptation
7. The nurse is teaching the parents of a child with sickle cell disease about the condition. Which statement would explain the circumstances that lead to sickle cell crisis?
   1. Cells lack sufficient Hgb to transport O_2.
   2. Sickled cells are unable to transport adequate O_2.
   3. Sickled cells form clumps that obstruct blood flow.
   4. The bone marrow stops producing RBCs.

   NCLEX Client Need: Physiological Integrity: Physiological Adaptation
8. Factors that can trigger a sickle cell crisis include which of the following? (Select all that apply.)
   1. Dehydration
   2. Infection
   3. Low iron intake
   4. Smoking
   5. Cold weather

   NCLEX Client Need: Physiological Integrity: Physiological Adaptation
9. A patient is being admitted in the acute phase of a sickle cell crisis. The nurse anticipates that pain management usually requires which of the following?
   1. NSAIDs
   2. Physical therapy
   3. Nerve blocks
   4. Opioid analgesics

   NCLEX Client Need: Physiological Integrity: Pharmacological Therapies
10. Overstimulation of the normal blood-clotting process can result in which of the following?
    1. DIC
    2. ITP
    3. TTP
    4. Hemophilia

    NCLEX Client Need: Physiological Integrity: Physiological Adaptation
11. Hemophilia A is treated with which factor?
    NCLEX Client Need: Physiological Integrity: Pharmacological Therapies

chapter 34

Immunologic Disorders

http://evolve.elsevier.com/Linton/medsurg

Stacey Young-McCaughan

Objectives

1. List the components of the immune system and describe their role in innate immunity, acquired immunity, and tolerance.
2. List the data to be collected when assessing a patient with a disorder of the immune system.
3. Describe the tests and procedures used to diagnose disorders of the immune system and nursing considerations for each.
4. Describe the nursing care for patients undergoing common therapeutic measures for disorders of the immune system.
5. Describe the pathophysiology, signs and symptoms, medical diagnosis, and medical treatment for selected disorders of the immune system.
6. Assist in developing a nursing care plan for a patient with a disorder of the immune system.

Key Terms

Acquired immunity
Antibody (ĂN-tī-bŏ-dē)
Antibody-mediated immunity
Antigen (ĂN-tī-gĕn)
Cell-mediated immunity
Compromised host precautions
Eicosanoid (ī-KŌ-săh-noid)
Immunity (ĭ-MŪ-nō-tē)
Immunoglobulin (ĭ-MŪ-nō-GLŎB-ū-lĭn)
Innate immunity
Pathogen (PĂTH-ō-gĕn)
Phagocytes (FĂG-ō-sīts)

The immune system is the body's defense network against infection. It is an inherently complex system that recognizes, isolates, and destroys **pathogens** as quickly as possible. Disorders of the immune system leave the patient susceptible to overwhelming, life-threatening infections. The nurse plays an important role in helping to assess, plan, and manage the care of patients with these disorders.

ANATOMY AND PHYSIOLOGY OF THE IMMUNE SYSTEM

ANATOMIC STRUCTURES AND COMPONENTS OF THE IMMUNE SYSTEM

Bone Marrow

The bone marrow is the spongy center of the bones where the white blood cells (WBCs) are made. The marrow of all bones produces these cells; however, in adults the majority of WBCs are produced in the vertebrae, ribs, sternum, skull, pelvis, and long bones of the legs.

Stem Cells

Stem cells are called *progenitor cells*, or *precursor cells*, because they are capable of developing into the various WBCs, red blood cells (RBCs), or platelets (Fig. 34-1). Although the majority of stem cells are located in the bone marrow, some stem cells circulate in the blood.

White Blood Cells (Leukocytes)

The bone marrow produces WBCs. Five major types of WBCs exist: (1) neutrophils, (2) monocytes, (3) eosinophils, (4) basophils, and (5) lymphocytes. Each type of WBC combats certain types of microorganisms. Normally, WBCs identify and destroy foreign **antigens** or proteins by ingesting them. Because this process destroys the WBCs themselves, the normal life span for a WBC is only a few hours to a few days. Neutrophils may live as little as 6 hours. Other cells called *macrophages* clean up the WBC debris. If the dead WBCs build up faster than the macrophages can clean them up, pus is formed. This is why pus is a classic sign of infection and should be reported to a nurse or a physician immediately and carefully monitored.

Neutrophils. Neutrophils fight bacterial infections. They are the most numerous of the WBCs, comprising approximately 60% of all WBCs. These cells are known by many names, including *polymorphonuclear neutrophils (PMNs, polys), neuts, granulocytes (grans)*, or *segmented neutrophils (segs)*. The bone marrow is capable of producing huge numbers of neutrophils to fight infection.

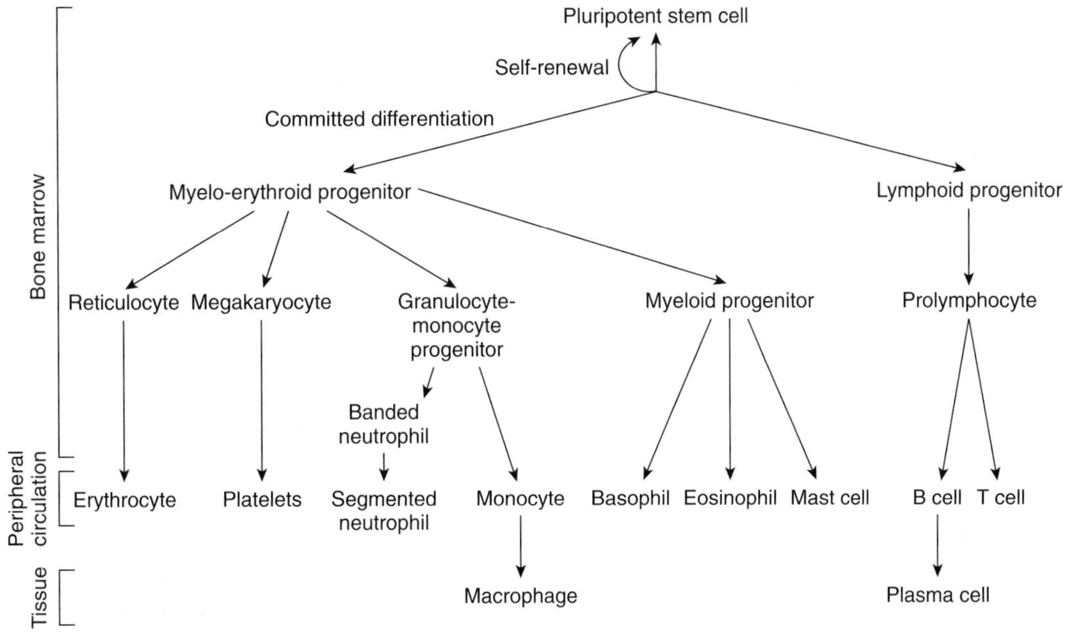

FIGURE 34-1 Maturation of cells constituting the hematologic and immune systems. (From Young-McCaughan S, Jennings BM: Hematologic and immunologic systems. In Alspach JG, editor: *Core curriculum for critical care nursing*, ed 5, Philadelphia, 1998, Saunders.)

Monocytes and Macrophages. Once released from the bone marrow, monocytes circulate in the bloodstream for approximately 1 day before leaving the peripheral circulation and entering tissue. When monocytes enter tissue, they are called *macrophages.* Some macrophages move throughout the body whereas others stay in one particular tissue monitoring for microorganisms. Unlike neutrophils, which are destroyed during phagocytosis, macrophages can ingest many foreign antigens and survive months to years.

Eosinophils. Eosinophils combat parasitic infections. They are also associated with allergic reactions and other inflammatory processes.

Basophils. Basophils can initiate a massive inflammatory response that quickly brings other WBCs to the site of infection. Basophils work in conjunction with **immunoglobulin** E (IgE). When IgE identifies a foreign antigen, it triggers basophils to release histamine from cell vesicles located in the basophils. Histamine is a potent vasodilator that increases blood circulation to the site, quickly bringing other WBCs to the site of infection.

Mast Cells. Like basophils, mast cells also store histamine in cell vesicles that can be released by IgE. Although basophils normally circulate in the blood, mast cells are located in the tissue.

B Lymphocytes (B Cells). B cells manufacture antigen-binding proteins, called immunoglobulin (Ig), on their cell membrane. When the B cell Ig binds with a particular antigen, the B cell is stimulated to produce plasma cells and memory B cells. Plasma cells are **antibody** factories that immediately produce large amounts of Ig. Memory B cells go into a resting state but can be reactivated quickly to produce plasma cells and antibodies if exposed to the same antigen in the future.

Once the Ig is released from the membrane of either the B cell or the plasma cell, it is called an *antibody.* Four major types of antibodies exist. IgM is the first Ig to be secreted during the primary immune response to an antigen.

IgG is secreted during the secondary immune response and is more specific to a particular antigen.

IgA is present in secretions such as mucus and mother's milk. IgE attaches to the cell membranes of basophils and mast cells, where it triggers the cell to release histamine.

T Lymphocytes (T Cells). Two major types of T lymphocytes exist: (1) T helper (T_H) cells and (2) T cytotoxic (T_C) cells. T_H cells are also called *CD4 cells* because of the protein complex CD4 found on their cell membranes. When T_H cells come in contact with foreign antigens, they secrete cytokines that activate other components of the immune system to facilitate the body's immune response. These are the cells that can become infected with the human immunodeficiency virus (HIV). T_C cells are also called *CD8 cells* because of the protein complex CD8 found on their cell membranes. When T_C cells come in contact with foreign antigens, they can directly destroy the invader.

Cytokines

Cytokines are hormones secreted by cells to signal other cells. Examples of cytokines include interferon, interleukin, tumor necrosis factor (TNF), granulocyte-macrophage colony-stimulating factor (GM-CSF), granulocyte colony-stimulating factor (G-CSF), and erythropoietin (EPO).

Eicosanoids

Eicosanoids are a class of fatty acids that regulate blood vessel vasodilation, temperature elevation, WBC activation, and other physiologic processes involved in **immunity**. Many commonly prescribed drugs, such as nonsteroidal antiinflammatory drugs (NSAIDs), disrupt eicosanoid production, thereby affecting a person's ability to mount an immunologic response.

Thymus

The thymus is a lymphoid organ located in the upper chest below the thyroid. Early in life, certain WBCs, called *lymphocytes*, migrate from the bone marrow where they are produced to the thymus where they mature into T lymphocytes, or T cells. Mature T lymphocytes are then released into circulation. After puberty, the T cell population has been maximized. These mature T cells continue to live and function throughout a person's life. At this point, the thymus stops growing and eventually shrinks because it is no longer needed to mature T cells.

Lymph, Lymphatics, and Lymph Nodes

When blood flows through the capillary beds to deliver oxygen (O_2) and pick up carbon dioxide (CO_2), not all of the plasma returns to the veins to be recirculated. The lymphatic system is a network of open-ended tubes—separate from the blood circulation system—that collects the plasma left behind in the tissues and returns it to the venous system. In addition, various WBCs that travel through tissues and organs to monitor for infection reenter the blood circulation via the lymphatic system. This mixture of plasma and cells is known as *lymph fluid.* Lymph fluid is propelled along the lymphatic system by the normal contraction of skeletal muscles. One-way valves located in the lymphatic vessels prevent the lymph fluid from pooling in the periphery. The lymphatic vessels empty into the venous system through the right lymphatic duct of the right subclavian vein and the thoracic duct of the left subclavian vein. Figure 34-2 shows a diagram of the lymphatic system. The lymphatic vessels can be damaged during surgery or following radiation therapy. As a result, lymph fluid can build up in the tissues distal to the affected area, resulting in lymphedema of the extremity.

Lymph nodes are small patches of lymphatic tissue located along the lymphatic system that filter microorganisms from the lymph fluid before it is returned to the bloodstream. Lymph nodes are located throughout the body, as shown in Figure 34-2. Individual lymph nodes can become swollen with infection and also with some cancers. The nodes closer to the surface of the body in the neck, under the arm, and in the groin can be palpated when they are swollen. Usually lymph nodes deeper in the body cannot be palpated but can be visualized with computed tomography (CT) if they are larger than 2 cm. During surgery for cancer, the surgeon usually will biopsy nearby lymph nodes and have the pathologist check the specimens to see if the cancer might have spread.

Liver

The liver is located in the upper right quadrant of the abdomen. One of the many functions of the liver is to filter microorganisms from the blood so that macrophages can destroy them.

Spleen

The spleen is located in the upper left quadrant of the abdomen. Like the lymph nodes, the spleen filters microorganisms from the blood. Once trapped in the spleen, microorganisms are destroyed by the WBCs that reside in the spleen.

Under some circumstances the spleen is surgically removed. Trauma from a motor vehicle accident can rupture the victim's spleen, necessitating removal. Patients newly diagnosed with Hodgkin disease, a form of cancer of the lymph nodes, may have their spleens removed and pathologically examined to help determine the best treatment. Anyone without a spleen is at increased risk for certain kinds of infections such as pneumococcal infections. If possible, patients should receive a Pneumovax vaccine before undergoing splenectomy so that the body can form its own antibodies against pneumococcal bacteria. Vaccinations are not always possible for the individual undergoing an emergency splenectomy.

Peyer Patches

Peyer patches are lymphoid tissue found in the small intestine where it transitions into the large intestine. Macrophages and both B and T lymphocytes found in this lymphoid tissue attach any foreign microorganisms that attempt to enter the bloodstream and could cause infection.

PHYSIOLOGIC FUNCTIONS OF THE IMMUNE SYSTEM

Innate Immunity

Innate immunity is operational at all times, whether or not a pathogen is present. At birth, innate immunologic defense systems are immediately functional. Innate immunologic systems include anatomic and physiologic barriers, inflammatory response, and the ability of certain cells to phagocytose foreign invaders.

Anatomic and Physiologic Barriers. The skin and mucous membranes are the body's first line of defense, acting as a protective covering and secreting substances that inhibit the growth of pathogens. Sweat glands secrete a lysozyme, an antimicrobial enzyme. The skin and the mucosa of the gastrointestinal (GI) and genitourinary systems are acidic, which inhibits the growth of many pathogenic organisms. Secretions from the respiratory and GI tracts contain

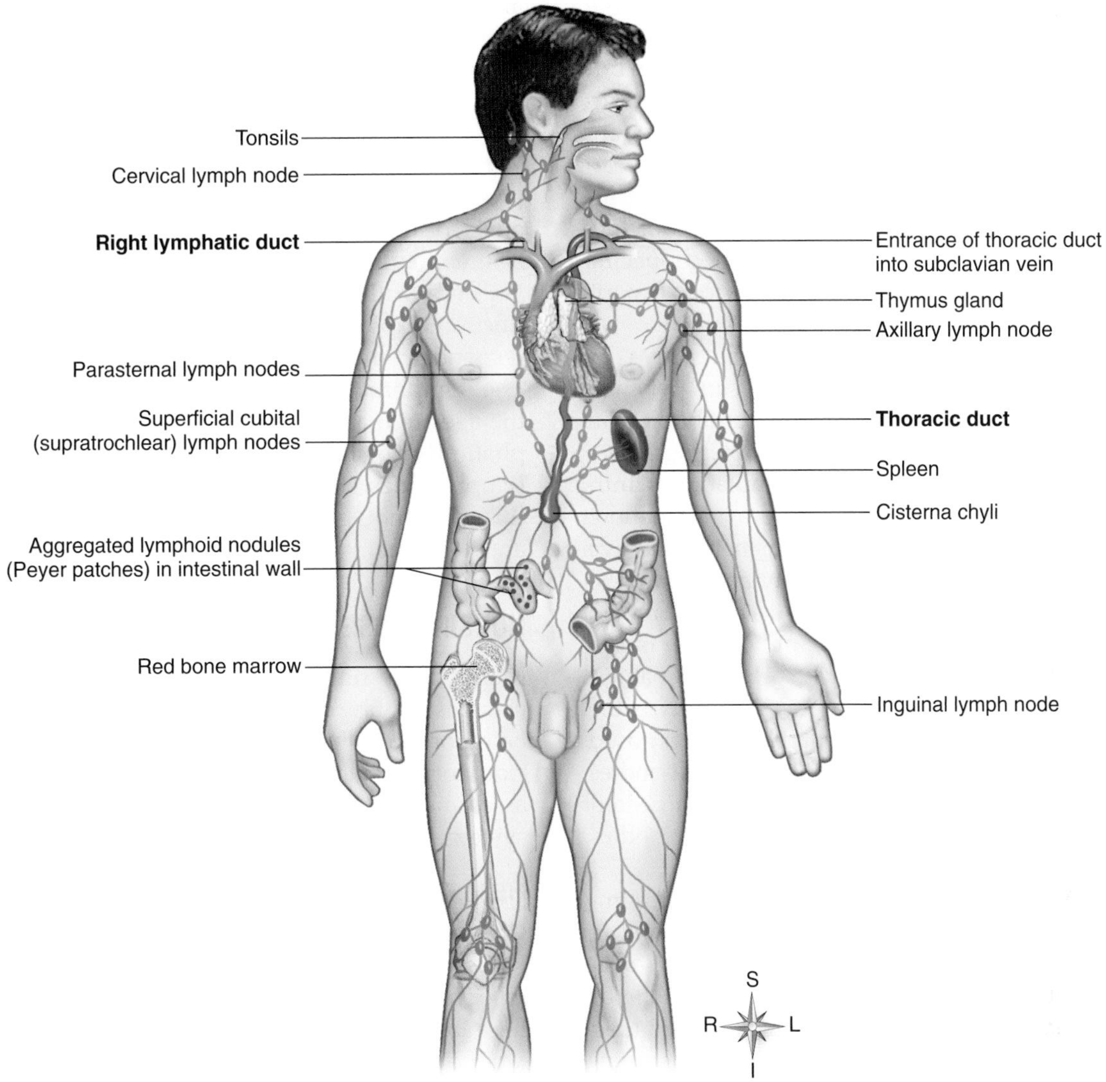

FIGURE 34-2 Diagram of the lymphatic system. (From Thibodeau GA, Patton, KT: *Anatomy and physiology*, ed 8, St. Louis, 2013, Mosby.)

the antibody IgA, as well as **phagocytes**. Skin and mucous membrane surfaces are colonized by normal bacterial flora, which prevents pathogens from attaching and gaining access to the body. Normal flora is a mixture of organisms regularly found at any anatomic site. In addition, coughing and sneezing, peristalsis in the GI tract, emptying the bladder, and sloughing of dead skin cells all serve to remove microorganisms from the body, thus preventing their invasion and overgrowth.

Inflammation. The body initially responds to an injury or infection by dilating the capillary bed and increasing the capillary permeability of the affected area. This brings WBCs to the site and allows them to enter the tissue to attack microorganisms. This multistep process is called *inflammation* and is recognized by rubor (redness), tumor (swelling), calor (heat), and dolor (pain) at the site of injury or infection.

Phagocytosis. Phagocytosis is the process of ingesting and digesting invading pathogens, dead cells, and cellular debris. Neutrophils, monocytes, and macrophages are capable of phagocytosis and are sometimes called *phagocytes*.

Acquired Immunity

Whereas innate immunity fights any type of invader and is operational at all times, **acquired immunity** is specific to a particular pathogen and is activated only when needed. The two types of acquired immunity are (1) antibody mediated and (2) cell mediated.

Antibody-Mediated Immunity. An **antibody-mediated immune** response is initiated when the IgM on the surface of B lymphocytes detects a foreign antigen. With the help of T_H cells, the B lymphocytes secrete additional IgM and differentiate to produce antibody-secreting plasma cells and memory B cells. The newly made plasma cells can produce and secrete large amounts of IgM antibody. When antibodies bind to an antigen, they do not actually destroy the pathogen but they make the antigen readily recognizable to neutrophils, monocytes, and macrophages, which can phagocytose the pathogen. If in the future this same pathogen tries to reenter the body, the memory B cells are triggered to immediately produce large amounts of IgG antibody. IgG is like IgM except that it is more specific to one particular pathogen, based on previous experience with that same pathogen.

Acquired antibody immunity can be active or passive. Active acquired immunity occurs when a person synthesizes his or her own antibodies in response to a pathogen. A person is exhibiting active acquired immunity when he or she manufactures antibodies in response to an infection or a vaccination. Active acquired immunity is permanent. Passive acquired immunity occurs when an antibody produced by one person or an animal is transferred to another person. For example, IgA antibodies in mother's milk confer passive immunity to breast-fed babies. Another example of passive acquired immunity is the gamma globulin that may be given to a person exposed to hepatitis. Gamma globulin contains IgG antibodies that help to destroy the hepatitis virus. Passive acquired immunity lasts only 1 to 2 months after the antibodies have been received.

Cell-Mediated Immunity. Antibody-mediated immune responses are aimed primarily at invading microorganisms such as bacteria. In contrast, **cell-mediated immunity** is aimed primarily at intracellular defects caused by viruses and cancer. Cell-mediated immunity is also responsible for delayed hypersensitivity reactions and rejection of transplanted tissue. T_C cells are the primary component of cell-mediated immunity. When T_C cells recognize foreign antigens in cells, they secrete cytotoxic substances that destroy the defective cells. Unfortunately, a transplanted tissue graft, such as a kidney transplant or a heart transplant, may be recognized by the organ recipient's immune system as foreign and is attacked by T_C cells in this same way.

Tolerance

As part of initiating an immunologic response, the immune system must be able to recognize its own proteins and not mount an immune response against itself. This process of self-recognition occurs as part of normal neonatal growth and development. Autoimmune diseases occur when a breakdown of tolerance takes place. The immune system inappropriately identifies its own proteins as foreign and mounts a response to destroy these self-proteins. Examples of autoimmune diseases include idiopathic thrombocytopenic purpura (ITP), thrombotic thrombocytopenic purpura (TTP), acute rheumatic fever, type 1 diabetes mellitus, systemic lupus erythematosus (SLE), rheumatoid arthritis, multiple sclerosis, Graves disease, and Hashimoto thyroiditis.

AGE-RELATED CHANGES

With advancing age, the bone marrow becomes less productive. Immunologic function is generally not affected unless a person is unusually stressed by trauma, a chronic infection, or treatment for cancer. Yet even with conditions necessitating a higher production of blood cells, the bone marrow usually can respond to the increased demand, given more time. The lymphatic tissue grows very quickly between the ages of 6 and 20 years. With advancing age, lymphatic tissue shrinks, resulting in fewer and smaller lymph nodes. However, as with the bone marrow, this does not generally affect the overall health of an individual.

NURSING ASSESSMENT OF THE IMMUNE SYSTEM

Many subtle findings in the assessment can suggest changes in the patient's immune system that should be reported to the registered nurse (RN) or the physician for evaluation. Box 34-1 outlines the nursing assessment of patients with disorders of the immune system.

HEALTH HISTORY

Chief Complaint and History of Present Illness

Pay special attention to the patient who remarks that he or she has frequent or persistent infections, bleeds for a long time when cut, bruises easily, or has chronic fatigue, because these symptoms may reflect an underlying immunologic disorder.

Past Medical History

A patient could have an underlying immunologic problem if he or she reports any of the following: cancer or prior treatment for cancer; HIV infection; history of splenectomy; history of organ transplant; or placement of an indwelling venous access device, indicating that the patient needed long-term venous access. Medications the patient is currently using or a recent change in medication may suggest an underlying immunologic problem. It is important to find out what over-the-counter (OTC) medications (including herbal products) the patient uses, because many of these products contain aspirin or NSAIDs, which may disrupt immunologic function. Ask the patient about any recent changes in medications and any recent immunizations.

Family History

Note any family history of immunologic disorders such as cancer. Death of a family member at a young age for reasons other than trauma may indicate a genetic immunologic disorder.

Box 34-1 Assessment of a Patient with Disorders of the Immune System

HEALTH HISTORY

History of Present Illness

Frequent or persistent infections, prolonged bleeding, easy bruising, chronic fatigue

Past Medical History

Cancer or prior treatment for cancer, human immunodeficiency virus (HIV) infection, history of splenectomy, history of organ transplant, placement of an indwelling venous access device indicating that the patient needed long-term venous access, recent infections, current medications (including over-the-counter [OTC] medications, recent changes in medication, herbal products), recent immunizations

Family History

Cancer, death of a family member at a young age for reasons other than trauma

Review of Systems

Integumentary

Rash, breaks in the skin, ulcers, lesions, or enlarged lymph nodes; red, swollen, or painful areas

Neurologic

Weakness, lethargy, malaise, restlessness, apprehension, headache

Respiratory

Sinus pain, dyspnea, cough

Gastrointestinal

Mouth ulcerations, sore throat, pain with swallowing, pain with defecation, unplanned weight loss or weight gain, diarrhea

Genitourinary

Pain or burning with urination

Musculoskeletal

Pain in bones or joints

Endocrine

Fatigue

Functional Assessment

Occupation and hobbies, changes in ability to do activities of daily living (ADL), roles at home and work, self-concept, activities and exercise, sleep and rest, nutrition, interpersonal relationships, stressors, coping style

PHYSICAL EXAMINATION

Vital Signs

Fever, tachycardia, tachypnea, hypotension

Height and Weight

General Survey

Responsiveness, mood, expression, posture

Skin

Color

Head and Neck

Enlarged, swollen, or draining areas; enlarged lymph nodes

Thorax

Enlarged lymph nodes, respiratory rate, breath sounds, heart rate

Abdomen

Organ enlargement, enlarged lymph nodes

Review of Systems

The review of systems is aimed at finding out what symptoms the patient has been experiencing over the past weeks or months. These symptoms might provide clues as to what specific medical disorder the patient may now have. The primary symptom of an immunologic disorder is infection. The patient should be carefully questioned about any reddened, swollen, painful, or unusually warm areas that might indicate an infectious process. Ask about fever, chills, or night sweats. Night sweats can occur when the patient's temperature rises at night but the patient does not awaken until the temperature falls, causing sweating. Night sweats can occur normally in women undergoing menopause. However, night sweats can also be a symptom of infection (e.g., tuberculosis, malaria), leukemia (cancer of the WBCs), or lymphoma (cancer of the lymph nodes).

Begin the review of systems with the integument. Ask about any red, swollen, or painful areas (which could be sites of infection) and any breaks in the skin, ulcers, lesions, or enlarged lymph nodes (which could indicate a site of infection). Relevant data about the neurologic system include weakness, lethargy, malaise, restlessness, apprehension, or headache, which could indicate a central nervous system (CNS) infection. In relation to the respiratory system, ask about sinus pain, dyspnea, or cough, which could indicate an infection. If the cough is productive, ask the patient to describe the sputum. When assessing the GI system, ask about sore throat, any pain with swallowing, and any pain with defecation. Ask about any unplanned weight loss or weight gain. When reviewing the genitourinary system, ask about any pain or burning with urination, any change in the frequency of urination, and any blood in or discoloration of the urine. Finally, when assessing the endocrine system, ask about any unusual fatigue.

Functional Assessment

Patients newly diagnosed with an immunologic disorder may not experience dramatic changes in their functional abilities. However, many immunologic disorders are chronic conditions that the patient has lived with—and been treated for—for many years.

Occupation and Hobbies. Knowing a patient's job and hobbies can alert the nurse to unusual chemical exposures. Because various chemicals can affect the bone marrow and blood, note any recent chemical exposure. For example, someone who builds models for a hobby may be exposed to unusual glues or paints that may affect the blood count.

Self-Concept. The patient's self-concept can be assessed by exploring the patient's feeling about himself or herself. For many people, one's self-concept depends on one's job. If the patient is unable to work because of an immunologic disorder, his or her self-concept can be adversely affected. In addition, medical insurance is often contingent on employment. Loss of medical insurance and the need to go on state or federal assistance can diminish a patient's self-concept. Another factor that can adversely affect the patient's self-concept is a change in appearance because of the disease or the treatment.

Activity and Exercise. Document the current activity level as well as the effects of the disease and treatment on the patient's usual pattern of activity and exercise. Ask about the layout of the patient's home, specifically the location of bathrooms in relation to living areas and bedrooms. Ask if the patient must climb stairs to enter the home or get to a second floor; stair climbing can quickly tire a patient with an immunologic disorder. Also ask what the patient does for recreation and whether these activities can still be done during times of decreased energy.

Sleep and Rest. Note the number of continuous hours the patient sleeps every night as well as whether any sleeping aids are used, what interrupts the patient's sleep, and whether the patient naps during the day.

Nutrition. Ask the patient to describe his or her usual diet and any recent changes in appetite or weight. Identify factors that might be interfering with eating, such as nausea, vomiting, and taste changes (see *Nutrition Considerations* box). Depression and loneliness can adversely affect a patient's nutritional status. Limited financial resources can also limit a patient's ability to maintain a nutritious diet.

Nutrition Considerations

1. Because food contains microorganisms, patients with low white blood cell (WBC) counts are often discouraged from eating raw fruits and vegetables and from drinking milk. However, it is not clear that this actually reduces infection in these patients.
2. Patients with human immunodeficiency virus (HIV) require high calorie and nutrient intake to combat wasting.

Interpersonal Relationships. Explore the patient's view of himself or herself as a husband or wife, partner, father or mother, son or daughter, friend, and co-worker. Discuss the effects of the disease on these relationships and the patient's roles in the home. Ask what household chores the patient is responsible for doing as well as who does the shopping, cooking, and cleaning. If the patient has children who need care, ask whether the patient is able to perform the usual child care activities.

Coping and Stress. Ask what worries the patient has and how he or she usually deals with stress. Explore sources of support, which might include family, support groups, and spiritual beliefs and practices.

Perception of Health. Discuss the patient's view of his or her own health and health practices. This might include measures taken to prevent complications from disease and keeping regular medical appointments.

PHYSICAL EXAMINATION

The physical examination begins with measurement of vital signs and height and weight. Be alert for fever, tachycardia, tachypnea, and hypotension.

General Survey

Note the patient's responsiveness, mood, expression, and posture. Throughout the examination, carefully inspect and describe any reddened, swollen, or painful areas the patient identifies.

Skin

Inspect the patient's skin from head to toe, noting the general color, texture, turgor, temperature, and integrity. Also palpate for any swollen or painful areas.

Head and Neck

When examining the eyes, ears, nose, mouth, and throat, it is important to note any enlarged, swollen, or draining areas that might indicate an infection. Examples might be swollen, draining sinuses; a canker sore in the mouth; or enlarged tonsils with exudate. The examiner with advanced skills may palpate the neck for enlarged lymph nodes.

Thorax

The examiner with advanced skills may palpate the axilla for enlarged lymph nodes.

Lungs. Document the patient's respiratory rate and effort and auscultate for wheezing, crackles, or rhonchi. Patients with a respiratory tract infection may have abnormal breath sounds or a cough.

Heart and Vascular System. Record the patient's heart rate and blood pressure. Patients with a severe infection may be tachycardic or hypotensive.

Abdomen

The examiner with advanced skills may palpate the abdomen for tenderness. The liver and spleen can become enlarged with blood cell disorders, causing abdominal fullness and tenderness. The advanced practice examiner may palpate the patient's groin for enlarged lymph nodes.

DIAGNOSTIC TESTS AND PROCEDURES

Various blood studies are used to screen the function of the patient's immunologic system. Blood studies, as well as other tests and procedures done to diagnose disorders of the immune system, are described in Tables 34-1 and 34-2. The laboratory performing the test should provide normal values for the various blood tests. Ranges of normal values can be found in various textbooks of laboratory and diagnostic tests.

Table 34-1 Diagnostic Tests and Procedures — Laboratory Studies to Evaluate the Immune System

TEST/STUDY	PURPOSE AND PROCEDURE	PATIENT PREPARATION	POSTPROCEDURE NURSING CARE
Blood tests (CBC, ANA, LE prep)	Used to measure various blood components. Different blood tests are collected in different laboratory tubes containing specific reagents or no reagents at all. Usually the tubes have color-coded tops. Be sure to collect the blood in the blood tube specific for the blood test ordered.	Choose the correct blood tube in which to collect the blood. Tell the patient that he or she will feel a needlestick as the needle goes through the skin.	Apply a bandage. Have the patient hold pressure on the site for 1 minute. The bandage may be removed in 1 hour.
Blood cultures	Used to detect and identify microorganisms in the blood.	Choose the correct blood culture bottles according to whether aerobic or anaerobic cultures are to be drawn. The vein is prepared with Betadine and allowed to dry. The tops of the blood culture bottles are prepared with Betadine and allowed to dry. Do not touch the draw site except with sterile gloves. Tell the patient that he or she will feel a needlestick as the needle goes through the skin. Draw enough blood so that 5 mL of blood can be placed in each culture bottle. Send the specimens to the laboratory immediately. Blood culture results are evaluated at 48 and 72 hours. Tell the patient not to expect any final results for 3–4 days.	Apply a bandage. Have the patient hold pressure on the site for 1 minute. The bandage may be removed in 1 hour.
Sputum cultures	Used to detect and identify microorganisms in the sputum.	Give the patient a sterile cup. Have the patient collect sputum the next time he or she coughs. Caution the patient not to collect saliva. Sputum comes from the lungs with coughing. Send the specimen to the laboratory immediately.	No special care is required after the procedure.
Urine cultures	Used to detect and identify microorganisms in the urine.	Give the patient wipes and a sterile container. Have the patient clean around the meatus of the urethra. Tell the patient to urinate a small amount into the toilet and stop. Then tell the patient to collect a urine specimen. If the patient is unable to collect the specimen, the physician may request a straight catheterization to collect the specimen. Follow the procedures for catheterizing a patient as described in Chapter 42. If the patient has an indwelling catheter, clamp the catheter. In approximately 15 minutes, prepare the withdrawal port on the catheter with Betadine and allow the Betadine to dry. Withdraw a sample of urine through the port with a sterile needle and syringe and transfer the specimen into a sterile collection cup. Send the specimen to the laboratory immediately.	No special care is required after the procedure.
Stool cultures	Used to detect and identify microorganisms in the stool.	Have the patient defecate into a clean bedpan or other container. Using a sterile tongue blade, collect a specimen in a sterile container. Send the specimen to the laboratory immediately. Some tests must be done while the specimen is still warm.	No special care is required after the procedure.

Data from Fischbach FT, Dunning MB: *A manual of laboratory and diagnostic tests*, ed 8, Philadelphia, 2009, Lippincott-Williams & Wilkins.
ANA, Antinuclear antibody; *CBC*, complete blood count; *LE prep*, lupus erythematosus preparation.

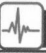

Table 34-2 Diagnostic Tests and Procedures **Special Procedures to Evaluate the Immune System**

TEST/STUDY	PURPOSE AND PROCEDURE	PATIENT PREPARATION	POSTPROCEDURE NURSING CARE
Lymphangiography (LAG)	LAG demonstrates the anatomy of the lymphatic vessels and nodes. The patient is taken to diagnostic radiology, where a 1- to 2-inch incision is made on the dorsum of each foot or hand. The lymphatic vessels are cannulated and dye is injected. Several radiographs are taken as the dye moves up the extremities. The patient returns to diagnostic radiology 12 to 24 hours later for more radiographs of the lymph nodes and higher lymphatic channels.	Explain the purpose and procedure to the patient and obtain signed consent. Ask the patient about any allergies to contrast media. No fasting is necessary. Some local discomfort may be experienced as the local anesthetic is injected to numb the top of the feet or hands. Incisions may stain blue from the dye. The procedure takes approximately 3 hours. The patient returns to diagnostic radiology 12 to 24 hours later for more radiographs.	Check the patient's vital signs every 4 hours (q4h) for 48 hours. Keep the incisions clean and dry after the procedure. The physician may order the legs or arms to be elevated. Stitches may be in place and should be removed in 5–7 days.
Spleen scan	A spleen scan is used to evaluate the size and function of the spleen. In the nuclear medicine department, a radioactive dye is injected into a vein. The amount of dye taken up by the spleen is measured by a machine 20–60 minutes after the dye is injected.	Explain the purpose and procedure to the patient. Ask the patient about any allergies to contrast media. No fasting is necessary. An intravenous line must be in place to inject the dye but may be discontinued after the injection. The procedure takes approximately 60 minutes.	No special care is required after the procedure.
Gallium scan	A gallium scan is used to detect the presence, location, and size of chronic infections, abscesses, and malignant tumors primarily of lymphoid origin. In the nuclear medicine department, a radioactive dye is injected into a vein. The amount of dye taken up by lymphoid tissues is measured by a machine 24–72 hours after the dye is injected.	Explain the purpose and procedure to the patient. Ask the patient about any allergies to contrast media. An intravenous line must be in place to inject the dye but may be discontinued after the injection. Scanning is usually done 24–72 hours after dye injection. If the abdomen is to be scanned, a laxative is usually given the evening before the scanning. However, the patient may eat breakfast the morning of the scan. During imaging the patient must lie quietly for 45–90 minutes.	No special care is required after the procedure.
Skin tests	Skin testing is done for several reasons: to detect sensitivity to allergens such as pollen, to determine sensitivity to microorganisms that cause disease (e.g., tuberculin), and to determine whether cell-mediated immune functions are normal. The inner side of the patient's forearm is cleaned. Generally, 0.1 mL of the test material is injected intradermally using a 26- or 27-gauge needle and tuberculin syringe.	Explain the purpose and procedure to the patient. Tell the patient that he or she will feel a needlestick as the needle goes through the skin.	No special care is required after the procedure. Tell the patient that he or she must be reexamined in 2–3 days to determine the results of the testing. Swelling at the site of injection indicates that the body's cell-mediated immune system is functioning.

Adapted from Fischbach FT, Dunning MB: *A manual of laboratory and diagnostic tests*, ed 8, Philadelphia, 2009, Lippincott-Williams & Wilkins.

BLOOD TESTS

The complete blood count (CBC) is a common blood test done in most laboratories; it reports the total number of WBCs as well as what percentage of the total number of WBCs are neutrophils, monocytes, eosinophils, basophils, and lymphocytes. Both the total number of WBCs in the body and the differential, or percentage of each of the specific types of WBCs in the body, are evaluated. Normal WBC counts range between 5000 and 10,000 WBCs per cubic millimeter (mm^3) of blood. The majority of the WBCs (60%) are neutrophils. Physicians and nurses are interested primarily in the number of neutrophils because these are the cells that fight bacterial infections. To calculate the absolute neutrophil count (ANC), one multiplies the percentage of neutrophils indicated on the differential of the CBC by the total number of WBCs. See Box 34-2 for a sample calculation.

Other blood tests are specific to the diagnosis of a particular disease. The antinuclear antibody (ANA) test detects antibodies in the blood that may be indicative of SLE or other autoimmune disorders. A lupus erythematosus preparation (LE prep) is a blood test more specific to SLE. An enzyme-linked immunosorbent assay and Western blot tests are used to diagnose HIV infection. T cell counts and viral load are tests used to determine the severity of the infection. Table 34-1 describes the procedures for collecting blood specimens for these tests.

CULTURES OF BLOOD, URINE, SPUTUM, AND STOOL

Cultures are done to detect infections in the blood, sputum, urine, or stool. When a patient has a fever without an obvious source of infection, all of these specimens are obtained to look for the source of the infection. Table 34-1 describes the procedures for collecting these specimens for culture.

SKIN TESTS

Skin tests can serve as a barometer of immune system functioning, pointing out either hyposensitivities or hypersensitivities to a particular antigen. Examples of allergens used in skin testing include dust, pollen, animal dander, purified protein derivative, tuberculin bacillus, and *Candida albicans.* Table 34-2 describes the procedure for skin tests.

Box 34-2 Calculating Absolute Neutrophil Count from Complete Blood Count

COMPLETE BLOOD COUNT REPORT	
White blood cells (WBCs) × 10^3	6.5
Red blood cells (RBCs) × 10^6	4.51
Hemoglobin (Hgb) in g/dL	14.0
Hematocrit (Hct) %	40.8
Mean corpuscular volume (MCV) in fl	90.5
Mean corpuscular hemoglobin (MCH) in pg	30.9
Mean cell hemoglobin concentration (MCHC) in g/dL	34.2
Platelet count (PLT) × 10^3	333
AUTOMATED DIFFERENTIAL	
Lymphocytes %	35.0
Monocytes %	10.3
Neutrophils %	46.3
Eosinophils %	7.3
Basophiles %	1.0
MANUAL DIFFERENTIAL	
Segmented neutrophils %	49.0
Banded neutrophils %	1.0
Lymphocytes %	32.0
Monocytes %	8.0
Eosinophils %	9.0
Basophils %	1.0

To calculate the absolute neutrophil count (ANC), use the *manual differential* because it is more accurate. Multiply the percentage of segmented neutrophils (49% in this example) plus the percentage of banded neutrophils (1% in this example) by the total number of WBCs (6500 in this example). Banded neutrophils are included in the calculations of the ANC because they are developmentally nearly mature neutrophils and can function as mature neutrophils (see Fig. 34-1). If a manual differential has not been done, the automated differential can be used; however, if the total WBC count is >10,000/mL or <3000/mL, a manual differential should be requested.

GENERIC CALCULATION

$$ANC = (\%\ Neutrophils + \%\ Banded\ neutrophils) \times WBCs$$

CALCULATIONS FOR THIS EXAMPLE

$$(0.49 + 0.01) \times 6500.00 = 3250.00$$

COMMON THERAPEUTIC MEASURES

NURSING ACTIONS FOR THE PATIENT AT RISK FOR INJURY FROM INFECTION

The lower a patient's WBC count is (in particular, the lower his or her neutrophil count is), the greater is the patient's risk of infection. Box 34-3 outlines typical nursing actions for the patient at risk for injury from infection.

BONE MARROW TRANSPLANTATION AND PERIPHERAL BLOOD STEM CELL TRANSPLANTATION

Bone marrow transplantation and peripheral blood stem cell transplantation are done to restore the hematologic and immunologic systems in patients with malignancies who have received extremely high doses of chemotherapy and radiation therapy. Bone marrow transplantation is also used in patients with genetic bone marrow defects and aplastic anemia in an attempt to repopulate the bone marrow with blood-producing

Box 34-3 Nursing Actions for the Patient at Risk for Injury from Infection: Compromised Host Precautions

1. The patient should have a private room. It does not have to be an isolation room. The door may be left open. A *Compromised Host Precaution* sign should be posted on the door.
2. All persons entering the patient's room must wash their hands before touching the patient for any reason. This is the most important way to prevent infection. The patient and family should be encouraged to remind all staff and visitors to wash their hands before touching the patient.
3. Monitor the patient's vital signs every 2 to 4 hours. Notify the physician immediately of a temperature >101°F to consider the need for an infectious fever workup and initiation or changing of antibiotics. An infectious fever workup usually includes two sets of blood cultures, a chest radiograph, sputum culture, urine culture, wound culture, and cultures of other sites suggestive of infection. Patients with a central line or permanent, indwelling venous access device usually have one set of specimens for culture drawn from the line and one set drawn from a peripheral site. Mark the culture bottles clearly regarding where the specimen was obtained to assist with localization of the infection. Blood cultures are more likely to yield the offending organism if the blood is drawn as the patient's temperature is rising instead of after the patient's temperature has peaked.
4. Invasive procedures should be kept to a minimum. Invasive devices such as catheters and tubes should be removed as soon as the patient's medical condition permits.
5. Careful attention to aseptic technique must be observed, especially when performing phlebotomy, handling intravenous lines, or performing other invasive procedures.
6. Designate a particular stethoscope and thermometer to be used exclusively in caring for the patient.
7. Masks are not required; in fact, they are discouraged. Staff with upper respiratory tract or other infections should not care for the patient.
8. Clean table tops, equipment, and the floor frequently with hospital-approved disinfectant, clean cloths, and clean mops.
9. The patient should be taught to wash his or her hands before and after eating, using the toilet, and doing any self-care procedure. If possible, the patient should shower every day. Liquid soap instead of bar soap should be used.
10. Encourage the patient to cough and deep breathe every 4 hours. Mobility should be encouraged. Smoking should be discouraged.
11. Only canned or cooked foods may be served. Raw fruits, raw vegetables, and milk products may not be served because of the risk of *Escherichia coli*, *Pseudomonas aeruginosa*, and *Klebsiella* spp. bacteria on or in these food items. The patient should be encouraged to choose appropriate foods from the menu. The diet roster should be annotated *compromised host precautions* so that the nutrition care staff can verify that appropriate choices are being made.
12. Tests, scans, and appointments away from the patient's room should be coordinated in advance to eliminate or minimize waiting time in common waiting areas.
13. The patient should wear a clean mask when outside the room, especially in heavily traveled public areas such as corridors, elevators, and waiting rooms. The mask may be removed when the patient is in less public areas. A new mask should be used for each trip out of the room.
14. Some hospitals allow flowers and plants in the patient's room; however, they should not be handled by the patient because of the possibility of *Escherichia coli* contamination of the water and soil.
15. No humidifiers with standing water should be used in the patient's room. If a wall humidifier is needed, the water should be changed every day.
16. Teach the patient and family about the underlying pathophysiology that puts the patient at risk for infection and about precautions to minimize the risk for infection.

cells. The donated bone marrow is administered to the patient just like a blood transfusion through an intravenous line. The infused bone marrow finds its way to the patient's bone marrow, where it starts growing and producing healthy WBCs, RBCs, and platelets.

Three main types of transplants exist: (1) allogeneic bone marrow transplant, (2) autologous bone marrow transplant, and (3) peripheral blood stem cell transplant. *Allogeneic bone marrow transplants* have been done the longest. They originally were used to treat people with leukemia, or cancer of the WBCs. High doses of chemotherapy and radiation therapy are given to destroy all of the cancerous bone marrow. Then bone marrow from a human leukocyte antigen (HLA)–matched donor is collected from the iliac crest much like a bone marrow biopsy is done, only under anesthesia with repeated extractions of the liquid marrow, which is then reinfused in the patient to restore bone marrow function. HLA typing is similar to blood typing but is much more specific. Because these HLAs are genetically determined, brothers and sisters of the patient are initially tested to determine whether they can be bone marrow donors for their sibling. A 25% chance exists that a sibling will be an HLA match to a patient needing a bone marrow transplant. A possibility exists that someone in the general population might be HLA matched to the patient but the chances of finding a matched unrelated donor (MUD) are very small. For many patients, an allogeneic bone marrow transplant is not possible because a matched donor cannot be found.

Another type of bone marrow transplant harvests the patient's own bone marrow before chemotherapy and radiation therapy. After therapy, the patient's own bone marrow is returned to the patient. This type of bone marrow transplant, called an *autologous bone marrow transplant*, is the best option for patients with a solid tumor that has not metastasized to the bone marrow—for example, patients with lymphoma. An autologous bone marrow transplant is generally not an option for patients with leukemia or those who have a cancer that has metastasized to the bone marrow, because healthy bone marrow must be reinfused in the patient after chemotherapy and radiation therapy to prevent cancer recurrence.

A third type of bone marrow transplant is a *peripheral blood stem cell transplant*. For this type of transplant, colony-stimulating factors are administered to the patient to stimulate the bone marrow to produce large numbers of WBCs. Then apheresis is performed to collect the patient's peripheral stem cells. Apheresis is a procedure similar to hemodialysis. A large-bore apheresis catheter is placed into the subclavian vein that allows simultaneous blood withdrawal and blood reinfusion. The patient's blood is first drawn off into the apheresis machine. The apheresis machine centrifuges, or spins, the blood, separating it into WBCs, RBCs, and plasma. The stem cells in the WBC layer are removed and stored and the rest of the WBCs, RBCs, and plasma are returned to the patient. When enough of these peripheral blood stem cells are harvested and stored, the patient is treated with chemotherapy and radiation therapy. After treatment, the peripheral blood stem cells are returned to the patient. Stem cells reengraft more quickly than bone marrow, reducing the duration of neutropenia and therefore the risk of infection. Often peripheral blood stem cell transplants are administered concurrently with autologous bone marrow transplants. Peripheral blood stem cell transplants have been so successful that they are quickly becoming the most common type of transplant.

Major complications of bone marrow transplantation and peripheral blood stem cell transplantation include infection, thrombocytopenia, renal insufficiency, hepatic veno-occlusive disease, and graft-versus-host disease. Infection is a constant concern in the care of patients undergoing bone marrow transplantation. For approximately 2 weeks after transplantation, when the new bone marrow is engrafting, patients are severely neutropenic and at very high risk for infection. Even when WBCs and neutrophil counts approach normal levels, the patient's cell-mediated immune function can be compromised for more than 1 year.

Thrombocytopenia can be profound and prolonged in the patient undergoing bone marrow transplantation or peripheral blood stem cell transplantation because of the high doses of chemotherapy and radiation therapy.

Renal insufficiency can occur if the kidneys are damaged with high doses of nephrotoxic drugs such as cisplatin chemotherapy or the antibiotic gentamicin. Kidney function can be further compromised if blood flow to and through the kidneys is not maintained.

Hepatic veno-occlusive disease can occur if the liver is damaged with high doses of chemotherapy and radiation therapy. Blood flow into and out of the liver can be obstructed, resulting in ischemia, ascites, and increasing serum bilirubin.

Graft-versus-host disease is a complication of allogeneic bone marrow transplants in which T lymphocytes in the transplanted bone marrow identify the patient's tissue as foreign and try to destroy the patient's tissues. The transplanted T lymphocytes attack primarily epithelial cells of the skin, GI tract, biliary ducts, and lymphoid system, resulting in a skin rash; large amounts of green, watery, heme-negative diarrhea; and elevated liver enzyme levels.

Patients undergoing bone marrow transplantation or peripheral blood stem cell transplantation as treatment for a hematologic or immune system disorder are frequently hospitalized in a specialized bone marrow transplant unit and need intensive nursing care and long-term follow-up to ensure that their new immune system is functioning and that the underlying disease does not recur.

Put on Your Thinking Cap!

Compare and contrast the three types of bone marrow transplants in relation to the following: patient preparation, source of cells, advantages, disadvantages, and complications.

WHITE BLOOD CELL DISORDERS OF THE IMMUNE SYSTEM

The main function of the WBCs is to protect the body against pathogens. Patients are at great risk for infection when the WBCs are not functioning properly.

NEUTROPENIA

Neutropenia occurs when the total number of neutrophils is abnormally low, putting the patient at increased risk of infection. Decreased bone marrow production (e.g., because of infiltration with malignant cells), chemotherapy, radiation therapy, certain drugs (e.g., zidovudine, clozapine), or an autoimmune reaction (e.g., SLE, rheumatoid arthritis) can cause neutropenia. The longer the patient is neutropenic, the greater is the chance of infection. Because these patients do not have adequate numbers of WBCs to mount an immunologic response, classic signs of infection (e.g., redness, swelling, pain) may be absent. Fever may be the only sign of infection.

The most common sites of infection in neutropenic patients are the lung (pneumonia), blood (septicemia), skin, urinary tract, and GI tract (mucositis, esophagitis, perirectal lesions). Usually bacteria cause infections in neutropenic patients; however, fungi and viruses can also infect these patients. The goal of antibiotic therapy is to support the patient until the patient's own WBCs are available to fight the infection. In addition to administering prescribed antibiotics, it is important to minimize the patient's exposure to infectious agents by instituting **compromised host precautions**, described in Box 34-3.

NON-HODGKIN LYMPHOMA

Non-Hodgkin lymphoma is a cancer of the lymph system. The American Cancer Society estimated that almost 70,000 new cases of non-Hodgkin lymphoma would be diagnosed in 2013, accounting for about 4% of all new cases of cancer diagnosed. Patients of any age and either gender may get non-Hodgkin lymphoma, although the disease is more commonly seen in older people. Non-Hodgkin lymphomas are staged as low grade, intermediate grade, or high grade. The higher the grade of lymphoma, the more aggressive the cancer. Medical treatment of non-Hodgkin lymphoma can include either radiation therapy or chemotherapy depending on the stage of the disease. High-dose therapy with bone marrow transplantation or peripheral blood stem cell transplantation is an option for some patients who suffer disease reoccurrence after standard treatment. Survival rates vary widely depending on the grade of the disease at diagnosis. The overall 5-year survival rate for patients with non-Hodgkin lymphoma is 68%.

HODGKIN DISEASE

Hodgkin disease is a type of lymphoma characterized by Reed Sternberg cells in the lymph nodes. According to American Cancer Society statistics, more than 9000 new cases of Hodgkin disease would be diagnosed in 2013, accounting for less than 1% of all new cases of cancer diagnosed. Incidence of the disease is highest for people in their 20s and their 50s. Men are more likely than women to have the disease. Medical treatment of Hodgkin disease can include either radiation therapy or chemotherapy depending on the stage of the disease. High-dose therapy with bone marrow transplantation or peripheral blood stem cell transplantation is an option for patients who suffer disease reoccurrence after standard treatment. Survival rates vary widely depending on the stage of the disease at diagnosis. The overall 5-year survival rate for patients with Hodgkin disease is 85%.

LEUKEMIA

Leukemia is a cancer of the WBCs in which the bone marrow produces too many immature WBCs. These nonfunctioning, immature WBCs leave the patient unprotected against microorganisms and at great risk for life-threatening infections. The American Cancer Society estimated that more than 52,000 cases of leukemia would be diagnosed in 2014, accounting for 3% of all new cases of cancer diagnosed in that year. Although for most cases no cause is identified, factors that may be associated with the development of leukemia are exposure to large doses of ionizing radiation or exposure to certain chemicals such as benzene, a compound found in gasoline. Persons with Down syndrome and certain other genetic abnormalities are at increased risk for developing leukemia.

Two main types of leukemia exist: (1) myelogenous and (2) lymphocytic. Each type of leukemia can be either chronic or acute. The chronic leukemias—chronic myelogenous leukemia (CML) and chronic lymphocytic leukemia (CLL)—occur most often in adults. In both types of chronic leukemias, the WBC count slowly increases over months or years. The disease usually can be controlled with oral chemotherapy for many years. Patients being treated for chronic leukemia generally feel healthy. They do not lose their hair and usually do not experience nausea. Most of these patients can continue to work. A new drug now available for patients with CML, imatinib mesylate (Gleevec), has revolutionized the treatment of this particular leukemia. Gleevec is a protein tyrosine kinase inhibitor that targets the leukemic cells while sparing normal cells. It is an oral medication taken once a day. Only minimal side effects have been reported. Research continues to determine the optimal length of treatment and follow-up needed for these patients. The average life expectancy after diagnosis for a patient with CML ranges from 3 to 8 years, depending on the stage of the disease. It is anticipated that life expectancy will increase with Gleevec treatment (but by how much is currently unknown). The average life expectancy for a patient with CLL ranges from 2 to 10 years, again depending on the stage of the disease when diagnosed. After this time, the chronic leukemias often transform into an acute leukemia that is very difficult to treat. Patients generally die shortly after they enter this accelerated phase.

Each of the chronic forms of leukemia—lymphocytic and myelogenous—also has an acute form. Acute lymphocytic leukemia (ALL) occurs most often in children between the ages of 2 and 6 years. Acute nonlymphocytic leukemia (ANLL), also called *acute myelogenous leukemia (AML)*, occurs more often in adults. The acute leukemias appear very suddenly. The patient's WBC count can skyrocket in days, crowding out the normal RBCs and platelets and leaving the patient at severe risk for infection and bleeding. Treatment with chemotherapy must be started as soon as possible. Between 70% and 80% of children diagnosed with ALL will be alive in 5 years. Only 20% of patients diagnosed with ANLL will be alive in 5 years.

Signs and Symptoms of Acute Leukemia

Patients with leukemia commonly have infections because their bone marrow is producing huge numbers of immature WBCs that cannot effectively fight infection; fevers and night sweats are in response to the infection. Because the leukemic WBCs crowd out the normal cells in the bone marrow, patients may have symptoms related to low RBC counts, such as fatigue, paleness, tachycardia, and tachypnea. Concurrently, patients may have symptoms related to low platelet counts, such as petechiae or purpura, epistaxis (nose bleeds), gingival bleeding (from the gums), melena (blood in the stool), or menorrhagia (heavy menstrual bleeding). Some patients may have bone pain because of the crowding created by rapidly dividing leukemic cells in the bone marrow. Patients may report weight loss and swollen lymph nodes.

Medical Diagnosis of Acute Leukemia

A CBC with an extremely high WBC count indicates that leukemia might be present. A bone marrow biopsy enables diagnosis of the specific type of leukemia. Tables 33-2 and 34-1 describe these diagnostic procedures.

Medical Treatment of the Patient with Acute Leukemia

The acute leukemias are initially treated using high doses of chemotherapy to destroy the diseased bone marrow and allow the body to regrow healthy bone marrow. Patients are at great risk for infection and bleeding while their healthy bone marrow is growing back but this is the only way the acute leukemias can be treated. Patients stay in the hospital during the chemotherapy treatments and afterward to receive antibiotic drugs and blood transfusions until their own bone marrow grows back. After the initial high doses of chemotherapy, called *induction therapy*, patients with ALL take lower doses of chemotherapy, called *maintenance therapy*, for 1 to 3 years. Patients with ANLL immediately receive the same high doses of chemotherapy two to four more times over the next 2 to 4 months but are then finished with treatment. Subsequent chemotherapy for ANLL is called *intensification* and *consolidation therapy*. Bone marrow transplantation is one form of intensification therapy.

❖ NURSING CARE of the Patient with Acute Leukemia

Patients with acute leukemia require intensive nursing care. Patients are normally hospitalized for only 2 to 3 weeks and are critically ill most of that time. Once a patient's vital signs stabilize and the patient has no signs or symptoms of infection, he or she can be discharged from the hospital and followed as an outpatient until normal bone marrow function returns and adequate numbers of WBCs, RBCs, and platelets are being made. The physical and psychologic nursing care of these patients is intensive.

■ Assessment

Infection is the leading cause of death in patients with leukemia. Therefore patients are frequently assessed for any signs or symptoms of infection. The most common sites of infection are the lungs, blood, skin, urinary tract, and GI tract. Take complete vital signs every 4 hours. Fever is the hallmark of infection. Other vital sign changes caused by sepsis or widespread infection include tachycardia, tachypnea, and hypotension. Auscultate the patient's breath sounds every shift and note changes. A cough, especially a productive cough, may indicate an early pulmonary infection. If sputum is produced, note the amount and color. The physician may want the sputum cultured. Each day, carefully inspect the patient's skin for any reddened, swollen, painful, or draining areas. This is most easily done when helping the patient to bathe. Because patients with leukemia do not have normal WBCs, pus may not be seen even though an infection may be present. Redness, swelling, pain, or a combination of these may be the only symptoms of a serious infection. Inspect the patient's mouth and pharynx, looking for any reddened, swollen, painful, or draining areas. In addition, ask the patient about any pain or burning on urination, indicating a possible bladder infection.

While monitoring for infection, also look for any evidence of bleeding. The lower the platelet count is, the greater is the patient's risk for bleeding. A platelet count below 50,000 cells/mm^3 is cause for concern. Note any petechiae, purpura, or ecchymoses. Patients may have or report epistaxis, gingival bleeding, melena, or menorrhagia. Perform a guaiac test to assess for blood on all bowel movements as directed.

In addition, note any side effects from the chemotherapy, such as nausea and vomiting or stomatitis, so that the appropriate interventions can be taken. Remember that most patients lose their hair from chemotherapy for acute leukemia beginning 1 to 2 weeks after treatment. While doing a physical examination, also assess how much the patient knows about the disease and his or her treatment, as well as how the patient is coping with this life-threatening disease and the side effects of treatment.

Nursing Diagnoses, Goals, and Outcome Criteria: Acute Leukemia

Nursing Diagnoses	Goals and Outcome Criteria
Risk for Injury related to infection, thrombocytopenia, and anemia	Absence of injury from infection, bleeding, and inadequate oxygenation: normal body temperature, no bruising or frank bleeding, pulse and respiratory rates within patient's norms
Fatigue related to the disease process and treatment	Reduction in fatigue: patient reports tolerance of activity has improved
Impaired Oral Mucous Membrane related to stomatitis	Intact mucous membranes: oral tissues normal in color without lesions

Continued

Nursing Diagnoses, Goals, and Outcome Criteria: Acute Leukemia—cont'd

Nursing Diagnoses	Goals and Outcome Criteria
Imbalanced Nutrition: Less Than Body Requirements related to nausea and vomiting	Adequate intake of nutrients: stable body weight
Anxiety related to the disease, treatment, and uncertain outcome	Reduced anxiety: patient reports anxiety is reduced, calm manner
Ineffective Self-Health Management related to lack of knowledge about the disease process and treatment	Patient manages side effects of treatment effectively: patient resumes self-care; verbalizes disease process, treatment, and implications

Interventions

Risk for Injury

Infection. Infection presents the greatest risk to patients with leukemia. Most hospitals institute compromised host precautions when a patient's ANC falls below 1000 cells/mm^3. Thorough hand washing is of extreme importance in caring for these patients. Microorganisms are transmitted by hospital personnel who do not diligently wash their hands. Encourage patients to shower every day to remove bacteria from the skin and perianal area. Because patients with low WBC counts often become infected with their own microorganisms through their GI tract, consider discouraging patients from eating fresh fruits or vegetables and from drinking milk products. Uncooked foods naturally contain the bacteria *Escherichia coli, Pseudomonas aeruginosa,* and *Klebsiella* spp. A normal immune system can destroy the bacteria in uncooked foods. However, patients undergoing treatment for leukemia are at high risk for infection after being exposed to even small amounts of these bacteria. Box 34-3 outlines typical compromised host precautions for patients with low WBC counts. Once the patient's ANC climbs above 1000 cells/mm^3, compromised host precautions can be discontinued and a regular diet resumed without restrictions.

Thrombocytopenia. In addition to infection, patients with leukemia are at great risk for bleeding related to thrombocytopenia (a low platelet count). The primary treatment for thrombocytopenia is a platelet transfusion. However, physicians try not to prescribe platelet transfusions for patients unless they are actively bleeding or their platelet count is below 20,000 cells/mm^3 because of the risks associated with blood product administration. Nursing considerations in administering platelet transfusions are outlined in Box 33-6. While patients are thrombocytopenic, take bleeding precautions as outlined in Box 33-4.

Anemia. Anemia, or hematocrit (Hct) below 30% and hemoglobin (Hgb) below 10 gm/dL, is a common finding in patients with leukemia. Expect anemia along with neutropenia and thrombocytopenia. As with neutropenia and thrombocytopenia, the leukemic cells crowding out the healthy red cells in the bone marrow may cause anemia, or it may be the result of chemotherapy. The primary treatment for anemia is a RBC transfusion. Nursing considerations in administering blood transfusions are outlined in Box 33-5. Other precautions for patients with anemia are outlined in Box 33-3.

Fatigue

Almost all patients with acute leukemia experience fatigue, which has been described as an overwhelming tiredness or exhaustion. Causes of fatigue in these patients can include a low RBC count (anemia) from both the disease and the treatment, the buildup of metabolic wastes as the leukemic cells are being destroyed and cleared from the body, disrupted sleep, and the psychologic stress of the disease and treatment. A discussion of fatigue is presented in the Nursing Care of the Patient With Cancer section in Chapter 25.

Impaired Oral Mucous Membrane

Stomatitis, or an inflammation of the mucous membranes, is also a common side effect of chemotherapy. A detailed discussion of the nursing management of stomatitis is presented in Chapter 25.

Imbalanced Nutrition: Less Than Body Requirements

Nausea, with or without vomiting, is a common side effect of chemotherapy. Persistent nausea and vomiting can adversely affect a patient's nutritional status and psychologic state. The licensed vocational nurse/licensed practical nurse (LVN/LPN) can play an important role in managing this most distressing side effect. A discussion of the nursing management of nausea and vomiting related to chemotherapy is presented in Chapter 25.

Anxiety

A diagnosis of leukemia is always a shock to patients and their families. Patients must deal not only with the disease and treatment but also with the feelings and emotions of facing a life-threatening illness. Encourage patients to ask questions and talk about their feelings. Often a patient's fears are due to a lack of knowledge about the disease and treatment. The oncology clinical nurse specialist or other specially trained oncology nurse can answer many of the patient's and family's questions. Often information is what the patient and family need to deal with their anxieties. However, a referral to a social worker, chaplain, or mental health counselor may be indicated if the patient and family are having continued anxiety and difficulty in coping.

It is important to know what the patient understands about the disease, the treatment, and the prognosis so that correct information can be reinforced.

Ineffective Self-Health Management

The patient must receive accurate, consistent information from all members of the health care team. An oncology clinical nurse specialist or other specially trained oncology nurse usually can provide comprehensive information about the disease and its treatment to the patient and family and answer questions as they arise during hospitalization. All nurses reinforce this teaching. The Leukemia & Lymphoma Society (www.lls.org; telephone: 1-800-955-4572) provides excellent, free literature on the different types of leukemia. The National Cancer Institute, through the Cancer Information Service, provides excellent, free literature on chemotherapy for people receiving treatment. It can be reached by calling 1-800-4CANCER or on the internet at www.nci.nih.gov. The American Cancer Society (www.cancer.org; telephone: 1-800-ACS-2345) offers various local support services for people with all forms of cancer, including leukemia.

OTHER IMMUNE SYSTEM DISORDERS

HYPERSENSITIVITY REACTIONS

Hypersensitivity reactions, or allergies, are exaggerated immune responses that can be uncomfortable and potentially harmful to the patient. The four types of hypersensitivity reactions are classified according to the time between exposure and reaction, the immune mechanism involved, and the site of reaction.

Type I immediate hypersensitivity reactions are mediated by IgE reacting to common allergens such as dust, pollen, animal dander, insect stings, or various drugs. Type I reactions can be either local (resulting in local swelling and discomfort) or systemic (resulting in anaphylaxis and possible death if not recognized and treated promptly). Type I anaphylactic (systemic) hypersensitivity reactions occur in the following way. After a first, sensitizing exposure to a specific allergen, subsequent exposures to the same allergen trigger an exaggerated antibody reaction. For example, in a person with a hypersensitivity reaction to insect stings, one insect sting results in the production of abnormally large amounts of IgE antibodies. When this person is stung again by the same type of insect, the circulating IgE immediately triggers the release of histamine and other cytokines from mast cells, causing bronchiole constriction, peripheral vasodilation, and increased capillary permeability. These individuals can experience airway obstruction, pulmonary congestion, peripheral edema, hypotension, shock, and circulatory collapse. Prompt diagnosis and treatment of anaphylaxis with epinephrine, antihistamines, steroids, and hemodynamic support are of paramount importance.

Type II immediate hypersensitivity reactions are mediated by antibody reactions. Type II hypersensitivity reactions can occur with a mismatched blood transfusion or as a response to various drugs.

Type III immediate hypersensitivity reactions result in tissue damage resulting from precipitation of antigen-antibody immune complexes. Type III hypersensitivity reactions can occur with autoimmune reactions, with some occupational diseases, or as a response to various drugs.

Type IV delayed hypersensitivity reactions result from immune cells migrating to the site of exposure days after the exposure to the antigen. Type IV hypersensitivity reactions can occur with contact dermatitis, measles rash, tuberculin skin testing, or various drugs. Transplanted graft rejection occurs because of a type IV hypersensitivity reaction. Hypersensitivity reactions to drugs, or drug allergies, are one of many possible adverse drug reactions. Drug-induced hypersensitivity reactions can be any of the four types of hypersensitivity.

IDIOPATHIC THROMBOCYTOPENIC PURPURA

ITP is an antibody-mediated autoimmune disorder in which IgG mistakenly helps to destroy the patient's own platelets. Drugs known to induce ITP include sulfonamides, thiazide diuretics, chlorpropamide, quinidine, and gold. Patients with HIV infection are at increased risk for developing ITP.

Treatment for ITP can include steroid drugs and intravenous immune globulin (IVIG). Approximately 75% of adult patients with ITP will sequester (store) platelets in the spleen and so splenectomy is done in some patients to remove this storehouse, thereby increasing the circulating blood levels of platelets. Immunosuppressive therapy with cytotoxic drugs (e.g., vincristine or cyclophosphamide) can be used in patients who do not respond to splenectomy. Platelet transfusions are *not* indicated because the underlying problem is platelet consumption, not platelet production. If platelets are transfused, they are immediately destroyed. Nursing actions for the patient who is at risk for injury from bleeding from ITP are outlined in Box 33-4.

Pharmacology Capsule

Advise patients taking steroids to take them early in the day because these drugs can disrupt sleep.

THROMBOTIC THROMBOCYTOPENIC PURPURA

TTP is an exaggerated immunologic response to vessel injury that results in extensive clot formation and decreased blood flow to the site. These patients become critically ill, developing fever, thrombocytopenia, hemolytic anemia, renal impairment, and neurologic symptoms.

The main treatment for TTP is plasmapheresis, which presumably removes the immunologic agent that triggered the TTP from the plasma. The patient's blood is centrifuged in an apheresis machine that separates the blood components so that the plasma can be selectively removed. The patient's own WBCs, RBCs, and platelets are reinfused during the treatment. Critically ill patients can become hemodynamically unstable during this procedure and need close monitoring and timely interventions to maintain cardiac output and blood pressure. Plasmapheresis usually is done daily or every other day for several weeks until the patient's hematologic parameters stabilize. Other treatments include steroids, antiplatelets (e.g., aspirin or dipyridamole [Persantine]), splenectomy, or all three. Platelet transfusions are usually contraindicated because they may contribute to the abnormal clotting process. Nursing actions for the patient who is at risk for injury from bleeding are outlined in Box 33-4.

AUTOIMMUNE DISEASES

As mentioned earlier in the description of tolerance and how the body learns to recognize itself, autoimmune diseases occur when a breakdown of tolerance occurs. The immune system inappropriately identifies its own proteins as foreign and mounts a response to destroy these self-proteins. Examples of autoimmune diseases are ITP, TTP, acute rheumatic fever, type 1 diabetes mellitus, SLE, multiple sclerosis, rheumatoid arthritis, Graves disease, and Hashimoto thyroiditis.

SYSTEMIC LUPUS ERYTHEMATOSUS

SLE is an autoimmune disease in which the person's immune system loses its ability to recognize itself and mounts an immune response against its own proteins. Damage results from antibodies and immune complexes directed against one or many organ systems. The cause of SLE is unknown. Ninety percent of cases occur in women, usually of childbearing age. The disease is much more common in African Americans, Latinos, and Asian Americans than in Caucasians (see *Cultural Considerations* box). Organ damage is progressive in this disease. The most common cause of death in these patients is infection and disease of the cardiovascular system, renal system, pulmonary system, and CNS. Factors associated with a poor outcome include increased creatinine, hypertension, large amounts of protein excreted in the urine, anemia, and low socioeconomic status.

Cultural Considerations

What Does Culture Have to Do with Lupus?

Although the cause of systemic lupus erythematosus (SLE) is unknown, a genetic predisposition may exist. The disease is more common in women and is three times more common in African-American women than in Caucasian women.

Signs and Symptoms

Patients with SLE can experience long periods of remission alternating with periods of symptom exacerbation. Almost every organ system can be affected. The most common symptoms, experienced by 95% of patients at some time during the course of their disease, are fatigue, malaise, fever, anorexia, nausea, and weight loss. Musculoskeletal symptoms, also experienced by 95% of patients at some time during the course of their disease, include arthralgias (joint pain) and myalgias (muscle pain). Joints are often swollen, tender, stiff, and painful with movement. Cutaneous symptoms can include a rash and photosensitivity. The classic skin lesion is a butterfly-shaped rash across the bridge of the nose and the cheeks. This rash can extend to the neck, upper trunk, and arms. Life- and organ-threatening symptoms can include inflammation of the kidneys, heart, and lungs resulting in organ failure. Inflammation of the retina of the eye can result in sudden-onset blindness, which can be very frightening to patients.

Medical Diagnosis

No one test confirms the diagnosis of SLE. Blood work may detect ANAs but a positive ANA assay is not specific for SLE. A negative ANA assay makes the diagnosis of SLE unlikely but not impossible. The LE prep is another blood test that can be used to help diagnose SLE. Rather than on blood tests, the diagnosis of SLE is based on the constellation of symptoms the patient is experiencing. Because symptoms come and go, the diagnosis of SLE can be very difficult to make and can take a long time. The American Rheumatism Association has established criteria for the diagnosis of SLE. If a patient experiences any four of the following symptoms, a diagnosis of SLE can be made:

- Characteristic rash
- Photosensitivity with exposure to sunlight
- Oral ulcers
- Arthritis
- Pleuritis or pericarditis (i.e., inflammation of the lungs or heart)
- Renal disorder (e.g., proteinuria)
- Neurologic disorder (e.g., seizures, psychosis)
- Hematologic disorder (e.g., anemia, leukopenia, thrombocytopenia)
- Immunologic disorder (as evidenced by detection of abnormal antibodies in the blood)
- Positive ANA

Medical Treatment

No cure for SLE exists. The medical treatment of SLE is symptomatic and aimed at minimizing symptoms, preventing organ damage, and maintaining quality of life. Fever, arthralgias, myalgias, and rash are managed with analgesics, NSAIDs, antimalarials, and corticosteroid drugs. If symptoms are not controlled with these drugs or if organ function is threatened, cytotoxic agents (e.g., azathioprine, cyclophosphamide, methotrexate) can be used to suppress the abnormal immune response.

NURSING CARE of the Patient with Systemic Lupus Erythematosus

The nursing care of the patient with SLE varies depending on the severity of the symptoms the patient may be experiencing. Patients are treated primarily as outpatients. Because patients with SLE are frequent consumers of medical care, they often become very knowledgeable about their disease and want to be fully informed about all treatments they are receiving as well as the possible side effects of the treatments. The goal of care is quality of life.

Assessment

The complexity of SLE requires a thorough health history and physical examination. It is critical to do a complete functional assessment to determine the effects of the symptoms on the patient's activities of daily living (ADL).

Nursing Diagnoses, Goals, and Outcome Criteria: Systemic Lupus Erythematosus

Nursing goals and diagnoses for the patient with SLE are extremely individualized but may include the following.

Nursing Diagnoses	Goals and Outcome Criteria
Fatigue related to the disease process and treatment	Decreased fatigue: patient manages daily routines without excessive tiring
Acute Pain related to inflammation of joints and muscles	Pain relief: patient states pain is relieved, appears relaxed
Disturbed Body Image related to skin rash, joint deformity	Improved body image: patient makes positive statements about self, takes measures to improve appearance
Ineffective Coping related to stress of chronic illness	Effective coping: patient uses positive coping skills to reduce stress
Ineffective Self-Health Management related to lack of knowledge about disease process and treatment	Patient resumes self-care: patient accurately describes disease process, treatments, and side effects of treatment

Interventions

Fatigue

Almost all patients with SLE report experiencing fatigue. Causes of fatigue in these patients can include a low RBC count from both the disease and the treatment, chronic pain, disrupted sleep, and the psychologic stress of the disease and treatment. The nursing management of fatigue is discussed in Chapter 25.

Acute Pain

Inflammation of muscles and joints, as well as inflammation of various organs, can cause pain. Closely monitor the patient's pain level and medication use. Keeping a flow sheet of patient reports of pain on a 10-point scale can be helpful, especially as different nurses care for the patient throughout the day. A *0* represents no pain while a *10* represents the worst pain a patient has ever experienced. The patient report of pain coupled with the amount of pain medication he or she is receiving can guide the nurse and physician as to the appropriate type and amount of pain medication. Pharmacologic and nonpharmacologic pain management strategies are presented in Chapter 15.

Disturbed Body Image

Encourage the patient to avoid prolonged exposure to the sun and to use sunscreen with a sun protection factor (SPF) rating greater than 15 to prevent the skin rash and exacerbation of symptoms.

Ineffective Coping

A diagnosis of SLE is always a shock to patients and their families. Patients must deal not only with the disease and treatment but also with the emotions of facing a chronic illness. Encourage patients to ask questions and to talk about their feelings. A referral to a social worker, chaplain, or mental health counselor may be indicated if the patient and family are having difficulty coping.

Ineffective Self-Health Management

It is very important that the patient receive accurate, consistent information from all members of the health care team. A clinical nurse specialist or other specially trained nurse usually can provide comprehensive information about the disease and its treatment to the patient and family and answer questions as they arise during hospitalization. It is important to know what the patient has been told about the disease, the treatment, and the prognosis so that correct information can be reinforced (see *Patient Teaching* box). The patient's interpretation and understanding of the information is essential. The Lupus Foundation of America (www.lupus.org; telephone: 202-349-1155) provides excellent, free literature on SLE and can help to locate support groups in specific regions of the country.

Patient Teaching

Systemic Lupus Erythematosus

- Know the names, dosages, schedule, and side effects of your drugs.
- Avoid prolonged exposure to the sun and use sunscreen with a sun protection factor (SPF) rating >15.
- You can get additional information from The Lupus Foundation of America.

Table 34-3 Drug Therapy: Drugs Used to Prevent Rejection of a Transplanted Organ

DRUG	USE AND ACTION	SIDE EFFECTS	NURSING INTERVENTIONS
Corticosteroids: for example, dexamethasone (Decadron), methylprednisolone (Solu-Medrol), prednisone, prednisolone, hydrocortisone (Solu-Cortef)	Used to prevent rejection of a transplanted organ because glucocorticoids interfere with eicosanoid production. Also used to treat type I immediate hypersensitivity reaction (anaphylaxis).	Side effects include glucose intolerance, muscle wasting, obesity, hyperlipidemia, redistribution of body fat, growth inhibition in children, increased capillary fragility, osteoporosis, stomach irritation and peptic ulcer disease, hypertension, sodium and water retention, and mood changes.	Give these drugs with meals. An H2 receptor antagonist such as ranitidine (Zantac) may be prescribed to decrease gastric acid production. If the patient takes these drugs for an extended period of time, the drug should not be stopped abruptly. Instead the drug dose should be gradually decreased over time under a physician's direction.
Purine and pyrimidine analogs: for example, azathioprine, mycophenolic acid, brequinar	Used to prevent rejection of a transplanted organ by interfering with deoxyribonucleic acid (DNA) synthesis in rapidly dividing cells such as T cells.	Side effects include bone marrow suppression, increased susceptibility to infection, stomach irritation, diarrhea, and hepatotoxicity.	Closely monitor the patient's complete blood count (CBC) and liver function studies.

TRANSPLANT REJECTION

When patients undergo kidney, heart, liver, or other organ transplantation, their own healthy immune systems may recognize the transplanted organ (or allograft) as foreign and try to destroy it. Rejections occur through various mechanisms. T_C lymphocytes can directly attack the allograft, resulting in acute transplant rejection within hours of the transplant. B lymphocytes can make antibodies against the allograft. Fibrin accumulates on the transplanted tissue, causing ischemia. In this way the allograft is slowly rejected over months to years. Tissue matching of donor to recipient minimizes the chance of the recipient's immune system attacking the allograft after transplantation.

Various combinations of drugs are also given to suppress the recipient's immune system and minimize the immune response to the allograft (see *Complementary and Alternative Therapies* box). However, these drugs also suppress the patient's ability to fight bacteria, viruses, fungi, and parasites, putting the patient at increased risk for infection. Combinations of steroid drugs (which inhibit the inflammatory response by inhibiting the production of prostaglandins), cyclosporine (which inhibits T lymphocytes), and azathioprine (which inhibits B cell and T cell proliferation) are commonly used to chronically suppress the immune system after an organ transplant. Table 34-3 describes the nursing care of patients taking these drugs. In addition, several newer drugs target the T cells while preserving B cell function and thus more of the patient's immune function. Patients who have undergone organ transplantation must take immunosuppressive therapy for the rest of their lives to preserve the allograft.

Complementary and Alternative Therapies

Patients with immunologic disorders should consult with their physicians prior to, because they have adverse effects and can interact with some medications.

Put on Your Thinking Cap!

Explain what would happen if transplant recipients did not take immunosuppressant drugs to prevent organ rejection.

Get Ready for the NCLEX® Examination!

Key Points

- The immune system is the body's defense network against infection; it provides the body with resistance to invading organisms and enables it to fight off invaders once they have gained access.
- Body organs that are part of a functioning immune system include the bone marrow, lymph nodes, spleen, and thymus.
- Antigens are foreign substances that stimulate a response from the immune system whereas antibodies are proteins that are produced by the immune system to help eradicate antigens.
- Innate immunity is present in the body at birth whereas acquired immunity develops after birth as a result of the body's immune response to specific antigens.
- Many types of leukocytes (WBCs) act as nature's cleanup mechanism by migrating to infected or

inflamed areas and engulfing and destroying antigens through a process known as *phagocytosis*.
- The two types of acquired immunity are antibody mediated and cell mediated.
- Acquired immunity depends on the proper development and functioning of specific WBCs called *B* and *T lymphocytes*.
- Immunodeficiency occurs when the body is unable to launch an adequate immune response, resulting in an increased risk for infection.
- Because the bone marrow becomes less responsive with age, the older person's immune response may be inadequate under stressful situations.
- The patient with a low WBC count is at risk for infection.
- Bone marrow transplantation and peripheral blood stem cell transplantation are procedures that reconstitute the hematologic and immunologic systems after certain cancer therapies.
- The two main types of leukemia are (1) myelogenous and (2) lymphocytic.
- Infection is the leading cause of death in patients with leukemia.
- Drugs used to suppress the immune response after organ or tissue transplantations also put the patient at risk for infection.
- Allergy or hypersensitivity occurs when a normally inoffensive foreign substance stimulates an atypical or exaggerated immune response.
- SLE is considered an autoimmune disorder.
- SLE can affect multiple body systems.

Additional Learning Resources

SG Go to your Study Guide for additional learning activities to help you master this chapter content.

evolve Go to your Evolve website (http://evolve.elsevier.com/Linton/medsurg) for the following learning resources and much more:
- Interactive Prioritization Exercises
- Fluid & Electrolyte Tutorial
- Pharmacology Tutorial
- Review Questions for the NCLEX® Examination

Review Questions for the NCLEX® Examination

1. A patient has a neutrophil count that is 70% of his total WBC count. You should suspect infection caused by ____________________.
   NCLEX Client Need: Physiological Integrity: Physiological Adaptation
2. Mr. B. had chickenpox as a child. When he was exposed to chickenpox years later, he did not become infected. His resistance was most likely the result of which type of acquired immunity?
   NCLEX Client Need: Physiological Integrity: Physiological Adaptation
3. Which of the following correctly describe(s) the effects of age-related changes in the immune system? (Select all that apply.)
   1. The bone marrow becomes less productive with advancing age.
   2. The immune system functions well under normal circumstances.
   3. Lymphatic tissue shrinks so that fewer and smaller lymph nodes exist.
   4. Older people have better immune function than most young adults.
   5. The bone marrow usually can respond to increased demand, given more time.

   NCLEX Client Need: Health Promotion and Maintenance.
4. Which of the following conditions are classified as *autoimmune disorders*? (Select all that apply.)
   1. Type 1 diabetes mellitus
   2. Graves disease
   3. Rheumatoid arthritis
   4. SLE
   5. Multiple sclerosis

   NCLEX Client Need: Physiological Integrity: Physiological Adaptation
5. Which of the following is a priority when collecting data about the patient with an immune disorder?
   1. Signs and symptoms of infection
   2. Unexplained changes in weight
   3. Increased blood pressure
   4. Characteristics of urine

   NCLEX Client Need: Physiological Integrity: Physiological Adaptation
6. During a report, it is noted that your patient's WBC is 20,000. What is the best interpretation of this laboratory finding?
   1. Your patient could have a mild infection.
   2. Your patient's infection is resolving.
   3. Your patient could have a severe infection.
   4. Your patient is producing excess neutrophils, artificially raising the WBC.

   NCLEX Client Need: Physiological Integrity: Physiological Adaptation
7. One of your patients who has leukemia is on compromised host precautions. You understand that which of the following precautions are required? (Select all that apply.)
   1. Visitors and staff should wash their hands before patient contact.
   2. The patient can have no fresh, raw fruits and vegetables.
   3. Staff should always wear masks when in the patient's room.
   4. Vital signs should be monitored at least every 8 hours.
   5. The patient will be placed in an isolation room.

   NCLEX Client Need: Physiological Integrity: Reduction of Risk Potential

8. Shortly after receiving an antibiotic, a patient experienced a type 1 immediate hypersensitivity reaction. Signs and symptoms would include which of the following? (Select all that apply.)
   1. Mental confusion
   2. Difficulty breathing
   3. Hypotension
   4. Nausea and vomiting
   5. Peripheral edema

   NCLEX Client Need: Physiological Integrity: Physiological Adaptation
9. A patient is scheduled for an autologous bone marrow transplant. Which of the following statements by the patient indicate that he correctly understands the procedure? (Select all that apply.)
   1. "A donor with tissue similar to mine is being sought."
   2. "Donor bone marrow will be injected into my hip bone."
   3. "Healthy bone marrow will be given to prevent cancer recurrence."
   4. "I will be given chemotherapy and radiation."
   5. "The physician will first remove a sample of my bone marrow."

   NCLEX Client Need: Physiological Integrity: Reduction of Risk Potential
10. The nurse collects all of the data listed below related to a patient with leukemia who is undergoing chemotherapy. Which data should be reported immediately?
    1. The patient states that he feels tired all the time.
    2. The patient's skin is pale and dry.
    3. The patient's oral temperature is 101°F.
    4. The patient eats only half of the food served at lunch.

    NCLEX Client Need: Physiological Integrity: Physiological Adaptation

chapter 35

Human Immunodeficiency Virus and Acquired Immunodeficiency Syndrome

Mark A. Meyer

http://evolve.elsevier.com/Linton/medsurg

Objectives

1. Describe the history of human immunodeficiency virus (HIV) and acquired immunodeficiency syndrome (AIDS).
2. Explain the pathophysiology and cause of HIV infection.
3. List risk factors associated with HIV infection.
4. Identify complications associated with HIV infection.
5. Identify criteria for diagnosis of AIDS.
6. Name the major HIV drugs, indications, side effects, and nursing considerations.
7. Describe appropriate nursing care and patient teaching of the patient with HIV and AIDS.

Key Terms

Acquired immunodeficiency syndrome (AIDS) (ĬM-myū-nō-dē-FĬ-shĕn-sē)
Highly active antiretroviral therapy (HAART) (ĂN-tē-rĕ-trō-vī-rŭl)
Human immunodeficiency virus (HIV)
Protease inhibitor (PRŌ-tē-ās ĭn-HĬ-bĭ-tĕr)

Few viruses have descended on human beings as swiftly and wreaked as much devastation as the **human immunodeficiency virus (HIV)**. The disease it causes, **acquired immunodeficiency syndrome (AIDS)**, has been seen in every country on the globe and claims victims without regard to age, race, class, gender, or sexual orientation.

Research and education on the prevention and treatment of HIV infection must continue unabated. Despite advances, a cure has not been found; however, reason for hope exists. In the developed world, the disease has come to be viewed less as a fatal illness and more as a manageable chronic condition. However, in the developing world, where access to health care and medications is often difficult, the picture is less optimistic. Worldwide, only about 1 in 5 people at risk of becoming infected with HIV has access to prevention services.

HISTORY

The origins of HIV and the disease it causes, AIDS, are difficult to pinpoint. According to the Centers for Disease Control and Prevention (CDC, 2013), scientists believe that a type of chimpanzee in West Africa was the original source of HIV infection in humans. The virus most likely jumped to humans who hunted these chimpanzees and came into contact with their blood. Over several years, the virus slowly spread across Africa and later into other parts of the world (CDC, 2013, HIV/AIDS Basic Questions. Retrieved on June 4, 2013 from www.cdc.gov/hiv/resources/qa/definitions.htm).

The earliest known case of infection with HIV in a human was detected in a man in Kinshasa, Democratic Republic of the Congo. (How he became infected is not known.) Genetic analysis of his blood sample suggested that HIV may have stemmed from a single virus in the late 1940s or early 1950s. The virus may have appeared as early as the 1940s but it was not recognized as a new pathogen until the early 1980s. Young men generally have normally functioning immune systems. Epidemiologists (physicians who study patterns of illness) began to take note when immune deficiency conditions such as oral candidal infection (thrush); herpes; *Pneumocystis jirovecii* pneumonia; and Kaposi sarcoma (KS), a rare type of cancer, began to show up in the United States, primarily among urban populations of men who have sex with men (MSM). In 1986 two types of the HIV (HIV-1 and HIV-2) were isolated as the viruses that cause AIDS. HIV-1 is the predominant type around the world while HIV-2 is mostly confined to West Africa. Within these types are multiple groups and subtypes. Some differences exist between the types with HIV-1 being more easily transmissible and more likely to be progressive than HIV-2. When references are made to HIV without specifying a type, it can be assumed to be HIV-1 because it is so much more common.

MSM were just the first population to be affected. Infection was soon seen in other populations, including the following:

- Individuals with hemophilia who must use blood products to treat the blood clotting disorder.
- Patients who received a transfusion with HIV-infected blood or blood products
- Newborns and breast-fed infants of HIV-infected mothers (perinatal transmission)
- Injection drug users
- Partners, including heterosexuals, who had unprotected sex with those infected with the virus

In some developing countries, such as those in sub-Saharan Africa, HIV infects more heterosexuals than homosexuals (see *Cultural Considerations* box). It is transmitted by exposure to body fluids (e.g., blood, semen, breast milk, vaginal secretions) that contain the virus, not by lifestyle or sexual orientation.

Cultural Considerations

What Does Culture Have to Do with Human Immunodeficiency Virus and Acquired Immunodeficiency Syndrome?

According to the Centers for Disease Control and Prevention (2011), the estimated number of persons in the United States living with diagnosed human immunodeficiency virus (HIV) infection is 872,990. The highest rate (1008.6 per 100,000 people) and the largest percentage (44%) are among African Americans. Among the remaining races and ethnicities, the rates are 325.2 for Latinos, 256.3 for persons of multiple races, 178.9 for Native Hawaiians and other Pacific Islanders, 149.7 for Caucasians, 140.8 for American Indians and Alaska Natives, and 65.7 for Asians. It appears that HIV is disproportionately represented in some cultural groups. Therefore prevention programs need to be culturally sensitive to reach target audiences.

According to the CDC (2013), approximately 50,000 newly diagnosed HIV infections occur annually in the United States. Since the disease was recognized in 1981, nearly 635,000 deaths in the United States have been attributed to AIDS, with 25 million deaths worldwide. In 2010, 15,500 people died from AIDS (Table 35-1).

DEMOGRAPHICS

Although HIV can infect anyone, infection rates are often reported by demographics, such as age, race, and gender.

- *Age group.* From 2008 through 2011, the rates of infection increased among persons aged 20 to 24 and 25 to 29 years. The rates of infection decreased among persons aged 30 to 34, 35 to 39, 40 to 44, 45 to 49, 55 to 59, and 60 to 64 years. The rates of infection remained stable for children (aged less than 13 years) and persons aged 13 to 14, 15 to 19, 50 to 54, and 65 years and older. In 2011, the highest rate of infection was among persons aged 20 to 24 years (36.4 per 100,000 people), followed by persons aged 25 to 29 years (35.2 per 100,000 people). Table 35-2 list the specific number of AIDS cases diagnosed within each of these exposure categories in the United States in 2011.
- *Young people.* Those aged 13 to 24 years are especially affected by HIV. They comprised 16% of the U.S. population but accounted for 26% of all new HIV infections in 2010. However, all young people are not equally at risk. Young MSM, for example, accounted for 72% of all new infections in people aged 13 to 24 years and young African-American MSM are especially at risk (CDC, 2011).
- *Race and ethnicity.* African Americans are most affected by HIV. In 2010, African Americans made up only 12% of the U.S. population but accounted for 44% of all new HIV infections. Likewise, Latinos made up 17% of the U.S. population but accounted for 21% of all new HIV infections (CDC, 2013, Basic Statistics). Table 35-3 list the specific number of AIDS cases diagnosed within each of these exposure categories in the United States in 2011.
- *Gender.* In 2011, males accounted for 79% of all diagnoses of HIV infection among adults and adolescents. The rate for adult and adolescent males was 30.8 per 100,000 people and the rate for females was 7.7 (CDC, 2011).

Another way of reporting HIV rates and AIDS diagnoses is by mode of transmission. The CDC has established five primary transmission categories:

1. Male-to-male sexual contact (greatest exposure category)
2. Injection drug use (third greatest exposure category)
3. Heterosexual (male-to-female) contact (second greatest exposure category)
4. Mother-to-child (perinatal) transmission
5. Other (includes blood transfusions and unknown causes; HIV has been found in low concentrations in the saliva, tears, and urine of infected individuals but no recorded cases of transmission from these fluids exist.)

Tables 35-4, 35-5, and 35-6 list the specific number of AIDS cases diagnosed within each of these exposure categories in the United States in 2011.

HIV is transmitted by blood and body fluids (i.e., breast milk, semen, and vaginal fluids). The risk of HIV transmission by various behaviors can be seen on a continuum from low risk to high risk. Table 35-7 identifies the levels of risk of HIV transmission associated with various behaviors.

PATHOPHYSIOLOGY

Infection with HIV causes destruction of immune cells. HIV falls into a category of viruses called *retroviruses.* In these viruses, transcription of genetic material is reversed. Ribonucleic acid (RNA) is made into

Table 35-1 HIV and AIDS Statistics by Geographical Region, 2001 and 2010

	ADULTS AND CHILDREN LIVING WITH HIV	ADULTS AND CHILDREN NEWLY INFECTED WITH HIV	PREVALENCE OF HIV INFECTION AMONG ADULTS (%)	ADULTS AND CHILDREN DYING FROM AIDS-RELATED CAUSES	PREVALENCE OF HIV INFECTION AMONG PEOPLE 15–24 YEARS OLD (%) MEN	WOMEN
Sub-Saharan Africa						
2010	22,900,000 [21,600,000–24,100,000]	1,900,000 [1,700,000–2,100,000]	5.0 [4.7–5.2]	1,200,000 [1,100,000–1,400,000]	1.4 [1.1–1.8]	3.3 [2.7–4.2]
2001	20,500,000 [19,100,000–22,200,000]	2,200,000 [2,100,000–2,400,000]	5.9 [5.6–6.4]	1,400,000 [1,300,000–1,600,000]	2.0 [1.6–2.7]	5.2 [4.3–6.8]
Middle East and North Africa						
2010	470,000 [350,000–570,000]	59,000 [40,000–73,000]	0.2 [0.2–0.3]	35,000 [25,000–42,000]	0.1 [0.1–0.2]	0.2 [0.1–0.2]
2001	320,000 [190,000–450,000]	43,000 [31 000–57,000]	0.2 [0.1–0.3]	22,000 [9700–38,000]	0.1 [0.1–0.2]	0.1 [0.1–0.2]
South and South-East Asia						
2010	4,000,000 [3,600,000–4,500,000]	270,000 [230,000–340,000]	0.3 [0.3–0.3]	250,000 [210,000–280,000]	0.1 [0.1–0.2]	0.1 [0.1–0.1]
2001	3,800,000 [3,400,000–4,200,000]	380,000 [340,000–420,000]	0.3 [0.3–0.4]	230,000 [200,000–280,000]	0.2 [0.2–0.2]	0.2 [0.2–0.2]
East Asia						
2010	790,000 [580,000–1,100,000]	88,000 [48,000–160,000]	0.1 [0.1–0.1]	56,000 [40,000–76,000]	<0.1 [<0.1–<0.1]	<0.1 [<0.1–<0.1]
2001	380,000 [280,000–530,000]	74,000 [54,000–100,000]	<0.1 [<0.1–0.1]	24000 [16,000–45,000]	<0.1 [<0.1–<0.1]	<0.1 [<0.1–<0.1]
Oceania						
2010	54,000 [48,000–62,000]	3300 [2400–4200]	0.3 [0.2–0.3]	1600 [1200–2000]	0.1 [0.1–0.1]	0.2 [0.1–0.2]
2001	41,000 [34,000–50,000]	4000 [3300–4600]	0.2 [0.2–0.3]	1800 [1300–2900]	0.1 [0.1–0.2]	0.2 [0.2–0.3]
Latin America						
2010	1,500,000 [1,200,000–1,700,000]	100,000 [73,000–140,000]	0.4 [0.3–0.5]	67,000 [45,000–92,000]	0.2 [0.1–0.4]	0.2 [0.1–0.2]
2001	1,300,000 [1,000,000–1,700,000]	99,000 [75,000–130,000]	0.4 [0.3–0.5]	83,000 [50,000–130,000]	0.2 [0.1–0.6]	0.1 [0.1–0.2]
Caribbean						
2010	200,000 [170,000–220,000]	12,000 [9400–17,000]	0.9 [0.8–1.0]	9000 [6900–12,000]	0.2 [0.2–0.5]	0.5 [0.3–0.7]
2001	210,000 [170,000–240,000]	19,000 [16,000–22,000]	1.0 [0.9–1.2]	18,000 [14,000–22,000]	0.4 [0.2–0.8]	0.8 [0.6–1.1]
Eastern Europe and Central Asia						
2010	1,500,000 [1,300,000–1,700,000]	160,000 [110,000–200,000]	0.9 [0.8–1.1]	90,000 [74,000–110,000]	0.6 [0.5–0.8]	0.5 [0.4–0.7]
2001	410,000 [340,000–490,000]	210,000 [170,000–240,000]	0.3 [0.2–0.3]	7800 [6000–11,000]	0.3 [0.2–0.3]	0.2 [0.1–0.2]
Western and Central Europe						
2010	840,000 [770,000–930,000]	30,000 [22,000–39,000]	0.2 [0.2–0.2]	9900 [8900–11,000]	0.1 [0.1–0.1]	0.1 [<0.1–0.1]
2001	630,000 [580,000–690,000]	30,000 [26,000–34,000]	0.2 [0.2–0.2]	10,000 [9500–11,000]	0.1 [0.1–0.1]	0.1 [0.1–0.1]

Continued

Table 35-1 HIV and AIDS Statistics by Geographical Region, 2001 and 2010—cont'd

	ADULTS AND CHILDREN LIVING WITH HIV	ADULTS AND CHILDREN NEWLY INFECTED WITH HIV	PREVALENCE OF HIV INFECTION AMONG ADULTS (%)	ADULTS AND CHILDREN DYING FROM AIDS-RELATED CAUSES	PREVALENCE OF HIV INFECTION AMONG PEOPLE 15–24 YEARS OLD (%)	
					MEN	WOMEN
North America						
2010	1,300,000 [1,000,000–1,900,000]	58,000 [24,000–130,000]	0.6 [0.5–0.9]	20,000 [16,000–27,000]	0.3 [0.2–0.6]	0.2 [0.1–0.4]
2001	980,000 [780,000–1,200,000]	49,000 [34,000–70,000]	0.5 [0.4–0.7]	19,000 [15,000–24,000]	0.3 [0.2–0.4]	0.2 [0.1–0.3]
Total						
2010	34,000,000 [31,600,000–35,200,000]	2,700,000 [2,400,000–2,900,000]	0.8 [0.8–0.8]	1,800,000 [1,600,000–1,900,000]	0.3 [0.3–0.3]	0.6 [0.5–0.6]
2001	28,600,000 [26,700,000–30,900,000]	3,100,000 [3,000,000–3,300,000]	0.8 [0.7–0.8]	1,900,000 [1,700,000–2,200,000]	0.4 [0.4–0.4]	0.8 [0.7–0.8]

From UNAIDS: *Global HIV/AIDS response: epidemic update and health sector progress towards universal access* (website): www.unaids.org/en/resources/publications/2011/name,64437,en.asp. Accessed February 11, 2014.
AIDS, Acquired immunodeficiency syndrome; *HIV*, human immunodeficiency virus.

Table 35-2 Acquired Immunodeficiency Syndrome Cases by Age, United States

AGE (IN YEARS)	ESTIMATED NUMBER OF AIDS CASES IN 2011	CUMULATIVE ESTIMATED NUMBER OF AIDS CASES, THROUGH 2011*
Under 13	16	9,945
Ages 13 to 14	49	1,510
Ages 15 to 19	5175	8,364
Ages 20 to 24	2,438	48,338
Ages 25 to 29	3,471	139,329
Ages 30 to 34	4,050	226,605
Ages 35 to 39	4,148	246,886
Ages 40 to 44	4,848	205,417
Ages 45 to 49	5,095	137,407
Ages 50 to 54	3,649	80,073
Ages 55 to 59	2,233	43,694
Ages 60 to 64	1,123	23,113
Ages 65 or older	923	20,038

*Includes persons with a diagnosis of acquired immunodeficiency syndrome (AIDS) from the beginning of the epidemic through 2011 (CDC, 2007b).
From Centers for Disease Control and Prevention: *HIV Surveillance Report* 23:1–84, 2011. www.cdc.gov/hiv/topics/surveillance/resources/reports/. Accessed June 5, 2013.

Table 35-3 Acquired Immunodeficiency Syndrome Cases by Race and Ethnicity, United States*

RACE OR ETHNICITY	ESTIMATED NUMBER OF AIDS CASES IN 2011	CUMULATIVE ESTIMATED NUMBER OF AIDS CASES, THROUGH 2011†
Caucasian, not Hispanic	8,304	435,744
African American, not Hispanic	15,966	486,763
Hispanic	6,849	236,410
Asian	492	9,088
Native American/Alaskan Native	146	3,788

*The Centers for Disease Control and Prevention (CDC) tracks human immunodeficiency virus (HIV)/acquired immunodeficiency syndrome (AIDS) information on five racial and ethnic groups: (1) Caucasian, (2) African American, (3) Hispanic (Latino), (4) Asian, and (5) Native American/Alaskan Native.
†Includes persons with a diagnosis of AIDS from the beginning of the epidemic through 2011.
From Centers for Disease Control and Prevention: *HIV Surveillance Report* 23:1–84, 2011. www.cdc.gov/hiv/topics/surveillance/resources/reports/. Accessed June 5, 2013.

Table 35-4 Acquired Immunodeficiency Syndrome Cases by Exposure Category, United States

	ESTIMATED NUMBER OF AIDS CASES IN 2011*		
EXPOSURE CATEGORY	MALE SUBJECTS	FEMALE SUBJECTS	TOTAL
Male-to-male sexual contact	16,812	—	16,812
Injection drug use	2,447	1,642	4,089
Male-to-male sexual contact and injection drug use	1,411	—	1,411
Heterosexual contact	3,638	6,330	9,968
Other†	134	129	261

*Includes persons with a diagnosis of acquired immunodeficiency syndrome (AIDS) for 2011.
†Includes hemophilia, blood transfusion, perinatal, and risk not reported or not identified.

Table 35-5 Cumulative Acquired Immunodeficiency Syndrome Cases by Exposure through 2011, United States*

EXPOSURE CATEGORY	MALE SUBJECT	FEMALE SUBJECT	TOTAL
Male-to-male sexual contact	560,860	—	560,860
Injection drug use	201,271	92,833	294,104
Male-to-male sexual contact and injection drug use	83,455	—	83,455
Heterosexual contact	81,477	142,153	223,630
Other†	12,157	6,567	18,724

*Includes persons with a diagnosis of acquired immunodeficiency syndrome (AIDS) from the beginning of the epidemic through 2011.
†Includes hemophilia, blood transfusion, perinatal, and risk not reported or not identified.
From Centers for Disease Control and Prevention: *HIV Surveillance Report* 23:1–84, 2011. www.cdc.gov/hiv/topics/surveillance/resources/reports/. Accessed June 5, 2013.

Table 35-6 Acquired Immunodeficiency Syndrome Cases among Children, United States*

EXPOSURE CATEGORY	ESTIMATED NUMBER OF AIDS CASES IN 2006	CUMULATIVE ESTIMATED NUMBER OF AIDS CASES, THROUGH 2011†
Perinatal	14	9,059
Other‡	2	887

*The term *children* refers to persons younger than age 13 years at the time of diagnosis.
†Includes persons with a diagnosis of acquired immunodeficiency syndrome (AIDS) from the beginning of the epidemic through 2011.
‡Includes hemophilia, blood transfusion, perinatal, and risk not reported or not identified.
From Centers for Disease Control and Prevention: *HIV Surveillance Report* 23:1–84, 2011. www.cdc.gov/hiv/topics/surveillance/resources/reports/. Accessed June 5, 2013.

deoxyribonucleic acid (DNA) rather than the normal pattern of DNA to RNA. Reverse transcriptase is an enzyme that is responsible for transcribing RNA into DNA (Bell, 2007).

LIFE CYCLE OF HUMAN IMMUNODEFICIENCY VIRUS

HIV first penetrates the body through blood and body fluids. HIV is spheric in shape and has two protein markers that protrude from the virus. These markers are like keys that attach themselves to protein markers found on macrophages and T4 helper cells or CD4

Table 35-7 Levels of Human Immunodeficiency Virus Transmission Risk Associated with Various Behaviors

No-risk behavior	Casual contact Shaking hands Hugging and kissing Eating in restaurants Using restrooms Swimming Insect bites and mosquitoes Donating blood
Little-risk behavior	Mutual masturbation, rubbing, cuddling, kissing, oral sex with condom, sex toys not shared with a partner, oral sex without contact with glans penis
Moderate-risk behavior	Oral sex with contact with glans penis Anal or vaginal sex with a condom and a water-based lubricant
Very high–risk behavior	Use of injection drugs, including steroids (needle sharing) Partners of injection drug users Unprotected, penetrative sex (anal, vaginal)

Data from Kirton C: Risk assessment, identification, and HIV counseling. In Kirton C, Talotta D, Zwolski K, editors: *Handbook of HIV/AIDS nursing,* St. Louis, 2001, Mosby.

Table 35-8 Normal Lymphocyte Counts

AGE	CD4 ABSOLUTE COUNT (CELLS/mm^3)	CD8 ABSOLUTE COUNT (CELLS/mm^3)	CD4:CD8 RATIO
18 years to 70 years	600–980	420–660	1.2–1.9

Data from Kirton C: Clinical application of immunological and virological markers. In Kirton C, Talotta D, Zwolski K, editors: *Handbook of HIV/AIDS nursing*, St. Louis, 2001, Mosby.

cells. Macrophages and T4 helper cells are distributed throughout the body, especially in mucous membranes and body orifices. Once HIV attaches to the macrophages and T4 helper cells, it infuses its genetic material into the host cell. The reverse transcriptase enzyme then transcribes HIV RNA into HIV DNA and inserts the HIV DNA into the host's DNA. Once the HIV DNA is incorporated into the host cell's DNA, billions of copies of HIV are made (Colagreco, 2003). Roughly 21 billion new HIV virions (complete viral particles) are produced daily compared with 1 to 2 billion new T4 helper cells. A person who is HIV positive may have an entire supply of T4 helper cells depleted every 15 days. Eventually, the body is unable to maintain a healthy immune response and the body will begin to show symptoms of HIV/AIDS (Colagreco, 2003).

BODY'S RESPONSE TO HUMAN IMMUNODEFICIENCY VIRUS INFECTION

Once infected with HIV, the body mounts a defense with antibodies and T cells. *Viral load* is a term used to describe how much virus is found in the blood. Especially high levels of viral load have been documented in the early phases of HIV infection. Approximately 12 weeks after infection, the body produces enough antibodies to be detected by standard HIV testing. Once a sufficient amount of antibodies is produced, the HIV viral load begins to drop, indicating partial effectiveness of the body to rid itself of HIV. Throughout the course of HIV infection, the body maintains high levels of HIV antibodies. However, CD8 cells and CD4 cells continue to decline throughout the course of the illness. Table 35-8 lists normal lymphocyte counts.

STAGES OF HUMAN IMMUNODEFICIENCY VIRUS INFECTION

The initial stage of HIV infection lasts 4 to 8 weeks from the time of exposure. High levels of the virus are in the blood. About 50% of people who become infected with HIV experience generalized flulike symptoms, which is called *acute retroviral syndrome*. The other 50% have no symptoms of infection. The virus then enters a latent stage during which it is inactive in the infected, resting CD4 host cells. When the resting CD4 host cells are activated for an immune response, the virus begins to replicate. Levels of virus are high in the lymph nodes where CD4 cells reside but are low in the blood. The latent stage can last 2 to 12 years, during which time the patient is asymptomatic although the number of CD4 cells declines. During the third stage of HIV infection, the patient begins to experience opportunistic infections. These infections are called *opportunistic infections* because one can say that these microbes take advantage of the opportunity to infect the person who is HIV positive when his or her T cells are low. Levels of CD4 cells are usually less than 500 cells/mm^3 and declining while levels of virus in the blood are increasing. This stage can last 2 to 3 years. Once the CD4 cell levels drop below 200 cells/mm^3, the patient is considered to have AIDS. Virus levels in the blood are high. With the development of **highly active antiretroviral therapy (HAART)** and improved treatment of HIV complications, 80% of those diagnosed with HIV have now survived 10 years after being diagnosed. HIV/AIDS is increasingly becoming a chronic, managed disease rather than a terminal illness.

SIGNS AND SYMPTOMS OF HUMAN IMMUNODEFICIENCY VIRUS INFECTION

Patients in the initial stage of HIV infection may experience only generalized flulike symptoms such as malaise, nausea and vomiting, decreased appetite, rash, and diarrhea. Because the symptoms are vague, HIV infection often is not diagnosed in the early stage. During the second, latent stage of the disease, patients may not experience any symptoms. Eventually they begin to experience frequent and persistent infections. Patients may present for medical care complaining of fever, night sweats, swollen lymph nodes, or other symptoms specific to the site of infection, such as headache, skin lesions that do not heal, sore throat, dyspnea, burning with urination, or diarrhea. Patients also may report extreme fatigue and weight loss. Any of these symptoms coupled with a history of unprotected sexual contact with persons possibly infected with HIV, a history of intravenous drug use with shared needles, or a history of a blood transfusion before 1989 warrants consideration of a diagnosis of HIV infection.

COMPLICATIONS

The major complications of HIV infection are opportunistic infections, wasting, secondary cancers, and dementia. Patients with AIDS are at very high risk for opportunistic fungal, parasitic, and viral infections. Infections that these patients commonly experience include oral candidiasis, *Pneumocystis jirovecii* (formerly *P. carinii*) pneumonia, herpes simplex, cytomegalovirus retinitis, *Cryptosporidium* enteritis, *Cryptococcus neoformans* meningitis, and toxoplasmosis (Fig. 35-1). Almost all patients with HIV infection experience a wasting syndrome characterized by weight loss and

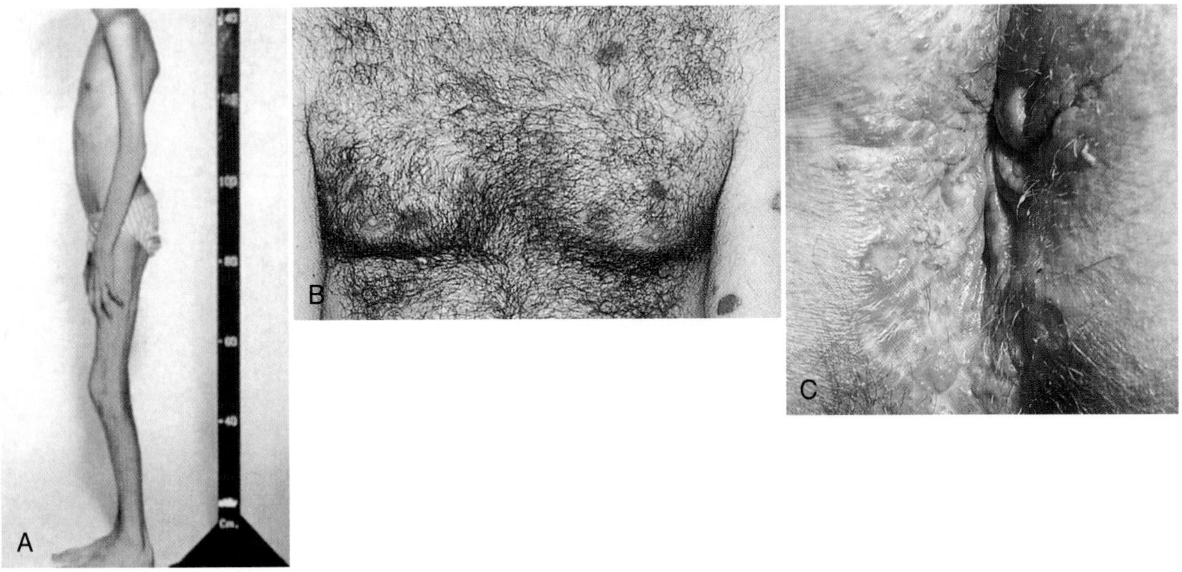

FIGURE 35-1 Clinical symptoms of acquired immunodeficiency syndrome (AIDS). **A,** Severe weight loss and anorexia. **B,** Biopsy-proven Kaposi sarcoma (KS) lesions. **C,** Perianal vesicular and ulcerative lesions of herpes simplex infection. (A from Taylor PK: *Diagnostic picture tests in sexually transmitted disease*, London, 1995, Mosby; B and C from Morse SA, Ballard BC, Holmes KK, et al., editors: *Atlas of sexually transmitted diseases and AIDS*, ed 3, London, 2003, Mosby.)

malnutrition. Reduced food intake, malabsorption of nutrients, and altered metabolic pathways all contribute to this wasting syndrome. Cancers such as KS, non-Hodgkin lymphoma (NHL), anal cancer, and cervical cancer occur in 40% of patients with HIV infection. Presumably this increased incidence of cancer is due to the inability of the patient's crippled immune system to identify and destroy cells that undergo malignant changes. The virus can affect the central nervous system (CNS), causing encephalopathy, cognitive impairment, and dementia.

OPPORTUNISTIC INFECTIONS

Once the body's CD4 cells, CD8 cells, or HIV antibodies (or a combination of these) fall below normal levels, infections and cancers that the body normally could resist take advantage of this opportunity and cause infection or cancer in the body. That is why these infections are called *opportunistic infections.* The leading cause of death in persons with AIDS is now non-AIDS-related cancers (Evans, 2011). Parasites, fungi, bacteria, and viruses can cause opportunistic infections. Figure 35-2 shows tissues that may be affected by HIV infection.

PARASITIC INFECTIONS

Opportunistic parasitic infections include cryptosporidiosis, isosporiasis, and toxoplasmosis.

Cryptosporidiosis and Isosporiasis

Cryptosporidium and *Isospora*, the causative agents for cryptosporidiosis and isosporiasis, respectively, are fairly common in the environment, particularly in developing countries. *Cryptosporidium* and *Isospora* pose a special threat when the CD4 cell count of the patient with HIV infection falls below 200 cells/mm^3. The main symptom of infection with these parasites is watery diarrhea that may be severe and persistent, resulting in severe dehydration and electrolyte imbalances. Diagnosis is based on laboratory examination of a stool specimen (Chimienti, Panther, & Graham, 2007).

Nursing care is directed toward preventing dehydration and maintaining fluid and electrolyte balance. Antidiarrheal drugs and intravenous fluids may be ordered. Antimicrobials are effective for some parasitic infections but others can be treated only symptomatically. To reduce the risk of transmission and reinfection, teach the patient to practice good hand washing and personal hygiene and to avoid ingestion of potentially contaminated water (Chimienti, Panther, & Graham, 2007).

Toxoplasmosis

Toxoplasma gondii, a protozoon that causes toxoplasmosis, has a worldwide distribution. Cats, mammals, and birds serve as hosts for the causative agent. Humans become infected by ingesting contaminated, undercooked meats or vegetables or by contact with cat feces. Toxoplasmosis can affect any tissue in the body but affects mostly the brain, lungs, and eyes. In immunosuppressed patients, toxoplasmosis encephalitis is the most common form. Unless detected and treated early, toxoplasmosis can be fatal. Symptoms include dull, constant headache, weakness, seizures, altered level of consciousness, hemiparesis, cerebellar tremor, and visual field defects. Pulmonary infections result in a feverish illness that mimics *P. jirovecii* pneumonia with shortness of breath and a nonproductive cough.

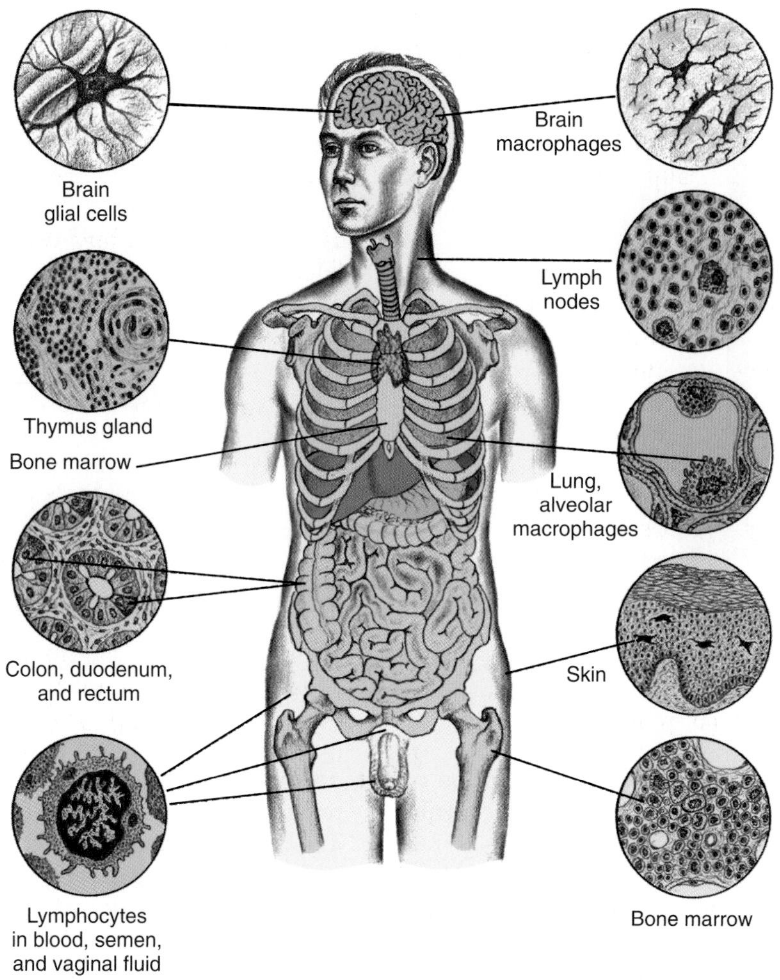

FIGURE 35-2 Distribution of tissues that can be infected by human immunodeficiency virus (HIV). Infection is closely linked to the presence of CD4 receptors on host tissue, with the possible exceptions of glial cells in the brain and chromaffin cells in the colon, duodenum, and rectum. (From Monahan F, Sands J, Neighbors M, et al.: *Phipps' medical-surgical nursing: health and illness perspectives*, ed 8, St. Louis, 2006, Mosby.)

When it affects the eyes, a loss of visual acuity, as well as photophobia, exists. Bactrim is used to treat toxoplasmosis. Teach patients to wash their hands, avoid undercooked and raw meats, and avoid cat litter boxes (Chimienti, Panther, & Graham, 2007).

FUNGAL INFECTIONS

Opportunistic fungal infections include microsporidiosis, *P. jirovecii* pneumonia, aspergillosis, candidiasis, coccidioidomycosis, cryptococcosis, and histoplasmosis. These infections may be treated with various antifungal drugs, including amphotericin B (Amphotec), itraconazole, nystatin, clotrimazole, fluconazole, ketoconazole, fluconazole, and flucytosine.

Pharmacology Capsule

Amphotericin B, which is administered intravenously, causes fever, rigors, and headache. Pretreatment with Benadryl, Demerol, and Tylenol as ordered will minimize this reaction. Amphotericin B can also cause electrolyte disturbances and is toxic to the kidneys. Other antifungal drugs are hepatotoxic.

Microsporidiosis

The source of human infection with microsporidiosis is unknown, although some believe that it is caused by the ingestion of *Microsporum* spores. Symptoms are watery diarrhea with weight loss, malabsorption, abdominal cramps, and flatulence. Management focuses on treating the symptoms because no curative therapy is available. Patients are encouraged to drink 3 L of fluid each day and milk products should be avoided. A diet low in fat and residue and high in protein and calories is recommended. The best way to avoid being infected with *Microsporum* is to practice good hand washing and good hygiene and to avoid ingestion of food or water contaminated with fecal matter (Chimienti, Panther, & Graham, 2007).

Pneumocystis jirovecii Pneumonia

P. jirovecii is a fungal organism acquired by inhalation that can cause *P. jirovecii* pneumonia (previously known as *Pneumocystis* pneumonia [PCP]). *P. jirovecii* pneumonia is the second leading cause of death among AIDS patients. By lodging in interstitial spaces of the lung tissue, *P. jirovecii* pneumonia cysts prevent the exchange of gases. This causes shortness of breath on exertion, fever, and a nonproductive cough. Treatment uses Bactrim, dapsone, clindamycin, and pentamidine. Patients considered at high risk for *P. jirovecii* pneumonia are treated prophylactically with Bactrim (Chimienti, Panther, & Graham, 2007).

Aspergillosis

Aspergillosis is caused by *Aspergillus*, which lives in soil, water, and air. Pulmonary infection can develop when *Aspergillus* spores are inhaled, especially by patients whose CD4 cell count has dropped below 50 cells/mm^3. Symptoms include fever, cough, dyspnea, chest pain, and hemoptysis. Despite antifungal treatment, aspergillosis is usually fatal within 8 weeks. To decrease the risk of aspergillosis, the patient should avoid wet, cool places. Potted plants, marijuana, wicker, and household dust are common sources of *Aspergillus* (Chimienti, Panther, & Graham, 2007).

Candidiasis

Candida albicans is a fungal yeast organism that is found in most foods, soil, and inanimate objects. Approximately 80% of patients with HIV infection will develop candidiasis, which usually affects the mouth, vagina, or anus (or a combination of these areas). Symptoms include thrush, which is an oral form of candidiasis. Unlike oral hairy leukoplakia (OHL), *Candida* plaques can be scraped off the skin. Any patient with oral or vaginal candidiasis who is not on antibiotic therapy should be tested for HIV. Inform the patient that candidiasis often reappears and that he or she must monitor for reinfection (Chimienti, Panther, & Graham, 2007).

Coccidioidomycosis

The causative agent for coccidioidomycosis is *Coccidioides immitis*, which is endemic in the southwestern United States and northern Mexico. Particles are inhaled into the lungs. Symptoms include fever, weight loss, fatigue, dry cough, or pleuritic chest pain. Dissemination to other organs may occur after infection of the lungs. Persons with HIV infection should avoid exposure to disturbed soils in endemic areas.

Cryptococcosis

Cryptococcosis is caused by a yeast *(Cryptococcus neoformans)* and is the most common systemic fungal infection in patients with AIDS. Symptoms appear approximately 30 days after exposure to the yeast and include fever, headache, malaise, nausea, vomiting, altered mental status, and a stiff neck (Chimienti, Panther, & Graham, 2007).

Histoplasmosis

Histoplasma is a fungus that is endemic in the central and southern parts of the United States. It is found in soil and bird droppings. Infection (histoplasmosis) usually involves the lungs after *Histoplasma* spores are inhaled. Once inhaled into the lungs, *Histoplasma* can be disseminated to other organs. Symptoms include fever, night sweats, weight loss, and shortness of breath. Patients with HIV infection should avoid areas where *Histoplasma* is common, such as disturbed soils, chicken coops, and caves. Teach patients to avoid cleaning out bird cages (Chimienti, Panther, & Graham, 2007).

VIRAL INFECTIONS

Opportunistic viral infections include various types of cytomegalovirus (CMV) infections, herpes simplex, herpes zoster, OHL, and progressive multifocal leukoencephalopathy (PML). Antiviral drugs are limited in number and work primarily by suppressing viral replication rather than killing the virus. Some of the antiviral drugs used are ganciclovir, foscarnet, and acyclovir.

Cytomegalovirus Infections

CMV is a virus found in semen, cervical secretions, saliva, urine, blood, and organs. It is transmitted mainly by blood and body fluids through unprotected sex. In patients with AIDS, complications of CMV infection include chorioretinitis, radiculopathy, subacute encephalitis, colitis, esophagitis, and pneumonia (Chimienti, Panther, & Graham, 2007). Specific types of CMV infections are described in Table 35-9.

Herpes Simplex and Herpes Zoster

More than 70% of patients who are HIV positive have previously been infected with herpes simplex virus-1 (HSV-1), herpes simplex virus-2 (HSV-2), or both. When herpes simplex virus (HSV) is reactivated in patients with HIV infection, it can cause serious disease and tissue destruction. HSV infection follows a predictable pattern: primary outbreak, latency, and possible reactivation at some later point in life. Most adults carry herpes zoster virus (HZV) because of exposure to the chickenpox virus as a child. Reactivation of HZV usually occurs as *shingles* and can be very painful and serious in the immunocompromised patient (Robinson, 2003; see *Patient Teaching* box).

Patient Teaching

Herpes Simplex Virus or Herpes Zoster Virus

When a patient has open sores on the skin, he or she should be instructed to do the following (Kirton, 2003):

- Maintain good hygiene without drying out the skin.
- Avoid deodorant astringent soap.
- Use tepid water; pat the skin dry and do not rub it.
- Apply lotion after bathing and at bedtime.
- Do not scratch.
- Use a separate cloth for affected areas.
- Remember that some wounds need special care.
- Avoid contact with people who have never had chickenpox.

Table 35-9 Cytomegalovirus

CYTOMEGALOVIRUS TYPE	SYMPTOMS	DIAGNOSIS
Cytomegalovirus (CMV) retinitis	Decreased visual acuity, presence of floaters, progression to visual field loss leading to blindness	Funduscopic examination
CMV radiculopathy	Spinal cord syndrome: lower extremity weakness, spasticity, areflexia, urinary retention	Cerebrospinal fluid (CSF) culture
CMV subacute encephalitis	Mental changes, somnolence, headache	Brain biopsy
CMV esophagitis	Painful swallowing	Endoscopic examination
CMV pneumonia	Dyspnea on exertion; dry, nonproductive cough	Radiograph examination and histologic findings
Colitis	Diarrhea, weight loss, fever	Endoscopic examination, ulcerated colon

Data from Zwolski K: Viral infections. In Kirton C, Talotta D, Zwolski K, editors: *Handbook of HIV/AIDS nursing,* St. Louis, 2001, Mosby.

Oral Hairy Leukoplakia

OHL is characterized by thick, white patches on the buccal mucosa, soft palate, floor of the mouth, and tongue. It is associated with Epstein-Barr virus and is more common among smokers. The mouth often is painful. Advise the patient to drink from a straw. Ice cream or Popsicles can be used to numb the area. Hot and spicy foods and alcohol may exacerbate mouth pain (Chimienti, Panther, & Graham, 2007).

Progressive Multifocal Leukoencephalopathy

PML, which is caused by the Jamestown Canyon virus (JC virus), develops in 2% to 4% of patients with AIDS and is recognized as an AIDS indicator illness. The JC virus causes progressive degeneration of the white matter of the brain; death ensues within 4 to 6 months after the onset of symptoms. Symptoms include weakness and progressively impaired speech, vision, and motor function. No proven effective therapy exists for treatment of PML. Intrathecal cytosine arabinoside (Ara-C) may be tried but it causes bone marrow suppression. Maintaining low viral loads through antiretroviral therapy seems to be the best strategy for preventing PML (Kirton, 2003). The family and the patient need support to accept and plan for the patient's approaching decline and death. Anticipate grief over loss and help the family to arrange nursing home care and advance directives (Chimienti, Panther, & Graham, 2007).

BACTERIAL INFECTIONS

Opportunistic bacterial infections include bacillary angiomatosis (BA), *Mycobacterium avium* complex (MAC), and tuberculosis. Treatments use various antibacterial drugs depending on the infecting organism. Patients need to understand the importance of taking antibacterials exactly as prescribed and completing the prescribed course of therapy. In persons with HIV infection, antiinfective drugs sometimes are ordered prophylactically when the CD4 cell count falls below specific levels.

Bacillary Angiomatosis

BA is a disease caused by bacteria (*Bartonella henselae* and *B. quintana*) that usually cause skin lesions. However, any organ may be affected. BA is usually transmitted by cats and their fleas. Most patients with BA have been bitten or scratched by a cat. Symptoms include papules and plaques that may occur anywhere on the skin. Patients with HIV should be warned about the risk of being around cats; the patient should avoid rough play with cats and ensure that cats are treated for fleas (Chimienti, Panther, & Graham, 2007).

Mycobacterium avium Complex

Mycobacterium avium, the causative agent for MAC, is found everywhere, including in most food, animal, and soil sources. MAC may affect any organ of the body, causing fever, fatigue, weight loss, night sweats, abdominal pain, and diarrhea. It is not contagious. Prophylactic treatment should be considered when CD4 cell counts drop below 50 cells/mm^3 (Chimienti, Panther, & Graham, 2007).

Tuberculosis

Patients with HIV infection are much more likely than healthy persons to develop tuberculosis if exposed to the causative agent *Mycobacterium tuberculosis.* This is particularly true if CD4 cell counts drop below 200 cells/mm^3 (Chimienti, Panther, & Graham, 2007). Tuberculosis is discussed in Chapter 32.

ONCOLOGIC CONDITIONS

Oncologic conditions that occur most often in persons with HIV infection include KS and lymphoma. Other cancer sites are the rectum and the vagina.

Kaposi Sarcoma

KS is a common type of neoplasm that develops in people with AIDS. It is thought to be caused by the sexual transmission of the human herpes virus 8 (HHV-8) (Moran, 2003). KS affects the skin first, appearing as a macular, painless, nonpruritic lesion. KS can vary in color—pink, red, purple, and brown. When KS is confined to the skin, no symptoms exist. However, symptoms develop when tumors spread to the gastrointestinal (GI) system and lungs. Sometimes when KS shows on the skin, it has already affected the body internally. When KS affects the GI system, bleeding may result, causing anemia. When KS affects the respiratory system, hypoxia may occur (Dezube, 2007).

Diagnosis. KS is diagnosed by clinical appearance but the most definitive method of diagnosis is a biopsy. No cure exists for KS and treatment is considered palliative.

Treatment. Treatment of KS includes simple observation, HAART, surgical removal, cryotherapy, radiotherapy, and chemotherapy. To help patients with self-care, see the *Patient Teaching* box.

Patient Teaching

Patient with Kaposi Sarcoma

- Tumor growth varies from patient to patient.
- Regardless of therapy, Kaposi sarcoma (KS) tends to reoccur.
- Various therapies are available; each has risks and benefits.
- For patients with cutaneous KS: report blood in stool or abdominal pain.

Data from Dezube BJ: Diagnosis and management of opportunistic cancers: Kaposi's sarcoma. In Libman H, Makadon H, editors: *HIV*, ed 3, Philadelphia, 2007, American College of Physicians.

Lymphoma

Lymphoma is a type of cancer that originates in lymphoid tissue—bone marrow, spleen, or thymus gland. Immunodeficient patients have a 14 times greater risk of getting lymphoma than the general population. The two types of lymphoma are (1) Hodgkin and (2) non-Hodgkin. NHL is the second most common malignancy found in patients with AIDS.

The prognosis with NHL is poor because the disease has spread widely by the time it is discovered. With chemotherapy, survival rates are as follows:

- 24 months with CD4 cell counts above 100 cells/mm^3
- 4½ months with CD4 cell counts less than 100 cells/mm^3
- 2 months if the CNS is affected

Symptoms typically are vague, vary according to the site involved, and include chills, fever, night sweats, and weight loss. Having a fever for more than 2 weeks strongly suggests lymphoma. Diagnosis is based on results of biopsy of lymphoid tissue. Other diagnostic testing includes radiography, computed tomography (CT) scan, bone marrow smear, and lumbar puncture. Treatment is with chemotherapy (Doweiko, 2007).

MEDICAL DIAGNOSIS OF HUMAN IMMUNODEFICIENCY VIRUS

To be diagnosed as HIV positive, the patient must test positive to an HIV *antibody* test (enzyme-linked immunosorbent assay [ELISA] or Western blot). The ELISA test is usually done first and has been shown to have 99% reliability. The Western blot test is used as a confirmation test and has been shown to have 99.99% reliability (Kirton et al., 2001). Persons who test negative initially should be retested in 3 to 6 months because of the lag time between exposure and a positive test. It is important to remember that some individuals never test positive for HIV because they never produce enough antibodies to the HIV virus to be detected.

The CDC (2013) criteria for a diagnosis of AIDS include the following:

- CD4 cell count of less than 200 cells/mm^3, asymptomatic
- CD4 cell count of less than 200 cells/mm^3, with category B symptoms (which include BA; candidiasis; oropharyngeal, vaginal, and cervical dysplasias; herpes zoster [shingles]; idiopathic thrombocytopenic purpura [ITP]; listeriosis; OHL; pelvic inflammatory disease [PID]; and peripheral neuropathy)
- Category C symptoms, regardless of CD4 cell count (these include candidiasis of bronchi, trachea, or lungs; esophageal or cervical cancer; coccidioidomycosis; cryptococcosis; cryptosporidiosis; CMV; encephalopathy; HSV; chronic ulcers of longer than 1 month's duration or bronchitis, pneumonitis, or esophagitis; histoplasmosis; isosporiasis; KS; lymphoma; *M. avium, M. tuberculosis,* or *P. jirovecii* pneumonia; pneumonia—recurrent; progressive multifocal leukoencephalopathy; salmonella; septicemia—recurrent; toxoplasmosis; and wasting because of HIV infection)

In 1996 the Home Access HIV-1 Test System was introduced; it allows individuals to collect a specimen at home and receive prompt results after submitting it by mail for analysis. The U.S. Food and Drug Administration (FDA) has approved a home-testing kit—OraQuick ADVANCE—that detects HIV-1 and HIV-2 in 20 minutes using a cheek swab. Home testing is controversial because of the risks of false-negative and false-positive results as well as the lack of professional counseling about the results. For example, a person in the early stage of infection who tests negative because not enough antibodies exist to be detected might assume that he or she is free of infection and fail to protect a sexual partner.

MEDICAL TREATMENT

No cure for HIV infection exists. The medical treatment of HIV infection is symptomatic and is aimed at reducing the viral load, preventing and treating infections, and treating malignancies. Patients also are encouraged to maintain a balanced diet, exercise regularly, maintain good dental hygiene, avoid smoking and using illicit drugs, limit alcohol intake, minimize stress, and practice safe sexual habits. The *Health Promotion* box addresses reducing the risk of perinatal transmission of HIV infection. Table 35-10 outlines the drugs used to treat HIV infection.

Health Promotion

WOMEN AND HUMAN IMMUNODEFICIENCY VIRUS

Women with human immunodeficiency virus (HIV) infection should be treated with antiretroviral drugs during pregnancy and delivery. As well, the newborn should be treated for the first 6 weeks of life to decrease the risk of transmission of the virus to the baby.

OLDER ADULTS AND HUMAN IMMUNODEFICIENCY VIRUS

Approximately 10% of acquired immunodeficiency syndrome (AIDS) cases through 2011 were people aged 50 years or older. Older adults are at increasing risk for HIV infection, AIDS, and other sexually transmitted infections (STIs). A growing number of people over age 50 years now have HIV/AIDS. Many factors contribute to the increasing risk of infection in this age group. In general, older Americans know less about HIV/AIDS because they have not been educated about STIs as much as younger people have. Additionally, older adults are less likely than younger people to discuss their sex lives or drug use with physicians and physicians do not tend to ask older patients about sex or drug use. Finally, older adults often mistake the symptoms of HIV/AIDS for the aches and pains of normal aging, so they are less likely to be tested for HIV infection (National Institute on Aging, 2009).

PHARMACOLOGY

Patients with HIV infection commonly are started on a medication regimen called HAART, which is recommended when the HIV viral load reaches certain levels. The usual combination of drugs is one **protease inhibitor** and two nucleoside reverse transcriptase inhibitors (NRTIs). A protease inhibitor interferes with the maturation of viral particles. Some protocols use NRTIs with one nonnucleoside reverse transcriptase inhibitor (NNRTI) or three NRTIs. Zidovudine (AZT) is a common NRTI that works by blocking an enzyme needed for viral replication. Efavirenz (Sustiva) is an example of an NNRTI, which also prevents viral replication. Enfuvirtide (Fuzeon) is a newer type of antiretroviral drug called a *fusion inhibitor.* A fusion inhibitor inhibits the binding of HIV with the human cell.

Before the patient with HIV infection is started on a medication regimen, it is important to assess the patient's ability and willingness to comply with the therapy. Once a medication regimen is started, the patient with HIV infection should not miss doses. When a dose is missed, the serum drug level falls, which allows the virus to mutate and build resistance to the HIV medications. Resistance is a very serious problem with HAART. If resistance to enough of the HIV medications builds up, the patient will have no medication options, which will ultimately end in his or her death. Therefore if the patient will not comply with the HIV medication regimen, it would be better to not start it. Some common side effects of HAART are as follows:

- Lipodystrophy
- Hepatitis
- Diabetes
- Increased cholesterol
- Increased low-density lipoproteins (LDLs)
- Increased triglycerides
- Pancreatitis
- Hemolytic anemia
- Peripheral neuropathy
- Nephrolithiasis and nephrotoxicity
- Stevens-Johnson syndrome
- Myopathy
- Hypersensitivity reaction
- Hepatotoxicity
- Nightmares
- Nausea, vomiting, and diarrhea

GI upset is a very common side effect of HAART and is one of the major reasons for noncompliance. The nurse should make the patient with HIV infection aware that many of the side effects of HAART are transitory and will subside within a few weeks. Table 35-10 summarizes the drugs used to treat HIV infection.

NURSING CARE of the Patient with Human Immunodeficiency Virus Infection

Care of the patient with HIV infection varies depending on the stage of infection the patient is experiencing (see Nursing Care Plan: Patient with Human Immunodeficiency Virus Infection). During the early stages of the disease, patients are treated primarily as outpatients. Because patients with HIV infection are frequent consumers of medical care, they often become very knowledgeable about their disease and treatment options and want to be actively involved in all treatment decisions. In the later stages of HIV infection, nursing care is much more intensive as the patient becomes more debilitated. Throughout the course of this disease, the goal of all treatments is good quality of life.

Assessment

Infection is the leading cause of death in patients with HIV infection. Therefore it is important to assess the patient frequently for any signs or symptoms of infection. The most common sites of infection are the lungs, mouth, GI tract, skin, blood, and CNS. Any change in the physical examination findings or any change in function should be reported to a registered nurse (RN) or physician. While collecting data about the patient's

Table 35-10 Medications Used to Treat Patients with Human Immunodeficiency Virus Infection

DRUG	USE AND ACTION	SIDE EFFECTS	NURSING INTERVENTIONS
Nucleoside Reverse Transcriptase Inhibitors			
Abacavir, lamivudine, and zidovudine (Trizivir) Didanosine, or ddI (Videx, Videx EC) Emtricitabine, or FTC (Emtriva) Lamivudine and zidovudine (Combivir) Lamivudine, or 3TC (Epivir) Stavudine, or d4T (Zerit) Tenofovir (Viread) Zalcitabine, or ddC (Hivid) Zidovudine, or AZT (Retrovir)	Used to slow the progression of human immunodeficiency virus (HIV) by interfering with replication inside the T helper/CD4 cell.	Headache, nausea and vomiting, fatigue, muscle aches, neutropenia, anemia, peripheral neuropathy, skin rash, elevated liver enzymes, pancreatitis, diarrhea, and lipodystrophy.	Some of these drugs should be taken on an empty stomach while others can be taken with or without food. Administration recommendations for specific drugs should be reviewed with the patient. A complete blood count (CBC) will be ordered periodically to monitor the patient's white blood cell (WBC) and red blood cell (RBC) counts. Liver function tests will also be monitored. Multiple drug interactions are possible between nucleoside reverse transcriptase inhibitors (NRTIs) and other drugs; therefore the patient's complete medication record must be reviewed before beginning these drugs and before adding other drugs to the patient's regimen after he or she is started on an NRTI.
Protease Inhibitors			
Atazanavir (Reyataz) Fosamprenavir (Lexiva) Indinavir (Crixivan), lopinavir and ritonavir (Kaletra) Nelfinavir (Viracept) Ritonavir (Norvir) Saquinavir mesylate (Invirase)	Used to slow the replication and progression of HIV by blocking protease enzymes so that infected cells cannot produce HIV proteins.	Diarrhea, nausea and vomiting, kidney stones, jaundice, abdominal pain, headache, skin rash, numbness and tingling around the mouth, drooling, dizziness, sleepiness, sore throat, sweating, altered taste, and lipodystrophy.	Some of these drugs should be taken on an empty stomach while others should be taken with food. Administration recommendations for specific drugs should be reviewed with the patient. Multiple drug interactions are possible between protease inhibitors and other drugs; therefore the patient's complete medication record must be reviewed before beginning these drugs and before adding other drugs to the patient's regimen after he or she is started on a protease inhibitor.
Nonnucleoside Reverse Transcriptase Inhibitors			
Delavirdine (Rescriptor) Efavirenz (Sustiva) Nevirapine (Viramune)	Used to slow the progression of HIV by interfering with replication inside the T helper/CD4 cell.	Skin rash, headache, nausea, diarrhea, and fatigue.	Can be taken with or without food. Multiple drug interactions are possible between nonnucleoside reverse transcriptase inhibitors (NNRTIs) and other drugs; therefore the patient's complete medication record must be reviewed before beginning these drugs and before adding other drugs to the patient's regimen after he or she is started on an NNRTI.
Fusion Inhibitors			
Enfuvirtide (Fuzeon)	Fusion inhibitors are a new class of antiretrovirals. Fuzeon is used in combination with other antiretroviral drugs in treatment-experienced patients. This drug prevents the HIV from fusing with the cell membrane.	Irritation at injection site, fatigue, nausea, insomnia, and peripheral neuropathy.	Reconstitute and store as directed. Inject subcutaneously as ordered and rotate sites.

Nursing Care Plan — Patient with Human Immunodeficiency Virus Infection

ASSESSMENT

HEALTH HISTORY A 25-year-old divorced mother of two children works as a freelance accountant and lives with her parents, who provide financial and emotional support. She was diagnosed with human immunodeficiency virus (HIV) infection during the pregnancy with her daughter, who is now 3 years old, and has shown no signs of HIV infection. The patient and her husband have been divorced since her infection was diagnosed. His HIV status is not known. She reports tiring easily but most days is able to work about 6 hours and care for her children. She is seen monthly by a nurse practitioner (NP) at a neighborhood clinic. Her medications are indinavir (Crixivan), stavudine (Zerit), and didanosine (Videx). She reports bouts of depression and anxiety about her own and her children's future. Her most recent blood studies show a decline in the number of T helper (CD4) cells. The CD4 cell count today is 480 cells/mm^3. She has been treated twice this fall for upper respiratory tract infections. She does not sleep well. She has experienced a 10-lb weight loss in the past 3 months and reports poor appetite and frequent diarrhea.

PHYSICAL EXAMINATION Healthy-looking young woman. Alert. Converses easily. Vital signs within normal limits (WNL). No fever. Skin intact; no lesions. Lungs clear on auscultation. No lymphadenopathy. Abdomen soft. Bowel sounds present in all four quadrants. Normal reflexes. Full range of motion in all joints.

Nursing Diagnosis	Goals and Outcome Criteria	Interventions
Ineffective Self-Health Management related to lack of knowledge about disease process and treatment, denial, and fear	Patient will effectively manage self-care, as evidenced by correctly taking prescribed medications and following medical advice for rest and protection from infection.	Provide written and verbal instructions for any prescribed drugs. Advise her of the kinds of side and adverse effects she might experience. Explain the importance of continuing the drugs under medical supervision. Discuss ways to conserve energy and to promote restful sleep at night. Explore options to obtain assistance with child care.
Anxiety related to disease and treatments	Patient will verbalize decreased anxiety and will appear more relaxed.	Encourage her to ask questions and talk about her feelings. Be accepting of feelings she may express (fear, anger, and depression are common). Provide information or refer her to a social worker, support groups, chaplain, or mental health counselor if needed.
Risk for Infection related to impaired resistance	Patient will remain free of infection, as evidenced by absence of fever, lesions, or signs of inflammation.	Encourage her to report any signs of infection immediately. If antibiotics are ordered, encourage her to take them as prescribed. Explain the need to avoid people with infections and crowded public places during seasons when upper respiratory tract infections are common.
Impaired Oral Mucous Membrane related to human immunodeficiency virus (HIV) infection and oral opportunistic infections	Patient will have intact oral mucous membranes with normal color and no lesions.	Teach the importance of regular dental care. Advise her to use a soft toothbrush and to avoid traumatizing oral tissues. Explain how maintaining good fluid intake keeps mucous membranes moist and reduces oral complications.
Imbalanced Nutrition: Less Than Body Requirements and **Deficient Fluid Volume** related to HIV infection, diarrhea, and gastrointestinal (GI) infections	Patient's intake of food and fluids will be adequate, as evidenced by stable body weight, moist mucous membranes, and normal blood pressure and pulse.	Suggest the addition of Carnation Instant Breakfast to her daily diet to increase calorie intake. Weigh her weekly. Talk to the nurse practitioner (NP) about prescribing antinausea medication, an appetite stimulant, and an antidiarrheal.

Critical Thinking Questions

1. How would you explain to the patient the importance of taking the prescribed drugs as ordered?
2. What other suggestions could you give this patient to help her increase her intake of food and liquids throughout the day?

physical status, determine how much the patient knows about the disease and treatment as well as how the patient is coping with this life-threatening disease. The complete assessment, as done by the RN, is outlined here. The licensed practical nurse/licensed vocational nurse (LPN/LVN) may collect some of these data.

Health History

A complete health and social history should be obtained from each patient with HIV infection. The history should include the following:

- STI history
- Surgical history
- Medication history: all current drugs, compliance, allergies, response to HIV drugs
- Immunization history
- Family history
- Sexual history—number of partners the patient has had in the past year
- Needle and blood exposure history—exposure to hepatitis B and C
- History of screening for hepatitis B and C
- Tobacco and alcohol use
- Illegal drug use history—use of intravenous drugs or unsafe behavior while using drugs
- Travel history—travel outside United States to locations where possible exposure to pathogens may have occurred
- Pet history—exposure to cats, birds, or exotic pets
- Occupational history—exposure to pathogens in the workplace
- Nutritional history—usual food and fluid intake
- Gynecologic history—number of pregnancies, knowledge of contraceptives

Physical Examination

A complete physical examination should be performed (review the Nursing Care Plan). The examination should include the following (Kirton, 2003):

- General examination—measurement of height, weight, vital signs
- Skin examination—signs of infections, lesions
- Head, ears, eyes, nose, and throat examination
- Lymphatic system—enlarged lymph glands
- Respiratory system—auscultation for quality of breath sounds
- Cardiovascular examination
- Abdominal examination
- Musculoskeletal examination
- Neurologic examination—orientation, alertness, sensory and cognitive functioning
- Genitourinary examination
- Laboratory profile
- CD4 cell count
- CD8 cell count
- HIV viral load
- Complete blood count (CBC)
- Chemistry profile
- Rapid plasma reagin (RPR) (syphilis)
- Lipid profile
- STI screening
- Purified protein derivative (PPD) tuberculosis screening
- Chest radiograph
- Hepatitis A, B, C antibody titers
- Toxoplasmosis antibody titers
- Titers for all immunizations received

Nursing Diagnoses, Goals, and Outcome Criteria: Human Immunodeficiency Virus Infection

Nursing Diagnoses	Goals and Outcome Criteria
Ineffective Self-Health Management related to lack of knowledge about disease process and treatment, denial, fear	Effective self-care management: patient correctly describes and demonstrates self-care measures
Anxiety related to the disease and treatment	Reduced anxiety: patient reports anxiety is lessened, more relaxed manner
Risk for Infection (lung, mouth, gastrointestinal [GI] tract, skin, blood, central nervous system [CNS], eye) related to decreased immunity	Patient remains free of infection: no fever, signs of inflammation, lesions
Impaired Oral Mucous Membrane related to the disease and oral infections	Intact oral mucous membranes: normal color of mouth tissues, no lesions
Imbalanced Nutrition: Less Than Body Requirements and **Deficient Fluid Volume** related to the disease, diarrhea, and GI infections	Adequate intake of nutrients and fluids: stable weight, intake and output approximately equal, moist mucous membranes
Acute Confusion or **Chronic Confusion** related to disease-induced dementia	Resolved confusion: patient's consciousness, attention, cognition, and perception improve to baseline Patient safety: absence of injuries associated with irreversible confusion
Acute Pain or **Chronic Pain** related to actual or potential tissue damage	Pain relief: patient states pain is relieved, appears relaxed
Ineffective Coping related to perceived lack of support, fear, anxiety	Effective coping: patient demonstrates strategies to cope with feelings about diagnosis in a positive way.

Interventions

Ineffective Self-Health Management

It is very important that the patient receive accurate, consistent information from all members of the health care team. A clinical nurse specialist or other specially trained nurse usually can provide comprehensive information about the disease and its treatment to the patient and family and answer questions as they arise during hospitalization. You can reinforce this teaching. Excellent sources of current information about HIV and AIDS for patients, families, and health care providers are available on the internet (e.g., www.thebody.com).

Anxiety

A diagnosis of HIV infection is always a shock to patients and their families. Patients must deal not only with the disease and treatment but also with the emotions of facing a life-threatening illness. Encourage patients to ask questions and to talk about their feelings. Often a patient's fears result from lack of knowledge about the disease and treatment. The clinical nurse specialist or other specially trained nurse can answer many of the patient's and family's questions. Often information will help the patient and family to deal with their anxiety. A referral to a social worker, chaplain, or mental health counselor may be indicated if the patient and family are experiencing continued anxiety and difficulty in coping. It is important for the nurse to know what the patient has been told about the disease, the treatment, and the prognosis so that correct information can be reinforced. The patient's interpretation and understanding of the information are essential.

Risk for Infection

As emphasized earlier, patients with HIV infection are at high risk for opportunistic infections. Early detection and prompt treatment of infections are vital. Many patients take antiinfective drugs (e.g., trimethoprim-sulfamethoxazole, pentamidine) prophylactically to prevent infections. Educate the patient about the importance of taking drugs exactly as prescribed. If a patient does develop an infection, stress the importance of taking antibiotics exactly as prescribed. Stopping antibiotic therapy early can result in incomplete treatment and the development of resistant organisms. Many of the antibiotics must be administered intravenously and require nursing coordination for intravenous access and either clinic or home administration.

Impaired Oral Mucous Membrane

Patients with HIV infection can experience altered oral mucous membrane integrity because of the disease and oral infections. Encourage patients to clean their teeth and mouth regularly with dental floss and a soft toothbrush. Debilitated patients may need assistance with mouth care. Encourage noncaffeinated fluids to maintain hydration and keep oral mucous membranes moist. Topical anesthetics to control pain can be applied before eating. Prescribed topical antibiotics should be reapplied after eating and routine mouth care. Regular dental evaluations can help to prevent and manage oral disease and infections in these patients.

Imbalanced Nutrition: Less Than Body Requirements

A referral to a dietitian for nutrition education and counseling should be made as soon as the patient is diagnosed with HIV infection. Strategies to maximize calorie and nutrient intake can be discussed. Oral supplements with Carnation Instant Breakfast, Ensure, Sustacal, or Resource can be added as indicated. Administer medications to improve appetite (e.g., megestrol, dronabinol), relieve nausea (e.g., prochlorperazine, metoclopramide), and control diarrhea (e.g., diphenoxylate hydrochloride with atropine sulfate) as prescribed.

In general, the patient's diet should be high in calories and proteins with supplemental vitamins. Advise the patient to avoid caffeine and food that might contain pathogens (e.g., undercooked meat, raw eggs, unpasteurized milk) (see *Nutrition Considerations* box).

Nutrition Considerations

Acquired immunodeficiency syndrome (AIDS) wasting is common among patients with AIDS. Wasting is caused by lack of nutritional intake or the inability of the body to absorb and use nutrition. Every patient with human immunodeficiency virus (HIV) infection should be seen by a nutritionist. Helpful nutrition teaching for the patient with HIV infection includes the following:

- Do not buy expired foods.
- Do not buy cracked eggs.
- Thoroughly cook meats and poultry.
- Wash hands thoroughly before preparing foods.
- Wash all fruits and vegetables before eating them.
- Thaw frozen foods in the refrigerator and not at room temperature.
- Avoid eating leftovers.
- If the CD4 cell counts drop below 100 cells/mm^3, boil water for 1 minute or use sterile water products.
- Remember that many HIV drugs cause hyperlipidemia. You should eat small, frequent meals that are low in fat and lactose and high in caloric intake.
- Abstain from alcohol and caffeine.
- Eat healthy meals with five to six servings of fruits and vegetables per day.
- Weigh yourself daily and report patterns of weight loss or weight gain to your physician.

Data from Winson G: HIV/AIDS nutritional management. In Kirton C, Talotta D, Zwolski K, editors: *Handbook of HIV/AIDS nursing*, St. Louis, 2001, Mosby.

Deficient Fluid Volume

Since many HIV patients develop infections or cancers related to the GI tract, they often experience diarrhea, nausea and/or vomiting, or a poor appetite. This will often lead to fluid and electrolyte imbalances. It is very important for the nurse to assess the patient's intake and output, daily weights, electrolytes, protein and albumin levels; and inform the provider of abnormal levels. HIV patients should be educated about the importance of maintaining a healthy, well-balanced diet, drinking 4-6 (8 oz) glasses of water daily and taking a daily multivitamin if not contraindicated.

Patients who are nauseated or who are vomiting may be prescribed an antiemetic. Patients who have a poor appetite may be prescribed appetite stimulants. It is vital that the nurse assesses the patient frequently for fluid volume and electrolyte and nutritional status.

Acute Confusion or Chronic Confusion

Patients with HIV-induced encephalopathy may experience cognitive and motor impairment. Patients may withdraw from social activities because of embarrassment. Patients may become angry and hostile with the onset of yet another disability. Many patients with HIV-induced encephalopathy improve with zidovudine therapy. In the hospital and at home, patient safety needs to be reevaluated constantly based on the patient's mental and physical capabilities.

Acute Pain or Chronic Pain

Pain has been an underrecognized problem for patients with HIV infection. Pain can be caused by opportunistic infections, viral invasion into the nerves and muscles, malignant tumors, and diagnostic procedures. Closely monitor the patient's pain level and medication use. Keeping a flow sheet of patient reports of pain on a 10-point scale can be helpful, especially as different nurses care for the patient throughout the day. A *0* represents no pain while a *10* represents the worst pain a patient has ever experienced. The patient's report of pain coupled with the amount of pain medication he or she is receiving can guide the nurse and physician as to the appropriate type and amount of pain medication. Pharmacologic and nonpharmacologic pain management strategies are presented in Chapter 15.

Ineffective Coping

A diagnosis of HIV/AIDS, with its life-threatening consequences, can overwhelm the patient's ability to cope. Patients and their significant others may experience many emotions, such as fear, anxiety, anger, shame, grief, depression, and loss of self-esteem. Fearing social stigma, patients may be reluctant to share the diagnosis with others. Other than sexual partners and health care providers, the patient is not obligated to inform other persons.

Nurses must be aware of their own feelings, and even fears, about caring for people with HIV infection. Education about self-protection and measures to take in the event of body fluid exposure can relieve some of the nurse's concerns. Sensitivity and touch can be very comforting to patients. When changes in a patient's emotional state are noted, encourage the patient to talk about his or her feelings. Provide information about support groups and mental health care as needed.

Get Ready for the NCLEX® Examination!

Key Points

- HIV is transmitted by high-risk behavior and body fluid exposure, including intrauterine exposure. HIV infection occurs in heterosexual and homosexual people of all races.
- Behaviors by which HIV may be transmitted include needle sharing, unprotected sex, and blood transfusions.
- HIV is a retrovirus that enters the body through blood, semen, vaginal fluids, or breast milk.
- HIV infection eventually exhausts the immune response to pathogens.
- CD8 cell count drops drastically in the late stage of HIV infection; CD4 cell count slowly declines throughout the course of the infection.
- A patient is considered to have AIDS when the CD4 cell count drops below 200 cells/mm^3.
- Initial symptoms of HIV infection are usually flulike symptoms.
- During the latent stage, which can last 2 to 12 years, patients may have no symptoms.
- During the later stages of HIV, patients may have fever, night sweats, swollen lymph glands, skin lesions, dyspnea, burning with urination, diarrhea, and other symptoms.
- The major complications of HIV infection are opportunistic infections, wasting, secondary cancers, and dementia.
- Parasites, viruses, bacteria, and fungi can cause opportunistic infections.
- The most common types of cancer associated with HIV infection are KS and lymphoma.
- Blood tests used to diagnose HIV infection are the ELISA and Western blot; both detect HIV antibodies.
- Infections are the leading cause of death in patients with HIV infection.
- The most commonly used types of drugs for HIV infection are NRTIs, protease inhibitors, NNRTIs, and fusion inhibitors.
- Failure to take HIV drugs as scheduled can encourage resistant strains of HIV.
- Nursing diagnoses for the patient with HIV infection may include ineffective self-health management; anxiety; risk for infection; impaired oral mucous membrane; imbalanced nutrition: less than body requirements; deficient fluid volume; acute confusion or

chronic confusion; acute pain or chronic pain; and ineffective coping.
- Inadequate nutritional intake or the inability of the body to absorb and use nutrition causes wasting.

Additional Learning Resources

SG Go to your Study Guide for additional learning activities to help you master this chapter content.

evolve Go to your Evolve website (http://evolve.elsevier.com/Linton/medsurg) for the following learning resources and much more:
- Interactive Prioritization Exercises
- Fluid & Electrolyte Tutorial
- Pharmacology Tutorial
- Review Questions for the NCLEX® Examination

Review Questions for the NCLEX® Examination

1. HIV can best be described as which of the following?
   1. DNA virus
   2. Messenger RNA (mRNA) virus
   3. Transfer RNA (tRNA) virus
   4. Retrovirus

   NCLEX Client Need: Physiological Integrity: Physiological Adaptation
2. During the latent stage of HIV infection, which of the following cells host the HIV?
   1. CD4 cells
   2. CD8 cells
   3. Antibodies
   4. Natural killer cells

   NCLEX Client Need: Physiological Integrity: Physiological Adaptation
3. Through which of the following does HIV enter the body?
   1. The respiratory tract
   2. Blood and body fluids
   3. Contaminated food
   4. Skin contact

   NCLEX Client: Physiological Integrity: Physiological Adaptation
4. What is the leading cause of death in persons with AIDS?

   NCLEX Client Need: Physiological Integrity: Physiological Adaptation
5. Under what circumstances is it possible for a person with HIV infection to have negative HIV blood tests?
   1. Prescribed antibiotics are effectively destroying the HIV.
   2. The patient has produced too few antibodies to be detected.
   3. Some strains of HIV do not induce antibody production.
   4. The patient did not fast for 24 hours before the test.

   NCLEX Client Need: Physiological Integrity: Reduction of Risk Potential
6. Which of the following tests is usually done first to screen for HIV antibodies?
   1. ELISA
   2. CD4:CD8 ratio
   3. Western blot
   4. CBC

   NCLEX Client Need: Physiological Integrity: Reduction of Risk Potential
7. In relation to risk for transmission of HIV, how is anal or vaginal sex with a condom classified?
   1. Very high–risk behavior
   2. Little-risk behavior
   3. Moderate-risk behavior
   4. No-risk behavior

   NCLEX Client Need: Health Promotion and Maintenance
8. AZT is classified as which type of drug?
   1. NNRTI
   2. Nucleotide reverse transcriptase inhibitor
   3. Protease inhibitor
   4. NRTI

   NCLEX Client Need: Physiological Integrity: Pharmacological Therapies
9. Side effects of AZT include which of the following? (Select all that apply.)
   1. Skin rash
   2. Elevated liver enzymes
   3. Nausea and vomiting
   4. Hyperlipidemia
   5. Constipation

   NCLEX Client Need: Physiological Integrity: Pharmacological Therapies
10. Types of cancer that occur most often in persons with HIV infection include which of the following? (Select all that apply.)
    1. Lung cancer
    2. Melanoma
    3. KS
    4. Lymphoma
    5. Rectal cancer

    NCLEX Client Need: Physiological Integrity: Physiological Adaptation
11. A patient with HIV infection has recently become confused. Which of the following explanations should you provide to the patient's partner?
    1. "Confusion with HIV is rare and irreversible."
    2. "The patient's confusion is probably related to something other than HIV."
    3. "The patient's mental status may improve with drug therapy."
    4. "Confusion usually occurs shortly before death."

    NCLEX Client Need: Physiological Integrity: Physiological Adaptation

chapter 36

Cardiac Disorders

Judy L. Maltas

http://evolve.elsevier.com/Linton/medsurg

Objectives

1. Label the major parts of the heart.
2. Describe the flow of blood through the heart and coronary vessels.
3. Name the elements of the heart's conduction system.
4. State the order in which normal impulses are conducted through the heart.
5. Explain the nursing considerations for patients who are having procedures to detect or evaluate cardiac disorders.
6. Identify nursing implications for common therapeutic measures, including drug, diet, or oxygen therapy; pacemakers and automatic implantable cardioverter defibrillators (AICDs); percutaneous coronary intervention (PCI); cardiac surgery; and cardiopulmonary resuscitation, defibrillation, and cardioversion.
7. Explain the pathophysiology, risk factors, signs and symptoms, complications, medical treatment, and nursing care for selected cardiac disorders.
8. List the data to be obtained in assessing the patient with a cardiac disorder.
9. Assist in developing nursing care plans for patients with cardiac disorders.

Key Terms

Afterload
Arteriosclerosis (ăr-tē-rē-ō-sklĕ-RŌ-sĭs)
Atherosclerosis (ăth-ĕr-ō-sklĕ-RŌ-sĭs)
Bradycardia (bră-dĕ-KĂR-dē-ă)
Contractility
Diastole
Dysrhythmia (dĭs-RĬTH-mē-ă)
Hemodynamic (hē-mō-dī-NĂ-mĭk)
Murmur (MŭR-mĕr)
Myocardial infarction (mī-ō-KĂR-dē-ăl ĭn-FĂRK-shŭn)
Palpitation (păl-pĭ-TĀ-shŭn)
Perfusion (pĕr-FYŪ-shŭn)
Preload
Regurgitation (rē-gŭr-jĭ-TĀ-shŭn)
Syncope (SĬN-kă-pē)
Systole
Tachycardia (tă-kĕ-KĂR-dē-ă)
Thromboembolism (thrŏm-bō-ĔM-bō-lĭzm)

The cardiovascular system carries oxygenated blood and nutrients to the cells and transports carbon dioxide (CO_2) and wastes from the cells. It requires a reservoir for blood coming from the tissues, pumping action to send blood to the lungs and the body, and an intact vascular system to transport the blood. A malfunction in any of these components may affect other body systems and may threaten the life and health of the person.

The heart is a hollow muscular pump located in the mediastinum (Fig. 36-1). The right and left sides of the heart receive blood from and send blood to different parts of the body. The heart is covered and protected by the sternum and the ribs anteriorly and flanked by the lungs laterally. The esophagus, the descending aorta, and the fifth through eighth thoracic vertebrae are directly behind the heart. The heart rests on the diaphragm, with two thirds of it to the left of the sternum. The right side of the heart is located under the sternum. The heart is approximately the size of the person's fist, weighs 10 to 14 oz in the adult, and is covered by membranes called the *visceral* and *parietal pericardium*. The space between the pericardial membranes contains fluid that lubricates the membranes and decreases friction.

ANATOMY AND PHYSIOLOGY OF THE HEART

CHAMBERS

The heart is divided into four chambers: two upper atria (right and left) and two lower ventricles (right and left). The four chambers are separated by septa (walls), with two chambers on the right (atrium and ventricle) and two chambers on the left (atrium and ventricle). Valves separate the atria from the ventricles.

The right atrium (RA) is a thin-walled reservoir and conduit for systemic blood. It receives blood from the

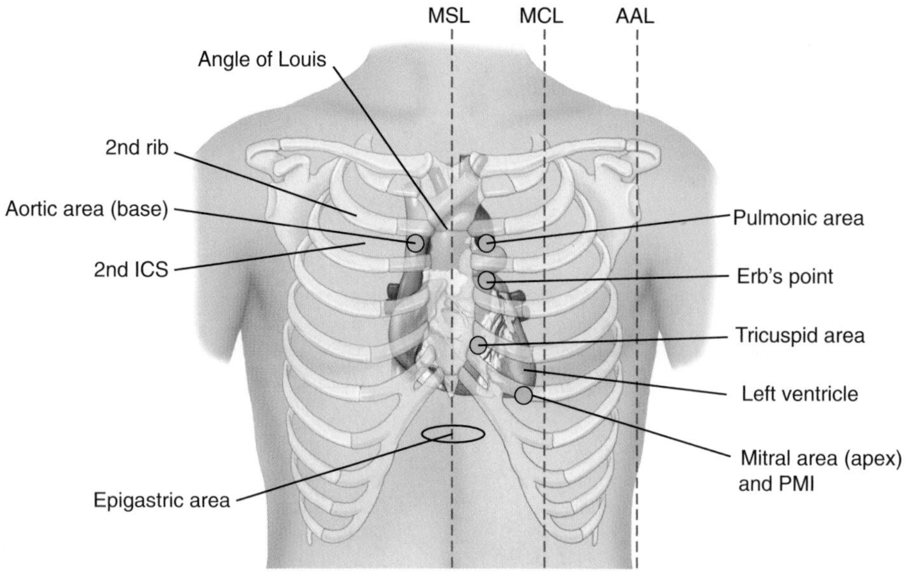

FIGURE 36-1 Anatomic location of the heart. *AAL*, anterior axillary line; *ICS*, intercostal space; *MCL*, midclavicular line; *MSL*, midsternal line; *PMI*, point of maximal impulse. (From Lewis SL, Dirksen SR, Heitkemper MM, et al: *Medical-surgical nursing: assessment and management of clinical problems*, ed 9, St. Louis, 2015, Mosby.)

inferior and the superior venae cavae and from the coronary sinuses. The right ventricle (RV) has thicker walls than the RA and receives blood from the RA through the tricuspid valve. Blood moves rather passively from the RA to the RV. When the RV contracts (**systole**), blood is ejected through the pulmonic valve into the pulmonary artery. The pulmonary artery carries the blood to the lungs, where it releases CO_2 as waste and picks up oxygen (O_2) to be taken to the tissues. Pulmonary veins carry the blood from the lungs to the left atrium (LA).

The blood passes from the LA through the mitral valve into the left ventricle (LV), the chamber with the thickest, strongest muscle. The LV is cone shaped and contains the apex of the heart located at the midclavicular line at the fourth or fifth intercostal space. An apical pulse is taken by auscultating the heartbeat at this location.

When the LV contracts (systole), blood is ejected through the aortic valve into the aorta and the systemic circulation. The systemic circulation carries O_2 and nutrients to all active cells and transports wastes to the kidneys, liver, and skin for excretion (Fig. 36-2).

The pressures in the RA and RV are very low compared with the pressures in the LA and LV. This is because the LV pumps blood out into the systemic circulation. The pressure in the LV is the highest of all the chambers.

MUSCLE LAYERS

Three layers of cardiac muscle tissue exist: (1) the endocardium, (2) the myocardium, and (3) the epicardium. The endocardium is the inner layer that lines the heart chambers. The middle layer, the myocardium, is made of muscle fibers. It is responsible for the pumping action of the heart. The thickness of the myocardium varies with each chamber. The outer layer, the epicardium, is also the visceral pericardium. The coronary arteries are embedded in the epicardium.

VALVES

Four valves exist in the heart: (1) the mitral, (2) the tricuspid, (3) the aortic, and (4) the pulmonic. Their purpose is to retain blood in one chamber until the next chamber is ready to receive it. The valves keep blood flowing in one direction. The valves open and close passively, in response to changes in pressure and volume. A valve opens when the pressure behind it is greater than the pressure ahead of it. A valve closes when the pressure ahead of it is greater than the pressure behind it.

Atrioventricular Valves

The mitral and tricuspid valves are called *atrioventricular (AV) valves* because they separate the atria from the ventricles. The mitral valve is between the LA and the LV. The tricuspid valve separates the RA from the RV. The cusps, or leaflets, are attached by chordae tendineae to the papillary muscles that line the floor of the ventricles. These valves are closed during systole and open during diastole.

Semilunar Valves

The semilunar valves, called *aortic* and *pulmonic*, separate the ventricles from the aorta and the pulmonary artery, respectively. These valves are open during systole and closed during diastole. The semilunar valves have three cusps (cup-shaped structures) each.

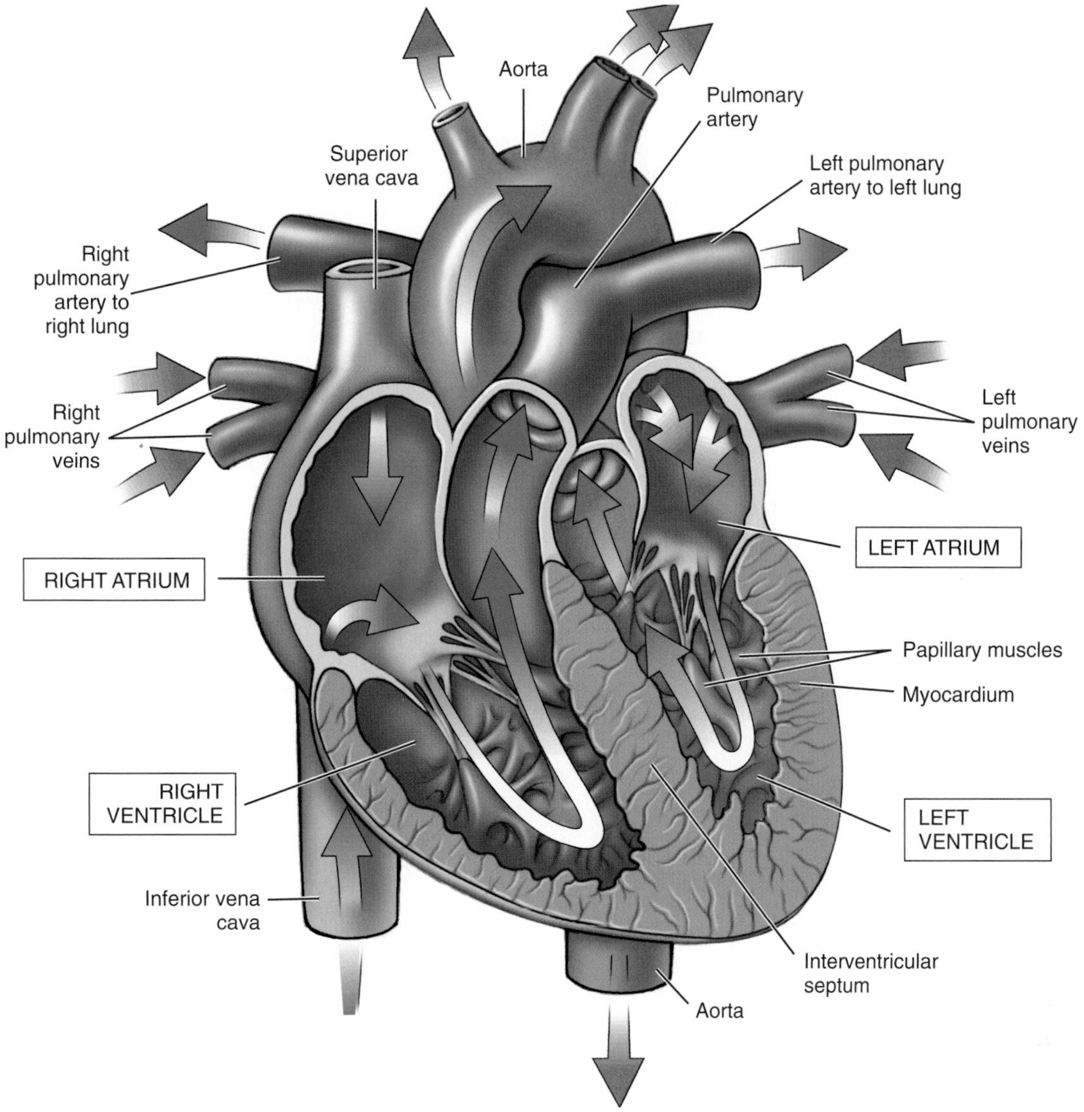

FIGURE 36-2 Normal circulation through the heart. (From Herlihy B: *The human body in health and illness*, ed 4, St. Louis, 2011, Saunders.)

Heart Sounds

Closure of the valves produces the heart sounds auscultated over the heart. The first heart sound (S_1), referred to as *lub*, occurs when the ventricles contract during systole and when the mitral and tricuspid valves close. The second heart sound (S_2), called *dub*, occurs during ventricular relaxation or diastole and is caused by the closing of the aortic and pulmonic valves.

CORONARY BLOOD FLOW

The coronary arteries are the first branches of the systemic circulation. These arteries supply blood to the myocardium and the conductive tissue of the heart. The two major coronary arteries, the left coronary artery and the right coronary artery, arise from the aorta just beyond the aortic valve. Blood flow through the coronary arteries occurs during diastole. The left coronary artery, which branches into the left anterior descending and circumflex arteries, supplies blood to the LA, most of the LV, and most of the septum between the two ventricles (interventricular septum). The right coronary artery branches to supply the sinoatrial (SA) and the AV nodes, the RA and RV, and the inferior part of the LV. Variations in the pattern of arterial branching are common.

Collateral arteries are connections between two branches of arteries. They are more common in certain areas of the heart. It is thought that collateral circulation protects the heart and that coronary collaterals develop over time as a result of gradual coronary occlusion.

In general, the venous system parallels the arterial system: the great cardiac vein follows the left anterior descending artery and the small cardiac vein follows the right coronary artery. The veins meet to form the coronary sinus (the largest coronary vein), which returns deoxygenated blood from the myocardium to the RA (Fig. 36-3).

CONDUCTION SYSTEM

For the heart to pump blood through the chambers, nerves must stimulate muscle contractions in an orderly fashion. The conduction pattern follows a particular route. The SA node, also called the *pacemaker*, initiates the impulse. The impulse is carried throughout the atria to the AV node, located on the floor of the RA. The impulse is delayed in the AV node and then transmitted to the ventricles through the bundle of His. The bundle is made up of Purkinje cells and is located where the atrial and ventricular septa meet. The bundle of His divides into the left and right bundle branches. The left bundle branch divides into anterior and posterior branches called *fascicles.* The terminal ends of the right and left branches are called the *Purkinje fibers.* When the impulse reaches the Purkinje fibers, the ventricles contract (Fig. 36-4).

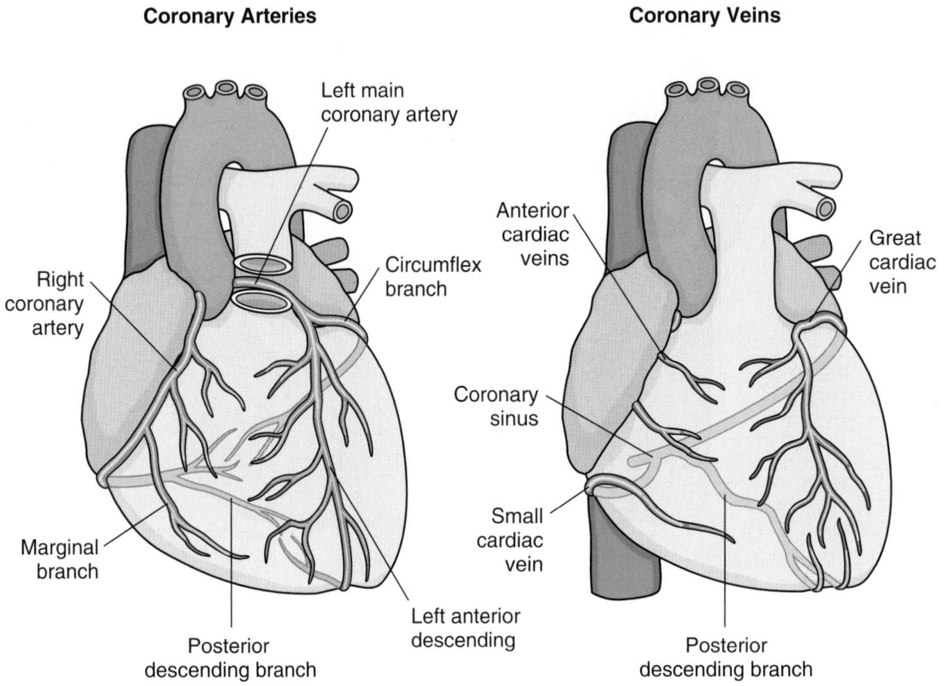

FIGURE 36-3 Coronary arteries and veins. (From Monahan F, Sands J, Neighbors M, et al: *Phipps' medical-surgical nursing: health and illness perspectives,* ed 8, St. Louis, 2007, Mosby.)

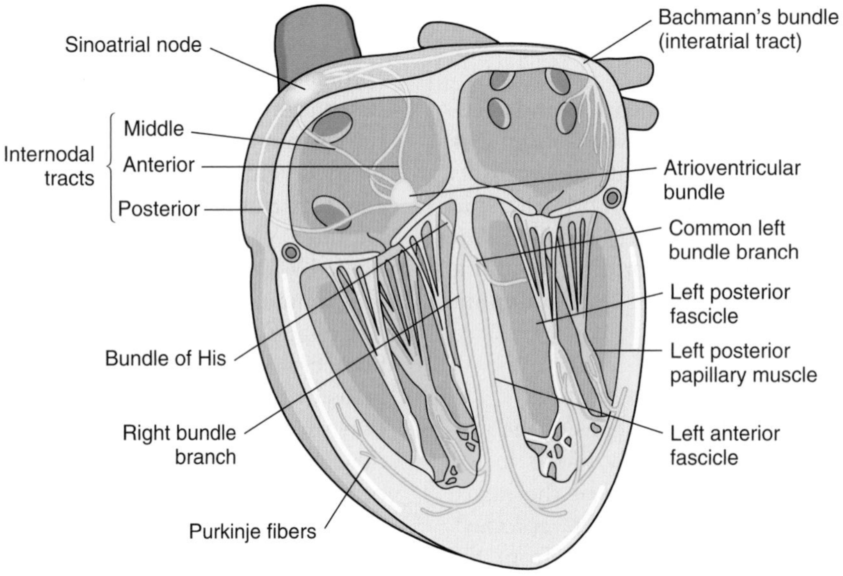

FIGURE 36-4 The conduction system of the heart. (From Monahan F, Sands J, Neighbors M, et al: *Phipps' medical-surgical nursing: health and illness perspectives,* ed 8, St. Louis, 2007, Mosby.)

The impulse produces a change in the movement of electrically charged ions across the membrane of cardiac cells. Cardiac cells at rest are electrically polarized, with the inside of the cell negatively charged and the outside of the cell positively charged. When stimulated, cardiac cells lose their internal negativity by a process called *depolarization.* Depolarization moves from cell to cell, producing a wave of electrical activity that is transmitted throughout the heart. Once depolarization is complete, the resting state (i.e., the inside of the cell more negative than the outside) is restored through a process called *repolarization.*

The SA node normally generates these impulses at a rate between 60 and 100 beats per minute (bpm). The SA node is called the *pacemaker of the heart.* The AV node is also capable of generating an impulse if the SA node should fail. The AV node rate is 40 to 60 bpm. The Purkinje network also can generate an impulse but it does so at less than 40 bpm, which could prevent cessation of heart function for a short time (Table 36-1).

Cardiac Innervation

Sympathetic and parasympathetic fibers of the autonomic nervous system innervate the heart. Sympathetic fibers are distributed throughout the heart. Sympathetic stimulation results in increased heart rate, increased speed of conduction through the AV node, and more forceful contractions. Parasympathetic fibers, which are part of the vagus nerve, are found primarily in the SA and AV nodes and the atrial tissue. Parasympathetic stimulation results in slowing of the heart rate, slowing of conduction through the AV node, and decreased strength of contraction.

CARDIAC FUNCTION

The primary function of the heart is to pump blood through the pulmonary and systemic circulations. This is accomplished by a continually repeating pattern of contraction and relaxation.

Cardiac Cycle

Contraction and relaxation of the heart make up one heartbeat and are called the *cardiac cycle.* When the ventricles are at rest (relaxation phase), they are filling up with blood coming from the atria. This is called **diastole**. At the end of diastole, the atria contract to eject more blood into the ventricles (called the *atrial kick*). Once the ventricles have filled with blood and the electrical impulse has reached the terminal fibers of the conduction system, the ventricles contract and eject blood into the pulmonary artery from the RV and into the aorta from the LV. This is called *systole.* A person with a heart rate of 60 bpm would have 60 cardiac cycles per minute.

Table 36-1 Intrinsic Heart Rates

INITIATION OF IMPULSE	RATE
Sinoatrial (SA) node	60–100 beats per minute (bpm)
Atrioventricular (AV) node	40–60 bpm
Ventricle	15–40 bpm

Cardiac Output

The volume of blood ejected by the heart each minute is determined by the stroke volume and the heart rate. Stroke volume is the amount of blood ejected with each ventricular contraction. The normal stroke volume is 60 to 100 mL. Cardiac output (CO) is the amount of blood (in liters) ejected by the heart per minute. It is calculated by multiplying the heart rate (HR) by the stroke volume (SV):

$$CO = HR \times SV$$

The normal cardiac output is 4 to 8 L/min. In the normal heart, cardiac output responds to the increased demands for O_2 and nutrients that occur with exercise, infection, or stress.

Three factors affect stroke volume: (1) preload, (2) contractility, and (3) afterload.

Preload. **Preload** is the amount of blood remaining in a ventricle at the end of diastole or the pressure generated at the end of diastole. Increased preload results in increased stroke volume and thus increased cardiac output. Factors that increase preload include increased venous return to the heart and overhydration. Factors that decrease preload include dehydration, hemorrhage, and venous vasodilation.

Contractility. **Contractility** is the ability of cardiac muscle fibers to shorten and produce a muscle contraction. *Inotropy* is a term used to refer to the contractile state of the cell. Factors that increase contractility are said to have a positive inotropic effect and factors that decrease contractility create a negative inotropic effect.

Afterload. **Afterload** is the amount of pressure the ventricles must overcome to eject the blood volume. It is determined primarily by the pressure in the arterial system. Afterload is decreased by vasodilation and increased by vasoconstriction.

Myocardial Oxygen Consumption

Myocardial tissue routinely needs 70% to 75% of the O_2 delivered to it by the coronary arteries. Skeletal muscles, by contrast, need 35% at rest and up to 75% during exercise. The only ways to increase O_2 supply to the myocardium are to (1) increase the coronary blood flow by coronary artery vasodilation or (2) increase the O_2 in the blood by administering supplemental O_2.

AGE-RELATED CHANGES

It is difficult to separate the normal age-related changes in the heart and blood vessels from the changes caused by disease. In general, age-related changes progress slowly whereas pathogenic changes are more likely to be sudden.

HEART

Changes in the heart muscle include increased density of connective tissue and decreased elasticity. Cardiac contractility may decline, making the heart less able to adapt to changes in circulating blood volume. The valves may thicken and stiffen. If they do not close properly, the patient may have a murmur. The valves may also partially block the path of blood flow, causing incomplete emptying of the chambers.

The number of pacemaker cells in the SA node decreases, as does the number of nerve fibers in the ventricles. The aging heart takes longer to respond to stress and then responds less dramatically. It also takes longer to return to normal after exercise or stress. Cardiac dysrhythmias are more common in older people but should still be evaluated because they can be dangerous.

BLOOD VESSELS

Changes in connective tissue and elastic fibers in arteries cause them to become stiffer. Physical activity can help to reverse or delay this process (see *Health Promotion* box). Pulse pressure (the difference between the systolic and diastolic pressures) and systolic blood pressure generally increase. Hypertension should not be considered a normal response to the aging process and should be treated. The veins stretch and dilate, leading to venous stasis and sometimes impaired venous return. Thrombophlebitis and varicosities are more common in older people.

Health Promotion

Long-Term Conditioning

Long-term conditioning with an exercise program may help to decrease arterial stiffening and improve the function of the left ventricle (LV) in older individuals. Physical exercise does not have to be strenuous to be helpful. Activity should become a part of an individual's regular routine.

The cardiovascular system adapts more slowly to changes in position; therefore postural hypotension may occur.

NURSING ASSESSMENT OF CARDIAC FUNCTION

HEALTH HISTORY

A complete assessment is important for the cardiac patient. However, if the patient is having acute symptoms, a detailed assessment must be deferred until the patient is stable.

Chief Complaint and History of Present Illness

Determine the patient's reason for seeking medical care. Common symptoms that may be related to cardiac disorders include fatigue, edema, **palpitations**, dyspnea, and pain. It is important to note when symptoms occur, what aggravates them, and what relieves them.

Medical History

Ask whether the patient has had specific conditions that may be related to cardiac disease. These include hypertension, kidney disease, pulmonary disease, diabetes mellitus, stroke, rheumatic fever, streptococcal sore throat, anemia, smoking, and alcoholism. Note previous cardiac disorders and hospitalizations and list recent and current medications, recording any allergies in the appropriate records. It is also important to ask whether the patient is taking any vitamins, herbs, or homeopathic remedies. It may be easier to ask something such as "What are you doing to stay healthy or to help you feel better?"

Family History

Because cardiovascular problems are often familial or hereditary, ask whether immediate relatives have had hypertension, coronary heart disease (CHD), other cardiac disorders, or diabetes mellitus.

Review of Systems

Inquire whether the patient has experienced the following specific symptoms: weight gain, fatigue, dyspnea (shortness of breath), cough, orthopnea (difficulty breathing in a supine position), paroxysmal nocturnal dyspnea (sudden dyspnea during sleep), palpitations, chest pain, **syncope** (fainting), concentrated urine, or leg edema.

If the patient has had dyspnea or orthopnea, it is important to determine when it occurred and whether the onset was gradual or sudden. Pain also requires detailed descriptions. The pain of heart problems may radiate or be referred to other areas. The pain may radiate down either arm, to the jaw, or to just below the sternum. The severity may range from mild, intermittent discomfort to severe, crushing chest pain. Ask the patient to rate the severity of the pain on a scale of 1 (mildest) to 10 (worst possible). Chest pain may be experienced differently in women, patients with diabetes, and the elderly and may be described as *indigestion, a feeling of anxiety, nausea,* or *a feeling of fatigue.* Document the exact description, location, and severity of the pain, as well as whether the pain is radiating, what events cause it, and what relieves the pain.

Functional Assessment

Determine how this illness has affected the patient's ability to carry out usual activities. Describe activity, rest patterns, and usual diet. It is especially important to record salt and fat intake. Ask the patient about sources of stress and coping strategies.

PHYSICAL EXAMINATION

Begin the physical examination with measurement of height and weight and recording of vital signs.

Vital Signs

Blood Pressure. The correct size of blood pressure cuff must be used. Position the patient's arm at the heart level and check the blood pressure in both arms. It is important to note the pulse pressure (difference between the systolic and diastolic pressures) because this is a noninvasive measure of cardiac output. Next, measure blood pressures and pulse rates in the lying, sitting, and standing positions. A blood pressure decrease of 20 mm Hg or more with a position change indicates decreased blood volume or an autonomic response. As blood pressure decreases, the pulse should increase as a compensatory mechanism.

Pulses. Palpate the radial pulses for rate, rhythm, quality, and equality and auscultate the apical pulse for rate and rhythm. Apical and radial pulses may be taken simultaneously to detect a pulse deficit. The normal heart rate is 60 to 100 bpm. A rate of less than 60 bpm is considered to be **bradycardia**; **tachycardia** is characterized by a heart rate in excess of 100 bpm. The rhythm is described as *regular, irregular*, or *regularly irregular*. The quality of a palpated pulse is graded on a 4-point scale: *0,* absent pulse (not palpable); *1,* weak or thready pulse (pulse easily obliterated by slight finger pressure, returning as pressure is released); *2,* normal pulse (easily palpable); and *3,* bounding pulse (forceful, not easily obliterated by finger pressure). With a stethoscope, listen at the fifth intercostal space at the midclavicular line to assess the apical pulse. In addition to the radial pulse, assess the carotid, brachial, femoral, popliteal, posterior tibial, and dorsalis pedis pulses at appropriate times during the physical examination.

Respirations. Observe the patient's respiratory effort and skin color; count the respiratory rate; and auscultate the breath sounds for crackles, rhonchi, and wheezes. If the patient produces sputum, describe the color, amount, and appearance.

Skin

Inspect the skin for color, hair distribution, and capillary refill and palpate for temperature. Skin color and temperature should be relatively the same over the entire body.

Heart Sounds

The heart sounds are systole (*lub*) and diastole (*dub*). To auscultate heart sounds, place the diaphragm of the stethoscope firmly on the bare anterior chest (not through clothing). Figure 36-5 shows where the heart sounds, made by closing of the valves, may be heard best. With practice, you can learn to distinguish these. The following pattern of auscultation is recommended:

1. Listen to the aortic area first and then to the pulmonic. As the aortic and pulmonic valves close, the *dub* should be louder than the *lub* in the aortic and pulmonic areas.
2. Listen to the tricuspid and mitral valves in the areas indicated. In these areas the *lub* should be louder than the *dub.*
3. After listening to each area with the diaphragm, repeat the pattern with the bell of the

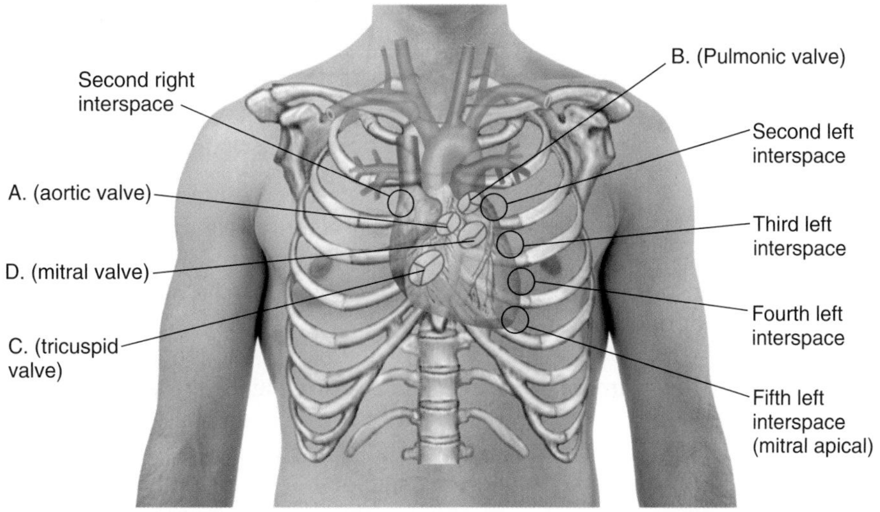

FIGURE 36-5 Auscultation of the heart. **A,** Aortic valve at the second intercostal space to the right of the sternum. **B,** Pulmonic valve at the second intercostal space to the left of the sternum. **C,** Tricuspid valve at the fifth intercostal space to the left of the sternum. **D,** Mitral valve at the fifth intercostal space in the midclavicular line. (From Seidel HM, Ball JW, Dains JE, et al: *Mosby's guide to physical examination*, ed 7, St. Louis, Mosby, 2011.)

Table 36-2 Grading of Heart Murmurs

GRADE	DESCRIPTION
I	Very faint
II	Faint but recognizable
III	Loud but moderate in intensity
IV	Loud and accompanied by a palpable thrill
V	Very loud, accompanied by a palpable thrill, and audible with the stethoscope partially off the client's chest
VI	Extremely loud; may be heard with the stethoscope slightly above the client's chest

From Ignatavicius DD, Workman ML: *Medical-surgical nursing: patient-centered collaborative care*, ed 7, Philadelphia, 2013, Saunders.

stethoscope. Note additional sounds of S_3 and S_4. The S_3 and S_4 sounds are heard best with the bell of the stethoscope placed at the apex when the patient is positioned on the left side. S_3, also called a *ventricular gallop*, occurs early in diastole. S_3 is normal in children and young adults and may be pathologic after age 30. S_4, also called an *atrial gallop*, occurs late in diastole. S_4 is an abnormal heart sound.

Heart Murmurs. A heart **murmur** is the sound produced by turbulent blood flow across the valves. Murmurs are recorded as having high, low, or medium pitch and they are located using the anatomic landmarks where they are heard best. The timing of a murmur relates to when it is heard in the cardiac cycle: systole or diastole. Murmurs are graded according to intensity or loudness (Table 36-2).

A *rub* is heard when the pericardium is inflamed. A scratchy or muffled sound may be heard best by having the patient sit upright and lean forward. This position brings the pericardium closer to the chest wall. A pericardial friction rub is best heard along the left sternal border throughout the cardiac cycle. It may help to ask patients to hold their breath briefly. If a rub is heard during this brief time, it is a pericardial rub rather than a pleural rub.

Extremities

Inspect and palpate the extremities for color, edema, warmth, temperature, pulse quality, and hair distribution.

Assessment of the cardiac patient is summarized in Box 36-1.

DIAGNOSTIC TESTS AND PROCEDURES

A number of tests or procedures may be used to assess cardiac structure and function. More common tests are described here. Patient preparation and postprocedure care are detailed in Table 36-3.

Box 36-1 Assessment of Patients with Cardiac Disorders

HEALTH HISTORY

Present Illness

Fatigue, edema, palpitations, pain; aggravating and relieving factors

Past Medical History

Hypertension, kidney disease, pulmonary disease, diabetes mellitus, stroke, rheumatic fever, streptococcal sore throat, scarlet fever, previous cardiac diseases or conditions, previous hospitalizations, recent and current medications, allergies

Family History

Hypertension, coronary heart disease (CHD) or other cardiac conditions, diabetes mellitus

Review of Systems

Weight gain, fatigue, dyspnea, cough, orthopnea, palpitations, chest pain, fainting, concentrated urine, leg edema

Functional Assessment

Effects of illness on usual activities, activity and rest pattern, lifestyle, diet, sodium and fat intake, sources of stress, coping strategies

PHYSICAL EXAMINATION

General Survey

Apparent distress

Height and Weight

Vital Signs

Blood pressure in both arms and while supine, sitting, standing; apical heart rate and rhythm; peripheral pulses: rate, rhythm, quality, equality; respiratory effort and rate

Skin

Color, hair distribution, capillary refill, temperature

Thorax

Heart sounds, heart murmurs, rubs; breath sounds, crackles, wheezes; presence and appearance of sputum

Extremities

Pulses, color, warmth, edema, hair distribution

ELECTROCARDIOGRAM

The electrocardiogram (ECG) allows study of the electrical activity (conduction system) through the heart muscle. An electrical impulse causes contractions as it passes through the heart muscle. Electrodes placed on the surface of the skin pick up the electrical impulses of the heart. The standard ECG records the electrical activity using 12 leads. Interpreting the 12-lead ECG allows detection of conduction disturbances, ischemia and infarction, electrolyte imbalances, and structural changes.

The ECG is graphed on standardized paper or viewed on an oscilloscope. Each cardiac cycle is represented by a series of P, Q, R, S, and T waves. The activity represented by each wave is explained in the section titled "Interpretation of Electrocardiograms." The ECG is interpreted to detect abnormalities in rate, rhythm,

Table 36-3 Diagnostic Tests and Procedures **Heart**

TEST	PURPOSE AND PROCEDURE	PATIENT PREPARATION	POSTPROCEDURE NURSING CARE
Electrocardiogram (ECG)	Electrodes are placed on the skin to detect electrical activity of the heart. Detects abnormalities in conduction of impulses, including changes caused by heart damage.	Tell the patient what to expect and that the procedure is painless. No special preparation is needed.	Remove the gel and electrode pads from the patient's skin. No special care is needed.
Holter monitor	Provides continuous ECG monitoring for 24–48 hours. Detects occasional dysrhythmias that may be correlated with specific activities noted in the patient's diary.	Tell the patient to wear loose clothing, take only a sponge bath, avoid magnets and metal detectors, and monitor placement of electrodes. Emphasize keeping an accurate diary of activities and to push "event button" if symptoms occur.	Return at the scheduled time. ECG recording will be retrieved for inspection.
Implantable loop recorder (ILR)	Provides ECG monitoring for longer periods and saves the information on a memory loop for analysis. Detects dysrhythmias causing syncopal episodes.	Tell the patient, family member, or significant other to activate the recorder when symptoms occur and to keep a written record of events.	Return at the scheduled time. ECG recording will be retrieved for inspection.
Echocardiogram	Uses ultrasound to create images of the heart. Gel is placed on the patient's skin and a transducer is moved over the area. Detects valve abnormalities, left ventricular hypertrophy, and hypertrophic cardiomyopathy (CMP).	Tell the patient what to expect and that the procedure is painless. No special preparation is needed.	Remove the gel from the patient's skin. No special care is needed.
Transesophageal echocardiogram (TEE)	Used when a conventional echocardiogram is not diagnostic. Probe is inserted through the esophagus into stomach (behind the heart). Has the same purpose as an echocardiogram.	Tell the patient what to expect: throat will be anesthetized, may have intravenous (IV) line installed. Signed consent is needed.	Monitor the patient's vital signs and gag reflex; if sedated, monitor the level of consciousness.
Stress test (exercise tolerance test [ETT])	Assesses the presence and severity of coronary heart disease (CHD) by having the patient exercise during ECG monitoring. Blood pressure is monitored. The test is stopped if symptoms of CHD occur.	Tell the patient what to expect. Nothing by mouth (NPO) for 2 hours before the test. Have the patient wear loose clothing and comfortable shoes. Give a beta-blocker if prescribed. Signed consent is needed.	No special care is needed.
Magnetic resonance imaging (MRI)	Creates images of body structures without radiation. The patient lies on a firm pad that rolls into a circular device. "Open MRI" is better tolerated by claustrophobic patients because the machine does not surround the patient. Clanging sounds are heard as the machine works.	Tell the patient what to expect. All metal must be removed. Sedation may be ordered if the patient is very anxious or unable to be still.	No special care is needed. Safety precautions should be taken if a sedative has been given.

Continued

Table 36-3 Diagnostic Tests and Procedures Heart—cont'd

TEST	PURPOSE AND PROCEDURE	PATIENT PREPARATION	POSTPROCEDURE NURSING CARE
Multiple-gated acquisition (MUGA) scanning	Radioactive material is injected intravenously and the heart is scanned to evaluate function. May be done at rest or during exercise.	Tell the patient what to expect. NPO for 2 hours before the procedure. Start IV infusion as ordered. Signed consent is needed.	No special care is needed.
Myocardial perfusion imaging • Positron emission tomography (PET) scan • Single photon emission computed tomography (SPECT)	Radioisotope(s) administered by IV route to assess perfusion of the heart. May be done with stress/exercise.	Tell the patient that one or two IVs may be inserted and that he or she may be asked to use an exercise bike or treadmill during scanning. The patient may be NPO for 4–6 hours before the test and should abstain from caffeine, alcohol, and tobacco for 24 hours before the test.	Encourage the patient to change positions slowly to avoid postural hypotension and to drink fluids, if not contraindicated, to help with excretion of the radioisotopes.
Ultrafast computed tomography (CT); also known as *electron beam tomography (EBT)*,	Imaging technology that provides images used to assess myocardial perfusion and right and left ventricular muscle mass and function, and to measure calcium deposits in the coronary circulation.	Tell the patient what to expect (e.g., lie on the table, hold very still, you may be asked to hold breath for a few seconds at a time). No special preparation is needed.	No special care is needed.
Cardiac catheterization	A catheter is passed through a vein or artery and dye is injected. Radiographs are taken to visualize heart structures and blood vessels. The procedure is done in a special room. Blood pressure, pulse, and ECG are monitored throughout test.	Tell the patient what to expect. Assess for allergies to seafood or iodine and inform the radiologist if they are present. NPO for specified time before procedure. Tell the patient to expect a flushing sensation when the dye is injected. Give a sedative if ordered. Signed consent is needed.	Check the puncture site; maintain pressure per protocol if a vascular sealing device is not used. Monitor vital signs and peripheral pulses on the affected extremity. Enforce bed rest as ordered.
Electrophysiology study (EPS)	A catheter with multiple electrodes is passed into the right side of the heart through the femoral vein. The electrodes record electrical activity of the conduction system and may be used to stimulate the patient's dysrhythmia.	Tell the patient what to expect. NPO for 6 hours before the procedure. Premedicate the patient with prescribed sedatives. Signed consent is needed.	Similar to cardiac catheterization (described above).
Arterial blood gases (ABGs)	Assesses acid-base balance by measuring pH, partial pressure of carbon dioxide in arterial blood ($PaCO_2$), partial pressure of oxygen in arterial blood (PaO_2), bicarbonate (HCO_3^-), and base excess.	Tell the patient about arterial puncture. Prepare a heparinized syringe and obtain a blood sample.	Remove air bubbles from the sample. Place the tube on ice and send it out for immediate analysis. Apply pressure to the puncture site for 5 minutes. Report any results.
Troponin	Measures protein released after myocardial injury: cardiac troponin T (cTnT) and cardiac troponin I (cTnI).	Tell the patient a blood sample will be drawn. No special preparation is needed.	Check the venipuncture site. Apply pressure if it is oozing.

Table 36-3 Diagnostic Tests and Procedures Heart—cont'd

TEST	PURPOSE AND PROCEDURE	PATIENT PREPARATION	POSTPROCEDURE NURSING CARE
Cardiac enzymes (creatine kinase [CK], creatine kinase-MB fraction [CK-MB], lactate dehydrogenase [LDH])	Measures enzymes that rise in a predictable pattern with myocardial damage.	Tell the patient a blood sample will be drawn. No special preparation is needed. To detect acute myocardial infarction (MI), draw a specimen before other invasive procedures.	Check the venipuncture site. Apply pressure if it is oozing.
Myoglobin	Measures myoglobin levels in the blood. Rises soon after myocardial injury. Also elevated by strenuous exercise, renal failure, and some other conditions.	Tell the patient a blood sample will be drawn. No special preparation is needed.	Check the venipuncture site. Apply pressure if it is oozing.
Complete blood count (CBC)	Counts white blood cells (WBCs) and red blood cells (RBCs), hemoglobin (Hgb) and hematocrit (Hct), RBC indices, and sometimes platelets. (Normal values are listed in Table 36-6.)	Tell the patient a blood sample will be drawn. No special preparation is needed.	Check the venipuncture site. Apply pressure if it is oozing.
Lipid profile	Measures common serum lipids (cholesterol, triglycerides, lipoproteins). Used to evaluate risk of CHD.	Tell the patient to expect venipuncture. NPO for 12 hours before the sample is drawn. Remind patient to eat usual diet for 2 weeks before the test.	Check the venipuncture site. Apply pressure if it is oozing.
B-type natriuretic peptide (BNP)	Measures naturally occurring BNP levels that are elevated in heart failure (HF) and CMP. Helps to differentiate dyspnea related to cardiac problems from noncardiac-related dyspnea.	Tell the patient a blood sample will be drawn. No special preparation is needed.	Check the venipuncture site. Apply pressure if it is oozing.
C-reactive protein (CRP)	Acute phase protein that is elevated in system inflammation. Elevated levels seen with acute coronary syndrome (ACS).	Tell the patient a blood sample will be drawn. No special preparation is needed.	Check the venipuncture site. Apply pressure if it is oozing.

or impulse conduction. The normal finding is called a *normal sinus rhythm*, which is characterized by the following:

1. A rate of 60 to 100 bpm
2. A regular rhythm
3. A P wave preceding each QRS complex
4. A PR interval that is within 0.12 to 0.20 seconds
5. A QRS complex that is less than 0.12 seconds

AMBULATORY ELECTROCARDIOGRAM (HOLTER MONITOR)

An ambulatory ECG uses a portable ECG machine with a memory to provide continuous cardiac monitoring for 24 to 48 hours. A complete record of the heart rhythm is stored and analyzed later. This type of monitoring is used to detect dysrhythmias that occur infrequently, to determine if symptoms correlate with any underlying cardiac disease, to assess the effects of medications, and for research purposes. The patient records in a diary all activity that occurs during the monitoring, such as walking, stair climbing, sleeping, and engaging in sexual activity. The monitor strip is computer scanned and then interpreted by a physician.

Even more sophisticated monitoring is accomplished by transtelephonic means. An audio signal is sent over telephone lines to a station operated by personnel trained to recognize potentially dangerous dysrhythmias.

IMPLANTABLE LOOP RECORDER

For longer monitoring periods, to record a patient's ECG during syncopal episodes, an implantable loop recorder (ILR) may be used. This device, implanted just under the patient's skin in the chest area, continually monitors the ECG activity of the patient in a memory loop. The patient, family member, or significant other is taught to activate the recorder when symptoms are felt. The ECG can then be analyzed and appropriate treatment implemented.

ECHOCARDIOGRAM (HEART SONOGRAM)

The echocardiogram visualizes and records the size, shape, position, and behavior of the heart's internal structures, especially wall motion and valve function. Ultrasonic waves are beamed into the heart and their echoes are recorded. This painless test may be performed at the bedside or in a laboratory. Gel is applied to the skin and a special device called a *transducer* is moved over the precordium. The transducer picks up sound waves and converts them to electrical impulses that are recorded as waveforms on an oscilloscope, a videotape, or a strip chart. Common echocardiogram types include motion mode (M-mode) and two-dimensional mode (2D mode). Echocardiograms can also be enhanced using Doppler technology (Doppler echocardiogram) and color-flow imaging.

TRANSESOPHAGEAL ECHOCARDIOGRAM

At times the echocardiogram is not diagnostic and a transesophageal echocardiogram (TEE) is used. A flexible endoscopic probe with an ultrasound transducer is passed down the back of the throat into the esophagus. A local anesthetic to the throat decreases the gag reflex. Occasionally, an intravenous (IV) sedative is needed to reduce patient anxiety. Images are obtained from behind the heart as the probe moves down into the stomach. The probe is down for approximately 15 to 20 minutes. The TEE provides information that is useful in the evaluation of ventricular wall motion and function and possible heart valve disorders.

STRESS TEST (EXERCISE TOLERANCE TEST)

The stress test is a noninvasive method of assessing the presence and severity of CHD by recording a person's cardiovascular response to exercise. It is also used to measure functional capacity for work, sport, or participation in a rehabilitation program. The stress test is not flawless and false-positive and false-negative results are common. A negative test result does not absolutely exclude CHD. However, the stress test is the best noninvasive screening procedure available. The alternative is the much more invasive cardiac catheterization.

For the stress test, a continuous ECG is monitored while the patient uses a treadmill or a stationary bicycle. Every 2 to 3 minutes the speed and incline angle of the treadmill are increased (or pedal resistance is increased with a bicycle) until (1) the patient cannot continue for whatever reason, (2) the patient's maximum heart rate is achieved (220 – patient's age = maximum heart rate), (3) symptoms intervene, or (4) significant changes are detected on the ECG. The target heart rate is 85% of the predicted maximum heart rate for the patient's age and sex. When patients are unable to exercise, a pharmacologic stress test can be performed using medications that dilate the coronary arteries (Dobutamine, Adenoscan, etc.).

Significant CHD limits blood flow to the myocardium. The increased demands of exercise may cause the patient to have symptoms of CHD, which are angina, dizziness, dyspnea, dysrhythmias, a falling blood pressure, and certain ECG findings. If these symptoms occur, the test must be stopped immediately.

Contraindications for the test include acute systemic illness, severe aortic stenosis, uncontrolled congestive heart failure (CHF), severe hypertension, angina at rest, and significant dysrhythmia. Although the mortality rate for test participants is very low, cardiopulmonary resuscitation (CPR) equipment must be available.

MAGNETIC RESONANCE IMAGING

A magnetic resonance imaging (MRI) scan provides high-resolution, three-dimensional images of body structures. Cardiac tissue is imaged without lung or bone interference. The patient is enclosed in a chamber for approximately 30 to 90 minutes for an MRI scan of the heart. No loose metallic objects are permitted in the chamber during the procedure. Patients with intracranial aneurysm clips, intraocular metal foreign bodies, and some middle ear prostheses should not have MRI scans because the devices may be affected by the magnetic field or may interfere with the MRI. Other implanted devices that contraindicate MRI include pacemakers, automatic implantable cardioverter defibrillators (AICDs), and implanted infusion pumps. For patients who are claustrophobic, an open MRI may be available.

MULTIPLE-GATED ACQUISITION SCAN

In a multiple-gated acquisition (MUGA) scan, the patient is injected with a radioactive tracer. The heart is then scanned to assess left ventricular structure and function, to evaluate myocardial wall motion, to assess valvular disease, and to identify location and size of a myocardial infarction (MI). Assessment of ventricular function can be done while the patient is resting or exercising. Sublingual nitroglycerin may be administered to assess its effect on ventricular function.

MYOCARDIAL PERFUSION IMAGING

Myocardial perfusion imaging (MPI) is a noninvasive study that shows how well blood is perfusing the heart. Areas that are not receiving enough blood flow will be evident. There are two types of MPI: the positron emission tomography (PET) scan or the single photon emission computed tomography (SPECT). Both of these scans are noninvasive and use a radioactive tracer and a gamma camera to assess the coronary arteries and how well blood is flowing to the cardiac muscle. The scans will show healthy and damaged cardiac muscle. Both scans are often used in conjunction with stress testing (exercise or drug induced) (American Heart Association-Myocardial Perfusion Imaging, 2012).

ULTRAFAST COMPUTED TOMOGRAPHY

Ultrafast computed tomography (CT), also known as *electron beam tomography (EBT)*, is a fast form of imaging technology that allows for high-quality images that are not affected by the movement of the heart as it contracts and relaxes. The images obtained are used to assess myocardial perfusion, along with right and left ventricular muscle mass and function. In addition, ultrafast CT can measure calcium deposits in the coronary arteries and a coronary calcium score can be derived. The greater the amount of coronary calcium is, the higher is the score and hence the risk of coronary occlusive disease.

CARDIAC CATHETERIZATION (CARDIAC ANGIOGRAPHY, CORONARY ARTERIOGRAPHY)

Cardiac catheterization is a procedure in which a catheter is inserted into a vein or artery and is threaded into the heart chambers, coronary arteries, or both under fluoroscopy (Fig. 36-6). A contrast dye is injected through the catheter and films are made of the visualized heart structures. Vital signs and ECG are monitored during the procedure.

In a catheterization of the right side of the heart, the catheter is inserted into a vein and threaded into the vena cava, RA, RV, and pulmonary artery. Pressures in the RA, RV, and pulmonary artery may be determined. The function of the pulmonic and tricuspid valves may be assessed.

In a catheterization of the left side of the heart, the catheter is inserted into an artery and threaded against the flow of blood into the coronary arteries or the LV. The function of the coronary arteries and the aortic and mitral valves may be assessed. Blood samples may be drawn and pressures in the various structures are

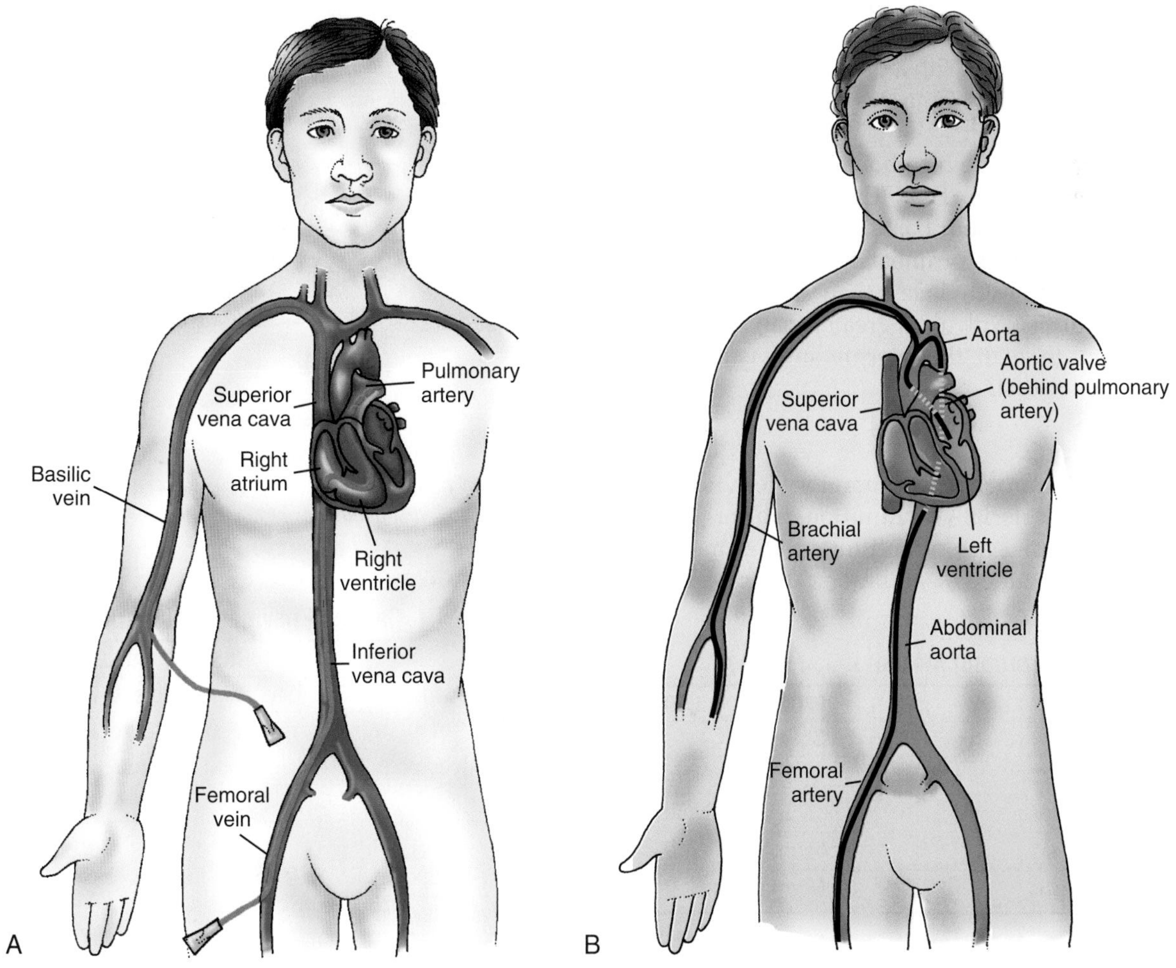

FIGURE 36-6 Right-sided (**A**) and left-sided (**B**) heart catheterization.

measured. The femoral vein and artery are the preferred insertion sites for cardiac catheterization.

Complications of cardiac catheterization include bleeding, hematoma formation, infection, and embolus or thrombus formation. Nursing care before and after the procedure is very important.

ELECTROPHYSIOLOGY STUDY

The electrophysiology study (EPS) is used to record the heart's electrical activity from within the heart using catheters with multiple electrodes inserted through the femoral vein into the right side of the heart. The electrodes record the electrical activity of the heart's conduction system. In addition, the electrodes can be used to stimulate dysrhythmias that will help to locate the source of the patient's dysrhythmia.

LABORATORY TESTS

Arterial Blood Gases

Arterial blood gases (ABGs) are analyzed to determine the body's ability to maintain the acid-base balance. Acidity or alkalinity is determined by pH. If the serum pH is less than 7.35, the blood is acidic; pH greater than 7.45 indicates alkalinity. Carbonic acid dissociates into CO_2 and water. The lungs regulate CO_2. A partial pressure of carbon dioxide in arterial blood ($PaCO_2$) greater than 45 with an acidic pH is a respiratory acidosis and indicates that the body is unable to excrete the excess CO_2 through the lungs. With a pH in excess of 7.45 and a $PaCO_2$ of less than 35, a respiratory alkalosis is present.

The kidneys regulate bicarbonate (HCO_3-) through excretion and retention. The HCO_3- (or base excess, a combination of all serum bases) is assessed to determine metabolic causes of imbalance. If the pH is less than 7.35 and the HCO_3- is less than 22, the body is in metabolic acidosis. With a pH greater than 7.45 and an HCO_3- greater than 26, the interpretation is metabolic alkalosis (Table 36-4).

Pulse Oximetry

Pulse oximetry, though not a laboratory test, noninvasively measures arterial O_2 saturation. Light is passed through a pulsating artery and interpreted mechanically to determine the O_2 saturation. The transdermal clip or patch may be applied to a digit (finger or toe), the ear, or the nose (Fig. 36-7).

Table 36-4 Interpreting Arterial Blood Gases

CONDITION	pH	$PACO_2$	HCO_3-
Normal range	7.35–7.45	35–45	22–26
Respiratory acidosis	↓	↑	Normal
Respiratory alkalosis	↑	↓	Normal
Metabolic acidosis	↓	Normal	↓
Metabolic alkalosis	↑	Normal	↑

↑, Elevated; ↓, decreased; HCO_3-, bicarbonate; $PaCO_2$, partial pressure of carbon dioxide in arterial blood. If the arrows are in the same direction, a metabolic problem exists. If arrows are in opposite directions, a respiratory problem exists.

Cardiac Markers

Cardiac markers are released when heart cells die as a result of damage. These markers (enzymes and other proteins) are measured in the serum and their values rise as indicators of damage to the heart cells. Table 36-5 lists normal cardiac marker levels.

Troponin. Troponin is a protein involved in the contraction of muscles. Two subtypes, cardiac troponin T (cTnT) and cardiac troponin I (cTnI), are specific to cardiac muscle and are released into the circulation after an MI. Troponin levels, generally not detectable in healthy individuals, will elevate significantly after an MI. Troponin levels rise in 3 to 6 hours from onset of symptoms, peak in 12 hours, and remain in the circulation for up to 10 to 14 days. This test is done in the emergency department because the results are available more quickly than the cardiac enzymes.

Creatine Kinase. The creatine kinase (CK) enzyme is found in high concentration in three tissues: (1) the brain, (2) the heart, and (3) the skeletal muscle. The type of CK specific to heart tissue is creatine kinase-MB fraction (CK-MB). Elevation of the CK-MB level

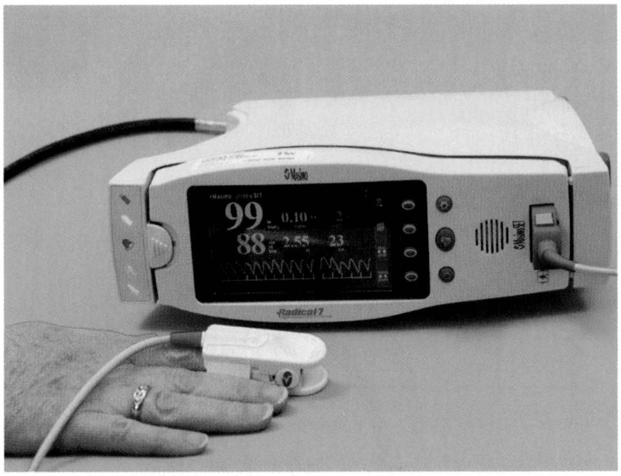

FIGURE 36-7 Pulse oximeter. (From Potter PA, Perry AG, Stockert P, Hall A, editors: *Fundamentals of nursing*, ed 8, St. Louis, 2013, Mosby-Elsevier.)

Table 36-5 Cardiac Enzymes and Markers

TEST*	NORMAL VALUES
Creatine kinase (CK)	Male subject: 55–170 U/L
	Female subject: 30–135 U/L
CK isoenzymes	MM fraction: 100%
	MB fraction: 0%
	BB fraction: 0%
Cardiac troponin T (cTnT)	<0.1 ng/mL
Cardiac troponin I (cTnI)	<0.03 ng/mL
Myoglobin	<90 mcg/mL

*Values may vary according to the laboratory equipment used.

indicates damage to the myocardial cells. The CK-MB level can be expected to rise 4 to 6 hours after an MI, peak in 18 to 24 hours at more than six times the normal value, and return to normal within 2 to 3 days if no new damage occurs. Serial trends should be observed. Musculoskeletal injuries (especially fractures and surgery) and recent excessive athletic activity can also elevate the total CK level.

Myoglobin. Myoglobin is another protein found in cardiac and skeletal muscle that is released into the circulation very quickly after an MI. Myoglobin levels increase in 1 to 4 hours after symptoms. Because it is also found in skeletal muscle, myoglobin levels may be elevated by such things as strenuous exercise, renal failure, and neuromuscular diseases. This makes interpreting myoglobin levels difficult in some circumstances.

Complete Blood Count

The complete blood count (CBC) is a basic screening test. Included in this test are the white blood cell (WBC) count, the red blood cell (RBC) count, the hemoglobin (Hgb) and hematocrit (Hct) measurements, the RBC indices, and (in some laboratories) the platelet count. Components of the CBC are presented in Table 36-6.

White Blood Cell Count. The WBC count indicates the body's ability to defend itself against infection and inflammation. The WBC level usually is elevated with inflammatory processes such as MI and bacterial infections but it may be below normal with viral infections and bone marrow depression.

Table 36-6 Complete Blood Count

TEST*	NORMAL VALUES
White blood cells (WBCs)	5000–10,000/mm^3
Differential	
Neutrophils	60.0%–70.0%
Eosinophils	1.0%–4.0%
Basophils	0.5%–1.0%
Lymphocytes	20.0%–40.0%
Monocytes	2.0%–6.0%
Red Blood Cells (RBCs)	
Male subject	4,200,000–5,400,000/mm^3
Female subject	3,600,000–5,000,000/mm^3
Hematocrit (Hct)	
Male subject	40.0%–54.0%
Female subject	37.0%–47.0%
Hemoglobin (Hgb)	
Male subject	13.5–17.5 g/dL
Female subject	12.0–16.0 g/dL
Platelets	150,000–350,000/mm^3

*Values may vary according to the laboratory equipment used.

Red Blood Cell Count. The RBC count is assessed to determine the ability of the blood to carry O_2 from the lungs to the tissues and CO_2 from the tissues to the lungs. The RBC level may be below normal with anemias and malignancies and may be elevated in dehydration.

Hematocrit. The hematocrit (Hct) is the percentage of packed red blood cells (PRBCs) in the total sample of whole blood. With severe dehydration, the plasma portion of the blood decreases and the Hct is elevated. In anemias and hemorrhage, the Hct is below normal. In general, the Hct is three times the Hgb measurement.

Hemoglobin. Hgb is the main component of the RBCs. Its function is to transport O_2 to the cells. The Hgb measurement may be below normal in anemias and hemorrhage. It is elevated in dehydration, chronic obstructive pulmonary disease (COPD), and CHF. An Hgb of less than 5 g/dL leads to heart failure (HF) and death if not corrected.

Platelet (Thrombocyte) Count. The platelets (thrombocytes) are the smallest of the formed elements in the blood. They are necessary for coagulation. The platelet count is below normal with anemias, bone marrow depression, and bleeding. The count may be increased in acute infections and some heart diseases. A count of less than 20,000 may result in spontaneous bleeding.

Lipid Profile

A lipid profile is a battery of tests that measure the most common serum lipids: cholesterol, triglycerides, and lipoproteins.

Cholesterol is a blood lipid produced by the liver. It is used to form bile salts for the digestion of fat and the production of adrenal, ovarian, and testicular hormones. The normal adult serum cholesterol level is less than 200 mg/dL. Elevated cholesterol levels (hypercholesterolemia) are associated with increased risk of CHD, hypertension, and MI. The cholesterol accumulates in the arterial lumen and in time results in decreased blood flow and occlusion.

Several forms of cholesterol are identified; however, the high-density lipoproteins (HDLs) and low-density lipoproteins (LDLs) are the two that most closely correlate with CHD. The HDLs are desirable because they promote the excretion of cholesterol; therefore higher levels of HDLs are encouraged. On the other hand, elevated LDL levels are associated with a higher risk of CHD; therefore lower LDL levels are encouraged. A good way to remember the difference is that HDLs are healthy and LDLs are lethal. Currently, the recommendations are for HDL levels greater than 40 mg/dL (for men) or greater than 50 mg/dL (for women) and for LDL levels less than 100 mg/dL (American Heart Association-What Your Cholesterol Means, 2013). See the *Health Promotion* box for advice on increasing HDL levels.

Health Promotion

Low High-Density Lipoprotein Levels

Low high-density lipoprotein (HDL) levels can be raised by being physically active at least 30 minutes every day, by not smoking, and by losing weight (or maintaining a healthy weight).

Triglycerides are a major contributor to CHD. They are produced in the liver. Triglyceride levels increase when LDL levels increase. The normal triglyceride level is less than 150 mg/dL.

B-Type Natriuretic Peptide

B-type natriuretic peptide (BNP) is a cardiac hormone released when ventricular dilation and stretch (such as occurs in HF) occur. Less than 100 pg/mL is considered a normal BNP level and elevated levels relate closely to the severity of HF (e.g., the higher the levels, the more severe the failure). In addition, BNP levels can be monitored to assess the effectiveness of treatment.

C-Reactive Protein

C-reactive protein (CRP) is an acute-phase protein and a marker for systemic inflammation. Elevated levels of CRP are present in patients with acute coronary syndrome (ACS). CRP can be used to predict an individual's risk for cardiovascular disease or events.

COMMON THERAPEUTIC MEASURES

DRUG THERAPY

Commonly used cardiac drugs are cardiac glycosides, antianginals, antidysrhythmics, and miscellaneous and emergency drugs. Examples of these drugs, their actions, and adverse effects, as well as associated nursing considerations, are provided in Table 36-7.

Cardiac Glycosides

The cardiac glycosides are also called *cardiotonics* or *digitalis glycosides*. Examples are digoxin (Lanoxin) and digitoxin. These drugs have several important pharmacologic actions on the heart. They slow the heart rate (negative chronotropic effect) and increase the force of myocardial contraction (positive inotropic effect), causing increased stroke volume and cardiac output. Cardiac glycosides are widely used in the treatment of HF. They are also used to treat some cardiac dysrhythmias.

When rapid effects are needed, a patient can be given a loading dose (called a *digitalizing dose*) of cardiac glycosides. Once therapeutic blood levels are obtained, a maintenance dose is prescribed to maintain the therapeutic effects. These drugs have high potential for toxicity and require close monitoring. Common practice is to count the apical pulse before giving each dose. If the rate is less than 60 bpm in adults, withhold the dose and contact the physician. Because patients are often on cardiac glycosides for long-term therapy, they must be taught to monitor their own pulse and to report symptoms of toxicity (anorexia, nausea, visual disturbances). Other specific nursing considerations are presented in Table 36-7.

Antianginals

Drugs used to treat angina (chest pain related to myocardial ischemia) include nitrates, beta-adrenergic blockers, and calcium channel blockers. Nitrates are used to treat actual anginal episodes and to prevent angina. Beta-adrenergic blockers and calcium channel blockers are used in the long-term management of angina. Examples of each classification and nursing considerations are presented in Table 36-7.

Antidysrhythmics

Drugs used to treat abnormal cardiac rhythms are called *antidysrhythmics* or *antiarrhythmics*. Four main classes of antidysrhythmics exist, each with various actions. In general, they work by slowing the rate of impulse conduction, depressing automaticity, or increasing resistance to premature stimulation. All antidysrhythmics have the potential to cause additional dysrhythmias. Specific drugs and nursing considerations are presented in Table 36-7.

Angiotensin-Converting Enzyme Inhibitors

Angiotensin-converting enzyme (ACE) inhibitors work against the renin-angiotensin-aldosterone (RAA) system to dilate arteries and decrease the resistance to blood flow in the arteries (reduced afterload). In addition, less fluid is retained because aldosterone release is blocked. ACE inhibitors are prescribed for patients with HF, in some cases of hypertension, and in some cases after myocardial infarction. Examples of these medications are captopril (Capoten), enalapril (Vasotec), and quinapril (Accupril). Information about these medications is presented in Chapter 38, Table 38-3. Some patients do not tolerate the ACE inhibitors. In these cases, angiotensin receptor blockers (ARBs) may be prescribed by the physician. Examples of ARBs are valsartan (Diovan), losartan (Cozaar), and telmisartan (Micardis).

Diuretics

Diuretics are often prescribed for cardiac conditions. Many patients with heart problems have fluid retention that is treated with diuretic drugs. The most frequently used diuretics are the loop diuretics such as furosemide (Lasix), the thiazide diuretics such as hydrochlorothiazide (Esidrix), and the potassium-sparing diuretics such as spironolactone (Aldactone). Information about these and other diuretics is presented in Chapter 42, Table 42-3.

Text continued on p. 702

Table 36-7 **Medications for Cardiovascular Disorders**

DRUG	USE AND ACTION	NURSING INTERVENTIONS
Cardiac Glycosides		
digoxin (Lanoxin)	Delays impulse conduction through the AV node to slow the heart rate (negative chronotropic effect). Increases strength or force of myocardial contraction (positive inotropic effect). Increases stroke volume and CO. Used for HF, atrial fibrillation and flutter, and paroxysmal atrial tachycardia.	Obtain baseline vital signs, ECG, and electrolytes before administering the first dose. Assess apical pulse for 1 minute; hold the drug and notify the physician if the patient's pulse is <60. Cannot be administered intramuscularly. Monitor potassium (K^+) levels because low potassium increases the risk of digitalis toxicity. Administer K^+ supplements as ordered. Decreased renal function may delay excretion and lead to toxicity. Toxic effects may be indicated by dysrhythmias, pulse <60 bpm, anorexia, nausea, syncope, visual disturbances, and abdominal pain. Therapeutic level: 0.8–2.0 ng/mL; toxic level: >2.0 ng/mL. Teach the patient the following: • Take your radial pulse for 1 minute at the same time each day.
Antianginal Agents		
nitroglycerin (available as sublingual tablets, ointment, transdermal patch, buccal tablets, mist, sustained-release oral tablets, and injectable [IV])	Acts as a vasodilator (arteries and veins). Relaxes all smooth muscles, especially vascular smooth muscle. Decreases preload, afterload, BP, CO, and systemic vascular resistance. Used to prevent and treat angina.	Assess the patient's BP and pulse before administration. Apply ointment in a uniform layer on the paper provided; apply to nonhairy skin (e.g., chest, back, upper arm); do not touch (causes headache); rotate sites. IV drug is delivered in glass containers with special tubing; use an infusion pump; monitor the patient closely. Teach the patient the following: • Sit or lie down at onset of chest pain. • Place the tablet under the tongue; the tablet causes tingling sensation if effective (older adults may not detect this). • Repeat every 5 minutes for a total of three doses; if chest pains are not relieved, have someone else drive to the emergency department. Note: Some sources advise to seek medical care if pain is not relieved by one tablet. • Keep the tablets in the containers in which they are supplied; the drug decomposes on exposure to light and air. • Headache decreases with tolerance. • Drug may be taken before activities likely to cause angina (e.g., exercise, sex).
isosorbide dinitrate (Isordil)	Acts as a vasodilator that works by relaxing smooth muscles. Decreases preload, afterload, left ventricular end-diastolic pressure, and myocardial oxygen (O_2) consumption. Used for acute angina and maintenance of chronic angina.	Assess vital signs before administration. Teach the patient: • Take the drug 1–2 hours before meals and at bedtime. • Sit when taking the sublingual or chewable medications. • Change positions slowly to avoid orthostatic hypotension. • Avoid hot showers, tubs, and saunas. • Headache decreases over time. • Alcohol potentiates hypotension. • If three sublingual or chewable doses do not relieve angina, go to the emergency department.

Continued

Table 36-7 Medications for Cardiovascular Disorders—cont'd

DRUG	USE AND ACTION	NURSING INTERVENTIONS
propranolol (Inderal)	Acts as a nonselective beta-adrenergic blocker. Decreases HR, myocardial irritability, and contractibility. Decreases BP in hypertension. Decreases CO. Used in dysrhythmia, myocardial infarction (MI), hypertension, migraines, and chronic stable angina.	Monitor vital signs. May be administered with diuretic to decrease sodium and water retention. May cause bronchial constriction. Use with caution in all patients with obstructive lung disease. Auscultate lungs for crackles and heart for S_3 and S_4. Monitor weight daily; check for peripheral edema. Monitor blood glucose with diabetes. Teach the patient: • Do not discontinue this drug abruptly; taper over 2 weeks. • Take the drug at the same time (or times) each day. • While on this drug, use alcohol only in moderation; refrain from smoking; decrease sodium intake. • The normal increase in HR does not occur with exercise and stress; increase activity slowly. • Weigh yourself daily; check for edema.
atenolol (Tenormin) and metoprolol tartrate (Lopressor)	Acts as a cardioselective beta-adrenergic blocker used to treat angina and hypertension. Reduces HR, BP, CO, and myocardial O_2 consumption.	Monitor vital signs. Provide continuous ECG monitoring with IV administration. Take apical pulse before each dose. Teach the patient: • Take the drug with or after meals. • Do not discontinue it abruptly. • Take your pulse and report to the physician if it is <60 bpm. • Avoid alcohol and smoking. • Avoid OTC cold remedies.
diltiazem hydrochloride (Cardizem)	Acts as a calcium channel blocker. Dilates coronary arteries; increases the availability of O_2 to the myocardium. Decreases total PVR, afterload, and systolic BP. Slightly decreases myocardial contractility. Prolongs AV node refractory period. Used in chronic stable angina, coronary artery spasm, and hypertension.	Dose may need to be reduced in older adult patients. Teach the patient: • Take your radial pulse for 1 minute. • Limit caffeine intake. • Change positions with caution to prevent postural hypotension. • Take the drug before meals and at bedtime.
nifedipine (Procardia)	Acts as a calcium channel blocker. Decreases myocardial O_2 consumption. Dilates coronary arteries. Decreases PVR. Increases CO. Used for angina, mild to moderate hypertension, vascular headaches, and coronary artery spasms.	Monitor BP during titration (i.e., during dose adjustment). Teach the patient: • Smoking is contraindicated (nicotine constricts coronary arteries). • Do not discontinue this drug abruptly. • Limit caffeine intake.
verapamil hydrochloride (Calan, Isoptin)	Acts as a calcium channel blocker. Slows AV conduction. Dilates peripheral and coronary arteries. Increases O_2 supply to the myocardium. Used to treat supraventricular tachycardias, atrial fibrillation and flutter, angina, hypertension, and vascular headaches.	Assess baseline vital signs as well as hepatic and renal function. Assess for signs of CHF (pulmonary or peripheral edema). Monitor pulse and BP before each dose. Administer an IV bolus more slowly to older adults. Teach the patient: • Take your radial pulse for 1 minute; report an irregular or slow pulse. • Avoid caffeine (opposes calcium channel blocking effect). • Change position slowly until tolerance develops. • Exercise with caution; drug's effects may give false impression of tolerance.

Table 36-7 Medications for Cardiovascular Disorders—cont'd

DRUG	USE AND ACTION	NURSING INTERVENTIONS
Antidysrhythmic Agents		
amiodarone hydrochloride (Cordarone)	Acts as an antidysrhythmic. Increases action potential duration and effective refractory period. Increases CO. Decreases PVR, coronary artery resistance, and HR. Used for severe tachycardia and supraventricular tachycardias.	Continuously monitor ECG for a decrease in dysrhythmia. Observe for thyroid dysfunction (each 200-mg tablet contains 75 mg of iodine) and neurologic effects (tremors, ataxia, headache, insomnia). Teach the patient the following: • Take your radial pulse daily. • Photosensitivity and photophobia may occur. • Pharmacologic action may have a delayed onset of 5 days to 3 months. • Skin discolorations fade with time.
disopyramide phosphate (Norpace)	Reduces the rate of spontaneous diastolic depolarization in pacemaker cells. Increases SVR. Decreases myocardial conductivity. Suppresses ectopic focal activity. Used to suppress and prevent recurrent PVCs and ventricular tachycardia.	Assess apical pulse before administration. Hold the drug if the pulse is <60 or >120 bpm and notify physician. Monitor BP. Monitor intake and output. Urinary retention and constipation may occur. Teach the patient: • Take your radial pulse daily. • Weigh yourself daily; observe for edema. • Change position slowly. • Do not drink alcohol (severely decreases BP). • Relieve dry mouth with sugarless gum or dry candy. • Avoid sunlight (photosensitivity).
flecainide acetate (Tambocor)	Acts as an antidysrhythmic. Decreases conduction velocity. Increases ventricular refractory period. Used to treat PVCs, atrial tachycardia, and other dysrhythmias not responsive to other antidysrhythmics.	Monitor ECG.
lidocaine (Xylocaine)	Increases the electrical stimulation threshold of the ventricular conduction system. Used for rapid control of ventricular dysrhythmias during MI, cardiac surgery, cardiac catheterization, and digitalis intoxication.	Administer the drug with an infusion pump. Monitor BP and ECG. May precipitate malignant hyperthermia (tachycardia, tachypnea, elevated temperature). Assess breath sounds for crackles.
mexiletine hydrochloride (Mexitil)	Acts as an antidysrhythmic structurally similar to lidocaine. Used to suppress symptomatic ventricular dysrhythmias.	Administer the drug with food or antacids. Monitor ECG. Mix the IV solution immediately before administration.
phenytoin sodium (Dilantin)	Used to treat paroxysmal atrial tachycardia and ventricular dysrhythmias.	May need a lower dose in older adults. Administer the drug only in normal saline (drug crystallizes in dextrose). Do not exceed 50 mg/min IV. Teach the patient: • Alcohol potentiates the action and therefore may precipitate toxicity.
propranolol (Inderal)	(See description under Antianginals.)	
quinidine	Acts as an antidysrhythmic. Depresses myocardial excitability, contractility, automaticity, and conduction velocity. Anticholinergic effects increase the ventricular rate. Relaxes muscles. Used for atrial and ventricular dysrhythmias.	If administered with digoxin, it may produce toxicity or unpredictable dysrhythmias. Administer the drug with meals to decrease gastric distress. Severe hypotension may occur with large doses. Monitor electrolytes; continuing diarrhea may indicate electrolyte imbalance.

Continued

Table 36-7 Medications for Cardiovascular Disorders—cont'd

DRUG	USE AND ACTION	NURSING INTERVENTIONS
tocainide hydrochloride (Tonocard)	Acts as an antidysrhythmic. It is a primary analog of lidocaine. Used for life-threatening ventricular dysrhythmias associated with prolonged QT interval.	Monitor ECG. Administer the drug with food or antacids to decrease gastrointestinal (GI) side effects. Monitor CBC for blood dyscrasias (agranulocytosis, leukocytosis, neutropenia).
Verapamil (Calan, Isoptin)	(See description under Antianginals.)	
Anticoagulant Agent **Direct Thrombin Inhibitor**		
dabigatran (Pradaxa)	Prevents blood clot formation. Used to prevent the risk of stroke and serious blood clots in patients with atrial fibrillation.	Monitor for bleeding. Teach the patient: • Take with or without food. • Do not stop the medication suddenly without the direction of the physician. • Check with your physician before beginning any OTC medications.
Antiplatelet Agents		
clopidogrel (Plavix)	Decreases platelet aggregation. Prolongs bleeding time. Used to prevent thromboembolic disorders such as stroke and MI.	Monitor bleeding time, CBC with differential, and platelet count. Avoid OTC medications with aspirin or NSAIDs unless prescribed by the physician. Teach the patient: • Report bleeding. • Keep appointments for blood work.
ticlopidine (Ticlid)	Same as Plavix.	Monitor liver function studies, CBC, and prothrombin time (PT). Teach the patient: • Report bleeding. • Take the drug with food. • Keep appointments for blood work.
abciximab (ReoPro)	Inhibits platelet aggregation. Given IV to reduce ischemic complications with angioplasty or atherectomy.	Used only in the hospital. Monitor vital signs, ECG, and level of consciousness. Assess hemoglobin (Hgb), hematocrit (Hct), platelet count, and clotting factors frequently. Watch for bleeding. Protect from trauma.
Lipid-Lowering Agents		
cholestyramine (Questran)	Prescribed when diet, exercise, and weight loss fail to bring cholesterol levels under control. Lowers LDL cholesterol. Increases HDL cholesterol.	Interferes with absorption of some other drugs, so check drug-drug interactions before giving this medication. To get the best effect, teach patients to: • Continue diet and exercise. • Increase fluid intake to counter constipating effects.
gemfibrozil (Lopid)	Decreases synthesis and secretion of VLDL by liver. Decreases triglyceride levels.	For best effect, teach the patient: • Continue diet and exercise. • Take the drug with meals.
nicotinic acid (niacin)	Decreases synthesis and secretion of VLDL and LDL by the liver. Increases HDL.	For best effect, teach the patient: • Continue diet and exercise. • Take the drug with meals to decrease GI side effects.
pravastatin (Pravachol), simvastatin (Zocor), lovastatin (Mevacor), atorvastatin (Lipitor)	Increases rate of removal of LDL from plasma. Decreases synthesis of LDL.	Monitor liver function tests. For best effect, teach the patient: • Continue diet and exercise. • Report muscle tenderness. • Take as single dose in the evening. • Have routine eye examinations.

Table 36-7 **Medications for Cardiovascular Disorders—cont'd**

DRUG	USE AND ACTION	NURSING INTERVENTIONS
Miscellaneous and Emergency Agents		
amrinone lactate (Inocor)	Acts as an inotropic medication and vasodilator. Increases myocardial contractions without increasing HR. Increases blood flow through collateral coronary vessels. Increases stroke volume and CO. Decreases preload and afterload. Used to treat HF refractory to other medications.	Administer the drug with an infusion pump. Titrate to target BP. Monitor intake and output. Avoid extravasation. Discard the solution 24 hours after preparation.
atropine sulfate	Acts as a vagal blocker. Increases HR and CO in heart blocks and severe bradycardia. Used in symptomatic bradycardia and bradydysrhythmias.	Assess HR, rhythm, and BP.
calcium chloride	Necessary for cardiac rhythm, tone, and contraction. Increases muscle tone and force of contraction. Used in cardiac resuscitation and in cardiac irregularities associated with hyperkalemia.	Monitor ECG, BP, and arterial blood gases (ABGs). Avoid extravasation; causes necrosis. Alkalosis decreases the absorption of calcium. Acidosis increases the absorption of calcium.
dobutamine (Dobutrex)	Acts as a synthetic catecholamine and beta-adrenergic agonist. Increases CO with less increase in HR and BP than other catecholamines. Used in CHF and after cardiac surgery to increase myocardial contractility, stroke volume, and CO.	Continuous monitoring of ECG, cardiac parameters, and urinary output; titrate to HR and BP. Urinary output should increase with improved CO and renal function. Often used with nitroprusside or dopamine for additive effects. Causes less increase in HR, PVR, and dysrhythmias than dopamine. At a rate <7 μg/kg/min, expect increased myocardial contraction, CO, and renal blood flow. At a rate of >7 μg/kg/min, expect peripheral vasoconstriction and increased MAP.
dopamine hydrochloride (Intropin)	Acts as a neurotransmitter (a precursor to norepinephrine). Increases CO and BP. Improves renal blood flow and therefore urine output with lower doses. Used for hemodynamic support in shock.	Avoid extravasation; causes necrosis. Monitor vital signs, ECG, urine output, and extremity color. Titrate to target BP; use an infusion pump. Peripheral vasoconstriction is noted with cold upper and lower extremities.
epinephrine hydrochloride (Adrenalin chloride)	Acts as a catecholamine. Strengthens myocardial contraction; increases BP, HR, and CO. Dilates bronchial tree. Used in anaphylactic shock and to restore cardiac rhythm in cardiac arrest.	Monitor vital signs and ECG continuously. Avoid extravasation; causes sloughing. Titrate to cardiac response. *Caution:* Drug is available in several concentrations (1:100, 1:1000, 1:10,000); be sure to check for the prescribed solution. May be administered by endotracheal tube because drug is rapidly absorbed from the lungs.

Continued

Table 36-7 **Medications for Cardiovascular Disorders—cont'd**

DRUG	USE AND ACTION	NURSING INTERVENTIONS
isoproterenol hydrochloride (Isuprel)	Acts as a cardiac stimulant (positive inotropic and chronotropic effects), a bronchodilator, and a peripheral vasodilator. Increases HR and contractility. Decreases PVR and diastolic BP, resulting in increased CO and systolic BP, decreased MAP, and increased myocardial O_2 consumption. Used as a cardiac stimulant in cardiac arrest, cardiogenic shock, ventricular dysrhythmias, and heart block.	Continuously monitor ECG. Monitor vital signs, urine output, and peripheral blood flow. Titrate to desired HR, BP, and urine output. Avoid extravasation.
sodium nitroprusside (Nipride)	Acts as a vasodilator. Decreases preload and afterload. Used in hypertensive crises.	Remember that this is a light-sensitive preparation and should be wrapped in aluminum foil. Administer the drug with an infusion pump. Titrate to maintain CO. Continuously monitor BP. Discard the solution 4 hours after preparation. Assess thiocyanate levels daily for patients on long-term therapy.
norepinephrine (Levophed)	Acts as a catecholamine (vasoconstrictor and cardiac stimulant). Produces increased BP, myocardial O_2, and coronary artery blood flow. Used in acute hypotensive states, MI, and cardiac arrest.	Mix the drug only with dextrose in water or dextrose in saline. Administer the drug with an infusion pump. Report decreased urine output immediately. Continuously monitor and titrate the drug to the desired BP. Monitor peripheral blood flow. Avoid extravasation.
sodium bicarbonate	Acts as a systemic alkalinizer. Used to correct metabolic acidosis in cardiac arrest.	Do not infuse the drug with calcium. Monitor ABGs. Avoid extravasation; causes severe tissue damage.
milrinone (Primacor)	Acts as an inotropic agent. Increases myocardial contractility and CO. Vasodilation decreases preload and afterload. Used to treat CHF that does not respond to usual therapy.	Monitor vital signs, intake and output, and daily weight during therapy. Monitor ECG continuously. Give potassium as ordered for hypokalemia.

AV, Atrioventricular; *BP,* blood pressure; *bpm,* beats per minute; *CBC,* complete blood count; *CHF,* congestive heart failure; *CO,* cardiac output; *ECG,* electrocardiogram; *HDL,* high-density lipoprotein; *HF,* heart failure; *HR,* heart rate; *IV,* intravenous; *LDL,* low-density lipoprotein; *MAP,* mean arterial pressure; *NSAIDs,* nonsteroidal antiinflammatory drugs; *OTC,* over-the-counter; *PVC,* premature ventricular contraction; *PVR,* peripheral vascular resistance; *SVR,* systemic vascular resistance; *VLDL,* very-low-density lipoprotein.

Anticoagulants

Anticoagulants are used to prevent clot formation. Heparin, low-molecular-weight heparin (LMWH), warfarin, and dabigatran (Pradaxa) are the most commonly used preventive anticoagulant drugs.

Heparin. Heparin interferes with factor III in the clotting process. It is administered by continuous IV drip or subcutaneously. When a patient has a clotting episode, a heparin bolus is administered and a continuous infusion is started. The infusion rate is set to deliver a prescribed number of heparin units per hour. The physician adjusts the heparin dose based on the activated partial thromboplastin time (aPTT). When the aPTT has stabilized (generally at 1.5 to 2.0 times the control level), the drug can be changed to the subcutaneous route. Because heparin cannot be administered orally, the patient must remain hospitalized during its administration. Heparin is recommended for use with ACS, during percutaneous coronary interventions (PCIs) and surgical revascularization, and in conjunction with fibrinolytic therapy.

Low-Molecular-Weight Heparin. LMWHs, such as enoxaparin (Lovenox), are fragments derived from heparin that work by blocking the formation of thrombin and preventing the development of a clot. The advantages of using LMWHs are that the anticoagulant effect is more predictable, they are administered subcutaneously once or twice a day, and they do not require such close monitoring of aPTT. LMWHs are recommended for patients with venous thromboembolism (VTE), for those with unstable angina, and in some cases of MI (before a thrombus occludes the coronary vessel).

Warfarin. The anticoagulant drug that may be administered orally, warfarin (Coumadin), is started as soon as possible. The warfarin dose is regulated by the prothrombin time (PT) and international normalized ratio (INR). The PT is kept in a therapeutic range of 1.5 to 2.0 times the normal level. The INR may be kept at 2.0 to 4.5. Patients who have had artificial valve replacements must remain on anticoagulant therapy for life.

All patients on anticoagulants must be monitored closely for any signs of bleeding. In addition, patients should be taught how to reduce the risk of bleeding, such as to use an electric razor and a soft-bristled toothbrush.

Dabigatran. Dabigatran (Pradaxa) and rivaroxaban (Xarelto) are two new oral anticoagulants classified as direct thrombin inhibitors. These drugs are used to prevent the development of blood clots and stroke in patients with atrial fibrillation (irregular heartbeat). Dabigatran and rivaroxaban do not require frequent monitoring of lab results or frequent visits to the physician. However, these medications are not recommended for patients with heart valve replacements and patients on these medications still need to be monitored closely for signs of bleeding (MedlinePlus [Dabigatran], 2013).

Pharmacology Capsule

Heparin dose is adjusted based on the patient's activated partial thromboplastin time (aPTT). Warfarin dose is adjusted based on the patient's prothrombin time (PT) and international normalized ratio (INR).

Antiplatelet Agents

Antiplatelet therapy is often used after an MI to prevent additional myocardial infarction and strokes. The dose of aspirin as an antiplatelet agent in MI and stroke prevention continues to be studied extensively in various groups (women, men, elderly, diabetics, etc.). Aspirin should be used under the direction of a health care provider so that each patient's unique situation can be taken into consideration (Park & Bavary, 2013). Ticlopidine (Ticlid) and clopidogrel (Plavix) also exhibit antiplatelet effects and may be prescribed for patients who are unable to tolerate aspirin.

Glycoprotein (GP) IIb/IIIa inhibitors block the platelet receptor sites that bind with fibrinogen and lead to platelet aggregation. GP IIb/IIIa inhibitors such as abciximab (ReoPro) and eptifibatide (Integrilin) are used in combination with heparin and aspirin as part of the medical treatment for unstable angina and MI. They are also being used after MI in conjunction with fibrinolytic therapy, PCIs, or both.

Pharmacology Capsule

Anticoagulants and antiplatelet agents prevent formation of new clots, but fibrinolytics destroy clots that have already formed.

Fibrinolytic Agents

Whereas anticoagulants and antiplatelet agents prevent the continued formation of clots, the fibrinolytic agents (also called *thrombolytic agents*) act to destroy clots that have already formed. Streptokinase, reteplase, and tissue plasminogen activator (t-PA) are examples of thrombolytics. They are best used as soon as evidence of clot formation is seen. They are administered intravenously when certain criteria have been met. Administration is continued until evidence of reperfusion is noted or until the maximum dose has been given. These medications are often referred to as *clot busters*.

Information about anticoagulants, antiplatelet, and fibrinolytic agents is presented in Tables 28-2 and Table 37-2. Selected antiplatelet agents are also listed in Table 36-7.

Lipid-Lowering Agents

Lipid-lowering drugs are frequently part of the overall treatment plan, along with diet and exercise, for many patients with heart disease. The goal of therapy is for the patient to have decreased serum triglyceride and LDL levels and an improved HDL level. Patients on this group of medications need to be encouraged to adhere to diet restrictions, exercise, and quit smoking (see *Complementary and Alternative Therapies* box). Serial laboratory tests (lipid profile and liver function) are closely monitored. Selected lipid-lowering medications are included in Table 36-7.

Complementary and Alternative Therapies

Some people use garlic to reduce plasma lipids and lower blood pressure. The best garlic preparation is an enteric-coated dried preparation that contains adequate allicin and allinase, the "active ingredients" in the preparation. Most of the allicin and allinase are destroyed when fresh garlic is cooked or eaten raw. Garlic irritates the gastrointestinal (GI) tract and increases the effects of anticoagulants and insulin.

Analgesics

Patients who are experiencing chest pain often require analgesic medications. Initially, sublingual nitroglycerin is administered to treat the chest pain. Nitroglycerin is a vasodilator. If the sublingual nitroglycerin is not effective, IV nitroglycerin and/or IV morphine may be administered. Morphine relieves pain, reduces anxiety, and reduces the workload of the heart by trapping some of the venous blood in the periphery of the body. An alternative to morphine is meperidine hydrochloride (Demerol). Meperidine is less effective in relieving anxiety and cardiac workload than morphine. Morphine and meperidine are most effective when administered intravenously.

DIET THERAPY

Reduction of body weight lessens the workload on the heart. A low-fat, high-fiber diet usually is recommended for cardiac patients. Patients are encouraged to eat a well-balanced diet that includes an emphasis on fruits, vegetables, grains, and proteins low in fat (fish, legumes, poultry, and lean meats). Cholesterol intake should be limited to 200 mg/day for individuals with heart disease or at high risk for heart disease. It is also recommended that foods with trans fatty acids be limited to less than 1% of total daily calories (American Heart Association-Know Your Fats, 2013). An exercise program may help the patient to achieve optimal weight.

Sodium

If fluid retention accompanies the cardiac problem, the physician may order sodium restriction. A diet containing less than 1500 mg/day is recommended. More severe restrictions of sodium intake are difficult to achieve and patients find it difficult to comply with the dietary regimen (FDA-Sodium in Your Diet, 2013; Whelton et al., 2012). Salt substitutes are available.

Potassium

Patients taking potassium-wasting diuretics (e.g., furosemide, hydrochlorothiazide) need to include adequate potassium in the diet to counteract the depletion. Patients taking large doses of potassium-wasting diuretics need to have potassium supplements prescribed.

Pharmacology Capsule

Potassium-wasting diuretics such as furosemide and hydrochlorothiazide may cause hypokalemia, which can lead to dangerous dysrhythmias.

OXYGEN THERAPY

The myocardium needs an adequate blood supply to function properly. Any patient complaining of chest pain unrelieved by nitroglycerin should have supplemental O_2 administered. A nasal cannula or face mask should be applied and set to deliver the prescribed liter flow; the patient's response to this therapy should be monitored.

PACEMAKERS

A pacemaker is a device used to restore regular rhythm and to improve cardiac output and tissue **perfusion**. Pacemakers may be temporary or permanent. Methods for temporary pacing are transcutaneous, transvenous, or epicardial. Transcutaneous pacemakers deliver impulses through the skin from externally placed electrode pads. A transvenous pacemaker has a pacing electrode that is threaded through a vein into the right side of the heart. Epicardial pacing wires are placed into the epicardial wall of the heart during cardiac surgery and the wires are brought through the chest wall. Temporary pacemakers all require an external pulse generator to provide the electrical energy needed to stimulate depolarization. A permanent pacemaker is a small device that is surgically placed subcutaneously in the wall of the chest, with the electrical leads placed into the heart through a vein. Impulses are conducted from the power source (external pulse generator or implanted pacemaker) to the heart to stimulate contraction of the myocardium.

Pacemakers can be used to stimulate the atrium or ventricle (called *single-chamber pacing*) or they can be used to stimulate both chambers (called *dual-chamber pacing*). Dual-chamber pacing produces conduction and contraction that is near normal. Pacemakers have multiple settings related to pacing and sensing.

Temporary Pacemakers

Temporary pacemakers can be used electively or for emergency situations. Elective uses include gaining control of very rapid supraventricular tachycardic rhythms, assessing the need for permanent pacing in patients with bradycardias, and after cardiac surgery.

Permanent Pacemakers

Permanent pacemakers are indicated in a number of patient situations in which conduction defects or dysrhythmias compromise the normal function of the heart. Several clinical conditions indicate the need for permanent pacing. A few of these conditions are acquired AV block, sinus node dysfunction, chronic bifascicular or trifascicular block, symptomatic tachycardias, and carotid sinus syndrome. A permanent implantable pacemaker is inserted under local anesthesia. The batteries, usually lithium, have an 8- to 10-year expected life. Permanent pacemakers are inserted in the operating room, catheterization laboratory, or special procedures area. The pacing lead(s) are positioned (through the subclavian or cephalic vein) in the RA, RV, LV, or a combination of these (depending on the patient's problem). The generator is placed in a subcutaneous pocket, usually under the clavicle or in the abdomen (Epstein et al., 2012).

NURSING CARE of the Patient with a Pacemaker

Patients with inserted pacemakers recover on a telemetry unit. Monitor the patient for proper pacemaker functioning by observing for the pacemaker "spike." The pacemaker spike is a mark observed on the ECG tracing that represents the impulse generated by the pacemaker. Malfunctions of the pacemaker include failure to pace, failure to sense, and failure to capture. Assess vital signs and inspect the incision frequently for bleeding. Once stable, most patients may be up and active but should limit movement of the arm and shoulder on the implanted side. Immobilization of the arm may be ordered by the physician. Limited arm and shoulder movement reduces the risk of lead dislodgement. Prophylactic antibiotics may be administered before and after insertion of a pacemaker. Monitor the patient for elevated temperature, signs of infection at the site, and an elevated WBC count.

After insertion of a temporary pacemaker, microshock precautions should be followed. Monitor the patient's ECG monitor and transport the patient with a portable cardiac monitor and a nurse in attendance. Assess the pacemaker for misfiring and plan a gradual increase in activities.

Three major problems can occur with pacing. The first problem, failure to pace, means that the pacemaker did not initiate the electrical stimulus when it was due to fire. Frequently caused by battery failure or lead wire displacement, it is recognized by the lack of a pacer spike on the ECG tracing. The second problem, failure to capture, means that the electrical stimulus from the pacemaker is not followed by electrical activity in the patient's heart. Caused by dislodgement of the lead or the pacemaker output setting set too low, failure to capture is recognized by noting the presence of a pacer spike without ECG activity after the spike. The third problem, failure to sense, means that the pacemaker does not sense the patient's cardiac rhythm and initiates an electrical impulse when it is not needed. Failure to sense is most often caused by displacement of the electrode and can be recognized by pacer spikes that fall too close to the patient's rhythm.

When a permanent pacemaker has been inserted, teach the patient how to count the pulse for 1 full minute daily and keep a record to share with the physician. Explain wound care and the healing process and advise the patient to notify the physician of symptoms of decreased cardiac output: dyspnea, dizziness, syncope, weakness, fatigue, and chest pain. In addition, instruct the patient to carry an identification card describing the type of pacemaker implanted.

Automatic Implantable Cardioverter Defibrillator (AICD)

The AICD is used to treat patients who have survived life-threatening recurrent ventricular tachycardia or fibrillation or who are at high risk for development of either of these. The device senses heart rate, identifies rhythm changes, and treats ventricular dysrhythmias. The AICD generator is implanted in the subcutaneous tissue over the pectoral muscle. The lead system is placed via a subclavian vein into the endocardium. The cardioverter recognizes ventricular fibrillation and ventricular tachycardia and uses the shocks to convert the dysrhythmia to normal sinus rhythm. When the AICD senses these lethal dysrhythmias, it delivers a shock of up to 25 joules to defibrillate. If the heart rhythm does not return to normal, the device can continue to deliver shocks. The patient is instructed to sit or lie down when experiencing a shock and to keep a record of the number of shocks delivered. Patients report that the shocks feel like a blow to the chest. In addition to defibrillation, AICDs can also function as antitachycardia and antibradycardia pacemakers (Epstein et al., 2012).

Complications. Complications associated with the AICD are inappropriate shocks, broken or displaced leads, and failure to deliver shocks as a result of battery failure or failure to recognize a dysrhythmia.

❖ NURSING CARE of the Patient with an Automatic Implantable Cardioverter Defibrillator

Postinsertion care is similar to that for pacemaker insertion described previously. In addition to postprocedure care, nurses can promote psychosocial adaptation in patients with AICDs. The patient may be concerned with body image change and develop a fear of shocks. It is important to decrease anxiety about being shocked. Some patients become very dependent on the device. These patients and families need teaching and support. People who touch the patient during a shock will feel a tingling sensation, which is not harmful. An established support group for the patient and family is very helpful. The family must be instructed in CPR. An identification bracelet and a card with instructions about the AICD setting are carried at all times. Patients and families should be instructed about what to do if the AICD fires. For example, the patient should sit or lie down if the device fires and if the device shocks more than one time or the patient is not feeling well. Emergency Medical Services (EMS) should be called. Advise patients to avoid strong magnetic fields (e.g., metal detectors, power plants, MRI). The device should be checked for correct function at appropriate intervals determined by the health care provider.

CARDIOVERSION

Cardioversion is the delivery of a synchronized shock to terminate atrial or ventricular tachydysrhythmias (rapid abnormal heart rhythms). It may be done as an emergency or elective procedure. The shock is synchronized with the R wave of the QRS complex on the ECG to avoid shocking during the vulnerable period of the T wave. A shock delivered during ventricular relaxation can initiate ventricular fibrillation.

If the patient is receiving digoxin, the drug is withheld for 24 hours before the procedure. Emergency drugs are made available and the patient has a patent intravenous line in place before the procedure. Explain the procedure and obtain informed consent. A short-acting sedative is usually given. The cardioverter is set to the synchronized mode and two electrodes are placed on the chest. One electrode is placed to the right of the sternum just below the clavicle and the other is placed at the apex of the heart. The initial impulse varies from 50 to 100 joules, depending on the type of dysrhythmia. If the initial impulse does not convert the dysrhythmia to normal sinus rhythm, the impulse energy is increased and the procedure is repeated.

After cardioversion, the patient usually recovers very quickly from the sedation and does not remember the event. Inspect the skin under the electrodes for irritation and monitor the patient's heart rate and rhythm, vital signs, and neurologic status. Transient dysrhythmias and a drop in blood pressure are common. Be especially alert for atrial fibrillation, which can contribute to the formation of atrial wall thrombus and emboli.

CARDIOPULMONARY RESUSCITATION

CPR is the restoration of heart and lung function after cardiac arrest. The procedure is used in basic cardiac life support and advanced cardiac life support. The reader is referred to materials prepared by the American Heart Association for current, in-depth coverage of the procedure.. Advanced cardiac life support (ACLS) incorporates CPR with defibrillation, advanced airway management, and cardiac dysrhythmia care. The ability to perform ACLS requires additional training and certification by the American Heart Association.

DEFIBRILLATION

Defibrillation is the delivery of an electrical shock to the heart in an effort to restore normal cardiac conduction and contraction in the patient experiencing ventricular fibrillation or pulseless ventricular tachycardia (American Heart Association-Defibrillation, 2012). Defibrillation needs to be used as soon as possible when one of these abnormal rhythms is detected. There are standard defibrillators (usually biphasic) available in acute care facilities and portable, automated defibrillators known as automated external defibrillators (AEDs) available in most locations where people gather (airports, malls, schools, etc.). The use of a standard defibrillator is taught in ACLS and the use of an AED is part of the CPR and ACLS courses.

CARDIAC SURGERY

The most common surgical procedures involving the heart are pacemaker or AICD insertion, heart surgery to repair or replace valves and remove tumors, and coronary artery bypass surgery. Pacemaker insertion is described earlier in this chapter. Coronary artery bypass surgery is described as a surgical treatment for MI under "Cardiac Disorders."

For some of the surgical procedures on the heart, the heart muscle must be at rest during the procedure. This requires placing the patient on a machine to direct the blood away from the heart and lungs and to maintain appropriate O_2 and CO_2 levels. The heart's rhythm is interrupted by an electrolyte solution and may be restarted after the surgery by electrical stimulation. During this type of surgery, the patient's core temperature usually is reduced to decrease the O_2 needs of the entire body, especially the brain.

PREOPERATIVE NURSING CARE of the Cardiac Surgery Patient

Assessment

Nursing assessment of the patient with cardiac disorders is summarized in Box 36-1. When a patient is facing cardiac surgery, the nurse must also assess the patient's fears and anxiety (see *Patient Teaching* box). Patients are usually upset and very concerned when heart surgery is recommended. It is important to determine what patients know about the surgery and what more they would like to know.

Patient Teaching

Cardiac Surgery, Preoperative

The specifics of the teaching plan depend on the exact procedure and agency or surgeon procedures. General content of the teaching plan includes the following:

- Preoperative routines: nothing by mouth (NPO), monitoring, diagnostic tests, any special preparation
- Where the patient will be after surgery: in intensive care unit after extensive procedures; in telemetry unit after pacemaker or AICD insertion
- The postoperative care setting: the room and the equipment
- Postoperative routines: how to turn, cough, deep breathe, and exercise the leg muscles; monitoring; procedures
- Postoperative pain: amount of pain to expect; relief measures such as splinting, positioning, medication
- Communication: means of communication established before surgery (because most patients are intubated for 4 to 8 hours after more extensive surgery)

Nursing Diagnoses, Goals, and Outcome Criteria: Preoperative Cardiac Surgery

Nursing Diagnoses	Goals and Outcome Criteria
Fear related to perceived threat of death or unfamiliarity with setting and procedures	Reduced fear: patient states is less fearful, demonstrates relaxed manner
Anxiety related to threat to health status or uncertain outcome	Reduced anxiety: patient states is less anxious, is calmer

Interventions

Fear and Anxiety

Encourage the patient to identify feelings and then explore the basis of those feelings. Do not assume that you know how the patient feels. Accept the patient's feelings and avoid trite reassurance (e.g., "Don't worry; everything will be fine."). Accurate information about what to expect helps to reduce fear of the unknown. Physical comfort measures such as a massage or back rub also may be soothing. If the patient's anxiety level remains high, notify the physician.

Good patient teaching is essential to address fear and anxiety. The physician reviews necessary diagnostic tests, the surgical procedure itself, and what to expect after surgery. Nevertheless, the nurse must be able to clarify and further explain what the patient will experience. If the surgery is done on an emergency basis, little time is available for preoperative teaching. However, planned cardiac surgery allows time for the patient to accept the need for surgery and to explore why the procedure is necessary. Include the family in the preoperative teaching to decrease their anxiety and allow them to participate in the patient's recovery. The patient teaching plan must be individualized for the type of surgical procedure.

Put on Your Thinking Cap!

A patient is scheduled for extensive cardiac surgery and will be on a ventilator for up to 8 hours postoperatively. What means of communication can you establish in advance? What if the patient is illiterate? What if the patient is deaf?

POSTOPERATIVE NURSING CARE of the Cardiac Surgery Patient

Nursing care needs vary considerably depending on the type of surgical procedure. Care specific to certain conditions is discussed with those conditions. In addition, see Chapter 17 for thorough coverage of care of the surgical patient. This section addresses needs common to many patients having cardiac surgery.

Assessment

Assessment of the cardiac patient is summarized in Box 36-1. After surgery, be especially alert to changes in the patient's vital signs, breath sounds, urine output, mental alertness, and color. In the intensive care unit, monitor cardiac rhythm, ABGs, and hemodynamic pressures. It is also important to assess chest tube function and frequently inspect all dressings for type and amount of drainage. Examine the patient's surgical wound site and the insertion sites of tubes and cannulas for increasing redness, swelling, and purulent drainage. In addition, assess urine amount, appearance, and odor.

Nursing Diagnoses, Goals, and Outcome Criteria: Postoperative Cardiac Surgery

Nursing Diagnoses	Goals and Outcome Criteria
Ineffective Breathing Pattern related to mechanical ventilation, general anesthesia, pain, or restrictive surgical dressings	Adequate oxygenation: arterial blood gases (ABGs) within normal limits for the patient
Acute Pain related to tissue trauma	Pain relief: patient states pain reduced or relieved, relaxed manner
Ineffective Thermoregulation related to cooling during surgery	Normal body temperature: temperature of at least 36.7°C (98°F) orally
Decreased Cardiac Output related to fluid loss or decreased fluid intake	Normal cardiac output: fluid intake equal to output
Risk for Infection related to altered skin integrity	Absence of infection: no fever; decreasing drainage, redness, and swelling of wound
Anxiety related to unfamiliar routines and stressful experience	Reduced anxiety: patient states anxiety is reduced

Interventions

Ineffective Breathing Pattern

Patients with open heart or bypass surgery are unresponsive on arrival in the intensive care unit. Ventilatory assistance is of primary importance. Reassess breath sounds and ABGs frequently and connect chest tubes to underwater seal drainage. (See Chapter 31 for the care of chest tubes.) Reposition the patient often to promote removal of pulmonary secretions and improve respiratory excursion.

When the patient is extubated, provide an O_2 mask or nasal cannula as ordered to provide supplemental O_2. Also assist the patient to cough and deep breathe frequently. A pillow or a blanket in a pillowcase can be used as an incisional splint during coughing. An incentive spirometer is usually ordered; monitor its use and remind the patient to use it. Assist the patient with early ambulation, as ordered, to reduce the risk of pulmonary complications.

Acute Pain

Effective pain relief makes it easier for the patient to turn, cough, and deep breathe. Assess the patient's pain: location, severity, aggravating factors, and relieving factors. Administer analgesics as ordered; intravenous morphine in small doses is most frequently prescribed for analgesia. You may also use independent measures, including position changes, back rubs, relaxation techniques, and imagery. Assess the effectiveness of the interventions in managing pain and provide for periods of rest and sleep after pain relief efforts.

Ineffective Thermoregulation

Warmed blankets, heating blankets, and warming lights may be used to assist with rewarming. Monitor the patient's body temperature continuously until the patient is stable.

Decreased Cardiac Output

While in the intensive care unit, the patient's cardiac pressures are monitored continuously until they stabilize. Prescribed medications are adjusted based on vital signs, hemodynamic pressures, and cardiac rhythms. Pacing wires are connected to a temporary pacemaker. It is important to monitor fluid and blood administration and assess urinary and other drainage outputs. Volume expanders (i.e., albumin) and vasoactive drugs may be necessary to maintain blood pressure. Oral fluids are ordered shortly after extubation.

Risk for Infection

The patient is at risk for incisional, respiratory tract, and urinary tract infections. In addition, the presence of multiple tubes and cannulas provides additional sites for potential nosocomial infection. To reduce the risk of infection, it is vital to practice good hand washing technique and use aseptic technique when handling dressings and invasive equipment. Provide wound care as ordered (or per agency policy) and administer antibiotics as ordered. Before discharge, begin teaching the patient how to care for the surgical wounds. Emphasize signs or symptoms that should be reported to the physician (e.g., fever, increasing or purulent wound drainage, increasing redness or swelling, separation of wound margins).

Anxiety

Tell the patient and family what is being done and how the patient is responding. Remember to talk to the patient and offer reassurance. When the patient is on a ventilator, use the previously established nonverbal means of communication. It is often necessary to repeat instructions because of the effects of pain, medications, and anxiety (see *Complementary and Alternative Therapies* box). As the patient improves, explain the importance of follow-up care and rehabilitation.

Complementary and Alternative Therapies

For pain relief, many complementary therapies are used with analgesics. Examples are massage, relaxation techniques, and imagery.

CARDIAC DISORDERS

CORONARY HEART DISEASE (CHD)

CHD, also referred to as *coronary artery disease (CAD)* and *ischemic heart disease (IHD)*, occurs when the major coronary arteries supplying the myocardium are partially or completely blocked. Blockage of the arteries is caused by coronary artery spasm, arteriosclerosis, or atherosclerosis and may result in ischemia or infarction of myocardial tissue. In 2010, 15.4 million Americans had CHD (see *Cultural Considerations* box). CHD is the largest single cause of death in Americans (male and female subjects). In 2009 the overall death rate for CHD in the U.S. was 116.1 per 100,000 population (Go et al., 2013). See the *Health Promotion* box.

Cultural Considerations

What Does Culture Have to Do with Heart Disease?

Native Americans and African Americans develop coronary heart disease (CHD) at an earlier age than other Americans. The incidence of CHD is highest among middle-aged Caucasian men. Latinos have lower death rates from CHD than non-Latinos. Nurses can educate high-risk patients about risk factors that can be modified: obesity, hypertension, and stress. Role models from the target population are especially influential.

Health Promotion

Risk Factor Modification

Risk factor modification will help to reduce an individual's chances for developing coronary heart disease (CHD), angina, and acute coronary syndrome (ACS). Controlling hypertension; reducing serum cholesterol and low-density lipoproteins (LDLs); quitting smoking; participating in regular, moderate exercise; obtaining and maintaining ideal body weight; and learning to handle stress are recommended lifestyle changes that can help to decrease risk.

Arteriosclerosis

Arteriosclerosis is an abnormal thickening, hardening, and loss of elasticity of arterial walls. Smooth muscle cells and collagen migrate to the tunica intima (innermost layer of the artery) and cause the arterial wall to stiffen and thicken and the lumen to decrease in diameter. Lipids, cholesterol, calcium, and thrombi adhere to the damaged arterial wall. This process limits the elasticity of the wall and decreases the flow of O_2-carrying blood to tissues. Some effects of arteriosclerosis are hypertension, impaired tissue perfusion, and aneurysms.

Atherosclerosis

Atherosclerosis, a form of arteriosclerosis, is an inflammatory disease that begins with endothelial injury and progresses to the complicated lesion seen in advanced stages of the disease process. Atherosclerosis begins with injury to the endothelial cells that line the wall of the arteries. Endothelial injury, which leads to inflammation and dysfunction of the endothelial cells, results in the deposit of LDL along the intima of arteries. These deposits are called *foam cells.* When enough foam cells accumulate, they progress to the lesions associated with atherosclerosis: fatty streaks, fibrous or stable plaque, and unstable plaque.

Progression of Lesions

Fatty Streak. The fatty streak is the earliest lesion to develop in atherosclerosis. Yellow-colored lipids (fat) fill smooth muscle cells, producing streaks of fat that cause no obstruction to the affected vessel. Fatty streaks may begin as early as infancy and continue to develop through childhood. No symptoms are associated with these lesions.

Fibrous Plaque. The fibrous plaque is the characteristic lesion of progressing atherosclerosis, which develops over time. Smooth muscle cells, chronically stimulated by LDLs and platelet-activated growth factors, proliferate, produce collagen, and migrate over the fatty streak. This forms a fibrous plaque that protrudes from the wall of the artery into the lumen. Other substances (WBCs, platelets, lipids, calcium) adhere to and collect within the plaque. The fibrous plaque is whitish or grayish in appearance, may develop in one portion of the artery or circle the entire lumen, and may have smooth or rough edges. Fibrous plaque, often referred to as stable plaque, contributes to the loss of arterial elasticity and impairs the vessel's ability to dilate to meet increased O_2 needs.

Unstable Plaque. The outer layer of the fibrous plaque often thins out, making the plaque unstable and increasing the risk of ulceration and rupture. When the plaque ruptures, platelets are activated and trigger the coagulation cascade with the development of a thrombus that partially or totally obstructs (occludes) the artery.

Collateral Circulation. If plaque formation occurs slowly, collateral circulation may develop. Collateral blood vessels are new branches that grow from existing arteries to provide increased blood flow.

Risk Factors. Factors that increase the risk of atherosclerosis include increased serum cholesterol, high blood pressure, tobacco smoke, diabetes mellitus, obesity and overweight, physical inactivity, age, gender, and heredity (American Heart Association-Coronary Artery Disease-Coronary Heart Disease, 2013). These risk factors are divided into two categories: (1) risk factors that can be modified and (2) risk factors that cannot be modified. Risk factors that *cannot* be modified are increasing age, gender, and heredity. The focus of patient education is on reducing the risk factors that *can* be modified. Other contributing factors for the development of CHD are stress, alcohol, and nutrition or diet (American Heart Association-Coronary Artery Disease-Coronary Heart Disease, 2013).

Healthy People 2020 has set several goals related to serum cholesterol levels. One of these is to reduce the mean total blood cholesterol in adults from 197.7 mg/dL to 177.9 mg/dL. In addition, efforts will be made to reduce the proportion of adults with high blood cholesterol, increase the proportion of adults who have had their blood cholesterol checked within the past 5 years, and increase the proportion of individuals with CHD who have LDL levels treated to at or below recommended levels (Healthy People 2020-Heart Disease and Stroke).

Signs and Symptoms

CHD usually is asymptomatic until the tissue's blood supply is reduced by at least 50%. Then the clinical manifestations of CHD include stable angina, ACS (unstable angina and MI), and sudden cardiac death. MI has been further categorized into non-ST segment elevation myocardial infarction (NSTEMI) and ST segment elevation myocardial infarction (STEMI).

ANGINA

Angina or chest pain, the most common symptom of CHD, results when the demand for O_2 by the myocardial cells exceeds the supply of O_2 delivered. Three different types of angina exist: (1) stable, (2) unstable, and (3) variant. Stable angina (also called *chronic angina* or *exertional angina*) occurs most often with exercise or activity and usually subsides with rest. Other precipitating factors are smoking, physical exertion, emotional stress, and heavy meals. The pain is usually substernal and described by the patient as viselike, burning, squeezing, or smothering. The pain may radiate to either arm, the shoulder, the jaw, the neck, or the epigastrium. Accompanying symptoms are diaphoresis, dyspnea, nausea, and vomiting. Stable angina occurs intermittently and is often predictable. Usually stable angina lasts only a few minutes and is relieved by rest or with nitroglycerin.

Unstable angina (categorized and treated as an ACS) is also called *crescendo angina* or *preinfarction angina.* The pain of unstable angina is more severe, occurs at rest or with minimal exertion, is often not relieved by nitroglycerin or requires more frequent nitroglycerin administration, and is not predictable. Unstable angina may occur in a patient with a history of stable angina; the patient may describe a change in the pain pattern or in the severity of the pain. On the other hand, unstable angina could be the first clinical manifestation of CHD that a patient experiences. In either case, unstable angina is considered more serious than stable angina and will be treated differently. Patients with unstable angina are at higher risk for MI and are often hospitalized for diagnostic workup and treatment.

Variant angina (also known as *Prinzmetal angina*) is caused by coronary artery spasm and may not be associated with CHD. This type of angina is unpredictable and often occurs at rest. When the coronary spasm occurs, the patient experiences angina and, if the patient is being monitored, transient ST segment elevation may be seen. When the spasm subsides, the pain goes away and the ST segment returns to normal. The treatment for variant angina is usually administration of calcium channel blockers to prevent the spasms from occurring.

Medical Treatment

Treatment of CHD includes diet therapy, drug therapy, and reduction of modifiable risk factors (e.g., smoking, overweight and obesity, high blood pressure). Recommendations for medical therapy have been developed for stable angina (Fihn et al., 2012) and unstable angina (Jneid et al., 2012). Initial therapy for patients with stable angina should be guided by the following mnemonic:

- A Antiplatelet, antianginal therapy, and ACE inhibitor
- B Beta-blocker and blood pressure
- C Cigarette smoking and cholesterol
- D Diet and diabetes
- E Education and exercise
- F Flu vaccine

Low-dose aspirin is administered to interfere with platelet aggregation and it may reduce the risk of MI (Ki & Bavry, 2013). If the patient cannot tolerate aspirin, another antiplatelet medication (e.g., Ticlid, Plavix) will be prescribed. Antianginal therapy includes nitrates, beta-adrenergic blockers, and calcium channel blockers. Nitrates such as nitroglycerin are used to treat actual episodes of angina and to prevent the occurrence of angina. Various forms of nitroglycerin are prescribed for treatment of angina. These are administered sublingually or buccally at the onset of pain. They are quickly absorbed and usually effective. Oral, topical, and transdermal nitrates may be ordered to prevent angina attacks. Beta-adrenergic blockers and calcium channel blockers are prescribed in the long-term management of angina.

After the initial relief and control of the anginal pain, the focus of therapy will turn to risk reduction to include optimizing blood pressure, smoking cessation, lipid control (diet alone or diet plus lipid-lowering medications), healthy diet and tight glucose control for diabetic patients, increasing physical activity, patient education (i.e., medication therapy, risk reduction, and what to do if symptoms of an MI occur), and yearly flu vaccine.

ACE inhibitors may also be prescribed to patients with stable angina to reduce the risk of MI. In addition, some patients may be recommended for further treatment with PCI, such as angioplasty, stent placement, or atherectomy.

Additional information about various drug therapies is presented in Table 36-7.

Unstable angina may be treated conservatively or more aggressively, depending on the situation. Because unstable angina may be a warning of more serious events, it has been classified as an ACS. In current recommendations, unstable angina and NSTEMI are addressed together because they are so closely related (Jneid et al., 2012). Patients with unstable angina should receive the A-B-C-D-E-Fs listed above. However, in addition to antiplatelet therapy, anticoagulation therapy with LMWH may be administered. For patients who will be undergoing cardiac catheterization and PCI, a platelet GP IIb/IIIa antagonist will also be administered.

Surgical Intervention

Surgical procedures to treat CHD are discussed under "Common Therapeutic Measures:—Preoperative and Postoperative Nursing Care of the Cardiac Surgery Patient." .

MYOCARDIAL INFARCTION

An MI is the death of myocardial tissue as a result of prolonged lack of blood and O_2 supply. Approximately 525,000 Americans have a new myocardial infarction every year and 190,000 Americans have recurrent attacks annually. Approximately 162,000 individuals in the United States will die each year from **myocardial infarction**. The average age for men having a first heart attack is 64.7 years and the average age for women having a first heart attack is 72.2 years (Go et al., 2013).

Risk Factors

Risk factors for MI include overweight and obesity, smoking, a high-fat diet, hypertension, family history, male gender, diabetes mellitus, physical inactivity, and excessive stress. Smoking, a high-fat diet, hypertension, physical inactivity, and stress are considered modifiable risk factors. This means that risk can be reduced by cessation of smoking, diet modification, management of hypertension, regular exercise, and stress reduction.

Pathophysiology

An MI begins with the occlusion of a coronary artery. Over a period of 4 to 6 hours, a process of ischemia, injury, and infarction develops. Ischemia results from a lack of blood and O_2 to a portion of the heart muscle. If ischemia is not reversed, injury occurs. Deprived of blood and O_2, the affected tissue becomes soft and loses its normal color. With continued ischemia, an infarction, or death of myocardial tissue, occurs. Ischemia lasting 20 minutes or more is sufficient to produce irreversible tissue damage.

Within 24 hours after an infarction, the healing process begins. By the third day, necrotic tissue has been broken down by enzymes and removed by macrophages. Collateral circulation develops to supply the injured area and scar tissue begins to form. About 10 to 14 days after the MI, the myocardium is especially vulnerable to stress because of the weakness of the healing tissue. Complete healing takes about 6 weeks.

An MI is considered an ACS, along with unstable angina, as mentioned earlier. For purposes of diagnosis and treatment, health care providers divide MI into two types: (1) NSTEMI and (2) STEMI. The ST segment of an ECG is usually flat or isoelectric (see "Interpretation of Electrocardiograms"). Because the ST segment can be displaced when partial or complete lack of O_2 flow to the myocardial cells occurs, the appearance of a patient's ST segment is an important component of the assessment of an MI. Patients with NSTEMI usually have transient or partial occlusion of a coronary artery whereas patients with STEMI have total occlusion of a coronary artery from coronary thrombosis.

Complications

The major complications of MI are dysrhythmias, HF, cardiogenic shock, **thromboembolism**, sudden cardiac death (SCD), and ventricular aneurysm and rupture.

Dysrhythmias. **Dysrhythmias** are disturbances in heart rhythm, including excessively rapid, slow, or irregular heartbeats. They occur in approximately 80% of all patients with MI. Because some dysrhythmias are life threatening, continuous cardiac monitoring is usually ordered for patients with MI. This permits early detection and prompt treatment of dysrhythmias. Recognition and treatment of specific dysrhythmias are addressed under "Electrocardiogram Monitoring" near the end of this chapter.

Heart Failure. The MI may cause the heart to fail as a pump if the injured LV is unable to meet the body's circulatory demands. The ventricle fails to empty efficiently. Increased preload leads to systemic and pulmonary edema. Initial signs and symptoms include dyspnea, restlessness, and increased heart rate. Cardiac output and blood pressure fall. Untreated HF progresses to cardiogenic shock and death. HF may become a chronic condition.

Cardiogenic Shock. Cardiogenic shock is the most frequent cause of death after an MI. It is usually related to extensive injury to the LV and is more common when the patient has had a previous infarction. Cardiogenic shock is marked by hypotension; cool, moist skin; oliguria; and decreasing alertness.

Thromboembolism. After an MI, thrombi may form in the injured heart chambers or in the veins of the legs. The thrombi may break loose, travel through the circulation, and lodge in the lung. Pallor, cyanosis, and HF may be caused by pulmonary emboli. Massive pulmonary embolism is characterized by sudden, severe dyspnea. It is usually fatal. Pulmonary emboli are discussed in detail in Chapter 31.

Sudden Cardiac Death. SCD occurs when heart activity and respirations cease abruptly. The most common underlying reason for sudden cardiac death is CHD and it can be a complication of MI.

The SCD event usually occurs during ordinary activity. It is often preceded by ventricular tachycardia or ventricular fibrillation and occasionally by severe bradydysrhythmias (slow, abnormal cardiac rhythms). Other causes include left ventricular dysfunction, cardiomyopathy (CMP), electrolyte imbalance, antidysrhythmics, electrocution, and pulmonary embolism.

Those who survive an episode of SCD need to undergo extensive testing to determine the nature and cause of the episode. Many of these people will need treatment of CHD (medical therapy, PCI, or coronary artery bypass graft [CABG]). Most of these patients have a lethal dysrhythmia that requires intervention. Diagnostic tests include 24-hour Holter monitoring or ILR (or both), stress testing, and electrophysiology study. During the electrophysiology study, pacing electrodes are placed in the heart and electrical stimuli are used to elicit the dysrhythmia. This helps the physician to determine appropriate medical therapy. In some patients, the dysrhythmia may be treated during the EPS with catheter ablation. The ablation (removal or "burning") of abnormal conduction pathways or irritable sites in the heart can prevent the dysrhythmia from recurring. Still other patients are treated effectively with antidysrhythmic agents such as amiodarone (Cordarone). Preventing the reoccurrence of SCD currently is accomplished with the use of an AICD.

Ventricular Aneurysm and Rupture. Weakened areas of the ventricular wall may bulge during contractions. If scar tissue is inadequate to strengthen the wall, an aneurysm may develop and rupture. Ventricular rupture is fatal.

Signs and Symptoms

Pain is the classic symptom of MI. It is typically a heavy or constrictive pain located below or behind the sternum, as described with angina. It may radiate to the arms, back, neck, or jaw. The pain may begin with or without exertion and lasts for more than 20 minutes. The pain is described as more severe than the pain of angina. The patient becomes diaphoretic and lightheaded and may experience nausea, vomiting, and dyspnea. The skin is frequently cold and clammy. The patient experiences great anxiety and often a feeling of impending doom. However, not all patients experience the more classic signs and symptoms. Women, older adults, and diabetic patients often have atypical symptoms. Women may complain of fatigue, shortness of breath, and atypical chest pain. Older adults and diabetic patients may not experience chest pain but will complain of other symptoms such as shortness of breath, dizziness, and nausea.

Medical Diagnosis

The diagnosis of MI is based primarily on the patient's history and the physical signs and symptoms. Laboratory evidence and ECG changes help to confirm the MI.

Cardiac Markers

Troponin. Cardiac troponin T (cTnT) and cardiac troponin I (cTnI) are proteins released from cardiac muscle when the muscle is damaged. Troponin levels elevate in 3 hours after myocardial injury, peak in 12 hours, and remain in the circulation for up to 10 to 14 days. Troponin levels may be drawn in the emergency department, helping to establish an early diagnosis.

Cardiac Enzymes. A blood sample is drawn from anyone with prolonged chest pain to measure cardiac enzymes. With sustained ischemia, the cell membrane is impaired and enzymes are released from their intracellular location into the interstitial fluid. These enzymes can be measured in the serum and are assessed at regular intervals to confirm MI. CK and its isoenzyme CK-MB (myocardial) elevate rapidly with infarction. Beginning 4 to 6 hours after infarction, the CK rises to five or more times the normal level within 18 to 24 hours and returns to normal in 2 to 3 days.

Myoglobin. Myoglobin is released within 1 to 4 hours after an MI and levels rise before CK-MB levels; therefore myoglobin levels can be helpful in the early diagnosis of MI. Myoglobin levels also will be increased after strenuous exercise or renal failure and in the presence of neuromuscular disease.

Electrocardiogram. Changes in the normal waveform and dysrhythmias can be seen on an ECG. With ischemia, the ST segment is often depressed and the T wave is inverted. If prolonged total occlusion of a coronary artery has occurred, the ECG will show ST segment elevation (STEMI). If transient or partial occlusion of the artery has occurred, the ECG may not show ST segment elevation (NSTEMI). After infarction, another change often seen on the ECG waveforms is a significant Q wave (Fig. 36-8). A significant Q wave is one that is greater than one third the height of the R wave. The most frequently observed dysrhythmias are premature ventricular contractions, ventricular tachycardia, and ventricular fibrillation.

Medical Treatment

The goals of medical therapy after MI are to limit the amount of cardiac muscle injury, to relieve symptoms, and to prevent or minimize complications (Jneid et al., 2012; O'Gara et al., 2012).

Drug Therapy. Sublingual or IV nitroglycerin is administered to dilate coronary arteries and increase blood flow to the damaged area. If the nitroglycerin relieves the pain, the infarction may not extend. Morphine sulfate is also used for chest pain. It has many effects in addition to analgesia. Morphine causes peripheral pooling of blood, which decreases the blood returning to the heart and lungs. It also diminishes anxiety, decreases tachypnea, and relaxes bronchial smooth muscles, thereby improving gas exchange. If the patient cannot tolerate morphine, meperidine (Demerol) may be ordered but it does not have all of the other beneficial properties of morphine and may increase the heart rate.

O_2 is administered at 4 to 6 L/min to assist in oxygenating myocardial tissue to support pumping activity and to repair damaged tissue. If the patient is not already on aspirin (or other antiplatelet medication), aspirin will be administered.

Fibrinolytic therapy is recommended for patients with STEMI (patients with total occlusion from thrombus formation) when PCI is not available (Levine, 2012). Fibrinolytics such as streptokinase and t-PA are administered intravenously to dissolve the thrombus. This treatment is most effective when initiated early (within 30 minutes of arrival to hospital) but may be administered up to 12 hours from the onset of chest pain. The patient must meet strict criteria (i.e., no recent surgery or active bleeding, no history of a stroke, no bleeding disorders) and provide informed consent before the administration of fibrinolytic agents. After administration of the fibrinolytic agents, heparin is administered to prevent further clot formation. To monitor the effectiveness of this therapy, nurses should assess for relief of chest pain and the return of the ST segment to baseline. Bleeding is the greatest risk associated with fibrinolytic therapy and the nurse should assess for signs of major bleeding: change in level of consciousness from intracerebral bleeding; decrease in Hgb and Hct; sudden decrease in blood pressure and increase in HR; and blood in stool, urine, or both.

Beta-adrenergic blockers should be administered as soon as the patient can tolerate them and if not contraindicated. Beta-adrenergic blockers improve survival rates by decreasing the heart rate, reducing the work of the heart, and lessening the O_2 demand of the myocardium. ACE inhibitors may be prescribed for some patients to minimize the abnormal shaping or ventricular remodeling that can occur in the damaged ventricular muscle. As the myocardium receives blood and O_2, reperfusion dysrhythmias that require treatment may be noted.

Dysrhythmias often occur as a result of either the MI or medication therapy; they should be treated if they are causing the patient symptoms.

Percutaneous Coronary Intervention. Emergency PCI is the first choice for treatment of an MI, if available (Levine, 2012). The goal is to reopen the occluded artery within 90 minutes of arrival to the emergency department. Several PCI procedures (American Heart Association-Cardiac Procedures, 2013) can be performed in the cardiac catheterization laboratory: percutaneous transluminal coronary angioplasty (PTCA, or balloon angioplasty), intracoronary stent placement, atherectomy, and laser angioplasty. PTCA

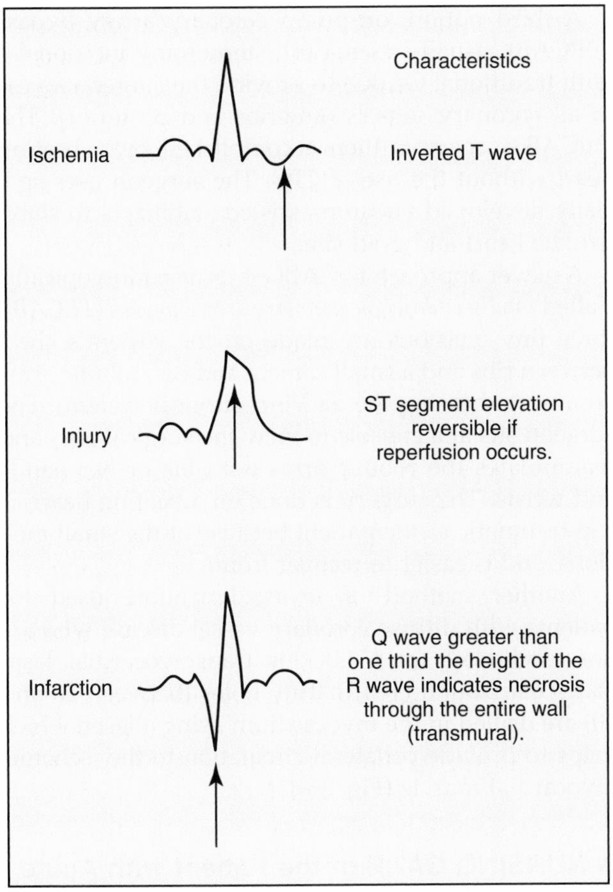

FIGURE 36-8 Electrocardiographic changes with myocardial infarction.

involves passage of a catheter through a peripheral artery (usually the femoral artery) into the occluded coronary artery. The tip of the catheter contains a balloon that is inflated to compress the atherosclerotic plaque and dilate the artery. PTCA is often used when single-vessel disease, noncalcified lesions, or lesions that are not at bifurcations are noted. The majority of PTCA procedures include the placement of intracoronary stents. Stents are devices that are positioned within the blockage through a balloon-tipped catheter, expanded into place, and left to support the arterial wall. Over time, endothelial cells will line the inner wall of the stent completely to produce a smooth inner lining (Fig. 36-9). After an intracoronary stent is placed, the patient will be on antiplatelet agents or anticoagulants to decrease the chance of occlusion in the stent. Stents are available coated with a medication that prevents overgrowth of the new inner lining and reduces the incidence of reocclusion (American Heart Association-Cardiac Procedures, 2013).

When appropriate, PTCA and/or intracoronary stent placement is preferred over coronary artery bypass surgery because it can be done under local anesthetic, it is less invasive, and the recovery time is faster. The procedure is safer than bypass surgery but is not without risks. Complications of PTCA and

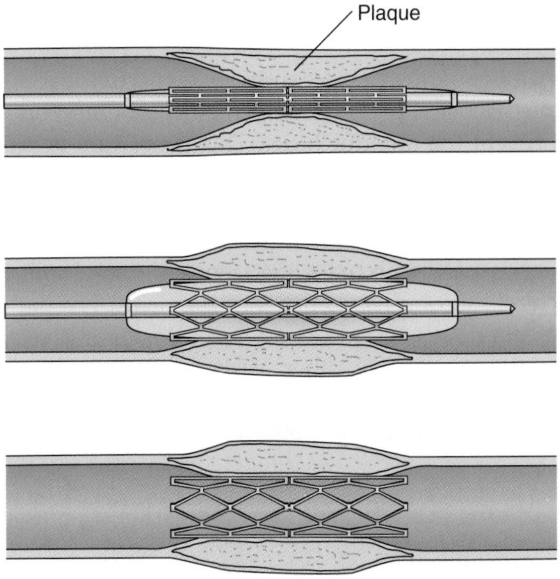

FIGURE 36-9 Intracoronary stent. (From Lewis SM, Heitkemper MM, Dirksen SR, et al: *Medical-surgical nursing: assessment and management of clinical problems*, ed 9, St. Louis, 2015, Mosby.)

intracoronary stents include coronary artery dissection, dysrhythmias, coronary spasm, hematoma at the catheter site, restenosis, and death. Coronary atherectomy is a procedure that widens the coronary artery by removing the atherosclerotic plaque using a device that shaves the plaque off the vessel walls. The laser angioplasty uses a catheter with a laser on its tip. The laser is used to widen the lumen of the artery by destroying atherosclerotic plaque.

Coronary Artery Bypass Graft Surgery. CABG surgery (also known as coronary revascularization surgery) may be performed to improve the blood supply to the myocardium (American Heart Association-Cardiac Procedures, 2013). Arterial bypass surgery uses the patient's own vasculature as bypasses for occluded coronary arteries. Multiple occluded sections may be bypassed during a single surgical procedure. The saphenous veins and the internal mammary artery are most commonly used. The saphenous veins are removed from one or both legs, inspected for patency, and reversed so that the valves do not inhibit blood flow. The bypass vessels are attached to the aorta and below the occlusions in the coronary arteries and serve as new conduits for oxygenated blood to the myocardium (Fig. 36-10). The internal mammary artery is left attached to the subclavian (point of origin), dissected from surrounding tissue, and attached to the coronary artery below the occlusion. This is major surgery that requires the heartbeat to be stopped and the patient to be placed on a cardiopulmonary bypass (CPB) machine during the surgery. Use of CPB supports the body's tissue needs during the surgery but several complications are associated with CPB. These include postoperative bleeding, hypothermia, dysrhythmias, unstable hemodynamics, and pulmonary dysfunction.

The survival rate is higher in patients who are in stable condition.

Another approach to surgical revascularization is being used on patients who require surgery on the arteries of the anterior heart. This procedure is called *minimally invasive direct coronary artery bypass grafting* and is performed through a small anterior thoracotomy incision. The patient's left internal mammary artery is used to bypass the stenosed vessel and the bypass is accomplished on a beating heart. The patient does not have to be placed on CPB. Postoperative care is similar to that of other cardiac surgery, although patients do not require as lengthy ventilatory support and total hospital stay is shorter.

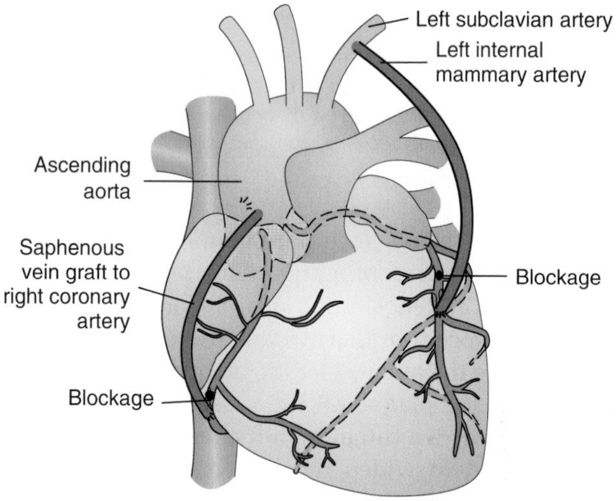

FIGURE 36-10 Coronary artery bypass graft (CABG) surgery. (From Lewis SL, Dirksen SR, Heitkemper MM, et al: *Medical-surgical nursing: assessment and management of clinical problems*, ed 8, St. Louis, 2010, Mosby.)

A third option, off-pump coronary artery bypass (OPCAB), usually uses a full sternotomy incision (as with traditional CABG) to provide the surgeon access to all coronary vessels (anterior and posterior). The OPCAB surgery is then accomplished on a beating heart without the use of CPB. The surgeon uses specially developed vacuum-assisted stabilizers to stabilize the heart and graft site.

A newer approach to CABG is done endoscopically. Called *totally endoscopic coronary artery bypass (TECAB)*, three tiny incisions are made on the patient's chest between ribs and a small camera and two robotic arms are inserted (using the da Vinci surgical system). The surgeon sits at a console to view the surgical area and manipulates the robotic arms with his or her hands and wrists. The surgery is done on a beating heart, is less traumatic to the patient because of the small incisions, and is easier to recover from.

Another method of revascularization, used for patients with diffuse coronary vessel disease who are not candidates for CABG, is transmyocardial laser revascularization (TMR). Tiny holes (between 10 and 50) are drilled in the myocardium using a laser, which helps to provide collateral circulation to the ischemic myocardial muscle (Fig. 36-11).

❖ NURSING CARE of the Patient with Acute Myocardial Infarction

■ Assessment

General assessment of the cardiac patient is summarized in Box 36-1. When a patient has an MI, be especially concerned with assessment of pain. When chest pain is present, early evaluation and treatment are paramount. Ask the patient to describe the pain,

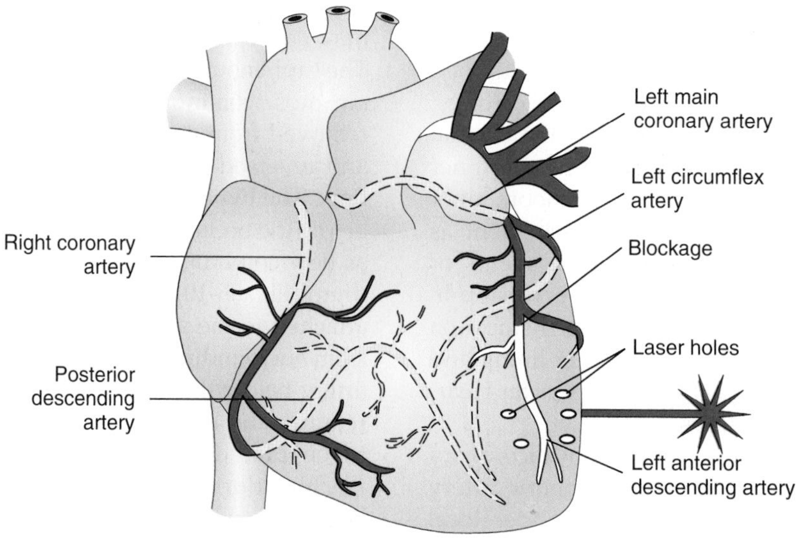

FIGURE 36-11 Transmyocardial laser revascularization (TMR). (From Ballard JC, Wood LL, Lansing AM: Transmyocardial revascularization: criteria for selecting patients, treatment, and nursing care, *Crit Care Nurs* 17(1):42–49, 1997. Reprinted with permission.)

including type, location, duration, and severity. It is recommended that chest pain be assessed using the mnemonic PQRST, as follows:

P Precipitating factors, palliative: What was the patient doing when the pain began? Did anything make the pain better? Worse?
Q Quality: Have the patient describe what the pain feels like (in his or her own words).
R Region, radiation: Where is the pain located? Does it hurt anywhere else?
S Severity, symptoms: Have the patient rate the pain. Use the 0 to 10 pain scale. Note other symptoms (e.g., nausea, diaphoresis).
T Time: When did the pain start? How long did it last?

Record what the patient was doing when the pain started, what action was taken, and the effects of any actions or treatments. In addition, inspect the patient's skin for color and palpate for temperature and moisture. Frequently assess vital signs and document the patient's mental status and level of anxiety. When cardiac monitoring is initiated, evaluate the rate and rhythm.

Nursing Diagnoses, Goals, and Outcome Criteria: Acute Myocardial Infarction

Nursing Diagnoses	Goals and Outcome Criteria
Acute Pain related to lack of oxygen (O_2) to the myocardium	Pain relief: patient statement of relieved pain, relaxed manner
Decreased Cardiac Output related to dysrhythmia and abnormal heart rate	Normal cardiac output: normal pulse, blood pressure, and cardiac rhythm
Anxiety related to feeling of impending doom, lack of understanding of routines	Reduced anxiety: patient statement of lessened anxiety, calm manner, and self-care

Interventions

Acute Pain

Administer analgesics as ordered and monitor for relief of pain. Morphine is usually administered in small amounts (2 to 4 mg) intravenously every few minutes until pain relief is evident. Provide supplemental O_2 as ordered through nasal cannula at 2 to 4 L/min to provide adequate O_2 to the heart muscle. The head of the bed is usually elevated at least 30 degrees. Inform the physician if the patient has an increasing respiratory rate or dyspnea.

Decreased Cardiac Output

Monitor the patient's vital signs hourly or more frequently until he or she is stable. Watch the ECG for changes from the normal waveform (inverted T wave, ST segment elevation, and Q wave) and for dysrhythmias. Notify the physician of changes in the rhythm. In an intensive care unit, standing orders prescribe drug therapy for specific dysrhythmias. An IV line is usually established so that emergency drugs can be administered quickly and directly. Prompt treatment of dysrhythmias may prevent fatal alterations in rhythm. Monitor the patient for fluid volume excess (crackles, cough, jugular vein distention) and report any such evidence to the physician.

Interventions to decrease demands on the heart include assisting the patient to rest; spacing activities and providing rest periods; providing adequate ventilation and oxygenation; relieving pain; and maintaining a calm, quiet environment.

Anxiety

Provide as calm an environment as possible and explain procedures and equipment to the patient and family, using simple terms. Keep family members informed of the patient's progress. They can be helpful in calming the patient during the acute episode.

During the acute phase of MI, provide simple explanations of the procedures and routines. Reinforce information given by the physician about the diagnosis and treatment. Patient teaching is especially important in the rehabilitation phase.

Cardiac Rehabilitation

As soon as the patient is stable, begin rehabilitation by teaching the patient and family about exercise, medications, and diet. If surgical intervention has been proposed, you may also teach the patient about that procedure.

The purpose of rehabilitation is to minimize the risk of repetition of adverse cardiac events. The goal of rehabilitation is to enable patients to attain the highest level of wellness and work ability.

The program is individualized to the patient for maximal success (see *Patient Teaching* box). The four phases of cardiac rehabilitation are (1) inpatient management; (2) immediately after discharge, using telemetry monitoring during exercise; (3) later rehabilitation, which is unmonitored; and (4) maintenance. A team of medical professionals (e.g., nurse, physician, physical therapist, nutritionist, social worker) plans the individual program. Education during the rehabilitation process should include normal anatomy and physiology of the heart; pathophysiology of CHD, angina, and MI; risk factor modification; activity and exercise; medications; diet; and when to seek medical advice. See the *Nutrition Considerations* box for a discussion of dietary considerations for patients with heart disease.

Nutrition Considerations

1. A major part of treatment for people with heart disease is reduction of fat and cholesterol in the diet.
2. When fats are used in cooking or eating, unsaturated fats (vegetable oil such as corn oil, canola oil, or olive oil) should be substituted for saturated fats (animal fat such as butter or lard).
3. Fats and oils used in cooking or eating should be limited to five to eight servings daily in normal adults.
4. Saturated fat can be limited by eating only 5 to 7 oz of meat daily.
5. Foods that contain omega-3 fatty acids (certain fish, walnuts, and soybeans) lower serum triglycerides and decrease the number of deaths resulting from heart disease.

Patient Teaching

Myocardial Infarction

After myocardial infarction (MI), the following are some key points in the discharge teaching plan:

- It is very important to take your medications as prescribed and to contact the physician if you have any problems. (Provide written information about drug names, dosages, purpose, interactions with other medications and foods, and adverse effects that should be reported.)
- Your physician may prescribe a low-fat, low-sodium diet to decrease weight and to reduce the workload on your heart.
- Participation in cardiac rehabilitation will help you to become active again in a safe manner.
- Stop smoking. Smoking stimulates the heart rate and causes blood vessels to constrict, which makes the heart work harder.
- Maintain normal weight (or lose weight if obese) to decrease the work of the heart.
- The local chapter of the American Heart Association is a helpful resource for information and guidance on diet, smoking cessation, and exercise.

Put on Your Thinking Cap!

A new patient is being seen in the physician's office. Basic information and health history data include the following: 58-year-old Caucasian man, blood pressure 152/84 mm Hg, pulse 82 beats per minute (bpm), respiration 14 breaths per minute, temperature 98°F (36.7°C) measured orally, height 5′9″, weight 190 lb.

SOCIAL HISTORY

Real estate salesman (describes himself as "pretty successful" and able to maintain a good quality of life). Plays tennis three times a week; walks 2 miles, four times a week. Divorced father of three adult children; one son who recently was admitted to rehabilitation for substance abuse has no insurance. Patient has conflict with ex-wife related to son's situation. Enjoys a "few beers" in the evening. Has eggs, bacon, biscuits, coffee for breakfast; has lunch (sandwich, fries) at a fast-food restaurant; and cooks dinner (usually "meat and potatoes"). Sleeps 7 to 8 hours; usually rested on arising. Some recent trouble sleeping because of son's problems. No current significant other.

HEALTH HISTORY

Hypertension for 5 years treated with daily antihypertensive drug; chronic sinusitis; arthritis in left knee related to sports injury.

FAMILY HISTORY

Mother, age 78, living and in moderately good health. Had mild stroke last year without permanent effects. Has diabetes. Father died suddenly at age 66 of myocardial infarction (MI). Two living brothers, ages 52 and 49. Both are hypertensive.

ANALYSIS

1. Based on the data available, identify modifiable and unmodifiable risk factors for coronary heart disease (CHD).
2. Identify one strategy to address each modifiable factor.
3. Identify current factors that reduce the patient's risk of CHD.

HEART FAILURE

HF is the inability of the heart to meet the metabolic demands of the body. The pumping ability of the heart is ineffective.

Cause and Risk Factors

Heart failure is the preferred term used to describe the clinical picture of failure. *Congestive heart failure* is a term commonly used for HF; it describes the symptoms seen when the heart fails to pump effectively and blood "backs up" into the vasculature of the lungs, producing congestion. The two terms (*HF* and *CHF*) are often used interchangeably in the clinical setting. Causes of HF are primarily of two types: (1) disorders that increase the workload of the heart and (2) disorders that interfere with the pumping ability of the heart. Therefore patients at risk for HF include those with CHD, MI, CMP, hypertension, COPD, pulmonary hypertension, anemia, disease of the heart valves, and fluid volume overload. Other conditions that increase metabolic needs, such as fever and pregnancy, also may precipitate HF. Approximately 5.1 million Americans have HF and HF is expected to increase by 25% by 2030 (Go et al., 2013). After age 65, 10 in 1000 individuals have HF and 75% of patients with HF have a history of hypertension (Go et al., 2013).

Pathophysiology

The LV, RV, or both fail as pumps. Usually the left side of the heart fails first. In time, the right side fails as a result of the left-sided failure. HF can be classified as *systolic HF resulting from ineffective pumping of the ventricles* or as *diastolic HF resulting from impaired filling of the ventricles.* With either classification, cardiac output is decreased. HF can occur acutely, with onset over several hours or days, or it can be chronic, with onset over months to years. In addition, patients with chronic HF can experience acute heart failure syndrome (AHFS).

Compensation. *Compensation* is a term used to describe the cardiac and circulatory adjustments that maintain or restore cardiac output to normal or near normal. Compensation occurs through several mechanisms, although the major mechanisms are sympathetic nervous system stimulation, regulation of blood volume by the kidneys, and enlargement of the ventricular myocardium.

Sympathetic Compensation. The sympathetic nervous system responds to decreased cardiac output and blood pressure. Catecholamines are released that increase heart rate, stroke volume, cardiac output, and venous tone. Increased venous tone increases systemic vascular resistance, venous return, and ventricular filling.

Renal Compensation. The second mechanism that responds to decreased cardiac output is renal compensation. When cardiac output falls, so does renal perfusion. This initiates the RAA mechanism. Renin, secreted by the kidneys, activates angiotensinogen to convert to angiotensin I. Angiotensin I is converted to angiotensin II, which causes vasoconstriction and triggers release of aldosterone. Vasoconstriction raises the blood pressure by increasing peripheral resistance to blood flow. Aldosterone causes the kidneys to retain sodium and water, which increases blood volume.

Natriuretic Peptides. Natriuretic peptides are neurohormonal substances released with HF. Atrial natriuretic peptide (ANP) is released in response to increased volume and stretch in the cardiac atria. BNP is released when the cardiac ventricles stretch, usually from increased blood volume. The natriuretic peptides are thought to counter the vasoconstrictive and volume-increasing effects of the sympathetic nervous system and the RAA system. BNP levels can be measured in the blood and can be used as a diagnostic tool for HF.

Ventricular Hypertrophy. The final mechanism is enlargement of the ventricular myocardium, called *ventricular hypertrophy*, which results from strain and initially increases contractility. The increased blood volume raises the pressure in the ventricles, which can also cause the ventricles to dilate. Eventually the ventricle changes in size and shape, which impairs pumping effectiveness. This process is called *ventricular remodeling*.

After a period, the compensatory mechanisms may no longer be able to meet the increased demands. AHFS, a gradual or rapid change in HF signs and symptoms, occurs when compensatory mechanisms are overwhelmed. Contractility decreases; the heart muscle can stretch only so far before becoming inefficient. The force of contraction of the LV decreases. Stroke volume and cardiac output decrease as pumping action fails. Afterload increases with left-sided HF. Blood backs up in the LA and then in the pulmonary veins. Because of the high pressure in the pulmonary veins (pulmonary hypertension), fluid leaks from the capillaries into the interstitial space and alveoli, causing pulmonary edema. Pulmonary hypertension eventually causes the right side of the heart to fail as well. Then blood returning to the right side of the heart from the body meets resistance from the pulmonary hypertension, which causes blood to back up into the venous system and organs. This results in peripheral edema and enlargement of the liver and spleen. If HF is not corrected, death eventually ensues.

With left-sided HF, the patient has increased left ventricular end-diastolic pressure, increased left atrial pressure, increased pulmonary pressure, and resulting pulmonary edema as the excess fluid leaks into the lung tissues. In right-sided HF, right ventricular pressure increases, right atrial pressure increases, and fluid accumulates in the systemic vasculature.

Put on Your Thinking Cap!

1. Explain why a patient with heart failure (HF) might (1) feel anxious and (2) gain weight.
2. A patient with HF is advised to try to lose 30 lb. What nursing strategies would help her to achieve this goal?
3. You suspect that a patient with HF and hypertension is not taking her blood pressure medication regularly as prescribed. What strategies might improve her compliance?

Signs and Symptoms

The patient with left-sided HF is typically very anxious, pale, weak, and tachycardic. Consecutive blood pressure readings may show a downward trend. Auscultation of the lung fields may reveal crackles, wheezes, dyspnea, and cough. When assessing heart sounds, S_3 and S_4 may be heard as a result of the backup of fluid and the heart's inability to handle the excess fluid. The exchange of O_2 and CO_2 in the lungs is impaired and patients are often restless and confused.

With right-sided HF, the patient has increased central venous pressure, jugular venous distention, abdominal engorgement, and dependent edema. Anorexia, nausea, and vomiting may result from the abdominal engorgement. Fatigue, weight gain, and decreased urinary output are common complaints.

Medical Diagnosis

The diagnosis of HF is made on the basis of the history, physical examination, radiographs, and laboratory test results. A chest radiograph may reveal hazy lung fields, distended vasculature, and cardiomegaly. An echocardiogram may reveal heart enlargement and ineffective ventricular contraction. Laboratory tests indicative of HF are decreased serum sodium and Hct from hemodilution and decreased saturated arterial oxygenation from poor pulmonary perfusion. The blood urea nitrogen (BUN) and creatinine are elevated with decreased renal function. BNP levels are elevated in HF and the higher the levels, the more severe the failure. Liver function test results are elevated with hepatomegaly (liver enlargement). The patient who is critically ill with HF may require more intensive monitoring of **hemodynamic** parameters.

Medical Treatment

Medical treatment of HF (Yancy et al., 2013) includes management of the underlying cause, drug therapy to improve cardiac output and eliminate excess fluid, conservative measures to decrease demands on the heart, and possibly cardiac resynchronization therapy (CRT). Sodium restriction is prescribed for most patients with HF.

Treatment of the underlying problem may involve such interventions as correction of dysrhythmias, management of hypertension, and valve replacement or repair.

Drug Therapy. A number of drugs are used to treat HF. Current recommendations include ACE inhibitors, diuretics, beta-adrenergic blockers, inotropic agents, cardiac glycosides, and nitrates. In addition, certain patients will benefit from BNP. ACE inhibitors decrease preload and afterload by blocking the RAA system, resulting in vasodilation, decreased blood volume, and lower blood pressure. In addition, ACE inhibitors are thought to limit the progression of ventricular remodeling. Diuretics are prescribed to decrease circulating fluid volume and decrease preload. Loop diuretics such as furosemide (Lasix) are usually used in HF. Spironolactone, a weak potassium-sparing diuretic drug, may be prescribed for some patients because it acts by blocking aldosterone and may slow the process of remodeling. Beta-adrenergic blockers improve survival rates by decreasing the heart rate, reducing the work of the heart, and lessening the O_2 demand of the myocardium. Inotropic agents such as dopamine, dobutamine, and amrinone are prescribed initially and in the short term to improve cardiac contractility, improve renal perfusion, and decrease fluid retention. Digoxin, a cardiac glycoside with inotropic effects, is prescribed in the long term to improve pump function by increasing contractility and decreasing heart rate. Nesiritide (Natrecor) is a recombinant human BNP that may be prescribed in patients with AHFS. Nesiritide counteracts the vasoconstriction and fluid retention of the RAA system and relieves the severe dyspnea seen in these patients. Nitrates, such as nitroglycerin, are venodilators that reduce preload for patients with HF. This helps to reduce the workload on the heart. Morphine may be used to decrease anxiety, dilate the vasculature, and reduce myocardial O_2 consumption in the acute stage. Table 36-7 provides additional information on drugs used to treat HF.

Other Therapies. Other therapies are available to decrease cardiac workload and increase myocardial oxygenation. The intraaortic balloon pump (IABP), ventricular assist devices (VADs), and CRT (also called biventricular pacing) may be used. The IABP is a temporary device used in the intensive care unit to increase cardiac output and coronary artery perfusion. VADs can partially or completely support a patient's failing heart. In some patients with HF, a VAD is considered a temporary intervention, used as a "bridge" to transplantation. Other patients may have long-term therapy with a VAD instead of transplantation; this is called destination therapy (Vallika & Cotts, 2012). CRT is useful in patients with HF who have conduction delays in the right or left bundle branch. These conduction delays result in the ventricles being depolarized and contracting out of synchrony. This reduces cardiac output and can contribute to the worsening of HF. In CRT, leads are placed in both ventricles and stimulated at the same time. Cardiac contraction occurs in both ventricles at the same time and cardiac output is improved.

Surgery. CABG surgery is recommended in patients with HF who experience angina. Valve repair or replacement is recommended when valve dysfunction contributes to the HF. Partial left ventriculectomy may be useful in some patients. Cardiac transplantation is often the last option for patients with end-stage HF whose symptoms are not responding to conventional therapy.

Complications

Dysrhythmias, pulmonary edema, renal failure, and cardiogenic shock are possible complications.

❖ NURSING CARE of the Patient with Heart Failure

■ Assessment

Complete assessment of the cardiac patient is outlined in Box 36-1 (see also Nursing Care Plan: Patient with Heart Failure). It is especially important to assess heart sounds, rate, and rhythm. The point of maximum impulse should be noted and the apical and radial pulses assessed frequently. The nurse should inspect for jugular vein distention. A baseline respiratory assessment of rate, rhythm, and breath sounds is vital. In addition, the patient's weight and blood pressure should be measured accurately and the skin inspected and palpated for turgor and edema. Intake and output records and daily weights may be done to evaluate fluid retention or loss. If ordered, central venous pressure and hemodynamic readings should be taken as well. If cardiac monitoring is done, the nurse should observe for dysrhythmias. Nurses who work in intensive care units routinely interpret ECGs. Interpretation is discussed under "Electrocardiogram Monitoring" near the end of this chapter.

Nursing Care Plan — Patient with Heart Failure

ASSESSMENT

HEALTH HISTORY A 73-year-old Chinese-American woman is admitted through the emergency department. She is a retired business owner who lives alone and has no immediate family in the area. She began having dyspnea and orthopnea that has become progressively worse over the past 3 days. Her past medical history includes a myocardial infarction 1 year ago and a 10-year history of hypertension treated with diet and verapamil 240 mg daily. In addition to the verapamil, she takes only an occasional laxative. She complains of fatigue, restlessness, nervousness, irritability, insomnia, anorexia, and a productive cough with pink sputum.

PHYSICAL EXAMINATION Vital signs: blood pressure 168/96 mm Hg, pulse 104 bpm with slight irregularity, respiration 24 breaths per minute, temperature 98°F (36.7°C) measured orally. Height 5′2″, weight 152 lb (a 7-lb increase in 1 week). She is alert but appears anxious. Her skin is pale and diaphoretic. An S_3 is present. Jugular vein distention is noted. Auscultation of the lungs reveals crackles in the lower lobes of both lungs. The abdomen is distended. Bowel sounds are present in all four quadrants and 3+ pitting edema exists in both feet and ankles.

She is being admitted to the telemetry unit for treatment, where she will have continuous ECG and be placed on O_2.

Nursing Diagnosis	Goals and Outcome Criteria	Interventions
Decreased Cardiac Output related to decreased myocardial contractility	The patient's cardiac output will improve, as evidenced by normal heart rate and rhythm, normal blood pressure, normal hemodynamic measures, and breath sounds clear to auscultation.	Monitor the patient's vital signs, heart and lung sounds, level of consciousness, and electrocardiography. Enforce bed rest, with the head of the bed elevated. Schedule activities to allow rest. Request small, frequent meals. Administer cardiotonics, vasodilators, and angiotensin-converting enzyme (ACE) inhibitors as ordered.
Impaired Gas Exchange related to pulmonary congestion	The patient's gas exchange will be evidenced by pulse oximetry >95%, normal skin color, absence of dyspnea, and clear lung sounds.	Assess lung sounds and respiratory status every 4 hours. Monitor her oxygen (O_2) saturation. Elevate the head of the bed. Administer O_2 as ordered. Assist to cough and deep breathe every 2 hours. Administer diuretics and morphine sulfate as ordered.
Excess Fluid Volume related to decreased glomerular filtration rate, increased aldosterone, sodium and water retention, and increased antidiuretic hormone (ADH) release	The patient will have normal fluid balance as evidenced by weight of 145 lb, absence of edema, absence of crackles and wheezes in lungs, and ability to participate in activities of daily living (ADL) without dyspnea.	Monitor for jugular venous distention and peripheral edema. Auscultate heart and lung sounds every 4 hours. Measure weight daily and record her intake and output accurately. Maintain intravenous lines and correct fluid infusion rate. Administer diuretics as ordered. Teach the patient about sodium restriction and the rationale behind it. Protect any edematous extremities from pressure or injury.
Activity Intolerance related to imbalance between O_2 supply and demand	The patient's activity tolerance will improve, as evidenced by performance of ADL without excessive fatigue or dyspnea.	Assess response to activity when permitted. Monitor her for dyspnea and changes in vital signs. Limit fatiguing activities. Gradually increase activity as her tolerance improves.
Anxiety related to hypoxia, life-threatening situation	The patient's anxiety will be reduced, as evidenced by calm demeanor and statement that she feels less anxious.	Explain the procedures and equipment used. Tell her about congestive heart failure (CHF) and how it is being treated. Point out signs of improvement. Visit often and respond to the call bell promptly. Offer to engage the help of a spiritual counselor if desired.
Deficient Knowledge of condition, treatment, self-care, and resources related to lack of exposure to information.	The patient will verbalize information about her condition, treatment, self-care measures, and resources.	Provide a simple explanation of CHF, its effects, and its treatment. As discharge nears, discuss diet, exercise, and drug therapy. Explain signs and symptoms that should be reported to her physician. Advise the patient of services offered by the American Heart Association. Explore sources of support and the need for a visiting nurse or home health services.

Critical Thinking Questions

1. What is the rationale behind sodium restriction in patients with heart failure (HF)?
2. Describe three signs of improvement in a patient with HF.

Nursing Diagnoses, Goals, and Outcome Criteria: Heart Failure

Nursing Diagnosis	Goals and Outcome Criteria
Decreased Cardiac Output related to mechanical failure	Improved cardiac output: normal heart rate and rhythm, fluid intake and output equal
Impaired Gas Exchange related to decreased pulmonary perfusion	Adequate oxygenation: clear breath sounds, respiratory rate 12 to 20 breaths/min without dyspnea
Excess Fluid Volume related to ineffective cardiac pumping	Normal fluid volume: no edema or dyspnea, blood pressure consistent with patient norms
Activity Intolerance related to inability to meet oxygen (O_2) demands	Increase activity tolerance: performance of activities of daily living (ADL) without fatigue
Anxiety related to edema and difficulty breathing	Reduced anxiety: patient statement of reduced anxiety, calm manner

Interventions

Decreased Cardiac Output

Give medications as ordered and monitor the patient for therapeutic and adverse effects. Older adult patients are more susceptible to adverse drug effects because they may metabolize and excrete drugs more slowly. This is especially true when the older patient is taking digitalis. Advise the patient to report early signs of digitalis toxicity: anorexia, nausea, and visual disturbances. Bed rest and stress reduction decrease the cardiac workload. When the patient is acutely ill, eliminate all unnecessary activity. Give partial baths rather than complete bed baths and assist the patient to change positions at least every 2 hours so that the skin can be inspected for signs of pressure. Visitors may be permitted but advise them to sit quietly with the patient for short periods.

Pharmacology Capsule

Before each dose of digitalis, the apical pulse is counted for 1 full minute. If the heart rate is less than 60 beats per minute (bpm), the drug is withheld and the physician is notified.

Pharmacology Capsule

The most common adverse effects of diuretic therapy are fluid and electrolyte imbalances.

Impaired Gas Exchange

Hypoxia is a common finding with left-sided HF because of pulmonary edema. It is common with right-sided HF because of decreased blood flow to the lungs. The patient with HF usually breathes more easily in a semi-Fowler or high Fowler position. Elevation of the upper body facilitates breathing by reducing pressure of the abdominal organs on the diaphragm. Supplemental O_2 is usually prescribed at 4 to 6 L/min per nasal cannula. The flow rate may be reduced to 2 L/min for patients with chronic hypoxia. Assess the patient's respiratory status and blood gases frequently.

Prescribed bed rest can lead to other pulmonary complications related to immobility (i.e., hypostatic pneumonia, pulmonary emboli). Teach the patient to cough and deep breathe at least every 2 hours to promote respiratory excursion and to mobilize secretions. Other interventions to prevent complications of immobility are detailed in Chapter 21.

On discharge, the physician may order portable O_2 for use at home. The nurse or a respiratory therapist instructs the patient in the use of the equipment and the safety precautions to take when using O_2 (see Chapter 31).

Excess Fluid Volume

Fluid retention is a response to HF (i.e., an attempt to maintain normal cardiac output). Unfortunately, it compounds the problem by increasing the workload on the heart. Therefore measures are taken to reduce the fluid volume to normal while improving the function of the heart. Administer diuretics as ordered and monitor the patient for adverse effects. The most common adverse effects of diuretic therapy are fluid and electrolyte disturbances. Signs and symptoms that may indicate fluid or electrolyte disturbances include cardiac dysrhythmias, muscle weakness or twitching, cramps, changes in mental status, and abdominal distention. Frequent serum electrolyte measurements are usually ordered. Note the results and inform the physician of any abnormal findings. If hourly urine output is being measured, report an output of less than 30 mL/h to the physician as well. The patient should be weighed daily.

An IV catheter is usually placed to provide a line for drug administration. If IV fluids are administered, monitor the rate of administration very carefully. If fluid retention is not relieved by other means, fluid restriction may be instituted. All staff should know the exact amount of fluid allowed and must record all intake. Fluid restriction can be very uncomfortable for the patient. Even with fluid volume excess, the patient may feel thirsty because of electrolyte imbalances. Present oral fluids in small containers and offer them at reasonable intervals. Provide frequent mouth care. The patient and family must understand why fluids are restricted so that the patient does not exceed the prescribed intake.

The most common therapeutic dietary measure for chronic HF is sodium restriction (see *Patient Teaching* box). The patient may be limited to 1.5 g of sodium per day. In severe cases, a limitation of 500 to 1000 mg/day may be prescribed. Reduced sodium intake decreases fluid retention, thereby reducing the cardiac workload. For a 1.5 g sodium diet, advise the patient to avoid foods high in sodium (a list should be provided), not to add salt before or after cooking, and to use no more than 2 cups of milk products daily. Patients often have difficulty changing their use of seasonings. Acknowledge the difficulty and explain how sodium limitation contributes to improvement of cardiac function.

Patient Teaching

Chronic Heart Failure

- Reducing sodium in your diet will help to control swelling and reduce the workload on your heart.
- Excess weight makes your heart work harder. Your physician may prescribe a weight loss diet for you.
- Take your medications as prescribed to improve your heart function. (Provide written information about drug names, actions, dose, schedule, side and adverse effects, special aspects of administration, and interactions with other medications and food.)
- Gradually increase your activity. Avoid activity that causes shortness of breath or severe fatigue.
- Weigh yourself each morning, before breakfast, on the same scale and wearing the same amount of clothing.
- Contact your physician if you gain 3 to 5 lb in 1 week, develop a persistent cough, or have shortness of breath or chest pain.
- Resources: The American Heart Association provides information about diet and exercise. The Visiting Nurses Association or a home health agency can monitor your condition and help you in your home.

It is best to identify the type of diet that will be prescribed on discharge as early as possible. This allows time for a dietary consultation to be arranged, which should be followed by reinforcement by the nurse. The person who prepares the patient's meals at home must be included in the teaching sessions.

Activity Intolerance

Frequent rest periods, pacing of activities, and relaxation techniques help the patient to conserve energy. As the fluid volume is decreased and the cardiac output is increased, the patient can expect to be less fatigued.

The patient may be referred to a rehabilitation facility for exercise training. In general, the patient is advised to plan rest periods before and after tiring activities. Activity should be increased gradually, with rest periods taken when fatigue or dyspnea occurs. The physician may prescribe vasodilators for patients who experience chest pain with some activities. If monitoring is indicated after discharge, request a referral to a home nursing agency.

Instruct the patient to notify the physician if the following problems develop: increasing dyspnea or edema, excessive fatigue, or pain that is not relieved by rest or prescribed medications. Early recognition of signs and symptoms that the patient's condition is deteriorating is crucial to avoiding rehospitalization (see *Health Promotion* box). In addition, advise the patient to avoid smoking and smoky environments as well as to refrain from wearing constricting clothing on the lower extremities.

Health Promotion

Heart Failure: Discharge Instructions

A major goal for patients with heart failure (HF) is to prevent rehospitalization. A critical factor in reaching this goal is for the patient and family members to recognize early signs and symptoms of worsening failure and to contact the health care provider. Examples of symptoms to call about are difficulty breathing (especially with activity); dry, hacking cough; weakness and increased fatigue; foot and ankle swelling; dizziness; and weight gain of 3 to 5 lb in 1 week or less.

Anxiety

Factors that may cause the patient to become anxious are dyspnea, unfamiliar setting and routines, and uncertainty about what is happening. Acknowledge the patient's anxiety and attempt to identify its basis. While taking immediate measures to relieve dyspnea, calmly explain what is being done. It may be helpful to tell the patient how specific measures help to relieve symptoms. The presence of family members may have a calming effect if the relatives understand that they, too, must remain calm.

Pharmacology Capsule

Older adults are more susceptible to adverse drug effects because they metabolize and excrete drugs more slowly.

CARDIOMYOPATHY

Cause and Risk Factors

CMP is disease of the heart muscle. The cause of CMP is often unknown or CMP may be secondary to another disease process. The disease usually leads to HF. Three major types of CMP are recognized: (1) dilated, (2) hypertrophic, and (3) restrictive (Fig. 36-12). Dilated CMP is the most common type. Many possible causes of dilated CMP exist, such as ischemia, hypertension, alcohol or drug abuse, infections, chemotherapy, pregnancy, and genetics. Hypertrophic CMP often results from valvular heart disease or hypertension. There also appears to be a hereditary link. Hypertrophic CMP is more common in younger individuals; many young athletes who die suddenly are found to have hypertrophic CMP (see *Cultural Considerations* box). Restrictive CMP is the least common type of CMP. Amyloidosis, sarcoidosis, and other immunosuppressive disorders may predispose individuals to restrictive CMP (Yancy et al., 2013).

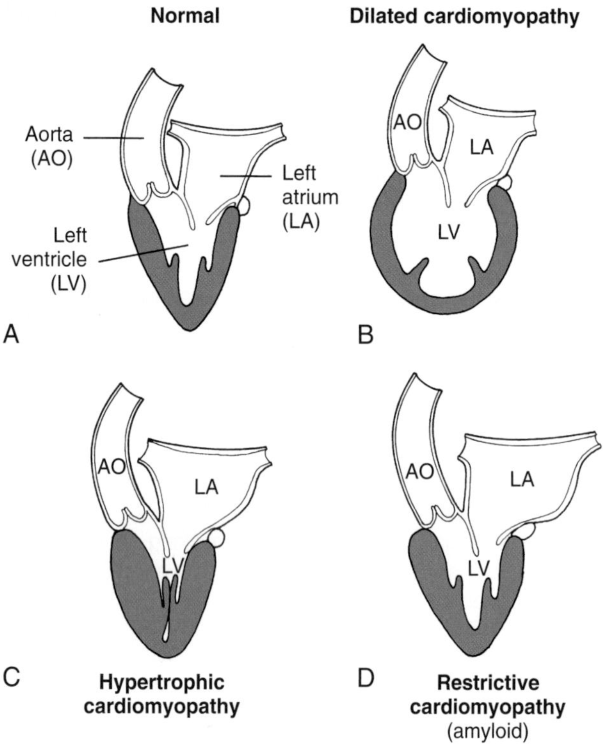

FIGURE 36-12 Cardiomyopathy (CMP). **A,** Normal heart. **B,** Dilated CMP. **C,** Hypertrophic CMP. **D,** Restrictive CMP. (From McCance KL, Huether SE: *Understanding pathophysiology*, ed 5, St. Louis, 2013, Mosby.)

Cultural Considerations

What Does Culture Have to Do with Cardiomyopathy?

African-American men are at increased risk for dilated cardiomyopathy (CMP). Be alert to complaints of decreasing exercise tolerance and dyspnea in this population.

Pathophysiology

With dilated CMP, the patient has dilation of the ventricular chamber and severely impaired systolic function. This causes decreased contractility, decreased ejection fraction and stroke volume, and increased left ventricular end-diastolic pressure. Pressure backup results in dilation of all four chambers and is most pronounced in the ventricles. Left ventricular failure and resulting HF are seen as the result of excessive back pressure (see Fig. 36-12, *B*).

In hypertrophic CMP, the LV hypertrophies and thickening of the ventricular septum occurs. The left ventricular capacity decreases and the outflow track of the LV is decreased in size. The size of the LA increases as a result of the back pressure. The exterior heart size may appear to be normal. Ventricular dysrhythmias are common (see Fig. 36-12, *C*).

In restrictive CMP, the myocardium becomes rigid and noncompliant. This reduces ventricular filling and cardiac output. Pulmonary and systemic congestion result (see Fig. 36-12, *D*).

Signs and Symptoms

Dilated CMP is a progressive, chronic disease. The onset is gradual, with dyspnea, fatigue, left-sided HF, and moderate to severe cardiomegaly. Mitral valve regurgitation and S_3 and S_4 sounds are evident.

With hypertrophic CMP, the progression of symptoms is slow. Dyspnea, orthopnea, angina, fatigue, syncope, palpitations, ankle edema, and S_4 sounds are found.

With restrictive CMP, the primary symptom is exercise intolerance. Dyspnea, fatigue, right-sided HF, S_3 and S_4 sounds, and mitral valve regurgitation are also noted.

Medical Diagnosis

Diagnosis of dilated CMP is made primarily on the basis of echocardiographic results. Cardiac enlargement may be noted on chest radiography. The echocardiogram and chest radiograph are also used to diagnose hypertrophic CMP. Other findings include a systolic murmur and atrial and ventricular dysrhythmias. An enlarged LV may be accompanied by left atrial enlargement. The diagnosis of restrictive CMP is demonstrated by decreased cardiac output and HF. It must be differentiated from pericarditis. An echocardiogram may show impaired diastolic function and decreased ventricular size.

Medical Treatment

Supportive measures are used for dilated CMP. Positive inotropic drugs to improve cardiac output, diuretics to decrease preload, and ACE inhibitors and vasodilators to decrease afterload provide this type of therapy. Anticoagulants may be used to prevent thrombi. If all other measures fail, the patient needs a heart transplant. Medical treatment for hypertrophic CMP includes antidysrhythmic agents, antibiotics, anticoagulants, calcium channel blockers, and beta-blockers. Surgical incision of the hypertrophied septal muscle and resection of some of the hypertrophied muscle may be considered for hypertrophic CMP. An alternative for select patients, nonsurgical reduction of the hypertrophied septum with alcohol ablation, may be done percutaneously in the cardiac catheterization laboratory. Some patients with hypertrophic CMP may benefit from an AICD placed to prevent SCD. Treatment of restrictive CMP is similar to that of HF therapy. Heart transplantation may be considered. Complications observed with all types of CMP are dysrhythmias, HF, and death. A poor prognosis exists with CMP. Mortality from CMP is highest in older adults, men, and African Americans (Yancy et al., 2013).

❖ NURSING CARE of the Patient with Cardiomyopathy

■ Assessment

These patients are primarily assessed for HF. Be alert for dyspnea, cough, edema, dysrhythmias, and decreased cardiac output.

Nursing Diagnoses, Goals, and Outcome Criteria: Cardiomyopathy

Nursing Diagnoses	Goals and Outcome Criteria
Decreased Cardiac Output related to ventricular failure	Improved cardiac output: normal pulse and blood pressure
Activity Intolerance related to poor tissue perfusion	Increased activity intolerance: performance of daily activities without excessive fatigue
Hopelessness related to poor prognosis	More positive outlook: patient's expression of feelings about condition and hopeful statements

Interventions

The care of these patients is similar to that of patients with HF. In addition, a hopeful atmosphere and a careful explanation of care requirements are necessary. Encourage the family to support the patient. The teaching plan guides the patient to make lifestyle changes. It is important to encourage the patient to make decisions and choices.

CARDIAC TRANSPLANTATION

The first heart transplantation was performed in 1967 in South Africa by Dr. Christiaan Barnard. Transplantation is considered for end-stage HF that is not responding to therapy, CMP, and severe inoperable CHD. Psychologic makeup is assessed carefully before transplantation. Patients with a history of depression, noncompliance, and inability to cope with stress are poor candidates. In the United States, federal regulations prohibit the sale of human organs.

The donor must meet the criteria for brain death, have no malignancies outside the central nervous system (CNS), be free of infection, and not have experienced severe chest trauma. Prolonged advanced life support measures are avoided. The donor and recipient organs must be carefully matched. The donor heart size must be sufficient to meet the needs of the recipient. The donor heart may be preserved for 4 to 6 hours before transplantation.

The recipient must be free of infection at the time of transplantation. The patient is prepared for surgery as with any open heart procedure. CPB is initiated and the recipient's heart is removed except for the posterior portions of the atria (Fig. 36-13). The donor heart is trimmed and anastomosed to the remaining native heart. The patient is removed from bypass, the heart is restarted, and the chest is closed.

Aftercare of the patient with a heart transplant is similar to that of the patient after coronary artery bypass surgery. Hemodynamic monitoring, mechanical ventilation, cardiac assessment, care of chest tubes, and accurate intake and output measurements are vital. Immediately after surgery, the patient is placed in a private room in the intensive care unit. Gowns, masks, and careful hand washing are often used to protect the patient from infection. Invasive lines and tubes (e.g., endotracheal tube, pulmonary artery catheter, Foley catheter, chest tubes) are removed as rapidly as possible to decrease the chance of infection. The prevention of postoperative infection is a major goal. Pulmonary infections are most frequently found after heart transplantations. Moving the patient from the intensive care unit to a private room and then to home as soon as possible decreases the incidence of nosocomial infections. Patients and families are taught the signs and symptoms of infection and to avoid crowds and others with infections.

In addition, the patient with a transplant receives immunosuppressive medications. Lifelong immunosuppression is administered to prevent the body from

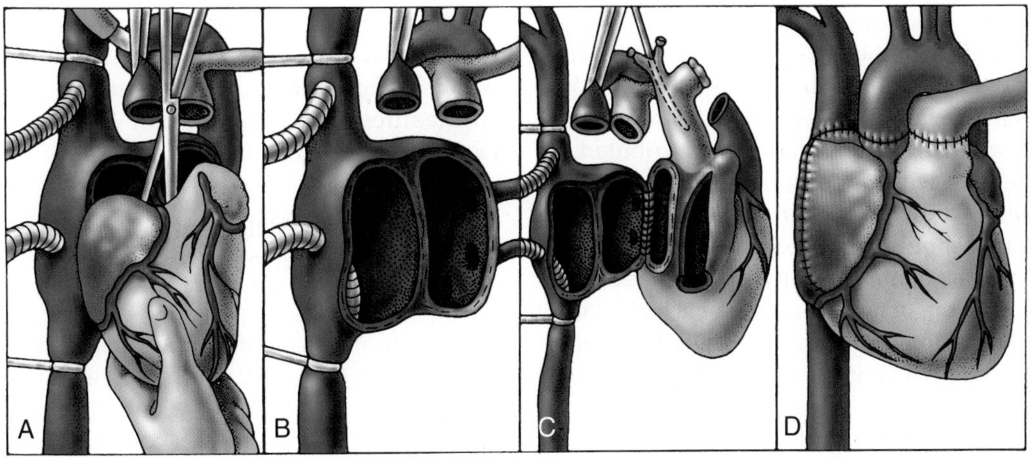

FIGURE 36-13 Heart transplantation. **A,** After the recipient is placed on cardiopulmonary bypass (CPB), the heart is removed. **B,** The posterior walls of the recipient's left and right atria are left intact. **C,** The left atrium (LA) of the donor heart is anastomosed to the recipient's residual posterior atrial walls and the other atrial walls, the atrial septum, and the great vessels are joined. **D,** Postoperative result.

rejecting the donated heart, which it recognizes as foreign tissue. Initially, large doses of corticosteroids are administered and the dose is decreased over time. At the first indication of rejection (increased temperature, infection, dyspnea, malaise, fatigue, dysrhythmia), the steroid dose usually is increased. Other drugs used to prevent and treat rejection are azathioprine (Imuran) and cyclosporine (Sandimmune). Protocols using several immunosuppressive agents are considered most effective. Reduced dosages of each drug provide for a lower incidence of toxicity.

Rejection is monitored through endomyocardial biopsies and the Heartsbreath test. These are performed frequently in the period immediately after transplantation and less frequently over time. Patients are taught to monitor their own progress and to report problems promptly. The transplant team monitors patients closely and observes them for infection, rejection, quality of life, and complications. Common complications noted after heart transplantation, other than rejection and infection, are hypertension, elevated cholesterol, obesity, and malignancies.

Pharmacology Capsule

Patients who are taking immunosuppressive drugs to prevent rejection of transplanted tissue have reduced resistance to infection.

INFLAMMATORY DISORDERS

Inflammation of the heart most often results from systemic infections. The endocardium, myocardium, and pericardium may be affected.

Infective Endocarditis

Cause and Risk Factors. Microbial infections of the endocardium primarily affect the valves. Organisms present in the blood easily colonize valves damaged by rheumatic heart disease or congenital defects or a mitral valve that is prolapsed.

Although the incidence of infective endocarditis (IE) has decreased with the use of antibiotic drugs, the problem has increased in IV drug abusers. The more frequent use of invasive intravascular catheters for severely compromised patients has also contributed to the frequency with which IE occurs.

Patients with known valvular disease are also at risk for IE. They should be treated with prophylactic antibiotics before dental or invasive procedures. Immunosuppression or any source of bacterial contamination (lacerations, pneumonia, invasive procedures, IV drug use with contaminated needles) places patients at risk.

Pathophysiology. Pathogens, usually bacteria, enter the bloodstream by any of the previously mentioned means. The pathogen accumulates on the heart valves, the endocardium, or both and forms vegetations. The mitral valve is the most common site for these vegetations. The turbulence of the blood flow through the heart weakens the vegetations and causes pieces to break off; these emboli can then obstruct circulation and impair tissue perfusion in the lungs, brain, kidneys, and heart.

Complications. Complications of IE include HF and embolization. HF is the most frequent cause of death with IE.

Signs and Symptoms. Patients usually have fever, chills, malaise, fatigue, and weight loss. The fever may be low grade (99°F to 102°F/37.2°C to 38.9°C) or higher (102°F to 105°F/38.9°C to 40.6°C). The fever is accompanied by chills and night sweats. Chest or abdominal pain may be reported, possibly indicating embolization. Vegetative fragments and microembolizations can produce petechiae inside the mouth and on the ankles, feet, and antecubital areas. Pea-sized, tender, red to purple lesions known as *Osler nodes* may be on the patient's fingertips or toes. Janeway lesions (flat, red, painless spots) may be noted on palms and soles. A new or changing heart murmur is noted in most patients (usually mitral or aortic).

Medical Diagnosis. The diagnosis of IE is based on the history, physical examination, and results of laboratory studies. A history of recent dental or surgical procedures may precede IE. Auscultation may reveal a heart murmur. Echocardiography helps to visualize vegetation and valvular regurgitation. Right-sided or left-sided HF may be evident. Serial blood cultures may give clues to the causative organism or organisms. The WBC count may be elevated.

Medical Treatment. Antimicrobial drugs, rest, and limitation of activities are the primary therapeutic measures for IE. Antimicrobials are given intravenously for 2 to 6 weeks, depending on the organism. The patient is usually hospitalized for at least 1 week and then receives home IV therapy if that is available. Prophylactic anticoagulants may be necessary. Surgery may be necessary to replace an infected valve. A key to prevention of IE is prophylactic antibiotics for patients with specific cardiac conditions who are undergoing dental, GI, genitourinary, or respiratory procedures (American Heart Association-Infective Endocarditis, 2013).

NURSING CARE of the Patient with Infective Endocarditis

Assessment

Complete assessment of the cardiac patient is summarized in Box 36-1. With IE, review the patient's history for risk factors, recent invasive procedures, known pathologic cardiac conditions, and onset of symptoms. It is also important to assess for temperature elevation, heart murmur, evidence of HF (cough, peripheral edema), and embolization.

Nursing Diagnoses, Goals, and Outcome Criteria: Infective Endocarditis

Nursing Diagnoses	Goals and Outcome Criteria
Decreased Cardiac Output related to impaired valve function	Normal cardiac output: normal pulse and blood pressure
Impaired Physical Mobility related to fatigue and prolonged intravenous therapy	Resumption of usual physical activities without symptoms: performance of activities of daily living (ADL) without fatigue
Risk for Decreased Cardiac Tissue Perfusion related to embolization	Normal tissue perfusion: absence of dyspnea or signs of circulatory obstruction

Interventions

Administer antibiotics as prescribed. Throughout the course of the illness, it is important to continue to assess cardiac output and monitor for complications. Teach the patient about the medications prescribed and any restrictions imposed. Encourage him or her to get adequate rest, which is necessary during the healing process. Range-of-motion exercises may be necessary during the acute stage and until the patient is ambulatory.

Pericarditis

Cause and Risk Factors. Pericarditis is an inflammation of the pericardium. It may be a primary disease or associated with another inflammatory process. The disease may be acute or chronic. Viruses, bacteria, fungi, trauma, or MI (Dressler syndrome) causes acute pericarditis. Tuberculosis, radiation, or metastases cause chronic pericarditis.

Pathophysiology. In acute pericarditis, the inflammatory process causes an increase in the amount of pericardial fluid and inflammation of the pericardial membranes. In chronic pericarditis (also called *constrictive pericarditis*), scarring of the pericardium fuses the visceral and parietal pericardia together. Loss of elasticity results from the scarring. This constrictive process prevents adequate ventricular filling.

Complications. The major complication of pericarditis is pericardial effusion or accumulation of fluid in the pericardial space. This may lead to cardiac tamponade when sufficient fluid accumulation decreases ventricular filling. The resulting drop in cardiac output is an emergency. It is treated with pericardiocentesis to remove the accumulated fluid.

Signs and Symptoms. Chest pain is the hallmark symptom of pericarditis. The pain is most severe on inspiration. It is most often sharp and stabbing but may be described as *dull* or *burning*. It is relieved by sitting up and leaning forward. Dyspnea, chills, and fever accompany pericarditis. ST segment elevation may be noted on the ECG. A pericardial rub may be present. Slowly progressing pericardial effusion does not result in hemodynamic compromise until 400 to 500 mL of fluid has accumulated. Rapidly accumulating fluid may precipitate sudden symptoms with only 250 mL of fluid.

Medical Diagnosis. The diagnostic challenge is to differentiate pericarditis from MI. Serial ECGs show that the ST segment elevation resolves in several weeks. QRS complex voltage may decrease because of the accumulated fluid in the pericardial space. An echocardiogram may show pericardial thickening and effusion. Atrial fibrillation may occur because of the irritation. The CK-MB and troponin may be elevated. Blood cultures may identify the causative organism or organisms. One differentiating feature to consider is that position change does not relieve ischemic chest pain or angina; however, the chest pain that accompanies pericarditis often is relieved by a change in position.

Medical Treatment. The patient is treated with analgesics, antipyretics, antiinflammatory agents, and antibiotics. With constrictive pericarditis, the patient would be treated as for HF. Pericardiocentesis to remove the accumulated fluid will be performed with cardiac tamponade. Surgical creation of a pericardial window (removal of a segment of parietal pericardium to allow continuous drainage of pericardial fluid) may be necessary to treat chronic pericarditis with effusion (American Heart Association-What is Pericarditis, 2013).

NURSING CARE of the Patient with Pericarditis

Assessment

General nursing assessment of the cardiac patient is summarized in Box 36-1. With pericarditis, assessment of heart sounds is especially important.

Nursing Diagnoses, Goals, and Outcome Criteria: Pericarditis

Nursing Diagnoses	Goals and Outcome Criteria
Acute Pain related to pericardial inflammation	Pain relief: patient statement that pain is reduced, relaxed manner
Decreased Cardiac Output related to pericardial constriction	Improved cardiac output: normal pulse and blood pressure
Anxiety related to illness	Decreased anxiety: patient statement that anxiety is reduced, calm manner

Interventions

Rest and reduction of activity decrease the workload of the heart. Administer medications and teach the patient about them. Emotional support from the nursing staff and significant others is vital. The patient can be instructed in relaxation techniques. Monitor vital signs and auscultate for a pericardial friction rub. The rub is heard during inspiration with the diaphragm of the stethoscope placed between the second and fourth intercostal spaces at the left sternal border. It is heard when no fluid accumulation is present. Distant heart sounds may be heard when fluid accumulation exists. It is important to note pain characteristics and response to analgesics and antiinflammatory agents. Also monitor the ECG for dysrhythmias.

VALVULAR DISEASE

The purpose of the heart valves is to maintain blood flow in one direction. If the valves are damaged through a congenital defect or acquired disease, their function is compromised. Stenosis and regurgitation are the two major valve problems. Stenosis is narrowing of the valvular opening. A stenotic valve limits the amount of blood ejected from one chamber to the next. **Regurgitation**, the inability of the valve to close completely, allows the blood to flow backward when a valve does not close efficiently. The left side of the heart is affected most often and the mitral valve is the most frequently affected of all the valves. The pulmonic valve in the right side of the heart is infrequently affected. Only left-sided valvular disease is discussed here.

Antibiotics have decreased the incidence of valvular disease from rheumatic fever but the incidence of nonrheumatic valvular disease has increased. Longer life span and IV drug abuse are the primary causes of the increasing incidence of nonrheumatic valvular disease.

Mitral Stenosis

Mitral stenosis is a narrowing of the opening in the mitral valve that impedes blood flow from the LA to the LV. The mitral valve leaflets become thickened and fibrotic. Rheumatic heart disease is the leading cause of mitral stenosis. Congenital malformations of the mitral valve occur but are not common. Other causes are calcium accumulation on valve leaflets and atrial myxomas (tumors).

Pathophysiology. The thickening of the valve structures reduces the outflow of blood from the LA to the LV. The LA dilates to accommodate the amount of blood not ejected and left atrial pressure increases. As left atrial pressure increases, the blood volume backs up into the pulmonary system, increasing pulmonary pressures. This increases the workload on the right side of the heart, leading to right ventricular hypertrophy. Eventually, the RV fails and cardiac output decreases because less blood is delivered to the LV.

Signs and Symptoms. Symptoms may begin soon after the disease process or may be delayed for many years. Dyspnea, fatigue, cough, chest pain, and activity intolerance are the most frequent symptoms. Exertional dyspnea and pulmonary edema occur as blood backs up in the pulmonary system and serous fluid leaks into the pulmonary tissues. Because stenosis causes turbulent blood flow through the valve, a murmur is present during diastole (best heard at the apex of the heart).

Medical Diagnosis. Diagnosis is made on the basis of the patient history, physical examination, and results of diagnostic procedures. The chest radiograph shows left atrial, right ventricular, and pulmonary vascular enlargement. Echocardiography, often TEE, is used to visualize the mitral valve. Cardiac catheterization is used to confirm the diagnosis and determine the extent of the disease process.

Medical Treatment. When symptomatic, the patient with mitral stenosis is treated as for HF with drug therapy, sodium and fluid restrictions, and activity restriction. Digoxin, diuretics, beta-blockers, and antidysrhythmic agents may be prescribed. If the patient has atrial fibrillation, anticoagulant agents also may be prescribed. Prophylactic antibiotics are prescribed before any invasive procedure for patients with mitral stenosis because bacteria tend to cluster on the damaged valves.

Surgical Treatment. Surgical treatment includes commissurotomy, mitral valve replacement, and balloon valvuloplasty. Commissurotomy is excision of parts of the leaflets to enlarge the opening. The mitral valve may be replaced with a biologic or synthetic valve (Fig. 36-14). Both commissurotomy and mitral valve replacement require major surgery with CPB.

Balloon valvuloplasty, a procedure done in the cardiac catheterization laboratory, has been very successful in dilating stenosed heart valves. It is less invasive than valve replacement or commissurotomy. To dilate the mitral valve, a balloon catheter (similar to the one used for PTCA) is threaded from the femoral artery to the mitral valve. The balloon is positioned in the valve and inflated until the valve opens sufficiently. After the procedure, the patient is observed closely in an intensive care unit for dysrhythmias and complications. Complications include valve regurgitation, restenosis, perforation of the myocardium, and, rarely, systemic embolization.

NURSING CARE of the Patient with Mitral Stenosis

Assessment

It is most important to obtain a complete history as summarized in Box 36-1 and a record of signs and symptoms being experienced. Take the patient's vital signs and auscultate for heart murmurs. The murmur of mitral stenosis is described as *rumbling* and *low pitched*. It is heard best at the apex of the heart. The ECG may show a notched P wave, indicating left atrial enlargement. Atrial fibrillation is frequently seen. Tachycardia and tachypnea are common signs. The pulse pressure may be decreasing, indicating low

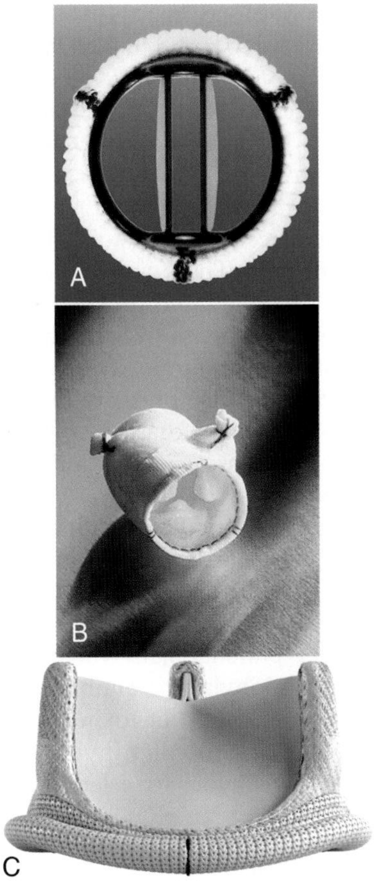

FIGURE 36-14 Types of prosthetic and tissue valves. **A,** St. Jude Medical Masters HP Series Mechanical Heart Valve. **B,** Freestyle Valve. **C,** Carpentier-Edwards PERIMOUNT Magna Ease aortic heart valve. (A, St. Jude Medical is a trademark of St. Jude Medical, Inc. or its related companies. Reprinted with permission of St. Jude Medical, Copyright 2014. All rights reserved. B, Copyright 2014 Medtronic, Inc. C, Used with permission from Edwards Lifesciences LLC, Irvine, Calif.)

cardiac output. Jugular venous distention and crackles are found with pulmonary congestion.

Interventions

See the section titled "Nursing Care of the Patient with Heart Failure" for the remainder of the nursing process.

Mitral Regurgitation

Mitral regurgitation (insufficiency) allows blood to flow back into the LA during diastole. The valve does not close completely because one or both of the valve leaflets becomes rigid and shortens.

The LA and LV hypertrophy as a result of the backflow of blood against the incompetent valve. Left ventricular hypertrophy is compensatory in an attempt to maintain cardiac output. Eventually, the left side of the heart fails and symptoms are then the same as with mitral stenosis.

Nursing Diagnoses, Goals, and Outcome Criteria: Mitral Stenosis

The nursing diagnoses and goals for mitral stenosis are the same as those for congestive heart failure (CHF) and for all valvular diseases.

Nursing Diagnoses	Goals and Outcome Criteria
Decreased Cardiac Output related to narrowing or insufficiency of valvular competence	Increased cardiac output: normal pulse and blood pressure
Impaired Gas Exchange related to pulmonary congestion	Improved gas exchange: clear breath sounds, normal arterial blood gases (ABGs)
Activity Intolerance related to imbalance between oxygen (O_2) supply and demand	Improved activity tolerance: performance of daily activities without excessive fatigue
Excess Fluid Volume related to decreased glomerular filtration rate, increased aldosterone, sodium and water retention, and increased antidiuretic hormone (ADH) release	Normal fluid balance: no edema, clear breath sounds, fluid output equal to or exceeds fluid intake

The murmur of mitral regurgitation is high pitched and blowing and occurs during systole. It is best heard at the apex and may radiate to the axilla. With severe disease, S_3 and S_4 sounds may be auscultated. Atrial fibrillation occurs as the LA enlarges.

Mitral regurgitation is treated with vasodilators to decrease the afterload and therefore the regurgitation. Other medical treatment includes activity restriction, dietary sodium limitation, diuretics, and digitalis. Surgical treatment includes annuloplasty and mitral valve replacement. Annuloplasty is reconstruction of the leaflets and the annulus.

Mitral Valve Prolapse

The mitral valve prolapses when one or both leaflets enlarge and protrude into the LA during systole. It has a tendency to run in families and may be caused by heart infections, rheumatic fever, or a wide variety of congenital anomalies. The disease is usually benign but may progress to mitral insufficiency.

In most patients, symptoms do not occur or may occur with stress. Symptoms include chest pain, palpitations, dizziness, and syncope. Some patients exhibit dysrhythmias. The ECG usually shows normal findings. Evidence of mitral valve prolapse may be found on echocardiography. The problem is often controlled with stress reduction techniques. Beta-blockers may be prescribed to decrease syncope, palpitations, and severe chest pain. Therapeutic management is matched to the degree of symptoms.

Aortic Stenosis

Cause and Risk Factors. Stenosis of the aortic valve occurs when the valve cusps become fibrotic and calcify. It may be caused by a congenital malformation or result from rheumatic fever, syphilis, or the aging process (atherosclerosis and calcification). When seen in younger patients, it is most often caused by a congenital malformation. The aortic valve is most commonly diseased in the aging population.

Pathophysiology. The valve opening decreases to one third its normal size before symptoms occur. As flow is impeded through the narrowed valve, the LV hypertrophies to compensate for the extra pressure needed to eject blood. The LA also compensates by delivering a strong atrial kick. These compensatory mechanisms allow normal function until atrial fibrillation disrupts the atrial kick or until the LV hypertrophies to the point of dysfunction, with decreased cardiac output and myocardial ischemia. With left ventricular dysfunction, blood backs up into the LA and the pulmonary system. If uncorrected, eventually the right side of the heart fails.

Signs and Symptoms. The patient complains of dyspnea on exertion, angina, and syncope. Fatigue, orthopnea, and paroxysmal nocturnal dyspnea are late symptoms and indicate HF. A systolic murmur may occur.

Medical Diagnosis. The chest radiograph shows atrial and ventricular enlargement, which are late signs. The murmur of aortic stenosis is heard best in the aortic area, the second intercostal space to the right of the sternum. The echocardiogram shows left ventricular wall thickening. An exercise tolerance test (ETT) may be ordered to evaluate heart function.

Medical Treatment. Prophylactic antibiotics are prescribed to prevent IE with dental and invasive procedures. HF is treated with digoxin, diuretics, a low-sodium diet, and activity restriction. Surgical treatment includes balloon valvuloplasty and aortic valve replacement.

❖ NURSING CARE of the Patient with Aortic Stenosis

The nurse should monitor for a bounding arterial pulse and widened pulse pressure. The nursing process is the same as for HF (see Nursing Care Plan: Patient with Heart Failure).

Aortic Regurgitation

Fibrosis and thickening of the aortic cusps progress until the valve no longer maintains unidirectional blood flow. Aortic regurgitation (insufficiency) is caused primarily by rheumatic fever. Other causes include IE, blunt chest trauma, calcification of the valve, and chronic hypertension.

Regurgitation of blood into the LV during diastole increases the amount of blood in the LV. The LV dilates and hypertrophies. Myocardial ischemia and left ventricular failure occur. Blood backs up into the pulmonary system and eventually right ventricular failure occurs.

The murmur of aortic regurgitation is high pitched and blowing and occurs in diastole. It is auscultated best at the aortic area. The point of maximal impulse may be shifted to the left and down. Tachycardia and palpitations are compensatory mechanisms. Later signs of HF such as fatigue, dyspnea, and ascites develop. A widened pulse pressure (increased difference between systolic and diastolic pressures) results from a low diastolic pressure. S_3 and S_4 sounds are often auscultated.

Left atrial and ventricular dilation are noted on chest radiography. The echocardiogram shows left ventricular dilation. Cardiac catheterization is used to determine the extent of incompetence.

As with other patients with valve disease, these patients have prophylactic antibiotics prescribed before invasive procedures. Digoxin and diuretics are prescribed for left ventricular hypertrophy. Aortic valve replacement provides long-term correction.

ELECTROCARDIOGRAM MONITORING

Nurses who work in critical care areas are responsible for monitoring and interpreting ECGs. Patients usually are monitored continuously at the bedside and have intermittent monitoring through a 12-lead ECG.

12-LEAD ELECTROCARDIOGRAM

A 12-lead ECG looks at the heart from 12 directions or perspectives. This permits more precise evaluation of the heart's electrical activity. Three leads are placed on the limbs (leads I, II, and III); three leads are augmented (aVR, aVL, and aVF); and six chest, or precordial, leads exist (V_1 to V_6). Electricity flows from the negative to the positive lead. If the depolarization wave flows toward the positive pole (electrode), the deflection is upright. If the wave flows away from the positive pole, the deflection is negative.

CONTINUOUS MONITORING

Most units that perform continuous monitoring use the five-lead system, with four limb electrodes and a chest electrode (which is placed at one of the V lead sites). The electrodes are held in place by adhesive pads. Thoroughly clean the electrode sites before applying the pads and change the pads according to agency policy. In addition, monitor the patient's skin for irritation or breakdown. The lead monitored depends on the purpose of the monitoring (e.g., to detect dysrhythmias, to detect ischemia).

INTERPRETATION OF ELECTROCARDIOGRAMS

To interpret an ECG strip, refer to Figure 36-15. The graph paper consists of horizontal and vertical small and large squares. The horizontal axis measures time; the vertical axis measures voltage. Each small square represents 0.04 second on the horizontal axis and 1 mm on the vertical axis. Each large square, bounded by heavy lines, is made up of five small squares and represents 0.20 second and 5 mm. The electrical activity of the heart is represented by deflections, positive and negative, from the baseline. A deflection is an upward or downward movement from the baseline. The baseline is called the *isoelectric line.* The first positive deflection (upward movement) is the small, rounded P wave that represents atrial depolarization. The second positive deflection is the peaked QRS complex that represents ventricular depolarization. The Q is the first negative deflection, meaning that the line moves below the isoelectric line. The R wave corresponds to the patient's pulse. Atrial repolarization occurs during ventricular depolarization and is obscured by the QRS complex. The third deflection is the rounded T wave, which represents ventricular repolarization. The fourth deflection, if present, is the U wave. It is small, rounded, and usually indicates electrolyte imbalance (hypokalemia).

The PR interval represents the time it takes the impulse to travel from the atria through the AV node to the ventricles. The PR interval is measured from the beginning of the P wave to the Q wave. The normal PR interval is 0.12 to 0.20 second. The QRS complex is measured from the point at which the Q leaves the isoelectric line to the point at which the S returns to the isoelectric line. The normal QRS complex is less than 0.12 second. The ST segment represents the time from ventricular depolarization to ventricular repolarization. The ST segment should be along the isoelectric

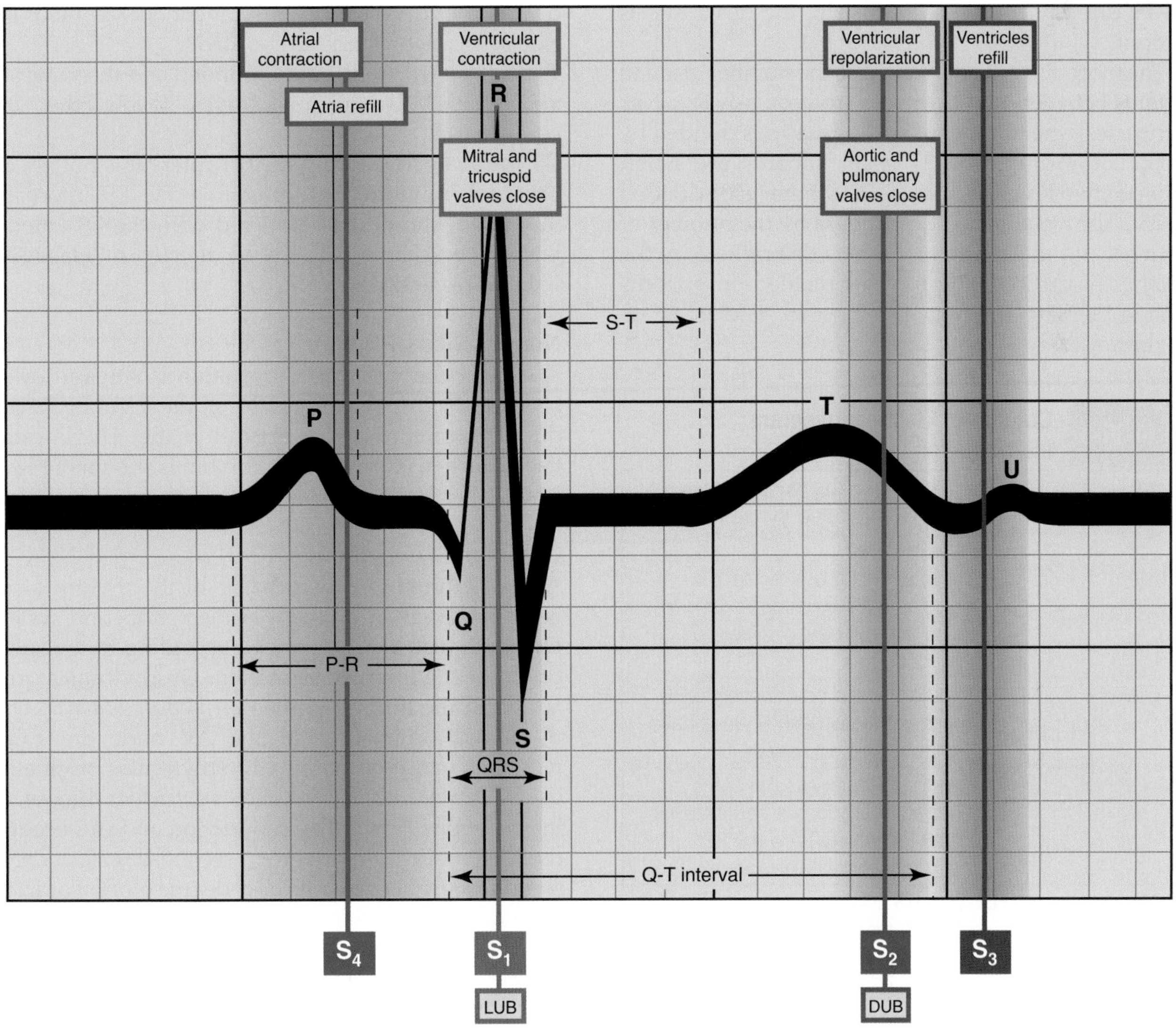

FIGURE 36-15 Relationship between the cardiac cycle and the heart sounds. (From Monahan FD, Drake DT, Neighbors M, editors: *Medical-surgical nursing: foundations for clinical practice*, ed 2, Philadelphia, 1998, Saunders.)

line. The QT interval represents ventricular refractory time. It is measured from the beginning of the QRS complex to the end of the T wave. The normal QT interval time range varies with heart rate; therefore it is necessary to compare the QT interval obtained with a table (QT tables are available in most textbooks dealing with dysrhythmias). The QT interval is affected by age, gender, and heart rate.

Criteria for Interpreting Electrocardiograms

Criteria have been established for interpreting an ECG strip. The ECG is evaluated for rate, regularity, P waves, PR interval, and QRS complexes (Table 36-8).

Rate Calculation. Most ECG strips have tic marks indicating 3-second time periods. Heart rate can be calculated from the ECG strip in several ways. The quickest but least accurate method is to count the number of P waves (for atrial rate) or R waves (for ventricular rate) in a 6-second strip (between three tic marks or 30 large squares) and multiply by 10 for the estimate of the number of bpm. For example, if six R waves are seen in a 6-second strip, the heart rate is 60 bpm.

The more accurate method uses the number of small squares between two P waves (atria) or two R waves (ventricles); the number of small squares is divided by 1500. For example, if 25 small squares are noted between two R waves, the rate is 60 bpm (1500 divided by 25). The atrial rate is determined by the number of P waves and the ventricular rate is determined by the number of QRS complexes. This method only works with a regular rhythm. The normal rate is 60 to 100 bpm.

Table 36-8 Criteria for Electrocardiogram Interpretation

Rate	Are the atrial and ventricular rates the same as measured by the P-P and R-R intervals?
Rhythm	Is the rate regular or irregular? If irregular, does a pattern exist? Are these ectopic beats? Where do they occur?
P waves	Is there a P wave before every QRS complex? Does each P wave have the same size and shape?
PR interval	Are all the PR intervals the same length? If not, does a pattern exist to the irregularity? Are the PR intervals within normal range?
QRS complexes	Do all QRS complexes look alike? Are all QRS complexes within the normal range (0.06–0.10 sec)?
ST segment	Is the ST segment isoelectric, depressed, or elevated?
T waves	Do all T waves look alike? Are the T waves upright or inverted?

Rhythm. The consecutive P-P intervals for the atria and the consecutive R-R intervals for the ventricles are measured for consistency. Using calipers or a blank piece of paper, the distance between P waves and R waves is noted. If the distances do not vary more than one small square, the rhythm is considered regular. If the distances are greater than one small square, the rhythm is irregular.

P Waves. The next evaluation is of P waves. Is a P wave noted before each QRS complex? If so, the rhythm originates in the SA node. Do all P waves appear to be the same size and shape? If so, the impulse originates in the SA node.

PR Interval. Does the PR interval fall within the normal range of 0.12 to 0.20 second? If so, no interference occurs in conduction from the SA node to the AV node.

QRS Complex. Does the QRS complex fall within the range of 0.06 to 0.10 second? If the QRS is prolonged (0.12 second or greater), a delay occurs in conduction through the ventricles.

ST Segment. Next the ST segment is examined. Is it isoelectric, depressed, or elevated?

T Waves. Are the T waves rounded and the same size and shape? Do the T waves follow the QRS complexes?

QT Interval. Measuring the QT interval is not always part of dysrhythmia interpretation. The QT interval, if measured, should be compared with the QT interval table. The QT interval may be affected by electrolyte imbalances and drugs.

Normal Sinus Rhythm

The most common cardiac rhythm is sinus in origin because the impulse originates in the SA node, is conducted normally, and meets all of the criteria established earlier. Normal sinus rhythm is shown in Figure 36-16.

Common Dysrhythmias

A dysrhythmia is a disturbance of the rhythm of the heart caused by a problem in the conduction system. Dysrhythmias are categorized according to the site of origin of the impulse formation. Dysrhythmias originating in the atria are called *atrial dysrhythmias.* Dysrhythmias originating in the AV node are called *junctional* or *escape rhythms.* Dysrhythmias originating below the AV node are called *ventricular.* Blocks are interruptions in impulse conduction and can occur at the AV node (first-degree, second-degree type I, second-degree type II, or third-degree blocks) or in the right or left bundle of His (right or left bundle branch blocks). Dysrhythmias and blocks have unique characteristics that are seen on the ECG and interpreted by specially trained technicians, nurses, and physicians. See Figures 36-17 through 36-23 for examples. Only more common dysrhythmias and lethal dysrhythmias are included in this text. For more in-depth

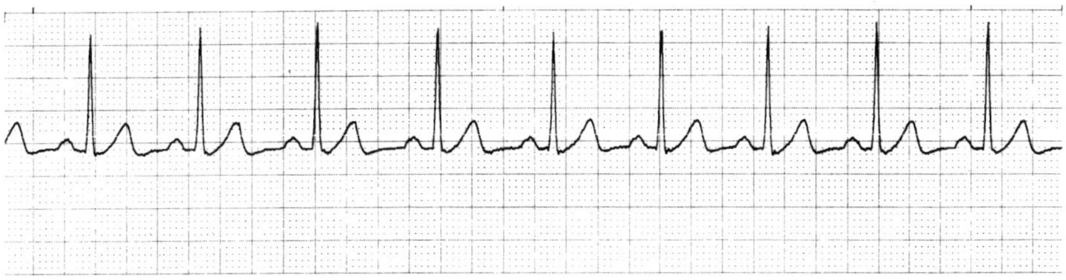

FIGURE 36-16 Normal sinus rhythm. Each segment between the dark lines (above the monitor strip) represents 3 seconds, when the monitor is set at a speed of 25 mm/sec. Characteristics: rate—60 to 100 beats per minute (bpm); regularity—essentially regular (P-to-P and R-to-R intervals are regular with only minor variation); P wave, PR interval—a P occurs before every QRS (each P wave is the same size and shape; PR interval is between 0.12 and 0.20 second); QRS—falls between 0.06 and 0.10 second; T wave—rounded, all the same shape. Interpretation: normal sinus rhythm. (From Ignatavicius DD, Workman ML: *Medical-surgical nursing: patient-centered collaborative care*, ed 6, St. Louis, 2010, Saunders.)

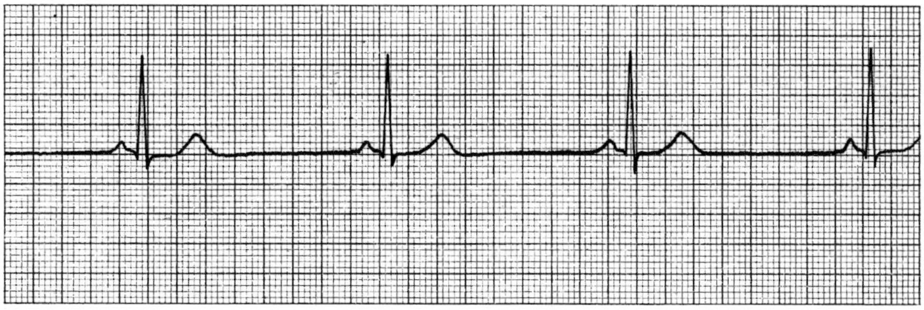

FIGURE 36-17 Sinus bradycardia. Characteristics: rate—less than 60 beats per minute (bpm); regularity—normal; P wave, PR interval—normal; QRS—normal; T wave—normal. Interpretation: All characteristics are within normal ranges except for the rate, which is slow. Causes: drugs, including digitalis and beta-blockers; vagal stimulation (Valsalva maneuver); severe pain; hyperkalemia; infection; and myocardial infarction (MI). Frequently seen in athletes as a result of conditioning. Symptoms: dizziness, syncope, chest pain, hypotension, sweating, nausea, dyspnea, and disorientation; sometimes no symptoms. Treatment: Not treated unless the patient is symptomatic. The underlying cause is treated. Atropine may be given to increase the heart rate. Isoproterenol is used with extreme caution. A pacemaker may be needed. (From Ignatavicius DD, Workman ML: *Medical-surgical nursing: patient-centered collaborative care*, ed 6, St. Louis, 2010, Saunders.)

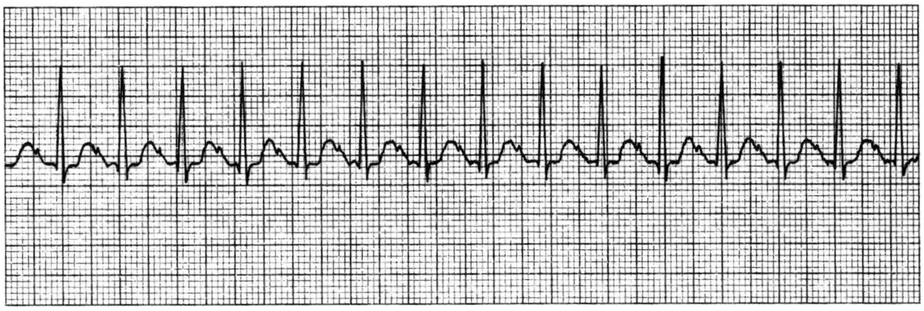

FIGURE 36-18 Sinus tachycardia. Characteristics: rate—greater than 100 beats per minute (bpm), usually less than 150 bpm; regularity—regular; P wave, PR interval—P waves may be buried in T wave of preceding beat with very rapid rates, more than 140 bpm; QRS—normal; T wave—normal. Interpretation: All characteristics are within normal range except for the rate, which is excessive. Causes: fever, dehydration, hypovolemia, increased sympathetic nervous system stimulation, stress, exercise, and acute myocardial infarction (MI). Symptoms: palpitations most common. Angina and decreased cardiac output from the decreased ventricular filling time also may occur. Treatment: correction of underlying cause; elimination of caffeine, nicotine, and alcohol; vagal stimulation may decrease the rate but does not treat the cause; beta-blockers. (From Ignatavicius DD, Workman ML: *Medical-surgical nursing: patient-centered collaborative care*, ed 6, St. Louis, 2010, Saunders.)

artery. The catheter is balloon tipped and flows with the blood. Different waveforms are seen on an oscilloscope as the catheter moves through the different areas of the heart. Pulmonary artery catheters have multiple lumens and are approximately 110 cm (44 inches) long. Various lumens are used to measure the pulmonary capillary wedge pressure, inflate the balloon, measure right atrial pressure, determine cardiac output, and administer fluids and drugs. Newer catheters incorporate fiberoptics for continuous monitoring of saturated venous oxygen (SvO_2), a measure of tissue perfusion or continuous cardiac output.

The purpose of a pulmonary artery catheter is to measure right-sided heart pressures and pulmonary artery pressures and to assess left-sided heart function. The proximal port is used to measure the right atrial pressure or central venous pressure (normal value: 2 to 6 mm Hg). The distal port measures the pulmonary artery pressure (normal value: 20 to 30/0 to 10). The lungs are low-pressure organs unless the patient has COPD.

The pulmonary capillary wedge pressure is used to assess the function of the left side of the heart. To determine the pulmonary capillary wedge pressure, the balloon is inflated with up to 1.5 mL of air. This allows the tip of the catheter to float into a pulmonary capillary until it occludes the capillary. This measures the pressure ahead of the catheter; therefore it measures the left ventricular heart function. The normal pulmonary capillary wedge pressure is 4 to 12 mm Hg. Once the pressure is recorded, the balloon is deflated. This pressure is lower when fluid is restricted, when diuretics are being administered, and when patients are receiving vasodilator drugs such as nitroglycerin or morphine. The pressure is elevated with excess fluid, when fluid volume expanders such as albumin are being administered, or in left heart dysfunction.

Cardiac Output

With a pulmonary artery catheter in place, cardiac output can be measured continuously or by the thermodilution method. The normal cardiac output is 4 to 8 L/min. Stress increases the cardiac output. Cardiac output may decrease with MI, HF, bradycardia, tachycardia, and some drugs. It is important for the nurse to use consistent technique in measuring cardiac output.

Mixed Venous Oxygen Saturation

Pulmonary artery catheters may have sensors in place that allow for measurement of mixed SvO_2 or, if the sensor is not part of the catheter, a blood sample can be obtained from the distal port (which opens in the pulmonary artery). Blood in the pulmonary artery is the blood returned from all of the organs and tissues in the body and mixed in the pulmonary artery. When the O_2 saturation of this mixed venous blood is measured (in a laboratory or through fiberoptics), the results reflect the degree of O_2 use by the body tissues. SvO_2 can be decreased when O_2 delivery is decreased or the body has increased the use of O_2 (fever, pain, stress). SvO_2 can be increased when O_2 delivery is increased or when O_2 use is decreased (hypothermia, general anesthesia). Normal SvO_2 is 60% to 75%.

ARTERIAL LINE

An arterial line may be inserted (most often in the radial artery) to provide a direct measurement of systolic and diastolic blood pressures. Once the line is inserted, it is connected to a pressurized solution to keep the catheter patent and to a transducer to assess pressure. The mean arterial pressure (MAP) is an indication of tissue perfusion. This pressure is elevated with sympathetic stimulation and increased heart rate.

Get Ready for the NCLEX® Examination

Key Points

- The primary function of the heart is to pump blood through the pulmonary and systemic circulation.
- The heartbeat has two phases: (1) systole (contraction) and (2) diastole (relaxation).
- Cardiac output is the amount of blood ejected per minute by each ventricle; stroke volume is the amount of blood ejected by a ventricle in a single contraction. The factors that affect stroke volume are preload, contractility, and afterload.
- The heart sounds are *lub*, heard during systole, and *dub*, heard during diastole.
- The most common cardiac surgical procedures are pacemaker or AICD insertion, valve repair or replacement, and coronary artery bypass surgery.
- Nursing concerns after cardiac surgery include ineffective breathing pattern, acute pain, ineffective thermoregulation, decreased cardiac output, risk for infection, and anxiety.
- Pacemakers are electronic devices that deliver impulses to stimulate contraction of the myocardium.
- An AICD is an implanted device that monitors cardiac activity, detects life-threatening dysrhythmias, and delivers a shock to convert the rhythm to a normal one.
- CHD is treated with drug therapy, diet modifications, lifestyle modifications, surgical intervention, or a combination of these.
- Risk factors for atherosclerosis are age, gender, heredity, diabetes mellitus, serum cholesterol, tobacco smoking, hypertension, overweight and obesity, and physical inactivity.
- Angina is the pain that results from myocardial ischemia. It is treated with vasodilators and rest.

- Procedures used to improve myocardial blood flow include percutaneous coronary balloon angioplasty, stent placement, laser angioplasty, atherectomy, CABG, and TMR.
- MI, caused by partial or complete occlusion of a coronary artery, can lead to dysrhythmias, HF, cardiogenic shock, thromboembolism, sudden cardiac death, and ventricular aneurysm and rupture.
- Nursing care of the patient with MI addresses anxiety, acute pain, and decreased cardiac output.
- Patients with acute cardiac conditions often have continuous cardiac monitoring to detect potentially fatal dysrhythmias for prompt treatment.
- Cardiac rehabilitation begins with a cardiac incident, lasts throughout life, and includes the patient and family in teaching about exercise, diet, and medications.
- HF, the inability of the heart to meet the metabolic demands of the body, may be caused by disorders that increase the heart's workload or interfere with its pumping action.
- Treatment of HF may include correction of underlying causes, drug therapy to improve cardiac function and eliminate excess fluid, and measures to decrease demands on the heart.
- Complications of HF are dysrhythmias, pulmonary edema, and cardiogenic shock.
- Nursing care of the patient with HF focuses on excess fluid volume, impaired gas exchange, anxiety, decreased cardiac output, and activity intolerance.
- CMP is a disease of the heart muscle that is treated with supportive measures but may lead to HF that eventually requires cardiac transplantation.
- Patients who have received heart transplants require immunosuppressive drugs for the remainder of their lives to prevent rejection of the foreign tissue.
- Signs and symptoms of cardiac transplant rejection are fever, dyspnea, fatigue, and dysrhythmias.
- Cardiac inflammatory conditions (endocarditis and pericarditis) are treated with drug therapy and rest.
- The primary disorders of the heart valves are stenosis, which interferes with blood movement from one chamber to the next, and regurgitation, which allows blood to flow backward.
- Valve disease may be treated with drug therapy to improve cardiac function, with balloon valvuloplasty to dilate stenosed valves, with commissurotomy to enlarge the opening, and with valve replacement using a biologic or synthetic valve.
- General measures to maintain perfusion of vital organs are O_2, IV fluids, and drugs to maintain or restore blood pressure.
- A dysrhythmia (also called an *arrhythmia*) is a disturbance of the heart rhythm caused by a problem in the conduction system.

Additional Learning Resources

SG Go to your Study Guide for additional learning activities to help you master this chapter content.

evolve Go to your Evolve website (http://evolve.elsevier.com/Linton/medsurg) for the following learning resources and much more:

- Interactive Prioritization Exercises
- Fluid & Electrolyte Tutorial
- Pharmacology Tutorial
- Review Questions for the NCLEX® Examination

Review Questions for the NCLEX® Examination

1. Normally, the impulse that stimulates a myocardial contraction begins at the ________.
   NCLEX Client Need: Physiological Integrity: Physiological Adaptation
2. Which statement correctly describes one of the three factors that affect stroke volume?
   1. Contractility is the ability of cardiac muscle fibers to shorten and produce a muscle contraction.
   2. Preload is the amount of blood remaining in the atria at the end of diastole.
   3. Cardiac output is the amount of blood ejected by the heart with each ventricular contraction.
   4. Afterload is the amount of blood remaining in the ventricles at the end of systole.

   NCLEX Client Need: Physiological Integrity: Physiological Adaptation
3. The nurse hears a murmur when auscultating the heart sounds of an 80-year-old patient. The nurse recalls that age-related changes in the circulatory system that can cause heart murmurs include which of the following? (Select all that apply.)
   1. Decreased elasticity of connective tissue in the heart muscle
   2. Arterial stiffening caused by changes in connective tissue and elastic fibers
   3. Heart valves that are stiff and do not close properly
   4. Stretching and dilation of veins resulting in impaired venous return
   5. The aging heart responds more slowly to increased demands

   NCLEX Client Need: Physiological Integrity: Physiological Adaptation
4. Before administering digoxin, the nurse counts a patient's apical heart rate and finds that it is 62 bpm. The patient's usual rate ranges from 65 to 75 bpm. Should the nurse administer the digoxin?
   NCLEX Client Need: Physiological Integrity: Physiological Adaptation
5. The licensed vocational nurse/licensed practical nurse (LVN/LPN) is administering medications to patients in long-term care. Three of the patients are taking various antidysrhythmic drugs. Which of the following is a potential adverse effect common to all antidysrhythmic drugs?
   1. Fluid and electrolyte imbalance
   2. Drowsiness
   3. Diarrhea
   4. Additional dysrhythmias

   NCLEX Client Need: Physiological Integrity: Pharmacological Therapies

6. The nurse is preparing a teaching plan for a cardiac patient who lives at home. The plan should include which of the following dietary recommendations? (Select all that apply.)
   1. Restrict sodium intake to 1 g/day.
   2. Avoid raw fruits and vegetables that are difficult to digest.
   3. Use unsaturated fats such as vegetable oil instead of butter.
   4. Limit saturated fats by eating no more than 12 oz of meat per day.
   5. Include foods that contain omega-3 fatty acids.

   NCLEX Client Need: Physiological Integrity: Basic Care and Comfort
7. Nurses in a retirement community are preparing a program to educate residents about risk factors for atherosclerosis that can be modified. Which of the following risk factors should be addressed? (Select all that apply.)
   1. Increased serum lipids
   2. Hypertension
   3. Heredity
   4. Physical inactivity
   5. Stress

   NCLEX Client Need: Physiological Integrity: Reduction of Risk Potential
8. Your neighbor was mowing his lawn when he began to have chest pain that radiated to his left shoulder. What is this type of pain called?

   NCLEX Client Need: Physiological Integrity: Physiological Adaptation
9. Which of the following drugs may be administered after MI to dissolve thrombi?
   1. Heparin
   2. t-PA
   3. Aspirin
   4. Lidocaine

   NCLEX Client Need: Physiological Integrity: Pharmacological Therapies
10. When cardiac output falls, compensatory mechanisms include which of the following? (Select all that apply.)
    1. Elimination of excess fluid by the kidneys
    2. Constriction of blood vessels in the extremities
    3. Stimulation of the parasympathetic nervous system
    4. Enlargement of the ventricular myocardium
    5. Increased heart rate

    NCLEX Client Need: Physiological Integrity: Physiological Adaptation
11. Discharge teaching for a patient with HF should include which of the following instructions?
    1. "Immediately begin a vigorous program of exercise."
    2. "Inform the physician if you gain more than 3 to 5 lb in 1 week."
    3. "Weigh yourself before going to bed each night."
    4. "Expect to continue having shortness of breath, chest pain, and cough."

    NCLEX Client Need: Physiological Integrity: Reduction of Risk Potential
12. Before invasive procedures, including dental work, patients with valvular heart disease usually are prescribed antibiotics to prevent ________________.

    NCLEX Client Need: Physiological Integrity: Reduction of Risk Potential
13. A patient who has had heart transplantation comes to the physician's office complaining of fever, fatigue, shortness of breath, and an irregular heartbeat. What problem should you suspect?

    NCLEX Client Need: Physiological Integrity: Physiological Adaptation
14. Which of the following findings would you expect in a patient with mitral stenosis?
    1. Increased left atrial pressure
    2. Decreased pulmonary pressure
    3. Increased cardiac output
    4. Decreased right ventricular pressure

    NCLEX Client Need: Physiological Integrity: Physiological Adaptation

chapter 37

Vascular Disorders

http://evolve.elsevier.com/Linton/medsurg

Objectives

1. Identify specific anatomic and physiologic factors that affect the vascular system and tissue oxygenation.
2. Indicate data to collect for assessment of a patient with peripheral vascular disease, aneurysm, and aortic dissection.
3. Discuss nursing care related to tests and procedures used to diagnose selected vascular disorders.
4. Describe the pathophysiology, signs and symptoms, complications, and medical or surgical treatments for selected vascular disorders.
5. Assist in developing a plan of nursing care for patients with selected vascular disorders.

Key Terms

Aneurysm (ĂN-yŭr-ĭzm)
Bruit (BRŪ-ē)
Embolism (ĔM-bō-lĭzm)
Hemoconcentration
Ischemia (ĭs-KĒ-mē-ă)
Paresthesia (păr-ĕs-THĒ-zhă)
Phlebitis (flĕ-BĪ-tĭs)
Poikilothermy (pŏy-kĕ-lō-THĔR-mē)
Thrombosis (thrŏm-BŌ-sĭs)
Vasoconstriction (vā-zō-kŏn-STRĬK-shŭn)
Viscosity (vĭs-KŎ-sĭ-tē)

The delivery of oxygen (O_2) and nutrients to the tissues depends on adequate perfusion (blood flow), which requires a functionally intact cardiovascular system. When the cardiovascular system is compromised by vascular disease, the homeostasis of the body is affected. Risk factors for vascular disease include advanced age, heredity, smoking, obesity, physical inactivity, hypertension, and diabetes mellitus. Vascular diseases can affect the arterial and venous components of the circulation, resulting in pain, impaired function, and even death.

Atherosclerosis is discussed in Chapter 36. Other peripheral vascular disorders, as well as aortic aneurysm and aortic dissection, are presented here.

ANATOMY AND PHYSIOLOGY OF THE VASCULAR SYSTEM

The peripheral vascular system comprises arteries, capillaries, veins, and the lymph vessels (Fig. 37-1). The function of this system is to maintain blood flow to supply adequate O_2 and nutrients to all tissues. Any interruption of the blood flow results in tissue hypoxia, which can lead to tissue necrosis (death) if untreated.

ARTERIES

Arteries are the vessels that carry the blood away from the heart toward the tissues. These vessels are normally elastic and have greater tensile strength than the veins. The aorta, which is the largest artery in the body, transports oxygenated blood from the left ventricle (LV) of the heart. Arteries that branch from the aortic arch supply the head and arms. The thoracic branch of the descending aorta supplies intercostal muscles, the esophagus, and some respiratory passages. The abdominal branch of the descending aorta supplies the gastrointestinal (GI) organs, the kidneys, the gonads, the lumbar area of the back, and the legs. Arteries branch into progressively smaller vessels as they travel away from the aorta. The smallest branches of the arteries are called *arterioles.*

Arteries and arterioles are thick-walled structures with three layers: (1) the intima, (2) the media, and (3) the adventitia (Fig. 37-2). The *intima* is composed of endothelial cells that form the smooth inner surface of the arteries, allowing the blood to flow with little resistance. The middle layer is the *media*, the primary structure of the artery. The media is composed of smooth muscle, elastic fibers, and connective tissue fibers.

Smooth muscles encircle and control the diameter of arteries and arterioles. Contraction of the muscles constricts the vessels whereas relaxation of the muscles results in vessel dilation. The autonomic nervous system and other chemical and hormonal factors govern smooth muscle contraction and relaxation.

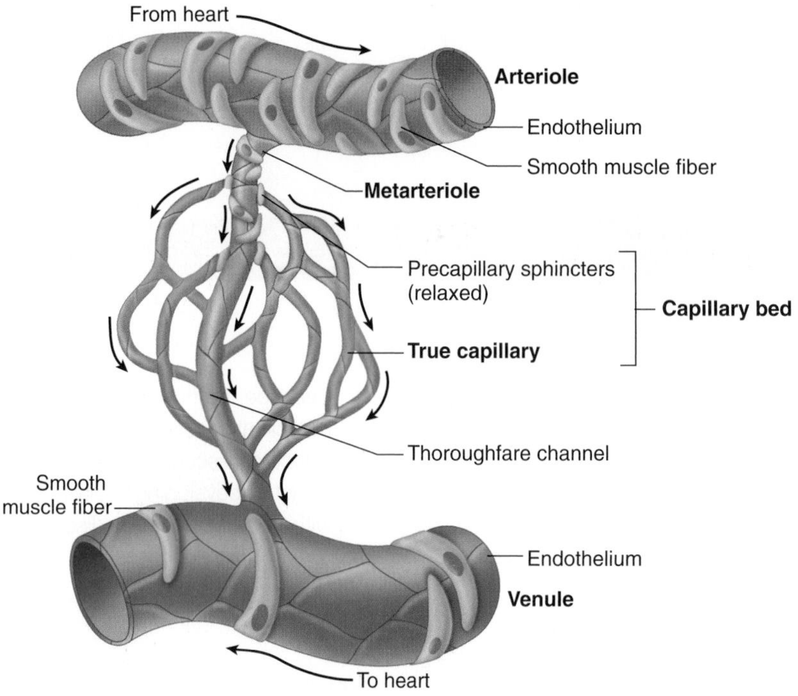

FIGURE 37-1 Capillary bed. Foods, nutrients, and oxygen (O_2) are delivered to tissues through the capillaries and wastes are collected from the capillaries for recycling or excretion. Precapillary sphincters help to regulate the flow. (From Patton KT, Thibodeau GA: *Anatomy and physiology*, ed 8, St Louis, 2014, Mosby.)

The outer layer of the arteries and arterioles is the *adventitia.* This layer, which is composed mostly of connective tissue, secures the artery or arteriole to the surrounding structures.

CAPILLARIES

Arterioles branch into progressively smaller and smaller vessels, until they form the capillaries. Capillaries consist of a single layer of endothelial cells that allow the efficient delivery of nutrients and O_2 into the tissues and the removal of metabolic wastes from the tissues. Transfer of O_2 and nutrients between the blood and the tissue cells occurs in the capillaries. Red blood cells (RBCs) must conform to the size of the capillaries by changing their shape to fit through the small diameter.

The tiny vessels that receive blood from the capillaries are venules, which are the smallest veins. The metabolic activity occurring in the tissue determines the distribution of capillaries. Tissues such as skeletal muscles and digestive tract lining have a rich capillary network whereas tissues such as bone and cartilage have a scanty capillary network.

Because capillaries have less smooth muscle than the arteries, the amount of blood in the capillary is controlled by sphincters on the arteriolar side of the capillary. Other factors such as chemical stimulation and hormonal changes also influence blood flow and fluid shifts in the capillaries. For example, histamine causes the capillary permeability to increase, allowing more fluid to shift into the tissues.

VEINS

The blood is returned to the heart by way of the venules and veins. These vessels are formed as the capillaries organize into larger and larger vessels. The venous system is less sturdy and more passive than the arterial system. The walls of veins and venules are composed of the same three layers as the walls of the arteries and arterioles but the layers are less defined (see Fig. 37-2). Because the walls of the veins and venules are thinner and less muscular, they can stretch more than those of the arterial system. Thus the venous system can store a large volume of blood under relatively low pressure. As much as 75% of the body's total blood volume is housed in the venous system.

Valves

The venous system is equipped with valves that are composed of endothelial leaflets (Fig. 37-3). Valves allow the blood to move in only one direction and prevent backflow of the blood in the extremities. Skeletal muscle contractions compress the veins, forcing blood back toward the heart. This action reduces venous pooling and increases the circulating blood volume. As deoxygenated blood moves toward the heart, carbon dioxide (CO_2) and other metabolic wastes are carried to the lungs and kidneys for elimination.

Innervation

The sympathetic nervous system innervates the venous system, acting on the musculature of the veins to

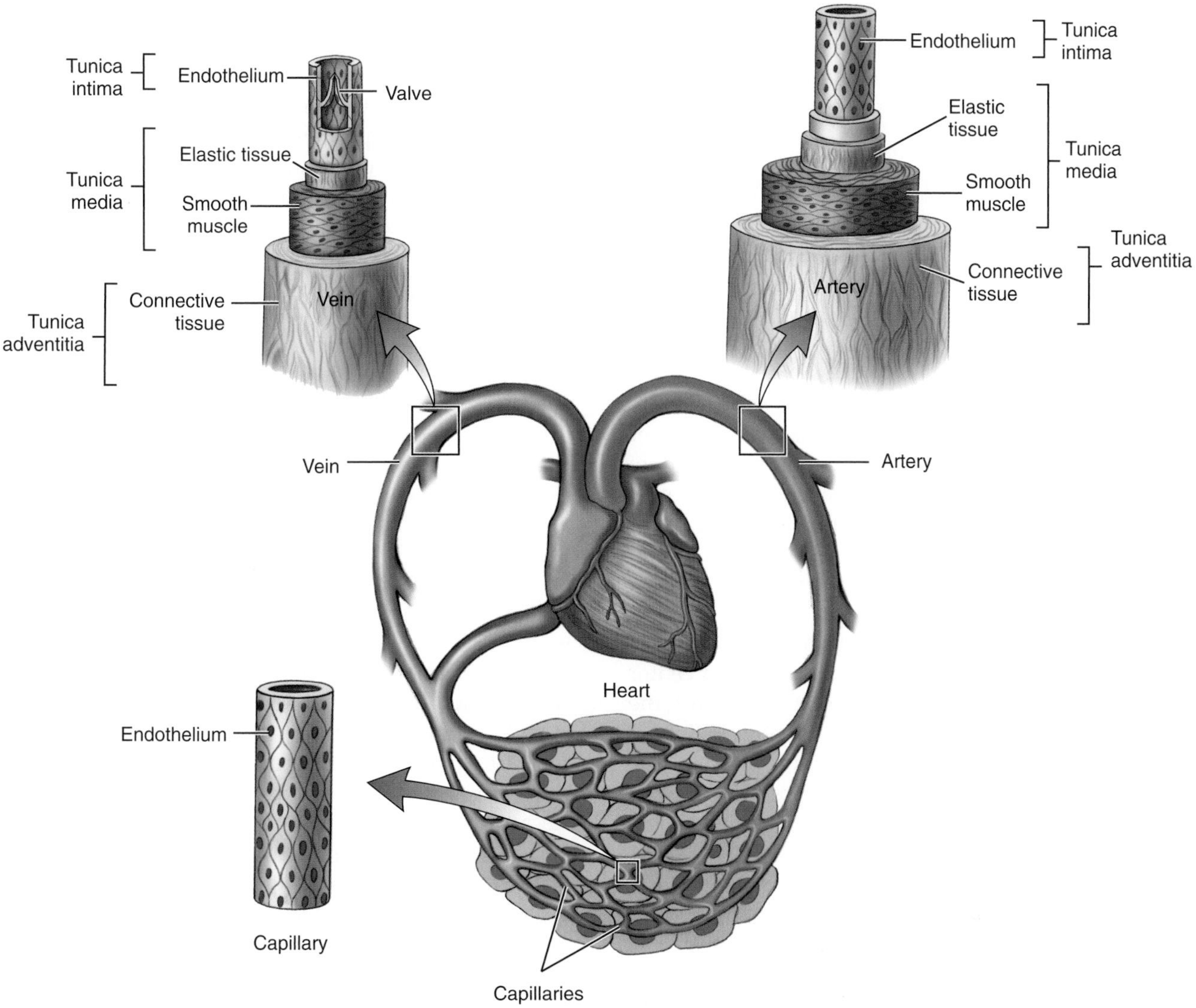

FIGURE 37-2 Tissue layers of veins and arteries. (From Herlihy B: *The human body in health and illness*, ed 4, St. Louis, 2011, Saunders.)

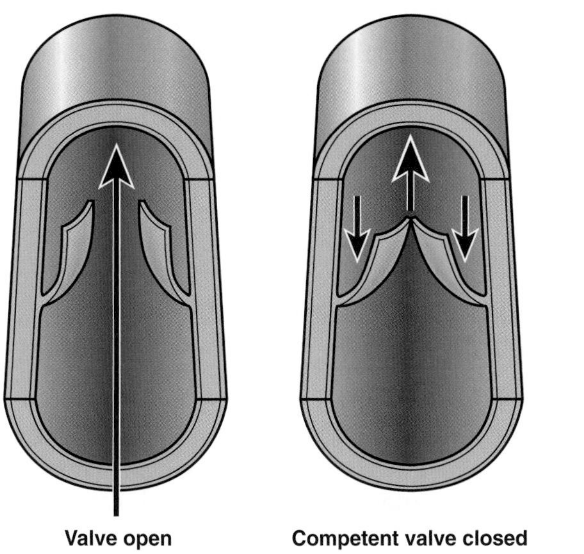

FIGURE 37-3 Veins contain bicuspid valves that open in the direction of blood flow but prevent regurgitation of flow when pockets become filled and distended.

stimulate venoconstriction. Blocking of sympathetic nerve stimulation permits venodilation.

LYMPH VESSELS

The lymph system is an organization of small, thin-walled vessels that resemble the capillaries. These vessels accommodate the collection of lymph fluid from the peripheral tissues and the transportation of the fluid to the venous circulatory system. Because the lymph system interacts with the venous system, it is classified as part of the cardiovascular system. The lymph system comprises two main trunks: (1) the thoracic duct and (2) the right lymphatic duct. Each of these trunks is responsible for collecting and draining fluid from specific areas of the body. (See Chapter 34 for additional information.)

Lymph fluid is composed of plasmalike fluid, large protein molecules, and foreign substances. Because these protein molecules are too large to enter the capillaries or the venules, the lymph fluid carries them to the lymphatic ducts, where they are emptied into the subclavian and internal jugular veins. The movement of lymph fluid is accomplished by the contraction of muscles that encircle the lymphatic walls and surrounding tissues.

FACTORS THAT AFFECT BLOOD FLOW

The body has multiple homeostatic mechanisms to control the systemic and local blood volume. These mechanisms work by changing resistance within the vessels or by changing the blood **viscosity**.

Resistance

Resistance within the vascular system is controlled by the diameter of the vessels. When vascular diameter increases, peripheral resistance falls and blood flow increases. When vascular diameter decreases, however, peripheral resistance increases, thereby reducing blood flow. As previously noted, the diameter of blood vessels is controlled by the central nervous system, hormones, some ions, and blood pH.

The sympathetic nervous system plays a major role in adjusting vascular resistance. The vasomotor center located in the medulla and the pons regulates the diameter of peripheral blood vessels. Stimulation of the sympathetic nervous system by either physiologic or psychologic stressors also triggers the adrenal glands to release norepinephrine and epinephrine, which cause **vasoconstriction**.

Other substances that cause changes in vascular resistance are angiotensin, serotonin, histamine, the kinins, and the prostaglandins. Angiotensin II is a potent chemical released by the kidneys that causes intense vasoconstriction and retention of salt and water by the kidneys. The kinins, histamine, and prostaglandins cause vasodilation, which decreases peripheral resistance. Serotonin, a chemical that is liberated from platelets when vessel walls are damaged, can cause vasoconstriction or vasodilation, depending on tissue conditions.

Blood Viscosity

In addition to changes in peripheral resistance, modification of blood viscosity helps to regulate blood flow to peripheral tissues. Viscosity describes the thickness of the blood. The blood viscosity is usually constant but can be affected by changes in the proportions of the solid or liquid components. An increase in RBCs or a decrease in body water produces **hemoconcentration**, which increases blood viscosity. When blood is concentrated, the kidneys usually begin to retain water and the movement of fluid out of the capillaries is restricted.

An important factor that affects blood viscosity is capillary permeability. Hydrostatic and osmotic pressures normally maintain balanced movement of fluids in and out of the capillaries. Any mechanism that alters capillary permeability changes the amount and direction of fluid movement, resulting in a change in blood viscosity. Factors that increase capillary permeability include histamine, bradykinin, leukotrienes, and prostaglandins. Certain muscle metabolites, hypoxemia, malnutrition, and pH imbalances can also increase capillary permeability. When the proportion of serum to solid components in the blood is greater than normal, blood is less viscous and the kidneys excrete excess fluid.

AGE-RELATED CHANGES

The primary age-related change in peripheral vessels is hardening of the vessel walls, called *arteriosclerosis*. As arteriosclerosis develops, the delivery of O_2 and nutrients to the tissues is compromised and a buildup of waste products occurs in the tissue.

The hardening of the peripheral vessels associated with aging occurs in both the intima and the media of the vessel wall. The intima is thickened and hardened by the proliferation of cells. It becomes roughened, which increases the risk of thrombus formation and emboli. The connective and elastic tissue fibers in the media become calcified. This process produces a thinner and fragmented layer within the peripheral vessels. Loss of elasticity in the peripheral vessels increases peripheral resistance, which impairs blood flow and results in increased left ventricular workload. As a result, the transportation of O_2 and nutrients to and the removal of wastes from the tissues are affected adversely. The same changes that affect peripheral blood vessels also occur in the aorta of the older adult. The aorta stiffens, thickens, and loses distensibility, which increases resistance to blood flow.

The transportation of O_2 also may be compromised by the decrease of hemoglobin (Hgb) seen in some older adults. A reduction of Hgb in the blood reduces the O_2-carrying capacity of the blood. Because the stiffening blood vessels decrease blood flow and because decreased Hgb compromises the O_2-carrying capacity, peripheral circulation can be substantially affected.

Overall, aging in the vascular system may cause a slowing of the heart rate and a decrease in the stroke volume, which may result in a 30% to 40% decrease in cardiac output. If cardiac output is altered, the older adult may adapt more slowly to changes in the peripheral vascular system.

NURSING ASSESSMENT OF THE VASCULAR SYSTEM

HEALTH HISTORY

Chief Complaint and History of Present Illness

The nursing assessment of a patient who may have a vascular disorder requires a thorough cardiovascular assessment by the registered nurse (RN), as described in Chapter 36. The licensed vocational nurse/licensed practical nurse (LVN/LPN) may assist by collecting relevant data. Assessment of the peripheral circulation focuses on the six classic *P*s characteristic of peripheral vascular disease (PVD): (1) pain, (2) pulselessness, (3) **poikilothermy**, (4) pallor, (5) **paresthesia**, and (6) paralysis. Each of these components needs to be evaluated.

Pain. A thorough pain history provides valuable information about vascular disease. Ask the patient to describe the nature of any pain or discomfort in the calf, thigh, hip, or buttock areas. Document the nature of the pain (e.g., sharp, throbbing, continuous, intermittent), the location and duration of the pain, the precipitating factors (e.g., exercise, lying down in bed), and any alleviating factors (whatever brings relief). Acute pain is associated with acute arterial obstruction. Intermittent claudication and pain at rest are considered chronic pain.

When pain is caused by a venous disorder, patients typically describe it as *tenderness, heaviness,* or *fullness in the extremity.* It is important to note whether the pain was alleviated by elevating the extremity or by wearing support stockings. Pain associated with an aortic aneurysm varies with the location of the aneurysm.

Intermittent Claudication. Intermittent claudication is pain associated with decreased perfusion that is aggravated by exercise and relieved by rest. Intermittent claudication can affect any major muscle group distal to (beyond) the point of arterial occlusion. The pain is described as a feeling of *tightness, burning, fatigue, aching,* or *cramping.* Exercise causes the muscle group to become ischemic because blood flow is inadequate to supply nutrients and O_2 and to remove wastes. This results in the development of pain. When the exercise is stopped, the metabolic demands of the muscle tissue decrease, wastes are removed from the tissues, and the pain is relieved.

Rest Pain. Rest pain indicates severe arterial occlusion (obstruction). By impeding blood flow, the occlusion causes tissue **ischemia** in the extremity. For example, a person with arterial occlusion in the lower extremities may experience severe, burning pain in the legs and feet after lying flat for a period of time. The pain is relieved when the extremity is dangled in a dependent position that promotes blood flow by gravity. Frequently, the patient sleeps best in a chair or with the feet in a dependent position.

Pulselessness. Palpate the peripheral pulses for rate, rhythm, and quality and compare pulses bilaterally to detect any differences.

Poikilothermy and Pallor. Poikilothermy is decreased temperature at an ischemic site, which is detected by palpating the affected and surrounding areas. The poikilothermic area feels cooler than the rest of the extremity. Pallor, meaning paleness, is apparent over an area of reduced blood supply. Pallor is detected by inspecting the affected site and comparing skin color with other parts of the body.

Paresthesia and Paralysis. Paresthesia, paralysis, or both should be noted. Paresthesia is an abnormal sensation such as numbness, tingling, a "pins-and-needles" sensation, or a crawling sensation. Paralysis is impairment of motor function. These symptoms may be associated with impaired conduction of nerve impulses caused by inadequate O_2 and nutrients to the nerve tissues and the accumulation of waste materials.

Past Medical History

The past medical history includes the cardiovascular assessment, as described in Chapter 36. Document a history of hypertension, coronary heart disease (CHD), myocardial infarction, or atherosclerosis. Because atherosclerosis affects the cerebral, renal, and respiratory blood vessels, it is important to include each of these areas in the discussion of past medical problems. It is especially significant if the patient has diabetes, because PVD is a common complication of diabetes.

Family History

The family history documents any cardiovascular disorders or other relevant conditions in immediate family members. Relevant diseases include hypertension, CHD, myocardial infarction, atherosclerosis, aneurysm, and diabetes.

Review of Systems

Changes in the integument provide important clues to the presence and severity of PVD. Changes that may be associated with PVD are thick and brittle nails; shiny, taut, scaly, and dry skin; skin temperature variations; skin ulcerations; muscle atrophy; localized redness and hardness; and hair loss on the extremities.

Another component of the review of systems is the assessment for chest pain and dyspnea. These symptoms are important because 10% of people with deep vein **thrombosis** (DVT) develop a pulmonary embolus.

Aneurysms are often asymptomatic. Depending on the location of the aneurysm, the patient may report hoarseness, dysphagia, dyspnea, abdominal or back pain, or swelling of the head and arms.

Functional Assessment

The functional assessment determines the effect of the disease process on the patient's life. The pain associated with PVD can interfere with work and recreation. Inactivity can reduce the patient's stamina. If the patient has had a limb amputated because of PVD, explore how the limb loss affects the patient's functioning. Other aspects of the functional assessment that are relevant to vascular disease are smoking history and dietary habits. Smoking causes vasoconstriction and a high fat intake can contribute to arteriosclerosis. Both are associated with PVD.

PHYSICAL EXAMINATION

The patient's vital signs, height, and weight all are relevant to the PVD assessment. The physical examination helps to determine whether the disease process is arterial or venous in nature. In general, arterial complications involve multiple areas whereas venous complications remain more localized, usually in the lower extremities. Inspect the skin for color and lesions. Pallor suggests peripheral vasoconstriction or inadequate arterial blood flow. A reddish-brown discoloration called *rubor* in a dependent lower extremity suggests the presence of arterial occlusive disease. In venous disorders, the affected areas of the skin may have a brownish discoloration and be cyanotic when the extremity is dependent. It is important to be alert for open ulcers and for scars around the ankles that may be associated with either arterial or venous disease. Note the presence of stasis dermatitis, a brown pigmentation with flaky skin over the edematous areas of the ankles. It may take on a bluish cast when the leg is in a dependent position. Arterial stasis dermatitis begins as ulcerations in the toes. The ulcers are painful, pale, crusty, and located over bony prominences. Venous stasis dermatitis begins as ulcers in the ankle area. The ulcers develop very slowly, are usually painless, and are difficult to heal.

Determine capillary refill time in the nail beds to determine the adequacy of peripheral perfusion. To do this, press the nail bed until it blanches (turns pale). Then release the pressure and note the number of seconds it takes for the color to return. Capillary refill time greater than 3 seconds denotes a reduction in peripheral perfusion.

Palpate the affected areas to evaluate the temperature, detect edema, and assess peripheral pulses. Skin temperature should be palpated bilaterally, moving proximally to distally (toward the feet), to detect any ischemic areas. A cool limb suggests an arterial problem and a warm limb suggests a venous problem. A pulsating mass detected on abdominal palpation may be an aneurysm.

Dependent edema develops as a result of systemic disorders, lymphatic dysfunction, DVT, or chronic venous insufficiency. To determine the severity of edema, the examiner presses the thumb into the edematous area for approximately 5 seconds. If the depression of the thumb remains in the edematous area, the edema is said to be *pitting*. The severity of pitting edema is graded from 1+ to 4+. A slight indentation with no apparent leg swelling is graded 1+. Moderate pitting that subsides rapidly is graded as 2+. A deep indentation that remains briefly, with swelling of the leg is graded 3+. Deep pitting that lasts a long time accompanied by gross leg swelling is graded 4+. The same area on both extremities should be compared.

Another aspect of the examination is the evaluation of peripheral pulses (Fig. 37-4). Palpate pulses for presence, symmetry, volume, and rhythm. The peripheral pulses to be palpated in the upper extremities include the brachial, ulnar, and radial arteries. The peripheral pulses appraised in the lower extremities are the femoral, popliteal, dorsalis pedis, and posterior tibial arteries. Pulses should be compared bilaterally and any absent or asymmetric pulses documented. The palpation of the arteries provides valuable information concerning the condition of the vessels. A sclerotic vessel feels stiff and cordlike whereas a normal vessel can be palpated as soft and springy.

Homans sign traditionally has been checked to evaluate for PVD. The assumption was that pain elicited by sharply dorsiflexing the patient's foot (*positive Homans sign*) indicated the presence of DVT in that leg. However, this test is not reliable and should *not* be included.

A test that can be beneficial in the assessment of the peripheral vascular system is the Allen test. The Allen test is used to determine the adequacy of arterial circulation to the hand. The patient is asked to clench the fist tightly while the nurse occludes the radial and ulnar arteries. The patient is then instructed to open the fist and the nurse releases pressure on the ulnar artery. If the ulnar artery is patent, the palm should promptly return to a normal color. A persistence of pallor in the palm area indicates an occlusion of the ulnar artery. The test can be repeated with the ulnar artery being occluded instead of the radial artery to detect occlusion within the radial artery (see Chapter 31, Fig. 31-6).

The nurse with advanced education can further evaluate peripheral vascular function by auscultating the sounds of blood flow through the arteries. **Bruits** sound like turbulent, fast-moving fluid. The presence of bruits can signal the presence of an aneurysm or the development of chronic arterial occlusive disease long before other signs appear.

Nursing assessment of the patient with PVD is summarized in Box 37-1.

DIAGNOSTIC TESTS AND PROCEDURES

Based on physical examination findings, the physician orders selected diagnostic studies to confirm the disease process and to determine the severity of the condition. The procedures and tests that may be used to diagnose PVD are ultrasonography, serum lipids, pressure measurements, stress testing, tomographic angiography, magnetic resonance angiography, and angiography, which includes arteriography and venography, as shown in Table 37-1. Procedures that are useful in the diagnosis of aneurysms include chest radiography, abdominal ultrasound, computed tomography (CT), and transthoracic echocardiography. When pulmonary embolism is suspected, diagnostic tools that might be used include the lung scan, pulmonary angiogram, and spiral CT scan.

ULTRASONOGRAPHY

Doppler ultrasound is used to facilitate the diagnosis of PVD and to monitor the changes in blood flow

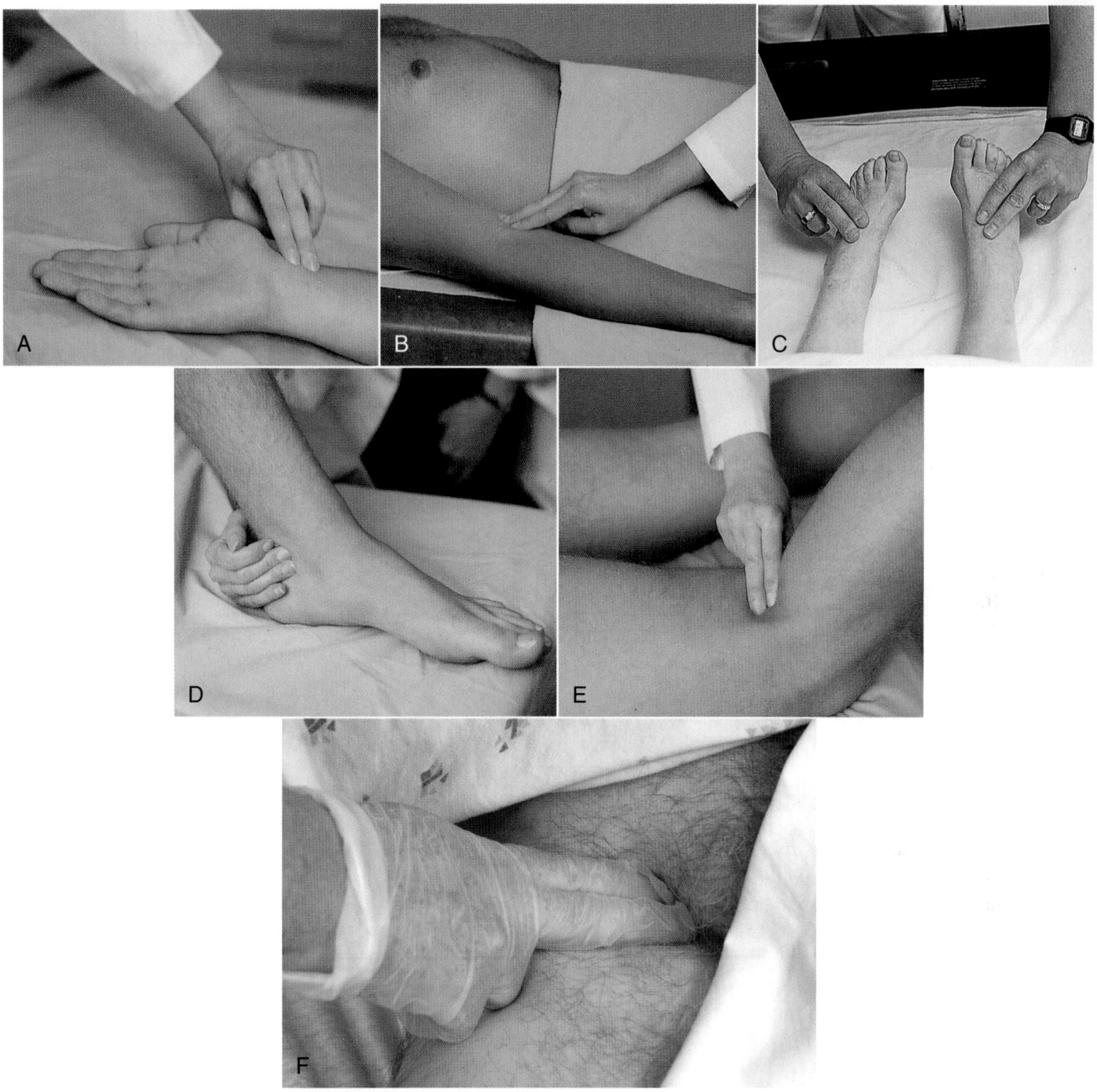

FIGURE 37-4 Palpating peripheral pulses. **A,** Radial. **B,** Brachial. **C,** Dorsalis pedis. **D,** Posterior tibial. **E,** Popliteal. **F,** Femoral. (From Perry AG, Potter PA, Ostendorf W: *Clinical nursing skills and techniques,* ed 8, St. Louis, 2014, Mosby.)

associated with vascular diseases. It is a noninvasive, inexpensive, highly reliable diagnostic tool. Low-intensity, high-frequency sound waves are directed toward the vessels being tested, primarily the posterior tibial, popliteal, and common femoral veins. These sound waves strike the moving blood cells and are reflected back to the receiver. Arteries reflect a high-pitched sound whereas veins produce sounds that vary with respirations and have a "blowing" tone. The sounds are diminished in the presence of an occluded or narrowed vessel. The test takes 10 to 20 minutes. Abdominal ultrasound may be used to screen for abdominal aneurysms. Duplex scanning combines two types of ultrasonography to evaluate blood flow and provide a two-dimensional image of the blood vessel and the blood flow.

PRESSURE MEASUREMENTS

Plethysmography is a noninvasive study used to measure blood flow in the extremities. Multiple blood pressure cuffs are applied to different parts of the extremities. Variations in pressure from one site to another can reveal vascular occlusions or obstructions. Although plethysmography is less accurate than

Box 37-1 Assessment of the Patient with Peripheral Vascular Disease or Aneurysm

HEALTH HISTORY

Present Illness

Complaints of pain, pulselessness, poikilothermy, pallor, paresthesia, and paralysis

Past Medical History

Hypertension, CHD, myocardial infarction (MI), amputations, atherosclerosis, diabetes mellitus

Family History

Hypertension, CHD, MI, atherosclerosis, diabetes mellitus, aneurysm

Review of Systems

Hairlessness on lower extremities; peripheral edema; discoloration of dependent areas; temperature changes in compromised areas; ulcerations on lower extremities; limb pain; thick, brittle toenails; temperature variation over involved area; muscle atrophy; localized redness and induration in affected extremity; chest pain; dyspnea; hoarseness; swelling of head, arms, or both; back or abdominal pain

Functional Assessment

Mobility restricted by pain, decreased stamina

PHYSICAL EXAMINATION

General Survey

Posture, gait, presence of pain in affected extremities, edema of face or arms (or both)

Cardiovascular

Symmetric peripheral pulses, capillary refill time

Integument

Temperature of affected area, edema in dependent area, color of affected extremity, rubor in lower extremities, stasis dermatitis or ulcers

Abdomen

Palpable pulsatile mass

Table 37-1 Diagnostic Tests and Procedures Peripheral Vascular Disease

TEST	USES	PATIENT PREPARATION	POSTPROCEDURE CARE
Duplex ultrasound: combines compression ultrasound with Doppler	Uses sound waves to facilitate diagnosis of PVD	Tell the patient the test is painless and has no risks. Patient may be asked to change the position of the extremity being evaluated and perform breathing exercises.	No special care is required.
Plethysmography	Used to detect DVT, to screen patients who are at risk for PVD, and to investigate the possibility of pulmonary emboli	Tell the patient the procedure is safe, painless, and takes about 30–45 minutes. Patient's leg will be elevated and a pressure cuff will be placed on the thigh. Electrodes record information about blood flow in the veins.	No special care is required.
Pressure measurement	Types include segmental limb pressures and pulse volume measurements	Tell the patient blood pressures will be measured in multiple sites over the extremities to assess the blood vessels. Pressures are measured during activity and while at rest. Test is noninvasive, painless, and safe.	No special care is required.
Exercise (treadmill) test	Evaluates the functional abilities of patients with PVD by measuring pulse volumes before, during, and after exercise	Tell the patient the test is noninvasive. Patient will be asked to walk for approximately 5 minutes on a treadmill. The test will be stopped if the patient has pain or dyspnea.	Carefully monitor the patient for any complications that may develop as a result of the test.
Angiography (venography: contrast, CT, MRI; arteriography, and radiographs)	Identifies vascular obstruction, aneurysm, and atherosclerotic plaques	Tell the patient dye will be injected and radiographs taken. Patient may briefly feel a burning sensation when the dye is injected. Signed consent is required. Patient should receive nothing by mouth (NPO) for 4 hours before the test. Inform the radiologist if the patient is allergic to iodine or seafood. Risks include hemorrhage at insertion site, dye-induced allergic reaction, thrombosis/embolism, renal insufficiency, and pseudoaneurysm.	Bed rest is required for several hours. Monitor the patient's vital signs and pulses hourly for 6 hours. Assess the injection site for bleeding, hematoma, and pulsating mass (pseudoaneurysm). Neurovascular checks (pulses, sensation, movement, color, warmth) should be conducted.

CT, Computed tomography; *DVT,* deep vein thrombosis; *MRI,* magnetic resonance imaging; *PVD,* peripheral vascular disease.

arteriography and venography, it is very safe and can be used to assess patients who are too ill to undergo arteriography.

EXERCISE TOLERANCE TEST

The exercise test is sometimes referred to as a *stress test* or exercise stress testing. This noninvasive procedure helps to evaluate the patient's tolerance for physical activity. Signed consent is required. The patient is asked to walk for on a treadmill while continuous electrocardiogram (ECG) and blood pressure monitoring is done. Several protocols exist with various durations, speeds, and incline elevations. Most continue the testing until the patient achieves 85% of his or her maximal heart rate. A gross estimate of maximal heart rate is obtained by subtracting the patient's age from 220. If the patient experiences distress, signs of myocardial ischemia, or claudication, the test is stopped immediately. After the test, the patient should be monitored until vital signs return to normal.

ANGIOGRAPHY

The purposes of angiography are to confirm the diagnosis of PVD, to distinguish clot formation from venous obstruction, and to locate a suitable vessel for grafting. Angiography is an invasive procedure that requires the injection of dye into the vascular system, which makes the vessels visible on radiographs. The two types of angiography are (1) arteriography, which examines arteries, and (2) venography, which examines veins. Abnormalities can be visualized and assessed during the procedure. The risks associated with these tests are hemorrhage at the intravenous insertion site, dye-induced allergic reactions, thrombosis at the insertion site, and emboli. The patient is exposed to relatively high doses of radiation.

COMMON THERAPEUTIC MEASURES

The primary goals for the patient with PVD are to increase the arterial blood supply to the extremities, reduce venous congestion, dilate blood vessels to increase arterial blood flow, prevent vascular compression, provide relief from pain, attain or maintain tissue integrity, and encourage adherence to the treatment plan.

Exercise programs, stress management, pain management, smoking cessation, elastic stockings, intermittent pneumatic compression units, body positioning, drug therapy, surgical interventions, and patient education are used in the management of the disease process.

EXERCISE

The simple act of walking stimulates the movement of blood from the dependent areas of the extremities toward the heart. Walking contracts the muscles of the lower extremities, pushing venous blood upward toward the heart and promoting the development of collateral circulation. For patients with vascular disease, the physician must prescribe any exercise program. Patients who have leg ulcers, gangrene, or acute thrombotic occlusion may be restricted to bed rest until the condition improves.

A specific type of exercise program that is effective in the management of PVD is the use of Buerger-Allen exercises or active postural exercises (Fig. 37-5) (see *Patient Teaching* box).

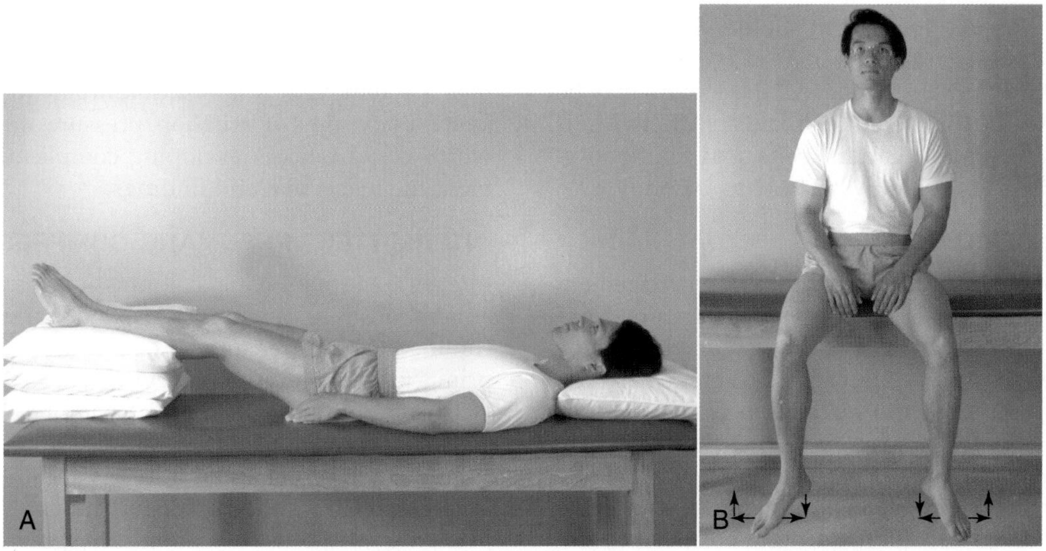

FIGURE 37-5 Buerger-Allen exercises for peripheral vascular disease (PVD). **A,** Elevate and support the legs at a 45- to 90-degree angle for 2 to 3 minutes, or until the skin blanches. **B,** Sit with feet in a dependent position so that the skin turns red. Support the legs in this position for 5 to 10 minutes, then flex, extend, pronate, and supinate each foot three times. Finally, lie flat in a supine position for 10 minutes. (From Monahan FD, Drake DT, Neighbors M, editors: *Medical-surgical nursing: foundations for clinical practice*, ed 2, Philadelphia, 1998, Saunders.)

Patient Teaching

Buerger-Allen Exercises

These exercises allow gravity to fill and empty the blood vessels.

- Lie flat on your back and raise your legs above the level of your heart for 2 minutes or until they become very pale.
- Lower the legs to a dependent position and flex and extend your feet for 3 minutes or until color returns to your legs.
- Keep your legs flat for 5 minutes.
- Go through the entire process six times in each session if you can tolerate it. Three to four sessions a day provide the best results.
- Stop the exercises immediately if you have pain or severe skin color changes.

STRESS MANAGEMENT

Emotional stress causes peripheral vasoconstriction, which is detrimental to a patient whose circulation is already compromised. Resistance to blood flow is increased, which reduces blood flow to the tissues. Emotional stress cannot be avoided entirely but can be reduced with a stress management plan, which may include lifestyle changes, massage, relaxation, or other stress-reducing activities.

PAIN MANAGEMENT

The patient with PVD often limits ambulation because of pain. However, immobility tends to worsen circulatory problems. Therefore pain management is an important aspect of care. Pain can be managed by promoting circulation to the affected area, by administering prescribed analgesics, or both. When intermittent claudication occurs, the patient should stop the exercise. Rest decreases circulatory demands and alleviates the pain. Once the pain is relieved, the activity may be resumed. Advise the patient to avoid constrictive garments such as girdles, garters, belts, and tight pantyhose that can cause pain by obstructing blood flow.

SMOKING CESSATION

Smoking cessation is critical to effective management of PVD because smoking causes vasoconstriction (constriction of the blood vessels). Vasoconstriction can be documented for up to 1 hour after a cigarette has been smoked. In addition, the nicotine in tobacco causes vasospasms, which drastically restrict the peripheral circulation. Measures to help the patient include encouragement; reinforcement; teaching about the nature of tobacco addiction, the harm of smoking, and the benefits of stopping; self-help materials or "Quit Kits" that are available from various agencies; and pharmacotherapy. Nicotine (patches, spray, gum, inhalers), varenicline (Chantix), and bupropion (Zyban) enhance the chances of success. Even though the best smoking cessation programs have about a 25% to 30% success rate, that rate is significant when one realizes that 45 million Americans smoke cigarettes and that smoking is responsible for about 430,700 preventable deaths in the United States annually.

Pharmacology Capsule

Drugs that help some people who are trying to quit smoking are nicotine, varenicline, and bupropion.

ELASTIC STOCKINGS

Another therapy that is useful in the management of PVD is the use of elastic stockings or antiembolism hose. These stockings provide sustained, evenly distributed pressure over the entire surface of the calves and thighs. The correct placement of elastic stockings compresses superficial veins, resulting in improved blood flow to the deeper veins. It is important to take care when applying these stockings because they can become tourniquets if applied incorrectly. The proper size of elastic stockings must be determined for each patient by using the instruction sheet provided by the manufacturer. Elastic stockings are best applied in the morning before rising from bed because swelling is usually at its lowest level at this time of the day. With the stocking inside out, begin by pulling the stocking onto the foot with firm, even support (Fig. 37-6). Once the elastic stocking is positioned over the heel, pull from the sides so that it distributes evenly over the entire length of the leg. The stockings should be smooth when the application process is completed. If the top is allowed to roll or turn down, circulatory stasis occurs. The stockings should be removed for 10 to 20 minutes twice a day, during which time it is best for the patient to be resting in bed or with the extremities in a nondependent position. When the elastic stockings are removed, it is also important to inspect the skin for any signs of irritation, pressure, or tenderness, which could reflect developing complications. Document the inspection and findings.

INTERMITTENT PNEUMATIC COMPRESSION

Intermittent pneumatic compression or a pulsatile antiembolism system may be used for patients who are confined to bed after surgery or a traumatic injury. The primary function of these devices is to prevent DVT. With intermittent pneumatic compression, elastic stockings are applied that are sequentially inflated from the ankles, calves, and thighs and then deflated. This expansion and contraction mimics the muscle pumping of the lower extremities, prevents venous pooling, and stimulates the circulation.

POSITIONING

Body positions play an important part in the management of PVD. Frequently, patients are restricted to bed

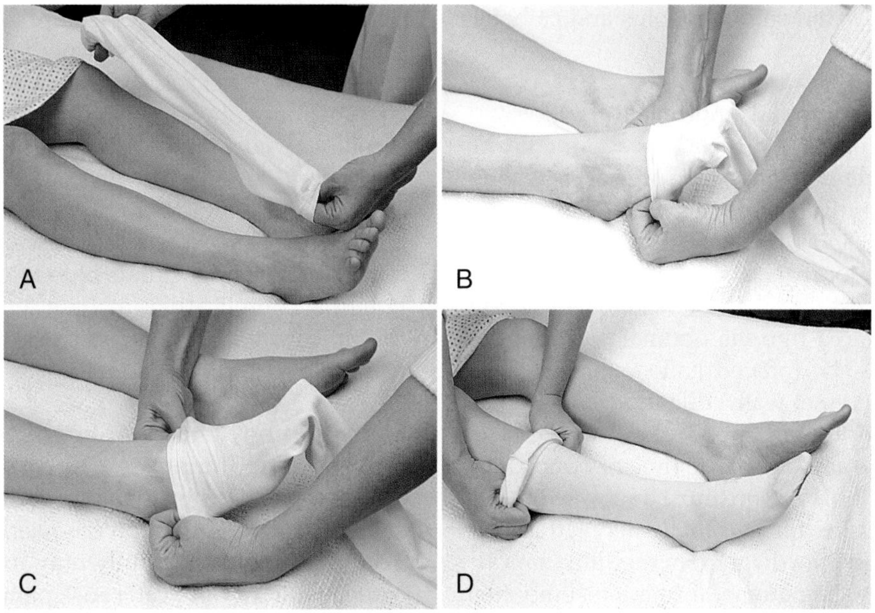

FIGURE 37-6 Elastic stockings provide sustained, consistently distributed pressure over the entire surface of the calves and thighs to promote venous return. (From Elkin MK, Perry AG, & Potter PA: *Nursing interventions and clinical skills*, ed 4, St. Louis, 2007, Mosby.)

during the acute phases of the disease process. It is important to use different positions to mobilize the blood volume that has become stagnant in the dependent areas. Lowering the extremities below the level of the heart enhances arterial blood supply. Elevating the lower extremities above the level of the heart promotes venous return and reduces venous stasis. For patients who are not restricted to bed, prolonged standing puts strain on the venous system. Instruct the patient to sit down and elevate the extremity to a nondependent position whenever possible.

THERMOTHERAPY

Thermotherapy (either warm or cold) can be used for its effects on the circulatory system. Heat, whether dry or moist, works as a vasodilator that promotes arterial flow to the peripheral tissues. Heat should be used cautiously, however, because patients with PVD may suffer burns because they have impaired sensation as a result of tissue ischemia. Blood vessels constrict in response to cold. Clothing can be used effectively to promote warmth and to prevent chilling and vasoconstriction.

PROTECTION

Affected extremities must be protected from trauma because the healing process is usually impaired with PVD. To prevent injury to poorly perfused tissues, the patient must avoid scratching and vigorous rubbing. Caution the patient to wear properly fitting shoes and clean socks or hose, to keep fingernails and toenails trimmed and smooth, and not to walk about barefoot. Inform the physician of ingrown toenails, blisters, or skin injuries so that prompt treatment can be initiated.

PATIENT TEACHING

Patient education is important in the management of PVD. The patient must understand the disease process and the prescribed therapies. The teaching plan should include cleanliness, warmth, safety, comfort measures, prevention of constricting blood flow, exercise, signs and symptoms that should be reported to the health care provider, drug therapy, and the importance of smoking cessation.

SURGICAL PROCEDURES

As PVD progresses, surgical intervention may become necessary. Embolectomy, percutaneous transluminal angioplasty (PTA), endarterectomy, sympathectomy, vein ligation and stripping, sclerotherapy, and laser or light therapy are procedures that may be used.

Embolectomy

Embolectomy is the removal of a blood clot located in a large vessel. An incision is made into the vessel and the clot is removed under direct visualization of the site or through a catheter. This procedure is used when an arterial **embolism** is present and the patient has complicating factors that restrict the use of thrombolytics. Another method for performing an embolectomy is the use of a Fogarty embolectomy catheter. The catheter, which has a soft, inflatable balloon near the tip, is positioned in the artery. The tip of the catheter is passed through the embolus and inflated. Once the balloon is inflated, a steady tension is placed on the catheter to withdraw the entire embolus and catheter from the vessel.

Percutaneous Transluminal Angioplasty

PTA is used to gain access to the arteries in the lower extremities in people who are poor surgical risks. The primary purpose of this technique is to relieve arterial stenosis in such areas as the superficial femoral and iliac arteries. Under local anesthesia, a balloon catheter is passed into the vessel to the stenotic area. Once the catheter is maneuvered into the optimal position, the balloon is inflated. The inflated balloon presses outwardly against the vessel walls, dilating the lumen of the artery and improving blood flow. Heparin is injected through the catheter at the time of removal to prevent clot formation. Pressure must be applied to the catheter insertion site for approximately 10 to 20 minutes to prevent hemorrhage from the site. Complications of PTA are hematoma formation, embolus, arterial dissection, and allergic reactions to the dye used in angiography.

Endarterectomy

An endarterectomy requires an incision in the obstructed vessel. The emboli and atherosclerotic plaque are stripped away from the intima of the vessel and the vessel is surgically closed.

Sympathectomy

A sympathectomy may be done to improve vascular circulation when the patient has intermittent claudication. The process involves the excision of the sympathetic ganglia, which results in arteriolar dilation and increased blood flow. When poor circulation is related to atherosclerotic vessels, a sympathectomy is not the treatment of choice because the hardened blood vessels have limited ability to dilate. To evaluate the capacity for vascular dilation, a lumbar sympathetic block may be done and the temporary effects monitored.

Vein Ligation and Stripping

Vein ligation and stripping are used primarily to treat varicose veins. The greater or lesser saphenous systems, or both, are the vessels removed in this manner. The surgeon must be certain that the deeper veins are patent before the varicosities are removed. Pressure and elevation are used during the procedure to reduce the bleeding. A disadvantage of this procedure is that removal of the saphenous vein means that it would not be available if the patient required coronary artery bypass graft (CABG) surgery in the future.

Sclerotherapy

Sclerotherapy is another method for managing varicose veins, primarily for cosmetic treatment of small, prominent varicosities. Sclerotherapy requires the injection of a chemical that irritates the venous endothelium, causing localized inflammation and fibrosis. One type of this treatment is ultrasound-guided foam sclerotherapy (UGFS). The vein becomes thrombosed and eventually closes. Sclerotherapy may be used in conjunction with vein ligation and stripping. The protocol followed after the procedure depends on the physician but usually involves wearing compression stockings or support stockings for a specified period of time. An exercise program of walking is emphasized to encourage and facilitate blood flow to the extremity. Potential complications include pulmonary embolism, thrombosis, injection site necrosis, vasospasm, hemolysis, and allergic reactions.

Laser Therapy and High-Intensity Pulsed Light Therapy

Laser or light therapy is an option for patients with small varicosities. It involves several treatments at 6- to 12-week intervals. Light therapy uses a slightly different technology. Both can cause pain, blisters, increased pigmentation in the treated area, and superficial ulcers.

❖ NURSING CARE Related to Peripheral Vascular Surgery

■ Preoperative Nursing Care

General preoperative care is discussed in Chapter 17. The patient with severe cardiovascular disease may have activity restrictions to reduce the demands on the circulatory system until the surgical procedure is done. The affected extremity should be maintained in a level or slightly dependent position as ordered. To optimize peripheral circulation, it is important to keep the extremity warm. Protect the limb from further injury.

■ Postoperative Nursing Care

The primary goal of the postoperative period is to stimulate circulation by encouraging movement and preventing stasis within the extremity. Closely monitor tissue perfusion in the postoperative period by assessing the affected extremity for color, temperature, complaints of pain or tenderness, capillary refill time, presence of edema, quality of peripheral pulses, and exercise tolerance. Anticoagulants are usually continued after surgery to prevent the formation of a thrombus at the operative site. If a peripheral pulse disappears, suspect a thrombus and immediately notify the RN or surgeon. Emphasize that the patient ! should not cross the legs or place the affected extremity in a dependent position for long periods of time. Elevating the extremity helps to prevent edema.

DRUGS

Drugs most often used to treat PVD include anticoagulants, thrombolytics, platelet aggregation inhibitors, vasodilators, nonsteroidal antiinflammatory drugs (NSAIDs), and analgesics. Table 37-2 contains information about these medications (see also *Complementary and Alternative Therapies* box).

Table 37-2 Medications for Peripheral Vascular Disorders

DRUG	ACTION AND USES	SIDE EFFECTS	NURSING INTERVENTIONS
Anticoagulant Agents: Most Effective Against Venous Thrombosis			
Unfractionated heparin	Interferes with blood clotting; prevents formation of new clots; does not affect existing clots. Rapid effect. Used to treat pulmonary embolism, evolving stroke, and massive DVT. Prevents clotting during open heart surgery and renal dialysis. May be used *with* a thrombolytic agent for AMI. Low-dose heparin may be used to prevent postoperative venous thrombosis.	Thrombocytopenia (reduced platelets and increased clotting), hemorrhage, nausea and vomiting, and local irritation at injection site. Allergic response: chills, fever, hives. Osteoporosis with long-term, high-dose use.	Regular blood testing must be done to monitor effect on clotting. Check aPTT before each dose (not necessary with low-dose therapy). Goal is aPTT 1.5–2.0 times normal (60–80 seconds). Monitor the patient for bleeding. Monitor platelet counts. Avoid trauma. Heparin should be given via IV or deep subQ route. Draw up with 20- to 22-gauge needle but use a 25-gauge needle for a subQ injection. After a subQ injection, apply pressure 1–2 minutes; do not massage. Rotate injection sites. Move heparin locks every 2–3 days. Protamine sulfate should be available as an antidote.
LMWH: enoxaparin (Lovenox), dalteparin (Fragmin), tinzaparin (Innohep)	Prevents formation of fibrin and thrombin. First-line therapy to prevent and treat thromboembolism. Approved to prevent DVT after some surgeries (e.g., hip or knee replacement), to treat DVT, and to prevent complications of specific cardiac conditions. Used off-label to prevent DVT after general surgery and in patients with multiple trauma or acute spinal injury.	Bleeding, thrombocytopenia, anemia, edema, nausea, fever, confusion, cardiac toxicity, and bruising. Severe neurologic injury in patients having spinal puncture.	Remember that this drug is given deep subQ only! Do not aspirate. Rotate sites. Leave a bubble in the syringe when administering the drug. Administer the drug at the same time each day. Do not give the drug IM. Teach the patient to report any bleeding, to use a soft toothbrush and electric razor, and to not take aspirin. Monitoring of aPTT is not necessary. Overdose is treated with protamine sulfate.
warfarin sodium (Coumadin)	Interferes with blood clotting; may prevent extension of existing clots and formation of new clots. Can be used long term to prevent thrombosisin patients with prosthetic heart valves and atrial fibrillation.	Bruising, hemorrhage, nausea, and anorexia. Long-term use may weaken bones.	May be required to report PT and INR to physician before each dose. Dose may be individualized based on PT and INR. Monitor the patient for bleeding. Teach the patient not to take aspirin with warfarin.
Direct thrombin inhibitor: dabigatran etexilate (Pradaxa, Pradax)	Inhibits thrombin. Used to prevent stroke with atrial fibrillation and, in Canada, to prevent VTE after knee or hip replacement surgery.	Safer than warfarin but can still cause serious bleeding and GI disturbances (nausea and vomiting, abdominal pain, GERD, gastritis, ulcer). No specific antidote exists.	Take with food to reduce GI distress. Swallow capsules intact. Drug is unstable when exposed to moisture, so keep in original container. Use within 60 days of opening.
Direct factor Xa inhibitor: rivaroxaban (Xarelto)	Inhibits production of thrombin. Used to prevent DVT and pulmonary embolism after knee and hip surgery and to prevent stroke related to atrial fibrillation.	Bleeding. Hematoma after spinal or epidural puncture. No specific antidote exists.	Compared with warfarin, has rapid onset, fixed dosage, lower bleeding risk, few drug interactions, and no need to monitor INR.

Continued

Table 37-2 Medications for Peripheral Vascular Disorders—cont'd

DRUG	ACTION AND USES	SIDE EFFECTS	NURSING INTERVENTIONS
Platelet Aggregation Inhibitors and Antiplatelet Agents: Primarily Used to Prevent Arterial Thrombosis			
Cyclooxygenase inhibitor: aspirin	Inhibits platelet aggregation, decreases inflammation and fever, and reduces pain.	GI irritation, tinnitus, pruritus, headache, and bleeding.	Assess the patient for bruising and bleeding. Give the drug with milk or food if GI irritation occurs.
cilostazol (Pletal)	Inhibits platelet aggregation. Pletal is used to treat intermittent claudication.	Cardiac dysrhythmias, headache, dizziness, and diarrhea.	Monitor the patient for bleeding and signs of heart failure. Blood work must be done during therapy. May take up to 12 weeks for effects.
Glycoprotein IIb/IIIa receptor antagonist: abciximab (ReoPro), eptifibatide (Integrilin), tirofiban (Aggrastat)	Intended for short-term use to prevent ischemia with acute coronary syndromes and to prevent reocclusion after certain angioplasty and atherectomy procedures. Usually given with low-dose heparin and aspirin.	Risk of major bleeding.	Immediately report GI, urinary, or puncture site bleeding. Infusion should be stopped if major bleeding occurs. Route of administration is IV.
Adenosine diphosphate receptor antagonist: clopidogrel (Plavix), ticlopidine (Ticlid)	Inhibits platelet aggregation. Plavix used to prevent blockage of coronary artery stents and to reduce thrombotic events in various cardiac conditions. Ticlid used to prevent thrombotic stroke.	Both can cause GI disturbances, rash, and TTP. A lower risk of bleeding exists with clopidogrel than with ticlopidine. Ticlopidine also can cause various blood dyscrasias.	Explain to the patient the importance of having regular blood tests and reporting any bleeding, bruising, or rash. Taking the drug with food decreases GI symptoms.
Thrombolytic Agents ("Clot Busters"): Used to Treat Existing Thrombi			
streptokinase (Streptase), urokinase (Abbokinase), alteplase (tissue plasminogen activator [t-PA]) (Activase), tenecteplase (TNKase), reteplase (Retavase)	Dissolves existing clots. Used to treat acute coronary thrombosis, DVT, and massive pulmonary embolism. Alteplase can be used for ischemic stroke. Urokinase is approved to clear IV catheters.	Minor to major bleeding; transient thrombocytopenia and alopecia, hypersensitivity and hypotension with streptokinase; and cardiac dysrhythmias with restored blood flow.	Monitor tests of clotting activity. Monitor ECG and vital signs. Assess the patient for bleeding and protect from trauma. Educate the patient that chest pain or other symptoms of MI should be evaluated immediately. Early thrombolytic therapy (within 4–6 hours) may reduce myocardial damage. To reduce the risk of bleeding, handle the patient gently and avoid IM and SubQ injections and invasive procedures.
Vasodilators			
Calcium Channel Blockers			
nifedipine (Procardia), amlodipine (Norvasc), diltiazem (Cardizem)	Dilates peripheral and coronary arteries. Used to treat hypertension, angina pectoris, and cardiac dysrhythmias.	Drowsiness, dizziness, cardiac dysrhythmias, CHF, MI, hypotension, and polyuria.	Monitor the patient's blood pressure and pulse. Check for edema. Tell the patient to limit caffeine, avoid alcohol, and swallow extended-release tablets and capsules whole. Teach the patient how to manage postural hypotension.

Table 37-2 **Medications for Peripheral Vascular Disorders—cont'd**

DRUG	ACTION AND USES	SIDE EFFECTS	NURSING INTERVENTIONS
Alpha-Adrenergic Blockers			
prazosin (Minipress), terazosin (Hytrin)	Decreases vascular resistance and lowers blood pressure. Used to treat hypertension, Raynaud disease, urinary symptoms associated with BPH	Dizziness, headache, drowsiness, nausea, orthostatic hypotension, edema, and palpitations.	Teach the patient to manage orthostatic hypotension, to take safety precautions if dizzy, and to monitor his or her weight daily. Take first dose or any increased dose at bedtime because of potential hypotension. Monitor blood pressure and pulse.
Hemorheologic Agent			
pentoxifylline (Trental)	Decreases blood viscosity, fibrinogen, and platelet aggregation; increases flexibility of RBCs to allow passage through small vessels; used to treat intermittent claudication	Dyspepsia, epistaxis, dizziness, nausea, vomiting, angina, tachycardia, cardiac dysrhythmias, leukopenia, headache, tremors, and rash.	Assess the patient's vital signs. Administer the drug with meals to decrease GI upset. Take safety precautions if the patient is dizzy. Tell the patient to report a rapid or irregular pulse. Explain how to manage epistaxis if it occurs. Monitor the patient's WBC count.

AMI, Acute myocardial infarction; *aPTT,* activated partial thromboplastin time; *BPH,* benign prostatic hypertrophy; *CHF,* congestive heart failure; *DVT,* deep vein thrombosis; *ECG,* electrocardiogram; *GERD,* gastroesophageal reflux disease; *GI,* gastrointestinal; *IM,* intramuscular; *INR,* international normalized ratio; *IV,* intravenous; *LMWH,* low-molecular-weight heparin; *MI,* myocardial infarction; *PT,* prothrombin time; *RBC,* red blood cell; *SubQ,* subcutaneous; *TTP,* thrombotic thrombocytopenic purpura; *VTE,* venous thromboembolism; *WBC,* white blood cell.

Complementary and Alternative Therapies

Many herbal remedies interact with conventional drugs. Feverfew, garlic, ginger root, and ginkgo enhance the effects of antiplatelet drugs. St. John's wort can decrease the effectiveness of warfarin. Caution patients against using herbal remedies while on prescribed anticoagulants.

Anticoagulant Agents

Anticoagulant therapy is used to prolong the clotting time, hinder the extension of a thrombus, and inhibit the formation of a thrombus during the postoperative period. The primary anticoagulant medications used are heparin, low-molecular-weight heparin (LMWH), and warfarin sodium (Coumadin) derivatives. Heparin is given intravenously for immediate response and subcutaneously for maintenance or prophylaxis. LMWH is given only subcutaneously and warfarin is given orally. The clinical indications for anticoagulant treatment are venous thrombosis, pulmonary embolism, and risk for embolism. When anticoagulant therapy is used, regular coagulation tests are done to assess the effectiveness of the treatment regimen. The effective range for the activated partial thromboplastin time (aPTT) during heparin treatment is 1.5 to 2.5 times the control. Warfarin dosage is based on the patient's prothrombin time (PT) and international normalized ratio (INR). The target PT and INR depend on the condition being treated. LMWH has advantages over heparin because a fixed dose can be administered, laboratory monitoring is not necessary, and one or two doses daily are sufficient.

The fundamental complication of anticoagulant therapy is spontaneous bleeding that can occur anywhere in the body and may be evident in the urine, stool, emesis, or integument. Because of the risk of bleeding, the antidotes for each type of anticoagulant should be accessible (see *Patient Teaching* box). The antidote for heparin and LMWH is protamine sulfate; for warfarin sodium it is vitamin K.

Patient Teaching

Anticoagulant Therapy

- Anticoagulants help to prevent blood clots from forming. Take your medications exactly as prescribed.
- Because these drugs can interfere with normal blood clotting, notify your physician of excessive bruising, bleeding gums, or blood in stools or urine.
- Consult your physician before taking any additional medications because some drugs affect the action of your anticoagulant.
- If taking heparin sodium or warfarin, keep appointments for regular blood tests that must be done to monitor the serum level of your drugs. Test results are used to ensure that your dosage is safe and effective.
- Wear a medical alert bracelet noting anticoagulant therapy.

Medications such as some antibiotics, mineral oil, NSAIDs, aspirin, and tolbutamide can intensify the anticoagulant effects of warfarin sodium. Some drugs that decrease the effectiveness of warfarin are antacids, barbiturates, oral contraceptives, and adrenal corticosteroids.

Pharmacology Capsule

Patients taking anticoagulant drugs must be monitored for bleeding.

Thrombolytic Agents

Thrombolytic therapy is given intravenously to dissolve an existing blood clot. Examples of thrombolytic medications are streptokinase (Streptase), urokinase (Abbokinase), alteplase (tissue plasminogen activator [t-PA]) (Activase), reteplase (Retavase), and tenecteplase (TNKase). Thrombolytic therapy is used to treat acute myocardial infarction (AMI), pulmonary embolism, DVT, and arterial thrombosis or embolism. Uncontrolled bleeding can result from thrombolytics; therefore the patient must be monitored continuously during the treatment regimen.

Pharmacology Capsule

Anticoagulants prevent the formation of blood clots; thrombolytics dissolve existing blood clots.

Other Medications

Many other types of medications are used to treat PVD. Vasodilators are used to relax the vascular smooth muscle, which reduces resistance in the vessels and results in increased blood flow. Commonly used vasodilators are calcium channel blockers and alpha-adrenergic inhibitors. Analgesics, including NSAIDs, are used to relieve the pain caused by ischemia. With less pain, a patient can participate more in exercises. Platelet aggregation inhibitors (antiplatelets), such as aspirin, are used to prevent clot formation by making the platelets less likely to clump together. Pentoxifylline is used to treat PVD by improving the passage of RBCs through small vessels.

In addition to drugs that prevent clot formation, patients also may be taking medications such as hypoglycemic agents for diabetes and antihypertensives for high blood pressure because those conditions contribute to the development of PVD.

Pharmacology Capsule

Monitor patients taking vasodilators for hypotension. Teach them how to manage orthostatic hypotension.

DIETARY INTERVENTIONS

The dietary interventions used with PVD are like those recommended for cardiovascular health. Atherosclerotic plaques create rough vessel walls and contribute to peripheral vascular complications. Low-fat diets reduce serum cholesterol levels, thereby reducing the risk of atherosclerotic plaque formation. A weight reduction diet may be prescribed if the patient is obese because obesity causes a strain on the heart, increases venous congestion, and reduces peripheral circulation. Adequate vitamin B, vitamin C, and protein are needed to promote healing and improve tissue integrity. (See the *Nutrition Considerations* box.)

DISORDERS OF THE PERIPHERAL VASCULAR SYSTEM

ARTERIAL EMBOLISM

Pathophysiology

The development of an arterial embolism is a potentially life-threatening event. The arterial embolus usually forms in the heart. However, a roughened atheromatous plaque in any artery can lead to thrombus formation. If a thrombus breaks loose, it becomes an embolus traveling through the circulatory system until it lodges in a vessel, blocking blood flow distal to the occlusion. Thrombi from the right side of the heart lodge in the lungs, causing a pulmonary embolism (addressed later), whereas thrombi from the left side usually affect a leg. The effects of arterial occlusion depend on the size of the embolus formed, the organs involved, and the extent to which collateral circulation can maintain sufficient blood supply to affected tissues.

Signs and Symptoms

Whereas some patients with arterial obstruction have no pain, others experience severe pain and other symptoms of tissue ischemia. When the collateral circulation cannot compensate for the compromised blood flow, the patient has distinct symptoms of reduced blood flow to the tissues. Signs and symptoms of inadequate blood supply in the lower extremities include:

1. Severe, acute pain
2. Gradual loss of sensory and motor function in the affected areas
3. Pain aggravated by movement or pressure
4. Absent distal pulses
5. Pallor and mottling (irregular discoloration)
6. A sharp line of color and temperature demarcation (tissue beyond the obstruction is pale and cool)

Medical and Surgical Treatment

Arterial embolism is managed with intravenous anticoagulants and thrombolytics. Thrombolytics can be delivered via one of several procedures. These medications cannot be used with active internal bleeding, cardiovascular accident, recent major surgery, uncontrolled hypertension, and pregnancy. Patients who cannot be treated with medications may be prepared for thrombectomy (surgical removal of the embolus). Failure to restore perfusion results in tissue death and requires amputation of the affected part. Patients at risk for future arterial emboli are often treated long term with oral anticoagulants.

❖ NURSING CARE of the Patient with Arterial Embolism

■ Assessment

The assessment of the patient with PVD is outlined in Box 37-1.

Nursing Diagnoses, Goals, and Outcome Criteria: Arterial Embolism

Nursing Diagnoses	Goals and Outcome Criteria
Ineffective Peripheral Tissue Perfusion related to compromised circulation	Improved tissue perfusion: normal skin color, palpable pulses, capillary refill time less than 3 seconds in affected extremity
Fear related to the treatments, environment, and risk of limb loss	Reduced fear: patient calm, states fear is reduced or relieved
Impaired Physical Mobility related to the surgical procedure and compromised circulation	Improved physical mobility: patient increases activity without discomfort
Impaired Skin Integrity related to ischemic changes from the impairment of peripheral circulation	Healthy skin in affected areas: skin intact
Ineffective Self-Health Management related to lack of knowledge of self-care, including drug therapy	Patient knows and practices prescribed self-care measures: patient correctly describes and demonstrates self-care measures and self-medication

■ Interventions

Nursing interventions are designed to improve circulation and prevent further damage to the affected tissue.

Ineffective Peripheral Tissue Perfusion

To promote circulation, maintain the affected extremities at or slightly below the horizontal position. Administer prescribed medications and perform range-of-motion exercises as ordered.

Fear

To decrease fear, orient the patient to the environment and the expected therapies using simple statements to explain the disease process and procedures. Encourage the patient to express feelings of helplessness and anxiety and to identify coping mechanisms that have worked in other situations.

Impaired Physical Mobility

Until the thrombus is removed, the affected limb may be immobilized. The physician will order the appropriate level of activity. Improved physical mobility requires instruction in range-of-motion exercises and the development of a progressive exercise plan. This exercise plan usually is limited to 15 minutes, three times a day, in the initial days after surgery or treatment. The progression of exercise is determined by the individual patient's response.

Impaired Skin Integrity

With arterial embolism, the affected tissue is highly susceptible to injury. Protect the limb from pressure, trauma, and extreme heat or cold. Edematous tissue is equally susceptible to injury and must be protected.

Ineffective Self-Health Management

Patient teaching enables the patient to participate in the plan of care during and after hospitalization. For information on teaching interventions for patients on anticoagulant therapy, see the *Patient Teaching* box, Anticoagulant Therapy.

Patient Teaching

Arterial Embolism

Discharge teaching should include the following:
- Protect affected limbs from pressure, trauma, and temperature extremes.
- Exercise to improve blood flow; gradually increase activity as you are able to tolerate it.
- Report pain, numbness, coolness, or pale or bluish skin color to your physician.

Table 37-3 compares features of arterial and venous disease.

PERIPHERAL ARTERIAL DISEASE OF LOWER EXTREMITIES

Pathophysiology

Peripheral arterial disease (PAD) is characterized by pathologic changes in the arteries, typically plaque formations that arise where the arteries branch, veer, arch, or narrow (Fig. 37-7). The most common sites for arterial occlusion are the distal superficial femoral and the popliteal arteries. Occlusions prevent the delivery of O_2 and nutrients to the tissues. Hypoxia affects all tissues distal to the occlusion. Peripheral nerves and muscles are more susceptible to harm from hypoxia than the skin and subcutaneous tissues. Severe O_2 deprivation may lead to ischemia and then to necrosis (tissue death).

Because PAD develops gradually, compensatory mechanisms attempt to maintain circulation. These compensatory mechanisms include the development of collateral blood vessels, vasodilation, and anaerobic

Table 37-3 Comparison of Arterial and Venous Disease in the Legs

CHARACTERISTIC	PERIPHERAL ARTERY DISEASE	VENOUS DISEASE
Peripheral pulses	Decreased or absent	Present; may be difficult to palpate with edema
Capillary refill	>3 seconds	<3 seconds
Edema	Absent unless leg constantly in dependent position	Lower leg edema
Hair	Loss of hair on legs, feet, toes	Hair may be present or absent
Skin color	Dark reddish color when in dependent position; pale when elevated	Bronze-brown pigmentation; varicose veins may be visible
Skin texture	Thin, shiny, taut	Thick, hardened, indurated
Skin temperature	Cool, temperature gradient down the leg	Warm, no temperature gradient
Pain	Intermittent claudication or rest pain in foot; ulcer may or may not be painful	Dull ache, heaviness in calf or thigh; ulcer often painful
Ulcers	Location: tips of toes, foot, lateral malleolus Margins: round, smooth Drainage: minimal Color: black or pale pink	Location: near medial malleolus Margins: irregular Drainage: moderate to large amount Color: yellow or dark red
Dermatitis and pruritus	Rate	Frequent

Modified from Lewis SM, Dirksen SR, Heitkemper MM, Bucher L, Camera IM: *Medical-surgical nursing: assessment and management of clinical problems,* ed 8, St. Louis, 2011, Elsevier-Mosby.

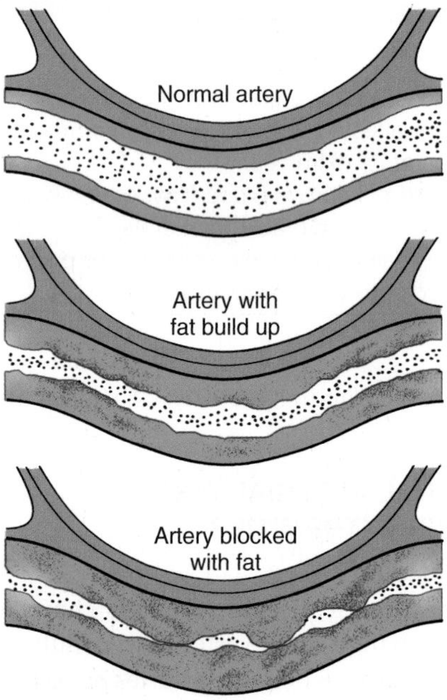

FIGURE 37-7 Development of atherosclerosis. (From Ignatavicius DD, Workman ML: *Medical-surgical nursing: patient-centered collaborative care*, ed 7, St. Louis, 2013, Saunders.)

metabolism. Collateral blood vessels are small, new vessels that branch out to supply blood to poorly perfused tissues. The extent of collateral circulation determines the severity of symptoms.

PAD is most common in men older than 50 years. Factors that contribute to the development of this disease include atherosclerosis, embolism, thrombosis, trauma, vasospasm, inflammation, and autoimmune responses. Other risk factors that are more controllable are hyperlipidemia, diabetes mellitus, hypertension, cigarette smoking, and stress.

Signs and Symptoms

The clinical manifestations of PAD develop gradually. Intermittent claudication is the classic sign. It is experienced as the aching, cramping, tiredness, and weakness in the legs that occur with walking and is relieved by rest. Another manifestation of PAD is the absence of peripheral pulses below the occlusive area. *Rest pain,* pain that develops during rest, is common. Rest pain is described as *persistent* and *aching.* Complaints of tingling or numbness (or both) in the toes are common. The affected extremity is cold and numb because of the reduction in the flow of blood to the area. Muscle atrophy may be evident. The skin of the affected area is pale because of reduced blood flow. When the extremity is in a dependent position, the color becomes red. Reduced blood supply to toenails can cause the nails to thicken. Other signs of arterial occlusion are shiny, scaly skin; subcutaneous tissue loss; hairlessness on the affected extremity; and ulcers with a pale gray or yellowish hue, especially at the ankles. If one extremity is affected more than the other, size differences between the extremities may be apparent.

Medical Diagnosis

The primary diagnostic tests used to confirm a diagnosis of PAD are duplex imaging, segmental blood pressures, and, if surgery is contemplated, angiography.

Medical and Surgical Treatment

The first step in managing PAD is for the patient to make lifestyle changes, including smoking cessation, exercise, and weight management. Smoking cessation is a high priority. Success may be enhanced with varenicline (Chantix), nicotine replacement therapy, or bupropion (Zyban). Exercise programs found to be most successful with PAD include at least three sessions of 30 to 60 minutes of exercise each week for 3 to 6 months. Training programs typically use a treadmill that allows gradual increases in speed and grade (incline). The benefits are sustained only as long as the patient continues regular exercise. Treatment should be initiated for hypertension, hyperlipidemia, and diabetes, if present. The angiotensin-converting enzyme (ACE) inhibitor ramipril improves outcomes. Among the drugs used to treat claudication are cilostazol (Pletal) and pentoxifylline (Trental), which prevent platelets from clumping and dilate blood vessels. Aspirin or clopidogrel (Plavix) is used for antiplatelet activity. Several new types of drugs under study include recombinant growth factor, immune modulators, and carnitine. Scientists hope that gene therapy will stimulate growth of new blood vessels.

Surgical interventions include stenting (to keep the vessel lumen open), endarterectomy, grafting, and catheter-based interventional radiology procedures. Endarterectomy is the surgical removal of the obstruction. Grafting is the surgical replacement of a diseased segment of an artery with a graft of some type, either synthetic or from another blood vessel. Interventional radiology is done in the catheterization laboratory, is highly successful, and requires a recovery period of only 24 to 48 hours. Percutaneous transluminal angioplasty (PTA) is one interventional radiology procedure. PTA enlarges the interior diameter of the blood vessel and is followed by stent placement. Possible complications of PTA are hematoma formation, embolus, arterial dissection, and allergic reaction.

❖ NURSING CARE of the Patient with Peripheral Arterial Disease

■ Assessment

Complete assessment of the patient with PAD is summarized in Box 37-1. When the patient has had surgical intervention, it is especially important to monitor the pulses distal to the surgical site and compare them with the same pulses in the unaffected extremity. Cessation of a pulse suggests possible arterial occlusion and the surgeon must be notified immediately. Other important aspects of the postoperative assessment are vital signs, color and temperature of the affected extremity, fluid intake and output, central venous pressure, and mental status. If the patient has pain, document the location, severity, and nature of the pain.

Nursing Diagnoses, Goals, and Outcome Criteria: Peripheral Arterial Disease

Nursing Diagnoses	Goals and Outcome Criteria
Activity Intolerance related to impaired blood flow to extremities	Improved activity tolerance: patient states is increasingly able to perform activities without pain
Chronic Pain related to ischemia	Reduced pain: patient states pain is reduced, relaxed manner
Impaired Skin Integrity related to inadequate circulation	Healthy skin: skin intact with normal color and warmth
Disturbed Body Image related to muscle atrophy, stasis ulcers, and skin discoloration	Positive body image: positive patient statements about self, patient makes effort to maintain good physical appearance
Ineffective Peripheral Tissue Perfusion related to vascular occlusion	Adequate tissue perfusion: palpable peripheral pulses, extremity warm with normal skin color
Ineffective Self-Health Management related to lack of knowledge of disease process, treatment, and self-care	Patient carries out proper self-care measures: patient describes and demonstrates self-care

If surgical intervention is performed, additional diagnoses and goals may include the following.

Nursing Diagnoses	Goals and Outcome Criteria
Risk for Infection related to surgical incision, graft placement	Absence of infection: normal body temperature, decreasing wound redness and drainage
Decreased Cardiac Output related to hemorrhage, diuresis, fluid shifts	Normal cardiac output: pulse and blood pressure consistent with patient norms
Ineffective Peripheral Tissue Perfusion related to graft thrombosis	Patent graft: operative extremity warm, with improved color and palpable pulses
Acute Pain related to surgical incision	Pain relief: patient relaxed, states that pain is relieved
Impaired Physical Mobility related to weakness, fear, surgical procedure	Increased physical mobility: increasing activity without pain

■ Interventions

Activity Intolerance

To monitor the patient's activity tolerance, assess the patient before, during, and after planned activities; then monitor progress as treatment progresses. When planning an exercise regimen, use the following guidelines:

1. Work with the patient to plan the activity schedule and goals.
2. Gradually increase the exercise time as tolerance increases.
3. Discontinue activity if the patient has chest pain, bradycardia, dyspnea, or intermittent claudication. After rest relieves the pain of intermittent claudication, the patient may resume activity.
4. Reduce the intensity of the activity if the pulse takes longer than 3 to 4 minutes to return to the baseline rate or if the patient has severe dyspnea.
5. For patients confined to bed, start exercises with range-of-motion exercises performed twice daily.
6. Patients should *not* exercise when they have leg ulcers, cellulitis, DVT, or gangrene.

Chronic Pain

The chronic pain associated with ischemia is exhausting and greatly reduces the patient's quality of life. Therefore pain management must be a priority. The most direct interventions are those that increase circulation or decrease metabolic demands of ischemic tissues. Resting the extremities in a dependent position may help to relieve the pain of arterial occlusive disease. Administer analgesics as prescribed, along with other comfort measures. Nonpharmacologic pain relief measures include relaxation techniques, warm baths, breathing exercises, and back rubs (see *Complementary and Alternative Therapies* box). See Chapter 15 for a detailed discussion of pain management.

Complementary and Alternative Therapies

Relaxation, warm baths, breathing exercises, and back rubs can help the patient with chronic pain.

Impaired Skin Integrity

The nursing interventions for maintaining skin integrity focus on improving circulation and avoiding tissue trauma. If the patient has an ulcerated area, keep it clean and free of pressure. Various wound care products may be prescribed to protect the wound and prevent infection. However, unless circulation is improved, healing is unlikely. The physician will prescribe any activity limitations.

The feet are especially susceptible to injury and require special care. Advise the patient not to go barefoot, to wear only shoes that fit properly, to inspect the feet daily for signs of pressure or lesions, and to keep the toenails neatly trimmed. Because of the risk of ingrown nails, nails should not be trimmed too short. Toenails should always be cut straight across rather than in a curved shape. The patient should see a peripheral vascular specialist promptly if any foot problems develop.

Disturbed Body Image

Encourage the patient to express any feelings that result from problems associated with PAD, such as activity intolerance, stasis ulcers, discoloration of the extremities, and, for some, amputations. It is important to be supportive and help the patient to identify coping strategies to deal with the feelings.

Ineffective Peripheral Tissue Perfusion

Administer vasodilators and other drugs that improve blood flow as ordered. Encourage exercise according to the individualized exercise plan. Maintain adequate warmth and discourage smoking. Elevation of the extremities usually is *not* recommended with arterial disease.

Additional interventions are indicated for the postoperative patient.

Ineffective Self-Health Management

To cope with PAD, the patient must understand the disease process and treatment. Include the family in patient teaching because their fears and concerns can have an enormous effect on the patient's perception of the situation. The patient teaching plan is the same as for the patient with arterial embolism. Adaptation to lifestyle changes is essential to good management of PAD. Additional interventions are indicated for the postoperative patient.

Risk for Infection

After surgery, patients are at risk for infection of the surgical incision and the grafts (especially synthetic grafts) that are used to replace the diseased blood vessel. An infected synthetic graft is very serious because it necessitates removal of the graft and often amputation. Monitor the patient's temperature and report fever to the surgeon. It is vital to inspect the incision for increasing redness, edema, and drainage that suggest infection. Antimicrobials are usually ordered before surgery and may be continued after surgery.

Decreased Cardiac Output

Monitor for signs and symptoms of deficient fluid volume: tachycardia, restlessness, decreased urine output, pallor, and hypotension. Provide intravenous and oral fluids as ordered and maintain records of fluid intake and output. Monitor daily weights and inspect the surgical dressing for bleeding, which must be reported immediately to the surgeon.

Ineffective Peripheral Tissue Perfusion

Thrombus formation can occur in the graft, causing occlusion and impaired blood flow. Monitor the pulses, warmth, and color of the operative extremity and promptly inform the surgeon of diminishing pulses, coolness, and pallor or cyanosis. Some patients are given anticoagulants or thrombolytics to decrease the risk of graft occlusion. Edema for 4 to 8 weeks is common after bypass surgery. The leg is usually wrapped in a light dressing or vascular boot and kept flat initially. Elastic stockings are not used immediately after a vein graft.

Acute Pain

Acute postoperative pain is treated with analgesics, positioning, and relaxation techniques as described in Chapters 15 and 17.

Impaired Physical Mobility

After surgery, the patient's activities are increased gradually. A specific program of exercises may be prescribed. Assist the patient and assess muscle strength and tolerance of activity.

THROMBOANGIITIS OBLITERANS

Thromboangiitis obliterans, also called *Buerger disease,* is an inflammatory thrombotic disorder of arteries and veins in the lower and upper extremities. It is not an atherosclerotic process. The exact cause is unknown but it occurs only in smokers (see *Cultural Considerations* box). Because patients often have periodontitis, it is thought that bacteria may be a contributing factor. Signs and symptoms may include intermittent claudication, rest pain, skin color and temperature changes in affected areas, cold sensitivity, abnormal sensation, ulceration, and gangrene. Diagnosis is based on a history of young age at onset, physical findings, and arteriography.

Cultural Considerations

What Does Culture Have to Do with Buerger Disease?

Buerger disease is very common in India, Korea, and Japan. It is relatively uncommon in the United States. When assessing patients, especially those of Indian, Korean, or Japanese heritage, be alert for related signs and symptoms.

The most important aspect of treatment is smoking cessation. Palliative treatments include sympathectomy, spinal cord stimulation, and drugs such as analgesics for pain and antibiotics if infected. The prostaglandin iloprost has shown some benefit in European studies. Gene therapy is under study. Ulcers may respond to treatment with vascular endothelial growth factor. If gangrene develops (most commonly below the knee), amputation is the only treatment option. Forty percent of patients who continue tobacco use eventually require amputations. Nursing care is similar to that of patients with PAD. Emphasis is on smoking cessation measures (see Chapter 32) and protection of the affected extremities.

RAYNAUD DISEASE

Pathophysiology

Primary and secondary Raynaud phenomenon are forms of an intermittent constriction of arterioles that affects the hands primarily, although it can affect the toes and tip of the nose. Increased or unusual sensations of coldness, pain, and pallor reflect temporary constriction of the arterioles in the affected areas. Gangrene is not common but can develop in the skin on the tips of the digits. The cause of primary Raynaud phenomenon is unknown but it may be related to hypersensitivity to cold or release of serotonin. Primarily women aged 16 to 40 years are affected, especially during the winter months or in northern areas where cold weather is more common. Stress seems to aggravate the disease process. Secondary Raynaud phenomenon follows the same general pattern but is typically secondary to connective tissue or collagen vascular disease. The term *primary Raynaud phenomenon* is synonymous with Raynaud disease; secondary Raynaud phenomenon is also called simply *Raynaud phenomenon.*

Signs and Symptoms

The cardinal signs and symptoms of Raynaud disease are chronically cold hands, numbness, tingling, and pallor. Finger involvement is not symmetric and the thumb is not usually affected. During an arterial spasm, the skin color changes from pallor to cyanosis to redness. Pallor is the result of sudden vasoconstriction. Cyanosis reflects inadequate oxygenation. As the spasm resolves, vasodilation allows blood flow to return, which produces a red color.

Medical Diagnosis

The diagnosis of Raynaud disease is usually based on the signs and symptoms and on the absence of evidence of occlusive vascular disease.

Medical and Surgical Treatment

The goals of the medical treatment plan for Raynaud disease are to prevent pain and to promote vasodilation in the extremities (see *Complementary and Alternative Therapies* box). The most commonly used drugs are calcium channel blockers or alpha-adrenergic blockers., Other drugs that have been used include transdermal nitroglycerin, an endothelin receptor antagonist (bosentan), phosphodiesterase inhibitors (e.g., sildenafil), and intravenous prostaglandins (e.g., iloprost, alprostadil). In severe cases the physician may resort to sympathectomy to interrupt the sympathetic nerves. This surgical procedure aids some patients but tends to have temporary effects and is not used routinely.

Complementary and Alternative Therapies

Biofeedback is sometimes helpful in controlling vasospastic episodes with Raynaud disease.

NURSING CARE of the Patient with Raynaud Disease

Assessment

Assessment of the patient with PVD is summarized in Box 37-1. With Raynaud disease, assessment of the hands is the priority.

Nursing Diagnoses, Goals, and Outcome Criteria: Raynaud Disease

Nursing Diagnoses	Goals and Outcome Criteria
Acute Pain related to the ischemia that develops from vasoconstriction	Reduced pain: patient states that pain has decreased, appears relaxed
Ineffective Peripheral Tissue Perfusion related to vasoconstriction	Improved oxygenation of peripheral tissue: improved warmth and color of affected areas
Fear related to the potential loss of work, difficulty performing activities of daily living (ADL)	Relief from fear: patient states fear is reduced, appears more relaxed

Interventions

Acute Pain and Ineffective Peripheral Tissue Perfusion

Nursing interventions to reduce pain and improve tissue perfusion focus on teaching the patient to avoid the stimuli that cause the vasoconstriction: exposure to cold, smoking, and excessive stress. Encourage the patient to take part in a smoking cessation program and to dress warmly when going outside in cold weather. Mittens are better than gloves for maintaining warmth. Sometimes the patient can interrupt an acute attack by placing the affected parts in warm water or by using a hair dryer or hand- and foot-warming devices. In addition to alcohol and caffeine, many over-the-counter (OTC) cold remedies contain vasoconstrictors that can aggravate Raynaud phenomenon. Patients should wear medical alert identification and inform all new health care providers of their diagnosis so that inappropriate medications will not be prescribed.

Pain can be managed by carefully warming the area when vasoconstriction occurs. However, the affected areas must be protected from trauma. Hot water should not be used to warm affected tissue because the lack of sensation during the period of vasoconstriction could result in serious burns.

Fear

Fear can be addressed in much the same manner as anxiety. Attempt to determine the actual cause of fear, which might be loss of work, loss of limb, or pain. Accept and explore the patient's feelings, provide factual information, encourage problem solving, and help the patient to learn to live with the condition and to manage the prescribed therapy.

ANEURYSMS

Pathophysiology

An **aneurysm** is a dilated segment of an artery caused by weakness and stretching of the arterial wall. Aneurysms can be congenital or acquired. Conditions associated with congenital aneurysms are Marfan syndrome and Ehlers-Danlos syndrome. Marfan syndrome is a disorder of connective tissue; Ehlers-Danlos syndrome affects the joints, the skin, and the capillaries. Acquired aneurysms can be caused by atherosclerosis, trauma, or infection. The most common cause is atherosclerosis. Hypertension and high cholesterol are contributing factors. Atherosclerosis weakens elastic fibers in the media, which allows a segment of the vessel to balloon outward. Infections, including syphilis, can also damage the media and result in the formation of aneurysms. The abdominal aorta is the most common site of aneurysm formation.

Signs and Symptoms

Signs and symptoms, if any, vary with the location of the aneurysm. People with thoracic aneurysms usually have no symptoms, though some report deep, diffuse chest pain. If the aneurysm puts pressure on the recurrent laryngeal nerve, the patient may complain of hoarseness. Pressure on the coronary arteries can cause angina and pressure on the esophagus may cause dysphagia (difficulty swallowing). If the superior vena cava is compressed, the patient may have edema of the head and arms. Signs of airway obstruction may be present if the aneurysm presses against pulmonary structures.

Abdominal aneurysms are usually detected during routine physical examinations or diagnostic procedures. The aneurysm may be palpated as a pulsating mass in the area slightly to the left of the umbilicus. Although most abdominal aneurysms are asymptomatic, pressure on abdominal organs and nerves may cause back pain, epigastric pain, or constipation.

Complications

Complications of aneurysms include rupture, thrombus formation that obstructs blood flow, emboli, and pressure on surrounding structures.

Medical Diagnosis

Diagnosis is made on the basis of physical findings and radiologic studies. Studies performed to obtain better visualization of the aneurysm include echocardiography, ultrasonography, CT, and aortography.

Medical and Surgical Treatment

Repair of aneurysms may be done by replacing the dilated segment of the artery with a synthetic graft or, in some cases, by suturing or patching the defective area. For the patient with an abdominal aneurysm, endovascular aneurysm repair (EVAR) may be an option. EVAR places an aortic stent graft in the aneurysm through a femoral artery cutdown. This minimally invasive procedure is less risky than open surgical repair. However, not all patients are candidates for EVAR. Repair is usually done as soon as possible but may be delayed until the patient is evaluated for other problems that increase surgical risk.

Decisions to attempt repair of aneurysms are based on the size of the defect and the patient's general status. For example, an abdominal aortic aneurysm smaller than 5 cm is usually monitored with periodic ultrasound studies. If it begins to enlarge, surgical repair may be recommended.

Complications of aneurysm surgery vary with the location of the defect. Complications of aortic abdominal aneurysm surgery include myocardial infarction, sexual dysfunction, renal failure, emboli, spinal cord ischemia with paralysis, bowel and bladder incontinence, and impaired sensation. Although EVAR is generally safer, complications can include graft leakage, stent migration, aneurysm rupture, bleeding, and infection.

❖ PREOPERATIVE NURSING CARE of the Patient with an Aneurysm

When surgical repair of an aneurysm is planned, the patient should be prepared physically and emotionally as described in Chapter 17. It is important to document chronic conditions such as emphysema or heart disease that increase the risk of postoperative complications. Marking pedal pulses will make it easier to locate them postoperatively.

❖ POSTOPERATIVE NURSING CARE of the Patient with an Aneurysm

After aortic aneurysm repair, the patient usually is kept in a critical care area for 24 to 48 hours. Mechanical ventilation may be used initially to maintain good oxygenation status. This section addresses the post–intensive care unit (ICU) recovery period. The recovery time following EVAR is typically much shorter than with open procedures.

■ Assessment

General postoperative assessment is outlined in Chapter 17, Box 17-4. After repair of an aortic aneurysm, it is vital to monitor vital signs, hemodynamic status, renal function, and fluid balance. The nurse should also inspect and palpate the extremities for color, warmth, and peripheral pulses.

■ Interventions

Impaired Urinary Elimination

During repair of an abdominal aneurysm, the aorta is clamped for a period of time. This poses a risk of renal damage and subsequent renal failure. Therefore fluid intake and urine output are measured hourly at first, then less often if output is satisfactory. Declining urine output must be reported promptly to the physician. In addition to daily weights, blood urea nitrogen (BUN), creatinine, and electrolyte levels are usually measured daily to detect increases associated with renal failure. Because fluid retention or circulatory obstruction may cause edema, its presence should be noted. Intravenous fluids should be administered as ordered.

Nursing Diagnoses, Goals, and Outcome Criteria: Aortic Aneurysm Repair

In addition to the routine problems of the postoperative patient (see Chapter 17), nursing diagnoses for the patient who has had an aortic aneurysm repair may include the following.

Nursing Diagnoses	Goals and Outcome Criteria
Impaired Urinary Elimination related to interrupted blood flow	Normal urinary function: urine output approximately equal to fluid intake
Risk for Injury related to ileus	Absence of injury related to ileus: wound margins intact, no abdominal distention, bowel sounds present
Ineffective Breathing Pattern related to abdominal incision or splinting	Effective breathing pattern: regular respirations, 12 to 20 breaths/min; clear breath sounds
Decreased Cardiac Output related to myocardial infarction, occlusion of blood vessels, graft leakage	Adequate cardiac output: pulse and blood pressure consistent with patient norms
Ineffective Peripheral Tissue Perfusion related to vascular occlusion	Normal peripheral circulation: warm extremities with palpable pulses

Risk for Injury

After abdominal surgery, peristalsis ceases temporarily. A nasogastric tube may be inserted and attached to suction to prevent gaseous distention of the bowel, which is uncomfortable and places stress on the abdominal incision. Ensure that the suction is working properly and monitor for distention and the return of bowel sounds.

Ineffective Breathing Pattern

Whether the patient has an abdominal or a thoracic incision, a risk of poor lung expansion exists. After thoracic surgery, patients are at especially high risk for atelectasis and pneumonia. Mechanical ventilation in the immediate postoperative period maintains adequate ventilation until the patient is able to breathe effectively. Thereafter, assist the patient to turn, deep breathe, and cough frequently. An incentive spirometer may be used to encourage lung expansion. It is important to support the patient's incision during the breathing exercises. Pain control measures include patient-controlled analgesia (PCA), an epidural catheter, as needed (PRN) parenteral analgesics, and other measures as appropriate. The patient can breathe more effectively if good pain relief is achieved. Monitor lung sounds frequently to assess for abnormalities.

Decreased Cardiac Output

Cardiac output may fall as a result of myocardial infarction, cardiac dysrhythmias, heart failure, or hemorrhage. Hemorrhage may occur in the incision or by separation of the graft. Closely monitor the patient's vital signs and hemodynamics. In addition, inspect wound dressing and drains for increasing bleeding. Early signs of circulatory failure are restlessness and tachycardia. Later signs are hypotension, cyanosis, and decreased alertness. Immediately notify the physician if evidence of decreasing cardiac output is seen.

Ineffective Peripheral Tissue Perfusion

A risk of impaired blood flow below the level of the repaired aneurysm exists. Monitor peripheral pulses and the color and warmth of the extremities. This assessment is especially important when a patient has had a femoral or popliteal aneurysm repair. Signs and symptoms of occlusion include pain, pallor or cyanosis, and coldness distal to the repair. If these manifestations occur, they must be reported to the physician at once.

!

AORTIC DISSECTION

Aortic dissection is different from an aneurysm. A small tear in the intima permits blood to escape into the space between the intima and the media. Blood accumulates between the layers, possibly causing the media to split lengthwise. The split may extend up and down the aorta, where it can occlude major arteries. The risk of life-threatening complications (e.g., rupture, stroke) is much greater when the ascending aorta is involved than when only the descending aorta is affected. If no complications occur, the patient may be managed with antihypertensive agents and drugs that decrease the strength of cardiac contractions. Otherwise, the affected area is replaced with a synthetic graft. A key aspect of postoperative care is keeping the blood pressure at the lowest possible level. In other respects, the care is similar to that of a patient who has had an aneurysm repair.

VARICOSE VEIN DISEASE

Pathophysiology

Varicose veins are referred to as *varicosities*. Varicosities are dilated, tortuous, superficial veins—often the saphenous veins in the lower extremities (Fig. 37-8). The dilation of the vessels results from incompetent valves in the veins; that is, the valves cannot prevent backflow of blood. Vein incompetence is a result of hereditary weakness made worse by aging, pregnancy, obesity, occupations requiring prolonged standing, or a combination of these. Restrictive clothing aggravates the condition. Varicose veins are classified as *primary* (only superficial veins are affected) and *secondary* (characterized by deep vein obstruction). In addition to peripheral veins, varicosities can occur in other areas such as the esophageal and hemorrhoidal veins. Incompetent valves cannot be repaired.

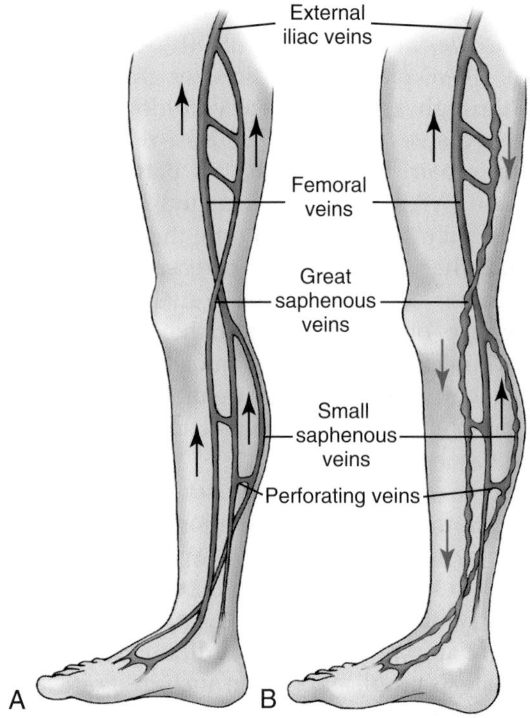

FIGURE 37-8 Venous return from the legs. **A,** Normal flow. **B,** Varicosities and retrograde venous flow. (From Monahan FD, Drake DT, Neighbors M, editors: *Medical-surgical nursing: foundations for clinical practice*, ed 2, Philadelphia, 1998, Saunders.)

Signs and Symptoms

The onset of varicose vein disease is gradual but the condition is progressive. When only the superficial veins are involved, the signs and symptoms are minimal except for the cosmetic changes that occur. The dilated veins are seen as oversized, discolored (purplish), and tortuous. Symptoms typically include dull aching sensations when standing or walking; a feeling of heaviness in the affected legs; muscle cramps, especially at night; increased muscular fatigue in the affected area; and ankle edema. Over time, some people develop postphlebitic syndrome, which is evidenced by persistent edema, brownish skin discoloration, and ulcers most commonly on the inner aspect of the ankle.

Medical Diagnosis

Varicose veins typically are diagnosed on the basis of their appearance. Duplex ultrasonography may be used to evaluate obstruction and reflux. Information about other diagnostic tests and procedures is presented in Table 37-1.

Medical and Surgical Treatment

Conservative treatments of varicosities are used whenever possible. Advise the patient to avoid restrictive garments, prolonged standing or sitting, crossing the legs or knees, and injury to the compromised areas. If the patient is obese, explain that weight reduction usually reduces pressure on the lower extremities. Support stockings often are ordered, although research on the benefits of this therapy has not consistently shown value. If the physician recommends support stockings, help the patient to learn how to put them on correctly.

Sclerotherapy, light therapy, or laser therapy may be effective in the treatment of superficial varicosities. Surgery may be recommended for cosmetic reasons or if stasis ulcers develop. The surgical procedure that removes large dilated veins is called *ligation and stripping*. It requires several incisions along the course of the affected vein. For some patients, a simpler procedure is possible in which the saphenous vein is ligated (tied shut) at the groin, requiring only one incision. Endovenous ablation uses a catheter that is threaded into the vein. The catheter emits energy that causes the vein to collapse and harden.

❖ NURSING CARE of the Patient with Varicose Vein Disease

■ Assessment

When a patient has varicose veins, the health history determines the presence of pain, edema, cramps, and muscle fatigue. Note a family history of varicose veins and document the patient's occupation and usual activities. When taking a pain and discomfort history, determine what measures the patient has used for pain control. The physical examination focuses on inspection of the legs for color, edema, turgor, and capillary refill. Palpate the legs for tenderness. Postoperative assessment is especially concerned with monitoring peripheral circulation and tissue perfusion.

■ Interventions

The primary nursing role in the care of the patient with varicose veins is teaching self-care. Interventions to improve activity tolerance and to manage pain are outlined in the *Patient Teaching* box. In general, measures that improve venous return also decrease pain.

For the surgical patient, patient teaching also is of paramount importance because the procedure is usually done as a same-day surgical procedure. While the patient is still in the surgical suite, pressure bandages are placed on the extremities. The surgeon orders specific aspects of postoperative care, such as when the pressure bandages should be removed, what types of stockings are recommended afterward, and how long they should be worn. Activity restrictions and positioning of the legs (usually 15 to 30 degrees for the first 24 hours) are also ordered at this time. Serious complications are rare; however, bleeding is most likely to occur in the groin area, so the dressing in that area should be monitored. After sclerotherapy or laser therapy, both of which are outpatient procedures, the patient is advised to wear compression stockings for as long as 6 weeks.

Nursing Diagnoses, Goals, and Outcome Criteria: Varicose Veins

Nursing Diagnoses	Goals and Outcome Criteria
Chronic Pain related to engorgement of the veins	Reduced pain: patient states that pain with activity has decreased
Activity Intolerance related to feelings of heaviness and fatigue	Improved activity tolerance: patient reports gradual increase in activity with less discomfort
Ineffective Self-Health Management related to management of the varicosities	Patient carries out appropriate self-care: patient correctly verbalizes and demonstrates self-care

Patient Teaching

Varicose Veins

- Exercise regularly to promote circulation.
- Avoid prolonged standing, sitting, and crossing your legs.
- Avoid restrictive clothing.
- Elevate extremities whenever possible.
- Obesity contributes to the development of varicose veins. People who are overweight usually see improvement with weight loss.
- Nonprescription analgesics and frequent position changes usually control pain.
- Wear antiembolism hose or support hose if recommended by your physician.

VENOUS THROMBOSIS

Pathophysiology

A variety of terms are used to describe inflammation and thrombus formation in the veins. **Phlebitis** is inflammation of a superficial vein. When a thrombus forms in the presence of phlebitis, the condition is called *venous thrombosis*. Depending on the depth of the affected veins, venous thrombosis is labeled *superficial vein thrombosis* (SVT) or *deep vein thrombosis* (DVT). The superficial vein that is most often the site of thrombus formation is the saphenous vein. The deep veins commonly involved are the femoral, popliteal, and small calf veins. *Venous thromboembolism* (VTE) is a term that includes both SVT and DVT. A grave complication of DVT is a pulmonary embolism.

Risk Factors

Some of the factors that place a person at risk for the development of thrombi are:

1. Prescribed bed rest
2. Surgery under general anesthesia for people older than 40 years
3. Leg trauma resulting in immobilization from casts or traction
4. Previous venous insufficiency
5. Obesity
6. Use of oral contraceptives
7. Malignancy

Research has identified three factors (called *Virchow's triad*) that contribute to venous thrombus formation: (1) stasis of the blood, (2) damage to the vessel walls, and (3) hypercoagulability.

Signs and Symptoms

The signs and symptoms of venous thrombosis vary with the size and location of the thrombus, the amount of obstruction, the collateral circulation, and the existence of other medical problems. SVT is characterized by a vein that feels firm and cordlike when palpated. The area around the vein may be warm, red, and tender. When obstruction occurs in a deep vein, the affected extremity may be edematous and painful with warmth and tenderness at the area of compromise. The patient may have a mild elevation in systemic temperature.

Medical Diagnosis

The primary diagnostic examinations used in the detection of venous thrombi are venography, Doppler ultrasonography, and duplex ultrasonography. These tests are instrumental in the confirmation of the disease process and determination of the treatment plan. A lung scan, pulmonary angiogram, or spiral CT scan may be done if pulmonary embolism is suspected.

Medical and Surgical Treatment

The goals of treatment are to prevent thrombus extension and pulmonary emboli, to reduce the risk of further thrombus formation, and to reduce discomfort. Anticoagulant or thrombolytic therapy (or both) is begun promptly after diagnosis. The treatment plan typically includes patient teaching about the disease; ongoing assessment for pulmonary emboli; bed rest; elevation of the extremity; warm, moist soaks to the affected area; and compression stockings. Ambulation is initiated after the acute phase. Surgery may be considered when the patient cannot receive anticoagulants or thrombolytic therapy or when the possibility of pulmonary emboli is high.

❖ NURSING CARE of the Patient with Venous Thrombosis

Assessment

Assessment of the patient with PVD is summarized in Box 37-1.

Nursing Diagnoses, Goals, and Outcome Criteria: Venous Thrombosis

Nursing Diagnoses	Goals and Outcome Criteria
Impaired Skin Integrity related to venous stasis	Intact skin: absence of redness, rash, pallor, lesions
Acute Pain related to impaired circulation and tissue ischemia	Pain relief: patient verbalizes pain relief, relaxed manner
Anxiety related to hospitalization and uncertainty of disease process	Reduced anxiety: patient states that anxiety is reduced, calm manner
Activity Intolerance related to leg pain or swelling	Improved activity tolerance: increasing activity without pain
Ineffective Peripheral Tissue Perfusion related to impaired peripheral circulation	Adequate tissue perfusion: pulses present and symmetric, normal skin color and warmth
Impaired Gas Exchange related to pulmonary emboli	Normal gas exchange: respiratory rate consistent with patient norms, no dyspnea or chest pain
Ineffective Self-Health Management related to the developing disease process, treatment, self-care	Patient adheres to prescribed plan of care: correctly describes and demonstrates self-medication, exercises, and precautions

Interventions

Impaired Skin Integrity

Maintaining intact skin is a priority. Carefully inspect the skin to detect early signs of breakdown and compare the extremities for symmetry in color, warmth, pulses, and circumference. Elevate affected extremities to promote venous return and improve circulation to the area. Because edematous tissue is easily injured and heals poorly, it must be protected from trauma, including pressure.

Acute Pain

The patient's pain must be reduced before activity tolerance can improve. Administer analgesics as prescribed and implement other prescribed comfort measures such as warm, moist soaks and elevation of the extremity. Massage is contraindicated because it may dislodge a thrombus. A "traveling" blood clot is called an *embolus.* It is very dangerous because it can !

obstruct blood flow with serious effects, including a potentially fatal pulmonary embolism.

Anxiety

Anxiety may be related to lack of knowledge about the disease and its treatment as well as to concerns about the effects of the condition on employment, activities of daily living (ADL), and quality of life. The patient may even restrict activities out of fear of pain. The relief of anxiety can help the patient to move toward an acceptable level of activity. Anxiety can be reduced by helping the patient to understand the condition and how it can best be managed.

Activity Intolerance

Initially the patient may be on bed rest. Because inactivity increases the risk of venous thrombosis, it is important to make an effort to get the inactive patient mobile again as soon as permitted (see *Patient Teaching* box). Work with the patient to establish a realistic exercise or activity plan. The plan should begin at the patient's current level and slowly add activities during a period of several weeks. Instruct the patient to stop any activity temporarily if pain occurs. Once the pain subsides, the activity may be continued.

Patient Teaching

Venous Thrombosis

- Protect your legs from pressure and trauma.
- Elevate your legs when sitting to improve circulation.
- Do not massage or rub affected areas.
- Gradually increase your activity; slow down or stop if you have pain during activity.
- Avoid prolonged standing and crossing your legs.
- Notify your physician if you have any chest pain or shortness of breath.

Ineffective Peripheral Tissue Perfusion

Improved peripheral circulation aids in tissue perfusion, which decreases pain, improves skin integrity, reduces anxiety, and increases physical activity. Administer prescribed anticoagulants or platelet aggregation inhibitors to prevent new clots or administer thrombolytics to dissolve existing clots and reestablish blood flow to the affected area. Check blood test results before giving anticoagulants and take action according to agency policy. Apply warm, moist packs to the affected area as ordered to improve circulation and assist the patient in the placement of antiembolism hose, if prescribed, to prevent stasis and improve circulation. Explain to the patient how stress reduction and smoking cessation can improve tissue perfusion by reducing vasoconstriction.

Impaired Gas Exchange

The possibility of a pulmonary embolus developing during the treatment of venous thrombosis is ever present. When an embolus lodges in the lung, the affected blood vessels can no longer exchange gases. Pressure builds in vessels behind the embolus. Symptoms of pulmonary embolism depend on the amount of tissue affected. Small emboli may produce no symptoms. Larger emboli can cause dyspnea, chest pain, tachycardia, cough, fever, anxiety, and a change in mental status. A massive embolus can cause heart failure and shock. Sixty percent of people do not survive massive emboli.

To improve oxygenation when a patient has a pulmonary embolism, elevate the head of the bed to a 45-degree angle and administer O_2 as ordered. It is also vital to monitor and document any changes in the patient's respiratory pattern, address anxiety, teach the patient deep-breathing and coughing techniques, and assist with position changes every 2 hours. Administer drugs as ordered to dissolve existing clots and prevent future clots. Surgical removal of the clot, called *pulmonary embolectomy*, is sometimes indicated. Additional discussion of pulmonary embolism is found in Chapter 31.

Ineffective Self-Health Management

To follow the long-term plan of care, the patient must understand the condition and how it can best be managed. Once the acute process has resolved, discharge planning must include patient teaching as outlined. In addition, for more on the care of a patient on anticoagulant therapy, see the *Patient Teaching* box, Anticoagulant Therapy.

CHRONIC VENOUS INSUFFICIENCY

Pathophysiology

Chronic venous insufficiency is the culmination of long-standing pressure that stretches the veins and damages the valves. Elevated venous pressure causes edema, primarily around the ankles. RBCs seep into the tissues and combine with metabolic wastes to impart a brownish color, called *stasis dermatitis*, around the ankles. Ulcers may form because of the pressure exerted by edema or as a result of trauma. The ulcers develop most often on the medial malleolus (the prominent bone on the inner aspect of the ankle). Because of the poor circulation, the ulcers are very resistant to healing and susceptible to infection. Some ulcers eventually necessitate amputation.

Signs and Symptoms

Signs and symptoms of chronic venous insufficiency include edema around the lower legs, pain, brownish skin discoloration (stasis dermatitis), and stasis ulcerations. Patients often describe pain as *heaviness* or *dull ache* in the calf or thigh. The skin temperature is cool and nails are normal. Peripheral pulses are present but may be difficult to palpate because of the edema. The feet and ankles often are cyanotic when in a dependent position.

Medical Diagnosis

The physical examination provides evidence of chronic venous insufficiency. Noninvasive screening may be done to confirm the diagnosis of chronic venous insufficiency or to assess its severity. A culture may be ordered to determine the infectious agent if the stasis ulcer is draining.

Medical and Surgical Treatment

The medical management of stasis ulcerations is constantly changing; however, compression, which promotes venous return, remains the key to healing existing ulcers and preventing new ones. Among the many options are elastic or compression stockings and pneumatic compression devices. However, high-pressure compression is contraindicated if the patient's arterial blood flow is poor.

If the patient has an ulcer, treatment typically includes special dressings along with compression. Topical debriding agents may be used to prepare a clean wound bed. Dressings that maintain a moist environment are believed to be superior to dry dressings. However, evidence supporting one type of dressing over another is limited. A wound, ostomy, continence (WOC) nurse can advise on the most current effective treatment for a specific situation. Infected ulcers are treated with systemic antibiotics, which are more effective than topical ointments. Skin grafting or surgical closure of the ulcer along with removal of the associated varicose veins is sometimes done. Hyperbaric O_2 therapy may be prescribed in an attempt to promote healing of the ulcer by reducing capillary pressure and hyperoxygenating the blood. The overall goal for medical management of ulcerations is to preserve the extremity by stimulating granulation tissue in the ulcer.

NURSING CARE of the Patient with Chronic Venous Insufficiency

Assessment

The complete general assessment of peripheral vascular status is summarized in Box 37-1. When the patient has chronic venous insufficiency, inspect the lower extremities for rubor and stasis dermatitis, palpate skin temperature, evaluate edema, and determine the presence of pain in the affected extremity (see Nursing Care Plan: Patient with a Venous Stasis Ulcer).

Nursing Diagnoses, Goals, and Outcome Criteria: Chronic Venous Insufficiency

Nursing Diagnoses	Goals and Outcome Criteria
Ineffective Peripheral Tissue Perfusion related to reduced vascular circulation	Improved peripheral circulation and venous return: absence of edema and lesions, improved skin color
Disturbed Body Image related to chronic, open stasis ulcerations	Patient adapts to changes in appearance: patient expresses concerns about changes, makes effort to maintain or improve appearance
Risk for Infection related to compromised circulation and impaired skin integrity	Decreased risk for infection: healed ulcer, intact skin. Absence of infection: normal body temperature, absence of local redness or drainage
Impaired Skin Integrity related to stasis dermatitis and ulcerations	Restored skin integrity: skin intact in affected areas

Interventions

Ineffective Peripheral Tissue Perfusion

To improve circulation in areas of compromised vascular function, the patient should elevate the legs when sitting and wear compression stockings. Stocking size is determined by patient leg measurements. The patient should put on the stockings before rising. The toe opening should be under the toes and the heel section in place. The thigh gusset should be on the inner thigh. The stocking must be smooth and not allowed to roll down at the top. The stocking should be removed for 10 to 20 minutes for bathing and skin care. Stockings should be replaced every 4 to 6 months. The patient should avoid standing still, crossing the legs, and wearing restrictive clothing, especially socks or hose with tight, narrow bands. When sitting, encourage the patient to exercise the feet, ankles, and knees to promote venous return.

Disturbed Body Image

Encourage the patient to share feelings about body image changes and be accepting and supportive. Encourage the patient to pay attention to grooming; he or she may prefer clothing that conceals stockings or dressings.

Risk for Infection

Carefully monitor for signs of infection such as elevated temperature; chills; general malaise; and localized redness, pain, and purulent drainage. Teach the patient thorough hand washing, good hygiene, and appropriate wound care. The fragile edematous tissue also must be protected from trauma to avoid creating portals for pathogens.

Impaired Skin Integrity

Inspect for dermatitis and ulcerations, especially in the ankle area. Apply a moisturizer to dry, intact skin. Patient education is critical because these ulcerations are frequently treated on an outpatient basis. Instruct the patient and family in the management of the

Nursing Care Plan — Patient with a Venous Stasis Ulcer

ASSESSMENT

HEALTH HISTORY A 75-year-old man is being seen in the community clinic for an ulcer on the medial malleolus of the right ankle. The ulcer is shallow and measures 1.5 cm × 2.5 cm. He describes a "heavy" burning sensation in the lower legs. He worked for many years as a tollbooth attendant and has had chronic venous insufficiency for 5 years. He reports having had hypertension in the past but is taking no medication for it. Otherwise he has been in good health and remains active. He is the caregiver for his wife, who has been disabled for 3 years because of a stroke. He has a daughter who helps with her care and who has been dressing his leg ulcer.

PHYSICAL EXAMINATION Vital signs: blood pressure 194/102 mm Hg, pulse 64 bpm respiration 16 breaths per minute, temperature 97°F (36.1°C) measured orally. Height 5′9″, weight 170 lb. Alert and oriented. Walks with slight limp. 2+ edema, both ankles. Varicosities noted in both legs. Stasis dermatitis in ankles and calves. Ulcer is 1.5 cm × 2.5 cm and shallow. Ulcer is slightly moist, pink, with no drainage or odor. Ankles and feet are cooler than calves. Pedal pulses faint but palpable, slightly stronger in left foot.

Nursing Diagnosis	Goals and Outcome Criteria	Interventions
Ineffective Peripheral Tissue Perfusion related to compromised circulation	Tissue perfusion will improve, as evidenced by reduced pain, redness, and edema; skin will be warm to the touch.	Instruct the patient in measures to improve circulation: exercise moderately each day, elevate the legs above the level of the heart when resting, avoid smoking, apply dressings and compression stockings as ordered, avoid prolonged periods of walking or standing still. Teach wound care as ordered. At each visit, assess the condition of his ulcer, peripheral pulses, skin color and warmth, pain, and edema.
Risk for Infection related to open wound	The patient will remain free of signs and symptoms of infection: fever, increasing redness, and purulent drainage.	Teach hygienic techniques of hand washing and wound care. Encourage him to choose a diet with adequate protein and vitamins. Teach the signs and symptoms of infection that should be reported to the physician. Instruct him in antimicrobial therapy if prescribed.
Chronic Pain related to circulatory impairment	The patient will report pain relief.	Encourage the patient to increase movement and maintain warmth to improve circulation. Teach pain relief measures including relaxation, deep-breathing techniques, cutaneous stimulation, and behavior modification. Explain the use of prescribed analgesics. Assess the effectiveness of pain control measures.
Impaired Skin Integrity related to circulatory impairment	The patient's wound will heal completely.	Assess and document the condition of the ulcer during each clinic visit. Advise the patient to use gentle soap for bathing, to avoid trauma, and not to rub the ulcer. Encourage good nutrition and adequate fluid intake. Discuss wound care with the physician or wound, ostomy, continence (WOC) nurse (specialist in wound care).
Ineffective Self-Health Management related to lack of knowledge of chronic venous insufficiency and treatment of stasis ulcer	The patient will correctly explain chronic venous insufficiency and demonstrate correct care of the ulcer.	Assess the patient's understanding of his condition and self-care. Advise him to avoid restrictive clothing, smoking, and weight gain. Explore sources of stress and coping strategies.
Ineffective Self-Health Management related to lack of knowledge of importance of treating hypertension	The patient will verbalize understanding of the need to have his blood pressure evaluated and will make an appointment for evaluation.	Explain the importance of detecting and treating hypertension. Refer the patient to the physician or blood pressure clinic for evaluation.

Critical Thinking Questions

1. What data will contribute to the assessment of the effectiveness of pain and infection control techniques?
2. What role does nutrition play in the therapeutic treatment of venous stasis ulcers?
3. What data should you collect related to the condition of the ulcer?

ulcerations while in the home setting. A referral for home health care may be appropriate.

LYMPHANGITIS

Pathophysiology

Lymphangitis is acute inflammation of the lymphatic channels. The inflammation is the result of an infectious process, usually caused by *Streptococcus.*

Signs and Symptoms

The primary characteristic of lymphangitis is enlargement of the lymph nodes along the lymphatic channel. Each node can be palpated along the course of the channel. The patient complains of tenderness as these nodes are assessed. A red streak from the infected wound extends up the extremity along the path of the lymphatics, as each node drains into the lymphatic system and the cardiovascular system. These nodes are located in the groin, the axilla, and the cervical regions. The symptoms of a generalized infection—elevated temperature and chills—are present. The infectious material can localize into an abscess with necrotic, suppurative discharge from the area.

Medical Diagnosis

The classic signs and symptoms, supported by wound culture results, are usually adequate to confirm lymphangitis. Lymphangiography, which uses a contrast medium for the radiologic visualization of the lymphatic system, will also provide evidence of lymphangitis.

Medical and Surgical Treatment

Antimicrobials are used to treat lymphangitis. When an abscess develops, the area is incised to drain the suppurative material. Other supportive measures that may be ordered are rest and elevation of the limb; warm, wet dressings; and elastic support hose.

NURSING CARE of the Patient with Lymphangitis

Assessment

Care of the patient with lymphangitis includes inspection of the skin for open wounds, signs of inflammation (redness, warmth, edema), and presence of red streaks along the paths of lymphatic channels (see *Nutrition Considerations* box). Palpate the lymph nodes in the groin and underarm areas for any enlargements.

Nutrition Considerations

1. Edema frequently is treated with a low-sodium diet; sodium-restricted diets vary from 4 g (least restrictive) to 250 mg (severe sodium restriction) daily.
2. Foods high in sodium include salt, monosodium glutamate, smoked or processed meats (ham, bacon, frankfurters, cold cuts), salted foods (potato chips, pretzels, salted nuts, popcorn), prepackaged frozen foods, and canned foods.
3. Older adults who take diuretics generally are not encouraged to restrict sodium intake because they are at risk for the adverse effects of low sodium.
4. Salt substitutes are a source of potassium, which is desirable in patients who are receiving potassium-wasting diuretics; however, salt substitutes should always be approved by a physician before they are used.

Nursing Diagnoses, Goals, and Outcome Criteria: Lymphangitis

Nursing Diagnoses	Goals and Outcome Criteria
Acute Pain related to the inflammatory process in the lymphatic system	Pain relief: patient verbalizes less pain, appears relaxed
Activity Intolerance related to pain with movement	Improved activity intolerance: patient increases activity without increased pain
Risk for Injury related to infection	Decreased risk for injury: protection of affected tissue Resolution of infection: absence of fever, normal white blood cell count, decreasing swelling and pain

Interventions

Nursing care of the patient with lymphangitis is essentially the same as that for chronic venous insufficiency.

Interventions to relieve pain include administration of the prescribed analgesics and antimicrobials and elevation of the extremity to reduce lymphedema. Nonpharmacologic measures should be used in addition to analgesics. The application of warm, moist soaks to the infected areas as prescribed improves the circulation to the area. As the circulation is improved, white blood cells (WBCs), nutrients, and O_2 are delivered, which aids in the recovery of the healthy tissue. Elastic support hose are used for several months after an acute attack of lymphangitis to prevent the formation of lymphedema.

Get Ready for the NCLEX® Examination!

Key Points

- The peripheral vascular system comprises arteries, capillaries, veins, and lymph vessels, each of which plays a critical role in the oxygenation and nourishment of body tissues.
- Risk factors for PVD include older age, heredity, smoking, obesity, physical inactivity, hypertension, and diabetes mellitus.
- Common age-related changes in the vascular system include arteriosclerosis (stiffening of blood vessel walls), decreased Hgb, slower heart rate, and decreased cardiac output.
- The six *P*s characteristic of PVD are (1) pain, (2) pulselessness, (3) poikilothermy, (4) pallor, (5) paresthesia, and (6) paralysis.
- Intermittent claudication is pain in any major muscle group that is precipitated by exercise and relieved by rest.
- Poikilothermy describes an area of the body that is cooler than the rest of the body because of local ischemia.
- Tests and procedures used to diagnose PVD include Doppler ultrasound, duplex ultrasonography, pressure measurement, exercise testing, and angiography.
- Common therapeutic measures used in the management of PVD are exercise programs, drug therapy, stress management training, pain management, smoking cessation, elastic stockings or intermittent pneumatic compression devices, positioning, thermotherapy, protection, and patient teaching.
- Common surgical interventions for PVD include PTA, stenting, endarterectomy, embolectomy, sclerotherapy, laser therapy, light therapy, and vein ligation and stripping.
- Blood flow may be improved with drug therapy using anticoagulants, thrombolytics, platelet aggregation inhibitors, and vasodilators. NSAIDs and other analgesics may be needed for pain and inflammation.
- For persons with vascular disorders, a low-fat diet is usually prescribed and a weight reduction program may be advised if appropriate.
- The most dangerous complication of venous thrombosis is pulmonary embolism.
- An arterial embolus, an unattached clot or other material in an artery, can lodge in an artery and obstruct blood.
- Nursing care of the patient with an arterial embolus focuses on ineffective peripheral tissue perfusion, fear, impaired skin integrity, impaired physical mobility, and ineffective self-health management.
- PAD impairs blood flow and may be treated surgically.
- Nursing care of the patient with PAD focuses on activity intolerance, chronic pain, impaired skin integrity, disturbed body image, ineffective peripheral tissue perfusion, and ineffective self-health management.
- Thromboangiitis obliterans (Buerger disease) is an inflammatory thrombotic disorder of arteries and veins in upper and lower extremities of smokers; atherosclerosis is not a factor.
- Primary and secondary Raynaud phenomenon are characterized by intermittent arteriolar vasoconstriction that is usually treated with vasodilators.
- An aneurysm is a dilated segment of an artery, most often the aorta, that can rupture, serve as a site for thrombus formation, and compress surrounding tissues.
- Aortic dissection results from a tear in the intima that allows blood to escape into the space between the intima and the media, which causes the media to split lengthwise.
- Varicose veins are dilated, tortuous, superficial veins that result from incompetent venous valves; they may lead to chronic venous insufficiency and are treated with conservative measures to improve venous return and sometimes with surgical intervention or laser therapy.
- Phlebitis is inflammation of a vein wall.
- Thrombosis is clot formation and DVT indicates that the clot is located in deep veins, a condition that poses a high risk for pulmonary emboli.
- Risk factors for thrombus formation are bed rest, surgery in people older than 40 years, leg trauma and immobilization, previous venous insufficiency, obesity, oral contraceptives, and malignancy.
- Nursing care of the patient with venous thrombosis addresses impaired skin integrity, acute pain, anxiety, activity intolerance, ineffective peripheral tissue perfusion, impaired gas exchange, and ineffective self-health management.
- Chronic venous insufficiency causes edema and stasis dermatitis around the ankles.
- Lymphangitis is an inflammation of the lymphatic channels that is treated with antimicrobials, analgesics, heat therapy, and rest.

Additional Learning Resources

SG Go to your Study Guide for additional learning activities to help you master this chapter content.

evolve Go to your Evolve website (http://evolve.elsevier.com/Linton/medsurg) for the following learning resources and much more:

- Interactive Prioritization Exercises
- Fluid & Electrolyte Tutorial
- Pharmacology Tutorial
- Review Questions for the NCLEX® Examination

Review Questions for the NCLEX® Examination

1. At which of the following levels does the exchange of O_2 and nutrients occur?
   1. Arteriole
   2. Capillary
   3. Venule
   4. Lymphatic

   NCLEX Client Need: Physiological Integrity: Physiological Adaptation

2. Nursing students in a gerontology course learn that the intima layer of blood vessels thicken and harden with age. The students recognize that such changes put the older adult at risk for which of the following?
   1. Anemia
   2. Bradycardia
   3. Emboli
   4. Hypotension

   NCLEX Client Need: Physiological Integrity: Physiological Adaptation
3. A patient complains of pain and cramping in the legs that occurs when walking and is relieved by rest. What term is used to describe this complaint?

   NCLEX Client Need: Physiological Integrity: Physiological Adaptation
4. When inspecting a patient's legs, you press your thumb into an edematous area around each ankle. Each time you remove your thumb, a moderate indentation appears that soon subsides. Which of the following should you document?
   1. 1+ edema noted
   2. Pitting edema, both ankles
   3. Mild edema, both ankles
   4. 2+ edema, both ankles

   NCLEX Client Need: Physiological Integrity: Physiological Adaptation
5. Which of the following is an invasive diagnostic procedure used to assess the vascular system?
   1. Ultrasound
   2. Plethysmography
   3. Angiography
   4. Exercise test

   NCLEX Client Need: Physiological Integrity: Reduction of Risk Potential
6. Measures used to improve venous return in the patient with PVD include which of the following? (Select all that apply.)
   1. Exercise
   2. Elastic stockings
   3. Thermotherapy
   4. Elevation of extremities
   5. Smoking cessation therapy

   NCLEX Client Need: Physiological Integrity: Reduction of Risk Potential
7. Mr. J. has been on warfarin (Coumadin) to prevent a stroke related to atrial fibrillation. Mr. J.'s doctor is changing him from warfarin to dabigatran (Pradaxa). When Mr. J. asks the home health nurse why he should change medications, what should he be told? (Select all that apply.)
   1. Dabigatran does not require regular blood testing.
   2. He will be able to take the same dose every day.
   3. Dabigatran is not affected by food or other drugs.
   4. Bleeding is less likely with dabigatran than with warfarin.
   5. An overdose of dabigatran can be readily reversed.

   NCLEX Client Need: Physiological Integrity: Pharmacological Therapies
8. Which of the following is included in discharge teaching for the patient with peripheral arterial disease affecting both legs?
   1. Elevate your feet when sitting
   2. Exercise is contraindicated
   3. Promptly report any injury to the feet or legs
   4. Take prescribed vasoconstrictors as ordered

   NCLEX Client Need: Physiological Integrity: Reduction of Risk Potential
9. Mrs. P. has had an open abdominal aneurysm repair. Her nurse knows that it is *especially important* to monitor:
   1. Reflexes in the lower extremities
   2. Intake and output
   3. Mental status
   4. ECG

   NCLEX Client Need: Physiological Integrity: Reduction of Risk Potential
10. Which of the following is the *most serious* complication of venous thrombosis?
    1. Pulmonary embolism
    2. Stasis dermatitis
    3. Ankle ulceration
    4. Pitting edema

    NCLEX Client Need: Physiological Integrity: Physiological Adaptation

chapter 38

Hypertension

Lark A. Ford

http://evolve.elsevier.com/Linton/medsurg

Objectives

1. Define hypertension.
2. Explain the physiology of blood pressure regulation.
3. Discuss the risk factors, signs and symptoms, diagnosis, treatment, and complications of hypertension.
4. Identify the nursing considerations when administering selected antihypertensive drugs.
5. List the data to be collected during the nursing assessment of a person with known or suspected hypertension.
6. Describe the nursing interventions for the patient with hypertension.
7. Identify the nursing diagnoses, goals, and outcome criteria for the patient with hypertension.

Key Terms

Dyslipidemia (dĭs-lĭp-ĭ-DĒ-mē-ă)
Epistaxis (ĕp-ĭ-STĂK-sĭs)
Hypertension (hī-pĕr-TĔN-shŭn)
Hypertrophy (hī-PĔR-trō-fē)
Orthostatic hypotension (ŏr-thō-STĂ-tĭk hī-pō-TĔN-shŭn)
Syncope (SĬN-kō-pē)
Thrombus (pl. thrombi) (THRŎM-bŭs, THRŎM-bī)

Hypertension, or high blood pressure (HBP), is defined as a persistent systolic blood pressure (SBP) greater than or equal to 140 mm Hg, diastolic blood pressure (DBP) greater than or equal to 90 mm Hg. Approximately 65 million American adults, or nearly 1 in 3, have HBP. The prevalence of hypertension among citizens in the United States and Canada is 32% and 22%, respectively. Hypertension and its management among various racial and ethnic groups in the United States demand special attention from health care providers. African Americans, as compared to other ethnic groups, have the highest prevalence of hypertension in the world. African Americans develop hypertension at a younger age than Caucasians. African-American women have a higher incidence of hypertension than African-American men (see *Cultural Considerations* box). The condition is usually detected in people ages 30 to 50 years; however, it is being found with increasing frequency in children. The development of hypertension in children and adolescents is due in part to the increasing prevalence of childhood obesity as well as to the growing awareness of this disease. Secondary hypertension is more common in preadolescent children, with most cases caused by renal disease. Primary or essential hypertension is more common in adolescents and has multiple risk factors, including obesity and a family history of hypertension. Hypertension is a known risk factor for coronary heart disease (CHD) in adults and the presence of childhood hypertension may contribute to the early development of CHD.

Cultural Considerations

Cultural and Ethnic Health Disparities for Hypertension

- African Americans, as compared to other ethnic groups, have the highest prevalence of hypertension in the world.
- African Americans develop hypertension at a younger age than Caucasians.
- African American women have a higher incidence of hypertension than African American men.
- Hypertension is more aggressive in African Americans and results in more severe end-organ damage.
- African Americans have a higher mortality rate related to hypertension than Caucasians.
- African Americans and Caucasians living in the southeastern United States have a higher incidence of hypertension than similar ethnic groups living in other parts of the United States.
- Mexican Americans have lower levels of awareness of hypertension and its treatment than other ethnic groups.
- Mexican Americans are less likely to receive treatment for hypertension than Caucasians and African Americans.
- Mexican Americans and Native Americans have lower rates of adequate blood pressure control than Caucasians and African Americans.

From Lewis SM, Dirksen S, Heitkemper MM, et al.: *Medical-surgical nursing: assessment and management of clinical problems*, ed 8, St. Louis, 2010, Mosby.

Hypertension is called "the silent killer" because it often has no symptoms and is not discovered until a serious complication develops. It is estimated that 30% of those with hypertension do not know they have it. Among individuals in the United States with hypertension, 59% are being treated but only 34% are considered to be in control of their condition. This is unfortunate because it is believed that hypertension can be controlled in most people. Prehypertension is diagnosed in adults when the average of two or more diastolic readings on at least two subsequent visits is between 80 and 89 mm Hg or when the average of multiple SBP readings on two or more subsequent visits is between 120 and 139 mm Hg. Hypertension exists when DBP readings are greater than 89 mm Hg and when SBP readings are greater than 139 mm Hg.

Complications of hypertension, including damage to the heart, blood vessels, kidneys, brain, and eyes, increase after age 50. As blood pressure (BP) rises, so does the risk of heart attack, heart failure (HF), stroke, kidney disease, and blindness. Men, especially African-American men, suffer serious complications more often than women. Cardiac disease is the leading cause of death in people with hypertension. Improved management of hypertension has significantly reduced the death rate from stroke in women age 50 and older.

DEFINITIONS

The *Eighth Report of the Joint National Committee on Prevention, Detection, Evaluation, and Treatment of High Blood Pressure (JNC 8)* defines normal BP as systolic pressure of less than 120 mm Hg and diastolic pressure of less than 80 mm Hg. People with systolic pressures between 120 and 139 mm Hg and with diastolic pressures between 80 and 89 mm Hg are said to have prehypertension. Readings classified as *Stage 1* and *Stage 2 hypertension* are outlined in Table 38-1. If the systolic and diastolic pressures fall into different stages, the higher measurement is used to classify the stage of hypertension. Complications and death increase directly with the stage of hypertension.

In addition to staging, patients with hypertension are classified as being in *Risk Group A, B,* or *C.* Individuals in Risk Group A have no major risk factors, no target organ damage, and no clinical cardiovascular disease. Individuals in Risk Group B have one or more risk factors, not including diabetes; no target organ damage; and no clinical cardiovascular disease. Individuals in Risk Group C have target organ damage and clinical cardiovascular disease, diabetes, or all of these conditions, with or without other risk factors.

Some people have only occasional elevations in BP and normal readings at other times. These findings are called *isolated pressure elevations.* Isolated SBP elevations of 160 mm Hg or more frequently occur in older adults. The elevations are usually caused by atherosclerosis.

TYPES OF HYPERTENSION

Hypertension is classified as *primary* (essential) or *secondary.* Primary hypertension accounts for 90% to 95% of all cases of hypertension. Even though the cause for primary hypertension is unknown, several contributing factors, including increased sodium intake, greater than ideal body weight, diabetes mellitus, and excessive alcohol consumption, have been identified. Secondary hypertension is caused by underlying factors such as kidney disease, certain arterial conditions, some drugs, and occasionally pregnancy.

ANATOMY AND PHYSIOLOGY OF BLOOD PRESSURE REGULATION

Two factors determine BP: cardiac output (CO) and peripheral vascular resistance (PVR):

$$BP = CO \times PVR$$

CARDIAC OUTPUT

CO is the volume of blood pumped by the heart in a specific period of time (usually 1 minute). It is

Table 38-1 Guidelines for Diagnosis of Hypertension in Persons Age 18 Years and Older*

CATEGORY	SYSTOLIC BLOOD PRESSURE (mm Hg)		DIASTOLIC BLOOD PRESSURE (mm Hg)
Normal†	<120	*and*	<80
Prehypertension	120–139	*or*	80–89
Hypertension‡			
Stage 1	140–159	*or*	90–99
Stage 2	≥160	*or*	≥100

From Joint National Committee on Prevention, Detection, Evaluation, and Treatment of High Blood Pressure: *The seventh report of the Joint National Committee on Prevention, Detection, Evaluation, and Treatment of High Blood Pressure*, Bethesda, Md, 2003, Department of Health and Human Services, National Institutes of Health, National Heart, Lung, and Blood Institute.

*Not taking antihypertensive drugs and not acutely ill.

†Optimal blood pressure (BP) with respect to cardiovascular risk is below 120/80 mm Hg. However, unusually low readings should be evaluated for clinical significance.

‡Based on the average of two or more readings taken at each of two or more visits after an initial screening.

determined by the strength, rate, and rhythm of the contraction of the left ventricle (LV) and by the blood volume.

PERIPHERAL VASCULAR RESISTANCE

PVR is the force in the blood vessels that the LV must overcome to eject blood from the heart. Resistance to blood flow is determined primarily by the diameter of the blood vessels and blood viscosity (thickness). Increased PVR results from a narrowing of the arteries and arterioles or an increased fluid volume in the blood vessels that results from sodium and water retention. Increased PVR is the most prominent characteristic of hypertension.

The diameter of blood vessels is regulated largely by the vasomotor center. The vasomotor center is located in the medulla of the brain. Sympathetic nervous system tracts from the medulla extend down the spinal cord to the thoracic and abdominal regions. Stimulation of the sympathetic nervous system causes release of the hormones *norepinephrine* and *epinephrine*. These hormones, called *catecholamine*, are vasoconstrictors, meaning that they cause the blood vessels to constrict, making their diameters smaller. By constricting blood vessels, norepinephrine increases PVR and raises BP. Epinephrine constricts blood vessels and increases the force of cardiac contraction, causing BP to raise.

Vasoconstriction decreases blood flow to the kidneys, which then release renin. Renin leads to the formation of angiotensin, another potent vasoconstrictor. Angiotensin stimulates the adrenal cortex to secrete aldosterone, a hormone that promotes sodium and water retention. This results in an increased blood volume. Vasoconstriction, cardiac stimulation, and retention of fluid all contribute to hypertension. Figure 38-1 illustrates how various factors raise BP.

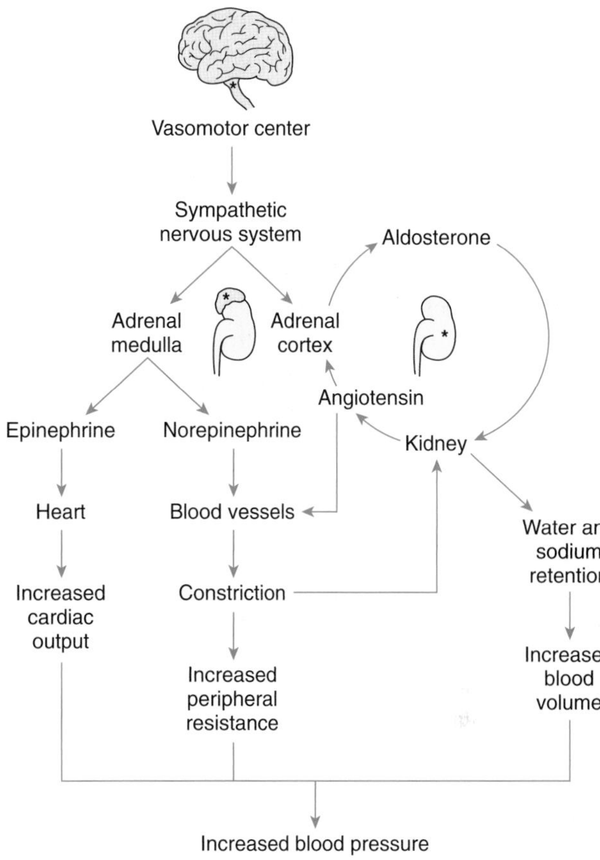

FIGURE 38-1 Factors that increase blood pressure (BP).

AGE-RELATED CHANGES AFFECTING BLOOD PRESSURE

Some age-related changes affect BP. With aging, atherosclerotic changes reduce the elasticity of the arteries, causing a decrease in CO and an increase in PVR. After age 60, PVR increases by approximately 1% per year. Systolic pressure rises in response to increased PVR. In addition, pulse pressure (the difference between the systolic and diastolic pressures) widens in response to a decreased ability of the aorta to distend (stretch).

Research has shown that older people do benefit from controlling hypertension; however, the 2014 JNC 8 recommends target rates of <150 for SBP and <90 for DBP in people ages 60 and older.

PRIMARY (ESSENTIAL) HYPERTENSION

RISK FACTORS

The most significant risk factors for primary (essential) hypertension are dyslipidemia, atherosclerosis, diabetes mellitus, tobacco use, age beyond 55 years for men or beyond 65 years for women, family history (i.e., father or brother diagnosed with heart disease before age 55; mother or sister diagnosed with heart disease before age 65), and sedentary lifestyle. Obesity, defined as weight 20% over ideal body weight, is also a risk factor. The additional weight and fat cause increases in the number of blood vessels, circulating blood volume, and cardiac workload. Atherosclerosis decreases the elasticity of the arteries and arterioles, causing increased PVR. Nicotine in cigarettes constricts blood vessels and stimulates the release of epinephrine and norepinephrine. As mentioned, these hormones also constrict blood vessels and raise heart rate and BP. Lack of physical activity leads to pooling of blood in the extremities and increases the workload of the cardiovascular system.

Other risk factors include stress; overstimulation; and a family history of obesity, hypertension, or **dyslipidemia**. Dyslipidemia refers to the abnormal amount of specific lipids and lipoproteins in the blood, a factor that contributes to atherosclerosis. Stress caused by such factors as a high-pressure job, financial worries, or family problems increases secretion of catecholamine. Stimulants that may contribute to or aggravate hypertension include caffeine, nicotine, and amphetamines. Caffeine is found in tea, coffee, and chocolate. Nicotine is obtained by smoking or chewing tobacco products.

SIGNS AND SYMPTOMS

Many people with hypertension have no symptoms. Symptoms that may accompany hypertension include occipital headaches that are more severe on arising, lightheadedness, and **epistaxis** (nosebleed). If hypertension has damaged blood vessels in the heart, kidneys, eyes, or brain, the patient may have symptoms of impaired function of those organs.

COMPLICATIONS

The most serious consequences of hypertension are heart attack, HF, stroke, kidney disease, and blindness. Complications occur because the long-term effect of prolonged hypertension is replacement of elastic arteriolar tissue with stiffer, fibrous collagen tissue. Thickening of the arteriolar wall decreases its ability to distend, resulting in increased PVR and decreased blood flow to various organs. The organs that are most sensitive to these changes are the heart, kidneys, brain, and eyes. Patients with hypertension must be assessed frequently for damage to these sensitive ("target") organs (Fig. 38-2).

Heart

CHD develops in patients with hypertension two to three times more frequently than in people with normal BP. CHD reduces blood supply to the myocardium, which can result in angina, myocardial infarction (MI), and congestive heart failure (CHF). MI, commonly called a *heart attack*, results when the blood supply to the heart muscle is inadequate and the myocardium is deprived of oxygen (O_2).

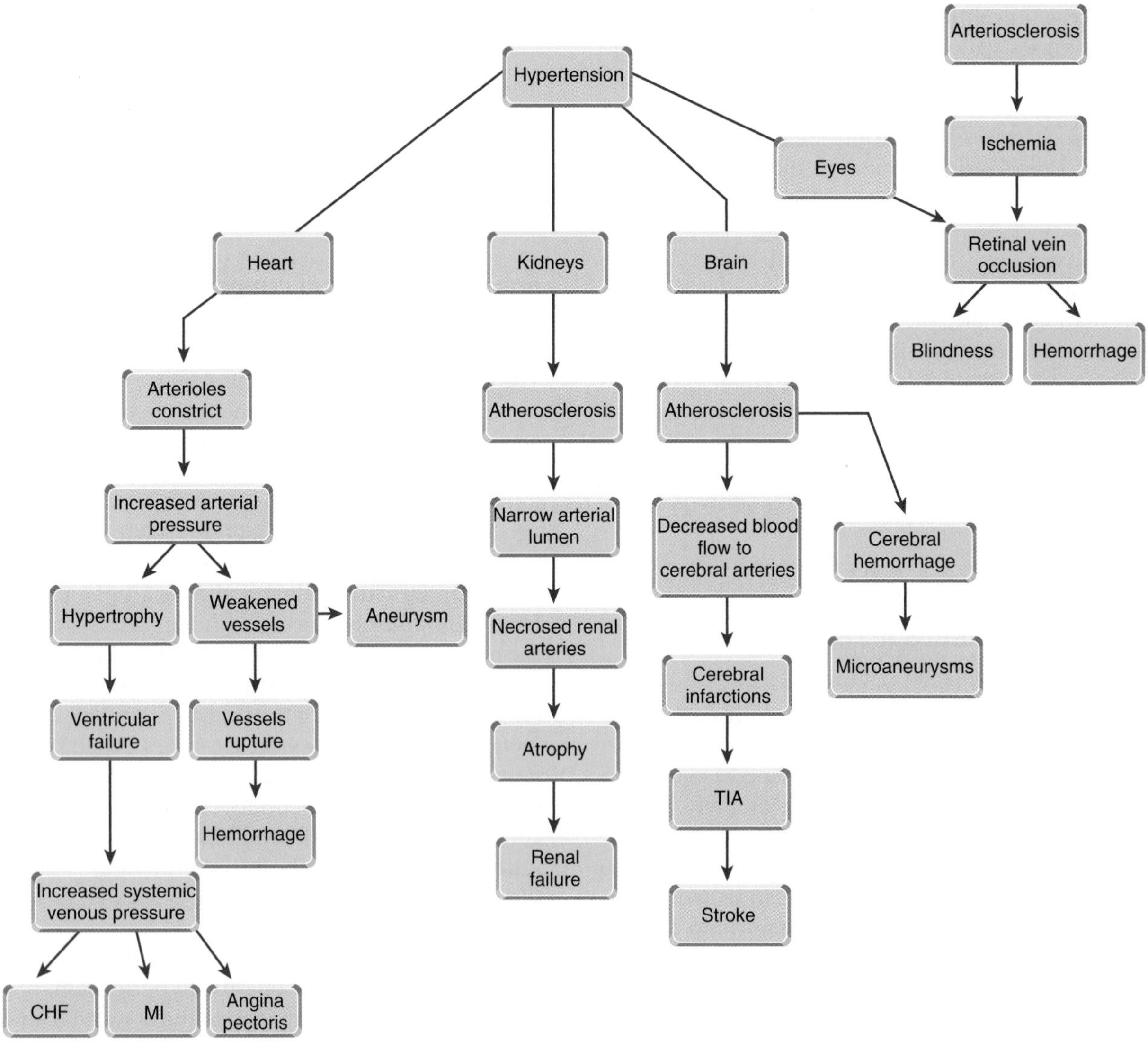

FIGURE 38-2 How hypertension affects major target organs. *CHF*, Congestive heart failure; *MI*, myocardial infarction; *TIA*, transient ischemic attack. (From Monahan FD, Drake DT, Neighbors M, editors: *Medical-surgical nursing: foundations for clinical practice*, ed 2, Philadelphia, 1998, Saunders.)

Sustained hypertension requires the LV to work harder to overcome increased peripheral resistance. The increased workload may cause the LV to **hypertrophy** (enlarge), and it may eventually fail.

Kidneys

Narrowing of the renal arteries may decrease renal function and lead to chronic renal failure. Initial indicators of renal failure are nocturia (need to urinate during the night) and azotemia (accumulation of nitrogen waste products in the blood). In addition, urinalysis may reveal protein (proteinuria), blood (hematuria), or both in the urine.

Brain

Prolonged hypertension constricts and damages cerebral arteries, putting the patient at risk for transient ischemic attacks (TIAs) and cerebrovascular accidents (CVAs). A TIA, sometimes called a *little stroke*, is a temporary neurologic dysfunction caused by cerebral ischemia.

A CVA, or stroke, results from interrupted blood flow in the brain caused by a **thrombus** (clot) that occludes the vessel or by a rupture of a blood vessel. People with hypertension have a sevenfold increased incidence of CVAs compared to those with normal BP.

Eyes

Damage to the eyes may include narrowing of the retinal arterioles, retinal hemorrhages, and papilledema (edema of the optic nerve). These changes may lead to blindness.

DIAGNOSTIC TESTS AND PROCEDURES

Diagnosis of hypertension is based on direct and indirect data. Hypertension is confirmed by repeated findings of average pressures equal to or greater than 140/90 mm Hg. When elevations are found in clinics or in screenings, the physician might have patients monitor their own BPs at home for comparison. In addition, ambulatory BP monitors, which can be programmed to record readings every 15 to 30 minutes for 24 hours, typically provide readings lower than clinic readings. These readings provide a better foundation for the diagnosis of hypertension than a few isolated readings. The process is not cost effective for all patients but is appropriate in selected situations.

On finding an elevated BP, the physician collects data about the patient's lifestyle, other cardiovascular risk factors, and other medical diagnoses such as diabetes. The patient is examined for effects of hypertension on the heart, eyes, kidneys, and brain. An electrocardiogram (ECG) and blood and urine studies should be ordered. Blood studies include glucose, hematocrit, potassium, calcium, creatinine, and a lipid profile. If kidney damage exists, the serum creatinine level is elevated. Abnormal serum lipids and lipoproteins may indicate atherosclerosis. A chest radiograph may show enlargement of the heart or pulmonary blood vessels.

Physicians disagree about the need to try to determine the cause of hypertension. If no evidence suggests an underlying disease process, the consensus is to limit diagnostic tests to those that are most significant. This reduces patient care costs.

MEDICAL TREATMENT

The goal of therapy for hypertension is to gradually reduce PVR and BP. Lowering BP to less than 140/90 mm Hg significantly decreases cardiovascular risks. For patients who have diabetes or renal disease, the medical goal is less than 130/80 mm Hg. Optimal BP is usually defined as a diastolic pressure of less than 80 mm Hg and a systolic pressure less than 120 mm Hg. Treatment of underlying conditions may lower the BP in people with secondary hypertension.

For treatment of primary hypertension, a conservative, nonpharmacologic (without drugs) method usually is tried first. Drug treatment may be added if needed.

Lifestyle Modifications

A nonpharmacologic approach includes weight reduction, smoking cessation, sodium and alcohol restriction, exercise, and relaxation techniques. Reduction of weight can reduce BP by reducing the cardiac workload. Stopping smoking eliminates vasoconstriction caused by nicotine. Reduction of sodium in the body reduces water retention and decreases the blood volume.

A planned program of exercise improves cardiac efficiency by increasing CO and decreasing PVR. Exercise also decreases the patient's blood glucose and cholesterol levels and promotes a sense of well-being. Isotonic exercises such as walking, bicycling, and swimming help to reduce weight and promote relaxation.

Relaxation therapy, biofeedback, and behavior modification techniques also may be used to reduce stress and lower BP (see *Complementary and Alternative Therapies* box). Alcohol intake should not exceed 2 oz per day because alcohol can increase BP and alter the effects of some antihypertensive drugs.

Complementary and Alternative Therapies

Complementary therapies such as relaxation, biofeedback, and behavior modification may be used along with traditional medical treatment of hypertension.

Lifestyle modifications are recommended for individuals with all stages of hypertension regardless of the risk group (Table 38-2).

Table 38-2 Principles of Lifestyle Modification

- Encourage healthy lifestyles for all individuals.
- Prescribe lifestyle modifications for all patients with prehypertension and hypertension.
  - Components of lifestyle modifications include weight reduction, DASH (Dietary Approaches to Stop Hypertension) eating plan, dietary sodium reduction, aerobic physical activity, and moderation of alcohol consumption.

Lifestyle Modification Recommendations

MODIFICATION	RECOMMENDATION	AVERAGE SYSTOLIC REDUCTION RANGE*
Weight reduction	Maintain normal body weight (body mass index [BMI] 18.5–24.9 kg/m^2).	5–20 mm Hg/10 kg
DASH eating plan	Adopt a diet rich in fruits, vegetables, and low-fat dairy products with reduced content of saturated and total fat.	8–14 mm Hg
Dietary sodium reduction	Reduce dietary sodium intake to ≤100 mmol per day (2.4 g sodium or 6 g sodium chloride).†	2–8 mm Hg
Aerobic physical activity	Engage in regular aerobic physical activity (e.g., brisk walking) at least 30 minutes per day, most days of the week.	4–9 mm Hg
Moderation of alcohol consumption	Men should be limited to ≤2 drinks‡ per day. Women and lighter-weight persons should be limited to ≤1 drink‡ per day.	2–4 mm Hg

From Joint National Committee on Prevention, Detection, Evaluation, and Treatment of High Blood Pressure: *The seventh report of the Joint National Committee on Prevention, Detection, Evaluation, and Treatment of High Blood Pressure*, Bethesda, Md, 2003, Department of Health and Human Services, National Institutes of Health, National Heart, Lung, and Blood Institute.
*Effects are dose and time dependent.
†National Research Council recommends daily sodium intake of 1500 mg with upper limit of 2300 mg per day.
‡1 drink = ½ oz or 15 mL ethanol (e.g., 12-oz beer, 5-oz wine, 1.5-oz 80-proof whiskey).

Pharmacologic Therapy

Drug therapy is indicated if the BP is very high initially (systolic ≥160, diastolic ≥100) or if conservative therapies for less severe hypertension are not effective within 3 to 6 months. Drug therapy must be individualized for each patient and may be recommended at earlier stages. The goal of drug therapy is to normalize BP using the smallest number of the safest drugs at the lowest effective dosages. A single agent is preferred if good control can be achieved, because patients are more likely to take one drug as prescribed than multiple agents. However, most patients require two or more drugs to achieve control. Antihypertensive drugs are listed in Table 38-3.

JNC 8 Recommendations for Treatment of Hypertension. Table 38-4 discusses the management guidelines for hypertension recommended by the *JNC 8*. If lifestyle modifications have not achieved the BP goal, initial drug choices are made on the basis of individual factors. Different recommendations are made depending on whether the patient has Stage 1 or Stage 2 hypertension. Stage 1 hypertension is defined as a SBP of 140 to 159 or a DBP of 90 to 99; Stage 2 hypertension is defined as a SBP of 160 or more or a DBP of 100 or more. Some patients have "compelling indications for individual drug classes." Specific classes of drugs are recommended for patients with HF, diabetes, and chronic kidney disease as well as for patients who have had an MI, are at high risk for cardiovascular disease, or are being treated to prevent a recurrent stroke.

Specific Antihypertensive Drugs. First-line antihypertensive drugs recommended by *JNC 8* include thiazide diuretics, angiotensin-converting enzyme (ACE) inhibitors, angiotensin II receptor blockers, and calcium channel blockers. Other categories that may be used are alpha$_1$-adrenergic blockers, beta blockers, central alpha$_2$ agonists and other centrally acting drugs, and direct vasodilators. A number of combination drugs are available and these reduce the number of tablets the patient must take.

Diuretics. Several types of diuretics may be used to treat hypertension. These include thiazide-type diuretics, loop (high ceiling) diuretics, and potassium-sparing diuretics. *JNC 8* recommends a thiazide-type diuretic such as hydrochlorothiazide (HydroDIURIL) for initial therapy. Thiazide-type diuretics decrease the reabsorption of sodium and water, which lowers BP by reducing blood volume. They also promote vasodilation by an unknown mechanism. Although they reduce blood volume initially, that effect stabilizes over time; however, the BP reduction persists. Diuretics are especially effective in treating African-American patients with hypertension.

Patients taking diuretics must be monitored for fluid and electrolyte imbalances, especially hypovolemia and potassium imbalances. Intake and output records may be kept on hospitalized patients who are taking diuretics. Hypokalemia is a potentially serious problem except with potassium-sparing diuretics (e.g., amiloride [Midamor]). Older patients are especially

Table 38-3 **Drug Therapy: Antihypertensive Drugs and Nursing Interventions**

General Considerations

1. Monitor blood pressure (BP) regularly with patient in supine, sitting, and standing positions.
2. Encourage patients to take medications and keep follow-up appointments even when they are feeling well.
3. Teach patients with orthostatic hypotension to rise slowly, avoid prolonged standing, and avoid hot baths and showers.
4. Advise patients to consult physician or pharmacist about safety of over-the-counter (OTC) drugs.
5. Do not stop drugs abruptly because rebound hypertension may occur.

DRUG CLASSES AND EXAMPLES	USE AND ACTION	SIDE EFFECTS	NURSING INTERVENTIONS
Centrally Acting Agents (Alpha$_2$-Agonists)			
clonidine (Catapres), methyldopa (Aldomet)	Acts on the central nervous system (CNS) to block vasoconstriction, which lowers BP; also reduces anxiety.	Drowsiness, dry mouth, weakness, depression, and retention of sodium and water. Orthostatic hypotension occurs with some drugs.	Monitor the patient's BP. Take safety precautions and encourage good oral hygiene. Assess the patient for edema. Teach the patient to manage orthostatic hypotension.
Alpha-Adrenergic Receptor Blockers (Antagonist)			
doxazosin (Cardura), prazosin (Minipress), terazosin (Hytrin)	Blocks the effects of norepinephrine, causing vasodilation.	Reflex tachycardia, palpitations, headache, dizziness, drowsiness, and nausea. Potentially severe orthostatic hypotension can occur with first or increased dose of prazosin.	Monitor the patient's pulse and BP. Advise the patient that most side effects diminish over time. Give the first or increased dose of prazosin at bedtime. Advise the patient of possible orthostatic hypotension. Change positions slowly.
Beta-Adrenergic Receptor Blockers			
propranolol (Inderal), atenolol (Tenormin)	Decreases cardiac stimulation.	Bradycardia, fatigue, drowsiness, depression, hypoglycemia, and bronchial constriction.	Monitor the patient's pulse, BP, and respiration. Assess the patient's emotional status. Monitor patients with asthma for dyspnea and patients with diabetes for low blood glucose.
Direct Vasodilators			
hydralazine (Apresoline)	Relaxes vascular smooth muscle, causing vasodilation.	Reflex tachycardia, headache, dizziness, nausea and vomiting, anorexia, and hypotension.	Monitor the patient's pulse and BP.
Calcium Channel Blockers			
verapamil (Calan), diltiazem (Cardizem), amlodipine (Norvasc), amlodipine and atorvastatin (Caduet), nifedipine (Procardia)	Decreases the force of cardiac contraction and dilates the peripheral blood vessels.	Bradycardia, flushing, dizziness, headache, edema, and palpitations.	Monitor the patient's pulse. Elevate the legs when sitting to reduce edema.
Angiotensin-Converting Enzyme Inhibitors			
captopril (Capoten), enalapril (Vasotec), lisinopril (Zestril, Prinivil)	Reduces aldosterone secretion and prevents the formation of angiotensin II, thus decreasing peripheral resistance and fluid volume.	Skin rash, headache, dizziness, neutropenia, and cough. Renal failure can occur in patients with renal artery stenosis.	Monitor the patient's blood cell counts. Report any changes in urine output to the physician.

Continued

Table 38-3 **Drug Therapy: Antihypertensive Drugs and Nursing Interventions—cont'd**

DRUG CLASSES AND EXAMPLES	USE AND ACTION	SIDE EFFECTS	NURSING INTERVENTIONS
Diuretics			
hydrochlorothiazide (HCTZ), furosemide (Lasix)	Reduces fluid volume; may cause vasodilation; sodium loss may reduce vasoconstriction.	Fluid volume deficit, hyponatremia, and hypokalemia (except with potassium-sparing diuretics).	Monitor the patient's fluid balance: hydration, urine output, mental status, and muscle tone. Recommend foods high in potassium (e.g., bananas, orange juice) unless potassium-sparing diuretics are being given.
Angiotensin II Receptor Antagonists			
losartan (Cozaar), valsartan (Diovan)	Blocks the action of angiotensin II; causes vasodilation; increases renal excretion of sodium and water.	Dizziness.	Take safety precautions to prevent injury to the patient who may experience dizziness.

Table 38-4 **JNC 8 2014 Hypertension Management Guidelines for Individuals Aged 18 and Older**

AGE	BP GOAL	DRUG THERAPY	LIFESTYLE MODIFICATIONS
≤ 60 years	SBP < 150 mm Hg DBP < 90 mm Hg	Thiazide diuretic or ACE inhibitor or ARB or CCB, alone or in combination	Yes
< 60 years	SBP < 140 mm Hg DBP < 90 mm Hg	Non-African American: Thiazide diuretic or ACE inhibitor or ARB or CCB, alone or in combination African American: Thiazide diuretic or CCB, alone or in combination	Yes
All ages with DM; no CKD	SBP < 140 mm Hg DBP < 90 mm Hg	Non-African American: Thiazide diuretic or ACE inhibitor or ARB or CCB, alone or in combination African American: Thiazide diuretic or CCB, alone or in combination	Yes
All ages with CKD; with or without DM	SBP < 140 mm Hg DBP < 90 mm Hg	ACE inhibitor or ARB, alone or in combination with another drug class	Yes

Data from 2014 Evidence-Based Guideline for the Management of High Blood Pressure in Adults: Report for the Panel Members Appointed to the Eighth Joint National Committee (JNC 8). *JAMA* (2014); 311(5): 507-520.
ACE, Angiotensin converting enzyme; *ARB,* angiotensin receptor blocker; *CCB,* calcium channel blocker; *DBP,* diastolic blood pressure; *SBP,* systolic blood pressure.

susceptible to hypokalemia. The nurse should monitor for signs of hypokalemia: confusion, irritability, muscle weakness, cardiac dysrhythmias, and anorexia. Severe hypokalemia can lead to respiratory arrest and disruptions in cardiac rhythm. To prevent hypokalemia, it is important to encourage the patient to consume additional dietary potassium. Sources of potassium include bananas and orange juice. After blood levels are drawn to determine the need for potassium supplementation, some patients require supplementary potassium as ordered.

Pharmacology Capsule

When patients are taking diuretics, monitor for signs and symptoms of hypokalemia: cardiac dysrhythmias, muscle weakness, and diminished bowel sounds.

Beta-Adrenergic Receptor Blockers. Beta-adrenergic receptor blockers, commonly called *beta-blockers,* reduce BP by blocking the beta effects of catecholamine. Examples of beta-blockers used to treat hypertension are atenolol (Tenormin), labetalol (Normodyne), metoprolol (Lopressor), and propranolol (Inderal). When beta receptors are stimulated, they stimulate the heart and relax bronchial smooth muscle. Beta-blockers prevent this stimulation, resulting in decreased heart rate, decreased strength of cardiac contraction, and bronchial constriction. A number of beta-blockers have slightly different effects. Some affect cardiac function more; others have an increased effect on the bronchi. Except for labetalol, beta-blockers are less effective than other types of antihypertensive drugs in African-American patients (see *Cultural Considerations* box).

Cultural Considerations

What Does Culture Have to Do with Antihypertensive Drugs?

Your genes affect the way you metabolize drugs. Therefore ethnicity and race explain some variations in effects of antihypertensive drugs. For example, Asians respond better to beta-blockers than do Caucasians. African Americans are best treated with thiazide diuretics and/or calcium channel blockers.

Common side effects of beta-blockers include bradycardia and hypotension, hypoglycemia, and increased low-density lipoprotein (LDL) in the blood. Beta-blockers usually are not recommended in patients with asthma, chronic obstructive pulmonary disease (COPD), or heart block. When a patient is taking a beta-blocker, the nurse should monitor for bradycardia and hypotension. People with diabetes should be watched carefully for hypoglycemia because beta-blockers lower blood glucose and suppress the usual signs of hypoglycemia. Diaphoresis (excessive perspiration) may be the only sign of hypoglycemia when people with diabetes are taking beta-blockers. Older adult patients are at increased risk compared to young patients for hypotension and bradycardia associated with beta-blockers. Therefore they should be started on low doses that are increased cautiously if needed.

Pharmacology Capsule

Monitor people with diabetes for low blood glucose if they are taking beta-blockers.

Calcium Antagonists. Calcium antagonists are called *calcium channel blockers* because they block the movement of calcium into cardiac and vascular smooth muscle cells. This action reduces the heart rate, decreases the force of cardiac contraction, and dilates peripheral blood vessels. Because dilated vessels present less resistance to blood flow, BP is reduced. Diltiazem (Cardizem), isradipine (DynaCirc), nicardipine (Cardene), nifedipine (Procardia), amlodipine (Norvasc), amlodipine and atorvastatin (Caduet), and verapamil (Calan) are examples of calcium channel blockers used for hypertension.

Common side effects of calcium channel blockers are flushing, dizziness, and headache. The nurse should also monitor for hypotension, bradycardia, and edema.

Angiotensin-Converting Enzyme Inhibitors. ACE inhibitors prevent the conversion of angiotensin I to angiotensin II, a potent vasoconstrictor. Blocking the production of angiotensin II decreases peripheral resistance. ACE inhibitors also decrease fluid retention by decreasing the production of aldosterone. Examples of ACE inhibitors are captopril (Capoten), lisinopril (Zestril, Prinivil), and enalapril (Vasotec). ACE inhibitors with diuretics are often effective for African-American patients. Adverse effects can include a chronic cough, dizziness, headache, fatigue, angioedema, hyperkalemia, and hypotension.

Angiotensin II Receptor Antagonists. Angiotensin II receptor antagonists prevent vasoconstriction in response to angiotensin. They also prevent the release of aldosterone, which increases excretion of salt and water, thereby reducing blood volume. Examples of angiotensin II receptor antagonists are losartan (Cozaar) and valsartan (Diovan). Unlike the ACE inhibitors, the only significant adverse effect of these drugs has been dizziness in some patients.

Central Adrenergic Blockers. Central adrenergic blockers inhibit impulses from the vasomotor center in the brain that maintain the muscle tone in blood vessels. The effect of this type of drug is to reduce peripheral resistance and lower BP. Examples of centrally acting adrenergic blockers are clonidine (Catapres) and methyldopa (Aldomet).

Alpha-Adrenergic Receptor Blockers. Stimulation of alpha receptors produces constriction of arterioles. Drugs such as doxazosin (Cardura) and prazosin (Minipress) block alpha receptor stimulation and lower BP by reducing peripheral resistance. The most important adverse effect is **orthostatic hypotension**, which is most severe with initial or increased dosages. Patients should lie down for 2 hours after taking a first or increased dose of this drug. For this reason, it is best given at bedtime. Alpha-blockers can also cause dizziness, headache, and drowsiness.

Direct Vasodilators. Direct vasodilators lower BP by relaxing arteriolar smooth muscle. Examples of direct vasodilators are fenoldopam (Corlopam), minoxidil (Loniten), hydralazine (Apresoline), diazoxide (Hyperstat IV), and sodium nitroprusside (Nipride). Fenoldopam, nitroglycerin, sodium nitroprusside, hydralazine, and diazoxide are used to treat hypertensive crisis. Most emergency vasodilators are diluted in intravenous fluids and administered at the rate needed for the desired results. Diazoxide is given by direct intravenous injection (IV push), usually in small, repeated doses until the BP reaches the target reading.

Nursing Implications. You must be familiar with the drugs commonly prescribed for hypertension. Nursing responsibilities include administering the drugs to inpatients, monitoring for therapeutic and adverse effects, and teaching patients about their drugs. Additional information about antihypertensive drugs and nursing interventions is presented in Table 38-3.

Older adults respond differently to drug therapy. Older patients are at increased risk for adverse effects of medications because of reduced liver and kidney function. They are especially susceptible to orthostatic hypotension because their blood vessels respond more slowly to position changes. This creates increased risk for falls. !

Older people may respond differently to beta-blockers and to diuretics. The effectiveness of beta-blockers may be reduced because beta receptor activity is lessened in older adults. In addition, diuretics may produce a more profound decrease in blood volume in these patients. Also older patients often are taking medications for other conditions. Drug interactions can alter therapeutic effects or enhance side effects. Dosages for antihypertensive medications may need to be reduced or adjusted depending on what conditions the patient has.

Put on Your Thinking Cap!

You have been asked to give a talk on hypertension to members of a senior center. The members are low income and have minimal education. Some speak limited English.

1. How might you explain the effects of hypertension on the body?
2. Select one lifestyle modification and explain how it reduces the risk of hypertension.

SECONDARY HYPERTENSION

Secondary hypertension, which has a specific known cause, is less common than primary hypertension. Causes include renal disease, excess secretion of adrenal hormones, narrowing of the aorta, increased intracranial pressure, and some drugs such as vasoconstrictors.

NURSING CARE of the Patient with Hypertension

Assessment

Early detection, education, and promotion of adherence to treatment are the keys to controlling BP. Periodic BP checks detect new or unknown people with hypertension and provide data to evaluate the effect of therapy in known people with hypertension.

The nursing assessment of the person with known or possible hypertension begins with a complete history and physical examination by the registered nurse (RN). The licensed vocational nurse/licensed practical nurse (LVN/LPN) may be involved in initial BP screenings and monitoring and provides important data to evaluate treatment effectiveness.

Health History

The patient's reason for seeking care should be noted. Because hypertension often has no symptoms, the visit may be related to some other problem. It is important to explore the patient's past medical history to determine whether he or she has ever had hypertension or renal, cardiac, or endocrine disorders. Note the date and readings of the last BP measurement. Ask the female patient about pregnancy and about hormone replacement therapy, if appropriate. List current medications, including over-the-counter (OTC) drugs. In the family health history, inquire about hypertension, MI, or CVAs among relatives.

Review the body systems for significant signs and symptoms, particularly headaches, epistaxis, dizziness, visual disturbances, dyspnea, angina, or nocturia. Information about the patient's usual functioning may detect some potential risk factors for hypertension. This includes occupation, exercise and activity, sleep and rest, nutrition, interpersonal relationships, and stressors.

Physical Examination

While taking the health history and beginning the physical examination, observe the patient's general appearance, noting any obvious distress. Measure height, weight, and vital signs. The nurse may be the first to detect elevated pressure, so accurate measurement of BP is very important. The patient should be seated comfortably in a chair with his or her feet on the floor. Position the arm on a surface at the level of the heart. The proper cuff size is essential; the bladder of the cuff should encircle at least 80% of the circumference of the patient's arm. A cuff that is too small may give a false high reading whereas a cuff that is too large may give a false low reading. For a more accurate reading, determine the systolic pressure first by palpation. To do this, palpate the radial or brachial pulse while inflating the cuff. The pressure when the last pulse is felt is the palpated systolic pressure. Then deflate the cuff and take the pressure by auscultation, being careful to reinflate the cuff above the palpated systolic pressure.

For the initial assessment, usually done by the RN or physician, multiple readings should be taken. The BP should be assessed in both arms first with the patient in the supine position, then with the patient sitting and finally standing. It is normal for the SBP to fall approximately 10 mm Hg and the DBP to rise approximately 5 mm Hg between the supine and standing readings. In general, BP readings obtained in the home are more valid measures because patients are more relaxed there than in a clinic or office.

In addition to BP and pulses, assess respiratory rate and effort and inspect extremities for edema and color. Note any abnormalities in neurologic or muscular function.

Nursing assessment of the patient with known or possible hypertension is summarized in Box 38-1.

When screening persons for hypertension, if the BP is elevated initially, reassess it after 1 to 5 minutes. If the pressure remains elevated, refer the patient for medical evaluation. Remember that a single elevated reading does not mean that the patient has hypertension. If the BP is severely elevated (diastolic pressure of 115 mm Hg or more), the patient is in imminent danger of a stroke and immediate medical care is needed.

Box 38-1 Assessment of the Patient with Known or Possible Hypertension

HEALTH HISTORY
Present Illness
Description of reason for seeking care
Past Medical History
Hypertension; last blood pressure (BP) reading; renal, cardiac, or endocrine disorders; pregnancy; current medications
Family History
Hypertension, myocardial infarction (MI), cerebrovascular accident (CVA)
Review of Systems
Headache, dizziness, epistaxis, visual disturbances, dyspnea, angina, nocturia
Functional Assessment
Occupation, activity and exercise, sleep and rest, nutrition, interpersonal relationships, current stressors
PHYSICAL EXAMINATION
General Appearance
Distress
Height and Weight
Vital Signs
BP: supine, sitting, standing
Pulse
Respiration
Temperature
Extremities
Edema
Neuromuscular
Abnormalities

Nursing Diagnoses, Goals, and Outcome Criteria: Hypertension

Nursing Diagnoses	Goals and Outcome Criteria
Ineffective Self-Health Management related to lack of knowledge about management of hypertension, drug side effects, difficulty maintaining lifestyle changes	Effective patient management of prescribed treatment: patient correctly explains hypertension and its treatment. Patient adheres to prescribed treatment plan: lowered blood pressure (BP), evidence of positive lifestyle changes (weight loss, cessation of smoking)
Risk for Injury related to orthostatic hypotension secondary to antihypertensive drug therapy, sedation	Lack of injury: no falls or other incidents associated with orthostatic hypotension or sedation
Ineffective Coping related to depression secondary to drug side effects	Effective coping: patient reports positive emotional state
Sexual Dysfunction related to drug side effects	Satisfactory sexual function: patient's statement of ability to manage effects of drug therapy on sexual function

Interventions

Ineffective Self-Health Management

Adherence to therapy requires commitment and active participation on the part of the patient. Lifestyle changes may be required and pharmacologic side effects may be unpleasant. Failure to follow the prescribed regimen is often referred to as *noncompliance.* Some people prefer the term *nonadherence* as being less judgmental. In counseling the patient, it must be stressed that hypertension is a chronic disease that requires long-term management. Sometimes patients discontinue drug therapy inappropriately because they have no symptoms and current BP readings (while on medications!) are normal.

Patient education is critical for effective management of hypertension. Education begins as soon as the condition is diagnosed and continues throughout life. As with any patient teaching, begin by finding out what the person already knows and is most interested in learning. Addressing the patient's immediate concerns first builds trust that should facilitate further teaching. It is important to present measures to manage hypertension as *health practices that are beneficial to everyone*, rather than as a long list of what the patient should or should not do. Include members of the patient's household, especially a spouse, in the teaching. Their understanding and cooperation can be very supportive to the patient.

It is hoped that teaching patients about their medications will promote adherence. Information in writing and a chart with times for medication administration may be helpful. Patients who do not take their medications as prescribed often cite the adverse side effects as reasons for noncompliance. It is important to teach patients to report unpleasant drug side effects to the physician promptly. A change in dosage or in the medication itself may reduce undesirable effects but the patient should not make changes unless advised to do so by the physician. Common side effects of antihypertensive drugs that may affect adherence are orthostatic hypotension, sedation, sexual dysfunction, and depression.

Diet Therapy. The goals of diet therapy for the person with hypertension are to maintain ideal body weight and prevent fluid retention. Total calorie intake may need to be adjusted to achieve these goals. A diet low in saturated fats with no more than 2 g of sodium is often prescribed. Sodium restriction is more effective for some patients than for others. According to the National Research Council, 1500 mg of sodium daily is an adequate intake. The upper limit of sodium intake should not exceed 2300 mg daily.

If the patient is taking a potassium-wasting diuretic, dietary potassium intake may need to be increased or potassium supplements may be recommended.

The nurse and the dietitian should cooperate in teaching patients about their prescribed dietary alterations. If someone other than the patient prepares the food at home, that person should be included in the dietary teaching (see *Cultural Considerations* box).

Cultural Considerations

What Does Culture Have to Do with Diet?

Cultural dietary practices affect the types of foods eaten and how they are prepared. These practices must be considered and incorporated when teaching patients about healthier dietary practices.

The DASH (Dietary Approaches to Stop Hypertension) eating plan helps to lower BP in those with hypertension and it decreases the risk of developing hypertension in those who currently have BP in the healthy range. Therefore it is a good plan for the whole family (Table 38-5).

The *Nutrition Considerations* box discusses diet and hypertension.

Nutrition Considerations

1. Diet and lifestyle changes, including weight reduction, exercise, and stress management, are important in the treatment of hypertension.
2. Weight loss in obese people lowers blood pressure (BP) at a rate of 1 mm Hg per kg (2.2 lb) of body weight.
3. Sodium-restricted diets help to lower BP in many people with hypertension.
4. A high potassium intake may help to lower BP and replace potassium lost with potassium-wasting diuretics. Foods particularly high in potassium are fresh fruits and vegetables.
5. An adequate calcium intake may help in preventing and treating hypertension. Two to three cups of milk or yogurt per day, 4 oz of low-sodium cheese, or calcium supplements (calcium carbonate, 1 to 2 g/day) can provide adequate calcium intake.

Table 38-5 DASH Eating Plan

The DASH (Dietary Approaches to Stop Hypertension) eating plan is based on 2000 calories a day. The number of daily servings in a food group may vary from those listed, depending on an individual's caloric needs.

FOOD GROUP	DAILY SERVINGS (EXCEPT AS NOTED)	SERVING SIZES
Grains and grain products	7–8	1 slice of bread 1 cup of ready-to-eat cereal* ½ cup of cooked rice, pasta, or cereal
Vegetables	4–5	1 cup of raw leafy vegetable ½ cup of cooked vegetable 6 oz of vegetable juice
Fruits	4–5	1 medium fruit ¼ cup of dried fruit ½ cup of fresh, frozen, or canned fruit 6 oz of fruit juice
Low-fat or fat-free dairy foods	2–3	8 oz of milk 1 cup of yogurt 1½ oz of cheese
Lean meats, poultry, and fish	2 or fewer	3 oz of cooked lean meat, skinless poultry, or fish
Nuts, seeds, and dry beans	4–5 per week	⅓ cup or 1½ oz of nuts 1 tablespoon or ½ oz of seeds ½ cup of cooked dry beans
Fats and oils†	2–3	1 teaspoon of soft margarine 1 tablespoon of low-fat mayonnaise 2 tablespoons of light salad dressing 1 teaspoon of vegetable oil
Sweets	5 per week	1 tablespoon of sugar 1 tablespoon of jelly or jam ½ oz of jelly beans 8 oz of lemonade

From U.S. Department of Health and Human Services, National Institutes of Health, National Heart, Lung, and Blood Institute: *Your guide to lowering blood pressure*, Bethesda, Md, 2003, National Institutes of Health.

*Serving sizes vary between ½ cup and 1¼ cup. Check the product's nutrition label.

†Fat content changes serving counts for fats and oils. For example, 1 tablespoon of regular salad dressing equals 1 serving, 1 tablespoon of low-fat salad dressing equals ½ serving, and 1 tablespoon of fat-free salad dressing equals 0 servings.

Exercise. Nutrition and exercise go hand in hand. It is very difficult to maintain or lose weight without engaging in some form of exercise. Walking is highly recommended as an exercise that increases cardiovascular functioning, burns calories, relieves stress, and promotes a sense of well-being. Thirty minutes of physical exercise on most days of the week can make a difference. An exercise program can benefit people of all ages, even older adults. Advise patients to ask their physicians before beginning new exercise programs and instruct them to increase their activities gradually over a period of time.

A program of good nutrition and exercise may allow a patient to eliminate or reduce medications used to control hypertension. This information may be motivating to some people.

Stress Management. Patients need to understand that stress can raise BP. Help patients to identify stressors in their lives and explore ways to reduce them. Referrals to professional counselors may be in order for patients with complicated or multiple stressors. Some agencies or community centers offer classes in stress management or relaxation techniques.

Drug Therapy. Patients need to be well informed about their medications. Review with the patient the name, dosage, purpose, and side effects of any prescribed medications. Advise patients to never discontinue their drugs or change the dosage without consulting with the physician, even if they feel well. BP can be very high with no symptoms. Suddenly stopping antihypertensive drugs may produce adverse effects, including rebound hypertension (sudden return of elevated BP), MI, and CVA. In addition, explain that many OTC drugs, such as cold remedies, contain vasoconstrictors that can counteract BP medications (see *Patient Teaching* box).

Patient Teaching

Hypertension

- Good control of hypertension reduces the risk of heart attack and stroke.
- A diet low in saturated fats and sodium may help to lower blood pressure (BP).
- Regular exercise as advised by your physician helps with weight control and reduction of BP.
- Smoking aggravates hypertension; the American Heart Association has programs to help you quit smoking.
- Relaxation techniques lower BP.
- Do not stop taking your medications unless instructed to do so by your physician. Suddenly stopping these drugs may cause BP to rise rapidly.
- Keep appointments for follow-up care; feeling better does not necessarily mean that your hypertension is under control.

Box 38-2 summarizes a variety of actions patients may take to help lower their BP.

Box 38-2 Action Items to Help Lower Blood Pressure

- Maintain a healthy weight:
  - Check with your health care provider to see if you need to lose weight.
  - If you do, lose weight slowly using a healthy-eating plan and engaging in physical activity.
- Be physically active:
  - Engage in physical activity for a total of 30 minutes on most days of the week.
  - Combine everyday chores with moderate-level sporting activities, such as walking, to achieve your physical activity goals.
- Follow a healthy-eating plan:
  - Set up a healthy-eating plan with foods low in saturated fat, total fat, and cholesterol and high in fruits, vegetables, and low-fat dairy foods such as the DASH eating plan.
  - Write down everything that you eat and drink in a food diary. Note areas that are successful or need improvement.
  - If you are trying to lose weight, choose an eating plan that is lower in calories.
- Reduce sodium in your diet:
  - Choose foods that are low in salt and other forms of sodium.
  - Use spices, garlic, and onions to add flavor to your meals without adding more sodium.
- Drink alcohol only in moderation:
  - In addition to raising your blood pressure (BP), too much alcohol can add unneeded calories to your diet.
  - If you drink alcoholic beverages, have only a moderate amount—one drink a day for women, two drinks a day for men.
- Take prescribed drugs as directed:
  - If you need drugs to help lower your BP, you still must follow the lifestyle changes just mentioned.
  - Use notes and other reminders to help you remember to take your drugs. Ask your family to help you with reminder phone calls and messages.

From U.S. Department of Health and Human Services, National Institutes of Health, National Heart, Lung, and Blood Institute: *Your guide to lowering blood pressure*, Bethesda, Md, 2003, National Institutes of Health.

Risk for Injury

The patient who is taking antihypertensive medications may be at risk for injury because of drug side effects. The effects that pose the greatest potential for injury are orthostatic hypotension and sedation.

Orthostatic Hypotension. Orthostatic or postural hypotension is a sudden drop in SBP, usually 20 mm Hg, when going from a lying or sitting position to a standing position. Monitor for lightheadedness, dizziness, and **syncope** (fainting) in patients who are at risk for orthostatic hypotension. In addition, instruct patients who are prone to orthostatic hypotension to exercise their legs and then to rise slowly from a lying or sitting position. They should avoid activities that cause BP to fall, such as prolonged standing in one place and taking very hot baths or showers.

Sedation. Sedation may be dealt with by taking medications at bedtime to promote sleep. If drowsiness from a medication is unavoidable during the day, the patient should not engage in activities that require alertness during times of peak drug effect.

Ineffective Coping

If depression occurs as a side effect of an antihypertensive drug, the patient should consult the physician so that another drug may be substituted. This side effect should be taken very seriously. Refer patients with severe depression to a mental health professional.

Sexual Dysfunction

A common side effect of many antihypertensive medications is sexual dysfunction. Dysfunctions may take the form of decreased libido, inability to achieve an erection, or delayed ejaculation. Many patients consider sexual function to be a very personal subject, so it must be handled in a sensitive manner. Some patients volunteer information about sexual changes; others may fail to relate the problem to their medications and not report it to the nurse or the physician. You can introduce the subject by saying, "Some people who take this medication have changes in sexual function. Has this been a problem for you?" If it is a problem for the patient, advise the physician so that an alternative medication or other intervention can be considered.

Pharmacology Capsule

Advise patients not to discontinue antihypertensive therapy simply because they feel well. Blood pressure (BP) can be very high with no symptoms.

Older Patients

Planning nursing care for older patients with hypertension requires additional considerations. Response to drug therapy is more difficult to predict and side effects are more common. Orthostatic hypotension and sedation are especially problematic for the older person, who is prone to fall and suffer serious injuries. Depression also must be taken very seriously because it lowers motivation, impairs quality of life, and can lead to suicide.

Health care providers tend to assume that older adults are not sexually active. Therefore they often fail to assess sexual function or dysfunction in older people. This is a real disservice to the older person whose sexual functioning is impaired as a result of antihypertensive drugs. The older patient should be treated just like a younger patient in the assessment and management of distressing drug effects.

HYPERTENSIVE CRISIS

Hypertensive crisis is a life-threatening medical emergency. The patient has severe headache, blurred vision, nausea, restlessness, and confusion. Along with a very elevated DBP (130 mm Hg or more), the heart and respiratory rates are increased. This episode may occur because the patient has decided to stop taking antihypertensive drugs or it may be caused by malignant hypertension, hypertensive encephalopathy, eclampsia, pheochromocytoma (adrenal tumor), or a CVA. Malignant hypertension is a specific type of hypertensive crisis in which the diastolic pressure exceeds 140 mm Hg. It has a sudden onset and is seen most often in African-American men aged 30 to 40 years.

Without appropriate treatment, the patient in hypertensive crisis may incur cardiac and renal damage. Death may ensue as a result of a CVA, renal failure, or cardiac failure.

Put on Your Thinking Cap!

Albert Smith, a 34-year-old African-American man, arrives at the emergency department complaining of severe headache and blurred vision. His blood pressure (BP) is 220/146 mm Hg. The physician diagnoses malignant hypertension. Mr. Smith is anxious and says that his father died of a stroke at age 39. Mr. Smith is a carpenter who reports no history of serious illness except thyroid deficiency. What is his primary risk factor for malignant hypertension?

MEDICAL DIAGNOSIS

Assessment in the emergency department reveals elevated BP, pulse, and respiratory rate. Retinal hemorrhage, papilledema, or both can be observed in the fundus (back, interior portion) of the eye.

The physician may order blood drawn for arterial blood gases (ABGs), complete blood count (CBC), electrolytes, blood urea nitrogen (BUN), creatinine, and cardiac enzymes. A chest radiograph may be requested. Direct BP monitoring through an arterial catheter is preferred.

MEDICAL TREATMENT

The goal of drug therapy is to rapidly reduce BP to a nonlife-threatening level and then to bring it slowly within normal range. This is done with diuretics and potent vasodilators. Drugs that may be ordered include fenoldopam, nitroglycerin, diazoxide, hydralazine, phentolamine, labetalol, and nitroprusside. An intravenous line is usually established because many drugs are given by that route. Oral options for the management of hypertensive crisis include captopril, clonidine, and nifedipine. Drugs used to treat hypertensive crisis are listed in Box 38-3.

NURSING CARE of the Patient in Hypertensive Crisis

Assessment

The patient in hypertensive crisis must be monitored closely. Frequently check the patient's BP, pulse,

Box 38-3 Emergency Antihypertensive Drugs

VASODILATORS
- sodium nitroprusside (Nipride)
- nitroglycerin
- fenoldopam (Corlopam)
- diazoxide (Hyperstat)*

CALCIUM CHANNEL BLOCKERS
- nicardipine (Cardene)

ADRENERGIC BLOCKERS
- labetalol (Normodyne)

ANGIOTENSIN-CONVERTING ENZYME INHIBITORS
- enalaprilat (Vasotec)
- captopril (Capoten)

From Lehne RA: *Pharmacology for nursing care*, ed 6, Philadelphia, 2007, Saunders.
*Obsolete when no intensive monitoring is available.

respiration, and level of consciousness. Some drugs are given in intravenous fluids, requiring continuous monitoring and adjustment. Maintain a careful record of fluid intake and output. Nausea and vomiting may indicate an impending seizure or coma.

Interventions

The nurse's role in caring for the patient in hypertensive crisis includes administering prescribed drugs, monitoring vital signs before and after each drug dose, monitoring cardiac and renal function, starting and maintaining intravenous therapy and O_2 as ordered, and comforting the patient.

Take appropriate safety measures if the patient shows signs of seizure activity or a decreasing level of consciousness. Bed side rails should be raised and padded if necessary, according to agency policy. Elevate the head of the bed to facilitate breathing and place an oral airway and suction equipment at the bedside. Offer brief explanations or words of encouragement to allay some of the patient's anxiety. Once the patient's condition improves, it is important to explain how to manage hypertension and prevent future crises from developing. !

Get Ready for the NCLEX® Examination!

Key Points

- Hypertension is called "the silent killer" because it often has no symptoms and is not discovered until a serious complication develops, such as damage to the blood vessels in the kidneys, eyes, heart, or brain.
- Hypertension is defined as a persistent elevation of arterial BP of 140/90 mm Hg or greater.
- Primary (essential) hypertension has no known cause whereas secondary hypertension is caused by an underlying factor such as kidney disease.
- The two factors that determine BP are CO and PVR.
- The primary risk factors for primary hypertension are dyslipidemia, obesity, atherosclerosis, use of tobacco, diabetes, sedentary lifestyle, age, and family history of early heart disease.
- BP tends to rise as people age but age is not a barrier to aggressive treatment of hypertension.
- Hypertension often has no symptoms but some people experience occipital headaches, lightheadedness, and epistaxis.
- A diagnosis of hypertension is usually based on multiple readings and is accompanied by tests to rule out possible correctable causes.
- Conservative measures to treat hypertension include weight reduction, smoking cessation, sodium restriction, exercise, relaxation techniques, and modified alcohol intake.
- Pharmacologic treatment is based on the stage of hypertension and presence of other factors such as kidney disease and HF.
- Types of drugs used to treat hypertension include diuretics, beta-adrenergic receptor blockers, calcium channel blockers, ACE inhibitors, angiotensin II receptor antagonists, central adrenergic blockers, alpha-adrenergic receptor blockers, and direct vasodilators.
- Ethnicity affects response to many antihypertensive drugs.
- Nursing care of the person with hypertension addresses ineffective self-health management, risk for injury, ineffective coping, and sexual dysfunction.
- Hypertensive crisis, defined as a DBP of 130 mm Hg or more, is a life-threatening medical emergency that is usually treated with diuretics and potent vasodilators.
- Complications of hypertensive crisis include stroke, HF, and kidney failure.

Additional Learning Resources

SG Go to your Study Guide for additional learning activities to help you master this chapter content.

evolve Go to your Evolve website (http://evolve.elsevier.com/Linton/medsurg) for the following learning resources and much more:
- Interactive Prioritization Exercises
- Fluid & Electrolyte Tutorial
- Pharmacology Tutorial
- Review Questions for the NCLEX® Examination

Review Questions for the NCLEX® Examination

1. Which of the following is a persistent BP of 144/99 mm Hg considered to be?
   1. Normal
   2. High normal
   3. Stage 1 hypertension
   4. Stage 2 hypertension

   NCLEX Client Need: Physiological Integrity: Reduction of Risk Potential
2. Which individuals are at greatest risk for severe complications of hypertension?
   1. Caucasian men
   2. Caucasian women
   3. African-American men
   4. African-American women

   NCLEX Client Need: Physiological Integrity: Reduction of Risk Potential
3. What is the cause of primary (essential) hypertension?

   NCLEX Client Need: Physiological Integrity: Physiological Adaptation
4. Complications associated with prolonged hypertension include which of the following? (Select all that apply.)
   1. Glaucoma
   2. Damage to heart valves
   3. Renal failure
   4. Heart attack
   5. Blindness

   NCLEX Client Need: Physiological Integrity: Reduction of Risk Potential
5. To detect hypokalemia in a patient who is taking hydrochlorothiazide, the nurse should monitor for which of the following? (Select all that apply.)
   1. Edema
   2. Confusion
   3. Irritability
   4. Irregular pulse
   5. Muscle weakness

   NCLEX Client Need: Physiological Integrity: Reduction of Risk Potential
6. Beta adrenergic blockers lower BP by which of the following?
   1. Eliminating excess body fluid
   2. Inhibiting cardiac stimulation
   3. Blocking the movement of calcium into myocardial cells
   4. Preventing the formation of angiotensin II

   NCLEX Client Need: Physiological Integrity: Pharmacological Therapies
7. The routine measurement of BP should include which of the following?
   1. Determine the systolic pressure first by auscultation and then by palpation
   2. Select a cuff with a bladder that encircles 50% of the circumference of the arm
   3. Position the patient's arm above the level of the heart
   4. Have the patient seated with the feet on the floor

   NCLEX Client Need: Physiological Integrity: Reduction of Risk Potential
8. A patient who takes antihypertensive drugs complains of feeling dizzy when first rising from a supine position. What should you advise the patient to do when this occurs?
   1. "Change positions slowly and exercise the legs before standing."
   2. "Discontinue all antihypertensive drugs immediately."
   3. "Go back to bed and call the physician."
   4. "Increase salt intake to bring BP up to normal."

   NCLEX Client Need: Physiological Integrity: Pharmacological Therapies
9. An 80-year-old patient who has been diagnosed with hypertension is not taking her prescribed medications. She says, "Wouldn't you expect my BP to be up a bit at my age?" Which of the following is the nurse's most appropriate reply?
   1. "BP tends to increase with age but treatment reduces the risk of complications regardless of your age."
   2. "As long as you are feeling well, it will not hurt for you to skip your medication."
   3. "High BP medications probably offer little benefit to someone your age."
   4. "Your physician is going to be pretty upset if you don't follow medical orders."

   NCLEX Client Need: Physiological Integrity: Reduction of Risk Potential
10. The DASH diet plan is low in which of the following? (Select all that apply.)
    1. Fat
    2. Poultry
    3. Potassium
    4. Red meat
    5. Dairy products

    NCLEX Client Need: Physiological Integrity: Reduction of Risk Potential

chapter 39

Upper Digestive Tract Disorders

Amanda Flagg

http://evolve.elsevier.com/Linton/medsurg

Objectives

1. Identify the nursing responsibilities in the care of patients who are undergoing diagnostic tests and procedures for disorders of the upper digestive tract.
2. List the data to be included in the nursing assessment of the patient with upper digestive tract disorders.
3. Describe the pathophysiology, signs and symptoms, complications, and treatment of selected upper digestive tract disorders.
4. Assist in developing nursing care plans for patients receiving treatment for upper digestive tract disorders.

Key Terms

Anorexia (ăn-ŏ-RĔK-sē-ă)
Dysphagia (dĭs-FĀ-jē-ă)
Emesis (ĔM-ĕ-sĭs)
Eructation (ĕ-rŭk-TĀ-shŭn)
Gingivitis (jĭn-jĭ-VĪ-tĭs)
Peritoneum (pĕ-rĭ-tō-NĒ-ŭm)
Peristalsis
Peritonitis (pĕ-rĭ-tō-NĪ-tĭs)
Regurgitation (rē-gŭr-jĭ-TĀ-shŭn)
Stomatitis (stō-mă-TĪ-tĭs)

To remain healthy, the human body must have a steady supply of nutrients and fluids. The primary role of the digestive tract is to extract the molecules essential for cellular function from food and fluids. Disorders of the upper digestive tract can threaten the patient's nutritional status, leading to disorders in the structure and functioning of other body systems.

ANATOMY AND PHYSIOLOGY OF THE UPPER DIGESTIVE TRACT

The digestive tract is also called the gastrointestinal (GI) tract and the alimentary tract (Fig 39-1). It is a muscular tube about 30 feet long. The main parts of the digestive tract are the mouth, pharynx, esophagus, stomach, small intestine, large intestine, and anus. Other organs that are outside the digestive tract but considered part of the digestive system are called accessory organs. Accessory organs include the salivary glands, liver, gallbladder, and pancreas. Each of these organs secretes fluid containing specialized enzymes into the digestive tract. These enzymes play a part in the breakdown or metabolism of foodstuffs. A two-layer membrane, the **peritoneum**, lines the abdominal cavity and covers the surfaces of the abdominal organs. Lubricating fluid between the two layers permits the organs to move without friction during breathing and digestive movements.

The functions of the digestive tract are ingestion, digestion, absorption of nutrients, and elimination of wastes. Digestion is the breakdown of food into simple nutrient molecules that can be used by the cells. The process of digestion requires (1) the adequate intake of food and fluids, (2) the mechanical and chemical breakdown of food, and (3) the movement of food through the digestive tract.

The upper digestive tract, addressed in this chapter, comprises the mouth, pharynx, esophagus, and stomach. The lower digestive tract is addressed in Chapter 40.

MOUTH

Food is ingested into the mouth, where the teeth, tongue, and salivary glands begin the process of food digestion. As the teeth cut and grind the food, the salivary glands secrete saliva—a watery solution that contains amylase (ptyalin). Amylase is an enzyme that initiates the breakdown of carbohydrates. The tongue helps by mixing saliva with the food and pressing it against the teeth. When the bolus is swallowed, the tongue forces the food into the pharynx.

PHARYNX

The pharynx is a muscular structure that is shared by the digestive and respiratory tracts. It joins the mouth and nasal passages to the esophagus. During

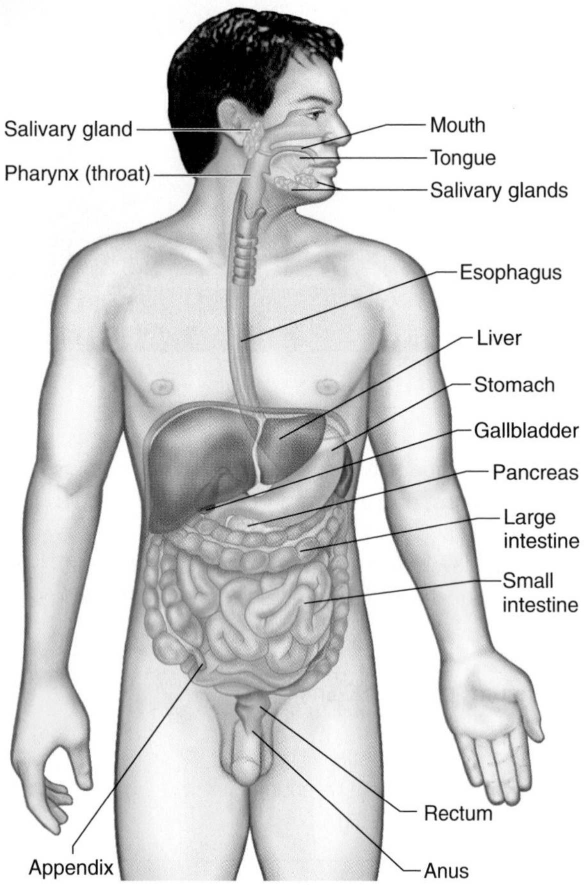

FIGURE 39-1 The digestive tract and associated structures. (From Thibodeau GA, Patton KT: *The human body in health and disease*, ed 6, St. Louis, 2014, Mosby.)

swallowing, the epiglottis covers the airway like a trapdoor to prevent food from entering the respiratory tract.

ESOPHAGUS

Food moves from the pharynx into the esophagus, a long muscular tube that passes through the diaphragm into the stomach. Gravity helps but is not essential for the movement of food through the esophagus. Circular, wavelike contractions of the muscles of the digestive tract propel food down the tract. This movement is called **peristalsis**.

STOMACH

The stomach is the widest section of the digestive tract. The stomach is not very large when empty but it expands considerably when food is present. It consists of three sections: (1) the fundus, (2) the body, and (3) the pylorus. A unique arrangement of muscle layers allows the stomach to churn the food, mixing it with gastric secretions until it becomes a semiliquid mass called chyme. Gastric secretions include rennin, pepsin, hydrochloric acid, and lipase. Rennin starts to break down milk proteins, lipase breaks down fats, and pepsin and hydrochloric acid partially digest proteins. The pyloric sphincter between the stomach and the small intestine keeps food in the stomach until it is properly mixed.

AGE-RELATED CHANGES

Normal aging generally does not significantly impair ingestion, digestion, absorption, or elimination. However, when acute or chronic illnesses occur, the older person is at increased risk for problems with digestion and elimination.

The teeth are mechanically worn down with age. They appear darker and somewhat transparent. The gingiva (gum) tends to recede. Although tooth loss is not a normal effect of aging, about 40% of all Americans ages 65 years and older are edentulous (toothless). The main reasons for tooth loss are caries and periodontal disease. Many older people have complete or partial dentures. The jaw may be affected by osteoarthritis. A significant loss of taste buds occurs with age. The older person may be able to detect sweet better than other tastes. Xerostomia (dry mouth) is common but may be caused more by poor hydration and drug side effects than by aging.

The walls of the esophagus and stomach become thinner with aging and secretions lessen. The lower esophageal sphincter that normally prevents the reflux of gastric contents is more relaxed. The production of hydrochloric acid and digestive enzymes decreases. Gastric motor activity slows; thus gastric emptying is delayed and hunger contractions diminish. No significant changes with age occur in the small intestine. The absorption of vitamin A may increase whereas the absorption of vitamin D, calcium, and zinc may be reduced. In the large intestine, the muscle layer and mucosa atrophy. Smooth muscle tone and blood flow decrease and connective tissue increases.

NURSING ASSESSMENT OF THE UPPER DIGESTIVE TRACT

HEALTH HISTORY

Chief Complaint and History of Present Illness

Although the registered nurse (RN) should perform the complete assessment, the licensed vocational nurse/licensed practical nurse (LVN/LPN) contributes to the database. The health history begins with a detailed description of the current complaints or symptoms. These symptoms or complaints may include weight changes, problems with food ingestion, descriptions of digestive disturbances such as vomiting or heartburn, or changes in bowel elimination. Past medical history may disclose recent surgery, trauma, burns, or infections. Note serious illnesses such as diabetes, hepatitis, anemia, peptic ulcers, gallbladder disease, Crohn disease, ulcerative colitis, liver dysfunction, and cancer. Identify any alternative methods of feeding or fecal diversion such as ileostomy or colostomy. Document any food allergy or intolerance, with a description of the reaction.

Pharmacology Capsule

Many drugs affect gastrointestinal (GI) function, causing anorexia, nausea, vomiting, and diarrhea or constipation.

Functional Assessment

The functional assessment focuses on nutrition, activity, and stressors. Information about general dietary habits should include the daily pattern of food intake (mealtimes, food eaten in a typical day, food likes and dislikes, and use of food supplements), attitudes and beliefs about food, and changes in dietary habits related to health problems. Describe the effects of the chief complaint on usual functioning and note whether the patient is able to obtain and prepare food and eat without difficulty.

PHYSICAL EXAMINATION

Begin the physical examination with the measurement of the patient's height, weight, and vital signs. Observe the patient's general appearance, noting skin color, texture, and turgor; posture; motor activity; and responses to instructions.

Head and Neck

Inspection of the mouth determines the condition of the lips, teeth, gums, tongue, and mucous membranes. Describe caries, moisture, color, and lesions and note any unpleasant or unusual odors of the mouth. If the patient has dentures, examine the mouth with and without the dentures in place. Assessment of the upper digestive tract is summarized in Box 39-1. Assessment of the lower digestive tract is detailed in Chapter 40.

Box 39-1 Assessment of the Patient with a Disorder of the Upper Digestive Tract

HEALTH HISTORY

Present Illness

Weight changes, problems with food ingestion, symptoms of digestive disturbances, changes in bowel elimination

Past Medical History

Recent surgery, trauma, infections, History of diabetes mellitus, hepatitis, anemia, peptic ulcer, gallbladder disease, cancer. Alternative methods of feeding: type, amount, schedule. Fecal diversion: type. Allergies: food, drugs.

Family History

Diabetes mellitus, cancer of the digestive tract, peptic ulcer disease, gallbladder disease, hepatitis, alcoholism, intestinal polyps, obesity

Review of Systems

General Health State: change in weight

Skin: color, pruritus

Oral Cavity: presence and condition of teeth, condition of gums, moisture, pain, abnormal tastes or odors, difficulty chewing

Appetite

Dysphagia

Digestive Disturbances: nausea, vomiting, dyspepsia, heartburn, pain, flatulence (gas), change in stool characteristics (frequency, amount, color, consistency, abnormal contents including blood and undigested food), painful defecation

Functional Assessment: dietary pattern, attitudes and beliefs about food, activity, stressors

PHYSICAL EXAMINATION

Height and weight, vital signs, general appearance, head and neck (condition of teeth, gums, tongue, mucous membranes, odors, uvula position).

DIAGNOSTIC TESTS AND PROCEDURES

ENDOSCOPIC EXAMINATION

Traditional endoscopic examinations permit direct inspection of hollow, interior organs through a lighted tube called an endoscope. Endoscopes may be rigid tubes or flexible fiberscopes. Endoscopic examinations of the upper gastrointestinal tract (UGI) include esophagoscopy, gastroscopy, gastroduodenoscopy, esophagogastroduodenoscopy, and endoscopic retrograde cholangiography.

Signed consent may be required before endoscopic examinations. Patients usually are not permitted food or fluids for 6 to 8 hours before the examination. A sedative may be ordered before the procedure to reduce anxiety. The most serious complication of endoscopy is perforation or puncture of the digestive tract.

An innovation in endoscopy uses a disposable video camera capsule that is about the size of a large vitamin tablet. The patient swallows the capsule. Leads are applied to the abdomen and connected to a recording device worn on a belt. Images are transmitted as the capsule moves through the digestive tract. The patient can go about usual activities while the capsule is in transit. It is especially useful for visualizing the small intestine, which is not accessible with traditional endoscopy. Patients fast overnight before swallowing the capsule. Bowel preparation may or may not be required, depending on institutional practice.

RADIOGRAPHIC STUDIES

The upper gastrointestinal (UGI or GI) series allows the radiologist to study the structure and function of the esophagus, stomach, and duodenum. This procedure includes esophagography, commonly called a barium swallow. Fluoroscopy and x-ray films outlines the upper digestive structures during and after the patient drinks a radiopaque barium solution. Preparation for the test includes fasting from food for 8 hours and from liquids for 4 hours before the test. Most drugs are withheld for 8 hours before the test as well. It is especially important to withhold drugs such as opioids and anticholinergics that affect intestinal motility. A laxative is given after the procedures to promote elimination of the barium. The barium causes stools to be white or gray until all is eliminated.

LABORATORY STUDIES

The most common laboratory studies related to the upper digestive tract are performed on blood and urine. Tests to detect *Helicobacter pylori* include analysis of the breath, urine, serum, stool, and gastric biopsy tissue. Studies that may be done to assess nutritional status include serum albumin, total lymphocyte count, urine creatinine/height index, mean corpuscular volume (MCV), and transferrin saturation. See Chapter 9 for details of the nutritional assessment.

Additional information about upper digestive tract diagnostic procedures is presented in Table 39-1.

COMMON THERAPEUTIC MEASURES

GASTROINTESTINAL INTUBATION

Tubes are inserted most often into the stomach or intestines to deliver feedings or to keep the digestive tract empty (decompression). Tubes that are passed through the nose are called nasogastric, nasoduodenal, or nasoenteric tubes, depending on whether the end is located in the stomach or the small intestine.

A variety of tubes exist for special purposes (Fig. 39-2). Nasogastric tubes such as the Levin and Salem sump tubes may be used for decompression. Nasoenteric tubes used for decompression of the small intestine include the Miller-Abbott, Cantor, and Harris tubes.

The Sengstaken-Blakemore esophageal-gastric balloon tube is a special tube used to control bleeding in the esophagus. It is generally used in patients with severe complications of liver disease and is therefore discussed in Chapter 41.

Gastrostomy tubes, used for feedings, are placed in the stomach through an opening (stoma) in the abdominal wall (Fig. 39-3). Levin and Dobhoff tubes are used for enteral feedings. The Dobhoff is a small nasoduodenal tube that is weighted so it passes through the stomach into the duodenum.

Care of the patient with tubes for feeding or decompression is discussed separately.

Tube Feedings

Patients who are unable to eat or swallow normally may have feeding tubes inserted. Once the tube is in place, exact feeding orders are written. Feedings may be delivered by gravity flow or by infusion pump. Without a pump, a syringe barrel or a packaged delivery set is used to put the feeding into the tube. Regardless of the method used, several key points must be remembered about this procedure.

1. It is critical to confirm that the tube is in the stomach or the duodenum before administering feedings. Radiographic confirmation is the most reliable method. Various other methods of checking placement have been used. Currently, observation of aspirated material and assessment of pH are thought to be the most reliable. Stomach contents are grassy green, clear and colorless, or brown; they normally have a pH of 5 or less. The intestinal pH is normally 6 or higher. Other measures that are being evaluated are checking the aspirated fluid for enzymes and bilirubin. Methods that lack scientific support are listening over the stomach area with a stethoscope while injecting air through the tube, placing the end of the tube in water to see if bubbles appear, testing the patient's ability to speak, and observing for respiratory symptoms. When a patient has continuous feedings, placement is usually checked at least once each shift.
2. Assist the patient into the Fowler position to reduce the chance of aspiration (regurgitation and passage of fluids into the respiratory tract). Keep the head and chest elevated for about 30 minutes after the feeding is completed.
3. Residual is monitored to help prevent overfilling of the stomach. Check for residual (formula remaining in the stomach from the previous feeding) before each feeding or according to agency procedure. Use a syringe to withdraw and measure the formula. Agency policy dictates what action should be taken based on the amount of residual formula. The RN or physician may need to be notified. The amount of the residual may be subtracted from the next feeding or feedings may be discontinued for a specified period of time. The residual formula should be returned through the tube to prevent loss of electrolytes.
4. Obtain the correct formula. In the hospital setting, feedings are commercially prepared. Many varieties of formulas exist. Be sure to give the right formula, in the right amount, at the right dilution, on the right schedule, to the right patient.
5. When tube feedings are first started, they often are diluted to one-half or one-fourth strength. If the patient tolerates the formula well, the concentration is gradually increased.
6. Stop the feeding and notify the health care provider if the patient has nausea or pain.
7. Rinse the tube by flushing it with at least 30 mL of water after each bolus feeding. Extra water may be ordered by the health care provider.
8. If diarrhea occurs, contact the health care provider regarding decreasing the concentration or the rate of delivery, or both, of the formula.
9. Dumping syndrome may occur with rapid feedings of concentrated formula. Signs and symptoms are cold sweat, abdominal distention, dizziness, weakness, rapid pulse rate, nausea, and diarrhea.

Table 39-1 Diagnostic Tests and Procedures **The Digestive Tract**

TEST AND PURPOSE	PATIENT PREPARATION	POSTPROCEDURE NURSING CARE
Radiographic Tests		
Upper gastrointestinal (UGI) or gastrointestinal (GI) series: Barium swallow detects abnormalities of esophagus and stomach.	Inform the patient that he or she will need to drink a solution containing contrast medium. Radiographs will be taken of the esophagus, stomach, and duodenum via fluoroscope. Films will be repeated 6 hours later to see how much barium has passed through the stomach. The patient should take nothing by mouth (NPO) 6–8 hours before the procedure, per agency protocol. Patient allergies should be noted prior to the procedure.	Monitor stools for at least 2 days for passage of white stools that show that barium is being eliminated (normal stool color returns in 3 days). Laxatives may be ordered to promote elimination. Provide food, extra fluids, and rest.
Small bowel series detects abnormalities of the small intestine.	The patient drinks a contrast solution. Films are taken at 20- to 30-minute intervals as the solution passes through the small intestine. The patient will be asked to assume various positions for the radiographs. The procedure may take several hours. Preparation is the same as for the UGI series.	Care is the same as for the UGI series.
Barium enema detects abnormalities of the large intestine.	A contrast solution is administered by enema and radiographs are taken with the patient in a variety of positions. The test may take as long as 1¼ hours to complete. The patient may be restricted to only clear liquids the day or evening before the procedure. A laxative and enemas are given on the previous day. Usually the patient is NPO after midnight. Enemas are given until the intestine is clear on the morning of the procedure.	Care is the same as for the UGI series.
Endoscopic Tests		
Upper Digestive Tract Esophagoscopy visualizes the esophagus. Gastroscopy visualizes the stomach. Gastroduodenoscopy visualizes the stomach and duodenum. Esophagogastroduodenoscopy visualizes the esophagus, stomach, and duodenum. Endoscopic retrograde cholangiography visualizes the bile ducts and gallbladder.	Upper digestive tract examinations include the following patient preparations: NPO for 6–8 hours. If ordered, give the patient a sedative shortly before the examination.	The patient should be NPO until the gag reflex returns. Monitor the patient for signs of trauma: bleeding from the throat or rectum. Monitor the patient for signs of perforation: fever, abdominal distention, cramping pain, and vague discomfort.
Capsule Endoscopy Capsule endoscopy transmits video images of the entire digestive tract to a recorder worn on a waistband. It is especially useful for the study of the small intestine and may detect obscure GI bleeding, inflammatory bowel disease (IBD), small bowel tumors, malabsorption disorders, and inflammation caused by nonsteroidal antiinflammatory drugs (NSAIDs) or radiotherapy.	A 10-hour overnight fast is required for the small bowel study. Bowel preparation, if any, varies with the agency and health care provider. Study of the esophagus requires a 2-hour fast. Simethicone may be given when the capsule is swallowed to reduce bubbles and improve visualization.	The capsule normally is eliminated painlessly in the stool. No special care is required. If the small intestine is obstructed, the capsule can become lodged at the site, requiring surgical removal. The patient returns to the office in 6–10 hours to turn in the recorder.

Continued

Table 39-1 Diagnostic Tests and Procedures The Digestive Tract—cont'd

TEST AND PURPOSE	PATIENT PREPARATION	POSTPROCEDURE NURSING CARE
Laboratory Tests		
Blood Tests		
Serum electrolytes measure electrolytes in the blood to detect imbalances.	Medications that affect results may be held until blood is drawn.	Resume medications after blood is drawn.
Serum protein electrophoresis measures serum protein, which may be decreased with peptic ulcers, acute cholecystitis, and malabsorption.	Medications that can alter test results (aspirin, isoniazid, neomycin, bicarbonate, sulfonamides) may be withheld until the blood sample is drawn.	Resume medications after blood is drawn.
Carcinoembryonic antigen (CEA) measures CEA in the blood that may indicate GI malignancy, although the test is not specific. This test is also used to monitor the patient's response to cancer therapy.	No special preparation is required. Note whether the patient smokes; if yes, he or she will most likely test positive for CEA.	No special care is required.
Esophageal Function Tests		
Esophageal pH monitoring is used to detect acid reflux. Manometry measures lower esophageal sphincter (LES) pressure and assesses esophageal swallowing waves. For the Bernstein test, hydrochloric acid and normal saline are alternately instilled in the esophagus to see if the patient experiences pain with the acid.	The patient should be NPO for 8 hours before the test. The procedure takes about 30 minutes. Tell the patient that it will be necessary to swallow several small tubes that will measure the pressure in the esophagus and record esophageal waves during swallowing. In some situations, the pH sensor is left in place for 24 hours.	No special aftercare is required. The patient may have a mild sore throat.
Stool Analysis		
Stool occult blood detects GI bleeding when blood is not readily seen.	Advise the patient of the need to obtain a stool specimen (see guidelines for specimen collection procedure in Chapter 40). If the test is done at home, explain the procedure.	No special care is required.
Stool ova and parasites detect parasitic infections.	Preparations are the same as for the stool occult blood test.	No special care is required.
Fecal fat tests for increased fat in stools that occurs with Crohn disease, malabsorption, and pancreatic disease.	Instruct the patient in how to observe a 60-g fat diet for 3–6 days, followed by collection of a stool specimen. No laxatives, enemas, or suppositories may be used for 3 days before the test. (See Chapter 40 for guidelines for specimen collection procedure.)	Tell the patient to resume a normal diet.

10. If using a syringe to give the feeding, do the following:
    - Remove the plunger from the barrel of the syringe.
    - Attach the barrel to the feeding tube.
    - Pinch or kink the tube while the syringe barrel is filled with formula to reduce the amount of air being forced into the stomach.
    - Hold the barrel about 12 inches above the level of the stomach and allow the fluid to flow by gravity.
    - Flush tubing with water per agency protocol.
11. If an infusion pump is used to deliver the feeding, fill the tubing with formula before connecting it to the feeding tube to reduce the amount of air forced into the digestive tract. Continuous feedings are usually given at a rate of 80 to 150 mL per hour. Bolus feedings are given at specified intervals. They usually consist of 200 to 300 mL over 30 to 45 minutes for each feeding. Oral drugs usually can be given through a nasogastric tube but some drugs should not be crushed. Prior to administering any medication, consult a drug reference. The tubing and bag must be changed every 24 hours.

Gastrointestinal Decompression

GI decompression is used for the relief or prevention of distention. A tube is passed through a nostril and into the stomach or intestines (or both) and attached

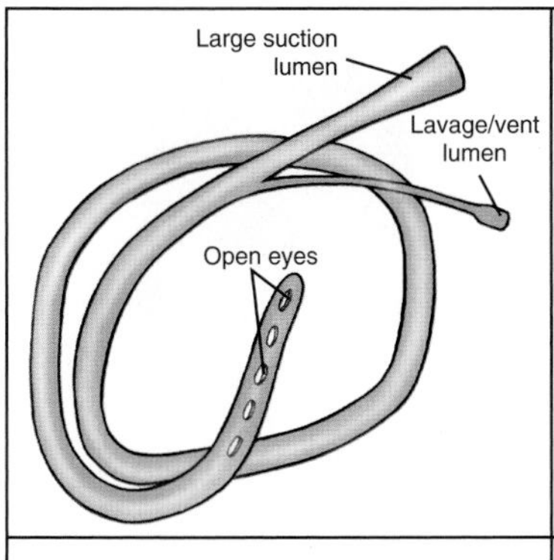

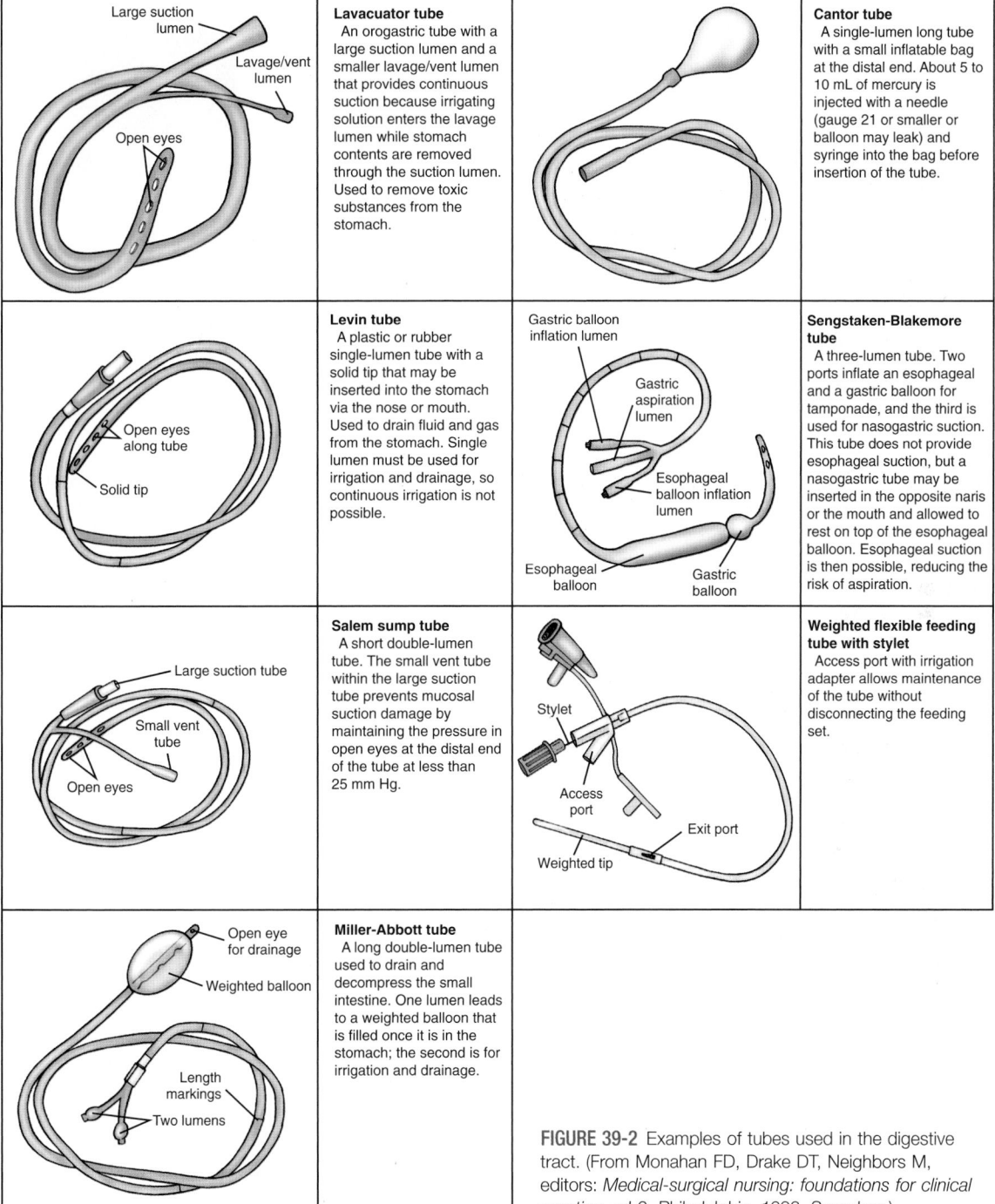

Lavacuator tube
An orogastric tube with a large suction lumen and a smaller lavage/vent lumen that provides continuous suction because irrigating solution enters the lavage lumen while stomach contents are removed through the suction lumen. Used to remove toxic substances from the stomach.

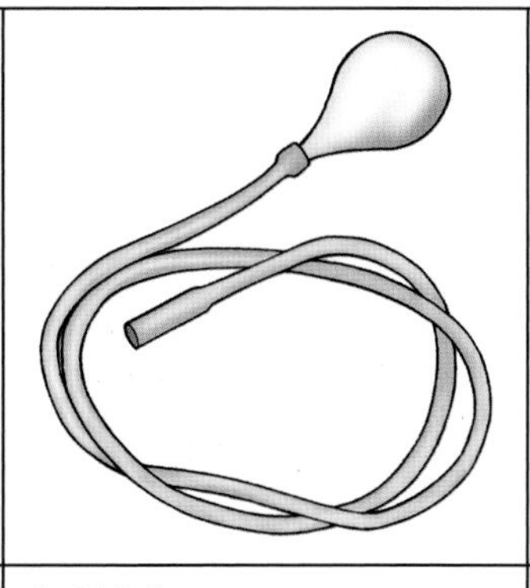

Cantor tube
A single-lumen long tube with a small inflatable bag at the distal end. About 5 to 10 mL of mercury is injected with a needle (gauge 21 or smaller or balloon may leak) and syringe into the bag before insertion of the tube.

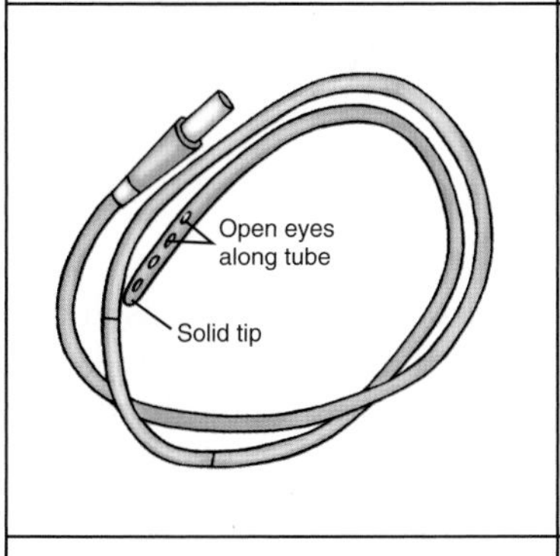

Levin tube
A plastic or rubber single-lumen tube with a solid tip that may be inserted into the stomach via the nose or mouth. Used to drain fluid and gas from the stomach. Single lumen must be used for irrigation and drainage, so continuous irrigation is not possible.

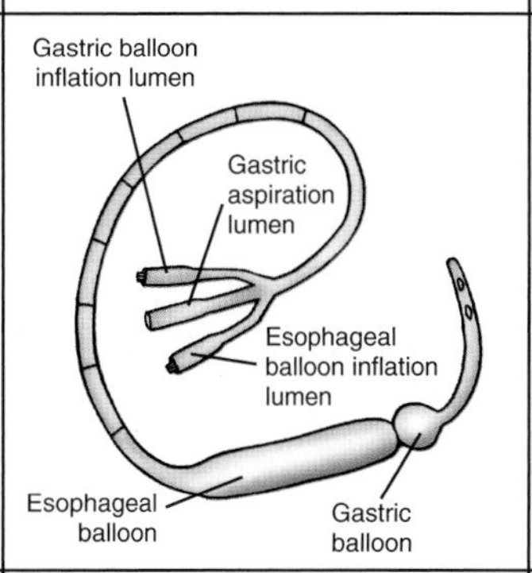

Sengstaken-Blakemore tube
A three-lumen tube. Two ports inflate an esophageal and a gastric balloon for tamponade, and the third is used for nasogastric suction. This tube does not provide esophageal suction, but a nasogastric tube may be inserted in the opposite naris or the mouth and allowed to rest on top of the esophageal balloon. Esophageal suction is then possible, reducing the risk of aspiration.

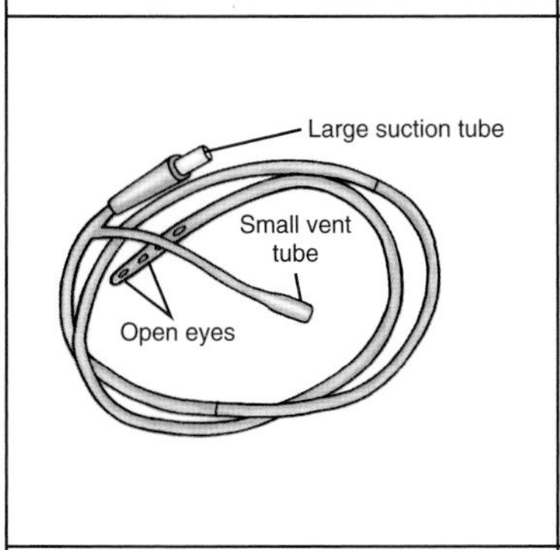

Salem sump tube
A short double-lumen tube. The small vent tube within the large suction tube prevents mucosal suction damage by maintaining the pressure in open eyes at the distal end of the tube at less than 25 mm Hg.

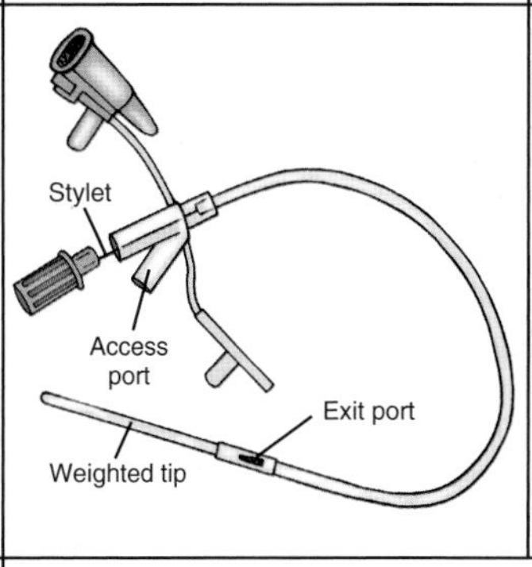

Weighted flexible feeding tube with stylet
Access port with irrigation adapter allows maintenance of the tube without disconnecting the feeding set.

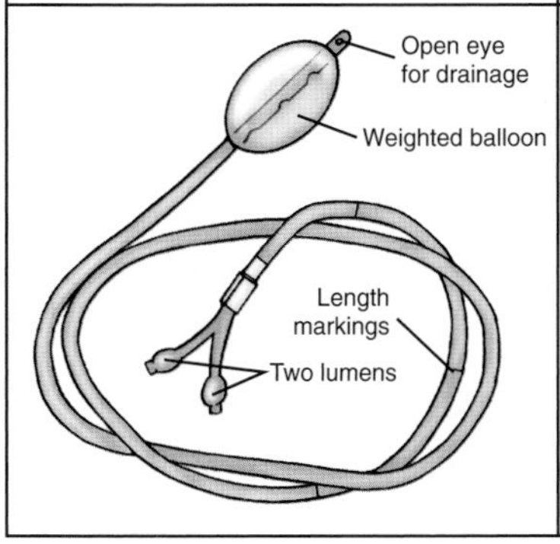

Miller-Abbott tube
A long double-lumen tube used to drain and decompress the small intestine. One lumen leads to a weighted balloon that is filled once it is in the stomach; the second is for irrigation and drainage.

FIGURE 39-2 Examples of tubes used in the digestive tract. (From Monahan FD, Drake DT, Neighbors M, editors: *Medical-surgical nursing: foundations for clinical practice,* ed 2, Philadelphia, 1998, Saunders.)

to suction. The suction removes fluid and gases that accumulate when GI motility is impaired or when a patient is intubated for respiratory failure. Conditions that slow motility include peritonitis, obstruction, and any type of surgery performed while the patient is under general anesthesia. Handling of the bowel during abdominal surgery often causes a temporary loss of peristalsis. Decompression may be ordered until bowel activity returns, usually in 3 to 5 days. The following are key points to remember when caring for the patient with GI suction:

1. Attach the tube to a suction apparatus as ordered.
2. Monitor the patency of the tube. Observe for the movement of fluids through the tubing into the suction container. If the tube does not seem to be draining, change the patient's position. Gently rotate the tube or pull it out very slightly. (Exception: Do not reposition tubes after gastric surgery.) Notify the health care provider if drainage does not resume.

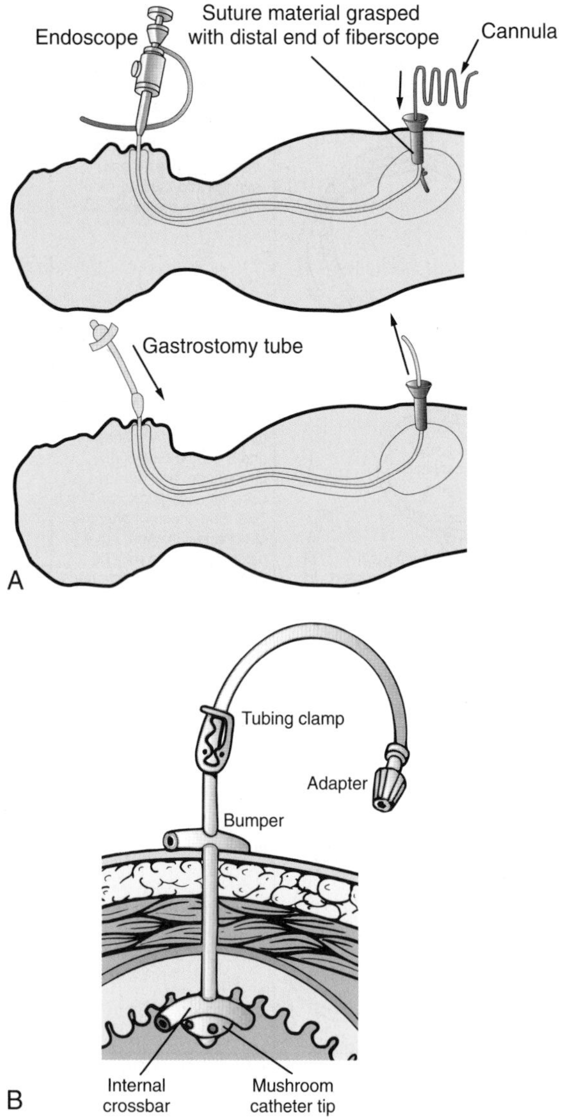

FIGURE 39-3 Percutaneous endoscopic gastrostomy (PEG). **A,** Placement of PEG tube. Using endoscopy, a gastrostomy tube is inserted through the esophagus into the stomach. A cannula is inserted through the abdominal wall into the stomach. The fiberscope grasps the cannula and the cannula and tube are pulled out through the abdominal wall. **B,** A retention disk and bumper keep the tube in place. (From Lewis SM, Heitkemper MM, Dirksen SR, et al: *Medical-surgical nursing: assessment and management of clinical problems*, ed 8, St. Louis, 2011, Mosby.)

3. Irrigations should not be done routinely but they may be ordered occasionally as needed. Frequent irrigations cause acid-base disturbances. For adults, irrigations are usually done with 20 to 30 mL of normal saline. Check the health care provider's order or the agency's procedure manual.
4. Monitor the suction output. Record the amount, color, and characteristics every shift. Monitor the patient for successful decompression. If distention is not being relieved effectively, the patient may have nausea and vomiting, shortness of breath, a feeling of fullness, and enlargement of the abdomen.

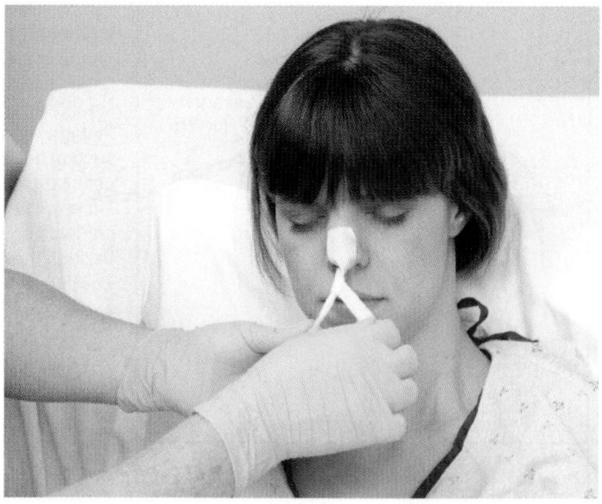

FIGURE 39-4 This method of taping a nasogastric tube anchors it securely while avoiding trauma to the nose. (From Potter PA, Perry AG, editors: *Fundamentals of nursing*, ed 8, St. Louis, 2013, Mosby.)

5. Assess for the return of peristalsis, indicated by the presence of bowel sounds and passage of flatus (gas) and stool through the rectum.
6. Provide comfort measures. The nasopharynx and throat are often very tender. Because the patient is placed on NPO (nothing by mouth) status, mouth dryness is another source of discomfort. Handle the tubing gently. Cleanse the nostrils and apply a water-soluble lubricant to reduce drying and irritation. Provide mouth care frequently. Moisturize the lips. Offer oral spray or lozenges as ordered to provide temporary relief of sore throat.
7. Once the tube is in place, tape it securely to the nose to prevent it from being pulled out. Tape should secure the tube to the upper lip and cheek or nose (Fig. 39-4). Do not tape the tubing to the forehead because this puts excessive pressure on the nasal tissues. During activity, move the tube carefully to avoid trauma to the nasopharynx. Wrapping the tube with a piece of tape that is pinned to the patient's gown may prevent accidental traction on the tube.

TOTAL PARENTERAL NUTRITION

Sometimes the digestive tract cannot be used for feedings. Total parenteral nutrition (TPN) bypasses the digestive tract by delivering nutrients directly to the bloodstream. A catheter such as a central venous catheter (Fig. 39-5) or peripherally inserted central catheter (PICC) is inserted into a large vein and is used for the feedings. The feeding passes directly into the superior vena cava and the right atrium (RA). This placement allows for rapid dilution of the concentrated feeding. The solution is never administered into a smaller vein because it would cause thrombophlebitis (inflammation of the vein).

When the catheter is inserted, it is sutured to the skin and the insertion site is covered with a sterile dressing. A radiograph is ordered to check placement before the catheter is used for feedings.

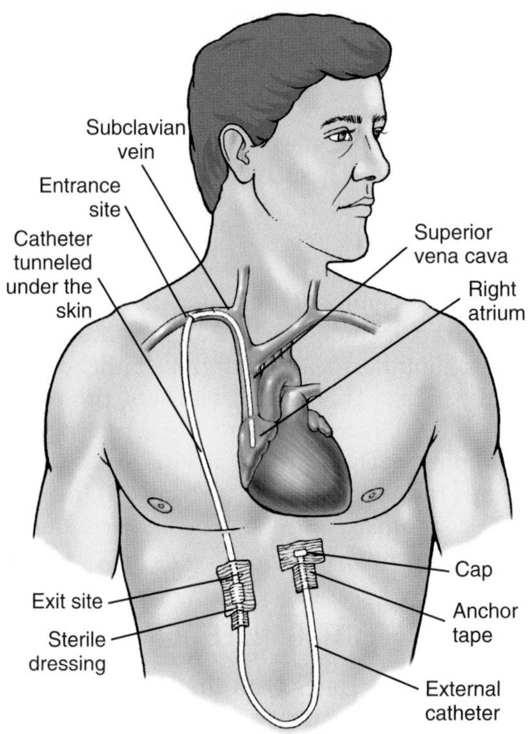

FIGURE 39-5 A catheter inserted into the right subclavian vein for total parenteral nutrition (TPN). A transparent waterproof dressing allows vapor to escape while maintaining sterility. (From Monahan FD, Drake DT, Neighbors M, editors: *Medical-surgical nursing: foundations for clinical practice*, ed 2, Philadelphia, 1998, Saunders.)

Regular intravenous feedings can provide only water, glucose, electrolytes, minerals, and vitamins. This is adequate for short-term problems but does not provide all of the nutrients necessary to maintain health or promote healing.

Two types of solutions are used for TPN therapy. The first is a concentrated solution of glucose, amino acids, vitamins, and minerals. It is administered using a special filter. A lipid solution also can be given through a peripheral vein. The lipids are not mixed with the TPN solution.

Important points to remember when caring for the patient receiving TPN include the following:

1. Take great care to prevent infection at the insertion site. Always use sterile technique for site care. The exact procedure should be ordered or written in the agency's procedure manual. With each dressing change, inspect the site for signs of infection (redness, swelling, foul odor, or purulent drainage). Monitor the patient's temperature for elevation.
2. Monitor the flow rate. If the solution is given too rapidly, the patient may have circulatory overload, changes in blood glucose, or excessive diuresis (urine output). If the feeding falls behind schedule, do not speed up the rate to catch up.
3. Monitor the patient for signs and symptoms of blood glucose changes. The concentrated glucose solution can raise the blood glucose excessively (hyperglycemia). Elevated glucose stimulates the pancreas to produce more insulin, which may then cause a drop in blood glucose (hypoglycemia). Blood should be monitored to detect abnormal glucose levels.
4. Label TPN lines and *never* use the TPN catheter to administer drugs.
5. Be sure that all staff who give medications differentiate TPN lines from small-bore enteral feeding tubes. Patient deaths have occurred as a result of oral medications being administered through a TPN line. !

Pharmacology Capsule

Never use a total parenteral nutrition (TPN) line to administer drugs.

GASTROINTESTINAL SURGERY

Conditions of the large intestine that may require surgery include cancer, diverticulosis, appendicitis, polyps, obstruction, and ulcerative colitis. General care of the surgical patient is discussed in Chapter 17.

PREOPERATIVE NURSING CARE of the Patient Having Gastrointestinal Surgery

Radiographic examinations of the digestive tract often are done before surgery. These may be done on an outpatient basis or after admission to the hospital. The digestive tract is usually cleansed before GI surgery. The extent of the cleansing depends on the exact site of the surgery. Oral preparations such as magnesium citrate or large-volume **cathartic** (laxative) solutions may be prescribed. Use of enemas until the returning fluid is clear also may be ordered. This process is tiring and may exhaust the very ill or older patient. The nurse should offer assistance with toileting and hygiene. Changes in vital signs (abnormal heart rate or rhythm, hypotension) or mental state during the bowel cleansing process should be reported to the health care provider.

Diet is usually limited to liquids for 24 hours before the surgery. The patient should have nothing to eat or drink for a specified period before surgery. Intravenous fluids may be ordered, especially if GI suction is being used. Oral antibiotics may be given to reduce the bacterial flora in the bowel, thereby decreasing the risk of contamination of the peritoneal cavity during surgery.

General anesthesia and abdominal surgery cause a temporary loss of peristalsis. Therefore, before or during surgery, a nasogastric tube may be inserted and attached to suction. This prevents the accumulation of fluid and gas in the digestive tract until peristalsis returns.

POSTOPERATIVE NURSING CARE of the Patient Who Has Had Gastrointestinal Surgery

Usual postoperative care, discussed in Chapter 17, includes measures to relieve pain; detect complications (hemorrhage, infection); and prevent adverse effects of immobility, anesthesia, and drug therapy. Immediately after surgery on the digestive tract, be especially concerned with preventing gastric or abdominal distention, replacing lost fluids, and maintaining urine elimination. The patient usually has a nasogastric tube in place for decompression. The intermittent removal of fluids and gas decreases the stimulation of the digestive tract and reduces pressure on the internal incisions. It is important to monitor GI suction to be sure it is functioning. Inspect, describe, and measure the drainage. Inspect and auscultate the abdomen for distention and bowel sounds. Follow the health care provider's orders regarding irrigation. After gastric surgery, do not irrigate or reposition the tube because of the possibility of traumatizing healing tissue. Notify the registered nurse (RN) or health care provider if the tube is not draining properly or if the abdomen becomes distended.

Intravenous fluids are given until GI suction is discontinued and oral intake is adequate. Maintain strict intake and output records. The patient is at risk for fluid and electrolyte imbalances when GI suction is used. Because patients often have difficulty voiding after abdominal surgery, an indwelling catheter is usually inserted during the procedure. If no catheter is present, nursing measures may be needed to promote voiding. These measures are discussed in Chapter 42.

DRUG THERAPY

Drugs that are commonly used for their effects on the digestive tract include emetics, antiemetics, laxatives, cathartics, antidiarrheals, antacids, anticholinergics, mucosal barriers, H2 receptor blockers, proton pump inhibitors, 5-HT receptor antagonists, prostaglandins, and antibiotics. These drugs are discussed with the conditions for which they are prescribed. In addition, Table 39-2 summarizes these drugs, their actions, and nursing interventions.

DISORDERS AFFECTING INGESTION

Anything that interferes with the ability to eat a balanced diet can cause nutritional deficiencies. Problems can be as basic as anorexia, inability to feed oneself, or dysphagia or they may occur secondary to other problems such as oral infection and inflammation, dental problems, oral cancer, and parotitis (inflammation of the parotid glands, as in mumps).

Table 39-2 Drug Therapy: Disorders of the Digestive Tract

DRUG	USE AND ACTION	SIDE EFFECTS	NURSING INTERVENTIONS
Antacids			
magnesium hydroxide, aluminum hydroxide, calcium carbonate, sodium bicarbonate	Used to reduce pain of peptic ulcers by neutralizing acid in the stomach, decreasing irritation of the stomach lining, and inhibiting production of pepsin.	Calcium and aluminum salts tend to cause constipation. Magnesium salts tend to cause diarrhea. Combinations may be used to neutralize these effects.	Teach patients that antacids are nonprescription drugs but still have side effects, interact with other drugs, and can be abused. Shake liquids before pouring. Follow the dose with water or milk to deliver antacid to the stomach. Antacids interfere with absorption of oral drugs if given within 1–2 hours of each other. Tablets should be chewed before swallowing.
H2 Receptor Blockers			
cimetidine (Tagamet), ranitidine (Zantac), famotidine (Pepcid), nizatidine (Axid)	Used to reduce secretion of gastric acid and promote healing of ulcers.	Diarrhea, muscle pain, rash, confusion, and drowsiness. Cimetidine can cause impotence and gynecomastia and impairs the metabolism of many common drugs. Other drugs have fewer side effects (and do not cause impotence or gynecomastia).	Give the drug with or after meals. Do not give ranitidine at the same time as antacids. Advise older patients of the risk of confusion and drug interactions with cimetidine.

Table 39-2 Drug Therapy: Disorders of the Digestive Tract—cont'd

DRUG	USE AND ACTION	SIDE EFFECTS	NURSING INTERVENTIONS
Proton Pump Inhibitors			
omeprazole (Prilosec), esomeprazole (Nexium), lansoprazole (Prevacid), pantoprazole (Protonix), rabeprazole (Aciphex)	Used to inhibit gastric acid secretion in the treatment of peptic ulcer disease, GERD, and Zollinger-Ellison syndrome.	Nausea, diarrhea, and headache.	Advise the patient to swallow the capsule whole. For patients who cannot swallow capsules, Prevacid capsules can be opened and the contents mixed in applesauce. A liquid preparation also is available.
Mucosal Barriers			
sucralfate (Carafate)	Used to permit healing of an ulcer by interacting with acid to form a protective gel that coats the ulcer surface.	Constipation, dry mouth, drowsiness, rash, and itching.	Give the drug on an empty stomach 1 hour before meals and antacids. The medication interferes with absorption of some other drugs.
Synthetic Prostaglandins			
misoprostol (Cytotec)	Used to decrease gastric acid secretion and protect the gastric mucosa. Often used to prevent gastric ulcers caused by NSAIDs.	Contraindicated during pregnancy. Diarrhea, abdominal pain, miscarriage, headache, flatulence, and nausea and vomiting.	Usually given with meals and at bedtime. Explain the importance of avoiding pregnancy during prostaglandin therapy because it can cause spontaneous abortion.
Anticholinergic Agents			
atropine, pirenzepine (Gastrozepin)	Used to block action of acetylcholine. Decreases salivary and gastric secretions. Reduces pain by reducing smooth muscle tone in GI tract.	Dry mouth, constipation, visual disturbance, and urine retention. Much milder side effects occur with pirenzepine than with atropine. Older adults may become confused, agitated, or drowsy.	Contraindicated with narrow-angle glaucoma, renal disease, prostatic hypertrophy, or intestinal obstruction. Best given ½ to 1 hour before meals and at bedtime. Provide oral hygiene for the patient and monitor stools and urine output. Report changes in behavior.
Laxatives and Stimulants			
bisacodyl (Dulcolax) tablets and suppositories, senna (Senokot), cascara sagrada, castor oil	Used to facilitate bowel elimination. Stimulates the GI tract by irritating the mucosa. Tends to produce diarrhea-like stools. Castor oil is too harsh for routine use.	Bisacodyl suppositories can irritate the anus. Cascara and senna can make the urine pink or brownish. Castor oil rapidly produces a watery stool. Oily laxatives are not recommended for older adults because of the risk for aspiration, which can cause lipid pneumonia.	Monitor the patient's stools. Encourage adequate fluids and fiber to reduce the need for laxatives. Laxatives are intended for temporary, relief and are contraindicated with undiagnosed abdominal pain and inflammatory conditions of GI tract. Chill castor oil and have the patient wash it down with fruit juice. Advise older adults to discuss most appropriate drugs to manage constipation with their health care provider.
Bulk-Forming Laxatives			
psyllium (Metamucil), methylcellulose (Citrucel)	Used to retain water in the stool to increase bulk and fluid, which stimulates peristalsis with the passage of the formed, soft stool.	One of safest laxatives for long-term therapy and during pregnancy. Obstruction can occur if it is not taken with adequate fluids or if passage through the intestine is arrested.	The patient must take adequate fluids or the mass can harden. It may take up to 3 days before the effect is evident, so it is used primarily for prevention of constipation.

Continued

Table 39-2 Drug Therapy: Disorders of the Digestive Tract—cont'd

DRUG	USE AND ACTION	SIDE EFFECTS	NURSING INTERVENTIONS
Saline (Osmotic) Laxatives			
magnesium citrate, magnesium hydroxide (milk of magnesia), sodium phosphate (Fleet Phospho-soda), polyethylene glycol (MiraLAX)	Used to draw water into bowel to distend and stimulate evacuation. It is intended for short-term use only.	Side effects include the risk of dehydration with frequent or prolonged use.	Most of these laxatives are contraindicated with kidney disease, heart failure, hypertension, and edema.
Lubricants			
mineral oil	Used to lubricate feces for easier passage.	Caution: there is a risk of lipid pneumonia if the product is aspirated.	Because mineral oil impairs absorption of fat-soluble drugs and nutrients, it should be given on an empty stomach.
Fecal Wetting Agents			
docusate calcium (Surfak), docusate sodium (Colace)	Used to soften fecal mass. Because it may take up to 3 days before effects are evident, these agents are used primarily for prevention of constipation.	Nausea, anorexia, cramps, diarrhea, rash, throat irritation.	Liquid forms can be given in milk or juice to mask taste.
Other Agents			
lactulose (Cephulac)	Used to increase fecal water content to stimulate evacuation. Promotes passage of ammonia through the rectum. Used in hepatic encephalopathy. Available for oral or rectal administration.	Cramps, flatulence, diarrhea, and hyperglycemia with diabetes.	Can be mixed with full glass of water, milk, or juice to disguise the taste. It is more effective on empty stomach. Report diarrhea because dosage needs to be reduced. For a retention enema, administer the agent with a rectal balloon catheter.
polyethylene glycol-electrolyte solution (GoLYTELY, HalfLytely, MoviPrep), glycerin suppository or enema	GoLYTELY, HalfLytely, and MoviPrep are used to cleanse the bowel before diagnostic procedures. HalfLytely and MoviPrep include other drugs that stimulate the bowel and require less fluid volume than GoLYTELY.	Nausea, bloating, abdominal discomfort.	GoLYTELY can be used with renal and cardiac disease because it does not disturb the patient's electrolyte balance. When prepared for administration, GoLYTELY comprises 4 L. The patient must drink 350–300 mL every 10 minutes over 2–3 hours. Glycerin, rarely used, but acts within 1 hour. With saline laxatives be sure the patient has immediate access to a toilet.
Antidiarrheal Agents			
Opiates			
morphine, diphenoxylate HCl, (Lomotil), loperamide HCl (Imodium)	Used to decrease intestinal motility so that the liquid portion of feces is reabsorbed.	CNS depression, drowsiness, dizziness, constipation, nausea, and dry mouth.	Do not exceed the maximum dosage. Use safety precautions and encourage good oral hygiene.
Adsorbents			
kaolin, aluminum hydroxide	Used to bind to substances that may cause diarrhea.		Shake the suspension before pouring. Do not administer it with other oral drugs because adsorbents will interfere with absorption.
Lactobacillus products	Used to replace normal bacterial flora of the bowel.		May require refrigeration.

Table 39-2 **Drug Therapy: Disorders of the Digestive Tract—cont'd**

DRUG	USE AND ACTION	SIDE EFFECTS	NURSING INTERVENTIONS
Antiemetics			
5-HT_3 Receptor Antagonists			
ondansetron (Zofran), granisetron (Kytril), palonosetron (Aloxi)	Used to prevent nausea and vomiting caused by chemotherapy. Aloxi has a very long half-life (40 hours), so a single dose usually controls initial and delayed chemotherapy side effects.	Medication is usually tolerated well. Most common side effects include the following: headache, constipation, diarrhea, abdominal pain, musculoskeletal pain, shivering, fever, hypoxia, and urinary retention.	After diluting the agent according to directions, it is given IV 30 minutes before a chemotherapy dose as ordered. Advise the patient that drowsiness may occur. Ask about constipation and difficulty voiding. Encourage fluids, fiber, and activity as appropriate. Stool softeners may be needed.
substance P/neurokinin 1 receptor blocker, aprepitant (Emend)	Used to prevent nausea and vomiting caused by chemotherapy. Used in combination with other antiemetics.	Common side effects include headache, dizziness, diarrhea, constipation, and nausea. Most serious side effects include thrombocytopenia and neutropenia.	Administer the agent as ordered: a 3-day course with the first dose 1 hour before therapy.
Antihistamines			
promethazine HCl (Phenergan), dimenhydrinate HCl (Dramamine)	Used to prevent and treat nausea. Decreases the sensitivity of the vestibular apparatus of the inner ear. Suppresses the vomiting center.	Drowsiness and confusion, especially if given with other CNS depressants.	Use these medications cautiously with asthma, glaucoma, and prostatic hypertrophy.
Sedatives			
hydroxyzine (Atarax)	Used to prevent perioperative nausea and vomiting; antianxiety effects.	Drowsiness, confusion, hypotension, dry mouth, nausea, diarrhea, urinary retention.	Monitor alertness, BP, urine output. Assist with ambulation. Bed in low position, Call bell in reach. Oral care.
Anticholinergics			
scopolamine (Transderm Scōp)	Used to suppress the vomiting center. Often used to prevent motion sickness.	Confusion, delusions and hallucinations, tachycardia, dry mouth, blurred vision, urinary retention	Transderm Scōp is a medicated adhesive disk that is placed behind the ear. Contraindicated with narrow-angle glaucoma and urinary tract obstruction
Prokinetic Agents			
metoclopramide (Reglan)	Used to speed up gastric emptying into the small intestine.	CNS depression, GI upset, and Parkinson-like symptoms.	Contraindications include the following: GI perforation, obstruction, hemorrhage, and epilepsy.
Antibacterials			
ciprofloxacin (Cipro), erythromycin (E-Mycin), metronidazole (Flagyl)	Used to treat diarrhea caused by pathogens. Cipro: *Escherichia coli, Campylobacter jejuni, Shigella* spp. E-Mycin: *Entamoeba histolytica* Flagyl: *Clostridium difficile*	Side effects vary with the specific drug.	Advise the patient to complete the entire course of therapy and to report worsening symptoms. Nursing care varies with specific agent.

Continued

Table 39-2 Drug Therapy: Disorders of the Digestive Tract—cont'd

DRUG	USE AND ACTION	SIDE EFFECTS	NURSING INTERVENTIONS
olsalazine (Dipentum)	Used to treat ulcerative colitis.	Abdominal pain, diarrhea, headache, and nausea.	Discontinue use if hives, rash, or wheezing occur. Encourage fluids.
amoxicillin (Amoxil)	Used to treat *Helicobacter pylori* when combined with omeprazole, prostaglandins, or bismuth subsalicylate (or a combination of these medications).	Rash, diarrhea, anaphylaxis, and superinfections (colitis).	Instruct the patient to take the full course of treatment.
Antifungals			
nystatin (Mycostatin)	Used as an effective treatment against *Candida albicans* (yeast) infections.	Nausea, vomiting, and diarrhea with nystatin.	Instruct the patient to dissolve lozenges in the mouth. Shake suspensions well. Swish in the mouth before swallowing.
clotrimazole (Mycelex)	Used to treat *Candida albicans* (yeast) infections.	Nausea, vomiting, and itching.	Vaginal preparations are available.

BP, Blood pressure; *CNS*, central nervous system; *GERD*, gastroesophageal reflux disease; *GI*, gastrointestinal; *IV*, intravenously; *NSAIDs*, nonsteroidal antiinflammatory drugs; *RN*, registered nurse.

ANOREXIA

The intake of food depends largely on having an appetite. Lack of appetite is called **anorexia**.

Causes

Anorexia can occur with many physical and emotional disturbances. Nausea, a decreased sense of taste or smell, mouth disorders, and medications are some physical factors that may decrease one's appetite. Emotional problems such as anxiety, depression, or disturbing thoughts also may cause anorexia. Older people often report decreased appetite. This may be attributed to diminished senses of taste and smell, drug effects, decreased activity, and social isolation.

Medical Diagnosis

The physician, nurse practitioner, or dietitian assess the patient for evidence of malnutrition. Weight may be monitored over several weeks. A complete history and physical examination are done to detect underlying problems and the effects of inadequate intake. Initial diagnostic tests that are likely to be ordered include measurements of serum hemoglobin (Hgb), iron, total iron-binding capacity (TIBC), transferrin, calcium, folate, vitamin B_{12}, and zinc. Tests of thyroid function may be ordered to detect metabolic disorders and skin tests may be ordered to evaluate allergic responses. A stool specimen may be tested for occult blood. If indicated, the health care provider may perform additional procedures to detect possible cancers of the digestive system, lungs, and breasts.

Medical Treatment

Correctable causes of anorexia are treated but sometimes no physical cause is found. Nutritional supplements may be ordered. The oral route is preferred but enteral feedings or TPN may be indicated in extreme cases. Some patients benefit from appetite stimulants such as megestrol (Megace).

NURSING CARE of the Patient with Anorexia

Assessment

The general assessment of the patient with digestive disturbances is summarized in Box 39-1.

Nursing Diagnosis, Goal, and Outcome Criteria: Anorexia

Nursing Diagnosis	Goal and Outcome Criteria
Imbalanced Nutrition: Less Than Body Requirements related to anorexia	Improved appetite and adequate food intake: patient states appetite is better, increased intake of food, stable or increased body weight

Interventions

It is helpful to identify factors that contribute to the patient's anorexia. If the patient has a dry mouth or bad taste in the mouth, assist with oral hygiene before and after meals. If the teeth or gums are in poor condition, teach proper oral hygiene and refer the patient for dental care. Poorly fitting dentures need to be relined for a tighter fit or replaced.

When a patient is nauseated, institute measures to relieve the nausea before presenting a meal tray. Nausea and anorexia can be related to unpleasant stimuli in the environment.

Many people enjoy meals more when they are in the company of others. Socialization during mealtime can greatly improve a person's appetite.

Before food is brought in by family or friends, advise them of any dietary restrictions. Small servings are more acceptable than large ones to the anorexic person. Additional nutrients can be provided by between-meal snacks.

FEEDING PROBLEMS

Patients may require assistance with meals because of temporary impairments or long-term disabilities. Patients with paralysis, arthritis, neuromuscular disorders, confusion, weakness, or visual impairment are likely to need assistance. Thorough assessments and individualized interventions are needed to ensure adequate nutrition despite disability.

Medical Diagnosis and Treatment

The medical diagnosis is directed at identifying the basic problems and prescribing treatment as appropriate. Patients often are referred to physical therapy and occupational therapy to help them regain basic self-care skills.

NURSING CARE of the Patient with Feeding Problems

Assessment

Determine the patient's ability to feed himself or herself independently. Determine the nature of the patient's difficulty and identify remaining abilities. Some patients are temporarily impaired because they are immobilized or confined to restricted positions as part of their medical treatment. Important aspects of the physical examination are visual acuity, range of motion and muscle strength in both arms, and range of motion and grip strength in both hands. Also, evaluate the patient's ability to follow instructions and to chew and swallow without choking or gagging.

Nursing Diagnoses, Goals, and Outcome Criteria: Feeding Problems

Nursing Diagnoses	Goals and Outcome Criteria
Self-Care Deficit, Feeding related to paralysis, weakness, poor coordination, confusion, visual impairment	Improved self-feeding: patient participates in feeding within his or her capabilities
Imbalanced Nutrition: Less Than Body Requirements related to inability to feed self	Adequate food intake: stable body weight or attainment of ideal body weight

Interventions

Encourage patients to be as independent as possible in feeding. For some, proper positioning and arrangement of the meal tray are all that is needed. Assistive devices designed for paralyzed and arthritic patients are available. These can be obtained through the physical therapy or occupational therapy department. Simple adaptations such as padding the handles of utensils may enable the patient with limited grasping ability to feed himself or herself. Thickening liquids also may be used to reduce the risk of choking.

Remember the following points when feeding a patient:

1. Check the diet and the patient's name for accuracy.
2. Seat the patient upright, with the head tilted slightly forward for easiest swallowing.
3. Tuck in a napkin or towel at the patient's chin to catch spills.
4. If the patient is able to communicate, ask in what order the food should be offered. The practice of mixing all food together to ensure that the patient gets a little of everything is unappetizing and not recommended.
5. Some patients do not open their mouths voluntarily. Touch the lips with the spoon or gently press just below the lower lip with a finger to encourage them to do so.
6. Pacing is important, so observe that the patient has swallowed before offering more food.
7. In stroke patients, food may accumulate in the affected side of the mouth. Check the mouth at intervals for accumulated food.
8. Offer fluids periodically.
9. At the completion of the meal, provide mouth care and record the amount of food taken.

Put on Your Thinking Cap!

Practice feeding a classmate a simple meal. Then reverse roles and permit the classmate to feed you. Assume that the person being fed is unable to speak clearly but understands what is said. Immediately afterward, write down (1) the steps you went through when feeding another person, (2) how you felt while being fed, and (3) what you learned from the experience that you could apply in patient care.

ORAL INFLAMMATION AND INFECTIONS OF THE ORAL CAVITY

Stomatitis

Stomatitis is a general term for inflammation of the oral mucosa. It may result from the mechanical trauma of poorly fitting dentures, the irritation of excessive tobacco or alcohol use, poor oral hygiene, inadequate nutrition, pathogenic organisms, radiation therapy, or drug therapy. Disorders of the kidney, liver, or blood also can cause stomatitis. Emotional tension and excessive fatigue seem to make people more susceptible to some types of stomatitis. Medical treatment is directed toward determining the cause and eliminating it. If specific pathogenic organisms are identified, appropriate antibiotics (usually topical) or antivirals may be prescribed.

Table 39-4 Complications of Peptic Ulcer Disease

COMPLICATION	SIGNS AND SYMPTOMS	TREATMENT	NURSING CARE
Hemorrhage	Thready pulse, restlessness, diaphoresis, chills, oliguria, hematemesis, tarry stools, hypotension	Saline lavage, vasopressin, arterial embolization	Assist with procedure; monitor effects of treatment; monitor for water intoxication: headache, coma, tremor, sweating, anxiety; monitor vital signs, intake and output; maintain patent NG tube; give IV fluids as ordered
Perforation	Sudden, sharp midepigastric pain that spreads over entire abdomen; rigid abdomen; absence of bowel sounds; shock	NG suction, IV fluids, antibiotics	Monitor vital signs, intake and output; enforce NPO order; give fluids and blood as ordered; keep NG tube patent
Obstruction	Feeling of fullness, nausea after eating, persistent vomiting	NG suction	Monitor vital signs, intake and output; keep NG tube patent

IV, Intravenous; *NG*, nasogastric; *NPO*, nothing by mouth.

Table 39-5 Surgical Treatment of Peptic Ulcer Disease

OPERATION	PROCEDURE	PURPOSE	ADVERSE EFFECTS
Truncal vagotomy	Vagus nerve that supplies the stomach is severed.	Decreases stimulation of gastric acid secretion.	Patient may experience delayed gastric emptying. Patient also may have a feeling of fullness, dumping syndrome, and diarrhea.
Selective or superselective vagotomy	Severs the part of the vagus nerve that stimulates acid production. Spares the nerve supply to the pyloric sphincter.	Decreases stimulation of gastric acid secretion.	Patient may experience delayed gastric emptying.
Pyloroplasty	Widens the pylorus.	Improves the passage of stomach contents into the duodenum. Procedure is usually done with a vagotomy to prevent gastric stasis.	Patient may experience dumping syndrome because of the rapid emptying of the stomach into the duodenum.
Simple gastroenterostomy	Creates a passage between the body of the stomach and the jejunum.	Permits passage of alkaline intestinal secretions into the stomach to neutralize gastric acid.	Patient may experience increased gastric acid secretion.
Antrectomy	Removal of the antrum of the stomach.	Reduces gastric acid by removing the source of acid secretion.	Patient may experience diarrhea, a feeling of fullness after eating, dumping syndrome, malabsorption, and anemia.
Subtotal Gastrectomy			
Gastroduodenoscopy (Billroth I)	Part of the distal portion of the stomach, including the antrum, is removed. Remaining stomach is anastomosed to the duodenum.	Reduces acid by removing the source of acid secretion.	Patient may experience dumping syndrome (less often than with other procedures), anemia, malabsorption, weight loss, and bile reflux.
Gastrojejunostomy (Billroth II)	Part of the distal portion of the stomach, including the antrum, is removed. Remaining stomach is anastomosed to the jejunum.	Removes the source of acid secretion.	Patient may experience dumping syndrome, weight loss, malabsorption, duodenal infection, pernicious anemia, and afferent loop syndrome (obstruction of the duodenal loop).
Total gastrectomy	Removal of the entire stomach. Esophagus anastomosed to the duodenum.	Removes the source of gastric acid secretion.	Patient can consume only small, frequent meals of semisolid foods. Patient may experience pernicious anemia and dumping syndrome.

Nursing Care Plan — Patient with a Peptic Ulcer

ASSESSMENT

HEALTH HISTORY A 47-year-old man has recently been diagnosed as having duodenal ulcers. He has a history of burning pain 2 to 3 hours after meals. The pain is located just beneath the xiphoid process and is relieved by antacid agents. Symptoms are sometimes accompanied by nausea but not vomiting. He noticed that his stools have been darker than usual this week. He describes his health as good but is being treated for hypertension.

He states that he rarely drinks alcoholic beverages but smokes 1½ packs of cigarettes daily. He is a truck driver who usually eats only two meals each day, at irregular hours.

PHYSICAL EXAMINATION Blood pressure, 136/82 mm Hg; pulse, 76 beats per minute; respiration, 16 breaths per minute; temperature, 97.6° F (36.4° C) measured orally. Height, 5′10″; weight, 210 lb. Alert and oriented. Abdomen soft. Bowel sounds present in all four quadrants.

Nursing Diagnosis	Goals and Outcome Criteria	Interventions
Chronic Pain related to ulceration of duodenum	Patient will verbalize pain relief and appear relaxed.	Administer drugs that decrease acid secretion, neutralize acid, or coat ulcer surfaces as ordered. Promote a restful environment and explain the importance of rest and teach relaxation techniques.
Imbalanced Nutrition: Less Than Body Requirements related to nausea, vomiting, anorexia, dietary restrictions	Patient will maintain adequate nutrition, as evidenced by stable body weight.	Provide diet as ordered: often bland, low-fat diet given in six small feedings. Administer antiemetic agents for nausea and vomiting. Monitor the patient's weight. Consult a dietitian if the patient is losing weight.
Risk for Injury related to hemorrhage, perforation, and obstruction	Patient will remain free of complications, as evidenced by normal vital signs and no vomiting, hematemesis, or tarry stools.	Monitor for signs and symptoms of bleeding. If hemorrhage occurs, notify the physician and monitor the patient's vital signs. Perform lavage via nasogastric tube as ordered. Keep the patient quiet, and enforce nothing by mouth (NPO) order. Maintain intravenous lines to ensure venous access in an emergency. Monitor for signs and symptoms of perforation. If perforation occurs, then notify the physician and monitor vital signs. Withhold oral fluids. Anticipate the need for nasogastric suction and intravenous fluids. Monitor for signs and symptoms of pyloric obstruction. Carry out orders, including nasogastric suction, intravenous fluids, and antibiotic agents.
Ineffective Coping related to prescribed alterations in lifestyle	Patient will express intent to implement lifestyle alterations.	Identify behaviors that aggravate peptic ulcer disease. Explain the effects of altering those behaviors on the disease. Offer information about resources that provide services to help patients give up tobacco.
Deficient Knowledge of self-care to manage peptic ulcer disease	Patient will correctly describe self-care measures to promote healing of duodenal ulcers and prevent recurrence.	Advise the patient to avoid substances that stimulate the release of gastrin: alcohol, tobacco, and caffeine. Stress the importance of taking drugs as prescribed. Explain the side effects and adverse effects and their management. List drugs that are contraindicated. Supplement verbal instruction with written information. Encourage follow-up care.

Interventions

Chronic Pain

The most important means of reducing pain associated with peptic ulcer disease are drug therapy, rest, and diet. Drugs reduce pain by neutralizing acid, decreasing acid secretion, or coating the ulcer surface. The environment should be as restful as possible. Encourage relaxation techniques and stress management strategies as described in Chapter 15.

Imbalanced Nutrition: Less Than Body Requirements

The patient is advised to avoid any foods that have caused gastric distress in the past. When nausea and vomiting are present, oral fluids may be restricted to clear liquids or the patient may be placed on NPO status. Administer antiemetics as ordered.

Risk for Injury

Monitor the patient for signs and symptoms of complications. Signs of bleeding are hematemesis (vomiting blood) and the presence of blood in the feces. Blood that has passed through the digestive tract is maroon to black and causes the stool to have a sticky or tarry quality. Stools and vomited fluid may be tested for occult blood. When blood loss is significant, the patient may go into shock. Early signs of shock are weakness, tachycardia, and pallor. Hypotension is a relatively late sign.

Nursing Diagnoses, Goals, and Outcome Criteria: Peptic Ulcer Disease

Nursing Diagnoses	Goals and Outcome Criteria
Chronic Pain related to ulceration of stomach or duodenum	Pain relief: patient states pain is reduced or relieved, relaxed manner
Imbalanced Nutrition: Less Than Body Requirements related to nausea, vomiting, anorexia, dietary restrictions, nothing by mouth (NPO) status	Adequate nutrition: stable body weight
Risk for Injury related to hemorrhage, perforation, obstruction	Absence of complications: vital signs within patient norms; no vomiting, hematemesis, or tarry stools
Ineffective Coping related to prescribed alterations in lifestyle	Effective coping: adjustment to prescribed changes in lifestyle, adherence to treatment regimen

If hemorrhage occurs, it is vital to notify the RN or health care provider immediately while continuing to monitor the patient's vital signs. Anticipate insertion of a nasogastric tube and saline lavage. Keep the patient quiet and give the patient nothing to eat or drink (NPO status). Maintain intravenous lines and record fluid intake and output. The patient may have to be prepared for transfer to intensive care or surgery.

Perforation is characterized by sudden, sharp pain starting in the midepigastric region and spreading across the entire abdomen. Digestive fluids in the abdomen cause peritonitis (inflammation of the peritoneum). With peritonitis, the abdomen is rigid and tender. The patient tends to draw the knees up toward the chest. When perforation is suspected, nursing care is much like that provided for hemorrhage.

Ineffective Coping

Explore what the patient thinks about prescribed treatments and how they will affect his or her lifestyle (see *Patient Teaching* box). Resources are available to help patients who have difficulty giving up alcohol or tobacco.

NURSING CARE of the Patient with Peptic Ulcer Managed Surgically

Preoperative nursing care is like the care outlined in Chapter 17 for any patient having major surgery. This section emphasizes the special postoperative needs of the patient who has undergone gastric surgery for peptic ulcer disease.

Patient Teaching

Peptic Ulcer

- It is important to know the name, dosage, schedule, and adverse effects of each drug taken.
- Avoid aspirin, nonsteroidal antiinflammatory drugs (NSAIDs), alcohol, and smoking because they aggravate peptic ulcer disease.
- The physician may recommend a specific diet that will decrease irritation to the stomach.
- Follow-up care is important to ensure that the ulcer is healing or has not recurred.
- Resources for stress management techniques and alcohol abuse (if appropriate) are available.

Assessment

Postoperatively, the patient should be assessed for pain, nausea, and vomiting. Measure vital signs at frequent intervals until the patient is stable. In addition, document the amount and type of intravenous fluids. If a nasogastric tube is present, document patency of the tube as well as the color and amount of drainage. Inspect the skin around the nostril where the tube is located for irritation, auscultate breath sounds, and inspect the wound dressing for bleeding. Once the dressing is removed, examine the incision for increased redness, swelling, drainage, and incomplete closure. Describe any drainage from the wound or from drains. Inspect the abdomen for distention and auscultate for bowel sounds. Finally, monitor urine output and palpate for bladder distention.

Nursing Diagnoses, Goals, and Outcome Criteria: Gastric Surgery

Nursing Diagnoses	Goals and Outcome Criteria
Risk for Injury related to gastric dilation, obstruction, perforation	Absence of complications: vital signs within patient norms, minimal vomiting
Imbalanced Nutrition: Less Than Body Requirements related to decreased capacity for intake of nutrients	Adequate nutrition: maintains or attains ideal body weight
Decreased Cardiac Output related to hypovolemia secondary to dumping syndrome	Normal cardiac output: no decrease in blood pressure after meals

Interventions

Risk for Injury

Potential complications of gastric surgery include gastric dilation, obstruction, and perforation. Gastric dilation results from accumulation of fluid in the stomach. Tachycardia, hypotension, and hiccups may develop. Obstruction can result from edema at the surgical site, causing pain and vomiting.

A nasogastric tube is usually inserted preoperatively and remains in place after surgery. Specific orders for suction will be written. It is very important to maintain suction and drainage as ordered.

! After gastric surgery, do not irrigate or reposition the tube. To do so may cause the suture line in the stomach to tear. Nasogastric drainage is usually bright red immediately after surgery. The color darkens over the first 24 hours and then turns yellow or green. The tube is removed when peristalsis returns, usually on the third to fifth postoperative day. Document the presence of bowel sounds and the passage of flatus through the rectum.

Imbalanced Nutrition: Less Than Body Requirements

After the tube is removed, the diet is gradually advanced from water or ice chips to clear liquids, full liquids, and then solid foods. Special dietary needs depend on the type of surgery (see *Patient Teaching* box).

Patient Teaching

Peptic Ulcer, Postoperative

- Know the name, dosage, schedule, and adverse effects of each medication taken.
- After subtotal gastrectomy, eat small, frequent meals until stomach capacity expands. After total gastrectomy, the need to eat small, frequent meals probably will be a requirement for life.
- Promptly inform the physician if nausea, vomiting, abdominal pain, or dark, tarry stools are present.
- Reduce the risk of recurrence by avoiding caffeine, alcohol, aspirin, and nonsteroidal antiinflammatory drugs (NSAIDs).
- If stressed, try stress management techniques such as relaxation exercises or seek personal counseling.

Gastric surgery can have serious effects on the patient's nutritional status. The absorption of vitamin B_{12}, folic acid, iron, calcium, and vitamin D may be impaired, so supplements will be needed. Without vitamin B_{12}, the patient develops pernicious anemia. Pernicious anemia is more common after a total gastrectomy but can follow a subtotal gastrectomy. As discussed earlier, the parietal cells in the stomach produce intrinsic factor, a substance that is needed to absorb vitamin B_{12}. Vitamin B_{12} is essential for the production of RBCs. When all or part of the stomach is removed, the patient develops a vitamin B_{12} deficiency and, eventually, severe anemia. The condition is easily treated with vitamin B_{12}.

Decreased Cardiac Output

Some patients experience dumping syndrome after gastric surgery. The symptoms of dumping syndrome may occur in stages. In the first stage, the patient experiences abdominal fullness and nausea within 10 to 20 minutes of eating. These symptoms are thought to be caused by distention of the small intestine by the consumed food and fluids and the shift of a modest amount of fluid from the circulation into the intestines. The patient feels flushed and faint, the heart rate races, and the patient breaks into a sweat as a result of pooling of blood in the abdominal organs. In the intermediate stage, the patient has abdominal bloating, flatulence, cramps, and diarrhea that occur 20 to 60 minutes after eating. These symptoms are probably related to the malabsorption of carbohydrates and other foodstuffs because of a deficiency of digestive enzymes. One to 3 hours later, the late stage may occur. The patient may perspire, feel weak, anxious, shaky, or hungry. These symptoms are blamed on hypoglycemia caused by an exaggerated rise in insulin secretion in response to the rapid delivery of carbohydrates into the intestine.

Dumping syndrome usually disappears within a few months. Meanwhile, the following directions for the patient will help:

1. Consume a diet low in carbohydrates and refined sugar, moderate in fat, and moderate to high in protein.
2. Smaller, more frequent meals may be better tolerated than three large meals.
3. Drink fluids between meals, not with them.
4. Lie down for about 30 minutes after meals.

STOMACH CANCER

Pathophysiology

Cancer of the stomach is diagnosed in more than 22,000 people in the United States each year. The incidence is highest among men, people older than 70 years, and people of lower socioeconomic status. Asians and Pacific Islanders, African Americans, and Latinos are at greater risk than non-Latino Caucasians (see *Cultural Considerations* box).

Stomach carcinoma begins in the mucous membranes, invades the gastric wall, and spreads to the regional lymphatics, liver, pancreas, and colon. Distant metastases are found in the lungs and bones. Unfortunately, no specific signs or symptoms are seen in the early stages. Late signs and symptoms are vomiting, ascites, liver enlargement, and an abdominal mass. By the time late signs appear, the cancer is advanced and the patient's chance of 5-year survival is poor.

Cultural Considerations

What Does Culture Have to Do with Stomach Cancer?

The incidence of stomach cancer in African-American men is greater than in Caucasians. In addition, culturally based dietary patterns (high intake of starch, salt, pickled foods, salted meats, and nitrates) increase the risk of stomach cancer.

Risk Factors

No specific cause of gastric cancer is known; however, various factors are known to increase a person's risk for this cancer. Risk factors include *H. pylori* infection, pernicious anemia, chronic atrophic gastritis, achlorhydria (lack of hydrochloric acid), type A blood, and a family history of stomach cancer. Some personal habits that seem to be related to stomach cancer are cigarette smoking and a diet high in starch, salt, pickled foods, salted meats, and nitrates. Patients who have had the Billroth II procedure (gastrojejunostomy) also have increased incidence of stomach cancer (see *Health Promotion* box).

Health Promotion

Breaking the Link between Diet and Digestive Tract Cancers

- People who have a poor diet, do not have enough physical activity, or are overweight may be at increased risk of several types of cancer. Overweight and obese individuals are two times more likely than people of healthy weight to develop a type of esophageal cancer called esophageal adenocarcinoma. A smaller increase in risk has been found for a specific type of stomach cancer that begins in the area of the stomach next to the esophagus.
- Having a healthy diet, being physically active, and maintaining a healthy weight may help to reduce cancer risk. The National Institutes of Health (NIH) recommends the following:
  - Eat well: A healthy diet includes plenty of foods that are high in fiber, vitamins, and minerals. This includes whole-grain breads and cereals and five to nine servings of fruits and vegetables every day. In addition, it is important to limit foods high in fat (e.g., butter, whole milk, fried foods, red meat).
  - Be active and maintain a healthy weight: Physical activity can help to control weight and reduce body fat. Most scientists agree that it is a good idea for an adult to engage in moderate physical activity (e.g., brisk walking) for at least 30 minutes on 5 or more days each week.

Data from National Cancer Institute: Cancer Trends Progress Report—2011/2012 Update. http://progressreport.cancer.gov/doc.asp?pid=1&did=2011&mid=vcol&chid=101.

Medical Diagnosis

Gastroscopy is used to examine the interior of the stomach and to take specimens for microscopic study. Other procedures that might be used to establish the diagnosis and extent of the cancer are endoscopic ultrasound, upper GI series, CT scan, bone scan, positron emission tomography (PET) scan, magnetic resonance imaging (MRI), and laparoscopy. Laboratory studies include Hgb and Hct, serum albumin, liver function tests, and carcinoembryonic antigen (CEA). Stool specimens may be tested for occult blood.

Medical Treatment

Stomach cancer may be treated with surgery, chemotherapy, and radiation therapy. If the cancer is detected early, surgical options include subtotal gastrectomy with lymph node dissection and total gastrectomy. Sometimes part of the esophagus or duodenum is resected. In more advanced cancer, the surgeon may remove as much of the tumor as possible to relieve or prevent obstruction without removing the entire stomach. In some cases, chemotherapy is given before and after surgery. Gene therapy and immune-based therapy are in early phases of study and may prove useful someday.

POSTOPERATIVE NURSING CARE of the Patient with Stomach Cancer

General preoperative and postoperative nursing care are discussed in Chapter 17. Chapter 25 discusses general care of the patient who has cancer. The special needs of patients having surgery for gastric cancer are discussed here.

Assessment

Data related to comfort, appetite, and nausea and vomiting are especially important after surgery for stomach cancer. Monitor the patient for weight changes and determine dietary preferences. Identify the patient's support system and coping strategies.

Nursing Diagnoses, Goals, and Outcome Criteria: Stomach Cancer: Postoperative Care

Nursing Diagnoses	Goals and Outcome Criteria
Acute Pain related to tumor, surgical trauma, or both	Pain relief: patient states less or no pain, relaxed manner
Imbalanced Nutrition: Less Than Body Requirements related to anorexia, pain, nausea and vomiting	Adequate nutrition: maintains or attains ideal body weight
Ineffective Coping related to diagnosis of cancer, poor prognosis	Effective coping: patient verbalizes concerns, seeks and uses resources as needed, makes realistic plans

Interventions

Acute Pain

Administer analgesics as ordered in addition to using nonpharmacologic measures to manage pain. Massage, relaxation techniques, and mental imagery are examples of complementary measures to help manage pain.

Imbalanced Nutrition: Less Than Body Requirements

Nutritional needs are much like those of the patient who has undergone surgery for peptic ulcer disease.

Ineffective Coping

The patient and family may need help in coping with this life-threatening illness. Encourage them to talk and to be accepting of the thoughts and feelings the patient expresses. Help the patient to think about changes in daily routines that may be necessary after discharge (see *Patient Teaching* box). If chemotherapy or radiation therapy is planned, the patient needs to know what to expect. Provide the patient with information about community resources such as home health agencies or the American Cancer Society (www.cancer.org).

If the patient is scheduled for chemotherapy or radiation therapy, explain what the patient can expect.

Patient Teaching

Stomach Cancer: Postoperative Care

- Know the name, dosage, schedule, and adverse effects of each medication.
- Eat six small meals a day and drink fluids between meals rather than with meals.
- Notify the health care provider if the wound shows increasing redness, swelling, pain, or drainage.

Get Ready for the NCLEX® Examination!

Key Points

- Any disorder of the digestive tract can cause nutritional deficiencies by disrupting one or more of its three functions: (1) digestion, (2) absorption, and (3) elimination.
- Anorexia, or lack of appetite, may be caused by illness, drugs, or emotional factors.
- Oral inflammations and infections can be caused by irritants, bacteria, viruses, and fungi and can interfere with food intake and enjoyment.
- Cancers inside the oral cavity are usually squamous cell carcinomas related to poor nutrition, chronic irritation, or combined tobacco and alcohol use.
- Cancers of the lip are usually basal cell carcinomas attributed to prolonged exposure to irritants, including sun, wind, and pipe smoking.
- Nursing care of patients being treated for oral cancers focuses on impaired oral mucous membranes; ineffective breathing pattern; acute pain; impaired verbal communication; imbalanced nutrition: less than body requirements; disturbed body image; risk for infection; and ineffective peripheral tissue perfusion.
- Cancer of the esophagus may be treated with surgery, radiotherapy, chemotherapy, or a combination of these or by palliative measures to maintain a patent esophagus.
- Vomiting, which can result in fluid and electrolyte imbalances, aspiration, and nutritional deficiencies, is treated with antiemetics, fluid and electrolyte replacement, and sometimes GI decompression.
- Treatment of hiatal hernia, the protrusion of the lower esophagus and stomach upward through the diaphragm, may include drug therapy, diet, measures to avoid increased intraabdominal pressure, or surgery.
- Gastritis is inflammation of the stomach lining usually caused by *H. pylori* and aggravated by alcohol, caffeine, and other irritants.
- Peptic ulcer is loss of tissue from the lining of the stomach or duodenum that can lead to hemorrhage, perforation, and obstruction.
- Nursing care of patients with peptic ulcer focuses on acute pain; imbalanced nutrition: less than body requirements; risk for injury; and ineffective coping.
- Dumping syndrome may occur after gastric surgery, causing weakness, dizziness, diaphoresis, and palpitations.
- Nursing care of the patient with stomach cancer, which is often advanced when diagnosed, focuses on acute pain; imbalanced nutrition: less than body requirements; and ineffective coping.

Additional Learning Resources

SG Go to your Study Guide for additional learning activities to help you master this chapter content.

evolve Go to your Evolve website (http://evolve.elsevier.com/Linton/medsurg) for the following learning resources and much more:

- Interactive Prioritization Exercises
- Fluid & Electrolyte Tutorial
- Pharmacology Tutorial
- Review Questions for the NCLEX® Examination

Review Questions for the NCLEX® Examination

1. The nurse is caring for patients with diseases that affect the stomach, small intestine, large intestine, and rectum. Which of these patients is at greatest risk for problems with absorption of nutrients?
   1. Stomach
   2. Small intestine
   3. Large intestine
   4. Rectum

   NCLEX Client Need: Physiological Integrity: Basic Care and Comfort
2. Inspection of the mouth of an older adult reveals all of the data listed below. Which findings should the nurse recognize as normal? (Select all that apply.)
   1. Worn chewing surfaces on the teeth
   2. Recession of the gingiva (gums)
   3. Loss of most of the natural teeth
   4. Teeth appear dark and transparent
   5. Whitish patches on the border of the tongue

   NCLEX Client Need: Health Promotion and Maintenance
3. Other than a radiograph, the most reliable way to assess placement of a nasogastric tube is to do which of the following?
   1. Auscultate the epigastrium while injecting air into the tube
   2. Examine and check pH of aspirated stomach contents
   3. Place the end of the tube in water and observe for bubbling
   4. Listen for air movement at the end of the tube

   NCLEX Client Need: Safe and Effective Care Environment: Safety and Infection Control

4. A patient who has had oral surgery complains of dry mouth. Your most appropriate action is to do which of the following?
   1. Tell the patient this is normal after oral surgery
   2. Provide a commercial mouthwash for rinsing the mouth
   3. Check the health care provider's orders for mouth care
   4. Suction the mouth after giving the patient sips of water

   NCLEX Client Need: Physiological Integrity: Basic Care and Comfort
5. You are reviewing the admission papers for a new resident of a long-term care facility. You note a medical diagnosis of achalasia. Which of the following should be included in the nursing care plan? (Select all that apply.)
   1. Determine the best position for the patient during meals
   2. Be sure clothing is not restrictive
   3. Place the patient on NPO status
   4. Auscultate bowel sounds in all four quadrants
   5. Maintain strict intake and output records

   NCLEX Client Need: Physiological Integrity: Reduction of Risk Potential
6. Which of the following types of antiulcer drugs work by inhibiting the secretion of gastric acid? (Select all that apply.)
   1. Antacids
   2. H2 receptor blockers
   3. Mucosal barriers
   4. Proton pump inhibitors
   5. Synthetic prostaglandins

   NCLEX Client Need: Physiological Integrity: Pharmacological Therapies
7. You have been assigned to care for a patient who was recently diagnosed with a hiatal hernia. The patient is experiencing chronic heartburn when eating a meal. You will teach the patient to *avoid* which of the following situations?
   1. Lying flat after eating a meal
   2. Ingesting small, frequent meals
   3. Raising the head of the bed on 6- to 8-inch blocks
   4. Taking the prescribed histamine receptor antagonist medications

   NCLEX Client Need: Physiological Integrity: Basic Care and Comfort
8. As the nurse, you are providing instructions to a patient who recently had a gastrectomy. You focus your teaching on prevention of dumping syndrome. Which instruction do you include in your teaching?
   1. Increase ambulation after each meal
   2. Eat high-carbohydrate meals
   3. Limit fluids taken with meals
   4. Remain in a high Fowler position while eating

   NCLEX Client Need: Physiological Integrity: Basic Care and Comfort
9. A patient with a diagnosis of chronic gastritis is at risk for which vitamin deficiency?
   1. Vitamin A
   2. Vitamin B_{12}
   3. Vitamin C
   4. Vitamin E

   NCLEX Client Need: Physiological Integrity: Reduction of Risk Potential
10. True or false: Among the outcomes of nursing care for patients with oral cancer are pain relief, effective communication, and adaptation to change in body image.

    NCLEX Client Need: Physiological Integrity: Basic Care and Comfort

chapter 40

Lower Digestive Tract Disorders

Amanda Flagg

http://evolve.elsevier.com/Linton/medsurg

Objectives

1. Identify the nursing responsibilities in the care of patients undergoing diagnostic tests and procedures for disorders of the lower digestive tract.
2. Describe the nursing care of patients with lower digestive tract surgery and drug therapy for lower digestive tract disorders.
3. Describe the pathophysiology, signs and symptoms, complications, and treatment of selected lower digestive tract disorders.
4. Assist in developing nursing care plans for patients who are receiving treatment for lower digestive tract disorders.

Key Terms

Cathartic (kă-THĂR-tĭk)
Flatus (FLĀ-tŭs)
Helminths (HĔL-mĭnthz)
Laxative (LĂK-să-tĭv)
Steatorrhea (stē-ĂT-ō-rē-ă)
Volvulus (VŌL-vyū-lŭs)

ANATOMY AND PHYSIOLOGY OF THE LOWER DIGESTIVE TRACT

As described in Chapter 39, the functions of the complete digestive tract are ingestion, digestion, absorption of nutrients, and elimination of wastes. The lower digestive tract assists in the further breakdown of food into molecules that can be used by the cells in our bodies. It also is needed to move food through the digestive tract and to eliminate waste materials. Parts of the lower digestive tract include the small intestine, large intestine, and anus.

SMALL INTESTINE

Gastric sections in the stomach mix with food to become a semiliquid mass called chyme. Chyme leaves the stomach and enters the small intestine, where chemical digestion and absorption of nutrients take place. The small intestine is approximately 20 feet long and consists of three sections: (1) the duodenum, (2) the jejunum, and (3) the ileum.

Liver and pancreatic secretions enter the digestive tract in the duodenum. Bile, produced in the liver and stored in the gallbladder, breaks down large fat globules. Pancreatic enzymes further reduce the fat to glycerol and fatty acids, which can be absorbed easily. The functions of the liver, gallbladder, and pancreas are discussed in more detail in Chapter 41.

Three layers of tissue make up the walls of the small intestine. The mucous membrane layer secretes the digestive enzymes sucrase, lactase, maltase, carboxypeptidase, aminopeptidase, dipeptidase, nucleosidase, lipase, and enterokinase. The inner layer is lined with thousands of microscopic projections called villi. Digested food molecules are absorbed through the villi into the bloodstream. Muscle layers contract to continue mixing the chyme, moving it toward the large intestine.

LARGE INTESTINE AND ANUS

Chyme enters the large intestine through the ileocecal valve. The first section of the large intestine is the cecum, where the appendix is located. The large intestine goes up the right side of the abdomen (the ascending colon), across the abdomen just below the waist (the transverse colon), and down the left side of the abdomen (the descending colon). The part of the descending colon between the iliac crest and the rectum is called the sigmoid colon. The last 6 to 8 inches of the large intestine is the rectum, which ends at the anus, where wastes leave the body. The presence of sphincters in the anus allows wastes to be stored until voluntary elimination occurs.

Unlike the small intestine, the large intestine has no villi and secretes no digestive enzymes. Its function is to absorb water from the chyme and to eliminate the remaining solid wastes in the form of feces.

AGE-RELATED CHANGES

As stated in Chapter 39, normal aging generally does not significantly impair ingestion, digestion, absorption, or elimination. When acute or chronic illnesses occur, however, the older person is at increased risk for problems with digestion and elimination.

No significant changes with age occur in the small intestine. The absorption of vitamin A may increase whereas absorption of vitamin D, calcium, and zinc may be reduced.

In the large intestine, the muscle layer and mucosa atrophy. Smooth muscle tone and blood flow decrease and connective tissue increases. Movements of contents through the colon are slower. The anal sphincter tone and strength decrease. Therefore constipation is a frequent complaint among older adults and they use **laxatives** more often than do young people. Many experts believe that constipation is not a normal age-related change but rather is caused by such factors as low fluid intake, lack of dietary fiber, inactivity, drugs, depression, and hypothyroidism.

NURSING ASSESSMENT OF THE LOWER DIGESTIVE TRACT

HEALTH HISTORY

The complete health history is detailed in Chapter 39.

PHYSICAL EXAMINATION

Abdomen

For the abdominal examination, the patient should be supine, with the head raised slightly and the knees slightly flexed. The areas of the abdomen are commonly described as quadrants. An imaginary line is drawn horizontally across the abdomen at the level of the umbilicus. A second imaginary line extends from the sternum to the pubic bone. This creates the four quadrants: (1) the right upper quadrant, (2) the left upper quadrant, (3) the right lower quadrant, and (4) the left lower quadrant. Findings can then be documented by anatomic location (Fig. 40-1).

Inspection. Inspect the skin of the abdomen for color, texture, scars, striae ("stretch marks"), rashes, lesions, and dilated blood vessels. Describe the general contour of the abdomen as flat, convex (rounded), concave (sunken), protuberant, or distended. Note the location and contour of the umbilicus. Aortic pulsations and peristalsis are sometimes observed, especially in thin people.

Auscultation. After inspecting the abdomen, auscultate the abdomen to assess bowel sounds. Auscultate *before* palpating because palpation can alter normal bowel sounds. Warm the diaphragm of the stethoscope and then use it to listen to each quadrant. Normal bowel sounds include clicks and gurgles that occur 5 to 30 times per minute. Listen to each quadrant for at least 2 minutes. If no sounds are heard, it is important to listen for a full 5 minutes before recording bowel sounds as absent. Bowel sounds may be described as present, absent, increased, decreased, high-pitched, gurgling, tinkling, or gushing. Loud gurgling sounds are called borborygmi. Note any facial grimacing during auscultation. Record the presence or absence of bowel sounds in each quadrant.

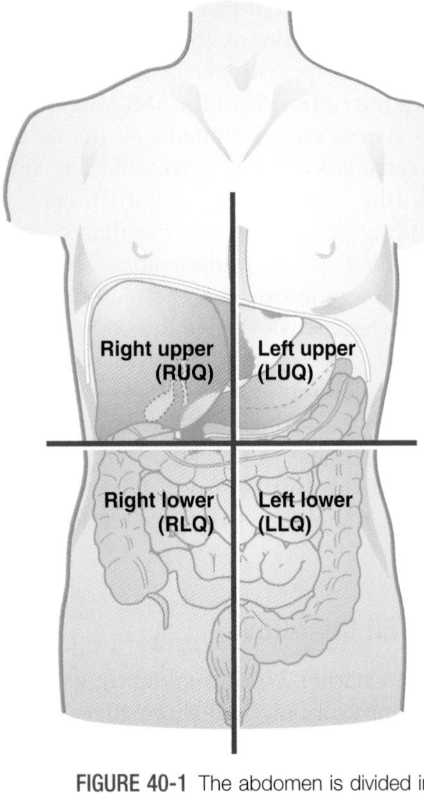

Quadrants of the abdomen and their underlying organs*

Right upper quadrant (RUQ) Adrenal gland (right) Colon (hepatic flexure and portions of ascending and transverse) Duodenum Kidney (portion of right) Liver (right lobe) Gallbladder Pancreas (head) Pylorus	Left upper quadrant (LUQ) Adrenal gland (left) Colon (splenic flexure and portions of transverse and descending) Kidney (portion of left) Liver (left lobe) Pancreas (body) Spleen Stomach
Right lower quadrant (RLQ) Appendix Bladder (if distended) Cecum Colon (portion of ascending) Kidney (lower pole of right) Ovary (right) Salpinx (uterine tube; right) Spermatic cord (right) Ureter (right) Uterus (if enlarged)	Left lower quadrant (LLQ) Bladder (if distended) Colon (sigmoid and portion of descending) Kidney (lower pole of left) Ovary (left) Salpinx (uterine tube; left) Spermatic cord (left) Ureter (left) Uterus (if enlarged)

*Small intestine loops in all quadrants.

FIGURE 40-1 The abdomen is divided into four quadrants. (From Black JM, Hawks JH: *Medical-surgical nursing: clinical management for positive outcomes*, ed 8, St. Louis, 2009, Saunders.)

Percussion. Nurses with advanced training in physical examination use percussion and palpation to collect additional data. Percussion is tapping on the skin to detect the presence of air, fluid, or masses in the underlying tissues. It also can be used to locate the margins of internal organs. Percussion over an air-filled organ produces a high-pitched, hollow sound called tympany. Tympany is similar to the sound made by a kettle drum. Percussion over a solid or fluid-filled structure sounds dull and flat. Normally, tympany is heard more often than dullness. All four quadrants of the abdomen should be percussed.

Palpation. Palpation is done to detect tenderness, sensitivity, masses, swelling, and muscular resistance. The examiner holds his or her fingers together and depresses the abdomen gently in all four quadrants. Light palpation depresses the abdominal wall only about 1 cm. Deep palpation uses more pressure. To assess for rebound tenderness, the abdomen is depressed and then quickly released. Grimacing or expressions of discomfort should be noted. Deep palpation and tests for rebound tenderness should be done only by people who are trained in these techniques.

Rectum and Anus

Gloves are worn when examining the anus and perianal area. Inspect the perianal skin for color, rashes, and lesions and note the presence of any external hemorrhoids. The rectal examination is performed by a trained examiner. The licensed vocational nurse/licensed practical nurse (LVN/LPN) may help to position, drape, and comfort the patient. The examiner inserts a gloved, lubricated finger into the rectum and points it toward the umbilicus. The patient is instructed to bear down as if to have a bowel movement. This relaxes the anal sphincter. The examiner palpates for lumps and tenderness in the rectum.

DIAGNOSTIC TESTS AND PROCEDURES

Diagnostic tests for lower gastrointestinal (GI) disorders include radiographic studies, endoscopic examinations, and laboratory studies. Always advise patients about the tests and procedures and ensure that required consent forms are signed.

For radiographs and imaging procedures, follow agency protocol regarding nothing-by-mouth (NPO) orders and any other preparation. If contrast media will be used, assess for allergy to the "dye," iodine, and shellfish. If the patient is allergic to any of these, the radiologist should be notified.

For laboratory blood tests, tell the patient that a blood sample will be taken and whether NPO is required. For a urine specimen, instruct the patient in the collection procedure.

RADIOGRAPHIC STUDIES

Radiographic studies include the upper gastrointestinal (UGI or GI) series (barium swallow), small bowel series, and barium enema examination. Radiographs of the gallbladder are obtained as well (discussed in Chapter 41). These studies allow the radiologist to study the structure and function of the digestive tract. A contrast medium is used in some studies. This is a substance, such as barium sulfate, that can be given orally or by enema. Sometimes air is introduced into the bowel for radiographic studies. This is called an air contrast procedure. When radiographs are taken, the contrast medium outlines the hollow organs of the digestive tract (Fig. 40-2).

Most hospitals and clinics have a specific protocol to follow before the examination to ensure that the GI tract is cleansed. If the patient is not properly prepared for the procedure, it may have to be repeated. Fluid restriction and bowel cleansing can be difficult for older or debilitated patients. If they become exhausted or if their vital signs change, the preparation should be stopped and the RN or physician notified. After the procedure, it is vital that the barium be cleared from the GI tract. See Figure 40-3 for an illustration of the time required for food and other substances to move through the digestive tract.

LABORATORY STUDIES

Occult Blood Test

Occult blood is blood that is not visible with the naked eye. Stool specimens are often tested for occult blood. To test for occult blood, a small sample of the stool is placed on a special type of paper that is then treated with a chemical. If blood is present, specific color changes are observed on the paper. Many facilities now require that specimens be sent to the laboratory for analysis. Nurses rarely perform this test on the unit.

Stool Examination

Stool specimens are examined most often for blood, bile, pathogenic organisms, and parasite ova (eggs). Fecal fat and the white blood cell (WBC) count may be determined in certain circumstances. Key points when stool examinations are ordered include the following:

1. Collect the specimen in a clean, dry container. Urine should not be in the container because it destroys parasites. Do not discard bathroom tissue in the container because the paper contains bismuth, which interferes with some tests.
2. It is best to deliver stool specimens to the laboratory immediately. If temporary storage is necessary, specimens for ova and parasites must be kept warm. Specimens for pathogens should be refrigerated.
3. When a stool specimen is being tested for occult blood, the patient should not eat red meat for 2

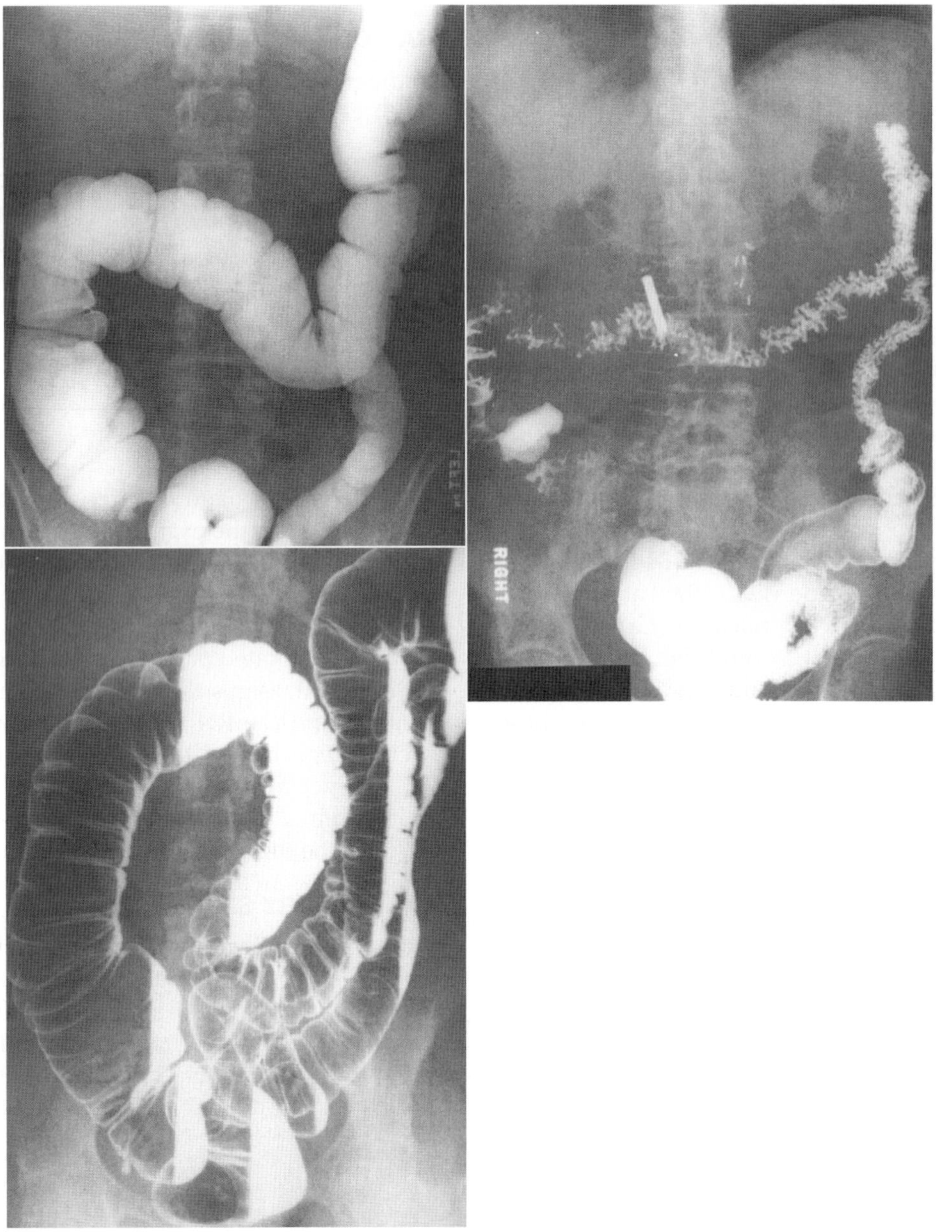

FIGURE 40-2 Contrast medium outlines the hollow organs of the digestive tract. (From Laufer I, Levine MC: *Double contrast gastrointestinal radiology*, ed 2, Philadelphia, 1992, Saunders.)

to 3 days before the specimen is collected. Red meat interferes with the test results.

4. Examples of drugs that may interfere with results are salicylates, ascorbic acid, anticoagulants, and steroids.
5. If visible blood or mucus is present in the stool, include it in the specimen sent to the laboratory.

Additional information about diagnostic tests and procedures is presented in Tables 39-1 and 40-1.

COMMON THERAPEUTIC MEASURES

DIGESTIVE TRACT SURGERY

Conditions of the large intestine that may require surgery include cancer, diverticulosis, appendicitis, polyps, obstruction, and ulcerative colitis. General care of the surgical patient is discussed in Chapter 17, and general care of patients having surgery on the digestive tract is addressed in Chapter 39.

DRUG THERAPY

Drugs that are commonly used for their effects on the digestive tract include emetics agents, antiemetics agents, laxatives agents, cathartics agents, antidiarrheals agents, antacids agents, anticholinergics agents, mucosal barriers, histamine$_2$ (H_2)-receptor blockers, proton pump inhibitors, 5-HT receptor antagonists agents, prostaglandins agents, and antibiotics agents. These drugs are discussed with the conditions for which they are prescribed. In addition, Table 39-23 in

Chapter 39 summarizes these drugs, their actions, and nursing interventions.

OBESITY

Obesity is defined as increased body weight caused by excessive body fat. The term *obesity* is used when a person's body mass index (BMI) is 30 kg/m^2 or more. This number is derived by dividing body weight in kilograms by height in meters squared. Although obesity is not classified as a disorder of the digestive tract, it is included here because the treatments affect the ingestion or absorption of food.

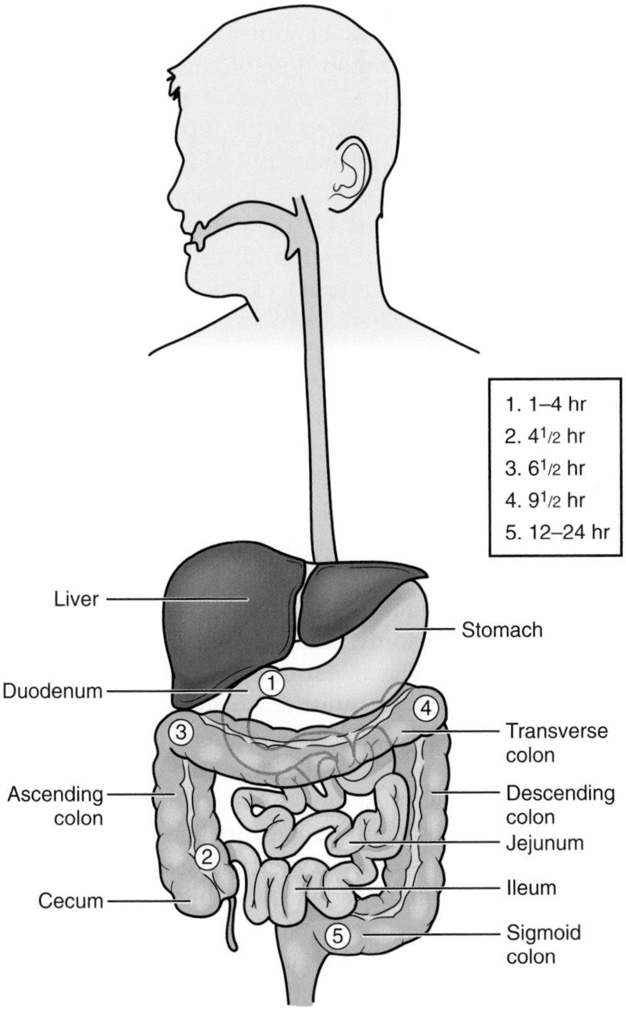

FIGURE 40-3 Time required for the passage of substances through the digestive tract.

CAUSES

Factors related to obesity include heredity, body build and metabolism, psychosocial factors, and some medications (e.g., some antipsychotic agents, antidepressants, antiepileptics, mood stabilizers, steroid hormones). Although many factors may contribute to obesity, the basic problem is that caloric intake exceeds metabolic demands. Excess food energy is converted to fat cells, which are capable of great expansion. When fat cells reach a certain size, they divide to form new fat cells. Fat cells decrease in size but not in number when a person loses weight.

Many attempts have been made to explain why some people become obese. A mechanism in the hypothalamus may regulate weight within a certain range. When a person's nutrient intake falls below the level required to maintain the set weight, the body conserves energy to maintain that weight. This may explain why some people always seem to return to a certain weight despite strict dieting and temporary weight loss.

COMPLICATIONS

Complications of obesity include cardiovascular and respiratory problems, polycythemia, diabetes mellitus, dyslipidemia, cholelithiasis (gallstones), infertility, endometrial cancer, and fatty liver infiltration. Obesity also aggravates degenerative joint disease. In addition, obesity can take its toll on the patient's emotional and social well-being. Very obese people may be ostracized and experience discrimination. Even health care providers sometimes treat obese patients as uncooperative and unmotivated.

MEDICAL DIAGNOSIS

Obesity may be defined using the formula in Box 40-1 or by comparison with standard weight tables. The amount of body fat can be estimated by measuring skinfold thickness at selected body sites. The health care provider may order tests of endocrine function to rule out correctable causes of obesity. Additional diagnostic tests and procedures may be done to detect complications associated with obesity.

Table 40-1 Diagnostic Tests and Procedures Lower Digestive Tract

TEST AND PURPOSE	PATIENT PREPARATION AND POSTPROCEDURE NURSING CARE
Colonoscopy visualizes the colon. Proctoscopy visualizes the rectum.	Lower digestive tract examinations include the following patient preparations: nothing by mouth (NPO) for 6–8 hours before the examination. The patient may be restricted to only liquids on the previous day or evening. Bowel cleansing may be done with cathartics, suppositories, and enemas.
Sigmoidoscopy visualizes the rectum and sigmoid colon.	Cathartics and suppositories are usually given on the evening before the test. Enemas may be ordered on the morning of the test until the colon is clear.

Box 40-1 Defining Obesity

FORMULA FOR BMI

$$\frac{\text{Weight (in kilograms)}}{\text{Height (in meters squared)}}$$

Normal: 18.5 to 24.9 kg/m^2
Overweight: 25.0 to 29.9 kg/m^2
Obese: 30.0 to 39.9 kg/m^2
Extremely obese: 40.0 kg/m^2 or more

MEDICAL AND SURGICAL TREATMENT

The primary treatment of obesity is a weight reduction diet accompanied by a planned exercise program. The ideal diet consists of foods from the four basic food groups and takes individual preferences into account (see *Patient Teaching* box). Very low–calorie diets are sometimes prescribed but have no greater long-term success than standard low-calorie programs. Sustained weight management requires changes in eating and activity patterns that are difficult for most people. A behavioral therapist can help the person to make gradual changes, achieve progressive goals, and overcome self-defeating thoughts. Drug therapy may be recommended under certain conditions when conservative treatment with diet and exercise has not been successful. Drugs that are available work by reducing appetite (sibutramine [Meridia]) or blocking the enzyme required for fat absorption (orlistat [Xenical]). To be effective, drugs must be used in combination with diet and exercise. Some antidepressants, including bupropion (Wellbutrin) and fluoxetine (Prozac), as well as the epilepsy drugs topiramate (Topamax) and zonisamide (Zonegran) have been shown to decrease the appetite (see *Complementary and Alternative Therapies* box).

Patient Teaching

Obesity

- A balanced, low-calorie diet is more effective over time than a faddish, quick weight loss program.
- Eating habits must be changed or any weight loss will be temporary.
- Goal weight should be determined with the health care provider and the dietitian. Realistic goals for weight loss should be set at 1 or 2 lb per week.
- A list of foods to include and those to avoid will be provided.
- Weighing food portions at the beginning of the diet makes you more aware of portion sizes.
- Physical activity is important for weight loss. With your health care provider's approval, gradually increase your activity as tolerance increases.

Complementary and Alternative Therapies

Ephedra sinica (ma huang) is prohibited in dietary supplements in the U. S. because it stimulates the body, especially the heart and central nervous system. The side effects can be most dangerous for people with hypertension, diabetes mellitus, prostate enlargement, and seizure disorders.

When extreme obesity (sometimes called morbid obesity) persists over a period of years despite conservative treatment, surgical intervention (bariatric surgery) may be recommended. Bariatric surgical procedures are either malabsorptive or restrictive. Malabsorptive procedures bypass a portion of the small intestine, which reduces food absorption. Restrictive surgery reduces the size of the stomach so that the patient feels full after eating only a small amount of food and takes in fewer calories. These procedures include Roux-en-Y gastric bypass (RNYGBP), sleeve gastrectomy (also called sleeve gastroplasty), duodenal switch with biliopancreatic diversion, and laparoscopic adjustable gastric banding.

RNYGBP is a common type of bariatric surgery. A small pouch that allows very small amounts of food and fluid to enter is created at the top of the stomach. The small intestine is then diverted from the main stomach below and connected to the pouch. Remember that the main part of the stomach remains and continues to make digestive juices. The portion of small intestine still attached to the main stomach is then reattached farther down to allow the digestive juices to flow into the small intestines. Sleeve gastrectomy does not affect the absorption of calories and nutrients in the same way as RNYGBP. Part of the stomach is removed. The smaller stomach cannot hold as much food, which lessens the production of the hormone called ghrelin. Less ghrelin may lessen the desire to eat, which in turn helps to decrease food intake.

Duodenal switch with biliopancreatic diversion, like sleeve gastrectomy, entails removal of a large part of the stomach. The distal end of the duodenum is attached to the large intestine so that food bypasses most of the small intestine, thereby reducing the absorption of calories and nutrients. The separated part of the small intestine is reattached to the duodenum to deliver bile and pancreatic digestive juices.

Lastly, laparoscopic adjustable gastric banding involves a band housing an inflatable balloon that is placed around the upper part of the stomach and is then held in place. This position creates a small stomachlike pouch above the band with a narrow opening into the rest of the stomach. The balloon can be deflated or inflated using a port placed under the skin of the abdomen. This procedure restricts the amount of food consumed but does not affect absorption.

NURSING CARE of the Obese Patient

Assessment

Assessment of the obese patient identifies factors that may contribute to obesity and explores the physical and psychosocial effects. If collecting data, record the patient's reason for seeking care. The past medical history documents pertinent chronic illnesses such as cardiac, respiratory, and orthopedic problems and diabetes mellitus. Ask about usual dietary practices and identify factors that trigger overeating and reactions to overeating. Inquire about interpersonal relationships, stresses, and coping strategies. In addition, collect data about previous efforts to lose weight and current interest in losing weight. Some aspects of the physical examination are more difficult when the patient is obese. For example, it may be difficult to auscultate heart, lung, and bowel sounds. Having the patient lean forward or lie on the left side may make it easier to hear heart sounds. Accurate measurement of blood pressure requires a large cuff. Scales must accommodate heavier patients.

When collecting these data, it is essential to convey an attitude of respect and concern. Be aware of your personal feelings about obese people and consider how these feelings affect the nurse-patient relationship.

Nursing Diagnoses, Goals, and Outcome Criteria: Obesity

Nursing Diagnoses	Goals and Outcome Criteria
Imbalanced Nutrition: More Than Body Requirements related to excessive calorie intake for metabolic needs	Appropriate nutrient intake: patient attains ideal body weight
Ineffective Peripheral Tissue Perfusion related to increased workload on heart	Adequate tissue perfusion: pulse and blood pressure within normal ranges
Ineffective Breathing Pattern related to restricted lung expansion	Effective ventilation: respiratory rate of 12 to 20 breaths/min without dyspnea
Disturbed Body Image related to excessive weight, perceived unattractiveness	Improved body image: positive patient statements about self, good grooming

Interventions for the Obese Patient Managed Nonsurgically

Imbalanced Nutrition: More Than Body Requirements

A registered dietitian should conduct the assessment of nutrition, development of a nutritional plan, and patient teaching for the obese patient. However, the nurse can reinforce what the patient has been taught. Before nutrition teaching begins, it is important to determine what the patient already knows and what he or she is motivated to learn.

Ineffective Peripheral Tissue Perfusion

Monitor the patient's tolerance of physical activity. Tachycardia and dyspnea suggest that the patient's tolerance has been exceeded. When an obese patient is hospitalized for a medical or surgical condition, take extra precautions to maintain circulation and respirations and to prevent skin breakdown. Position changes, deep breathing, and leg exercises reduce the risk of cardiopulmonary complications.

The obese patient is at increased risk for deep vein thrombosis (DVT) and pulmonary emboli when immobilized. Therefore early ambulation usually is ordered and the patient usually is treated with low-molecular-weight heparin (LMWH). Compression devices for the legs may be ordered. For the obese patient, the foot device may fit better than the long-leg device. Be sure to have adequate help when assisting the patient out of bed. Facilities that specialize in bariatric surgery usually are equipped and designed for safe movement of obese persons.

Ineffective Breathing Pattern

Monitor the patient's respiratory rate, effort, and breath sounds. During hospitalization, position changes and breathing exercises are especially important. The patient often breathes easier with the head of the bed elevated.

Disturbed Body Image

Demonstrate acceptance of obese patients by spending time with them, avoiding judgmental comments, and touching. Encourage the patient to identify solutions for overcoming perceived limitations imposed by weight. Acknowledge and compliment good grooming and attention to appearance and attributes other than physical size.

Interventions After Bariatric Surgery

After bariatric surgery, patients need the same care as any postoperative patient, as discussed in Chapter 17. However, the needs of the obese surgical patient that require special attention are covered here.

Nursing Diagnoses, Goals, and Outcome Criteria: Postoperative Bariatric Surgery

Nursing Diagnoses	Goals and Outcome Criteria
Impaired Gas Exchange related to weight of fatty tissue on chest	Effective gas exchange: vital signs and O_2 saturation within normal limits; breath sounds clear
Impaired Skin Integrity related to poor blood supply to adipose tissue, pressure and moisture of body tissue folds.	Skin warm, dry, intact, free of excess pressure: no redness, blanching, or breaks in skin; wound margins closed.
Imbalanced Nutrition: Less Than Body Requirements related to surgically reduced food ingestion and/or absorption.	Appropriate nutrient and supplement intake: patient loses weight at prescribed rate

Impaired Gas Exchange

Some obese people cannot expand the lungs fully because of the weight of fatty tissue on the chest. This increases the risk of postoperative atelectasis and pneumonia and makes breathing exercises and spirometry especially important. Elevating the head of the bed 30 to 45 degrees decreases pressure on the diaphragm. If the patient normally uses continuous positive airway pressure (CPAP) or bilevel positive airway pressure (BiPAP) equipment for sleep apnea, it will be needed during hospitalization as well. Monitor the results of serum electrolytes, blood urea nitrogen (BUN), and creatinine studies.

Impaired Skin Integrity

Skin and wound care is especially important for several reasons. The blood supply to adipose tissue is relatively poor, so healing is slow and pressure ulcers develop more readily. In addition, tissue folds tend to stay moist, so the patient may develop candidiasis. Therefore keep the skin clean and dry. Inspect the wound for intact margins. Instruct the patient to avoid strain on incision. Support abdomen with pillow for coughing and deep breathing. Avoid use of talcum powder and cornstarch; instead, place soft fabric between tissue layers to absorb moisture. Moisture barriers may be needed in the perineal area.

Imbalanced Nutrition: Less Than Body Requirements

Before the patient can be fed, imaging studies may be done to ensure that no leaks exist in the surgical sites in the digestive tract. The patient is advanced from water to clear liquids and then to full liquids. Initially the stomach or pouch will hold only 15 to 30 mL. Once solid food is permitted, the typical diet is 800 to 1200 calories per day in four to six small meals. The meals are high in protein and low in fat and carbohydrates. Multivitamin, calcium, and vitamin B_{12} supplementation may be needed. Dumping syndrome, described in Chapter 39, is a common problem. The patient can learn to avoid it by selecting appropriate foods in the proper amount.

DISORDERS AFFECTING ABSORPTION AND ELIMINATION

Malabsorption

Malabsorption is a term used to describe a condition in which one or more nutrients are not digested or absorbed. Among the many causes of malabsorption are bacteria, deficiencies of bile salts or digestive enzymes, alterations in the intestinal mucosa, and absence of all or part of the stomach or intestines. The specific effects of malabsorption depend on the type of deficiency that is present. Likewise, treatment is directed at replacing deficient enzymes or avoiding substances that cannot be absorbed. Two examples of malabsorption are (1) sprue and (2) lactase deficiency.

Two types of sprue exist: (1) celiac (nontropical) and (2) tropical. Celiac disease is caused by a genetic abnormality. It is characterized by severe changes in the intestinal mucosa and impaired absorption of most nutrients. Tropical sprue is caused by an infectious agent and results in malabsorption of fats, folic acid, and vitamin B_{12}.

People with lactase deficiency do not have adequate lactase to metabolize lactose. These people are said to have lactose intolerance. Lactase deficiency may be inherited or acquired. Causes of acquired lactase deficiency include inflammatory bowel disease (IBD), gastroenteritis, and sprue syndrome (see *Cultural Considerations* box).

Cultural Considerations

What Does Culture Have to Do with Malabsorption?

Inherited lactase deficiency is most prevalent among African Americans, Asians, and South Americans. The dietitian should be contacted to help the patient design a culturally appropriate diet.

Signs and Symptoms. A common sign of malabsorption is **steatorrhea**, the presence of excessive fat in the stool. Stools are large, bulky, foamy, and foul smelling. Patients also may have weight loss, fatigue, decreased libido, easy bruising, edema, anemia, and bone pain. Bloating, cramping, abdominal cramps, and diarrhea are symptoms of lactase deficiency that commonly occur within several hours of consuming milk products.

Medical Diagnosis. The diagnosis of sprue and celiac disease is based on laboratory studies, endoscopy with biopsy, and radiologic imaging studies. Lactase deficiency is diagnosed on the basis of the health history, the lactose tolerance test, a breath test for abnormal hydrogen levels, and, if necessary, biopsy of the intestinal mucosa.

Medical Treatment. Sprue is treated with diet and drug therapy. Foods that aggravate the patient's symptoms are eliminated from the diet. Celiac disease is treated by avoiding products that contain gluten (i.e., wheat, barley, oats, rye). Severe symptoms may be treated with corticosteroids. Tropical sprue is treated with antibiotics, oral folate, and vitamin B_{12} injections.

Lactase deficiency can be treated by eliminating milk and milk products from the diet, although many adults can tolerate small amounts of lactose without symptoms. Lactase enzyme can be mixed with milk or taken before drinking milk to avoid symptoms. Some milk and milk products that have been treated with lactase also are available. If milk products are limited, the diet must be assessed for adequacy of calcium, vitamin D, and riboflavin. Supplements may be advised.

NURSING CARE of the Patient with Malabsorption

Document the patient's symptoms and note stool characteristics. In the case of celiac sprue, it is helpful to teach the patient how to eliminate gluten from the diet. Today there are many products that are free of gluten and can be purchased from specialty food stores and supermarkets. Administer antibiotics as ordered for tropical sprue. If folic acid therapy is to be continued, instruct the patient in self-medication. The effect of therapy is evaluated by the return of normal stool consistency. Advise the patient with lactase deficiency of dietary restrictions and alternative products.

Diarrhea

Diarrhea is defined as the passage of loose, liquid stools with increased frequency. The patient also may have cramps, abdominal pain, and a feeling of urgency before bowel movements.

Causes. Many factors can cause diarrhea. They include spoiled foods, allergies, infections, diverticulosis, malabsorption, cancer, stress, fecal impactions, and tube feedings. Diarrhea is an adverse effect of some medications.

Complications. Diarrhea is usually temporary and causes no serious problems. However, it does pose an increased threat to the very old, the very young, and those in poor health. These individuals are more likely to become dehydrated and experience electrolyte imbalances and metabolic acidosis. Chronic diarrhea interferes with absorption of nutrients and can lead to malnutrition and anemia.

Medical Treatment. Acute diarrhea is usually treated by resting the digestive tract and giving antidiarrheal drugs. In the outpatient setting, the patient is advised to consume only clear liquids (see *Complementary and Alternative Therapies* box). A variety of liquids, such as broth, gelatin, and clear fruit juices, provide water, electrolytes, and some calories. Hospitalized patients may be placed on NPO status and given intravenous fluids. Severe, persistent diarrhea may require total parenteral nutrition (TPN). When diarrhea begins to improve, the diet gradually is expanded to include full liquids, bland solids, and then all other food.

Complementary and Alternative Therapies

Natural substances that can help to control diarrhea include rice water (made by boiling rice and straining the water), potatoes, and unpeeled apples. An herbal remedy is goldenseal, which is effective for diarrhea caused by some bacteria. However, high doses of this herb can cause dangerous central nervous system (CNS) stimulation and uterine contractions, which contraindicate its use during pregnancy.

NURSING CARE of the Patient with Diarrhea

Assessment

Nursing assessment of the patient with diarrhea can help to determine possible causes, the severity and progress of the condition, the complications, and the effect of treatment. Therefore the data that the nurse collects are very important. The history should record the presence of diarrhea and detail the onset, severity, precipitating factors, and measures that bring relief. Describe the pain that accompanies diarrhea and ask the patient about stool characteristics, including amount, color, odor, and unusual contents such as blood, mucus, or undigested food. The functional assessment focuses on usual diet, dietary changes, recent and current medications, and recent travel to a foreign country. It is also important to assess the patient's ability to get to the toilet independently or to call for assistance with toileting.

Important aspects of the physical examination include vital signs, weight, and tissue turgor. Tissue turgor is often assessed by gently pinching the tissue on the forearm. If the pinched tissue flattens as soon as it is released, tissue turgor is generally considered good. This test is not a good indicator of hydration in older adults because their tissue is less elastic, regardless of hydration. Palpate the abdomen for distention or tenderness and inspect the perianal area for irritation. A rectal examination should be performed as agency policy permits if the nurse believes that the patient may have fecal impaction.

Diarrhea is a nursing diagnosis but other related diagnoses, as outlined in the following box, also may be appropriate for the patient with diarrhea.

Nursing Diagnoses, Goals, and Outcome Criteria: Diarrhea

Nursing Diagnoses	Goals and Outcome Criteria
Deficient Fluid Volume related to fluid loss from diarrhea	Adequate hydration: pulse and blood pressure within patient norms, moist mucous membranes, urine output equal to fluid intake
Imbalanced Nutrition: Less Than Body Requirements related to failure to absorb nutrients	Adequate nutrition: patient attains and maintains normal body weight
Acute Pain related to abdominal cramping and rectal irritation	Pain relief: patient states less or no pain, relaxed manner
Impaired Skin Integrity related to irritation of diarrhea stool	Intact skin: no perianal redness, lesions
Self-Care Deficit, Toileting related to weakness or decreased level of consciousness	Improved self-care ability: patient uses toilet independently and without injury

Interventions

Deficient Fluid Volume and Imbalanced Nutrition: Less Than Body Requirements

The prevention of serious fluid and electrolyte imbalances requires careful monitoring and replacement of fluid losses. When patients have severe diarrhea, keep intake and output records. Whenever possible, measure liquid stools. Stool characteristics are also important and should be recorded. Signs and symptoms that suggest possible fluid imbalances include unequal fluid intake and output; decreased blood pressure; changes in pulse rate or rhythm; changes in respiratory rate or depth; confusion; muscle weakness, tingling, or twitching; dry mucous membranes; and poor tissue turgor. These changes may indicate serious imbalances in water and electrolytes. They should be recorded and reported promptly.

The daily fluid intake should be 2000 to 3000 mL of various fluids. Carefully monitor the flow rates of intravenous fluids. Excessive or rapid fluid replacement can cause heart failure, especially in older adults.

Acute Pain

Abdominal cramping associated with diarrhea is often relieved by antidiarrheal drugs that reduce intestinal activity. Record the severity, duration, and location of the pain as well as the effects of drug therapy.

Impaired Skin Integrity

Liquid stool is very irritating to the anal and perianal areas. With frequent bowel movements, skin breakdown may occur. If necessary, assist the patient with perianal care after each stool. Wash the area thoroughly and gently with warm water and mild soap, rinse, and then pat dry with a soft towel. Protective creams, sprays, or lotions can be applied.

Self-Care Deficit, Toileting

Older persons or those who are acutely ill may have difficulty with toileting during diarrhea episodes. If possible, they should be placed in rooms close to the nurses' station. Staff should be aware of the need to respond promptly to call bells. A bedside commode is recommended if the toilet is too far from the bed. Patients who are unable to call for help must be checked frequently for the presence of diarrhea stools (see *Coordinated Care* box).

> **Coordinated Care**
>
> **Helping Certified Nursing Assistants Assist with Toileting**
>
> Because certified nursing assistants (CNAs) usually assist patients with personal care, they are most likely to assist with toileting. The CNAs should inform the nurse if the patient has difficulty with defecation or has abnormal stools such as diarrhea or stools containing blood, mucus, or undigested food.

Constipation

The frequency of defecation varies among healthy people. Bowel movements may occur as often as two or three times daily or as seldom as once a week. If the stool is soft and is passed without difficulty, the patient is not constipated. Constipation is a condition in which a person has hard, dry, infrequent stools that are passed with difficulty.

> **Pharmacology Capsule**
>
> Laxatives, cathartics, enemas, and suppositories usually relieve constipation promptly but the effects of stool softeners are not seen for several days.

Causes. Many factors can contribute to constipation. When stool is present in the rectum, the urge to defecate occurs. If the urge is ignored, stool remains in the rectum longer than usual and becomes dry. It is then more difficult, and sometimes painful, to have a bowel movement. People who frequently ignore the urge to defecate may become chronically constipated. The frequent use of laxatives or enemas also may contribute to chronic constipation. These agents keep the lower digestive tract empty and eventually interfere with the normal pattern of elimination.

Because physical activity promotes normal bowel elimination, people who are inactive are at risk for constipation. Inadequate water intake can lead to constipation because more water will be reabsorbed from the stool in the large intestine. Diet significantly affects the stool. A diet that is low in fiber and high in foods such as cheese, lean meat, and pasta promotes constipation.

Drugs that slow intestinal motility or increase urine output also contribute to constipation. Examples of these drugs are those used for anesthesia, pain relief, and cold symptoms. Medical conditions that may be related to constipation include diseases of the colon or rectum as well as brain or spinal cord injury. Abdominal surgery causes a loss of intestinal activity but it should be temporary.

Many people believe that constipation is normal for older people. Normal age-related changes in the large intestine do not explain the frequent complaints of constipation by older adults. More likely, when constipation does occur, it is related to inactivity, drug therapy, long-term laxative or enema abuse, or some medical condition.

Many older adults grew up believing that a daily bowel movement was necessary for health. If a day passed without a bowel movement, they used laxatives or enemas to produce one. Over time, this practice fosters laxative or enema dependence. Eventually the person is unable to have a bowel movement without the laxative or enema. This dependence, established over many years, is very difficult to correct.

Complications. When people are constipated, they have to strain to have bowel movements. Straining occurs when a person attempts to exhale with the glottis closed, causing increased pressure in the chest and abdominal cavities. This is called the Valsalva maneuver. The pressure slows the flow of circulating blood back into the chest, causing a brief drop in pulse and blood pressure. Relaxation allows a rush of blood back into the chest, with a resulting rise in pulse and blood pressure. The rapid changes in blood flow can be fatal to a patient with heart disease. Therefore prevention of constipation and straining is very important in the care of cardiac patients.

Chronic constipation also contributes to the development of hemorrhoids. Another complication of constipation is fecal impaction, which is discussed below.

Medical Treatment. Treatment of constipation is directed toward immediate relief of the problem and prevention of future episodes. Laxatives, suppositories, enemas, or a combination is ordered to get prompt results. The health care provider may prescribe stool softeners as well. Stool softeners, as the name suggests, promote normal elimination by allowing more water to be held in the stool so that it is softer and more easily passed. It takes several days for the effects of stool softeners to be seen, so they are not used for acute constipation. They are relatively safe drugs that are often prescribed over a long period of time. The trade names of some stool softeners are Colace, Surfak, and Metamucil.

Metamucil is an example of a bulk-forming stool softener. In the intestinal tract, it absorbs water to produce a gel-like mass to aid in the passage of a soft stool. If the patient does not take adequate fluids, the mass can harden and cause obstruction in the intestine. Table 39-2 provides additional information about drugs used to treat constipation.

NURSING CARE of the Patient with Constipation

Assessment

The assessment of bowel elimination may detect constipation or risk factors that may cause it. Data that contribute to the assessment include the patient's usual pattern of bowel elimination, including frequency, amount, color, unusual contents (blood, mucus, undigested food), and pain associated with defecation. Note recent changes in any of these factors. Information about diet, exercise, and drug therapy is helpful in revealing potential risk factors for constipation. If any aids to elimination (laxatives, stool softeners, enemas, suppositories) are used, record the type and frequency of use.

Examine the abdomen for distention or visible peristalsis and auscultate for bowel sounds in all four quadrants. When severe constipation is accompanied by mild diarrhea, a rectal examination should be done to detect a fecal impaction if agency policy permits.

Nursing Diagnosis, Goal, and Outcome Criterion: Constipation

Nursing Diagnosis	Goal and Outcome Criterion
Constipation related to drug therapy, diet, inadequate fluid intake, inactivity, neuromuscular disorders, or laxative abuse	Establishment of normal bowel elimination: regular passage of formed stools without straining

Interventions

Constipation

The first action is directed at relieving the patient's constipation. Sometimes the health care provider will write an order for a laxative or an enema as needed. An enema or suppository is preferred if the patient is very uncomfortable because it usually acts within 1 hour. A laxative may take as long as 8 to 10 hours.

When a laxative is truly needed, it should be given. However, laxatives are often abused. Frequent use can lead to physical and psychologic dependence. Laxatives also can produce diarrhea, which may lead to excessive loss of fluids and electrolytes (see *Complementary and Alternative Therapies* box).

Complementary and Alternative Therapies

Herbs that have a laxative effect include aloe, cascara sagrada, and senna. Other complementary therapies include abdominal massage in a circular pattern with essential oil of rose, marjoram, fennel, or rosemary.

Nurses are often responsible for managing the bowel elimination of severely disabled people. This is especially true in long-term care facilities. It is critical to record and describe all stools so that problems can be found and treated early. Teach certified nursing assistant (CNAs) the importance of keeping accurate records. If detected early, constipation may be treated easily with a mild laxative or suppository. Severe constipation may require repeated enemas and laxatives for relief (see *Patient Teaching* box).

Patient Teaching

Constipation

- Include high-fiber foods such as fruits, raw vegetables, greens, and whole grains in the diet.
- Drink six to eight 8-oz glasses of water each day unless the health care provider has restricted fluid intake for some reason.
- Exercise daily. It need not be strenuous; walking is excellent exercise.
- Go to the bathroom promptly in response to the urge to have a bowel movement.
- Contrary to popular opinion, it is not necessary to have a bowel movement every day. A bowel movement every 2 or 3 days without pain or straining is normal for some people.
- Use a toilet that is comfortable. Feet should touch the floor, causing the hips to bend slightly. Use a footstool if necessary. This helps use of the abdominal muscles.
- Laxatives can be used safely for occasional constipation. If they are used frequently, however, they can interfere with normal elimination. Consult your health care provider for a recommended laxative.

In many cases, bowel elimination can be maintained with diet, fluids, exercise, and regular toilet habits. Occasional use of elimination aids is not harmful. However, some patients require nursing interventions to promote elimination over a long period.

Megacolon. Megacolon is a condition in which the large intestine loses the ability to contract effectively enough to propel the fecal mass toward the rectum. These patients usually need regular enemas for bowel cleansing. Other measures are generally not adequate. Patients who have special problems with constipation are those with neurologic conditions such as spinal cord injuries and cerebrovascular accident (CVA). The management of bowel elimination in these patients and the process of bowel retraining are discussed in Chapters 28 and 29.

Fecal Impaction. All nursing staff should understand the possibility of fecal impaction in the physically or mentally impaired person. Fecal impaction refers to the retention of a large mass of stool in the rectum that the patient is unable to pass. Some liquid stool trickles around the impaction and may be mistaken for diarrhea.

Consider possible impaction when a patient who has not had a bowel movement for several days has repeated episodes of mild diarrhea. If agency policy permits, assess for impaction by inserting a gloved, lubricated finger into the rectum. The fecal mass is usually easily felt. It may be very hard or soft.

The impaction should be removed following agency protocol or the health care provider's specific orders. This process usually requires administration of a mineral oil enema to soften hard stool, followed by a soapsuds enema. It may be necessary to break up and remove the mass manually. This procedure is painful and embarrassing for the patient. With good nursing care, manual extraction should rarely be necessary.

Intestinal Obstruction

Causes. Intestinal obstruction can be caused by many factors, including strangulated hernia, tumor, paralytic ileus, stricture, **volvulus** (twisting of the bowel), intussusception (telescoping of the bowel into itself), and postoperative adhesions. When the bowel is obstructed, digestive contents cannot progress. Volvulus and intussusception are illustrated in Figure 40-4.

Signs and Symptoms. Symptoms are most acute when an obstruction is located in the proximal portion of the small intestine. Early symptoms of obstruction are vomiting (possibly projectile), abdominal pain, and constipation. Gastric contents are vomited first, followed by bile and then fecal matter. Blood or purulent drainage may be passed rectally. Abdominal distention may develop, especially with colon obstruction.

Complications. If blood supply to the intestine is impaired, gangrene and perforation of the bowel may occur. Untreated obstruction can result in shock and death.

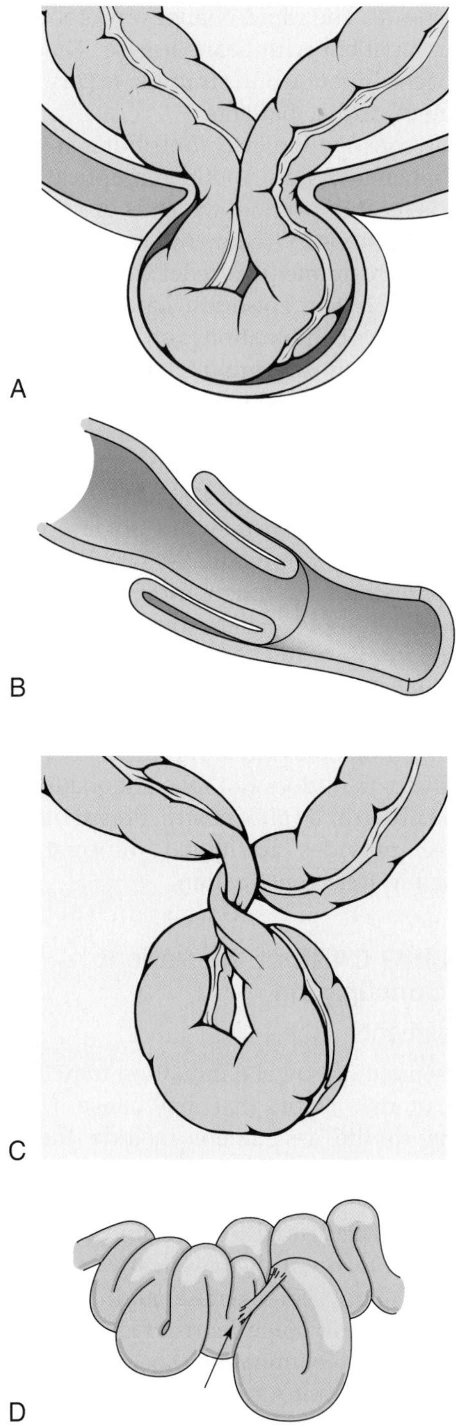

FIGURE 40-4 Causes of mechanical bowel obstruction. **A,** Incarcerated hernia. **B,** Intussusception. **C,** Volvulus. **D,** Adhesions. (From McCance KL, Huether SE: *Understanding pathophysiology*, ed 5, St. Louis, 2013, Mosby.)

Medical Diagnosis. Intestinal obstruction is considered possible based on the patient's history, physical examination, and laboratory studies. It is confirmed by radiologic studies.

Medical Treatment. The initial treatment of obstruction is GI decompression. A nasoenteral tube is passed and connected to suction. Intravenous fluids are provided. Depending on the cause of the obstruction, surgical intervention may be necessary.

NURSING CARE of the Patient with Intestinal Obstruction

Assessment

Ask about the patient's symptoms, including pain and nausea, and describe the onset and progression of those symptoms. The past medical history should include potentially related conditions, such as hernia, cancer of the digestive tract, and abdominal surgeries. Ask when the patient's last bowel movement was and if the characteristics were normal.

Take vital signs to detect signs of infection (e.g., fever, tachycardia) and impending shock (e.g., tachycardia, hypotension). Assess skin moisture and tissue turgor along with moisture of the mucous membranes. Inspect the patient's abdomen for distention and visible peristalsis. Auscultate for rapid, high-pitched tinkling bowel sounds and gently palpate for tenderness and guarding. Note any rectal bleeding or drainage.

Nursing Diagnoses, Goals, and Outcome Criteria: Intestinal Obstruction

Nursing Diagnoses	Goals and Outcome Criteria
Acute Pain related to distention	Pain relief: patient states less or no pain, relaxed manner
Deficient Fluid Volume related to vomiting, intestinal suction	Normal hydration: pulse and blood pressure within patient norms, moist mucous membranes, equal fluid intake and output
Risk for Infection related to complications of obstruction	Absence of infection: no fever, normal white blood cell (WBC) count
Ineffective Breathing Pattern related to abdominal distention	Effective ventilation: respiratory rate of 12 to 20 breaths/min without dyspnea
Anxiety related to pain, anticipated surgery	Decreased anxiety: patient states less or no anxiety, calm manner

Interventions

Acute Pain

Give analgesics as ordered and assess effectiveness. If the health care provider is withholding analgesics while making a diagnosis, inform the patient of this and use other pain relief strategies, such as massage and relaxation.

Deficient Fluid Volume

Promote fluid balance by providing intravenous fluids as ordered. Monitor the patient's vital signs, intake, and output. If a nasoenteral tube is ordered, place it per protocol, monitor output, and ensure free drainage at all times.

Risk for Infection

Monitor the patient's temperature. Signs of intestinal rupture (i.e., increasing tenderness, sudden sharp pain, abdominal rigidity) must be reported to the health care provider immediately.

Ineffective Breathing Pattern

Elevate the patient's head to relieve pressure on the diaphragm. Encourage deep breathing and coughing and administer oxygen as ordered. When surgery is planned, carry out preoperative orders, which often include giving an enema and intravenous fluids.

Anxiety

Give simple explanations of what is being done and what the patient should expect postoperatively if surgery is scheduled. Stress the importance of deep breathing, turning, coughing, and leg exercises.

POSTOPERATIVE NURSING CARE of the Patient with Intestinal Obstruction

Postoperative care depends on the surgical procedure performed.

Appendicitis

Pathophysiology. The appendix is a blind pouch in the cecum. Appendicitis is an inflammation of the appendix. Inflammation occurs when the opening of the appendix to the large intestine is blocked by feces, tumors, **helminths** (a worm classified as a parasite), or indigestible substances such as seeds. The tissue becomes infected by bacteria in the digestive tract. Pus accumulates, the blood supply is impaired, and the appendix may rupture. A ruptured appendix allows digestive contents to enter the abdominal cavity, causing peritonitis—a life-threatening surgical emergency. Early detection of appendicitis may permit treatment before the appendix ruptures.

Signs and Symptoms. The initial symptom of appendicitis is usually pain in the epigastric region or around the umbilicus, which then shifts to the right lower quadrant. The classic symptom of appendicitis is pain at McBurney point, which is located midway between the umbilicus and the iliac crest (Fig. 40-5). The patient may have temperature elevation and nausea and vomiting. Because of the pain, the patient may assume a position of hip flexion. The right leg cannot be straightened without pain. An elevated WBC count indicates the presence of infection.

Signs and symptoms of peritonitis are absence of bowel sounds, severe abdominal distention, increased pulse and temperature, nausea, and vomiting. The abdomen may be rigid, although this sign is often absent with peritonitis in older patients. Consider

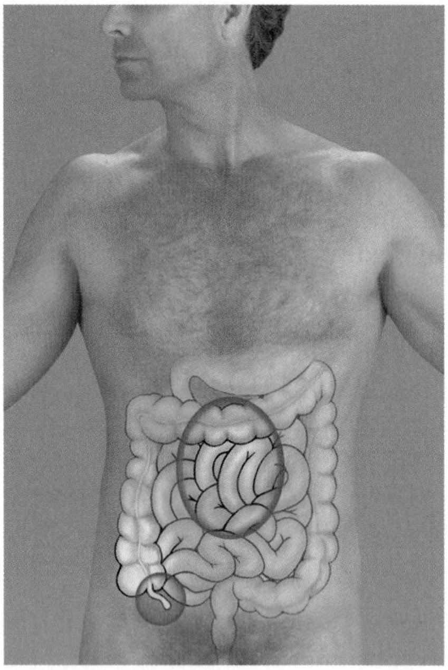

FIGURE 40-5 McBurney point is located in the right lower quadrant, midway between the anterior iliac crest (*in smaller circle*) and the umbilicus (*in larger circle*). Localized tenderness here is typical of appendicitis. (From Monahan FD, Drake DT, Neighbors M, editors: *Medical-surgical nursing: foundations for clinical practice*, ed 2, Philadelphia, 1998, Saunders.)

possible shock if the patient begins to lose consciousness and is cool and pale.

Medical Diagnosis. A diagnosis of appendicitis is based on classic signs and symptoms and a WBC count of 10,000 to 15,000/mm^3.

Medical Treatment. When appendicitis is suspected, the patient is placed on NPO status. A cold pack to the abdomen may be ordered. Laxatives and heat applications should never be used for undiagnosed abdominal pain. If the appendix is inflamed, heat or laxatives may cause it to rupture.

If rupture has not occurred, immediate surgical treatment is indicated. With a ruptured appendix, surgery may be delayed 6 to 8 hours while antibiotics and intravenous fluids are given.

NURSING CARE of the Patient with Appendicitis

Assessment

The patient's chief complaint is usually pain. Describe the location, severity, onset, duration, precipitating factors, and alleviating measures in relation to the pain. In the past medical history, note previous abdominal distress, chronic illnesses, and surgeries. Record allergies and any medications the patient may be taking. Review of systems assesses the presence of nausea and vomiting. Significant data in the physical examination are temperature; abdominal pain, distention, and tenderness; and the presence and characteristics of bowel sounds.

Nursing Diagnoses, Goals, and Outcome Criteria: Appendicitis

Nursing Diagnoses	Goals and Outcome Criteria
Risk for Infection (peritonitis) related to appendix rupture	Absence of infection: normal body temperature and vital signs, bowel sounds present, abdomen soft
Deficient Fluid Volume related to nausea, vomiting, medical restriction of fluid intake	Normal fluid balance: pulse and blood pressure within patient norms, moist mucous membranes, serum electrolytes within normal limits, fluid intake equal to output
Acute Pain related to inflammation of appendix or surgical tissue trauma	Pain relief: patient states less or no pain, relaxed manner
Ineffective Breathing Pattern related to incisional pain or anesthesia	Effective ventilation: respiratory rate of 12 to 20 breaths/min, clear breath sounds
Fear related to sudden emergency status, minimal preoperative teaching	Reduced fear: patient states less or no fear, calm manner

Preoperative Interventions

Before surgery, the patient probably will be most comfortable in a semi-Fowler or side-lying position with the hips flexed. Because the pain location and pattern help the health care provider to make a diagnosis, analgesics may be withheld initially. This should be explained to the patient. If rupture is suspected, elevate the patient's head to localize the infection.

Postoperative Interventions

Postoperatively the patient receives antibiotics, intravenous fluids, and possibly GI decompression. Assist the patient in turning, coughing, and deep breathing to promote expansion of the lungs. Incentive spirometry also can be useful. Show the patient how to splint the incision during deep breathing using a pillow or blanket. Early ambulation is usually ordered to reduce the risk of postoperative complications. Inspect the abdominal wound for redness, swelling, and foul drainage and provide wound care as ordered or according to agency policy.

If no complications occur, the patient is usually discharged in a day or two. Initially, lifting objects is usually limited to 5 to 10 pounds. Normal activities can be resumed in 2 to 3 weeks.

Peritonitis

Pathophysiology. Peritonitis is inflammation of the peritoneum caused by chemical or bacterial contamination of the peritoneal cavity. Chemical contamination may follow rupture of a digestive tract structure, including the appendix. Bacterial contamination may be caused by rupture of a digestive tract structure or fallopian tube or from nonsterile, traumatic wounds.

When a chemical or bacterial contaminant is present, the body's defenses attempt to wall off the area to contain the injury. Fluid shifts out of the bloodstream into the peritoneal cavity. Peristalsis slows or stops. If defenses are adequate, the offending fluid remains localized and is eventually eliminated. Complications of peritonitis include abscesses, adhesions, septicemia, hypovolemic shock, paralytic ileus, and possible organ failure.

Signs and Symptoms. Signs and symptoms of peritonitis include pain over the affected area, rebound tenderness, abdominal rigidity and distention, fever, tachycardia, tachypnea, nausea, and vomiting. The older patient may have more subtle symptoms with less pain and the absence of abdominal rigidity.

Medical Diagnosis. A diagnosis of peritonitis is suspected on the basis of the patient's history and physical examination. Diagnostic tests and procedures done to confirm the inflammation include a complete blood count (CBC), serum electrolyte measurements, abdominal radiography, computed tomography (CT), and ultrasound. Paracentesis may be done to obtain a specimen of fluid for culture.

Medical Treatment. A nasogastric tube is inserted for GI decompression. Intravenous fluids, antibiotics, and analgesics are ordered. Surgery may be done to close a ruptured structure and to remove foreign material and fluid from the peritoneal cavity.

NURSING CARE of the Patient with Peritonitis

Assessment

Begin by asking about the patient's present illness. Because pain is the prominent symptom, record the onset, location, and severity of the pain and any related symptoms. When peritonitis is suspected, record a history of abdominal trauma, including surgery. It is also important to take and record vital signs, inspect the abdomen for distention, and auscultate for the presence of bowel sounds. Evaluate fluid status, including tissue turgor, moisture of mucous membranes, and intake and output.

Interventions

Acute Pain

Administer opioid analgesics as ordered for pain. Position the patient with the head elevated and offer comfort measures, such as massage and relaxation techniques. Notify the health care provider if pain relief is not achieved.

Decreased Cardiac Output

The shift of fluid from the blood into the peritoneal cavity may be so great that the patient develops deficient intravascular fluid volume. Cardiac output falls and perfusion of vital organs is reduced. Administer intravenous fluids as ordered and monitor fluid intake and output. Monitor vital signs and immediately report increasing pulse, restlessness, pallor, and decreasing blood pressure. In addition to deficient fluid volume, the patient may go into shock because of septicemia (the presence of bacteria in the blood). This patient requires intense monitoring and probably will be placed in the intensive care unit. Report findings immediately to the health care provider.

Nursing Diagnoses, Goals, and Outcome Criteria: Peritonitis

Nursing Diagnoses	Goals and Outcome Criteria
Acute Pain related to inflammation	Pain relief: patient states pain is reduced or relieved, has relaxed manner
Decreased Cardiac Output related to decreased blood volume	Normal cardiac output: pulse and blood pressure within patient norms, skin warm and dry, fluid output equal to intake
Imbalanced Nutrition: Less Than Body Requirements related to nausea, vomiting, nothing-by-mouth (NPO) status	Adequate nutrition: stable body weight
Anxiety related to threat of serious illness and invasive treatment	Decreased anxiety: patient states anxiety is reduced or relieved, calm manner

Imbalanced Nutrition: Less Than Body Requirements

GI decompression usually eliminates nausea and vomiting but antiemetics may be ordered as needed. Check to ensure that the nasogastric tube is draining at all times.

Anxiety

The patient is likely to be anxious because of pain and uncertainty about what is happening. Even when a sense of urgency exists in caring for the patient, give simple explanations for procedures and tell the patient what to expect. Encourage the patient to ask questions. If surgery is planned, essential preoperative teaching may have to be done quickly. Explain to the patient the importance of breathing and leg exercises after abdominal surgery. The health care provider may order sedatives to calm the patient.

POSTOPERATIVE NURSING CARE of the Patient with Peritonitis

Postoperative care is like that for any major surgery and is described in Chapter 17. Care specific to surgery on the digestive tract is addressed in Chapter 39 under "Common Therapeutic Measures."

Abdominal Hernia

Pathophysiology. Muscles play an important role in keeping the abdominal organs in place. Weakness in those muscles may allow a portion of the large intestine to push through the abdominal wall. The bulging portion of intestine through the weak muscle is called a hernia. Hernias occur most often in areas where the abdominal wall is already weak. Weak locations include the umbilicus and the lower inguinal areas of the abdomen (Fig. 40-6). Hernias also may develop at the site of a surgical incision.

Hernias are classified as reducible or irreducible. A reducible hernia slips back into the abdominal cavity with gentle pressure or when the patient lies on his or her back. When the hernia cannot be manipulated back into place, it is said to be irreducible, or incarcerated. An irreducible hernia may impair blood flow to the trapped loop of intestine, causing it to become gangrenous. A hernia that is trapped and deprived of blood is said to be strangulated. This is treated as a medical emergency.

Signs and Symptoms. Hernias are usually diagnosed when a patient reports a smooth lump on the abdomen. The lump may disappear when the patient is lying down or at rest but returns when standing or straining. Heavy lifting or coughing usually causes the hernia to appear.

Hernias usually are not painful unless they become incarcerated. With incarceration, the patient has severe abdominal pain and distention, vomiting, and cramps.

Medical Diagnosis. Hernias are diagnosed on the basis of the health history and physical examination.

Medical Treatment. Surgical repair of hernias is usually recommended even if they are reducible. Repair prevents the possibility of incarceration. Two surgical procedures are used to repair hernias. Herniorrhaphy is the repair of the muscle defect by suturing. If additional measures are needed to strengthen the abdominal wall, a hernioplasty is done. Strong materials are used to cover and reinforce the defect.

Some patients cannot tolerate the stress of surgical hernia repair. For them, a truss may be advised, although trusses are not used as widely as in the past (see *Patient Teaching* box). A truss consists of a pad that is placed over the hernia and a belt that holds it in place. It provides support for the weak muscles.

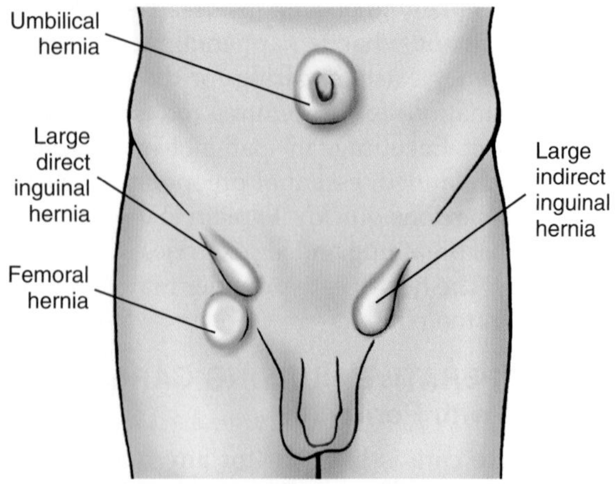

FIGURE 40-6 Abdominal hernias. (From Monahan FD, Drake DT, Neighbors M, editors: *Medical-surgical nursing: foundations for clinical practice*, ed 2, Philadelphia, 1998, Saunders.)

Patient Teaching

Truss

- Put the truss on before rising each morning.
- Check under the pad and belt several times daily for skin irritation.
- The truss does not cure a hernia, so you still should avoid straining.

NURSING CARE of the Patient with Abdominal Hernia

Assessment

Begin the assessment with the patient's chief complaint, usually a smooth lump in the abdomen that appears and disappears with various activities and positions. Ask about pain and vomiting, which may be present if the hernia is strangulated. Have the patient explain his or her work and home responsibilities to identify the type of physical exertion required. The most relevant aspect of the physical examination is the assessment of the abdomen. Inspect for abnormalities and listen for bowel sounds in all four quadrants. If the patient wears a truss, examine the skin underneath it for signs of irritation.

Nursing Diagnoses, Goals, and Outcome Criteria: Abdominal Hernia

Nursing Diagnoses	Goals and Outcome Criteria
Risk for Injury related to hernia strangulation or distention	Absence of injury (strangulation): normal pulse and temperature without abdominal pain
Impaired Skin Integrity related to pressure created by the truss	Absence of complications caused by truss: intact skin without redness under truss

Preoperative Interventions

Risk for Injury

Monitor the patient for signs and symptoms of strangulation (i.e., nausea, vomiting, pain, abdominal distention, fever, tachycardia). If these symptoms develop, it is vital to notify the health care provider immediately. It is important for the nonsurgical patient to know that these symptoms should be reported.

Determine what restrictions the patient has in relation to physical exertion and provide verbal and written instructions to the patient.

Impaired Skin Integrity

Teach patients who use a truss what measures to take to avoid injury to the skin.

1. Step into the truss and pull it up over the hips. If a belt is provided, wrap the belt around the abdomen surrounding the area of the hernia.
2. Insert the hernia pad or pads into the truss (if the truss does not already have pads attached). If there are hernias on both sides of the abdomen, insert a second pad.
3. Gently press the pads to push the hernia or hernias back into the abdominal cavity. Secure straps or tighten the belt to hold the pads in place and maintain compression on the hernia or hernias.

Remember, a truss should be worn only for a short period of time. It must be properly fitted and worn to be effective. Wearing a truss is not an alternative form of treatment. Patients should be advised to follow the guidelines and recommendations of their health care provider. Surgical intervention is the usual course of action taken to repair hernias.

Nursing Diagnoses, Goals, and Outcome Criteria: Abdominal Hernia Repair

Nursing Diagnoses	Goals and Outcome Criteria
Impaired Urinary Elimination related to abdominal surgery, anesthesia	Normal urinary function: urine output approximately equal to fluid intake, no bladder distention
Constipation related to immobility, effects of anesthesia, and abdominal surgery	Normal bowel elimination: formed stools at regular intervals without pain or straining
Acute Pain related to scrotal swelling	Pain relief: patient states there is less or no pain, relaxed manner
Risk for Injury (wound dehiscence) related to stress on wound margins	Well-healed wound: margins intact, decreasing redness and swelling

■ Postoperative Interventions

The general postoperative care of patients who have undergone surgery is discussed in Chapter 17. In addition to the routine postoperative assessments, after hernia repair the nurse should be especially concerned with assessing bowel and bladder elimination, wound healing, and the patient's knowledge about ways to avoid placing stress on the healing surgical wound.

Impaired Urinary Elimination

Many patients have temporary problems with urination after hernia repair surgery. Keep intake and output records, document voiding, and palpate for bladder distention.

Constipation

Bowel activity also may cease temporarily in response to the anesthesia and manipulation of the bowel during surgery. Therefore monitor bowel sounds and note the passage of **flatus**. Like any other patients having major surgery, patients undergoing hernia repair need to keep their lungs clear to prevent complications. Encourage them to turn and deep breathe but they should not cough or sneeze. Coughing and sneezing put tension on the surgical incision and repaired tissues.

Acute Pain

Scrotal swelling is common after inguinal hernia repair. A scrotal support and an ice pack can greatly reduce the painful swelling.

Risk for Injury

Activities are usually restricted for 2 to 6 weeks. Reinforce the health care provider's instructions about refraining from exertion and lifting. Advise the patient to report fever or wound drainage to the health care provider.

Inflammatory Bowel Disease

Pathophysiology. IBD refers to ulcerative colitis and Crohn disease. Crohn disease is also known as regional enteritis. In both conditions, inflammation and ulceration of the lining of the intestinal tract occurs. With ulcerative colitis, the inflammation typically begins in the rectum and gradually extends up the bowel toward the cecum. The progression of Crohn disease is different in that it can affect any area of the GI tract. Although the terminal ileum is most often affected, there may be multiple sites interspersed with healthy segments of bowel.

The two conditions have similar symptoms and are treated in much the same way medically. However, surgical options are different.

A patient with IBD may have a few isolated attacks or may have a chronic condition. With chronic IBD, attacks may last for days or even months, followed by periods of remission lasting several weeks to several years.

Causes. The exact cause of IBD is unknown. Possible causes that are being studied include infectious agents, autoimmune reactions, allergies, heredity, and foreign substances (see *Cultural Considerations* box). In the past, it was thought that IBD might be caused by stress. However, current thinking suggests that stress is a result of IBD rather than its cause.

Cultural Considerations

What Does Culture Have to Do with Inflammatory Bowel Disease?

Inflammatory bowel disease (IBD) is more common among Caucasians and people of Middle-Eastern origin than among African Americans and Asian Americans.

Signs and Symptoms. The symptoms of IBD vary with the extent of the disease. When ulcerative colitis affects only the rectum, the patient may be constipated. More commonly, however, patients have diarrhea with frequent bloody stools and abdominal cramping. In severe cases, the patient also may have fever and weight loss.

Symptoms of Crohn disease are even more variable, depending on the areas affected. If the stomach and duodenum are involved, symptoms include nausea, vomiting, and epigastric pain. Involvement of the small intestine produces pain, abdominal tenderness, and cramping. An inflamed colon typically causes abdominal pain, cramping, rectal bleeding, and diarrhea. Systemic signs and symptoms include fever, night sweats, malaise, and joint pain.

Complications. The local complications of IBD include hemorrhage, obstruction, perforation (rupture), abscesses in the anus or rectum, fistulas, and megacolon. Patients who have had ulcerative colitis for 10 years have a greatly increased risk of cancer of the large intestine. Patients with Crohn disease also are thought to have an increased risk of colon cancer, although the relationship is less clear.

Systemic complications also may be found with ulcerative colitis. These are conditions outside the intestine but related to the colitis. They include inflammation of the joints and eyes, skin lesions, urinary stones, and liver disease. Of course, severe or prolonged diarrhea can result in malnutrition, anemia, and fluid and electrolyte imbalances.

Medical Diagnosis. IBD is suspected on the basis of the history and physical examination. Abdominal radiography may be done to rule out obstruction before additional tests are done. To confirm the diagnosis, the health care provider may order a colonoscopy with biopsy, a barium enema examination with air contrast, ultrasonography, CT, and cell studies. The video capsule that is swallowed by the patient provides a view of the small intestine that is not accessible by endoscopy.

Medical Treatment. Treatment of IBD addresses the local and the systemic effects of the disorders. Intestinal inflammation is treated with drug therapy, diet, and rest. The following drugs may be used alone or in combination, depending on the specific situation:

- Corticosteroids—to decrease inflammation in mild to moderately severe episodes (not for maintenance therapy)
- Immunosuppressant agents—to inhibit the immune response
- Antidiarrheal agents—to control diarrhea (except in severe colitis)
- Anticholinergics—to reduce pain and GI motility and secretions
- Antibiotics—to treat mild to moderately severe attacks of Crohn disease (usually sulfasalazine, mesalamine, olsalazine; sometimes metronidazole, ciprofloxacin, cephalexin, or sulfamethoxazole/trimethoprim); antibiotics are not very useful for ulcerative colitis.
- Aminosalicylates—specifically 5-ASA (mesalamine oral, suppository, or enema; or sulfasalazine) to reduce symptoms
- Iron supplements and vitamin B_{12}—to treat anemia
- Infliximab (Remicade)—to block the inflammatory process in Crohn disease for patients who do not respond well to azathioprine (may be given in combination with azathioprine)
- Antidepressants—sometimes helpful

Patients with ulcerative colitis are usually maintained between acute episodes with aminosalicylates; however, 6-MP is appropriate in some circumstances. Crohn disease is less responsive to aminosalicylates, so the patient may be maintained on azathioprine or 6-MP.

Research is underway to assess the effects of other drugs, including monoclonal antibodies and cytokine interleukin-10. Based on the low incidence of IBD among smokers, therapy with nicotine transdermal patches or gum also is being studied.

A low-roughage diet without milk products is prescribed for mild to moderate IBD. Intravenous fluids or TPN may be needed to provide fluid, electrolytes, and nutrients when symptoms are severe.

Although most patients respond to medical treatment, some require surgery. Removal of the colon (colectomy) is curative for ulcerative colitis. When the colon is removed, an artificial opening from the small intestine through the abdominal wall is needed to allow elimination of digestive wastes. The opening is called an ileostomy. Although good health is usually restored after this surgery, an ileostomy is permanent and requires special care. Therefore surgery is not usually done unless all other measures have failed. Care of the patient with an ostomy is covered in Chapter 26.

Surgical treatment of Crohn disease is more likely to involve removal of the diseased portion of the intestine. Recurrence is so common that surgery is not usually done unless necessitated by serious complications. Postoperatively the disease typically reappears at the site of anastomosis within 1 year. Newly affected areas also may appear in other sections of the intestine.

Pharmacology Capsule

Corticosteroids suppress the immune and inflammatory responses, so the patient is more susceptible to infection.

NURSING CARE of the Patient with Inflammatory Bowel Disease

The nursing care of a patient during an acute attack of IBD is concerned with ongoing assessment, comfort measures, skin care, emotional support, and administering drugs and monitoring the effects. The nursing needs of the patient with IBD who undergoes surgery are like those of other patients who have undergone GI surgery, as discussed under "Common Therapeutic Measures" in Chapter 39.

Assessment

Assessment of the patient with IBD should identify the symptoms that caused the patient to seek care—usually pain and diarrhea. Record the onset, location, severity, and duration of pain. Note factors that contribute to the onset of pain, such as specific foods or stressors, as well as the onset and duration of diarrhea and the presence of blood. Explore the effect of the illness on the patient's life and how the patient copes.

Important aspects of the physical examination are vital signs, height and weight, and measures of hydration (tissue turgor, mucous membrane moisture). Inspect the perianal area for irritation or ulceration. Maintain accurate intake and output records, measuring and counting diarrhea stools as output if possible.

Nursing Diagnoses, Goals, and Outcome Criteria: Inflammatory Bowel Disease

Nursing Diagnoses	Goals and Outcome Criteria
Acute Pain related to abdominal cramping, perianal irritation	Pain relief: patient states pain is reduced or relieved, manner is relaxed
Diarrhea related to intestinal inflammation	Cessation of diarrhea: stools formed, less frequent
Deficient Fluid Volume related to diarrhea	Adequate hydration: pulse and blood pressure within patient norms, moist mucous membranes
Imbalanced Nutrition: Less Than Body Requirements related to malabsorption	Adequate nutrition: stable body weight

Nursing Diagnoses, Goals, and Outcome Criteria: Inflammatory Bowel Disease—cont'd

Nursing Diagnoses	Goals and Outcome Criteria
Ineffective Coping related to chronic illness	Effective coping: patient reports strategies to deal with inflammatory bowel disease (IBD), patient sees disease as manageable
Risk for Injury related to adverse drug effects	Absence of adverse drug effects: normal urine output, electrolyte and blood glucose levels within normal limits, no bruising

Interventions

Acute Pain

Perianal pain is treated with gentle cleansing, sitz baths, and skin protectants. Measures to relieve abdominal pain include administration of analgesics and antispasmodics and application of heat to the abdomen as ordered. Positioning, massage, relaxation, imagery, and other strategies, as described in Chapter 15, also may be used.

Put on Your Thinking Cap!

Compare and contrast ulcerative colitis and Crohn disease. How are they similar and how are they different?

Diarrhea

Easy access to a toilet and prompt response to calls for help reduce the chance of episodes of bowel incontinence. After each stool, gently clean and inspect the perianal area. If bedpans or bedside commodes are used, remove and clean them immediately and use room deodorizers to eliminate odors.

Prescribed drugs for diarrhea usually include antidiarrheals, antispasmodics, anticholinergics, antibiotics, and corticosteroids. The patient may be placed on NPO status or may be given only clear liquids when diarrhea is severe. Bed rest may be prescribed or the patient may be encouraged simply to rest (see *Patient Teaching* box).

Patient Teaching

Inflammatory Bowel Disease

Topics for patient teaching include the following:

- Stress reduction measures are recommended to help control your symptoms.
- Because people with inflammatory bowel disease (IBD) have increased risk of cancer, you should have regular colon screening.
- You can facilitate digestion by taking small bites, eating slowly, and chewing well.
- Avoid caffeine and other irritating fluids and foods; consume a high-calorie, low-residue diet.

Continued

Patient Teaching—cont'd

- You need to know the names, dosages, and schedules of your prescribed drugs and know what effects should be reported to the health care provider.
- Resources: National Foundation for Ileitis and Colitis: www.worldcat.org/identities/lccn-n83209215

Deficient Fluid Volume

Severe diarrhea can quickly deplete the patient's fluid volume. Assess fluid status on an ongoing basis. Signs of fluid volume deficit are dry mucous membranes, hypotension, tachycardia, and decreased urine output. Intravenous fluids and TPN should be administered as ordered.

Imbalanced Nutrition: Less Than Body Requirements

The patient with ulcerative colitis needs to avoid only foods that worsen symptoms. For the patient with Crohn disease, TPN and elemental enteral diets (e.g., Ensure) may be prescribed. The patient who is able to take solid food is usually placed on a low-residue diet without caffeine, pepper, or alcohol. Foods that are not allowed include whole grains, nuts, and raw fruits and vegetables. Consult a dietitian to teach the patient about the prescribed diet. Monitor the patient's weight on a routine basis.

Ineffective Coping

IBD is painful and stressful and can interfere with the patient's everyday life. Try to establish a trusting relationship with the patient. Encourage independence, participation in care and decision making, and realistic goal setting. People who have IBD may benefit from therapy that assists them with stress management. With the patient's approval, initiate a referral to a mental health professional or spiritual counselor. Report sadness and discouragement to the RN or health care provider.

Risk for Injury

Nursing responsibilities in relation to drug therapy for IBD include administering the drugs, monitoring their effects, and teaching the patient about long-term drug therapy. Sulfasalazine is the antibiotic most often prescribed for patients with ulcerative colitis. It is useful in treating acute attacks and preventing future attacks. After an acute attack has subsided, the drug dosage is gradually reduced. A low-maintenance dose may be given for as long as 1 year. Teach the patient that discontinuing the drug early may result in another acute attack.

Sulfasalazine can cause crystals to form in the urine (crystalluria), which can damage the kidneys. Therefore patients taking this drug should take enough fluids to maintain a urine output of 1500 mL/day. A high urine output reduces the risk of crystalluria.

Corticosteroids are used in IBD for their ability to reduce inflammation. Unfortunately this action also decreases the ability of the body to resist infection. Patients on steroids must be monitored for any signs and symptoms of infections. Instruct these patients to avoid unnecessary exposure to others with infectious conditions.

Long-term steroid therapy can have many other serious side effects. These include fluid and electrolyte imbalances, ulcers, increased blood glucose, weight gain, elevated blood pressure, acne, capillary fragility, and hirsutism (abnormal growth of hair).

Diverticulosis

Pathophysiology. Diverticulosis is a condition characterized by small, saclike pouches in the intestinal wall called diverticula. Diverticula occur when weak areas of the intestinal wall allow segments of the mucous membrane to herniate outward (Fig. 40-7). Most diverticula are found in the sigmoid colon and usually more than one exists.

Risk Factors. Because diverticulosis is most common in developed countries, it is thought that lack of dietary residue is a contributing factor. Other related factors are older age, constipation, obesity, and emotional tension.

Signs and Symptoms. Diverticulosis is often asymptomatic but many people report changes in bowel habits. The change may be constipation, diarrhea, or periodic bouts of each. Other symptoms might include

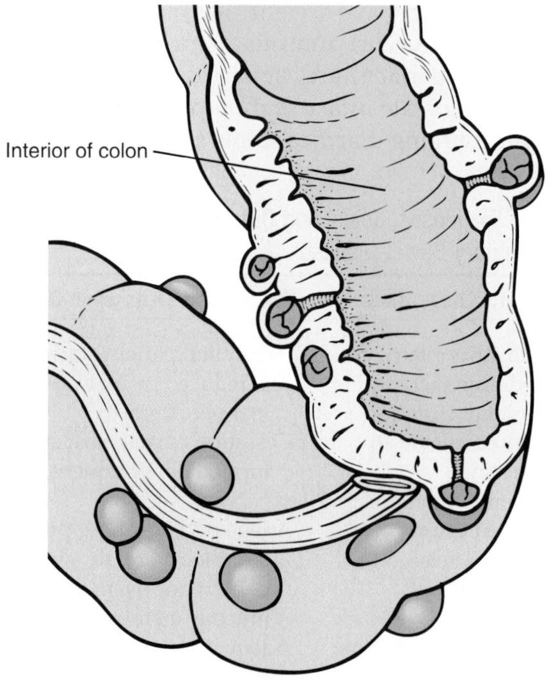

FIGURE 40-7 Diverticula in the sigmoid colon. (From Lewis SM, Heitkemper MM, Dirksen SR, et al.: *Medical-surgical nursing: assessment and management of clinical problems*, ed 9, St. Louis, 2015, Mosby.)

rectal bleeding, pain in the left lower abdomen, nausea and vomiting, and urinary problems.

Complications. Intestinal contents can lodge in diverticula, causing inflammation or infection. The patient is then said to have diverticulitis. Diverticulitis may be related to irritating foods, alcohol, chronic constipation, and persistent coughing. Symptoms of pain and bleeding are more severe with diverticulitis. The patient also may have a fever.

Possible complications of diverticulitis are severe bleeding, obstruction, perforation (rupture), peritonitis, and fistula formation. A fistula is an abnormal opening. In this case, it is most likely to develop between the colon and the bladder or vagina. The fistula permits bowel contents to pass into these other structures.

Medical Diagnosis. Diverticulosis may be suspected on the basis of the patient's symptoms. The stool is tested for occult blood. Abdominal CT and barium enema examination allow the health care provider to confirm the presence of diverticula. Because these procedures are invasive, they are delayed if signs and symptoms of acute inflammation exist.

Medical Treatment. Diverticulosis is currently treated with a high-residue diet without spicy foods. Stool softeners or bulk-forming laxatives are used to treat constipation and antidiarrheal agents are prescribed for those who have diarrhea. If pain is severe, it may be treated with analgesics. Opioids, especially morphine, should not be given because they cause constipation and may increase pressure in the sigmoid colon. Broad-spectrum antibiotics are often prescribed. Anticholinergics may be given to decrease spasms in the colon.

During periods of acute inflammation, the patient is placed on bed rest and NPO status. Intravenous fluids are ordered. GI decompression also may be instituted.

If symptoms persist and complications occur, surgical intervention may be necessary. The affected portion of the colon is removed. A temporary colostomy may be created to rest the colon while the surgical incisions heal. Sometimes elective surgery is recommended because the risk of surgical complications is much lower than it is with emergency surgery.

NURSING CARE of the Patient with Diverticulosis

Monitor the patient's comfort and stool characteristics. Note any nausea and vomiting, monitor the patient's temperature, and examine the abdomen for distention and tenderness.

Interventions

Provide fluids as permitted and monitor the patient's intake and output. Give antiemetics as ordered for nausea. Analgesics and anticholinergics may be given as ordered for pain. Be alert for signs of perforation

Nursing Diagnoses, Goals, and Outcome Criteria: Diverticulitis

Nursing Diagnoses	Goals and Outcome Criteria
Deficient Fluid Volume related to diarrhea and vomiting	Adequate hydration: pulse and blood pressure within patient norms, urine output approximately equal to fluid intake, moist mucous membranes
Acute Pain related to inflammation	Pain relief: patient states pain is decreased or relieved, has relaxed manner
Risk for Infection related to perforation	Absence of infection: no fever, normal white blood cell (WBC) count, abdomen soft and not tender

(i.e., fever, abdominal distention, rigidity). Teach the patient about diverticulosis, including the pathophysiology, treatment, and symptoms of inflammation.

If surgery is performed, the nursing care is similar to that described for any major abdominal surgery. General surgical care is discussed in Chapter 17 and care of the patient with an ostomy is discussed in Chapter 26.

Colorectal Cancer

Pathophysiology. Colorectal cancer, or cancer of the large intestine, is the third most common cancer. People at greater risk for colorectal cancer are those with histories of IBD or family histories of colorectal cancer or multiple intestinal polyps. Some evidence indicates that a high-fat, low-fiber diet and inadequate intake of fruits and vegetables also may contribute to the development of this type of cancer.

Colorectal cancer can develop anywhere in the large intestine. Three fourths of all colorectal cancers are located in the rectum or lower sigmoid colon.

Signs and Symptoms. Signs and symptoms of colorectal cancer depend on the location of the disease. In the early stages, symptoms are usually mild. If the cancer is located on the right side of the abdomen, the patient may have only vague cramping until the disease is advanced. Unexplained anemia, weakness, and fatigue related to blood loss may be the only early symptoms of right-sided colon cancer.

Cancers on the left side or in the rectum cause more obvious changes in bowel function. Patients may develop diarrhea or constipation and may notice blood in the stool. Stools may become very narrow, causing them to be described as pencil-like. This is because of pressure on the bowel from the growing tumor, which causes a narrowed lumen. The patient may report a feeling of fullness or pressure in the abdomen or rectum. If left untreated, obstruction of the bowel eventually occurs regardless of the tumor site.

Medical and Surgical Treatment. Colorectal cancers usually are treated surgically. The exact surgical procedure depends on the location and extent of the cancer. For cancers above the rectum, the diseased portion of the intestine often can be removed. The healthy ends of the remaining intestine are then anastomosed (connected).

Rectal cancers often require more extensive surgery, with incisions in the abdomen and the perineum (abdominoperineal resection). With removal of the rectum, a permanent colostomy may be created for fecal elimination. However, relatively new procedures may be used to attach the rectal stump to the anus in patients with certain rectal cancers. When this is possible, normal bowel elimination can be maintained and a colostomy can be avoided.

Combination chemotherapy may be recommended postoperatively if the tumor extends through the bowel wall or if lymph nodes are involved. Early-stage rectal cancer is sometimes treated with radiation and surgery.

❖ NURSING CARE of the Patient with Colorectal Cancer

Because the primary treatment for colon cancer is surgery, nursing care focuses on the surgical patient. Preoperative care includes bowel preparation, hydration, emotional support, and teaching postoperative routines to prevent surgical complications. Care of the patient with an ostomy is discussed in Chapter 26 and care of patients who are receiving radiation or chemotherapy is discussed in Chapter 25.

■ Assessment

In the postoperative period, assess vital signs, intake and output, breath sounds, bowel sounds, and pain. Describe the appearance of wounds and wound drainage. If the patient has a colostomy, measure and describe the fecal drainage. Assess the patient's reactions to the surgical procedure and any other anticipated therapies.

■ Interventions

Risk for Injury

The nursing care of a patient after an abdominoperineal resection is very demanding. The patient has three incisions: one on the abdomen, a second for the colostomy, and a third on the perineum. Check all three incisions for bleeding or drainage. The perineal wound normally drains a large amount of serosanguineous fluid. Serosanguineous fluid is made up of serum and blood. It is a pinkish color and thin in consistency. The wound may be open and packed, partly closed with Penrose drains, or closed and drained with a suction device. An example of a suction drainage system is the Jackson-Pratt drain and fluid collection device. Dressings should initially be reinforced when saturated. Disposable waterproof pads under the patient's hips protect bedding and can be changed easily. A T-binder holds the perineal dressing securely in place.

With so many wounds, especially open ones, these patients are at great risk for infection. Any handling of wound dressings should be done wearing sterile gloves. Always assess the wound for signs of infection (i.e., unusual odor, excessive redness or swelling around the wound, purulent drainage).

If packing has been placed in a wound, it will be removed gradually. Once the packing has been removed completely, the health care provider may order the wound to be irrigated on a regular schedule. Gentle irrigations promote healing by keeping the wound clean. It is important to use strict sterile technique during wound irrigation.

Ineffective Peripheral Tissue Perfusion

Because the abdominoperineal resection requires several incisions and is a lengthy procedure, the patient is at risk for respiratory and circulatory complications. Coughing, deep breathing, and incentive spirometry help to prevent fluid accumulation in the lungs. Encourage and help the patient to change positions at least every 2 hours. Leg exercises are important because the pressure on abdominal blood vessels during the long surgery may contribute to the formation of blood clots in the legs.

Acute Pain

Pain is severe for several postoperative days. Give opioid analgesics as ordered. Inform the health care provider if the drugs do not provide relief. In addition to drug therapy, implement comfort measures such as position changes and back rubs. At first, the patient

Nursing Diagnoses, Goals, and Outcome Criteria: Colorectal Cancer

Nursing Diagnoses	Goals and Outcome Criteria
Risk for Injury related to extensive surgical trauma, open wounds	Wound healing without infection: no fever, intact wound margins without excessive redness
Ineffective Peripheral Tissue Perfusion related to effects of anesthesia, immobility	Adequate tissue perfusion: vital signs consistent with patient baseline norms
Acute Pain related to tissue trauma	Pain relief: patient states less or no pain, relaxed manner
Sexual Dysfunction related to perineal surgery	Patient understanding of potential sexual dysfunction: patient describes possible problems and corrective measures
Ineffective Coping related to life-threatening illness	Effective coping: patient uses strategies that promote adaptation to illness

will probably be most comfortable in a side-lying position. Later, he or she will be able to tolerate being supine as well.

When the patient is allowed to be up, sitz baths may be ordered several times a day. The warm water cleans, soothes, and increases circulation to the perineum. Supervise the patient in the sitz bath the first few times in case of dizziness or faintness.

Sexual Dysfunction

Extensive perineal surgery can cause various types of sexual dysfunction. Be open and sensitive to questions that the patient may bring up about sexual function. Refer questions about the specific effects of particular surgical procedures on sexual function to the health care provider. The nurse should not dismiss or ignore patient concerns about sexuality but the information given must be accurate. Once the correct answers are known, the nurse can reinforce them.

Ineffective Coping

Patients with colorectal cancer and their families often face a difficult period of adjustment. For many people, the thought of having cancer brings up fears of pain, suffering, and a lingering death. These fears may not surface until after the patient recovers from the acute postoperative period. The nurse can help by encouraging the patient to express fears and ask questions and by being a kind listener. Referral to mental health or spiritual counselors or to support groups can be helpful (see *Patient Teaching* box).

Patient Teaching

Colorectal Cancer

As the patient improves, the nurse needs to consider long-term needs. The teaching plan should include the following:

- Wound care
- Colostomy care (see Chapter 26)
- Information about resources for treatment of sexual dysfunction (if appropriate)
- Diet (Your diet should be high in fiber. Avoid irritating foods and alcohol.)
- Medications (For each of your medications, know the drug names, dosages, schedule, and adverse effects.)
- Symptoms of inflammation (Promptly notify the health care provider if these symptoms of inflammation occur: bleeding, fever, and increased pain.)
- Resources: Enterostomal therapist (a nurse who is expert in the care of patients with ostomies); United Ostomy Association, www.ostomy.org.

While learning to deal with changes in body image and the threat of a potentially deadly disease, the patient may be faced with receiving chemotherapy as well. Most patients have heard about the side effects of the powerful drugs used in chemotherapy and they may be justifiably fearful of the treatments. The nursing care of patients who are receiving chemotherapy is discussed in detail in Chapter 25.

Polyps

Polyps are small growths in the intestine. Most are benign but they can become malignant. Two inherited syndromes, familial polyposis and Gardner syndrome, are characterized by multiple colorectal polyps and almost always lead to cancer. Polyps are usually asymptomatic and are found on routine testing. Potential complications are bleeding and obstruction. Polyps are diagnosed by a barium enema examination or an endoscopic examination. Some of the growths can be removed during the endoscopic examination. Colectomy may be advised for patients with familial polyposis or Gardner syndrome because of the high risk of malignancy.

Patients who are at risk for cancer should be encouraged to seek medical attention. If the patient has surgery, the postoperative care is similar to that of the patient with cancer of the colon. If a colostomy is created, the patient needs special support and teaching, as described in Chapter 26.

Hemorrhoids

Hemorrhoids are dilated veins in the rectum. They may be above the sphincter muscles of the anus (internal hemorrhoids) or below these muscles (external hemorrhoids) (Fig. 40-8). If blood clots form in external hemorrhoids, they become inflamed and very painful. Hemorrhoids containing clotted blood are said to be thrombosed.

Risk Factors. A key factor in the development of hemorrhoids is increased pressure in the rectal blood vessels. Pressure is increased by constipation, pregnancy, and prolonged sitting or standing.

Signs and Symptoms. The most common symptoms of hemorrhoids are rectal pain and itching. Bleeding may occur with defecation, especially if the hemorrhoids are internal. External hemorrhoids are easy to see and appear red or bluish.

Medical Diagnosis and Treatment. Hemorrhoids are diagnosed on visual inspection. Nonsurgical treatment of hemorrhoids attempts to relieve pain, swelling, and pressure. Topical medications such as creams, lotions, or suppositories may be ordered to soothe and shrink inflamed tissue (see *Complementary and Alternative Therapies* box). Sitz baths are often comforting. The health care provider may order heat or cold applications. Sometimes, especially with thrombosed hemorrhoids, ice packs may be applied for a few hours, followed by warm packs.

Complementary and Alternative Therapies

Witch hazel compresses applied to the anus after each bowel movement are soothing.

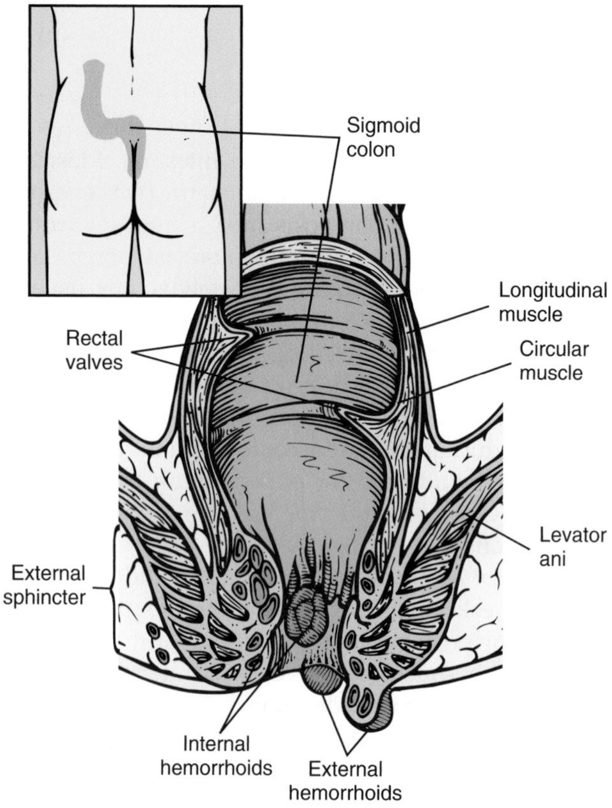

FIGURE 40-8 Internal and external hemorrhoids. (From Monahan F, Sands J, Neighbors M, et al.: *Phipps' medical-surgical nursing: health and illness perspectives*, ed 8, St. Louis, 2007, Mosby.)

A hemorrhoidectomy is the surgical excision (removal) of hemorrhoids. It is necessary when symptoms are very severe. After the hemorrhoids are removed, the wound may be closed with sutures or packed and left open to heal.

Outpatient procedures for removing hemorrhoids include the following:

- Ligation—tying off with rubber bands. The bands cut off the blood supply so that the vessels shrink and die. Dead tissue eventually breaks off and is eliminated.
- Sclerotherapy—the injection of an agent into the tissue around the hemorrhoids that causes them to shrink. Results often are temporary.
- Thermocoagulation and electrocoagulation—use of different types of devices to remove the hemorrhoid.
- Laser surgery—effective but more expensive and risky.

❖ NURSING CARE of the Patient with Hemorrhoids

Medical management of hemorrhoids usually does not require hospitalization. Therefore this section emphasizes the care of the surgical patient. Preoperative care includes bowel preparation and patient teaching of postoperative measures to prevent complications of immobility and anesthesia.

■ Assessment

After hemorrhoidectomy, monitor vital signs, intake and output, and breath sounds. Inspect the perianal area for bleeding and drainage.

Nursing Diagnoses, Goals, and Outcome Criteria: Post-Hemorrhoidectomy

Nursing Diagnoses	Goals and Outcome Criteria
Acute Pain related to tissue trauma	Pain relief: patient states less or no pain, relaxed manner
Impaired Skin Integrity related to surgical procedure	Healthy wound healing: surgical incision healed, no signs of infection (excessive redness, purulent drainage, continued pain)
Constipation related to patient fear of pain with defecation	Normal defecation: patient passes stool with minimal pain

■ Interventions

Acute Pain

Hemorrhoidectomy patients have severe postoperative pain that requires opioid analgesics for relief. Cold packs over the rectal dressing may be ordered initially. Imagery and relaxation techniques also may help to control pain.

Impaired Skin Integrity

The health care provider removes the wound packing a day or two after surgery. After the packing is removed, it is important to assess for rectal bleeding. Sitz baths may then be ordered to soothe and clean the area and to promote circulation. Provide a soft pad or cushion for more comfortable sitting.

Constipation

It is especially important to assess and record any stools passed after rectal surgery. The patient probably will dread the first bowel movement, expecting severe pain. Stool softeners probably will be ordered to reduce the trauma of defecation. Pain medication can be given as ordered before the patient tries to defecate (see *Patient Teaching* box). Someone should stay close by in case the patient feels weak or faint.

Patient Teaching

Hemorrhoids, Postoperative Care

- Notify your surgeon if you have fever or bleeding.
- To prevent recurrence, avoid constipation, prolonged sitting or standing, and straining to have a bowel movement.
- Ingest a high-fiber diet with plenty of fluids to promote regular, soft stools.
- Use stool softeners if prescribed.
- Follow a regular pattern of bowel elimination and do not delay defecation when the urge occurs.
- Follow the activity limitations prescribed by your health care provider.

Anorectal Abscess

An anorectal abscess is an infection in the tissue around the rectum. Signs and symptoms are rectal pain, swelling, redness, and tenderness. The patient often reports a history of diarrhea. If the abscess becomes chronic, it causes bleeding, itching, and discharge.

Anorectal abscess is treated with antibiotics followed by incision and drainage. The procedure may be done under local or general anesthesia, depending on how extensive the abscess is. Preoperatively, pain is treated with ice packs, sitz baths, and topical agents as ordered. Postoperatively, the nursing care is similar to that after hemorrhoidectomy. Pain is treated with opioid analgesics. Patient teaching emphasizes the importance of thorough cleansing after each bowel movement. Advise the patient to consume adequate fluids and a high-fiber diet to promote soft stools.

Anal Fissure

An anal fissure is a laceration between the anal canal and the perianal skin. Fissures may be related to constipation, diarrhea, Crohn disease, tuberculosis, leukemia, trauma, or childbirth. Sometimes a cause is not apparent. Signs and symptoms include pain before and after defecation and bleeding on the stool or tissue. If the fissure becomes chronic, the patient may experience pruritus, urinary frequency or retention, and dysuria. Fissures usually heal spontaneously but they can become chronic. Conservative treatment of anal fissures uses sitz baths, stool softeners, and analgesics. Surgical excision may be necessary. Postoperatively, instruct the patient to cleanse the perianal area after defecation. Pain relief measures and stool softeners are continued.

Anal Fistula

An anal fistula is an abnormal opening between the anal canal and the perianal skin. Fistulas can develop from anorectal abscesses or may be related to IBD or tuberculosis. The patient typically complains of pruritus and discharge. Sitz baths provide some comfort. The surgical treatment is excision of the fistula and surrounding tissue. Sometimes a temporary colostomy is done to allow the surgical site to heal. Postoperative care includes analgesics and sitz baths for pain.

Pilonidal Cyst

A pilonidal cyst is located in the sacrococcygeal area. It appears to result from an infolding of skin causing a sinus that is easily infected because of its closeness to the anus. Once infected, it is painful and swollen and may form an abscess. Surgical excision is usually recommended. Care is similar to that for the patient having a hemorrhoidectomy.

PATIENT EDUCATION TO PROMOTE NORMAL BOWEL FUNCTION

Nurses often have the opportunity to teach patients how to promote normal bowel function and detect problems early (see the *Nutrition Considerations* box below). Acute GI disorders can be caused by irritants or infectious agents. It is helpful for patients to identify and avoid foods that create distress

Good hand washing and proper food handling reduce the ingestion of infectious agents. Food poisoning can be acquired from food that has been improperly stored, poorly cooked, or exposed to contaminated containers or utensils.

Food poisoning is often a problem for frail older adults who live at home. Poor vision and smell can make food management difficult. It is a good idea for the home health nurse to check the patient's refrigerator and food cabinets to identify potential problems.

People who recognize that stress affects their GI function may benefit from relaxation techniques and stress management training.

Signs and symptoms of possibly serious digestive problems should be reported for prompt diagnosis and treatment if indicated. GI symptoms that could indicate gastric cancer include persistent gastric distress, anorexia, and weight loss. Rectal bleeding, a change in bowel habits, or both often occur with intestinal cancer. As part of the annual physical examination for people older than 40 years, many health care providers do a rectal examination and test the stool for occult blood. For men and women, the American Cancer Society recommends periodic sigmoidoscopy and fecal occult blood tests at intervals beginning at age 50 (see Chapter 25).

Teaching patients what is normal, how to promote normal bowel function, and how to detect problems can help to avoid serious GI dysfunction (see *Nutrition Considerations* Box).

Nutrition Considerations

1. Diarrhea is caused by pathogenic organisms, diet, intestinal lesions, or irritations associated with various diseases or conditions.
2. Replacement of lost fluids is the goal of nutritional therapy for diarrhea.
3. Constipation is caused by insufficient fiber intake, insufficient fluid intake, lack of exercise, some drugs, and the habitual use of laxatives.
4. The dietary treatment of constipation consists of increasing fluid (8 to 10 glasses of water a day) and fiber intake.
5. A hot drink such as coffee or tea enhances peristalsis and promotes defecation.

Get Ready for the NCLEX® Examination!

Key Points

- Various types of malabsorption (a condition in which one or more nutrients are not digested or absorbed) exist.
- Diarrhea is the frequent passage of loose or liquid stools. It can lead to fluid and electrolyte imbalances, metabolic acidosis, and malnutrition.
- Constipation is the difficult passage of hard, dry stools. It may be related to inactivity, dehydration, laxative dependence, a low-fiber diet, some drugs, and a variety of medical conditions.
- Fecal impaction is the retention of a large mass of stool in the rectum that the patient cannot pass and that may require removal with enemas and manual extraction.
- Factors that can cause intestinal obstruction include strangulated hernia, tumor, paralytic ileus, stricture, volvulus, intussusception, and postoperative adhesions.
- Appendicitis is inflammation of the appendix that requires surgical treatment to prevent rupture and peritonitis.
- A hernia is a portion of intestine that bulges through a weak area in the muscles of the abdominal wall and can become incarcerated (trapped) and obstructed.
- IBD, characterized by inflammation and ulceration of the lining of the intestines, includes ulcerative colitis and Crohn disease.
- Nursing care of the patient with IBD focuses on acute pain; diarrhea; deficient fluid volume; imbalanced nutrition: less than body requirements; ineffective coping; and risk for injury.
- Diverticulosis is characterized by small, saclike pouches in the intestinal wall that can become inflamed, causing obstruction, perforation, peritonitis, and fistula formation.
- Nursing care of the patient with colorectal cancer, which is usually treated surgically, focuses on risk for injury, ineffective peripheral tissue perfusion, acute pain, sexual dysfunction, and ineffective coping.
- Polyps are small growths in the intestine that are usually benign but may be removed because they may bleed, cause obstructions, or become malignant.
- Hemorrhoids are dilated rectal veins that can become inflamed and thrombosed; they are treated with topical medications, sitz baths, heat or cold, sclerotherapy, or surgical excision.
- Anal disorders include abscesses, fissures, and fistulas, all of which may be treated surgically.

Additional Learning Resources

SG Go to your Study Guide for additional learning activities to help you master this chapter content.

evolve Go to your Evolve website (http://evolve.elsevier.com/Linton/medsurg) for the following learning resources and much more:

- Interactive Prioritization Exercises
- Fluid & Electrolyte Tutorial
- Pharmacology Tutorial
- Review Questions for the NCLEX® Examination

Review Questions for the NCLEX® Examination

1. Prioritize the assessment techniques below in the order they should be performed.
   1. Palpation
   2. Auscultation
   3. Inspection
   4. Percussion

   NCLEX Client Need: Health Promotion and Maintenance
2. A patient who was admitted with severe abdominal pain is being evaluated for possible appendicitis. The physician should be notified immediately if the nurse's assessment reveals which of the following?
   1. The patient's WBC count is 15,000/mm^3.
   2. Palpation at McBurney point causes pain.
   3. The patient keeps both hips flexed.
   4. The patient's abdomen is rigid.

   NCLEX Client Need: Physiological Integrity: Physiological Adaptation
3. A patient asks if surgery would cure her Crohn disease. She states that her friend's ulcerative colitis was cured with surgery. The nurse should explain that surgery is used to treat Crohn disease less often than to treat ulcerative colitis for what reason?
   1. Crohn disease usually returns near the site of the anastomosis.
   2. Crohn disease typically involves the entire small and large intestines.
   3. Crohn disease usually can be cured with combination drug therapy.
   4. Crohn disease is associated with an increased risk of surgical complications.

   NCLEX Client Need: Physiological Integrity: Reduction of Risk Potential
4. The nurse is asked to speak at a support group for people with ulcerative colitis. Which content should be included in the presentation? (Select all that apply.)
   1. Stress management may help to control symptoms.
   2. Ulcerative colitis is caused by a bacterial infection.
   3. Avoid caffeine and any food that causes symptoms.
   4. Have regular colon screening examinations.
   5. Medications are needed only when acute symptoms occur.

   NCLEX Client Need: Physiological Integrity: Reduction of Risk Potential
5. A 16-year-old female presents to the camp clinic with abdominal pain in the right lower quadrant. She has a low-grade fever. The camp nurse should suspect which of the following?
   1. Colon cancer
   2. Pancreatitis
   3. Appendicitis
   4. Ascites

   NCLEX Client Need: Physiologic Integrity

6. Which gastrointestinal cancer has the highest rate of incidence and is responsible for the highest number of deaths?
   1. Esophageal
   2. Stomach
   3. Pancreatic
   4. Colorectal

   NCLEX Client Need: Health Promotion and Maintenance
7. The nurse is reviewing the record of a female client with Crohn disease. Which stool characteristics should the nurse expect to find in the patient's history?
   1. Diarrhea
   2. Chronic constipation
   3. Constipation alternating with diarrhea
   4. Stools constantly oozing form the rectum

   NCLEX Client Need: Safe and Effective Care Environment
8. The nurse recognizes the need for additional teaching when a patient with celiac disease states:
   1. "I should suggest that my sister be screened for celiac disease."
   2. "If I do not follow the gluten-free diet, I may develop a lymphoma."
   3. "I really don't need to restrict my diet of gluten-containing foods, as I am not having diarrhea."
   4. "It will be difficult to find gluten-free foods, as gluten is part of so many types of food."

   NCLEX Client Need: Safe and Effective Care Environment
9. As the nurse, you teach your patient with diverticulosis to: (Select all that apply.)
   1. Use anticholinergic medications to prevent bowel spasm
   2. Get an annual colonoscopy to detect any possible changes that may be cancerous
   3. Keep eating a high-fiber diet and using bulk laxatives to increase fecal volume
   4. Not consume whole-grain breads and cereals to prevent further irritation of the bowel

   NCLEX Client Need: Safe and Effective Care Environment
10. A patient in the clinic is prescribed an immunosuppressant drug for treatment of inflammatory bowel disease (IBD). Which patient teaching point related to this drug is appropriate?
    1. Always take your medication with food or milk
    2. Avoid people with active infections
    3. Stop the medication if you have diarrhea
    4. Take this medication only when you have symptoms

    NCLEX Client Need: Physiological Integrity: Pharmacological Therapies
11. Residents of an assisted living facility have asked how they can reduce the risk of colon cancer. The nurse should recommend a high intake of which of the following? (Select all that apply.)
    1. Vegetables
    2. Fruits
    3. Fat
    4. Fiber
    5. Proteins

    NCLEX Client Need: Physiological Integrity: Reduction of Risk Potential

chapter

41 Liver, Gallbladder, and Pancreatic Disorders

http://evolve.elsevier.com/Linton/medsurg

Objectives

1. Identify nursing assessment data related to the functions of the liver, gallbladder, and pancreas.
2. Identify the nurse's role in tests and procedures performed to diagnose disorders of the liver, gallbladder, and pancreas.
3. Explain the pathology, signs and symptoms, diagnosis, complications, and medical treatment of selected disorders of the liver, gallbladder, and pancreas.
4. Describe the care of the patient who has an esophageal balloon tube in place.
5. Assist in developing a nursing care plan for the patient with liver, gallbladder, or pancreatic dysfunction.

Key Terms

Ascites (ă-SĪ-tēz)
Cholecystectomy (kō-lē-sĭs-TĔK-tō-mē)
Cholecystitis (kō-lĕ-sĭs-TĪ-tĭs)
Choledocholithiasis (kō-lĕd-ō-kō-lĭ-THĪ-ă-sĭs)
Cholelithiasis (kō-lĕ-lĭ-THĪ-ă-sĭs)
Cirrhosis (sĭr-RŌ-sĭs)
Endocrine gland (ĔN-dŏ-krĭn)
Eructation (ĕ-rŭk-TĀ-shŭn)
Gluconeogenesis (glū-kō-nē-ō-JĔN-ĕ-sĭs)
Glycogenesis (glī-kō-JĔN-ĕ-sĭs)
Glycogenolysis (glī-kō-jĕ-NŎL-ĭ-sĭs)
Hepatic (hĕ-PĂ-tĭc)
Hepatitis (hĕ-pă-TĪ-tĭs)
Hepatomegaly (hĕ-pă-tō-MĔG-ă-lē)
Icterus (ĬK-tĕr-ŭs)
Jaundice (JĂWN-dĭs)

LIVER

The liver is the largest internal organ in the body. It is located under the diaphragm in the right upper quadrant of the abdomen (Fig. 41-1). The term *hepatic* refers to the liver.

ANATOMY AND PHYSIOLOGY OF THE LIVER

The liver can be divided into four lobes that are made up of many lobules (Fig. 41-2). Blood from the aorta is delivered to the liver via the hepatic artery. The portal vein delivers blood from the intestines to the liver. Portal blood circulates through the liver and is transported to the inferior vena cava by the hepatic veins. Figure 41-3 illustrates hepatic circulation.

Specialized **hepatic** cells allow the liver to carry out many critical functions. Reticuloendothelial cells, called *Kupffer cells,* ingest old red blood cells (RBCs) and bacteria. Parenchymal cells carry out various metabolic functions, including metabolism of carbohydrates, fats, proteins, and steroids and detoxification of potentially harmful substances.

BILE PRODUCTION AND EXCRETION

Bilirubin is a product of the normal breakdown of old RBCs in the liver. The initial breakdown product is unconjugated or indirect bilirubin. The liver then converts unconjugated bilirubin into conjugated bilirubin and secretes it into the bile. Bile produced in the liver passes through the cystic duct into the gallbladder for storage.

When fats pass into the duodenum, the gallbladder and the liver respond by delivering bile through the common bile duct into the small intestine. Bile emulsifies fat, meaning that it breaks it into small particles that can be absorbed easily. It also neutralizes the acidic chyme as it leaves the stomach. Bile plays a role in the absorption of fat-soluble vitamins and the removal of some toxins.

Bile travels through the intestines with the chyme. In the large intestine, it is converted to urobilinogen and then to stercobilin. This final breakdown product of bilirubin gives stool its characteristic brown color.

METABOLISM

Glucose Metabolism

The liver helps to maintain the blood glucose within a certain range. After a meal, excess glucose molecules

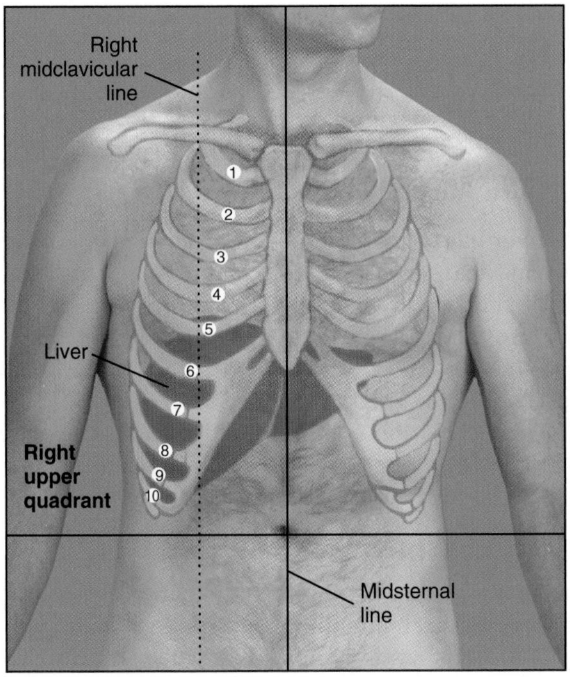

FIGURE 41-1 The liver is located under the diaphragm in the right upper quadrant of the abdomen. Anatomic landmarks are noted. (From Monahan FD, Drake DT, Neighbors M, editors: *Medical-surgical nursing: foundations for clinical practice*, ed 2, Philadelphia, 1998, Saunders.)

are taken up by the liver, combined, and then stored as glycogen. This process is called **glycogenesis**. When the glucose level in the blood falls, the process is reversed by **glycogenolysis** and the glucose molecules are returned to the blood. **Gluconeogenesis** is the third process by which the liver maintains blood glucose. Fats and protein are broken down in response to low blood glucose levels and the molecules are used to make new glucose.

Protein Metabolism

Some nonessential amino acids, plasma proteins (albumin and globulin), and clotting factors are synthesized in the liver. Another important liver function in relation to protein metabolism is the conversion of ammonia to urea. Ammonia is a byproduct of the metabolism of amino acids. If ammonia accumulates in the blood, it has toxic effects on brain tissue.

Lipid Metabolism

The liver synthesizes lipids from glucose, pyruvic acid, acetic acid, and amino acids. It also synthesizes fatty acids, breaks down triglycerides, and synthesizes and breaks down cholesterol.

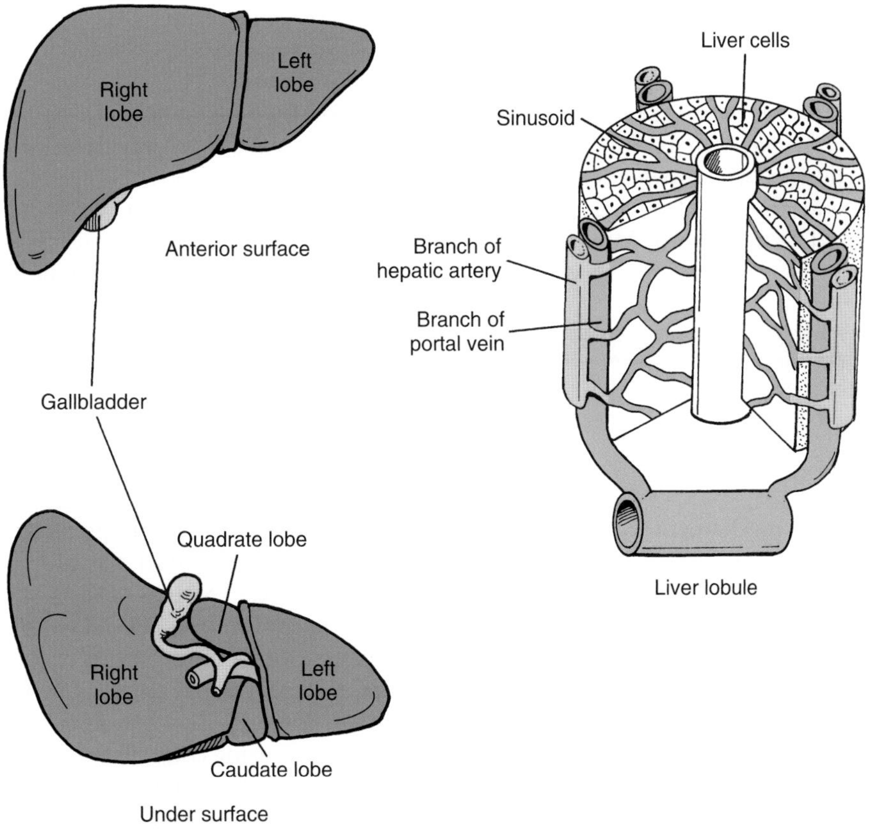

FIGURE 41-2 The liver has four lobes, each made up of many lobules.

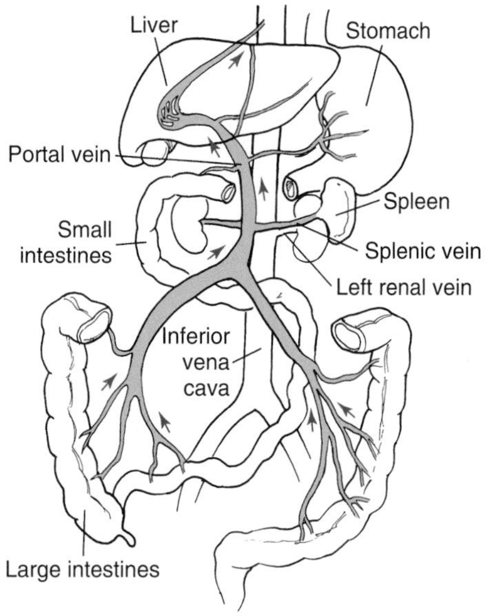

FIGURE 41-3 Hepatic circulation. Venous blood from the digestive tract and spleen passes through the liver via the portal vein and is delivered through the hepatic veins to the inferior vena cava.

Blood Coagulation

Normal blood coagulation (clotting) is a complex process. Two essential elements for coagulation, prothrombin and fibrinogen, are synthesized by the liver.

Detoxification

The liver filters the blood and inactivates many chemicals, including most medications. Therefore medications are prescribed very cautiously for patients with poor liver function. Patients with liver disease are at increased risk for toxic effects of drugs (see *Complementary and Alternative Therapies* box). With age, some decrease in liver function occurs, so lower drug dosages may be adequate. Especially with long-term therapy, the older person should be monitored closely for signs of toxicity.

> **Complementary and Alternative Therapies**
>
> Inform patients that the following herbs can harm the liver: comfrey, borage, coltsfoot, chaparral, and germander.

Immunity

An important protective mechanism is the development of antibodies to resist pathogens. Antibodies and other substances that help to resist infection are produced in the liver.

Hormone Metabolism

The liver plays an important role in the metabolism of adrenocortical hormones, estrogen, testosterone, and aldosterone. If these hormones are not metabolized, they accumulate, causing an exaggerated effect on target organs.

> **Pharmacology Capsule**
>
> Because many drugs are metabolized in the liver, patients with liver disease are at increased risk for toxic effects of drugs.

NURSING ASSESSMENT OF THE LIVER

The liver has so many important functions that alterations may cause a number of systemic signs and symptoms. The health history and physical examination may provide clues to liver dysfunction and may be used to assess responses to the treatment of liver disorders. Even though the registered nurse (RN) is responsible for the complete patient assessment, the licensed vocational nurse/licensed practical nurse (LVN/LPN) contributes data.

HEALTH HISTORY

The health history begins with the patient's reason for seeking medical attention. The patient may report various signs and symptoms related to the liver, including change in the color of skin, urine, or stools; abdominal pain, nausea, and vomiting; and fatigue.

Past Medical History

The past medical history documents any previous or chronic liver disorders. Record any surgical procedures, injuries, and blood transfusions because they sometimes expose the patient to the **hepatitis** virus. List all of the patient's medications, including over-the-counter and herbal products, because many of these are toxic to the liver.

Family History

Document whether any of the patient's family members have had cancer of the liver or colon, hepatitis, or alcoholism.

Review of Systems

Inquire about the patient's general health status and systematically assess for signs and symptoms related to liver dysfunction. General fatigue is a common complaint among people who have impaired liver function. They may have had personality or behavior changes but the patients are not always aware of these changes. Inquire about any changes in weight or skin color, itching, easy bruising, headaches, enlarged lymph nodes, breast enlargement in men, or dyspnea.

Gastrointestinal (GI) symptoms are common with liver disease. Therefore ask about the presence of anorexia, abdominal pain, nausea and vomiting, diarrhea, or GI bleeding. Note the color of stools because clay-colored (white) stools are characteristic of bile obstruction and black stools can indicate GI bleeding. Changes in urine color also may be significant because patients with liver disease often have dark urine.

In addition, ask whether the patient has had any numbness, tingling, or edema in the extremities.

Functional Assessment

Explore the patient's daily routines, including dietary intake and patterns of activity and rest. Because liver disease may be associated with exposure to toxins, assess the patient's exposure to chemicals, potentially toxic drugs such as acetaminophen, and alcohol use. Some people are reluctant to discuss alcohol use, so the subject must be handled tactfully. People tend to understate the amount of alcohol they typically consume. Note use of street drugs, especially those taken intravenously.

The last part of the functional assessment is the identification of stressors, usual coping strategies, and sources of support.

PHYSICAL EXAMINATION

The physical assessment begins with the measurement of vital signs, height, and weight, as well as observation of the patient's general appearance. Skin color is especially important in relation to the liver. **Jaundice** is a golden-yellow skin color associated with liver dysfunction or bile obstruction. It is relatively easy to recognize in fair-skinned people.

Inspect the sclera of the eyes. Like the skin, the sclera may turn yellow, a condition called scleral **icterus**. This sign is especially useful when jaundice cannot be seen elsewhere in dark-skinned people.

Observe for enlargement of breast tissue in men. Such enlargement is called *gynecomastia*. When inspecting the chest, also look for spider angiomas. Spider angiomas are small, visible vessels shaped like spiders.

The examination of the abdomen is especially important in detecting liver disease. Inspect the shape of the abdomen. Note the presence of prominent veins. If significant **ascites** (fluid accumulation in the peritoneal cavity) is present, the abdomen appears distended. Measure the abdomen at the largest circumference to permit comparative measurements later (Fig. 41-4).

Palpate the abdomen for distention and tenderness. Experienced examiners may be able to palpate the liver but unless it is enlarged, it is difficult to locate under the right rib cage. An enlarged, diseased liver may be felt well below the rib margin. Liver enlargement is called **hepatomegaly**.

Examine the extremities for bruising, edema, muscle wasting, and impaired sensation. Inspect the hands for palmar erythema (redness of the palms).

The assessment of a patient with a liver disorder is summarized in Box 41-1. Findings associated with liver disease are illustrated in Figure 41-5.

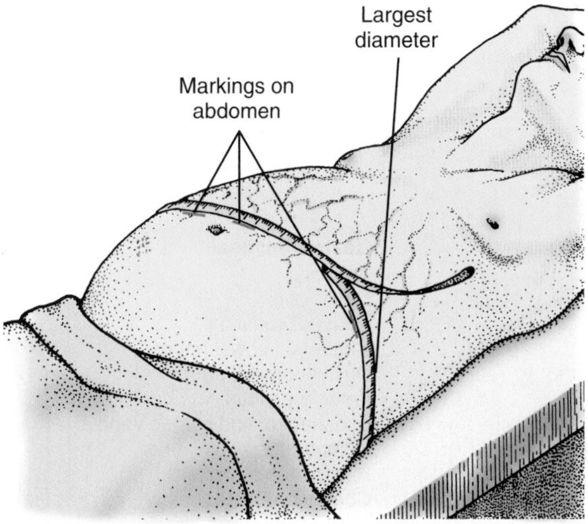

FIGURE 41-4 How to measure abdominal girth. Marks are made on the abdominal midline and on both sides so that subsequent measurements can always be made at the same place.

Box 41-1 Assessment of the Patient with Liver Disease

HEALTH HISTORY

Present Illness
Fatigue, weight changes, digestive disturbances, skin changes

Past Medical History
Previous liver disease, hepatitis B immunization, recent and current medications taken

Review of Systems
Weakness, fatigue, pruritus, dyspnea, anorexia, abdominal pain, nausea and vomiting, diarrhea, bloody stools, changes in urine or stool color, numbness or tingling of extremities

Functional Assessment
Diet, alcohol intake, occupation, exposure to toxins, stress, coping strategies, interpersonal relationships

PHYSICAL EXAMINATION

Vital Signs
Hypertension, tachypnea

Height and Weight

Skin
Dryness, scratches, jaundice, bruises

Eye
Scleral icterus

Thorax
Spider angiomas

Breasts
Gynecomastia

Abdomen
Distention, prominent veins, girth, liver enlargement

DIAGNOSTIC TESTS AND PROCEDURES

The physician uses a number of tools to assess liver function, including endoscopy, laboratory studies, imaging studies, and biopsies. Endoscopy was addressed in Chapter 39. Nursing care of patients who are having specific tests and procedures related to the liver is presented in Table 41-1.

LABORATORY STUDIES

Laboratory studies of specimens are done to measure bilirubin, urinary and fecal urobilinogen, serum proteins, ammonia, vitamin K production, prothrombin

Text continued on p. 855

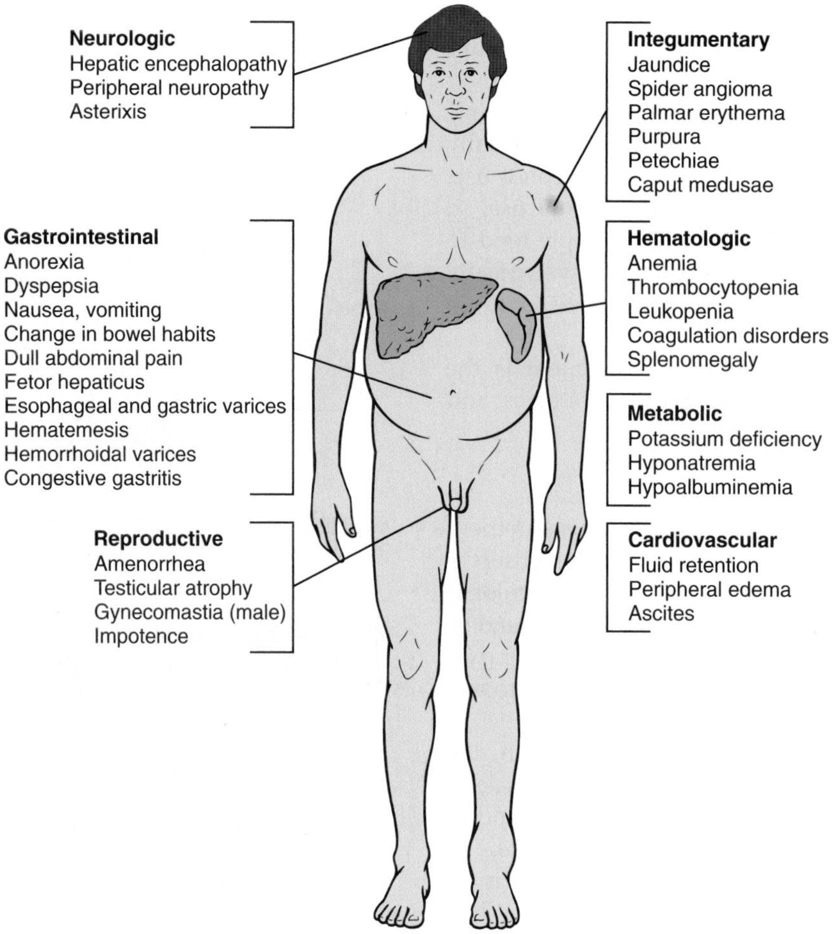

FIGURE 41-5 Findings associated with liver disease. (From Lewis SM, Heitkemper MM, Dirksen SR: *Medical-surgical nursing: assessment and management of clinical problems*, ed 5, St. Louis, 2000, Mosby.)

Table 41-1 Diagnostic Tests and Procedures Liver and Gallbladder

General Interventions: Check your agency procedure manual for diagnostic tests and procedures. Always tell the patient what to expect when tests are ordered. Explain if nothing-by-mouth (NPO) status is necessary. Document the care provided and relevant assessment data. If venipuncture is done, apply a dressing and check the site oozing. Apply pressure and elevate arm if patient's blood clotting is impaired.

TEST OR STUDY	PURPOSE AND PROCEDURE	PATIENT PREPARATION	POSTPROCEDURE NURSING CARE
Laboratory Studies			
Blood Studies			
Serum bilirubin	Assesses liver function. Normal values are total bilirubin 0.2–1.0 mg/dL or 3.4–17.1 μmol/L, conjugated bilirubin 0.0–0.2 mg/dL or 0.0–3.4 μmol/L, unconjugated bilirubin 0.2–0.8 mg/dL.	Fast at least 4 hours before blood sample drawn. Avoid yellow foods for 3–4 days before the test. Wait at least 24 hours after a contrast medium has been given.	No special care is required.
Alkaline phosphatase	Detects elevation associated with liver or bone disease. Normal value varies with method.	A 10- to 12-hour fast may be required. Some drugs may be withheld for 12 hours.	No special care is required.

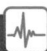

Table 41-1 Diagnostic Tests and Procedures Liver and Gallbladder—cont'd

TEST OR STUDY	PURPOSE AND PROCEDURE	PATIENT PREPARATION	POSTPROCEDURE NURSING CARE
Serum enzymes: alkaline phosphatase; gamma-glutamyl transpeptidase (GGT); alanine aminotransferase (ALT), also known as serum glutamic-pyruvic transaminase; aldolase; aspartate aminotransferase (AST), also known as serum glutamic-oxaloacetic transaminase; and lactate dehydrogenase (LDH).	Detects elevations in enzymes related to liver diseases. Normal values vary with gender and age. See laboratory manual.	Consult agency guidelines to see if fasting is necessary. Some require listing of patient's medications on request form.	No special care is required.
Prothrombin time (PT) and international normalized ratio (INR)	Measure clotting ability; may be prolonged due to liver disease, vitamin K deficiency, or anticoagulant therapy. Normal values are PT 11.0–14 seconds and INR 1.0–1.3.	No coffee or alcohol for 24 hours before the test. Many natural remedies affect the results.	Use pressure and arm elevation if needed to control bleeding at puncture site. Immediately report PT >46 seconds or INR ≥5.
Serum protein	Electrophoresis helps to diagnose conditions that affect serum proteins.	Avoid a high-fat diet for 8 hours before the test. Some medications may need to be withheld for several days before a blood sample is drawn.	No special care is required.
Radiographic Studies			
***General Interventions When Contrast Dye Used. Before Procedure:** Assess patient allergy to dye, iodine, or shellfish. If patient reports allergy, notify radiology. Tell patient that injection of contrast dye can create a feeling of warmth, a salty taste, and nausea. **After Procedure:** Inform the physician of any signs of allergic response to the contrast dye. Administer antihistamines as ordered for allergy.			
Computed tomography (CT)	CT creates cross-sectional images of liver and other organs to reveal abnormalities. Contrast dye may be used. The patient lies still on a stretcher while a donut-shaped machine moves around him or her. Contrast dye may be injected intravenously.	*Dye precautions. Inform the patient that the procedure is painless and noninvasive. NPO status may be ordered but routine drugs usually can be taken. Sedation can be ordered if the patient has difficulty lying still.	*Dye precautions. In most cases, no special care is required.
Cholangiography: T-tube, intravenous, percutaneous transhepatic, surgical, magnetic resonance cholangiopancreatography	Provides images of hepatic and biliary ducts through various procedures. A contrast agent may be injected and images obtained. The test takes 4–6 hours.	*Dye precautions. Food and fluids should be withheld as ordered. The patient is usually NPO after midnight before the study. A laxative also may be ordered the night before.	*Dye precautions. A fatty meal helps to eliminate dye, if used. After percutaneous transhepatic cholangiography, watch for signs of bleeding and respiratory distress.
Portal venography and hepatic arteriography	The tests use intravenous contrast dye followed by radiographs to study blood vessels in liver.	*Dye precautions.	*Dye precautions. Care is the same as for T-tube cholangiography.

Continued

Table 41-1 Diagnostic Tests and Procedures Liver and Gallbladder—cont'd

TEST OR STUDY	PURPOSE AND PROCEDURE	PATIENT PREPARATION	POSTPROCEDURE NURSING CARE
Liver scan	A radioactive substance that collects in the liver is given intravenously and radiographs are taken with the patient in various positions. A scanner maps uptake of radiation, revealing tumors and abscesses.	Assure patient that a small dose of radiation is harmless. A fast of 4–6 hours is required.	The patient must wash his or her hands thoroughly after voiding for 24 hours. Report any allergic symptoms.
Gallbladder scan, hepatobiliary scintigraphy, hepatobiliary imaging, biliary tract radionuclide scan, cholescintigraphy	A radionuclide is injected and images are taken of the biliary tract to assess patency and to detect cholecystitis. Takes about 90 minutes. Repeat imaging may be needed 24–48 hours later.	NPO at least 2 hours before the procedure.	Encourage the patient to drink fluids to promote elimination of radionuclide, to wash hands after voiding, and to flush immediately. Caregivers should wear gloves to handle urine. Wash gloved hands before removing gloves; wash hands after removing gloves. Dispose of gloves as you would other nuclear waste.
Other Imaging Procedures			
Ultrasonography	Ultrasonography uses high-frequency sound waves to create an image of the liver, spleen, pancreas, gallbladder, and biliary system. The patient lies on a table. A technician applies gel to the abdomen and moves an instrument called a *transducer* over the abdomen. Images are projected onto a screen. It is not painful.	The patient may be NPO for 8–12 hours before the procedure.	No special care is required after the procedure.
Magnetic resonance imaging (MRI)	MRI creates cross-sectional images of the liver and other organs without radiation. MRI is a painless, noninvasive procedure but the machine is noisy. The patient must remain still on a narrow surface.	All metal must be removed before the MRI. Older MRI devices are circular and surround the body like a tunnel. Closing the eyes reduces claustrophobia (open MRI eliminates claustrophobia).	No special care is required.
Tissue Examination			
Liver biopsy	A biopsy removes a small specimen of liver tissue for examination.	Baseline vital signs and blood coagulation studies should be obtained.	With *all* liver biopsies, do the following: Monitor vital signs for indications of bleeding (i.e., tachycardia, tachypnea, restlessness, hypotension) and pneumothorax (i.e., dyspnea, tachycardia).

Table 41-1 Diagnostic Tests and Procedures Liver and Gallbladder—cont'd

TEST OR STUDY	PURPOSE AND PROCEDURE	PATIENT PREPARATION	POSTPROCEDURE NURSING CARE
Needle biopsy	The specimen is obtained by inserting a special needle into the liver through the abdominal wall.	The patient is positioned supine with the right arm behind the head.	Check the pressure dressing for bleeding. Position the patient on the right side as ordered.
Open biopsy	An open biopsy is done in the operating room. An incision is made and a tissue sample is obtained under general anesthesia.	Requires standard preoperative procedures. Informed consent must be obtained from the patient.	Monitor for bleeding. Position as ordered.
Endoscopy			
Cholangiopancreatography, endoscopic retrograde cholangiopancreatography (ERCP)	Medication is used to suppress the gag reflex. A flexible endoscope is passed after injection of dye. The study permits visualization of pancreatic, hepatic, and common bile ducts as well as the ampulla of Vater. It is used to diagnose pancreatic disease. The study takes 30–60 minutes.	*Dye precautions. NPO for 8–12 hours.	*Dye precautions. Advise warm gargles or an ice pack to the neck for a sore throat. The patient may have belching and bloating. Immediately notify the physician of severe pain, fever, dyspnea, and hematemesis. NPO until gag reflex returns.

time (PT), international normalized ratio (INR), and serum enzymes. Table 41-1 explains the significance of these laboratory tests. Some patients are able to use an INR monitor at home.

Because GI bleeding is sometimes a problem with liver disease, gastric fluids and stools may be tested for the presence of occult blood. Urine specimens also may be tested for bilirubin and urobilinogen and stool specimens tested for urobilinogen.

IMAGING STUDIES: RADIOLOGIC STUDIES

Radiologic studies are used primarily to visualize the circulatory and biliary systems in the liver. They include computed tomography (CT), magnetic resonance imaging (MRI), hepatobiliary scintigraphy (HIDA), and abdominal ultrasound. CT and MRI are used to obtain scans of internal organs, including the liver. They are noninvasive, painless procedures. HIDA is a nuclear imaging scan that uses a radioactive substance. After being injected into a vein, the substance accumulates in the liver. Radiographs are then taken to reveal the size, shape, and position of the liver as well as tumors, cirrhosis, and abscesses. Ultrasonography uses sound waves to create an image of the liver, spleen, pancreas, gallbladder, and biliary system. It is a noninvasive, painless procedure.

LIVER BIOPSY

A liver biopsy involves removal of a small specimen of liver tissue for examination. The specimen can be obtained through an incision under general anesthesia (open biopsy). Another method (needle biopsy) involves the use of a special type of needle inserted through the abdominal wall to obtain the specimen.

Before either procedure, baseline vital signs should be obtained and blood coagulation studies done. The patient's blood should be typed and crossmatched because of the risk of bleeding. Signed consent is required. Tell the patient what to expect during the procedure. For a needle biopsy, position the patient supine with the right arm behind the head. Place a pad under the right chest. The physician instructs the patient to take a deep breath and hold it during the actual puncture. A sample of liver tissue is aspirated for study.

Afterward, a pressure dressing is placed over the puncture. It should be checked for bleeding every 15 minutes for the first hour, every 30 minutes for the next hour, and then hourly or according to agency protocol. Monitor vital signs at the same time for signs of blood loss (tachycardia, restlessness, hypotension) or pneumothorax (restlessness, tachypnea). The physician usually orders the patient kept on the right side for at least 2 hours to maintain pressure on the puncture site. After being allowed to change positions, the patient may still be kept flat for up to 14 hours.

The primary complications of liver biopsy are hemorrhage and pneumothorax. Bleeding is a possibility because of the liver's rich blood supply and the potential for impaired coagulation in the patient with liver disease. Pneumothorax occurs if the lung is accidentally punctured during the biopsy. Air escapes into the pleural cavity and the lung on the affected side collapses.

DISORDERS OF THE LIVER

HEPATITIS

Hepatitis is inflammation of the liver. It is estimated that more than 250,000 cases of viral hepatitis are reported in the United States each year. Although many patients have uneventful recoveries, others develop chronic conditions that eventually can lead to liver failure and death.

Pathophysiology

Hepatitis has local and systemic effects. Locally, the inflammatory process causes the liver to swell. If swelling is severe, two important effects occur. First, the bile channels are compressed, damaging the cells that produce bile. This results in an elevation in serum bilirubin and jaundice. Second, blood flow through the liver is impaired, causing pressure to rise in the portal circulation (see Fig. 41-3).

Systemic effects are related to altered metabolic functions normally performed by the liver and to the infectious response in viral hepatitis. Systemic signs and symptoms of hepatitis include rash, angioedema, arthritis, fever, and malaise.

Types of Hepatitis

Hepatitis can be classified as *infectious* or *noninfectious*. Viruses known to cause infectious hepatitis are classified as *types A, B, C, D*, and *E*. Other viruses that may cause hepatitis include the recently described hepatitis G and hepatitis GB. Noninfectious hepatitis is caused by exposure to toxic chemicals, including drugs. Key features of each type of hepatitis are summarized in Table 41-2.

Hepatitis A. Hepatitis A has been called *infectious hepatitis* and *epidemic hepatitis*. It is caused by the hepatitis A virus (HAV), which is transmitted from one person to another by way of water, food, or medical equipment that has been contaminated with infected fecal matter. Hepatitis A is the most common type of viral hepatitis. Fortunately, it is rarely fatal and infected persons do not become asymptomatic carriers.

Hepatitis B. Hepatitis B is caused by the hepatitis B virus (HBV). Because HBV is found in all body fluids of infected persons, modes of transmission include intimate contact with carriers as well as contact with contaminated blood or medical equipment. Current screening procedures make it highly unlikely that hepatitis will be transmitted in a blood transfusion. Hepatitis B can be transmitted from an infected mother to her baby. About 6% of those infected after age 5 develop chronic hepatitis and become carriers, meaning that they can transmit the infection to others. Chronic hepatitis B also increases the risk of cirrhosis, liver failure, and liver cancer. Vaccination of children and high-risk groups, including health care workers, has dramatically decreased the incidence of hepatitis B.

Hepatitis C. Hepatitis C is transmitted by contact with contaminated blood or medical equipment or by contact with infected body fluids. Like hepatitis B, it can be transmitted from an infected mother to her baby during birth; however, that is rare. While some individuals recover completely from acute hepatitis C, a significant proportion of people with hepatitis C develop chronic infections and become carriers. Many of these people will develop cirrhosis or cancer of the liver.

Hepatitis D. Hepatitis D is caused by a virus known as the *delta agent*, which is a defective ribonucleic acid (RNA) virus that can survive only in the company of HBV. Hepatitis D is transmitted percutaneously (through the skin or mucous membranes) with or following HBV infection. The presence of hepatitis D greatly increases the risk that the patient will progress to chronic hepatitis and possible liver failure.

Hepatitis E. Hepatitis E is similar to hepatitis A and is most commonly transmitted via water or food contaminated with infected fecal matter. Hepatitis E infection is rare in the United States, except among people who have traveled in developing countries where the virus is more common. No long-term, chronic form of hepatitis E infection exists.

Hepatitis G. Hepatitis G has been identified in some blood donors and can be transmitted by blood transfusion. Hepatitis G virus (HGV) appears to exist only with other viral infections but does not appear to cause chronic hepatitis by itself.

Noninfectious Hepatitis. Although the cause is not always identifiable, noninfectious hepatitis can be the result of exposure to toxins such as mercury and arsenic and drugs such as alcohol and acetaminophen.

Signs and Symptoms

Regardless of the cause, the signs and symptoms of hepatitis are similar. Differences occur in the number and severity of the symptoms from one person to the next. Many patients have no symptoms at all. For those who are symptomatic, the course of the disease is marked by three phases: (1) preicteric, (2) icteric, and (3) posticteric.

Preicteric Phase. Common findings in the preicteric phase include malaise, severe headache, right upper quadrant abdominal pain, anorexia, nausea, vomiting, fever, arthralgia (joint pain), rash, enlarged lymph nodes, urticaria, and enlargement and tenderness of the liver. The preicteric phase lasts 1 to 21 days and is the period when the patient is most infectious.

Icteric Phase. The icteric phase is characterized by jaundice, light- or clay-colored stools, and dark urine typical of impaired bile production and secretion. The

Table 41-2 Key Features of Each Type of Viral Hepatitis

TYPE	CAUSE	TRANSMISSION ROUTE	PREVENTION	TREATMENT
Hepatitis A	Hepatitis A virus (HAV)	Fecal-oral route (often via contaminated water or food). Infected food handler, poor sanitation. Incubation period: 15–50 days	Wash hands after toileting. Use clean water and food supplies. Use gloves to handle stool specimens and soiled articles. A vaccine is recommended for travel in certain countries. After exposure: HAV vaccine should be given to adults under age 40. Immune globulin (IG) is given instead to adults over age 40.	No drug therapy is available.
Hepatitis B	Hepatitis B virus (HBV)	Contaminated blood introduced through the skin or mucous membranes (often via contaminated needles or other medical or dental equipment). Sexual contact. Newborns may be infected before, during, or after birth. Incubation period: 45–180 days	Use disposable needles. Avoid contaminated articles. Screen blood donors. Use caution with body fluids. A vaccine is given to people, including nurses, who are at risk for exposure. Hepatitis B immune globulin (HBIG) is given after exposure.	*Acute* hepatitis B: no drugs are available. Treated with rest, good nutrition and hydration, and avoidance of alcohol. *Chronic* hepatitis B: may be treated with interferon alfa-2b, peginterferon alfa-2a, and antiviral such as lamivudine.
Hepatitis C	Hepatitis C virus (HCV)	Contaminated blood introduced through the skin or mucous membranes (often via contaminated needles or other medical or dental equipment). Although rare, it can be transmitted via sexual intercourse. Unborn babies may be infected by their mothers. Incubation period: 14–180 days	Use disposable needles. Avoid contaminated articles. Screen blood donors. Avoid risky sexual practices with people who may have hepatitis C. Do not share personal items such as razors. Use caution with body fluids. No vaccine is available.	Treated with peginterferon, ribavirin, and either boceprivir or telaprevir. Side effects of interferon include flulike symptoms, hair loss, low blood count, depression, and thinking difficulties. Success varies with the genotype of HCV.
Hepatitis D	"Delta agent" hepatitis D virus (HDV)	Contaminated blood or equipment or sexual contact. Can cause infection only when HBV is present. Incubation period: 2–26 weeks	The hepatitis B vaccine is given. Hepatitis D cannot infect unless hepatitis B is present.	Treated with pegylated interferon.
Hepatitis E	Hepatitis E virus (HEV)	Fecal-oral route (often via contaminated water or food). Incubation period: 15–64 days	Wash hands after toileting. Use clean water and food supplies. Use gloves to handle stool specimens and soiled articles. A vaccine has been developed but is not yet available for general use. For prevention, IG can be given before or within 48 hours after exposure.	Usually resolves in several weeks to months without treatment.

accumulation of bile salts under the skin may cause pruritus. GI symptoms from the preicteric phase often persist. The icteric phase lasts 2 to 4 weeks. Hepatitis patients who do not develop jaundice are said to have *anicteric hepatitis*.

Posticteric Phase. In the posticteric phase, fatigue, malaise, and liver enlargement persist for several months.

Complications

Most people recover fully from hepatitis A or B but residual damage and complications can occur. Some patients with hepatitis B or C become carriers. About one fourth of those who become carriers will have chronic active hepatitis, which can lead to cirrhosis. Carriers also are at increased risk for liver cancer. People who have had hepatitis cannot donate blood because of the risk of transmitting the disease to a recipient.

Complications of hepatitis include chronic hepatitis, fulminant hepatitis, cirrhosis of the liver, and liver cancer. Chronic hepatitis is characterized by a prolonged recovery with continuing fatigue and liver enlargement that eventually resolves. Signs and symptoms persist for more than 6 months. Liver damage continues and may lead to cirrhosis. If necrosis of damaged cells occurs without regeneration, fulminant hepatitis results. Severe liver failure may follow and is often fatal unless a liver transplant is done.

Medical Diagnosis

A diagnosis of hepatitis is based on the presence of viral antigens and antibodies specific to each type of hepatitis. The effects of the infection on the liver may cause liver function tests to be abnormal. Typical findings consistent with hepatitis include elevated levels of serum enzymes (aspartate aminotransferase [AST], alanine aminotransferase [ALT], gamma-glutamyl transpeptidase [GGT]), serum and urinary bilirubin, and urinary urobilinogen. The PT may be prolonged. Albumin may be normal or low and gamma globulin may be normal or high. A liver biopsy may be done to evaluate harm caused by chronic hepatitis B or C.

Medical Treatment

Because no cure for hepatitis exists, treatment is designed to promote healing and to manage symptoms. Chronic hepatitis B is treated with a course of an alpha-interferon and a combination of antiviral drugs. The most effective treatment for hepatitis C at this time uses peginterferon alfa-2a, ribavirin, and a protease inhibitor (boceprivir or telaprivir). Unfortunately, relapse is common after the drugs are stopped. The physician usually orders antipyretics for fever and antiemetics for nausea. The selection of drugs is important because hepatotoxic drugs (those that are toxic to the liver) should not be given. Suggested antiemetics are dimenhydrinate (Dramamine) and trimethobenzamide (Tigan). Phenothiazines are contraindicated. If a sedative is needed, chloral hydrate or diphenhydramine (Benadryl) is recommended. Corticosteroids, although controversial, may be ordered if the patient is very ill or if fulminant hepatitis is suspected.

The prescribed diet is usually high-calorie, high-carbohydrate, moderate- to high-protein, and moderate- to low-fat with supplementary vitamins, depending on the disease severity. Recommended activity depends on the patient's signs and symptoms and liver function tests. Bed rest may be ordered during the icteric phase but practices vary.

Pharmacology Capsule

Hepatotoxic drugs are contraindicated for the patient with hepatitis because they can cause further damage to liver cells.

Prevention

Vaccines are available to immunize people against hepatitis A and B. At this time no vaccine is available to prevent other types of hepatitis, although a hepatitis E vaccine is being studied. All care providers can reduce their risk of exposure by strict adherence to Standard Precautions. The Centers for Disease Control and Prevention (CDC) recommends that adults up to age 40 who are exposed to hepatitis A be given the HAV vaccine within 2 weeks of exposure to prevent infection. In adults over age 40, immune globulin (IG) should be given rather than the HAV vaccine. Active disease may be averted in patients who have been exposed to HBV by administering the HBV vaccine and hepatitis B immune globulin (HBIG), preferably within 24 hours after exposure.

NURSING CARE of the Patient with Hepatitis

Assessment

Nursing assessment of the patient with liver disease is outlined in Box 41-1. When taking a health history of the person with hepatitis, essential data include information about general health state; drug and alcohol use; chemical exposure; dietary habits; blood transfusions; recent travel; GI disturbances; and changes in skin, urine, or stools.

Ongoing physical assessment includes vital signs, inspection of skin, weight changes, and mental status.

Interventions

Activity Intolerance and Impaired Physical Mobility

Most patients with acute viral hepatitis are treated at home, so instructions about activity limitations are needed. The extent of activity limitation depends on the severity of symptoms. While the patient is symptomatic, bed rest may be advised. Explain that

Nursing Diagnoses, Goals, and Outcome Criteria: Hepatitis

Nursing Diagnoses	Goals and Outcome Criteria
Activity Intolerance and **Impaired Physical Mobility** related to fatigue, impaired metabolism, prescribed bed rest	Improved activity tolerance: patient reports less fatigue and improved activity tolerance.
	Absence of complications of immobility: skin intact, breath sounds clear, no calf tenderness
Imbalanced Nutrition: Less Than Body Requirements related to anorexia, nausea, and vomiting	Adequate dietary intake: stable body weight
Deficient Fluid Volume related to inadequate intake, vomiting	Normal fluid status: fluid output equal to intake, vital signs consistent with patient norms, moist mucous membranes
Risk for Impaired Skin Integrity related to pruritus and scratching	Intact skin: no abrasions
Disturbed Body Image related to jaundice	Improved body image: patient expresses acceptance of skin discoloration
Anxiety related to hospitalization, unfamiliar procedures, serious illness	Decreased anxiety: patient states that anxiety is decreased or absent, calm manner
Deficient Knowledge of treatment plan and self-care related to lack of exposure to information	Enhanced knowledge: patient describes therapy and identifies measures to care for self

rest allows the liver to heal by regenerating new cells to replace those damaged by hepatitis. Plan care activities to permit times when the patient is not disturbed. Offer diversions such as reading or television to combat boredom.

Unless the patient has severe complications, complete bed rest is usually not necessary. If complete bed rest is ordered, the patient is at risk for complications of immobility. Inspect the skin for early signs of pressure (redness, especially over bony prominences). If the patient is unable to turn independently, assist with turning at least every 2 hours. Moisturizing lotions protect the skin and can help to relieve itching associated with jaundice. Teach the patient to cough and deep breathe every 2 hours to reduce the risk of pneumonia. Gentle exercise of the legs promotes circulation and discourages the formation of thrombi. Discourage crossing of the legs. Inactivity tends to lead to constipation and may cause urinary stasis. Therefore record bowel movements and urine output and describe any abnormal characteristics of stool and urine. Care of the immobilized patient is discussed in detail in Chapter 21.

Imbalanced Nutrition: Less Than Body Requirements

Good nutrition is essential to decrease demands on the liver (see *Nutrition Considerations* box). Specific dietary orders depend on the extent of liver dysfunction. With uncomplicated hepatitis, protein requirements are the same or slightly higher than that for healthy adults. Fat intake may be restricted. Provide written information about dietary needs to the home caregiver.

Unfortunately, anorexia is a common symptom of hepatitis. Measures to manage anorexia include small, frequent meals, a pleasant eating environment, frequent oral hygiene, and explanations of the need for a balanced diet. Occasionally, a feeding tube is inserted to increase nutritional intake.

Nausea and vomiting also can contribute to nutritional deficits and fluid and electrolyte imbalances. Best results are usually obtained by administering an antiemetic as soon as nausea is reported. A cool, damp cloth applied to the face and neck is sometimes helpful. When the patient vomits, note the amount and contents of vomitus (emesis) as well as any visible or occult blood. Measure emesis and record the volume as output. Remove soiled clothing, linens, and basins promptly and handle them according to agency infection control guidelines.

Deficient Fluid Volume

The patient with hepatitis needs to maintain a fluid intake of 2500 to 3000 mL/day unless contraindicated. If the patient is hospitalized, maintain intake and output records. If the patient's fluid intake is low or if vomiting is present, also monitor for dehydration. Signs of dehydration include dry mucous membranes, tachycardia, concentrated urine, and confusion. Patients who are at risk for dehydration may receive intravenous fluids as prescribed. Patients with liver disease are also at risk for fluid volume excess. Signs of fluid retention include edema, increasing abdominal girth, and rising blood pressure (BP).

Risk for Impaired Skin Integrity

Pruritus, or itching, is an annoying symptom. Patients naturally respond by scratching, which may cause breaks in the skin. Nursing measures are designed to reduce dryness and irritation. The patient should bathe in tepid water and pat dry. Mild soap may be used unless it seems to increase symptoms. Lubricating lotions or topical antipruritics may be applied. Use light strokes in the direction of the heart. Select older, soft sheets. You can suggest that the patient gently pat the skin instead of scratching to reduce the itching sensation. If a patient is confused, trim the fingernails as agency policy permits. Mittens may be needed to prevent skin injury. If conservative measures are not effective, consult the physician about ordering an antihistamine.

Disturbed Body Image

The patient may be self-conscious about his or her appearance because of jaundice. Demonstrate acceptance of the patient and explain that the skin color usually returns to normal in 2 to 4 weeks.

Anxiety

Diagnostic tests and procedures and possible hospitalization can provoke anxiety in the patient with hepatitis. The patient also may be fearful about the expected course of the disease and the risk of complications. Encourage questions and find out what the patient wants to know. Explain what to expect to reduce the fear of the unknown. Explore how patients usually deal with stress and help them to identify coping strategies. If the patient has a history of drug or alcohol abuse, provide information about support groups such as Alcoholics Anonymous and Narcotics Anonymous.

Deficient Knowledge

It is particularly important for the patient with chronic hepatitis to learn how to live with the disease (see *Patient Teaching* box). Good nutrition, exercise, adequate sleep, and avoidance of illicit drugs and alcohol can slow the progression of the disease. In addition to the general teaching plan, explain the patient's specific treatment and the importance of taking medications as prescribed. If the patient is a sexually active female who is taking immune globulins or ribavirin, explain that these drugs can cause birth defects. Oral contraceptives may be ineffective, so condoms, spermicidal jelly or foam, or a diaphragm also should be used.

Patient Teaching

Hepatitis

Take precautions to avoid exposing others to the virus. Precautions vary with the type of hepatitis but the following guidelines are helpful:

- People who have had close contact with you should see a physician immediately. A vaccine or immune globulin (IG) may be available to protect them from infection.
- Do not share personal items or utensils with others.
- Wash your hands thoroughly after toileting.
- If you have active hepatitis B, use condoms for sexual intercourse; your partner should be vaccinated against the hepatitis B virus (HBV).
- Do not expose others to your blood.

Staff Protection

When patients are hospitalized, Standard Precautions are implemented. Nurses are at risk for exposure to hepatitis because they often handle body fluids. The Occupational Safety and Health Administration (OSHA) requires hepatitis B vaccination for nurses and other health care providers. The vaccine is given in a series of three injections and confers long-term immunity on most people. Follow-up testing may be done to assess the titer level, which is a measure of immunity. If the antibody titer is inadequate, up to three booster doses may be given. Vaccination has significantly decreased hepatitis B among health care providers; however, no vaccine exists for hepatitis C.

Table 41-2 summarizes precautions to be used to prevent transmission of hepatitis.

ALCOHOL-INDUCED LIVER DISEASE

Pathophysiology

The three kinds of liver disease related to alcohol consumption are (1) fatty liver, (2) alcoholic hepatitis, and (3) alcoholic cirrhosis.

Fatty Liver

Most people who drink alcohol in excess develop fatty liver characterized by a buildup of fat cells in the liver. Patients may experience discomfort in the upper abdomen caused by liver enlargement but many people have no symptoms. Fatty liver is reversible if alcohol intake ceases. The accumulation of fat in the liver not associated with alcohol, hepatitis, or autoimmune disease is called nonalcoholic fatty liver disease (NAFLD).

Alcoholic Hepatitis

Inflammation of the liver is fairly common with heavy alcohol consumption. It may be acute or chronic. In some cases life-threatening complications develop. Clinical manifestations may include fever, anorexia, nausea and vomiting, abdominal pain and tenderness, and jaundice.

Alcoholic Cirrhosis

Eventually 10% to 20% of those who ingest excessive amounts of alcohol develop alcoholic cirrhosis, a condition in which normal liver cells are replaced by scar tissue. The risk is increased for individuals who have alcohol-induced liver disease and another chronic liver disease such as hepatitis C. Although cirrhosis is not exclusively related to alcohol use, alcohol is the most common contributing factor. Cirrhosis is discussed next.

CIRRHOSIS

Pathophysiology

Cirrhosis is a chronic, progressive disease of the liver. It is characterized by degeneration and destruction of liver cells. Fibrotic bands of connective tissue impair the flow of blood and lymph and distort the normal liver structure.

As cirrhosis progresses, significant disruption of many physiologic processes occurs. The effects of liver disease include metabolic disturbances, blood abnormalities, fluid and electrolyte imbalances, decreased resistance to infection, accumulation of drugs and toxins, and obstruction of blood vessels and bile ducts in the liver.

Cirrhosis is described as *compensated* or *decompensated*. Both types are characterized by fibrosis and nodules but the presence of ascites, bleeding varices, encephalopathy, or jaundice defines decompensated cirrhosis.

Incidence

The highest incidence of cirrhosis is in people between the ages of 40 and 60. It is the twelfth leading cause of death in the United States (see *Cultural Considerations* box). It is more common in men than in women. The pathology is most often related to alcohol-induced liver disease (as described previously) or chronic viral infection.

Cultural Considerations

What Does Culture Have to Do with Cirrhosis?

Latinos have the highest rate of deaths from cirrhosis of the liver, followed by African Americans and Caucasians.

Types of Cirrhosis

Four major types of cirrhosis are classified based on cause: (1) alcoholic cirrhosis, (2) postnecrotic cirrhosis, (3) biliary cirrhosis, and (4) cardiac cirrhosis. Several other types occur infrequently.

- **Alcoholic Cirrhosis.** This type of cirrhosis is caused by exposure to alcohol. The liver enlarges, becomes "knobby," and then shrinks. Alcoholic cirrhosis is not reversible.
- **Postnecrotic Cirrhosis.** Postnecrotic cirrhosis can be a complication of hepatitis in which massive liver cell necrosis occurs.
- **Biliary Cirrhosis.** Biliary cirrhosis develops as a result of obstruction to bile flow.
- **Cardiac Cirrhosis.** Cardiac cirrhosis follows severe right-sided heart failure. Venous congestion and hypoxia lead to necrosis of liver cells.

Signs and Symptoms

In the early stage, signs and symptoms of cirrhosis are usually subtle. The patient may report slight weight loss, unexplained fever, fatigue, and dull heaviness in the right upper quadrant of the abdomen. These symptoms are probably the result of inflammation and enlargement of the liver. The liver may be palpable below the right rib margin.

As the disease progresses, impaired metabolism of carbohydrates, fats, and proteins causes GI disturbances such as anorexia, nausea, vomiting, diarrhea or constipation, flatulence, and dyspepsia (heartburn). Resistance to blood flow from the intestines to the liver causes circulation to become congested in the intestines, stomach, and esophagus. Elevated pressure in veins in the GI tract causes them to dilate and bulge. Dilated veins in the esophagus are called *esophageal varices* and those in the rectum are called *hemorrhoids*. Prominent veins may be visible on the abdomen.

Anemia, leukocytopenia, thrombocytopenia, and prothrombin deficiency are hematologic disorders associated with cirrhosis. As a result, patients tend to tire quickly and are more susceptible to infections. They bruise easily and may bleed excessively from minor trauma. Epistaxis (nosebleed) is common.

Later signs and symptoms of cirrhosis reflect the liver's inability to perform normal functions. Jaundice develops because of elevated serum bilirubin levels. Two factors contribute to jaundice in the patient with cirrhosis. First, diseased liver cells may be unable to conjugate and excrete bilirubin. Second, structural changes in the liver prevent the normal flow of bile out of the liver. Another effect of impaired bilirubin excretion, as previously mentioned, is the deposition of bile salts under the skin that can cause intense pruritus.

The diseased liver is unable to metabolize estrogen, testosterone, aldosterone, and adrenocortical hormones. Therefore the patient exhibits signs and symptoms of hormone excesses. Testicular atrophy, impotence, and gynecomastia may be noted in men and amenorrhea may be noted in women. Palmar erythema and spider angiomas also are attributed to hormone excess. Excess aldosterone contributes to sodium and water retention. The failing liver is also unable to metabolize ammonia, a product of protein metabolism. Excess ammonia affects the central nervous system (CNS), leading to confusion and decreasing consciousness.

Cirrhosis impairs the liver's ability to manufacture albumin. Albumin plays a critical role in creating the colloid osmotic pressure that retains water in the vascular compartment. With low serum albumin levels, water leaks from the capillaries, causing decreased blood volume and edema. Ascites is the accumulation of fluid in the peritoneal cavity.

Peripheral neuropathy, characterized by tingling or numbness in the extremities, is common with cirrhosis. This is thought to be caused by dietary deficiencies of vitamin B_{12}, thiamine, and folic acid.

Figure 41-5 illustrates the clinical picture of the patient with liver disease.

Complications

The patient with cirrhosis is at risk for many complications related to portal hypertension and liver insufficiency. They include esophageal varices, ascites, hepatic encephalopathy, hepatorenal syndrome (HRS), and spontaneous bacterial peritonitis.

Portal Hypertension. The portal vein delivers blood from the intestines to the liver. Changes in the liver with cirrhosis obstruct the flow of incoming blood, causing blood to back up in the portal system. High portal pressure, or portal hypertension, causes collateral vessels to develop. Collateral vessels commonly form in the esophagus, the anterior abdominal wall, and the rectum.

Esophageal Varices. Distended, engorged vessels in the esophagus are called *esophageal varices*. They are fragile and bleed easily, with the potential for fatal hemorrhage. Circumstances that may trigger bleeding include irritation and increased intraabdominal pressure. Sources of irritation are alcohol, coarse foods, and stomach acid. Intraabdominal pressure is increased by vomiting, coughing, heavy lifting, and straining to defecate.

Ascites. Ascites is an accumulation of fluid in the peritoneal cavity. Factors that contribute to the development of ascites with cirrhosis include portal hypertension, leaking of lymph fluid and albumin-rich fluid from the diseased liver, low serum albumin levels, increased aldosterone levels, and water retention.

Hepatic Encephalopathy. The failing liver is unable to detoxify ammonia, a breakdown product of protein metabolism. Excessive ammonia in the blood causes neurologic symptoms, including cognitive disturbances, declining level of consciousness, and changes in neuromuscular function. If the condition is not reversed, the patient lapses into unconsciousness, referred to as *hepatic coma*.

Factors that may precipitate hepatic encephalopathy are infection, fluid and potassium depletion, GI bleeding, constipation, and some drugs.

Hepatorenal Syndrome. HRS is renal failure in the patient with cirrhosis that often follows excessive diuresis, paracentesis without albumin infusion, or GI hemorrhage. Vasodilation associated with portal hypertension triggers a physiologic response that constricts renal blood vessels.

Spontaneous Bacterial Peritonitis. This infection is fairly common among patients with cirrhosis. While some patients have no symptoms, others have fever, jaundice, and abdominal pain.

Medical Diagnosis

When the patient's history and physical examination suggest cirrhosis, blood and urine tests, imaging procedures, and liver biopsy may be done to confirm or rule out the disease. Results of laboratory tests that are consistent with cirrhosis include elevated serum and urine bilirubin, elevated serum enzymes, decreased total serum protein, decreased cholesterol, and prolonged PT. The complete blood count (CBC) may reveal deficiencies of RBCs, white blood cells (WBCs), and platelets. The liver biopsy is performed to obtain a tissue specimen for microscopic study. Typical cellular changes occur with cirrhosis. Imaging procedures outline the liver features. Transient elastography is a newer study that uses ultrasound technology to measure liver stiffness.

Table 41-1 summarizes tests and procedures used to diagnose liver disorders.

Medical Treatment

The goals of medical treatment for cirrhosis are to limit deterioration of liver function and to prevent complications but no specific medical treatment exists. The approach is to promote rest so that the liver can regenerate. The earlier the condition is diagnosed and measures are taken to promote healing, the better is the chance of recovery. Compensated cirrhosis is managed with treatment of any underlying disease (e.g., antiviral treatment of hepatitis B or C), avoidance of liver toxins, and monitoring for varices and liver cancer.

If the patient is in liver failure, bed rest is usually ordered. Malnutrition is common and the specific diet depends on individual patient factors. A diet high in carbohydrates and vitamins with moderate to high protein intake is typically ordered unless the patient's blood ammonia level is elevated. In that case, protein is restricted until the ammonia level falls. Supplementary iron and vitamins also may be ordered. The amount of fat allowed in the diet varies with the patient's condition. Anorexia is frequently a problem with cirrhosis, so small, semisolid or liquid meals may be better received. Enteral feedings may be needed to provide adequate nutrients.

Other medical treatments may be ordered to correct the complications of cirrhosis. Intravenous fluids may be needed to correct fluid and electrolyte imbalances. Anemia may require blood transfusions. Water and sodium are likely to be restricted in patients with severe fluid retention. Cathartics and antibiotics may be used for hepatic encephalopathy. Beta-adrenergic blockers such as propranolol may be prescribed to reduce portal pressure, which decreases the risk of varices and hemorrhage.

Ascites. The medical management of ascites aims to promote reabsorption and elimination of the fluid by means of sodium restriction and diuretics, usually spironolactone, furosemide, or both. Combinations of various types of diuretics may yield better results than one alone. Salt-poor albumin may be given intravenously to help maintain blood volume and to increase urinary output. Albumin raises the serum colloid osmotic pressure, causing water to be drawn back into the bloodstream. Table 41-3 lists drugs used to treat the patient with ascites.

If ascites does not respond to conservative treatment, fluid can be removed with a needle, a procedure called *paracentesis*. Alternatives include the placement of a peritoneal-venous shunt or a transjugular intrahepatic portosystemic shunt (TIPS).

Paracentesis. Paracentesis is the removal of ascitic fluid from the peritoneal cavity. A special instrument

Table 41-3 Medications for Cirrhosis

General Nursing Implications

1. No drug can cure cirrhosis.
2. Drug therapy treats symptoms: fluid retention, portal hypertension, encephalopathy, and bleeding.
3. Patients with liver dysfunction may not metabolize drugs normally, so be alert for adverse effects.

DRUG	USE AND ACTION	SIDE EFFECTS	NURSING INTERVENTIONS
Diuretics			
Potassium-sparing diuretics: spironolactone (Aldactone), amiloride (Midamor), triamterene (Dyrenium) Loop diuretic: furosemide (Lasix) Thiazide diuretic: chlorothiazide (Diuril)	Used to promote excretion of excess fluid in edema and ascites.	Fluid and electrolyte imbalances, including fluid volume deficit, hyperkalemia, and hyponatremia. Most diuretics can cause hypokalemia. Potassium-sparing diuretics (e.g., spironolactone) can cause hyperkalemia.	Monitor the patient's intake, output, and abdominal girth. Check laboratory values for electrolyte imbalances.
Hormones			
sandostatin (Octreotide) vasopressin (VP)	Used to reduce pressure in the portal veins to treat bleeding esophageal varices.	Bradycardia, hyperglycemia, and hypoglycemia. VP: decreased coronary blood flow, increased blood pressure (BP), dysrhythmias. Nitroglycerin may be given with VP to minimize adverse effects.	Monitor the patient's pulse and notify the physician if it is below 60 beats per minute (bpm). Monitor glucose levels in patients with diabetes.
Beta-Adrenergic Blockers			
propranolol (Inderal)	Used to reduce pressure in the portal veins to reduce the risk of bleeding. Target heart rate is 50–55 bpm.	Bradycardia, hypotension, and bronchoconstriction. The drug masks signs of hypoglycemia.	Monitor the patient's pulse and notify the physician if it is below the target rate. Monitor blood glucose in patients with diabetes.
Antibiotics			
neomycin sulfate	Prevents or treats hepatic encephalopathy. Decreases gastrointestinal (GI) bacterial flora, which decreases ammonia.	The drug is toxic to the kidney and eighth cranial nerve (hearing and balance). It increases the action of neuromuscular blockers such as anesthetic drugs.	Monitor the patient's intake and output. Assess for hearing impairment, tinnitus (i.e., ringing in ears), nausea, and loss of balance.
Laxatives			
lactulose (Cephulac)	Prevents or treats hepatic encephalopathy by promoting elimination of ammonia in feces.	Cramps, distention, flatulence, eructation, and hyperglycemia with diabetes.	Drug may be ordered every hour at first and can be mixed with fruit juice, water, or milk. Monitor patients with diabetes for high blood glucose.
Vitamins			
B-complex vitamins	Needed for the production of red blood cells (RBCs) and for normal growth and development.	Allergic reaction to thiamine (anaphylaxis). Adverse effects are rare.	Intradermal test dose may be ordered to detect sensitivity to thiamine. Check the site for reaction (i.e., redness and swelling). Check medication reference material for incompatibility with other intravenous drugs.

Continued

Table 41-3 Medications for Cirrhosis—cont'd

DRUG	USE AND ACTION	SIDE EFFECTS	NURSING INTERVENTIONS
Vitamin K: phytonadione (AquaMEPHYTON)	Used to treat serious bleeding disorders caused by deficiency of prothrombin (given cautiously to patients with severe liver disease).	Gastric upset (oral route only), rash, urticaria, flushing, hemolytic anemia, pain and swelling at the injection site.	Check laboratory results for prothrombin time (PT). Report any abnormalities to the physician. Monitor complete blood count (CBC). Assess for bleeding. Apply pressure to needle puncture sites for 5 minutes.
Blood Derivative			
Albumin	Off-label use: Prevents renal dysfunction caused by spontaneous bacterial peritonitis.	Fluid volume excess: elevated BP, distended neck veins, dyspnea, headache.	Monitor vital signs. Must be reconstituted to prepare for intravenous administration.

called a *trocar* is inserted through the abdominal wall and a catheter is placed to allow the fluid to drain. This procedure is indicated only when ascites interferes with the patient's breathing. It is not used frequently because it removes essential protein and electrolytes. In addition, it provides a potential portal of entry for pathogens.

If paracentesis is done to remove ascites, your role is to prepare the patient, assist and support the patient during the procedure, and provide aftercare. The physician should explain what will be done and obtain patient consent. Reinforce explanations and obtain the written consent as agency policy permits. Obtain baseline vital signs, weight, and abdominal girth. Instruct the patient to void.

The procedure is often done at the bedside with the patient in a sitting position. During paracentesis, you should support and encourage the patient. The physician may request monitoring of vital signs during the process. Usually, 2 to 3 L of fluid is removed slowly. Rapid removal of ascitic fluid could result in circulatory collapse. After paracentesis, a sterile dressing is applied to the puncture site. Monitor vital signs every 15 minutes until the patient is stable and check the dressing for bleeding. Measure the fluid obtained and send a specimen for laboratory analysis. Document the procedure, including the amount and color of the fluid. Monitor for blood in the urine. Intravenous albumin may be ordered based on the amount of fluid removed.

Shunts. Shunts provide a mechanism to collect ascitic fluid and return it to the circulation. Advantages to shunting ascitic fluid rather than removing it are (1) protein-rich serum is retained and returned to the vascular compartment; and (2) urine output increases, which eliminates excess sodium and water. Two types of shunts are the peritoneal-venous shunt and the TIPS.

Peritoneal-venous shunts may be implanted permanently. Two types of peritoneal-venous shunts are (1) the LeVeen shunt and (2) the Denver shunt. The LeVeen shunt (Fig. 41-6) is a tube that is placed in the abdomen, running from the peritoneal cavity to the jugular vein or superior vena cava. The tube has a one-way valve that permits excess fluid to drain into the venous circulation when pressure rises in the abdomen. When the patient inspires, intraabdominal pressure rises, causing the valve to open. The Denver peritoneal-venous shunt involves a manual pump placed under the skin. It can be compressed to cause fluid to flow from the peritoneum to the venous system. Potential complications of peritoneal-venous shunts are peritonitis, tubing obstruction, circulatory overload, disseminated intravascular coagulation (DIC), variceal hemorrhage, and embolism.

Because of the complications encountered with peritoneal-venous shunts, the TIPS is often a preferred treatment. A catheter is threaded through the jugular vein and the inferior vena cava to the hepatic vein. The hepatic vein is punctured and connected to the portal vein with a stent. This procedure reduces pressure in the portal system with fewer complications.

The portacaval shunt and the distal splenorenal shunt are surgically created to reduce portal system pressure while maintaining liver perfusion. The patient with a portacaval shunt is at risk for hepatic encephalopathy because ammonia accumulates in the blood. The incidence of hepatic encephalopathy is lower with distal splenorenal shunts.

Bleeding Esophageal Varices. Several techniques can be used to control bleeding esophageal varices. These include drug therapy, sclerotherapy, and endoscopic ligation. Although now uncommon, placement of esophageal-gastric balloon tubes may still be useful to control severe hemorrhage.

Acute bleeding episodes may be treated with intravenous octreotide, which constricts blood vessels and lowers pressure in the hepatic circulation. In addition to blood transfusions, vitamin K and proton pump inhibitors (PPIs) such as pantoprazole (Protonix) may be ordered. Lactulose may be administered to prevent

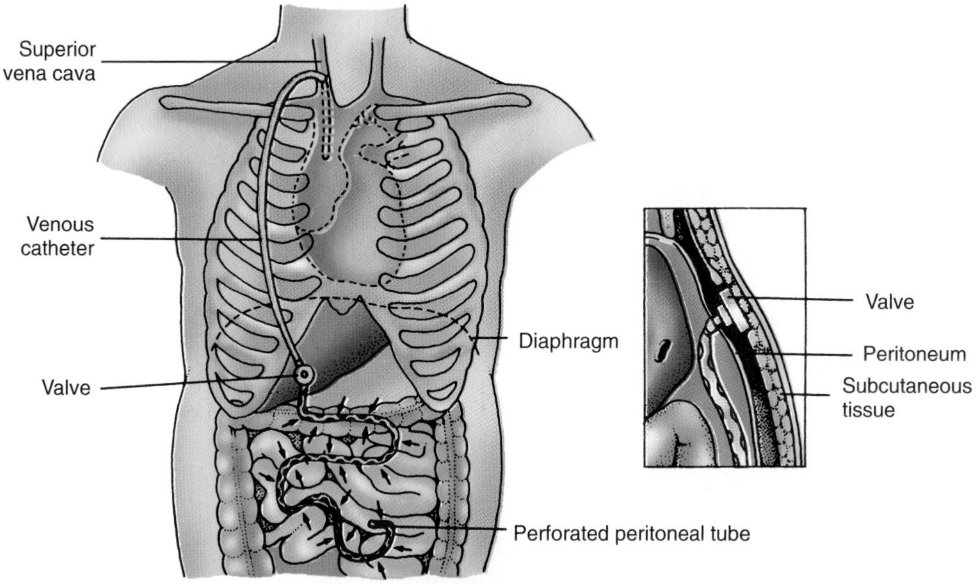

FIGURE 41-6 A peritoneal-venous shunt drains ascitic fluid from the abdominal cavity into the superior vena cava. (From Ignatavicius DD, Workman ML, Mishler MA: *Medical-surgical nursing across the health care continuum*, ed 3, Philadelphia, 1999, Saunders.)

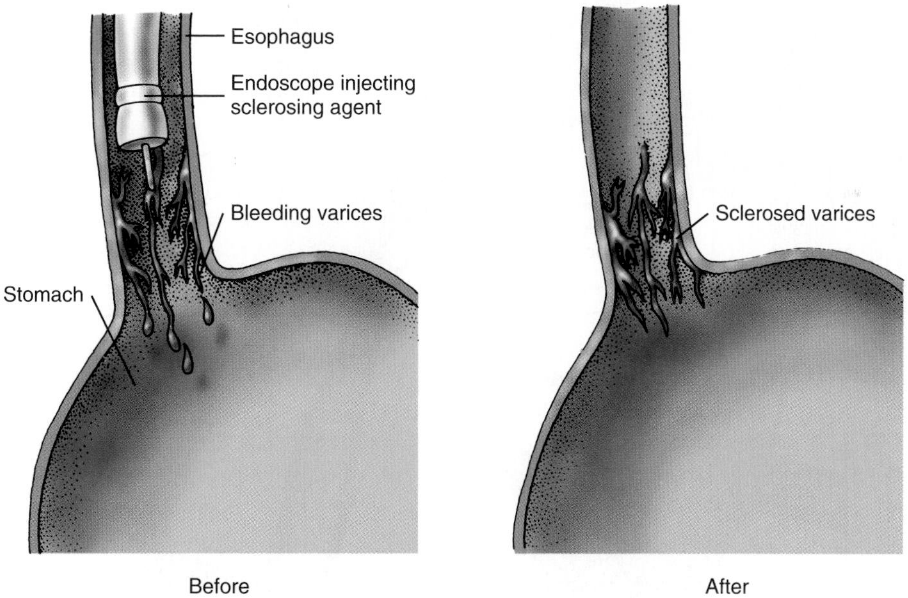

FIGURE 41-7 Injection sclerotherapy. (From Monahan FD, Drake DT, Neighbors M, editors: *Medical-surgical nursing: foundations for clinical practice*, ed 2, Philadelphia, 1998, Saunders.)

the breakdown of blood in the intestines that would release ammonia, contributing to hepatic encephalopathy. Beta-adrenergic blockers may be used to reduce BP in the long-term management of patients after acute bleeding episodes.

Surgical Treatment of Bleeding Varices. In an emergency situation, the surgeon may ligate (i.e., tie off) bleeding varices directly through an endoscope. The patient can then be stabilized before a more extensive corrective procedure. Corrective procedures surgically shunt blood from engorged varices to other veins. Shunting the blood reduces pressure in the portal venous system and the esophageal varices.

Sclerotherapy. Sclerotherapy is a procedure in which a solution is injected into the varices or into the veins that supply them, causing the varices to harden and close (Fig. 41-7). The procedure can be done through an endoscope or through a small surgical incision. Sclerotherapy can be done to prevent or to treat bleeding.

After sclerotherapy, patients often report chest discomfort for several days. The physician usually orders a mild analgesic. If it does not relieve the pain, the physician should be notified, because persistent pain may indicate perforation of the esophagus. Once a patient has had sclerotherapy, extra care must be taken in the insertion of nasogastric tubes.

Esophageal-Gastric Balloon Tube. Although uncommon, esophageal-gastric balloon tubes may be used to apply direct pressure to bleeding veins in the esophagus and stomach if ligation and sclerotherapy fail. Examples of tubes used for this purpose are the Sengstaken-Blakemore esophageal-gastric balloon tube and the Minnesota tube (Fig. 41-8). These tubes include balloons that are inflated in the esophagus and the stomach to apply pressure to varices. They also have a lumen that permits gastric suction to remove old blood from the stomach. The tube usually is left inflated for 24 to 48 hours. It then is deflated but left in place so that it can be reinflated if needed.

Hepatic Encephalopathy. Many factors can precipitate hepatic encephalopathy, including constipation, GI bleeding, hypokalemia, infection, opioids, dehydration, and renal failure. Treatment is aimed at correcting the cause and reducing the amount of ammonia being produced in the digestive tract. This reduction may be achieved with lactulose. Lactulose is a cathartic that promotes elimination of ammonia from the colon and discourages bacterial growth by making the intestinal contents more acidic.

If the patient has been bleeding into the GI tract, laxatives and enemas may be ordered to remove

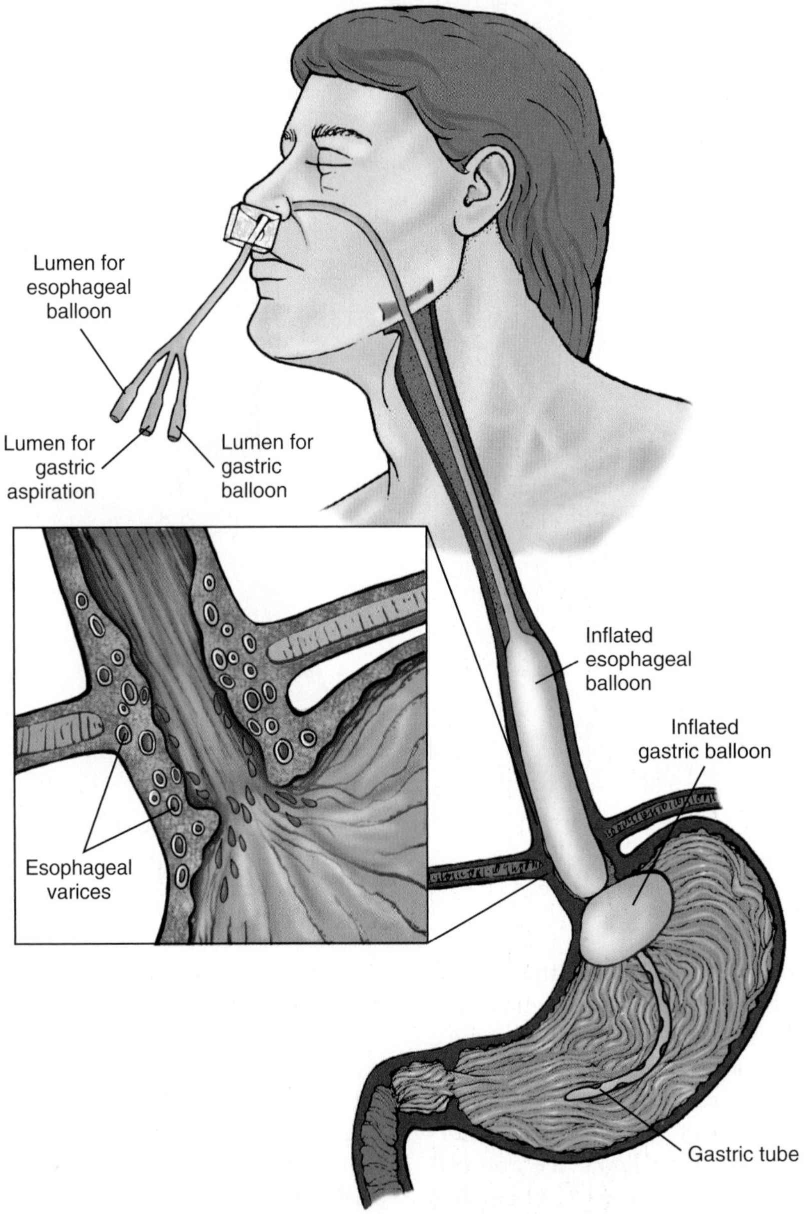

FIGURE 41-8 Sengstaken-Blakemore tube in place to compress bleeding esophageal varices. (From Ignatavicius DD, Workman ML, Mishler MA: *Medical-surgical nursing across the health care continuum*, ed 3, Philadelphia, 1999, Saunders.)

old blood and protein. Patients with recurring hepatic encephalopathy may be candidates for liver transplantation.

Hepatorenal Syndrome. HRS is renal failure accompanying cirrhosis. Precipitating factors include paracentesis, diuresis, and GI hemorrhage. It may be treated with a vasoconstrictor (octreotide with midodrine), albumin, and a TIPS. Extracorporeal albumin dialysis is an experimental procedure that is under study. Patients should not receive nephrotoxic drugs such as nonsteroidal antiinflammatory drugs (NSAIDs). Medical management is used primarily to support the patient until liver transplantation is available.

Spontaneous Bacterial Peritonitis. Spontaneous bacterial peritonitis is treated with antibiotics. Intravenous albumin is given to prevent renal dysfunction associated with this infection. Long-term prophylactic antibiotic therapy is reserved for a few circumstances because it leads to antibiotic resistance.

Drug Therapy. A variety of drugs may be used to treat the effects of cirrhosis. These drugs and nursing implications are summarized in Table 41-3. Because most drugs are metabolized by the liver and many drugs are hepatotoxic, the physician is cautious in the selection of drugs.

❖ NURSING CARE of the Patient with Cirrhosis

■ Assessment

Ongoing assessment of the cirrhosis patient should include daily measurements of weight, intake and output, and abdominal girth. Patients are monitored for signs and symptoms of complications—bleeding, ascites, encephalopathy, and renal failure.

Nursing Diagnoses, Goals, and Outcome Criteria: Cirrhosis

Nursing Diagnoses	Goals and Outcome Criteria
Imbalanced Nutrition: Less Than Body Requirements related to anorexia, metabolic imbalances	Adequate nutrition: stable body weight, consumes meals
Activity Intolerance related to fatigue	Improved activity tolerance: performs activities of daily living (ADL) without excessive fatigue
Risk for Impaired Skin Integrity related to edema, immobility, pruritus, hypoproteinemia	Intact skin: no redness or breaks in skin, no scratching
Ineffective Breathing Pattern related to ascites	Effective breathing: respiratory rate of 12 to 20 breaths/min without dyspnea

Nursing Diagnoses, Goals, and Outcome Criteria: Cirrhosis—cont'd

Nursing Diagnoses	Goals and Outcome Criteria
Risk for Injury related to impaired coagulation	Absence of bleeding: no blood in emesis or stool, vital signs consistent with patient norms
Acute Confusion related to elevated blood ammonia	Normal cognitive function: mentally alert, oriented
Deficient Fluid Volume (hypovolemia) or **Excess Fluid Volume** (in third space) related to hypoproteinemia, increased aldosterone	Normal fluid distribution in body fluid compartments: balanced fluid intake and output without edema or ascites; pulse and blood pressure (BP) consistent with patient norms
Risk for Infection related to liver dysfunction, impaired response to infection, malnutrition	Absence of infection: oral temperature less than 100°F (37.8°C)
Fear related to dyspnea, life-threatening illness	Reduced fear: patient states no or less fear, calm manner

■ Interventions

Imbalanced Nutrition: Less Than Body Requirements

Good nutrition is essential for regeneration of liver tissue. However, it is a challenge for the patient with cirrhosis, who often has anorexia, indigestion, nausea, and vomiting. Furthermore, the diet may be made less palatable by protein or salt restriction.

Explain the need for adequate food intake to the patient and encourage the patient to eat even when he or she is not hungry. Small, frequent meals may be more acceptable to the anorexic patient. Arrange a dietary consult for the patient to report likes and dislikes (see *Patient Teaching* box).

Make mealtimes as pleasant as possible. Put bedpans, emesis basins, and drainage collection devices out of sight. Ventilate the room to reduce odors. Do not schedule tiring activities immediately before meals. Record daily weights as ordered to monitor both nutritional and fluid status.

Activity Intolerance

Some activity limitations are usually imposed, depending on the patient's overall status. Schedule nursing care to allow some periods of undisturbed rest. The patient can generally assume any position that is comfortable.

If the patient spends all or most of the day in bed, there is a risk of complications related to immobility.

Patient Teaching

Cirrhosis

- A balanced diet will help to prevent additional injury to the liver and reduce the risk of complications.
- Avoid specific foods (as advised by the physician, the dietitian, or both).
- Notify your physician if you have increasing fluid retention, black tarry stools, bloody vomitus, increasing fatigue, or confusion.
- Alcohol is discouraged because of the toxic effects on the liver. Community resources you can use for information and assistance include Alcoholics Anonymous (if appropriate), the American Liver Foundation, and home health nursing services.
- Do not take medications except as approved by your physician. Many drugs, including acetaminophen, can be harmful to the liver.

Assist the patient to change positions, deep breathe, and exercise extremities regularly.

Risk for Impaired Skin Integrity

The patient with cirrhosis is at risk for skin breakdown for several reasons. Bile salts that are normally processed by the liver may be deposited under the skin, causing intense pruritus. Loss of muscle and fat tissue with advanced disease reduces the padding that normally protects the skin from pressure. Also, many patients have edema, which makes tissue more fragile and impairs healing.

Nursing measures to relieve the itching of pruritus include gentle bathing with mild soap and tepid water, thorough rinsing, and application of moisturizing lotions. The patient's nails should be kept short to reduce trauma from scratching. If scratching persists, put soft cotton mittens or gloves on the patient's hands. If itching is severe, consult the physician about ordering a medication to relieve the discomfort. Cholestyramine (Questran) may be ordered to increase the excretion of bile salts.

Ineffective Breathing Pattern

Ascitic fluid can cause the abdomen to become greatly distended. While in bed, the patient breathes easier with the head of the bed elevated. Sitting in a chair with the feet elevated, if allowed, may be even more comfortable.

Risk for Injury

The patient with cirrhosis is at great risk for injury or hemorrhage due to impaired coagulation and fragile varices. Handle the patient gently to avoid trauma. Use a soft toothbrush or swab for mouth care. Apply firm pressure to injection sites to minimize oozing. Pad side rails if the patient is restless.

An uncommon but effective treatment for bleeding esophageal varices is an esophageal-gastric balloon tube placement. The patient with this type of tube is usually in an intensive care unit, since close monitoring is necessary. The tube is uncomfortable and the patient is likely to be frightened about both the bleeding and the treatment. When the tube is in place, monitor the patient for signs of continued or renewed bleeding, including restlessness, increasing pulse and respirations, and falling blood pressure. Note stool characteristics. Bleeding from the esophagus or stomach usually produces a sticky (tarry), maroon to black stool. Examine aspirated stomach and esophageal contents for evidence of fresh bleeding. Old blood in the stomach is usually brownish and may be described as *resembling coffee grounds*. Fresh blood is bright to dark red.

Because the esophagus and the trachea are adjacent to each other, upward movement of the esophageal balloon can cause airway obstruction. Therefore when the balloon tube is in place, monitor the patient for sudden respiratory distress. If this occurs, both balloon ports must be cut promptly and the tubes removed by a properly trained person.

Acute Confusion

Cognitive changes in the patient with cirrhosis are usually due to hepatic encephalopathy. Nursing care of the patient with hepatic encephalopathy includes monitoring mental and neurologic status. Inform the RN or physician of changes in status. The patient who is confused or unconscious requires close attention to prevent injury or complications of immobility. Talk to the patient to provide basic information and reassurance. The family also may need an explanation of the patient's behavior. Administer prescribed drugs that decrease ammonia-producing bacteria in the intestines (e.g., lactulose). Be alert for adverse effects of drug therapy, which may include diarrhea or vitamin K deficiency.

Deficient Fluid Volume or Excess Fluid Volume

Fluid needs vary with the patient's condition. Sodium and water are likely to be restricted if marked edema or ascites exist. Despite the excess in total body water, the patient's blood volume may be dangerously low. Adequate water is present but it is not distributed appropriately. Without adequate albumin in the serum, colloid osmotic pressure falls and water shifts out of the capillaries into the tissues. Administer intravenous fluids and albumin 25% as ordered. In addition to monitoring vital signs, evaluate fluid intake and output.

Risk for Infection

The patient with cirrhosis is at risk for infection for several reasons. The liver is no longer able to filter bacteria from the blood as it comes from the intestines. The function of the spleen also is impaired, which lowers resistance to infection. In addition, these patients tend to be malnourished, so they lack the building materials necessary for tissue repair. Monitor for fever and malaise, which suggest infection. Protect the patient from others with infections. Practice good hand washing and use aseptic technique for invasive procedures.

Fear

Patients with cirrhosis can experience frightening complications, including confusion, dyspnea, and hemorrhage. With advanced cirrhosis, the prognosis is poor and patients often have repeated emergency admissions. Treatments and diagnostic procedures may be painful and anxiety producing. The nurse can help by recognizing the patient's fear and acknowledging it.

To provide emotional support to cirrhosis patients, you must be aware of your personal reaction to these patients. There is a stigma attached to cirrhosis because it is often associated with alcohol abuse. Health care providers must treat patients in a nonjudgmental manner. Nurses must realize that alcoholism is a complex chronic disease that is not easily controlled and that cirrhosis can be caused by factors other than alcohol (see *Complementary and Alternative Therapies* box).

> **Complementary and Alternative Therapies**
>
> Some patients have found acupuncture helpful for the treatment of alcoholism.

> **Put on Your Thinking Cap!**
>
> Identify three functions of the healthy liver. Describe how cirrhosis affects those functions. State one nursing implication related to the change with cirrhosis in each function.

Information can help to reduce fear. When the patient is acutely ill, give simple explanations and answer questions. When the patient improves, explore what he or she knows about cirrhosis and determine what additional information is needed. General teaching points are noted in the following *Patient Teaching* box.

> **Patient Teaching**
>
> **Cirrhosis**
>
> - A balanced diet will help prevent additional injury to the liver and reduce risk of complications.
> - Avoid specific food as advised by the physician and the dietitian.
> - Notify your physician if you have increasing fluid retention, black tarry stools, bloody vomitus, increasing fatigue, or confusion.
> - Alcohol is discouraged because of the toxic effects on the liver. Community resources you can use for information and assistance include Alcoholics Anonymous (if appropriate), the American Liver Foundation, and home health nursing services.
> - Do not take medications except as approved by your physician. Many drugs, including acetaminophen, can be toxic to the liver.

END-STAGE LIVER DISEASE

End-stage liver disease can result from injury or chronic disease. Hepatic injury may result from acute hepatitis, drug toxicity, or obstruction of the hepatic vein. Liver failure associated with injury is commonly called *fulminant liver failure*.

CANCER OF THE LIVER

Cancer rarely begins in the liver but the liver is a frequent site of metastasis. Cirrhosis is a predisposing factor for liver cancer. Signs and symptoms of liver cancer include liver enlargement, weight loss, anorexia, nausea, vomiting, and dull pain in the right upper quadrant of the abdomen. As the disease progresses, the signs and symptoms are essentially the same as those of cirrhosis. Because the early signs and symptoms of liver cancer are vague, the condition is often not diagnosed until it is advanced.

Tests and procedures used to diagnose liver cancer are liver scan, CT or MRI, biopsy, hepatic angiography, endoscopy, and measurement of alpha-fetoprotein levels. If the cancer is confined to one area, a lobectomy may be done; otherwise, chemotherapy is the primary treatment. Chemotherapy is generally considered to be palliative, meaning that it may slow the progress of the cancer and increase patient comfort but is unlikely to be curative. Transarterial chemoembolization is a procedure in which the chemotherapy drug and a drug that obstructs the blood vessels are injected into the blood vessels that supply the tumor. Other options are liver transplantation and ablation (destruction) of the tumor using heat, cold, alcohol, or acetic acid. Transplantation is an option unless the cancer is widespread.

During the course of the illness, the patient's needs are much like those of the patient with cirrhosis (discussed previously). Additional aspects of nursing care of the patient with cancer are discussed in Chapter 25.

LIVER TRANSPLANTATION

The only possible cure for end-stage liver disease is liver transplantation. Transplantation is also appropriate for patients with cancer that is confined to the liver and for patients with certain congenital disorders.

Donors may be deceased or living. When a living donor is available, a segment or lobe is transplanted. Patients who are recommended for transplantation but do not have a living donor are ranked by standard criteria and entered in a national computer network. When a liver becomes available by donation, the best recipient can then be identified. Patients awaiting transplantation must be on standby status in the event that a donor is located. This is a time of alternating hope and fear for patients and families.

After liver transplantation, the patient is cared for in a specialized unit. A transplant patient often has a

T-tube, wound drainage devices, a nasogastric tube, and a central line for total parenteral nutrition (TPN). Mechanical ventilation also is used initially.

Nursing assessments focus on neurologic status, vital signs, central venous pressure, respiratory status, and indicators of bleeding. If stable, the patient is moved out of the specialized unit after 3 or 4 days. Continue to monitor vital signs, intake and output, and neurologic status. Provide usual postoperative care, including assistance with turning, coughing and deep breathing, and progressive activity.

Prednisone usually is given during the surgery and continued for 2 weeks to 3 months. Thereafter, lifelong drug therapy, most often with cyclosporine or tacrolimus, is needed to prevent rejection of the donor liver. Some of the other available options are the monoclonal antibody OKT3, interleukin-2 receptor antagonists, and azathioprine. All have significant adverse effects. OKT3 is a newer agent that may prove to be highly effective and less toxic than other antirejection drugs.

The transplant recipient must be monitored for signs of rejection. These signs include fever, anorexia, depression, vague abdominal pain, muscle aches, and joint pain. Fever is sometimes the *only* sign of rejection. Rejection may be treated with corticosteroids or other immunosuppressant medications. If this treatment is unsuccessful, retransplantation may be needed.

Before discharge, the patient should know the signs and symptoms of transplant rejection and infection, wound care, dietary restrictions (usually sodium restriction), and self-medication.

Pharmacology Capsule

Drugs that suppress rejection of transplanted organs reduce the patient's ability to resist infection.

BILIARY TRACT

ANATOMY AND PHYSIOLOGY OF THE BILIARY TRACT

Bile is a yellow-green liquid that has several important functions. It contains bile salts, which are essential for the emulsification and digestion of fats. It also provides a medium for the excretion of bilirubin from the liver.

The biliary tract is made up of the gallbladder and the bile ducts. The function of the biliary tract is to deliver bile from the liver to the duodenum. Bile is produced in the liver and channeled into the common hepatic duct. The common hepatic duct joins the cystic duct to form the common bile duct. The cystic duct leads to the gallbladder, a saclike organ beneath the liver. Bile flows from the liver to the gallbladder, where it is stored and concentrated (Fig. 41-9).

When fats enter the duodenum, the gallbladder contracts and delivers bile to the intestine through the common bile duct.

NURSING ASSESSMENT OF THE BILIARY TRACT

The nursing assessment of the GI system is outlined in Chapter 39. Data that are especially important in a

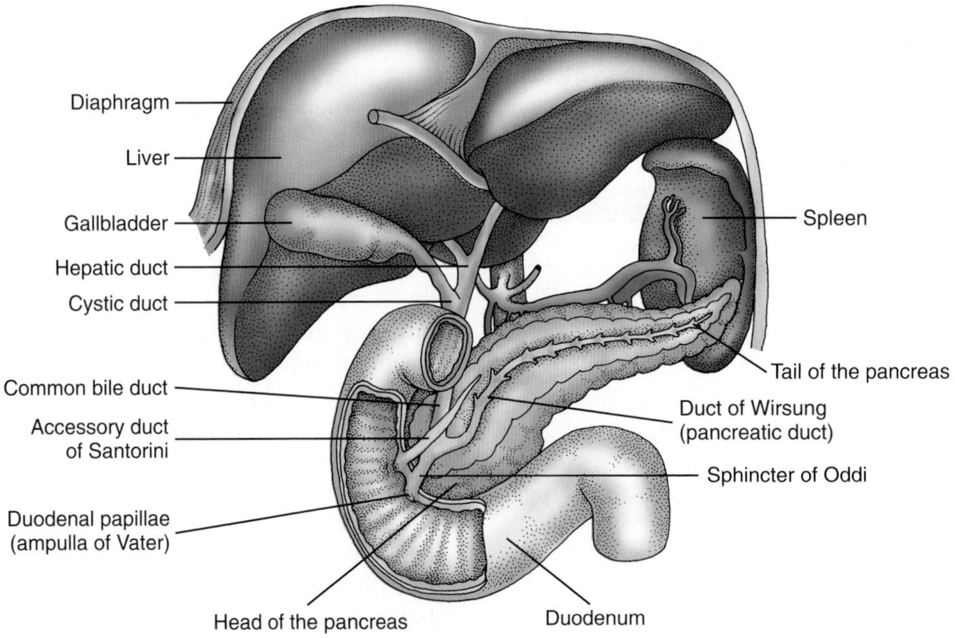

FIGURE 41-9 Anatomy of the liver, gallbladder, and pancreas. (From Ignatavicius DD, Workman ML: *Medical-surgical nursing: patient-centered collaborative care*, ed 6, St. Louis, 2010, Saunders.)

Box 41-2 Assessment of the Patient with Gallbladder Disease

HEALTH HISTORY
Present Illness
Digestive disturbances; pain: location, onset, intensity, duration, relationship to meals, aggravating and relieving factors
Past Medical History
Gallbladder disease, pregnancy, surgery, recent and current medications
Family History
Gallbladder disease
Review of Systems
Pruritus, indigestion, fat intolerance, dyspepsia, nausea, vomiting, light-colored stools, dark urine
PHYSICAL EXAMINATION
Vital Signs
Tachycardia, tachypnea, fever
Skin
Dryness, jaundice
Abdomen
Guarding, distention

patient with known or suspected gallbladder dysfunction are identified here.

HEALTH HISTORY

Digestive disturbances and pain are common complaints among persons with biliary problems. Obtain a complete description of these symptoms. Note factors that seem to bring on or relieve the symptoms. The relationship between symptoms and meals may be significant. Record the use of estrogen or oral contraceptives. Inquire about factors known to be associated with gallbladder disease: family history, obesity, Native American ancestry, and inactivity (see *Cultural Considerations* box). In the review of systems, ask whether the patient has had dry skin, indigestion, fat intolerance (foul stools after high-fat meals), dyspepsia, nausea, vomiting, light-colored stools, or dark urine.

Cultural Considerations

What Does Culture Have to Do with Gallbladder Disease?

Native Americans and Caucasians are at increased risk for gallbladder disease.

PHYSICAL EXAMINATION

When a patient has gallbladder disease, significant findings on the physical examination include dry skin, fever, jaundice, tachycardia, tachypnea, and abdominal guarding and distention. Assessment of the patient with a biliary tract disorder is summarized in Box 41-2.

DIAGNOSTIC TESTS AND PROCEDURES

Tests and procedures used to diagnose biliary tract disorders are ultrasonography, oral cholecystography, intravenous cholangiography, T-tube cholangiography, endoscopic retrograde cholangiopancreatography (ERCP), and percutaneous transhepatic cholangiography. Laboratory studies include liver function tests, serum and urine bilirubin measurements, alkaline phosphatase (ALP), aminotransferase, and CBC. Table 41-1 describes common diagnostic tests and nursing implications.

DISORDERS OF THE GALLBLADDER

Gallbladder disease is one of the most common health problems in the United States. The two most common gallbladder disorders are (1) cholecystitis and (2) cholelithiasis. Carcinoma of the gallbladder occurs but is unusual.

Risk factors for gallbladder disease include obesity, familial tendency, a sedentary lifestyle, and the use of estrogen or oral contraceptives. Women are at greater risk than men, especially women who have had multiple pregnancies. The "five Fs" are sometimes used to describe those at greatest risk for gallbladder disease: (1) female, (2) fat, (3) fair, (4) forty, and (5) fertile.

CHOLECYSTITIS AND CHOLELITHIASIS

Cholecystitis is inflammation of the gallbladder. It is caused most often by the presence of gallstones but can be the result of bacteria, toxic chemicals, tumors, anesthesia, starvation, and opioids. The inflamed gallbladder and cystic duct become swollen and congested with blood. The cystic duct actually may become occluded.

When gallstones are present, the patient is said to have **cholelithiasis**. Most gallstones are composed of cholesterol mixed with bile salts, bilirubin, calcium, and protein. It is not known exactly why gallstones form but the process is associated with high concentrations of cholesterol. The concentration of cholesterol rises when stasis of bile exists (as occurs with pregnancy, immobility, and inflammation of the biliary tract). Many patients with gallstones have no symptoms; the condition is often diagnosed incidentally during imaging procedures for unrelated complaints.

Gallstones may be found anywhere in the biliary tract: the gallbladder, the cystic duct, or the common bile duct (Fig. 41-10). The stones may move through the biliary tract with bile flow. If a stone cannot pass through the tract, it lodges and causes an obstruction. Ducts respond to obstruction with spasms in an effort to move the stone. This is responsible for an intense, spasmodic pain, called *biliary colic*.

If the cystic duct is obstructed, bile cannot leave the gallbladder and inflammation develops. Cystic duct obstruction does not prevent the flow of bile into the duodenum from the liver. However, if the common bile duct is obstructed (**choledocholithiasis**), bile is unable to flow into the duodenum.

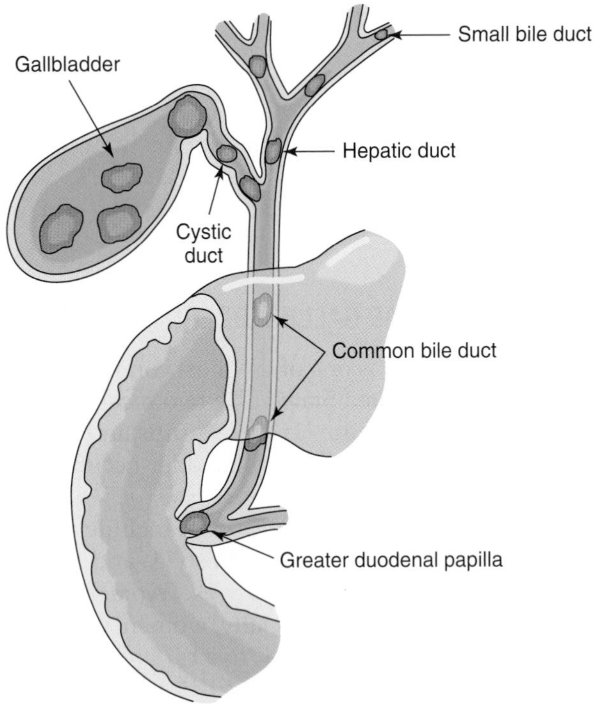

FIGURE 41-10 Gallstones within the gallbladder that could obstruct the common bile duct and the cystic duct. (From Monahan F, Sands J, Neighbors M, et al., editors: *Phipps' medical-surgical nursing: health and illness perspectives*, ed 8, St. Louis, 2007, Mosby.)

Signs and Symptoms

Signs and symptoms of cholecystitis vary from one patient to the next. Some have only mild indigestion whereas others have severe pain, fever, and jaundice. Other symptoms are nausea, **eructation** (belching), fever, chills, and right upper quadrant pain that radiates to the shoulder. Symptoms typically occur about 3 hours after a meal, especially if the food had high fat content.

When bile flow is obstructed, bile production in the liver decreases and the serum bilirubin rises, leading to obstructive jaundice. Some excess bilirubin is excreted in the urine, creating a dark-amber color. Digestion of fats is impaired, causing intolerance of fatty foods and steatorrhea (i.e., excess fat in feces). The absence of urobilinogen in the stool causes it to be a characteristic clay color. The patient is unable to absorb fat-soluble vitamins and may show signs of vitamin deficiencies. Vitamin K deficiency interferes with normal blood clotting and thus the patient bleeds and bruises easily.

Complications

The most serious complications of cholecystitis and cholelithiasis are pancreatitis, abscesses, cholangitis (i.e., inflammation of the biliary ducts), and rupture of the gallbladder.

Medical Diagnosis

Ultrasonography usually confirms a tentative diagnosis of cholelithiasis based on patient history and physical examination findings. Other diagnostic procedures include radiographs and radionuclide imaging. A technetium-labeled hepatobiliary iminodiacetic acid (HIDA) scan is a specific test for acute cholecystitis.

Blood and urine studies provide additional information. With inflammation or infection, the WBC count is elevated. If bile flow is obstructed, levels of serum and urinary bilirubin and serum enzymes may be elevated. Nursing considerations associated with specific diagnostic tests and procedures are summarized in Table 41-1.

Medical Treatment

Acute cholecystitis is managed symptomatically. Analgesics and anticholinergic agents are ordered to relieve pain and muscle spasms. Antibiotics are given to treat infection. Intravenous fluids are selected to maintain fluid balance, especially if the patient has been vomiting. A nasogastric tube may be inserted and attached to suction to rest the bowel. This relieves nausea and vomiting and reduces the stimulation of the gallbladder by intestinal contents.

Among the options available for the treatment of cholelithiasis or choledocholithiasis are drug therapy, shock wave lithotripsy, endoscopic sphincterotomy, and **cholecystectomy**. Patients with asymptomatic gallstones usually require no treatment except in special circumstances.

Drug Therapy. Drugs that dissolve gallstones include bile salts and dissolution agents. Bile salts include chenodeoxycholic acid (Chenodal) and ursodeoxycholic acid (UDCA) (Actigall). These drugs may be prescribed when the patient has only small cholesterol stones or for those who are poor surgical risks. However, they are expensive and typically require continuous treatment for as long as 2 years. Some patients require continuous therapy to prevent recurrence.

Methyl tertiary-butyl ether (MTBE) and ethyl propionate are dissolution agents. MTBE is instilled into the gallbladder through a transhepatic catheter. The physician instills and aspirates the drug repeatedly until fluoroscopy shows that the stones either have dissolved or are not responding to the treatment.

Drugs used to treat conditions of the biliary tract are described in Table 41-4.

Extracorporeal Shock Wave Lithotripsy. Extracorporeal shock wave lithotripsy (ESWL) uses sound waves to break up gallstones in patients with few stones and mild to moderate symptoms. Fragments that remain in the gallbladder are dissolved with UDCA. Gallstones recur in about half of patients successfully treated with ESWL. Laparoscopic cholecystectomy has largely replaced ESWL. For general information about lithotripsy, see the section titled "Renal Calculi" in Chapter 42.

Endoscopic Sphincterotomy. Endoscopic sphincterotomy involves the use of endoscopic instruments to

Table 41-4 **Drugs Used to Dissolve Gallstones**

General Nursing Implications

1. Drugs are effective only against small cholesterol stones.
2. Drug therapy is successful in only about one third to one half of patients treated.

DRUG	SIDE EFFECTS	NURSING INTERVENTIONS
Oral Bile Salts		
chenodeoxycholic acid (Chenix), ursodeoxycholic acid (UDCA) (Actigall)	Diarrhea; cramps; nausea; vomiting; elevated levels of serum enzymes, low-density lipoproteins (LDLs), and cholesterol. UDCA has milder side effects but is very expensive. Contraindications include biliary tract infection, pancreatitis, and pregnancy.	If the patient is a woman, advise her not to become pregnant while taking this drug. Stress the importance of periodic blood tests to determine liver enzyme and serum cholesterol levels.
Dissolution Agents		
methyl tertiary-butyl ether (MTBE)	Abdominal pain and nausea during treatment.	Oral contrast dye is given the previous evening. Position the patient on the right side after the procedure to reduce bleeding. Monitor for hemorrhage, shock, and pneumothorax. Measure the patient's vital signs every 15 minutes until stable; then 3 times at 4-hour intervals. The patient should be kept on bed rest for 24 hours.

incise the sphincter of Oddi and extract stones from the common bile duct, as illustrated in Figure 41-11. The patient is given a sedative but remains conscious during the procedure. Lidocaine spray is used to deaden the gag reflex so that the endoscope can be passed through the mouth. A choledochoscope also can be inserted through a T-tube into the common bile duct. A special basket (e.g., Dormia basket) is used to extract the stones.

After endoscopic sphincterotomy, the patient is usually kept on bed rest for 6 to 8 hours. Nothing is given by mouth until the gag reflex returns. The patient is monitored for signs of complications. Bloody stools and tachycardia may indicate hemorrhage secondary to trauma. Fever and abdominal pain may indicate pancreatitis or perforation of the duodenum.

Cholecystectomy. Cholecystectomy is the most frequently used treatment for cholelithiasis. The two procedures that may be used are via laparoscopy or through a right subcostal incision. For laparoscopic cholecystectomy, the surgeon inserts a laparoscope with a camera through a small abdominal incision. Using the camera, the surgeon guides forceps and a laser toward the gallbladder through other small abdominal incisions. The gallbladder is grasped with the forceps, cut free with the laser, and pulled out through one of the small incisions. Stones remaining in the common bile duct can be removed endoscopically. The most serious complication, although rare, is injury to the bile duct, which requires endoscopic repair. Patients usually are discharged the same day or on the day after surgery and resume regular activities within a week.

In the classic procedure, an incision is made below the right rib margin. The gallbladder is removed and the common bile duct is explored for stones. Exploration of the bile duct may cause it to swell and obstruct bile flow from the liver. A T-tube may be placed in the common bile duct to maintain bile flow until swelling in the duct subsides (Fig. 41-12). One part of the tubing is brought through the patient's skin and connected to a closed-gravity drainage receptacle. Wound drains also may be present.

When the patient first returns from surgery, the drainage from the T-tube may be bloody but it should soon become greenish brown. Drainage should gradually decrease as edema subsides in the common bile duct. Measure and record the amount of drainage and notify the physician if it exceeds 1000 mL in 24 hours.

Place the patient in a low Fowler position with the tube arranged to drain freely. Protect the tube during movement to prevent dislodging it. The physician specifies the level of the drainage bag and when it should be clamped. If the patient experiences pain, fever, chills, nausea, or distention, the tube should be unclamped. The physician removes the T-tube when the patient tolerates clamping for a prolonged period of time. Cleanse the area around wound drains using aseptic technique and dress per agency protocol.

If the patient is discharged with the T-tube in place, you must teach the patient to care for the tube, including emptying the receptacle, caring for the insertion site, and recognizing when to clamp and unclamp it.

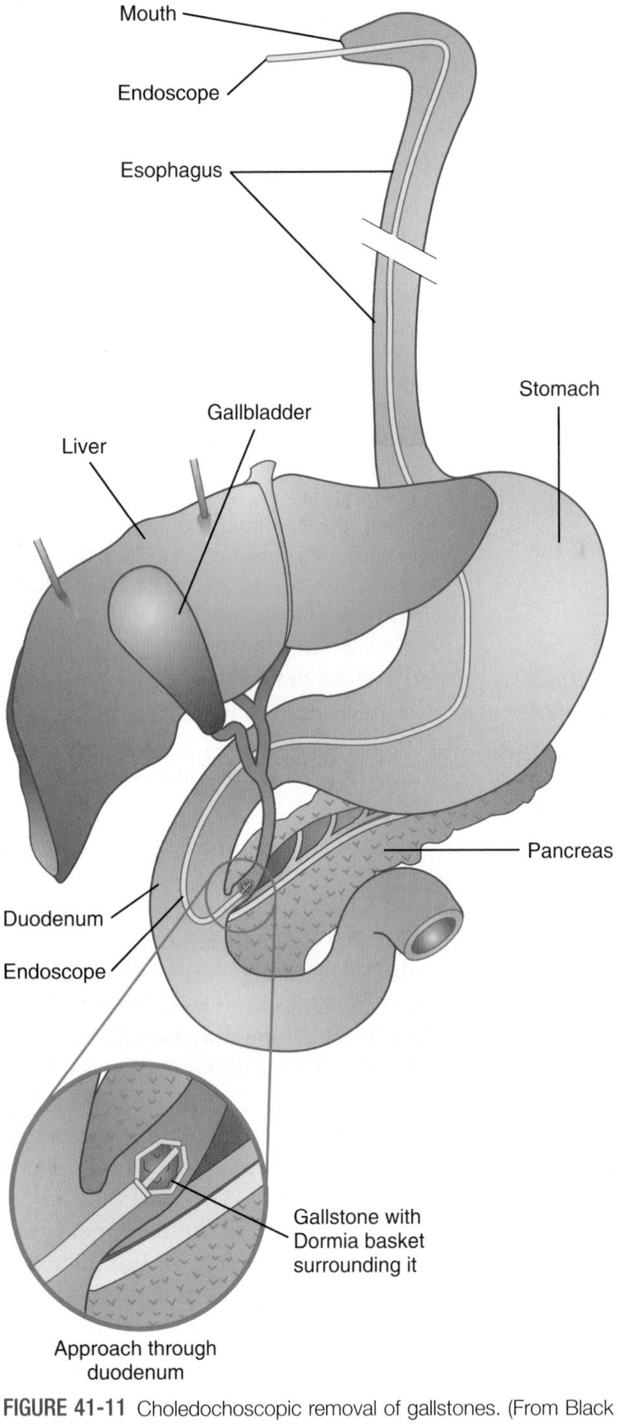

FIGURE 41-11 Choledochoscopic removal of gallstones. (From Black JM, Hawks JH: *Medical-surgical nursing: clinical management for positive outcomes*, ed 8, St. Louis, 2009, Saunders.)

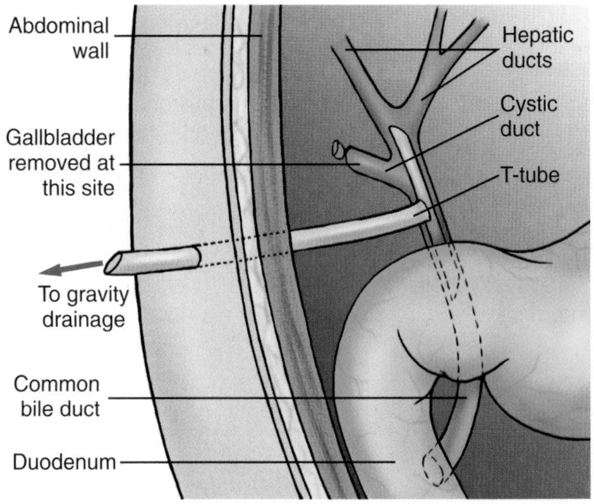

FIGURE 41-12 A T-tube in the common bile duct. (From Monahan FD, Drake DT, Neighbors M, editors: *Medical-surgical nursing: foundations for clinical practice*, ed 2, Philadelphia, 1998, Saunders.)

Nursing Diagnoses, Goals, and Outcome Criteria: Cholelithiasis

Nursing Diagnoses	Goals and Outcome Criteria
Acute Pain related to biliary colic	Reduced pain: patient states pain is reduced or relieved, rates pain lower on pain scale
Deficient Fluid Volume related to vomiting, inadequate intake	Adequate hydration: balanced fluid intake and output, vital signs consistent with patient norms
Risk for Impaired Skin Integrity related to pruritus	Decreased itching: no scratching, patient states less or no itching
Anxiety related to disease, anticipation of invasive procedures	Reduced anxiety: patient states anxiety relieved or reduced, relaxed manner
Risk for Injury (bleeding) related to vitamin K deficiency	Absence of bleeding: no abnormal bruising or bleeding

❖ NURSING CARE of the Patient with a Gallbladder Disorder

Assessment

General assessment of patients with problems of the biliary tract is outlined in Box 41-2.

Interventions

Acute Pain

The degree of pain with cholecystitis varies but many patients experience severe pain. Meperidine (Demerol) may be ordered because morphine causes spasms in the common bile duct, which would increase the patient's pain. However, some experts believe that morphine provides better pain control and that spasms can be controlled by giving atropine with the morphine. Evaluate comfort often and medicate the patient as soon as pain is reported instead of waiting for it to become severe. When opioid analgesics are given, take safety precautions because the drugs cause drowsiness. In addition to medications, use position changes, smooth linens, back rubs, and mouth care to promote comfort.

Attacks of biliary colic are caused by stimulation of the gallbladder, most often by fats in the duodenum.

A low-fat diet is recommended to decrease the incidence of acute symptoms.

Deficient Fluid Volume

If nausea and vomiting are present, the patient is at risk for fluid and electrolyte imbalances. Administer antiemetics as ordered. Keep intake and output records. Monitor for signs of deficient fluid volume (hypovolemia): tachycardia, hypotension, dry skin, concentrated urine, decreased urine output.

If vomiting is severe, a nasogastric tube may be inserted and attached to suction. Fluids are provided intravenously. Note the amount and characteristics of aspirated fluid. A problem associated with nasogastric decompression is the continuous removal of gastric secretions. When the fluid is continuously drained, the patient loses significant water, electrolytes, and acid. This puts the patient at risk for deficient fluid volume, potassium deficit, sodium excess, and metabolic alkalosis. Serum electrolytes are monitored and specific intravenous fluids are ordered to maintain or restore balance.

Risk for Impaired Skin Integrity

Patients who have obstructive jaundice due to blockage of the bile ducts often have pruritus caused by accumulated bile salts under the skin. Measures to promote comfort include tepid baths with baking soda or oily lotions, use of soft linens, and maintaining a comfortable room temperature. Patients should be advised not to scratch but that can be difficult. Short fingernails or even cotton gloves may be suggested to avoid skin injury from scratching. The physician may order a drug such as cholestyramine (Questran) to reduce the discomfort.

Anxiety

Acute pain and unexpected hospitalization can be anxiety provoking for patients and their families. Provide clear explanations about what is being done and what they can expect. Acknowledge their anxiety and take time to answer questions and offer reassurance.

Risk for Injury

A patient who has obstructed bile flow may have a deficiency of vitamin K because absorption of this vitamin in the digestive tract requires bile salts. Vitamin K is needed for the production of prothrombin, an essential element for clotting. Indications of vitamin K deficiency include bleeding gums and oozing of blood at injection sites. Minimize trauma by using a soft toothbrush or swab for mouth care and by applying gentle pressure to injection sites (see *Patient Teaching: Cholelithiasis* box).

Pharmacology Capsule

Caution patients that supplementary bile salts interfere with the effectiveness of oral contraceptives.

Patient Teaching

Cholelithiasis

- You need to have a low-fat diet with supplementary fat-soluble vitamins (or as ordered by the physician). The dietitian will explain the details of the diet to you.
- Notify your physician of signs of bile duct obstruction: light stools, dark urine, jaundice, and itching.
- If you are taking bile salts, report gastric upset.
- Keep medical appointments to have blood drawn to monitor liver function.
- Do not rely on oral contraceptives; bile salts interfere with their effectiveness.

❖ NURSING CARE of the Patient after Surgery for Cholelithiasis

Common nursing interventions for the patient who has undergone incisional surgery for cholelithiasis are presented here. Detailed assessment and care of the surgical patient are discussed in Chapter 17. Nursing care after laparoscopic cholecystectomy is much simpler because patients usually recover quickly and are discharged on the same day or within 24 hours. They usually do not need postoperative nasogastric intubation or T-tubes.

■ Assessment

Postoperatively, take the patient's vital signs until he or she is stable. Observe chest expansion and auscultate breath sounds. Inspect the dressing for bleeding. If a T-tube is present, note the color and amount of drainage. Examine passive drains to ensure that they are functioning properly. Inspect the skin around the incision or the drain for redness or breakdown. If a nasogastric tube is in place, observe the characteristics and amount of the drainage and ensure that the suction is operational. Inspect the patient's nares for irritation or pressure from the tube.

■ Interventions

Acute Pain

When the patient undergoes a procedure that requires a surgical incision, pain is expected. In addition to administering ordered analgesics, reposition the patient for comfort and check to ensure that any drainage tubes are functioning. Show the patient how to support the incision with the hands or a pillow during coughing and deep breathing. Other pain relief measures are described in Chapter 15. If pain continues despite these measures, notify the physician.

The patient who has a nasogastric tube in place has an additional source of discomfort. The nose and throat may become very sore. Secure the tube to the patient's upper lip or nose so that it is not moved or tugged easily. Gently cleanse the nares and provide frequent mouth care.

Nursing Diagnoses, Goals, and Outcome Criteria: Incisional Cholecystectomy

Nursing Diagnoses	Goals and Outcome Criteria
Acute Pain related to surgical incision, nasogastric tube	Pain relief: patient states pain relieved or reduced, relaxed manner
Ineffective Breathing Pattern related to splinting of the surgical incision	Effective breathing pattern: breath sounds clear on auscultation, respiratory rate of 12 to 20 breaths/min
Impaired Skin Integrity related to wound drainage, surgical incision	Wound healing without skin breakdown: clean wound margins without excessive redness
Deficient Fluid Volume related to gastrointestinal (GI) suction	Normal fluid and electrolyte status: electrolytes within normal limits, balanced fluid intake and output
Risk for Infection related to surgical incision, invasive procedure	Absence of infection: normal temperature and white blood cell (WBC) count

Ineffective Breathing Pattern

Potentially ineffective breathing patterns are most likely to be a problem when the patient has a subcostal incision. The incision is located close to the diaphragm, so full lung expansion is painful. The patient tends to guard the surgical area by not breathing deeply. Explain the importance of deep breathing and coughing to prevent atelectasis and pneumonia. Also demonstrate how splinting the area makes breathing and coughing more comfortable. Adequate pain management enables the patient to breathe more effectively. Monitor respiratory rate and breath sounds.

Impaired Skin Integrity

Patients who have subcostal incisions often have wound drains in place. These drains allow for removal of fluids that collect at the surgical site. A Penrose drain diverts fluids directly onto the wound dressings. This requires frequent dressing changes to prevent skin irritation. It is especially important if bile is present in the drainage because bile contains digestive enzymes, which are even more irritating. A pouch collection device like those used for stomas can be applied if needed to protect the skin. A passive drain such as the Jackson-Pratt drain has a fluid collection device that keeps fluid away from the skin.

Deficient Fluid Volume

Postoperatively, measure fluid intake and output. Until oral fluids are permitted, administer intravenous fluids as ordered. Blood studies may be ordered to assess serum electrolytes. If nasogastric suction is ordered, check frequently to ensure that it is working properly. Otherwise, the patient may have distention that causes vomiting and further loss of fluids and electrolytes.

Risk for Infection

The patient who has undergone gallbladder surgery is at risk for infection of the surgical wound. Draining wounds provide a moist environment for bacterial growth. Meticulous wound care can reduce that risk.

A complication of endoscopic sphincterotomy is pancreatitis caused by accidental injury to the pancreatic duct. Early signs of pancreatitis are pain and fever (see *Patient Teaching: Cholecystectomy* box).

Patient Teaching

Cholecystectomy

- After laparoscopic cholecystectomy, usual instructions include the following:
  - Avoid fatty foods for several weeks.
  - Remove the dressings and bathe or shower normally the next day.
  - Notify the physician if redness, drainage, or pus from the incision is noted.
  - Report any signs of peritonitis: severe abdominal pain, chills and fever, and vomiting.
  - A low-fat diet may be recommended for 4 to 6 weeks.
  - In general, avoid heavy lifting for 4 to 6 weeks or as prescribed. Other activities, including sexual intercourse, usually can be resumed when you feel well enough.
- After incisional cholecystectomy, you may have a T-tube: we will teach you how to care for the T-tube before you go home.

CANCER OF THE GALLBLADDER

Cancer of the gallbladder is rare and is thought to be related to chronic cholecystitis and cholelithiasis. The diagnosis is often delayed because early signs and symptoms are essentially the same as those of cholecystitis and cholelithiasis.

Cholecystectomy is the only treatment option; however, the prognosis is generally poor. Often only supportive, symptomatic care is given. Nursing care is similar to that for other patients with gallbladder disease. You also need to focus on the needs of the patient with cancer, as discussed in Chapter 25.

PANCREAS

The pancreas is a gland that has endocrine and exocrine functions. As an **endocrine gland**, it secretes into the blood hormones that regulate the blood glucose level. The exocrine function is the production of digestive enzymes that are secreted into the duodenum through a duct. This section focuses on disorders of the pancreas, with the exception of diabetes mellitus, which is discussed in Chapter 48.

ANATOMY AND PHYSIOLOGY OF THE PANCREAS

The pancreas is a fish-shaped organ located in the left upper quadrant of the abdomen behind the stomach. The head of the pancreas lies against the duodenum and the tail lies next to the spleen. The pancreatic ducts connect the pancreas to the duodenum. One duct goes directly to the duodenum and the other merges with the common bile duct, as shown in Figure 41-10.

EXOCRINE FUNCTION

The exocrine function of the pancreas is carried out by acinar tissue. Acinar tissue is composed of tiny grape-like clusters of cells that produce pancreatic fluid. Pancreatic fluid contains enzymes needed for the digestion of proteins, fats, and carbohydrates. It is secreted into the duodenum through the pancreatic duct.

The pancreatic enzymes trypsin, amylase, and lipase act on partially digested foods in the small intestine. Trypsin plays a role in the digestion of protein by breaking proteases and peptones into small polypeptides. Normally, trypsin is not activated until it enters the duodenum. Otherwise, it would digest the protein tissue of the pancreas itself. Amylase acts with intestinal enzymes to reduce starch, sucrose, and fructose to glucose, fructose, and galactose. Lipase acts on emulsified fats to yield fatty acids, glycerides, and glycerol.

ENDOCRINE FUNCTION

The endocrine function of the pancreas is carried out by clusters of specialized cells scattered throughout the pancreas. These cells are called *islets of Langerhans*. The islets contain alpha, beta, delta, and PP cells. Alpha cells produce and secrete glucagon. Beta cells produce and secrete insulin. Delta cells produce somatostatin, which inhibits the release of glucagon and insulin. PP cells secrete pancreatic polypeptides, a family of peptides known chiefly for their inhibitory functions.

Glucagon is secreted when the blood glucose level falls. It stimulates the liver to convert glycogen into glucose. Insulin is secreted when the blood glucose rises, as after a meal. It stimulates the use of glucose by the cells so that a normal blood glucose level is maintained. The endocrine function of the pancreas is discussed more thoroughly in Chapter 48.

NURSING ASSESSMENT OF THE PANCREAS

Assessment of the patient with a disorder of the pancreas is outlined in Box 41-3. The assessment focuses on digestive and metabolic functions.

HEALTH HISTORY

Inquire about the patient's general health status because pancreatic disorders are often accompanied by weakness and fatigue. The past medical history may reveal previous disorders of the biliary tract or duodenum, abdominal trauma or surgery, and metabolic disorders such as diabetes mellitus. The medication history should be detailed and specifically include the use of thiazide diuretics, furosemide, oral contraceptives, corticosteroids, sulfonamides, and NSAIDs. Note a family history of pancreatic disorders. In the review of systems, obtain a complete description of any pain in the upper abdomen or epigastric area. Other symptoms that may be important in relation to pancreatic disorders are dyspnea, nausea, and vomiting. The functional assessment includes data about the patient's dietary habits and use of alcohol.

Box 41-3 Assessment of the Patient with a Pancreatic Disorder

HEALTH HISTORY

Present Illness
General well-being, digestive disturbances, pain

Past Medical History
Disorders of the biliary tract or duodenum; abdominal trauma or surgery; metabolic disorders; medication history, especially thiazides, furosemide, estrogens, corticosteroids, sulfonamides, opiates, oral contraceptives, NSAIDs

Family History
Pancreatic disorders

Review of Systems
Pruritus, respiratory distress, nausea and vomiting, abdominal pain

Functional Assessment
Dietary habits, alcohol intake

PHYSICAL EXAMINATION

General Survey
Restlessness, flushing, diaphoresis

Vital Signs
Low-grade fever, tachycardia, tachypnea, hypotension

Skin
Jaundice, dryness, scratches

Abdomen
Distention, tenderness, diminished bowel sounds, discoloration

PHYSICAL EXAMINATION

Note any restlessness, flushing, or diaphoresis during the examination. Vital signs may disclose low-grade fever, tachypnea, tachycardia, and hypotension. Inspect the skin for jaundice. Assess the abdomen for distention, tenderness, discoloration, and diminished bowel sounds.

DIAGNOSTIC TESTS AND PROCEDURES

Tests and procedures used to diagnose pancreatic disorders include laboratory analyses of blood, urine, stool, and pancreatic fluid as well as imaging studies (chest and abdominal radiographs, CT scan, endoscopic ultrasonography, MRI, positron emission tomography [PET], ERCP).

Specific blood studies used to assess pancreatic function include measurements of serum amylase, lipase, glucose, calcium, and triglycerides. Urine amylase and renal amylase clearance tests also may be ordered. Stool specimens may be analyzed for fat content.

The secretin stimulation test measures the volume and bicarbonate concentration of pancreatic fluid after secretin is given intravenously to stimulate the production of pancreatic fluid.

If cancer is suspected, blood levels of cancer antigen (CA) 19-9 and carcinoembryonic antigen (CEA), which are considered "markers" for cancer, may be measured. Unfortunately, levels of these antigens are elevated with many types of cancer, so their presence does not specifically indicate pancreatic cancer.

Additional information about diagnostic tests and procedures for the pancreas is provided in Table 41-5.

Table 41-5 Diagnostic Tests and Procedures The Pancreas

TEST	PURPOSE AND PROCEDURE	PATIENT PREPARATION	POSTPROCEDURE NURSING CARE
Laboratory Studies			
General Interventions: Check your agency procedure manual for diagnostic tests and procedures. Always tell the patient what to expect when tests are ordered. Explain if nothing-by-mouth (NPO) status is necessary. Document the care provided and relevant assessment data. If venipuncture is done, apply a dressing and check the site oozing. Apply pressure and elevate arm if patient's blood clotting is impaired.			
Serum amylase	Increases with pancreatitis, parotitis, cholecystitis.	See General Interventions.	See General Interventions.
Serum enzymes	Lipase increases with pancreatic inflammation and carcinoma. Normal values vary with the type of test used.	See General Interventions.	See General Interventions.
Serum calcium	Decreases with many conditions, including pancreatic disorders.	See General Interventions.	See General Interventions.
Serum triglycerides	Increase with pancreatitis and many other conditions.	See General Interventions.	See General Interventions.
Tumor Markers			
Carcinoembryonic antigen (CEA), pancreatic oncofetal antigen (POA)	Increase with many types of cancer, including pancreatic cancer. Pancreatitis, cirrhosis, hepatitis, and chronic cigarette smoking also cause an increase in these antigens.	See General Interventions.	See General Interventions.
Secretin stimulation test	Secretin is given intravenously. Gastric and duodenal fluids are aspirated through a double-lumen tube. Fluid is analyzed. Decreased volume of secretions and bicarbonate is consistent with pancreatitis.	Tell the patient that a medication will be given in a vein and that a tube will be passed through the nose and into the stomach so that fluid can be removed from the stomach for study.	Remove tube unless instructed otherwise. Provide comfort measures.
Urine amylase	Increases with acute pancreatitis, peptic ulcer, and choledocholithiasis. Test may be ordered for a 1-hour, 2-hour, or 24-hour specimen.	Advise the patient of time for collection of specimens. Encourage fluids during the test if not contraindicated.	No special care is required.
Imaging Studies			
***General Interventions When Contrast Dye Used. Before Procedure:** Assess patient allergy to dye, iodine, or shellfish. If patient reports allergy, notify radiology. Tell patient that injection of contrast dye can create a feeling of warmth, a salty taste, and nausea. **After Procedure:** Inform the physician of any signs of allergic response to the contrast dye. Administer antihistamines as ordered for allergy.			

Table 41-5 Diagnostic Tests and Procedures The Pancreas—cont'd

TEST	PURPOSE AND PROCEDURE	PATIENT PREPARATION	POSTPROCEDURE NURSING CARE
Abdominal ultrasound	Uses sound waves to visualize the pancreas directly. Test is noninvasive. The patient will lie on the back on an examination table. A gel or oil is applied to the skin and an instrument is moved over upper abdomen. Images are seen on a screen and recorded.	Some laboratories require the patient to be placed on nothing-by-mouth (NPO) status before the procedure. Study cannot be done if barium or excessive gas is in the digestive tract.	No special care is required.
Computed tomography (CT)	Provides detailed information about the internal organ position and structure. Tell the patient to expect to lie on a narrow stretcher. Scanner is a donut-shaped machine that moves back and forth and around the stretcher; it makes clicking noises. Contrast medium may be given orally or intravenously	*Dye precautions if contrast media used. NPO status is needed before some CT scans. CT is contraindicated during pregnancy.	*Dye precautions if contrast media used.
Endoscopic retrograde cholangiopancreatography (ERCP)	Uses an endoscope to examine the gallbladder and pancreas to evaluate bile obstruction and to confirm pancreatic disease. Contrast medium is injected into bile duct.	*Dye precautions. A consent form must be signed. Patient will be NPO as long as 12 hours. Physician may order the patient to gargle with a topical anesthetic. An intravenous line may be started to administer sedatives.	*Dye precautions. Monitor the patient's vital signs for 4 hours. Check the gag reflex before giving fluids or food. Monitor for urinary retention. Report any temperature elevation that may indicate inflammation.

DISORDERS OF THE PANCREAS

PANCREATITIS

Pancreatitis is inflammation of the pancreas. It may be acute or chronic. Chronic pancreatitis may follow the acute condition but often develops independently.

Pancreatitis is most often associated with alcoholism or obstruction of the pancreatic duct by a gallstone. Other causes include viral infections; peptic ulcer disease; cysts; metabolic disorders (i.e., renal failure, hyperparathyroidism); and trauma from external injury, surgery, or endoscopic procedures. A high-fat diet and cigarette smoking may play a role as well. In addition, chronic pancreatitis is sometimes associated with cancer of the duodenum or pancreas.

Normally, pancreatic enzymes are activated in the small intestine. With pancreatitis, digestive enzymes (trypsin, elastase, and phospholipase A) are activated by some unknown mechanism and begin to digest pancreatic tissue (a process called *autodigestion*), fat, and elastic tissue in blood vessels. Pancreatic fluid may leak into the surrounding tissues. The effect of this escaped fluid has been compared to an internal chemical burn and it can be devastating.

Chronic pancreatitis is often related to alcohol abuse. It is usually characterized by obstruction of the pancreatic duct, leading to progressive destruction of the pancreas.

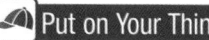

Put on Your Thinking Cap!

The term *autodigestion* is used to describe the effects of pancreatitis. Explain what this means.

Signs and Symptoms

Abdominal pain is the most prominent symptom of pancreatitis. The pain is typically severe with a sudden onset, is centered in the left upper quadrant or the epigastric region, and radiates to the back. Severe vomiting, flushing, cyanosis, and dyspnea often accompany the pain. Other signs and symptoms are low-grade fever, tachypnea, tachycardia, and hypotension.

The abdomen may be tender and distended. Bowel sounds may be absent, suggesting an ileus. Trypsin may damage blood vessels, causing pancreatic hemorrhage and discoloration of the abdomen. Cyanosis or greenish discoloration of the abdominal wall, the flanks, and the area around the umbilicus may be present. Enzymes released into the abdominal cavity increase capillary permeability, permitting protein-rich serum to leak from blood vessels. Bleeding and shifting of fluid reduce blood volume and may lead to shock. Early signs and symptoms of shock are restlessness and tachycardia. Hypotension is a late sign.

Symptoms of chronic pancreatitis are similar to those of the acute disease but usually appear as periodic attacks that become more and more frequent. In addition, patients with chronic pancreatitis may develop diabetes mellitus and malabsorption with steatorrhea.

Complications

Complications of pancreatitis include pseudocyst; abscess; hypocalcemia; and pulmonary, cardiac, and renal complications.

A pseudocyst is a fluid-filled pouch attached to the pancreas. It contains products of tissue destruction and pancreatic enzymes. The fluid can leak into the digestive tract or the abdominal cavity. Symptoms of pseudocyst include abdominal pain, nausea, vomiting, and anorexia. Sometimes a mass can be palpated in the epigastric area. Necrosis within the pancreas can lead to pancreatic abscess, a fluid-filled cavity in the pancreas. Symptoms are similar to those of pseudocyst. Patients usually run a high fever.

Hypocalcemia (low serum calcium) is caused by the action of fatty acids on calcium and increased loss of calcium in the urine. The pulmonary complications of pancreatitis are pneumonia and atelectasis. Pancreatitis can be fatal. In the early stage of acute pancreatitis, cause of death is usually cardiovascular, renal, or pulmonary failure. Later, sepsis and abscesses are the leading causes of death.

A person may recover completely from an attack of acute pancreatitis, have repeated acute episodes, or experience chronic pancreatitis.

Medical Diagnosis

The most important diagnostic findings in acute pancreatitis are elevated serum amylase, serum lipase, and urinary amylase levels. When the kidneys clear amylase more rapidly than they clear creatinine, acute pancreatitis is strongly suspected. Other findings with acute pancreatitis are elevated WBC count, elevated serum lipid and glucose levels, and decreased serum calcium level. Ultrasonography and ERCP may reveal the presence of gallstones, cysts, or abscesses and help to rule out other disorders that might be causing the patient's symptoms.

Tests for chronic pancreatitis include the secretin stimulation test and fecal studies in addition to the tests used for acute pancreatitis. Findings consistent with chronic pancreatitis are decreased volume and bicarbonate concentration of pancreatic fluid, low serum trypsinogen, and high fecal fat content. Imaging procedures reveal the structure of the pancreas and the pancreatic duct.

Medical Treatment

The patient with acute pancreatitis is usually allowed nothing by mouth (NPO). This removes the stimulus for secretion of pancreatic fluid. If the patient is vomiting or if an ileus is suspected, a nasogastric tube is inserted and connected to suction. Intravenous fluids are ordered to restore and maintain fluid balance. Blood or plasma expanders are given if the blood volume is low. Urine output is monitored and should be at least 40 mL/hour. A nasogastric or jejunal feeding tube or TPN may be needed to provide adequate nutrients. Once food is permitted, the patient is usually started on a bland, high-carbohydrate, low-fat diet divided into frequent, small meals. Because the inflamed pancreas is susceptible to infection, some physicians order prophylactic antibiotics. Sometimes peritoneal lavage or laparoscopy is used to remove toxic fluid from the peritoneum.

Drug Therapy. Drug therapy for pancreatitis commonly includes analgesics, antispasmodic agents, anticholinergic agents, and gastric acid inhibitors. Pain control is a major problem with pancreatitis. Opioids (e.g., morphine) traditionally have been avoided because they are thought to cause more spasm in the pancreatic ducts. However, dilaudid or morphine is gaining favor because the pain relief lasts longer and spasms can be managed with the antispasmodic drugs such as nitroglycerin. Anticholinergic agents decrease secretions, which also can reduce spasms and pain. Reducing the secretion of gastric acid decreases the stimulus for pancreatic secretions.

With chronic pancreatitis, acetaminophen or ibuprofen is tried initially for pain control. If these nonopioid agents do not provide relief, hydrocodone may be prescribed.

The patient with chronic pancreatitis is likely to need to take pancreatic enzymes to digest food. The enzymes can be taken with meals or snacks. The effect of the enzymes can be determined by examining the stools. Steatorrhea (i.e., bulky, frothy stools with a high fat content) results from inadequate enzymes. If diabetes mellitus develops, insulin or oral hypoglycemic drugs are needed and the patient requires diabetes education.

Other drugs that may be needed are antacids, anticholinergic agents, and histamine blockers to decrease hydrochloric acid in the stomach. Bile salts also may be needed to enhance absorption of fat-soluble vitamins. Drugs used to treat pancreatitis are described in Table 41-6.

Surgical Intervention. Various surgical procedures may be indicated. For example, if gallstones are present, endoscopic sphincterotomy followed by cholecystectomy may be done. If an abscess, pseudocyst, or severe peritonitis develops, surgical intervention is indicated. Debridement involves resection of necrotic tissue and irrigation of the cavity to remove harmful fluid. The procedure may need to be repeated more than once. After surgical debridement, multiple sumps may be placed in the abdomen for continuous postoperative irrigation. Each sump tube is connected to a separate suction apparatus. Irrigations may be alternated as ordered. Endoscopic or percutaneous debridement may be used in patients who are poor surgical risks.

NURSING CARE of the Patient with Pancreatitis

Assessment

General nursing assessment of the patient with a disorder of the pancreas is outlined in Box 41-3 (see also Nursing Care Plan: Patient with Pancreatitis). When a

Table 41-6 Drugs Used to Treat Pancreatitis

DRUG	USE AND ACTION	SIDE EFFECTS	NURSING INTERVENTIONS
Acute Pancreatitis			
Opioid analgesics: meperidine (Demerol) Morphine	Relieve pain. If morphine is ordered, an antispasmodic is usually ordered to prevent spasm of bile duct.	Sedation, confusion, hypotension, nausea, vomiting, constipation.	Monitor the patient's BP, pulse, and respiration. Assess bowel elimination. Observe safety precautions. Give antiemetics as ordered.
NSAIDs ketorolac (Toradol)	Relieve pain.	Headache, abdominal pain, GI bleeding, nephrotoxicity.	Assess emesis and stools for blood. Monitor urine output.
Smooth muscle relaxants: nitroglycerin	Relieve spasm, reduce pain.	Headache, dizziness, flushing, tachycardia, hypotension.	Monitor the patient's BP and pulse. Use special containers and tubing for IV administration.
Antispasmodics: propantheline bromide (Pro- Banthine)	Decrease bicarbonate and pancreatic enzyme secretion.	Tachycardia, dry mouth, constipation, urinary retention/ hesitancy, drowsiness.	Administer the drug 30 minutes before meals. Do not give the medication within 1 hour of antacids or antidiarrheals. Observe safety precautions if the patient is drowsy. Provide good mouth care and monitor stools.
Antacids	Neutralize gastric acid (indirectly decreases production of pancreatic secretions).	Constipation with aluminum and diarrhea with magnesium.	Monitor the patient's electrolytes. Give the drug 1 hour apart from other oral drugs and on an empty stomach. Have the patient chew the tablets and drink a full glass of water. Shake liquids well.
Carbonic anhydrase inhibitors: acetazolamide (Diamox)	Reduce bicarbonate concentration in pancreatic secretions.	Rash, drowsiness, nausea, vomiting, renal calculi, hypercalcemia, aplastic anemia, leukopenia, seizures, hypokalemia.	Encourage the patient to drink 2000–3000 mL fluid per day unless contraindicated. Give the drug with food to decrease GI distress. Observe safety precautions. Monitor electrolytes and blood cell counts.
Histamine-2 receptor blockers: cimetidine (Tagamet), ranitidine, (Zantac), famotidine (Pepcid)	Decrease production of HCl so that pancreatic enzymes cannot be activated.	Confusion, nausea, diarrhea, constipation, drowsiness, headache, rash, agranulocytosis.	Administer with or immediately after meals. Discourage smoking, which counteracts drug benefits. Observe safety precautions. Report a sore throat or fever to the physician. Cimetidine is not recommended for older adults due to risk of confusion and interaction with many other drugs.

Continued

Table 41-6 Drugs Used to Treat Pancreatitis—cont'd

DRUG	USE AND ACTION	SIDE EFFECTS	NURSING INTERVENTIONS
Vitamin and mineral supplements	Supplement poor dietary intake or impaired absorption (calcium treats hypocalcemia).	Potential for overdose of fat-soluble vitamins and calcium (calcium potentiates cardiac glycosides).	No special care required.
Adrenocortical steroids	Decrease inflammation.	Fluid retention, hypokalemia, hyperglycemia, hypocalcemia, decreased resistance to infection, mood swings.	Monitor the patient's BP, pulse, and blood glucose. Assess for edema. Protect the patient from infection. Explain that emotional and personality changes are temporary.
Chronic Pancreatitis			
Pancreatic enzymes: pancreatin pancrelipase (Cotazym, Viokase, Pancrease)	Supplement normal pancreatic enzyme secretion and aid in the digestion of fats, carbohydrates, and proteins. Goal is less frequent stools with lower fat content.	Diarrhea, nausea, stomach cramps, abdominal pain.	Give the drug with meals or snacks. Capsule contents can be sprinkled on food but should not be chewed. Mix powders with fruit juice or applesauce to mask the taste. Do not mix with protein foods. Have patient wipe the lips with a wet cloth to prevent skin irritation. Evaluate the drug effect by noting the number and consistency of stools.
Hypoglycemic agents: insulin, oral hypoglycemic agents	Used when the pancreas is unable to produce sufficient insulin.	Hypoglycemia.	See Chapter 48 for details on hypoglycemic drug therapy.

BP, Blood pressure; *GI*, gastrointestinal; *HCl*, hydrochloric acid; *IV*, intravenous; NSAIDs, nonsteroidal antiinflammatory drugs.

patient has acute pancreatitis, it is especially important to report signs of hypovolemic shock: restlessness, tachycardia, tachypnea, hypotension, and decreased urinary output. The abdomen should be inspected for discoloration, distention, tenderness, and diminished bowel sounds. The flanks also should be examined for discoloration. In addition, the patient's mental status should be monitored. Altered mental status may be the result of metabolic imbalances. The alcoholic patient may develop confusion and agitation because of alcohol withdrawal.

If the patient has surgery, general postoperative assessment should include the data covered in Chapter 17.

Nursing Diagnoses, Goals, and Outcome Criteria: Pancreatitis

Nursing Diagnoses	Goals and Outcome Criteria
Acute Pain related to inflammation, infection, biliary obstruction, autodigestion	Pain relief: patient states pain is reduced or relieved, relaxed manner
Deficient Fluid Volume related to vomiting, bleeding, fluid shift from the blood to the abdominal cavity	Normal fluid balance: balanced fluid intake and output, pulse and blood pressure (BP) consistent with patient norms

Nursing Diagnoses, Goals, and Outcome Criteria: Pancreatitis—cont'd

Nursing Diagnoses	Goals and Outcome Criteria
Risk for Infection related to tissue necrosis	Absence of infection: normal body temperature and white blood cell (WBC) count
Impaired Gas Exchange related to pain, pulmonary complications	Adequate gas exchange: breath sounds clear to auscultation, respiratory rate 12 to 20 breaths/min
Imbalanced Nutrition: Less Than Body Requirements related to anorexia, vomiting, digestive disturbance	Adequate nutrition: stable body weight
Anxiety related to unfamiliar setting and procedures, acute illness	Reduced anxiety: patient states anxiety is lessened, calm manner
Deficient Knowledge of therapy and measures to reduce risk of recurrence related to lack of exposure to information, acute illness	Enhanced knowledge: patient understands care while acutely ill; patient states understanding of self-care to prevent recurrence

Nursing Care Plan Patient with Pancreatitis

ASSESSMENT

HEALTH HISTORY Mrs. Sanchez is a 57-year-old Latino woman admitted with repeated attacks of severe pain in the left upper quadrant that radiates to her back. She reports having vomited repeatedly over the past 24 hours. When the pain is severe, she reports feeling flushed, faint, and short of breath. She has no other related symptoms. Mrs. Sanchez reports having had a gallbladder attack several months ago that resolved without surgery. She is a high school teacher who lives with her husband.

PHYSICAL EXAMINATION Vital signs: blood pressure 144/84 mm Hg, pulse 92 bpm, Ht 5′2″, Wt 150 lbs, respiration 24 breaths per minute, temperature 100.2°F (37.9°C), measured orally. The patient appears to be in acute distress but is alert and oriented. Abdomen is tender and distended, with hypoactive bowel sounds in all four quadrants.

Nursing Diagnosis	Goals and Outcome Criteria	Interventions
Acute Pain related to inflammation, biliary obstruction, autodigestion	The patient will report decreased pain and will appear more relaxed.	Document painful episodes. Treat the patient promptly with analgesics and antispasmodic drugs as ordered. Use distraction, imagery, and relaxation techniques to enhance drug therapy. Advise the physician if pain is unrelieved.
Deficient Fluid Volume related to vomiting, bleeding, fluid shift from bloodstream to abdominal cavity	The patient's fluid status will stabilize, as evidenced by stable blood pressure (BP) and pulse, normal skin color, and urine output equal to fluid intake.	Insert a nasogastric tube and connect it to low suction as ordered. Initiate intravenous fluid therapy and administer medications as ordered. Monitor the patient's vital signs, intake and output, weight, and electrolyte studies. Report any signs of fluid volume deficit (i.e., tachycardia, hypotension, dry skin, concentrated urine) to the physician.
Risk for Infection related to tissue necrosis	The patient will be free of signs and symptoms of infection: fever, tachycardia, and increased white blood cell (WBC) count.	Monitor the patient's vital signs and blood cell counts. Report any signs of infection. Administer antimicrobials as ordered. Use Standard Precautions for invasive procedures.
Impaired Gas Exchange related to pain, pulmonary complications	The patient will remain free of pulmonary complications, as evidenced by absence of dyspnea, tachypnea, and abnormal breath sounds.	Assess the patient's respirations and breath sounds. Assist her to change positions, to cough, and to deep breathe at least every 2 hours. Use a semi-Fowler position to promote lung expansion.
Imbalanced Nutrition: Less Than Body Requirements related to anorexia, vomiting, digestive disturbances	The patient's body weight will remain stable.	Administer total parenteral nutrition (TPN) if ordered. Monitor the patient for hyperglycemia and administer insulin as ordered. Take daily weights. When oral intake is permitted, monitor the patient's tolerance. Discourage spicy foods, caffeine, and alcohol.
Anxiety related to acute symptoms	The patient will report decreased anxiety and will be calm.	Check on the patient often. Respond to her needs promptly. Ask what questions she has and provide explanations of the condition and the treatment she is receiving.

Critical Thinking Questions

1. Explain why the patient with pancreatitis has severe pain.
2. Explain why it is necessary to monitor respiratory status in the patient with pancreatitis.

Interventions

Acute Pain

Describe the patient's pain and provide ordered analgesics and antispasmodics promptly. Reposition the patient for comfort. Other nursing measures for pain are described in Chapter 15 and include distraction, imagery, and cutaneous stimulation (see *Complementary and Alternative Therapies* box). Evaluate and record the effectiveness of pain control measures. The physician should be informed if pain is not relieved.

Complementary and Alternative Therapies

Distraction, imagery, relaxation, and cutaneous stimulation can enhance the effects of analgesics to promote pain relief.

Deficient Fluid Volume

If ordered, insert a nasogastric tube and connect it to suction. Administer prescribed intravenous fluids. Monitor the patient's fluid status by measuring vital signs, intake and output, and weight. Signs of fluid volume deficit include tachycardia, hypotension, dry skin, concentrated urine, and decreased urine output. The physician should be informed if the urine output falls below 40 mL/h. Depletion of blood volume causes hypovolemic shock and leads to death if not corrected. Other potential fluid imbalances are metabolic alkalosis from severe vomiting, hypokalemia, hyponatremia, hypocalcemia, and hypochloremia.

Risk for Infection

Necrosis of the pancreas and surrounding tissue provides a site for infection. If a surgical procedure is done, there also is risk for wound infection. Inform the physician of fever, purulent drainage, or separation of wound margins—all signs of infection. Take special care to maintain asepsis during wound care. Administer antibiotics as ordered.

Impaired Gas Exchange

Fluid accumulation in the peritoneal cavity puts upward pressure on the diaphragm, thereby limiting lung expansion. Because the acutely ill patient is inactive, secretions may pool in the lungs. Poor lung expansion and inactivity combine to invite pneumonia and atelectasis. Monitor for tachypnea, dyspnea, and abnormal breath sounds.

Measures to prevent pulmonary complications in the patient with pancreatitis include frequent turning, coughing, and deep breathing. The semi-Fowler position promotes lung expansion.

Imbalanced Nutrition: Less Than Body Requirements

Initially, the patient will be NPO because food and fluids stimulate pancreatic fluid secretion. When oral intake is resumed, small feedings of a bland, high-carbohydrate, low-fat diet are provided. Spicy foods, caffeine, and alcohol should be avoided (see *Patient Teaching* box). TPN (see Chapter 9) is usually needed only with severe malnourishment. Daily weights are used to evaluate the adequacy of the nutrition plan.

The patient with chronic pancreatitis commonly requires pancreatic enzyme replacement taken with meals and supplemental vitamins. If the pancreas is severely damaged, insulin secretion will be deficient. The patient will have to be managed like a person with diabetes mellitus (see Chapter 48).

Anxiety

Attempt to determine the reasons for the patient's anxiety. Some concerns can be alleviated by telling the patient what is happening and what to expect. Respond promptly to the patient's needs and offer comforting reassurance by checking on the patient frequently. Anxiety can be related to pain or hypoxia as well as to emotional distress, so assess comfort and oxygenation status and take appropriate corrective actions. During acute attacks, answer questions and give simple explanations. As the patient improves, implement your teaching plan.

Deficient Knowledge

The patient with acute pancreatitis is too ill for systematic teaching. Explain simply what you are doing and why. Answer any questions the patient may ask. As the patient improves, the teaching plan should address the importance of avoiding alcohol to prevent recurrences. Explain the rationale for the prescribed diet.

Patient Teaching

Pancreatitis

- Your prescribed diet (usually bland, high carbohydrate, low fat) will avoid stimulating your pancreas and will promote healing.
- At first, you may tolerate small, frequent meals better than large meals.
- Abstaining from alcohol decreases your risk of recurrence.
- Community resources such as Alcoholics Anonymous can assist if it is hard for you to abstain from drinking alcohol (www.aa.org; telephone: 1-212-686-1100).

CANCER OF THE PANCREAS

Cancer of the pancreas is extremely serious. Pancreatic cancer quickly spreads to the duodenum, stomach, spleen, and left adrenal gland. About 42,000 new cases are diagnosed each year in the United States. Only 24% of these people will survive for 1 year; 4% will be alive after 5 years (see *Cultural Considerations* box). Among persons diagnosed early, about 17% are alive after 5 years. The risk factors for pancreatic cancer include chronic pancreatitis and smoking. Other probable risk factors are a high-fat diet and exposure to certain toxic chemicals. Tumors may develop in the head, body, or tail of the pancreas.

Cultural Considerations

What Does Culture Have to Do with Pancreatic Cancer?

African-American heritage and a high-fat diet are two risk factors for pancreatic cancer.

Signs and Symptoms

Signs and symptoms of pancreatic cancer vary with the stage and location but often include pain, jaundice with or without liver enlargement, weight loss, and glucose intolerance. When located in the head of the pancreas, tumors typically obstruct the common bile duct, causing jaundice. In the early stage of the disease, jaundice may be the only sign present. If the patient seeks medical care early, the chance of survival is somewhat better. Other signs and symptoms may be weight loss, upper abdominal pain, anorexia, vomiting, weakness, and diarrhea.

When the tumor is in the body or the tail of the pancreas, the patient may not have any symptoms until the disease is advanced. Then the liver, gallbladder, and spleen may be enlarged. Pressure on the portal veins may cause esophageal and gastric varices (dilated veins) that bleed easily into the GI tract. Pressure on nerves may cause back pain.

Medical Diagnosis

The most useful diagnostic tests and procedures when pancreatic cancer is suspected are transabdominal ultrasound, CT, MRI, ERCP, magnetic resonance cholangiopancreatography (MRCP), and endoscopic ultrasonography. Blood studies and other imaging procedures can be helpful as well. Blood values associated with pancreatic cancer include elevated serum amylase, lipase, bilirubin, and enzyme levels. The tumor marker CA 19-9 is usually elevated with pancreatic cancer. Percutaneous transhepatic cholangiography and ERCP allow the physician to detect obstructed pancreatic ducts and to take samples of pancreatic fluid and tissue.

Medical Treatment and Surgical Treatment

Treatment depends on the location and extent of the malignant tissue. If the tumor is confined to the head of the pancreas, surgery may be an option. A variety of procedures may be used for pancreatic cancer. The most common are side-to-side pancreaticojejunostomy, caudal pancreaticojejunostomy, and radical pancreaticoduodenectomy (Whipple procedure), as illustrated in Figure 41-13. Potential complications of the Whipple procedure are listed in Table 41-7.

Sometimes surgical procedures are done primarily to relieve obstruction and improve patient comfort. Opioid analgesics are ordered for pain management. At times, a jejunostomy tube is placed below the obstruction so that the patient can be given tube feedings.

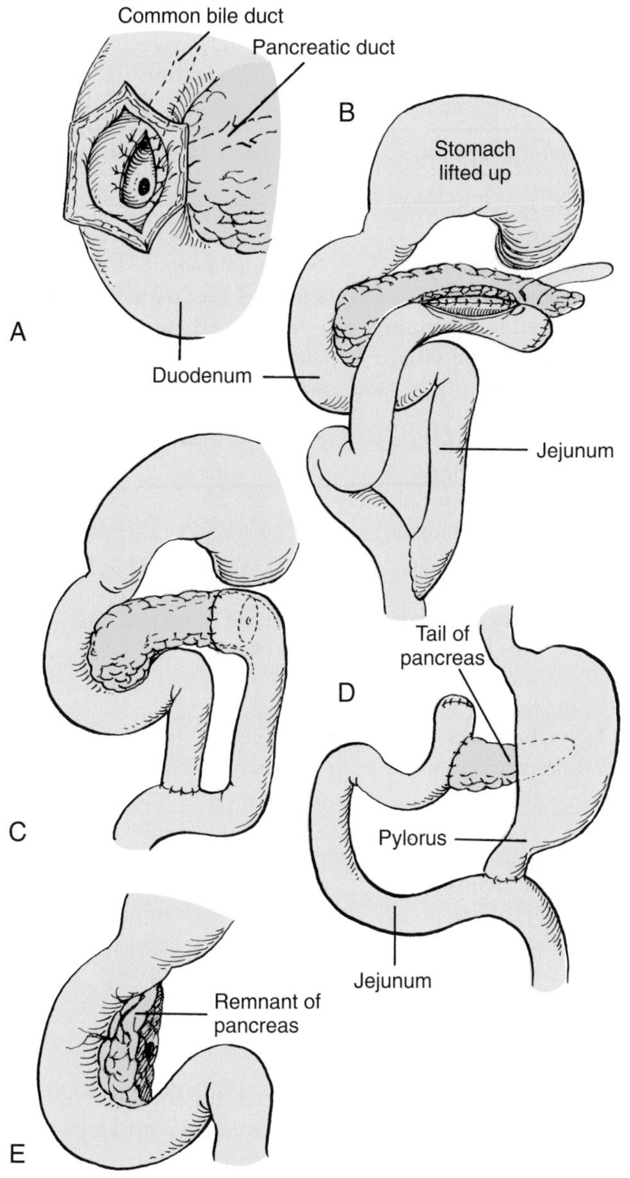

A. **Sphincteroplasty (ampullary)**
Indicated for stenosis of the sphincter of Oddi with dilation of the pancreatic duct. This procedure has limited application in pancreatitis and its use is decreasing.

B. **Side-to-side pancreaticojejunostomy (ductal drainage)**
Indicated when gross dilation of the pancreatic ducts is associated with septa and calculi. The most successful procedure, with rates of 60% to 90%.

C. **Caudal pancreaticojejunostomy (ductal drainage)**
Indicated for the uncommon cases of isolated proximal pancreatic ductal stenosis not involving the ampulla.

D. **Radical pancreaticoduodenectomy (ablative) (with preservation of pylorus) (Whipple procedure)**
Indicated when major changes are confined to the head of the pancreas. Preservation of the pylorus avoids the usual sequelae of gastric resection.

E. **Subtotal pancreatectomy (ablative)**
Indicated when other operations fail and when ducts are unsuitable for decompression. Because metabolic sequelae are significant, this procedure is declining in popularity.

FIGURE 41-13 Surgical procedures for pancreatic cancer. (From Black JM, Hawks JH, Keene AM: *Medical-surgical nursing: clinical management for continuity of care*, ed 6, Philadelphia, 2001, Saunders.)

Table 41-7 Potential Complications of the Whipple Procedure

COMPLICATION	NURSING INTERVENTIONS
Hemorrhage	Monitor vital signs for tachycardia and falling blood pressure (BP). Assess for restlessness. Check dressings and drains for excess bleeding.
Fluid and electrolyte imbalances	Assess for cardiac dysrhythmias, muscle weakness or twitching, and changes in mental status. Monitor intake and output as well as tissue turgor. Check laboratory reports and notify the physician of abnormalities.
Respiratory failure	Monitor respiratory rate and effort, skin color, and breath sounds.
Circulatory failure	Monitor for dysrhythmias, tachycardia, and falling BP.
Renal failure	Measure intake and urine output. Report output of less than 30 mL/h. Assess for edema. Maintain prescribed fluid intake.
Hepatic failure	Assess for jaundice, fatigue, confusion, and digestive disturbances.
Wound infection, dehiscence, and fistulas	Assess dressing and drains for excess bleeding, foul odor, and purulent drainage. Check the patient's temperature for fever. Note any elevation in the white blood cell (WBC) count.
Hyperglycemia	Monitor blood glucose as ordered. Note drowsiness, thirst, polyphagia, and polyuria.

Research is continuing to find the best strategy for this challenging cancer. Radiation therapy and chemotherapy may be advised either preoperatively or postoperatively. Radiation does not appear to improve survival but may reduce pain. The value of chemotherapy still is in doubt. Some physicians believe that a combination of surgery, radiation, and chemotherapy may be the best approach. These therapies are discussed in detail in Chapter 25.

NURSING CARE of the Patient with Pancreatic Cancer

Assessment

General assessment of the patient with a pancreatic disorder is outlined in Box 41-3. With pancreatic cancer, pay particular attention to GI function, pain, and emotional state. If surgery is planned, determine the patient's knowledge about preoperative and postoperative care.

Interventions

In many ways, the care of the patient with pancreatic cancer is like that discussed under "Nursing Care of the Patient with Pancreatitis." Chapter 25 also provides details of caring for the patient with cancer. Areas that require special attention with pancreatic cancer are discussed here.

Acute Pain

Assess and record pain severity, nature, and location. Opioid analgesics are usually needed for severe pain management; however, nonopioids may be effective for mild to moderate pain. Radiation therapy and chemotherapy can reduce pain by shrinking the tumor. A celiac plexus nerve block can be done during surgery or percutaneously and provides excellent pain control for several months. Other options for intolerable pain are patient-controlled analgesia (PCA) and epidural opioids. The effectiveness of drug therapy may be enhanced by distraction, imagery, and cutaneous stimulation, as discussed in Chapter 15.

Nursing Diagnoses, Goals, and Outcome Criteria: Cancer of the Pancreas

Nursing Diagnoses	Goals and Outcome Criteria
Acute Pain related to obstruction, extensive malignancy	Pain relief: patient states pain is reduced or relieved, more relaxed
Fear and **Grieving** related to diagnosis or poor prognosis	Reduced fear: patient states is less fearful, calm manner Family coping: family and patient make realistic plans, support each other
Imbalanced Nutrition: Less Than Body Requirements related to anorexia, nausea, vomiting	Adequate nutrition: stable body weight
Impaired Skin Integrity related to pruritus, inactivity, nutritional deficiencies	Healthy skin: skin intact without reddened area or abrasions
Disturbed Body Image related to jaundice, weight loss	Effective coping with physical changes: patient makes effort to improve appearance, attends to grooming and dress
Deficient Knowledge of symptom management, self-care, and sources of support	Adequate knowledge: patient and family demonstrate understanding of patient care and resources

Fear and Grieving

You can help the patient by recognizing and acknowledging his or her fear, showing compassion, teaching, and providing attentive care. A referral to a mental health professional or spiritual counselor can be made with the patient's consent.

Imbalanced Nutrition: Less Than Body Requirements

Monitor the patient's dietary intake and weight. If intake is poor, consult the dietitian. Small, frequent meals may be ordered. Pancrelipase tablets are needed if the patient has malabsorption. Sometimes a jejunostomy tube is placed and feeding is delivered by pump. Feedings are usually started with dilute formula given at a slow rate. Both the concentration and the rate are gradually increased. Inform the physician if the patient develops diarrhea. Some patients require TPN for adequate nourishment (see *Nutrition Considerations* box).

Impaired Skin Integrity

If pruritus is a problem, special skin care and protection are needed. Eliminate bath soaps and apply emollient lotions. Keep the fingernails short to reduce trauma from scratching. Supply mittens if the patient is unable to avoid scratching. The physician may order diphenhydramine (Benadryl) to reduce pruritus. If a patient has drains or fistulas, irritating digestive fluids may come in contact with the skin. Carefully cleanse the exposed skin. Skin barriers and pouches may be effective in protecting the skin. An enterostomal therapist may be consulted for advice on skin care.

Disturbed Body Image

Weight loss and jaundice alter the patient's appearance and may be distressing. Assist patients with grooming and encourage them to look their best.

Deficient Knowledge

People under stress retain only part of what they hear, so information often must be repeated and reinforced. Provide written material in addition to verbal instruction. The patient's family also may need information and support when dealing with a diagnosis of pancreatic cancer. Refer questions about medical decisions and prognosis to the physician. The specific teaching plan will depend on the diagnostic and therapeutic measures prescribed. You should advise the patient of community resources, including the American Cancer Society and home health nursing services.

Surgical Complications and Postoperative Nursing Care

In general, the postoperative care of the patient with pancreatic cancer is like that of any patient undergoing major abdominal surgery. If the Whipple procedure is performed, the patient is at risk for many complications. These include hemorrhage; fluid and electrolyte imbalances; respiratory, circulatory, renal, and hepatic failure; wound infection and dehiscence; fistulas; and hyperglycemia. Therefore ongoing nursing assessments are critical. Closely monitor vital signs, intake and output, and blood glucose values. Assess the wound for bleeding, infection, and separation of margins. Evaluate mental status to detect changes associated with electrolyte imbalances, poor circulation, and hepatic or renal failure.

Nutrition Considerations

1. People with gallbladder disease should follow a low-fat diet because fat intake usually causes pain.
2. For a person with hepatitis, the diet should be high in calories and vitamins with moderate to high protein and moderate to low fat.
3. When the liver is damaged by cirrhosis, protein may be restricted to lower blood ammonia.
4. In hepatitis and cirrhosis, carbohydrates should provide most of the calories.
5. A bland, high-carbohydrate, high-protein, low-fat diet is recommended for pancreatitis.
6. Pancreatitis patients must avoid alcohol and spicy foods that stimulate the pancreas.

Get Ready for the NCLEX® Examination!

Key Points

- The liver plays an important role in bile production and excretion; glucose, protein, and lipid metabolism; blood coagulation; detoxification; immunity; and hormone metabolism.
- Signs of liver dysfunction include jaundice (a golden-yellow skin color) and scleral icterus (yellowing of the sclera of the eyes).
- Hepatitis is liver inflammation caused by a viral infection or exposure to toxic substances; it can lead to hepatic failure.
- Nursing care of the patient with hepatitis addresses activity intolerance; impaired physical mobility; imbalanced nutrition: less than body requirements; acute pain; impaired skin integrity; deficient fluid volume; disturbed body image; and anxiety.
- Health care providers should be vaccinated against hepatitis B because it can be spread through contact with body fluids.
- Cirrhosis is chronic, progressive liver failure that disrupts metabolism and causes blood abnormalities, fluid and electrolyte imbalances, decreased resistance

to infection, accumulation of drugs and toxins, and obstruction of blood vessels and bile ducts in the liver.
- Cirrhosis may be caused by nutritional deficiencies, toxins (including alcohol), hepatitis, biliary obstruction, and heart failure.
- Complications of cirrhosis include portal hypertension, esophageal varices, ascites, spontaneous bacterial peritonitis, hepatic encephalopathy, and hepatorenal syndrome.
- Nursing care of the patient with cirrhosis addresses imbalanced nutrition: less than body requirements; activity intolerance; risk for impaired skin integrity; acute pain; ineffective breathing pattern; risk for injury; acute confusion; deficient fluid volume; excess fluid volume; risk for infection; and fear.
- The only cure for end-stage liver disease is liver transplantation, which requires lifelong treatment with antirejection drugs that suppress the immune system and put the patient at risk for infection.
- Signs and symptoms of transplanted organ rejection are fever, anorexia, depression, vague abdominal pain, muscle aches, and joint pain.
- Bile is produced in the liver, stored in the gallbladder, and delivered to the intestine, where it is essential for emulsification and digestion of fats.
- Cholecystitis is inflammation of the gallbladder, usually caused by gallstones; the gallstones may obstruct bile flow, causing symptoms from mild indigestion to nausea, chills and fever, and right upper quadrant pain that radiates to the shoulder.
- Cholelithiasis (stones in the bile) may be treated with cholecystectomy, oral bile salts, dissolution agents, lithotripsy, or endoscopic sphincterotomy.
- Nursing care of the patient with cholecystitis and cholelithiasis focuses on acute pain, deficient fluid volume, risk for impaired skin integrity, anxiety, risk for injury, and, *for surgical patients*, ineffective breathing pattern and risk for infection.
- The pancreas has an endocrine function (insulin and glucagon secretion) and an exocrine function (secretion of digestive enzymes).
- Pancreatitis is inflammation of the pancreas; it can lead to pseudocyst; abscess; hypocalcemia; and pulmonary, cardiac, and renal complications.
- Nursing care of the patient with pancreatitis addresses acute pain; deficient fluid volume; risk for infection; impaired gas exchange; imbalanced nutrition: less than body requirements; anxiety; and deficient knowledge.
- Most patients with pancreatic cancer die within 1 year, especially if the cancer is in the body or tail of the pancreas.
- Nursing care of the patient with pancreatic cancer usually focuses on acute pain; fear; grieving; imbalanced nutrition: less than body requirements; impaired skin integrity; and disturbed body image.

Additional Learning Resources

SG Go to your Study Guide for additional learning activities to help you master this chapter content.

evolve Go to your Evolve website (http://evolve.elsevier.com/Linton/medsurg) for the following learning resources and much more:
- Interactive Prioritization Exercises
- Fluid & Electrolyte Tutorial
- Pharmacology Tutorial
- Review Questions for the NCLEX® Examination

Review Questions for the NCLEX® Examination

1. Your focused assessment of a patient with hepatitis reveals jaundice, light-colored stools, and dark urine. These findings are typical of which phase of hepatitis?
   NCLEX Client Need: Physiological Integrity: Physiological Adaptation
2. A patient who has hepatitis reports that she is itching and cannot resist scratching. Which measures should help to control the itching? (Select all that apply.)
   1. Apply lubricating lotion
   2. Administer prescribed antihistamine
   3. Use tepid water for bathing
   4. Vigorously massage affected areas
   5. Administer prescribed antibiotics

   NCLEX Client Need: Physiological Integrity: Reduction of Risk Potential
3. Nursing students are required to have certain immunizations. Vaccination for which of the following is required because health care providers are often in contact with body fluids?
   1. Hepatitis A
   2. Hepatitis B
   3. Hepatitis C
   4. Hepatitis D

   NCLEX Client Need: Physiological Integrity: Reduction of Risk Potential
4. A patient with cirrhosis has esophageal varices and hemorrhoids. The nurse understands that varices and hemorrhoids are caused by:
   1. Blood vessels weakened by malnutrition
   2. Inability to conjugate and excrete bilirubin
   3. Elevated pressure in GI blood vessels
   4. Fluid retention associated with excess aldosterone

   NCLEX Client Need: Physiological Integrity: Physiological Adaptation
5. A patient comes to the clinic for follow-up 1 month after liver transplantation. Which of the following assessment findings would concern you *most*?
   1. Heartburn
   2. Constipation
   3. Pale urine
   4. Fever

   NCLEX Client Need: Physiological Integrity: Reduction of Risk Potential
6. Which of the following structures comprise the common bile duct? (Select all that apply.)
   1. Duodenum
   2. Cystic duct
   3. Hepatic bile ducts
   4. Main pancreatic duct
   5. Ductus arteriosis

   NCLEX Client Need: Physiological Integrity: Physiological Adaptation

7. A patient returns from surgery for an incisional cholecystectomy with a T-tube. The nurse understands that the purpose of the T-tube is to:
1. Maintain bile flow in the common bile duct
2. Relieve pressure on the liver
3. Divert intestinal contents from the surgical site
4. Prevent bile leakage into the abdomen
NCLEX Client Need: Physiological Integrity: Reduction of Risk Potential

8. The endocrine functions of the pancreas include which of the following? (Select all that apply.)
1. Storage and secretion of insulin in response to high blood glucose levels
2. Conversion of excess blood glucose to glycogen for storage
3. Breakdown of excessive fats and carbohydrates in the intestine
4. Production and secretion of digestive enzymes into the duodenum through a duct
5. Manufacture and storage of bile
NCLEX Client Need: Physiological Integrity: Physiological Adaptation

9. A patient with chronic pancreatitis is taking pancreatic enzyme tablets. To assess the effectiveness of the tablets, the nurse should:
1. Monitor daily weights
2. Examine the stools for steatorrhea
3. Record intake and output
4. Ask whether pain is relieved
NCLEX Client Need: Physiological Integrity: Physiological Adaptation

10. The nurse is teaching a health promotion class. The participants should be told that they can reduce the risk of pancreatic cancer by:
1. Smoking cessation
2. Increased dietary protein
3. Regular exercise
4. Stress reduction activities
NCLEX Client Need: Physiological Integrity: Reduction of Risk Potential

chapter 42

Urologic Disorders

http://evolve.elsevier.com/Linton/medsurg

Elizabeth Anderson

Objectives

1. List the data to be collected when assessing a patient who has a urologic disorder.
2. Describe the diagnostic tests and procedures for patients with urologic disorders.
3. Explain the nursing responsibilities for patients who are having tests and procedures to diagnose urologic disorders.
4. Describe the nursing responsibilities for common therapeutic measures used to treat urologic disorders.
5. Explain the pathophysiology, signs and symptoms, complications, and treatment of disorders of the kidneys, ureters, bladder, and urethra.
6. Assist in developing a nursing care plan for patients with urologic disorders.

Key Terms

Anuria (ă-NŪ-rē-ă)
Azotemia (ă-zō-TĒ-mē-ă)
Calculus (pl. calculi) (KĂL-kŭ-lŭs, KĂL-kŭ-lī)
Cystectomy (sĭs-TĔK-tō-mē)
Diuresis (dī-ŭ-RĒ-sĭs)
Diuretic (dī-ŭr-RĔ-tĭc)
Dysuria (dĭs-Ū-rē-ă)
Hematuria (hĕm-ă-TŪ-rē-ă)
Incontinence (ĭn-KŎN-tĭ-nĕns)
Lithotomy (lĭ-THŎT-ō-mē)
Lithotripsy (LĬTH-ō-trĭp-sē)
Nephrotoxic (nĕf-rō-TŎK-sĭk)
Nocturia (nŏk-TŪ-rē-ă)
Oliguria (ŏlĭ-GŪ-rē-ă)
Polyuria (pŏl-ē-Ū-rē-ă)
Uremia (ū-RĒ-mē-ă)

The urinary tract plays a vital role in maintaining homeostasis and removing metabolic wastes. Because body systems are interdependent, disease processes in other body systems may have a direct and harmful effect on the urinary system. Similarly, urinary system diseases may affect the respiratory and circulatory systems significantly. Serious alterations in urinary function eventually affect all other systems. A person can live with one functioning kidney but the body cannot support life with the loss of both kidneys.

ANATOMY OF THE URINARY SYSTEM

The urinary system consists of two kidneys, two ureters, the bladder, and the urethra (Fig. 42-1).

KIDNEYS AND URETERS

The kidneys are bean-shaped organs located just under and below the twelfth rib near the waist in an area of the body trunk called the *flank* (Fig. 42-2). They each are surrounded by fibrous capsules and layers of fat. They are tightly wedged between the peritoneum, a membrane that separates them from the digestive system, and a layer of muscle in the back.

The hilus, or entry, to the kidney is located on the concave surface of the kidney near the spine (Fig. 42-3). The right and left renal arteries branch off from the abdominal artery and enter the kidneys at the hilus. The entire blood supply circulates through the kidneys every 4 to 5 minutes. Each renal vein returns filtered blood directly to the inferior vena cava. The kidney is divided into an outer layer called the *cortex* and an inner layer called the *medulla*. The cortex receives a large blood supply and is very sensitive to changes in blood pressure (BP) and blood volume. The medulla is organized into 8 to 18 pyramid-shaped structures that concentrate and collect urine and drain it into the calices. The calices then drain urine into the renal pelvis. The renal pelvis is at the center of the kidney and forms the funnel-shaped proximal end of the ureter. The ureter carries urine from the renal pelvis to the bladder.

The nephron is the functional unit of the kidney. Each kidney has 1 to 1.25 million nephrons. The nephron is a vascular tubular system consisting of a glomerulus, a Bowman capsule, and a tubule. The glomerulus is a mass of blood vessels tucked into the cuplike Bowman capsule. Each tubular system consists

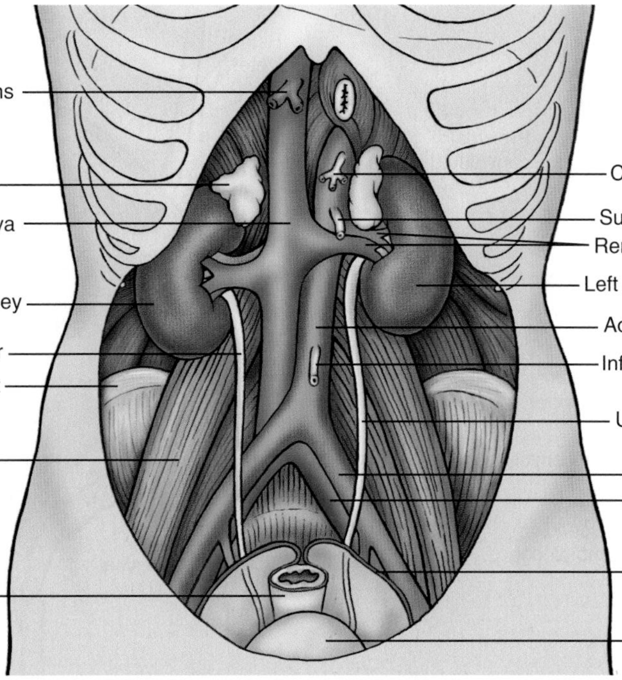

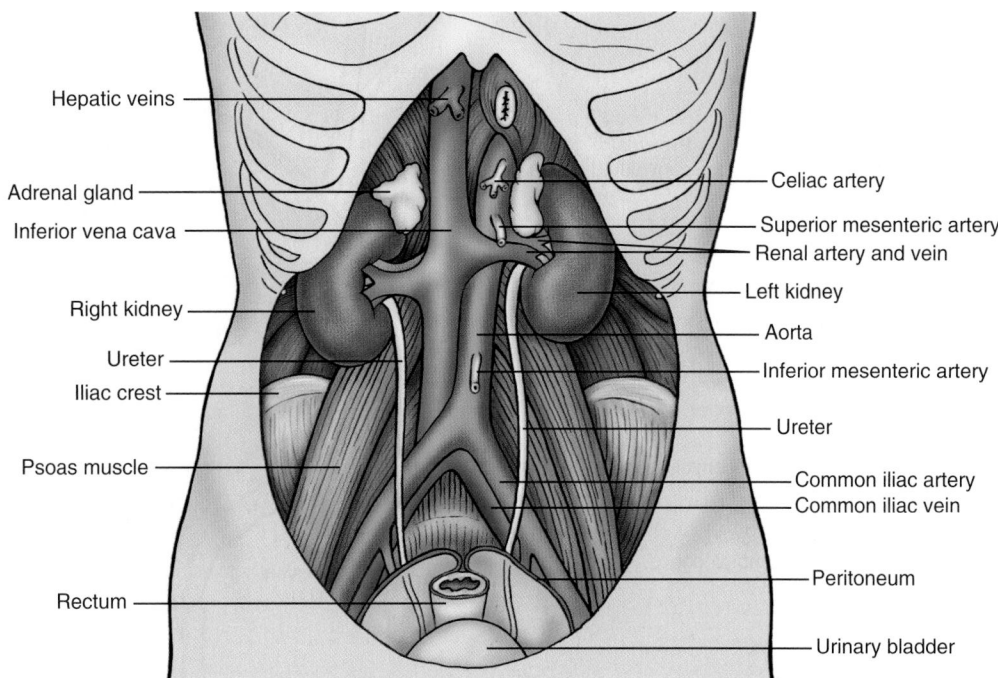

FIGURE 42-1 The kidneys and related structures. (From Monahan FD, Drake DT, Neighbors M, editors: *Medical-surgical nursing: foundations for clinical practice*, ed 2, Philadelphia, 1998, Saunders.)

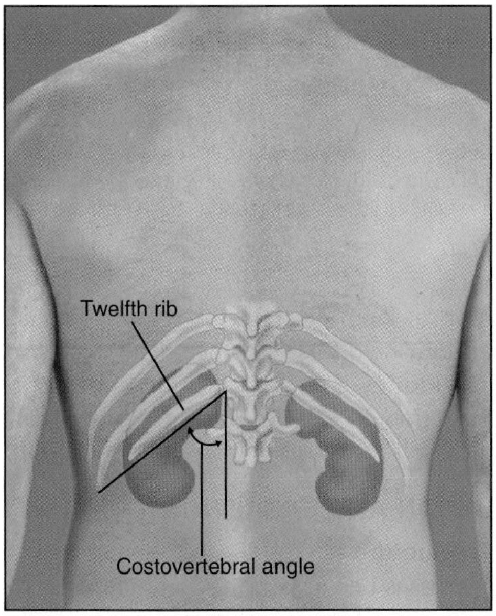

FIGURE 42-2 The kidneys are located just under and below the twelfth rib. The costovertebral angle is illustrated here. (From Monahan FD, Drake DT, Neighbors M, editors: *Medical-surgical nursing: foundations for clinical practice*, ed 2, Philadelphia, 1998, Saunders.)

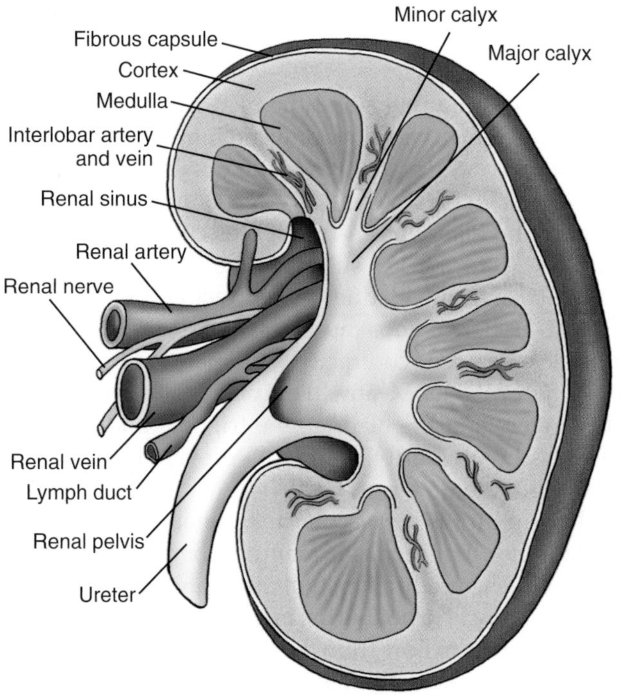

FIGURE 42-3 View of interior kidney structures. (From Monahan FD, Drake DT, Neighbors M, editors: *Medical-surgical nursing: foundations for clinical practice*, ed 2, Philadelphia, 1998, Saunders.)

of a proximal tubule, the loop of Henle, a distal tubule, and collecting tubules (Fig. 42-4). The nephron is located mostly in the cortex of the kidney, with the loop of Henle dipping into the medulla. A single collecting duct is formed by several tubules and travels through the medulla to the calices.

BLADDER AND URETHRA

The bladder is a muscular sac that readily stretches to store urine. The bladder rests on the floor of the pelvic cavity behind the peritoneum. It is located in front of the rectum in men and in front of the vagina and uterus in women. The upper portion of the bladder is called the *apex* and the base, or *fundus*, is close to the pelvic floor. The bladder neck, containing the internal sphincter, is the most inferior portion. The trigone is a triangular-shaped area on the posterior wall, as seen in Figure 42-5. The trigone muscles help to close the

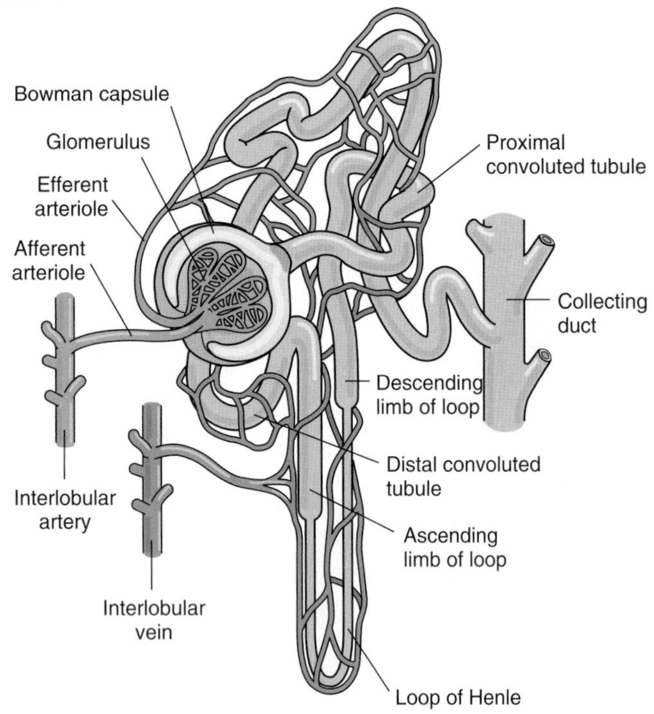

FIGURE 42-4 Details of a nephron. (From Monahan F, Sands J, Neighbors M, et al.: *Phipps' medical-surgical nursing: health and illness perspectives*, ed 8, St. Louis, 2007, Mosby.)

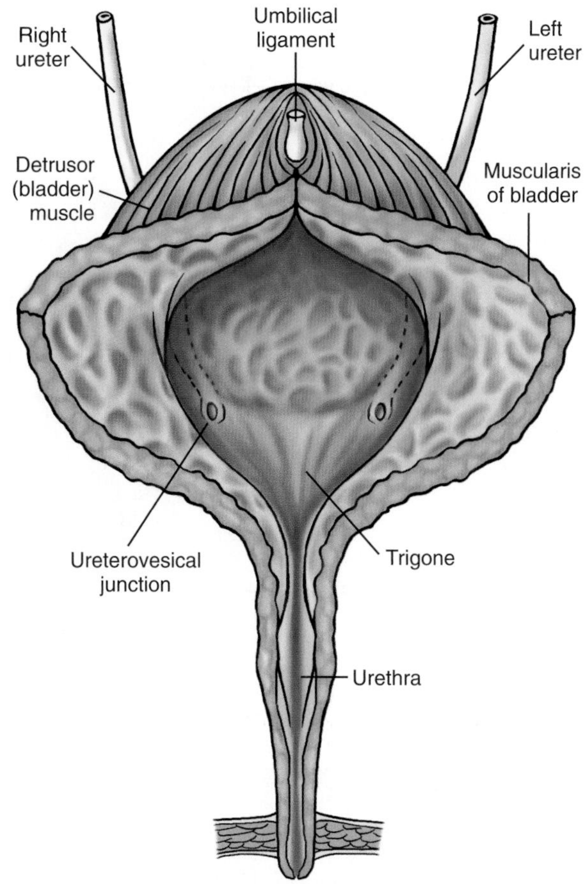

FIGURE 42-5 The urinary bladder cut to reveal the interior. (From Monahan FD, Drake DT, Neighbors M, editors: *Medical-surgical nursing: foundations for clinical practice*, ed 2, Philadelphia, 1998, Saunders.)

junction of the ureters and the bladder during urination, preventing backflow of urine into the ureters.

Control of the bladder is made possible by sensory and motor nerves. When 200 to 400 mL of urine collects in the bladder, sensory nerves cause the urge to urinate. Motor nerves stimulate the detrusor muscles in the base of the bladder to contract and empty (see Fig. 42-5). Pelvic floor muscles and external sphincter muscles can be contracted voluntarily to control outflow of urine. Meanwhile, back at the junction of the ureters and the bladder, the trigonal and ureteral muscles involuntarily contract to prevent backflow of urine into the ureters.

The urethra is a muscular tube lined with mucous membranes that carries urine from the bladder out of the body. The urethra functions as a sphincter, meaning that it contracts to hold urine in the bladder and relaxes to allow urine to flow from the bladder. Approximately 3 cm of the proximal male urethra is encircled by the prostate gland. The urethra is about 20 cm long in men and 3 to 5 cm long in women. The short length and proximity of the urethra to the female anus are two reasons for the increased incidence of bladder infections in women.

PHYSIOLOGY OF THE URINARY SYSTEM

The functions of the urinary system are regulatory, excretory, and hormonal. Regulatory functions are performed by the formation of urine and the secretion of renin, which affects BP. Regulatory processes maintain fluid balance, keep electrolytes within normal range, and maintain acid-base balance. The excretory function of the kidney is the elimination of urine. The hormonal function is to stimulate red blood cell (RBC) production.

REGULATION AND EXCRETION

Urine Production

Three processes occur in urine production: (1) glomerular filtration, (2) tubular reabsorption, and (3) tubular secretion.

Glomerular Filtration. Glomerular filtration is an ultrafiltration process in the glomerular capsule. Fluids, electrolytes, and other substances are filtered out of the blood as it passes through the glomerulus. Plasma proteins are too large to pass through the glomerulus and therefore remain in the blood. The ultrafiltration process requires adequate blood volume and BP. The product of glomerular filtration is called the *glomerular filtrate*. It contains water, electrolytes (i.e., sodium, potassium, calcium, magnesium, chloride, bicarbonate, phosphate, other anions), glucose, urea, creatinine, uric acid, and amino acids. Glomerular filtrate and blood plasma are essentially the same, except that the filtrate does not have proteins. Most of the filtrate is returned to the blood from the tubules by reabsorption.

Tubular Reabsorption. Water, some electrolytes, and nonelectrolytes are reabsorbed from the tubules of the kidney into the blood as needed to maintain normal fluid balance. Reabsorption occurs through diffusion, active transport, and osmosis. Some nonelectrolytes (i.e., urea, creatinine, uric acid) are not readily reabsorbed and are excreted in the urine. The reabsorption of water reflects the ability of the kidney to concentrate or dilute urine as necessary. The amount of water reabsorbed is influenced by antidiuretic hormone (ADH) and aldosterone. ADH, stored in the posterior pituitary, affects the amount of water reabsorbed in the distal tubules and the collecting ducts. If blood volume decreases or blood osmolality (concentration) increases, ADH is secreted from the posterior pituitary. The distal tubules and collecting ducts of the kidney become more permeable to water so that reabsorption into the circulating blood increases and urine becomes more concentrated.

Tubular Secretion. Potassium and hydrogen ions are secreted into the tubules from the blood. This secretion process regulates serum potassium levels and is the basis for the kidney's acid-base regulating mechanism. The normal pH of urine is 4.5 to 8.0.

The kidneys and lungs work together to maintain the acid-base balance of the body. The lungs excrete carbon dioxide (CO_2), a volatile acid, and the kidneys excrete fixed acids produced by normal metabolism. Base levels are maintained by renal conservation of bicarbonate, excretion of sodium for hydrogen, and excretion of ammonia.

The end product of glomerular filtration, tubular reabsorption, and tubular excretion is urine. Urine is composed mostly of water, sodium, potassium, chloride, urea, creatinine, and uric acid. The body normally excretes 1 to 2 L of urine each day, which is approximately 1% of the blood filtered by the glomeruli in the same period of time. Glucose and proteins are substances present in blood but not normally present in the urine. Normally, glucose is completely reabsorbed in the tubules. The presence of proteins in urine indicates glomerular damage. Urine is delivered to the renal pelvis, where it flows into the ureter. The production of urine is illustrated in Figure 42-6.

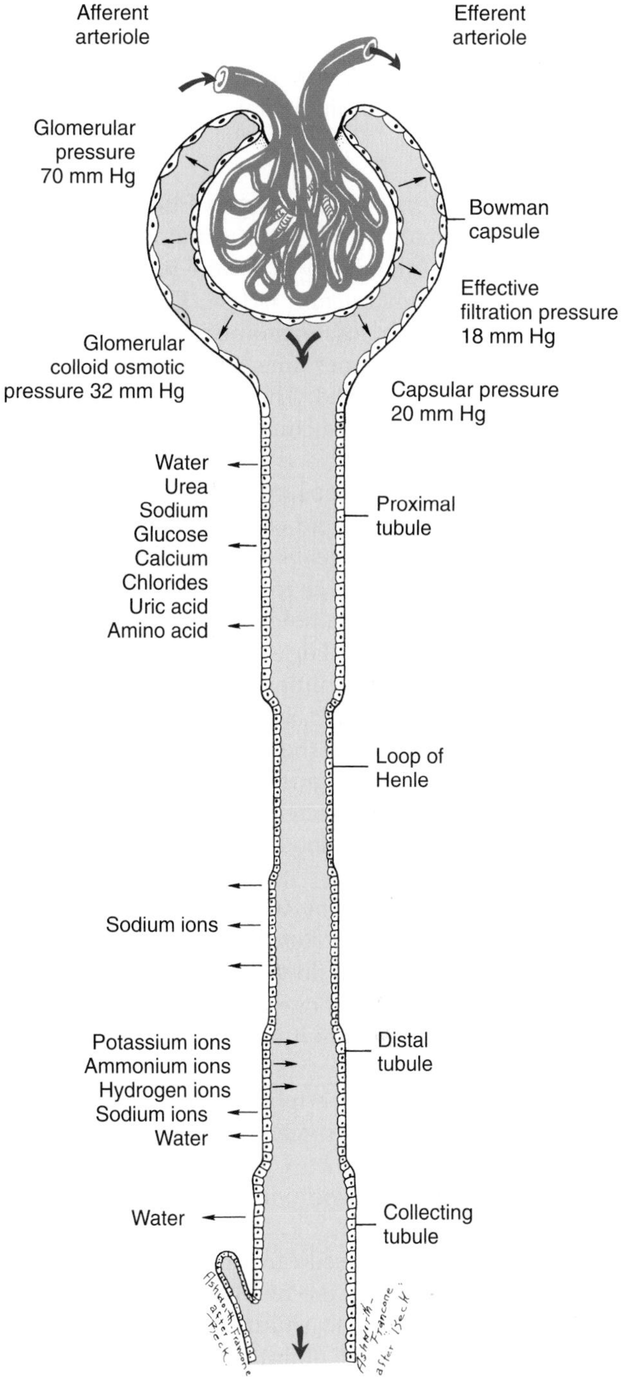

FIGURE 42-6 Urine production. (From Jacob WW, Francone CA: *Elements of anatomy and physiology*, ed 2, Philadelphia, 1989, Saunders.)

Urine Elimination

Peristaltic waves move urine from the kidney through the ureter to the bladder. The presence of 200 to 250 mL of urine in the bladder causes the urge to urinate, although the bladder can distend to hold several times that amount. Urination is a complex process that is under a variety of neural controls and is voluntary for the toilet-trained person with intact motor and sensory nerve pathways. Urination generally occurs five to six times a day and may occur once at night. The amount of urine produced is affected by fluid intake, temperature, diaphoresis, vomiting, diarrhea, and medications such as **diuretics**.

A series of events allow the release of urine from the bladder. The pelvic floor muscles and the urethral sphincter relax. The trigonal muscles contract, closing the ureters to prevent backflow of urine into the ureters. The bladder muscle (detrusor) contracts and urine is forced through the urethra. After the bladder empties, the bladder muscle relaxes, the bladder neck closes, the trigonal muscles relax, and the perineal muscles resume resting tone. Voiding is primarily an involuntary reflex act. Voluntary control of voiding is exhibited in the initiation, restraint, and interruption of urine flow.

Regulation of Serum Calcium and Phosphate

Parathyroid hormone (PTH) is a hormone secreted by the parathyroid glands to maintain serum calcium levels. When serum calcium is low, PTH is secreted and acts on the tubules to promote reabsorption of calcium ions. At the same time, tubular reabsorption of phosphate is decreased. This mechanism helps to maintain normal serum calcium and phosphate levels.

Regulation of Blood Pressure

BP is regulated through fluid volume maintenance and release of the hormone *renin* from the kidneys. One way to raise or lower BP is to change blood volume. This can be done by retaining additional fluid or by eliminating excess fluid. For example, suppose that a patient has had severe vomiting and diarrhea resulting in dehydration and low BP. Hypertonic plasma caused by dehydration stimulates the release of ADH from the posterior pituitary. ADH causes reabsorption of water from the renal tubules, decreasing urine volume. The retained fluid expands blood volume, with a subsequent rise in BP.

A second mechanism by which the kidneys affect BP is the secretion of renin. Renin is released in response to inadequate renal blood flow or low arterial pressure. Renin acts on angiotensinogen, a hormone produced by the liver, and converts it to angiotensin I. A lung enzyme converts angiotensin I to angiotensin II. Angiotensin II is a powerful peripheral vasoconstrictor. In addition, angiotensin II triggers the release of aldosterone from the adrenal cortex. Aldosterone stimulates tubular reabsorption of sodium and water and plasma volume is expanded.

With severely decreased cardiac output, as seen in hemorrhage and shock, the renal arteries constrict to prevent fluid loss and to shunt blood to more vital organs (i.e., heart, lungs, brain). This vasoconstriction limits renal blood flow. If blood flow is not restored, death of renal tissue may occur.

HORMONAL STIMULATION OF RED BLOOD CELL PRODUCTION

Erythropoietin is secreted in the kidneys and stimulates the bone marrow to produce RBCs. This process is triggered by decreased oxygen (O_2) in renal blood. Patients in renal failure have a deficiency of erythropoietin, which causes them to become anemic.

AGE-RELATED CHANGES IN THE URINARY SYSTEM

As people age, significant changes occur in the urinary system. Fortunately, the kidneys have enough reserve that normal function is usually maintained. However, when older people are stressed, the kidneys do not adapt as well as they do in younger people.

Structural changes in the kidney include loss of nephrons, thickening of membranes in nephrons, and sclerosis of renal blood vessels. Because of these changes, renal blood flow and glomerular filtration decline. In addition, plasma renin and aldosterone levels fall and tubules are less responsive to ADH. As a result of all of these changes, the older person's kidneys are less able to concentrate and dilute urine in response to changes in serum osmolality (concentration).

Creatinine clearance decreases with age. This means that the rate at which the kidneys are able to remove creatinine from the blood is diminished. Creatinine clearance is a better indicator of kidney function than serum creatinine. Some decline also occurs in erythropoietin, a factor that may contribute to anemia. In an older person, serum glucose may be considerably elevated before it is detected in the urine.

In younger people, urine production peaks during waking hours. This pattern is lost with age such that urine production does not decrease at night. Therefore older people often have **nocturia**, meaning that they awaken from sleep to void.

The bladder also undergoes changes with age. Bladder muscles weaken and connective tissue increases. The effect is decreased capacity and incomplete emptying. The mechanism that prevents the reflux of urine from the bladder into the ureters is less effective and can contribute to kidney infections.

Incontinence is not a normal consequence of age but it is common. Female urinary incontinence is often caused by relaxed pelvic muscles related to childbirth trauma and lack of estrogen after menopause. For detailed information on incontinence, see Chapter 23. In men, urethral obstruction is more often a problem. It is often caused by the enlarged prostate closing in on the urethra. Prostate enlargement is discussed in Chapter 50.

NURSING ASSESSMENT OF THE URINARY SYSTEM

Elimination is considered to be a very personal activity and some people are not accustomed to discussing it with others. Therefore assessment of urinary function and problems may be embarrassing for the patient. Privacy and a calm, accepting manner help to put the patient at ease.

HEALTH HISTORY

Chief Complaint

Patients with urinary problems most often report changes in urine quality or quantity, pain, or changes in urination.

History of Present Illness

Ask about the patient's normal or usual pattern of urination. Important data include volume of urine, frequency of voiding, and appearance of urine. The patient may have difficulty estimating the amount of urine voided but usually can recognize an increase or decrease from normal. If intake and output records are available, note the recent pattern. Terms used to describe urine volume are *polyuria, oliguria*, and *anuria*. **Polyuria** refers to a large urine output, **oliguria** to a low output, and **anuria** to the absence of output. Urine characteristics to record include color, clarity (clear or cloudy), presence of particles, and odor. **Hematuria** is the presence of blood in the urine.

Pain may or may not occur but it is more common with acute conditions. Painful urination is called **dysuria**. Inquire about the presence of pain or discomfort. Describe the characteristics of the pain: intensity, location, distribution, onset, duration, frequency, relationship to urination, precipitating factors, and measures that provide relief. Urologic conditions also may cause pain in the flank, abdomen, pelvic area, and genitalia. The pain may be so severe that it causes nausea and vomiting.

Include questions about any problem the patient has had with initiating or controlling urination. Document circumstances under which these problems occur. For example, involuntary loss of urine with laughing or sneezing is typical of stress incontinence. Urge incontinence is the inability to hold urine when feeling the urge to void.

Past Medical History

After the present illness has been fully described, the patient's past medical history should be explored. Significant findings include a history of streptococcal infections, recurrent urinary tract infections (UTIs), renal **calculi** ("stones"), diabetes mellitus, gout, or hypercalcemia. Ask if the patient has had urologic surgery, catheterization, examination (e.g., cystoscopy, radiography), or trauma and if the patient uses any type of urinary diversion or collection device. Document recent and current medications, including prescription and over-the-counter (OTC) drugs and herbal remedies, because some medications are **nephrotoxic** (harmful to the kidneys). Note exposure to toxic chemicals in the home or the workplace.

Family History

Describe the patient's family medical history. Important conditions to note are congenital kidney problems such as polycystic kidneys or urinary tract malformations, diabetes mellitus, and hypertension.

Review of Systems

Review the body systems to detect other problems that may be related to the urinary tract complaints. Ask if the patient has had changes in skin color, respiratory distress, edema, fatigue, nausea, vomiting, chills, and fever.

Functional Assessment

The functional assessment includes information about habits and practices that might affect or contribute to urinary tract disorders. Ask about daily fluid intake because urine production varies with fluid intake. It is also helpful to determine the patient's usual exercise pattern because excessive exercise or prolonged immobility affects the urinary system. Determine the effects of the chief complaint on daily life as well.

> **Pharmacology Capsule**
>
> Nephrotoxic drugs are harmful to the kidneys.

PHYSICAL EXAMINATION

The physical examination begins with inspection of the skin for color (i.e., ashen, yellow) and the presence of crystals on the skin (i.e., uremic frost). Evaluate tissue turgor to detect dehydration or edema. Examine the area around the eyes for periorbital edema, which suggests fluid retention. Inspect the mouth for moisture and odor. Patients in renal failure may have an odor of urine on their breath.

Observe respiratory rate, pattern, and effort. Respirations may be rapid with metabolic acidosis, infection, and fluid overload. Kussmaul respirations, seen with metabolic acidosis, are rapid and deep. Dyspnea may be evident with fluid overload. Auscultate the lungs for crackles or rhonchi that may indicate fluid overload. Heart rhythm irregularities may be noted with potassium imbalances.

Inspect the abdomen for scars and contours and palpate for tenderness and bladder distention. Auscultate the kidney area over the costovertebral angle (see Fig. 42-2) to detect renal bruits (swishing sounds caused by turbulent blood flow). Renal bruits indicate renal artery stenosis (narrowing). Then percuss the abdomen. A dull sound may be heard over a full bladder. Pain may be elicited over one or both kidneys.

Observe for edema throughout the examination. With renal failure, edema is generalized, not dependent. The skin may be dry, flushed, and shiny over the edematous area.

The last part of the physical examination is inspection of the genitalia. Standard Precautions should be observed. Examine the penis for lesions, scars, or discharge. If there are penile lesions or urethral discharge, smears should be obtained for culture. A nurse with advanced skills or the physician also may perform rectal and pelvic examinations, especially if symptoms suggest problems of the reproductive system. The pelvic examination may reveal gynecologic rather than urologic problems. The male rectal examination helps to detect prostate enlargement, which often creates

Box 42-1 Assessment of the Patient with a Urologic Disorder

HEALTH HISTORY

Present Illness
Changes in urine quality or quantity, voiding pattern, pain

Past Medical History
Streptococcal infections, urinary tract infections (UTIs) or calculi, gout, hypercalcemia, urologic surgery or instrumentation, urinary diversion, recent and current medications

Family History
Urinary disorders, diabetes mellitus, hypertension

Review of Systems
Fatigue, pruritus, dyspnea; urine quantity: polyuria, oliguria, anuria; urine quality: color, odor, components; frequency of voiding; pain: onset, intensity, frequency, location, duration, precipitating and relieving factors

Functional Assessment
Fluid intake, diet, activity

PHYSICAL EXAMINATION

General Appearance
Level of consciousness, orientation

Vital Signs

Height and Weight

Skin
Color, moisture, turgor, crystals

Respirations
Rate, pattern, effort, breath sounds

Circulation
Dysrhythmias, blood pressure (BP) alterations

Abdomen
Scars, contour, tenderness, bruits

Genitalia
Lesions, scars, discharge

problems with voiding. Nursing assessment of urologic function is outlined in Box 42-1.

DIAGNOSTIC TESTS AND PROCEDURES

Diagnostic tests and procedures for urinary disorders are described here. Related nursing care is presented in Table 42-1.

URINE TESTS

Urinalysis

A urine specimen is examined for color, pH, specific gravity, glucose, protein, blood, ketones, and bilirubin. Normal urine is straw colored and slightly acidic. Microscopic examination is used to assess for cells, casts, bacteria, and crystals. Chemical examination to assess electrolytes and osmolality (concentration) of the urine determines the ability of the kidneys to excrete or conserve electrolytes and water. By comparing the osmolality of urine with serum osmolality, it is possible to know if the kidneys are functioning appropriately. If serum osmolality is elevated, the kidneys should reabsorb or conserve water to dilute the serum and excrete more concentrated urine (i.e., urine with high osmolality). If serum osmolality is low (urine is dilute), the kidneys should reduce reabsorption of water to increase serum concentration and produce more dilute urine (i.e., urine with low osmolality). Specific gravity is a measure of osmolality. Data reported from a routine urinalysis are summarized in Table 42-2.

Urine Culture and Sensitivity

Normal urine is sterile. A urine culture permits identification of microorganisms present in the urine. Sensitivity testing determines which antibiotics will be effective against the specific organisms. The specimen can be obtained by the patient, if able, or the nurse. If an antibiotic is ordered, collect the urine specimen before starting the antibiotic drug. Instructions are given in Table 42-1.

Creatinine Clearance

Creatinine clearance, the rate at which the kidney removes creatinine from the blood, is the best test of overall kidney function. It serves as an estimate of glomerular filtration rate. This test requires collection of all urine for 12 or 24 hours, as ordered. Normal levels vary for men and women. Because values depend on muscle mass, they are usually lower in women. Urine and serum creatinine levels are compared to determine kidney function. If serum creatinine rises and urine creatinine falls, it is an indication of decreased kidney function and glomerular filtration rate.

BLOOD TESTS

Blood Urea Nitrogen

The blood urea nitrogen (BUN) test is a general indicator of the kidneys' ability to excrete urea, an end product of protein metabolism. In addition to renal failure, factors that increase BUN are a high-protein diet (especially with renal disease), gastrointestinal (GI) bleeding, dehydration, and some drugs (aspirin, chemotherapeutic drugs, diuretics, gentamicin, lithium carbonate, morphine, corticosteroids, sulfonamides, tobramycin).

Serum Creatinine

Creatinine is a waste product of skeletal muscle breakdown. The level of creatinine in the blood is an indication of the kidneys' ability to excrete wastes. Serum creatinine is elevated only in renal disorders and is a better measurement of kidney function than BUN. Unlike BUN, creatinine is not influenced by diet, hydration, nutritional status, or liver function. With normally functioning kidneys, the serum creatinine level is very low and the urine level is high. The normal ratio of BUN to creatinine is 12:1 to 20:1.

Serum Electrolytes

Serum electrolytes must be monitored in the renal patient because imbalances can have very serious consequences. In renal failure, sodium and potassium levels are elevated and calcium levels are decreased.

Table 42-1 Diagnostic Tests and Procedures **Urinary Disorders**

TEST AND PURPOSE	PATIENT PREPARATION	POSTPROCEDURE CARE
Laboratory Studies		
General Considerations: Check agency manual for specific instructions. Tell the patient that a sample (e.g., blood, urine) is needed and why. Determine whether the patient needs to fast before the sample is obtained. For blood studies, apply a small dressing to venipuncture site. Apply pressure if oozing persists or if the patient's blood does not clot normally. For urine samples, instruct the patient or assist in sample collection. Urine specimens should be sent to the laboratory promptly; refrigerate if a delay occurs.		
Urine culture and sensitivity: Culture identifies microorganisms in urine. Sensitivity determines which antibiotic will be effective. Normal: No growth occurs; results are obtained in 24–36 hours.	Collect a specimen of the first voided urine of the day. Instruct the patient in the midstream, clean-catch technique: cleanse the penis or vulva thoroughly, void a small amount, stop the urine stream, and then void into a sterile container. Collect the specimen before starting antibiotic therapy. If catheterization is necessary, collect the specimen after discarding a small amount of urine.	Unless the specimen container has a preservative, cap the specimen and refrigerate it or send it to the laboratory.
Blood urea nitrogen (BUN): Indicates the kidneys' ability to excrete urea, an end product of protein metabolism. Increases with renal failure, gastrointestinal (GI) bleeding, dehydration, and some drugs. Decreases with alcohol abuse, acromegaly, inadequate protein, hemodialysis, and some drugs.	No special preparation is required.	No special care needed. See General Considerations.
Urine creatinine clearance: Estimates glomerular filtration rate. Decreases with renal disease. Normal value: Varies with patient gender and age (usually lower in women).	Provide a specimen container. Document the first void and save all urine for the next 12 or 24 hours as ordered. Keep the specimen refrigerated. If the patient has a Foley catheter, place the drainage bag in a basin of ice and empty it into a refrigerated container hourly.	No special care needed. See General Considerations.
Serum creatinine: Measures the kidneys' ability to excrete waste based on the amount of creatinine in the blood. Normal values: Varies with the method used; should be small. Increased with impaired renal function, urinary obstruction, and muscle disease. Decreased with muscular dystrophy.	Usually no preparation is needed.	No special care needed. See General Considerations.
Serum electrolytes: Detects alterations reflecting the inability of kidneys to retain or excrete electrolytes. Sodium and potassium are elevated and calcium is decreased in renal failure. Normal values: See Chapter 14.	No special preparation is required.	Check laboratory reports and notify the physician of abnormalities. Electrolyte imbalances can be life threatening. See Chapter 14 for details on specific electrolytes.

Continued

Table 42-1 Diagnostic Tests and Procedures Urinary Disorders—cont'd

TEST AND PURPOSE	PATIENT PREPARATION	POSTPROCEDURE CARE
Ultrasound		
Abdominal and renal ultrasound: Uses sound waves to detect cysts, tumors, urinary calculi, and urinary tract malformations or obstructions. Can be used to guide needle insertion for closed biopsy.	Patient may have to drink a specified amount of water (typically three to four 8-oz glasses of water within 2 hours of the procedure) so that the bladder will be full during ultrasound. Tell the patient that the procedure is painless except for discomfort of full bladder; it takes about 15 minutes. An enema is usually given if the transrectal route is used. For the transabdominal route, gel is applied to the skin and an instrument is moved over the lubricated skin surface. Images are recorded for study. Patient instructions will vary if other routes are used.	Wash gel off the skin if the transabdominal route is used.
Radiographic Studies		
General Interventions: Explain the test to the patient. Radiation exposure is generally contraindicated during pregnancy. Patients should be questioned about allergies, especially any previous reactions to contrast dye. Special premedication may be ordered for those patients reporting an allergy to iodine. Itching, hives, wheezing, and respiratory distress are symptoms of an allergic reaction. Allergic reactions are treated by discontinuing the administration of the contrast, giving antihistamines, and administering cardiopulmonary resuscitation (CPR) if necessary. The patient can expect a flushed, warm feeling; a salty taste in the mouth; and maybe nausea when the contrast medium is injected. The procedure takes about 45 minutes.		
KUB provides radiographic view of the kidneys, ureters, and bladder	No special preparation is required. Schedule this test before studies that use contrast media.	No special care is required.
Intravenous pyelogram (IVP): Uses radiographs and a fluoroscope to outline the kidneys. Uses contrast medium to show urine flow and obstructions. Detects urinary abnormalities, calculi, ureters, and bladder. Laxatives can cause gas that obscures the visualization of stones.	Tell the patient that "dye" will be injected and radiographs taken to study the urinary tract. Give laxatives and enemas as ordered before the test. The patient should be placed on nothing-by-mouth (NPO) status 8–10 hours before the test.	Encourage fluids to flush contrast medium from the body. Monitor the patient for signs of iodine allergy: urticaria, rash, nausea, and swollen parotid glands. Check the injection site for inflammation.
Arteriogram: Uses radiographs and contrast medium to examine blood vessels of kidney.	Tell the patient that the physician will insert a catheter into the blood vessel (usually in the groin) and inject "dye." Radiographs are then taken as the dye circulates through the kidneys. Usual preparation: Patient is NPO for 8–12 hours and laxatives and enemas are given. Anticoagulant drugs are withheld before the test to reduce the risk of bleeding. Signed consent is required. Premedicate the patient if ordered to do so. Have the patient void before sedation.	Assess the patient for signs of bleeding: tachycardia, dyspnea, restlessness, and abdominal or flank pain. Check the injection site for bleeding. A pressure dressing should be in place. Monitor the patient's respiratory status if sedated. Electrocardiogram (ECG) monitoring may be ordered. Monitor the patient's pulse, color, warmth and sensation of the extremity in which the catheter was inserted. Maintain bed rest as ordered. Encourage fluids to eliminate the dye. Measure intake and output.

Table 42-1 Diagnostic Tests and Procedures Urinary Disorders—cont'd

TEST AND PURPOSE	PATIENT PREPARATION	POSTPROCEDURE CARE
Computed tomography (CT): Creates cross-sectional images of the kidneys and other organs to reveal abnormalities.	Inform the radiologist if the patient is allergic to contrast media, iodine, or shellfish. Inform the patient that the procedure is painless and noninvasive. NPO status may be ordered.	No special care is usually needed. Inform the physician of any signs of allergic response to the contrast dye. Give antihistamines as ordered for allergy (but routine drugs usually can be taken). The patient will lie still on a stretcher while a donut-shaped machine moves around him or her. Contrast dye is sometimes injected intravenously. It can create a feeling of warmth, a salty taste, and nausea. Sedation can be ordered if the patient has difficulty lying still.
Magnetic resonance imaging (MRI): Creates soft-tissue images using magnets and radio waves.	Tell the patient that the procedure is painless; he or she must lie still for 30 minutes or more. Some equipment has videos that the patient can view to reduce anxiety. Ask whether the patient is claustrophobic. Give sedation if ordered for agitated or anxious patients. Remove any metallic objects such as jewelry. Inquire whether the patient has any implanted devices such as cardiac pacemaker or intracranial aneurysm clips and notify the radiologist. Procedure is contraindicated with some implants. Metal may not be a problem with some newer equipment.	No special postprocedure care is required. Safety precautions should be taken if the patient is sedated.
Renal scan: Uses radioisotopes and radiographs to study renal blood flow. Detects infarctions, trauma, atherosclerosis, transplant rejection, and some renal diseases.	Tell the patient that an isotope will be injected and radiographs taken. Takes about 1 hour. Radiation dose is small and quickly eliminated.	No special care is required unless the patient is incontinent. If so, wear gloves to handle urine and change linens and discard per agency protocol. Continent patients can use a toilet. Pregnant caregivers should avoid these patients for 24 hours.
Invasive Procedures		
Renal biopsy: Excision of a small amount of kidney tissue is done for examination. May be obtained through an incision (open biopsy) or with a special needle (closed biopsy).	Physician explains the procedure selected. For closed biopsy, the patient is positioned prone with a rolled blanket under the abdomen for approximately 45 minutes. Ensure that reports of clotting studies (i.e., prothrombin time [PT], partial thromboplastin time [PTT], platelets) are on the chart. Report elevated blood pressure (BP), which increases the risk of bleeding. Patient should be NPO for 6 hours or as ordered. Signed consent is required.	Check the pressure dressing for bleeding. Monitor the patient's vital signs for hemorrhage: tachycardia, restlessness, and flank pain radiating to abdomen. Position the patient supine with a blanket roll or sandbag under the flank area. Patient should be on bed rest for 24 hours. Advise the patient to do no heavy lifting, exercise, or sports for 1–2 weeks. Hemoglobin (Hgb) and hematocrit (Hct) are checked at 6 and 24 hours after the biopsy.

Continued

Table 42-1 Diagnostic Tests and Procedures Urinary Disorders—cont'd

TEST AND PURPOSE	PATIENT PREPARATION	POSTPROCEDURE CARE
Cystoscopy: Uses lighted cystoscope inserted through the urethra to see urethra, bladder, and ureteral openings. Allows diagnosis of problems, removal of bladder calculi, biopsy, and some treatments. Local or general anesthesia may be used. Dye may be injected into the kidneys through ureters (retrograde pyelography).	Signed consent is required. Tell the patient that the procedure is done in the operating room or special room under sterile conditions. For local anesthesia, liquids may be allowed; patient should be NPO before general anesthesia. Give laxatives or enemas as ordered. Give medications as ordered to reduce anxiety and bladder spasms. Antibiotics may be ordered 2–3 days before procedure and continued several days afterward.	Safety precautions should be used the first time because orthostatic hypotension is common. Monitor the patient's intake and output, vital signs, and urine color; urine may be pink tinged to wine colored but lighten to its usual color in 24–48 hours. Report severe pain to the physician. Advise patient: (1) analgesics or antispasmodics may be prescribed for pain, (2) sitz baths help to relieve pain and urinary frequency, (3) drink 2–3 liters of fluids daily unless contraindicated, and (4) urine will be pink tinged for 1–2 days.
Urodynamic Studies		
Cystogram and cystourethrogram: Uses dye injected into the bladder through a catheter followed by radiographs to outline the bladder and demonstrate reflux of urine from bladder to ureters.	For a voiding cystourethrogram, the bladder and urethra are radiographed during urination. Rate of urine flow is measured. Tell the patient that a catheter will be inserted and dye instilled into the bladder.	Monitor urine output and vital signs. Encourage increased fluids unless contraindicated. Observe for allergic reaction to dye. Assess for urinary retention.
Cystometrogram: Evaluates bladder tone.	Tell the patient fluid will be instilled into the bladder through a urethral catheter. When the patient feels the urge to void, the catheter will be removed. After the patient voids, residual urine is measured. Drugs may be given to test bladder response.	Encourage increased fluids unless contraindicated. Monitor the patient's intake and output. Administer drugs as ordered for bladder spasms.

RADIOGRAPHIC TESTS AND PROCEDURES

Kidneys, Ureters, and Bladder

A KUB (for kidneys, ureters, and bladder) is a radiograph that provides a general outline of the kidneys, revealing their approximate size and contour. Tumors, malformations, and calculi may be found with this type of radiograph. This procedure requires no special preparation or aftercare. It is not done on pregnant patients and it should be done before any other studies that require contrast media.

Intravenous Pyelogram

An intravenous pyelogram (IVP) is a diagnostic procedure in which a radiographic contrast medium ("dye") is injected intravenously. Radiographs of the KUB are taken at 5- to 15-minute intervals. As the contrast is concentrated by the kidneys and excreted through the ureters into the bladder, kidney function and structures, ureter size and patency, bladder size and shape, and presence of calculi (stones) or other obstructions can be assessed. The procedure is contraindicated in older adult patients with known renal insufficiency and in patients with diabetes mellitus or multiple myeloma.

Renal Arteriogram

A renal arteriogram permits study of the renal blood vessels. It is used to diagnose renal artery stenosis, aneurysms, vascular tumors, renal cysts, and renal infarctions. A catheter is inserted through the femoral artery and threaded into the aorta. A contrast medium is injected into each renal artery and radiographs are taken as the contrast passes through the kidneys.

Cystogram

Contrast media can be instilled in the bladder using a catheter or a cystoscope. Films are then taken to visualize the bladder. This procedure is useful in detecting reflux of urine from the bladder into the ureters.

Renal Scan

A renal scan indicates the size, shape, and location of the kidneys; detects renal infarction, atherosclerosis, trauma, or rejection of a transplant; and identifies primary renal disease. An intravenous radioisotope is injected and radiographs are taken to demonstrate blood flow to each kidney. The test is not done on pregnant women but can be used for patients who are allergic to contrast that contains iodine.

Table 42-2 Urinalysis Data

COMPONENTS	NORMAL VALUES	IMPLICATIONS OF ABNORMAL VALUES
Color	Light yellow to amber	Dilute, colorless: overhydration, diabetes insipidus, diabetes mellitus, chronic renal failure Concentrated dark amber: dehydration, some medications or foods Bright red: gross hematuria in acid urine Tea colored: gross hematuria in alkaline urine
Appearance	Clear	Cloudy, hazy: bacteria, pus, small amount of blood
pH	4.0–8.0	<4.0: acidosis, starvation, diarrhea >7.0: alkalosis, bacteriuria, UTI
Specific gravity	1.003–1.030	<1.003: diabetes insipidus, overhydration, renal disease, severe hypokalemia >1.030: dehydration, diabetes mellitus
Protein	24-hour protein (quantitative): <150 mg/dL; reagent strip 0–trace	Persistent proteinuria: exercise, severe stress, fever, renal disease, malignancy
Glucose	Negative	Positive: diabetes mellitus, stroke, Cushing syndrome, anesthesia, severe stress
Ketones	Negative	Positive: diabetes mellitus, starvation, excessive protein ingestion
Bilirubin	Negative	Positive: liver disease (jaundice)
Microscopic Examination		
RBCs	0–4.0	>4.0 (hematuria): kidney trauma, renal disease, anticoagulants
WBCs	0–5.0	>5.0: UTI, strenuous exercise
Casts	Negative to occasional hyaline casts	Positive: fever, renal disease, heart failure
Crystals	Negative	Positive: renal stone formation
Bacteria	Negative	Positive: UTI

RBCs, Red blood cells; *UTI*, urinary tract infection; *WBCs*, white blood cells.

Computed Tomography and Magnetic Resonance Imaging

A computed tomography (CT) scan is useful in detecting kidney size, tumors, abscesses, obstruction, and adrenal masses and tumors. Contrast media may be used to clarify details; assess the patient for iodine sensitivity. Magnetic resonance imaging (MRI) also may be used to visualize the kidneys.

RENAL ULTRASOUND

Ultrasonography (ultrasound) uses high-frequency sound waves to create images of the bladder. It is used to detect urinary tract malformations and obstructions, tumors, renal calculi, perineal fluid accumulation, and cysts. Ultrasound also may be used to guide a needle inserted to aspirate specimens from cysts or tumors. The bladder should be full for visualization of organs and tissues. The procedure may be done through the abdominal wall (transabdominal), the rectum (transrectal), the urethra (transurethral), or the vagina (transvaginal). Preparation and patient instructions are specific for each approach.

INVASIVE PROCEDURES

Renal Biopsy

A renal biopsy is performed to obtain a specimen of renal tissue for direct microscopic examination. It is usually done to evaluate conditions leading to renal failure. The procedure may be done through open or closed methods. The open method is a surgical procedure in which an incision is made in the flank and a specimen of kidney tissue is removed. The closed procedure involves insertion of a needle under fluoroscopy or ultrasonography to aspirate the tissue specimen. For the closed procedure, the patient must be able to lie in the prone position with a blanket roll under the lower abdomen for up to 45 minutes. Patients with breathing problems may not be able to tolerate this position or alter their breathing patterns as needed during the procedure.

The most serious complication of a renal biopsy is hemorrhage. If bleeding is suspected, the patient is given intravenous fluids to restore fluid volume. Persistent bleeding may require surgery.

Cystoscopy

Cystoscopy is the direct visualization of the interior of the urethra, bladder, and ureteral orifices. The procedure may be done in the physician's office for diagnostic reasons or in an outpatient facility for diagnostic or treatment purposes under local or general anesthesia. As a diagnostic procedure, the cystoscopy allows the physician to observe lesions, locate sources of bleeding, and take biopsy samples. Treatments that can be performed with this procedure include cauterization of lesions; removal of calculi, tumors, or foreign materials; implantation of radium seeds; insertion of ureteral catheters; and control of bleeding. A lighted tube called a *cystoscope* is inserted through the urethra into the bladder under sterile conditions. Retrograde pyelography, which involves injecting contrast into the ureters, also can be done during cystoscopy.

Back pain, bladder spasms, urinary frequency, and burning on urination are common after cystoscopy. Mild analgesics may bring relief. Belladonna and opium suppositories may be ordered to reduce bladder spasms. Bladder perforation is rare but should be suspected if the patient has severe abdominal pain.

URODYNAMIC STUDIES

Urodynamic studies are performed to determine the physiology of urination. The studies assess innervation of the bladder, incontinence, and other variations in urinary patterns. Urodynamic studies measure the rate and volume of urine flow during voiding. The rate of flow is decreased with obstruction or decreased innervation.

Cystogram and Voiding Cystourethrogram

The cystogram outlines the contour of the bladder and shows reflux or backflow of urine from the bladder into the ureters. Cystograms are useful in diagnosing neurogenic bladders, fistulas, tumors, and ruptured bladders. For a cystogram, a catheter is inserted into the bladder, contrast is injected, and then radiographs are taken.

A voiding cystourethrogram gives the physician additional information on urethral disorders during voiding. The bladder is filled with contrast and radiographs are taken during and after urination. This procedure may be embarrassing for the patient. Explain the need for the test and provide as much privacy as possible during the procedure.

Cystometrogram

The cystometrogram is used to evaluate bladder tone in the patient with incontinence or with a neurogenic bladder. A catheter is inserted in the bladder and fluid is instilled until the patient reports the urge to void. When the patient feels urgency, the catheter is removed, the patient voids, and residual urine is measured. Drugs may be given to see if they effectively enhance or relax bladder tone in the individual patient.

COMMON THERAPEUTIC MEASURES

CATHETERIZATION

Catheterization is the introduction of a catheter through the urethra into the bladder for the purpose of draining urine. Catheters are inserted when patients are unable to void as a result of the effects of anesthesia, paralysis, trauma, unconsciousness, certain surgical procedures, and other factors that inhibit voiding. The major concern with catheterization is the potential for introduction of bacteria in the normally sterile bladder. Catheterization is the primary cause of health care–associated infections (HAIs). Therefore it is essential that strict aseptic techniques be followed when catheterization is necessary.

Urinary catheters are available in a variety of sizes for adults. The most commonly used sizes for adult urethral catheterization range from the small 12 French to the larger 18 French. Catheters may be of a retaining or nonretaining design. Examples of retaining catheters are the coudé, Foley, Malecot, and Pezzer. A retaining catheter is one that has a device, such as an inflatable balloon, that anchors the catheter in the bladder. Robinson and whistle-tip catheters are nonretaining or straight catheters. Nurses are most familiar with Foley catheters that have either double or triple lumina. Malecot and Pezzer catheters are used most often as suprapubic catheters.

To determine whether a patient is emptying his or her bladder, the amount of urine remaining in the bladder after voiding (residual urine) must be measured. A bladder scanner can be used to measure postvoid residual (PVR). This procedure may be diagnostic but it is often part of a bladder training program for patients who have lost control over bladder function. Residual volume should be measured immediately after voiding. Occasionally, patients are catheterized to measure residual urine. Less than 50 mL of residual urine is considered normal.

The reader should refer to a fundamentals textbook for detailed information on the insertion and care of urethral catheters. Key points to remember when catheterization is necessary are the following:

1. Catheterize only after other noninvasive measures have failed or when absolutely necessary for diagnostic purposes. If possible, have the patient shower or bathe before catheterization.
2. Wash hands thoroughly and use sterile technique and equipment to insert the catheter.
3. With an indwelling catheter, do the following:
   a. Secure the tubing to the female patient's inner thigh or the male patient's upper thigh or lower abdomen.
   b. Handle the catheter gently to avoid trauma to the urethra.
   c. Keep the urine collection bag below the level of the patient's bladder and the tubing in a circular fashion *on* the bed.
   d. Keep the drainage system closed as much as possible.
   e. Empty the bag *before* it is full. A full bag inhibits urine drainage, which could cause bladder spasms.
   f. Provide perineal care twice daily. (Note: Antibiotic ointments are not recommended.)

g. Use Standard Precautions before and after handling the catheter.

URETERAL CATHETER

A ureteral catheter is threaded through a ureter into the renal pelvis. It can be inserted through the bladder during cystoscopy or through an abdominal incision. A ureteral catheter permits urine to flow through the swollen ureter after traumatic surgery. The catheter is connected to a drainage system and output is measured every 1 to 2 hours. Record output from this catheter separately from other urine output. Make certain that the catheter is not kinked or clamped because pressure would build up in the kidney, causing tissue damage. The capacity of the renal pelvis is only 3 to 5 mL. If irrigation is ordered, slowly instill no more than 5 mL (or less, as ordered) of lukewarm, sterile normal saline. Use strict aseptic technique for the irrigation. Unless both ureters are completely obstructed, urine continues to drain into the bladder. Remember to record urine from each source on the output record.

The patient with a ureterostomy tube is usually kept on bed rest unless a double-J catheter is used. The double-J catheter has one coiled end in the renal pelvis and the other coiled end in the bladder.

NEPHROSTOMY TUBE

When a ureter is completely obstructed, the physician may insert a nephrostomy tube through a flank incision directly into the kidney pelvis. The tube is connected to a drainage system and assessed frequently. You must ensure that the tube is not kinked or clamped at any time because drainage must be continuous. Some urine usually leaks around the tube and flows through the flank incision. Perform sterile dressing changes and skin care as needed. Irrigation with a small amount of sterile normal saline may be ordered. Because of the small capacity of the renal pelvis, no more than 5 mL of irrigating fluid is used. You must use strict aseptic technique.

URINARY STENT

A stent is a hollow tube that is placed in a structure to give it support and allow fluid to flow through. A urinary stent may be placed in the ureter to maintain alignment or to provide a route for urine drainage. The physician inserts the stent; it may be completely internal or it may extend through the urethra or skin. Several types of stents are available.

UROLOGIC SURGERY

Urologic surgery may be done on any part of the urinary tract. *Nephrectomy* is removal of the kidney because of cancer, massive trauma or bleeding, severe chronic failure with infection, or polycystic kidney disease, or for donation. Many types of surgery are used to remove calculi, depending on their location. A surgical opening may be made in the renal tissue, renal pelvis, ureter, or bladder. *Lithotripsy* is a noninvasive procedure used to break up calculi but patient care is similar to that of the surgical patient. Bladder surgery may be necessitated by bleeding, functional problems, or cancer. Removal of the bladder is a **cystectomy**; an incision in the bladder is a *cystotomy*. Some surgical procedures can be done through a cystoscope, so no external incision exists. Surgical procedures that reroute the flow of urine are called *urinary diversions*. A *cystostomy* is the formation of an opening or stoma on the abdomen for catheterization or to enable the collection of urine in an external reservoir. Prostate surgery is discussed in Chapter 50.

Preoperative Care

Preparation for urologic surgery includes a complete diagnostic workup to rule out other medical problems. Fluid status is evaluated and any imbalances are corrected. Usual preoperative care measures are taken as described in Chapter 17. Bowel cleansing may be ordered before some procedures. If the patient will have a stoma for urine drainage, an enterostomal therapist is usually consulted to identify the optimal stoma site as well as for patient counseling and teaching.

Postoperative Care

After surgery, particular attention is given to urine output, respirations, and bowel function. Output is closely monitored, with drainage from various tubes recorded separately. Urine output of less than 30 mL/h should be reported to the physician. Flank or abdominal incisions cause pain on deep breathing. Adequate pain management and support of the patient for coughing and deep breathing decrease the risk of atelectasis and pneumonia. Auscultate lungs frequently to assess breath sounds. Urologic surgery often involves manipulation of the bowel, which can lead to paralytic ileus. Therefore food and fluids are usually withheld until bowel sounds are present.

DRUG THERAPY

A number of drugs are available to treat urinary tract disorders. Major classifications of commonly used drugs are diuretics, antihypertensives, phosphate binders, hormones, vitamin and mineral supplements, and immunosuppressants (see *Complementary and Alternative Therapies* box). These classifications, specific drugs, their actions and adverse effects, and nursing interventions are summarized in Table 42-3. Immunosuppressant drugs are addressed separately in Table 42-4.

Complementary and Alternative Therapies

Herbal remedies, like medications, can be harmful to the kidney. For example, aloe can cause nephritis and ephedra (*má huáng*) can cause kidney stones. Teach patients to always include alternative remedies in their medication histories.

Table 42-3 Medications for Urinary Disorders

General Considerations

1. Drugs are selected carefully because many drugs are nephrotoxic.
2. Drug dosages need to be reduced if renal function is impaired and the drug is excreted in the urine.

DRUG	USE AND ACTION	SIDE EFFECTS	NURSING INTERVENTIONS
Diuretics and Antihypertensive Agents			
Diuretics: General Information. Specific classes follow.	Cause kidneys to excrete water and sodium and lower blood pressure (BP).	Dehydration, electrolyte imbalances	Monitor the patient's intake and output, BP, and weight. Administer the drug in the morning to avoid nocturia. Assess for electrolyte imbalances. Monitor serum potassium level. Potassium supplements may be ordered except with potassium-sparing drugs.
Osmotic diuretics: mannitol (Osmitrol)		Edema, dehydration, electrolyte imbalances	Monitor for circulatory overload and extravasation during infusion. Administer only freshly prepared solutions.
Thiazide diuretics: hydrochlorothiazide (HydroDIURIL), metolazone (Zaroxolyn)		Hypokalemia, hypercalcemia, hypotension, hyponatremia	Monitor patients with diabetes for hyperglycemia. Monitor patients taking digoxin for low potassium levels. Encourage potassium-rich foods.
High ceiling (loop) diuretics: furosemide (Lasix)		Orthostatic hypotension, hypokalemia, hyponatremia, hearing loss	Monitor patients with diabetes for hyperglycemia. Encourage potassium-rich foods. Teach patients to cope with orthostatic hypotension.
Potassium-sparing diuretics: spironolactone (Aldactone), triamterene (Dyrenium), amiloride (Midamor)		Hyperkalemia, drowsiness, gynecomastia in men on long-term therapy, menstrual irregularities, impotence	Safety measures. Assess for hyperkalemia: diarrhea, muscle twitching, and dysrhythmias. Caution with angiotensin-converting enzyme inhibitors (ACEIs), angiotensin receptor blockers, and direct renin inhibitors.
Antihypertensive Agents: General Information. See specific classes below.	Lower BP.	Orthostatic hypotension. Reflex tachycardia and fluid retention with some types. Rebound hypertension if stopped suddenly.	Monitor the patient's BP. Do not discontinue the drug suddenly. For orthostatic hypotension, teach patients to change position slowly and avoid prolonged standing.
Centrally acting alpha$_2$ agonists: methyldopa (Aldomet), clonidine (Catapres)	Reduce sympathetic stimulation	Drowsiness, hemolytic anemia, liver damage	Sedation—administer the drug at bedtime. Dry mouth. Take safety precautions. Advise the patient to discontinue the drug only under medical direction.
Alpha$_1$ adrenergic antagonists: prazosin (Minipress)	Increase kidney perfusion; block sympathetic stimulation of blood vessels, permitting vasodilation	Orthostatic hypotension (especially with initial dose)	Give the first dose or increased dose at bedtime. Teach the patient to manage orthostatic hypertension.
Beta-adrenergic blockers/antagonists: propranolol (Inderal)	Inhibit the renin-angiotensin-aldosterone system.	Bronchoconstriction, bradycardia, hypoglycemia, heart failure. Masks symptoms of low blood glucose.	Monitor respirations in asthmatics and patients with chronic obstructive pulmonary disease. Assess for edema. Monitor glucose levels.

Table 42-3 **Medications for Urinary Disorders—cont'd**

DRUG	USE AND ACTION	SIDE EFFECTS	NURSING INTERVENTIONS
Direct-acting vasodilators: hydralazine (Apresoline)	Relaxation of blood vessels lowers peripheral resistance	Tachycardia, palpitations, headache, lupuslike syndrome	Report lupuslike signs: fever, sore throat, skin rash.
Phosphate Binder			
aluminum hydroxide gel (Amphojel)	Binds with phosphate in the intestines to prevent absorption. Given to prevent renal osteodystrophy. Raises serum calcium.	Hypophosphatemia: muscle weakness, anorexia, bone pain, constipation	Monitor the patient for hypophosphatemia. Record bowel movements. Give laxatives and stool softeners as ordered.
Vitamin and Mineral Supplements			
ferrous sulfate	Treats iron deficiency anemia.	Constipation or diarrhea, dark stools	Administer the drug on an empty stomach with water. Can give the liquid with water or fruit juice to disguise taste.
folic acid, calcium gluconate	Supplements dietary intake. Treats hypocalcemia.	Although few adverse effects are produced by these medications, occasional side effects include hypercalcemia and constipation.	Monitor the patient for occasional hypersensitivity. Monitor blood studies. Administer the drug in divided doses with or after meals. Do not give the medication with other drugs.
Erythropoietic growth factors: erythropoietin	Improve red blood cell (RBC) formation. Reverse anemia. Require adequate serum iron and ferritin to be effective.	Headache, tachycardia, hypertension, dyspnea, diarrhea, hyperkalemia, nausea, vomiting, clotted vascular assess, seizures	Monitor the patient's BP. Contraindicated in uncontrolled hypertension. Dosage is adjusted to maintain hemoglobin between 10 and 11 gm/dL.
Antibiotics			
Sulfonamides			
sulfisoxazole (Gantrisin)	In combination with trimethoprim. Treats urinary tract infections (UTIs).	Drowsiness, dizziness, agranulocytosis, anemia, thrombocytopenia. Nausea, vomiting, diarrhea. Liver dysfunction. Crystalluria leading to renal tubular damage. Photosensitivity. Allergy. Infertility.	Tell the patient that his or her urine will be orange. Monitor blood cell counts. Give the drug with a full glass of water. Maintain urine output of 1500 mL/day to prevent crystalluria. Have the patient avoid excessive sun exposure. Do not give the drug if the patient has history of sulfonamide allergy.
trimethoprim* (Trimpex)	In combination with sulfamethoxazole. Used to treat acute or chronic UTIs. Especially effective against recurrent UTIs in men.	Nausea, vomiting, glossitis. Skin rash.	Tell the patient to report any skin rash (which may be an allergic response).
Aminoglycosides: gentamicin (Garamycin)	Effective against gram-negative bacilli.	Ototoxicity, hepatotoxicity, nephrotoxicity, neurotoxicity	Assess the patient's hearing. Drug should be stopped if patient has tinnitus or subjective hearing loss. Monitor intake and output. Check blood urea nitrogen (BUN) and creatinine.

Continued

Table 42-3 Medications for Urinary Disorders—cont'd

DRUG	USE AND ACTION	SIDE EFFECTS	NURSING INTERVENTIONS
Penicillins: ampicillin	Effective against most gram-positive and some gram-negative pathogens.	Anaphylaxis, gastrointestinal (GI) distress, rash, blood dyscrasias	Monitor the patient for allergic reaction: rash, itching, wheezing. Report any evidence of an allergic reaction to the physician immediately.
Fluoroquinolones: ciprofloxacin	A broad-spectrum antibiotic that is effective against many gram-positive and gram-negative pathogens.	Drowsiness, headache, agitation, seizures, cardiac dysrhythmias, hepatotoxicity, pseudomembranous colitis. Anaphylaxis, severe skin reactions, crystalluria.	Observe the patient closely for an allergic reaction: rash, pruritus, urticaria, wheezing. Notify the physician immediately if one occurs. Monitor the patient's liver function tests. Advise the patient to drink 1500–2000 mL of fluid each day to prevent crystal formation. Do not give the drug within 2 hours of antacids, iron, or zinc. Check for many other drug-drug interactions. Use safety measures for drowsiness.
Urinary Antiseptics			
methenamine (Mandelamine)	An antibacterial agent that is effective only in chronic lower urinary tract infections.	Nausea, vomiting, diarrhea	Give the drug with meals to reduce GI effects. Encourage adequate fluids. Discourage large intake of milk products. Do not use in combination with sulfonamides.
nitrofurantoin (Furadantin, Macrodantin)	Treat acute and chronic UTIs.	Dyspnea. Nausea and vomiting. Numbness and tingling of legs. Hematologic reactions. Headache, vertigo, drowsiness.	Administer with food or milk to reduce gastric distress.
fosfomycin (Monurol)	Treats uncomplicated UTI.	Diarrhea, headache, vaginitis, nausea	Single dose regimen: 3-g water-soluble packet.

*Trimethoprim/sulfamethoxazole is a combination drug. Trade names include Bactrim and Septra.

URINARY TRACT INFLAMMATION AND INFECTIONS

UTIs are common, especially among women. They can involve any part of the urinary tract (upper or lower) and can be acquired through the blood or lymph or may enter through the urethra. UTIs are the most common HAIs (i.e., infections associated with health care). Most UTIs are bacterial but they can be caused by viruses, yeasts, and fungi. It is important to treat UTIs to prevent renal scarring that can lead to failure. Risk factors for UTI are listed in Box 42-2.

URETHRITIS

Urethritis is inflammation of the urethra. Inflammation may be caused by microorganisms, trauma, or hypersensitivity to chemicals in products such as vaginal deodorants, spermicidal jellies, or bubble bath detergents. The most frequently identified causative microorganisms are *Escherichia coli, Chlamydia, Trichomonas, Neisseria gonorrhoeae*, and herpes simplex virus type 2.

Signs and Symptoms

Signs and symptoms of urethritis include dysuria, frequency, urgency, and bladder spasms. A urethral discharge may be noted.

Medical Diagnosis

Urethritis is diagnosed based on patient signs and symptoms, urinalysis, and urethral smear. Cystitis may be present at the same time.

Table 42-4 Drugs for Suppressing Immunity

General Considerations

1. Patients on immunosuppressant drugs have reduced resistance to infection, so they must be monitored for subtle signs of infection.
2. Protect patients from infections.
3. Teach patients the importance of taking drugs as prescribed and keeping follow-up appointments.
4. Immunosuppressants increase the risk of malignancies.

DRUG	USE AND ACTION	SIDE EFFECTS	NURSING INTERVENTIONS
Corticosteroids			
prednisone (Deltasone), methylprednisolone (Medrol), methylprednisolone sodium succinate (Solu-Medrol)	Antiinflammatory agents that prevent movement of leukocytes into transplanted tissue	Retention of water and sodium; loss of potassium, elevated blood glucose, hypertension, GI bleeding, mood swings, psychosis, infections, and impaired healing	Monitor intake and output. Assess for fluid and electrolyte imbalances: edema, increased BP, cardiac dysrhythmias, muscle weakness, confusion. Antacids are often ordered to protect the stomach.
Cytotoxic Agents			
cyclophosphamide (Cytoxan)	Alkylating neoplastic agent	Diarrhea, bone marrow suppression, vomiting, sepsis, sterility, hemorrhagic cystitis	Ensure negative pregnancy test before starting therapy. Assess patient for thrombocytopenia (i.e., bruising, bleeding) and leukopenia (i.e., frequent infections).
Monoclonal Antibodies			
muromonab-CD3 (Orthoclone OKT3), basiliximab (Simulect), daclizumab (Zenapax)	Reacts with T cell antigens and destroys them. Used to treat acute rejection in renal transplant recipients.	Fever, chills, headache, tremor, dyspnea, flushing, anaphylaxis, nausea, vomiting, diarrhea, chest pain. Potentially fatal anaphylaxis.	Monitor closely for anaphylaxis, especially with the first dose. Monitor for fluid overload. Check the infusion site. Have the site changed if evidence of extravasation exists.
T Cell Suppressors			
cyclosporine (Sandimmune and Neoral are *not* interchangeable!), tacrolimus (Prograf)	Interferes with T-lymphocyte activity. Enhances transplant survival with less risk of infection.	Nephrotoxicity (elevated serum creatinine), fluid retention, hypertension, hyperkalemia, hirsutism, venous thrombosis, gingival hyperplasia, tremors, infections, anemia, leukopenia, thrombocytopenia, anaphylaxis with intravenous administration, hepatotoxicity	Monitor serum creatinine and electrolytes. Check for edema. Monitor BP. Have epinephrine available during intravenous administration. Monitor liver function studies. Mix the oral form with food or chocolate to disguise unpleasant oiliness.
azathioprine (Imuran), mycophenolate (CellCept)	Inhibits B and T lymphocytes.	Teratogenic. Neutropenia, thrombocytopenia, diarrhea, sepsis.	Assess CBC results, bleeding. Ensure pregnancy is ruled out before starting therapy.

BP, Blood pressure; *CBC,* complete blood count; *GI,* gastrointestinal.

Box 42-2 Risk Factors for Urinary Tract Infections

- Foreign bodies (urinary stone, catheters)
- Compromised immunity
- Female gender
- Vaginal infections
- Bubble baths and vaginal deodorant sprays
- Dehydration
- Tight-fitting, synthetic undergarments
- Infrequent voiding
- First trimester of pregnancy
- Trauma during delivery

Medical Treatment

Antimicrobials are used to treat the condition when it is caused by microorganisms. If the patient is sexually active, the patient and the sexual partner may be treated with antimicrobials to prevent reinfection.

NURSING CARE of the Patient with Urethritis

Assessment

Assessment of the patient with a urologic disorder is outlined in Box 42-1. Important aspects of assessment when a patient has urethritis are comfort, possible causative factors, and understanding of treatment and prevention.

Nursing Diagnoses, Goals, and Outcome Criteria: Urethritis

Nursing Diagnoses	Goals and Outcome Criteria
Acute Pain related to tissue inflammation	Pain relief: patient states pain is relieved, relaxed manner
Ineffective Self-Health Management related to lack of knowledge of cause, treatment, and prevention of urethritis	Patient manages treatment plan effectively: patient accurately describes treatment and preventive measures, has no recurrence

Interventions

Sitz baths are soothing and may reduce the pain of urethritis. Instruct female patients to wipe from front to back after toileting and to void before and after sexual intercourse as a means of preventing urethritis. Discourage bubble baths and vaginal deodorant sprays. Instruct uncircumcised male patients to clean the penis under the foreskin regularly. Advise patients to void after swimming.

CYSTITIS

Cystitis is inflammation of the urinary bladder. The most common cause is bacterial contamination. Other risk factors for cystitis are prolonged immobility, renal calculi, urinary diversion, indwelling catheters, radiation therapy, and some chemotherapy. Women are more susceptible than men to cystitis because the female urethra is shorter and closer to the vagina and rectum. The longer urethra and antibacterial substances in prostatic fluid are thought to decrease the incidence of UTIs in men. Cystitis in the absence of other pathology of the urinary tract is said to be *uncomplicated. Recurring* UTIs are more likely to be associated with urinary tract pathology.

Signs and Symptoms

Symptoms of cystitis include urgency, frequency, dysuria, hematuria, nocturia, bladder spasms, incontinence, and low-grade fever. Urine may be dark, tea colored, or cloudy. Fever, fatigue, and pelvic or abdominal discomfort are common. Bladder spasms may be manifested by pain behind the symphysis pubis. Spasms may occur during or after urination. Some patients have bacteria in the urine but no symptoms at all, a situation that does not warrant the use of antibiotics.

Medical Diagnosis

A urine specimen is obtained for urinalysis, culture, and sensitivity. The presence of bacteria does not mean that the patient has an infection unless the patient also has white blood cells (WBCs) in the urine. The presence of WBCs reflects bacterial tissue invasion—an indicator of infection. Other diagnostic procedures may be indicated to rule out pathology that might be responsible for the infection.

Medical Treatment

Cystitis is treated with antibiotics that concentrate in the urine. The physician may order an antibiotic while awaiting the results of the culture and sensitivity. The order is changed if the results show that another antibiotic would be more effective. For uncomplicated cystitis, treatment may be given in a single dose or in a 1- to 3-day regimen. Patients with recurrent cystitis may be placed on continuous prophylactic antibiotics. A mild analgesic such as acetaminophen is useful for relieving discomfort. Phenazopyridine (Pyridium) may be ordered for 2 to 3 days to decrease discomfort and bladder spasms. Hyoscyamine (Cystospaz) and flavoxate (Urispas) also may be ordered to decrease bladder spasms.

NURSING CARE of the Patient with Cystitis

Assessment

General assessment of the patient with a urinary tract disorder is outlined in Box 42-1. The nursing assessment of the patient with cystitis focuses on patient symptoms, possible causative factors, and understanding of treatment and prevention.

Nursing Diagnoses, Goals, and Outcome Criteria: Cystitis

Nursing Diagnoses	Goals and Outcome Criteria
Acute Pain related to tissue inflammation	Pain relief: patient states pain is relieved, relaxed manner
Ineffective Self-Health Management related to lack of knowledge of cause, treatment, and prevention of cystitis	Patient effectively manages treatment plan: patient accurately describes treatment and preventive measures, has no recurrence

Interventions

Cystitis usually is treated on an outpatient basis. Therefore patient teaching is essential. Advise the patient to take analgesics as ordered for pain. Warm sitz baths also are comforting. Patient teaching emphasizes the need for a high fluid intake, instructions about prescribed drugs, and measures to avoid future infections (see *Patient Teaching* box). The patient needs to consume at least 30 mL/kg of fluid per day and void frequently. Fluids should be consumed during the day and at night so that the urinary tract is continually flushed. Instruct the patient to complete the entire course of prescribed antibiotics. Also advise the patient taking phenazopyridine, a drug that relieves burning on urination, that the drug causes an orange-red urine color that may stain clothing.

Put on Your Thinking Cap!

Using the recommended fluid intake for a person with cystitis, calculate how much fluid you would need to take in 24 hours based on your body weight.

Patient Teaching

Cystitis

To reduce the risk of future infections, patients should be told the following:

- Wear cotton undergarments because they keep the perineum drier than synthetic materials. Moisture encourages bacterial growth.
- Avoid tight-fitting clothing in the perineal area.
- Take showers instead of tub baths.
- Avoid coffee, tea, carbonated beverages with caffeine, and apple, grapefruit, orange, and tomato juices, because these irritate the bladder.
- Maintain a high fluid intake and empty the bladder often.
- Cranberry juice is sometimes recommended to make the urine more acidic and discourage bacterial growth. Although some disagreement exists regarding the value of this juice and the amount needed to be effective, it is a safe, simple measure to try.
- Women should wipe from front to back after bowel movements or voiding.
- Drink a glass of water after swimming and before and after intercourse to "flush" the urethra.
- It is important to keep appointments for follow-up urinalyses to ensure that the infection has been eliminated.

Pharmacology Capsule

Instruct patients to complete the entire course of antimicrobial therapy to ensure that the infection is eradicated.

INTERSTITIAL CYSTITIS

Pathophysiology and Diagnosis

Interstitial cystitis is an inflammatory disease of the bladder that usually is chronic. The cause of the disease, which usually affects female subjects, is unknown. The patient typically reports moderate to severe bladder and pelvic pain and urinary frequency and urgency. Chronic inflammation can cause the bladder to become scarred and stiff, which reduces its capacity. Ulcers may form in the bladder lining and bleeding may occur. The condition is diagnosed by cystoscopy. Other diagnostic measures may be performed to rule out other pathologic conditions such as cancer.

Medical Treatment

Treatment is directed toward symptom management and attempts to treat possible causes. Among the drugs that sometimes are helpful are tricyclic antidepressants, antispasmodics, bladder anesthetics, calcium channel blockers, urine alkalinizers, and nonsteroidal antiinflammatory drugs (NSAIDs). A drug that brings symptomatic relief to many is pentosan polysulfate (Elmiron). Other treatments include stretching the bladder under anesthesia; instillation of various medications, including dimethyl sulfoxide, into the bladder; and electrostimulation. Some sources advise dietary and activity changes and heat application. Cystectomy (surgical removal of the bladder) is an extreme measure that is necessary in some cases (see *Complementary and Alternative Therapies* box).

Complementary and Alternative Therapies

Biofeedback may help some patients to deal with the symptoms of interstitial cystitis.

NURSING CARE of the Patient with Interstitial Cystitis

Patients are usually treated as outpatients, so you are more likely to encounter them in clinic or home settings than in hospitals. It is important to show acceptance of the patient and empathy for the disruption of lives caused by this disease. It is a physiologic illness, not a psychologic one. Your primary role is teaching and support. The Interstitial Cystitis Association (www.ichelp.com) is a source of general information as well as dietary advice to avoid bladder irritation (see *Patient Teaching* box).

PYELONEPHRITIS

Pyelonephritis is inflammation of the renal pelvis. It may affect one or both kidneys. Acute pyelonephritis most often is caused by an ascending bacterial infection but it may be bloodborne. Chronic pyelonephritis may be persistent or recurrent and results in damage

Patient Teaching

Interstitial Cystitis

- Avoid acidic foods, coffee, tea, citrus products, aged cheeses, nuts, vinegar, curry, hot peppers, alcohol, and carbonated drinks.
- Calcium glycerophosphate (Prelief) is an over-the-counter (OTC) urinary alkalinizer that your physician may suggest.
- Wear clothing that fits loosely around the waist and lower abdomen.
- A local support group may be available for education and encouragement.

to the renal parenchyma (functional tissue). It most often is the result of reflux of urine from inadequate closure of the ureterovesical junction during voiding. Progressive scarring results in atrophy of the affected kidneys and hypertension and renal ischemia develop.

Chronic pyelonephritis, usually caused by long-standing UTIs with relapses and reinfections, may lead to chronic renal failure. If the patient progresses to renal atrophy and end-stage renal disease, dialysis or transplantation is the only means of keeping the patient alive.

Signs and Symptoms

Signs and symptoms of acute pyelonephritis include high fever, chills, nausea, vomiting, and dysuria. Severe pain or a constant dull ache occurs in the flank area. The patient with chronic pyelonephritis often complains of bladder irritation, chronic fatigue, and a slight aching over one or both kidneys.

Medical Treatment

The goal of treatment for pyelonephritis is to prevent further damage. Mild symptoms usually can be managed on an outpatient basis. Severe symptoms commonly are treated in the hospital. Antibiotics, urinary tract antiseptics, analgesics, and antispasmodics may be ordered. Long-term antibiotic therapy may be prescribed for patients who have repeated acute infections or chronic infection. Additional medications may be needed to treat hypertension. Adults are advised to drink at least eight 8-oz glasses of fluids daily. Intravenous fluids may be ordered if the patient has nausea and vomiting. Dietary salt and protein restriction may be imposed on the patient with chronic disease. If an obstruction or congenital anomaly is present, it should be treated. Urine samples must be obtained for follow-up cultures to determine whether the infection has been resolved.

NURSING CARE of the Patient with Pyelonephritis

Assessment

General assessment of the patient with a urinary tract disorder is outlined in Box 42-1. When caring for the patient with pyelonephritis, record the presence of related signs and symptoms, a history of previous urinary tract disorders, any predisposing factors, and the effects of the infection on activities of daily living (ADL).

Nursing Diagnoses, Goals, and Outcome Criteria: Pyelonephritis

Nursing Diagnoses	Goals and Outcome Criteria
Acute Pain related to inflammation	Pain relief: patient states pain relieved, relaxed manner
Activity Intolerance related to fatigue	Improved activity tolerance: completes activities of daily living (ADL) without excessive fatigue
Deficient Fluid Volume related to vomiting, anorexia	Adequate hydration: fluid intake and output equal, pulse and blood pressure (BP) consistent with patient norms
Imbalanced Nutrition: Less Than Body Requirements related to anorexia, nausea, vomiting	Adequate nutrition: stable body weight
Ineffective Self-Health Management related to lack of knowledge of treatment and future prevention of pyelonephritis	Patient effectively manages treatment plan: patient accurately describes prescribed treatment and preventive measures, has no recurrence

Interventions

Acute Pain

Administer analgesics as ordered when the patient reports pain. Antibiotics and antiseptics do not provide direct pain relief but eventually help by eliminating the cause of the inflammation.

Activity Intolerance

The pain and systemic symptoms of infection contribute to fatigue and activity intolerance. Assist with ADL and schedule activities to allow for periods of uninterrupted rest. If the patient is being treated at home, advise family members of the patient's need for additional rest. Encourage the family to relieve the patient of some responsibilities until recovered.

Deficient Fluid Volume and Imbalanced Nutrition: Less Than Body Requirements

Adequate food and fluids are very important for the patient with pyelonephritis. If nausea and vomiting occur, inform the physician and administer antiemetics as ordered. Record food and fluid intake and fluid output. If the patient is unable to take the recommended 2 to 3 L of fluid daily, intravenous fluids may be prescribed. Be careful when forcing fluids to avoid circulatory overload. In the older patient, a sudden increase in fluid volume may result in heart failure (HF). Possible signs of this complication are bounding pulse, rising blood pressure, dyspnea, and edema

Ineffective Self-Health Management

If the patient will be taking medications at home, review the drugs and stress the importance of taking them as prescribed. Explain the importance of follow-up evaluation to assess effects of treatment and the need to report suspected recurrence to the physician immediately (see *Patient Teaching* box). Patients with chronic pyelonephritis must be adequately prepared for self-care.

Patient Teaching

Pyelonephritis

- Take your medications exactly as prescribed. Report adverse effects (for specific drugs) to your physician. Be sure to complete the course of therapy.
- Limit your physical activity and exercise as advised by your physician.
- Even after this infection has been treated, drink at least eight 8-oz glasses of fluids each day to dilute urine and to reduce the risk of recurrence.
- If advised, follow dietary protein and sodium restrictions.

HEREDITARY RENAL DISEASE

POLYCYSTIC KIDNEY DISEASE

Polycystic kidney disease is a hereditary disorder. Two types exist: (1) childhood and (2) adult. In adults, it usually is manifested by age 40. It is characterized by grapelike cysts in place of normal kidney tissue (Fig. 42-7). The cysts enlarge, compress functional renal tissue, and eventually result in renal failure. They also may create pressure on nearby organs. As the kidneys lose the ability to concentrate urine, hypertension and HF develop. Often, cystic lesions are found on other organs. Chronic infection contributes to progressive loss of function.

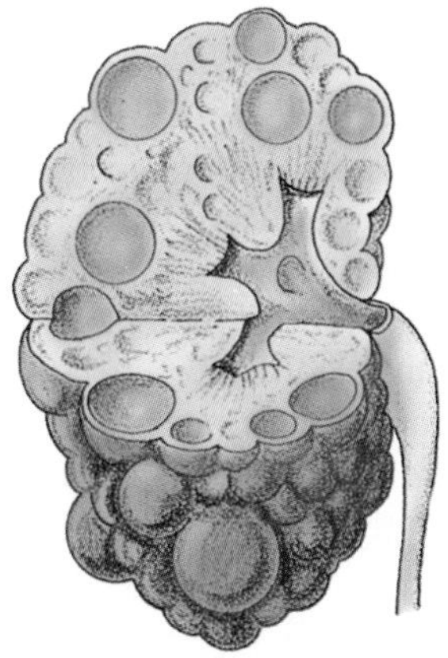

FIGURE 42-7 Polycystic kidney. (From Black JM, Hawks JH, Keene AM: *Medical-surgical nursing: clinical management for continuity of care*, ed 6, Philadelphia, 2001, Saunders.)

Signs and Symptoms

This slowly progressive disorder begins with various types of pain: dull, aching abdominal, lower back, or flank pain (or it begins with colicky pain that begins abruptly).

Medical Treatment

Supportive treatment is recommended to preserve kidney function, treat UTI, and control hypertension. Infections should be treated promptly with appropriate antibiotics. As the disease progresses, kidney function decreases and end-stage renal disease develops. Dialysis, nephrectomy, and transplantation are then treatment options. Genetic counseling is advised for these patients because each of their children has a 50% chance of having the condition.

NURSING CARE of the Patient with Polycystic Kidney Disease

See the sections on nursing care of patients with end-stage renal disease and those having renal surgery, dialysis, and transplantation in this chapter.

IMMUNOLOGIC RENAL DISEASE

ACUTE GLOMERULONEPHRITIS

Pathophysiology

Glomerulonephritis is an immunologic disease characterized by inflammation of the capillary loops in the glomeruli. Several immunologic mechanisms can cause acute glomerulonephritis. For example, the patient may develop antibodies against antigens in the glomeruli. A common type of glomerulonephritis follows an infection of the respiratory tract caused by group A–negative hemolytic streptococcus. An antigen-antibody reaction results in inflammation of the glomeruli and scar tissue forms. Glomerular permeability increases, allowing proteins to leak into the urine. The glomerular filtration rate decreases and nitrogenous wastes accumulate in the blood. Both BUN and serum creatinine levels rise. Acute glomerulonephritis usually resolves completely but some patients develop chronic glomerulonephritis or progress to irreversible renal failure.

Signs and Symptoms

Urine becomes tea colored as output decreases. Peripheral and periorbital (around the eyes) edema is evident. As glomerular filtration decreases, mild to severe hypertension occurs and hypervolemia (increased blood volume) results.

Medical Diagnosis

Diagnosis is based on patient assessment and laboratory tests. A urinalysis is done to detect proteinuria and RBC casts. Blood studies measure BUN, creatinine, and albumin. Streptococcal antibody tests indicate whether the patient has had a streptococcal infection. Findings in blood and urine studies tend to vary from one patient to another. Renal ultrasound, renal biopsy, or both also may be ordered.

Medical Treatment

Acute glomerulonephritis is treated with diuretics and, for severe hypertension, antihypertensive medications. Antibiotics are indicated if evidence of current streptococcal infection exists. In the acute phase, bed rest is ordered to prevent or treat heart failure and severe hypertension from fluid overload. Activity restriction usually is continued as long as urine tests show blood or protein or if BP is elevated. Fluids, sodium, potassium, and protein may be restricted until sufficient recovery of kidney function occurs. When fluid overload has been corrected, moderate activity is permitted but the patient still needs sufficient rest to allow the kidneys to heal.

Because some patients with acute glomerulonephritis develop renal insufficiency, follow-up is very important. If renal failure develops, dialysis is necessary. Patients who progress to chronic glomerulonephritis acquire end-stage renal disease in 1 to 30 years. (See the section titled "Chronic Kidney Disease.")

NURSING CARE of the Patient with Acute Glomerulonephritis

Assessment

Assessment of patients with urinary tract disorders is outlined in Box 42-1. For the patient with acute glomerulonephritis, it is especially important to note signs and symptoms, recent infections (especially sore throat or skin lesions), and changes in urine characteristics.

During the physical examination, inspect the area around the eyes, the extremities, and the abdomen for fluid accumulation. Assess tissue turgor. Evaluate respiratory and cardiac function for evidence of excess fluid volume: dyspnea, tachycardia, hypertension. Accurate intake and output records and daily weights help to assess the kidneys' ability to excrete excess fluid.

Interventions

Excess Fluid Volume

Administer diuretics as ordered. Maintain careful records of fluid intake and output. Instruct patients and family members about the importance of accurate records. If fluids are restricted, explain the need for the restriction and help the patient to plan the timing and amounts of allowed fluids. Fluid restriction can be very distressing. It helps to present fluids in small containers rather than serving an ounce or two in a large glass. If the patient has edema, special skin care is needed. Handle the patient gently because taut, swollen tissue is damaged easily and heals slowly.

Nursing Diagnoses, Goals, and Outcome Criteria: Acute Glomerulonephritis

Nursing Diagnoses	Goals and Outcome Criteria
Excess Fluid Volume related to renal dysfunction	Restoration of normal fluid balance: balanced fluid intake and output, vital signs consistent with patient norms, no edema
Activity Intolerance related to retention of chemical wastes, fatigue, prescribed bed rest	Improved activity tolerance: patient reports less fatigue with physical activity
Ineffective Self-Health Management related to prescribed bed rest, lack of knowledge of treatment measures of care	Patient adheres to plan of care: self-care is accomplished within activity restrictions, patient adheres to plan
Anxiety related to possibility of chronic illness	Reduced anxiety: patient states anxiety is lessened, appears calm

Activity Intolerance

Activity intolerance may be due to infection, accumulated toxins, or anemia. During the acute illness, discourage activity to allow the kidneys to heal. Explain the importance of rest for recovery. Schedule activities to allow for periods of uninterrupted rest. Of course, the patient on bed rest is at risk for complications of immobility: skin breakdown, pneumonia, muscle weakness, joint stiffness, constipation, and thrombus formation. Therefore have the patient change positions, cough and deep breathe, and gently exercise joints periodically. Nursing measures to prevent the complications of immobility are discussed in Chapter 21.

Ineffective Self-Health Management

The patient needs to understand that rest, dietary restrictions, and medications promote recovery. Provide assistance with ADL. Emphasize the need for follow-up care. When the patient is discharged, reinforce the importance of reporting any signs of recurrence such as changes in urine characteristics or edema. Instruct the patient to increase activities gradually as the edema and fatigue resolve.

Anxiety

The patient with acute glomerulonephritis may be very concerned about the possibility of developing a chronic, life-threatening condition. Give the patient an opportunity to ask questions and share concerns. Helpful interventions may include empathetic listening, providing factual information, and referrals to other professionals.

URINARY TRACT OBSTRUCTIONS

RENAL CALCULI

Urolithiasis is the formation of calculi (stones) in the urinary tract. The prevalence of urolithiasis in the United States has been rising. In their lifetime, 12% of men and 6% of women are predicted to have stone formation. It is most common among Caucasian men and has a high incidence of recurrence (see *Cultural Considerations* box).

Cultural Considerations

What Does Culture Have to Do with Urinary Calculi?

The incidence of uric acid stones is high among Jewish men. Caucasians have an increased risk of urinary calculi compared with African Americans. Cultural factors such as diet, as well as genetic factors, probably explain some of these differences.

Pathophysiology

Most calculi are precipitations of calcium salts (calcium phosphate or calcium oxalate), uric acid, magnesium ammonium phosphate (struvite), or cystine. All of these substances are normally found in the urine. Factors that foster the development of calculi are the following:

- Concentrated urine
- Excessive intake of vitamin D, animal protein, oxalates, sodium, sucrose, vitamin C, calcium-based antacids
- Low dietary calcium intake
- Familial history
- Hyperparathyroidism, gout, diabetes, obesity, gastric bypass procedure, Crohn disease, renal tubular acidosis
- Immobility, urinary stasis
- Sedentary lifestyle
- Altered urine pH
- Lack of kidney substance that inhibits calculi formation

In the past it was assumed that a high calcium intake would contribute to calculi formation. Evidence now indicates that *low* calcium intake is associated with calculi formation. Urine is normally acidic, with a pH ranging from 4.5 to 8.0. Some substances tend to precipitate in acid urine, causing **calculus** formation; others precipitate in alkaline urine. UTIs, particularly those caused by *Proteus, Klebsiella*, and *Pseudomonas*, are associated with calculi because these organisms cause the urine to become alkaline. The kidneys excrete substances that are believed to inhibit calculi formation, so a decrease in these substances may contribute to calculus formation.

Most calculi originate in the kidney (nephrolithiasis) and travel through the ureters to the bladder (urolithiasis).

Signs and Symptoms

The patient's chief complaint is usually pain. The location and characteristics of the pain may provide clues to the site of the calculus. Dull flank pain suggests a calculus in the renal pelvis or stretching of the renal capsule from urine retention (hydronephrosis). If a calculus lodges in a ureter, the patient usually has excruciating pain in the abdomen that radiates to the groin or the perineum. The ureter goes into spasm (colic) in an attempt to move the calculus along and relieve the obstruction. Nausea, vomiting, and hematuria may accompany the pain. The patient also may show signs and symptoms of UTI.

Medical Diagnosis

A helical CT scan is the preferred imaging procedure when stones are suspected. A routine urinalysis and culture and sensitivity usually are ordered as well. If a calculus can be obtained, its composition can be determined by laboratory analysis. Other diagnostic procedures may be done to rule out other causes of pain such as acute cholecystitis, pyelonephritis, musculoskeletal pain, duodenal ulcer, and abdominal aortic aneurysm.

Medical Treatment

Most calculi are passed spontaneously. Ambulation may facilitate the passage of many calculi. Opioid analgesics or parenteral NSAIDs and antispasmodics are ordered to relieve the intense, colicky pain. Intravenous fluids commonly are given, although no evidence indicates that hydration enhances the passage of existing stones. Antibiotics are ordered if infection is present or if internal manipulation of the calculus is necessary. If the calculus does not pass and symptoms continue, several procedures may be used to destroy or remove it. Options include the placement of a ureteral stent, lithotripsy, cystoscopic stone removal, and percutaneous nephrostolithotomy.

Lithotripsy. **Lithotripsy** (shattering of the calculus) may be accomplished by extracorporeal shock wave lithotripsy (ESWL), which uses sound, laser, or dry shock wave energy (electrohydraulic, electromagnetic, piezoelectric) to shatter the stones. ESWL uses a device called a *lithotripter* to deliver a series of shock waves to disintegrate the calculi. Guided by an ultrasound probe, the energy is directed to the stone through a water-filled cushion. Depending on the type of energy used, conscious sedation, preoperative sedation, or analgesics may be given because the series of 1000 to 1500 shocks is painful (Fig. 42-8). The shocks are coordinated with the patient's cardiac cycle. The pulverized calculus is excreted in the urine over 1 to 4 weeks. After lithotripsy, the urine is often a bright-red color at

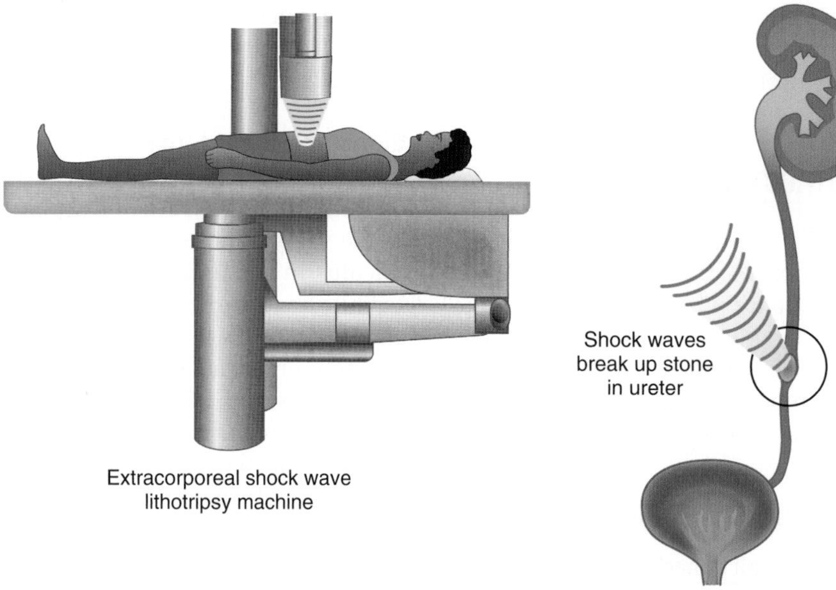

FIGURE 42-8 Extracorporeal shock wave lithotripsy (ESWL). (From Monahan FD, Drake DT, Neighbors M, editors: *Medical-surgical nursing: foundations for clinical practice*, ed 2, Philadelphia, 1998, Saunders.)

first, gradually turning to a dark-red or smoky shade. A stent may be placed in the ureter before treatment to facilitate passage of the stone fragments. The stent is usually removed in several weeks. Bruising and hemorrhage are possible complications of lithotripsy. However, most patients are able to resume normal activities on the day after the procedure. Antibiotics are generally given for about 2 weeks to prevent UTI.

Endourologic Procedures. Stones in the bladder often can be crushed and removed using cystoscopic techniques. An instrument called a *ureteroscope* can be passed through the bladder to reach stones located in the renal pelvis and ureters. Along with the ureteroscope, instruments that shatter the stones may be used. For example, with lasertripsy, the calculus is visualized and destroyed with a laser. Like ESWL, fragments are usually passed in the urine. General anesthesia is used but premedication is commonly omitted because radiographs must be obtained immediately before the procedure. When stones are large or cannot be broken with lithotripsy, a percutaneous nephrolithotomy may be done. The surgeon creates a tunnel directly through the skin into the kidney and then uses ultrasound or electrohydrolysis to break the stone into pieces. Some pieces are removed through the tunnel with a nephroscope. A nephrostomy tube is placed and left for 1 to 2 weeks to promote healing. The urine will be blood tinged for several days. Encourage oral fluid intake and record intake and output, including urine passed through the tube.

Surgical Procedures. With the advent of endoscopic procedures, surgical procedures are seldom needed. However, if calculi are not passed spontaneously or crushed with a lithotriptor, surgery may be necessary. The incision of an organ or a duct to remove a calculus is a **lithotomy**. A nephrolithotomy is the surgical procedure used if the calculus is in the kidney. The removal of a calculus from the renal pelvis is a pyelolithotomy. A ureterolithotomy is removal of a calculus from a ureter (Fig. 42-9).

Prevention

An important medical goal is to prevent recurrence of renal calculi. Long-term medical management of these patients includes a high fluid intake to keep urine dilute, dietary restrictions for specific elements depending on the type of stones (e.g., animal protein, purines), regular exercise, and occasionally medications to alter the urine pH. An appropriate fluid intake is judged by a urine output of at least 2 L a day. Fluid intake may need to be increased during hot weather because of the fluid loss through perspiration. Drugs that may be used include thiazide diuretics for elevated urine calcium and allopurinol for elevated urine uric acid. For individuals with oxalate stones, potassium citrate and magnesium supplement may be ordered. Medications are less effective than dietary management.

❖ NURSING CARE of the Patient with Renal Calculi

■ Assessment

Assessment of the patient with a urinary tract disorder is summarized in Box 42-1 (see also Nursing Care Plan: Patient with Renal Calculi). When the patient has known or suspected urinary calculi, pay particular attention to a personal or family history of calculi. Describe the patient's usual fluid intake and diet, including vitamin and mineral supplements. If pain is present, describe the location, severity, and nature of the pain. Also record any changes in urine amount or characteristics. Take the temperature to detect fever. A

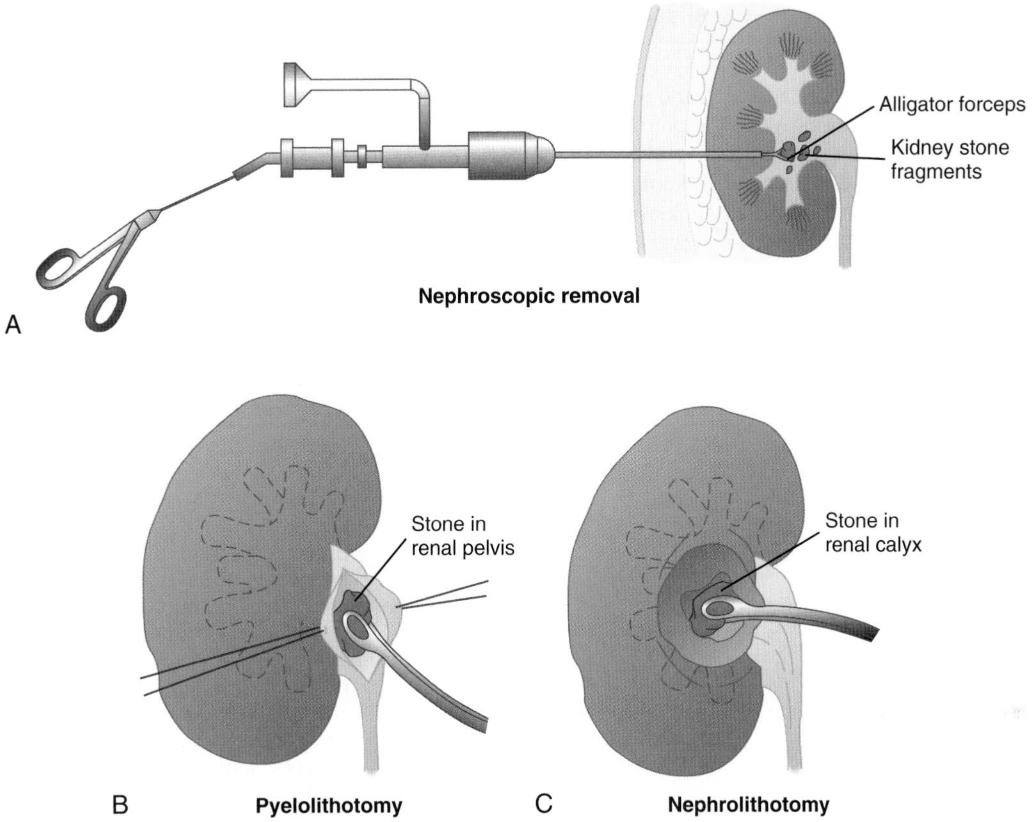

FIGURE 42-9 Surgical procedures for renal calculi. **A,** Nephroscopy. **B,** Pyelolithotomy. **C,** Nephrolithotomy. (From Black JM, Hawks JH: *Medical-surgical nursing: clinical management for positive outcomes*, ed 8, St. Louis, 2009, Saunders.)

nurse who is trained in physical examination palpates and percusses the flanks and the abdomen, noting the presence of pain, tenderness, or a distended bladder.

Nursing Diagnoses, Goals, and Outcome Criteria: Renal Calculi

Nursing Diagnoses	Goals and Outcome Criteria
Acute Pain related to obstruction, trauma, and renal colic	Pain relief: patient states pain has been relieved, relaxed manner
Impaired Urinary Elimination related to obstruction	Unobstructed urine elimination: urine output equal to fluid intake
Risk for Electrolyte Imbalance related to anorexia, nausea, and vomiting	Normal fluid balance: fluid intake and output approximately equal, pulse and blood pressure (BP) consistent with patient norms
Ineffective Self-Health Management related to lack of knowledge of prevention and treatment of calculi	Patient effectively manages treatment plan and takes preventive measures: patient accurately describes prevention and treatment, adheres to preventive measures, has no recurrences

Nursing Diagnoses, Goals, and Outcome Criteria: Renal Calculi—cont'd

If surgery is performed, additional nursing diagnoses and goals include the following.

Nursing Diagnoses	Goals and Outcome Criteria
Risk for Infection related to invasive procedures	Absence of infection: normal body temperature and white blood cell (WBC) count, clear urine
Decreased Cardiac Output related to blood loss	Adequate cardiac output: pulse and BP consistent with patient norms
Ineffective Breathing Pattern related to splinting of painful incision	Effective breathing patterns: clear breath sounds throughout lung fields, respiratory and depth consistent with patient norms

Interventions

Acute Pain

Because calculi in the urinary tract can cause excruciating pain (renal colic), pain relief is a major nursing concern. Initially it may be necessary to administer opioid analgesics intravenously or parenteral NSAIDs

Nursing Care Plan Patient with Renal Calculi

ASSESSMENT

HEALTH HISTORY Mr. Scarpino, age 43 years, was admitted with excruciating abdominal pain radiating to the groin. He experienced nausea and vomiting with the pain. Review of systems revealed a history of hypertension controlled with captopril. He also has had repeated urinary tract infections (UTIs), most recently 1 month ago. At that time he was treated with antibiotics and the symptoms subsided. Radiologic studies detected a calculus lodged in the right ureter. Extracorporeal shock wave lithotripsy (ESWL) was done to shatter the calculus. Mr. Scarpino returned to his hospital room 3 hours ago. He is complaining of soreness in the right lower abdomen.

PHYSICAL EXAMINATION Vital signs: blood pressure 138/74 mm Hg, pulse 88 bpm, respiration 20 breaths per minute, temperature 100°F (37.8°C) measured orally. Ht. 5′11″, Wt. 195 lbs. Patient is fully oriented but drowsy. His abdomen is soft but tender. No bladder distention exists. He voided 350 mL of pink-tinged urine. Intravenous fluids are infusing at 150 mL/h.

Nursing Diagnosis	Goals and Outcome Criteria	Interventions
Acute Pain related to obstruction, trauma, renal colic	Patient will report pain relief and will appear more relaxed.	Assess pain characteristics. For severe pain, administer analgesics as ordered. Administer antispasmodics as ordered. Assist with ambulation when permitted to promote passage of calculus fragments. Milder pain may be treated with nonopioid analgesics. Position changes, back rubs, relaxation, and imagery may be used to enhance analgesia. Document effects of pain relief interventions.
Impaired Urinary Elimination related to obstruction	Patient's urine output will be approximately equal to fluid intake.	Measure all fluid intake and output. Report low output to physician. Strain all urine to collect calculi fragments. Send fragments to laboratory for analysis. Maintain intravenous fluids.
Risk for Electrolyte Imbalance related to nothing-by-mouth (NPO) status, nausea, and vomiting, IV therapy	Patient will be adequately hydrated as evidenced by moist mucous membranes, dilute urine, and vital signs consistent with patient's norms.	Administer intravenous fluids as ordered. Assess for deficient fluid volume: hypotension, tachycardia, sticky mucous membranes, and concentrated urine. Encourage oral fluids when permitted. Administer antiemetics as ordered for nausea and vomiting.
Ineffective Breathing Pattern related to abdominal pain, splinting	Patient's breath sounds will be normal throughout the lung fields.	Assess respiratory status: rate, effort, breath sounds. Encourage deep breathing and coughing every 2 hours until fully ambulatory.
Decreased Cardiac Output related to blood loss	Patient's cardiac output will remain normal, as evidenced by vital signs consistent with patient's norms and by absence of tachycardia, hypotension, or restlessness.	Assess the abdomen and groin area for bruising; some is expected. Note red color and increased viscosity of urine associated with bleeding. Report increased redness. Monitor vital signs to detect decreasing cardiac output: tachycardia, restlessness, and hypotension.
Ineffective Self-Health Management related to lack of knowledge of prevention and treatment of calculi, self-care after lithotripsy	Patient will effectively manage self-care, as evidenced by correct description of self-care after lithotripsy and measures to prevent recurrence of calculi.	Tell the patient that the fragments are usually passed in the urine over a period of several weeks and may cause some pain. Administer antibiotics as ordered and emphasize the importance of treating any new urinary tract infections (UTIs) to reduce the risk of calculi formation. Advise the patient to consume enough fluid daily to produce 2 L of output, unless the physician prescribes less. Fluids should be taken around the clock to prevent concentration during the night. If any dietary restrictions are imposed, request a dietary consultation to explain them to the patient.

Critical Thinking Questions

1. Why would the patient continue to have pain after the stones have been shattered with lithotripsy?
2. When might 3 to 4 L/day of fluid intake be contraindicated?

to relieve the pain. Antispasmodics are usually ordered to reduce the smooth muscle spasms in the ureters. If pain is intermittent, the patient may be permitted to ambulate when comfortable. Ambulation actually may help the calculus to move through the urinary tract. Of course, safety precautions are needed if opioids have been given. The pain may resolve suddenly if the calculus moves into the bladder or is passed through the urethra.

Impaired Urinary Elimination

Depending on its size and location, a calculus may obstruct urine flow. If urine backs up into the kidney, hydronephrosis may develop. Hydronephrosis is distention of the kidney with urine, a condition that can cause permanent damage (Fig. 42-10). Maintain accurate records of fluid intake and output and report low output to the physician. In addition, all urine is strained and examined for calculi. If any calculi are recovered, send them to the laboratory for analysis.

Risk for Electrolyte Imbalance

Renal colic is often accompanied by nausea and sometimes vomiting. Give antiemetics promptly as ordered. The physician will probably order intravenous fluids to maintain dilute urine and to flush the urinary tract. A fluid intake to maintain an output of 2 L/day is recommended. Large volumes of fluids must be given carefully to the older patient, in whom fluid volume excess can develop easily. Monitor for signs of circulatory overload (tachycardia, bounding pulse, dyspnea, edema, hypertension). Although dilute urine decreases the risk of stone formation, increased fluids do not appear to facilitate the passage of existing stones.

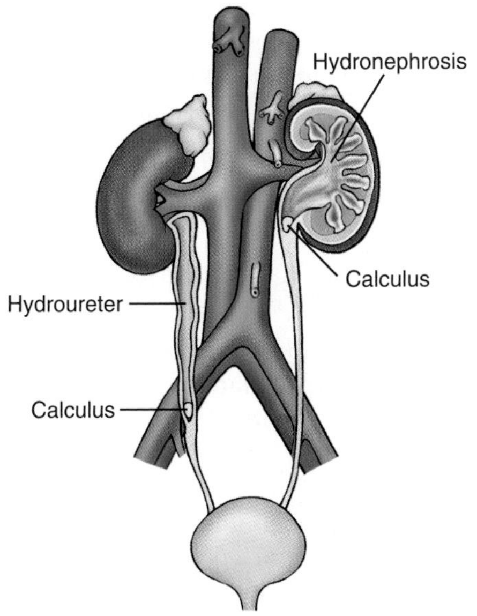

FIGURE 42-10 Hydronephrosis caused by obstruction of the upper portion of the ureter. Hydroureter caused by obstruction of the lower portion of the ureter. (From Monahan FD, Drake DT, Neighbors M, editors: *Medical-surgical nursing: foundations for clinical practice*, ed 2, Philadelphia, 1998, Saunders.)

Ineffective Self-Health Management

When the patient is discharged, reinforce the need to continue to consume adequate amounts of fluid daily. The fluid needs to be consumed over the 24-hour period so that urine does not become concentrated at night. Advise the patient to drink two glasses of water before bed and another two glasses when awakening at night to void. This pattern should be followed for life to reduce the risk of calculus formation in the future. If the physician has prescribed a special diet or dietary restriction, provide instructions or have the dietitian do so.

Postoperative Care

Before surgery, explain the expected procedure to the patient and answer any questions. Goals of postoperative care are maintenance of urine drainage, prevention of UTI, and prevention of pulmonary and circulatory complications.

Risk for Infection

To maintain alignment and urine flow, the patient is apt to have drains, catheters, a ureteral stent, or a combination of these. Each tube is connected to its own closed drainage system. Position tubes for free flow of urine at all times. Keep accurate accounts of drainage from each tube. If the patient has a flank incision, frequently check the area around the dressing for drainage because urine tends to leak from the incision. A large amount of serosanguineous drainage is normal immediately after surgery. In approximately 2 days, the drainage changes to serous. Frequent dressing changes using sterile technique may be required. In some cases, an ostomy appliance is used to collect drainage and to permit accurate measurement of the drainage.

Some patients have nephrostomy tubes placed directly in the kidney. The tube is placed for drainage or for instillation of irrigating fluid. It also diverts urine flow from the ureter until adequate healing has occurred. If irrigations are ordered, use strict aseptic technique and not more than 5 mL of warm, sterile normal saline at a time.

Decreased Cardiac Output

The patient is at risk for the same postoperative complications as any surgical patient. Be especially alert for any signs of excessive bleeding, infection, or pulmonary complications. To detect bleeding, inspect the dressing and drainage hourly for the first 24 hours. Immediately report bright red blood, excessive serosanguineous drainage, increasing pulse, restlessness, or decreasing blood pressure to the physician. Indications of infection such as odor, cloudy drainage, or temperature above 100°F also should be reported.

Measures to reduce the risk of infection include maintaining closed drainage systems, changing wet dressings promptly, and using strict aseptic technique when handling tubes or dressings.

Ineffective Breathing Pattern

Monitor the patient's pulmonary status carefully. A flank incision makes taking a deep breath very painful. Assist the patient to turn, cough, and deep breathe at least every 2 hours. An incentive spirometer helps to determine how much the patient is able to inflate the lungs. When the patient coughs, the incision needs to be splinted with pillows or folded blankets. For the first 1 or 2 postoperative days, administer analgesics before turning, coughing, and deep breathing to make these activities more comfortable. Adequate fluid intake thins respiratory secretions and makes them easier to expectorate. Early and frequent ambulation promotes improved respiratory function. All of these efforts help to prevent atelectasis and pneumonia, a primary treatment goal.

UROLOGIC TRAUMA

The kidneys sustain 50% of all urologic injuries. Trauma may be penetrating or blunt. Penetrating injuries most often result from knives or guns. Blunt trauma occurs when a force is applied to the abdominal wall and the energy is diffused into the abdominal cavity. Examples of blunt force are motor vehicle accidents, contact sports injuries, falls, and intentional injuries. Blunt injuries to the kidneys produce lacerations or contusions. The ureters are rarely injured with blunt trauma; they are disrupted most often by penetration and require surgical anastomosis. The bladder may rupture from blunt trauma if full but it is rarely harmed when empty. The urethra is most apt to be injured in men because of its unprotected anatomic location.

When blunt trauma is suspected, the patient is observed for bruising on the abdomen or in the flank area. Assess for signs of shock (tachycardia, restlessness, hypotension, pallor), pain, and a palpable abdominal or flank mass. Bruising over the flank and lower back that occurs with retroperitoneal bleeding is called *Grey Turner sign*.

The physician may order a KUB, urography, CT scan, or ultrasound to determine the extent of injury. Diagnostic peritoneal lavage may be performed to determine whether there is bleeding in the peritoneal cavity. A positive finding necessitates surgery to find and eliminate the source of bleeding.

The most common indication of urologic trauma is hematuria. It is best if the patient can void but this may not be possible with other injuries. Before catheterizing a patient with suspected trauma, carefully inspect the urethral meatus. If there is blood in or around the meatus, a urologist should perform the catheterization or insert a suprapubic catheter.

If the injury is not severe, if there is little bleeding, and if there are no signs of shock, monitor the patient closely. More severe injuries most likely require surgery to repair damage. Postsurgical care of these patients is similar to the care of the patient with a nephrectomy, urinary calculi, or cystectomy.

CANCERS OF THE URINARY SYSTEM

Care of the patient with cancer is discussed in Chapter 25. This section focuses on the specific needs of the patient with cancer of the urinary tract.

RENAL CANCER

Malignancies of the kidney account for approximately 57,000 new cases of cancer in the United States each year. Eighty percent of renal malignancies are adenocarcinomas. Primarily men aged 50 to 70 years are affected. The incidence is increased in African Americans and American Indians/Alaska Natives compared with Caucasians. Risk factors include cigarette smoking, obesity, hypertension, and environmental exposures (asbestos, gasoline).

A renal tumor may reach considerable size before it is detected. Renal malignancies metastasize to the liver, lungs, long bones, and the other kidney. Direct extension of the tumor may be found in the ureter. Early symptoms are anemia, weakness, and weight loss. Painless, gross hematuria is the classic sign but it usually occurs in the advanced stage. A dull ache in the flank area also is a late symptom.

Medical Diagnosis

The physician may be able to palpate a mass in the flank area. CT scan is the primary diagnostic tool for renal cell cancer. Diagnostic tests and procedures to study the mass may include ultrasonography and MRI and provide additional information that helps in making treatment decisions. Care of the patient undergoing these procedures is detailed in Table 42-1.

Medical Treatment

Removal of a kidney is called a *nephrectomy*. Radical nephrectomy involves removal of the kidney and its adjacent tissue, adrenal gland, renal artery and vein, and local lymph glands. Nephrectomy is the treatment of choice for renal cancer. Before nephrectomy, the renal artery may be occluded to reduce the blood supply to the tumor. Partial nephrectomy may be an option when the tumor is small. Laparoscopic complete or partial nephrectomy is becoming very common, replacing open surgical approaches. In general, renal tumors are not responsive to radiation or chemotherapy but radiation is sometimes used as a palliative measure for inoperable cancer. Biotherapy with alfa-interferon and high-dose interleukin-2 may be used for the patient with metastatic disease.

NURSING CARE of the Patient with Renal Cancer

Assessment

Nursing assessment of the patient with a urologic disorder is outlined in Box 42-1. When a patient has a suspected or confirmed renal malignancy, very few signs and symptoms may exist. Inquire about weakness, fatigue, and any changes observed in the urine. Explore the patient's emotional state, usual coping strategies, and support systems.

Preoperative Care

General preoperative nursing care is discussed in detail in Chapter 17. Before renal surgery, the patient's primary nursing diagnoses are *ineffective coping* related to potentially fatal disease and *deficient knowledge* of tests, procedures, and effects of renal surgery. The goals of nursing care are *effective patient use of coping mechanisms* and *understanding of what is being done and what to expect.*

Thorough explanations of diagnostic tests and preoperative teaching provide needed information. Assure the patient that one functioning kidney can sustain adequate kidney function. Tests are done to confirm that the unaffected kidney functions adequately before a nephrectomy. Serum and urine laboratory tests are usually ordered to serve as baseline data for postoperative comparison. Older patients are more likely to have renal insufficiency and they eventually may need renal dialysis after nephrectomy. The teaching plan includes what to expect in the postoperative period and how to turn, cough, and deep breathe. Other preoperative care is the same as that for any other major surgery.

Postoperative Care

Common aspects of postoperative care are discussed in Chapter 17. After nephrectomy, monitor vital signs to detect fluid volume alterations related to blood loss or fluid retention. Record intake and output as another measure of fluid balance and renal function. Routinely check drains and tubes to ensure proper function. Monitor dressings for drainage. Once the dressings have been removed, inspect the wound for intactness and signs of infection (excessive redness or swelling, purulent drainage). Determine the patient's comfort level. Auscultate breath sounds and bowel sounds. Anticipate some emotional distress and encourage the patient to express thoughts and feelings about having cancer.

Nursing Diagnoses, Goals, and Outcome Criteria: Renal Cancer, Postoperative

Nursing Diagnoses	Goals and Outcome Criteria
Acute Pain related to incisional tissue trauma	Pain relief: patient states pain is relieved, relaxed manner
Risk for Deficient Fluid Volume related to dehydration, blood loss	Normal hydration and blood volume: pulse and blood pressure (BP) consistent with patient norms, normal skin turgor
Ineffective Breathing Pattern related to proximity of incision to diaphragm	Effective breathing patterns: clear breath sounds throughout lung fields
Risk for Injury related to decreased peristalsis caused by bowel manipulation during surgery	Absence of abdominal distention: active bowel sounds, abdomen soft
Risk for Infection related to break in skin	Absence of infection: normal body temperature and white blood cell (WBC) count
Ineffective Coping related to diagnosis of cancer	Effective coping: patient practices strategies that reduce anxiety but do not interfere with therapeutic plan
Deficient Knowledge of postoperative limitations related to lack of information	Patient understands postoperative restrictions and accurately describes and adheres to activity limitations

Interventions

Acute Pain

Obtain a complete description of the patient's pain. Incisional pain is intense at first and requires prompt administration of prescribed analgesics. Because of the patient's position during surgery, there may be muscle aches in the opposite side and flank area. Medication can be supplemented with position changes and back rubs. Other comfort measures are described in Chapter 15.

Risk for Deficient Fluid Volume

Intravenous fluids are given initially. The physician normally orders approximately 3 L of fluid daily. Maintain accurate intake and output records. At first, the urine may be measured every 1 to 2 hours. Notify the physician if less than 30 mL is produced in an hour. When the patient is able to weighed, daily weights are an even better measure of fluid balance than intake and output. BUN, serum creatinine, serum electrolytes, and urine specific gravity are assessed and compared with preoperative values.

Also monitor the nephrectomy patient for bleeding. Frequently check the dressing drainage. Be careful to check *under* the patient because blood flows to the most dependent area. Sometimes the dressing is dry and intact but the patient is lying in a pool of blood. !

Ineffective Breathing Pattern

The location of the flank incision causes pain with expansion of the thorax. Patients tend to protect the area by not breathing deeply. This may lead to pneumonia and atelectasis. It is especially important to have the patient turn, cough, and deep breathe every 1 to 2 hours. You can help by supporting the incision during respiratory exercises. Supervise use of an incentive spirometer to encourage deeper inspiration. As soon as ambulation is permitted, assist the patient out of bed. Be careful not to place tension on tubes and drains. Gradually increase the time and distance walked.

Risk for Injury

Anesthesia and manipulation of abdominal organs cause temporary cessation of peristalsis in the intestines. Until peristalsis returns, the patient is not permitted to take anything by mouth. If peristalsis does not return within 3 to 4 days, the patient is said to have *paralytic ileus*. Because paralytic ileus is fairly common after nephrectomy, a nasogastric tube may be inserted and attached to suction during surgery. Suction keeps the stomach empty, reducing the risk of nausea and abdominal distention. The return of peristalsis is detected by active bowel sounds and the passage of flatus (gas). Auscultate the abdomen for bowel sounds and observe for abdominal distention. Ambulation promotes the return of peristalsis.

Risk for Infection

During dressing changes, use strict aseptic technique. Montgomery straps may decrease irritation from the adhesive tape if frequent dressing changes are required.

Ineffective Coping

The patient facing cancer fears the possibility of death, mourns the loss of an organ, and may dread additional cancer therapy. You can help by encouraging the patient to talk and clarify concerns, listening empathetically, providing requested information, and referring the patient to expert counselors. Explore usual coping strategies and sources of support. Chapter 25 provides additional details on nursing care of the patient with cancer.

Deficient Knowledge

Before discharge, caution the patient not to lift or participate in strenuous activities for 8 weeks. Contact sports are prohibited for life because trauma to the remaining kidney could eliminate all kidney function.

BLADDER CANCER

Cancer of the bladder is the most common malignancy of the urinary tract, with more than 70,000 new cases diagnosed each year in the United States. It occurs most often in men 60 to 70 years old. The ureteral orifices and the bladder neck are the most common sites of bladder cancer. Over the years, chemical agents have been suspected as carcinogens (see *Cultural Considerations* box). The tars found in smoking tobacco, aniline dyes found in industrial compounds, and tryptophan all have been implicated in the development of bladder cancer.

> **Cultural Considerations**
>
> **What Does Culture Have to Do with Bladder Cancer?**
>
> Risk factors for bladder cancer include cigarette smoking and exposure to chemicals used in the rubber and cable industries. Historically, men have been more likely than women to smoke and to work in industry, which might help to explain why this cancer is three times as common among men as among women.

Signs and Symptoms

The most common sign of bladder cancer is painless, intermittent hematuria. Other signs and symptoms include bladder irritability; infection, with dysuria, frequency, and urgency; and decreased stream of urine.

Medical Diagnosis

When the patient's signs and symptoms suggest bladder cancer, the physician may order a urinalysis with urine cytology and cystoscopy. Cystoscopy is done to visualize the bladder and permit biopsy of any observable lesions. Depending on the initial findings, additional studies may be done, including CT, MRI, IVP, CT-urogram, chest radiograph, and radionuclide bone scan. Details of these tests and procedures and nursing implications are provided in Table 42-1.

Medical Treatment

Bladder malignancies respond more favorably to chemotherapy than do kidney tumors but surgery is the treatment of choice. The type of surgery depends on whether the cancer is superficial, invasive, or metastatic. Superficial cancers involve only the bladder mucosa or submucosa, or sometimes both. Superficial lesions with low recurrence rates may be treated with cystoscopic resection and fulguration or with laser photocoagulation. Cystoscopic resection is the removal of tissue through a cystoscope with a special cutting instrument. Fulguration is the use of electric current to burn and destroy tissue. Laser photocoagulation is the use of an intense beam of light (argon laser) to destroy tissue.

Two other surgical procedures for bladder cancer are segmental bladder resection and radical cystectomy with pelvic lymphadenectomy (excision of lymph nodes). A segmental bladder resection is done for a single, primary tumor too large to remove by cystoscopic resection. It involves removal of the tumor and adjacent bladder muscle, a procedure that decreases the size of the bladder. A radical cystectomy is removal of the entire bladder and adjacent structures with diversion of the ureters. In men, the prostate is removed. In women, the urethra, uterus, fallopian tubes, ovaries, and anterior vaginal wall are removed. This procedure is reserved for malignancies that are untreatable with less conservative measures. Because this is a very extensive surgery, an optimal state of health before surgery is desirable. Chemotherapy, radiation, or both may be done before or after surgery, depending on the extent of the malignancy. Sometimes chemotherapeutic drugs or immune-stimulating agents are instilled directly into the bladder. This procedure is called *intravesical therapy*. A drug such as bacillus Calmette-Guérin (BCG) or mitomycin-C is administered into the bladder through a urinary catheter. The patient's position is changed at 15-minute intervals to ensure that the drugs reach the site of the lesion. After about 2 hours, the drugs are drained from the bladder. Treatment may be repeated weekly for 6 to 12 weeks, followed by a program of maintenance therapy.

Urinary Diversion. When the bladder and urethra must be removed completely, urine must be allowed to drain through another route, called *urinary diversion*. Several types of urinary diversions exist: ileal and sigmoid (colon) conduits, continent reservoir, cutaneous ureterostomy, and nephrostomy. These diversions are illustrated in Figure 42-11 and Figure 26-6 and discussed in detail in Chapter 26. Another option is the orthotopic neobladder. The neobladder is a reservoir that is attached to the urethra so that the patient voids through the urethra.

To form an ileal conduit, a portion of the ileum is resected from the small bowel. The ureters are implanted in the ileum, one end of the ileum is closed, and the open end is implanted on the abdominal surface as a stoma. Urine is excreted through the ileal conduit rather than the urethra. A urinary drainage pouch is attached to the skin to collect the urine. A sigmoid conduit is formed by the same procedure, except that a section of sigmoid colon instead of ileum is used. A continent reservoir is an internal pouch created from a segment of bowel. Urine collects in the pouch and is drained with a catheter at intervals. A ureterostomy brings the ureter to the abdominal

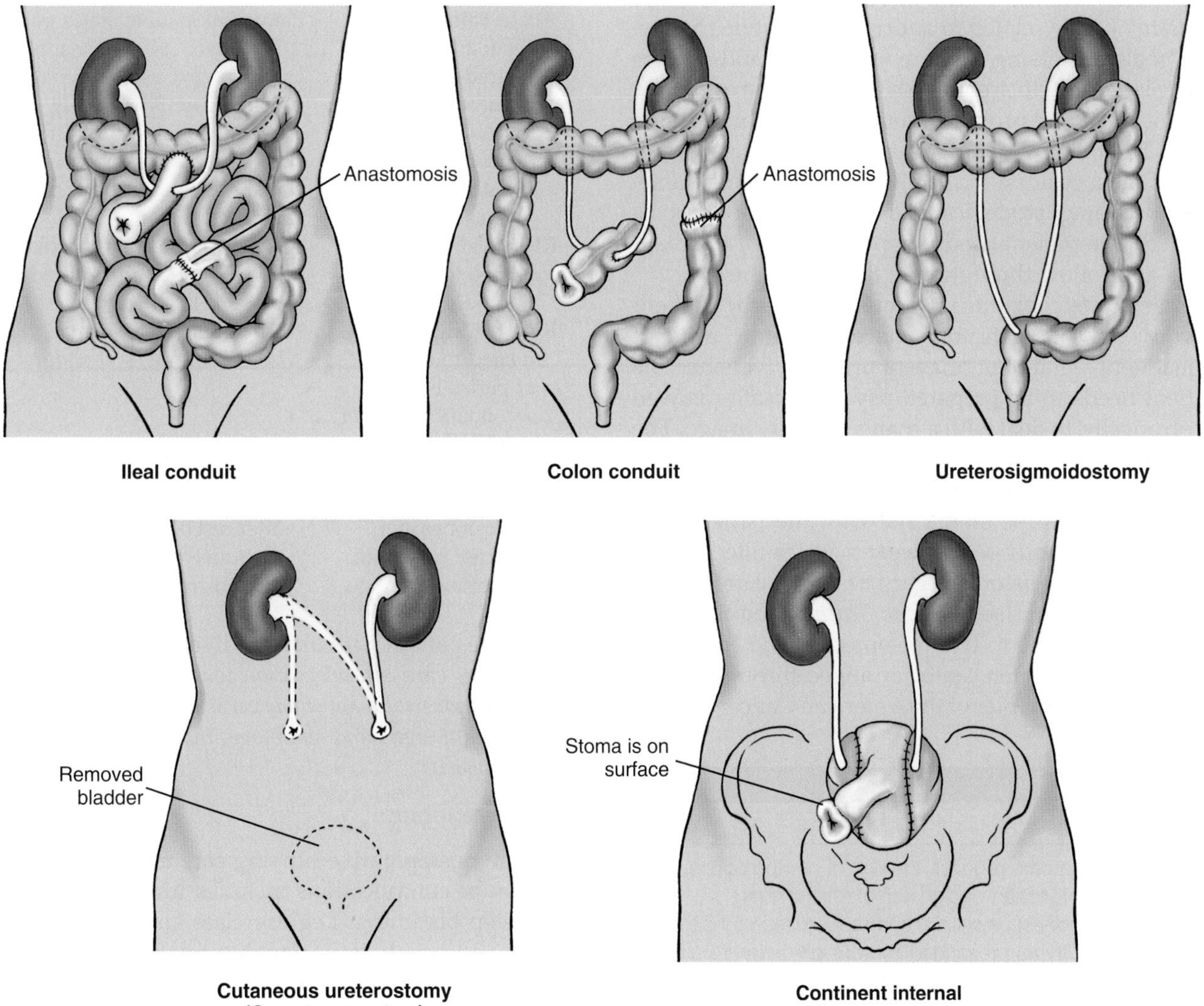

FIGURE 42-11 Types of urinary diversion procedures. (From Monahan FD, Drake DT, Neighbors M, editors: *Medical-surgical nursing: foundations for clinical practice*, ed 2, Philadelphia, 1998, Saunders.)

surface, where urine is eliminated through a stoma. A nephrostomy is the placement of a tube in the kidney so that urine may drain through the tube into an external collection device. Detailed information about urinary diversion is presented in Chapter 26.

NURSING CARE of the Patient with Bladder Cancer

Assessment

Assessment of the patient with possible or confirmed bladder cancer includes a complete description of urinary signs and symptoms. Fatigue and weight loss are significant and should be noted. The health history may reveal use of tobacco or exposure to carcinogenic chemicals. Explore the patient's emotional state, coping strategies, and sources of support.

Preoperative Care

In addition to the common nursing care described in Chapter 17, important preoperative nursing diagnoses for the patient facing segmental resection for cancer may be *fear* related to life-threatening diagnosis and *ineffective coping* related to anticipated lifestyle change. The goals of nursing care are *reduced fear* and *effective coping strategies*. To accomplish these goals, explore the patient's fear and provide information and encouragement. The thought of having cancer is frightening and nurses must educate the public that it is often curable. Assess coping strategies and provide resources as needed. The patient needs support to accept the diagnosis and follow through with the treatment.

Unless a neobladder is constructed, the patient having radical cystectomy faces a more difficult adjustment—that of permanent urinary diversion. The patient needs to be prepared psychologically, as well as physically, to deal with a change in body image. The enterostomal therapist is a valuable resource to both you and the patient in preparing for this surgery. The therapist selects the stoma site with the patient. The patient may be advised to wear a water-filled pouch for several days before surgery to help ensure proper stoma placement (see *Patient Teaching* box). If the patient would like to talk to someone who has had a cystectomy, this often can be arranged through a local ostomy club or chapter of the American Cancer Society.

Patient Teaching

Urinary Diversion

- Proper stoma care reduces the risk of complications.
- Notify your physician of signs of infection: fever; increasing redness, swelling, and tenderness of incisions.
- Restrict activity as prescribed by your physician to avoid strain on the surgical site.
- Resources include the enterostomal therapist, the American Cancer Society, and the United Ostomy Association (email: info@uoaa.org; telephone: 1-800-826-0826).

Preoperative care for an ileal or sigmoid conduit includes thorough preparation of the intestinal tract. Bowel preparation requires several days. The patient begins with a low-residue diet and then a clear-fluid diet. Oral neomycin, an antibiotic that is not absorbed from the intestinal tract, is ordered to reduce bacteria in the bowel. Enemas also are ordered before surgery.

The patient who has received effective preoperative nursing interventions demonstrates reduced fear and realistic problem solving.

Postoperative Care

Postoperative assessment includes vital signs, intake and output, patency of tubes, bowel sounds, comfort, and appearance of the drainage, stoma, and wound.

Additional nursing diagnoses such as *disturbed body image* and *deficient knowledge* of stoma care are appropriate if the patient has ostomy surgery.

Nursing Diagnoses, Goals, and Outcome Criteria: Bladder Surgery, Postoperative

Nursing Diagnoses	Goals and Outcome Criteria
Acute Pain related to tissue trauma	Pain relief: patient states pain is relieved, relaxed manner
Impaired Urinary Elimination related to urinary diversion	Unobstructed urine drainage: urine clear, flows freely, output equal to fluid intake
Impaired Skin Integrity related to surgical incision	Well-healed incision: wound margins intact, decreasing redness and swelling
Risk for Infection related to tissue trauma	Absence of infection: normal body temperature and white blood cell (WBC) count
Risk for Injury related to absence of peristalsis secondary to bowel manipulation during surgery	Normal peristalsis: active bowel sounds, soft abdomen
Deficient Knowledge of postoperative self-care related to lack of information	Patient understands self-care after discharge: patient accurately describes and demonstrates care

For the patient with urinary diversion, the outcomes of nursing care are *adaptation to disturbed body image, patient demonstration of stoma care,* and *patient knowledge of significant signs and symptoms that should be reported to the physician.*

Interventions

Routine postoperative nursing care aimed at the prevention of complications includes turning, coughing, and deep breathing. Leg exercises and early ambulation are especially important to prevent edema associated with excision of lymph nodes.

Acute Pain

Administer prescribed analgesics and use other comfort measures to control pain.

Impaired Urinary Elimination

Inspect urethral and suprapubic catheters and provide wound care as detailed in Chapter 17. Urine should be free of sediment, blood, or casts. Once the catheters are removed, encourage frequent voiding in the patient who has had a segmental resection. Bladder capacity will increase up to 250 to 300 mL over several months.

If a patient has had a radical cystectomy with urinary diversion, inspect the stoma for inflammation and irritation. Details of stoma care are provided in Chapter 26. The patient with a neobladder will have a catheter and a suprapubic drain. Irrigations are ordered to remove mucus. The catheter is left in place for several weeks. Once the catheter is removed, the patient is taught to empty the bladder by relaxing the external sphincter and straining to increase abdominal pressure. The patient is also taught self-catheterization in case the bladder cannot be emptied by voiding.

Impaired Skin Integrity

Monitor the surgical incision to ensure that it is healing without increasing redness, swelling, or purulent drainage. Provide wound care as ordered or per agency protocol. Sites of urine drains and the stoma also must receive care to prevent skin irritation and breakdown.

Risk for Infection

These patients are at risk for infections in the surgical incisions, drain sites, and urinary tract. Monitor the patient's vital signs, blood work, and wounds for evidence of infection (fever, elevated WBC count, foul odor). Use strict aseptic technique when providing wound care.

Risk for Injury

Withhold oral fluids as ordered until bowel sounds provide evidence that peristalsis has returned. Administer intravenous fluids as ordered. When oral intake is permitted, encourage an adequate fluid intake (2500 to 3000 mL/day).

Deficient Knowledge

Patient teaching must begin in the early postoperative period because the patient needs to learn self-care before discharge. Allow time for the patient or a caregiver to practice self-care procedures.

KIDNEY FAILURE

Kidney failure describes any condition that decreases the kidney's ability to function normally. Kidney failure is classified as *acute kidney injury* (formerly known as *acute kidney failure*) or *chronic kidney disease* based on onset and reversibility. Acute kidney injury has a rapid onset (1 to 7 days) and may be reversible. However, the mortality rate ranges from 35% to 65% depending on the presence of other diseases or complications. Chronic kidney disease has a slow onset (months to years) and is characterized by progressive, irreversible damage.

ACUTE KIDNEY INJURY

Causes

Causes of acute kidney injury (AKI) can be prerenal, intrarenal, or postrenal. Prerenal failure results from decreased blood flow to the glomeruli. A systolic BP of 70 mm Hg or greater is necessary to sustain glomerular filtration. If the systolic pressure drops to less than 70 mm Hg and is not corrected, renal failure may develop.

Intrarenal failure may be caused by nephrotoxic drugs, kidney infections, occlusion of intrarenal arteries, hypertension, diabetes mellitus, or direct trauma to the kidney. Antibiotics (particularly the "mycins"), heavy metals (lead and mercury), cleaning compounds, pesticides, and poisonous mushrooms may be toxic to the kidneys. Pyelonephritis, glomerulonephritis, renal tuberculosis, and polycystic kidney disease are examples of kidney conditions that may lead to kidney failure. The arteries in the renal parenchyma may become narrowed as a result of atherosclerosis, hypertension, nephrosclerosis, or blood components (sickled red cells, hemoglobin [Hgb], or myoglobin). Trauma from motor vehicle accidents, contact sports injuries, and other direct blows also may be intrarenal causes of failure.

Postrenal causes of AKI are obstructions beyond the kidneys causing urine to back up into the renal pelvis, resulting in *hydronephrosis*. Ureteral calculi, benign prostatic hypertrophy, prostate cancer, and trauma are the most common causes.

Patients at risk for AKI include those having major surgery, experiencing major trauma, or receiving large doses of nephrotoxic drugs. These patients should have their BP and fluid balance assessed more frequently than usual. Older people also are at risk for AKI because they are less able to adapt to alterations in fluid balance or cardiac output. Renal function should always be assessed with any acute condition in the older patient. Early detection and treatment may significantly decrease the risk of death from AKI.

Pharmacology Capsule

Nephrotoxic antibiotics can lead to acute kidney injury (AKI).

Stages of Acute Kidney Injury

The four stages of AKI are (1) initial, (2) oliguria, (3) **diuresis** (increased production of urine), and (4) recovery.

Initial Stage. The initial stage is short (1 to 3 days) and characterized by increasing BUN and serum creatinine with normal to decreased urine output. The primary treatment goal during this stage is reversal of failing renal function to prevent further damage.

Oliguric Stage. During the oliguric stage, the urine output decreases to 400 mL/day or less. The serum values for BUN, creatinine, potassium, and phosphorus increase. Serum calcium and bicarbonate decrease. The oliguric stage follows the onset stage and continues for up to 14 days. Urine specific gravity becomes fixed at 1.010 (normal range: 1.003–1.030), indicating the inability of the tubules to concentrate urine. The patient becomes hypervolemic, meaning that the blood volume is greater than normal. Urine osmolality decreases and serum osmolality increases as waste products are retained.

Diuretic Stage. The diuretic stage begins when urine output exceeds 400 mL/day and may rise above 4 L/day. Despite the production of large quantities of urine, few waste products are excreted and wastes accumulate in the blood. Toward the end of the diuretic stage, the kidneys begin to excrete BUN, creatinine, potassium, and phosphorus and retain calcium and bicarbonate. This is an indication of return of kidney function.

Recovery Stage. As renal tissue recovers, serum electrolytes, BUN, and creatinine return to normal. This recovery stage lasts 1 to 12 months. If complete recovery does not occur, renal insufficiency or chronic renal failure may develop. Renal insufficiency is indicated by loss of approximately 80% of function. It is possible to lead a relatively normal life with renal insufficiency unless other illnesses place an additional burden on kidney function.

Medical Treatment

The primary goal of treatment for AKI is to prevent further damage. Supportive measures aim to control symptoms and to prevent complications. Support measures include fluid and dietary restrictions, restoration of electrolyte balance, and dialysis if needed. Nephrotoxic drugs and drugs that reduce renal blood flow must be avoided. Additional treatment depends on the cause of the failure. For prerenal AKI, BP and blood volume must be restored. Treatment of intrinsic AKI is based on efforts to stimulate urine production with intravenous fluids and with dopamine, furosemide, or both. Postrenal AKI is treated by removal of the cause (typically an obstruction).

Drug Therapy. Oliguria is treated with diuretics, most often an osmotic diuretic such as mannitol or a loop diuretic such as furosemide (Lasix) or ethacrynic acid (Edecrin). Hyperkalemia, which typically accompanies oliguria, is treated aggressively because it can be life threatening. Drugs given intravenously to lower serum potassium include hypertonic glucose and insulin, sodium bicarbonate, and calcium gluconate. Sodium polystyrene sulfonate (Kayexalate), given orally or rectally, also lowers serum potassium.

Pharmacology Capsule

Oliguria may be treated with diuretics such as mannitol or furosemide.

Diet. Dietary modifications for AKI are based on consideration of serum electrolytes and urea. Sodium and potassium allowances are determined individually. Adequate carbohydrates and fats are provided to prevent the breakdown of fat and protein. Essential amino acid supplements may be ordered. If the patient's nutritional needs are not being met by oral intake, enteral nutritional support is instituted. If the GI tract is not functioning, total parenteral nutrition (TPN) is necessary.

Fluids. Daily fluid needs usually are calculated by adding 600 mL to the previous day's fluid output. The extra 600 mL represents the daily insensible loss (through breathing and perspiration). For example, an oliguric patient who has an output of only 400 mL today would be allowed 400 plus 600 mL, for a total of 1000 mL tomorrow.

Hemodialysis and Peritoneal Dialysis. Conditions that warrant hemodialysis when conservative measures fail include hyperkalemia, severe metabolic acidosis, pulmonary edema, and rising BUN. A temporary cannula can be placed in the jugular, femoral, or subclavian vein. A disadvantage of a femoral cannula is that the patient must be immobile between dialysis treatments. However, if the cannula is removed and replaced repeatedly, a risk of hematoma formation exists. A subclavian cannula can be left in place between treatments but can cause thrombosis, stenosis, pneumothorax, hemothorax, and brachial nerve damage. The disadvantage of leaving the cannula in place is that the risk of infection increases. Per agency policy, only trained dialysis staff should draw blood or administer medications through the temporary cannula. Peritoneal dialysis is also an option, especially for the patient in HF. The section titled "Chronic Kidney Disease" describes these procedures in more detail.

Continuous Renal Replacement Therapy. Continuous renal replacement therapy (CRRT) offers additional options for treating the patient with AKI. A cannula placed in an artery and a vein (arteriovenous therapy) or two veins (venovenous therapy) is connected to tubing that contains a blood filter and a collection device. The patient's blood flows through the tubing and excess fluids, electrolytes, and wastes are filtered into the collection device. The blood is then returned to the patient. This procedure does not require dialysate, has little effect on cardiovascular stability, and is continuous. It can be used alone or with hemodialysis (Fig. 42-12).

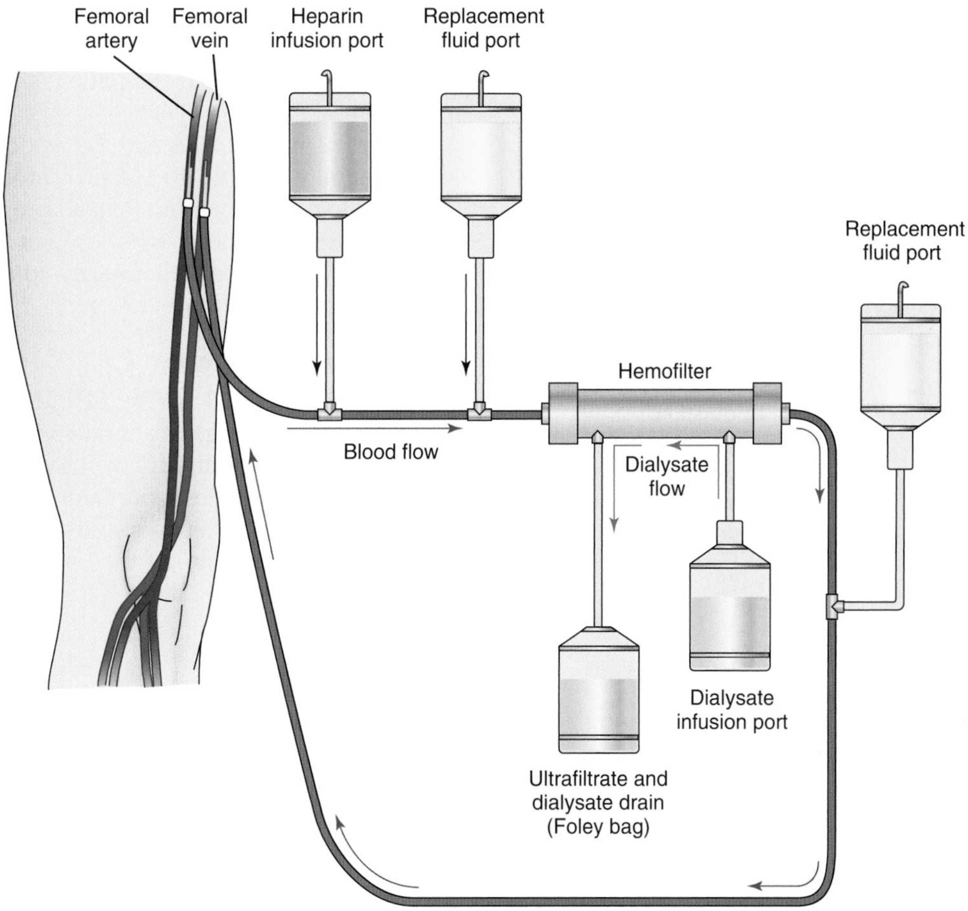

FIGURE 42-12 Continuous renal replacement therapy (CRRT). (From Lewis SM, Heitkemper MM, Dirksen SR: *Medical-surgical nursing: assessment and management of clinical problems*, ed 5, St. Louis, 2000, Mosby.)

NURSING CARE of the Patient with Acute Kidney Injury

Assessment

Complete assessment of the patient with a urinary disorder is summarized in Box 42-1. For the patient with AKI, monitoring fluid status is critical. Intake and output records must be kept carefully. Daily weights are an effective means of assessing changes in fluid status (500 mL of fluid weighs approximately 1 lb). To be useful, daily weights must be done at the same time each day, using the same scale, and with the patient wearing the same amount of clothing. Because hypervolemia (fluid volume excess) is a major problem during the oliguric stage, assess for signs and symptoms of impending heart failure: hypertension, bounding pulse, edema, cough, dysrhythmias.

Electrolyte imbalances can include alterations in serum potassium, sodium, calcium, phosphate, and magnesium. Signs and symptoms of each of these imbalances are discussed in Chapter 14. General assessment of electrolyte balance includes cardiac rate and rhythm, neuromuscular status, edema, and mental status. The acutely ill patient also must be monitored for signs and symptoms related to immobility (i.e., pressure sores, impaired circulation, constipation, atelectasis).

One final area of assessment is the patient's understanding of the condition and its treatment. Identify fears, anxiety, coping strategies, and sources of support.

Nursing Diagnoses, Goals, and Outcome Criteria: Acute Kidney Injury

Nursing Diagnoses	Goals and Outcome Criteria
Excess Fluid Volume related to impaired kidney function (oliguric stage)	Normal fluid and electrolyte balance: normal tissue turgor, absence of dyspnea, normal serum electrolyte values
Decreased Cardiac Output and **Deficient Fluid Volume** related to high-output renal failure (diuretic stage)	Normal cardiac output: pulse and blood pressure (BP) consistent with patient norms

Continued

Nursing Diagnoses, Goals, and Outcome Criteria: Acute Kidney Injury—cont'd

Nursing Diagnoses	Goals and Outcome Criteria
Anxiety related to life-threatening illness	Decreased anxiety: patient states anxiety is reduced, calm manner
Risk for Disuse Syndrome related to immobility	Absence of complications associated with immobility: intact skin, regular bowel movements without difficulty, breath sounds clear to auscultation
Deficient Knowledge of condition, treatment, and self-care related to lack of information	Patient understands condition, treatment, and self-care: patient accurately describes and participates in self-care as allowed

Interventions

Excess Fluid Volume

Assess and document fluid status on an ongoing basis. In the oliguric stage, fluid is likely to be restricted. Explain and reinforce fluid restrictions. The fluid allowance during the oliguric stage may be very limited. Measures to help the patient cope with fluid limitations include considering patient preferences in fluid selection and carefully planning fluid intake throughout waking hours. Remember to plan for fluids needed to take medications. When only a few ounces of fluids are allowed at a time, a small juice cup should be used rather than a large glass that is only one-quarter full. This creates an illusion of volume that may make the patient feel less deprived. To obtain patient cooperation, it is essential for the patient and family to understand the importance of adhering to the fluid restriction.

Give diuretics as ordered and monitor the patient for adverse effects. A fluid challenge of normal saline may be rapidly infused while diuretics are given to promote improved renal perfusion.

Decreased Cardiac Output and Deficient Fluid Volume

In the diuretic stage, patients produce large volumes of dilute urine. Deficient fluid volume becomes a possibility. The heart rate must increase to make up for the diminished blood volume. Because eventually the heart may fail, it is important to monitor for cardiac dysrhythmias, changes in blood pressure, and shortness of breath. Give oral and intravenous fluids as ordered with careful monitoring of output at the same time

Anxiety

Anxiety is understandable when a vital organ fails. The patient may fear death or chronic illness, with the potential for financial ruin, loss of vitality, and dependence on medical care. Provide honest responses to questions about renal failure and its treatment. Refer specific questions about the patient's prognosis to the physician.

The patient with AKI may have a complete recovery. This may take up to 1 year. Unfortunately, some patients do not recover but instead progress to chronic kidney disease. Those who do not improve need special support to help them learn to accept and deal with this major health deviation.

Risk for Disuse Syndrome

The patient with AKI is very ill and may be immobilized. Therefore you must attend to prevention of complications of immobility as well as to the acute renal problem. This includes skin care, turning, coughing, deep breathing, leg exercises, and measures to promote bowel elimination. Care of the immobilized patient is described in Chapter 21.

Deficient Knowledge

When the patient is acutely ill, provide basic information about the disease, diagnostic tests and procedures, and treatments. Explain the reasons for interventions such as fluid restrictions, turning, deep breathing, and leg exercises. As the patient improves, patient teaching should include management of fluids, diet, drug therapy, activity, and signs and symptoms that should be reported to the physician (i.e., dyspnea, edema, fever).

CHRONIC KIDNEY DISEASE

Chronic kidney disease is characterized by progressive destruction of the nephrons of both kidneys. The severity is described in stages, with the final stage (stage 5) being end-stage renal disease. The healthy kidneys comprise far more nephrons than needed. Therefore a person can lose about 80% of the nephrons before kidney function becomes impaired. Creatinine clearance is an important measure of renal function. When it falls below 15 mL/min, dialysis or transplantation becomes necessary.

Chronic kidney disease is characterized by **azotemia** (i.e., increased nitrogenous waste products in the blood). **Uremia** is the term used when the condition advances to the point that the kidneys are unable to maintain fluid and electrolyte or acid-base balance. Uremia is also called *end-stage renal disease.* All of the causes of AKI listed earlier may lead to chronic kidney disease. In addition, chronic renal infections may predispose the patient to progressive renal failure. However, the most common causes are hypertension, diabetes mellitus, and atherosclerosis.

Signs and Symptoms

Azotemia. The first function lost in chronic kidney disease is the ability to concentrate urine. This results in an increase of waste products in the blood, despite producing large amounts of dilute urine. As the disease progresses, urine output typically declines until very little to no urine is produced.

BUN is an approximate estimate of the glomerular filtration rate (GFR). It is affected by protein breakdown. Normal BUN ranges from 10 to 20 mg/dL. When BUN reaches or exceeds 70 mg/dL, dialysis is needed to reduce it.

Serum creatinine is a waste product of skeletal muscle breakdown. It is a more reliable measure of kidney function than BUN. It is not affected by diet, hydration, hepatic function, or metabolism. Normal serum creatinine is 0.5 to 1.5 mg/dL. A serum creatinine level that is twice the normal level reflects a 50% loss of function. When the value reaches or exceeds 10 times normal, 90% of function has been lost. The kidneys are able to adapt to a loss of up to 80% of function. The kidneys increase in size in an attempt to maintain function.

Creatinine clearance (a urine test) is the best indicator of renal function. It is ordered less often than serum creatinine, however, because it requires collection of all urine in a 12- or 24-hour period. Normal creatinine clearance exceeds 100 mL/min.

Insulin Resistance. In renal failure, cells become resistant to the action of insulin. As a result, blood insulin and glucose levels rise. Hyperinsulinemia (high blood insulin) stimulates the liver to produce triglycerides. Patients with chronic kidney disease have high serum levels of very-low-density lipoproteins (VLDLs). Elevated lipids in the blood contribute to atherosclerosis.

Electrolyte and Acid-Base Imbalances

Hyperkalemia. The primary means of potassium excretion is through the kidneys. As kidney function fails, potassium is retained, which results in hyperkalemia, the most life-threatening effect of renal failure. The normal range for serum potassium is 3.5 to 5.0 mEq/L. Elevated serum potassium interferes with normal cardiac function, causing cardiac dysrhythmias. Dysrhythmias are potentially fatal. The patient becomes apathetic and confused and may have nausea, abdominal cramps, muscle weakness, and numbness of the extremities. Serum potassium greater than 6 mg/dL requires cardiac monitoring. If the serum potassium is not reduced, bradycardia (pulse ≤50 beats per minute [bpm]) or asystole (no heartbeat) may develop.

Hyperkalemia is treated with intravenous glucose and insulin or intravenous 10% calcium gluconate. These drugs drive potassium back into the cells, reducing the serum potassium level. They are used as temporary emergency measures. Kayexalate, given orally or rectally, causes potassium to be drawn into the bowel and eliminated in the feces. The method used most often to reduce elevated serum potassium is dialysis.

Hypocalcemia. Diseased kidney tissue lacks the enzyme that activates vitamin D. Without active vitamin D, calcium absorption from the bowel decreases. The body tries to compensate by shifting calcium from the bones to the blood. Serum phosphate binds with calcium, further depleting calcium levels. The normal serum calcium level is 9 to 11 mg/dL or 4.5 to 5.5 mEq/L. Abnormally low serum calcium is called *hypocalcemia*. Patients with hypocalcemia experience tingling sensations, muscle twitches, irritability, and tetany. Tetany is sustained, painful muscle contraction. Hypocalcemia is treated with calcium supplements, active vitamin D, and phosphate binders. Phosphate binders include calcium carbonate, calcium acetate, or sevelamer (Renagel). Side effects of phosphate binders include hypophosphatemia and constipation. Antacids with aluminum or magnesium, such as milk of magnesia, magnesium carbonate, magnesium oxide, and magnesium trisilicate, should be avoided.

Metabolic Acidosis. Failure of the renal tubules to excrete acid ions and acid waste products causes the body's acid level to rise. Decreased bicarbonate reabsorption renders the body unable to neutralize the excess acid. Excess acid leads to metabolic acidosis. The lungs attempt to compensate by eliminating more CO_2 through hyperventilation. Manifestations of metabolic acidosis are headache, lethargy, and delirium.

Fluid Balance. Most patients with chronic kidney disease retain sodium and water, causing hypernatremia and hypervolemia. Elevated BP and edema are signs of hypervolemia. HF may develop in the hypervolemic patient because the patient's heart cannot handle the high fluid volume. Prevention and treatment of hypervolemia include fluid restriction, diuretics, and dialysis if necessary. A few patients are sodium wasters. These patients lose excess sodium and water in the urine and become hyponatremic and hypovolemic.

Hematologic System

Anemia. Kidneys of patients with chronic kidney disease produce less erythropoietin, a hormone necessary for RBC production. Even the RBCs that are produced have a shorter life span than usual because of the toxic environment in which they live. Therefore patients with chronic kidney disease have anemia. Iron supplements and folic acid may be ordered. Transfusions may be required if the hematocrit (Hct) drops below 20% (normal values: 35% to 45% for women and 45% to 55% for men). A genetically engineered erythropoietin (epoetin alfa) can be administered intravenously after hemodialysis or subcutaneously for patients on peritoneal dialysis. This product improves RBC formation and has reversed anemia and the need for transfusions in some patients with chronic kidney disease.

Infection. Because the inflammatory response diminishes with chronic kidney disease, fewer WBCs gather at the site of an infection or injury. The general immune response is suppressed and antibody production declines. Therefore the patient has a reduced ability to resist infections.

Cardiovascular System. The cardiovascular system is affected by hypervolemia, hyperkalemia, and hypocalcemia. Hypervolemia increases the workload of the heart, possibly leading to HF. Manifestations of HF are moist breath sounds, bounding pulse, dependent edema, and dyspnea. Dysrhythmias may be caused by hyperkalemia or hypocalcemia.

Neurologic System. Neurologic effects of chronic kidney disease are mental status changes (i.e., lethargy, irritability, confusion) and peripheral neuropathy. Peripheral neuropathy may be evident initially as a restless feeling and later as foot drop, loss of feeling in the legs, or paralysis of the legs. Many physicians treat the development of peripheral neuropathy as a signal to begin dialysis.

Disequilibrium syndrome may occur with hemodialysis. The rapid removal of urea from the blood leaves an increased concentration of solutes in the brain and the cerebrospinal fluid (CSF). The solutes increase the osmotic pressure, which draws fluid from the bloodstream into the CSF and brain tissue. Confusion, lethargy, headache, nausea, and vomiting may progress to coma or seizures if not treated. Disequilibrium is corrected with the administration of hypertonic glucose.

Integumentary System. The integumentary system is also affected by the accumulation of waste products. Calcium phosphate crystals and urea accumulate in the skin, causing itching. Dryness results from decreased oil gland production and decreased perspiration. A pale gray to yellow color may result from anemia and from unexcreted bilirubin and uremic pigments. Hair and nails become dry and brittle. *Uremic frost* is the term used when whitish crystals composed of urea and other salts precipitate on the skin. Uremic frost is most often noted around the mouth. It is a very late sign in chronic kidney disease.

Gastrointestinal System. Ammonia is a breakdown product of urea. When ammonia accumulates in the GI tract, it causes irritation, nausea, vomiting, a metallic taste in the mouth, and bleeding. Antacids administered every 2 hours help to relieve the irritation. A diet high in carbohydrates and low in protein is prescribed to reduce the accumulation of urea. Other common GI disturbances with chronic kidney disease are stomatitis (i.e., inflammation of the mouth), anorexia, nausea, vomiting, constipation, and diarrhea.

Musculoskeletal System. The term *renal osteodystrophy* refers to the skeletal changes characteristic of chronic kidney disease. The three major changes are (1) metastatic calcification, (2) bone demineralization, and (3) osteitis fibrosa. Metastatic calcification is deposition of calcium phosphate complexes in blood vessels and in joints, lungs, muscles, and eyes. Deposits in blood vessels can impair blood flow so severely that fingers and toes may become gangrenous. Bone demineralization is directly related to hypocalcemia. Low serum calcium triggers increased production of parathyroid hormone by the parathyroid glands. Parathyroid hormone mobilizes calcium from the bone and shifts it into the blood. Over time, loss of bone mass can be significant. When calcium is lost from bones, it is replaced with fibrous tissue. This condition is called *osteitis fibrosa*.

Reproductive System. Chronic kidney disease affects the male and female reproductive systems. The production of sex hormones declines and libido is diminished. Ovulation and menstruation usually cease in women. Men typically have low sperm counts and erectile dysfunction. The general effects of a chronic illness undoubtedly affect sexual desire and function as well.

Endocrine Function. Patients with chronic kidney disease usually appear hypothyroid. Hyperparathyroidism occurs in response to the chronically low serum calcium and high serum phosphates. Patients with diabetes require less exogenous insulin because the enzyme that normally breaks down insulin (renal insulinase) is reduced. Oral hypoglycemics also place the patient at risk for hypoglycemia because the drugs are normally excreted by the kidneys.

Emotional and Psychologic Effects. Emotional and psychologic effects of chronic kidney disease include emotional lability, depression, anxiety, and slowed intellectual functioning.

Medical Treatment

Treatment of chronic kidney disease aims to promote elimination of wastes, maintenance of fluid balance, and management of the systemic effects of the disease. Conservative treatment of the systemic effects of chronic kidney disease includes:

- Intravenous glucose and insulin, calcium carbonate, calcium acetate, or sodium polystyrene sulfonate to treat hyperkalemia
- Statins in the early stages of renal failure to decrease the risk of cardiovascular complications
- Calcium, active vitamin D, and phosphate binders to treat hypocalcemia
- Fluid and sodium restriction to treat hypervolemia
- Diuretics, angiotensin-converting enzyme inhibitors (ACEIs), angiotensin receptor blockers (ARBs), and calcium channel blockers to treat hypertension
- Water-soluble vitamins to replace those lost in dialysis
- Iron supplements, folic acid, and synthetic erythropoietin to treat anemia
- Hypertonic glucose to treat disequilibrium syndrome

- Diet tailored to chronic kidney disease stage and type of dialysis treatment

Dialysis. When kidney failure no longer can be managed conservatively, dialysis is required to sustain life. Dialysis is the passage of molecules through a semipermeable membrane into a special solution called *dialysate solution*. Dialysis operates like the kidney. Small molecules such as urea, creatinine, and electrolytes pass out of the blood, across a membrane, and into a solution.

The goals of dialysis are to do the following:

- Remove the end products of protein metabolism from the blood
- Maintain safe concentrations of serum electrolytes
- Correct acidosis and replenish the body's bicarbonate buffer system
- Remove excess fluid from the blood

Dialysis enables many patients to maintain or regain self-esteem and to be productive members of society. However, initial positive feelings about dialysis sometimes turn to depression as the reality of "being tied to a machine" is recognized. Two primary means of dialysis are (1) hemodialysis and (2) peritoneal dialysis.

Hemodialysis. Hemodialysis is a process by which blood is removed from the body and circulated through an "artificial kidney" for removal of excess fluid, electrolytes, and wastes. The dialyzed blood is then returned to the patient (Fig. 42-13). Hemodialysis requires vascular access (i.e., access to the patient's bloodstream). This may be accomplished by catheter, cannula, graft, or fistula. Subclavian or femoral catheters can be used for temporary access for dialysis during acute renal failure while a graft or fistula matures (dilates and toughens) or for patients on peritoneal dialysis who need immediate access for hemodialysis.

Internal connections between veins and arteries do not require dressings. An internal connection between the patient's artery and vein is called a *fistula*. A fistula requires approximately 6 to 8 weeks to mature and may be used for 3 to 5 years. Connections also may be made using bovine or synthetic grafts that require 2 to 4 weeks to heal before use and last for 7 to 9 years. Grafts have an increased rate of thrombosis and infection compared with fistulas.

An arteriovenous shunt or cannula is an external connection between an artery and a vein (Fig. 42-14). By connecting the external ends of the synthetic tubing for dialysis, venipuncture is not necessary. However, because the cannula is external, danger of hemorrhage, risk of skin breakdown, restriction of activities, and risk of site infection exist. The arteriovenous shunt is very rarely used because of the potential complications.

All vascular access sites must be assessed for patency. Check pulses below the shunt to ensure that circulation is adequate. *Steal syndrome* occurs when too much arterial blood is diverted from the extremity by the access device. Palpate the venous side of the shunt for a *thrill* or *rippling sensation* caused by movement of blood through a changed pathway. A *bruit* or *swoosh* may be heard through a stethoscope with each heartbeat. Absence of these signs may indicate occlusion of the vessel, making it unsuitable for hemodialysis.

Once vascular access is established, the patient may be hemodialyzed. Blood flows from the artery through the vascular access device, circulates through the

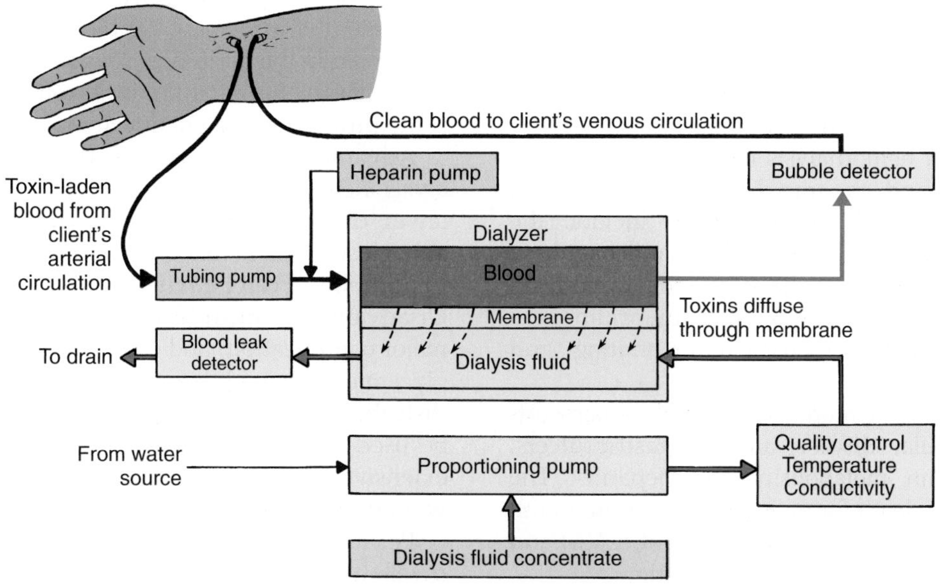

FIGURE 42-13 Schematic diagram of hemodialysis. As the patient's blood passes through the dialyzer, toxins diffuse into the dialysis fluid. (From Black JM, Hawks JH: *Medical-surgical nursing: clinical management for positive outcomes*, ed 8, St. Louis, 2009, Saunders.)

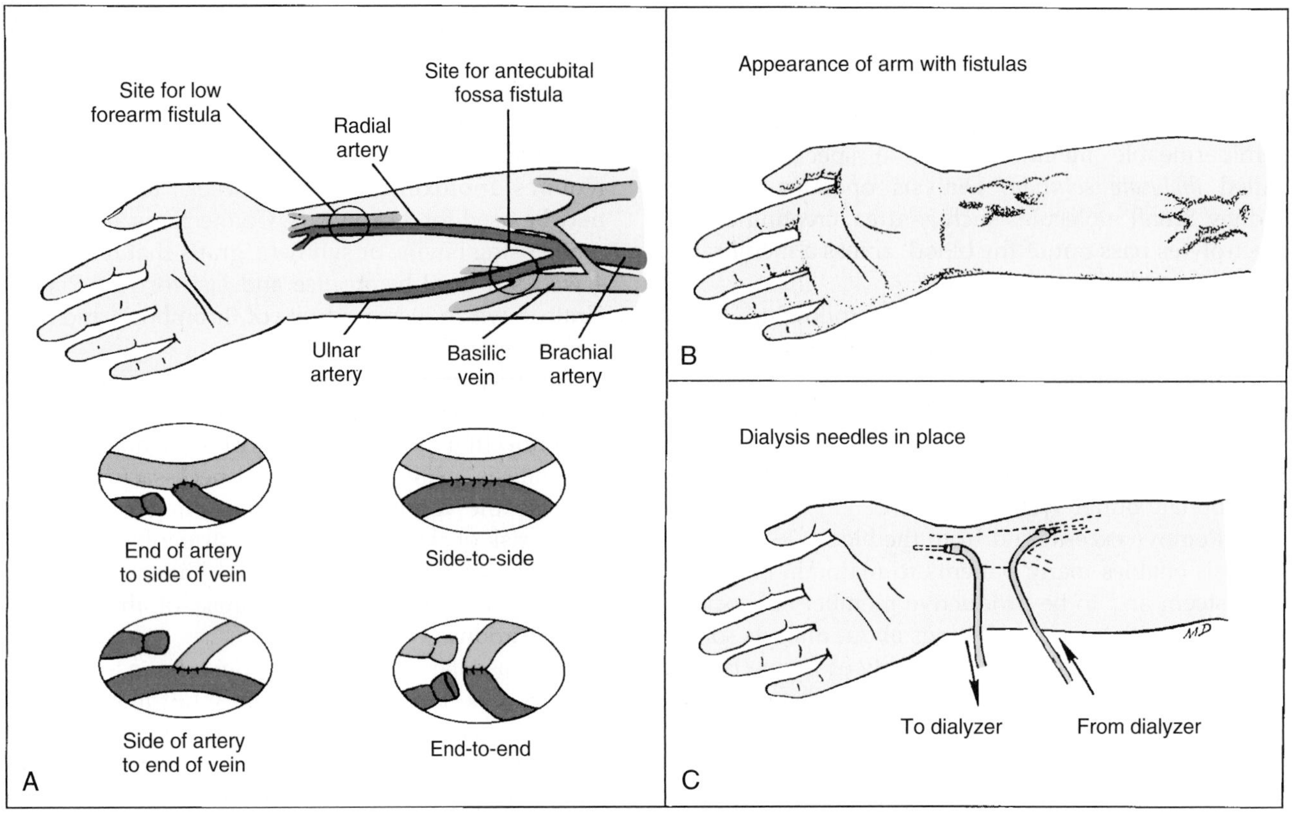

FIGURE 42-14 An internal arteriovenous fistula created by joining an artery and a vein. The fistula will be used for hemodialysis. **A,** Types of fistulas. **B,** The appearance of the arm with fistulas. **C,** Dialysis needles in place in the fistula. (From Black JM, Hawks JH: *Medical-surgical nursing: clinical management for positive outcomes*, ed 8, St. Louis, 2009, Saunders.)

dialyzer, and returns through the venous line. Heparin is used as an anticoagulant to prevent blood from clotting. Hemodialysis requires specially trained personnel and expensive equipment. Although dialysis for chronic kidney disease is usually performed in a dialysis center, home dialysis is available. The hemodialysis process takes approximately 4 hours and is usually done three times weekly. Certain medications, such as antihypertensive agents may be withheld.

Advantages of hemodialysis include its usefulness in emergencies and the rapid removal of wastes, electrolytes, and fluid. Disadvantages include the need for vascular access, the use of an anticoagulant, and the potential for hemorrhage, anemia, rapid fluid and electrolyte shifts (dialysis disequilibrium syndrome), muscle cramps, nausea and vomiting, and air emboli.

Complications of hemodialysis include atherosclerotic cardiovascular disease, anemia, gastric ulcers, disturbed calcium metabolism, and hepatitis. The leading causes of death for patients being treated with hemodialysis are cerebrovascular accident (CVA) and myocardial infarction, followed by infection.

Peritoneal Dialysis. Peritoneal dialysis uses the patient's own peritoneum as a semipermeable dialyzing membrane. Fluid is instilled into the peritoneal cavity; waste products are drawn into the fluid, which is then drained from the peritoneal cavity (Fig. 42-15).

Peritoneal dialysis may be done on either a temporary or a permanent basis. For temporary use, a catheter is inserted in the peritoneal cavity through the abdominal wall. For long-term use, a catheter is implanted in the peritoneal cavity. Over time, a fibrous tissue barrier forms at the insertion site and provides some protection against infection.

Advantages of peritoneal dialysis over hemodialysis include less anemia, reduced cost of equipment, fewer dietary and fluid restrictions, independence, and closer resemblance to normal kidney function. In addition, it can be initiated in almost any hospital. Disadvantages include the risk of peritonitis (the major complication) and catheter site infection, hyperglycemia, elevated serum lipids, and body image disturbance. In addition, peritoneal dialysis cannot be used for patients with recent abdominal surgery, extensive abdominal trauma, or open abdominal wounds.

Peritoneal dialysis has three phases: (1) inflow, (2) dwell, and (3) drain. The three phases comprise one exchange. During inflow, fluid (commonly 2 L) is allowed to drain into the peritoneal cavity through an established catheter over about 10 minutes. During the

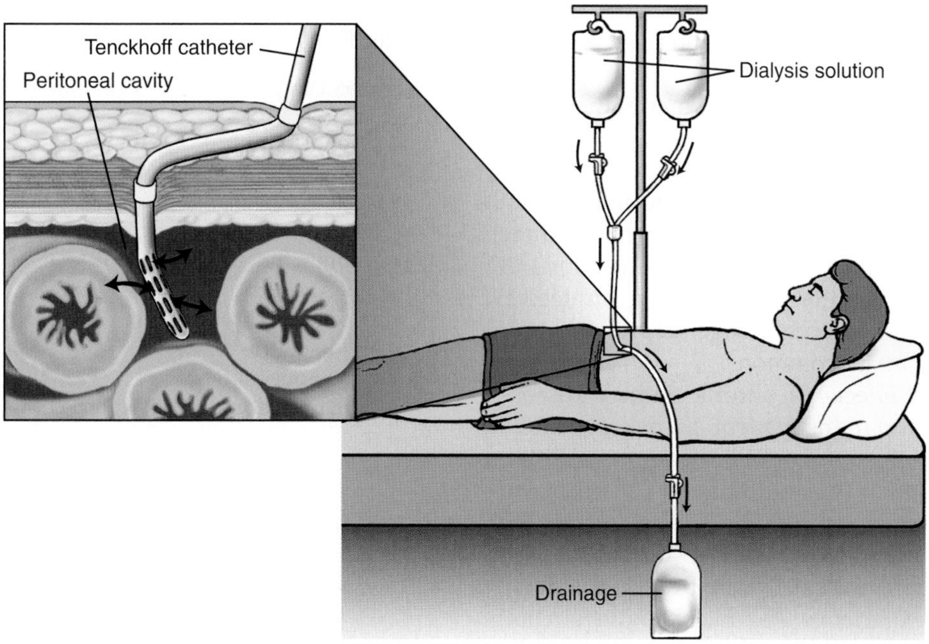

FIGURE 42-15 Peritoneal dialysis. (From Monahan FD, Drake DT, Neighbors M, editors: *Medical-surgical nursing: foundations for clinical practice*, ed 2, Philadelphia, 1998, Saunders.)

dwell time, fluid remains in the cavity for a specified period of time while ultrafiltration, osmosis, and diffusion occur. The fluid bearing wastes and excess water is then drained from the cavity over 20 to 30 minutes.

Continuous ambulatory peritoneal dialysis (CAPD) allows the patient freedom from a machine and the independence to perform dialysis alone. The exchange process usually is repeated four times each day by outpatients. It may be done more often in patients who are acutely ill and hospitalized. Strict aseptic technique must be used with the initiation of the process and with each exchange. The patient or a reliable caregiver must be taught the process by someone who understands it well.

Automated peritoneal dialysis (APD) uses a device called a *cycler* to perform the exchanges during the night. This allows the patient freedom during the day. It also reduces the risk of infection because the system is interrupted less often. Several variations of this procedure exist that may be done from five to seven times a week and may or may not leave the fluid in the abdomen during the waking hours.

Peritonitis (i.e., infection of the peritoneum) is the most serious complication of peritoneal dialysis. Infections also may develop at the catheter exit site and tunnel where the catheter is placed under the skin. Cloudiness and particles in the fluid in the outflow container are evidence of infection. Redness, swelling, and purulent drainage are signs of infection at the exit site. Immediately report any signs of infection to the physician. Peritonitis is usually treated with antibiotics administered through the peritoneal catheter. Other complications include bleeding, abdominal pain, hernias, low back pain, respiratory distress, and decreased serum albumin. Encapsulating sclerosing peritonitis is a condition in which a thick membrane develops around the bowel. The thickened membrane can obstruct the intestines and interfere with ultrafiltration.

❖ NURSING CARE of the Patient with Chronic Kidney Disease

■ Assessment

General assessment of the patient with a urologic disorder is outlined in Box 42-1. For the patient with chronic kidney disease, frequent monitoring for changes in status is especially important. Fluid balance is evaluated closely. During hospitalization, accurate intake and output records must be kept. Be alert for signs and symptoms of excess fluid volume that can lead to cardiac failure. Warning signs include increasing edema, dyspnea, tachycardia, bounding pulse, and rising BP.

Serum electrolytes are measured frequently but you must still be alert for signs and symptoms of electrolyte imbalances. With chronic kidney disease, the nurse is most concerned with detecting hyperkalemia, hypocalcemia, and metabolic acidosis. Hyponatremia and hypovolemia are less common. Assessment of fluid and electrolyte imbalances includes characteristics of pulse and respirations, BP, mental status, and neuromuscular activity.

Assessment of nutrition includes appetite, usual daily intake, weight gain or loss pattern, and prescribed diet. Determine how well the patient understands and follows the prescribed diet (see *Nutrition Considerations* box).

Do not overlook mental and emotional status when assessing the patient with chronic kidney disease. Increasing confusion or loss of consciousness can be due to accumulated toxins or electrolyte imbalances. Emotional responses to a diagnosis of chronic kidney disease vary. Determine the patient's perceptions of the situation and identify usual coping strategies. Anxiety, fear, disturbed body image, depression, and lowered self-esteem are common.

The long-term effects of chronic kidney disease and its treatment put the patient at risk for many complications. Monitor bowel elimination for either constipation or diarrhea. Monitor for signs and symptoms of local or systemic infections (redness, swelling, foul drainage, fever, increased WBC count). Inspect the skin for bruising, bleeding, or trauma. Evaluate sensation in the extremities. Ask if sexual dysfunction has been a problem and obtain a description of the problem.

Explore patient understanding about chronic kidney disease, its treatment, and self-care measures. Document the patient's ability to perform ADL.

Specific nursing diagnoses and goals vary based on the individual patient data. Many diagnoses and interventions discussed in the section titled "Acute Kidney Injury" also apply to the patient with chronic kidney disease. The emphasis in this section is on the common problems experienced by the patient with chronic failure.

Nursing Diagnoses, Goals, and Outcome Criteria: Chronic Kidney Disease

Nursing Diagnoses	Goals and Outcome Criteria
Excess Fluid Volume related to fluid retention	Reduced fluid volume and absence of symptoms of heart failure: normal tissue turgor, blood pressure (BP) within patient norms, no dyspnea
Imbalanced Nutrition: Less Than Body Requirements related to anorexia, nausea, vomiting, stomatitis, dietary restrictions	Adequate nutrition: consumption of prescribed diet, serum albumin and total protein within acceptable limits
Risk for Acute Confusion related to effects of uremia on the nervous system	Normal sensory perception: alert and oriented
Ineffective Coping related to multiple life changes	Effective coping: patient uses coping strategies that decrease anxiety without compromising care

Nursing Diagnoses, Goals, and Outcome Criteria: Chronic Kidney Disease—cont'd

Nursing Diagnoses	Goals and Outcome Criteria
Situational Low Self-Esteem related to self-worth, change in appearance, loss of kidney function, venous access devices, inability to fulfill usual roles and responsibilities	Improved self-esteem: positive statements of confidence
Risk for Infection related to impaired immune response, malnutrition, break in skin integrity	Absence of infection: normal body temperature and white blood cell (WBC) count
Risk for Injury related to coagulation disorder, impaired wound healing, bone demineralization, peripheral neuropathy	Absence of injury: no bruises, bleeding, fractures
Constipation related to inactivity, drug side effects, fluid restriction, electrolyte imbalances	Normal bowel elimination: regular formed stools passed without straining
Diarrhea related to electrolyte imbalances, drug side effects	Normal bowel elimination: formed stools
Sexual Dysfunction related to fatigue, drug side effects, hormone deficiencies, altered self-image	Satisfactory sexual function: patient states intimate relationship is satisfactory
Ineffective Self-Health Management related to lack of knowledge, confusion, anemia, fatigue	Accomplishment of self-care: patient performs activities of daily living (ADL) within limitations imposed by renal failure and treatments

Interventions

Excess Fluid Volume

As renal failure progresses, the patient's ability to excrete excess fluids continually declines. In the early stages, diuretics may be used to treat fluid retention but they are not used once dialysis is begun. Fluid intake may be restricted. If intravenous fluids are ordered, closely monitor the rate of infusion. Antihypertensive drugs may be needed to control blood pressure and digitalis may be given to support cardiac function. Dosage adjustments often are needed because kidney failure affects the ability to excrete these drugs. Administer medications, monitor for side effects, and teach the patient how to take them after discharge and what adverse effects to report.

Patients with excess fluid volume require comfort and safety measures. Edematous legs are injured easily and heal slowly. Protect them from pressure or trauma. If cardiac failure and dyspnea develop, position the patient with the head elevated to ease breathing. Cerebral edema causes confusion and decreasing consciousness. Implement safety measures to protect the confused or semiconscious patient from injury.

Pharmacology Capsule

Because most drugs are excreted in the urine, people with impaired renal function are at risk for drug toxicity.

Imbalanced Nutrition: Less Than Body Requirements

Adequate nutrition can be a challenge for the patient with chronic kidney disease. Anorexia, nausea, vomiting, and stomatitis interfere with food intake. In addition, sodium, potassium, protein, and sometimes fat restrictions make the diet less appealing. Measures to encourage food intake include frequent mouth care and small feedings. Explain the importance of good nutrition to the patient and family. The dietitian can help the patient learn to cope with the diet. The person who prepares the patient's food at home should be included in dietary instructions. Vitamin supplements are routinely ordered because of dietary restrictions. Monitor weight to evaluate both fluid and nutritional status. Teach the patient and the caregivers about medications and status monitors.

Nutrition Considerations

1. Renal failure results in an inability of the kidneys to excrete wastes and maintain fluid and electrolyte balance.
2. With renal failure, the nutritional goal is to modify the diet so that the work of the kidneys is reduced.
3. Fluid intake may be restricted to 1000 to 1500 mL/day for patients with renal disease.
4. Sodium and potassium intakes are restricted (including medications) to maintain electrolyte balance in patients who require dialysis.
5. Protein is restricted in patients with renal disease and any protein ingested should be high in essential amino acids. Examples of these proteins are eggs, meat, poultry, fish, and milk products.
6. People with renal calculi should increase fluid intake to maintain at least 2 L of urine output daily and should avoid foods that lead to the formation of calculi.
7. Contrary to previous beliefs, people with *low* serum calcium are at increased risk for formation of calculi.

Risk for Acute Confusion

Renal failure affects the central nervous system (CNS) and the peripheral nervous systems. Cerebral edema and elevated metabolic wastes in the blood can cause confusion, slowed thought processes, lethargy, and loss of consciousness. Protect confused patients and orient them to person, place, and time. Present information simply and repeat as needed. Avoid sensory overload by reducing environmental stimuli and demands on the patient. For safety reasons, assign the patient to a room close to the nurses' station. Put the bed in the low position and keep the call bell within reach.

The effects of renal disease on the peripheral nerves can lead to loss of sensation in the extremities (peripheral neuropathy). These patients are at risk for injury. Inspect the affected areas daily for any signs of injury. Pressure, ill-fitting shoes, or external heat or cold can cause serious injury before the patient is aware of it. Teach the patient about peripheral neuropathy and how to prevent injuries.

Ineffective Coping

Patients with chronic kidney disease often experience anxiety and fear. They face life-threatening illness, endure invasive treatments and procedures, and undergo radical changes in lifestyle. Explore the patient's coping strategies, and identify factors that interfere with adjustment to renal disease. It helps for the patient to have a regular primary nurse so that a therapeutic relationship can develop. Nurses can help by talking to patients and having them focus on the sources of their distress. It is important to be accepting of the patient's thoughts and feelings. Do not give false reassurance or tell patients not to worry! Explain routines and procedures and provide practical advice on the management of everyday problems. Many patients benefit from talking to a mental health professional or attending support groups with people with similar problems. While encouraging patients to accept treatment, respect their rights to be informed and to refuse treatment.

People on dialysis typically go through stages of adjustment. When dialysis is first started, they usually feel much better. They feel encouraged and view dialysis positively. This might be described as a "honeymoon period." At this stage, the patient is most receptive to teaching. It is wise to take advantage of this opportunity to educate the patient.

After several months of treatment, patients tire of the routine. Depression and disappointment are common. Some cope by denying the need for treatment. They may omit medications or fail to keep appointments for follow-up. Be accepting of the patient but not the behavior at this stage. Confront the patient when ineffective coping behaviors are identified.

Eventually, most patients accept the need for ongoing treatment. They may try to resume their former levels of activity. At this point, you may need to guide them in realistic goal setting.

Situational Low Self-Esteem

The patient's self-esteem may suffer because of changes in body image and role performance. Encourage patients to talk about the changes they are experiencing and what they mean. Therapeutic communication and touch convey acceptance to patients. Help the patient with grooming to enhance appearance.

Encourage patients to examine their daily routines and look for ways to conserve time and energy. Sources of help and support need to be identified (see *Complementary and Alternative Therapies* box). Family functions may have to be redistributed. It is important for the patient to continue to have roles in the family and to be seen as a contributing family member.

> **Complementary and Alternative Therapies**
>
> Patients with irreversible chronic diseases are vulnerable to claims of miracle cures. Caution patients to discuss alternative therapies with the physician to prevent potentially harmful outcomes.

Risk for Infection

Patients with chronic kidney disease must avoid exposure to others with infections. Be sure that they know how to take their own temperatures. Instruct them to report fever or other signs of infection to the physician. Practice good hand washing and aseptic technique for invasive procedures.

Risk for Injury

The patient is susceptible to injury because of impaired coagulation and wound healing, bone demineralization, and peripheral neuropathy. Calcium, vitamin D, and phosphate binders are ordered to reduce loss of calcium from the bones. Encourage ambulation, which helps to strengthen bones. Assess and protect body parts that lack sensation. Provide an environment with adequate support equipment and few obstacles that might cause bruises or falls.

Constipation

Constipation is a common problem with chronic kidney disease because of inactivity, fluid restriction, electrolyte imbalances, and drug side effects. Encourage activity within the patient's tolerance level. Stool softeners often are ordered to prevent constipation.

Diarrhea

Diarrhea may be caused by drugs or anxiety. Measure liquid stools and count as fluid output. Give antidiarrheals as ordered. Provide perianal care after each stool.

Sexual Dysfunction

Sexual dysfunction is attributed to physical and emotional causes. At first you may feel uncomfortable discussing sexual function with patients but they need to know that it is acceptable to express concerns. Explain how kidney disease affects sexual function and explore what this means to the patient. Referral to a counselor who specializes in treatment of sexual dysfunction may be appreciated. Alternative means of sexual expression may enable the patient to continue to feel loved and to be intimate with another person.

Ineffective Self-Health Management

Patients with chronic kidney disease spend more time at home than they do in the hospital. Nurses need to prepare them for self-care.

RENAL TRANSPLANTATION

KIDNEY DONATION

In 2010, 17,500 kidney transplants were done in the United States, with high rates of success. A healthy kidney may be obtained from a live donor (usually a relative) or from a cadaver. When a kidney is obtained from a living related donor, the 1-year recipient survival rate is 97.6%. Among the transplanted kidneys, 95% are functioning well 1 year later. Among patients who receive transplants from cadavers, 94% are alive 1 year later and 90% of those transplanted kidneys survive at least 1 year. The tissues of the donor and the recipient must match or the recipient will reject the new kidney. Matching is based on ABO blood groups and human leukocyte antigens. Crossmatching between the blood of the prospective donor and recipient reveals any cytotoxic preformed antibodies that would certainly result in organ rejection. A national network maintains lists of people awaiting donor kidneys. When a cadaver kidney is available, the network tries to locate the best match for the kidney to improve the chances of success.

Kidney donors must be at least 18 years of age, be free of systemic disease or infection, have no history of cancer or renal disease, have normal renal function, and be without major medical problems. People older than 60 years may be considered as candidates for donation on an individual basis. Unfortunately, many older people have advanced cardiac or respiratory disease that makes them ineligible.

Cadavers must meet the same criteria as living donors. Many people carry signed donor cards indicating their willingness to have organs used for transplantation in the event of brain death. If brain death does occur, written permission is still sought from the family of the potential donor before organs are removed. The vital organs of the brain-dead person must be kept functioning until the kidney is removed.

PREOPERATIVE NURSING CARE of the Renal Transplant Recipient

In some respects, preoperative care of the renal transplant recipient is similar to that of any other patient facing major surgery (see Chapter 17). The patient must be prepared mentally and physically for the procedure. The unique aspect of this situation is that the patient awaits an organ from another human being. If a relative is the donor, the surgery can be planned and both people prepared emotionally. Counseling is advised for both the donor and the recipient. The patient may be ambivalent about receiving a relative's organ. The gift of a kidney can restore health but the recipient may feel guilty about asking a loved one to endure surgery and to give up an organ. The donor faces the stress of surgery and a future with only one kidney. The donor also has to accept that the kidney could be rejected. Both recipient and donor face the threat of surgical complications.

If awaiting a cadaver kidney, the patient must face the idea that someone must die for a kidney to become available. These potential recipients are on call and must be ready to report to the hospital at any time. In a given year, only about 1 in 4 of the 75,000 patients on waiting lists receives a kidney.

The recipient and the live donor have complete diagnostic workups to rule out other medical problems and to evaluate the function of the urinary tract. Normal function of both of the donor's kidneys must be affirmed. The recipient is given medications to bring BP within normal limits. Immunosuppressant drugs are started to control the body's response to foreign tissue (i.e., the donated kidney; see Table 42-3). The recipient also may be given a transfusion of the donor's blood, a measure that has been found to reduce rejection. If the recipient has severe hypertension or a UTI, bilateral nephrectomies may be done before transplantation. The patient is dialyzed shortly before transplantation.

Assessment

In the preoperative period, a complete assessment is done as outlined in Chapter 17. Before renal transplantation, explore the patient's understanding of the surgery. Record baseline vital signs. Identify any specific fears or questions that need to be addressed.

Nursing Diagnoses, Goals, and Outcome Criteria: Renal Transplantation, Preoperative

Nursing Diagnoses	Goals and Outcome Criteria
Fear related to perceived threat of death	Reduced fear: patient states fear is lessened
Deficient Knowledge of surgical routines related to lack of information	Patient understands surgical routines: patient verbalizes accurate information, cooperates in care

Interventions

To achieve these goals, acknowledge and encourage the patient to discuss concerns. Accept fear as understandable and natural. Factual information helps the patient to cope by reducing fear of the unknown. Involve the patient in planning and self-care. When patients are active participants in their care, they feel less helpless and less anxious. Preoperative teaching begins when the patient is identified as a candidate for transplantation. Reinforce information when the actual surgery is imminent. It is somewhat more difficult to teach the patient who is awaiting a cadaver kidney because one never knows when, or if, the transplantation will take place.

SURGICAL PROCEDURE

The donor kidney is removed from the live donor in an operating room and taken to an adjacent room where the recipient has been prepared to receive it. A cadaver kidney is removed under sterile conditions and transported to the hospital where the recipient is waiting. The donor kidney is placed in the recipient's abdomen and anastomosed (attached) to the bladder via the ureter and also to the blood vessels (Fig. 42-16).

Complications

Complications after renal transplantation include acute tubular necrosis (ATN), rejection, renal artery stenosis, hematomas, abscesses, and leakage of ureteral or vascular anastomoses. When the time between organ harvest and implantation is delayed, a risk of ATN exists. With ATN, urine output may decline or water but not metabolic wastes may be eliminated. This condition requires dialysis until renal function improves (it usually does). Rejection of the new organ by the recipient is a major problem with most tissue

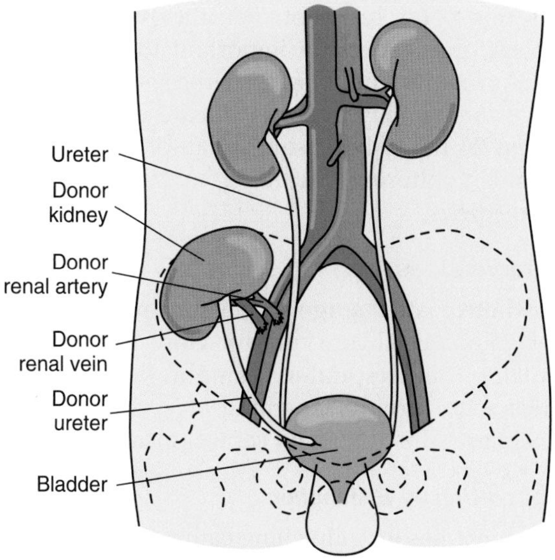

FIGURE 42-16 Placement of a transplanted kidney. (From Monahan F, Sands J, Neighbors M, et al.: *Phipps' medical-surgical nursing: health and illness perspectives*, ed 8, St. Louis, 2007, Mosby.)

transplants. Rejection is characterized by fever, elevated BP, and pain over the location of the new kidney. Three types of rejection can occur: (1) hyperacute, (2) acute, and (3) chronic. Hyperacute rejection occurs within 48 hours after transplantation. It is not reversible and the kidney must be removed. Acute rejection develops between 1 week and 2 years after transplantation and is treated with increased immunosuppressant drugs. Chronic rejection develops and progresses slowly. Chronic rejection eventually mimics chronic kidney disease and dialysis may become necessary.

Immunosuppressant drugs, begun before surgery, are continued in the postoperative period to reduce the risk of rejection. These drugs include (1) T cell suppressors: cyclosporine, tacrolimus, or sirolimus; (2) cytotoxic drugs: cyclophosphamide; and (3) corticosteroids. Antibodies are drugs that are used primarily for short periods to prevent or reverse acute rejection. Those used for transplant patients include polyclonal antibodies (antithymocyte globulin, antilymphocyte globulin) and monoclonal antibodies (muromonab-CD3, daclizumab). Examples of immunosuppressant agents, their actions and adverse effects, and nursing interventions are provided in Table 42-4. They are called *immunosuppressants* because they inhibit the body's immune response to foreign tissue. This action is intended to prevent the donor kidney from being destroyed by the recipient's defenses. Unfortunately, the action of immunosuppressants also reduces the body's response to pathogens. Therefore patients who take these drugs are at increased risk for infection.

❖ POSTOPERATIVE NURSING Care of the Renal Transplant Recipient

■ Assessment

General postoperative care is described in Chapter 17. This section emphasizes care that is unique to the renal transplant recipient. For the renal transplant recipient, it is especially important to monitor fluid intake, urine output, weight changes, and vital signs. Patients are usually in a critical care unit for at least the first 24 hours because circulatory status requires constant monitoring, including central venous pressure readings.

■ Interventions

Immediately after surgery, the transplant patient is taken to a special care unit for close monitoring for circulatory and respiratory complications. Assist the patient with turning, coughing, deep breathing, and leg exercises. Institute pain control measures.

Impaired Urinary Elimination

The patient has an indwelling catheter for 3 to 5 days to permit constant observation of urine output. Urine is pink to bloody initially and then gradually clears. Maintain catheter patency at all times. You may have an order to gently irrigate the catheter if obstruction by blood clots is suspected. Closely monitor the patient for signs that the transplanted organ is functioning: increasing urine output, normal BP, decreasing BUN and serum creatinine, stable weight. Commonly, the patient begins to diurese (i.e., eliminate excess fluid) as soon as blood flow to the donor kidney is established. The output may be as high as 1 L/h until BUN and serum creatinine return to normal.

If the patient is oliguric, a fluid challenge and diuretics are prescribed. In addition to the possibilities of renal failure and rejection, be alert for signs and symptoms of cardiac failure related to excess fluid volume (i.e., dyspnea, edema, bounding pulse, cardiac dysrhythmias).

Nursing Diagnoses, Goals, and Outcome Criteria: Renal Transplantation, Postoperative

Nursing Diagnoses	Goals and Outcome Criteria
Impaired Urinary Elimination related to rejection of transplanted kidney, renal failure	Adequate urine elimination: fluid intake and output equal
Deficient Fluid Volume related to diuresis, blood loss	Normal fluid volume: pulse and blood pressure (BP) consistent with patient norms
Risk for Infection related to suppression of immune response	Absence of infection: normal body temperature and white blood cell (WBC) count
Ineffective Self-Health Management of immediate and long-term postoperative care related to lack of information	Effective management of self-care: patient accurately describes and carries out plan of care
Anxiety related to possibility of organ rejection	Reduced anxiety: patient states anxiety is lessened, calm manner

Put on Your Thinking Cap!

What are some measures that you can take to maintain catheter patency in the posttransplant patient?

Deficient Fluid Volume

Massive postoperative diuresis causes fluid volume deficit in some patients. With excessive fluid loss, the patient is at risk for electrolyte imbalances and decreased cardiac output. A thready pulse, low BP, and poor tissue turgor suggest dehydration. Serum electrolyte studies are ordered to identify specific imbalances. Intravenous fluid orders must be carefully individualized.

Risk for Infection

Because the immunosuppressant drugs that protect the new kidney also inhibit the body's ability to resist pathogens, you must monitor the transplant recipient carefully for signs and symptoms of infection (i.e., fever, elevated WBC count, cough, purulent wound drainage). Signs and symptoms may be very subtle despite a major infection. Use good hand washing and aseptic technique when working with the patient. Separate the patient from others who have infections. Teach the patient and family members the importance of protecting the patient from exposure to infections. Give prophylactic antibiotics as prescribed. The physician prescribes any restrictions on diet, fluids, and activity. Clarify and reinforce these orders. It is critical that the patient knows the signs and symptoms of infection, rejection, and renal failure.

Ineffective Self-Health Management

Ideally, patient teaching begins before the transplant so that it can be reinforced after the procedure (see *Patient Teaching* box).

Anxiety

Anxiety may lessen as renal function improves but the patient always lives with the possibility of rejection. It is helpful for the patient to talk about feelings and explore ways to deal with them. Some patients find comfort in a support group of people who have had similar experiences or in spiritual resources. Others may need referral to a mental health professional to help them deal constructively with their stress.

Patient Teaching

Kidney Transplant

- Take your medication exactly as prescribed to control rejection and prevent other complications.
- Report adverse effects (specific to your drugs) to the physician.
- Follow the diet prescribed by your physician.
- Avoid people with infections because your resistance is lowered.
- Increase activity as allowed by your physician.
- Immediately notify your physician of signs and symptoms of infection (i.e., fever, cough, increasing wound drainage) and rejection (i.e., fever, pain in kidney area).

KIDNEY DONOR

In the excitement over the patient finally receiving a kidney, never forget the role of the donor at this dramatic time. Physical care of the donor is similar to that described earlier for nephrectomy. The nephrectomy may be conventional or laparoscopic. Pain is considerably worse with the conventional approach, so be sure to provide good pain control measures. With the conventional approach, the patient will be hospitalized 4 to 7 days and return to work in 6 to 8 weeks. With the laparoscopic approach, the donor is hospitalized 2 to 4 days and can return to work in 4 to 6 weeks.

Emotionally, the donor usually feels very good about the experience because of the value of the kidney to the recipient. If the kidney fails, however, the donor may be very disappointed. Be sensitive to the emotional needs of the donor.

Get Ready for the NCLEX® Examination!

Key Points

- The urinary system eliminates metabolic wastes in urine; stimulates RBC production; and maintains fluid, electrolyte, and acid-base balance.
- Age-related changes in the urinary system include reduced ability to concentrate or dilute urine, nocturia, and decreased bladder capacity.
- Untreated or repeated UTIs can result in renal scarring and lead to renal failure.
- Inflammatory conditions of the urinary tract include cystitis (bladder inflammation), urethritis (urethral inflammation), glomerulonephritis (glomerular inflammation), and pyelonephritis (inflammation of the renal pelvis).
- Risk factors for UTI include prolonged immobility, renal calculi, urinary diversion, and indwelling urinary catheters.
- UTIs are treated with antibiotics, urinary tract antiseptics, analgesics, and antispasmodic agents.
- Acute glomerulonephritis commonly follows a streptococcal respiratory infection and results in an immune response that scars the glomeruli.
- Patients with renal disorders are at risk for excess fluid volume, hypertension, and heart failure.
- Management of renal disorders requires attention to pain management, fluid balance, activity intolerance, and patient education.
- Urinary obstructions anywhere in the urinary tract can lead to hydronephrosis and kidney damage.
- Urinary calculi (stones) form in the urinary tract and may move through the tract with the flow of urine.
- Although most calculi pass spontaneously, some require surgical removal or disintegration by lithotripsy.
- Nursing care of the patient with renal calculi focuses on acute pain, impaired urinary elimination, risk for electrolyte imbalance, and ineffective self-health management.
- Complications of urinary tract surgery include urinary tract and wound infection, atelectasis, paralytic ileus, and hemorrhage.
- Renal tumors are often large before they are detected because early symptoms are subtle.
- Cystectomy (bladder removal) requires urine to be diverted to an alternate drainage or collection system. Types of urinary diversion used now are ileal and sigmoid conduits, ureterostomy, and nephrostomy.

- A neobladder is created from a segment of bowel and connected to the urethra for normal voiding.
- Nursing care after bladder surgery focuses on pain management, unobstructed urine flow, skin integrity, bowel function, and self-care.
- Renal failure can result from hypotension, toxins, infections, impaired blood flow, trauma, and obstructions.
- The four stages of acute renal failure are (1) onset, (2) oliguria, (3) diuresis, and (4) recovery.
- Management of AKI emphasizes fluid and dietary restrictions, restoration of fluid balance, waste elimination, and maintenance of cardiac output.
- When 90% to 95% of kidney function is lost, the patient is considered to have chronic kidney disease.
- Effects of chronic kidney disease include excess fluid volume, hyperkalemia, hypocalcemia, hyperuricemia, and anemia.
- Dialysis uses a semipermeable membrane to draw excess water, electrolytes, and wastes into a special solution called *dialysate*.
- Renal transplantation is the only alternative to dialysis for the patient with end-stage renal disease.
- Signs and symptoms of rejection of a transplanted kidney are fever, increased BP, and pain over the location of the new kidney.

Additional Learning Resources

SG Go to your Study Guide for additional learning activities to help you master this chapter content.

evolve Go to your Evolve website (http://evolve.elsevier.com/Linton/medsurg) for the following learning resources and much more:

- Interactive Prioritization Exercises
- Fluid & Electrolyte Tutorial
- Pharmacology Tutorial
- Review Questions for the NCLEX® Examination

Review Questions for the NCLEX® Examination

1. An 88-year-old woman was seen in the clinic three times last year for kidney infections. Which of the following age-related factors may be contributing to these frequent infections? (Select all that apply.)
   1. Incomplete bladder emptying
   2. Decreased renal blood flow
   3. Decreased creatinine clearance
   4. Reflux of urine into the ureters
   5. Decreased bladder capacity

   NCLEX Client Need: Physiological Integrity: Physiological Adaptation
2. A patient tells you that she has a painful, burning sensation during urination. The term you should use to record this symptom is ____________________.

   NCLEX Client Need: Physiological Integrity: Physiological Adaptation
3. The first time that a patient voids after cystoscopy, you notice pink-tinged urine. What is the nurse's most appropriate response?
   1. Promptly notify the physician
   2. Encourage additional fluids
   3. Recognize that this is normal
   4. Assess the patient's BP

   NCLEX Client Need: Physiological Integrity: Reduction of Risk Potential
4. The procedure that most often causes health care–associated infections is ____________________.

   NCLEX Client Need: Physiological Integrity: Reduction of Risk Potential
5. Patient teaching to reduce the risk of cystitis in women should include which of the following? (Select all that apply.)
   1. Avoid caffeine
   2. Tub baths are recommended over showers
   3. Drink a glass of water before and after intercourse
   4. Cleanse the perineum from front to back after elimination
   5. Wear synthetic undergarments that serve as a barrier to moisture

   NCLEX Client Need: Health Promotion and Maintenance
6. Glomerulonephritis is caused by which of the following?
   1. Bacteria
   2. Viruses
   3. Urinary obstruction
   4. Immunologic processes

   NCLEX Client Need: Physiological Integrity: Physiological Adaptation
7. Which of the following is a procedure that uses sound, laser, or dry shock wave energy to break up renal calculi?
   1. Lithotripsy
   2. Lithotomy
   3. Nephrolithotomy
   4. Ureterolithotomy

   NCLEX Client Need: Physiological Integrity: Reduction of Risk Potential
8. The maximum amount of fluid that can be used to irrigate a nephrostomy tube is __________ mL.

   NCLEX Client Need: Physiological Integrity: Reduction of Risk Potential
9. After a nephrectomy, a patient's urine output was 25 mL in the past hour. Which of the following actions should the nurse take?
   1. Have the patient change positions
   2. Give the patient an 8-oz glass of water every 2 hours
   3. Increase the flow rate of the patient's intravenous fluids
   4. Notify the physician that the patient's urine output is too low

   NCLEX Client Need: Physiological Integrity: Reduction of Risk Potential
10. A patient with chronic kidney disease becomes confused. He complains of nausea, abdominal cramps, and lack of sensation in his legs. His heart rhythm is irregular. Which of the following should you suspect?
    1. Increased BUN
    2. Hyperkalemia
    3. Metabolic acidosis
    4. Hypocalcemia

    NCLEX Client Need: Physiological Integrity: Physiological Adaptation

chapter 43

Connective Tissue Disorders

http://evolve.elsevier.com/Linton/medsurg

Objectives

1. Define connective tissue.
2. Describe the function of connective tissue.
3. Identify the data to be collected in the nursing assessment of a patient with a connective tissue disorder.
4. Describe the nurse's responsibilities for diagnostic tests and procedures used for assessing patient with connective tissue diseases.
5. Discuss the drugs used to treat connective tissue diseases.
6. Describe the pathophysiology and treatment of osteoarthritis (degenerative joint disease), rheumatoid arthritis, osteoporosis, gout, progressive systemic sclerosis, polymyositis, bursitis, carpal tunnel syndrome, ankylosing spondylitis, polymyalgia rheumatica, Reiter syndrome, Behçet syndrome, and Sjögren syndrome.
7. Describe the characteristics and prevalence of connective tissue diseases.
8. Assist in developing a nursing care plan for a patient whose life has been affected by a connective tissue disease.

Key Terms

Ankylosis (ăng-kĭ-LŌ-sĭs)
Arthroplasty (ĂR-thrō-plăs-tē)
Crepitus (KRĔP-ĭ-tŭs)
Goniometer (gō-nē-ŎM-ĕ-tĕr)
Hyperuricemia (hī-pĕr-ŭr-ĭ-SĒ-mē-ă)
Intraarticular (ĭn-tră-ăr-TĬK-ū-lăr)
Rheumatoid nodule (ROO-mă-toyd NŎD-ūl)
Tophi (TŌ-fī)
Vasculitis (văs-kū-LĪ-tĭs)

More than 50 million people in the United States report having been diagnosed with a condition that affects the joints, including osteoarthritis, rheumatoid arthritis (RA), gout, lupus, and fibromyalgia. Among adults age 65 and older, 50% report a diagnosis of arthritis. However, two thirds of Americans with arthritis are younger than age 65. Often called *rheumatoid disorders*, these conditions affect women more frequently than men. Although common in all racial and ethnic groups, arthritis is more disabling among individuals from racial and ethnic minorities. Most arthritic conditions are chronic and are characterized by alternating exacerbations and remissions, with progressive deterioration. Many have no known cause or cure. Rheumatoid disorders challenge the spirit and body of the patient. They can dramatically alter the patient's lifestyle, self-image, employability, and hope for the future.

A number of the conditions discussed in this chapter are classified as *autoimmune disorders*. They are included here because their primary effects are on connective tissue. For a thorough explanation of autoimmunity, see Chapter 34.

ANATOMY AND PHYSIOLOGY OF CONNECTIVE TISSUES

Connective tissues bind structures together, providing support for individual organs and a framework for the body as a whole. They also store fat, transport substances, provide protection, and play a role in repair of damaged tissue. The types of connective tissue are loose (areolar, adipose, reticular), dense (tendons, fascia, dermis, gastrointestinal [GI] tract submucosa, fibrous joint capsules), elastic (aortic walls, vocal cords, parts of trachea and bronchi, some ligaments), hematopoietic (blood), and strong supportive (cartilage, bone, ligaments).

This chapter is concerned primarily with disorders that affect bone, cartilage, ligaments, and tendons. Although selected autoimmune disorders that significantly affect the musculoskeletal system are included in this chapter, see Chapter 34 for a detailed discussion of autoimmune disorders. Blood disorders are addressed in Chapter 33, and skin disorders other than scleroderma are discussed in Chapter 52.

BONE

Bone is the hard tissue that makes up most of the skeletal system. The functions of the bones are support, protection, movement, storage of calcium and other ions, and manufacture of blood cells.

CARTILAGE

Cartilage is a specialized fibrous connective tissue. It provides firm but flexible support for the embryonic skeleton and part of the adult skeleton. Cartilage differs from bone in that its matrix has the consistency of a firm plastic or gristlelike gel. Cartilage cells are called *chondrocytes* and are located in tiny spaces that are distributed throughout the matrix.

LIGAMENTS

Ligaments are strong and flexible fibrous bands of connective tissue that connect bones and cartilage and support muscles. Yellow ligaments and white ligaments have distinctively different functions. Yellow ligaments, located in the vertebral column, are elastic and allow for stretching. White ligaments, found in the knee, do not stretch but provide stability.

TENDONS

Tendons are composed of very strong and dense fibrous connective tissue. They are in the shape of heavy cords and anchor muscles firmly to bones. One of the most prominent tendons is the Achilles tendon, which can be felt at the back of the ankle just above the heel.

JOINT STRUCTURE AND FUNCTION

Connective tissue disorders are often manifested as joint disorders because joint mobility depends on functional connective tissue. A joint is the site at which two or more bones of the body are joined. Joints permit motion and flexibility of the rigid skeleton. The only bone in the human body that does not articulate with at least one other bone is the hyoid bone, to which the tongue is attached.

Classified on the basis of the extent of movement, joints include synarthroses (fixed joints), amphiarthroses (slightly movable joints), and diarthroses (freely movable joints). Synarthroses, such as those in the skull, allow no movement at all. An example of a slightly movable joint, an amphiarthrosis, is the juncture of the ulna and radius in the forearm. Diarthroses, such as those in the elbows, shoulders, fingers, hips, and knees, allow considerable movement. Diarthroses are sometimes called *synovial joints*. They are encased in a fibrous capsule made of strong cartilage and lined with synovial membrane.

The synovial membrane is very smooth, thus permitting structures to move without friction. Ligaments are tough fibrous cords that bind the capsule. A smooth layer of cartilage also covers the ends of the bones, where it serves as a type of shock absorber. Synovial fluid fills and lubricates the space in the middle of the joint. Bursae are sacs of synovial fluid found in joints that also promote smooth articulation of joint structures. The bursae permit tendons to slide easily with movement of the bones.

AGE-RELATED CHANGES

Age-related changes in connective tissue can affect function significantly. A loss of bone mass and bone strength occurs. The progressive loss of bone density during later adult life accounts for the decline in bone strength. Significant bone loss, called *osteoporosis*, is more common in women but affects men as well. These changes put the older patient at risk for fractures.

Age-related joint changes occur primarily due to the changes in cartilage. With age, cartilage gradually loses elasticity and then becomes soft and frayed. Water content decreases and cartilage may ulcerate. Friction between unprotected bony joint surfaces promotes the growth of osteophytes (bony spurs). These joint changes result in pain and limited mobility and can contribute to a loss of independence.

NURSING ASSESSMENT OF CONNECTIVE TISSUE STRUCTURES

HEALTH HISTORY

The nursing assessment requires a detailed health history, because many of the signs and symptoms of connective tissue disorders are insidious. In addition, patients with chronic conditions may come to accept their symptoms as a way of life and fail to report them to the nurse. Therefore it may be helpful to have a family member present to assist the patient as historian. The family member may provide a clearer picture of how the changes in health have evolved.

Chief Complaint and History of Present Illness

It is important to determine why the patient is seeking health care. Complaints that suggest possible problems related to connective tissue disorders are aches, pain, joint swelling or stiffness, generalized weakness, a change in ability to work or to enjoy leisure activities, a change in appearance that is significant to the patient, and a change in ability to carry out activities of daily living (ADL).

Past Medical History

The past medical history provides information about the patient's prior state of health. Inquire about major childhood and adult illnesses, operations, and current medications and allergies. Ask whether a history of tuberculosis, poliomyelitis, diabetes mellitus, gout, arthritis, rickets, infection of bones or joints, autoimmune diseases, and neuromuscular disabilities exists. Record the dates of immunizations for polio and tetanus because postpolio syndrome and tetanus are characterized by musculoskeletal symptoms. Finally, document dietary pattern and use of vitamin and mineral supplements.

Accidents and Injuries. Accidents and injuries, even in the distant past, may be significant because they could be related to the patient's current problem. For example, low back pain in the present may be the result of an injury sustained several years ago. Inquire about participation in sports and the type of work the patient has done. Many types of sports injuries result in osteoarthritis later in life.

Current and Past Medications. Record the patient's use of prescription and over-the-counter (OTC) drugs. Self-medication is common with musculoskeletal pain and patients may fail to report it unless specifically asked. Inquire about the use of alternative therapies, including herbal supplements and home remedies. Some drugs, including corticosteroids and antiseizure drugs, can contribute to bone loss. Many herbal supplements interact with traditional medications and have significant side effects. It is important to list all medications prescribed previously and describe their effectiveness. Note any problems associated with current medications and whether the patient thinks that these medications are effective. Also record any allergies.

Family History

Ask whether the patient or any relative has had osteoporosis, osteoarthritis, RA, gout, or scoliosis, because these conditions appear to have some genetic basis. In addition, note any history of other autoimmune diseases, such as thyroid disorders.

Review of Systems

Collect data about each body system for significant symptoms. It is helpful to ask about the patient's general health status to determine the patient's perception of well-being. Specifically ask whether the patient has had fatigue, malaise, anorexia, weight loss, pain, stiffness, dysphagia, or dyspnea. With joint pain and stiffness, it is especially important to determine whether the symptoms are present on arising in the morning and how long they persist. Be aware that many cultures react differently to pain and disability; some may be stoic whereas others are very expressive. The loss of ability to perform certain daily functions can have a significant effect on the role in the family and therefore can cause emotional distress and frustration. For example, a breadwinner who can no longer work to support his or her family because of crippling arthritis will be greatly affected both physically and psychologically.

Functional Assessment

The following questions may be used to determine the patient's functional status and the significance of any changes to the patient.

- How does this problem affect the way you live?
- Have you had to change your everyday activities?
- How do you feel about any changes that you have had to make?
- What have you found helpful in adapting to these changes?
- How do you carry out the treatment program prescribed by your physician?
- Has your treatment plan been effective for you?
- What kind of support systems do you have at home?

PHYSICAL EXAMINATION

The physical examination begins with measurement of the patient's vital signs, height, and weight. Be aware that many patients with arthritis have limited physical abilities to stand, step up, or get onto an examination table. A chair scale is very useful for these patients. Compare findings with the patient's norms, if available. Significant data include fever, tachycardia, tachypnea, weight loss, and loss of height.

Inspect the skin for color, rashes, lesions, scars, or any signs of injuries. Palpate the skin for warmth, edema, and moisture and palpate the lymph nodes for enlargement and tenderness. Inspect joints for swelling and deformity and palpate for warmth, swelling, and tenderness. Assess joint pain and range of motion by asking the patient to move each extremity through the normal range of motion. Take care not to extend joints beyond their range or point of comfort. Inflamed joints are extremely sensitive to movement and pressure. During the movement, watch for signs of pain and listen for the crackling sound called **crepitus**. The physician or other advanced health care provider may make a more precise measurement of joint motion using an instrument called a **goniometer**, which measures the range of movement of the joints. Measurement of limb length and muscle strength also may be done. Nursing assessment of the patient with a connective tissue disorder is outlined in Box 43-1.

DIAGNOSTIC TESTS AND PROCEDURES

Procedures used to diagnose connective tissue diseases are mainly laboratory studies of blood and urine and radiologic imaging studies of the bones and joints.

Routine blood studies that are useful in diagnosing connective tissue disorders include a complete blood count (CBC), the erythrocyte sedimentation rate (ESR), and C-reactive protein (CRP) determination. These studies help to determine whether a disorder is inflammatory or noninflammatory. Other blood studies are the Venereal Disease Research Laboratory (VDRL),

Box 43-1 Assessment of the Patient with a Connective Tissue Disorder

HEALTH HISTORY

Present Illness

Changes in movement, activities of daily living (ADL); areas of pain, swelling, or tenderness; fatigue

Past Medical History

Tuberculosis, poliomyelitis, diabetes mellitus, gout, arthritis, rickets, neuromuscular disabilities

Family History

Rheumatoid arthritis (RA), degenerative arthritis (need for joint replacement surgery), gout, scoliosis, other autoimmune disorders

Review of Systems

Pain or swelling in joints, limitation of movement, weakness, malaise, change in general appearance of skin

Functional Assessment

Past or recent injuries because of accidents or falls, use of assistive devices

PHYSICAL EXAMINATION

General Survey

Posture, balance, gait, skin condition

Joints

Warmth, redness, swelling, tenderness, nodules, range of motion, crepitus, function of hands

Skin

Color, scars, bruising, warmth, swelling, nodules

Upper Extremities

Symmetry, swelling, tenderness, pain, range of motion, posture

Lower Extremities

Movement of hips, knees, and ankles; pain; skin condition

rheumatoid factor (RF), creatinine, and antinuclear antibody (ANA) tests. Urine may be tested for creatinine and uric acid levels. Fluids aspirated from joints may be studied to detect uric acid crystals or white blood cells (WBCs). Most laboratory tests are not diagnostic for a single condition; that is, many factors could cause measures of inflammation to increase. The physician may rely on multiple diagnostic procedures along with the health history and physical examination to reach a diagnosis.

Radiologic imaging studies include radiography, ultrasonography, arthrography, nuclear scintigraphy, magnetic resonance imaging (MRI), discography, tomography, and computed tomography (CT). Other useful measures are biopsy and arthroscopy. Table 43-1 summarizes commonly used diagnostic studies and related nursing care. Agency procedure manuals will provide more specific information on preparation and postprocedure care.

COMMON THERAPEUTIC MEASURES

Management of the patient with a connective tissue disorder often requires the services of a team that includes the patient, nurse, physician, social worker, nutritionist, physical therapist, and occupational therapist. The goals of therapy are to reduce inflammation and pain and to promote adaptation to the condition. Therapeutic measures may include physical and occupational therapy, modification of ADL, patient education and support, nutritional counseling, drug therapy, and surgical intervention. Although none of these measures is curative, they can greatly enhance the patient's function and quality of life. Various sources suggest dietary modifications for inflammatory conditions; research is ongoing to determine valid recommendations. Some patients report that specific foods increase or decrease their symptoms.

PHYSICAL AND OCCUPATIONAL THERAPY

Physical therapy uses exercise and positioning to help preserve functional capability and minimize disability. For many patients, braces and splints will be ordered to help support inflamed joints, protect the patient from further injury, and relieve discomfort. Occupational therapy assists the patient in making adaptations in work and personal life that allow maximal possible function.

EDUCATION AND SUPPORT

Education emphasizes the treatment plan and how it will benefit the patient. Team members must be sensitive to the inconvenience and discomfort that the disease has caused and also must help the patient to identify ways to cope with the condition. Patients and their families need information about community support groups that can offer encouragement, information, and resources. A patient's attitude is very important in the successful treatment and management of a disease; psychologic support should be provided. Many research studies have shown the connection between a patient's positive attitude and a successful outcome with chronic diseases.

DRUG THERAPY

Drug therapy for connective tissue disorders has traditionally included glucocorticoids and nonsteroidal antiinflammatory drugs (NSAIDs) to reduce inflammation (Table 43-2). When glucocorticoids are indicated, occasional local injections or short-term systemic therapy is preferred over long-term therapy. For many patients already on NSAIDs, acetaminophen is often prescribed as a safe analgesic. Other less-safe drugs are gold salts, azathioprine, penicillamine, and cyclosporine.

Three categories of drugs are used in the treatment of arthritis: (1) NSAIDs, (2) glucocorticoids, and (3) disease-modifying antirheumatic drugs (DMARDs). NSAIDs are the safest type of these; they relieve pain and reduce inflammation but do not prevent joint damage or slow the progress of the disease. First-generation NSAIDs include salicylates (e.g., aspirin)

Text continued on p. 949

Table 43-1 Diagnostic Tests and Procedures Connective Tissue Disorders

Common Nursing Interventions

General Interventions: Check your agency procedure manual for diagnostic tests and procedures. Always tell the patient what to expect when tests are ordered. Explain if nothing-by-mouth (NPO) status is necessary. Document the care provided and relevant assessment data. If venipuncture is done, apply a dressing and check the site oozing. Apply pressure and elevate the arm if patient's blood clotting is impaired.

TEST AND PURPOSE	PATIENT PREPARATION	POSTPROCEDURE NURSING CARE
Blood Studies		
Antinuclear Antibodies (ANAs) Positive in SLE, RA, SSc, Raynaud phenomenon, Sjögren syndrome, and necrotizing arteritis.	Fast 8 hours before test.	See General Interventions.
C-Reactive Protein (CRP) Detects active inflammation as in RA and disseminated lupus erythematosus.	Restrict food and fluids for 4 hours.	See General Interventions.
Creatinine Assesses renal function. Increased with SLE, SSc, and polyarteritis.	Fasting is not required.	See General Interventions.
Erythrocyte Sedimentation Rate (ESR) Determines the presence of inflammation. Increased with RA and rheumatic fever; decreased with osteoarthritis.	Fasting is not required.	See General Interventions.
Red Blood Cell (RBC) Count Detects and differentiates blood dyscrasias. Decreased in RA and SLE.	Fasting is not required.	See General Interventions.
Rheumatoid Factor (RF) Detects antibodies in patients with RA.	Fasting is not required.	See General Interventions.
Venereal Disease Research Laboratory (VDRL) Test Measures antibodies to syphilis. Sometimes decreased in SLE.	Fasting is not required.	See General Interventions.
White Blood Cell (WBC) Count Increased in infection, tissue necrosis, and inflammation; may decrease in SLE.	Fasting is not required.	See General Interventions.
Urine Studies		
24-Hour Urine for Creatinine Measures renal function and status of muscle diseases.	Instruct the patient to collect a 24-hour urine specimen. Discard the first morning specimen. Save the rest of urine voided over a 24-hour period in a clean, refrigerated 3-L container with or without preservative. Include urine voided at end of 24-hour period. Fasting not required.	See General Interventions.
Urinary Uric Acid (24-Hour Collection) Measures uric acid metabolism; increased in gout, liver disease, chronic myelogenous leukemia, and fever.	Requires 24-hour urine specimen (as described above). Fasting not required.	See General Interventions.
Radiologic Studies		

***General Interventions When Contrast Dye Used. Before Procedure:** Assess patient allergy to dye, iodine, or shellfish. If patient reports allergy, notify radiology. Tell patient that injection of contrast dye can create a feeling of warmth, a salty taste, and nausea. **After Procedure:** Inform the physician of any signs of allergic response to the contrast dye. Administer antihistamines as ordered for allergy.

Continued

Table 43-1 Diagnostic Tests and Procedures Connective Tissue Disorders—cont'd

TEST AND PURPOSE	PATIENT PREPARATION	POSTPROCEDURE NURSING CARE
Arthrography Uses contrast medium to show soft-tissue joint structures.	*Dye precautions. Tell the patient that needle insertion may cause discomfort and swelling that lasts several days.	*Dye precautions. Assess and document discomfort and swelling. Instruct the patient to avoid strenuous activity for 12–24 hours after test. Joint may be wrapped.
Computed Tomography (CT) Detects tumors and some spinal fractures.	Tell the patient that the procedure may be lengthy (up to 30 minutes per body part). Patient lies on a stretcher while a machine scans the area being studied.	See General Interventions.
Discography Visualizes the vertebral disk after contrast medium is injected into the disk.	Same as for arthrography.	Same as for arthrography.
Magnetic Resonance Imaging (MRI) Visualizes soft tissue. May detect avascular necrosis, disk disease, tumors, osteomyelitis, and torn ligaments.	Tell the patient that the procedure is painless; must lie still for 30 minutes or more. Some equipment includes videos that the patient can view to reduce anxiety. Ask whether the patient is claustrophobic. Give sedation if ordered for agitated or anxious patients. Remove any metallic objects such as jewelry. Inquire whether the patient has any implanted devices such as cardiac pacemaker or intracranial aneurysm clips and notify the radiologist. Procedure is contraindicated with some implants. Metal may not be a problem with some newer equipment.	See General Interventions. Take safety precautions if the patient is sedated.
Nuclear Scintigraphy (Bone Scan) Detects bone malignancies, osteoporosis, osteomyelitis, and some fractures.	Contraindicated during pregnancy. Tell the patient that a small amount of radioactive material will be injected intravenously; then a scanner will move slowly back and forth over the body as the patient lies on a stretcher. May take 1 hour. Procedure is painless except for venipuncture. Radioactive isotopes are not harmful except to fetus. Empty bladder immediately before procedure for comfort and to prevent blocked view of pelvis.	See General Interventions. No special precautions are required for handling urine or stool.
Radiography Shows density, texture, and alignments of bones; reveals soft tissue involvement.	Tell the patient to expect to lie on a radiograph table or to stand next to a special device while films are taken. Remove any radiopaque objects (e.g., jewelry) that can interfere with results. Advise radiology of the patient's physical limitations related to moving, turning, and climbing.	See General Interventions.
Tomography Provides details of structures otherwise hidden by bone.	Requires lying in a cylindric scanner; assess for claustrophobia and inform the radiologist.	See General Interventions.

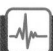

Table 43-1 Diagnostic Tests and Procedures Connective Tissue Disorders—cont'd

TEST AND PURPOSE	PATIENT PREPARATION	POSTPROCEDURE NURSING CARE
Ultrasonography Reveals masses or fluid in soft tissue.	No preparation is required.	See General Interventions.
Special Tests		
Arthroscopy A surgical procedure to visualize a joint cavity and structure and to obtain fluid, tissue, or both for study.	Inform the patient that the procedure is performed in an operating room under local or general anesthesia.	The patient will have a sterile dressing applied to the wound, which will also be wrapped with a compression dressing. Report any drainage of blood or fluid to the physician. Instruct the patient to limit activity for a few days.
Joint Aspiration Examination of fluid taken from a joint to diagnose inflammation.	Procedure is usually done at bedside or in examination room. Tell the patient that a local anesthetic is used to minimize discomfort.	Apply pressure dressing to the joint. Instruct the patient to rest the joint for 8–24 hours. Record on patient's chart and report to the physician or nurse supervisor any leakage of blood or fluid. Apply a pressure dressing to the affected area and keep it immobilized for 12–24 hours.
Bone Densitometry (DXA and DPA) Determines bone mineral content and density to detect osteoporosis. Screening procedures may scan the finger, heel, or radius. If abnormal, the more conclusive scan of the pelvis and hips is advised.	No special advance preparation is required. Patient will need to remove any metallic objects (e.g., zippers, belts) in the area being examined. Explain that the patient will be positioned on an imaging table and an instrument will pass over the pelvic and hip region. A computer will record density measurements. Radiation exposure is minimal. The procedure is painless.	See General Interventions.
Muscle Biopsy A sample of muscle tissue is taken to detect inflammatory reaction, as in polymyositis or myopathic disease.	May be performed under local or general anesthesia.	Apply a pressure dressing to the affected area and keep it immobilized for 12–24 hours.
Skin Biopsy Studies excised skin to confirm inflammatory connective tissue diseases such as SLE and SSc.	Tell the patient a local anesthetic will be injected; slight discomfort may be felt when the skin sample is obtained.	Keep the biopsy site clean and dry with a small adhesive bandage until a scab develops. Patients who are taking aspirin or NSAIDs are at risk for bleeding, bruising, or both at the biopsy site.

DPA, Dual-photon absorptiometry; *DXA,* dual-energy x-ray absorptiometry; *NSAIDs,* nonsteroidal antiinflammatory drugs; *RA,* rheumatoid arthritis; *SLE,* systemic lupus erythematosus; *SSc,* systemic sclerosis.
Note: See agency laboratory manual for specific preparation and norms. Results vary with different types of tests and may be reported in different units of measurement.

Table 43-2 Drugs Used to Treat Connective Tissue Disorders

DRUG	USE AND ACTION	SIDE EFFECTS	NURSING INTERVENTIONS
First-Generation Nonsteroidal Antiinflammatory Drugs (NSAIDs)			
aspirin diclofenac sodium (Voltaren) ibuprofen (Motrin, Rufen) indomethacin (Indocin) naproxen (Naprosyn) nabumetone (Relafen)	Analgesic. Antipyretic. Antiinflammatory (inhibits prostaglandin synthesis). Decreases pain and deformity. Inhibits platelet aggregation (clumping).	Gastrointestinal (GI) upset, GI bleeding may be silent in older adults. Ototoxicity. Bleeding because of anticoagulation. Some may cause drowsiness. Increased blood pressure (BP) because of fluid retention.	Instruct patient to take with food or to take enteric-coated aspirin and report ringing in ears (tinnitus), abdominal pain, dark stools. Assess for bruising and bleeding. Caution patient not to take aspirin and NSAIDs concurrently and not to drive if drowsy.
Second-Generation NSAIDs: Selective COX-2 Inhibitor			
celecoxib (Celebrex)	Analgesic. Antipyretic. Antiinflammatory (inhibits prostaglandin synthesis).	GI bleeding (less risk than first-generation NSAIDs), fatigue, dependent edema, nausea, increased BP because of fluid retention. Dizziness. FDA is studying for possible increased risk of MI, CVA, and death.	Administer with food or full glass of water. Remain in upright position 15–30 min after taking. Safety precautions if dizzy. Do not confuse with Celexa (antidepressant) or Cerebyx (injectable fosphenytoin to treat seizures). Do not use with aspirin, alcohol, or acetaminophen concurrently.
Glucocorticoids			
hydrocortisone (Cortef, Hydrocortone) hydrocortisone sodium succinate (Solu-Cortef, cortisol) cortisone acetate (Cortone) prednisone (Deltasone) prednisolone (Delta-Cortef)	Suppress normal immune response and inflammation. Used in inflammatory and allergic conditions.	Muscular weakness, nausea, anorexia, hypotension; sodium retention, hypokalemia; insomnia; nervousness; euphoria; rise in serum glucose. Osteoporosis. Increased susceptibility to infections.	Highest dose usually given in early morning; lowest dose given later in day to mimic normal secretion in body. Stress to patient need to adhere to prescribed schedule. Remember that glucocorticoids mask signs of infection. Observe for any unusual drainage, odors, and elevated temperatures. Must be tapered off rather than stopped abruptly.
Disease-Modifying Antirheumatic Drugs (DMARDs)			
Nonbiologic (First Choice) DMARDs			
methotrexate (Folex)	Treats rheumatoid and psoriatic arthritis (RA). Mild immunosuppressant.	Anorexia, nausea, vomiting, diarrhea. Toxic effects on oral tissues, liver, lungs, bone marrow, skin, and kidneys. Hemorrhage; hair loss.	Monitor periodic blood and urine studies to detect abnormalities of toxicity. Encourage fluid intake. Tell patient to avoid because of risk of bleeding; to avoid people with infections; and to report bruising, bleeding, or signs of infection promptly.
hydroxychloroquine sulfate (Plaquenil)	Basis of antirheumatic effects unknown; may suppress antigens that trigger hypersensitivity reactions.	Headache, nausea, vomiting, anorexia. Ocular toxicity. With prolonged therapy: bone marrow suppression, psychosis. Instruct patient to see an eye doctor while taking this drug.	Ask about known allergy to drug. Tell patient to report visual or hearing disturbances promptly. Monitor complete blood cell count (CBC) and liver function studies.

Table 43-2 **Drugs Used to Treat Connective Tissue Disorders—cont'd**

DRUG	USE AND ACTION	SIDE EFFECTS	NURSING INTERVENTIONS
sulfasalazine (Azulfidine)	Antimicrobial, anti-inflammatory. Used to treat RA.	Anorexia, nausea, vomiting, headache, oligospermia. Toxic effects on bone marrow, liver, kidneys. Rarely: anaphylaxis.	Monitor liver and kidney function. Ensure urine output of at least 1500 mL/day. Assess for bruising, jaundice, fever, sore throat. Tell patient to avoid direct sunlight.
leflunomide (Arava)	Treats active RA, retards structural damage. Slows disease progression.	Diarrhea, liver toxicity, hair loss. Teratogenic.	Monitor liver studies. Tell patient to report severe diarrhea. Known to cause fetal harm; women of childbearing age should avoid conception. Avoid alcohol consumption while on medication.
cyclosporine (Neoral)	Treats RA and psoriasis. Also used to prevent rejection of transplanted organs. Works by suppressing immune response.	Tremors, oral candida, gum hyperplasia, hirsutism, infection, renal failure, electrolyte imbalances.	Monitor renal and liver function studies. Carefully follow directions for preparation of oral dose. Do not give with grapefruit juice. IV drug must be administered via glass container only. Advise patient to report any signs of infection, even if minor. Avoid pregnancy during and 12 weeks after therapy.
Biologic DMARDs (BRMs)			
etanercept (Enbrel)	Used to treat severe RA in adults who do not respond to other DMARDs. Binds tumor necrosis factor (TNF), which is involved in immunity and inflammation.	Injection site reaction, abdominal pain, heartburn, headache, dizziness, upper respiratory infections, cough.	Reconstitute supplied diluent, add to powder, swirl to mix (do not shake), and administer immediately. Use only clear, colorless solution. Do not mix with other drugs. Administer SC in upper arm, abdomen, or thigh. Rotate sites. Check injection site for redness, itching. Caution in people with recurring infections or people at risk for infections.
infliximab (Remicade)	A monoclonal antibody that neutralizes activity of TNF, which decreases inflammation. Used to treat RA, Crohn disease.	Anaphylaxis, anemia, tachycardia, GI distress, skin rash, headache, dizziness, depression, upper respiratory infections, muscle aches, painful urination, chest pain, hypotension, hypertension.	Given IV every 1–2 months in combination with methotrexate. 2-hour infusion. Reconstitute and use immediately. Monitor for signs of infection, especially upper respiratory tract infections. Cannot be infused in IV line with other agents.
adalimumab (Humira)	A monoclonal antibody that inhibits structural damage by blocking the action of TNF. Used to treat rheumatoid and psoriatic arthritis.	Injection site reaction (swelling and pain at injection site may last 4–5 days), flulike symptoms, infection, headache, sinusitis, abdominal pain, nausea.	Stop treatment and notify physician if any signs of infection occur. For SC injection, do not mix with other drugs, do not use filter. DO protect from light. Rotate injection sites between abdomen, upper arms, and thighs; inject at 45-degree angle. Caution patient not to take immunizations while on Humira therapy.

Continued

Table 43-2 Drugs Used to Treat Connective Tissue Disorders—cont'd

DRUG	USE AND ACTION	SIDE EFFECTS	NURSING INTERVENTIONS
anakinra (Kineret)	Decreases cartilage damage and bone loss by blocking action of interleukin-1. Used to treat severe RA.	Injection site reaction (swelling and pain for 4–5 days), flulike symptoms, infection, headache, sinusitis, abdominal pain, nausea, worsening of RA symptoms.	For SC injection, do not mix with other drugs, do not use filter. DO protect from light. Rotate injection sites between abdomen, upper arms, and thighs. Do not use if cloudy or discolored. No concurrent immunizations.
abatacept (Orencia)	Inhibits activation of T lymphocytes, which are necessary for inflammatory process in RA.	Headache, dizziness, cough, back pain, nausea, hypertension. Serious infections.	Monitor for hypersensitivity (rare): dyspnea, hypotension. IV and SC routes. Prefilled syringes should be refrigerated. SC injection in anterior thigh, outer upper arm, or abdomen.
Antigout Medications			
allopurinol (Zyloprim) febuxostat (Uloric)	Inhibits synthesis of uric acid.	Drowsiness. Toxicity: maculopapular rash, fever, chills, joint pain. Rarely: bone marrow depression, nausea, diarrhea.	Tell patient to drink 8–10 glasses of fluid daily to maintain output of at least 2000 mL/day. Assess urine for abnormal characteristics. Safety precautions if drowsy. Tell patient it takes several weeks for full effects. Assess and record response.
probenecid (Benemid)	Increases urinary excretion of uric acid.	Headache, urinary frequency, GI distress. Rarely: anaphylaxis. Toxicity: maculopapular rash, fever, joint pain, leukopenia, GI distress. Urinary calculi (stones).	Assess allergies. Do not give with penicillin. Use caution with renal impairment. Encourage fluid intake to maintain output of at least 2000 mL/day. Tell patient it takes several weeks for full therapeutic effect.
Uricolytic			
pegloticase (Krystexxa)	Breaks uric acid down to readily excreted end product.	Gout flare during initial treatment. Anaphylaxis. Infusion reaction: urticaria, dyspnea, pruritis, chest discomfort.	Administer only in a setting equipped to handle emergencies. Premedicate with an antihistamine and glucocorticoid to prevent anaphylaxis. If mild or moderate infusion reaction occurs, slow rate of infusion. If severe reaction, stop infusion.
Bone Resorption Inhibitors			
ibandronate sodium (Boniva)	Used to prevent and treat osteoporosis in postmenopausal women.	Abdominal pain, hypertension, dyspepsia, arthralgia, nausea, diarrhea.	Main advantage is monthly dosing. Instruct patient to take on empty stomach upon arising. Do not eat or drink anything and remain upright for at least 60 minutes after each dose. Does not replace the need for adequate calcium and vitamin D intake. Contraindicated with uncorrected hypocalcemia.
alendronate sodium (Fosamax)	Increases bone mineral density by impairing bone resorption.	Abdominal pain, muscle pain, diarrhea, constipation, severe GI disturbances with overdose, hypocalcemia.	Take with 6–8 oz water upon arising, nothing else by mouth for 30 min. Patient should not lie down for 30 min after taking.

Table 43-2 Drugs Used to Treat Connective Tissue Disorders—cont'd

DRUG	USE AND ACTION	SIDE EFFECTS	NURSING INTERVENTIONS
calcitonin (Miacalcin)	Impairs bone resorption.	With injections: hypotension, flushing, nausea, vomiting, sweating. With oral form: constipation, edema.	Monitor for hypercalcemia (dry mouth, constipation, headache, depression, weakness). Take tablets with full glass of water ½ to 1 hour after meals. Not to be taken with other oral medications, alcohol, or foods with fiber. Patient must avoid excess tobacco use and caffeine.
raloxifene (Evista)	Prevents bone loss and lowers cholesterol without stimulating endometrium. Used to prevent osteoporosis in postmenopausal women.	Frequent side effects: infection, flu syndrome, nausea, hot flashes, weight gain, joint pain, sinusitis, thrombosis.	Seek medical care for chest pain, dyspnea, changes in vision. Should not be taken during pregnancy, before menopause, or during periods of immobility.

BRM, Biologic response modifier; *CVA*, cerebrovascular accident; *FDA*, U.S. Food and Drug Administration; *IV*, intravenous; *MI*, myocardial infarction; *SC*, subcutaneous.

and nonsalicylates such as ibuprofen. The only available second-generation NSAID, also called a selective COX-2 inhibitor, is celecoxib (Celebrex). Although celecoxib is less likely to cause stomach ulcers and bleeding than first-generation NSAIDs, it appears to increase the risk of myocardial infarction and stroke.

Glucocorticoids relieve symptoms, reduce inflammation, and may slow disease progression. Oral glucocorticoids such as prednisone are used for generalized symptoms whereas intraarticular injections may be used when only one or two joints are affected. Long-term glucocorticoid therapy is discouraged because of many adverse effects.

DMARDs reduce joint destruction and slow disease progression. They are classified as nonbiologic DMARDs or biologic DMARDS. DMARDs may be prescribed with a COX-2 inhibitor to obtain rapid symptom relief as well as joint preservation. The first choice among the DMARDs is usually the nonbiologic methotrexate. Other choices are leflunomide, hydroxychloroquine, cyclosporine, and sulfasalazine. Although all can have serious side effects, they generally are the safest of the DMARDs. The biologic DMARDs (biologic response modifiers, or BRMs) are immunosuppressive drugs that usually are given in combination with methotrexate. Biologic DMARDs work by interfering with some aspect of the inflammatory process. Examples of these drugs are etanercept (Enbrel), infliximab (Remicade), adalimumab (Humira), rituximab (Rituxan), and abatacept (Orencia). The nonbiologic agents are far less expensive than the biologic agents. Additional drugs will be noted with the conditions for which they are used. The DMARDs generally can have very serious adverse effects. Drugs that suppress the immune response put the patient at risk for overwhelming infection, so patients must be monitored for even mild symptoms. Patients should have immunizations updated before beginning therapy and should not receive immunizations while taking these drugs. Many of these drugs can be harmful to a developing embryo, so pregnancy should be avoided during and for a specified time after therapy.

SURGICAL TREATMENT

Surgical intervention may be indicated in some musculoskeletal disorders, such as degenerative joint disease and arthritis. Specific surgical interventions are discussed with the particular conditions.

A device used after some types of joint replacement surgery is the continuous passive motion (CPM) machine. This device moves the joints through a set range of motion at a set rate of movements per minute. The movement prevents formation of scar tissue and promotes flexibility of the new joint. The affected extremity may be placed in the CPM machine in the postanesthesia care unit or on the first postoperative day. The CPM machine is used for specific intervals and the time and degree of flexion and extension are gradually increased. The part of the machine that cradles the limb is padded to prevent pressure or abrasions. Be sure that the machine settings are correct as ordered and the limb is properly aligned. It is also important to keep the machine clean, because it could be a possible source of contamination. Several types of CPM machines are illustrated in the section titled "Nursing Care after Total Joint Replacement".

DISORDERS OF CONNECTIVE TISSUE STRUCTURES

OSTEOARTHRITIS

Osteoarthritis is the most common form of arthritis. Osteoarthritis may be classified as *primary* or *secondary*, depending on the cause. In primary osteoarthritis, some unknown factor triggers the release of chemicals that break down joint cartilage. Osteoarthritis that occurs with aging is generally considered to be primary and may have a genetic basis (see *Cultural Considerations* box). Secondary osteoarthritis may be associated with trauma, infection, congenital deformities, corticosteroid therapy, and a variety of other conditions including diabetes mellitus and obesity. The incidence of osteoarthritis increases with age, with persons older than 50 years most often affected.

Cultural Considerations

What Does Culture Have to Do with Osteoarthritis?

The sites affected most often by osteoarthritis vary with ethnic background. For example, osteoarthritis of the hips is more common among people who live in Japan and Saudi Arabia than among Caucasians living in the United States.

Osteoarthritis generally affects joints under pressure, especially the spine, fingers, knees, hips, and shoulders. People who are obese, who have poor posture, or who experience occupational stress are at greatest risk for the disease. The most common source of major disability is osteoarthritis of the knee.

Pathophysiology

Osteoarthritis is characterized by the degeneration of articular cartilage with hypertrophy of the underlying and adjacent bone. Normally, the articular cartilage provides a smooth surface for one bone to glide over another (Fig. 43-1). The cartilage transfers the weight of one bone to another so that the bones do not shatter. In osteoarthritis, deterioration of the articular cartilage means that the shock-absorbing protection is gradually lost. New bone growth is stimulated by exposed bone surfaces, causing bone spurs to develop. Although osteoarthritis is generally classified as a *noninflammatory condition*, inflammation of the joint is common in advanced conditions because of tissue breakdown.

Signs and Symptoms

Many people with osteoarthritis have no symptoms but others have pain ranging from mild to severe. The pain is what usually brings the patient to the physician. Pain is commonly associated with activity but relieved by rest. Along with pain in the affected joint, the patient with osteoarthritis may complain of stiffness, limitation of movement, mild tenderness, swelling, and deformity or enlargement of the joint (Fig. 43-2). Sometimes the symptoms subside for long periods of time and then return. The disease usually affects a single joint or only a few joints.

Medical Diagnosis

The diagnosis of osteoarthritis is usually based on the health history and radiographic studies. In the early stages of the disease, the patient may have no symptoms, even though radiographs reveal classic joint changes. From radiographic evidence, 68% of women older than 65 years have osteoarthritis. The incidence is slightly lower for men of the same age. The extent of the disease process is not necessarily related to the severity of symptoms.

Because plain radiographs do not always reveal cartilage abnormalities, arthroscopy, MRI, scintigraphy, and ultrasonography may be used as well. Synovial fluid may be aspirated to assess the presence of

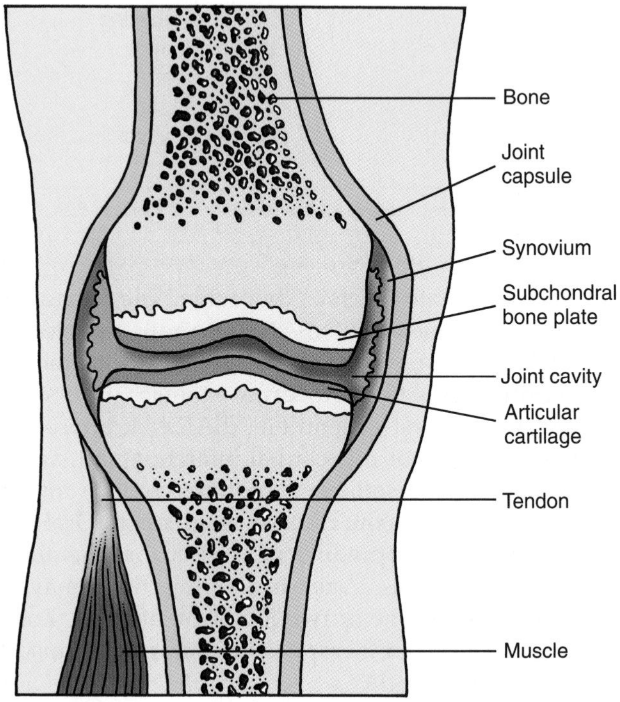

FIGURE 43-1 The structure of a diarthrodial joint. Synovium lines the joint capsule but does not extend into the articular cartilage. (From Ignatavicius DD, Workman ML: *Medical-surgical nursing: patient-centered collaborative care*, ed 6, St. Louis, 2010, Saunders.)

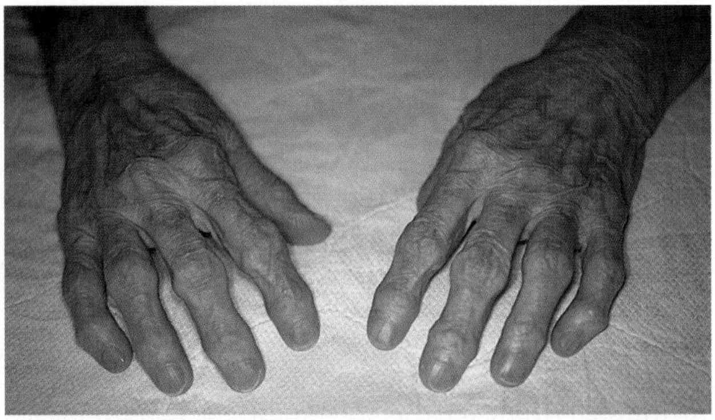

FIGURE 43-2 Osteoarthritis (degenerative joint disease): Heberden nodes at the distal interphalangeal joints and Bouchard nodes at the proximal interphalangeal joints. (From Swartz M: *Textbook of physical diagnosis: history and examination*, ed 6, Philadelphia, 2009, Saunders.)

leukocytes. A normal ESR, negative RF assay, and synovial fluid with few or no leukocytes are expected. However, it is not unusual for a healthy older person to have a slightly elevated ESR and low titers of RF and ANA.

Medical Treatment

No known cure exists for osteoarthritis but much can be done to make the patient more comfortable. The goals of patient therapy are to reduce the pain to a manageable level, maintain as much mobility as possible, and minimize disability.

The medical treatment regimen can include physical measures, education, drug therapy, and surgery. For some patients, diet and counseling are indicated. Referral to a pain specialist may be indicated if conservative measures are not effective. The course of the treatment is dictated by the individual patient's condition and response.

Physical Measures. The physical therapy program uses measures to improve range of motion and to maintain muscle mass and strength. Maintaining muscle mass reduces the load on joint cartilage. Most patients, especially those with mild osteoarthritis, benefit from such a program. Isometric exercises are recommended over isotonic exercises because isotonic movements place increased strain on the joints. Exercise should be followed by periods of rest during the day. When the hips or knees are affected, some activity restriction may be advised. Wearing cushioned shoes and using a cane to walk reduces the stress on the affected joints.

Moist heat and occasionally cold can be used to help relieve pain. Heat also prepares the muscles and joints for exercise. However, heat may be contraindicated in patients who have had arthroplasty or who have metal prostheses, because it may lead to deep thermal burns. Transcutaneous electrical nerve stimulation (TENS) devices are especially effective for treating back pain.

Drug Therapy. Although drug therapy is not curative, the pain of osteoarthritis usually can be controlled with nonopioid analgesics such as acetaminophen or NSAIDs. NSAIDs may decrease pain and improve mobility in patients with osteoarthritis but their side effects are more dangerous than those of acetaminophen. NSAIDs are especially effective when the patient shows signs of inflammation, such as warmth, swelling of joints, and erythema (redness). Similar to NSAIDs, indomethacin (Indocin) is effective in reducing inflammation but may cause serious adverse effects (see Table 43-2).

Salicylates are relatively inexpensive but a risk of toxicity exists. The symptoms of salicylate intoxication in older adults may be atypical. Instead of the common GI complaints or ototoxicity, the older person may exhibit confusion, slurring of speech, agitation, or seizures. Although systemic glucocorticoids are not indicated for the treatment of osteoarthritis, **intraarticular** injections can be beneficial. These injections can be given only three or four times a year because the drug may cause breakdown of cartilage with frequent use. The injection of hyaluronate into knee joints has improved symptoms in some patients.

A popular dietary supplement widely used for osteoarthritis is glucosamine often combined with chondroitin sulfate. Studies of these products have yielded conflicting results as to pain relief and slowing of joint damage. Some patients report relief of localized pain with the topical application of capsaicin.

Complementary and Alternative Therapies

Although glucosamine and chondroitin are popular with the public, studies of its effectiveness in treating osteoarthritis have had inconsistent results.

Pharmacology Capsule

First-generation nonsteroidal antiinflammatory drugs (NSAIDs) can cause significant gastrointestinal (GI) ulcers and bleeding.

Pharmacology Capsule

Salicylate toxicity may be manifested by tinnitus or, in older adults, by confusion, agitation, slurred speech, or seizures.

Surgical Management. Surgical management is usually reserved for persons with persistent pain and disability despite conservative treatment. Arthroscopic surgery that removes loose bodies and repairs defects may be useful for patients with osteoarthritis of the knee, shoulder, and ankle. The surgical treatment of choice for osteoarthritis of the hip or knee is total joint replacement (**arthroplasty**) (see Nursing Care Plan: Patient with a Total Hip Replacement). The primary indication for total joint replacement is intractable pain that disrupts sleep and daily activities. Total hip or knee arthroplasty usually relieves pain and restores function to the joint (Fig. 43-3). Some experts recommend delaying joint replacement until age 60 because of the risk of prosthesis failure during the expected lifetime. Others believe that most modern prostheses are durable enough to be implanted in younger persons. Prosthesis failure is most often characterized by loosening of the joint implant. Revision arthroplasty has a high rate of failure. A recent development is minimally invasive joint replacement surgery. This type of procedure requires a much smaller incision than the traditional approach. Some minimally invasive joint replacement procedures are done in outpatient surgical settings.

NURSING CARE of the Patient with Osteoarthritis

Assessment

General nursing assessment of the patient with a connective tissue disorder is summarized in Box 43-1.

Nursing Care Plan — Patient with a Total Hip Replacement

ASSESSMENT

HEALTH HISTORY A 74-year-old homemaker has had osteoarthritis for 10 years, with progressive loss of function in both hips. She had a left total hip replacement (arthroplasty) 2 days ago. Her past medical history reveals no other major health problems except poor vision. She lives with her daughter and helps with household chores, which gives her some satisfaction. Postoperatively she is alert and participates in her exercises. She was assisted out of bed this morning. She was somewhat weak but was able to walk a short distance.

PHYSICAL EXAMINATION Vital signs: blood pressure 148/66 mm Hg, pulse 82 bpm, respiration 16 breaths per minute, temperature 98°F (36.7°C) measured orally. Height 5′9″, weight 162 lb. Patient is positioned on her right side with an abductor cushion in place. Breath sounds are clear on auscultation. Abdomen is soft and bowel sounds are present. No bladder distention or redness exists over bony prominences on back and left side. Warmth, color, and peripheral pulses are symmetric in both legs. She has good sensation in affected leg. The dressing on the surgical incision is dry and intact.

Nursing Diagnosis	Goals and Outcome Criteria	Interventions
Ineffective Peripheral Tissue Perfusion related to deep vein thrombosis (DVT), decreased mobility, and surgical trauma	The patient will have adequate circulation in the affected extremity, as evidenced by warmth, normal color, and palpable pulses.	Assess neurologic and circulatory status. Check vital signs at least every 4 hours (q4h). Report and record any abnormalities. Observe for excess swelling or bleeding at operative site. Assist with exercises as prescribed by physical or occupational therapist. Record and report any change in condition of skin at operative site and pressure areas.
Risk for Injury related to unsteady gait	The patient will experience no falls during hospitalization.	Assist patient in and out of bed. Place call bell within easy reach. Check frequently for patient's need to toilet and need for change of position. Provide assistive devices as ordered.
Risk for Injury related to subluxation (dislocation) of joint prosthesis because of improper position, movement, or activity	The patient will maintain proper body alignment and hip positioning and will not exhibit signs of prosthesis dislocation: sudden, severe pain; abnormal position.	Instruct patient to keep legs slightly abducted. May place pillows between legs to achieve abduction while supine and during turning. Turn only to unaffected side. Tell patient not to cross legs or put on own shoes, socks, or stockings for 2 months. Assess for pain and loss of function. Make home health referral if needed to facilitate transition to home setting.
Risk for Infection related to break in skin integrity from surgical hip replacement procedure	The patient will be free of infection during hospitalization, as evidenced by orientation to person, place, and time; normal body temperature, intact wound with decreasing redness, minimal edema, and no purulent drainage.	Encourage fluids and activity when appropriate. Observe for change in mental status or confusion, which may be first signs of infection in older adults. Keep in mind that previous administration of prednisone may mask symptoms of infection. Turn at least every 2 hours (q2h) from back to unaffected side only. Use aseptic technique for wound care. Offer fluids at least q2h.

Critical Thinking Questions

1. Describe at least two behaviors that could reflect a change in this patient's mental status.
2. What data would suggest the need for a home health referral?

When a patient has osteoarthritis, ask about joint pain or tenderness and examine the joints for crepitus, enlargement, deformity, and decreased range of motion. It is helpful to compare affected and unaffected joints to detect abnormalities. Gently support joints during the examination to minimize the patient's discomfort. Observe the patient's movements and gait, noting abnormalities, and record the location and severity of any problems. It is also important to determine how the disease affects the patient's mobility and ability to perform ADL.

Interventions

Chronic Pain

With good pain management, a patient can be more active and have a better quality of life. Administer analgesic and antiinflammatory drugs as prescribed or instruct the patient in self-medication. In addition, instruct the patient in heat or cold treatments as ordered and monitor and record the effects of interventions designed to relieve pain. It is important to inform the physician if pain relief measures are ineffective.

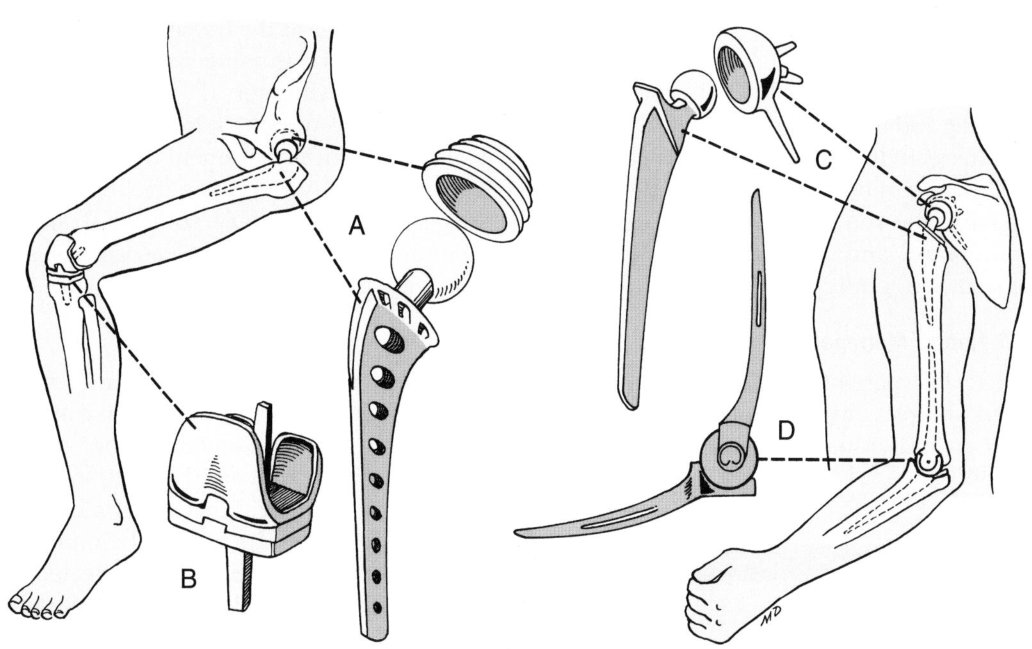

FIGURE 43-3 Total joint replacements. **A,** Hip. **B,** Knee. **C,** Shoulder. **D,** Elbow. (From Black JM, Matassarin-Jacobs E: *Luckmann and Sorenson's medical-surgical nursing: a psychophysiologic approach*, ed 4, Philadelphia, 1993, Saunders.)

Nursing Diagnoses, Goals, and Outcome Criteria: Osteoarthritis

Nursing Diagnoses	Goals and Outcome Criteria
Chronic Pain with motion related to loss of smooth joint surfaces	Pain relief: patient states pain is reduced or relieved, relaxed manner
Impaired Physical Mobility related to pain, limited range of motion	Improved functional mobility: patient accomplishes activities of daily living (ADL) with minimal discomfort
Ineffective Coping related to pain, discomfort, disability	Effective coping: patient states is able to make adaptations to cope with condition, makes positive comments about ability to manage
Ineffective Self-Health Management related to lack of understanding of osteoarthritis management and self-care	Patient manages disease appropriately: patient demonstrates self-care measures and describes prescribed regimen

Measures that protect the joint, discussed in the next section ("Impaired Physical Mobility"), also help to reduce chronic pain. Although it is not unusual for hospitalized patients to have osteoarthritis, most patients manage their own symptoms at home (see *Cultural Considerations* box). Therefore everyday management depends on good patient teaching.

Cultural Considerations

What Does Culture Have to Do with Chronic Illness?

How people react to chronic illness, disability, and dependence is related to their cultural values and beliefs. Consider the older Japanese-American patient who values family interdependence over independence, the Mexican-American patient who accepts illness as God's will, or the person of German heritage who faces pain stoically. Each of these may handle osteoarthritis differently. Nurses must consider these factors when planning patient care.

Impaired Physical Mobility

Impaired physical mobility can significantly interfere with the patient's ability to carry out usual activities in the home or work setting. Modification of daily activities and joint protection measures can help to maintain function. Recommend a regular program of exercise to maintain muscle mass. Aerobic, muscle-strengthening, and water-based exercises are appropriate. The patient who is overweight will benefit from weight loss to reduce stress on joints. Stress the importance of balancing rest and activity to avoid becoming overly tired. The household may need to be reorganized to reduce demands on the patient. Everyday tasks such as dressing and bathing may be affected by the disorder. If the patient's hands are affected, suggest clothing with Velcro closures rather than buttons, pants with an elastic waist, and slip-on shoes. Bathroom grab bars, a shower seat, and a raised toilet seat may promote independence and safety for the patient with poor hip mobility.

Ineffective Coping

Give the patient an opportunity to discuss concerns about osteoarthritis and its effects on lifestyle. Help the patient to prioritize activities and plan how to continue those activities that are most valued. Practical suggestions for managing the condition help the patient to feel a sense of control and confidence in his or her ability to live with the condition.

Ineffective Self-Health Management

Determine what the patient already knows about osteoarthritis and correct any misconceptions. Design and implement an individualized teaching plan (see *Patient Teaching* box).

Patient Teaching

Osteoarthritis

To reduce joint strain and pain, tell the patient the following:

- Maintain proper posture and body alignment.
- Attain and maintain a healthy body weight.
- Identify activities that take a long time to do or for which you need assistance.
- Plan activities when help is available or when time is not a major concern and take periodic rest breaks.
- Wear splints or support devices that rest or relieve painful, unstable joints.
- Push or slide heavy objects rather than pull them.
- Wear shoes with low heels and shock-absorbent soles to help decrease stress on the knee joints.
- Avoid stairs whenever possible.
- Sit rather than stand.
- Use high stools when sitting at a counter.
- Use higher chairs rather than low sofas.
- When rising from a chair, inch to the edge of the seat and then use the armrests to push up from the seat.
- Use large-diameter pencils and pens and use eating utensils with large, round handles.
- Self-medication:
  - Analgesics are usually more effective if taken routinely as prescribed rather than only when you have pain.
  - Know the side effects of your medications and notify your physician if they occur (provide specific list).
- Resource: Arthritis Foundation (www.arthritis.org; telephone: 1-800-283-7800).

❖ NURSING CARE after Total Joint Replacement

Joints that can be replaced include the elbow, shoulder, phalangeal finger joints, hip, knee, and ankle. Preoperative care prepares the patient for the surgical procedure and the postoperative period. Nurses and physical therapists may instruct the patient in postoperative exercises. It is helpful to advise the patient and family of postoperative limitations and encourage planning to adapt the home and work environment as needed. General nursing care of the surgical patient is discussed in Chapter 17. This section describes the postoperative nursing care needs of the patient who has had a joint replacement. Surgical orders or protocols are usually very specific for each type of joint surgery and may vary somewhat among surgeons. Common postoperative measures for specific procedures are presented in Box 43-2.

■ Assessment

Routine postoperative care includes monitoring vital signs, level of consciousness, intake and output, respiratory and neurovascular status, urinary function, bowel elimination, wound condition, and comfort and preventing complications of immobility. After total joint replacement, it is especially important to monitor circulation and sensation in the affected extremity and to determine the need for assistance with ADL.

Nursing Diagnoses, Goals, and Outcome Criteria: Total Joint Replacement, Postoperative

Nursing Diagnoses	Goals and Outcome Criteria
Acute Pain related to tissue trauma	Pain relief: patient states pain is reduced, relaxed expression
Risk for Injury related to improper alignment, dislocated prosthesis, weakness	Decreased risk for injury: patient maintains proper alignment of operative joint
Impaired Physical Mobility related to immobilization, pain, weakness	Physical mobility without complications of immobility: patient is increasingly mobile without excess fatigue or injury, absence of pressure sores
Ineffective Peripheral Tissue Perfusion related to trauma, hemorrhage, thrombi, compression of blood vessels	Normal circulation to affected extremity: symmetric color and warmth of extremities, palpable pulse in affected limb
Risk for Infection related to invasive procedure, prosthesis placement	Absence of infection: normal body temperature, decreasing wound redness, normal white blood cell (WBC) count
Anxiety or Fear related to outcome of procedure	Reduced anxiety and fear: patient states anxiety and fear are reduced, calm manner
Deficient Knowledge related to postoperative self-care	Patient understands self-care: patient describes and demonstrates self-care

Box 43-2 Guidelines for Nursing Care after Replacement of Specific Joints

HIP REPLACEMENT
1. Do not flex hip more than 90 degrees.
2. Avoid flexion, adduction, and internal rotation.
3. Place a large pillow between the patient's legs when turning the patient, when the patient is supine, and when the patient is lying on unaffected side.
4. Advise the patient not to cross the legs or feet and not to put on his or her own shoes, socks, or stockings for 6 weeks to 2 months, as directed by the surgeon.
5. Apply leg abductor splints as ordered.
6. Do not turn onto the operative side unless specifically ordered to do so by the surgeon.
7. Have the patient sit in a chair that has arms to facilitate rising without extreme hip flexion.
8. Arrange for a raised toilet seat to allow toileting without extreme hip flexion.
9. Permit weight bearing as ordered, depending on type of prosthesis used and whether cement was used.
10. Encourage the patient to exercise the unaffected extremities to maintain strength.

KNEE REPLACEMENT
1. Encourage quadriceps-setting exercises and straight leg lifts beginning on postoperative day 2 to 5, as ordered.
2. Use a continuous passive motion (CPM) machine as ordered; check the alignment and settings.
3. Monitor weight bearing with walker or crutches as ordered.

FINGER JOINT REPLACEMENT
1. Instruct the patient to elevate the affected hand.
2. Assess sensation and warmth in the affected fingers.
3. Instruct the patient to use splints during sleep as ordered.
4. Reinforce exercises taught by the physical therapist—must be continued for 10 to 12 weeks.
5. Advise the patient not to lift heavy objects with the affected hand.

Interventions

Acute Pain

To assist with assessment of the patient's pain, ask about pain location, nature, and severity. Surgical pain is expected but the patient with osteoarthritis also may have pain in other joints. If the patient has patient-controlled analgesia, reinforce instructions for its use. Administer analgesics as ordered and document their effects. Reposition the patient as permitted by physician's orders. Use massage, relaxation techniques, imagery, or other strategies described in Chapter 15 to help the patient deal with pain. Notify the surgeon of any sudden, severe pain in the surgical area, which may signal prosthesis dislocation. Uncontrolled pain may make the patient reluctant to participate in rehabilitation measures. Administer analgesics 30 minutes to 1 hour before painful exercises to improve patient participation.

Risk for Injury

Prosthetic joints can become dislocated if they are not maintained in proper alignment. For example, after hip replacement the affected leg must be kept in a position of abduction to prevent dislocation. Instruct patients not to cross the legs or flex the hip more than 90 degrees. Splints or traction may be used if ordered to maintain the desired position. Progressive exercises are usually prescribed and may be done by the physical therapist. As the patient's activity is increased, teach and reinforce precautions. Instruct the patient to recognize signs and symptoms of dislocation, including an audible *pop*, pain in the affected joint, loss of function, and shortening or deformity of the extremity.

Impaired Physical Mobility

The degree of mobility impairment depends on which joints are affected as well as on the patient's general physical state. In general, early mobility is encouraged. When mobility is severely impaired, the patient is at risk for pulmonary and circulatory complications, urine retention, constipation, and skin breakdown. In addition, unused muscles weaken and unused joints stiffen. Reposition the patient as allowed, carefully inspecting pressure areas for redness caused by circulatory impairment. In addition, coach and support the patient during coughing and deep-breathing exercises and use of the incentive spirometer. Auscultate for breath sounds to detect atelectasis or retained secretions and inspect and palpate the abdomen for bladder or bowel distention. Administer intravenous fluids as ordered until the patient takes adequate oral fluids. Give stool softeners and laxatives as ordered.

The patient may have self-care deficits related to mobility impairments or restrictions. It is vital to identify activities the patient cannot do alone and to provide appropriate assistance. As the patient progresses, encourage increasing independence. Rehabilitation requires patient participation in the prescribed exercise program. The patient may need reassurance that the joint can and should be exercised. A patient generally exercises better if pain control is adequate. A CPM machine may be used to reduce scar tissue formation and improve range of motion (Fig. 43-4). Some patients are discharged as soon as 3 days after joint replacement surgery. Individuals who will have difficulty at home may go to a rehabilitation facility initially.

Ineffective Peripheral Tissue Perfusion

Deep vein thrombosis (DVT) is the most serious postoperative complication of hip and knee replacement surgery. Signs and symptoms of DVT include tenderness, swelling, redness, warmth, and firm, palpable blood vessels called *cords*. Monitor body areas distal to the operative joint for circulatory adequacy by collecting data about skin temperature, color, and peripheral

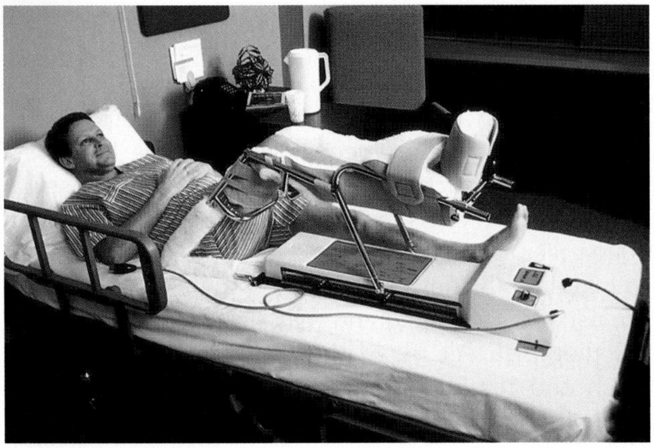

FIGURE 43-4 A continuous passive motion (CPM) machine in use. (Courtesy Chattanooga Group, Hixon, Tenn.)

pulses. To reduce the risk of DVT in the legs, antiembolic stockings or pneumatic compression devices may be ordered in addition to anticoagulant drugs. It is important to check splints, dressings, and stockings to ensure that they are not restricting circulation. Do not place pillows or pads under the legs. Determine the specific exercises that may be done, based on the physician's orders and protocols. For example, after hip replacement the patient should flex and extend the toes, feet, and ankles hourly to promote venous return. Coach the patient in prescribed exercises.

The patient is at risk for hemorrhage after joint replacement. Check the dressings and wound drainage for increasing bleeding. In addition, monitor vital signs for tachycardia and hypotension and observe for restlessness and anxiety. Inspect and measure wound drainage in suction devices at least every 8 hours. A risk of fat embolus exists, which can produce signs of local or cerebral blood vessel occlusion (i.e., petechial [pinpoint] hemorrhage of the upper chest and conjunctiva, fat globules in the urine, headache, irritability, confusion, loss of consciousness).

Pressure caused by edema or constrictive dressings can cause nerve damage, which may be manifested by anesthesia (lack of sensation) or paresthesia (abnormal sensation). Therefore monitor sensation distal to the joint and report symptoms of impairment to the surgeon. In addition, check dressings, stockings, and splints to ensure that they are not too tight.

Supervise ambulation until the patient is steady and clearly understands his or her limitations. Keep the environment free of clutter to prevent falls.

Risk for Infection

Monitor the patient's temperature for elevation that may indicate infection. Check the surgical wound for redness, swelling, warmth, and foul-smelling drainage. Use strict sterile technique when handling the wound, drains, or dressings and keep wound dressings clean and dry. Administer antimicrobials as ordered and instruct the patient in hand washing and wound care.

Anxiety or Fear

Total joint replacement is usually done after conservative treatments have failed to maintain joint mobility. The patient is typically hopeful but anxious about the outcome of the surgery. Tell the patient what to expect, explain procedures and equipment, and offer to answer questions. Responding promptly to the patient's needs and checking on him or her frequently are reassuring.

Deficient Knowledge

From admission through discharge, teach the patient about self-care, wound care, and signs of possible infection (see *Patient Teaching* box). Ensure understanding by having patients repeat important information in their own words. Before teaching, assess for pain, fatigue, or communication barriers. Recognizing cultural differences in lifestyle, diet, and care issues is important. You can assist patients in planning for care at home and involve family members in teaching sessions.

Patient Teaching

Total Joint Replacement

Specifics of the teaching plan depend on which joint was replaced but all patients need to know the following:

- What activities are permitted
- What activities are contraindicated
- Directions for drug therapy
- Wound care
- Signs and symptoms to be reported to the surgeon
- When to return for follow-up care
- Sources of assistance such as home health care

RHEUMATOID ARTHRITIS

RA is a chronic, progressive inflammatory disease. Although it is a systemic disorder, the most notable effect of RA is on diarthroses (synovial joints). The disease may occur at any time but has a peak onset in people 30 to 60 years of age and is more common in women than in men. It affects an estimated 1% of the population all over the world. The course of the disease is variable, ranging from minimal symptoms to severe debilitation.

Pathophysiology

No single cause of RA is known but it is considered an autoimmune disorder. Among the proposed triggers for RA are antigens in the patient's system, viruses or bacteria, genetic predisposition, environmental factors, and hormonal factors. Smoking appears to be a factor for people with a certain antigen. Research to determine the exact cause continues but many recent discoveries have improved the lives of RA patients.

Onset of the disease symptoms is characterized by synovitis (inflammation of the synovial tissues, which hold the lubricating fluid of the joints). In RA, the synovium thickens and fluid accumulates in the joint space. Vascular granulation tissue, called *pannus*, forms in the joint capsule and breaks down cartilage and bone. Fibrous tissue invades the pannus, converting it first to rigid scar tissue and finally to bony tissue. These changes result in **ankylosis** (loss of joint mobility) (Fig. 43-5). Other than joint effects, RA can be manifested in rheumatoid nodules, diminished lacrimal and salivary secretions, inflammation of the eye, enlargement of the spleen and lymph nodes, pulmonary disease, and blood dyscrasias. Rheumatoid nodules are firm, nontender masses that develop on the fingers, elbows, base of the spine, back of the head, sclera, and lungs.

Signs and Symptoms

The most common symptom of RA is pain in the affected joints that is aggravated by movement. Morning stiffness lasting more than 1 hour is almost always a feature of RA, unlike the stiffness of osteoarthritis, which is relieved within minutes. Other symptoms include weakness, easy fatigability, anorexia, weight loss, muscle aches and tenderness, and warmth and swelling of the affected joints. Joint changes are usually symmetric, meaning that the same joints in both extremities are affected simultaneously. The distal interphalangeal and metacarpophalangeal joints are affected most often. The wrist, elbow, knee, and ankle are other possible areas affected. **Rheumatoid nodules**, which are subcutaneous nodules over bony prominences, also may be present (Fig. 43-6).

Any organ of the body may be affected by RA. If blood vessels are affected, they become inflamed, a condition called **vasculitis**. With vasculitis, the blood supply to body organs is impaired, with possible ischemia or infarction of affected organs. Ischemic lesions of the skin are brownish spots most often seen around the nail beds. Large lesions that tend to ulcerate may appear on the legs. Secondary effects on bone can

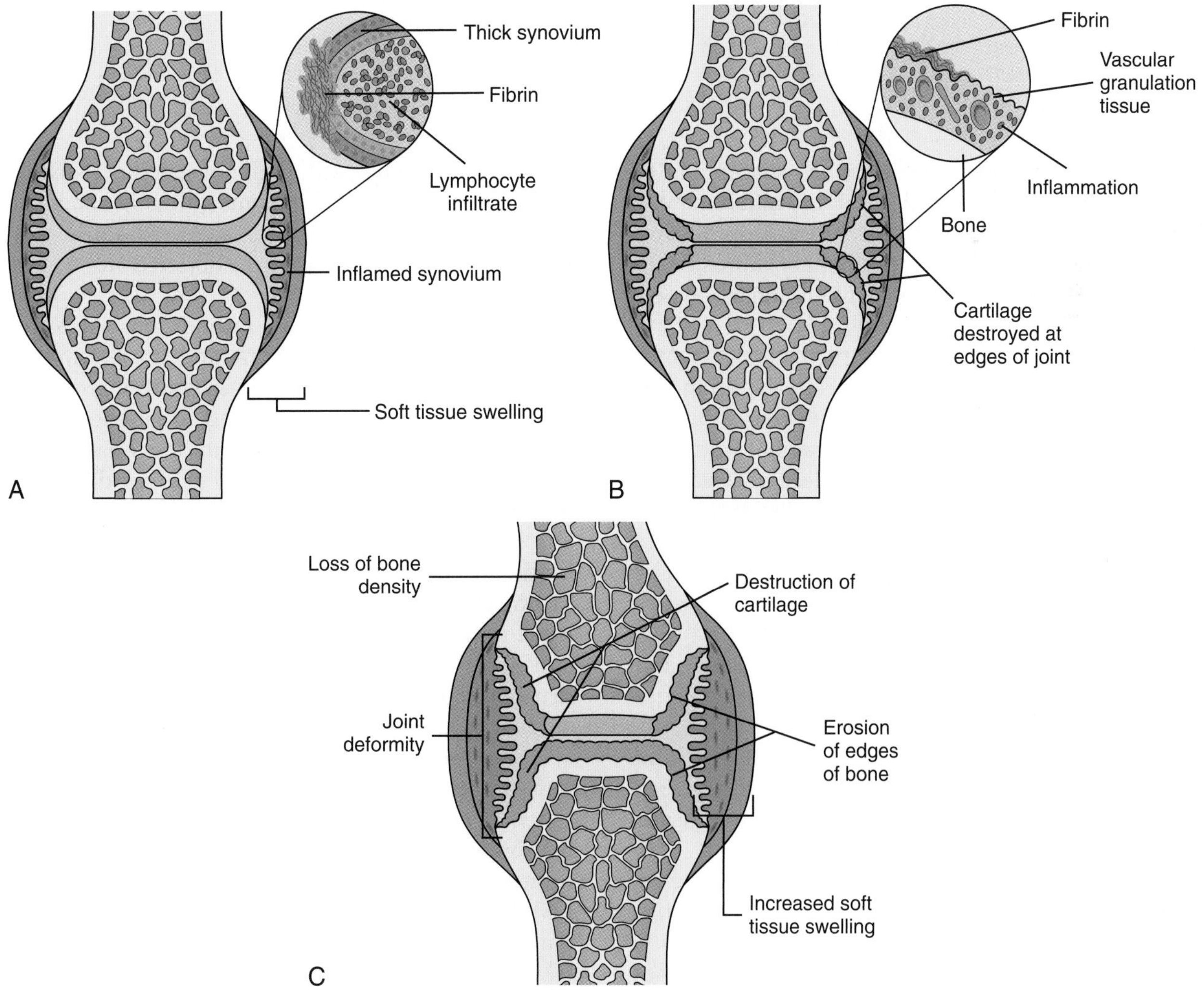

FIGURE 43-5 Phases in the progression of rheumatoid arthritis (RA). **A,** Early phase: leukocytes increase in inflamed synovium. **B,** Pannus grows over the cartilage; bone edges erode; destruction of articular tissue. **C,** Destruction of bone. (From Stevens A, Lowe J: *Pathology: illustrated review in color*, ed 2, London, 2000, Mosby.)

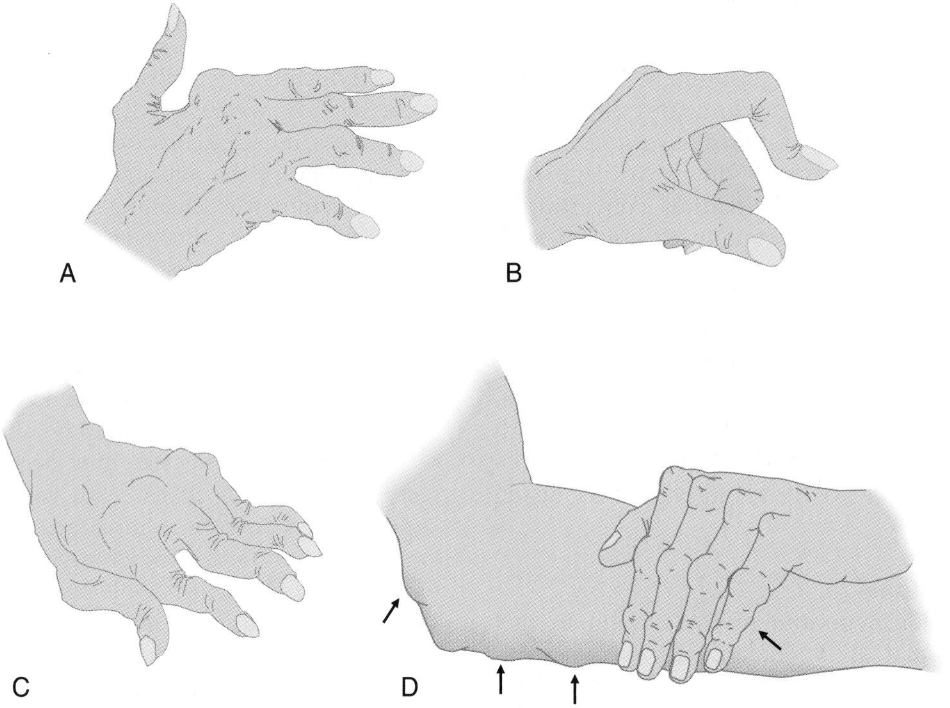

FIGURE 43-6 Four types of hand deformity characteristic of patients with rheumatoid arthritis (RA). **A,** Ulnar drift. **B,** Boutonnière deformity. **C,** Swan-neck deformity. **D,** Rheumatoid nodules. (From Black JM, Hawks JH, Keene AM: *Medical-surgical nursing: clinical management for continuity of care*, ed 6, Philadelphia, 2001, Saunders.)

cause osteoporosis, making the bones susceptible to fractures. The disease may produce inflammatory changes in the tissues of the heart, lungs, kidneys, and eyes. Pleural effusions and pulmonary fibrosis can lead to respiratory impairment or pulmonary hypertension and eventual heart failure.

Some patients with RA develop clusters of symptoms, including Sjögren syndrome, Felty syndrome, or Caplan syndrome. Sjögren syndrome is characterized by dryness of the mouth, eyes, and vagina. Felty syndrome, characterized by liver and spleen enlargement and neutropenia, is less common. Caplan syndrome, marked by rheumatoid nodules in the lungs, occurs most often in coal miners and asbestos workers.

Medical Diagnosis

The diagnosis of RA is based on the health history and physical examination, laboratory findings, and changes detected on radiographic and other imaging studies. No single test diagnoses RA but groups of tests and radiographic findings help to confirm the disorder. See Table 43-1 for common studies for connective tissue disorders.

Laboratory studies that are likely to be ordered include RF, ESR, CRP, anti-citrullinated protein antibodies (ACPA), and anti-cyclic citrullinated peptide (anti-CCP) antibodies. The presence of RF does not establish the diagnosis of RA; however, its presence may support a diagnosis in persons who have other signs and symptoms. The CRP level, ESR, and anti-CCP antibodies, although not specific, also help to support the diagnosis in patients with other suggestive symptoms. Synovial fluid is analyzed for viscosity, WBCs, and glucose and is subjected to a mucin clot test.

The primary purpose of radiographs is to detect changes brought about by RA and to determine the potential usefulness of disease-modifying drugs or surgery. MRI, bone scans, and dual-energy x-ray absorptiometry (DXA) scans provide more detailed information that may be used to monitor disease progression and response to treatment.

Medical Treatment

The treatment of RA involves combined efforts of medicine, nursing, physical therapy, occupational therapy, and social services. Treatment options include rest, drug therapy, physical and occupational therapy, and surgery.

Drug therapy is aimed at controlling the local inflammatory process and providing symptomatic relief. Aggressive therapies are used to relieve inflammation within a 3-month period and to prevent deformities. Combinations of NSAIDs, glucocorticoids, and DMARDs are prescribed to meet the individual patient's therapeutic goal. Leflunomide (Arava) is a DMARD that reportedly can slow the progression of the disease. Etanercept (Enbrel) and infliximab (Remicade) have shown great success in rheumatoid patients, with some patients having a remission of the disease. Joint injections of corticosteroids also can be given two or three times a year and may provide significant symptomatic relief. A nonbiologic DMARD such as methotrexate sodium (Folex) is often very effective in the symptomatic treatment of RA. Systemic glucocorticoids are used to control inflammation initially; then they are gradually reduced to the lowest effective dose as the DMARDs take effect. Maximal effects of DMARDs may require 2 to 6 months of therapy. Patients on glucocorticoid therapy should receive bisphosphonates to prevent osteoporosis associated with glucocorticoid therapy. (See Table 43-1 for details.)

In addition to drug therapy, supportive treatments may be used—including rest, splinting joints to reduce motion that aggravates the inflammation, orthotic devices to support deformed joints, and assistance in modifying ADL. Afternoon rest periods may reduce the fatigue often felt late in the day. Temporary immobilization may be prescribed during acute episodes. However, long-term immobilization contributes to decreased joint flexibility. Types of exercise that may benefit the patient with RA include walking, cycling, aerobics, yoga, and aquatics. The physical therapist can recommend the exact exercise program for each patient. Some resources recommend heat treatments before exercise. Because vitamin D is thought to play a role in reducing inflammation, some physicians may recommend supplements.

Surgical management of RA is reserved for those patients with severe pain and deformities. Among the options are arthroplasty (total joint replacement), synovectomy, tenosynovectomy, and arthrodesis (joint fusion). The most successful procedures are those performed on the knees and hips (see the "Osteoarthritis" section).

NURSING CARE of the Patient with Rheumatoid Arthritis

Assessment

General assessment of the patient with a connective tissue disorder is summarized in Box 43-1. When a patient has RA, collect data related to pain, joint swelling, tenderness, joint deformities and limitation of movement, fatigue, and decreased ability to perform ADL (e.g., dressing, grooming, eating, toileting).

Interventions

Chronic Pain

Chronic pain imposes a terrible burden on the patient. Administer prescribed drugs and teach outpatients about their drug therapy. Teach the patient other measures to control pain, including application of heat or cold and administration of medications as ordered. A warm shower on arising may relieve morning pain and stiffness (see *Complementary and Alternative Therapies* box). Maintaining a program of exercise and rest also can help to manage joint pain and relieve stress. Care of the patient with pain is discussed in Chapter 15.

Nursing Diagnoses, Goals, and Outcome Criteria: Rheumatoid Arthritis

Nursing Diagnoses	Goals and Outcome Criteria
Chronic Pain related to swelling and tenderness	Reduced pain: patient reports decreased pain, relaxed manner
Activity Intolerance related to fatigue	Improved activity tolerance: performance of small tasks without needing a rest period
Ineffective Coping related to frustration, embarrassment, inability to do activities independently	Effective coping: patient identifies ways to deal with physical changes
Social Isolation related to physical impairment and poor body image	Increased social activity: patient resumes at least one social activity that had been abandoned, has realistic view of physical abilities
Ineffective Self-Health Management related to lack of understanding of rheumatoid arthritis (RA), its treatment, and self-care	Patient effectively manages self-care: patient describes and demonstrates correct self-care

Pharmacology Capsule

Aspirin and nonsteroidal antiinflammatory drugs (NSAIDs) prolong bleeding time; thus patients must be monitored for bruising and bleeding.

Complementary and Alternative Therapies

Nonpharmacologic approaches to pain management include application of heat or cold, balanced exercise and rest, relaxation exercises, meditation, imagery, and music.

Activity Intolerance

With the patient, develop a plan of activities around periods of rest and activity. Provide assistance as needed with getting in and out of bed and going to the bathroom. Patients who are severely disabled may need help with all ADL. If needed, help the patient to change positions and provide assistance with meals. Physical and occupational therapy may be ordered. Encourage the patient to follow the prescribed therapy program.

Ineffective Coping

A trusting, collaborative relationship is a prerequisite to providing therapeutic care. Spend time with the patient exploring concerns, answering questions, teaching skills, and planning care. It is vital to emphasize the patient's strengths and explore previously used coping skills. Some patients respond to their physical and functional losses with demanding behavior that others see as manipulative. Patients from some cultures may deal with the pain and disability differently; some are more stoic and reserved while others are demanding or helpless (see *Cultural Considerations* box). Caregivers must recognize this as an attempt by the patient to maintain some control in his or her life. An important part of coping is learning to maintain maximal possible independence despite the crippling effects of RA. Adaptations in the home and workplace and the use of appropriate assistive devices can promote independence and an improved sense of well-being.

Cultural Considerations

What Does Culture Have to Do with Pain?

The way in which people deal with pain is culturally based. For example, people of German, Japanese, and Irish heritage try to be stoic and are reluctant to express pain whereas people from Italy and the Dominican Republic are more likely to express pain openly. Nurses should not make assumptions about a patient's pain based only on his or her behavior.

Because a chronic illness affects the family and the patient, it is important to reach out to the family, offering information, encouragement, problem solving, and resources. Recognize that the family structure differs from one culture to another; the patient's role in the family plays an important part in how he or she views the effects of the disease. Provide information about community resources, such as the local chapter of the Arthritis Foundation. If indicated, consult with the registered nurse (RN) or physician about a referral to a home care agency to help the patient learn to manage better at home.

Social Isolation

Physical deformities that alter appearance and impair function evoke a great sense of loss in the patient with RA. The resulting depression, irritability, and feelings of helplessness can have a devastating effect on the patient's interpersonal relationships. In addition, patients who take corticosteroids often have mood swings, which make their behavior unpredictable. These emotional changes may discourage visits from staff and family, which increases the patient's isolation. Visit the patient often so that he or she does not feel isolated and lonely. Explain the patient's irritability and mood swings to family and friends. In addition, emphasize the importance of their continued support to the patient and encourage the patient to identify appropriate social activities in which he or she can remain involved.

Ineffective Self-Health Management

The teaching plan should include information about the disease process, drug therapy, and the need for balanced rest and activity (see *Patient Teaching* box).

Patient Teaching

Rheumatoid Arthritis

- Take your medications exactly as prescribed and notify your physician of any adverse effects (provide drug names, dosage, schedule, side and adverse effects).
- Keep follow-up appointments; the effects of many drugs need to be monitored with periodic blood studies.
- You must balance your activity and rest.
- Avoid prolonged bed rest, which can lead to further loss of function.
- Use assistive devices as needed to maintain safe mobility.
- Support your joints in functional positions to reduce the risk of contractures.
- Continue to do as much as you can for yourself but do not hesitate to ask for help with difficult tasks.
- Avoid straining your joints with heavy lifting.

Put on Your Thinking Cap!

A 30-year-old mother of a 6-month-old infant and a 5-year-old child has just been diagnosed with rheumatoid arthritis (RA). She is married and works full time as a teacher. Identify ways in which she can modify strain on her joints in both the home setting and the work setting.

OSTEOPOROSIS

Pathophysiology

Bone is constantly being formed and absorbed. Until adolescence, bone formation exceeds bone absorption so that bones grow and strengthen. The processes remain equal through a person's 20s but beginning around age 30, bone absorption surpasses bone formation. Loss of trabecular bone, the innermost layer, occurs first. The loss of cortical bone, the hard outer shell, begins later in life. The loss of cortical bone begins earlier and progresses faster in women than in men. The net result is loss of bone mass, which leaves the patient susceptible to fractures. The most common sites of fractures because of osteoporosis are the wrist, vertebrae, and hip, followed by the pelvis and the humerus. Most cases of osteoporosis are related to aging and estrogen deprivation without other apparent causes. Other cases of osteoporosis are secondary to a wide range of disorders and other variables.

Risk Factors

Many factors appear to increase the risk of osteoporosis. At greatest risk are older women who have small frames, who are Caucasian or of northern European heritage, and who have fair skin and blond or red hair (see *Cultural Considerations* box). Other risk factors are estrogen deficiency; physical inactivity; low body weight; inadequate calcium, protein, or vitamin D intake; long-term therapy with corticosteroids or heparin; and excessive use of cigarettes, caffeine, and alcohol. A number of disorders, such as Cushing disease, hyperparathyroidism, hypogonadism, cirrhosis, leukemia, and diabetes mellitus, also are associated with osteoporosis.

Cultural Considerations

What Does Culture Have to Do with Osteoporosis?

Small, fair-skinned women of northern European descent are at greatest risk for osteoporosis. These women should be targeted early for bone-building dietary and exercise programs.

Signs and Symptoms

Signs and symptoms of osteoporosis may include back pain, fractures, loss of height because of vertebral compression, and kyphosis. Bone deterioration in the jaw can cause dentures to fit poorly. Collapsed vertebrae can cause chronic pain and decline in function. Often the patient has no symptoms of osteoporosis until a fracture occurs.

Medical Diagnosis

A variety of noninvasive tools can be used to assess bone mineral density. The most accurate and precise diagnostic study is DXA of the spine, hip, radius, finger, or total body. Radiographs show bone fractures but do not reveal decreased bone density until loss of 30% to 50% of the bone mass occurs. Blood studies are usually normal with primary osteoporosis but a battery of tests may be ordered to rule out possible secondary causes of osteoporosis. Several markers of bone turnover have been identified in the blood and urine but these are not routinely assessed.

Medical Treatment

Prevention of osteoporosis employs calcium and vitamin D supplementation, physical activity, smoking cessation, limited alcohol intake, and, in some cases, estrogen replacement.

It is generally accepted that calcium supplementation and estrogen replacement for postmenopausal women slow bone loss. The recommended elemental calcium intake is 1000 mg/day for premenopausal women and for postmenopausal women who are on estrogen replacement therapy. Postmenopausal women who are not on estrogen replacement therapy need 1200 to 1500 mg/day of calcium. The only contraindications to supplementary calcium are hypercalcemia, hypophosphatemia, or a history of kidney stones. Vitamin D supplements are also advised. Estrogen replacement in women is controversial but if it is not contraindicated, it may have beneficial effects on the bones for up to 15 years after the onset of menopause. The patient should discuss the issue with her physician. A physical therapist may be consulted to develop an appropriate exercise program for the patient. Although osteoporosis is more common in women, it affects men as well. Treatment options might include androgen replacement, hydrochlorothiazide, and alendronate.

Medical treatment has long been aimed at preventing fractures and stimulating bone formation but until recently there were no drugs that actually reversed the progression of osteoporosis. Drugs that may be used to prevent or treat osteoporosis include antiresorptive agents, selective estrogen receptor modulators (SERMs), bisphosphonates, calcitonin, strontium ranelate, and anabolic agents. Examples of bisphosphonates are alendronate sodium (Fosamax), risedronate (Actonel), and ibandronate (Boniva). Raloxifene (Evista) is a SERM. Synthetic parathyroid hormone (teriparatide) has been found to be effective in reducing the risk of fractures but its use is limited because osteosarcoma has been observed in laboratory animals. Researchers believe that regular exercise promotes bone formation and improves strength, balance, and reaction time, thereby reducing the risk of falls and fractures. Aerobic exercise at least three times a week is encouraged. The incidence or severity of osteoporosis may be reduced by identifying high-risk people and taking steps to promote healthy bone development.

Patients who have spinal fractures caused by osteoporosis may be considered for percutaneous vertebroplasty, which requires that a needle be inserted into the vertebra so that a special type of cement can be injected directly into the vertebra. This procedure is reported to prevent additional compression of the vertebra and to relieve pain caused by compression. Because percutaneous vertebroplasty is minimally invasive, risks are minimized and the recovery time is short. However, reinforced vertebrae may place additional stress on adjacent vertebrae. In addition, recent research found no differences between patients who had vertebroplasty and those who had a sham procedure.

❖ NURSING CARE of the Patient with Osteoporosis

■ Assessment

Nursing assessment of the patient with a connective tissue disorder is summarized in Box 43-1. When a patient has osteoporosis, collect data specifically about the patient's diet, calcium intake, and exercise pattern. In the reproductive history, note whether the patient is menopausal or has had an oophorectomy (i.e., surgical removal of the ovaries) and if she is taking estrogen replacement therapy. Measure the patient's height and compare it with previous measurements. Describe the patient's posture, clearly noting the presence and degree of deformity. Finally, assist the patient with changes in position during the examination for safety and comfort.

Nursing Diagnoses, Goals, and Outcome Criteria: Osteoporosis

Nursing Diagnoses	Goals and Outcome Criteria
Risk for Trauma related to loss of bone strength	Absence of trauma: performance of daily activities without falls or other injuries
Chronic Pain related to fractures, pressure on nerves because of vertebral compression	Pain relief: patient states pain is relieved, relaxed manner
Ineffective Self-Health Management related to lack of understanding of measures to promote bone formation and prevent bone loss	Effective patient management of condition: patient describes and demonstrates activities to improve bone mass

Interventions

Risk for Trauma

Determine the patient's ability to carry out ADL and provide assistance if necessary. Tell ambulatory patients to wear good supportive shoes and provide canes or walkers to improve balance if needed. Keep the environment free of hazards that might cause the patient to fall. Place personal articles within the patient's reach. In the home setting, look for possible hazards and take steps to provide a safer environment. Evaluate the patient's gross visual acuity. To maneuver safely, the patient must be able to see. If indicated, recommend an eye examination.

Chronic Pain

Obtain a complete description of the patient's pain. Administer analgesics as ordered but consider nonpharmacologic interventions as well (see Chapter 15). Some patients, especially those with vertebral compression, may have chronic pain that is difficult to manage. A referral to a clinic that specializes in pain management may be suggested. Document the effects of pain management strategies.

Ineffective Self-Health Management

Patient teaching is key to helping the patient learn to manage osteoporosis (see *Patient Teaching* box).

Patient Teaching

Osteoporosis

- Before menopause and while on hormone replacements, you need 1000 mg of calcium daily.
- After age 50, women need 1200 mg of calcium daily.
- Men require 1000 mg every day up to age 71, when the amount should be increased to 1200 mg per day.
- About 300 mg of calcium are found in each of the following: 1 cup of milk, 1 cup of yogurt, 1 oz of Swiss cheese.
- Nonfat and skim milk have as much calcium as whole milk.
- If you take calcium supplements, increase your fluid intake unless advised not to do so by your physician.
- You need at least 600 IU of vitamin D every day up to age 71, when your physician may advise an increase.
- Taking excessive amounts of calcium and/or vitamin D can cause kidney stones.
- Limit your intake of alcohol and caffeine.
- If Fosamax is prescribed, take it in the morning with a full glass of water on an empty stomach; sit or stand for 30 minutes after taking it.
- Regular weight-bearing exercise helps to maintain bone strength.
- Avoid activities that might lead to falls and fractures.

Put on Your Thinking Cap!

List two ways in which a premenopausal woman can obtain her recommended daily calcium intake without supplements.

GOUT

Gout is an inflammatory arthritis characterized by the deposition of urate crystals in the joints and other body tissues. Put simply, gout occurs when uric acid accumulates in the tissues due to an overproduction of inadequate excretion by the kidneys. When uric acid reaches a certain concentration in the body, it forms crystals that are deposited in connective tissue. When crystals are deposited in and around joints, painful inflammation known as gouty arthritis results. Gout is more prevalent among men than women, with a peak onset in men in their 40s and 50s. Women are rarely affected before menopause. Although the cause of most cases of gout is unknown, genetic and environmental factors appear to contribute to the development of this condition. The risk increases with hyperuricemia, obesity, and a high intake of alcohol, red meat, and fructose. A variety of drugs, including thiazide and loop diuretics and low-dose salicylates, can also play a role.

Pathophysiology

Gout is characterized by **hyperuricemia** (i.e., excess uric acid in the blood) and is related either to an excessive rate of uric acid production or to decreased uric acid excretion by the kidneys. Features of gout may include (1) increased serum urate levels; (2) recurring acute attacks of arthritis; (3) the clumping of urate clusters around the joints of the extremities, causing crippling deformities; (4) renal disease involving blood vessels and interstitial tissues; and (5) uric acid kidney stones.

Three stages of gout exist: (1) asymptomatic hyperuricemia, (2) acute gouty arthritis, and (3) chronic tophaceous gout. Infection may develop if the skin breaks open. Kidney stones develop in about 20% of patients with gout.

Signs and Symptoms

In the first stage, the patient's blood uric acid level is elevated but no other symptoms exist. Many people with asymptomatic hyperuricemia never progress to the next stage. The onset of stage 2, acute gouty arthritis, is abrupt, usually occurring at night. The patient is suddenly afflicted with severe, crushing pain and cannot bear even the light touch of bed sheets on the affected joint. The joint commonly affected is that of the great toe. The attack may be precipitated by trauma, diuretics, increased alcohol consumption, or a high-purine diet (food high in proteins). The symptoms usually disappear within a few days and joint function is completely restored until the next attack. Patients with advanced gout have **tophi**, which are deposits of sodium urate crystals that are visible as small white nodules under the skin (Fig. 43-7).

Medical Diagnosis

Gout is usually suspected on the basis of the history and physical examination and confirmed by the finding of urate crystals in synovial fluid. A 24-hour urine specimen may be ordered to measure urinary uric acid and a fasting blood sample may be drawn to measure the blood uric acid level.

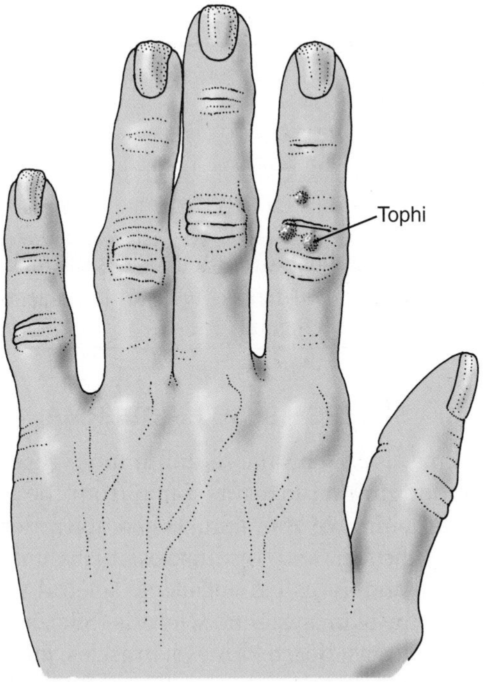

FIGURE 43-7 Typical appearance of tophi, which may occur in chronic gout, on an index finger. (From Ignatavicius DD, Workman ML, Mishler MA: *Medical-surgical nursing across the health care continuum*, ed 3, Philadelphia, 1999, Saunders.)

Medical Treatment

Asymptomatic hyperuricemia usually requires no medical treatment. The primary drugs used to treat attacks of acute gouty arthritis are NSAIDs, oral colchicine, and corticosteroids. If colchicine is used, it may be given hourly until the acute symptoms ease or until the patient develops diarrhea or vomiting. Patients taking NSAIDs may be given a proton pump inhibitor to prevent gastric ulcers and bleeding. When a single joint is affected, prednisone may be injected into the joint. Some sources recommend indomethacin and NSAIDs instead of colchicine in older adults. To manage chronic tophaceous gout and prevent future attacks, three types of drugs are available. Uricostatic agents which include allopurinol and febuxostat prevent urate formation. Probenecid is a uricosuric agent, meaning that it increases the renal excretion of uric acid. Pegloticase is a uricolytic agent; that is, it breaks down uric acid to a soluble product for elimination (see Table 43-2).

Patients who are on antigout medications do not have to severely restrict their diets. They are advised to avoid foods high in purines (liver, kidney, sweetbreads, etc.) and to limit animal proteins, alcohol, and fructose. Fructose is commonly used as a sweetener in prepared foods and drinks. If the patient is obese, weight loss will be recommended.

Pharmacology Capsule

Patients taking antigout drugs need to maintain urine output of at least 2000 mL/day to reduce the risk of urinary calculi formation.

NURSING CARE of the Patient with Gout

Assessment

Complete assessment of the patient with a connective tissue disorder is summarized in Box 43-1. When the patient has gout, collect data specifically about pain; joint swelling; tophi; uric acid stones; fever; and a history of trauma, injury, or surgery.

Interventions

Acute Pain

Nursing care to decrease discomfort includes elevating the affected extremity, administering prescribed medications, encouraging rest, and avoiding pressure on the area. Because even bed sheets may cause pain, a bed cradle should be used. Hot or cold packs may be ordered. Splints or bandages may be used to immobilize the affected joint. When a patient is taking

Nursing Diagnoses, Goals, and Outcome Criteria: Gout

Nursing Diagnoses	Goals and Outcome Criteria
Acute Pain related to joint inflammation	Pain relief: patient states there is pain reduction, relief, or both; appears relaxed
Impaired Physical Mobility related to painful joint movement	Improved mobility: patient gradually resumes activities without unbearable pain
Impaired Urinary Elimination related to urate kidney stones	Normal urine output without symptoms of urinary obstruction: fluid intake and output equal, no flank or abdominal pain, no hematuria
Ineffective Self-Health Management related to lack of knowledge of gout, its treatment, and self-care measures	Patient effectively manages condition: correctly describes and follows plan of care

colchicine, always check laboratory results for abnormalities in blood cell counts. Fatal blood dyscrasias have occurred in patients taking this drug.

Impaired Physical Mobility

Bed rest is usually recommended during the acute period. It is important to provide assistance with ADL as needed. When ambulation is permitted, advise the patient to protect affected joints from trauma by wearing supportive, firm shoes and by keeping walking pathways clearly lighted and free of obstacles that might cause falls.

Impaired Urinary Elimination

When the serum uric acid level is elevated, the excess acid is excreted in the urine, where it may form uric acid stones. Urinary stones can obstruct urine flow from the kidney, causing renal damage. To prevent this complication, advise the patient to drink eight to sixteen 8-oz cups of fluid daily unless contraindicated. Drugs may be prescribed to make the urine alkaline, because uric acid stones precipitate in acid urine. During hospitalization, intravenous fluids may be given. Monitor intake and urine output and promptly report signs and symptoms of urinary stones (i.e., pain in the flank, lower abdomen, or genitals; fever; hematuria; decreased urine output) to the RN or the physician.

Ineffective Self-Health Management

Instruct the patient in measures to prevent or decrease future attacks (see *Patient Teaching* box).

Box 43-3 Purine Content of Selected Foods

HIGH PURINE CONTENT

Avoid these foods during both acute and remission stages of gout:

Anchovies	Bouillon	Brains	Broth
Consommé	Goose	Gravy	Heart
Herring	Kidney	Mackerel	Meat extracts
Mincemeat	Mussels	Partridge	Roe
Sardines	Scallops	Sweetbreads	Yeast (baker's and brewer's as supplement)

MODERATE PURINE CONTENT

One serving (2–3 oz) meat, fish, or poultry or one serving (½ cup) of vegetable from these groups is allowed daily (depending on condition) during remissions:

- Fish, poultry, meat, shellfish
- Asparagus, dried beans, lentils, mushrooms, dried peas, spinach

Modified with permission from Mahan LK, Escott-Stump S, Raymond JL: *Krause's food and the nutrition care process,* ed 13, St. Louis, 2012, Elsevier-Saunders.

Patient Teaching

Gout

Consult a dietitian to help the patient plan a well-balanced diet and give the patient the following instructions:

- Your diet should limit animal protein, alcohol, and fructose. Avoid foods that are very high in purines (Box 43-3). Maintain a fluid intake of eight to sixteen 8-oz glasses daily to reduce the risk of uric acid stone formation in the urinary tract.
- Take your drugs as prescribed (provide specific dosage, schedule, list of side effects).
- To prevent severe attacks, report early joint or urinary symptoms to the physician. Severe attacks may be averted if treatment is begun soon after symptoms develop.
- If you are overweight, weight loss may help by reducing stress on joints.

Put on Your Thinking Cap!

Explain how increased fluid intake will help to prevent kidney stones in the patient with gout.

SYSTEMIC SCLEROSIS (SCLERODERMA)

Scleroderma is a chronic autoimmune disease of unknown origin that takes its name from the characteristic hardening of the skin. When scleroderma is confined to the skin and/or muscles, it is usually relatively mild and is called localized scleroderma. In addition to the skin, systemic sclerosis (SSc) can affect the GI tract, lungs, heart, kidneys, muscles, joints, and blood vessels. The course of the disease varies among individuals, depending on the severity of involvement of the internal organs. The onset of disease is usually between 30 and 50 years of age, with more women than men affected. Death may occur because of infection or cardiac or renal failure. An estimated 300,000 individuals in the United States have SSc.

Two types of SSc exist: (1) diffuse sclerosis and (2) limited sclerosis, also called CREST syndrome. Diffuse sclerosis is characterized by thickening of the skin and systemic effects, specifically hardening of internal organs. CREST syndrome consists of five features: (1) calcinosis (calcium deposits in the tissues), (2) Raynaud phenomenon (vascular spasms), (3) esophageal dysfunction, (4) sclerodactyly (scleroderma of the digits), and (5) telangiectasis (dilated superficial blood vessels).

Pathophysiology

SSc is thought to be the result of environmental factors and genetic susceptibility. Environmental factors that may serve as triggers include infectious agents and occupational, dietary, medical, and lifestyle exposures. The manifestations of the disease follow a chain of events from inflammation to degeneration of tissues that results in decreased elasticity, stenosis, and occlusion of vessels.

Signs and Symptoms

The signs and symptoms of SSc reflect problems of the blood vessels, skin, joints, and internal organs. Common manifestations are Raynaud phenomenon; symmetric, painless swelling or thickening of the skin; taut and shiny skin; morning stiffness; frequent reflux of gastric acid; difficulty swallowing; weight loss; dyspnea; pericarditis; and renal insufficiency. Raynaud phenomenon is manifested by episodes of vasoconstriction in the extremities, especially in response to cold exposure. Affected areas appear pale, then cyanotic, and finally red as blood flow returns.

Medical Diagnosis

Findings in the health history and physical examination may lead the physician to suspect SSc. However, it is difficult to differentiate from other autoimmune conditions at the earliest stage. A positive ANA assay result supports the diagnosis.

Medical Treatment

Even though no cure exists for SSc, treatment with immunosuppressive (e.g., cyclophosphamide, methotrexate) and antifibrotic drugs (e.g., D-penicillamine) may help. Low-dose, short-term corticosteroid therapy alleviates joint pain and stiffness but glucocorticoids are discouraged because they present a risk for renal complications. Various drugs are used to treat the symptoms of SSc, although results have been variable. The management of Raynaud phenomenon is aimed at eliminating anything that causes vasospasm: smoking, cold environmental temperature, and vasoconstricting drugs. Angiotensin II receptor blockers such as losartan are often effective. A variety of other vasodilators may be employed if losartan is not sufficient. Angiotensin-converting enzyme (ACE) inhibitors are used to control hypertensive crisis and to avert sclerodermal renal crisis.

Additional aims of treatment are management of symptoms and prevention of complications. Treatment includes physical therapy to maintain joint mobility and preserve muscle strength. Esophageal reflux may be treated with proton pump inhibitors to decrease the acidity of gastric secretions, periodic dilation of the esophagus, and other measures, such as small, frequent feedings and elevation of the head of the bed.

NURSING CARE of the Patient with Progressive Systemic Sclerosis

Assessment

General assessment of the patient with a connective tissue disorder is summarized in Box 43-1. When a patient has SSc, the health history should document pain and stiffness in the fingers and intolerance for cold. In the review of systems, record signs and symptoms suggestive of cardiovascular, respiratory, renal, and GI problems.

During the physical examination, inspect for skin rash, loss of wrinkles on the face, limitations of joint range of motion, muscle weakness, and dry mucous membranes. Carefully examine the hands for contractures of the fingers and for color changes or lesions on the fingertips. Palpate the fingers to determine warmth.

Nursing Diagnoses, Goals, and Outcome Criteria: Systemic Sclerosis

The nursing diagnoses and goals for patients with systemic sclerosis (SSc) are similar to those of patients with other connective tissue diseases. The following are the major diagnoses.

Nursing Diagnoses	Goals and Outcome Criteria
Impaired Skin Integrity related to thickening of tissues	Optimal skin integrity: warm, intact skin with normal color and texture
Self-Care Deficits (Bathing, Feeding, Toileting) related to pain, contractures of fingers, discomfort	Independent self-care: patient performs activities of daily living (ADL) without excessive discomfort
Chronic Pain related to swelling and stiffness, vasospasm	Pain relief: patient states pain is relieved, relaxed manner
Social Isolation related to poor self-concept, changes in physical appearance	Decreased social isolation: patient maintains or increases social interactions

Continued

Nursing Diagnoses, Goals, and Outcome Criteria: Progressive Systemic Sclerosis—cont'd

Nursing Diagnoses	Goals and Outcome Criteria
Imbalanced Nutrition: Less Than Body Requirements related to esophageal dysfunction	Adequate nutrition: stable body weight, maintains weight within standards recommended for height
Risk for Injury related to diminished renal blood flow	Decreased risk for renal injury: blood pressure (BP) consistent with patient norms, urine intake and output equal
Ineffective Self-Health Management related to lack of understanding of SSc, medical management, and self-care	Effective management of condition: patient correctly describes and follows plan of care

Interventions

Impaired Skin Integrity

Keep the patient's skin clean and dry. Encourage the patient to wear protective clothing as needed to maintain warmth and reduce skin discomfort. Cool baths with mild soaps followed by emollient skin lotions may be soothing. Meticulous mouth care is warranted to prevent oral lesions. Administer antifibrotic and vasodilating drugs if ordered and advise the patient to avoid practices that trigger vasospasm, such as exposure to cold and smoking.

Self-Care Deficits (Bathing, Feeding, Toileting)

Encourage the patient to participate in self-care as much as possible. Monitor the patient's tolerance for activity and provide assistance as needed. Schedule rest periods after activities to prevent overtiring. Encourage the hospitalized patient to maintain independence in activities within his or her abilities.

Chronic Pain

The patient with SSc usually has chronic joint pain and episodes of severe pain in the hands and feet associated with Raynaud phenomenon. Measures to treat joint pain are like those described for RA. During acute episodes of Raynaud phenomenon, the patient may be unable to tolerate anything touching the affected skin. A bed cradle can be used to keep the linens off the body. Adjust the room temperature to prevent chilling, which could provoke vasospasm, and ensure that the patient is aware that smoking and severe stress can also trigger vasospasm.

Social Isolation

Swelling of the hands and facial changes can create a birdlike appearance that may cause the patient to withdraw from social interactions (Fig. 43-8). Explore the patient's concerns about the altered appearance and help the patient to anticipate how to deal with various social situations. Demonstrate acceptance of the patient by expressing concern and using touch.

Imbalanced Nutrition: Less Than Body Requirements

If the patient has esophageal involvement, suggest smaller, more frequent meals, which may be better tolerated. A relaxing environment before and after meals is helpful. Spicy foods, alcohol, and caffeine are discouraged because they stimulate gastric secretions. Because esophageal reflux is common, a proton pump inhibitor may be ordered to reduce the risk of

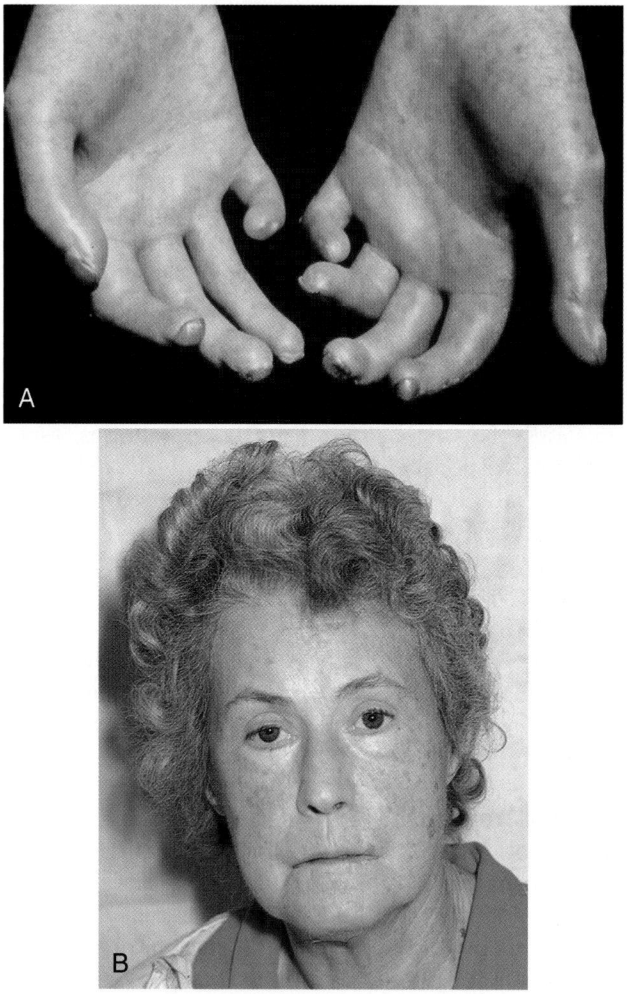

FIGURE 43-8 Late-stage skin changes seen in patients with progressive systemic sclerosis (SSc). **A,** Edema of the hands and fingers. **B,** Typical facial appearance. (A, From Ignatavicius DD, Workman ML, Mishler MA: *Medical-surgical nursing across the health care continuum*, ed 3, Philadelphia, 1999, Saunders. B, From Swartz M: *Textbook of physical diagnosis: history and examination*, ed 6, Philadelphia, 2009, Saunders.)

esophagitis and ulceration. After meals, the head of the bed should remain elevated for 1 to 2 hours to discourage reflux. Monitor and assess the adequacy of nutritional intake.

Risk for Injury

Scleroderma renal crisis is a life-threatening complication of SSc. Changes in blood vessels with SSc gradually reduce the renal blood flow. Increased renin secretion triggers vasoconstriction in a cycle that can result in malignant hypertension. This is a medical emergency that requires hospitalization and treatment with ACE inhibitors. Teach patients to monitor their blood pressure (BP) and to seek medical care if there is a sudden increase in BP.

Ineffective Self-Health Management

As with other chronic illnesses, the patient must learn to implement the medical plan and manage the signs and symptoms of the condition. Patient teaching with SSc includes the nature of the disease, measures to prevent episodes of Raynaud phenomenon, measures to maintain good nutrition and prevent esophageal reflux, signs and symptoms that should be reported to the physician, and self-medication. (Key points are listed in the *Patient Teaching* box.)

Patient Teaching

Systemic Sclerosis

- To prevent vasospasm, keep your hands warm and reduce stress and exhaustion.
- Take drugs as prescribed and report adverse effects to your physician (provide specific information about drug names, dosage, schedule, and adverse effects).
- Esophageal reflux can be managed with drug therapy; relaxing meals; avoiding spicy foods, caffeine, and alcohol; and maintaining an upright position for 1 to 2 hours after eating.

DERMATOMYOSITIS AND POLYMYOSITIS

Dermatomyositis and polymyositis are relatively rare acute or chronic inflammatory diseases that affect primarily the skeletal muscle. The term *polymyositis* is applied to the condition when no skin involvement exists and the term *dermatomyositis* is used when a characteristic skin rash occurs. No known cause for these conditions exists but they are frequently seen in patients with scleroderma, RA, vasculitis, systemic lupus erythematosus (SLE), or Sjögren syndrome.

Pathophysiology

The major activity producing pathology in polymyositis is infiltration of inflammatory cells, causing destruction of muscle fibers. Inflammation of tissues surrounding blood vessels is an outstanding pathologic feature of the disease. The condition is sometimes associated with malignancy.

Signs and Symptoms

The primary symptom of polymyositis is muscle weakness, reflected in inability to do normal activities like climbing stairs, raising the arms over the head, and turning over in bed. Other symptoms are Raynaud phenomenon and joint pain and inflammation. Patients with dermatomyositis typically have periorbital edema (i.e., swelling around the eyes) as well. The onset may be abrupt or slow.

Medical Diagnosis

The diagnosis is based on the presence of proximal muscle weakness, a muscle biopsy positive for muscle degeneration, elevated muscle enzymes, and myopathic electromyographic changes.

Medical Treatment

Drug therapy includes high-dose glucocorticoids such as prednisone and chemotherapeutic drugs such as methotrexate. Supportive treatment centers on the balancing of rest and exercise to prevent contractures. This goal is difficult to achieve because range-of-motion exercises may aggravate the condition.

NURSING CARE of the Patient with Polymyositis

Because polymyositis is seen in conjunction with other connective tissue diseases, see earlier sections of the chapter for applicable nursing interventions.

Nutrition Considerations

Connective Tissue Disorders

1. A daily intake of 1000 to 1200 mg/day of calcium and 600 IU/day of vitamin D is important for the prevention of osteoporosis.
2. Eight ounces of milk (whole, low fat, or skim) provides 300 mg of calcium.
3. A well-balanced diet, including foods high in vitamin E and zinc, is recommended for persons with rheumatoid arthritis (RA).
4. A weight loss program for persons with arthritis reduces stress on weight-bearing joints.
5. Patients with gout are advised to limit intake of animal foods, alcohol, and fructose.
6. The patient with esophageal involvement of systemic sclerosis (SSc) needs small, frequent meals and limited spicy foods, alcohol, and caffeine.

OTHER CONNECTIVE TISSUE DISORDERS

Other connective tissue disorders described in Table 43-3 are bursitis, carpal tunnel syndrome, ankylosing spondylitis, polymyalgia rheumatica, Reiter syndrome, Behçet syndrome, Sjögren syndrome, and periarteritis nodosa. SLE is an important autoimmune disorder that is discussed in Chapter 34. The term *mixed* (or *overlapping*) *connective tissue disease* may be used when patients have features of multiple rheumatic diseases. These patients typically progress to develop SLE, SSc, or polymyositis.

Table 43-3 Other Connective Tissue Disorders

DISORDER	PATHOPHYSIOLOGY	MANAGEMENT
Bursitis	Description: Acute or chronic inflammation of the bursae caused by trauma, strain, or infection. Calcification of bursae may occur. Cause: Usually excessive use of joint. Signs and symptoms: Pain and limited movement in affected joints. Shoulder and hip most often affected.	NSAIDs, rest, and splinting; cold compresses for the first 24 hours and heat thereafter; lidocaine injections for temporary pain relief. Once pain resolves, progressive range of motion, such as "walking" the fingers of the affected arm up the wall, is helpful.
Carpal tunnel syndrome	Description: Common condition in which the median nerve in the wrist becomes compressed, causing pain and numbness. Cause: Caused by pressure on median nerve as it passes through structures of the wrist. People who do repetitive wrist movements such as typing are at risk. Signs and symptoms: Pain and numbness in palmar side of fingers, weakness of thumb.	Splinting to prevent flexion and hyperextension, glucocorticoid injections, and surgical release of transverse carpal ligament. Postoperatively, assess color and temperature of hand. Notify surgeon of pallor, cyanosis, or numbness.
Ankylosing spondylitis	Description: Chronic inflammatory disease that affects vertebral column, causing spinal deformities. Cause: Unknown but appears to be linked to HLA-B27 antigen. Signs and symptoms: First symptom usually dull, aching pain in buttocks. In addition, low-back morning stiffness of several hours' duration that improves with activity; fatigue. Complications: Spinal fractures, iritis (inflammation of the iris of the eye), arthritis.	NSAIDs, DMARDs, monoclonal antibodies. Physical therapy.
Polymyalgia rheumatica and giant cell arteritis (GCA)	Description: Rheumatic disease. Cause: Unknown but likely has hereditary link. Signs and symptoms: Aching and morning stiffness in neck, shoulders and hips, proximal extremities, and torso. Symptoms resolve in 1–2 hours and return after a period of inactivity. Fatigue, weight loss, low-grade fever, anemia. Risk of vision loss with GCA.	Corticosteroids.
Reactive arthritis (Reiter syndrome)	Description: Connective tissue disease. Cause: Often follows infection of GI or GU tract (esp. *Chlamydia trachomatis*); incidence increased in people with certain familial tendencies. Signs and symptoms: Triad of arthritis, urethritis, conjunctivitis. Fever, malaise, fatigue, anorexia, weight loss, conjunctivitis, heel pain, skin lesions.	Antibiotic, NSAIDs, and physical therapy.
Behçet syndrome	Description, signs and symptoms: Chronic systemic autoimmune syndrome. Classic signs: oral and genital ulcers, eye inflammation. Other: large joint arthritis, GI lesions. Cause: Not considered hereditary but there seems to be a familial link.	Treatment varies based on specific manifestations. May include colchicine, thalidomide, anticoagulants, glucocorticoids, cyclosporine, tumor necrosis factor inhibitors (e.g., infliximab), chlorambucil, azathioprine, methotrexate, and retinal proteins.

Table 43-3 Other Connective Tissue Disorders—cont'd

DISORDER	PATHOPHYSIOLOGY	MANAGEMENT
Sjögren syndrome	Description: Inflammatory disease that obstructs secretory ducts in the eyes, mouth, and vagina. Cause: Autoimmune disorder; often seen with rheumatoid arthritis (RA), polymyositis, scleroderma, or systemic lupus erythematosus (SLE). Classic signs and symptoms: Dry eyes, mouth, and vagina. Can affect joints, lung, liver, nervous system, blood, and kidney.	Artificial tears and lubricant ointments; artificial saliva, pilocarpine hydrochloride to stimulate salivary flow, and dental care; vaginal lubricants, perineal hygiene; and glucocorticoids. Other agents based on additional manifestations.
Polyarteritis nodosa	Description: A form of systemic necrotizing vasculitis. Inflammation of small- and medium-sized arteries; can result in thrombosis, infarction, hemorrhage. Affects mainly skin, peripheral nerves, GI tract, and kidneys. May be associated with hepatitis B. Signs and symptoms: Onset insidious. Fever, weight loss, skin lesions, hypertension, joint swelling, malaise, abdominal pain, change in urinary pattern, anemia, ischemia of fingers, pleuritis. Symptoms of renal, GI, and cardiac involvement.	Glucocorticoids, methotrexate, cyclophosphamide, antihypertensive agents, lamivudine or entecavir, and diuretics. Other drugs are prescribed for specific manifestations of the disorder.

DMARDs, Disease-modifying antirheumatic drugs; *GI,* gastrointestinal; *GU,* genitourinary; *NSAIDs,* nonsteroidal antiinflammatory drugs.

Get Ready for the NCLEX® Examination!

Key Points

- The major connective tissues are bone, blood, cartilage, ligaments, skin, and tendons.
- Age-related changes in connective tissue can have a significant effect on function and quality of life.
- Osteoarthritis is characterized by degeneration of articular cartilage, hypertrophy of underlying and adjacent bone, and inflammation of surrounding synovium that leads to pain with joint movement.
- Osteoarthritis may be treated with drug therapy, education, physical therapy, modification of daily activities, and surgery.
- Nursing care of the patient with osteoarthritis focuses on chronic pain, impaired physical mobility, ineffective coping, and ineffective self-health management.
- Total joint replacement can be done on the elbow, shoulder, phalangeal finger joints, hip, knee, and ankle.
- Nursing care after total joint replacement addresses acute pain, risk for injury, impaired physical mobility, ineffective peripheral tissue perfusion, risk for infection, anxiety or fear, and deficient knowledge of postoperative self-care.
- RA, a chronic, progressive inflammatory disease that leads to deformity and loss of joint mobility, is treated with drug therapy, supportive treatments, and modification of ADL.
- Gout, a systemic disease characterized by the deposition of urate crystals in the joints and other body tissues, usually responds to drug therapy that lowers the serum uric acid level.
- SSc, commonly called *scleroderma*, is characterized by thickening of the skin and may affect the blood vessels, GI tract, lungs, heart, and kidneys.
- Nursing care for the patient with SSc addresses impaired skin integrity; self-care deficits (bathing, feeding, toileting); chronic pain; social isolation; imbalanced nutrition: less than body requirements; ineffective self-health management; and risk for injury.
- Less common connective tissue disorders are polymyositis, ankylosing spondylitis, polymyalgia rheumatica, Reiter syndrome, Behçet syndrome, Sjögren syndrome, and periarteritis nodosa.
- Most connective tissue disorders are chronic and, although they are not specifically curable, can be improved with symptomatic treatment.

Additional Learning Resources

SG Go to your Study Guide for additional learning activities to help you master this chapter content.

evolve Go to your Evolve website (http://evolve.elsevier.com/Linton/medsurg) for the following learning resources and much more:
- Interactive Prioritization Exercises
- Fluid & Electrolyte Tutorial
- Pharmacology Tutorial
- Review Questions for the NCLEX® Examination

Review Questions for the NCLEX® Examination

1. The joints between the bones of the skull are classified as which type of joint?
   NCLEX Client Need: Physiological Integrity
2. Age-related changes in connective tissue include which of the following? (Select all that apply.)
   1. Hardening of bone tissue
   2. Decreased water content
   3. Loss of cartilage elasticity
   4. Growth of bony spurs
   5. Softening of cartilage
   6. Loss of bone mass

   NCLEX Client Need: Health Promotion and Maintenance

3. A patient who has gout calls the clinic to report having flank pain and blood in her urine. Which of the following actions should you take?
   1. Report signs and symptoms of urinary stones to the physician immediately
   2. Tell her that these symptoms are normal with gout and that they will improve soon
   3. Make an appointment for her to see the physician within 1 week
   4. Document her complaints in her record and ask her to call the next day if symptoms continue

   NCLEX Client Need: Physiological Integrity: Physiological Adaptation
4. Following total knee replacement, a continuous passive motion (CPM) machine is ordered. The nurse should explain to the patient that the purpose of the CPM machine is to: (Select all that apply.)
   1. Promote joint flexibility
   2. Prevent scar tissue formation
   3. Lubricate the prosthesis
   4. Restore muscle strength
   5. Test the prosthetic joint

   NCLEX Client Need: Physiological Integrity: Reduction of Risk Potential
5. One week after total hip replacement surgery, a patient complains of sudden severe pain in the affected hip and inability to bear weight on that leg. Which of the following should be suspected?
   1. Wound dehiscence
   2. Prosthesis rejection
   3. A new hip fracture
   4. Prosthesis dislocation

   NCLEX Client Need: Physiological Integrity: Reduction of Risk Potential
6. The licensed vocational nurse/licensed practical nurse (LVN/LPN) is assisting in developing a care plan for a patient with RA. Which nursing diagnoses are likely to be appropriate? (Select all that apply.)
   1. Activity intolerance related to fatigue
   2. Social isolation related to physical impairment and poor body image
   3. Ineffective tissue perfusion related to vasoconstriction
   4. Chronic pain related to joint inflammation and swelling
   5. Risk for trauma related to loss of bone strength

   NCLEX Client Need: Physiological Integrity: Physiological Adaptation
7. A women's club has asked the nurse to explain how osteoporosis can be prevented. The nurse should inform the club members that recommended daily calcium intake for women ages 50 and older is:
   1. 200 mg
   2. 500 mg
   3. 1000 mg
   4. 1200 mg

   NCLEX Client Need: Health Promotion and Maintenance
8. When probenecid (Benemid) is prescribed for a patient with gout, patient teaching should include which of the following points? (Select all that apply.)
   1. Avoid people who have infections because your immune system is depressed.
   2. Drink enough fluid each day to maintain urine output of at least 2 L.
   3. It takes several weeks for this medication to be fully effective.
   4. Go to an emergency room if your blood pressure suddenly increases.
   5. Remain in an upright position for at least 30 minutes after taking this medication.

   NCLEX Client Need: Physiological Integrity: Pharmacological Therapies
9. Which statement should be included in the teaching plan for a patient with SSc (systemic scleroderma)?
   1. Keep the temperature in your home below 70 degrees.
   2. Remain upright for 1 to 2 hours after meals.
   3. This is an acute condition that will improve over time.
   4. SSc affects only the skin.

   NCLEX Client Need: Physiological Integrity: Physiological Adaptation
10. A patient being admitted for surgery reports that she has Sjögren syndrome. The nurse should anticipate a need for:
    1. Dim lighting in her room
    2. Oral moisturizer
    3. Assistance with meals
    4. Hand splints

    NCLEX Client Need: Physiological Integrity: Physiological Adaptation

chapter 44

Fractures

http://evolve.elsevier.com/Linton/medsurg

Objectives

1. Identify the types of fractures.
2. Describe the five stages of the healing process.
3. Discuss the signs and symptoms of the major complications of fractures.
4. Compare the types of medical treatment for fractures, particularly reduction and fixation.
5. Describe common therapeutic measures for fractures, including casts, traction, crutches, walkers, and canes.
6. Discuss the nursing care of a patient with a fracture.
7. Describe specific types of fractures, including hip fractures, Colles fractures, and pelvic fractures.

Key Terms

Bone remodeling
Closed reduction *or* manipulation
Comminuted fracture (KŎM-ĭ-nūt-ĕd)
Compartment syndrome
Complete fracture
Delayed union
Fat embolism (ĔM-bō-lĭzm)
Fixation (fĭx-SĀ-shŭn)
Fracture
Greenstick fracture
Incomplete fracture
Malunion (măl-ŪN-yŏn)
Nonunion (nŏn-ŪN-yŭn)
Open *or* compound fracture
Open reduction
Reduction
Stress fracture

A **fracture** is defined as a break or disruption in the continuity of a bone. When a fracture occurs, surrounding soft tissue is injured also. The severity of soft tissue injury depends on the location and severity of the break.

All fractures are either complete or incomplete. A **complete fracture** is one in which the break extends across the entire bone, dividing it into two separate pieces. An **incomplete fracture** is one in which the bone breaks only partway across, leaving some portion of the bone intact. The term **greenstick fracture** has been used to describe the incomplete fractures most commonly seen in children. In this case the bone is splintered on one side but only bent on the other.

CLASSIFICATION OF FRACTURES

Fractures may be classified as *open* or *closed*, depending on the type and extent of soft tissue damage. A closed or simple fracture is one in which the broken bone does not break through the skin. In an **open** or **compound fracture**, the fragments of the broken bone break through the skin. Open fractures have three grades of severity:

- Grade I: least severe injury, with minimal skin damage
- Grade II: moderately severe injury, with skin and muscle contusions (bruises)
- Grade III: most severe injury (wound larger than 6 to 8 cm), with skin, muscle, blood vessel, and nerve damage

Fractures also may be classified as *stress* or *pathologic fractures*, depending on their cause. A **stress fracture** is caused by either repeated or prolonged stress. Stress fractures are often related to sports such as track or basketball. A pathologic fracture occurs because of a pathologic condition in the bone such as a tumor or disease process that causes a spontaneous break. Figure 44-1 illustrates common types of fractures.

CAUSE AND RISK FACTORS

Fractures are most commonly caused by trauma to the bone, especially as a result of automobile accidents and falls. Bone disease such as bone cancer also can lead to a fracture. Hip fractures in older adults usually are associated with falls. Risk factors for hip fractures include osteoporosis, advanced age, Caucasian race, and female gender (see *Cultural Considerations* box). Certain drugs contribute to osteoporosis, including glucocorticoids, cyclosporine, methotrexate, heparin, and anticonvulsants.

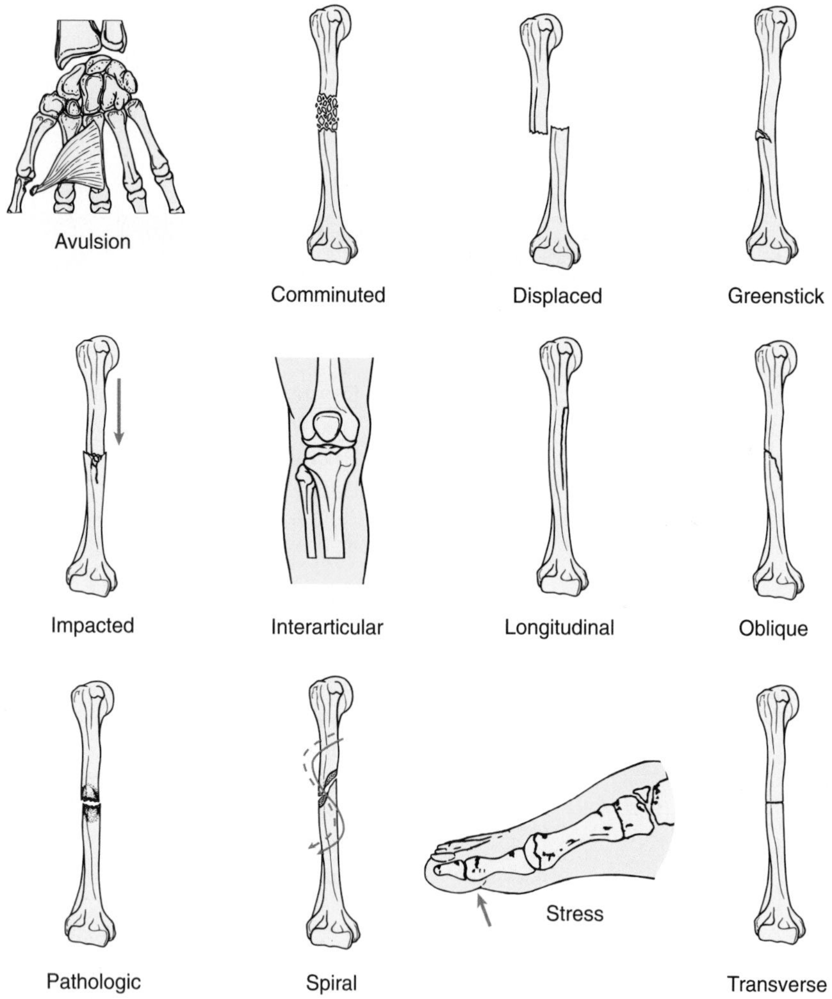

FIGURE 44-1 Common types of fractures. (From Lewis SM, Heitkemper MM, Dirksen SR, et al.: *Medical-surgical nursing: assessment and management of clinical problems*, ed 7, St. Louis, 2007, Mosby.)

Cultural Considerations

What Does Culture Have to Do with Fractures?

Older Caucasian women have a high incidence of osteoporosis and therefore are at increased risk for fractures. This risk can be reduced by targeting these women for preventive measures throughout life. Osteoporosis is easier to prevent than to treat.

In adults, the bones most commonly fractured are the ribs. Fractures of the femur are most common in young and middle-aged adults whereas hip, wrist, and vertebral fractures are most common in older adults. In 2010, hip fractures accounted for more than 258,000 hospital admissions among persons aged 65 and older.

FRACTURE HEALING

A bone begins to heal as soon as an injury occurs. New bone tissue is formed to repair the fracture, resulting in a sturdy union between the broken ends of the bone. Healing occurs in the following five stages:

- Stage 1: *Hematoma formation.* Immediately after a fracture, bleeding and edema occur. In 48 to 72 hours, a clot or hematoma forms between the two broken ends of the bone.
- Stage 2: *Fibrocartilage formation.* The hematoma that surrounds the fracture does not resorb, as does a hematoma in other parts of the body. Instead, other tissue cells enter the clot and granulation tissue forms, replacing the clot. The granulation tissue then forms a collar around each end of the broken bone, gradually becoming firm and forming a bridge between the two ends.
- Stage 3: *Callus formation.* Within 1 to 4 weeks after injury, the granulation tissue changes into a callus formation. Callus is made up of cartilage, osteoblasts (i.e., bone cells that form new bone), calcium, and phosphorus. The callus is larger than the diameter of the bone and serves as a temporary splint.
- Stage 4: *Ossification.* Within 3 weeks to 6 months after the break, a permanent bone callus, known as *woven bone*, forms. It is during this stage that the ends of the broken bone begin to knit.
- Stage 5: *Consolidation and remodeling.* Consolidation occurs when the distance between bone

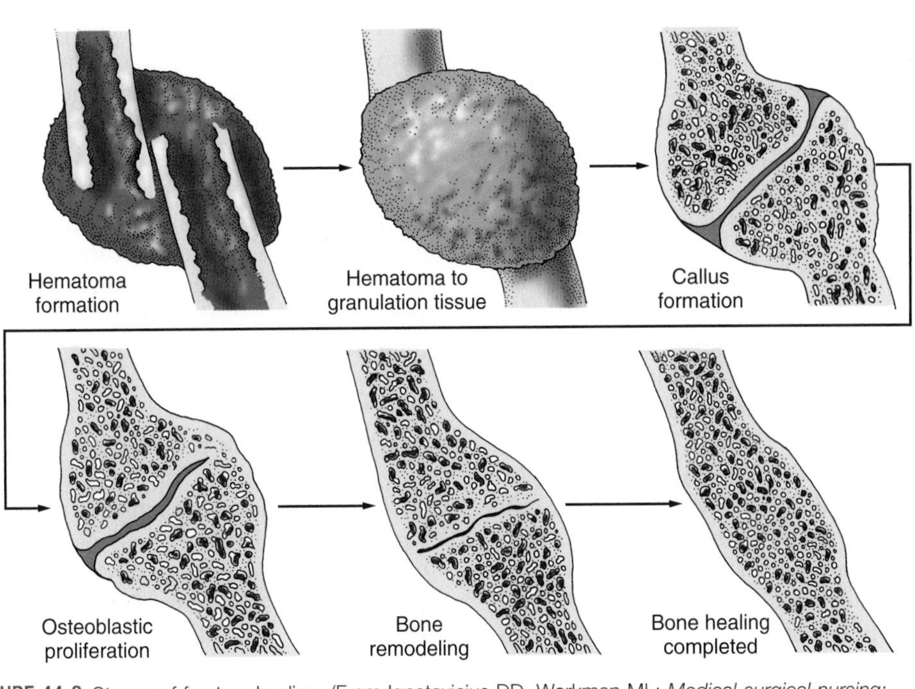

FIGURE 44-2 Stages of fracture healing. (From Ignatavicius DD, Workman ML: *Medical-surgical nursing: patient-centered collaborative care*, ed 6, St. Louis, 2010, Saunders.)

fragments decreases and eventually closes. During **bone remodeling,** the immature bone cells are gradually replaced by mature bone cells. The excess bone is naturally chiseled away by stress to the affected part from motion, exercise, and weight bearing. The bone then takes on its original shape and size (Fig. 44-2).

Healing is affected by many factors, including the location and severity of the fracture, the type of bone, other bone pathology, blood supply to the area, infection, and the adequacy of immobilization. Other factors that affect healing include age, endocrine disorders, and some drugs. The healing time for fractures increases with age and it may take six times as long for the same type of fracture to heal in an older adult as in an infant. In the absence of bone disease, most older adults eventually heal as well as younger adults. However, many older adults, especially women, have a loss of bone mass.

COMPLICATIONS

Complications of a fracture can delay or impede healing and may even be life threatening. Short-term complications include infection, fat embolism, deep vein thrombosis (DVT), compartment syndrome, and shock. Long-term complications include joint stiffness and contractures, malunion, nonunion, delayed union, posttraumatic arthritis, avascular necrosis, and complex regional pain syndrome.

INFECTION

Infection of the bone, called *osteomyelitis*, can result from contamination of the open wound associated with a fracture, from contamination of the indwelling hardware used to repair the broken bone, or through the blood from a distant infection. When an infection is inadvertently introduced by surgery or other treatment, it is known as an *iatrogenic* or *health care–associated infection.* Any infection can interfere with normal healing. Osteomyelitis occurs most commonly after an open fracture and surgical repair and may become chronic. In deep, grossly contaminated wounds, gas gangrene may develop.

Signs and symptoms of bone infection are local pain, redness, purulent wound drainage, chills, and fever. With gas gangrene, a foul-smelling watery drainage is seen, with significant redness and swelling of affected tissue. A diagnosis is based on clinical findings supported by culture of drainage or material obtained by needle aspiration. Imaging procedures—computed tomography (CT), magnetic resonance imaging (MRI), positron emission tomography (PET) scan—may be helpful. Radiographic changes typically are not seen until 10 to 14 days after the onset of infection.

Osteomyelitis requires aggressive antibiotic therapy. Intravenous antibiotics may be given for 4 to 8 weeks, followed by an additional 4 to 8 weeks of oral drug therapy. Chronic infection may require continuous, long-term antimicrobials. Wound care may include irrigation, treatment with antibiotic beads, and surgical removal of dead bone tissue, hardware, or both.

FAT EMBOLISM

Fat embolism is a condition in which fat globules are released from the marrow of the broken bone into the bloodstream. Once the fat droplets enter the circulation, they migrate to the lungs. Because they are too large to pass through the pulmonary circulation, they lodge in the capillaries and obstruct blood flow. The fat particles break down into fatty acids, which inflame the pulmonary blood vessels, leading to pulmonary edema.

Fat embolism syndrome is most commonly associated with fractures of the long bones, multiple fractures, and severe trauma. It occurs 24 to 72 hours after injury, most often in young men ages 20 to 40 years and in older adults ages 70 to 80 years. An older patient with a hip fracture is at highest risk. The most important preventive action is careful immobilization of fractures.

Respiratory distress is the first sign of a fat embolism, followed by tachycardia, tachypnea, fever, confusion, and decreased level of consciousness. Another characteristic feature is petechiae, a measles-like rash over the neck, upper arms, chest, or abdomen. Treatment of fat embolism consists of bed rest, gentle handling, oxygen (O_2), and ventilatory support. Other specific interventions will be needed if the patient develops hypovolemic shock, acidosis, and/or pulmonary edema. Though controversial, corticosteroids sometimes are used. The prognosis is generally good; however, the condition can be fatal.

DEEP VEIN THROMBOSIS

Venous stasis, vessel damage, and altered clotting mechanisms all contribute to the formation of blood clots (thrombi), most commonly in the deep veins of the legs. This complication is increased with immobility often associated with a fracture. Like fat particles, thrombi can break off and travel to the lungs, causing a pulmonary embolism. The prevention and treatment of DVT and pulmonary embolism are discussed in Chapter 31.

COMPARTMENT SYNDROME

Compartment syndrome is a serious complication that results from internal or external pressure on the affected area. Compartments are located in the muscles of the extremities. They are enclosed spaces made up of muscle, bone, nerves, and blood vessels wrapped by a fibrous membrane, or fascia. External pressure caused by a cast or tight dressing can decrease blood flow to the area. Internal pressure can be caused by edema or bleeding into a compartment. Fluid trapped in the compartment puts pressure on the tissues, nerves, and blood vessels, decreasing blood flow and resulting in pain and tissue damage.

Although compartment syndrome is relatively rare, it is a serious condition and can create an emergency situation. Within 4 to 6 hours after the onset of compartment syndrome, irreversible muscle and nerve damage can occur. Paresis (i.e., partial paralysis) can result if the condition is not treated within 24 hours. In 24 to 48 hours, the limb can become useless.

A primary symptom of compartment syndrome is pain, especially with touch or movement that cannot be relieved with opioid analgesia. Other signs and symptoms are edema, pallor, weak or unequal pulses, cyanosis, tingling, numbness, and paresthesia.

The goal of treatment is to relieve pressure. When internal pressure exists, a surgical fasciotomy, which entails making linear incisions in the fascia, may be done to relieve pressure on the nerves and blood vessels. For external pressure, the cast or dressings are removed and replaced.

SHOCK

After a fracture, a risk of excessive blood loss exists. Tissue trauma may rupture local blood vessels and vascular internal organs may be punctured, with resultant internal bleeding. Loss of blood leads to shock, which is evidenced by tachycardia, anxiety, pallor, and cool, clammy skin. Careful immobilization of fractures reduces the risk of hemorrhage. If severe external bleeding is evident, external pressure should be applied and medical assistance summoned immediately. Management of hypovolemic shock is discussed in Chapter 19.

Put on Your Thinking Cap!

A 16-year-old male patient was admitted after a motorcycle accident. He had a compound fracture of the femur with severe soft tissue injury. After surgery, he has an external fixation device on the affected leg. A Jackson-Pratt drain is in place. Daily wound care is ordered. List all potential sources of bone infection.

JOINT STIFFNESS AND CONTRACTURES

Joint fractures or dislocations may be followed by stiffness or contractures, especially in older persons, because of immobility often associated with a fracture. Prevention requires appropriate positioning and progressive exercise programs as prescribed. Treatment may include the use of splints, traction, casts, surgical manipulation, and aggressive physiotherapy.

MALUNION, NONUNION, AND DELAYED UNION

Malunion is when expected healing time is appropriate but unsatisfactory alignment of bone results in external deformity and dysfunction. **Nonunion** occurs when a fracture never heals. Failure of a fracture to heal in the expected time is called **delayed union**. With delayed union, the bone usually heals eventually—it may just be slower. These complications may be caused by inadequate immobilization or excess movement, poor alignment of the bone fragments, infection, or poor nutrition.

When nonunion of a fracture exists, a variety of methods may be used to stimulate fracture healing. The implantation of bone grafts is an *osteogenic method*. *Osteoconductive methods* use synthetic materials to provide a matrix for bone growth. The use of substances such as platelet-derived growth factor is called *osteoinduction.* In addition, devices that deliver electric stimulation or pulsed electromagnetic fields may be used to stimulate bone growth. The stimulation may be internal or external and is done up to 10 hours a day for 3 to 6 months. Although the procedure is time consuming, it can prevent further surgery and bone grafts. Hyperbaric oxygen therapy has been used but the value in treatment of nonunion has not been confirmed.

POSTTRAUMATIC ARTHRITIS

Weight-bearing joints are most vulnerable to posttraumatic arthritis. Excessive stress and strain on the joint or fracture must be avoided to reduce the risk of this complication. Posttraumatic arthritis can be a result of nonunion of a fracture.

AVASCULAR NECROSIS

A fracture or bone infection can interfere with the blood supply to the bone. Once bone cells are deprived of O_2 and nutrients, they die and their cell walls collapse. This condition is called *avascular necrosis.* Signs and symptoms include increasing pain, instability, and decreased function in the affected area. Treatment measures include relief of weight bearing and removal of part of the bone to decrease pressure. If conservative measures fail, a variety of surgical procedures may be recommended. Sometimes amputation is necessary.

COMPLEX REGIONAL PAIN SYNDROME

Complex regional pain syndrome Type 1 (CRPS Type 1) is usually precipitated by a fracture or other trauma. It is characterized by severe pain at the injury site despite no detectable nerve damage, edema, muscle spasm, stiffness, vasospasms, increased sweating, atrophy, contractures, and loss of bone mass. Symptoms persist longer than expected with the type of injury suffered. The condition is treated with nerve blocks; physical therapy; transcutaneous electrical nerve stimulation (TENS); and drugs, including analgesics, antiseizure drugs, antidepressants, and alpha-1 adrenergic agonists. Various nonopioid infusions such as lidocaine and ketamine have been used with some success. The effects and treatment of CRPS Type 2, also called *causalgia,* are similar but nerve damage can be detected.

SIGNS AND SYMPTOMS

The signs and symptoms of a fracture depend on the type and location of the break. Some fractures have so few clinical manifestations that they can be detected only with a radiograph. The most common signs and symptoms are swelling, bruising, pain, tenderness, loss of normal function, abnormal position, and decreased mobility. Box 44-1 lists various signs and symptoms of fractures and their causes.

Box 44-1 Signs and Symptoms of Fractures and Their Causes

PAIN
Immediate, severe pain is felt at the time of injury. After injury, pain may result from muscle spasm, overriding of the fractured ends of the bone, or damage to adjacent structures.

DEFORMITY
Strong muscle pull may cause bone fragments to override; therefore alignment and contour changes occur, such as (1) angulation, rotation, and limb shortening; (2) bone depression; or (3) altered curves in the injured site, especially when compared with the opposite site. Swelling (edema) may appear rapidly from localization of serous fluid at the fracture site and extravasation of blood into adjacent tissues. Bruising (ecchymosis) may result from subcutaneous bleeding. Muscle spasms—involuntary muscle contractions near the fracture—may occur.

TENDERNESS
Tenderness over the fracture site is due to underlying injuries.

IMPAIRED SENSATION (NUMBNESS)
Sensation may be impaired as a result of nerve damage or nerve entrapment from edema, bleeding, or bony fragments.

LOSS OF NORMAL FUNCTION
Normal function may be lost because of instability of the fractured bone, pain, or muscle spasm.

PARALYSIS
Paralysis may be caused by nerve damage.

ABNORMAL MOBILITY
Movement of a part that is normally immobile is due to instability when the long bones are fractured.

CREPITUS
Crepitus results from broken bone ends rubbing together. Grating sensations or sounds are felt or heard if the injured part is moved.

HYPOVOLEMIC SHOCK
Hypovolemic shock may result from blood loss or other injuries.

Modified from Black JM, Hawks JH, Keene AM: *Medical-surgical nursing: clinical management for positive outcomes*, ed 6, Philadelphia, 2001, Saunders.

DIAGNOSTIC TESTS AND PROCEDURES

A thorough history and physical are important when fracture is suspected because they may provide valuable information, such as mechanism of injury, and often help to direct treatment. The most common diagnostic tests used to confirm the presence of a fracture are radiologic studies. Standard radiographs are used first to reveal bone disruption, deformity, or malignancy. CT may be used to detect fractures of complex structures, such as the hip and pelvis, or compression fractures of the spine. MRI aids in the assessment of soft tissue damage. A bone scan may be useful for detecting small bone fractures or fractures caused by stress or disease. Diagnostic tests for fractures are the same as those for connective tissue disorders described in Chapter 43, Table 43-1.

MEDICAL TREATMENT

The goals of medical treatment for a fracture are to realign the bone fragments, establish a sturdy union between the broken ends of the bone, and restore function. The most common therapeutic techniques to accomplish these goals are closed or open reduction and internal or external fixation.

REDUCTION

Reduction is the process of bringing the ends of the broken bone into proper alignment. **Closed reduction** or **manipulation** is the nonsurgical realignment of the bones that returns them to their previous anatomic position. No surgical incision is made; however, general or local anesthesia is given. Closed reduction may be done by using traction, manual pressure, or a combination of these (Fig. 44-3). After reduction of a fracture, a radiograph is taken and the injured part is immobilized.

Open reduction is a surgical procedure in which an incision is made at the fracture site. It is usually done for open (i.e., compound) or **comminuted fractures** (i.e., bone is broken or crushed into small pieces) to clean the area of fragments and debris.

Effective pain management of a fracture is essential for patient mobilization and healing. Once the fracture is aligned, immobilization is necessary for healing to occur. Immobilization of the bones is important because it prevents movement and increases union. It can be accomplished in many ways such as fixation, casts, splints, and traction.

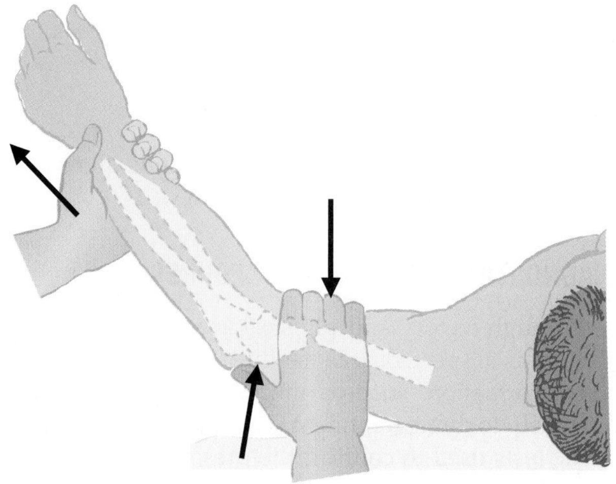

FIGURE 44-3 Closed (manipulative) reduction to realign a fracture of the arm. (From Black JM, Hawks JH: *Medical-surgical nursing: clinical management for positive outcomes*, ed 8, St. Louis, 2009, Saunders.)

FIXATION

Fixation is an attempt to attach the fragments of the broken bone together when reduction alone is not feasible because of the type and extent of the break. Internal fixation is done during the open reduction surgical procedure. Internal fixation includes the use of rods, pins, nails, screws, or metal plates to align bone fragments and keep them in place for healing (Fig. 44-4). Figure 44-4, *C*, illustrates an open reduction and internal fixation of a fractured femur in which a nail is used to maintain alignment. Internal fixation promotes early mobilization and is often preferred for older adults who have brittle bones that may not heal properly or who may suffer the consequences of immobility.

External fixation is similar to internal fixation but the pins are inserted directly into the bone, above and below the fracture. The pins are then attached to an external frame and adjusted to align the bone (Fig. 44-5). When extensive soft tissue damage or infection occurs, external fixation allows easier access to the site and facilitates wound care. In addition, the device allows for early ambulation and mobility while relieving pain. Pin track infection occurs in approximately 10% of patients with external fixation. Pin care is extremely important to prevent the migration of organisms along the pin from the skin to the bone. Patients

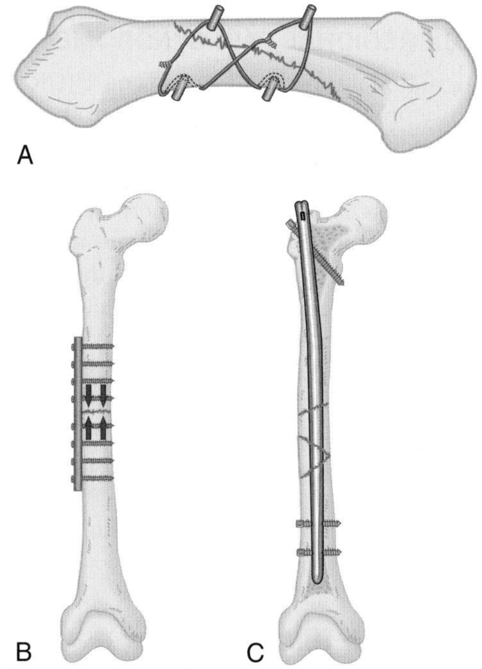

FIGURE 44-4 Examples of different types of internal fixation devices. **A,** Tension band wiring technique using Kirschner wires for fracture of a phalanx. **B,** Compression plate applied to the lateral aspect of the femur. **C,** Intramedullary nail fixed to both proximal and distal fragments of the femur. (From Black JM, Hawks JH: *Medical-surgical nursing: clinical management for positive outcomes*, ed 8, St. Louis, 2009, Saunders.)

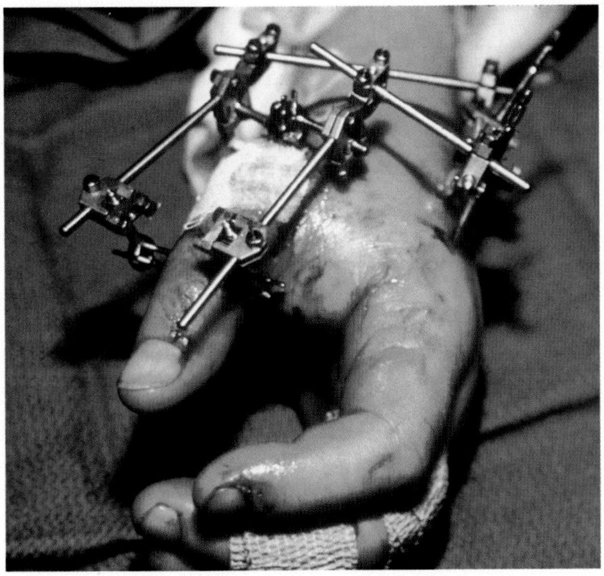

FIGURE 44-5 External fixators. Mini Hoffman system in place on hand. (Courtesy Stryker, Howmedica Osteonic, Inc., Mahway, NJ.)

should be taught to do their own pin care and to recognize signs of infection.

COMMON THERAPEUTIC MEASURES

CASTS, SPLINTS, AND IMMOBILIZERS

Casts, splints, and other immobilizers are used to secure the position of the body parts being treated. They hold the bone in alignment while allowing enough movement of other parts of the body to carry out activities of daily living (ADL). Types of materials used for a cast are plaster of Paris, fiberglass, thermoplastic resins, thermolabile plastic, and polyester-cotton knit impregnated with polyurethane. A variety of materials are used to make splints and immobilizers.

Plaster of Paris consists of anhydrous calcium sulfate embedded in gauze. It is the least expensive type of cast to use. After a well-fitting stockinette has been applied, the gauze is immersed in water and wrapped around the affected part. The stockinette must not be too tight because it may impair circulation. A stockinette that is too loose can wrinkle and result in pressure sores. The strength of the cast is determined by the number of layers of wrapped gauze and the technique of application.

Initially the wet cast is hot and the heat may cause edema of the underlying tissues from the increased circulation. The cast quickly becomes damp and cool. It dries after about 24 to 72 hours, depending on the size and location. When the cast is dry and strong, it can withstand weight bearing and other stresses. The underlying stockinette covers the edges of the cast to prevent scratching and irritation from the rough plaster. Short pieces of tape are sometimes placed over the edges of the casts to prevent skin irritation by rough edges and to protect the cast from moisture and soiling. This is referred to as *petaling*.

Fiberglass is a synthetic material used for casts that is lighter and has a shorter drying time than plaster of Paris. Drying time is 10 to 15 minutes and the cast can withstand weight bearing 30 minutes after application. Sometimes physicians use plaster of Paris casts on lower extremities for heavier weight bearing and fiberglass casts on upper extremities.

Other types of synthetic materials are thermolabile plastic (Orthoplast) and thermoplastic resins (Hexcelite). They are heated in warm water and molded to fit the torso or extremity. Polyurethane is formed from chemically treated polyester and cotton fabric. The fabric is immersed in cool water to start the chemical process for wrapping.

Sometimes the cast is split down the front to allow the casting material and padding to spread. This is referred to as a *univalved cast*. A *bivalved cast* is cut down both sides so that the front portion can be removed while the back portion maintains immobilization. When an opening is cut into the cast to allow inspection of the body area or to relieve pressure, it is said to be a *windowed cast*. It is important to save the cut out "window" because it may be reinserted later.

The four main groups of casts are (1) upper extremity, (2) lower extremity, (3) cast brace, and (4) body or spica cast. Various types of casts are illustrated in Table 44-1. An upper extremity cast is used for breaks in the shoulder, arm, wrist, and hand. A patient who is wearing an arm cast should keep the arm elevated above the heart when lying in bed to prevent swelling. The arm is kept in a sling for support when the patient is up and out of bed.

Lower extremity casts are used for breaks in the upper and lower leg, ankle, and foot. A leg cast is used to allow mobility and may be used with crutches. A cast shoe or rubber walking pad protects the cast and prevents falls. The affected leg should be elevated on several pillows during the first few days after the break to prevent swelling.

After an adequate amount of healing has taken place and edema has subsided, cast braces may be used for injury to the knee. A cast brace supports the affected part while allowing the knee to bend. This is accomplished by applying a cast above and below the knee and connecting them with a hinge.

Body or spica casts are used when a fracture is located somewhere in the trunk of the body. A body cast encircles the trunk whereas a spica cast encases the trunk plus one or two extremities. When both legs are casted, a bar joins the two at knee level. Body or spica casts severely limit mobility and may cause complications related to lack of movement, such as skin breakdown, respiratory problems, constipation, and joint contractures. Turning a patient in a spica cast usually requires several people. Never use the bar for turning because it can break and disrupt the

Table 44-1 Cast Types and Common Uses

TYPE	ILLUSTRATION	COMMON USES
Short arm cast	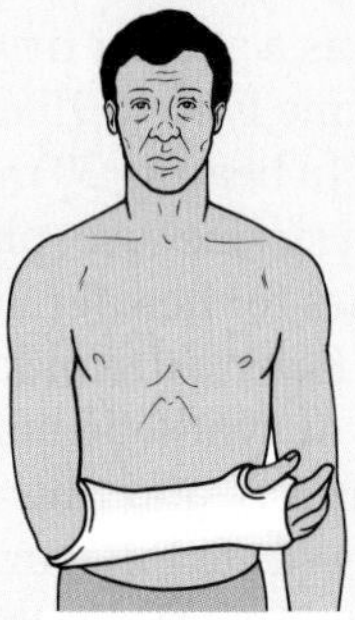 Short arm cast	Fracture of hand or wrist Postoperative immobilization after open reduction and internal fixation
Long arm cast	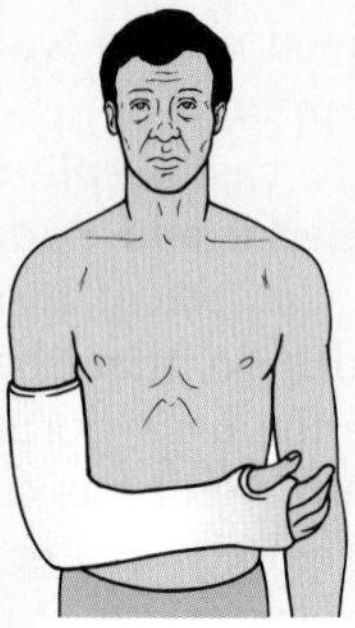 Long arm cast	Fracture of forearm, elbow, or humerus Postoperative immobilization after open reduction and internal fixation Can be weighted to create traction
Body jacket cast	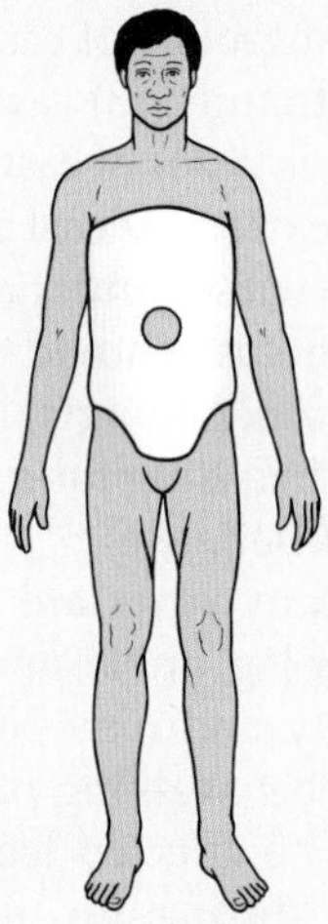 Body jacket cast	Stable spine injuries of the thoracic or lumbar spine
Bilateral long leg hip spica cast	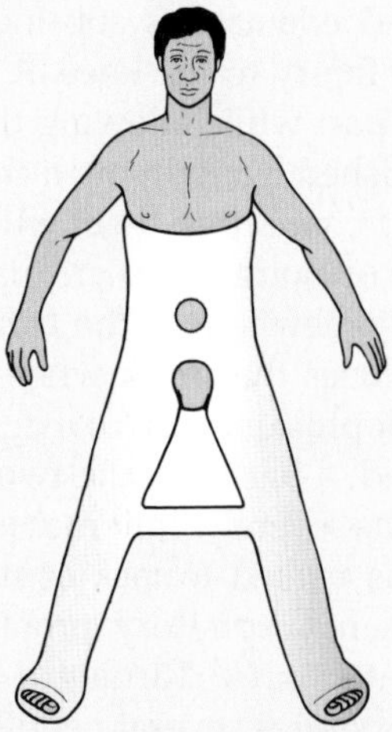 Double hip spica	Fractures of femur, acetabulum, or pelvis Postoperative immobilization after open reduction and internal fixation

Table 44-1 Cast Types and Common Uses—cont'd

TYPE	ILLUSTRATION	COMMON USES
Long leg cast	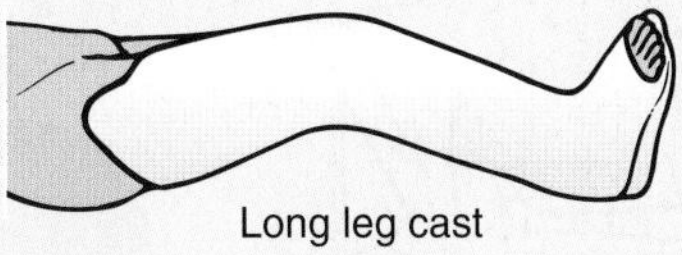 Long leg cast	Fracture of distal femur, knee, or lower leg Soft tissue injury to knee or knee dislocation Postoperative immobilization after open reduction and internal fixation
Short leg cast	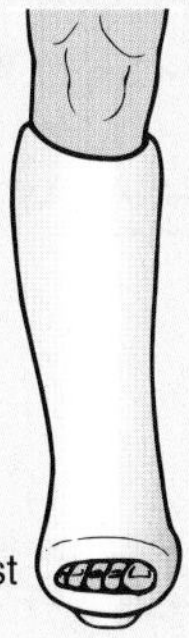 Short leg cast	Fracture of foot, ankle, or distal tibia or fibula Severe sprain or strain Postoperative immobilization after open reduction and internal fixation Correction of deformity, such as talipes equinovarus

Illustrations from Lewis SM, Dirksen SR, Heitkemper MM, Dirksen SR, Bucher L, Camera IM: *Medical-surgical nursing: assessment and management of clinical problems*, ed 8, St. Louis, 2011, Mosby.

immobilization. In addition, a condition known as *cast syndrome* is caused by compression of a portion of the duodenum between the superior mesenteric artery and the aorta and vertebral column. Signs and symptoms of cast syndrome include nausea and abdominal distention (see *Patient Teaching* box).

Patient Teaching

Cast Care

- Keep plaster casts dry; follow the physician's instructions regarding wetting synthetic casts.
- Do not remove any padding.
- Do not insert any foreign object inside the cast.
- Do not bear weight on a new plaster cast for 48 hours (with synthetics, may be less than 1 hour).
- Do not cover the cast with plastic for prolonged periods.
- *Do report the following to a health care provider:* swelling, discoloration of toes or fingers, pain during motion, and burning or tingling under the cast.

The cast is removed only on physician's orders. A special device called a *cast cutter* is used to cut the plaster. Blunt scissors are then used to cut the padding. Tell the patient that the cutter blade is noisy but will not cut the skin. When the cast is removed, the skin that was under the cast will be tender and dry and may have crusts of dry skin. Gently wash the area and explain that the skin will regain its normal appearance after a few days. Muscle atrophy may be apparent. Assure the patient that muscle mass will be restored with use of the limb.

TRACTION

Traction exerts a pulling force on a fractured extremity to provide alignment of the broken bone fragments. It also is used to prevent or correct deformity, decrease muscle spasm, promote rest, and maintain the position of the diseased or injured part.

Traction may be applied directly to the skin (i.e., skin traction) or attached directly to a bone by means of a metal pin or wire (i.e., skeletal traction). Examples of skin traction, such as Buck traction, are shown in Figure 44-6. It is used for hip and knee contractures, muscle spasms, and alignment of hip fractures. Weight used during skin traction should not be more than 5 to 10 lb to prevent injury to the skin.

Skeletal traction provides a strong, steady, continuous pull and can be used for prolonged periods of time. Examples of skeletal traction are Gardner-Wells, Crutchfield, and Vinke tongs and a halo vest, in which pins are inserted into the skull on either side (see Figs. 29-6 and 29-7). Heavier weights can be used with skeletal traction, usually from 15 to 30 lb. Crutchfield traction and a halo vest are used for reduction and immobilization of fractures of the cervical or high thoracic vertebrae.

Traction may involve complications such as impaired circulation, inadequate fracture alignment, skin breakdown, and soft tissue injury. As noted earlier, pin track infection and osteomyelitis can occur with skeletal traction. The following are important points to remember when patients are in traction:

- Weights always must hang freely.
- Ensure that the amount of weight used is correct as ordered, clamps are tight, and ropes move freely over pulleys.

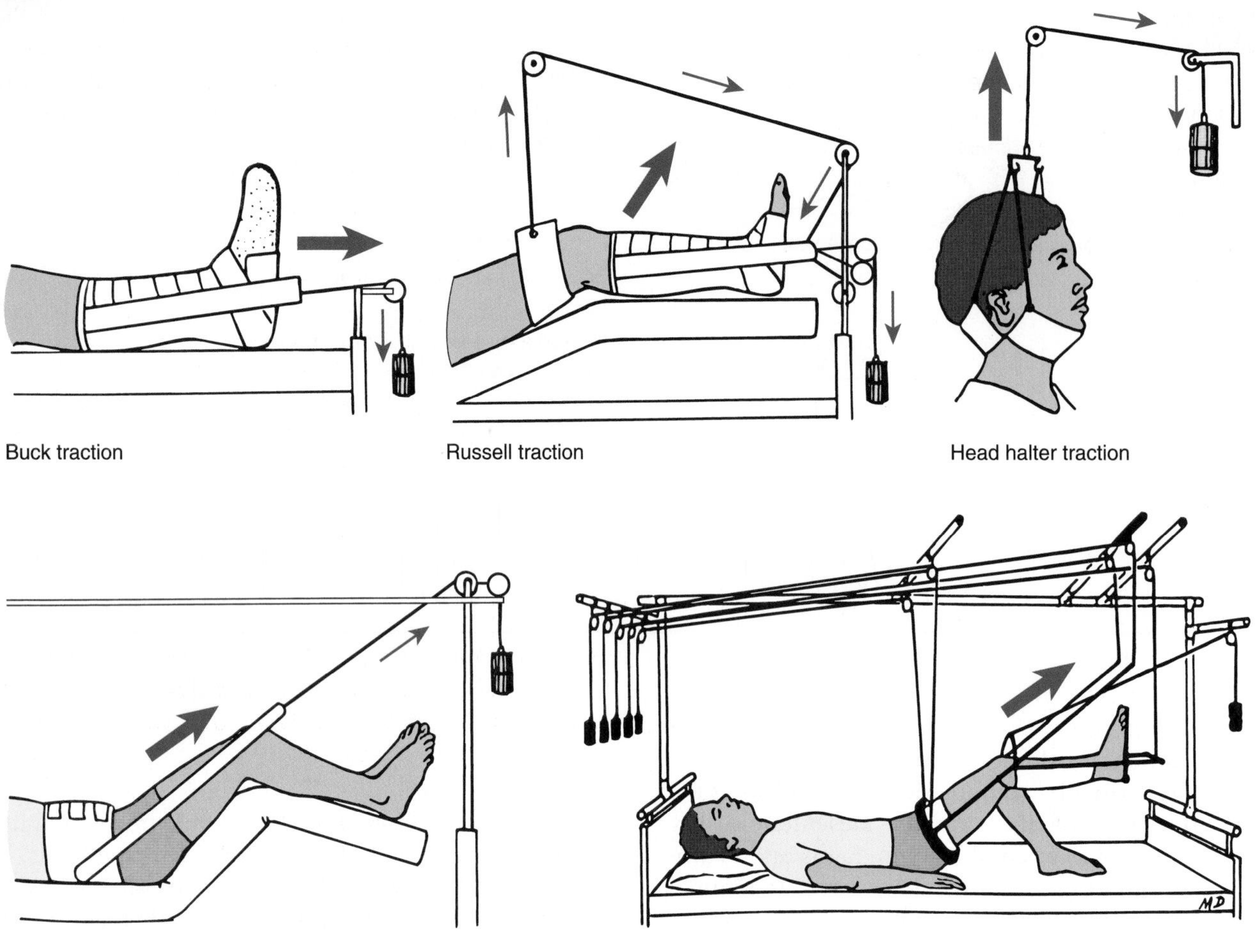

FIGURE 44-6 Examples of skin traction. (Redrawn from Polaski AK, Tatro SE: *Luckmann's core principles and practice of medical-surgical nursing*, Philadelphia, 1996, Saunders.)

- Maintain good body alignment so that the line of pull is correct.
- Use padding to prevent trauma to skin where traction is applied. Report skin breakdown or irritation to the physician.
- Assess affected extremities for temperature, pain, sensation, motion, capillary refill time, and pulses.
- With skeletal traction, assess pin sites for redness, drainage, or odor, which may indicate infection.

ELECTRICAL STIMULATION AND PULSED ELECTROMAGNETIC FIELDS (PEMFS)

Electrical stimulation may be used to promote bone healing by promoting bone growth. An electrical current is delivered through a surgically implanted device, a device applied to the skin, or a device that uses pins inserted through the skin. Electrical bone stimulators are successful in approximately 80% of cases, with an average healing time of 16 weeks. PEMFs are noninvasive devices that include a control box and a pad that induces electrical changes around and within the cell. In theory, the electrical changes activate and regenerate cells, which promotes healing and reduces pain.

ASSISTIVE DEVICES

CRUTCHES

Crutches increase mobility and assist with ambulation after a fracture of the lower extremity. Success in crutch walking depends on many factors, including the patient's motivation, age, interests and activities, and ability to adjust to the crutches. Crutch use requires good upper body strength, so it may not be appropriate for older or frail patients.

In most cases, a physical therapist measures the patient for proper fit and instructs the patient in crutch-walking techniques. The nurse reinforces the instructions and evaluates whether the crutches are being used properly. A properly fitted crutch should reach to 3 to 4 fingerbreadths below the axilla to avoid pressure on the axilla and nerves when walking (Fig. 44-7). Axillary pressure could result in temporary or permanent numbness in the hands. When walking, the patient's weight should be put on the hand grips. The hand grips are adjusted so that the elbow is flexed no more than 30 degrees when the patient is standing in the tripod position, which is the basic crutch stance: feet parallel, crutches 6 inches in front of and 6 inches to the side of each foot.

Gait Patterns

Several types of gait patterns are used with crutches. The type of gait used depends on the severity of the patient's disability and the patient's physical condition, trunk strength, upper and lower extremity strength, and balance. All of the gaits begin with the tripod position.

The five types of gait patterns used with crutches are as follows:

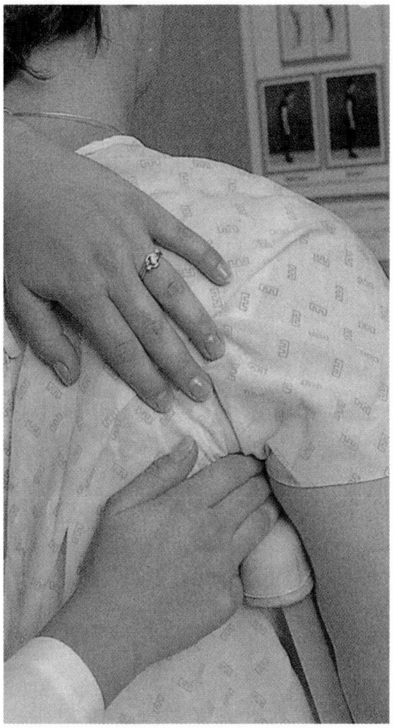

FIGURE 44-7 The distance between the crutch pad and the patient's axilla should be 3 to 4 fingerbreadths. (From Potter PA, Perry AG, editors: *Fundamentals of nursing*, ed 7, St. Louis, 2009, Mosby.)

1. *Two-point gait:* The crutch on one side and the opposite foot are advanced at the same time. This gait is used with partial weight-bearing limitations and with bilateral lower extremity prostheses.
2. *Three-point gait:* Both crutches and the foot of the affected extremity are advanced together, followed by the foot of the unaffected extremity. This gait requires strength and balance. It is used for partial weight bearing or no weight bearing on the affected leg.
3. *Four-point gait:* The right crutch is advanced, then the left foot, then the left crutch, and then the right foot. This gait is used if weight bearing is allowed and one foot can be placed in front of the other.
4. *Swing-to gait:* Both crutches are advanced together and then both legs are lifted and placed down again on a spot behind the crutches. The feet and crutches form a tripod.
5. *Swing-through gait:* Both crutches are advanced together and then both legs are lifted through and beyond the crutches and placed down again at a point in front of the crutches. This gait is used when adequate muscle power and balance in the arms and legs exist.

To sit down after walking with crutches, the patient walks up to a chair, turns using the crutches, and backs up until the unaffected leg touches the seat of the chair. One hand then grips both crutches by the hand grips and the crutches are placed to the unaffected side. The patient bends at the waist, places the hand on the affected side on the seat, moves the affected leg forward, and lowers onto the seat slowly (Fig. 44-8). To get up from a sitting position, the patient pushes off against the chair with the hand of the affected side and

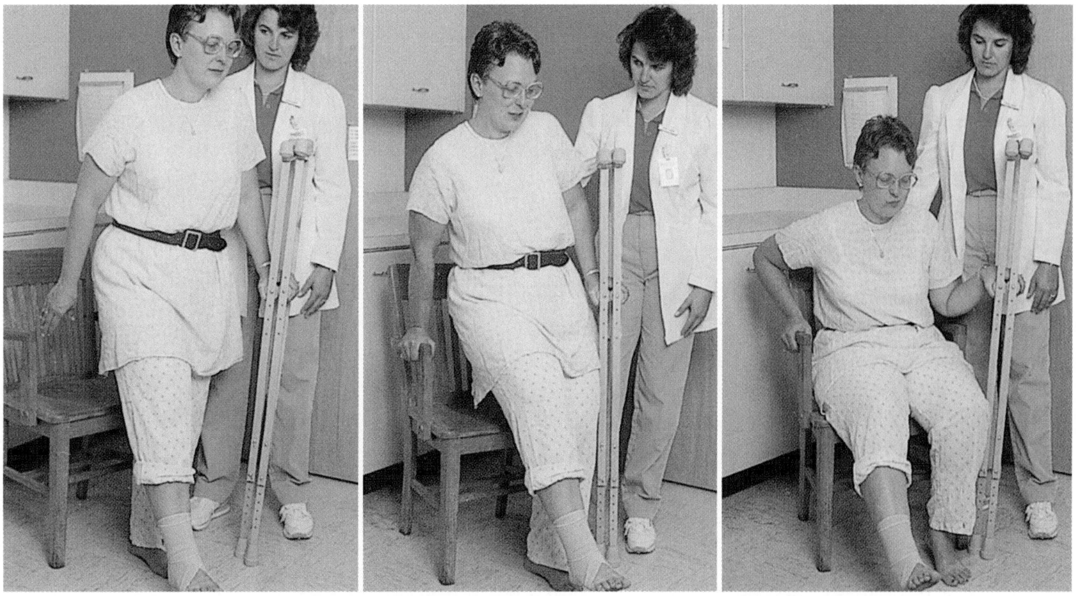

FIGURE 44-8 Standing to sitting with crutches. (From Potter PA, Perry AG, editors: *Fundamentals of nursing*, ed 7, St. Louis, 2009, Mosby.)

pushes down with the other hand, which is holding both crutches by the hand grips.

Going up and down stairs on crutches is challenging. For stair climbing, the unaffected leg goes up the step first while the body is supported by the crutches. The full body weight is transferred to the unaffected leg, followed by movement of the crutches and the affected leg to the step. To descend stairs, the affected leg and the crutches move down one step first and then the unaffected leg follows. So, when climbing stairs, the good leg goes first and when descending stairs, the bad leg goes first. ("The good leads up and bad leads down.")

WALKERS

A walker is used for support and balance, usually by older clients. A modified swing-to gait is used with a walker so that the walker is pushed or lifted forward and then the legs are brought up to it. Rather than lifting both legs forward together, as with crutch walking, one foot is brought forward at a time.

CANES

Canes are used to provide minimal support and balance and to relieve pressure on weight-bearing joints. The cane is placed on the unaffected side with the top of the cane even with the patient's greater trochanter. The elbow should be flexed to approximately 30 degrees. A two-point or four-point gait is used with a cane. The cane should be held close to the body on the unaffected side and advanced along with the affected leg. When walking, it is better to lift the cane rather than slide it along to prevent catching the cane tip and tripping or falling.

Nursing Care Plan — Patient with a Fracture

ASSESSMENT

HEALTH HISTORY Mrs. Jacobson, age 80, was admitted for a Colles fracture in the left wrist 2 days ago. Before the injury, she lived alone and cared for herself. She was active, alert, and independent. Since the fracture repair, she has complained of pain over the area of the break but has had no signs of infection. Her physician is ready to discharge her to her home.

PHYSICAL EXAMINATION Vital signs: blood pressure 165/95 mm Hg, pulse 98 bpm with slight irregularity, respiration 20 breaths per minute, temperature 97.4°F (36.3°C) measured orally. Height 5′3″, weight 132 lb. Alert and oriented to time, place, and person. Needs assistance with activities of daily living (ADL), particularly bathing, dressing, and toileting. Cast on left arm from above her elbow to her fingers.

Nursing Diagnosis	Goals and Outcome Criteria	Interventions
Acute Pain related to bone fracture, edema, soft tissue damage, muscle spasm	The patient's pain will be relieved, as evidenced by absence of verbal complaints, anxiety, and moaning or wincing; patient confirms pain relief.	Provide adequate pain relief using medications and other comfort measures such as positioning and massage.
Ineffective Peripheral Tissue Perfusion related to decreased blood flow caused by injury	The patient will have adequate tissue perfusion, as evidenced by normal skin color in areas distal to the fracture, adequate capillary refill, and adequate sensation.	Relieve edema by elevating the affected limb above the level of the patient's heart while she is lying in bed and applying cold for brief periods of time; encourage patient to wiggle fingers to increase circulation to the area.
Impaired Physical Mobility related to pain and treatment modalities for fracture	The patient will maintain as much mobility as possible, as evidenced by independence in ADLs and absence of secondary complications.	Encourage regular movement, including passive or active range-of-motion exercises. Reinforce activity and exercise program for the patient. Seek referral to home health for assistance at home.
Risk for Impaired Skin Integrity related to cast	The patient will maintain skin integrity, as evidenced by intact skin.	Inspect the skin around cast edges for pressure or irritation. Monitor circulation and sensation in the fingers.
Deficient Knowledge related to lack of experience with immobilization devices (e.g., casts)	The patient will demonstrate understanding of the immobilization device and will describe its proper care and complications that could arise.	Teach the patient interventions that promote bone and tissue healing; teach the patient to recognize signs and symptoms of complications that should be reported to the physician. Instruct the patient in cast care.
Self-Care Deficit (Bathing, Feeding, Dressing, Toileting) related to immobilization of wrist	The patient performs ADL independently or with assistance.	Assess the patient's ability to do ADL and to perform tasks such as cooking and grocery shopping. Determine whether she has anyone to assist her if needed. If not, request a home health or social work evaluation so that home care or assistance can be provided.

Critical Thinking Questions

1. What activities can the patient perform that will promote bone and tissue healing?
2. What signs and symptoms require physician intervention?

❖ NURSING CARE of the Patient with a Fracture

Once the initial emergency treatment and medical management of a patient with a fracture have been provided, nursing care becomes very important. The focus of nursing care is on preventing complications and restoring the patient to independent function. (See Nursing Care Plan: Patient with a Fracture. For a discussion of emergency care, see Chapter 16.)

■ Assessment

Health History

Even after the initial medical care has been given and the fracture has been set, it is helpful to gather information on the cause, type, and extent of the injury. This information is important because it allows you to observe for complications or other injuries that may have been overlooked during the emergency situation. Ask the patient, family members, or witnesses about the events leading up to the accident and exactly what happened during it. In addition, describe symptoms associated with the injury, including the type and extent of pain, the presence of numbness or tingling or both, the loss of motion and sensation, and the complaint of muscle spasms.

Document the number and types of prescription and over-the-counter (OTC) medications taken by the patient to determine whether they played any role in the development of the fracture or will affect recovery and rehabilitation. It is also helpful to find out about other medical problems that either may have been related to the cause of the fracture, such as a pathologic fracture, or may affect healing. Determine the patient's occupation and usual roles and responsibilities and discuss with the patient and family the effects of the injury on usual activities.

Physical Examination

Because fractures usually involve some type of accidental injury, be alert for signs of serious complications, such as head, thoracic, or abdominal injuries. In addition, examine the patient for associated tissue trauma, such as bleeding, bruising, and lacerations.

When inspecting the suspected fracture area, observe for deviations in bone alignment. The limb may appear to be deformed. The length of the extremity may change, usually becoming shorter. Inspect the skin over the fracture for lacerations, bruising, or swelling.

Compare the affected extremity with the unaffected extremity. Do neurovascular checks (i.e., pulse, skin color, capillary refill time, sensation) in the areas distal to the wound to compare circulation and sensation. Assess pulse rate and volume as well as capillary refill time in the nails distal to the injury. Observe capillary refill time by applying pressure to the nail and checking the time required for color to return to the area. Skin color is a good indication of circulation to the extremity and pallor indicates poor circulation. Determine sensation by pinprick, especially in the web space between the first and the second toes or between the thumb and the forefinger.

Nursing Diagnoses, Goals, and Outcome Criteria: Fracture

Nursing Diagnoses	Goals and Outcome Criteria
Acute Pain related to bone fracture, edema, soft tissue damage, or muscle spasm	Pain relief: relaxed manner, patient statement of pain relief
Ineffective Peripheral Tissue Perfusion related to tissue trauma or pressure caused by edema, bone fragments, hemorrhage, or therapeutic devices	Adequate circulation: affected tissue warm, normal pulses, normal skin color, minimal edema
Risk for Infection related to break in skin, bone trauma, soft tissue damage	Absence of infection: normal body temperature and white blood cell (WBC) count, clear wound drainage, decreasing edema and redness
Impaired Physical Mobility related to pain and immobilization	Improved physical mobility: patient performs daily activities as permitted while protecting fracture
Risk for Impaired Skin Integrity related to injury, immobility, and immobilizing devices	Intact or healing skin: absence of open wounds, redness, or pallor because of pressure; skin warm
Activity Intolerance related to prolonged immobilization	Improved activity intolerance: performance of daily activities without fatigue

Nutrition Considerations

1. Calcium in the diet and calcium supplements are recommended to help *prevent* fractures because of osteoporosis in older age.
2. Prolonged immobilization, which often is required after multiple fractures, contributes to the loss of calcium and protein.
3. Essential nutritional elements for optimal bone healing are protein, calcium, and vitamins D, B, and C.
4. Supplemental feedings that are high in calories, protein, and calcium, such as milkshakes, may be served between meals to promote healing.
5. During periods of immobilization, a daily fluid intake of 2000 to 3000 mL is recommended (unless contraindicated) to promote bowel and bladder function.
6. Advise the patient in a hip spica that overeating may cause abdominal pressure and cramping.

Additional nursing diagnoses may include *imbalanced nutrition: less than body requirements* related to additional metabolic needs of healing bone and soft tissues (see *Nutrition Considerations* box); *constipation* related to prolonged immobility and pain medication; *self-care deficit* related to pain and immobility; *ineffective coping* related to prolonged immobility, hospitalization, or altered lifestyle; *disturbed sleep pattern* related to pain or immobility; and *deficient diversional activity* related to immobility.

Interventions

Acute Pain

Fractures are painful. The degree of pain experienced depends on the extent and type of injury and the pain tolerance of the patient. The primary method of pain relief is immobilization of the affected part. Elevating the affected area will help to manage edema. Analgesic medications and muscle relaxants, as well as cold therapy, are used. Other methods of pain relief include repositioning, massage, and diversion. General pain management is discussed in more detail in Chapter 15.

Ineffective Peripheral Tissue Perfusion

Factors that cause ineffective peripheral tissue perfusion are soft tissue injury resulting from trauma, fracture fragments, hemorrhage, edema, compartment syndrome, and positioning. The treatment of the fracture also can interfere with peripheral circulation, including moving or splinting the fracture, manipulation during reduction, and application of a cast, a splint, traction, or a brace.

Frequent neurovascular checks determine whether circulation is adequate and detect signs of pressure on nerves. For patients at risk for circulatory impairment, elevate the affected part above the level of the heart, apply cold packs as ordered to minimize edema, and encourage finger and toe movement. Evidence of impaired circulation includes abnormal coolness or warmth, weak or absent pulses, pale or bluish skin color, and sluggish capillary refill. Pressure on a nerve can cause pain, tingling, numbness, or motor impairments. Immediately report signs of impaired circulation to the physician. If a cast is too tight, it may need to be cut or replaced.

Risk for Infection

Disruption of skin may occur with a fracture and when there is open reduction with external fixation, the potential for infection always exists. Infection can delay healing and rehabilitation. Bone infections are especially difficult to treat. Use strict aseptic technique for dressing changes, wound irrigations, and care of pins and drains. Observe wounds and pin sites for signs of infection, such as drainage, redness, swelling, and warmth, and monitor the patient's temperature for fever. If an infection develops, employ standard infection control precautions and administer antibiotics as prescribed. The management of infection is discussed more completely in Chapter 13.

Impaired Physical Mobility

Interventions for immobility are aimed at promoting independence and preventing related complications. Patients may experience anxiety and powerlessness when their activity is restricted because of the enforced immobilization related to traction, casts, or other equipment. In addition, they may experience secondary complications of immobility such as DVT; pulmonary embolism; contractures or muscular atrophy; skin breakdown; and gastrointestinal (GI) problems, especially constipation. Older individuals are particularly vulnerable to the effects of immobility. Adequate hydration and nutrition are important.

Encourage all patients with fractures to engage in regular movement of some kind. Passive or active range-of-motion exercises are helpful for both bedridden and ambulatory patients. Support the joints above and below the injury in functional positions. Periodic elevation of the affected limb promotes venous return and reduces edema. Gait training with crutches, walkers, and canes promotes mobility and independence. A physical therapist usually works out an activity and exercise program for patients recovering from fractures and the role of the nurse is to reinforce and encourage patients to carry out the program. More discussion of immobility appears in Chapter 21.

If patients are unable to care for themselves independently at home, assistance from formal agencies such as home health services or social services may be needed. Areas to be assessed for home care needs include ability to carry out ADL, mobility, mental status, and skilled nursing needs. If you think home care will be needed, consult the case manager or social worker about the appropriate referral.

Risk for Impaired Skin Integrity

Skin integrity may be impaired as a result of the injury itself or the treatment of the injury. A compound fracture causes a break in the skin and soft tissue injury occurs with almost every kind of fracture. Treatment measures such as immobilization or devices such as casts or traction may cause pressure on areas of the skin and result in pressure sores. In addition, the improper use of equipment can cause pressure on certain areas of the skin. Individuals who are at highest risk for skin breakdown are older adults, people with preexisting conditions such as diabetes mellitus, and people whose general condition was poor before the injury.

To prevent skin breakdown, patients should begin moving around as soon as possible after the fracture has been treated. Proper positioning and frequent turning are essential for the prevention of skin breakdown. Guidelines for proper positioning are listed in

Table 44-2 Tips on Positioning

FRACTURE	POSITIONING
Cervical	Before treatment: with victim supine, immobilize neck with sandbags or Philadelphia collar If patient *must* be turned, be sure head and neck alignment is maintained
Thoracic spine	Position of comfort
Lumbar spine	Avoid high sitting positions, logroll
Pelvis	Stable fracture or after fixation: turn to side opposite fracture Unstable: do not turn
Hip	Before surgical treatment: turn toward fracture (avoid dislocation or further displacement of fragments) with pillows between legs Postoperatively: turn away from fracture until comfortable enough to turn on operative side, with pillows between legs Arthroplasty: maintain abduction at all times with abduction pillow or regular pillows between legs
Shoulder/humerus	Elevate head of bed to comfort Turn to side opposite fracture
Forearm/foreleg	Elevate distal portion of extremity higher than heart

From Maher AB, Salmond SW, Pellino TA: *Orthopedic nursing,* Philadelphia, 1994, Saunders.

Table 44-2. Good nutrition and fluid intake help to maintain healthy tissues.

Put on Your Thinking Cap!

Assume that you are going home with a walker. Assess the barriers in your home and modifications that would be needed for you to get around safely in it.

Activity Intolerance

With prolonged immobility, people become weaker and their ability to participate in activities diminishes. Encourage patients to keep their strength up by carrying out range-of-motion exercises, resistance exercises of the unaffected extremities, and, when possible, ambulation. Participation in ADL and recreational activities also is helpful. Rest periods between activities help to preserve strength.

Teaching should take place in the hospital immediately after the fracture is treated to prepare for the patient's discharge home. Assess the patient and family members for their readiness and ability to learn. Patient teaching after fractures should include the types of medical and nursing interventions that will be carried out to promote bone and tissue healing, signs and symptoms of complications that should be reported to a physician, how to use equipment and assistive devices, and techniques for managing ADL.

Pharmacology Capsule

Patients who administer their own pain medications are more in control and better able to manage their pain successfully.

MANAGEMENT OF SPECIFIC FRACTURES

HIP FRACTURE

By age 90, 17% of men and more than 30% of women have sustained a hip fracture. Most hip fractures are in the femoral neck and intertrochanteric regions (Fig. 44-9). The most common direct cause is a fall on a hard surface; however, it is thought that many fractures in older individuals result from decreased bone mass or brittle bones associated with osteoporosis (see *Health Promotion* box). Among older adults, 3% to 5% of all falls result in fractures. Signs and symptoms of a hip fracture are a history of a fall, severe pain and tenderness in the region of the fracture site, evidence of soft tissue trauma, the affected leg being shorter than the unaffected leg, and the hip on the affected side being rotated externally.

Medical Diagnosis

Hip fracture should be suspected any time an older adult falls on a hard surface. The first health care provider on the scene should assess for external rotation (turning outward) of the hip, muscle spasm, shortening of the affected extremity, and severe pain and tenderness at the affected site. The diagnosis of hip fracture is confirmed by radiography. Other studies, such as a complete blood count (CBC), a urinalysis, and electrocardiography, may be done in preparation for surgery.

Medical Treatment

Traction and surgical repair (internal fixation, femoral head replacement, or total hip replacement) are the standard treatments for hip fracture. For older patients, surgical repair of the fracture is often the treatment of choice because it allows them to move around sooner

Health Promotion

Once Is Enough: Preventing Future Fractures in Patients with Osteoporosis

Osteoporosis is a public health threat that affects 9% of Americans aged 50 years and older. The disease makes bones more prone to fractures, especially of the hip, spine, and wrist. One in two women and one in four men will have an osteoporosis-related fracture in their lifetime. Women near or past menopause who have sustained a fracture in the past are twice as likely to experience another fracture. However, unfortunately only 5% of patients with osteoporotic fractures are referred for an osteoporosis evaluation and medical treatment.

Ensure that your patients receive the necessary referrals for bone mineral density testing and other appropriate evaluations. Patients may be reluctant to exercise for fear of breaking another bone. Explain that engaging in weight-bearing exercises and resistance exercises preserves bone density and prevents falls by enhancing balance, flexibility, and strength. As appropriate, you can recommend the following activities to your patients:

- Walking
- Strength training
- Dancing
- Tai Chi
- Stair climbing
- Hiking
- Bicycling
- Swimming
- Gardening

Adapted from National Institute of Arthritis and Musculoskeletal and Skin Diseases: *Once is enough: a guide to preventing future fractures*, January 2012 (website): www.niams.nih.gov/bone/ hi/prevent_fracture.htm. Accessed November 5, 2013.

and results in fewer complications related to immobility. Traction may require 12 to 16 weeks of immobilization for healing.

Postoperatively, patients may begin physical therapy as early as 1 day after surgery, depending on the type of repair. They may begin by sitting in a chair and then progress to walking with a walker. After internal fixation, weight bearing on the affected side is limited initially and then gradually increased as tolerated. After total hip replacement, weight bearing can begin almost immediately.

POSTOPERATIVE NURSING CARE of the Patient with a Hip Fracture

Assessment

Patients with a hip fracture are assessed in the same way as patients with other types of fractures. Monitor for pain, impaired peripheral circulation on the affected side, complications of immobility, skin breakdown, and ability to carry out ADL. Older patients are particularly prone to developing delirium after a broken hip, particularly from the use of anesthesia during surgery; therefore note mental status and problem behaviors related to confusion.

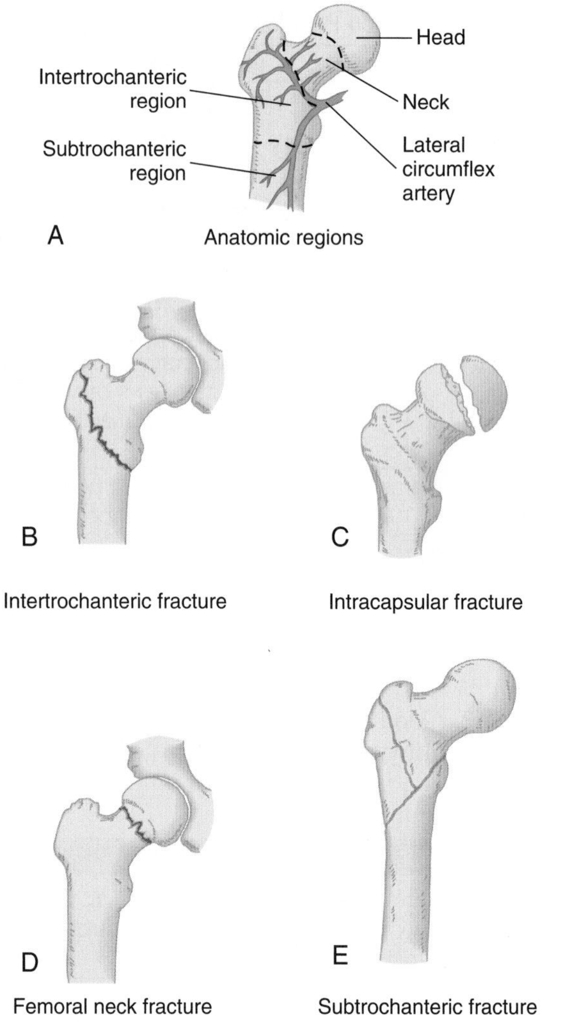

FIGURE 44-9 Femoral fractures. **A,** Anatomic regions of the proximal end of femur. **B,** Intertrochanteric fracture. **C,** Intracapsular fracture. **D,** Femoral neck fracture. **E,** Subtrochanteric fracture. (From Black JM, Hawks JH, Keene AM: *Medical-surgical nursing: clinical management for continuity of care*, ed 6, Philadelphia, 2001, Saunders.)

Nursing Diagnoses, Goals, and Outcome Criteria: Hip Fracture

General nursing diagnoses, goals, and outcome criteria for the patient with a fracture were presented earlier under "Nursing Care of the Patient with a Fracture." The special needs of the patient with a hip fracture are discussed here.

Interventions

Nursing interventions are geared toward relieving pain, promoting mobility and independence, and preventing complications. Older patients have special nursing care needs because they are vulnerable to complications of immobility and confusion. Pain management is of utmost importance. Confused patients may not be able to tell you the extent or degree of their pain and, many times, they may be undermedicated. Problem behaviors such as agitation, trying to climb out of bed, pulling out intravenous tubes or other tubes, and alterations in sleep patterns may be related to pain. Employ comfort measures such as repositioning, body massage, and diversional activities to enhance the effect of medications.

Proper body alignment is extremely important in preventing injury to the fracture area after it has been treated. Turn patients from side to side as ordered. After total hip replacement, the affected hip must not be adducted and must not be flexed more than 90 degrees because excessive flexion or adduction can dislocate the prosthesis. Instruct these patients to use elevated toilet seats, sit in supportive chairs with straight backs and seats, and avoid crossing their legs even at the feet. Care of the patient who has undergone joint replacement surgery is detailed in Chapter 43. Fall prevention is discussed in Chapter 20.

COLLES FRACTURE

Colles fracture is a break in the distal radius (wrist area). Colles fractures often occur in older adults, particularly older women, when an outstretched hand is used to break a fall. The major signs and symptoms are pain and swelling in the area of the injury and a characteristic displacement of the bone in which the wrist has the appearance of a dinner fork. The most common complication is impaired circulation in the area resulting from edema.

Medical Diagnosis

The diagnosis is confirmed by the characteristic bone deformity of the wrist and by radiography.

Medical Treatment

Colles fractures are managed by closed reduction or manipulation of the bone and immobilization in either a splint or a cast. The elbow is immobilized as well, to prevent misalignment.

❖ NURSING CARE of the Patient with a Colles Fracture

■ Assessment

Assess patients for pain and swelling following medical treatment of the fracture.

■ Nursing Diagnoses, Goals, and Outcome Criteria: Colles Fracture

General nursing diagnoses, goals, and outcome criteria for the patient with a fracture were presented earlier under "Nursing Care of the Patient with a Fracture." The special needs of the patient with a Colles fracture are discussed here.

■ Interventions

Interventions are aimed at relieving pain and preventing or reducing edema. The extremity should be supported and protected and can be elevated on a pillow during the first few days. Encourage patients to move their fingers and thumb to promote circulation and reduce swelling and to move their shoulders to prevent stiffness and contracture. In addition, teach proper cast care.

PELVIC FRACTURE

Although pelvic fractures account for a small percentage of total fractures (3%), they are the second leading cause of death from trauma, after head injury. Motor vehicle accidents are the most common cause of pelvic fractures in young adults and falls are the main cause in older adults. The extent of the injury can range from minimal to life threatening. Internal trauma, such as laceration of the colon, hemorrhage, or rupture of the urethra or bladder, often accompanies a pelvic fracture. The patient may have local swelling, tenderness, bruising, and deformity. Pelvic fractures typically heal within 6 to 8 weeks.

Medical Diagnosis

As with other fractures, the diagnosis and severity of the injury are confirmed by radiography.

Medical Treatment

Medical treatment depends on the severity of the fracture. A less severe nondisplaced fracture is usually treated with bed rest on a firm mattress or bed board for a few days to 6 weeks. A more severe fracture may require one or more of the following: a pelvic sling, skeletal traction, a double hip spica cast, or external fixation.

❖ NURSING CARE of the Patient with a Pelvic Fracture

■ Assessment

Observe for signs of bleeding, swelling, infection, thromboembolism, and pain. Because of the high risk of internal trauma, closely monitor the patient so that specific injuries can be treated immediately. Check for the presence of blood in the urine and stool and assess the abdomen for any signs of rigidity or swelling. Assess urine output because the absence of urine may indicate a perforated bladder.

■ Nursing Diagnoses, Goals, and Outcome Criteria: Pelvic Fracture

General nursing diagnoses, goals, and outcome criteria for the patient with a fracture were presented earlier under "Nursing Care of the Patient with a Fracture." The special needs of the patient with a pelvic fracture are discussed here.

■ Interventions

Interventions are designed to alleviate pain, promote mobility, and prevent complications. When handling patients, take extreme care to prevent displacement of fracture fragments. Move the patient gently and turn *only* as ordered by the physician. Have the patient pull up on the trapeze so that back care can be given. Encourage ambulation as soon as ordered to prevent the serious consequences of immobility. !

Get Ready for the NCLEX® Examination!

Key Points

- A fracture is a break or disruption in the continuity of a bone, usually causing injury to surrounding soft tissue.
- Open or compound fractures have three grades of severity, ranging from least severe injury with minimal skin damage to most severe injury with skin, muscle, blood vessel, and nerve damage.
- Fractures of the femur are most common in young and middle-aged adults and fractures of the hip, wrist, and vertebrae are most common in older adults.
- Fractures are usually caused by trauma to the bone, especially as a result of falls and automobile accidents.
- Risk factors for hip fractures include osteoporosis, advanced age, Caucasian race, use of psychotropic drugs, and female gender.
- The most common signs and symptoms of a fracture are swelling, bruising, pain, tenderness, loss of normal function, and abnormal mobility.
- Bone healing occurs in five stages: (1) hematoma formation, (2) fibrocartilage formation, (3) callus formation, (4) ossification, and (5) consolidation and remodeling.
- Healing time for fractures increases with age; it may take six times as long for the same type of fracture to heal in an older person as it does in an infant.
- Complications of a fracture include infection, fat embolism, DVT and pulmonary embolism, joint stiffness and contractures, posttraumatic arthritis, compartment syndrome, malunion, nonunion, delayed union, avascular necrosis, and complex regional pain syndrome.
- The goals of medical treatment for a fracture are to realign the bone fragments, establish a sturdy union between the broken ends of the bone, and restore function.
- The most common therapeutic techniques used to treat a fracture are closed and open reduction and internal and external fixation.
- Casts are used for external fixation of extensive fractures and fractures of the extremities.
- Traction provides alignment of the broken bone fragments, prevents or corrects deformity, decreases muscle spasm, promotes rest and exercise, and maintains the position of a diseased or injured part.
- Crutches increase mobility and assist with ambulation after a fracture of the lower extremity.
- A walker is used for support and balance, usually by older patients.
- Canes provide minimal support and balance and relieve pressure on weight-bearing joints.
- Common nursing diagnoses for the patient with a fracture include acute pain, ineffective peripheral tissue perfusion, risk for infection, impaired physical mobility, risk for impaired skin integrity, and activity intolerance.

Additional Learning Resources

SG Go to your Study Guide for additional learning activities to help you master this chapter content.

evolve Go to your Evolve website (http://evolve.elsevier.com/Linton/medsurg) for the following learning resources and much more:

- Interactive Prioritization Exercises
- Fluid & Electrolyte Tutorial
- Pharmacology Tutorial
- Review Questions for the NCLEX® Examination

Review Questions for the NCLEX® Examination

1. A patient is brought to the emergency department with an injury to his arm that was incurred in a fall. A bone end protrudes from his forearm. The surrounding skin is bruised and swollen. Exposed muscle tissue is also swollen. The patient has normal sensation in his fingers. His injury is best described as which of the following?
   1. Closed complete fracture
   2. Grade III incomplete open fracture
   3. Grade I complete closed fracture
   4. Grade II complete open fracture

   NCLEX Client Need: Physiological Integrity: Physiological Adaptation
2. The ends of a broken bone begin to knit during which stage of healing?

   NCLEX Client Need: Physiological Integrity: Physiological Adaptation
3. A patient with a femoral fracture suddenly complains that he cannot catch his breath. His pulse is 106 bpm and respiration is 30 breaths per minute. You notice a measleslike rash on his neck and chest. You should suspect which of the following?
   1. Shock
   2. Fat embolism
   3. Avascular necrosis
   4. Compartment syndrome

   NCLEX Client Need: Physiological Integrity: Physiological Adaptation
4. A patient's femoral fracture is not healing as rapidly as hoped. Methods that might be used to stimulate bone growth and healing include: (Select all that apply.)
   1. Traction
   2. Pulsated electromagnetic fields
   3. Bone grafts
   4. Fixation
   5. Electrical stimulation

   NCLEX Client Need: Physiological Integrity: Physiological Adaptation
5. A patient is being discharged with a plaster of Paris cast on her arm. Patient teaching should include which of the following? (Select all that apply.)
   1. Notify the physician if your fingers become discolored.
   2. Do not insert any objects under the cast.
   3. After the cast dries, you can take a shower without damaging it.
   4. Loss of sensation is normal; it will return when the cast is removed.
   5. The cast dries completely within 8 hours.

   NCLEX Client Need: Physiological Integrity: Reduction of Risk Potential

6. A patient with a foot injury is leaving the clinic with crutches. The nurse knows that the crutches are properly fitted when:
   1. The patient says that he or she is comfortable
   2. The elbows are bent at 45-degree angles
   3. The crutch is 75% of the patient's height
   4. The crutch pad is 3 to 4 fingerbreadths below the axilla

   NCLEX Client Need: Physiological Integrity: Reduction of Risk Potential
7. Which of the following is the main advantage of surgery over traction for older patients with hip fractures?
   1. Traction is more expensive because a longer hospitalization is required.
   2. Surgery allows earlier mobilization, which results in fewer complications.
   3. After a few days, surgical treatment is generally less painful than traction.
   4. Bones of older people heal better with surgery than with traction.

   NCLEX Client Need: Physiological Integrity: Reduction of Risk Potential
8. Which of the following is the most common cause of Colles fracture?
   1. Using an outstretched hand to break a fall
   2. Jumping from a high place onto a hard surface
   3. Landing in a sitting position after falling
   4. Falling with the leg in a position of outward rotation

   NCLEX Client Need: Physiological Integrity: Physiological Adaptation
9. Mr. J. was recently discharged to home health care after treatment for a pelvic fracture. The nurse is encouraging a diet to promote healing of the fracture, which should include: (Select all that apply.)
   1. Reduced fat and calories to prevent weight gain
   2. High-calorie meal supplements
   3. Increased protein and calcium to build new bone
   4. Supplementary doses of vitamins B, C, and D
   5. Decreased fluid intake to prevent bladder distention

   NCLEX Client Need: Physiological Integrity: Basic Care and Comfort
10. A patient comes to the clinic after a fall at home. When he moved his injured arm, a grating sound was heard. How should the nurse document this sound?

    NCLEX Client Need: Physiological Integrity: Physiological Adaptation

chapter

45 Amputations

http://evolve.elsevier.com/Linton/medsurg

Objectives

1. Identify the clinical indications for amputations.
2. Describe the different types of amputations.
3. Discuss the medical and surgical management of the patient undergoing amputation.
4. Identify appropriate nursing interventions during the preoperative and postoperative phases of care.
5. Assist in developing a nursing care plan for the amputation patient.

Key Terms

Amputation (ăm-pū-TĀ-shŭn)
Amputee (ăm-pū-TĒ)
Closed amputation
Congenital amputation (kŏn-JĔN-ĭ-tăl ăm-pū-TĀ-shŭn)
Gangrene (găng-GRĒN)
Guillotine amputation (GĬL-ō-tēn ăm-pū-TĀ-shŭn)
Open amputation
Phantom limb
Replantation (rē-plăn-TĀ-shŭn)
Residual limb (rē-ZĬ-dū-ăl lĭm)
Staged amputation
Stump

Derived from the Latin word meaning *cutting around*, the term **amputation** refers to the removal of body limbs or parts of limbs. Amputations have been performed since the beginning of humankind, according to findings by archaeologists. Ancient amputations were originally performed to remove gangrenous or damaged limbs; they also were performed for ritual sacrifice, punishment, exorcism of evil spirits, and, in some cases, beautification.

In the past 2 decades, many advances have been made in surgical amputation and **replantation** (i.e., limb reattachment) techniques, prosthetic devices (i.e., artificial limbs), and rehabilitation programs. Limb transplantation has been done on a limited basis. Advances have allowed many **amputees** (i.e., people with amputations) to remain active and productive despite their disabilities. In the United States, the vast majority of amputees have had lower extremity amputations.

AMPUTATION

Amputation can occur through a joint (between the bones) or through a bone itself. *Disarticulation* is the term used for an amputation through the joint. The general site of the amputation is described by the joint nearest to it. For example, removal of the lower leg at the middle of the shin or calf is called a *below-knee amputation.* Some of the most common sites of amputation are shown in Figure 45-1.

INDICATIONS AND INCIDENCE

Conditions or situations that lead to the need for an amputation generally can be grouped into four categories: (1) trauma, (2) disease, (3) tumors, and (4) congenital defects.

Trauma

In some serious accidents, part or all of a limb may be removed. This often is referred to as a *traumatic amputation.* In other situations the limb may be damaged so severely that it must be removed surgically. Common types of accidents and injuries leading to amputation include those involving motorcycles and automobiles, farm machinery, firearms and explosives, electrical equipment, power tools, and frostbite. Trauma tends to be the most common reason for upper extremity amputations. Because these accidents are typically occupational hazards, the victims are usually young men.

Disease

Vascular diseases account for the majority of the estimated 185,000 lower extremity amputations performed in the United States each year. In these cases, blood supply to the tissues is inadequate and the tissues become deprived of oxygen (O_2) and other important nutrients. Without these nutrients, necrosis or death of the tissue occurs. Some examples of diseases leading to impaired circulation are peripheral vascular disease, diabetes mellitus, and arteriosclerosis. These problems

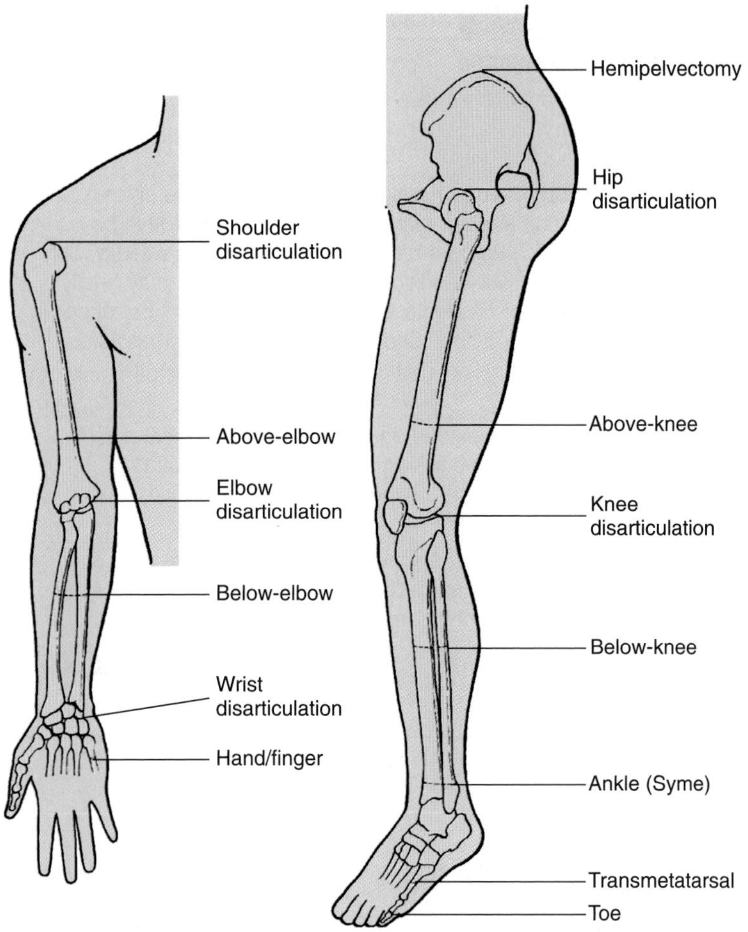

FIGURE 45-1 Common sites of amputation in the upper and lower extremities. (From Monahan FD, Drake DT, Neighbors M, editors: *Medical-surgical nursing: foundations for clinical practice*, ed 2, Philadelphia, 1998, Saunders.)

also can be complicated by infection, because wounds sustained by limbs without a good blood supply do not heal well and **gangrene** can set in quickly. Gangrene is the death of tissue caused by inadequate circulation and followed by infection. Circulation problems are more common among older adults and in the lower extremities. Chronic osteomyelitis, an infection of the bone, bone marrow, or surrounding soft tissue, can also lead to amputation. Sometimes when disease leads to severe necrosis, auto amputation can occur. *Auto amputation* is when the limb, most often a toe, self-amputates itself without surgery.

Tumors

Amputations also may be performed for bone tumors that are very large and invasive. Treatment may require amputation and disarticulation of an entire limb. Primary bone tumors occur most frequently in adolescents but can occur at any age. Approximately one third of these individuals are 11 to 20 years of age.

Congenital Defects

In some situations, a limb or part of a limb may be absent or deformed at birth. These are sometimes called **congenital amputations**. They result from factors that affect the developing fetus in such a way that the infant is born with a missing, deficient, or abnormal limb. Sometimes surgery is performed to convert a deformed limb into a more functional one that can be fitted with a prosthetic device.

DIAGNOSTIC TESTS AND PROCEDURES

The types of diagnostic studies done for a patient requiring amputation depend on the underlying disease or injury. For example, in a patient with vascular disease, tests to assess circulation are indicated. An elevated white blood cell (WBC) count is consistent with infection. Table 45-1 lists examples of diagnostic findings associated with some of the contributing factors in amputations.

Vascular Studies

Vascular studies may be done for a patient with compromised circulation, such as in trauma or vascular disease. Angiography is a procedure that involves the injection of a radiopaque dye into blood vessels, which are then viewed radiographically to determine their patency.

Table 45-1 Diagnostic Tests and Procedures Indications for Amputation

TEST AND PURPOSE	PATIENT PREPARATION	POSTPROCEDURE CARE
White blood cell (WBC) count detects elevation associated with infection.	Tell patient a blood sample will be drawn. Fasting not necessary.	Apply small dressing to site. Assess for bleeding.
Arteriography detects arterial occlusion.	Inquire about allergy to contrast medium or iodine. Inform radiologist if allergic. Mark peripheral pulses. Nothing by mouth (NPO) 8 hours before. Signed consent required. Tell patient "dye" will be injected into arm or groin; may briefly feel flushed or nauseated. Then radiographs will be taken to assess blood flow. Should void just before procedure. Remove jewelry and metal objects. Must remain still during test.	Maintain pressure dressing on puncture site as ordered. Assess for bleeding. Frequent neurovascular checks on extremity used to inject dye. Encourage increased fluid intake if permitted.
Pulse volume recording (plethysmography) used to evaluate arterial blood flow to an extremity.	Pressure cuffs are placed on extremities and arterial pressure is measured during inflation and deflation. Explain procedure to patient. Signed consent not required.	No special care.
Doppler ultrasound used to assess pulses, patency of blood vessels.	Tell patient procedure is noninvasive and painless. Conductive gel is applied and a sensor is passed over the extremity to detect pulses.	Cleanse gel from skin.
Bone biopsy usually done after imaging procedures reveal suspicious lesions.	Signed consent required. Sample of bone surgically excised for study.	Inspect site for bleeding. Administer analgesics as ordered.

Pulse Volume Recording

Pulse volume recording uses a noninvasive device that gives general information about the volume of blood flow to an extremity. Another name for this procedure is *plethysmography.*

Thermography

Thermography involves the use of a device that detects and records heat in various parts of the body. Relatively hot or cold spots are revealed, indicating the amount of blood flow to that part of the body. Cool areas generally indicate a decreased blood flow as compared with warm areas.

Doppler Ultrasound

Doppler ultrasound uses sound waves to determine the presence of pulses in the extremities. This technology is much more sensitive than using the fingertips to try to palpate a pulse. The adequacy of circulation can also be assessed with transcutaneous tissue O_2 measurement.

Biopsy

In patients with tumors, a biopsy is often done to determine the nature of the tumor. A biopsy involves removing a small portion of tissue, which is then examined for malignancy.

MEDICAL AND SURGICAL TREATMENT

The management of amputations requires both medical and surgical approaches by the physicians involved in the care of the patient.

Medical Treatment

The medical care of the patient undergoing amputation must include the appropriate treatment and control of any underlying diseases or injuries. For example, diet, medication, and exercise are used to help patients with diabetes and poor peripheral circulation attain good control of their diabetes. Patients with peripheral vascular disease are encouraged to stop smoking because nicotine causes vasoconstriction. The patient who has experienced trauma may have to be stabilized with measures that will maintain his or her heart rate and blood pressure (BP) within a normal range.

Surgical Treatment

Amputation is recommended only when other options are not possible or have failed. In an effort to avoid amputation, the physician may perform angioplasty or surgical bypass of obstructed vessels.

Surgical management of the patient aims for amputation at the lowest level that will still preserve healthy tissue and favor wound healing. The surgeon chooses one of two basic types of surgical procedures, depending on the condition of the extremity and the reason for the surgery. These two types are **closed amputations** and **open amputations**.

Closed Amputations. Closed amputations are usually performed to create a weight-bearing **residual limb** or **stump**, which is especially important for lower extremity amputations. In this procedure, a long skin flap with soft tissue and muscle is positioned over the severed end of the bone and sutured in place. The sutures are placed so that they do not bear the full

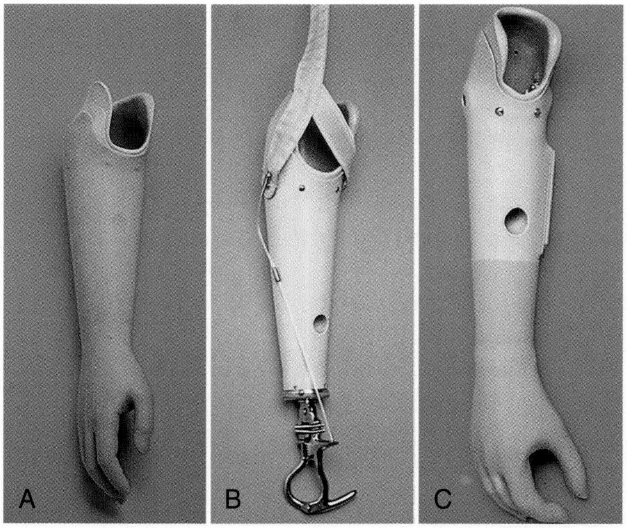

FIGURE 45-2 Upper extremity prostheses. **A,** Cosmetic. **B,** Cable activated. **C,** Myoelectrically controlled. (Copyright Otto Bock Healthcare LP, Minneapolis, Minn.)

weight of the patient. This technique has many variations.

Open Amputations. In open amputations, the severed bone or joint is left uncovered by a skin flap. This type of amputation is required when an actual or potential infection exists, as may occur with gangrene or trauma. The wound is left open for 5 to 10 days, sometimes longer, and is closed surgically when infection no longer poses a problem. Another term for this procedure is a **staged amputation** or **guillotine amputation**.

Prostheses. Prostheses are artificial substitutes for missing body parts. A prosthetist creates the prosthesis, fits the patient, and instructs the patient in its use. In some situations, a limb prosthesis may be placed while the patient is still in the operating room. In other cases, particularly with lower extremity amputations, older or debilitated patients, and infection, fitting of the prosthesis is delayed until the residual limb heals. Provided that no problems occur, a patient can usually bear full weight on a permanent prosthesis approximately 3 months after amputation. Various prostheses are depicted in Figures 45-2 and 45-3. Advances in prosthesis design and surgical muscle reinnervation are allowing significant improvements in function.

COMPLICATIONS

Complications associated with amputations include hemorrhage and hematoma, necrosis, wound dehiscence, gangrene, edema, contracture, pain, infection, phantom limb sensation, and phantom limb pain. Factors contributing to each of these complications are listed in Table 45-2.

❖ PREOPERATIVE NURSING CARE of the Patient Having Amputation Surgery

Routine preoperative and postoperative care is detailed in Chapter 17. This section focuses on the specific needs of the patient having an amputation (see also

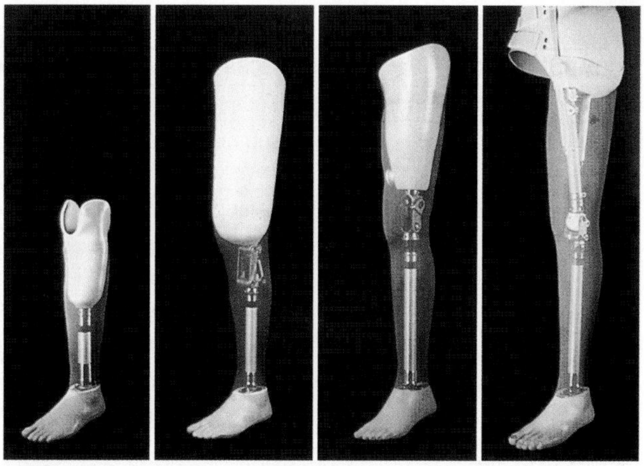

FIGURE 45-3 Lower extremity prostheses. (Copyright Otto Bock Healthcare LP, Minneapolis, Minn.)

Nursing Care Plan: Patient with an Upper Extremity Amputation). The preoperative nursing assessment is summarized in Box 45-1.

■ Assessment

Health History

The licensed vocational nurse/licensed practical nurse (LVN/LPN) collects data to assist the registered nurse (RN) with a comprehensive assessment that is described here. Record the conditions that resulted in the need for an amputation (e.g., diseases such as diabetes mellitus or peripheral vascular insufficiency, traumatic injuries, neoplasms, birth defects). Take a complete health history, including information on the patient's past medical and surgical conditions. Note preexisting cardiovascular problems because hypertension, coronary artery disease (CAD), congestive heart failure (CHF), and cardiac defects can greatly affect the patient's ability to tolerate surgery and recover successfully. Also, determine whether the patient has ever had phlebitis, varicosities, thromboses, emboli, or stasis ulcers in either the affected or the unaffected extremities.

Record relevant disorders in the family history including diabetes, hypertension, and vascular diseases.

Document signs and symptoms that relate to the vascular condition or other chronic and acute problems. Significant signs and symptoms are pain (location, severity, type, precipitating factors, alleviating factors), loss of sensation or abnormal sensations, intolerance of local heat or cold, color changes in the extremities, leg ulcers, and sexual dysfunction.

Significant data in the functional assessment are usual diet and fluid intake, intake of salt and alcohol, and use of tobacco. Describe exercise and rest and sleep habits as well as the effects of the current symptoms on the patient's usual activities. Identify the patient's occupation and responsibilities to determine how amputation will affect that aspect of his or her life.

A review of the patient's psychosocial background may offer insight into how the patient will tolerate

Table 45-2 Complications of Amputation

COMPLICATION	DESCRIPTION AND CONTRIBUTING FACTORS
Hematoma and hemorrhage	Bleeding into tissue in and around residual limb because of inadequate hemostasis
Necrosis	Tissue destruction and death because of ongoing disease; requires surgical debridement or revision, or both
Wound dehiscence	Opening of suture line because of early removal of sutures or trauma; requires reclosure
Gangrene	Death of tissue associated with inadequate blood supply and bacterial destruction of tissue; requires reamputation
Edema	Swelling and discomfort in residual limb because of dependent position or incorrect wrapping; requires elevation and rewrapping
Contracture	Flexion of joints with loss of range of motion because of prolonged elevation or immobilization of extremities; may be prevented by frequent position changes and range-of-motion exercises
Pain	Extreme, sharp pain at incision site because of scar formation on nerve fibers (neuroma); may require surgical treatment
Infection	Redness, warmth, swelling, and exudate formation at residual limb site because of invasion of tissues by pathogens; may require antibiotics and surgical drainage
Phantom limb sensation	Patient experiences sensations (tingling, numbness, itching, warmth/cold) as if the limb were still present; caused by stimulation along a nerve pathway in which sensory endings were in the amputated part
Phantom limb pain	Patient experiences pain as if the limb were still present; more common when patient had pain in limb before amputation; pain may be enhanced by anxiety and depression; usually diminishes over time but may become chronic

Nursing Care Plan: Patient with an Upper Extremity Amputation

ASSESSMENT

HEALTH HISTORY A 32-year-old man sustained an injury in an industrial accident that required amputation of his right forearm just below the elbow. The patient's right hand was his dominant hand. He has had no other serious physical injuries or illnesses. He is a machinist who is a senior employee in his department. He is married and is the father of three children. His wife is a homemaker who has never worked outside the home.

PHYSICAL EXAMINATION Vital signs: blood pressure 126/68 mm Hg, pulse 80 bpm, respiration 16 breaths per minute, temperature 98.2°F (36.8°C) measured orally. Alert. A bulky dressing is in place on the residual limb of the right arm; dressing is dry and intact. A Jackson-Pratt drain is in place and the receptacle contains approximately 30 mL of sanguineous fluid. Intravenous fluids are infusing into the left arm. Up in chair for breakfast. Using left arm for self-feeding. Expresses intent to remain independent.

Nursing Diagnosis	Goals and Outcome Criteria	Interventions
Decreased Cardiac Output related to blood loss	The patient's blood volume will remain normal, as evidenced by stable vital signs, urine output equal to fluid intake, and absence of restlessness or frank bleeding.	Reinforce dressing, apply pressure, and elevate residual limb if bleeding is apparent. Monitor for signs of hypovolemia: tachycardia, restlessness, and decreased urine output. Check brachial pulse on the affected arm if dressing allows.
Acute Pain related to surgical incision, trauma, edema	The patient will state that pain is relieved and will appear more relaxed.	Have the patient describe pain nature, location, and severity. Administer analgesics as ordered. Provide comfort measures such as back rub, distraction, and imagery. Inform the surgeon if pain is not relieved.
Risk for Infection related to surgical wound, traumatic injury	The patient will remain free of infection, as evidenced by normal body temperature and absence of foul drainage, excessive redness, warmth, or edema.	Monitor temperature for elevation. Assess the dressing for foul drainage. When the dressing is removed, inspect the residual limb for excessive redness, warmth, or edema. Use Standard Precautions when handling the dressing and residual limb. Teach the patient good hygiene to decrease the risk of infection. Administer antimicrobials as ordered.

Nursing Care Plan Patient with an Upper Extremity Amputation—cont'd

Nursing Diagnosis	Goals and Outcome Criteria	Interventions
Impaired Skin Integrity related to incision	The patient's residual limb will heal completely.	Keep the residual limb dressing smooth and snug to mold the residual limb for future prosthesis use. Use caution not to impair blood flow. Check the residual limb for irritation or signs of pressure. Maintain elevation as ordered to minimize edema and pressure on the suture line. Apply cold to the residual limb dressing as ordered. After the first week, massage the residual limb as ordered to promote circulation.
Deficient Knowledge of phantom limb sensation or phantom limb pain related to lack of information	The patient will report phantom limb sensations or pain if they occur.	Tell the patient that these sensations sometimes follow amputation. Notify the surgeon. Medicate as ordered. Advise the patient that several therapies are available for the treatment of this problem.
Risk for Injury related to loss of part of limb, weakness	The patient will identify activities requiring adaptation and will avoid dangerous activities.	Help the patient to identify usual activities that cannot be done safely without the dominant hand or that require modification. Discuss strategies to adapt activities or to learn to use the left hand. Consult a rehabilitation specialist for adaptation in work setting.
Readiness for Enhanced Self-Care related to expressed desire to perform self-care independently	The patient will accomplish self-care with minimal assistance from others.	Assist the patient with self-care but encourage increasing effort on his part. Praise efforts. Organize the environment to facilitate self-care (e.g., place bedside objects on the patient's left).
Anxiety related to perceived threat of disability	The patient will verbalize concerns about injury.	Explore the patient's fears and anxiety. Encourage the patient to talk about the loss. Express concern but not pity. Request the services of a mental health or spiritual counselor if the patient desires. Include family in care and explore their needs as well.
Ineffective Coping related to overwhelming injury	The patient will demonstrate realistic goal setting and express intent to participate in rehabilitation program.	Explain the importance of proper residual limb care in preparing for rehabilitation. Consult a social worker to assist the patient in obtaining rehabilitation services.
Disturbed Body Image related to loss of body part	The patient will express feelings about loss of the hand and will consider strategies to improve function and appearance.	Gradually encourage the patient to take more responsibility for care of the residual limb. Counsel family members to demonstrate acceptance of the injury and not to promote excessive dependence. Facilitate a meeting with prosthetist to discuss cosmetic and functional options.
Readiness for Enhanced Self-Care related to expressed interest in gaining independence	The patient will verbalize personal role in recovery and rehabilitation.	Teach the patient to care for the residual limb and any prosthesis. 1. Wash residual limb with soap and water daily, rinse, and dry. 2. Inspect residual limb daily for irritation, redness, and edema. 3. Keep prosthetic socket and residual limb sock clean and dry. 4. Do not apply lotions, powders, or creams except as prescribed by the physician. 5. If residual limb is red or irritated, temporarily remove the prosthesis; see physician. 6. Prosthesis will require periodic adjustments.

Critical Thinking Questions

1. What data should you collect to assess the patient's pain?
2. What sensations might this patient feel after the amputation?
3. List three activities that are likely to require modification after loss of the dominant hand.
4. How would you help this patient to explore his fears and anxieties?

Box 45-1 Assessment of the Patient Undergoing an Amputation

HEALTH HISTORY

Chief Complaint and History of Present Illness
Condition or incident leading to amputation

Past Medical History
Previous illnesses, operations, hospitalizations, trauma, hypertension, coronary artery disease (CAD), congestive heart failure (CHF), cardiac murmurs or defects, phlebitis, varicosities, thromboses, emboli, stasis ulcers, diabetes mellitus

Family History
Diabetes mellitus, hypertension, vascular diseases

Review of Systems

Pain
Nature, location, severity, precipitating factors, alleviating factors

Sensation
Loss or change, abnormal perception of heat and cold

Skin
Color, lesions, ulcers

Leg Ulcers
Location, size, color, drainage

Sexual
Dysfunction

Functional Assessment
Usual diet and fluid intake; intake of salt and alcohol; use of tobacco; exercise, rest, and sleep habits; occupation, roles, and responsibilities

Coping Strategies

Fears and Concerns

PHYSICAL ASSESSMENT

Height and Weight

Vital Signs

Skin
Color, texture, temperature, turgor, lesions

Peripheral Pulses
Presence, quality, symmetry

Capillary Refill

Sensation

Mental Status
Level of consciousness, emotional state

Cognition
Ability to follow directions

treatments and procedures. Knowledge of how the patient copes with stress may help in planning care to reduce anxiety and fear. The patient about to undergo an amputation will undoubtedly have a number of fears and concerns about the surgical procedure, the loss of a body part, the potential loss of independence, and pain and disfigurement. Open discussion of these concerns may help to alleviate those fears.

Physical Examination

A total physical examination should be done, with special attention to the neurologic, cardiovascular, and integumentary systems. Measure height and weight and vital signs to uncover factors that may affect circulation, including obesity and hypertension. Throughout the examination, evaluate neurovascular status. Record the patient's skin color, texture, temperature, and turgor. The overall color, condition, and temperature of the skin are good indicators of blood supply to the extremities. Cool or cold, clammy, mottled skin that is pale or cyanotic may indicate a poor blood supply. Palpating both legs simultaneously makes it easier to detect circulatory differences between the two legs. In addition, there may be open areas on the skin. Describe any skin lesions and drainage from them. Wounds to the extremities are common when blood supply is inadequate.

Palpate the peripheral pulses for presence, quality, and symmetry. If pulses are not palpable, a Doppler ultrasound device can be used. Determine capillary refill by applying pressure to the nail bed of a finger or toe until it blanches (i.e., turns white). When the pressure is released, the nail bed normally regains its normal pink color within 3 seconds. In extremities with a diminished supply of blood, capillary refill may take 5 seconds or longer. Check sensation by asking the patient to identify touch on the extremities. Experienced examiners may evaluate the patient's ability to sense sharp, dull, warm, and cold stimuli.

Collect data about the patient's mental and emotional status and general cognitive abilities to determine the patient's understanding of the condition and its implications.

Nursing Diagnoses, Goals, and Outcome Criteria: Amputation, Preoperative

Nursing Diagnoses	Goals and Outcome Criteria
Anxiety related to anticipated change in body image and in function	Decreased anxiety: relaxed manner, patient statement that anxiety is reduced
Grieving related to expected loss of body part and function	Progress toward grief resolution: patient expresses feelings about impending losses, demonstrates healthy coping strategies

Interventions

Anxiety

Emotional support is important throughout all phases of care of the patient with an amputation. The patient needs time to prepare psychologically and emotionally for the surgery. Encourage the patient to express thoughts and concerns about the impending amputation. Accept the patient's responses. Allow the patient to express anger or to cry without being judged or given false reassurances. Tell the patient about physical and occupational therapy programs designed to restore maximal independent function.

Grieving

Recognize that the loss of a limb or part of a limb as well as the loss of functional abilities is stressful. Patients commonly experience *anticipatory grief* and mourn the impending loss. The patient may be concerned about altered physical appearance as well as loss of function. Explore the patient's expectations and fears about these changes. Gently encourage the patient to focus on what he or she will be able to do despite physical limitations. Allowing patients to grieve is an important part of their recovery and rehabilitation. Nursing care of the grieving patient is discussed in Chapter 24.

❖ POSTOPERATIVE NURSING CARE of the Patient Having Amputation Surgery

The postoperative phase begins immediately after the surgical amputation and includes immediate postoperative care as well as the long-term rehabilitation that is necessary for these patients. Priorities for the postoperative patient are (1) pain relief, (2) restored function, and (3) avoidance of complications.

■ Assessment

Monitor vital signs frequently in the first 48 hours postoperatively to detect early signs of problems. Inspect the dressing frequently for any bleeding. Some nurses try to monitor the amount of oozing by marking the stained area on the dressing with a pen, although this is a very rough assessment of bleeding. Sometimes the dressing is dry but blood is draining around the dressing and under the patient. If a drain receptacle is present, note the color and amount of the drainage. The drainage should gradually decrease in amount and lighten in color. Monitor the patient's temperature for elevations that may indicate infection. Also note any foul odor from the dressing. After the dressing is removed, inspect the residual limb for edema. Document the patient's pain, including type, location, severity, and response to treatment. Other aspects of postoperative assessment are detailed in Chapter 17.

■ Interventions

Decreased Cardiac Output

Hemorrhage is the greatest danger in the early postoperative period. It may be detected by observations of excessive bleeding or changes in vital signs and behavior. Restlessness and increasing pulse and respiratory rates may be early signs of hemorrhage. Hypotension and cyanosis are late signs. If an immediate prosthesis had been applied, you cannot see the

Nursing Diagnoses, Goals, and Outcome Criteria: Amputation, Postoperative

Nursing Diagnoses	Goals and Outcome Criteria
Decreased Cardiac Output related to blood loss	Normal cardiac output: pulse and blood pressure (BP) consistent with patient norms, skin warm and dry
Acute Pain related to surgical wound	Pain relief: relaxed manner, patient statement that pain is relieved
Risk for Infection related to surgical disruption of skin integrity	Absence of infection: normal body temperature, decreasing redness and edema of wound margins, drainage that decreases in volume and becomes clear
Impaired Skin Integrity related to incision	Healed wound: incision margins intact without drainage, excessive swelling, or warmth
Risk for Impaired Skin Integrity related to advanced age and decreased mobility	Absence of new skin lesions: skin intact, no redness because of pressure
Deficient Knowledge about phantom limb sensations or phantom limb pain related to lack of information	Patient understands phantom limb sensation/pain: patient acknowledges that phantom limb sensation/pain is normal after amputation, states that pain or other sensation is reduced
Risk for Injury related to loss of a limb or part of a limb, weakness, debilitation	Absence of injury: no falls or evidence of injury because of weakness or problems with balance
Impaired Physical Mobility related to loss of a limb or part of a limb	Restored mobility: patient performs activities of daily living (ADL), gradually returns to preoperative level of functioning
Activity Intolerance related to weakness	Improved activity tolerance: patient carries out daily activities without excessive fatigue, gradual increase in activity level
Readiness for Enhanced Self-Care related to expressed need to function independently after loss of limb	Resumed self-care: patient performs self-care within limits imposed by limb loss, learns new ways to care for self
Anxiety or Fear related to perceived threat of disability, possibility of death	Decreased anxiety, fear, or both: calm manner; patient statement of lessened anxiety, fear, or both
Ineffective Coping related to inadequate support system, use of inappropriate coping mechanisms	Effective coping with loss: patient talks about loss, participates in rehabilitation efforts and self-care
Disturbed Body Image related to loss of a body part or residual limb	Positive body image: patient accepts limb loss, demonstrates proper care, makes positive remarks about self and abilities

dressing well so monitoring vital signs is even more critical.

A portable wound suction system, such as a Jackson-Pratt drain, may be placed to collect drainage. Inspect the dressing and the bed linens under the patient. Bright red bleeding, either from the drains or from the dressing itself, is *not* normal. If this is observed, apply a pressure dressing over the existing dressing, elevate the residual limb (also called a stump), and notify the surgeon immediately. A large BP cuff may be placed at the bedside for emergency use as a tourniquet.

Put on Your Thinking Cap!

Sometimes an immediate postoperative prosthesis is applied to the residual limb while the patient is in surgery. The surgical site is heavily covered and makes it difficult to assess the condition of the wound, so you must rely on other assessment data. What data would cause you to suspect excessive blood loss in that situation?

Acute Pain

Postoperatively, the patient has incisional pain that is treated with prescribed pain medications, usually opioid analgesics. After giving analgesics, document the effects and notify the physician if pain is not relieved. For a thorough discussion of pain management, see Chapter 15.

Risk for Infection

Use aseptic technique when handling the residual limb, the dressing, and the drains to help reduce the risk of infection. Monitor for signs and symptoms of infection. The incision should be dry, intact, and only slightly red. Suspect infection if a foul or unpleasant odor comes from the dressing, if the patient has a sudden temperature elevation, or if the residual limb is red, excessively warm, or edematous. Laboratory results also may detect an elevated WBC count. Treatment for infection may include antibiotics and incision and drainage of the infected residual limb. In severe cases, the infection may cause further tissue damage and require reamputation at a higher level. Therefore it is very important to take measures to prevent infection and to act promptly if there is evidence of infection.

Impaired Skin Integrity and Risk for Impaired Skin Integrity

The care of the residual limb depends on the overall condition of the patient and the type of prosthesis. If the amputation is closed, some type of compression dressing with elastic bandages is used, as well as a cast in some cases. The residual limb is bandaged to promote healing and to shrink and shape the residual limb to a tapered, round, smooth end that will fit the prosthesis. Wrap the bandage smoothly with even, moderate tension to all parts of the residual limb. Rewrap the residual limb as needed to maintain pressure. It is very important to avoid a tourniquet-like effect caused by pulling the bandage too tightly or unevenly. Figure 45-4 illustrates the correct bandaging of a residual limb. Commercial "shrinker socks" are available that maintain compression; however, they

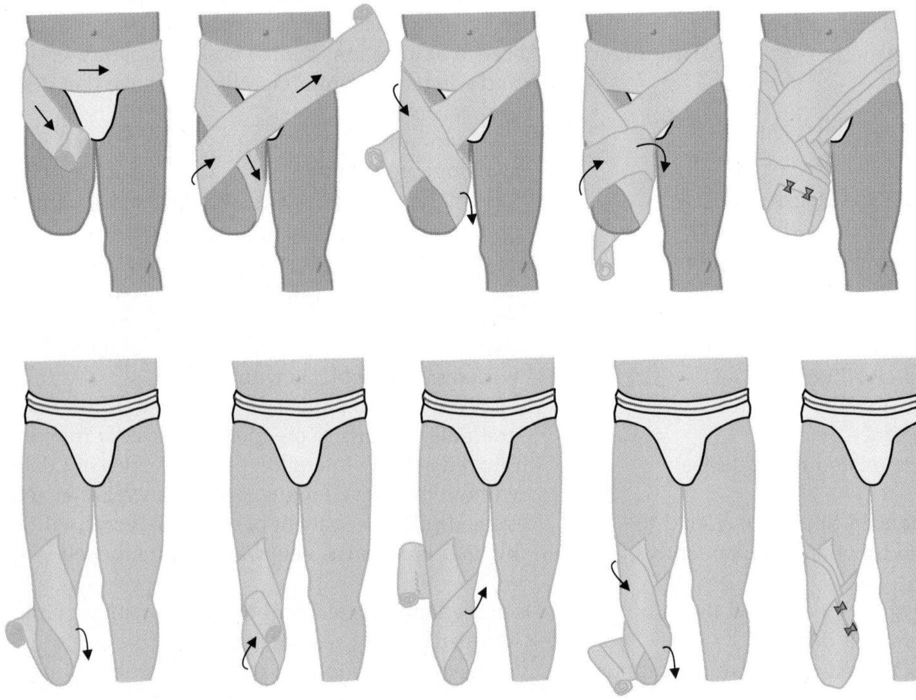

FIGURE 45-4 Proper techniques for wrapping a lower extremity residual limb. (From Black JM, Hawks JH, Keene AM: *Medical-surgical nursing: clinical management for continuity of care*, ed 6, Philadelphia, 2001, Saunders.)

are expensive and it is difficult to find the right size and length for many patients.

Inspect the residual limb frequently for irritation and edema. Edema in the residual limb is most common during the first 24 hours postoperatively. To minimize this, a heavy cast or pressure dressing is applied in the operating room. Elevate the affected lower extremities by raising the foot of the bed. Pillows can be placed under a below-knee amputation, although the use of pillows is discouraged with lower extremity amputations because it can cause contractures of the hip. For the same reason, position the patient in a low Fowler rather than a high Fowler position. After the fifth to seventh postoperative day, the residual limb can be massaged to promote circulation. If permitted, a patient with a lower extremity amputation should lie prone for 30 minutes three or four times a day.

Deficient Knowledge

As mentioned earlier, **phantom limb** sensation or pain is common. It is often described as a burning, stinging, or crushing pain. It tends to lessen with activity, weight bearing, and exercise. If the patient reports such pain, notify the surgeon. Reassure the patient that this is common after amputation and that various treatments are available. Treatment for this type of pain may include diversional activities, whirlpool, massage, injection of the residual limb with an anesthetic, or transcutaneous electrical nerve stimulation (TENS). A properly fitting dressing helps some patients. Drugs that are sometimes helpful include beta-blockers, anticonvulsants, neuroleptics, benzodiazepines, and antidepressants (see *Complementary and Alternative Therapies* box).

Complementary and Alternative Therapies

Many complementary therapies may be used with analgesics to control pain. Examples are imagery, relaxation, meditation, and acupuncture.

Put on Your Thinking Cap!

The home health nurse is visiting an older woman who had a lower leg amputation 1 month ago. The wound appears to be well healed but the woman complains of pain that is sometimes severe in the amputated limb. She asks if she is going crazy. What would you tell her?

Risk for Injury

The patient must learn to function without the amputated limb (see *Patient Teaching* box). He or she must also learn to compensate for the lost extremity in unexpected ways, such as maintaining balance in sitting and standing positions. After lower extremity amputation, safe mobility is a priority. Reinforce the proper use of assistive devices (e.g., crutches, walkers) as taught by the physical therapist. Also encourage and assist the patient to do exercises to strengthen remaining limbs. Keep the environment free of clutter to prevent tripping. Patients with upper limb amputations must learn adaptations to perform activities of daily living (ADL). Everyday activities such as cooking may result in injury. The occupational therapist helps the patient learn to perform these tasks safely. Rehabilitation centers typically have demonstration homelike settings that allow patients to practice meal preparation and other daily activities. Occupational therapy services also extend to the home, where the therapist helps the patient and family to plan for any needed environmental alterations.

Patient Teaching

Amputation

- A rehabilitation team, including a prosthetist (if applicable), physical therapist, and occupational therapist, will work with you to help you regain the best function possible.
- If a prosthetic device is appropriate for you, the prosthetist will fit the device and teach you about it.
- Many modern prostheses are nearly lifelike in appearance and function.
- Phantom limb sensations are sensations perceived in the limb that has been removed; they are commonly experienced by amputees and may disappear spontaneously or continue for years.
- Medications and other treatments can be used to treat phantom pain.
- With lower extremity amputation (if applicable), upper body training is important to strengthen your arms.
- If you will be using crutches, we will teach you crutch walking and you will need to practice.
- We can arrange for a person who has recovered after an amputation like yours to visit, if you would like that.

Impaired Physical Mobility

The physical therapist usually initiates an exercise program. An important goal is the prevention of contractures. These are most common in the knee, hip, and elbow. The patient with a lower extremity amputation may be instructed to lie prone (if tolerable), with the head turned away from the affected side for 30 minutes three or four times a day. Traction, trochanter rolls, and a firm mattress may keep the body in alignment while the patient is in bed. An overbed trapeze may be ordered to facilitate moving back and forth between the bed and the chair. Avoid prolonged flexion of the hip (as when propped on a pillow). Prolonged sitting can lead to hip and knee contractures. Active and passive range-of-motion exercises also are an important part of maintaining mobility and preventing debilitation. Explain the value of exercises to the patient to encourage cooperation and participation.

The patient may have either an immediate or a delayed prosthetic fitting. An immediate fitting allows the patient to become accustomed to weight bearing, ambulation, and balance shortly after surgery. A delayed fitting is usually performed in above-knee amputations, bilateral extremity amputations, or cases of infection in which an open amputation has been performed. The appropriate time frame for fitting a prosthesis in these situations depends on the healing of the residual limb and the overall condition of the patient. When the residual limb has healed well, the patient is fitted for a prosthesis. A suitable choice for a prosthesis is based on the site of the amputation and the age, intelligence, health, motivation, occupation, and financial status of the patient.

Activity Intolerance

Surgery and bed rest may adversely affect the patient's tolerance for any type of sustained activity. It is extremely important to plan care to avoid too much patient exertion. Encouraging the patient to resume the preoperative level of activity too soon can impair physical and psychologic healing. A typical activity order is for the patient to be assisted out of bed two or three times on the first postoperative day for 1 hour at a time. Over the next few days, the patient with a lower extremity amputation is usually encouraged to remain out of bed for longer periods and to begin to practice ambulation gradually. This may initially involve only a few steps but these will gradually be increased over time. The patient's level of activity and the rate at which he or she regains endurance depend on many individual factors.

Readiness for Enhanced Self-Care

During the immediate postoperative period, assist the patient in performing ADL as needed. Gradually, guide the patient to adapt to the lost limb and encourage more independence. Patients feel less helpless when they regain the ability to provide self-care.

Anxiety or Fear and Ineffective Coping

Provide opportunities for patients to talk about their concerns. Explore how the patient's usual coping strategies can be employed in this situation. Encourage and support effective coping strategies. Identify inappropriate behaviors and attempt to help the patient find alternatives. Referral to a local amputee support group may be helpful. As mentioned earlier, it is normal for the patient to experience a grieving process, especially if the amputation is traumatic.

Disturbed Body Image

The patient may have difficulty looking at and caring for the affected extremity (see *Cultural Considerations* box). It takes time for the patient to incorporate the change into his or her body image. Encourage the patient to talk about the change and the effects it will have. Emphasize ways to adapt to the loss and, if the patient wishes, to conceal it. Gradually encourage the patient to participate more in care of the residual limb. Patient instruction for residual limb care is extremely important (see *Patient Teaching* box). Counsel family and friends to support the patient and not to encourage excessive dependence.

Cultural Considerations

What Does Culture Have to Do with Amputations?

Values related to body appearance, function, and independence are culturally influenced and will affect the way in which individuals react to amputation. In addition, religious beliefs may dictate the disposal of amputated body parts by burial or cremation. For example, Orthodox Jews require that such body parts be made available for burial.

Patient Teaching

Care of Residual Limbs and Prostheses

RESIDUAL LIMBS

- Wash the residual limb with soap and water every night. Rinse and dry the skin thoroughly.
- Each day use a mirror to inspect the entire residual limb, especially the incision, for irritation, redness, and edema.
- Expose the residual limb to air when possible.
- Residual limb socks should be hand washed, rinsed well, and dried flat. A clean sock should be used every day. Having several socks will allow time for the socks to dry between washings.
- Do not wear mended socks because a seam is irritating and creates pressure.
- Shoes with uneven heels will change the weight distribution of the residual limb and lead to irritation and possible skin breakdown.
- Do not use lotions, ointments, or powders unless prescribed by the physician.
- If redness or irritation develops on the residual limb, discontinue use of the prosthesis until you have the area checked.

PROSTHESES

- Keep the prosthetic socket (the opening in which the residual limb is seated) clean.
- The residual limb may shrink in size for up to 2 years after surgery. Annual visits to the prosthetist are recommended for necessary adjustments (these visits are more frequent for children, as their residual limb grows in size with them).
- Each day, wipe the inside of the prosthesis socket with a damp, soapy cloth, then remove the soap with a clean, damp cloth. Dry thoroughly.
- Consult a prosthetist if any problems occur with the prosthesis. Do not attempt to make adjustments yourself.

OLDER ADULT WITH AN AMPUTATION

The older adult with an amputation may have some additional needs that should be considered when planning and providing care. For example, when constructing a teaching plan for the older adult, keep in mind that the healthy older person is completely capable of learning but often requires smaller units of information, more repetition, and more time. Skip unnecessary details and make sure that patients with glasses or hearing aids have them in place during the teaching process.

It is also important to clearly explain phantom sensations to older adults. Some may not wish to report phantom sensations or phantom pain for fear of seeming foolish. Reminding the older patient that phantom sensations are not uncommon or bizarre can reduce the fear or anxiety that these sensations can cause.

Many older adults have one or more chronic health problems. This factor should be considered in the selection of a prosthetic device. For example, a patient with diabetes is prone to circulation problems and poor wound healing and may need a prosthesis with extra padding or support. Poor vision and decreased sensation may keep the older person from recognizing complications.

Because many older adults have decreased appetites, their nutritional status may be poor. Emphasizing high-calorie and high-protein intake is essential to promote healing and to maintain or build strength (see *Nutrition Considerations* box).

Nutrition Considerations

1. A nutritional assessment should be made preoperatively for patients undergoing surgical amputation, especially for older, immobilized, or chronic alcoholic patients.
2. Patients undergoing surgical amputation should be well hydrated; intravenous fluids may be given if oral fluids are not tolerated.
3. Surgical amputation is accompanied by a stress response, resulting in an increased need for calories and protein for healing.
4. Dietary supplements may be needed for patients whose intake of regular foods is inadequate for healing.
5. Patients are encouraged to become mobile as soon as possible after an amputation to prevent loss of calcium and protein.
6. Dietary choices high in protein, zinc, and vitamin C promote wound healing.

Remembering that the loss of a limb or part of a limb can be especially difficult for older adults is important in providing psychologic support. This is because many older individuals have had to deal with other losses in their lives, such as the loss of loved ones, the loss of independence, and the loss of income associated with retirement. Older people may lack confidence that they can adapt and gain strength.

If the patient is unable to participate fully in his or her care, instruct family members along with the older patient. Home health nursing services may be arranged to facilitate adaptation in the home setting and to monitor for complications. Empathy, patience, and respect are essential in approaching older patients. Building strength and activity tolerance is vital to walking with a lower extremity prosthesis. Some frail older adults will need to use a wheelchair rather than a prosthesis.

REPLANTATION

In some amputation injuries, a type of surgical technique called *replantation* may be performed. This involves the use of a microscope and highly specialized instruments to reanastomose (reconnect) blood vessels and nerve fibers in a severed limb. The limb is then sutured into its correct anatomic position. Advances in microsurgical techniques and preservation of severed limbs have made this technique increasingly successful. Attachment of donor limbs (transplantation) is gaining acceptance and success as more effective drugs are being developed to control rejection. However, lifelong immunosuppression creates new risks and challenges.

INDICATIONS

A number of factors are considered by the surgeon before performing replantation surgery—for example, the type of injury and location and the extent of limb ischemia. Replantation surgery is most likely to be performed for amputations through the hand or wrist. Amputated thumbs are reattached whenever possible because of the thumb's importance in total hand function. In a severely injured hand in which two or more fingers are detached, an attempt is made by the surgeon to restore as many fingers as possible. In general, the greater the muscle mass injury, the less likely that replantation will be successful or even possible.

EMERGENCY CARE

Proper handling of amputated parts is extremely important for successful replantation. Current preservation techniques include wrapping the amputated parts in a clean cloth saturated with normal saline or lactated Ringer solution. These parts are then placed in a sealed plastic bag that is placed in ice water. Direct contact between the amputated part and the ice can lead to further tissue damage and cell death. Partially amputated parts should remain attached to the patient and also should be kept cool if possible. Extra care should be taken to avoid detaching any parts because even small connections increase the chances for successful repair.

The patient may require treatment for shock because of blood loss. This may include intravenous fluids and blood products. Blood loss from the residual limb may be minimized by using a clean, dry dressing, which can be reinforced as needed. Tourniquets should not be used unless absolutely necessary, because they can cause ischemia of the residual limb.

PREOPERATIVE NURSING CARE of the Patient Having Replantation Surgery

Assessment

General preoperative care of the replantation patient includes careful assessment of circulatory status, close monitoring of vital signs, and inspection of the residual limb (or dressing) for bleeding. Ask about pain at the site of the injury and at other locations. Measure and record fluid intake and output. Note the patient's emotional status and assess understanding of the preoperative activities and postoperative routines. Identify sources of support.

Nursing Diagnoses, Goals, and Outcome Criteria: Replantation, Preoperative

Nursing Diagnoses	Goals and Outcome Criteria
Decreased Cardiac Output related to decreased blood volume	Normal cardiac output: pulse and blood pressure (BP) within patient norms, skin warm and dry
Fear related to severe injury or possible failure of replantation	Reduced fear: calm manner, patient statement of less fear
Anxiety related to lack of knowledge of surgical routines	Decreased anxiety: relaxed manner, patient statement of reduced anxiety
Acute Pain related to tissue trauma	Decreased pain: patient statement of less pain, relaxed manner, pulse and BP within patient norms

Interventions

Administer intravenous fluids and blood as ordered. If the dressing becomes saturated with blood, reinforce the dressing. Report continued or excessive bleeding to the physician. Even though preparations for replantation are hurried, be sensitive to the patient's fear and anxiety. Accept the patient's feelings. Provide brief, simple explanations. Administer analgesics as ordered for pain.

POSTOPERATIVE NURSING CARE of the Patient Having Replantation Surgery

Routine postoperative care is discussed in detail in Chapter 17. This section emphasizes the special needs of the replantation patient.

Assessment

Postoperative assessment includes monitoring vital signs, intake and output, and level of consciousness. An essential aspect of care after replantation is hourly neurovascular assessment of the replanted limb. A Doppler device or pulse oximeter may be used to evaluate circulation. When the patient arrives on the nursing unit, immediately assess and document circulatory status to establish a baseline for comparison. Note and record the limb's color, capillary refill, turgor, temperature, and sensation. Signs of arterial occlusion are pale or blue color, slow capillary refill, shriveled appearance, and coolness. Signs of venous congestion are cyanosis, rapid capillary refill, edema, and warmth. Assess the limb for edema, because massive edema often accompanies replantation.

Nursing Diagnoses, Goals, and Outcome Criteria: Replantation, Postoperative

Nursing Diagnoses	Goals and Outcome Criteria
Ineffective Peripheral Tissue Perfusion related to trauma, edema, compensatory vasoconstriction	Adequate circulation to replanted limb: warmth, normal skin color, arterial pulses
Acute Pain related to tissue trauma	Pain relief: relaxed expression, statement of less pain
Disturbed Body Image related to disfigurement, loss of function	Improved body image: patient touches and looks at affected part, makes positive statements about self

Interventions

Measures to promote circulation to the replanted limb include elevation of the limb and microvascular precautions. Elevation of the limb promotes venous and lymphatic drainage. Take care not to elevate the limb above the level of the heart, because this may impair arterial flow. Several soft pillows or a stockinette connected to an intravenous pole may help to achieve this. Microvascular precautions include avoiding any substances or conditions that contribute to blood vessel spasm or constriction. Encourage the patient to abstain from nicotine- and caffeine-containing products for 7 to 10 days postoperatively. In addition, maintain room temperature at 80°F to prevent compensatory vasoconstriction of the peripheral tissues in response to cold. Loosen tight or restrictive gowns or pajamas. Explain the importance of these measures to the patient and family (see *Patient Teaching* box).

Patient Teaching

Postoperative Replantation

- Avoid nicotine and caffeine for 7 to 10 days or as directed by the surgeon.
- Avoid tight clothing that could impair circulation to the replanted limb or digit.
- Keep the limb positioned as instructed.
- A rehabilitation team will teach you proper care to promote improved function.
- Immediately advise your surgeon of changes in the color or warmth of the replanted limb or digit.

Administer intravenous low-molecular-weight dextran (Dextran 40), aspirin, or heparin as ordered to reduce the risk of thrombosis. Monitor for adverse effects. Inadequate arterial blood flow to the replanted limb is a medical emergency. If evidence of inadequate arterial circulation exists (i.e., no pulse, pallor or cyanosis, cool skin), immediately notify the surgeon and prepare the patient for a return to the operating suite. In some facilities, venous congestion is treated with leeches (hirudotherapy). Leeches are attached to a selected area of the replanted limb. The saliva of the leeches contains an anticoagulant, a local vasodilator, and a local anesthetic. The leech extracts excess blood, reducing venous congestion.

Provide the patient with an opportunity to discuss thoughts and feelings about the replantation, disfigurement, and loss of function. It may take time before the patient is able to look at and touch the replanted limb. Support the patient and demonstrate acceptance of him or her. Your comfort with handling the limb can help the patient to feel accepted. The rehabilitation team works with the patient to restore maximum possible function.

If the replantation is not successful, the limb is surgically removed. This represents a significant loss to the patient. Recognize this loss and support the patient.

Other essential aspects of care include routine postoperative measures such as frequent position changes, pulmonary toilet, and pain management.

Put on Your Thinking Cap!

What could you do or say to support the patient whose replanted limb must be amputated?

Get Ready for the NCLEX® Examination!

Key Points

- Amputation is the surgical removal of body limbs or parts of limbs.
- Conditions or situations that can lead to an amputation include trauma, disease, tumors, and congenital problems.
- The medical management of patients who have amputations involves the appropriate treatment and control of underlying diseases such as diabetes mellitus and peripheral vascular disease.
- Complications of amputation include hemorrhage, hematoma, necrosis, wound dehiscence, gangrene, edema, contracture, pain, and infection.
- Preoperatively, the patient needs to prepare physically and psychologically for an impending amputation.
- Postoperative nursing care focuses on decreased cardiac output, acute pain, risk for infection, impaired skin integrity, risk for impaired skin integrity, deficient knowledge, risk for injury, impaired physical mobility, activity intolerance, readiness for enhanced self-care, anxiety or fear, ineffective coping, and disturbed body image.
- Replantation of severed limbs is sometimes possible.
- Before replantation, nursing and medical care focus on preserving the severed part and managing the patient's blood loss.
- Priorities after replantation include assessing for and managing ineffective tissue perfusion, acute pain, and disturbed body image.
- If evidence of inadequate arterial circulation in a replanted limb exists, immediately notify the surgeon and prepare the patient for a return to the operating suite.

Additional Learning Resources

SG Go to your Study Guide for additional learning activities to help you master this chapter content.

evolve Go to your Evolve website (http://evolve.elsevier.com/Linton/medsurg) for the following learning resources and much more:

- Interactive Prioritization Exercises
- Fluid & Electrolyte Tutorial
- Pharmacology Tutorial
- Review Questions for the NCLEX® Examination

Review Questions for the NCLEX® Examination

1. Which of the following is the most common cause of lower extremity amputation?
   1. Trauma
   2. Vascular disease
   3. Tumors
   4. Congenital defects

   NCLEX Client Need: Physiological Integrity: Physiological Adaptation
2. The nurse is teaching a patient who had a finger replanted. The teaching plan should explain that smoking is contraindicated after replantation because nicotine causes ______________.

   NCLEX Client Need: Physiological Integrity: Reduction of Risk Potential
3. In which of the following situations would an *open* amputation be most likely?
   1. A teenager with bone cancer
   2. A diabetic patient with poor arterial blood flow
   3. A child with a congenital deformity
   4. An accident victim with a crushing injury

   NCLEX Client Need: Physiological Integrity: Reduction of Risk Potential

4. A patient complains that her amputated foot itches and feels hot. The nurse should recognize that this represents which of the following?
   1. Poor psychological adjustment
   2. Phantom limb sensation
   3. Early symptoms of infection
   4. Denial of the amputation

   NCLEX Client Need: Physiological Integrity: Physiological Adaptation
5. In the early postoperative period, what is the greatest danger to the patient who has had an amputation?
   1. Pneumonia
   2. Pain
   3. Hemorrhage
   4. Anxiety

   NCLEX Client Need: Physiological Integrity: Physiological Adaptation
6. A patient who had a below-knee amputation this morning has a cast on the residual limb. The nurse knows that the purpose of the cast in this case is to:
   1. Reduce pain
   2. Shape the residual limb
   3. Prevent wound contamination
   4. Prevent stimulation of nerve endings

   NCLEX Client Need: Physiological Integrity: Reduction of Risk Potential
7. When caring for a patient who has had an above-knee amputation, the nurse implements measures to prevent contractures in the residual limb. These measures should include: (Select all that apply.)
   1. Keep the patient up in a chair as much as possible
   2. Guide the patient through active range-of-motion exercises
   3. Have the patient lie supine for 30 minutes three or four times a day
   4. Prop the residual limb on a pillow when the patient is supine
   5. Encourage the patient to sleep on the side of the amputation

   NCLEX Client Need: Physiological Integrity: Reduction of Risk Potential
8. Patient teaching related to care of a residual limb and prosthesis should include which of the following statements? (Select all that apply.)
   1. Wear a clean residual limb sock every day.
   2. Wash, rinse, and dry the prosthetic socket every day.
   3. Apply lotion to the residual limb only if ordered to do so.
   4. Redness and irritation of the residual limb are normal.
   5. Wash the residual limb with soap and water daily.

   NCLEX Client Need: Physiological Integrity: Reduction of Risk Potential
9. While on a camping trip, a camper accidentally cut off a finger while chopping wood. A nurse provided first aid and summoned emergency medical care. Meanwhile, how should the amputated finger be handled for possible replantation?
   1. Cover the finger with ice
   2. Wrap the finger in a clean, dry cloth
   3. Wash the part carefully, dry it, and wrap it in plastic
   4. Seal the part in a plastic bag and put it in ice water

   NCLEX Client Need: Physiological Integrity: Reduction of Risk Potential
10. When you examine a patient's replanted hand, it is slightly bluish, swollen, and warm. These findings indicate which of the following?
    1. Arterial occlusion
    2. Rejection of the replanted hand
    3. Venous congestion
    4. That the replantation was successful

    NCLEX Client Need: Physiological Integrity: Physiological Adaptation

chapter 46

Pituitary and Adrenal Disorders

Maria Danet Sanchez Lapiz-Bluhm, Adrianne Dill Linton

http://evolve.elsevier.com/Linton/medsurg

Objectives

1. Identify data to be collected for the nursing assessment of adrenal and pituitary function.
2. Describe the tests and procedures used to diagnose disorders of the adrenal and pituitary glands.
3. Describe the pathophysiology and medical treatment of adrenocortical insufficiency, excess adrenocortical hormones, hypopituitarism, diabetes insipidus, and pituitary tumors.
4. Assist in developing nursing care plans for patients with selected disorders of the adrenal and pituitary glands.

Key Terms

Acromegaly (ăk-rō-MĔG-ă-lē)
Addison disease (ĂD-ĭ-sŏnz dĭ-ZĒZ)
Adrenaline (ă-DRĔN-ă-lĭn)
Androgens (ĂN-drō-jĕnz)
Catecholamines (kăt-ĕ-KŌL-ă-mēnz)
Cushing disease (KŬSH-ĭng dĭ-ZĒZ)
Cushing syndrome (KŬSH-ĭng SĬN-drōm)
Diabetes insipidus (DI) (dī-ă-BĒ-tēz ĭn-SĬP-ĭ-dŭs)
Dwarfism (DWORF-ĭ-zm)
Endocrine glands (ĔN-dŏ-krĭn)
Estrogens (ĔS-trō-jĕnz)
Gigantism (JĪ-găn-tĭzm)
Glucocorticoid (gloo-kō-KŎR-tĭ-koyd)
Hypophysectomy (hī-pō-fĭ-SĔK-tŏ-mē)
Mineralocorticoids (mĭn-ĕr-ăl-ō-KŎR-tĭ-koyd)
Syndrome of inappropriate antidiuretic hormone (SIADH) (ăn-tĭ-dī-ū-RĔT-ĭk HŎR-mōn)

The endocrine system is a complex communication network composed of glands and glandular tissue that make, store, and secrete chemical messengers called *hormones*. It affects virtually every cell in the human body. Hormones are delivered to tissues by the bloodstream to target organs and body. The **endocrine glands** are depicted in Figure 46-1.

Another class of glands includes the exocrine glands. The exocrine glands pass secretions through ducts or tubes that empty outside the body or into the lumen or opening of other organs. Examples of this type of gland are sweat glands and the portion of the pancreas that secretes digestive enzymes.

HORMONE FUNCTIONS AND REGULATION

The term *hormone* was coined in 1905. It is derived from the Greek word meaning "I arouse to activity." This definition is appropriate because hormones are normally released in response to the body's needs. Hormones are responsible for important functions related to reproduction, fluid and electrolyte balance, host defenses, responses to stress and injury, energy metabolism, and growth and development. The overall mission of the endocrine system is to maintain homeostasis. Homeostasis is the maintenance of physiologic stability despite the constant changes that occur in the environment. A hormone is a substance composed of amines, peptides, or steroids. These substances bind to receptors located inside the cell nucleus or on the cell membranes of target organs or tissues. Receptors are specific for certain kinds of hormones. Once the hormones bind with their receptors, they exert their effects on the organ or tissue.

Regulation of endocrine activity is controlled by mechanisms, called *feedback mechanisms*, that either stimulate or inhibit hormone synthesis and secretion. Feedback mechanisms are triggered by blood levels of specific substances. These substances may be hormones or other chemical compounds regulated by hormones. Feedback may be either positive or negative (Fig. 46-2).

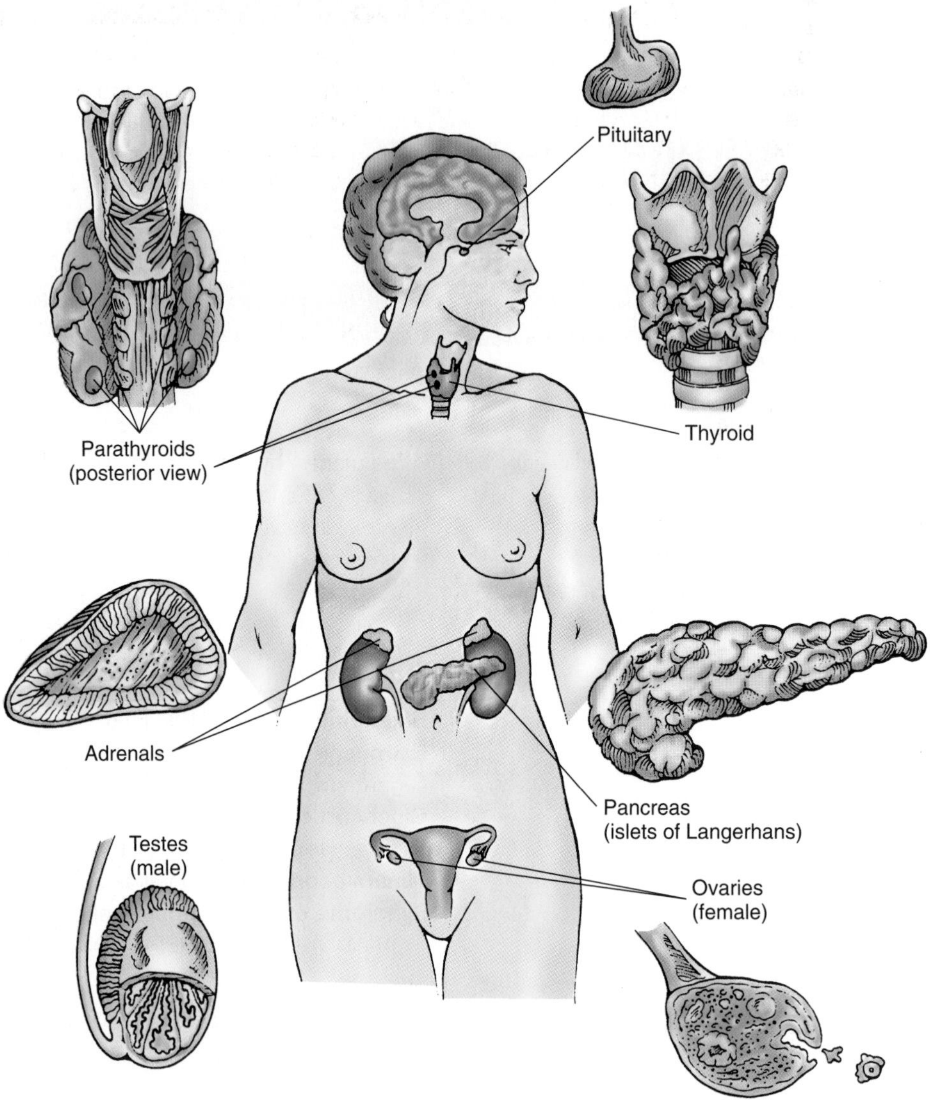

FIGURE 46-1 The endocrine system. The organs of the endocrine system include the pituitary gland, thyroid gland, parathyroid glands, adrenal glands, pancreas, testes (in the man), and ovaries (in the woman). (From Ignatavicius DD, Workman ML, Mishler MA: *Medical-surgical nursing across the health care continuum*, ed 3, Philadelphia, 1999, Saunders.)

In negative feedback, high levels of a substance inhibit hormone synthesis and secretion whereas low levels stimulate hormone synthesis and secretion. A simple example of this is the household thermostat. As the environmental temperature rises, the production of heat is decreased or stopped; however, as the temperature drops, heat production increases. In positive feedback, high levels of a substance stimulate hormone synthesis and secretion whereas low levels inhibit additional hormone synthesis and secretion.

Hormones have specific rates and rhythms of secretion. Three basic secretion patterns are (1) circadian or diurnal pattern, (2) pulsatile and cyclic patterns, and (3) patterns that depend on levels of circulating substances (e.g., calcium, sodium, potassium, or the hormones themselves).

PITUITARY GLAND

ANATOMY AND PHYSIOLOGY OF THE PITUITARY GLAND

The pituitary gland, also called the *hypophysis*, is a structure that weighs approximately 0.6 g and is located in the sella turcica, a small indentation in the sphenoid bone at the base of the brain. It is connected to the hypothalamus by the infundibular (hypophyseal) stalk. The pituitary gland is small and oval and has a diameter of approximately 1 cm. It consists of two parts, or lobes. The larger of the two lobes, which accounts for 70% to 80% of the gland's weight, is the anterior lobe. The anterior lobe is also called the *adenohypophysis*. The hormones of the anterior pituitary and their actions are as follows:

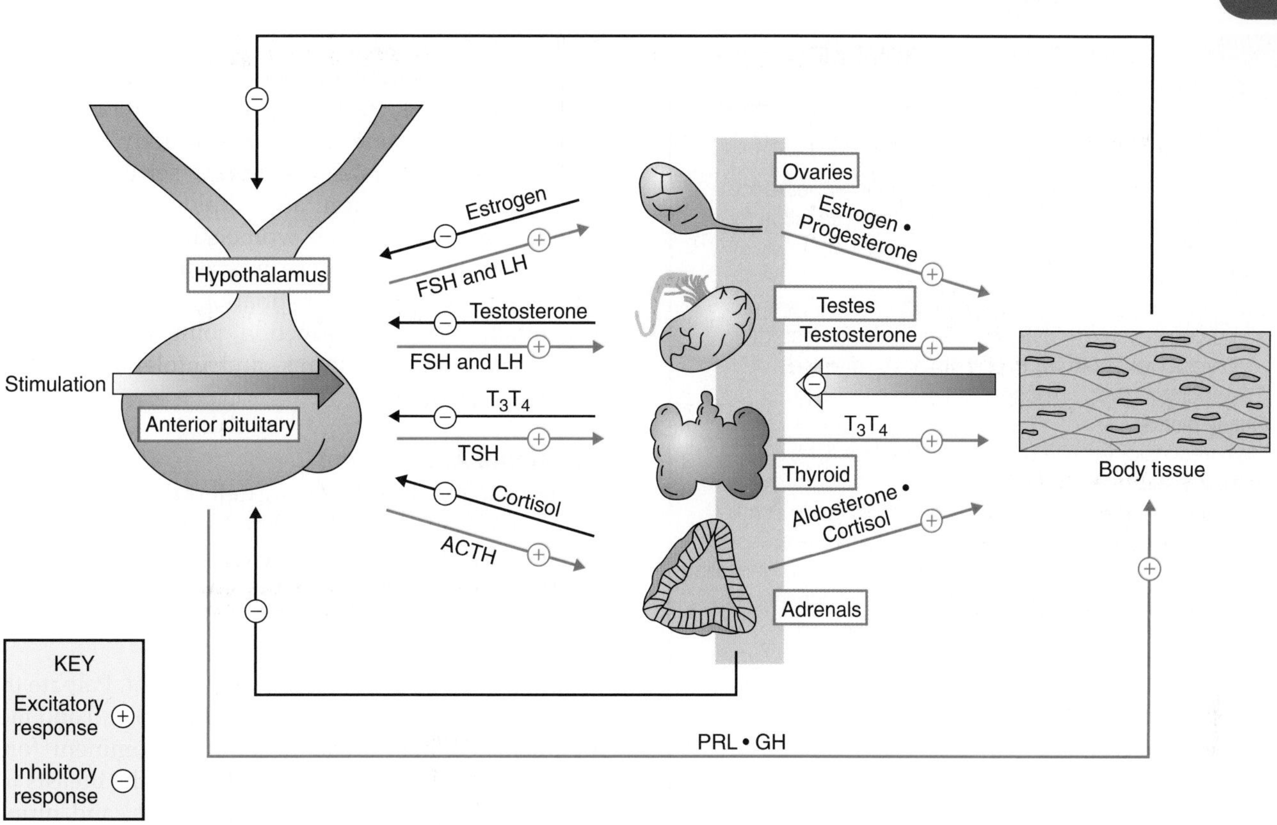

FIGURE 46-2 The feedback system of the hypothalamus, pituitary, and target glands. *ACTH*, Adrenocorticotropic hormone; *FSH*, follicle-stimulating hormone; *GH*, growth hormone; *LH*, luteinizing hormone; *PRL*, prolactin; T_3, triiodothyronine; T_4, thyroxine *TSH*, thyroid-stimulating hormone. (From Ignatavicius DD, Workman ML, Mishler MA: *Medical-surgical nursing across the health care continuum*, ed 3, Philadelphia, 1999, Saunders.)

1. Growth hormone (GH), or somatotropic hormone: stimulates the growth and development of bones, muscles, and organs. GH stimulates the release of insulin-like growth factor 1 (IGF-1) by the liver and other tissues. IGF-1 promotes tissue growth.
2. Adrenocorticotropic hormone (ACTH): controls the growth, development, and function of the cortex of the adrenal glands; controls release of glucocorticoids and adrenal androgens; necessary for secretion of aldosterone but does not control rate of aldosterone secretion.
3. Thyroid-stimulating hormone (TSH), or thyrotropic hormone: controls the secretory activities of the thyroid gland.
4. Follicle-stimulating hormone (FSH): stimulates the development of the eggs in the ovaries and estrogen production in the woman; stimulates sperm production in the man.
5. Luteinizing hormone (LH): controls progesterone production and ovulation or egg release in the woman; controls testicular growth and testosterone production in the man.
6. Prolactin, or lactogenic hormone: stimulates breast milk production in the woman.
7. Melanocyte-stimulating hormone (MSH): promotes pigmentation.

The smaller lobe of the pituitary is known as the *posterior pituitary* because it is located behind the anterior lobe in the sella turcica. It is sometimes referred to as the *neurohypophysis.* The hormones secreted by the posterior pituitary and their actions are as follows:

1. Antidiuretic hormone (ADH), or arginine vasopressin: causes the reabsorption of water from the renal tubules of the kidney. By doing so, water excretion from the body in the form of urine is decreased.
2. Oxytocin: causes contractions of the uterus in labor and the release of breast milk.

NURSING ASSESSMENT OF THE PATIENT WITH A PITUITARY DISORDER

The nursing assessment of the patient with a pituitary disorder is outlined in Box 46-1. The licensed vocational nurse/licensed practical nurse (LVN/LPN) assists with the collection of relevant data.

HEALTH HISTORY

Present Illness

Some problems related to pituitary function that may cause the patient to seek medical care are slowed or accelerated growth; visual disturbances; headache;

Box 46-1 Assessment of the Patient with a Pituitary Disorder

HEALTH HISTORY

Chief Complaint and Present Illness

Slowed or accelerated growth; change in appearance, urine output, and secondary sex characteristics (or a combination)

Past Medical History

Brain tumors; pituitary surgery; head trauma, central nervous system (CNS) infection; vascular disorders; chronic renal failure; hypothyroidism; diseases of the pancreas, liver, or bone

Family History

Diabetes insipidus (DI) or diabetes mellitus (DM)

Review of Systems

Fatigue, restlessness, agitation, skin moisture and hair distribution, vision disturbances, changes in breasts, chest pain, constipation, polyuria, changes in genitalia, sexual dysfunction, joint pain, abnormal sensations, edema, seizures, intolerance of heat or cold

Functional Assessment

Sleep pattern, usual diet, effects of disease on self-concept and daily life

PHYSICAL EXAMINATION

General Survey

Body proportion, behavior, mental and emotional state

Vital Signs

Height and Weight

Skin

Moisture and edema

Head and Face

Thickened lips, broad nose, prominent forehead and jaw

Neck

Jugular venous distention

Eyes

Visual acuity

Breasts

Enlargement, discharge

Extremities

Edema, range of motion, crepitus

Neurologic

Slow reflexes

Genitalia

Loss of pubic hair, testicular atrophy

and changes in urine output, appearance, skin, and secondary sex characteristics.

Past Medical History

A history of brain tumors, pituitary surgery, head trauma, central nervous system (CNS) infection, vascular disorders, chronic renal failure, and hypothyroidism, as well as disease of the pancreas, liver, or bone, should be documented.

Family History

Note a family history of **diabetes insipidus (DI)**.

Review of Systems

Ask about the patient's general health state and note fatigue, weakness, restlessness, or agitation. Inquire about skin moisture and changes in body hair distribution. Note reports of significant sensory changes such as blurred vision and diplopia (i.e., double vision). For both men and women, ask about changes in the breasts. Also inquire whether the patient has experienced chest pain, constipation, polyuria, changes in genitalia, sexual dysfunction, joint pain, abnormal sensations, edema, seizures, and intolerance of heat or cold.

Functional Assessment

In the functional assessment, determine whether the patient has had sleep disturbances. Obtain a description of usual diet and note the effects of symptoms on the person's self-concept and usual activities.

PHYSICAL EXAMINATION

Measure vital signs and height and weight. Palpate the skin for moisture and edema. Inspect the head and face for thickened lips, broad nose, and prominent forehead and jaw. Test visual acuity. Inspect the breasts for enlargement in men, atrophy in women, and nipple discharge. Inspect and palpate the extremities for edema. Perform joint range of motion, noting any limitations or crepitus. Test reflexes for slowness of response. Inspect the male genitalia for loss of hair and palpate for testicular atrophy. The ophthalmologist may test the visual fields.

AGE-RELATED CHANGES

In healthy older adults, pituitary function remains adequate. However, the *response* to ADH is diminished so that the older person is less able to compensate for inadequate fluid intake or excessive fluid loss and is at risk for dehydration. GH and IGF-1 decline, resulting in reduced protein synthesis, decreased lean body and bone mass, and reduced immune function. Although some scientists have hoped that GH supplementation would slow or reverse the aging process, the benefits have been limited and the side effects troubling.

DIAGNOSTIC TESTS AND PROCEDURES

RADIOGRAPHIC STUDIES

Conventional radiographs, computed tomography (CT) scans, and magnetic resonance imaging (MRI) may be used to detect a pituitary tumor. Cerebral angiography, in which a radiopaque dye is injected into the cerebral arteries, may reveal the presence of vascular anomalies that can interfere with the supply of blood in the brain and lead to pituitary damage.

LABORATORY STUDIES

Because hormones are circulating in very small quantities, tests to identify normal levels must be sensitive and precise. The radioimmunoassay and the enzyme-linked immunosorbent assay (ELISA) are tests that measure levels of hormones in the blood.

Hormone reserve activity also can be measured using a number of "suppression" or "stimulation" tests. In these tests, hormone levels are measured after administration of an agent that stimulates or suppresses hormonal function. Stimulation will cause a healthy endocrine gland to increase hormone production. Suppression will cause a healthy endocrine gland to decrease hormone production. The response helps the physician to determine whether the target gland (e.g., thyroid, adrenal, gonads) or the hypothalamic-pituitary regulatory mechanism is responsible for abnormal hormone levels.

A GH suppression test may be done by measuring blood glucose levels before and after a dose of a glucose solution. The glucose will suppress GH levels through a negative-feedback process. In normal patients, GH levels fall to less than 5 mg/mL. However, in patients with hyperpituitarism, large decreases in GH occur. This constitutes a positive result. Other studies measure serum levels of GH, IGF-1, and gonadotropins (FSH, LH). A 6-hour water deprivation test is done to determine the cause of DI. ADH is administered and urine and blood samples are taken at intervals. Additional information about diagnostic tests and procedures for pituitary disorders and related nursing care is presented in Table 46-1.

Table 46-1 Diagnostic Tests and Procedures Pituitary Disorders

TEST AND PURPOSE	PATIENT PREPARATION	POSTPROCEDURE NURSING CARE
Imaging Studies		
General Interventions When Contrast Dye Used. Before Procedure: Assess patient allergy to dye, iodine, or shellfish. If patient reports allergy, notify radiology. Tell patient that injection of contrast dye can create a feeling of warmth, a salty taste, and nausea. **After Procedure:** Inform the physician of any signs of allergic response to the contrast dye. Administer antihistamine as ordered for allergy.		
Cerebral CT scan: Uses radiographs to create images of internal structures; detects tumors, edema, and structural abnormalities.	Tell the patient he or she will lie still on a stretcher while a circular scanner moves around the head. Clicking sounds are heard but no sensations are felt. Remove jewelry and hairpins. Contrast precautions.	If contrast medium is used, assess for side effects: nausea, vomiting, headache, and delayed allergic reaction.
MRI scan with gadolinium infusion. Gadolinium is a contrast medium used with MRI to enhance brain imaging.	The patient will be given an IV injection. All metal, including medication patches with metallic backing, must be removed. No food or fluid restrictions exist, although the patient might wish to void in advance to avoid discomfort of a full bladder. During the scan, the patient must remain still. A loud thumping noise will be heard during the procedure.	No special care is required except to check the venipuncture site for bleeding.
Cerebral angiogram: Radiographs are taken to study cerebral blood flow and blood vessels.	Signed consent is required. Contrast precautions. General anesthesia needed for patients who cannot cooperate. Tell patient there may be a burning sensation when contrast medium is injected. Stress importance of lying still. Remove jewelry and hairpins.	Apply pressure to arterial puncture site for 15 min. Assess for bleeding afterward. Record VS per agency protocol. Immobilize extremity as ordered. Bed rest 12–24 h. Neurologic checks hourly 4 times, then every 4 h 20 times.
Laboratory Studies		
***General Interventions:** Check agency procedure manual for diagnostic tests and procedures. Always tell the patient what to expect when tests are ordered. Explain if NPO status is necessary. Document the care provided and relevant assessment data. If venipuncture is done, apply a dressing and check the site for oozing. Apply pressure and elevate arm if patient's blood clotting is impaired.		

Continued

Table 46-1 Diagnostic Tests and Procedures Pituitary Disorders—cont'd

TEST AND PURPOSE	PATIENT PREPARATION	POSTPROCEDURE NURSING CARE
GH suppression test (glucose loading test): Evaluates response to glucose dose to detect abnormally high level of GH consistent with hormone hypersecretion.	Tell patient fasting blood glucose will be measured; then a glucose solution will be given and blood samples taken to measure glucose levels at specified intervals. Enforce NPO.	*General Interventions. Provide ordered diet.
Dexamethasone suppression tests: Measure cortisol, which increases with adrenal hyperplasia, Cushing syndrome, oat cell carcinoma; decreases with histoplasmosis and tuberculosis.	Tell patient that baseline serum and urine cortisol will be measured. For overnight test, a dose of dexamethasone is given, usually around 11 PM, and a blood sample is drawn for cortisol level at 8 AM. Alternative tests are the low-dose test and high-dose test with various schedules for obtaining blood and urine specimens. Explain 24-h urine collection, if ordered.	Send blood sample to laboratory within 30 min. *General Interventions.
Pituitary hormone levels (LH, FSH, GH, ACTH, TSH, prolactin): Serum levels are measured to detect elevations or deficiencies of pituitary hormones.	*General Interventions.	*General Interventions.
Hypertonic saline test: An infusion of hypertonic saline is given to stimulate release of ADH; used to detect DI.	Tell patient IV fluids will be given. Urine output and specific gravity will be measured hourly. Explain urine collection process.	*General Interventions.
Fluid deprivation: Detects changes in specific gravity and osmolality after aqueous vasopressin is given subcutaneously. Specific gravity and osmolality decrease with primary and secondary DI. No response with nephrogenic DI.	NPO for specified time. Tell patient VS will be taken, urine specimens collected, body weight measured hourly. A medication will be given and additional measurements done. Administer ordered medication and collect designated specimens.	No special care is required.

ACTH, Adrenocorticotropic hormone; *ADH,* antidiuretic hormone; *CT,* computed tomography; *DI,* diabetes insipidus; *FSH,* follicle-stimulating hormone; *GH,* growth hormone; *IV,* intravenous; *LH,* luteinizing hormone; *MRI,* magnetic resonance imaging; *NPO,* nothing by mouth; TSH, thyroid-stimulating hormone; VS, vital signs.

DISORDERS OF THE PITUITARY GLAND

Dysfunction of the pituitary gland can result from a problem in the gland itself or from a problem in the hypothalamus. The hypothalamus is an organ in the brain that secretes factors that can directly inhibit or stimulate the pituitary (see Fig. 46-2). Pituitary disease is usually manifested by excess or deficient production and secretion of a specific hormone. These hormone imbalances lead to disorders that can be manifested in a variety of ways, including changes in physical appearance, emotional state, mental status, metabolism, and homeostatic mechanisms essential for survival. The pituitary disorders discussed in this chapter are hyperpituitarism, hypopituitarism, DI, and **syndrome of inappropriate antidiuretic hormone (SIADH)**.

HYPERPITUITARISM

Cause

Hyperpituitarism is a pathologic state caused by excess production of one or more of the anterior pituitary hormones. GH, prolactin, FSH, LH, and ACTH are the hormones most often produced in excess. GH is responsible for the growth and development of the body's muscles, bones, and other tissue. Overproduction of GH can lead to gigantism or acromegaly. Overproduction of prolactin causes hyperprolactinemia.

The most common factor in hyperpituitarism is the presence of a pituitary adenoma. An adenoma is a benign tumor composed of epithelial tissue. It may vary in size and invasiveness. Those that are larger than 10 mm are called *macroadenomas;* those that are smaller than 10 mm are called *microadenomas.* Adenomas tend to occur most commonly in young women in their teens through early 30s. Pituitary adenomas that secrete hormones may cause amenorrhea, galactorrhea (i.e., abnormal milk secretion), hyperthyroidism, and Cushing syndrome, in addition to gigantism or acromegaly.

GH, in addition to regulating tissue growth, mobilizes stored fat for energy. As a result of lipolysis of body adipose, excess levels of GH elevate free fatty acids in the bloodstream. This can stimulate the development of atherosclerosis, which causes coronary artery disease (CAD) and cerebrovascular disease over time. Excess GH also antagonizes insulin and interferes with its effects, leading to hyperglycemia and possibly diabetes mellitus (DM).

Prolactinemia. Excess prolactin can cause prolactinemia, characterized by abnormal lactation (galactorrhea), amenorrhea, decreased vaginal lubrication, impotence and decreased libido in men, depression, anxiety, and visual loss.

Gigantism. **Gigantism** occurs in early childhood or puberty, while the long bones of the body are still growing. The long bones consist of epiphyses, which are the end portions of the bone, and a diaphysis, which is the middle or shaft of the bone. Toward the end of puberty or in early adulthood, the line between these structures seals or closes, preventing further growth. Before the epiphyseal plates on the ends of these bones close, the diaphysis or long shaft of the bone may continue to grow to great lengths when stimulated by excess GH. The growth in these bones is usually proportional and may cause affected people to reach heights of up to 8 feet and weights of more than 300 lb. These people tend to have multiple health problems and often die in early adulthood. Figure 46-3 illustrates gigantism.

Acromegaly. **Acromegaly**, although rare, is more common than gigantism. Most patients with acromegaly are found to have pituitary macroadenomas that secrete excess GH. Symptoms usually appear in the fourth or fifth decade of life and affect men and women equally. In these people, excess GH production occurs after epiphyseal closure. The closed epiphyses prevent longitudinal growth of the bones; instead, bones increase in thickness and width. Acromegaly also affects the cardiovascular, digestive, nervous, and genitourinary systems.

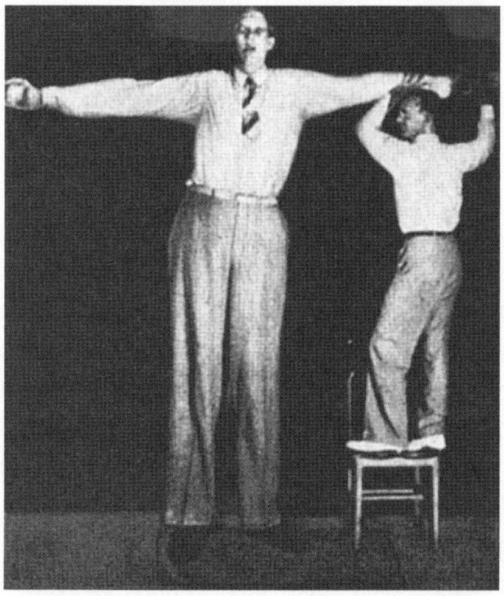

FIGURE 46-3 Clinical features of growth hormone (GH) excess. Robert Wadlow, nicknamed the Alton Giant, weighed 9 lb at birth but grew to 32 lb by 6 months of age. By his first birthday, he weighed 62 lb. He died at age 22 because of complications from cellulitis of the feet. At the time of his death, he was 8 feet, 11 inches tall and weighed 475 lb. (Courtesy Charles CM, Macbryde CM.)

Signs and Symptoms

Visual deficits and headaches are common in hyperpituitarism and may be the first symptoms of a problem. Visual problems are most often a result of pressure on optic nerves where they are joined near the pituitary gland. Physical features of the disease include enlargement of the hands, feet, and paranasal and frontal sinuses and deformities of the spine and mandible. In addition, soft tissues may become enlarged, especially the tongue, skin, liver, and spleen. This may in turn lead to speech impediments, coarse or distorted facial features, abdominal distention, and sleep apnea. People with acromegaly also may report excessive perspiration (diaphoresis), oily skin, peripheral neuropathies, degeneration of the joints, and proximal muscle weakness. The effects of excess GH impede the activity of insulin, causing patients to have symptoms of DM.

In addition to the features just described, patients with gigantism and acromegaly initially have increased strength, progressing rapidly to complaints of weakness and fatigue. The skilled examiner also may detect organomegaly (i.e., enlargement of internal organs), hypertension, dysphagia, and a deep voice because of hypertrophy of the larynx. Those patients who also have elevated levels of prolactin may have galactorrhea (in women) or hypogonadism (in men). A dramatic example of acromegaly is shown in Figure 46-4.

Medical Diagnosis

The diagnosis of hyperpituitarism is based on a number of data sources, including physical assessment, radiographic studies, and laboratory findings.

Radiographic Studies. Radiographic films of the skull may show a large sella turcica and increased bone density. Enhanced CT scans using a water-soluble dye or MRI scans with gadolinium infusion may be performed to locate and evaluate potential intracellular or extracellular lesions or tumor formation. Angiography also may be of use to rule out any vascular abnormalities such as aneurysms or arteriovenous malformations.

Laboratory Studies. As mentioned earlier, in hyperpituitarism usually only one pituitary hormone, such as GH or prolactin, is produced in excess. Pathologic conditions producing elevated levels of LH or FSH are extremely rare. In patients with possible hyperpituitarism, levels of anterior pituitary hormones are measured. Elevation of any hormone level requires further evaluation and follow-up. It is normal for LH and FSH to be slightly elevated in postmenopausal women. The GH suppression test is the most reliable test for acromegaly. While the GH concentration normally falls in response to glucose, it is unchanged in the patient with acromegaly.

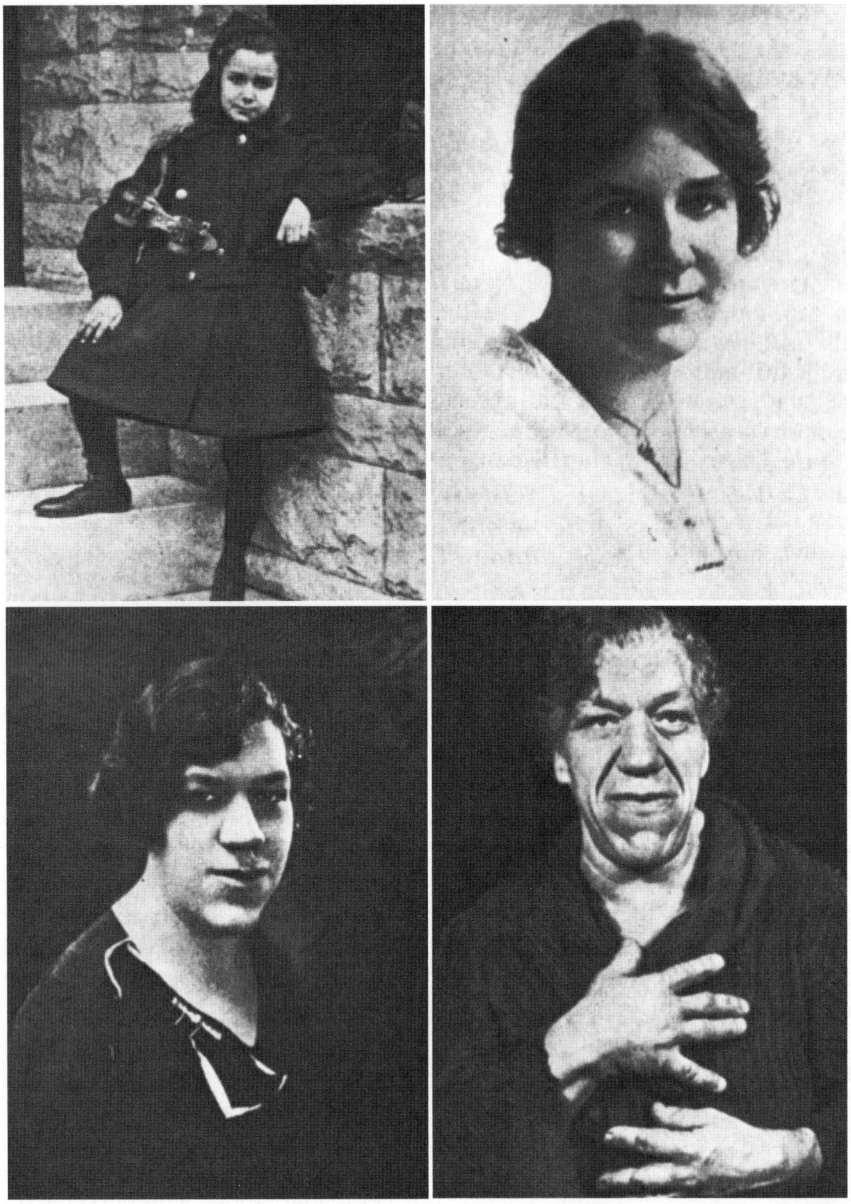

FIGURE 46-4 The progression of acromegaly. A series of photographs of the same person over the course of her lifetime depict the physical changes that occurred. The woman was affected after reaching maturity. (From Mendeloff A, Smith DE, editors: Acromegaly, diabetes, hypermetabolism, proteinuria and heart failure, *Am J Med* 20:133, 1956.)

Dexamethasone suppression tests are used to rule out problems related to dysfunction of the adrenal glands (see detailed discussion in the section titled "Disorders of the Adrenal Glands").

Medical Treatment

Hyperpituitarism that is manifested as acromegaly or gigantism has skeletal changes and disfigurement that cannot be reversed with treatment. However, soft tissue hypertrophy can improve with treatment. Treatment options to prevent further changes include surgery, radiation, and drug therapy.

Surgical Management. For patients diagnosed with pituitary tumors, the surgical removal of the adenoma or of the pituitary itself (**hypophysectomy**) is the treatment of choice. A transsphenoidal approach is the most commonly used surgical method. A transsphenoidal hypophysectomy is a microsurgical procedure performed under general anesthesia with the patient in the semi-Fowler position. An incision is made at the inner aspect of the upper lip through the maxillary bone and the sella turcica is entered through the sphenoid sinus (Fig. 46-5). A newer procedure is performed endoscopically through the nasal cavity. After the gland or a portion of it is removed, a small piece of adipose tissue is harvested from the abdomen and is used to pack the dura mater (one of the meningeal layers) to prevent leakage of cerebrospinal fluid (CSF). An absorbent gauze or similar dressing is used to pack the nasal passages and an external nasal dressing is

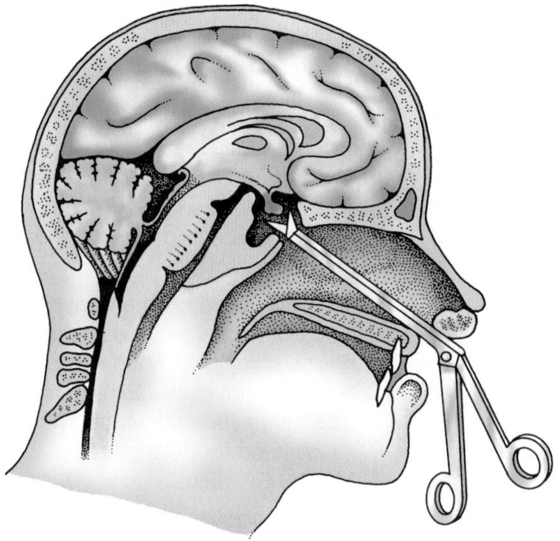

FIGURE 46-5 The transsphenoidal surgical approach to the pituitary gland. (From Ignatavicius DD, Workman ML: *Medical-surgical nursing: patient-centered collaborative care*, ed 6, St. Louis, 2010, Saunders.)

applied to keep the packing in place. If the entire pituitary is removed, the patient will require lifelong replacement of glucocorticoids, thyroid hormone, and sex hormones.

An earlier surgical approach, called a *transfrontal craniotomy*, is sometimes used if a tumor is especially large or is invading other structures. This is a more invasive procedure that involves the removal of a portion of the frontal bone of the skull. The cranial vault is then entered and structures superior to the pituitary gland are displaced to reach it. This involves manipulation of the meningeal layers and the frontal and temporal lobes of the cerebrum as well as the optic nerve. As a result, the risk of complications and brain damage is much increased.

Radiation. Radiation therapy is sometimes used to treat tumors that produce excess GH but the overall response is slow and numerous complications, such as hypopituitarism, optic nerve damage, cognitive dysfunction, and visual defects, can occur. It may be used in combination with surgery or drug therapy. Gamma Knife radiosurgery (stereotactic radiosurgery), which uses radiation delivered to the site from multiple angles, may be used to treat acromegaly. Patients usually require hormone replacement after radiosurgery.

Drug Therapy. Several types of drugs are effective in the treatment of acromegaly. These include somatostatin analogs, dopamine agonists, and GH receptor antagonists. Octreotide (Sandostatin), a somatostatin analog, is the most commonly prescribed drug for patients with acromegaly. It is given three times weekly by subcutaneous injection. Common side effects of octreotide acetate are nausea, vomiting, diarrhea, abdominal pain, and pain at the injection site. Because this drug also suppresses insulin secretion, the patient's blood glucose must be monitored. Blood pressure (BP) and weight are monitored to detect fluid retention. Newer drugs in this category are given intramuscularly every 2 to 4 weeks. Dopamine agents such as cabergoline (Dostinex) suppress the secretion of GH. Pegvisomant (Somavert) is a GH receptor antagonist. It is most often used after radiotherapy. Bromocriptine (Parlodel) once was the primary drug but it has been largely replaced by the newer options that have fewer side effects. Some of the most common side effects of bromocriptine are headache, dizziness, drowsiness, confusion, nausea, vomiting, dry mouth, and urticaria.

Table 46-2 provides additional information about drugs used to treat hyperpituitarism.

Pharmacology Capsule

Drugs used to treat gigantism and acromegaly decrease hormone secretion but do not reverse the existing skeletal effects of the condition.

NURSING CARE of the Patient with Hyperpituitarism

Education and emotional support are vital components in the nursing care of the patient with hyperpituitarism. Patients with hyperpituitarism need to know that many body changes, such as visual disturbances and visceral enlargement, are not reversible. Surgical treatment is aimed primarily at preventing further symptoms and complications.

Assessment

Assessment of the patient with a pituitary disorder is summarized in Box 46-1. When a patient has gigantism or acromegaly, areas that merit special attention are energy level, height and weight, vital signs, contours of the face and skull, visual acuity, speech, voice quality, and abdominal distention. If surgical intervention is planned, determine what the patient knows and expects.

Interventions

Disturbed Body Image

Demonstrate acceptance of the patient and provide opportunities for the patient to share feelings and concerns. Encourage the patient to pay attention to grooming. If he or she has difficulty adjusting, a referral to a support group or mental health professional may be appropriate.

Activity Intolerance

Because the patient with acromegaly tires quickly, plan activities to allow for adequate rest periods. Help the patient to develop a daily schedule that permits achievement of necessary activities balanced with rest requirements.

Table 46-2 **Drug Therapy for Pituitary Disorders**

DRUG	USE AND ACTION	SIDE EFFECTS	NURSING INTERVENTIONS
ADH Hormone Preparations			
	All promote conservation of water.	All can cause water intoxication, inadequate tissue perfusion because of vasoconstriction.	Monitor for early signs and symptoms of water intoxication: drowsiness, listlessness, headache. Patient should reduce fluid intake first few days of treatment.
lypressin (Diapid) nasal spray	Treats DI.	Rhinorrhea, nasal irritation, and congestion. Rarely: dyspnea, hypertension, coronary vasoconstriction.	Teach patient use of intranasal inhaler: hold bottle upright, place nozzle in nostril, spray prescribed number of times, do not inhale. Explain how to monitor intake and output. With DI, stress need for lifelong therapy. Monitor BP, pulse.
desmopressin (DDAVP) nasal spray, parenteral, oral preparations	Treats DI, hemophilia (increases production of clotting factor VIII), nocturnal diuresis, headache.	Same as lypressin.	Same as lypressin.
vasopressin (Pitressin) synthetic for SC and IM	Treats DI, postoperative abdominal distention. Used to dispel gas before abdominal radiography. Powerful vasoconstrictor.	May cause angina, MI in patients with CAD.	Same as lypressin. Also assess cardiac and peripheral circulation. Extreme caution with cardiac disease.
Pituitary Hormone Suppressants			
octreotide acetate (Sandostatin), lanreotide (Somatuline Depot)	Suppresses secretion of growth hormone. Most effective drug for acromegaly.	Nausea, vomiting, diarrhea, headache, flushing, edema, dizziness, altered blood glucose, drowsiness, orthostatic hypotension, visual disturbances, cholelithiasis.	Monitor weight, BP, pulse, respirations, urine output. Assess for edema. Refrigerate ampules. Discard if discolored or contains visible particles. Teach patient to give self-injections; advise to take exactly as prescribed and never take double doses. Assess for changes in blood glucose. Caution about drowsiness and dizziness. Very expensive.
bromocriptine (Parlodel)	Inhibits release of prolactin from anterior pituitary. Suppresses lactation. Restores ovulation. Treats acromegaly.	Nausea, vomiting, constipation, hypotension, drowsiness, MI, pulmonary infiltrates, nasal stuffiness, vasoconstriction, anorexia, headache. Rarely: visual disturbances, confusion.	Safety measures if dizzy. Monitor BP. Record bowel movements and stool consistency. Assess effects. Teach patient to report chest pain and/or dyspnea immediately, to rise slowly to standing position, that driving may be dangerous because of drowsiness and dizziness, and that the drug may restore fertility.
Dopamine agonist: cabergoline (Dostinex)	Prevents/inhibits secretion of prolactin. May lower GH secretion in some patients with acromegaly.	Nausea, constipation, abdominal pain, headache, dizziness, asthenia, fatigue, drowsiness.	Contraindicated with uncontrolled hypertension.
GH receptor antagonist: pegvisomant (Somavert)	Used to treat acromegaly. Prevents GH from exerting effects on body tissues.	Infection, pain, injection site reaction, chest pain, back pain, flu syndrome, abnormal liver function tests, diarrhea, dizziness, edema, sinusitis.	Contraindicated with latex allergy because vial stopper contains latex. Each patient or family member to prepare and give SC injections. Do not shake vial when reconstituting drug. Solution should be clear. Discard leftover reconstituted drug.

Table 46-2 **Drug Therapy for Pituitary Disorders—cont'd**

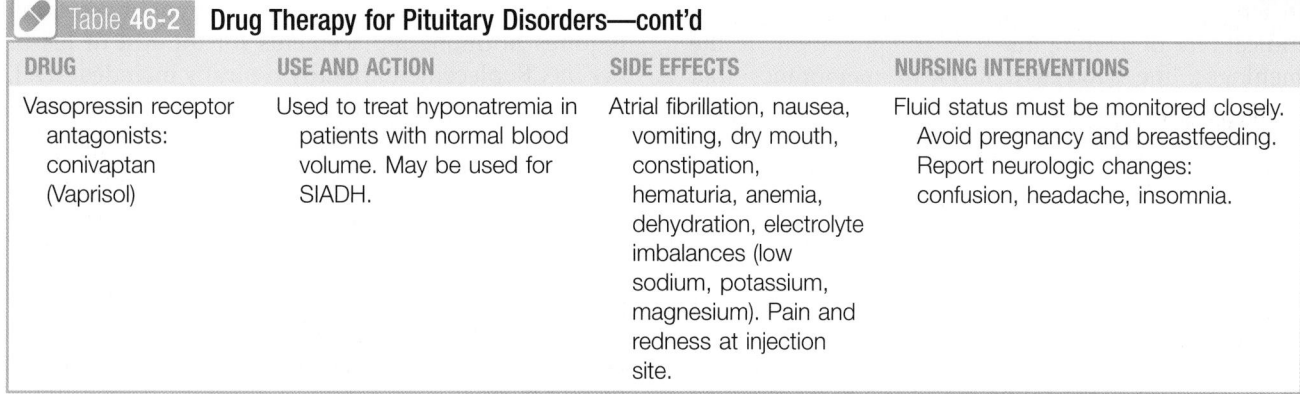

DRUG	USE AND ACTION	SIDE EFFECTS	NURSING INTERVENTIONS
Vasopressin receptor antagonists: conivaptan (Vaprisol)	Used to treat hyponatremia in patients with normal blood volume. May be used for SIADH.	Atrial fibrillation, nausea, vomiting, dry mouth, constipation, hematuria, anemia, dehydration, electrolyte imbalances (low sodium, potassium, magnesium). Pain and redness at injection site.	Fluid status must be monitored closely. Avoid pregnancy and breastfeeding. Report neurologic changes: confusion, headache, insomnia.

ADH, Antidiuretic hormone; *BP,* blood pressure; *CAD,* coronary artery disease; *DI,* diabetes insipidus; *GH,* growth hormone; *IM,* intramuscular; *MI,* myocardial infarction; *SC,* subcutaneous; *SIADH,* syndrome of inappropriate antidiuretic hormone.

Nursing Diagnoses, Goals, and Outcome Criteria: Hyperpituitarism

Nursing Diagnoses	Goals and Outcome Criteria
Disturbed Body Image related to changes in physical appearance	Adjustment to physical changes: patient verbalizes feelings about body and indicates acceptance of changes
Activity Intolerance related to fatigue	Improved activity tolerance: accomplishment of daily activities without excessive tiring
Chronic Pain related to musculoskeletal overgrowth, headache	Pain relief: patient verbalizes relief of pain, appears relaxed
Ineffective Self-Health Management related to lack of knowledge of condition, treatment, and expected outcomes	Patient manages own treatment with realistic expectations: patient correctly describes self-medication, therapeutic effects, and drug adverse effects

Chronic Pain

Monitor and document pain. Teach relaxation techniques as discussed in Chapter 15 (see *Complementary and Alternative Therapies* box). Administer prescribed analgesics and evaluate effects.

Put on Your Thinking Cap!

Explain why some people with excess growth hormone (GH) develop gigantism and other people with excess GH develop acromegaly.

Ineffective Self-Health Management

Advise patients on drug therapy to take medications exactly as prescribed and not to take double doses if a dose is missed. Other nursing implications are noted in Table 46-2.

POSTOPERATIVE NURSING CARE of the Patient with Hyperpituitarism

If the patient has surgery (in this case, hypophysectomy), general preoperative and postoperative care is provided, as described in Chapter 17. This section describes specific nursing care of the patient having pituitary surgery. The patient may be admitted to a critical care unit for the first 24 hours after surgery because of the risk for a number of complications.

Assessment

Even though the registered nurse (RN) is responsible for the complete assessment, the LVN/LPN collects data that are essential to caring for the patient during the postoperative period. Neurologic status and vision must be monitored closely, with particular attention to level of consciousness, pupil size and equality, and vital signs. Changes in data that may indicate edema caused by the manipulation of tissues or intracranial bleeding are decreasing alertness, slow pupil response to light, and decreased or asymmetric muscle strength.

Strict documentation of intake and output and measurement of specific gravity are important because these patients are at risk for DI or possibly SIADH. These disorders are discussed in detail in the sections titled "Diabetes Insipidus" and "Syndrome of Inappropriate Antidiuretic Hormone."

Inspection of the nasal dressing for drainage is important because CSF leaks may sometimes occur. Document clear, colorless drainage and notify the surgeon. To confirm whether the drainage is CSF, a specimen of the drainage should be sent to the laboratory for glucose testing. A high level of glucose supports the diagnosis of a CSF leak. A bedside test using a testing strip is no longer recommended. CSF leaks often resolve within 72 hours with rest and head elevation; however, severe, persistent headaches may be treated with a spinal tap to reduce CSF pressure. A return to surgery is rarely indicated.

Monitoring the patient for signs and symptoms of infection also is an important aspect of nursing care. An elevated white blood cell (WBC) count, sudden rise in temperature, headache, or nuchal rigidity may be indications of meningitis (i.e., inflammation of the meninges, the protective layer of membranes that cover the brain and spinal cord). When meningeal inflammation is present, the patient experiences severe head or neck pain when touching the chin to the chest.

The patient who has had Gamma Knife radiosurgery (stereotactic radiosurgery) will return from the procedure with a stereotactic frame in place. Because the frame is secured to the skull with pins, pin care is needed. If the patient has a history of seizures, he or she is at increased risk for seizures for at least 24 hours. In an emergency, the frame may have to be removed quickly by trained personnel. The nursing unit should have a protocol for this procedure.

Nursing Diagnoses, Goals, and Outcome Criteria: Hypophysectomy, Postoperative

Nursing Diagnoses	Goals and Outcome Criteria
Anxiety related to lack of knowledge of surgical postoperative care and routines	Reduced anxiety: patient calm, states he or she feels less anxious
Decreased Intracranial Adaptive Capacity related to tissue trauma and swelling	Absence of visual disturbances associated with swelling brain tissue: patient reports no change in vision
Acute Pain related to tissue trauma	Pain relief: patient statement of pain relief, relaxed manner
Impaired Oral Mucous Membrane related to surgical incision	Healed surgical incision: incision closed, minimal swelling and redness
Risk for Injury related to disruption of packing	Absence of cerebrospinal fluid (CSF) drainage: no clear nasal drainage
Excess Fluid Volume or **Deficient Fluid Volume** related to abnormal antidiuretic hormone (ADH) production	Normal fluid balance: fluid intake and output approximately equal, normal tissue turgor
Risk for Infection related to impaired tissue integrity, pins for stereotactic frame	Absence of infection: normal white blood cell (WBC) count; no neck stiffness, fever, or headache; pin insertion sites clean without drainage or excessive redness or swelling

Interventions

Anxiety

Orient the patient to the environment and explain all procedures. Give drugs as ordered to replace pituitary hormones. When the patient is well enough, provide information about drug therapy and self-medication. The patient who has a complete hypophysectomy requires hormone replacements for the rest of his or her life. Replacement therapy typically includes ADH, cortisol, and thyroid medication (see the section titled "Disorders of the Adrenal Glands" for a more detailed discussion of glucocorticoids).

Decreased Intracranial Adaptive Capacity

Be aware of existing visual disturbances and collect data to identify new disturbances that might indicate increased intracranial pressure. Treatment usually does not correct existing disturbances but can prevent further harm.

Acute Pain and Impaired Oral Mucous Membrane

The immediate postoperative period is uncomfortable, especially when nasal packing is present and the patient is forced to breathe through the mouth. Administer analgesics as ordered and follow up to see if the medication was effective. The presence of a "mustache" dressing also may make the patient feel uncomfortable. Frequent mouth care with moistening of the lips increases comfort. If a gingival incision was done, tooth brushing is not permitted until the incision heals. With Gamma Knife radiosurgery, the pin insertion sites may cause discomfort.

Risk for Injury

To prevent dislodgment of the fat pad or adipose graft at the surgical site, instruct the patient to avoid any activities that can cause a Valsalva maneuver. Coughing, straining, vomiting, or sneezing can create enough intracranial pressure to disrupt the surgical site and cause CSF leakage or even bleeding. Stool softeners and laxatives may be ordered to prevent straining. Instead of coughing, incentive spirometry and deep-breathing exercises help to maintain pulmonary function without increasing intrathoracic and intracranial pressure. Advise the patient to avoid lifting heavy objects and bending from the waist. Instruct patients to avoid these activities at home as the physician directs (usually for 2 to 3 months after surgery) (see *Patient Teaching* box).

Patient Teaching

Hypophysectomy, Postoperative

- If the anterior pituitary is removed, you will need hormone replacements for the rest of your life.
- For 3 months (or as advised by your physician), avoid any activities that cause straining, heavy lifting, and bending from the waist.
- It is important to prevent constipation because straining increases intracranial pressure.
- Numbness of the incision area and decreased sense of smell are temporary.
- Follow-up care is essential to monitor for any signs of tumor recurrence.

Excess Fluid Volume or Deficient Fluid Volume

Provide intravenous fluids as ordered and monitor pulse, BP, and intake and output. Monitor for transient DI (i.e., large volume of dilute urine). Notify the physician of excessive fluid retention or diuresis. Changes in vital signs, mental status, and neuromuscular status suggest fluid and electrolyte imbalances.

Risk for Infection

Administer antibiotics as ordered. Monitor body temperature. Be especially alert for stiffness of the neck and headache because these are symptoms of meningitis. The patient with a stereotactic frame will require pin care. If the patient will be discharged with the frame in place, teach a family member how to perform pin care.

HYPOPITUITARISM

Cause and Pathophysiology

When inadequate secretion of GH occurs during preadolescence, a syndrome called **dwarfism** may result. Dwarfism is defined as attainment of a maximum height that is 40% below normal. In addition, chronic diseases associated with inadequate growth may be present. The causes of dwarfism may be hereditary or may be related to damage to the anterior portion of the pituitary gland. The anterior pituitary may be damaged by necrosis after hemorrhage, trauma, infection, radiation, or autoimmune disorders. Inadequate secretion of GH or an inability of the target organs to respond to GH is usually considered to be the major cause. In rare instances, hypothalamic dysfunction can lead to dwarfism as well. It is important to note that although an actual or relative deficiency of GH may exist, other anterior pituitary hormones also may be deficient.

Complementary and Alternative Therapies

Imagery, relaxation exercises, and massage all can be used with analgesics to manage pain.

If growth has been completed and some pathologic process impairs the function of the pituitary, a syndrome known as *panhypopituitarism* can occur. In this situation, all hormones of the anterior pituitary are usually affected. A number of causes exist for panhypopituitarism, which are identified as follows:

1. Sheehan syndrome: shock and hypotension during the postpartum period leading to infarction of the pituitary gland
2. Tumors of the pituitary gland itself or cranial tumors that impinge on the pituitary
3. Chronic recurrent infections
4. Total or subtotal destruction or removal of the pituitary as a result of trauma, surgery, or radiation therapy
5. Suppression of pituitary tropic hormones by excess target gland hormones (e.g., as seen in patients on prolonged corticosteroid therapy)

Signs and Symptoms

The manifestations of hypopituitarism depend on the stage of life when the deficiency occurs and which hormones are deficient. In dwarfism, which occurs early in life, the person is remarkably short in stature, sometimes as short as 36 inches, but with proportional physical characteristics. These people often have delayed or absent sexual maturation. An increased frequency of mental retardation exists compared with the population at large. Dwarfs also have an accelerated pattern of aging and thus have a shorter life span than the general population, by as much as 20 years.

When a state of panhypopituitarism exists, a syndrome called *Simmonds cachexia* is present. The patient has muscle and organ wasting and disruptions of digestion and metabolism. Decreased muscle and organ size is attributed to decreased GH. An absence of ACTH affects the person's ability to cope effectively with stress. (See the section titled "Adrenal Hypofunction.") This in turn affects the person's ability to metabolize glucose and hypoglycemia may result. Because TSH is depleted, the thyroid is not stimulated to produce thyroid hormone. A lack of thyroid hormone produces a state referred to as *hypothyroidism.* In hypothyroidism, insufficient thyroid hormone is available for normal metabolism and thermogenesis, or heat production. Consequently, people who are hypothyroid may be unable to maintain a normal basal metabolic rate (BMR) or body temperature.

If a lack of MSH exists, decreased pigmentation of the skin occurs. This results in extreme pallor. Finally, with the absence of gonadotropins, gonads may become atrophied. In both men and women, loss of libido, decreased body hair, and sexual dysfunction may occur; in women, amenorrhea (i.e., absence of menstruation) may be seen.

General signs and symptoms may include fatigue, weakness, malaise, cold intolerance, and lethargy. Again, the type and degree of symptoms depend on specific hormones affected. If the pituitary dysfunction is caused by a tumor, the patient may have headaches, vision disturbances, seizures, and loss of the sense of smell.

Medical Diagnosis

A diagnosis of dwarfism or panhypopituitarism is based on the health history, physical examination, and diagnostic tests. In cases of dwarfism, the physical examination findings are fairly diagnostic. Diagnostic tests and procedures may include conventional radiographs and CT scans to detect pituitary or cranial tumors. Cerebral angiography may be ordered to detect malformed blood vessels. Serum levels of pituitary hormones may be measured as well.

Medical and Surgical Treatment

Deficient hormones are replaced as needed, depending on the specific deficiencies of the patient. Deficiency of TSH necessitates thyroid replacement with drugs such as levothyroxine (Synthroid) or liothyronine (Cytomel), usually for the rest of the person's life. Gonadotropin deficiency requires lifelong therapy. To produce or maintain libido, secondary sexual characteristics, and well-being, men also should receive testosterone and women should receive estrogen. In patients for whom childbearing is desirable, FSH and LH are administered to both men and women. However, gonadotropin replacement is contraindicated is some conditions, including breast cancer in women and prostate cancer in men. GH replacement is necessary for growth in children. In most instances, GH is administered until the epiphyses (endplates) of the long bones close or the person no longer responds to the drug. Replacement of GH in adults with a GH deficiency produces improved energy, increased lean body mass, and a general feeling of well-being. The use of human GH produced by bacteria through recombinant deoxyribonucleic acid (rDNA) technology such as somatropin (Humatrope and others) is considerably safer than products used previously. The annual cost of therapy with GH is very expensive. Another option for children with GH deficiency is mecasermin (Increlex), which is identical to endogenous IGF-1. If a tumor is causing hypopituitarism, surgery or radiation is the treatment of choice. (See "Surgical Management" in the Hyperpituitarism section.) Table 46-2 provides additional information about drug therapy for hypopituitarism.

NURSING CARE of the Patient with Hypopituitarism

Assessment

The general assessment of the patient with a pituitary disorder is summarized in Box 46-1. When collecting data for assessment of the patient with hypopituitarism, be especially aware of mental acuity, emotional stability, and affect. Document the patient's general sense of well-being, energy level, and appetite. In reviewing the systems, ask the patient about changes in skin texture, body temperature, hair, and libido. Determine the patient's usual activities and whether there has been any difficulty carrying out those activities.

In the physical examination, measure height and weight and compare with previous measurements. Inspect the hair for distribution, texture, and thickness. Inspect and palpate the skin and nails for color, texture, and moisture. Document the development of secondary sex characteristics, including axillary and pubic hair, genital maturity, breast development, and onset of menarche.

Nursing Diagnoses, Goals, and Outcome Criteria: Hypopituitarism

Nursing Diagnoses	Goals and Outcome Criteria
Disturbed Body Image related to lack (or loss) of secondary sex characteristics	Improved body image: patient makes positive statements about self and takes measures to improve appearance
Sexual Dysfunction related to hormone deficiency	Enhanced sexual development and function: secondary sex characteristics and satisfying sexual function
Imbalanced Nutrition: More or **Less Than Body Requirements** related to hormone imbalance	Adequate nutrition: body weight normal for height
Deficient Fluid Volume related to hormone deficiency, impaired homeostasis	Normal fluid balance: normal tissue turgor, pulse, and blood pressure (BP)
Ineffective Self-Health Management related to lack of understanding of condition, treatment, and self-care	Patient follows prescribed treatment regimen: correctly demonstrates self-care, diminishing signs and symptoms of hormone deficiency

Interventions

Patient education is the most important aspect of nursing care because disturbances in body image, sexual function, nutritional status, and fluid balance all can be improved if the patient understands and follows the prescribed therapy. Meanwhile, acknowledge the patient's feelings and encourage expression of concerns (see *Patient Teaching* box). Referral to a mental health counselor is appropriate if the patient has difficulty dealing with the effects of the disease. Good teaching is essential for patients and families to understand hypopituitarism and to participate in the treatment plan.

Patient Teaching

Hypopituitarism

- It will be necessary for you to take medications for the rest of your life to replace the pituitary hormones.
- You must become familiar with the signs and symptoms of inadequate or excessive hormone replacement (provide written descriptions) and appropriate actions.
- You must have periodic follow-up care.
- Wear a medical alert bracelet or necklace so that your condition can be recognized quickly in an emergency.
- Carry a card that lists prescribed drugs and dosages and your physician's name and phone number.

POSTERIOR PITUITARY DISORDERS

Disorders of the posterior pituitary or neurohypophysis are characterized by deficient or excess ADH production. Another name for ADH is *vasopressin.* ADH helps to maintain fluid balance by promoting reabsorption of water in the renal tubules when body water is decreased or very concentrated. The amount of ADH secreted is reflected in the amount of water retained by the kidneys. Increased ADH release causes increased water retention. This results in increased intravascular volume and decreased urine output.

Two disorders are associated with dysfunction of the neurohypophysis: (1) DI and (2) SIADH. DI is the more common of the two disorders.

DIABETES INSIPIDUS

Cause

DI is characterized by excessive output of dilute urine. It can be caused by a number of factors. Thus DI is classified as nephrogenic, neurogenic (central or hypothalamic), or dipsogenic DI (primary polydipsia). Nephrogenic DI is an inherited defect in which the renal tubules of the kidney do not respond to ADH, resulting in inadequate water reabsorption by the kidneys. In this case, ADH is produced in sufficient amounts but the kidneys do not respond to it appropriately. Some cases are caused by drugs such as lithium carbonate (Eskalith-CR) or demeclocycline (Declomycin), which affect the kidney by inhibiting its response to ADH. In neurogenic DI, a defect in either the production or the secretion of ADH exists. Neurogenic DI can result from hypothalamic tumors, head trauma, infection, surgical procedures (hypophysectomy), or metastatic tumors originating in the lung or breast. It also can be triggered by a cerebrovascular accident (CVA), aneurysm, or intracranial hemorrhage. Dipsogenic DI is a disorder of thirst stimulation. When the patient ingests water, serum osmolality decreases, which causes reduced vasopressin secretion. Other factors that may be associated with dipsogenic DI are habitual excessive water intake and psychiatric conditions. The severity of symptoms in dipsogenic DI varies.

Pathophysiology

ADH deficiency or an inability of the kidneys to respond to ADH results in the excretion of large volumes of very dilute urine, a symptom referred to as *polyuria.* The distal tubules and collecting ducts do not reabsorb sufficient water. Massive diuresis occurs, resulting in increased plasma osmolarity, which stimulates the osmoreceptors. The osmoreceptors in turn relay information to the cerebral cortex, causing the person to feel thirsty. Increased thirst serves as a compensatory mechanism in that it causes the person to increase water ingestion. Unfortunately, this compensatory mechanism cannot keep up with the demand for water and diuresis continues. Massive dehydration ensues, which leads to decreased intravascular volume, hypotension, and circulatory collapse. This is accompanied by neurologic changes such as a decreased level of consciousness and severe electrolyte imbalances. Electrolyte imbalances contribute to circulatory collapse by causing dysrhythmias and impaired contractility of the heart. If left untreated, severe cases of DI can lead to cardiac arrest and death.

When DI follows intracranial surgery, a typical pattern occurs. The initial acute phase is marked by the sudden onset of polyuria. In the next phase, urine volume returns to normal. Then the third phase, which occurs 10 to 14 days postoperatively, results in permanent DI. When DI is associated with head trauma, it is more likely to resolve with treatment.

Signs and Symptoms

Common signs and symptoms of DI are massive diuresis, dehydration, and thirst. Dehydration is characterized by hypotension, tachycardia, dizziness, decreased skin turgor, weakness, and possible fainting episodes. Additional findings include malaise, lethargy, and irritability. An irregular heartbeat may be detected.

Medical Diagnosis

The diagnosis of DI is made primarily on the basis of the health history, physical examination, and laboratory findings. A history of any known cause, such as surgery, infection, injury, or medication ingestion, should be noted.

The loss of free water is apparent in laboratory studies of blood and urine. An initial diagnosis of DI is made based on a 24-hour urine output greater than 4 L, without food or fluid restrictions. Patients with DI can excrete up to 30 L/day, depending on the severity of the ADH deficiency or relative deficiency. Because the urine is very dilute, the specific gravity is also extremely low and the osmolarity of the urine is decreased. For the water deprivation test, water is withheld for 8 to 16 hours during which time BP, weight, and urine osmolality are measured each hour. The test is stopped when the osmolalities stabilize, the patient loses 5% of his or her body weight, or the patient develops orthostatic hypotension. A dose of ADH is then given and the urine osmolality is measured 1 hour later. If the patient has neurogenic DI, the urine osmolality should increase (i.e., the urine is more concentrated).

Management of DI is geared to controlling the signs and symptoms of the disease and possibly reversing the cause of the syndrome. Intravenous fluid volume replacement and vasopressors often are required to maintain adequate BP. Treatment also includes a variety of pharmacologic therapies. A list of these agents can be found in Table 46-2. Most of these agents act by augmenting existing ADH or replacing it. The most common hormone replacement drug for neurogenic DI is desmopressin acetate (DDAVP), which can be given orally, intravenously, or by nasal inhalation. Short-term therapy is usually managed with subcutaneous injections of aqueous vasopressin. This is usually indicated in situations in which the cause of DI is reversible, such as infection- or medication-related DI. Patients on long-term therapy are placed on nasal spray (lypressin), which may be required for life. This long-term therapy may be necessary after hypophysectomy or other surgical procedures. Patients with primary polyuria related to a psychiatric condition may require ADH supplementation while psychotherapy is used to treat the underlying disorder.

The administration of ADH does not help with nephrogenic DI because the kidneys do not respond to the hormone. Sodium intake may be restricted and thiazide diuretics prescribed for nephrogenic DI. This depletes sodium and decreases the glomerular filtration rate, which increases the reabsorption of water in the proximal tubules.

A variety of other drugs such as chlorpropamide (Diabinese), clofibrate (Atromid-S), carbamazepine (Tegretol), and indomethacin (Indocin) may be used to treat DI, depending on the circumstances.

Pharmacology Capsule

Adverse effects of vasopressin administered as a nasal spray are mucous membrane ulcers, chest tightness, and upper respiratory infections.

NURSING CARE of the Patient with Diabetes Insipidus

Assessment

A complete history of the patient's symptoms, medical history, and drug history should be obtained by the RN. The LVN/LPN can assist by monitoring for thirst, change in urine appearance or volume, dizziness, weakness, fainting, and palpitations. The physical examination focuses on the symptoms of DI. Monitor hydration, including skin turgor, moisture of mucous membranes, pulse rate and quality, BP, and mental status. Maintain records of intake and output, daily weights, and urine specific gravities.

Interventions

The patient with a pituitary disorder may be experiencing mild to moderate symptoms or may be critically ill. Specific nursing care depends largely on the type of DI, the severity of the symptoms, and the needs identified in the nursing assessment.

Anxiety and Disturbed Body Image

The patient who is able must be allowed adequate time to express feelings and discuss the disorder. Changes in body function can be very disturbing. Assure the patient that some changes can be controlled with proper treatment. Be alert to the patient's emotional status and provide support and make referrals as necessary.

Nursing Diagnoses, Goals, and Outcome Criteria: Diabetes Insipidus

Nursing Diagnoses	Goals and Outcome Criteria
Anxiety related to physical symptoms and diagnosis	Decreased anxiety: patient states anxiety is reduced, appears calm
Disturbed Body Image related to altered function	Adaptation to physical changes: patient adjusts routines to minimize symptoms
Deficient Fluid Volume related to excessive urine output	Normal fluid balance: fluid intake approximately equal to fluid output
Activity Intolerance related to fatigue and weakness	Improved activity tolerance: patient performs activities of daily living (ADL) without tiring
Ineffective Self-Health Management related to lack of understanding of symptom management and treatment of diabetes insipidus (DI)	Effective self-care: patient describes and demonstrates self-care and self-medication

Deficient Fluid Volume

Carefully measure intake and output. When the urine output is excessive, as in DI, the physician may order measurement of output at 15- to 30-minute intervals. Because adequate hydration is essential, administer intravenous fluid replacements as ordered. Encourage oral intake, with the prescribed amount based on the volume of urinary output. In addition, weigh the patient at least once daily to identify significant weight loss secondary to water loss.

In situations in which the patient is experiencing excessive fluid loss, administer exogenous ADH as ordered (see Table 46-2). Be familiar with routes of administration, side effects, and contraindications associated with the use of these agents. Be aware that reversal of the fluid volume deficit with ADH can result in water intoxication. Continued monitoring of urine output and osmolality is essential.

Activity Intolerance

Extreme fatigue or muscle weakness can interfere with the patient's ability to participate in activities of daily living (ADL), such as hygiene and grooming. Frequently observe the functional ability of these patients and address the amount of assistance required in the patient's care plan.

Ineffective Self-Health Management

Patients who require long-term treatment of DI must learn to manage their symptoms and medications. If the patient has difficulty doing this, a family member or friend may be included in the teaching sessions. Some patients are taught to adjust dosages based on urine output, specific gravity (using a hydrometer), and thirst. If the patient's self-care abilities are in doubt, initiate a referral to a home nursing service (see *Patient Teaching* box).

Patient Teaching

Irreversible Diabetes Insipidus

- Continue your prescribed drug therapy and notify your physician of any side or adverse effects (provide written details).
- Notify your physician if you have increased urine output, thirst, weight loss, and general feelings of malaise or weakness. You may need additional treatment.
- Prolonged use of nasal sprays can cause ulceration of mucous membranes, chest tightness, upper respiratory infections, and respiratory problems.
- Keep office or clinic appointments to identify any changes in pituitary function.
- Schedule activities and regular rest periods to avoid excessive fatigue.
- Wear a medical alert bracelet.
- Drowsiness, listlessness, and headache are signs of water intoxication, which may result from vasopressin therapy.

SYNDROME OF INAPPROPRIATE ANTIDIURETIC HORMONE

Cause

SIADH is characterized by a water imbalance related to an increase in ADH synthesis, ADH secretion, or both. Factors that may cause or contribute to the development of SIADH include brain trauma, surgery, tumors, and infection; some drugs, including vasopressin, general anesthetics, oral hypoglycemics, and tricyclic antidepressants; some pulmonary diseases; hypothyroidism; lupus erythematosus; and some types of cancer, including small cell lung cancer, duodenal cancer, and pancreatic cancer.

Pathophysiology

When ADH is elevated despite normal or low serum osmolality, the kidneys retain excessive water. Plasma volume expands, causing the BP to rise. Body sodium is diluted (hyponatremia) and water intoxication develops. Several types of SIADH exist, with various patterns of abnormal ADH secretion.

Signs and Symptoms

The main symptoms of SIADH initially reflect the effects of dilutional hyponatremia and water retention: weakness, muscle cramps or twitching, anorexia, nausea, diarrhea, irritability, headache, and weight gain without edema. When the CNS is affected by water intoxication, the level of consciousness deteriorates. The patient may have seizures or lapse into a coma.

Medical Diagnosis

The diagnosis of SIADH is confirmed by laboratory tests of serum and urine electrolytes and osmolality. Simultaneous measurements of urine and serum osmolality are especially useful. When measured simultaneously, urine osmolality much higher than that of the serum indicates SIADH. In this case, the serum is very dilute and the urine is very concentrated. Major characteristics include hyponatremia, hypochloremia, hypouricemia, reduced blood urea nitrogen (BUN) and creatinine clearance, increased urine sodium, and fluid volume excess without edema. Urine osmolality may be high, considering the level of serum osmolality, or it may be extremely dilute. Radiographic studies of the brain and lungs also may be done to detect causative factors.

Medical Treatment

Treatment is intended to correct the cause, if possible, and promote elimination of excess water. Acutely ill patients (i.e., those with neurologic symptoms and serum sodium of 120 mEq/L) are treated with hypertonic saline given very slowly over a 4- to 6-hour period. Once neurologic symptoms resolve, principles of chronic therapy are instituted. One approach is to restrict fluids to 800 to 1000 mL/day with a high intake of dietary sodium. For severe hyponatremia, normal saline may be administered with loop diuretics. A diuretic can be used only if the serum sodium is at least 125 mEq/L because the diuretic will cause further loss of sodium. Patients on diuretic therapy may require sodium and potassium supplements. Patients who cannot adhere to fluid restriction with high sodium intake may be given demeclocycline or lithium carbonate, which blocks the effects of ADH on the renal tubules, thereby increasing water excretion. Adverse effects of these drugs can cause complications (see Table 46-2). A class of drugs that induces water elimination while conserving sodium is the vasopressor receptor antagonist, called *vaptans*. Vaptans include tolvaptan, lixivaptan, and conivaptan.

❖ NURSING CARE of the Patient with Syndrome of Inappropriate Antidiuretic Hormone

■ Assessment

The health history records the presence of anorexia, nausea, vomiting, diarrhea, headache, irritability, and muscle cramps and weakness. Document a history of cancer, pulmonary disease, nervous system disorders, hypothyroidism, or lupus erythematosus. Note any prescription drugs the patient is taking. Measure the patient's vital signs, weight, intake and output, and urine specific gravity. Palpate the skin for moisture. Test muscle strength by having the patient grip your hands and push and pull against resistance. Document seizures and muscle weakness, twitching, or cramps. Describe mental status (level of consciousness, orientation) at least every 4 hours in the alert, oriented patient and hourly if there is evidence of impairment.

Nursing Diagnoses, Goals, and Outcome Criteria: Syndrome of Inappropriate Antidiuretic Hormone

Nursing Diagnoses	Goals and Outcome Criteria
Risk for Injury related to confusion associated with hyponatremia, fluid retention, cerebral edema	Absence of injury: no seizures or associated trauma
Excess Fluid Volume related to excess antidiuretic hormone (ADH) secretion	Normal fluid balance: normal tissue turgor, fluid intake and output approximately equal
Ineffective Self-Health Management related to lack of understanding of management of chronic syndrome of inappropriate antidiuretic hormone (SIADH)	Patient effectively manages prescribed therapy: takes drugs correctly, monitors for and reports adverse effects

Interventions

Risk for Injury

If the patient becomes confused, take measures to ensure safety, including putting the bed in a low position and checking on the patient frequently. If intravenous normal saline is needed to treat severe hyponatremia, the solution must be infused very ! slowly using an infusion pump. Rapid infusion could cause hypernatremia. In general, the head of the bed should be elevated no more than 10 degrees. This position improves the return of blood to the heart and reduces the release of ADH. However, in the presence of cerebral edema, position the patient with the head elevated 30 to 45 degrees or as specified by the physician. Institute seizure precautions per agency policy.

Excess Fluid Volume

Advise the physician of declining neurologic status or weight gain in excess of 2 lb/day. Enforce fluid restrictions, which may be as little as 500 mL/24 h. Explain the restriction to the patient and family. Remove the large water pitcher. Space fluids over waking hours to reduce thirst and feelings of deprivation. Serve oral fluids in small containers to create the illusion of volume. Encourage frequent mouth care.

Ineffective Self-Health Management

Although SIADH is usually temporary, it may not resolve during hospitalization and the patient may need to learn how to manage the condition at home. Provide verbal and written information about prescribed drugs, dosages, and adverse effects. Be sure the patient has a scale at home to monitor weight (see *Patient Teaching* box).

Patient Teaching

Syndrome of Inappropriate Antidiuretic Hormone

- Weigh daily and notify the physician if you gain 2 lb or more in 1 day.
- In addition to weight gain, signs and symptoms of excessive water retention (water intoxication) are drowsiness, listlessness, and headache.
- Do not take any nonprescription drugs without consulting your physician or pharmacist.
- See your physician on a regular basis.
- If taking demeclocycline or lithium carbonate, report adverse effects to your physician (provide specifics).
- Maintain a daily fluid intake of 800 to 1000 mL/day or as advised by your physician.
- Ice chips and sugarless chewing gum may help you to manage thirst.

ADRENAL GLANDS

ANATOMY AND PHYSIOLOGY OF THE ADRENAL GLANDS

The adrenal glands are a pair of small, highly vascularized, triangular-shaped organs. They are located in the retroperitoneal cavity on the superior poles of each kidney, lateral to the lower thoracic and upper lumbar vertebrae. Each gland weighs approximately 4 g and measures 3.3 cm in length. The adrenal gland itself is composed of two parts: (1) an outer portion called the *cortex* and (2) an inner portion called the *medulla*. The cortex and medulla have very different, independent functions.

MEDULLA

The medulla constitutes 20% of the gland and contains sympathetic ganglia (i.e., groups of nerve cell bodies) with secretory cells. Stimulation of the sympathetic nervous system causes the medulla to secrete two types of **catecholamines**: (1) norepinephrine (i.e., noradrenaline) and (2) epinephrine (i.e., **adrenaline**). Both of these substances act as neurotransmitters. They are released into the circulation and transported to target organs or tissues, where they exert their effects by binding to adrenergic receptors. Catecholamine effects vary depending on the specific receptor in the cell membrane of the target organ. Multiple adrenergic

Table 46-3 **Receptors and Effects of Adrenal Medullary Hormones on Selected Organs and Tissues**

ORGAN OR TISSUE	RECEPTOR	EFFECT
Heart	β_1	Positive inotropic action (increases myocardial contractility) Positive chronotropic action (increases heart rate)
Blood vessels	α β_2	Vasoconstriction (except in cardiac and skeletal muscles) Vasodilation
Gastrointestinal (GI) tract	α, β	Increased sphincter tone, decreased motility
Kidney	β_2	Increased renin release
Bronchioles	β_2	Relaxation, dilation
Bladder	α β_2	Sphincter contractions, urinary retention Relaxation of detrusor muscle
Skin	α	Increased sweating, piloerection
Adipose tissue	β	Increased lipolysis
Liver	α	Increased gluconeogenesis and glycogenolysis
Pancreas	α β	Decreased glucagon and insulin release Increased glucagon and insulin release
Eyes	α	Dilation of pupils

α, Alpha; β, beta.

receptors exist, including $alpha_1$-, $alpha_2$-, $beta_1$-, and $beta_2$-receptors. Norepinephrine binds to alpha-adrenergic receptors whereas epinephrine affects primarily beta-adrenergic receptors. Table 46-3 lists the specific effects of these catecholamines and the types of receptors with which they bind. The major function of these substances is adaptation to stress, as characterized by the "fight-or-flight response," and maintenance of homeostasis.

CORTEX

The adrenal cortex, which comprises 80% of the adrenal gland, is the outer portion of the gland. This is the portion that is considered to be a part of the endocrine system. The cortex is essential for maintenance of many life-sustaining physiologic activities. The cells of the cortex are organized into three distinct layers or zones. Proceeding from the outermost to innermost layers, they are (1) the zona glomerulosa, (2) the zona fasciculata, and (3) the zona reticularis. The hormones synthesized and secreted by the cortex are known as *steroids* and consist of mineralocorticoids, glucocorticoids, and androgens or estrogens.

FUNCTION OF THE ADRENAL GLANDS

MINERALOCORTICOIDS

The zona glomerulosa produces **mineralocorticoids**, the most abundant of which is aldosterone. Mineralocorticoids play a key role in maintaining an adequate extracellular fluid volume. Aldosterone functions at the renal collecting tubule to promote the reabsorption of sodium and the excretion of potassium by the kidney. The secretion of aldosterone is regulated by several factors: serum levels of potassium, the renin-angiotensin mechanism, and ACTH.

RENIN, ANGIOTENSIN, AND ALDOSTERONE

Renin is produced by the juxtaglomerular cells of renal afferent arterioles. Its release is stimulated by a decrease in extracellular fluid volume. Any factor that can cause this decrease (blood or fluid loss, sodium depletion, or changes in body position or posture) can stimulate renin release. Renin acts on plasma proteins to release angiotensin I, which is catalyzed in the lung to angiotensin II. Angiotensin II stimulates the secretion of aldosterone, which results in sodium and water retention. Retention of sodium and water preserves or increases extracellular fluid volume and subsequently increases BP. This compensatory mechanism plays a very important role in maintaining intravascular volume in shock states.

GLUCOCORTICOIDS

The **glucocorticoids** are produced by the zona reticularis and zona fasciculata. The most abundant and potent of the glucocorticoids is cortisol. Approximately 92% of circulating cortisol is bound to a plasma protein. Free cortisol (8%) binds with receptors in the cytoplasm and nuclei of target cells. Cortisol has a permissive effect on other physiologic processes, meaning that the glucocorticoid must be present for other processes, such as catecholamine activity and excitability of the myocardium, to occur. Glucocorticoid functions include control of carbohydrate, lipid, and fat metabolism; regulation of antiinflammatory and immune responses; and control of emotional states by the following:

- Increasing hepatic gluconeogenesis and inhibiting peripheral glucose use to maintain glucose levels

- Increasing lipolysis and release of glycerol and free fatty acids
- Increasing protein catabolism
- Degrading collagen and connective tissue
- Increasing polymorphonuclear leukocytes released from bone marrow
- Decreasing capillary permeability, movement of WBCs into the injured tissue, and phagocytosis
- Stabilizing lysosomal membranes
- Suppressing lymphocyte reproduction
- Maintaining behavioral and cognitive functions

SEX HORMONES

Adrenal **androgens** are another class of steroids produced in the zona fasciculata and zona reticularis of the adrenal cortex. Their primary function is masculinization in men. Other sex hormones include estrogen and progesterone. In men, these substances contribute little to reproductive maturation. In women, however, **estrogens** are supplied by the ovaries and the adrenal glands. In postmenopausal women, the adrenal cortex is the primary source of endogenous estrogen.

NURSING ASSESSMENT OF THE PATIENT WITH AN ADRENAL DISORDER

HEALTH HISTORY

Present Illness

Symptoms of adrenal dysfunction that may cause the patient to seek medical attention include decreased energy, mental changes (e.g., depression, anxiety, nervousness, confusion), sexual dysfunction, gastrointestinal (GI) disturbances, and abnormal skin pigmentation.

Past Medical History

Aspects of the past medical history that may be significant include radiation to the head or abdomen, intracranial surgery, and recent and current medications. Tuberculosis is the most common cause of primary adrenal insufficiency.

Review of Systems

Determine the patient's perception of his or her general state of health. Ask about changes in skin color, especially bronzed or smoky pigmentation, and increased facial hair in women. Note changes in weight and appetite. Symptoms that may be related to adrenal dysfunction are headache, lightheadedness with position changes, muscle weakness, nausea, vomiting, abdominal pain, anorexia, menstrual dysfunction, and erectile dysfunction.

Functional Assessment

Document usual dietary and activity patterns and disruptions in lifestyle.

PHYSICAL EXAMINATION

Measure the patient's height, weight, and vital signs. Take the BP when the patient is reclining and after the patient has moved to an upright position to detect a significant decrease. Note patient responses and ability to follow instructions. Inspect the skin for a bronzed or smoky pigmentation (especially in surgical scars, the skin over the knuckles, skinfolds, and the areola), bruising, petechiae, vitiligo (i.e., loss of pigmentation), and pallor. Inspect the face of the female patient for excess facial hair. Examine the oral mucous membranes for color changes. Inspect the anterior thorax for fat pads under the clavicles and the posterior thorax for the "buffalo hump." Note obesity of the trunk. Examine the breasts for striae and darkening of the areola. Inspect the abdomen for striae and the extremities for muscle wasting and edema. During examination of the external genitalia, assess for atrophy, hair loss, and appropriateness for age.

Assessment of the patient with an adrenal disorder is summarized in Box 46-2.

AGE-RELATED CHANGES

Under normal circumstances, adrenal function remains adequate in the older person. Some older adults have a decline in cortisol secretion but this is balanced by a decrease in cortisol metabolism such that blood levels remain normal. Secretion of aldosterone and plasma renin activity decline with age and thus the abilities to conserve sodium and adapt to position changes become less efficient.

DIAGNOSTIC TESTS AND PROCEDURES

Because only two deviations from normal adrenal function are covered here, the appropriate diagnostic tests and procedures are discussed with each condition.

DISORDERS OF THE ADRENAL GLANDS

ADRENAL HYPOFUNCTION (ADDISON DISEASE)

Cause

Adrenal insufficiency may be classified as either *primary* or *secondary*. Primary adrenal insufficiency, which is also called **Addison disease**, is frequently the result of a destructive disease process affecting the adrenal glands that causes deficiencies of cortisol and aldosterone. The most common cause of Addison disease is idiopathic atrophy, an autoimmune disease in which adrenal tissue is destroyed by antibodies formed by the patient's own immune system. Other causes of Addison disease are tuberculosis, hemorrhage related to anticoagulant therapy, fungal infections (i.e., histoplasmosis, coccidioidomycosis), acquired immunodeficiency syndrome

Box 46-2 Assessment of the Patient with an Adrenal Disorder

HEALTH HISTORY

Present Illness

Decreased energy, mental changes, sexual dysfunction, gastrointestinal (GI) disturbances, abnormal skin pigmentation

Past Medical History

Radiation to head or abdomen, intracranial surgery, recent and current medications

Review of Systems

General well-being, bronzed or smoky skin color, increased facial hair in women, headache, lightheadedness with position changes, muscle weakness, nausea, vomiting, abdominal pain, anorexia, menstrual dysfunction, erectile dysfunction

Functional Assessment

Changes in height and weight, changes in diet, salt craving, disruption of lifestyle by symptoms

PHYSICAL EXAMINATION

Height and Weight

Vital Signs

Mental Status

Skin

Smoky or bronzed pigmentation prominent on surgical scars, knuckles, in skin folds, areola; bruising, petechiae, vitiligo, pallor

Head and Face

Excess facial hair

Mouth

Color change of oral mucous membranes

Thorax

Supraclavicular fat pads, buffalo hump

Trunk

Obesity

Breasts

Striae, darkening of areola

Abdomen

Striae

Extremities

Muscle wasting, edema

Genitalia

Atrophy, loss of hair, appropriate development for age

(AIDS), metastatic cancer, gram-negative sepsis (Waterhouse-Friderichsen syndrome), adrenalectomy, adrenal toxins, and abrupt withdrawal of exogenous steroids.

Secondary adrenal insufficiency is a result of dysfunction of the hypothalamus or pituitary (decreased corticotropin, ACTH), which leads to decreased androgen and cortisol production. Unlike primary adrenal insufficiency, in which all steroids are affected, aldosterone may or may not be affected. Causes of secondary adrenal insufficiency include pituitary tumors; postpartum necrosis of the pituitary (Sheehan syndrome); hypophysectomy; radiation therapy; pituitary or intracranial lesions; or high-dose, long-term glucocorticoid treatment, which suppresses the adrenal glands' intrinsic activity.

Pathophysiology

Insufficiency of adrenocortical steroids causes defects associated with the loss of mineralocorticoids and glucocorticoids. Impaired secretion of cortisol results in decreased gluconeogenesis and decreased liver and muscle glycogen. This in turn decreases supplies of available glucose, causing hypoglycemia. In addition, the glomerular filtration rate of the kidneys and gastric acid production by the parietal cells of the stomach both slow significantly. The cumulative effects of these processes cause decreased urea nitrogen excretion, irritability, anorexia, weight loss, nausea, vomiting, and diarrhea.

Decreased levels of aldosterone alter the clearance of potassium, water, and sodium by the kidney. Potassium excretion is decreased and hyperkalemia may occur. Because hyperkalemia promotes hydrogen ion retention, metabolic acidosis also can occur. Hypovolemia and hyponatremia may result from accelerated sodium and water excretion.

Other manifestations of adrenal insufficiency are progressive weakness, lethargy, unexplained abdominal pain, and malaise. Skin hyperpigmentation, particularly in sun-exposed areas, pressure points, joints, and creases of the body, is another possible sign. It is most likely the result of increased secretion of a betalipoprotein or a MSH, which is released by a part of the pituitary. This is a direct result of hypercortisolism and a lack of negative feedback.

If adrenal androgen levels are lowered, a decrease or loss of body, axillary, and pubic hair may occur. In prepubescent people, facial, pubic, and axillary hair may fail to grow entirely. The severity of these symptoms is linked to the degree of hormone deficiency. This lack of secondary sex characteristics tends to be seen in primary adrenal insufficiency rather than in secondary adrenal insufficiency.

Symptoms of chronic insufficiency are generally less dramatic and life threatening than symptoms presented during acute adrenal crisis, which is discussed following.

Put on Your Thinking Cap!

Explain how a pituitary disorder could cause adrenal insufficiency.

Acute Adrenal Crisis (Addisonian Crisis). Patients with either primary or secondary adrenal insufficiency are at risk for episodes of acute adrenal crisis, also called *addisonian crisis*, which is a life-threatening emergency. This usually results from a sudden marked decrease in available adrenal hormones. Precipitating factors are adrenal surgery, pituitary destruction, abrupt withdrawal of steroid therapy (often a result of a patient unwittingly stopping medications), and stress. Any factor that causes stress in the person can initiate a crisis. Examples of stressors include infection,

Table 46-4 Emergency Medical Care for Acute Adrenal Crisis

INTERVENTION	RATIONALE
1. Blood sample collected to determine plasma cortisol level	1. To establish a baseline and obtain data to guide treatment
2. Intravenous (IV) infusion of normal saline with 5% dextrose	2. To provide access for administration of fluids and drugs
3. Initial dose of hydrocortisone (Solu-Cortef) IV push, followed by infusion of saline and dextrose over 8 h	3. To provide a loading dose and maintenance infusion
4. Additional doses of hydrocortisone per infusion at rate of 100 mg every 8 h	4. To ensure continuous source of glucocorticoids

illness, trauma, and emotional or psychiatric disturbances.

Manifestations of an addisonian crisis include more severe symptoms of mineralocorticoid and glucocorticoid deficiency: hypotension, tachycardia, dehydration, confusion, hyponatremia, hyperkalemia, hypercalcemia, and hypoglycemia. If left untreated, fluid and electrolyte imbalances can lead to circulatory collapse, cardiac dysrhythmias, cardiac arrest, coma, and death. The management of an addisonian crisis is outlined in Table 46-4.

Pharmacology Capsule

When steroid therapy is discontinued, the drug is tapered gradually. An abrupt decline in adrenal hormones could precipitate acute adrenal crisis.

Medical Diagnosis

Laboratory Studies. Addison disease is diagnosed on the basis of clinical manifestations and a variety of laboratory findings, including a low serum and urinary cortisol level, decreased fasting glucose, hyponatremia, hyperkalemia, and increased BUN. In addition, 24-hour urine tests may be performed. This type of testing reflects steroid secretion over a 24-hour period and is the most accurate measurement of steroid secretion, which varies with the diurnal rhythm. Urinary 17-hydroxycorticosteroids also are sometimes measured as an indicator of glucocorticoid metabolites and are specific for this category of steroids. Androgen metabolites can be determined by measurement of 17-ketosteroids. Both of these substances are low or borderline low in adrenal hypofunction. See Box 46-3 for a list of drugs that interfere with urine tests for 17-hydroxycorticosteroids and 17-ketosteroids.

Measurement of plasma ACTH concentration before treatment helps to define the basis of the patient's symptoms. If the plasma ACTH level is low, the pituitary is at fault for not producing adequate ACTH. An increased plasma ACTH level suggests that the adrenal glands are at fault because they are unable to respond to stimulation to produce corticoids. An ACTH stimulation test is necessary for a definitive diagnosis of hypoadrenalism. One common technique used in this test is the administration of a dose of synthetic ACTH (cosyntropin), which is given intramuscularly or intravenously. Plasma cortisol levels are measured at onset of administration and at 30 and 60 minutes after administration. In primary adrenal insufficiency, the cortisol response is absent or markedly decreased. In secondary insufficiency, a decrease in serum cortisol levels occurs; however, it is not as significant a decrease as in cases of primary insufficiency. An eosinophil count may be performed during ACTH stimulation. The eosinophil count drops significantly after ACTH administration in normal people. Patients with Addison disease show little or no change in the number of circulating eosinophils. If a glucose fasting test is performed, the serum glucose does not rise as high as it would in normal people and returns to a fasting level more rapidly.

Electrocardiogram. Alterations in electrolyte levels often are reflected as deviations in the normal electrocardiogram (ECG). For example, hyperkalemia results in peaked T waves, a widened QRS complex, and an increased PR interval.

Box 46-3 Drugs That Interfere with Urine Tests for 17-Hydroxycorticosteroids and 17-Ketosteroids

acetaminophen	medroxyprogesterone
acetazolamide	meperidine
acetylsalicylic acid	metyrapone
amphetamines	mitotane
ascorbic acid	morphine
barbiturates	nalidixic acid
calcium gluconate	oral contraceptives
carbon disulfide	paraldehyde
chloral hydrate	penicillin
chlordiazepoxide	pentazocine
chlorthalidone	perphenazine
colchicine	phenobarbital
corticotropin	phenothiazines
cortisone	phenylbutazone
dexamethasone	phenytoin
diazepam	promazine
digoxin	propoxyphene
diphenhydramine	quinidine
erythromycin	quinine
estrogens	reserpine
fructose	secobarbital
glutethimide	spironolactone
hydralazine	testosterone
iodides	vitamin K

Modified from Ignatavicius DD, Workman ML, Mishler M: *Medical-surgical nursing: a nursing process approach*, ed 3, Philadelphia, 1999, Saunders.

Radiographic Studies. Skull films, an arteriogram, CT scan, and MRI may be performed to rule out causative factors in secondary adrenal insufficiency. They may reveal intracranial lesions that impinge on the pituitary, aneurysms, or other defects. Abdominal imaging may detect atrophy of the adrenal glands and identify a possible cause of primary insufficiency.

Medical Treatment

The mainstay of treatment of patients with Addison disease is replacement therapy with glucocorticoids and mineralocorticoids. Hydrocortisone commonly is used because it contains both. If glucocorticoids such as cortisone are given, they may be given in a single morning dose or divided into doses with two thirds of a daily dose taken in the morning and one third taken in the evening. The divided dosage schedule is based on human hormonal variations. Glucocorticoids normally peak in the early morning and are at their lowest level in the afternoon. A mineralocorticoid (fludrocortisone), if needed, is typically given each morning or every other morning. See Table 46-5 for details. Secondary adrenal insufficiency is treated with glucocorticoids but mineralocorticoids are usually unnecessary. If the patient has an acute illness, additional glucocorticoids are needed to prevent a life-threatening condition (i.e., addisonian crisis). Addisonian crisis is treated with intravenous fluids, hydrocortisone, electrolytes, and dextrose to restore normal BP.

Patients with Addison disease are not at great risk for harmful side effects of corticosteroids because the goal is only to restore the blood level to normal.

Pharmacology Capsule

Addison disease is treated with glucocorticoids given in a single morning dose or in divided doses to mimic the body's normal hormonal cycles.

NURSING CARE of the Patient with Addison Disease

Assessment

Assessment of the patient with an adrenal disorder is summarized in Box 46-2 (see also Nursing Care Plan: Patient with Addison Disease). Details of the health history that are especially relevant to Addison disease are weight loss, salt craving, nausea and vomiting, abdominal cramping and diarrhea, muscle weakness and aches, poor stress response, decreased libido, and amenorrhea. The patient may be irritable or confused. The physical examination may reveal pale skin with bronzed areas, emaciation, sparse body hair, poor skin turgor, hypotension, and muscle wasting. The patient with acute episodes of Addison disease requires ongoing monitoring of fluid and electrolyte levels and measurement of daily weights.

Nursing Diagnoses, Goals, and Outcome Criteria: Addison Disease

Nursing Diagnoses	Goals and Outcome Criteria
Ineffective Peripheral Tissue Perfusion related to electrolyte imbalance, hypovolemia, cardiac dysrhythmias	Improved tissue perfusion: warm, dry skin with strong peripheral pulses
Risk for Injury related to acute adrenal insufficiency, postural hypotension, impaired physiologic response to stress	Decreased risk for injury: blood pressure (BP) within patient norms, absence of faintness with position changes
Imbalanced Nutrition: Less Than Body Requirements related to impaired metabolism, inability to ingest sufficient nutrients, lack of interest in eating	Adequate nutrition: weight within 5 lb of patient's baseline
Fatigue related to fluid, electrolyte, and glucose imbalances	Improved stamina: patient states fatigue is lessened, performs activities of daily living (ADL) without tiring
Disturbed Body Image related to changes in appearance and function	Adaptation to physical changes: patient makes efforts to improve appearance, makes positive comments about self
Ineffective Self-Health Management of long-term glucocorticoid and mineralocorticoid replacement therapy	Patient manages self-care and prescribed treatment: patient explains disease process and treatment with stated intent to adhere to prescribed regimen

Interventions

Ineffective Peripheral Tissue Perfusion

Monitor for signs and symptoms of inadequate tissue perfusion: confusion, disorientation, tachycardia, apical-radial pulse deficit, general weakness and malaise, and hypotension (including orthostatic changes). Administer prescribed intravenous normal saline, plasma expanders, and vasopressors to maintain blood pressure. The patient whose fluid output is greater than intake is at risk for hypovolemia. Because the patient is at risk for hyperkalemia, monitor serum electrolytes and assess for weakness, paresthesia, dizziness, and electrocardiogram changes. Promptly report these signs and symptoms of hyperkalemia to the physician (see *Patient Teaching* box).

Risk for Injury

Be alert for postural hypotension and other signs of hypovolemia. Instruct the patient who has dizziness

Table 46-5 Drug Therapy for Adrenal Disorders

DRUG	USE AND ACTION	SIDE EFFECTS	NURSING INTERVENTIONS
Glucocorticoids			
cortisone acetate (Cortone Acetate) prednisolone (Delta-Cortef, Prelone) prednisolone acetate (Econopred) hydrocortisone (Cortef)	All stimulate formation of glucose, promote storage of glucose as glycogen, affect fluid and electrolytes, increase hemoglobin, suppress inflammation. Used to treat adrenal insufficiency. Some also have mineralocorticoid effects.	All: hypokalemia, hypocalcemia, nausea and vomiting, edema, hypertension, increased risk of infection, hyperglycemia, muscle wasting, osteoporosis, ulcer development, acne, pathologic fractures. May cause death if suddenly discontinued.	Monitor weight, intake and output, BP, blood glucose. Assess for edema. Protect from sources of infection. Report signs of infection even if subtle. Assess for hypocalcemia: muscle weakness and twitching. Assess for hypokalemia: muscle weakness and tingling, cardiac dysrhythmias, irritability. Protect from falls and possible fractures. Give oral drugs with food or milk. Many patients with adrenal insufficiency manage with only glucocorticoids.
Mineralocorticoids			
fludrocortisone (Florinef Acetate)	Stimulates reabsorption of sodium and excretion of potassium and hydrogen ions in renal tubules. Used to treat adrenal insufficiency.	Hypokalemia, nausea and vomiting, edema, hypertension, muscle weakness, dizziness, tendon contractures, CHF.	Monitor weight, intake and output, BP, heart rate and rhythm, serum electrolytes. Assess for hypokalemia-prescribed sodium intake. Do not discontinue suddenly. Tell patient to carry drug identification card.
Adrenocortical Cytotoxics			
mitotane (Lysodren)	Suppresses adrenocortical function.	Nausea and vomiting, diarrhea, lethargy, dizziness, hypouricemia, hearing and vision disturbances, BP changes, dyspnea.	Monitor BP. Report infections or trauma so drug can be discontinued temporarily. Tell patient not to have immunizations without physician approval and to avoid contact with people who have recently had polio or DPT vaccine. Increase fluid intake and monitor uric acid.
Antifungals			
ketoconazole (Nizoral)	Fungistatic. Suppresses adrenocortical function.	Nausea and vomiting, pruritus, diarrhea or constipation, GI bleeding, lethargy, headache, dizziness, adrenocortical insufficiency. Occasionally: thrombocytopenia, hemolytic anemia, hepatotoxicity.	Monitor stools. Administer antipruritics or apply topical agents as ordered. Safety measures if dizzy or drowsy. Monitor liver function tests and assess for pale stools, dark urine, fatigue, and anorexia. Avoid alcohol.

BP, Blood pressure; *CHF*, congestive heart failure; *DPT*, diphtheria, pertussis, and tetanus; *GI*, gastrointestinal.

Nursing Care Plan — Patient with Addison Disease

ASSESSMENT

HEALTH HISTORY A 52-year-old Caucasian man is admitted with Addison disease. He considers himself healthy but has had some joint pain in his knees. He had an appendectomy 20 years ago. The patient complains of weight loss, anorexia, weakness, and darkening of the skin on his face and arms. His usual weight is 170 lb. He has had bouts of nausea, vomiting, and diarrhea accompanied by vague abdominal pain. The patient is a salesman and reports that his symptoms are making it difficult for him to keep up with his work. He is embarrassed about the change in his skin color.

PHYSICAL EXAMINATION Vital signs: blood pressure 110/80 mm Hg (sitting) and 88/42 mm Hg (standing), pulse 102 bpm with slight irregularity, respiration 20 breaths per minute, temperature 98°F (36.7°C) measured orally. Height 5′8″, weight 155 lb. The patient is oriented but somewhat lethargic. The skin on his face and arms and his abdominal scar are darkly pigmented. His body hair is sparse. The patient's oral mucous membranes are slightly dry.

Nursing Diagnosis	Goals and Outcome Criteria	Interventions
Ineffective Peripheral Tissue Perfusion related to electrolyte imbalance, fluid volume deficit, and cardiac dysrhythmias	The patient will have improved tissue perfusion, as evidenced by warm, dry skin, strong peripheral pulses, and fluid output equal to fluid intake.	Monitor for signs and symptoms of inadequate tissue perfusion: confusion, disorientation, tachycardia, hypotension, apical-radial pulse deficit, fluid output exceeding intake. Administer intravenous fluids (normal saline, plasma expanders) and vasopressors, as ordered. Monitor for hyperkalemia: weakness, paresthesia, dizziness. Report evidence of inadequate tissue perfusion or hyperkalemia to the physician.
Risk for Injury related to acute adrenal insufficiency, impaired stress response, postural hypotension	The patient will remain free of injury because of hypotension, shock, or falls.	Monitor for postural hypotension. If the patient has dizziness with position changes, instruct him to exercise his legs before rising, to rise slowly, and to call for help when getting out of bed. Administer fluids and hormones as ordered.
Imbalanced Nutrition: Less Than Body Requirements related to impaired metabolism, inability to ingest sufficient nutrients, and lack of interest in eating	The patient will be adequately nourished, as evidenced by weight within 5 lb of baseline.	Weigh daily to monitor fluid balance and nutritional status. Request dietary consult for patient education so that his food preferences can be respected. Provide a high-protein, low-carbohydrate diet as ordered. Tell the patient that salt may be used freely. Provide a pleasant atmosphere for meals. Report signs of hypoglycemia: headache, trembling, tachycardia, sweating.
Fatigue related to fluid, electrolyte, and glucose imbalances	The patient will report improved stamina.	Explain medically prescribed activity limitations. Plan care to allow for periods of rest. Discuss energy conservation after discharge.
Disturbed Body Image related to changes in appearance and function	The patient will adapt to altered physical appearance and function, as evidenced by efforts to improve appearance and positive comments about self.	Explore how the patient feels about skin changes. Discuss strategies to deal with changes: long sleeves, avoidance of excess sunlight. Advise the patient to arrange work with rest periods. Encourage attention to grooming. Compliment his efforts.
Ineffective Self-Health Management related to lack of understanding of long-term glucocorticoid therapy	The patient will manage self-care and prescribed treatment; correctly explain the disease, its treatment, and medication therapy; state intent to adhere to prescribed regimen.	Implement a teaching plan for Addison disease to include the following: • Wear a medical alert tag and carry an emergency kit with dexamethasone. • Take glucocorticoids as directed, either a single morning dose or in divided doses in the morning and afternoon with food. • Increase medication dosage as ordered when under stress. • Notify the physician or go to the emergency room if unable to take oral medications for more than 24 hours. • Remember that lifelong therapy and monitoring are needed. • Report signs and symptoms of inadequate and excessive hormone replacement.

Critical Thinking Questions

1. Name three strategies for energy conservation.
2. How might you encourage the patient to share his feelings about the skin changes?

Patient Teaching

Addison Disease

- Wear a medical alert tag and carry an emergency kit with dexamethasone.
- Take glucocorticoids as ordered as a single morning dose or in divided doses in the morning and afternoon with food.
- Increase your medication dosage as ordered when under stress.
- Notify the physician or go to the emergency department if you are unable to take oral medications for more than 24 hours.
- Remember that lifelong therapy and monitoring are needed.
- Report signs and symptoms of inadequate and excessive hormone replacement.

with position changes to call for help when getting out of bed and to rise slowly to prevent falls. Exercising the legs before standing promotes venous return and may minimize the drop in BP.

Sudden profound weakness with postural hypotension is characteristic of acute addisonian crisis and leads to shock and death if not corrected. Administer fluid replacement and hormones as ordered to treat addisonian crisis.

Imbalanced Nutrition: Less Than Body Requirements

Daily weights provide important data to assess fluid balance. Weight changes also provide information about the adequacy of the patient's diet (see *Nutrition Considerations* box). If nutrition is a problem, consult the dietitian. Salt is not restricted because patients with Addison disease tend to lose sodium. People who live in hot climates may actually need to increase their salt intake to make up for losses through perspiration. Respect the patient's food preferences as much as possible. The mealtime atmosphere should be conducive to eating.

Hypoglycemia may develop as a result of decreased cortisol secretion. Encourage frequent rest periods to avoid depletion of glycogen stores. Meals should be taken regularly and between-meal snacks may be needed to maintain blood glucose. Monitor for (and teach) the patient symptoms of hypoglycemia: headache, tachycardia, trembling, and sweating. Periodic laboratory studies are done to assess nitrogen balance, liver function, serum albumin, glucose, electrolytes, BUN, and creatinine.

Fatigue

Explain any prescribed activity limitations to the patient. Plan specific rest periods to conserve energy. Provide assistance with ADL as needed. If the patient is on bed rest, intervene to prevent complications of immobility as described in Chapter 21.

Disturbed Body Image

Explore the patient's reaction to the physical changes experienced. Discuss strategies to cope with changes. When the patient's condition has stabilized, encourage attention to grooming and compliment the patient's efforts.

Ineffective Self-Health Management

Care of the patient with a chronic disease requires in-depth education and information about stress management. It is critical for the patient to understand Addison disease and to know how to recognize the effects of the disease as well as those of overmedication. The patient must learn to make adjustments in replacement hormones depending on various stressors. Provide written material to supplement the teaching sessions.

ADRENAL HYPERSECRETION (CUSHING SYNDROME)

Cause

Hypersecretion of the adrenal cortex may result in the production of excess amounts of corticosteroids, particularly glucocorticoid. The condition that results from excessive cortisol is called **Cushing syndrome**. The overproduction of adrenocortical hormones may result from endogenous (internal) as well as exogenous (external) causes.

Endogenous causes include corticotropin-secreting pituitary tumors, a cortisol-secreting neoplasm within the adrenal glands, and excess secretion of corticotropin by a carcinoma of the lung or other tissues. Excessive production of ACTH because of a pituitary tumor is called **Cushing disease**. The incidence of Cushing syndrome caused by disease is infrequent, affecting women eight times more often than men. Approximately 25% of cases of Cushing syndrome are due to adrenal tumors.

The single exogenous cause of Cushing syndrome is prolonged administration of high doses of corticosteroids. This is also the most common cause of Cushing syndrome.

Pathophysiology

Clinical manifestations of Cushing syndrome affect most body systems and are related to excess levels of circulating corticosteroids. In some instances, signs and symptoms of mineralocorticoid and androgen excess may appear; however, signs and symptoms of glucocorticoid excess usually predominate.

Hyperadrenalism produces marked changes in the personal appearance of the affected person, including obesity, facial redness, hirsutism (i.e., excess hair), menstrual disorders, hypertension of varying degrees, and muscle wasting of the extremities (Fig. 46-6). Additional findings include delayed wound healing, insomnia, irrational behavior, and mood disturbances

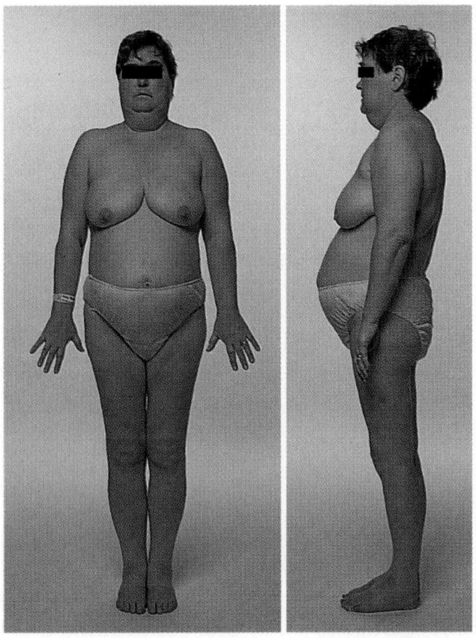

FIGURE 46-6 Clinical manifestations in a patient with Cushing syndrome. (From Forbes CH, Jackson WF: *Color atlas and text of clinical medicine*, ed 3, St. Louis, 2003, Elsevier Science Limited/Mosby.)

such as irritability and anxiety. The following are hallmark findings that lead to a diagnosis of Cushing syndrome:

- Truncal obesity (excess adipose in body trunk)
- Protein wasting (slender extremities and very thin and friable skin)
- Facial fullness, often called a *moon face*
- Purple striae on the abdomen, breasts, buttocks, or thighs
- Osteoporosis (a significant finding in premenopausal women)
- Hypokalemia of uncertain cause

Medical Diagnosis

In addition to physical signs and symptoms, some laboratory, radiographic, and imaging results may be useful in determining a diagnosis.

Laboratory Studies. When Cushing syndrome is suspected, a 24-hour urine collection for free cortisol usually is ordered. A low-dose dexamethasone suppression test may be done as well. In normal people, the cortisol and 17-hydroxycorticosteroid levels are suppressed. If these levels are not suppressed (compared with the baseline sample), the test is repeated using a higher dose of dexamethasone.

Abnormal laboratory findings include polycythemia, hypokalemia, hypernatremia, hyperglycemia, leukocytosis, glycosuria, hypocalcemia, and elevated plasma cortisol. ACTH may be high or low, depending on whether the basic problem lies in the adrenals or in the pituitary. In some cases, malignant tumors, especially small cell cancer of the lung, can secrete ACTH, which stimulates excess cortisol secretion.

Radiographic Studies. If a tumor is suspected as a causative factor in Cushing syndrome, a CT scan and MRI may be done to localize the site of the tumor. Radiographic films also may reveal osteoporosis of the spinal column, especially in women.

Medical Treatment

Depending on the specific patient and the cause of the disease, various therapies may be used. These include drug therapy, radiation, and surgery. If Cushing syndrome is caused by administration of synthetic glucocorticoids, the physician may gradually withdraw them. Most patients affected with hyperadrenalism because of a single benign adrenal tumor undergo surgical intervention. Bilateral benign tumors more often are treated with an aldosterone antagonist agent (i.e., a drug that reduces aldosterone secretion or blocks its effects). An example of an aldosterone antagonist is the potassium-sparing diuretic spironolactone (Aldactone). Patients with metastatic adrenal cancer are usually treated with surgery and chemotherapy. However, a cure for metastatic adrenal cancer is yet to be found. When Cushing syndrome is caused by a pituitary tumor, removal of part of the pituitary or radiation may reduce ACTH secretion without disturbing other pituitary functions. If this fails, the remaining pituitary tissue may be removed.

Drug Therapy. When surgery is contraindicated, certain agents that interfere with ACTH production or adrenal hormone synthesis may be administered. One example is mitotane (Lysodren), a cytotoxic substance that is used as a palliative treatment for inoperable adrenal tumors. Agents that interfere with cortisol production include ketoconazole (Nizoral), aminoglutethimide (Cytadren), and metyrapone (Metopirone). Metyrapone is also used in combination with mitotane for enhanced effects. A risk of acute adrenal crisis occurs when patients are on drugs that suppress adrenal function. In addition, the drugs must be promptly discontinued if trauma or shock occurs because the patient's ability to adapt is diminished. Table 46-5 provides additional information.

Pharmacology Capsule

Drugs that suppress adrenal function can lead to acute adrenal crisis and must be promptly discontinued if shock or trauma occurs.

Radiation. In cases in which a pituitary adenoma causes excessive secretion of ACTH, the adenoma may be treated with radiation therapy. Radiation can be administered either externally or internally. Internal radiation involves the transsphenoidal implantation of a radioactive material that remains in place for a specified period of time. Radiation therapy is not always effective, requires a long period of treatment, and can destroy healthy tissue. If radiation therapy is being used to treat a patient with a pituitary adenoma, you must be alert for any significant changes in the patient's neurologic status, such as a complaint of headache or a change in mental status or pupillary responses. In addition, the patient may experience side effects associated with radiation therapy. These include alopecia (i.e., hair loss) and dry, red, or irritated skin. The patient must be educated about these drug effects.

Surgical Management. The surgical treatment of hyperadrenalism depends on the specific cause of the disorder. For example, if adrenal hypersecretion is due to a pituitary adenoma that is producing ACTH, a transsphenoidal hypophysectomy is performed (see "Surgical Management" in the Hyperpituitarism section). If adrenal adenoma or carcinoma is the cause of the adrenal hypersecretion, an adrenalectomy (i.e., removal of the adrenal gland) is performed. If only one gland is removed, the procedure is referred to as a *unilateral adrenalectomy*; the removal of both glands is called a *bilateral adrenalectomy*. An adrenalectomy may be performed in situations in which drug and radiation therapies are unsuccessful. Patients who are undergoing a unilateral adrenalectomy can expect to require replacement therapy for up to 2 years after surgery. A bilateral adrenalectomy necessitates lifelong replacement of both glucocorticoids and mineralocorticoids. Depending on the tumor size, a laparoscopic procedure may be an option. Surgery and chemotherapy are indicated for metastatic adrenal cancer. These treatments may induce remission but are not curative.

NURSING CARE of the Patient with Cushing Syndrome

Assessment

Initial assessment of the patient with Cushing syndrome includes a detailed history and physical examination done by the RN. The LVN/LPN may collect specific information about the onset of symptoms, prior treatments, drug allergies, and current medications (see *Complementary and Alternative Therapies* box). The complete nursing assessment of the patient with an adrenal disorder is summarized in Box 46-2.

Complementary and Alternative Therapies

Patients with Cushing syndrome should be cautioned that long-term use of some herbs, including celery, juniper, licorice, and parsley, can cause hypokalemia.

Interventions

Risk for Infection

Exposure to people with infections should be avoided because of the patient's decreased resistance to infection. Minor symptoms, such as a low-grade fever (99.5°F or higher), sore throat, or aches, can indicate the onset of a potentially serious infection. Any symptoms indicative of a cold or other problem should be brought to the attention of the physician.

Nursing Diagnoses, Goals, and Outcome Criteria: Cushing Syndrome

Nursing Diagnoses	Goals and Outcome Criteria
Risk for Infection related to high serum cortisol levels	Absence of infection: normal body temperature and white blood cell (WBC) count
Anxiety related to depression, mood swings, anxiety, irrational behavior	Decreased anxiety: stable mood, calm demeanor
Risk for Impaired Skin Integrity related to changes in skin and connective tissue and edema	Absence of injury to skin: skin intact with minimal or no bruising
Risk for Injury (fracture) related to osteoporosis	Absence of fractures: no skeletal trauma or fractures
Disturbed Body Image related to changes in physical appearance and function	Adaptation to altered body image: patient attends to appearance, grooming; makes positive comments about self
Ineffective Self-Health Management related to lack of understanding of disease, drug therapy, diet, and self-care	Patient follows prescribed treatment: verbalizes and demonstrates self-care, condition stabilizes

Anxiety

Personality changes often accompany adrenal disorders. When they do occur, discuss them with the patient and the family. Understanding that mood swings are a part of this disorder may help the patient and family to cope more effectively. If the emotional changes, particularly depression, become severe, carefully monitor the patient. A psychiatric referral may be necessary.

Risk for Impaired Skin Integrity

The skin of the patient with Cushing syndrome is extremely fragile. Inspect the skin daily to detect early signs of pressure or injuries. Assist the patient with limited mobility to change positions at least every 2 hours. Keep bed linens clean and dry. Advise the patient to wear shoes when out of bed to reduce the risk of foot injuries. During transfers and position changes, be careful to prevent trauma to the skin.

Risk for Injury

Because fractures occur very easily, protect the patient with Cushing syndrome from falls or trauma. Keep the bed in low position and the call bell within reach. If the patient is very weak or confused, raise the side rails. Instruct the patient to call for assistance when getting in and out of bed.

Disturbed Body Image

Bruises, abnormal fat distribution, and hirsutism may embarrass the patient. Provide an opportunity for the patient to share thoughts and concerns about these changes. If they are distressing, suggest clothing to conceal them. Encourage and assist patients to be well groomed. Women may choose to shave or to use depilatories to remove unwanted hair. Reassure the patient that physical changes usually improve gradually after medical or surgical treatment.

Ineffective Self-Health Management

To manage Cushing syndrome, the patient must understand the condition, complications, treatment, and self-care. Provide written information to supplement verbal teaching about drugs, including drug names and dosages, schedules, and adverse effects. A referral may be made to the dietitian for nutritional counseling. The diet is typically low in calories with sufficient protein and calcium. (For key teaching points, see the *Patient Teaching* box.)

Patient Teaching

Cushing Syndrome

- Avoid people with infections because you have increased risk of infections; report any temperature elevation to your physician.
- Mood swings and changes in appearance are usually corrected with treatment.
- Avoid activities that could result in trauma because you have increased risk of bleeding and fractures.
- It is critical that you continue drug therapy under medical supervision.

NURSING CARE of the Adrenalectomy Patient

General nursing care of the surgical patient is discussed in Chapter 17. This section addresses the specific needs of the adrenalectomy patient.

Preoperative Nursing Care

Preoperative care of the patient undergoing an adrenalectomy involves monitoring for and correcting any existing electrolyte imbalances. Strict hand washing and observance of aseptic technique are key in the prevention of infections in these susceptible patients. Preoperative education involves a discussion of glucocorticoid replacement therapy, including dosage, side effects, and complications.

Postoperative Nursing Care

After adrenalectomy, the patient is sent to a critical care unit for at least 1 to 2 days for close observation and assessment. During this period, monitor vital signs for signs and symptoms of impending shock, which may be evident as hypotension, a weak or thready pulse, decreased urinary output, and changes in level of consciousness. Pulse and BP may be unstable for 24 to 48 hours after surgery and vasopressors may be needed to maintain BP in the immediate postoperative period.

A nursing diagnosis specific to the adrenalectomy patient is *risk for injury* related to addisonian crisis as a result of the sudden decrease in adrenal hormone secretion. Assess for signs and symptoms of acute adrenal insufficiency: vomiting, weakness, hypotension, joint pain, pruritus, and emotional disturbances. Closely monitor fluid and electrolyte balance. Intravenous fluids may be prescribed to restore or maintain balance. High doses of cortisol are given intravenously during and for several days after surgery to enable the patient to deal with the physical stress of surgery. The dosages are adjusted on the basis of the BP, blood glucose, serum electrolytes, and serum cortisol levels. Later, glucocorticoids are administered orally.

Because the patient's resistance to infection is lowered, be especially careful to protect the patient by using strict aseptic technique for wound care and invasive procedures. Signs of infection may be very subtle.

Assess comfort at frequent intervals and treat pain with opioid analgesics. Document the effects of treatment. To minimize the risk of pulmonary complications, such as stasis of secretions and pneumonia, instruct the patient to turn, cough, deep breathe, or use an incentive spirometer.

Nutrition Considerations

1. Early symptoms of Addison disease may include anorexia, nausea, vomiting, diarrhea, and weight loss, resulting in impaired nutrition.
2. Patients with Addison disease are advised not to restrict salt intake.
3. Patients with Cushing syndrome may experience sodium and water retention.
4. Diet therapy for Cushing syndrome may include decreased caloric and sodium intake and increased potassium intake.
5. Reducing sodium intake can decrease edema and related weight gain with Cushing syndrome.
6. Patients with diabetes insipidus (DI) usually experience excessive thirst or urination, so they must drink liquids almost continuously to avoid dehydration and hypovolemic shock.

PHEOCHROMOCYTOMA

A pheochromocytoma is a tumor, usually benign, of the adrenal medulla that causes secretion of excessive catecholamines (i.e., epinephrine, norepinephrine). Patients with a pheochromocytoma exhibit episodes of severe hypertension, hypermetabolism, and hyperglycemia. The classic clinical findings are hypertension with a diastolic pressure of 115 mm Hg or higher; severe, pounding headache; and diaphoresis (profuse sweating). Other signs and symptoms include pallor, dilated pupils, orthostatic hypotension, and blurred vision. Episodes may be triggered by emotional distress, exercise, manipulation of the tumor, postural changes, and major trauma, including surgery.

The condition is treated by surgical removal of the tumor, usually via laparoscopy. Before surgery the surgeon attempts to normalize vital signs with adrenergic antagonists (i.e., drugs that block the effects of catecholamines) and stabilize the patient's fluid status. The nurse monitors cardiovascular status and prepares the patient for surgery as detailed in Chapter 17. Postoperative nursing care is generally the same as that described for the patient having an adrenalectomy. However, special postoperative problems in the patient with pheochromocytoma include a greater risk for fluctuations in blood pressure and hypoglycemia. These problems require close monitoring and treatment. Patients who are not candidates for surgery may be treated with metyrosine (Demser), which reduces catecholamine production.

Get Ready for the NCLEX® Examination!

Key Points

- The endocrine system secretes hormones—chemical messengers that affect target organs and body tissues.
- Endocrine activity is regulated by feedback mechanisms that either stimulate or inhibit hormone synthesis and secretion.
- Pituitary hormones affect growth, fluid and electrolyte balance, metabolism, ovulation, milk production, uterine contractions, and skin pigmentation.
- Pituitary and adrenal function usually remain adequate in older people.
- Hyperpituitarism, caused by excess anterior pituitary hormones, leads to gigantism or acromegaly.
- Hyperpituitarism is treated with drugs or surgery to remove the tumor or the entire pituitary (hypophysectomy).
- Treatment of hyperpituitarism can prevent further changes and complications. Soft tissue hypertrophy may be reduced but existing skeletal changes are not reversible.
- Dwarfism is the result of inadequate GH.
- Panhypopituitarism is a deficiency of all anterior pituitary hormones and is treated with replacement hormones.
- DI, caused by a deficit in ADH, results in massive diuresis and is treated with vasopressin.
- SIADH, caused by excess ADH, results in fluid retention and is treated with diuretics and demeclocycline.
- The adrenal medulla secretes the catecholamines epinephrine and norepinephrine, which promote adaptation to stress.
- The adrenal cortex secretes steroids in the form of mineralocorticoids, glucocorticoids, and androgens or estrogens.
- Primary adrenal insufficiency (Addison disease) causes hypoglycemia, hyperkalemia, hyponatremia, and hypovolemia and requires lifelong replacement of glucocorticoids and mineralocorticoids.
- Acute adrenal crisis is a life-threatening emergency caused by a sudden marked decrease in adrenal hormones that can lead to circulatory collapse and death.
- Cushing syndrome results from hypersecretion of cortisol, a glucocorticoid, or from prolonged administration of corticosteroids.
- Cushing syndrome is characterized by polycythemia, hypokalemia, hyperglycemia, leukocytosis, and glycosuria.
- Cushing syndrome is treated with drug therapy, radiation, and hypophysectomy or adrenalectomy.
- Nursing care for the patient with Cushing syndrome is concerned with risk for infection, anxiety, risk for impaired skin integrity, risk for injury, disturbed body image, and ineffective self-health management.
- All chronic pituitary and adrenal conditions require patient teaching to enable the patient to manage the condition by taking medications properly and recognizing the need for medical intervention.
- A pheochromocytoma is an adrenal tumor that increases secretion of catecholamines, causing hypertension, hypermetabolism, and hyperglycemia.

Additional Learning Resources

SG Go to your Study Guide for additional learning activities to help you master this chapter content.

evolve Go to your Evolve website (http://evolve.elsevier.com/Linton/medsurg) for the following learning resources and much more:

- Interactive Prioritization Exercises
- Fluid & Electrolyte Tutorial
- Pharmacology Tutorial
- Review Questions for the NCLEX® Examination

Review Questions for the NCLEX® Examination

1. Which of the following is the overall mission of the endocrine system?
  1. To maintain electrolyte balance
  2. To control metabolic rate
  3. To maintain homeostasis
  4. To resist infection
  NCLEX Client Need: Physiological Integrity: Physiological Adaptation

2. Hormones secreted by the anterior pituitary include which of the following? (Select all that apply.)
  1. ADH
  2. ACTH
  3. GH
  4. LH
  5. TSH
  NCLEX Client Need: Physiological Integrity: Physiological Adaptation

3. A patient who has recently started treatment for acromegaly says, "I will be so glad to look like myself again!" Which of the following is the most appropriate response?
   1. "I know you are looking forward to that."
   2. "The process of reversing the effects of acromegaly is very slow."
   3. "Treatment will keep your symptoms from getting worse but will not reverse all of them."
   4. "These drugs can slow down the progression of acromegaly but you will have additional bone enlargement."

   NCLEX Client Need: Physiological Integrity: Physiological Adaptation
4. After surgery to remove a pituitary adenoma, a patient complains of neck stiffness. Which of the following actions should you take?
   1. Give a gentle neck massage
   2. Administer a prescribed analgesic
   3. Lower the head of the bed
   4. Look for other signs of infection

   NCLEX Client Need: Physiological Integrity: Reduction of Risk Potential
5. Patients with hypopituitarism who wish to have children must be treated with which of the following hormones? (Select all that apply.)
   1. LH
   2. Thyroid hormone
   3. FSH
   4. Prolactin
   5. ACTH

   NCLEX Client Need: Physiological Integrity: Pharmacological Therapies
6. Which of the following is the main symptom of SIADH?
   1. Increased blood glucose
   2. Water retention
   3. Generalized edema
   4. Hypotension

   NCLEX Client Need: Physiological Integrity: Physiological Adaptation
7. To regulate drug dosages for the patient with DI, which of the following records must be maintained?
   1. Daily diet
   2. Sodium intake
   3. Urine specific gravity
   4. BP and pulse

   NCLEX Client Need: Physiological Integrity: Reduction of Risk Potential
8. Fluid and electrolyte imbalances associated with Addison disease include which of the following? (Select all that apply.)
   1. Hyperkalemia
   2. Hyponatremia
   3. Hypervolemia
   4. Metabolic alkalosis
   5. Hypercalcemia

   NCLEX Client Need: Physiological Integrity: Physiological Adaptation
9. A patient who is brought to the emergency department has BP 88/40 mm Hg; pulse 108 bpm, thready; and dry skin and mucous membranes. He is confused. A medical alert card in his wallet states that he takes drugs for Addison disease. You recognize the signs and symptoms of which of the following?
   1. Acute adrenal crisis
   2. Cushing syndrome
   3. Diabetic ketoacidosis
   4. Cushing disease

   NCLEX Client Need: Physiological Integrity: Physiological Adaptation
10. Nursing care of the patient with Cushing syndrome should include which of the following?
    1. Apply moisturizers to dark, toughened areas of skin
    2. Protect the patient from visitors and other patients with infections
    3. Tell the patient that mood swings and irritability will lessen with treatment
    4. Encourage the patient to use salt liberally to offset excessive loss in the urine

    NCLEX Client Need: Physiological Integrity: Physiological Adaptation and Reduction of Risk Potential

chapter

47 Thyroid and Parathyroid Disorders

http://evolve.elsevier.com/Linton/medsurg

Objectives

1. Identify nursing assessment data related to the functions of the thyroid and parathyroid glands.
2. Describe tests and procedures used to diagnose disorders of the thyroid and parathyroid glands as well as the nursing responsibilities relevant for each.
3. Describe the pathophysiology, signs and symptoms, complications, and treatment of hyperthyroidism, hypothyroidism, hyperparathyroidism, and hypoparathyroidism.
4. Assist in the development of nursing care plans for patients with disorders of the thyroid or parathyroid glands.

Key Terms

Chvostek sign (KVŎS-tĕks)
Cretinism (KRĒ-tĭn-ĭzm)
Exophthalmos (ĕk-sŏf-THĂL-mŏs)
Goiter (GOI-tĕr)
Goitrogen (GOI-trō-jĕn)
Laryngospasm (lă-RĬNG-gō-spăzm)
Myxedema (mĭk-sĕ-DĒ-mă)
Nodule (NŎD-ūl)
Parotiditis (pă-rŏt-ĭ-DĪ-tĭs)
Tetany (TĔT-ă-nē)
Thyroiditis (thī-roid-Ī-tĭs)
Thyrotoxicosis (thī-rō-tŏk-sĭ-KŌ-sĭs)
Trousseau sign (troo-SŌZ)

THYROID GLAND

ANATOMY AND PHYSIOLOGY OF THE THYROID GLAND

The thyroid gland is located in the lower portion of the anterior neck. It consists of two lobes, one on each side of the trachea. The lobes are connected in front of the trachea by a narrow bridge of tissue called the *isthmus* (Fig. 47-1).

The thyroid gland plays a major role in regulating the body's rate of metabolism and growth and development. When the metabolic rate falls, the hypothalamus stimulates the pituitary gland to secrete thyroid-stimulating hormone (TSH). This hormone in turn stimulates the thyroid gland to secrete hormones that affect the production and use of energy.

The hormones produced by the thyroid gland are thyroid hormone, triiodothyronine, and calcitonin. Each of these is known by several names. Thyroid hormone also is called *thyroxine, tetraiodothyronine,* or T_4. Triiodothyronine is referred to as T_3. Both T_4 and T_3 increase the body's metabolic rate. Calcitonin, or thyrocalcitonin, plays a role in regulating the serum calcium level. It is secreted when serum calcium levels are high, limiting the shift of calcium from the bones into the blood.

AGE-RELATED CHANGES IN THYROID FUNCTION

In the healthy older person, serum levels of T4 and T3 remain approximately the same as in younger adults. The incidence of hypothyroidism increases with age, especially among women. Thyroid **nodules** are more common among older persons. Thyroid conditions are often overlooked in older adults because signs and symptoms may be subtle, with an atypical presentation, and attributed to the aging process. The word *atypical* means that the patient does not have the most common signs and symptoms of a condition. Weight changes may not occur in the older person as they do with younger people with thyroid disorders. In general, hypothyroidism in older adults is associated with a gradual decrease in mental and physical function. Symptoms of hyperthyroidism include irregular cardiac rhythms, heart failure (HF), weight loss, and muscular weakness. Although treatment of thyroid disorders can have a profound positive effect on the patient's quality of life, there continues to be debate regarding whether mild elevations in TSH require treatment. Mild thyroid dysfunction may, in fact, reflect the body's decreased use of thyroid hormone because of the age-related decline in lean body mass. Details about thyroid dysfunction and treatment are provided later in this chapter.

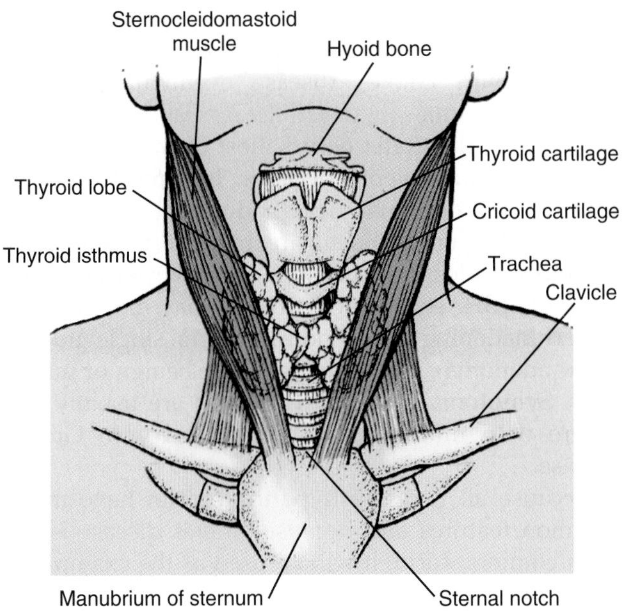

FIGURE 47-1 The thyroid gland. (From Monahan FD, Drake DT, Neighbors M, editors: *Medical-surgical nursing: foundations for clinical practice*, ed 2, Philadelphia, 1998, Saunders.)

Pharmacology Capsule

Any older adult who is taking more than 0.15 mg of L-thyroxine daily is at risk for hyperthyroidism.

NURSING ASSESSMENT OF THE THYROID GLAND

Thyroid disorders may escape detection until they are rather severe because the symptoms are often vague. Periodic assessment of the patient with a thyroid disorder is necessary for the physician to evaluate the response to treatment and make adjustments if necessary. Data collected by the registered nurse (RN) and the licensed vocational nurse/licensed practical nurse (LVN/LPN) contribute to this assessment and evaluation.

HEALTH HISTORY

To elicit information about common symptoms of thyroid disorders, ask if the patient is aware of any changes in energy level, sleep patterns, personality, mental function, or emotional state. Fatigue may be found with both hypothyroidism and hyperthyroidism. Because thyroid hormones affect the metabolic rate, patients may have unexplained weight changes. Hormone deficiency lowers the metabolic rate, so patients may gain weight. At the other extreme, hormone excess increases the metabolic rate, often causing weight loss.

In the review of systems, pay particular attention to changes in menstrual cycles, sexual function, hydration (i.e., thirst, changes in urine output, tissue turgor, moisture of mucous membranes), bowel elimination pattern, and tolerance of heat and cold.

Box 47-1 Assessment of the Patient with a Thyroid Disorder

HEALTH HISTORY

Present Illness

Fatigue, weight changes, mental and emotional changes

Past Medical History

Recent surgery or trauma, radiation of the head or neck, recent and current medications, history of thyroid or renal disorders

Review of Systems

Fatigue, changes in hair or skin, voice changes, palpitations, edema, constipation or diarrhea, polyuria, nervousness, weight loss, temperature intolerance, excessive perspiration, changes in libido or sexual function

Functional Assessment

Sleep disturbances, usual dietary intake, anorexia, ability to cope with stress

PHYSICAL EXAMINATION

Vital Signs

Abnormal heart rate and rhythm, blood pressure (BP) changes, tachypnea

Height and Weight

Skin

Changes in moisture, temperature, and texture

Hair

Changes in texture

Eyes

Exophthalmos

Neck

Enlargement

Hands

Tremor

PHYSICAL EXAMINATION

Measure the patient's vital signs and height and weight. Note the facial expression and characteristics as well as the mental alertness. Vital signs are important because they reflect the metabolic rate. Thyroid disorders may cause increased or decreased heart rate, respirations, blood pressure (BP), and temperature as well as irregular heart rhythms. Inspect and palpate the skin for moisture, temperature, and texture. In the head and neck examination, note the hair texture. Examine the eyes for **exophthalmos** (bulging). Inspect the neck for enlargement typical of goiter. Observe the hands for tremor. Nurses with advanced physical examination skills may palpate the neck for thyroid enlargement or nodules.

Key components of the nursing assessment of the patient with a thyroid disorder are outlined in Box 47-1.

DIAGNOSTIC TESTS AND PROCEDURES

Diagnostic studies of the thyroid gland include laboratory blood tests and studies employing radioactive iodine (RAI). Table 47-1 summarizes the use of each test and identifies nursing implications.

The most useful tests of thyroid function are measurements of serum TSH and free T4. The thyroid-releasing hormone (TRH) stimulation test measures the blood level of TSH after administration of TRH. This test shows whether thyroid hormone abnormalities are caused by a disorder of the thyroid gland itself or by altered production of stimulating hormones by the hypothalamus or the pituitary. Additional blood tests may help to determine the type of dysfunction.

The thyroid gland uses iodine to manufacture hormones. Therefore RAI isotopes (iodine-131 [^{131}I], iodine-123 [^{123}I], and technetium-99m [99mTc]) are useful for diagnostic purposes because they concentrate in the thyroid. The amount of iodine taken up by the thyroid is measured to assess the activity level of the gland. This test is called a *RAI uptake test.*

For a thyroid scan, the patient ingests RAI; then a specialized instrument is used to scan the area of the thyroid gland. It creates an image of the gland based on the distribution of the iodine. The image aids in diagnosing cancer because the patterns of iodine concentration in normal and malignant tissue are different. The scan may be repeated at specific intervals. The low dose of radiation used for diagnostic purposes poses no danger to the patient or others. However, pregnancy is a contraindication because of possible harm to the fetus.

Thyroid ultrasonography yields very clear images of the thyroid gland and any nodules present. This technology can be used to guide a needle for aspiration of samples from the nodules. For evaluation of metastatic disease or to image the portion of the thyroid concealed by the sternum, magnetic resonance imaging (MRI) or computed tomography (CT) is used.

Put on Your Thinking Cap!

A patient's blood studies show a high level of TSH and a low level of T_4. Explain what this finding means.

DISORDERS OF THE THYROID GLAND

HYPERTHYROIDISM

Hyperthyroidism, or thyrotoxicosis, is characterized by abnormally increased synthesis and secretion of thyroid hormones. The most common types of hyperthyroidism are Graves disease (also called *toxic diffuse goiter*) and multinodular goiter (also called *toxic nodular goiter*).

Graves disease is thought to be an autoimmune disorder triggered by genetic and environmental factors. Antibodies activate TSH receptors, which in turn stimulate thyroid enlargement and hormone secretion. Graves disease develops most often in women. Whether treated or not, the condition tends to have periods of remission and exacerbation. Some patients with Graves disease eventually develop hypothyroidism.

Multinodular goiter occurs most often in women in their sixth and seventh decades. It is most likely to develop in people who have had goiter for a number of years. Hyperthyroidism in this case is caused by thyroid nodules that secrete excess thyroid hormone without TSH stimulation. There may be multiple hyperfunctioning small nodules or a single nodule (toxic adenoma). The nodules can be benign or malignant. Symptoms of hyperthyroidism are usually less severe with multinodular goiter than with Graves disease.

Because all types of hyperthyroidism have many common features and because Graves disease is the most common form, it will be used as the example of hyperthyroidism.

Signs and Symptoms

Many of the signs and symptoms of hyperthyroidism are caused by an increased metabolic rate and can range from mild to severe. Weight loss and nervousness may be the only symptoms in patients with a mild form of the disease. In more severe cases, the patient's history may reveal restlessness, irritable behavior, sleep disturbances, emotional lability, personality changes, hair loss, and fatigue. Weight loss, even when the patient is eating well, is common. Some patients overcompensate for the increased metabolism, overeat, and gain weight. Many patients report poor tolerance of heat and excessive perspiration. Changes in menstrual and bowel patterns may occur. Examination findings may include warm, moist, velvety skin; fine tremors of the hands; swelling of the neck; and exophthalmos (protruding eyeballs). Exophthalmos is a classic sign of Graves disease. It is caused by fat accumulation, edema, and inflammation of the orbital contents. Tearing, light sensitivity, decreased visual acuity, and swelling around the orbit of the eye occur as well (Fig. 47-2).

Excess thyroid hormones stimulate the heart, causing tachycardia, increased systolic BP, and sometimes atrial fibrillation. The heart rate may be as rapid as 160 beats per minute (bpm). Even during sleep, the pulse may remain above 80 bpm.

Complications

If untreated, hyperthyroidism may lead to **thyrotoxicosis** (thyroid storm or crisis). Thyrotoxicosis is excessive stimulation caused by elevated thyroid hormone levels that produce dangerous tachycardia and hyperthermia. A risk of heart failure exists. The patient is restless and agitated and may lapse into a coma. Thyrotoxicosis is a medical emergency. Fortunately, modern treatment of hyperthyroidism makes this complication rare.

Table 47-1 Diagnostic Tests and Procedures Thyroid Disorders

TEST AND PURPOSE	PATIENT PREPARATION	POSTPROCEDURE CARE
Laboratory Studies		
***General Interventions:** Check your agency procedure manual for diagnostic tests and procedures. Always tell the patient what to expect when tests are ordered. Explain if nothing-by-mouth (NPO) status is necessary. Document the care provided and relevant assessment data. If venipuncture is done, apply a dressing and check the site oozing. Apply pressure and elevate arm if patient's blood clotting is impaired.		
Serum T3 (triiodothyronine) and serum T4 (thyroxine): measurements of free and total T4 detect abnormal levels of thyroid hormones. Elevated T3 indicates possible Graves disease, toxic adenoma, and toxic nodular goiter. Elevated T4 indicates hyperthyroidism or excessive thyroid hormone replacement. T3 and T4 decrease with hypothyroidism.	*General Interventions. No fasting required. Some medications may be withheld before blood is drawn.	*General Interventions.
Serum thyroid-stimulating hormone (TSH): increases with hypothyroidism and decreases with hyperthyroidism.	*General Interventions.	*General Interventions.
Thyroid-releasing hormone (TRH) stimulation test: assesses the response of the pituitary to TRH and differentiates the types of hypothyroidism. TRH normally increases after TRH is given intravenously.	Tell the patient that a drug will be given intravenously; then several blood samples must be drawn.	*General Interventions.
Uptake and Imaging Procedures		
Radioactive iodine (RAI) uptake test: After RAI is given orally, the amount of iodine-131 (131I) taken up by thyroid is measured with a special instrument. High uptake is seen with hyperthyroidism and low uptake is seen with hypothyroidism.	Tell the patient that the procedure is painless. Ask about pregnancy, in which case radiation is contraindicated. Advise the patient that the radiation dose is small and will not harm others.	For 24 hours after the test, the patient should be sure to wash his or her hands thoroughly with soap and water after voiding. If a caregiver discards the patient's urine, gloves should be worn; the used gloves should be washed, removed, and the caregiver's bare hands washed. Pregnant women should avoid patient contact for 24 hours.
Thyroid scan: ^{131}I, iodine-123 (^{123}I), or technetium-99m (99mTc) is given orally and a scanner is used to detect the pattern of uptake by the thyroid gland. This test can differentiate benign and malignant nodules as well as other abnormalities.	Tell the patient that if ^{131}I is used, he or she will be given the isotope in liquid form and will return to radiology 24 hours later for the scan. With ^{123}I, the scan is done after 3 to 6 hours. The patient will have to lie still on his or her back for 20 minutes during the scan. For 1 week before the test, the patient should not consume iodine. Iodine is in radiographic dyes, some oral contraceptives, weight control drugs, multivitamins, all thyroid drugs, and some food (especially seafood).	Postprocedure care is the same as for the RAI uptake test.
Thyroid ultrasonography: provides high-quality images of the thyroid and any nodules.	Advise the patient that the procedure is painless and noninvasive. An instrument is moved over the neck area and uses sound waves to create an image of the gland.	No special care is needed.
Fine-needle aspiration biopsy: Material from thyroid nodules can be aspirated using a needle and guided by ultrasonography.	Give the patient the same instructions as for thyroid ultrasonography. Tell the patient that the physician will use a small needle to remove a tissue sample.	Assess the patient for any signs of bleeding: swelling in the area of the biopsy site, bleeding from the puncture site, increasing pulse.

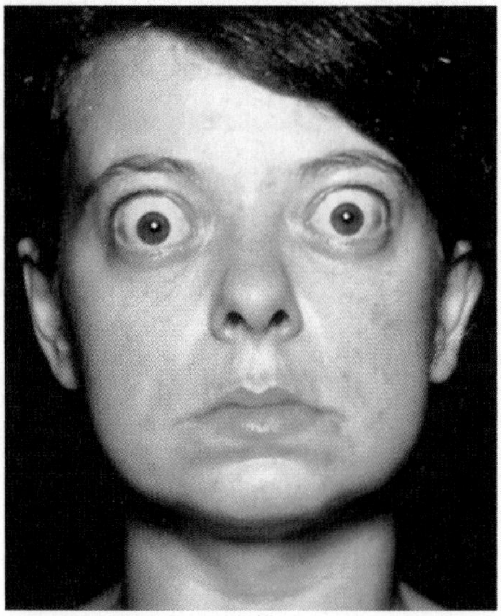

FIGURE 47-2 This patient has exophthalmos, bulging eyes, associated with Graves disease. (From Ignatavicius DD, Workman ML: *Medical-surgical nursing: patient-centered collaborative care*, ed 6, St. Louis, 2010, Saunders.)

Medical Diagnosis

Laboratory findings consistent with Graves disease are decreased TSH and elevated serum T4. TSH can be so low that it cannot be detected in the blood. Measurement of thyroid-stimulating antibodies and results of an RAI uptake test are useful in specifically diagnosing Graves disease.

Medical Treatment

Three methods are used to treat hyperthyroidism: (1) drug therapy, (2) radiation therapy, and (3) surgery. In addition, beta-adrenergic blockers such as propranolol (Inderal) may be given to relieve some of the cardiovascular symptoms associated with hyperthyroidism.

Drug Therapy. Hyperthyroidism may be treated initially with antithyroid drugs (i.e., drugs that block the synthesis, release, or activity of thyroid hormones). Thionamides and iodides are antithyroid drugs. Although these drugs can be used for long-term treatment of hyperthyroidism, they often are used temporarily to lower the level of hormones in the blood before surgery or radiation therapy. This process reduces the risk of bleeding and lowers the danger of releasing large amounts of thyroid hormones into the bloodstream during surgery. When a patient is on drugs that interfere with T4 secretion, monitor for symptoms of hypothyroidism (e.g., cold intolerance, edema, weight gain).

Pharmacology Capsule

Patients on antithyroid drugs must be monitored for hypothyroidism.

Thionamides. Examples of thionamides are propylthiouracil (PTU) and methimazole (Tapazole). It usually takes several weeks before the effects of thionamides are noticeable. The drugs may be given for months or years. The goal is to induce a remission that will allow the drugs to be discontinued. A disadvantage of thionamides is that they can cause agranulocytosis, a condition in which the production of neutrophils is suppressed. Without adequate neutrophils, the patient is unable to resist infection. Any signs of infection, such as sore throat or fever, should be reported to the physician immediately.

Iodides. Iodides are useful because iodine inhibits the synthesis of thyroid hormones. They are used most often after a course of PTU to suppress hormone secretion before thyroidectomy. The iodides also may be used to treat thyrotoxicosis. Saturated solution of potassium iodide (SSKI) can be given to people who have been exposed to radiation to prevent damage to the thyroid gland.

The iodides most often used to treat hyperthyroidism are Lugol iodine (5% iodine and 10% SSKI) and SSKI. Iodides may bring some relief within 24 hours but it takes several weeks for maximum effect. The effect does not last as long as that of thionamides; therefore iodides are not generally used as the sole treatment for hyperthyroidism.

Iodine solutions can cause discoloration of the teeth and gastric upset. These effects are minimized if the iodine solution is diluted with milk, fruit juice, or some other beverage and sipped through a straw. Signs of iodine toxicity include swelling and irritation of the mucous membranes and increased salivation.

Pharmacology Capsule

Iodine solutions can stain the teeth! They should be mixed with a beverage and sipped through a straw.

Radioactive Iodine. RAI (iodine-131) can be used alone or with antithyroid drugs to treat hyperthyroidism. It quickly accumulates in the thyroid gland, where it destroys thyroid tissue. However, the resulting decrease in thyroid hormone production is not evident for several months. Meanwhile, beta-adrenergic blockers can be given to control cardiac symptoms.

The radiation dose used to treat hyperthyroidism does not pose a threat to others. However, it should not be used during pregnancy because it affects the thyroid gland of the fetus. Side effects of the treatment are minimal. Inflammation of the thyroid gland (**thyroiditis**) and the parotid glands (**parotiditis**) may occur. Parotiditis causes the mouth to be dry and irritated. Hypothyroidism may develop years after treatment. Drugs used to treat thyroid disorders are summarized in Table 47-2.

Surgical Treatment. Graves disease is often treated by removing most of the thyroid gland. This procedure is called a *subtotal thyroidectomy.* The procedure may be done endoscopically or through a larger incision across

Table 47-2 **Drug Therapy: Thyroid Conditions**

DRUG	USE AND ACTION	SIDE EFFECTS	NURSING INTERVENTIONS
Thyroid Hormone Replacement Drugs			
levothyroxine (Synthroid), liothyronine (Cytomel), liotrix (Thyrolar)	Treat hypothyroidism and thyroiditis (increases the metabolic rate).	Overdose: irritability, insomnia, nervousness, tachycardia, diarrhea, and weight loss may occur.	Older patients are more susceptible to toxicity. Low doses are given initially and gradually increased. Lifelong therapy usually required. Monitor the pulse and blood pressure (BP) of older patients. Withhold the medication and notify the physician if the patient's pulse is greater than 100 beats per minute (bpm). Thyroid preparations interact with many other drugs by affecting the metabolic rate.
Antithyroid Drugs			
Thionamides			
methimazole (Tapazole), propylthiouracil (PTU)	Treat hyperthyroidism by interfering with the synthesis of thyroid hormones.	Agranulocytosis, rash, thrombocytopenia, skin discoloration, fever, headache, drowsiness, diarrhea, nausea, and vomiting.	Avoid during pregnancy. Monitor for bleeding because of decreased platelets and prothrombin, signs of liver toxicity (e.g., jaundice, abdominal pain), agranulocytosis (e.g., fever, sore throat, malaise), and hypothyroidism (e.g., weight gain, fatigue). Tell the patient to report any of these signs and symptoms to the physician. Safety precautions if drowsy. Stress importance of appointments.
Iodides			
Strong iodine solution (Lugol iodine), saturated solution of potassium iodide (SSKI)	Reduce size and vascularity of the thyroid gland in hyperthyroidism. May be used before thyroidectomy.	Excess iodine: fever, rash, oral lesions, metallic taste, diarrhea, parotitis, hypothyroidism.	Dilute liquids in water, fruit juice, or milk. Give SSKI after meals. Reduce the unpleasant taste and tooth-staining potential by having the patient use a straw. Monitor for symptoms of excess iodine.
Radioactive iodine (RAI): iodine-131 (^{131}I) and iodine-123 (^{123}I)	Used in thyroid scans (concentrates in thyroid tissue). A higher therapeutic dose destroys thyroid tissue in hyperthyroidism and thyroid malignancies.	Diagnostic dose: no side effects. Therapeutic dose: nausea, vomiting.	Diagnostic dose usually requires no radiation precautions except precautions with urine for 24 hours after the test (see Table 47-1). Therapeutic dose requires isolation measures. Monitor the patient for signs of hypothyroidism (e.g., fatigue, weight gain).

the top of the clavicles. As mentioned earlier, patients are commonly given antithyroid drug therapy for several weeks before surgery. Before these drugs were commonly used, patients often had dramatic postoperative responses because of the escape of thyroid hormones into the bloodstream during surgery. This severe episode of hyperthyroidism, called *thyroid storm* or *thyroid crisis*, is a medical emergency because it is potentially fatal.

❖ NURSING CARE of the Nonsurgical Patient with Hyperthyroidism

Most patients with hyperthyroidism are treated as outpatients. Therefore the nurse in the community or long-term care setting may need to help the patient learn to adapt until treatment brings relief (see Table 47-2).

■ Assessment

Complete assessment of the patient with a thyroid disorder is summarized in Box 47-1. Data collected by the LVN/LPN help to provide a detailed picture of the patient's status. For the patient with hyperthyroidism, significant data would include activity tolerance, heat tolerance, bowel elimination pattern, appetite, weight changes, and food intake. Also consider the patient's mental-emotional state, adaptation to the condition, and understanding of the treatment. Measure vital signs and height and weight. Document skin texture and edema.

Nursing Diagnoses, Goals, and Outcome Criteria: Hyperthyroidism

Nursing Diagnoses	Goals and Outcome Criteria
Decreased Cardiac Output related to cardiac dysrhythmias or heart failure caused by excessive thyroid hormone stimulation	Normal cardiac output: pulse and blood pressure (BP) within patient norms, no edema or dyspnea (signs and symptoms of heart failure)
Disturbed Sleep Pattern related to metabolic disturbance	Improved sleep pattern: absence of insomnia, patient describes feeling rested on awakening
Hyperthermia related to increased metabolic energy production	Improved heat tolerance: patient statement of comfort in relation to environmental temperature, no excess perspiration
Imbalanced Nutrition: Less Than Body Requirements related to increased metabolic requirements	Adequate nutrition: stable body weight if no significant recent loss, weight gain if underweight
Risk for Injury related to exophthalmos	Decreased risk of eye injury: lids cover eyeball, eyeball is moist, no pain associated with corneal injury
Impaired Comfort related to ophthalmopathy	Improved comfort: patient reports less eye pain, photosensitivity
Diarrhea related to excessive thyroid hormone stimulation	Normal bowel elimination: formed stools at regular intervals

Put on Your Thinking Cap!

Explain why people with hyperthyroidism do not tolerate heat well.

Interventions

When a person is treated as an outpatient, teaching should focus on self-care. In the unlikely event that a patient is hospitalized for hyperthyroidism, the nurse provides more direct care.

Decreased Cardiac Output

Monitor the patient's pulse and blood pressure for elevations. Give beta-adrenergic blockers as ordered to counteract the stimulant effects of the elevated thyroid hormones. Signs of heart failure include tachycardia, tachypnea, dyspnea, confusion, and edema. Older adults require especially careful monitoring because they are more susceptible to cardiovascular stress with thyroid disease. Immediately report any signs of heart failure to the RN or physician. Medical treatment of heart failure usually includes oxygen, intravenous fluids, sedatives, and cardiac drugs.

Disturbed Sleep Pattern

Despite fatigue and weakness, the hyperthyroid patient often feels restless and has trouble sleeping. Encourage the patient to arrange the day to allow periods of rest. Caffeine should be avoided because of its stimulating effects. Encourage bedtime rituals, which may be helpful in preparing for sleep. For the hospitalized patient, provide a restful environment and a soothing back rub to promote relaxation. Give sedatives as ordered to promote sleep.

In addition to physical rest, patients need emotional rest. The patient and the family may be able to cope better if they understand the reason for the patient's irritability and nervousness. Patients need to recognize stressful situations and avoid them.

Hyperthermia

Hyperthyroid patients usually have some heat intolerance because of their high metabolic rate. They tend to feel too warm even when others are comfortable. Only light clothing may be needed. Adjust the environmental temperature as much as possible for comfort. A private room allows the patient more freedom to select the room temperature. If the patient perspires heavily, frequent bathing and clothing changes help to promote comfort.

Imbalanced Nutrition: Less Than Body Requirements

Despite a normal dietary intake, the patient may not be meeting the increased caloric needs (see *Nutrition Considerations* box). Weigh daily to monitor nutritional adequacy. A diet high in calories, vitamins, and minerals is recommended. Depending on the severity of the condition, the patient may need additional full meals or between-meal snacks. Some patients require as many as 4000 to 5000 calories daily to maintain body weight. The physician may order supplementary vitamins. Additional fluids are recommended to replace fluids lost through increased insensible loss (i.e., fluid lost through the skin and the lungs).

Nutrition Considerations

1. Hypothyroid and hyperthyroid patients may require adjustments in calorie intake that are appropriate to metabolic needs.
2. Lack of iodine is associated with the development of a goiter (enlargement of the thyroid gland) in adults and cretinism in infants.
3. Iodized salt is the best way to obtain an adequate amount of iodine in the diet.
4. Another important source of iodine is saltwater seafood.
5. Parathyroid hormone (PTH), secreted by the parathyroid gland, and thyrocalcitonin, secreted by the thyroid gland, maintain serum calcium levels.

Risk for Injury

Exophthalmos is a condition in which deposits of fat and fluid behind the eyeballs make them bulge outward (see Fig. 47-2). Both eyes are usually affected. If the condition is severe, the eyelids do not cover the eyeballs. The eyeballs are not kept moist and are susceptible to injury. It may be necessary to tape the lids shut. Lubricated eye pads or artificial tears may be used. Raising the head of the bed at night and limiting salt intake may be helpful.

The patient with exophthalmos has a startled appearance. This may make the person self-conscious and embarrassed. Dark glasses help to conceal the eyes. For these patients, *disturbed body image* is an important additional nursing diagnosis. Reassure the patient that the condition usually goes away after treatment of hyperthyroidism.

Impaired Comfort

In addition to exophthalmos, the hyperthyroid patient has a variety of eye symptoms that may include double vision, periorbital edema, tearing, photosensitivity, and a feeling of "sand" in the eyes. It helps to elevate the head of the bed, reduce bright lighting, and advise use of tinted glasses. Methylcellulose eye drops and diuretics may be ordered to decrease inflammation and swelling. Severe inflammation is treated with a 2- to 4-week course of prednisone. After acute inflammation subsides, surgical procedures on the eyeball muscles and the eyelids may be needed to eliminate double vision and to restore coverage of the eye.

Diarrhea

If the patient has diarrhea, electrolyte imbalances and skin irritation may result. Give antidiarrheal medications as ordered and monitor the effect. Thorough perianal cleansing after each stool reduces the risk of skin breakdown.

Patient Teaching

Hyperthyroidism

- This is a chronic condition that requires long-term care.
- You must take your medications exactly as prescribed.
- Notify your physician of excessive fatigue and depression, which may indicate hypothyroidism caused by your antithyroid drug.

❖ NURSING CARE of the Patient Having a Thyroidectomy

General care of the surgical patient is discussed in Chapter 17. This section covers the special needs of the patient having a thyroidectomy.

■ Assessment

Preoperative Care

The preparation of the patient undergoing thyroid surgery is essentially the same as for any major surgery. Ask what the patient knows about surgery and what to expect before and after the procedure. Nursing diagnoses may include those listed earlier for hyperthyroidism but the condition is usually brought under control before surgery is scheduled. In addition, identify and address learning needs (see *Patient Teaching* box). Teaching is the primary preoperative nursing intervention. The goals of preoperative teaching are patient understanding of the usual preoperative and postoperative procedures and decreased anxiety. Tell the patient to expect a dressing on the front of the neck. The size of the incision will depend on the surgical approach used. Demonstrate how to avoid straining the neck incision by supporting the head when rising. To evaluate the effectiveness of preoperative teaching, ask the patient to repeat the information presented. Ask patients to return demonstrations of activities such as deep breathing and supporting the head during position changes.

Postoperative Care

The patient usually recovers quickly from a thyroidectomy and may be discharged in 1 or 2 days. Rare but serious complications are airway obstruction, recurrent laryngeal nerve damage, hemorrhage, and tetany (a sign of hypocalcemia associated with damage to the parathyroids). One other complication, thyroid crisis, is usually prevented by preoperative treatment with antithyroid drugs.

If part of the thyroid gland is left (i.e., subtotal thyroidectomy), it should eventually regenerate and produce adequate hormones. The patient may be somewhat hypothyroid at first but replacement therapy is not recommended. Giving thyroid hormone would interfere with the regeneration of thyroid tissue.

Immediately after thyroidectomy, it is especially important to *assess* and *document* respiratory status, level of consciousness, wound drainage or bleeding, voice quality, comfort, and neuromuscular irritability (muscle twitching, spasms).

■ Interventions

Ineffective Airway Clearance

Turning and deep breathing are recommended to prevent respiratory complications, as with any other surgical patient. However, the surgeon may not want the patient to cough because of possible stress on the suture line.

It is especially important to monitor and document the rate and ease of respirations after thyroidectomy. Respiratory distress can result from compression of the trachea or from a spasm of the larynx because of nerve damage or hypocalcemia. Before the patient returns

Nursing Diagnoses, Goals, and Outcome Criteria: Thyroidectomy

Nursing Diagnoses	Goals and Outcome Criteria
Ineffective Airway Clearance related to airway obstruction, laryngeal nerve damage, laryngeal spasm	Effective airway clearance: normal breath sounds, respiratory rate of 12 to 20 breaths per minute, no dyspnea
Decreased Cardiac Output related to blood loss, heart failure (HF) secondary to thyroid crisis	Normal cardiac output: pulse and blood pressure (BP) within normal limits, no edema
Disturbed Body Image related to surgical scar	Adaptation to change in appearance: looks at scar, verbalizes acceptance of scar
Acute Pain related to tissue trauma	Pain relief: patient statement of less or no pain, relaxed manner
Risk for Infection related to impaired skin integrity	Absence of infection: wound margins intact, minimal redness, no purulent drainage, normal body temperature

from surgery, suction equipment, a laryngoscope, an endotracheal tube, oxygen (O_2), and an emergency tracheotomy tray must be available. Your agency may require the tracheotomy tray at the bedside. Elevate the head of the bed to decrease edema. Use pillows to prop and support the head to avoid stress on the suture line.

Because of the location of the thyroidectomy incision, edema or bleeding can cause pressure on the trachea. Signs and symptoms of poor oxygenation because of airway obstruction or blood loss include restlessness, increasing pulse and respiratory rates, and dyspnea. Without prompt intervention, the patient with airway obstruction could die.

The laryngeal nerve innervates the vocal cords. If it is damaged during surgery, vocal cord paralysis can occur. Paralysis of both cords may cause spasms (**laryngospasm**) that close the airway. An emergency tracheotomy is needed to restore the airway. Signs of laryngeal nerve damage are hoarseness and inability to speak. This is more severe than the usual hoarseness most people have after general anesthesia. Ask the patient to respond verbally to simple questions to determine voice quality.

Before the function of the parathyroid glands was understood, patients having a thyroidectomy often experienced unexplained muscle contractions and respiratory difficulty that sometimes led to death. Eventually, it was determined that the symptoms were caused by hypocalcemia because of a deficiency of parathyroid hormone (PTH). Surgeons are now careful to locate and spare the small parathyroid glands. Occasionally, however, the parathyroid glands are injured or accidentally removed during thyroidectomy.

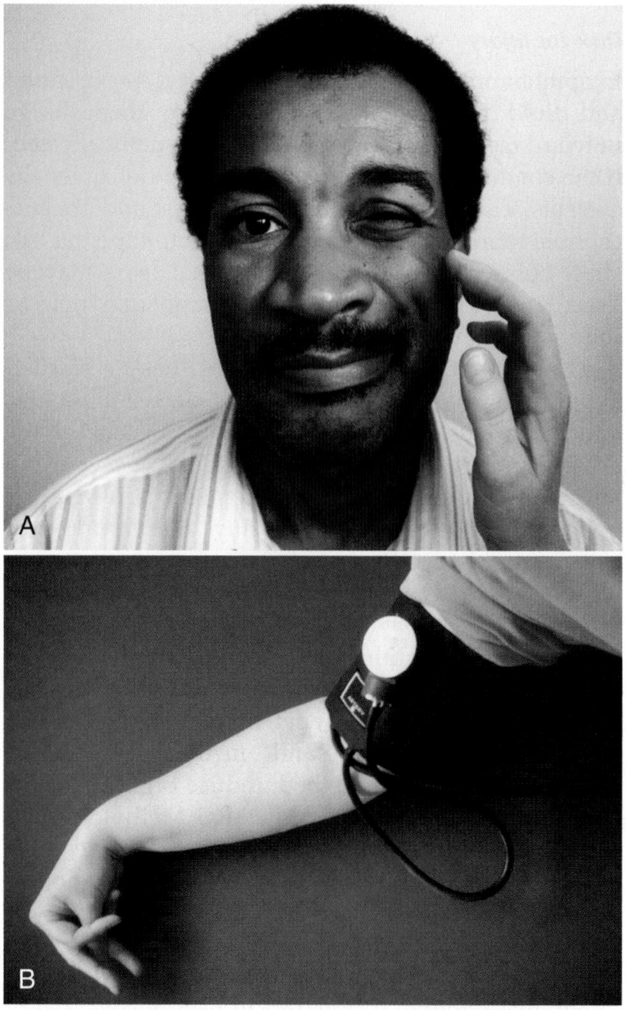

FIGURE 47-3 Signs of hypocalcemia. **A,** Chvostek sign (facial twitch). **B,** Trousseau sign (carpopedal spasm). (From Ignatavicius DD, Workman ML: *Medical-surgical nursing: patient-centered collaborative care*, ed 6, St. Louis, 2010, Saunders.)

Without PTH, the serum calcium level falls, thus causing **tetany**. Muscle contractions begin as twitches around the mouth and eyes. The face, fingers, and toes begin to tingle. The patient may have painful "cramps," including the classic signs depicted in Figure 47-3. The most serious effect of hypocalcemia is spasm of the larynx. As the larynx closes, the patient has difficulty breathing and can suffocate. Cardiac dysrhythmias and seizures also can occur.

Tetany is treated with calcium salts given intravenously or orally. The condition usually improves as the injured parathyroid glands recover. Rarely is hypoparathyroidism permanent. If it is, lifetime treatment is required, as described later in the section on "Hypoparathyroidism."

Decreased Cardiac Output

Frequently inspect the dressing to detect bleeding and take the vital signs. Because the dressing is on the front of the neck, blood might flow under the dressing to the back of the neck. Therefore be sure to check behind the patient's neck and upper back to detect this.

Complementary and Alternative Therapies

Position changes and back rubs enhance the effects of prescribed analgesics.

Thyroid crisis (thyroid storm) can develop when large amounts of thyroid hormone enter the bloodstream during surgery or when patients with severe hyperthyroidism develop a severe illness or infection. This postoperative complication is rare because surgery is typically delayed until serum hormone levels are reduced. However, a brief description follows. Approximately 12 hours after surgery, the patient in thyroid crisis shows signs of severe hyperthyroidism (e.g., tachycardia, cardiac dysrhythmias, vomiting, fever, confusion).

If not treated promptly, the patient will die as a result of HF. Early detection of thyroid crisis requires careful monitoring of vital signs during the first postoperative day. Treatment of thyroid crisis consists of antithyroid drugs, intravenous sodium iodide, corticosteroids, beta-adrenergic blockers, antipyretics, intravenous fluids, O_2, and a hypothermia (cooling) blanket or other measures to reduce body temperature.

Disturbed Body Image

The patient may be worried about the appearance of the surgical scar. Thyroidectomy incisions follow the natural contours of the neck. Once the scar fades, it usually is not noticeable. Meanwhile, it is easy to conceal the fresh scar with clothing. If an endoscopic procedure is used, the incisions will be very small.

Acute Pain

Frequently inquire about the postoperative patient's comfort level. Promptly administer prescribed analgesics and evaluate and document effects. Chapter 15 discusses pain management in detail.

Risk for Infection

Whenever the skin is broken, the potential for infection exists. Practice good hand washing and use aseptic technique when handling dressings. Tell the patient to avoid touching the fresh incision and to report any signs and symptoms of infection (i.e., fever, increasing wound redness and swelling, foul drainage). Protect the incision from strain and possible dehiscence by supporting the neck when arising and reclining (see *Patient Teaching* box).

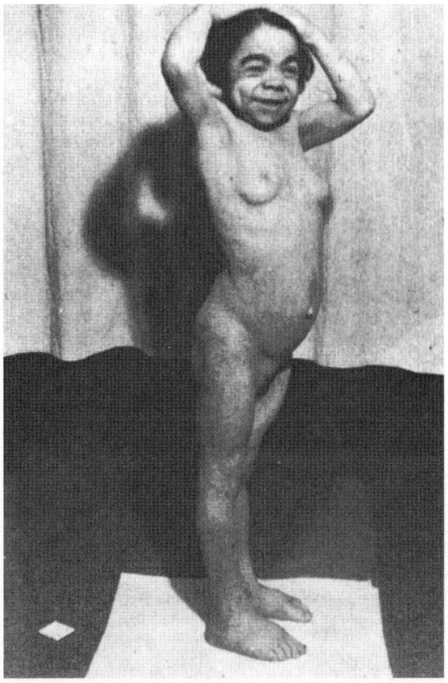

FIGURE 47-4 Cretinism is a condition of permanent physical and mental retardation resulting from untreated hypothyroidism in infancy. (From Ignatavicius DD, Workman ML, Mishler M: *Medical-surgical nursing across the health care continuum*. Philadelphia, 1991, Saunders.)

Patient Teaching

Thyroidectomy

- If all of your thyroid gland was removed, you will need lifelong replacement of thyroid hormones.
- If only part of your thyroid gland was removed, you may feel tired for a while; however, this should improve as the remaining gland increases hormone production.
- Thyroidectomy scars usually heal so that they are eventually barely noticeable; they are easily concealed with clothing.
- Take your drugs exactly as prescribed.
- Nervousness and palpitations may be adverse effects of thyroid replacement drugs (hyperthyroidism); notify the physician if they occur.

HYPOTHYROIDISM

Hypothyroidism is the result of inadequate secretion of thyroid hormones. It is seen in infants, children, and adults. If not treated early, hypothyroidism during infancy causes permanent retardation of physical and mental development (**cretinism**) (Fig. 47-4) (see *Cultural Considerations* box). The effects in adults can be quite serious but usually are reversible with treatment. The term **myxedema** sometimes is used for hypothyroidism. Myxedema actually refers to edema that develops in the hands, face, feet, and area around the eyes with severe, long-term hypothyroidism (Fig. 47-5). Not all hypothyroid patients have myxedema.

Cultural Considerations

What Does Culture Have to Do with Cretinism?

Neonatal hypothyroidism, which causes cretinism if not corrected early, is much more common among Caucasians than among those of African heritage.

Cause and Risk Factors

Hypothyroidism has many causes, including atrophy of the thyroid gland after years of Graves disease or thyroiditis, treatment for hyperthyroidism, dietary iodine deficiency, high intake of **goitrogens**, and defects in thyroid hormone synthesis. These are examples of *primary hypothyroidism.* They account for 90% to 95% of all cases of hypothyroidism. Some foods and drugs act as goitrogens, meaning that they suppress thyroid hormone production. Examples of foods that are goitrogens if taken in large quantities are soybeans, turnips, and rutabagas. Goitrogenic drugs that often are used to treat hyperthyroidism are propylthiouracil, methimazole, and iodine (see *Cultural Considerations* box).

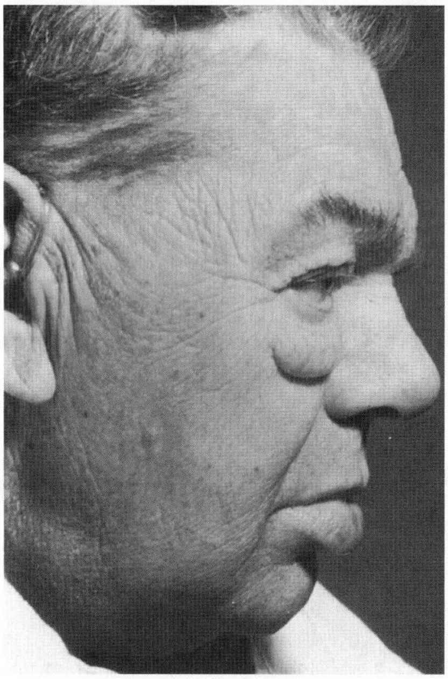

FIGURE 47-5 Typical appearance of the patient with myxedema. (From Jacob WW, Francone CA: *Elements of anatomy and physiology*, ed 2, Philadelphia, 1989, Saunders.)

Cultural Considerations

What Does Culture Have to Do with Hypothyroidism?

The incidence of hypothyroidism is 10 to 20 times higher in iodine-deficient parts of the world (e.g., Zaire, Nepal) than in the United States.

Hypothyroidism caused by pituitary or hypothalamic disorders is called *secondary hypothyroidism.* Deficiency of TSH lowers the secretion of thyroid hormones even though the thyroid gland itself remains normal. Of course, patients who have had their entire thyroid or pituitary gland surgically removed also will be hypothyroid. Hypothyroidism also can result from tissue resistance to thyroid hormone—that is, the hormone is present but the body cells are unable to use it normally.

Signs and Symptoms

The signs and symptoms of hypothyroidism in general are the opposite of those of hyperthyroidism (Table 47-3). The onset is usually gradual. The metabolic rate slows, often causing weight gain even with decreased food intake. Hypothyroid patients commonly report

Table 47-3 Comparison of Signs and Symptoms of Hypothyroidism and Hyperthyroidism

SYSTEM	HYPOTHYROIDISM	HYPERTHYROIDISM
Integumentary	Coarse, dry skin and hair; thick nails	Smooth, moist skin; silky hair; diaphoresis
Musculoskeletal	Muscle aches and pains, weakness, slow movements	Weakness
Cardiovascular	Bradycardia, dysrhythmias, hypotension, anemia, capillary fragility	Tachycardia, dysrhythmias, palpitations, systolic hypertension, angina
Respiratory	Hypoventilation, dyspnea	Increased respiratory rate, dyspnea
Gastrointestinal (GI)	Anorexia, nausea and vomiting, constipation, weight gain	Increased appetite, increased bowel sounds, diarrhea, weight loss
Neurologic	Apathy, lethargy, slowed mental function, depression, slow speech, paresthesias, decreased tendon reflexes	Nervousness and irritability, insomnia, personality change, agitation, inability to concentrate, fine tremor of fingers and tongue, hyperreflexia
Reproductive	Women: amenorrhea or prolonged menses, infertility, decreased libido Men: decreased libido, erectile dysfunction	Women: menstrual irregularities, decreased libido Men: decreased libido, erectile dysfunction, gynecomastia
Other	Cold intolerance, decreased body temperature, facial puffiness or coarseness, thick tongue, nonpitting edema of hands and feet, sensitivity to central nervous system (CNS) depressants	Increased body temperature, exophthalmos, goiter, sensitivity to CNS stimulants

lethargy, forgetfulness, and irritability. They may experience frequent headaches, constipation, menstrual disorders, numbness and tingling in the arms and legs, and intolerance to cold. The pulse tends to be slow and dyspnea may be present.

Examination may reveal swelling of the lips and eyelids; dry, thick skin; bruising; thin, coarse hair; and hoarseness. Generalized nonpitting edema and facial edema may be present. The patient may seem slow, depressed, or apathetic. Pallor may be present, associated with anemia. Signs and symptoms may be more subtle in the older patient or may be masked by signs and symptoms of other acute or chronic disorders. Therefore thyroid function in older adults should be assessed as part of routine checkups.

Medical Diagnosis

Hypothyroidism is diagnosed based on the laboratory determination of free T4 and TSH. A TRH stimulation test also may be ordered. Free T4 is low with hypothyroidism, except when the problem is tissue resistance to the hormone. TSH level enables the physician to determine whether the basic problem is primary or secondary hypothyroidism.

Complications

Severe, untreated hypothyroidism can progress to myxedema coma. Infection, trauma, excessive chilling, and some drugs (opioids, sedatives, and tranquilizers) may precipitate myxedema coma in a hypothyroid patient. The main signs of this life-threatening condition are hypothermia, hypotension, and hypoventilation.

Medical Treatment

Hypothyroidism is treated with hormone replacement therapy, most commonly levothyroxine (Synthroid). Patients should be monitored periodically to evaluate the response to therapy. A patient with heart disease may have difficulty adapting to a sudden increase in metabolic rate. For that reason, replacement therapy for older patients or those with heart disease is usually started with a very low dose and gradually increased. If these patients have any chest pain once therapy is started, the physician should be notified immediately. Because of variations between brands, patients should consistently take the same brand. If a brand change is required, the serum TSH should be checked in 6 weeks and dosage adjusted as needed.

Pharmacology Capsule

Opioids, sedatives, and tranquilizers can precipitate potentially fatal myxedema coma in a severely hypothyroid person.

NURSING CARE of the Patient with Hypothyroidism

Hypothyroidism usually does not require hospitalization but it may be detected when patients are hospitalized for other reasons. Because the onset of symptoms is often subtle, the nurse in the community or long-term care setting must be alert for signs and symptoms of hypothyroidism (see Nursing Care Plan: Patient with Hypothyroidism).

Assessment

General assessment of the patient with a thyroid disorder is summarized in Box 47-1. Relevant data include

Nursing Diagnoses, Goals, and Outcome Criteria: Hypothyroidism

Nursing Diagnoses	Goals and Outcome Criteria
Activity Intolerance related to decreased metabolic energy production	Improved activity tolerance: patient report of less fatigue with daily activities
Imbalanced Nutrition: More Than Body Requirements related to intake greater than metabolic needs	Balanced nutrition: stable body weight or gradual return to weight before thyroid disorder
Hypothermia related to cold intolerance	Improved cold tolerance: warm hands and feet, no complaints of coldness
Constipation related to decreased peristalsis	Normal bowel function: regular stools without difficulty
Risk for Impaired Skin Integrity related to dryness and edema	Decreased risk of skin breakdown: skin moist, intact
Decreased Cardiac Output related to cardiovascular changes secondary to hypothyroidism	Normal cardiac output: improved stamina, pulse and blood pressure (BP) within normal limits; no dyspnea, edema, or dysrhythmias
Disturbed Body Image related to altered physical appearance, disturbed thought processes, lack of energy	Improved body image: patient makes positive statements about appearance, tends to personal appearance
Fatigue related to slow metabolism	Less fatigue : patient gradually resumes responsibility for personal care, completes care with less fatigue
Deficient Knowledge of effects of hypothyroidism and self-care related to lack of information	Improved knowledge: patient describes therapy, self-care, and intent to comply with instructions; patient understands that changes in mental and emotional status are symptoms of his or her condition and that they will improve with treatment

measurement of vital signs, height, and weight. In addition, ask about activity and temperature tolerance, voice quality, bowel elimination pattern, and changes in weight and dietary intake. Inspect and palpate the skin for turgor, texture, and moisture. Note level of consciousness and emotional state. Ask if the patient has noticed a change in mental alertness. Also explore the patient's understanding of hypothyroidism and its treatment.

Interventions

Activity Intolerance

The hypothyroid patient lacks energy and tires easily. Arrange the schedule to allow for rest periods. Sedatives and barbiturates should be avoided because they may cause excessive sedation. If they are given, lower dosages are recommended. Monitor and document the patient's respirations and level of consciousness.

Nursing Care Plan: Patient with Hypothyroidism

ASSESSMENT

HEALTH HISTORY A 53-year-old woman comes to the physician's office complaining of fatigue and irritability. Her symptoms have gradually worsened and are now interfering with her work as an executive assistant. She reports that her health has generally been good, with only one hospitalization for an appendectomy 7 years ago. The review of systems reveals frequent headaches, anorexia, constipation, menstrual irregularity, numbness and tingling in the legs, and intolerance to cold. She has noticed a 10-lb weight gain over the past 6 months without a change in diet or exercise.

PHYSICAL EXAMINATION Vital signs: blood pressure 90/60 mm Hg, pulse 56 bpm, respiration 18 breaths per minute, temperature 97°F (36.1°C) measured orally. Height 5′5″, weight 155 lb. Patient's record indicates that her previous blood pressure was 128/76 mm Hg and previous pulse was 74 bpm. She is oriented but lethargic. Her hair is coarse and her skin is dry.

Nursing Diagnosis	Goals and Outcome Criteria	Interventions
Activity Intolerance related to decreased metabolic energy production	The patient will report less fatigue with activities of daily living (ADL).	Advise the patient to schedule additional rest periods until the condition improves. Assure her that these symptoms are temporary.
Imbalanced Nutrition: More Than Body Requirements related to intake greater than metabolic needs	The patient's weight will stabilize within 2 lb of her usual 145 lb.	Weigh the patient during each office visit. Encourage a balanced diet. Tell her that her weight should normalize when the condition is corrected.
Hypothermia related to cold intolerance	The patient will report adequate warmth and increased tolerance of cool temperatures.	Advise the patient to adjust the room temperature for comfort. Provide adequate covering during physical examination.
Constipation related to decreased peristalsis	The patient will have regular bowel movements passed without straining.	Encourage increased fluid intake and a high-fiber diet with fresh fruits and raw vegetables. Instruct the patient in taking stool softeners if advised by physician. Encourage a gradual increase in physical activity as tolerance improves.
Risk for Impaired Skin Integrity related to dryness	The patient's skin will remain intact and usual moisture will be restored.	Advise the patient to decrease bathing frequency and to use moisturizing creams or lotions. Advise her to avoid scratching.
Decreased Cardiac Output related to cardiovascular changes secondary to hypothyroidism	The patient's cardiac output will improve, as evidenced by improved stamina, regular pulse between 60 and 100 beats per minute (bpm), blood pressure (BP) consistent with patient norms, and no dyspnea.	Monitor the patient for tachycardia, hypertension, and dysrhythmias after hormone replacement therapy is begun. Tell her to notify the physician if she has palpitations.
Deficient Knowledge of mental and emotional effects of hypothyroidism related to lack of information	Improved knowledge: The patient acknowledges that her mental and emotional symptoms will improve with treatment; patient will identify strategies to reduce workplace demands.	Explain that mental slowness is related to hypothyroidism and that it will improve with treatment. Do not overload the patient with information. Teach only the critical information initially and supplement it with written information. Ask her how her work expectations could be adjusted temporarily to accommodate her symptoms.
Fatigue related to slow metabolism	Less fatigue: The patient's ADL will be accomplished with only normal fatigue.	Ask the patient to consider her daily activities and set priorities. Encourage rest periods. Delay difficult or strenuous tasks until her condition improves.

Critical Thinking Questions

1. What is the most critical information you should teach the patient about hypothyroidism?
2. How can you help the patient to set priorities and determine daily activities?

Families and employers need to understand the patient's fatigue and make adjustments until the patient recovers. Improvement is gradual but is usually evident after 2 to 3 weeks.

Imbalanced Nutrition: More Than Body Requirements

Despite having a poor appetite, the patient may have gained weight. Weekly weights are helpful in evaluating the effects of hormone replacement therapy. Calorie reduction may be prescribed for the patient who is overweight. Encourage a balanced diet.

Hypothermia

Cold intolerance is a very uncomfortable effect of hypothyroidism. Provide extra clothing and blankets as needed. Maintain the room temperature at a level comfortable to the patient. This is easier to manage if the patient has a private room. Once thyroid replacement is initiated, cold intolerance gradually improves.

Constipation

Constipation is a common problem. Until the hypothyroidism is corrected, take measures to promote normal elimination. Adequate fluids, dietary fiber, and physical activity all help to reduce constipation. Bulk laxatives or stool softeners may be indicated if other measures do not solve the problem. Remember that adequate fluids are essential to prevent bowel obstruction with bulk laxatives. Older patients should increase activity levels gradually to avoid excessive stress on the heart.

Risk for Impaired Skin Integrity

Dry skin, which is common with hypothyroidism, is prone to breakdown. Liberally apply lotions and creams to help maintain moisture and control itching. Reduce the frequency of bathing to prevent additional drying of the skin.

Decreased Cardiac Output

Atherosclerosis and heart disease develop in patients whose hypothyroidism is uncorrected for a long time. Monitor these patients for any signs and symptoms of HF, such as dyspnea and increasing edema. After hormone replacement therapy is begun, some risk of excessive cardiac stimulation exists. Tell the patient that any chest pain should be reported promptly. Monitor the pulse to detect potentially serious changes in rhythm or rate. Remember that the older adult's circulatory system adapts more slowly to increased thyroid hormone.

Acute Confusion

Mental dullness and depression can significantly affect the patient's life. Explain that these symptoms are related to hypothyroidism and that correction of hypothyroidism usually results in marked improvement. (An exception is the person who has cretinism caused by untreated hypothyroidism during fetal development or early infancy. The mental retardation of cretinism is not reversible.) Until mental function improves, be careful not to demand too much of the patient. Break teaching into small units and reinforce at intervals.

Disturbed Body Image

The puffy, apathetic look and weight gain associated with hypothyroidism can be very distressing to the patient. Be accepting of the patient's concerns but encourage good grooming and attention to appearance. Tell the patient that treatment will gradually eliminate these changes.

Fatigue

Encourage the patient to examine daily activities in order to make a schedule that conserves energy. Assure him or her that fatigue gradually lessens with treatment. Educate the family about the patient's need for extra rest and relief from some responsibilities at this time.

Deficient Knowledge

The hypothyroid patient can expect to need lifelong hormone replacement therapy. Explain this to the patient and stress the need for periodic medical evaluation. Describe the name, dosage, and adverse effects of the prescribed drug therapy. Teach the patient the symptoms of hyperthyroidism that might occur with excessive hormone replacement (tachycardia, weight loss, nervousness). Document patient teaching.

Put on Your Thinking Cap!

A patient who was recently diagnosed with hypothyroidism complains that she has no appetite but has gained 20 lb over the past few months. How would you explain this to her?

GOITER

Goiter is the term used to describe enlargement of the thyroid gland. Enlargement may be caused by simple goiter, thyroid nodules, or thyroiditis.

Simple Goiter

Thyroid enlargement with normal thyroid hormone production is called *simple goiter* (Fig. 47-6). Causes include iodine deficiency and long-term exposure to goitrogens. The gland may enlarge to compensate for hypothyroidism. Sometimes the enlarged gland produces excess hormones, making the patient hyperthyroid.

The type of treatment depends on the degree of enlargement and level of thyroid hormone production. If enlargement is mild and hormones are normal, no intervention is required. Some patients need hormone replacement therapy. Surgery is indicated if pressure is noted on the trachea or esophagus or if the condition is disfiguring.

Nodules

Multinodular goiter is discussed earlier with "Hyperthyroidism." As noted, nodules can be benign or malignant. To help determine whether cancer is present, the physician may order a scan that uses RAI. Nodular goiters are usually removed surgically. In benign conditions, only the nodule may be removed.

THYROID CANCER

Thyroid cancer is not common. It is fatal in less than 1% of all cases. In the early stages, the only sign may be a nodule that can be felt on the thyroid gland. Later, if the cancer spreads, enlarged lymph nodes are felt in the neck. The patient may not show dramatic changes in thyroid hormone levels. Total thyroidectomy is the usual treatment. Nursing care of the thyroidectomy patient is covered in the section on "Hyperthyroidism." If the malignancy has spread beyond the thyroid gland, more radical surgery may be indicated.

Surgery may be followed with RAI treatment to destroy any remaining tissue that might harbor malignant cells. This is the same type of iodine used in diagnostic studies but a larger dose is used. The patient needs to be isolated and on radiation precautions. Body fluids must be handled according to radiation precaution guidelines because they are contaminated. The care of the patient receiving internal radiation therapy is discussed in Chapter 25.

The patient will be alarmed at the diagnosis of cancer. He or she may find some comfort in knowing that the 5-year survival rate for thyroid cancer is among the highest of all types of cancer. Long-term care after thyroid cancer includes management of hypothyroidism and monitoring for recurrence. Scans using RAI are sometimes ordered at intervals to detect the presence of any remaining cancerous tissue. Periodic TSH and thyroglobulin tests may be ordered. Thyroglobulin rises if thyroid cancer recurs. Thyroid replacement therapy is based on the TSH level.

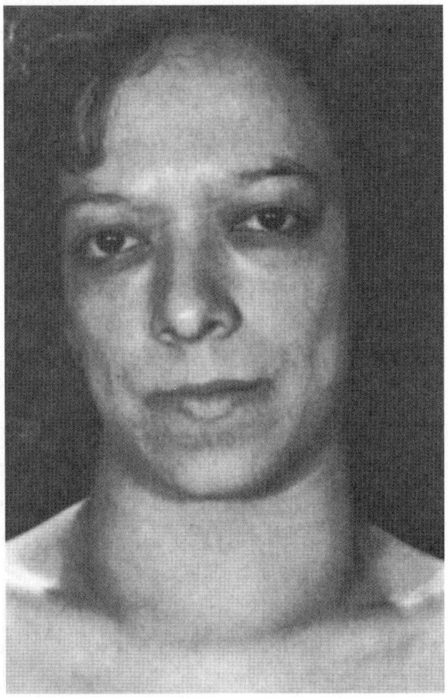

FIGURE 47-6 Goiter. (From Wilson J, Foster D: *Williams textbook of endocrinology*, ed 7, Philadelphia, 1985, Saunders.)

PARATHYROID GLANDS

ANATOMY AND PHYSIOLOGY OF THE PARATHYROID GLANDS

The parathyroid glands are small glands usually located on the back of the thyroid gland (Fig. 47-7). Occasionally some glands are found in the mediastinum as well. Most people have four parathyroids but some people have more. Even though they are typically embedded in the thyroid, the parathyroids function independently. They secrete only one hormone but it is a vital one. PTH, also called parathormone, plays a critical role in regulating the serum calcium level.

Calcium is an essential component of strong bones and plays a vital role in the functions of nerve and muscle cells. When the serum calcium level falls, PTH is secreted. PTH increases the absorption of calcium from the intestines, transfers calcium from the bones to the blood, and signals the kidneys to conserve calcium. In general, calcium retention by the kidney is balanced by phosphate loss.

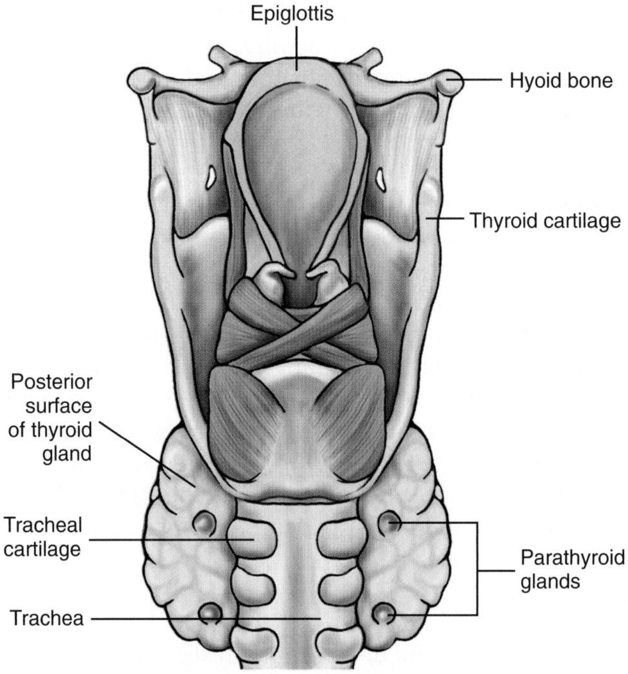

FIGURE 47-7 Posterior view of the neck and thyroid gland, showing the approximate location of the parathyroid glands. (From Monahan FD, Drake DT, Neighbors M, editors: *Medical-surgical nursing: foundations for clinical practice*, ed 2, Philadelphia, 1998, Saunders.)

NURSING ASSESSMENT OF PARATHYROID FUNCTION

HEALTH HISTORY

Although the RN is responsible for the complete assessment, the LVN/LPN may assist with data collection. Relevant data from the health history include changes in mental and emotional status, such as memory problems, irritability, or personality changes. Ask about a history of musculoskeletal problems, including weakness, skeletal pain, backache, and muscle twitching or spasms. Note if the patient has experienced urinary frequency, polyuria, urinary calculi (stones), or constipation. Document a past medical history of head or neck radiation, renal calculi, or chronic renal failure. List medications, including calcium and vitamin D supplements.

PHYSICAL EXAMINATION

Important data in the physical examination include heart rate and rhythm, BP, respiratory effort, muscle strength, muscle twitching, and hair and skin texture. Simple tests are used to elicit **Chvostek sign** and **Trousseau sign**, which are both indicative of hypocalcemia. Chvostek sign is a spasm of the facial muscle when the face is tapped over the facial nerve. Trousseau sign is a carpopedal spasm that occurs when a BP cuff is inflated above the patient's systolic BP and left in place for 2 to 3 minutes (see Fig. 47-3).

Nursing assessment of the patient with a parathyroid disorder is outlined in Box 47-2.

Box 47-2 Assessment of the Patient with a Parathyroid Disorder

HEALTH HISTORY

Present Illness
Changes in mental and emotional status, neuromuscular symptoms

Past Medical History
Head or neck radiation, renal calculi, chronic renal failure, recent and current medications (including calcium and vitamin D supplements)

Review of Systems
Fatigue, irritability, muscle tremors or spasms, bone pain, urinary frequency, polyuria, constipation or diarrhea, depression, personality changes

PHYSICAL EXAMINATION

Vital Signs
Dysrhythmias, hypertension or hypotension

Skin and Hair
Changes in moisture and texture

Urologic
Flank pain

Musculoskeletal
Weakness, tremors

Neurologic
Abnormally active or depressed reflexes, irritability, headache, confusion, positive Chvostek sign, positive Trousseau sign

DIAGNOSTIC TESTS AND PROCEDURES

The diagnosis of parathyroid disorders is based on blood and urine studies and skeletal radiographs. Blood tests include measurements of calcium, phosphate, creatinine, uric acid, magnesium, alkaline phosphatase, and PTH. The presence of parathyroid antibodies also may be identified through blood studies. A 24-hour urine specimen may be collected to determine how much calcium is being excreted in the urine.

If excessive calcium has been drawn from bones, demineralization will be apparent on radiographs. Bone cysts and tumors may be found. A dental examination may be done to detect changes in the teeth consistent with parathyroid dysfunction. An electrocardiogram (ECG) also may be ordered because calcium imbalances can cause alterations in the electrical activity in the heart.

DISORDERS OF THE PARATHYROID GLANDS

HYPERPARATHYROIDISM

The secretion of excess PTH is called *hyperparathyroidism.* It is caused most often by a tumor called an *adenoma.* The tumors can be benign or malignant. Other factors that may stimulate excess PTH secretion are vitamin D deficiencies, malabsorption, chronic renal failure, exposure to neck radiation in childhood, and elevated serum phosphate. People who receive a kidney transplant after having been on dialysis for a long time also may have hyperparathyroidism.

The most notable effect of hyperparathyroidism is elevation of serum calcium (i.e., hypercalcemia). High levels of PTH cause calcium to shift from the bones into the bloodstream. Excess PTH also promotes retention of calcium and loss of phosphate by the kidneys. If hyperparathyroidism is untreated, severe demineralization of bone tissue occurs. Bones can become brittle, resulting in serious fractures. The high level of calcium in the urine can lead to the formation of urinary calculi. Obstruction of the urinary tubules by calculi can quickly cause severe kidney damage. The effects of hyperparathyroidism on the heart can cause dysrhythmias and hypertension.

Signs and Symptoms

Because hyperparathyroidism usually develops gradually, symptoms are vague at first. The patient may report weakness, lethargy, depression, anorexia, and constipation. Other findings might include mental and personality changes, cardiac dysrhythmias, weight loss, and urinary calculi. Additional signs and symptoms of hyperparathyroidism are outlined in Table 47-4.

Table 47-4 Comparison of Signs and Symptoms of Hypoparathyroidism and Hyperparathyroidism

SYSTEM	HYPOPARATHYROIDISM	HYPERPARATHYROIDISM
Musculoskeletal	Fatigue, weakness, cramps, twitching	Poor muscle tone, weakness, bone pain, demineralization, fractures
Urinary	Frequency	Polyuria, renal calculi
Cardiovascular	Decreased cardiac output, dysrhythmias	Hypertension, dysrhythmias
Neurologic	Hyperactive reflexes, memory impairment, depression, anxiety, irritability, personality changes, confusion, numbness and tingling of hands and feet and around mouth, muscle spasms	Depressed reflexes, decreased mental function, depression, mood swings, confusion, coma, poor coordination
Gastrointestinal (GI)	Abdominal cramps	Anorexia, nausea and vomiting, constipation
Integumentary	Brittle nails, dry skin	Moist skin
Temperature tolerance	Cold intolerance	Heat intolerance

Medical Diagnosis

The diagnosis of hyperparathyroidism is based primarily on blood and urine studies. Typical findings include elevated serum calcium and decreased serum phosphate, elevated PTH, and elevated 24-hour urine calcium. Skeletal radiographs and bone density studies reveal bone demineralization if the condition is severe. Sometimes the condition is not recognized until the patient has a spontaneous fracture. Other procedures that may be used include renal CT and ultrasound, MRI, fine-needle aspiration, and selective arteriography.

Medical Treatment

Surgical Intervention. If a tumor is causing hyperparathyroidism, it usually is removed surgically. In some cases, more than one gland is removed. The surgeon attempts to leave some parathyroid tissue to prevent hypoparathyroidism. It often is possible for the procedure to be done with an endoscope. However, parathyroidectomy can be a complicated procedure because some parathyroid glands may be located in the mediastinum. Sometimes the patient's normal parathyroid tissue is transplanted to a muscle in the forearm or the neck where it will continue to secrete PTH.

Drug Therapy. If the condition is mild or the patient is not a good candidate for surgery, medical treatment is aimed at lowering the serum calcium level. The patient is instructed to maintain a high fluid intake to dilute the urine. Calcium intake may be restricted. Sodium and phosphorus replacements may be ordered. When it is necessary to lower the calcium level quickly, an infusion of normal saline is often prescribed. Several drugs can be used to treat hypercalcemia. Calcitonin (Calcimar), bisphosphonates (zoledronate), and estrogen inhibit the release of calcium from bones. Cinacalcet suppresses PTH secretion. Oral phosphates inhibit the absorption of calcium from the digestive tract. Furosemide (Lasix) may be given to promote the excretion of calcium in the urine. If hypercalcemia is caused by vitamin D intoxication, glucocorticoids are highly effective. Drugs used to treat parathyroid disorders are described in Table 47-5.

Pharmacology Capsule

Furosemide (Lasix) is a diuretic that promotes the excretion of calcium in the urine.

NURSING CARE of the Patient with Hyperparathyroidism

Assessment

When caring for the patient with hyperparathyroidism, monitor vital signs, urine output, weight, muscle strength, neuromuscular irritability, bowel elimination, and digestive disturbances.

Nursing Diagnoses, Goals, and Outcome Criteria: Hyperparathyroidism

Nursing Diagnoses	Goals and Outcome Criteria
Activity Intolerance related to weakness and fatigue	Improved activity tolerance: patient reports performing daily activities with less fatigue
Risk for Injury related to weakness and decreased bone mass	Reduced risk for injury: improved muscle strength, no falls
Impaired Urinary Elimination related to urinary calculi	Normal urinary output: urine output equal to fluid intake
Constipation related to altered intestinal motility	Normal bowel elimination: regular stools without straining
Deficient Knowledge of mental and emotional effects of hypercalcemia related to lack of information	Improved knowledge of effects of hypercalcemia: patient understands that irritability and depression are symptoms that will improve with treatment.
Imbalanced Nutrition: Less Than Body Requirements related to nausea and vomiting	Adequate nutrition: stable body weight, no nausea or vomiting

Table 47-5 Drug Therapy: Parathyroid Conditions

DRUG	USE AND ACTION	SIDE EFFECTS	NURSING INTERVENTIONS
Oral Calcium Salts			
calcium carbonate (highest % calcium) calcium citrate (most soluble) calcium chloride calcium gluconate calcium lactate	Correct calcium deficiency due to hypoparathyroidism.	Overdosage (hypercalcemia): weakness, hypertension, dysrhythmias, polyuria, bone pain.	Take with food. Serum calcium levels should be monitored. Notify physician of signs of hypercalcemia.
Vitamin D			
calcitriol dihydrotachysterol ergocalciferol	Promote calcium absorption from digestive tract.	Overdosage (hypercalcemia): weakness, hypertension, dysrhythmias, polyuria, bone pain.	Serum calcium levels should be monitored. Notify physician of signs of hypercalcemia.
Bisphosphonates			
zoledronate (Reclast, Zometa)	Inhibits bone resorption and osteoclasts. Reduces serum calcium.	Magnesium and phosphate deficiencies. Nausea, vomiting, constipation. Flu-like symptoms. Hypotension. Renal toxicity if given over less than 15 minutes. Osteonecrosis of jaw, usually after invasive dental procedures.	Monitor pulse, BP, fluid intake, and urine output. Patient should be well hydrated before zoledronate is given. Patient should have dental examination and needed treatment before starting zoledronate.
Other			
furosemide (Lasix)	Promotes excretion of excess calcium in hypoparathyroidism.	Fluid and electrolyte imbalances: metabolic alkalosis, hypovolemia, dehydration, hyponatremia, hypokalemia. Dizziness, headache, tinnitus, hyperglycemia.	Monitor intake and output, serum calcium and potassium levels, pulse, BP, blood glucose.
parathormone teriparatide (Forteo)	Short-term treatment of hypoparathyroidism.	Overdosage (hypercalcemia): dysrhythmias, hypertension, weakness, polyuria, bone pain. Risk of osteosarcoma.	Available only for parenteral use.
calcitonin (Calcimar, Cibacalcin)	Treats hypercalcemia caused by hyperparathyroidism.	Nausea, vomiting, injection site reactions, facial flushing, anaphylaxis.	Monitor for tachycardia due to hypocalcemia. Have epinephrine, antihistamines, and O_2 available. Sensitivity test should be done before giving. Tell patient that flushing is temporary. Teach self-medication. Encourage adequate fluid intake.
cinacalcet (Sensipar)	Treats severe hypercalcemia by decreasing PTH.	Nausea, vomiting, diarrhea. Muscle aches. Dizziness. Hypocalcemia.	Take with or shortly after food. Report muscle cramps to physician.

BP, Blood pressure; *O_2*, oxygen; *PTH*, parathyroid hormone.

Interventions

Activity Intolerance and Risk for Injury

Determine the patient's ability to perform self-care safely and provide help as needed. Move and handle the patient gently. Evaluate the environment for any safety hazards and take corrective measures. Plan care to allow for periods of rest. If the patient is being treated at home, stress the need to plan for rest periods. Assure the patient that weakness and fatigue are caused by the parathyroid disorder and will improve as the condition is corrected.

Impaired Urinary Elimination

Maintain accurate intake and output records because hypercalcemia can cause urinary calculi and serious kidney damage. Decreasing urine output; sharp pain in the flank (kidney area), lower abdomen, or genitalia; and hematuria are consistent with urinary calculi and should be reported to the physician. A high fluid intake, sometimes as much as 4000 mL/day, may be ordered. Closely monitor urine output and vital signs when large volumes of fluid are administered. Older adults and people with heart disease are at risk for excess fluid volume and HF. Patients with cardiac or renal disease may be unable to tolerate this much fluid. Urine may be strained and examined for crystals or calculi. A low-calcium diet and urine acidifiers may be ordered to decrease the risk of calculi formation.

Constipation

Chart bowel movements, including frequency and characteristics of stools. Constipation can often be managed with adequate fluids and fiber in the diet. If these measures are not effective, the physician may order bulk laxatives or stool softeners. It is especially important to monitor bowel elimination in the older patient. Illness, inactivity, and multiple medications combine to increase their risk of constipation and even fecal impaction.

Deficient Knowledge

Recognize that irritability, personality changes, and depression are common with hyperparathyroidism. Patients and their families appreciate knowing that these symptoms are caused by an elevated blood calcium lever and that they will improve with treatment (see *Patient Teaching* box).

Imbalanced Nutrition: Less Than Body Requirements

Take measures to control nausea and vomiting if present. Monitor weight to detect inadequate nutrition if the patient's intake is poor. Small feedings may be better tolerated. Provide a pleasant mealtime environment.

Patient Teaching

Hyperparathyroidism

- Take drugs exactly as ordered and report adverse effects to the physician.
- Eat a balanced diet with moderate calcium and high fluid intake. Notify the physician of bloody urine or pain in the kidney area or groin.
- Increase fluid intake to the amount recommended by the physician.

Postoperative Care

After parathyroidectomy, the patient requires the same care as any surgical patient, as detailed in Chapter 17. Two potential complications specific to parathyroidectomy are (1) airway obstruction and (2) hypocalcemia. When the patient has a neck incision, accumulated fluid and blood in the surgical site can compress the trachea and cause airway obstruction. Monitor and document the respiratory rate and effort and the pulse rate. Increasing pulse and respiratory rates, especially accompanied by restlessness, suggest inadequate oxygenation. Notify the physician of any indications of respiratory distress. Keep an emergency tracheotomy tray at the bedside in the event of acute obstruction.

A second possible cause of airway obstruction is related to severe hypocalcemia. Be alert for tetany, a symptom of hypocalcemia, caused by the postoperative decrease in PTH. A tingling sensation around the mouth and in the fingers is an early symptom of tetany. It may progress to severe muscle spasms or cramps and even to laryngospasm. To prevent this from happening, calcium and other electrolytes are monitored closely in the postoperative period. Promptly inform the RN or physician of signs of tetany or abnormal electrolyte values. Tetany is treated with oral or intravenous calcium supplements. Treatment of hypocalcemia is discussed in detail in the Hypoparathyroidism section below.

The classic incision is on the front of the neck, the upper chest, or both and usually it is covered with a bulky pressure dressing. As with the thyroidectomy patient, this patient's suture line should be protected from stress. Show the patient how to support the head when changing positions. The incisions created by an endoscopic surgical procedure are much smaller. Inspect the dressing and the back of the patient's neck for bleeding. Elevate the patient's head to help reduce swelling.

HYPOPARATHYROIDISM

Hypoparathyroidism is a deficiency of PTH. It is an uncommon condition, usually caused by unintentional removal of or damage to parathyroid glands during surgery. Primary hypoparathyroidism can be caused by an autoimmune process and by several conditions, including Wilson disease (copper overload). Inadequate secretion of PTH leads to hypocalcemia. Severe hypocalcemia can progress to convulsions and respiratory obstruction because of spasms of the larynx. Laryngospasm can be fatal.

Signs and Symptoms

The possibility of parathyroid dysfunction requires close monitoring after thyroid surgery. Trauma or accidental removal of one or more parathyroid glands may lead to symptoms of hypoparathyroidism, as discussed in the section titled "Nursing Care of the Patient Having a Thyroidectomy."

Signs and symptoms of hypocalcemia are painful muscle cramps, fatigue and weakness, tingling and twitching of the face and hands, mental and emotional changes, dry skin, and urinary frequency. With severe hypocalcemia, the patient may have difficulty breathing, convulsions, and cardiac dysrhythmias.

Medical Diagnosis

The diagnosis of hypoparathyroidism is based on patient signs and symptoms and blood studies. Typical findings include low serum calcium, elevated serum phosphate, low urine calcium, and sometimes low serum magnesium. Two classic signs of hypocalcemia that support a diagnosis of hypoparathyroidism are Chvostek sign and Trousseau sign.

Medical Treatment

Acute hypoparathyroidism is sometimes treated with parenteral PTH, which is not practical for chronic management. Severe hypocalcemia is treated with intravenous calcium salts. Other electrolyte imbalances must be treated as well.

On a long-term basis, the patient with chronic hypoparathyroidism is treated with oral calcium salts and a form of vitamin D. Chronic hypoparathyroidism that normally is well controlled may be affected when the patient is under severe stress or is very ill. If the patient is unable to take oral calcium, hypocalcemia can develop quickly. Temporary intravenous calcium may be needed.

Pharmacology Capsule

Lifelong calcium supplementation is required to treat chronic hypoparathyroidism.

❖ NURSING CARE of the Patient with Hypoparathyroidism

■ Assessment

Assessment of the patient with hypoparathyroidism is summarized in Box 47-2.

Nursing Diagnoses, Goals, and Outcome Criteria: Hypoparathyroidism

Nursing Diagnoses	Goals and Outcome Criteria
Risk for Injury related to hypocalcemia	Decreased risk for injury: serum calcium level within normal limits; no muscle spasms, convulsions, or respiratory distress; negative Chvostek and Trousseau signs
Decreased Cardiac Output related to dysrhythmias and heart failure (HF) secondary to hypocalcemia	Normal cardiac output: normal pulse rate and rhythm, normal blood pressure (BP), no dyspnea or edema

■ Interventions

Administer drugs as ordered for hypoparathyroidism and hypocalcemia. When administering calcium salts intravenously, monitor the infusion site carefully because the leakage of calcium salts into body tissues causes inflammation. The infusion site should be changed if extravasation occurs. Frequently assess the patient for signs and symptoms of calcium imbalances. Hypocalcemia may appear as a result of inadequate calcium supplementation. Hypercalcemia can result from excessive calcium intake.

If there has been any recent seizure activity or if the patient shows severe neuromuscular irritability, follow seizure precautions. Any signs of respiratory distress may suggest laryngospasm and should be documented and reported to the physician immediately. Monitor the pulse and BP to detect dysrhythmias and HF. Report cardiac irregularities, edema, and dyspnea to the physician.

Teach patients with chronic hypoparathyroidism the signs and symptoms of calcium imbalances and provide instructions for self-medication. Advise them to carry medical identification cards to alert health care providers to the disorder in the event of an emergency.

Get Ready for the NCLEX® Examination!

Key Points

- Thyroxine (T4), triiodothyronine (T3), and calcitonin are hormones produced by the thyroid gland that affect metabolic rate, growth and development, and serum calcium regulation.
- Hyperthyroidism is the abnormally increased production of thyroid hormones that may be treated with antithyroid drugs, surgery, or radiation therapy.
- Nursing care of the patient with hyperthyroidism may address disturbed sleep pattern; hyperthermia; imbalanced nutrition: less than body requirements; decreased cardiac output; risk for injury; and diarrhea.
- Nursing care after thyroidectomy is concerned with ineffective airway clearance, decreased cardiac output, disturbed body image, acute pain, and risk for infection.

- Hypothyroidism is inadequate secretion of thyroid hormones that is treated with hormone replacement therapy.
- Nursing care of the patient with hypothyroidism addresses activity intolerance; imbalanced nutrition: more than body requirements; hypothermia; constipation; risk for impaired skin integrity; decreased cardiac output; disturbed body image; and deficient knowledge.
- Goiter is enlargement of the thyroid gland that may be associated with hypothyroidism or hyperthyroidism.
- The parathyroid glands secrete PTH, which regulates the serum calcium level.
- Hyperparathyroidism raises the serum calcium level and may cause bone demineralization and obstruction of kidney tubules.
- Nursing care of the patient with hyperparathyroidism focuses on activity intolerance; risk for injury; impaired urinary elimination; constipation; deficient knowledge; and imbalanced nutrition: less than body requirements.
- Hypoparathyroidism, a deficiency of PTH that sometimes follows thyroidectomy, causes the serum calcium level to fall, producing neuromuscular irritability that can progress to seizures, cardiac dysrhythmias, and laryngospasm.
- Nursing diagnoses for the patient with hypoparathyroidism are risk for injury and decreased cardiac output.

Additional Learning Resources

SG Go to your Study Guide for additional learning activities to help you master this chapter content.

evolve Go to your Evolve website (http://evolve.elsevier.com/Linton/medsurg) for the following learning resources and much more:

- Interactive Prioritization Exercises
- Fluid & Electrolyte Tutorial
- Pharmacology Tutorial
- Review Questions for the NCLEX® Examination

Review Questions for the NCLEX® Examination

1. The primary function of thyroid hormones is to regulate ____________.
   NCLEX Client Need: Health Promotion and Maintenance
2. You are notified that a patient with severe hypothyroidism is being admitted to your nursing unit. Which of the following actions are appropriate? (Select all that apply.)
   1. Obtain an emergency tracheostomy tray
   2. Close the blinds to dim the light in the room
   3. Have extra blankets put in the room
   4. Pad the side rails on the bed
   5. Set the room temperature to 68°F

   NCLEX Client Need: Physiological Integrity: Basic Care and Comfort
3. Which of the following findings are most likely in a patient with severe hyperthyroidism? (Select all that apply.)
   1. Respiratory rate of 12 breaths per minute
   2. Heart rate of 120 bpm
   3. Fine tremors of the hands
   4. BP of 160/90 mm Hg
   5. Oral temperature of 96°F

   NCLEX Client Need: Physiological Integrity: Physiological Adaptation
4. You observe that a hyperthyroid patient has prominent, bulging eyeballs. What term is used to describe this condition?
   NCLEX Client Need: Physiological Integrity: Physiological Adaptation
5. A 6-week course of treatment with propylthiouracil (PTU) is prescribed for a patient who is scheduled for a thyroidectomy. The patient asks why she has to take this medication. Which of the following is the best response?
   1. "PTU will help you to eliminate excess thyroid hormone."
   2. "It reduces your thyroid activity, which makes surgery safer for you."
   3. "PTU will provide replacement thyroid hormones after your thyroid gland is removed."
   4. "This drug will cause your thyroid gland to shrink, which will reduce pressure on your airway."

   NCLEX Client Need: Physiological Integrity: Pharmacological Therapies
6. In the immediate postoperative period after thyroidectomy, which of the following is the *first* priority?
   1. Maintain a patent airway
   2. Inspect for hemorrhage
   3. Monitor for hypocalcemia
   4. Prevent strain on the suture line

   NCLEX Client Need: Physiological Integrity: Reduction of Risk Potential
7. Which of the following is the purpose of measuring serum thyroglobulin in a patient who has had thyroid cancer?
   1. To determine adequacy of thyroid hormone replacement
   2. To detect any recurrence of the thyroid cancer
   3. To see whether all RAI has been eliminated
   4. To determine whether parathyroid function is normal

   NCLEX Client Need: Physiological Integrity: Reduction of Risk Potential
8. A patient who is hypoparathyroid after thyroidectomy asks what the parathyroids do and why she needs calcium. Which of the following statements by the nurse accurately describe the relationship between PTH and serum calcium? (Select all that apply.)
   1. The secretion of PTH increases when serum calcium is low.
   2. Increased secretion of PTH causes the kidneys to retain calcium.
   3. Chronically decreased PTH can lead to bone demineralization.
   4. Decreased serum PTH causes calcium to shift from the bones to the blood.
   5. PTH regulates the level of calcium in the blood.

   NCLEX Client Need: Physiological Integrity: Physiological Adaptation

9. A patient had a parathyroid adenoma removed 2 days ago. She is now complaining of muscle cramps in her hands and feet. Which of the following should you suspect?
   1. Poor circulation
   2. Thyroid storm
   3. Hypocalcemia
   4. Metabolic acidosis

   NCLEX Client Need: Physiological Integrity: Physiological Adaptation

10. Nursing implications in administering iodide solutions to a patient include which of the following?
    1. Dilute in milk or juice and provide a straw
    2. Take the patient's pulse and BP before each dose
    3. Tell the patient to report any changes in hearing acuity
    4. Carefully maintain accurate intake and output records

    NCLEX Client Need: Physiological Integrity: Pharmacological Therapies

chapter

48 Diabetes Mellitus and Hypoglycemia

http://evolve.elsevier.com/Linton/medsurg

Lisa Hooter, MSN, RN-BC

Objectives

1. Explain the pathophysiology of diabetes mellitus and hypoglycemia.
2. Explain the difference between type 1 and type 2 diabetes mellitus.
3. Describe the role of insulin in the body.
4. Describe the signs and symptoms of diabetes mellitus and hypoglycemia.
5. Describe the complications of diabetes mellitus.
6. Differentiate between acute hypoglycemia and diabetic ketoacidosis.
7. Describe the treatment of a patient experiencing acute hypoglycemia or diabetic ketoacidosis.
8. Identify nursing interventions for a patient diagnosed with diabetes mellitus or hypoglycemia.
9. Explain tests and procedures used to diagnose diabetes mellitus and hypoglycemia.
10. Discuss treatment of diabetes mellitus and hypoglycemia.
11. Assist in developing a nursing care plan for patients with diabetes mellitus, hypoglycemia, or ketoacidosis.

Key Terms

Endogenous (ĕn-DŎJ-ĕn-ŭs)
Exogenous (ĕks-ŎJ-ĕn-ŭs)
Glycosuria (glī-kō-SŪ-rē-ă)
Hyperglycemia (hī-pĕr-glī-SĒ-mē-ă)
Hypoglycemia (hī-pō-glī-SĒ-mē-ă)
Ketoacidosis (kē-tō-ă-sĭ-DŌ-sĭs)
Ketone bodies (KĒ-tōn)
Lipoatrophy (lĭp-ō-ĂT-rō-fē)
Lipohypertrophy (lĭp-ō-hī-PĔR-trō-fē)
Macrovascular (MĂK-rō-văs-cū-lăr)
Microvascular (MĪK- rō-văs-cū-lăr)
Nephropathy (nĕ-FRŎP-ă-thē)
Neuropathy (nū-RŎP-ĕ-thē)
Polydipsia (pŏl-ē-DĬP-sē-ă)
Polyphagia (pŏl-ē-FĂ-jē-ă)
Polyuria (pŏl-ē-Ū-rē-ă)
Retinopathy (rĕt-ĭ-NŎP-ă-thē)

DIABETES MELLITUS

Symptoms of diabetes mellitus (DM) have been reported in the literature throughout history but the cause was not identified until the early twentieth century. In an experiment, the pancreata of several sheep were removed, resulting in the development of diabetes. Through this experiment, insulin and the role it plays in the body was discovered. The search then began for a way to provide insulin to people whose bodies did not produce enough. Before insulin became available for commercial use in 1921, people with diabetes were placed on high-protein diets until they went into acidosis and died, usually a short time after the onset of the disease.

The National Diabetes 2012 statistics estimate that 29.1 million people in the United States have DM, which is 9.3% of the total population. This estimate includes 8.1 million people with undiagnosed diabetes. It is estimated that an additional 86 million have prediabetes. Diabetes is a major health problem and a leading cause of death by disease. People with diabetes are at increased risk for heart disease, renal disease, blindness, amputation, and complications during pregnancy. Fortunately, with early diagnosis and better management, it is possible to reduce the risk of serious complications.

PATHOPHYSIOLOGY

DM is a chronic disorder characterized by impaired metabolism and by vascular and neurologic complications. A key feature of diabetes is elevated blood glucose, called **hyperglycemia**. The blood glucose level is normally regulated by insulin, a hormone produced by the beta cells in the islets of Langerhans located in the pancreas. In healthy individuals, small amounts of insulin are secreted continuously (basal secretion) into the bloodstream. The ingestion of carbohydrates triggers the secretion of a larger volume of insulin (bolus secretion). Insulin that is produced in one's own body is called **endogenous**, meaning that it is produced internally. Insulin that is obtained from other sources and administered to a person is called

exogenous, meaning that it comes from an external source.

DM is classified as *type 1* (previously called *insulin-dependent diabetes mellitus [IDDM]*) or *type 2* (previously referred to as *noninsulin-dependent diabetes mellitus [NIDDM]*). Both types have a genetic component but many people with diabetes have no genetic predisposition.

Type 1 DM, characterized by the absence of endogenous insulin, was previously called *juvenile-onset diabetes* because it occurs most commonly in juveniles and young adults. However, it can also occur in middle-aged and older adults. An autoimmune process, possibly triggered by a viral infection, causes destruction of the beta cells, the development of insulin antibodies, and the production of islet cell antibodies (ICAs). Affected people require exogenous insulin for the rest of their lives.

Type 2 DM is characterized by inadequate endogenous insulin and the body's inability to use insulin properly. Initially, beta cells respond inadequately to hyperglycemia, resulting in chronically elevated blood glucose. The continuous high glucose level in the blood desensitizes the beta cells so that they become progressively less responsive to the elevated glucose. In relation to the use of insulin, specific receptor sites become insensitive to insulin (i.e., "insulin resistance"), preventing glucose from entering the cells. Although type 2 DM is more common among adults, it is increasingly found in children as well. One inherited form (maturity-onset diabetes of the young) causes type 2 DM among all age groups in affected families.

Type 2 DM may be controlled by diet and exercise alone or may require oral hypoglycemic agents or exogenous insulin. Some patients are treated with insulin initially to normalize blood glucose and then are treated with diet, exercise, and perhaps oral agents.

Gestational diabetes mellitus (GDM) is diagnosed when a woman is found to have glucose intolerance for the first time during pregnancy. After delivery, the condition resolves. (See a maternity nursing text for information on the management of GDM.)

Role of Insulin

Insulin is considered a critical hormone for glucose metabolism. However, insulin also is needed for the synthesis of fatty acids and proteins (Box 48-1).

Glucose. Insulin stimulates the active transport of glucose into the cells. When insulin is absent, glucose cannot enter most cells, so it remains in the bloodstream. The blood then becomes thick with glucose, which increases the osmolality of the blood. Increased osmolality stimulates the thirst center, causing the patient to experience **polydipsia** (i.e., excessive thirst) and take in additional fluid. The increased fluid does not pass into body tissues, however, because the high serum osmolality retains the fluid in the bloodstream. As the blood passes through the kidneys, some excess glucose is eliminated. The osmotic force created by the glucose draws extra fluid and electrolytes with it, causing abnormally increased urine volume (**polyuria**).

Because most cells are not able to use glucose without insulin, stored fat is broken down in an effort to provide fuel for heat and energy. Tissue breakdown and loss of lean body mass send hunger signals to the hypothalamus. The patient experiences excessive hunger (**polyphagia**). The patient may take in more food but unfortunately the cells of the body cannot use the extra glucose without insulin. Weight loss often occurs despite increased appetite and food ingestion.

Insulin is needed to transport glucose into resting muscle cells. During heavy exercise, however, muscle fibers are highly permeable to glucose even in the absence of insulin. Therefore exercise must be considered in the regulation of serum glucose levels. Other tissues that can use glucose without insulin are the brain, nerves, heart, and lens of the eye.

Insulin regulates the rate of glucose metabolism. The greater the insulin response to carbohydrate ingestion, the faster carbohydrates are metabolized. In a healthy person, when blood glucose falls, insulin production is inhibited and stored glycogen is converted to glucose by a process called *glycogenolysis.* When blood glucose rises, insulin production is stimulated and the conversion of glycogen to glucose is inhibited. This process usually maintains the blood glucose within a normal range. However, when insulin secretion is inadequate, glycogen is converted to glucose in an attempt to nourish glucose-starved tissues; yet hyperglycemia occurs because cells cannot use the glucose.

Fatty Acids. Insulin promotes fatty acid synthesis and the conversion of fatty acids into fat, which is stored as adipose tissue. Insulin also spares fat by inhibiting the breakdown of adipose tissue and the mobilization

Box 48-1 Insulin: Actions and Effects of Deficiency

INSULIN
- Increases the transport of glucose into the resting muscle cell
- Regulates the rate at which carbohydrates are used
- Promotes the conversion of glucose to glycogen
- Inhibits the conversion of glycogen to glucose
- Promotes fatty acid synthesis
- Spares fat
- Inhibits the breakdown of adipose tissue
- Inhibits the conversion of fats to glucose
- Stimulates protein synthesis in the tissues
- Inhibits the conversion of protein into glucose

LACK OF INSULIN
- Stimulates the conversion of glycogen to glucose
- Permits fat stores to break down
- Increases triglyceride storage in the liver
- Halts the storage of proteins
- Causes protein to be dumped into the bloodstream

of fat and by inhibiting the conversion of fats to fatty acids and glycerol.

Without adequate insulin, fat stores break down and increased triglycerides are stored in the liver. The liver can store up to one third of its weight as fat. Increased fatty acids in the liver can triple the production of lipoproteins, which promotes the development of atherosclerosis. This helps to explain why people with DM have a high incidence of cardiovascular disease.

Protein. Insulin enhances protein synthesis in tissues and inhibits the conversion of protein into glucose. Amino acids are allowed into cells, which enhances the rate of protein formation while preventing the degradation of proteins. Without adequate insulin, the storage of proteins halts and large amounts of amino acids are dumped into the bloodstream. High levels of plasma amino acids place people with diabetes at risk for development of gout. Changes in protein metabolism lead to extreme weakness and poor organ functioning.

CAUSE

Type 1 DM has been attributed to genetic, immunologic, and environmental (i.e., viruses, toxins) factors. The tendency toward type 1 DM is found in families with a genetic predisposition. Evidence of a strong genetic component in type 2 DM is seen as well.

It is possible that an autoimmune disorder triggers the sudden onset of diabetes. Our bodies are guarded by an elaborate and extensive immune system. When a microbe and its antigen enter the blood, they encounter white blood cells (WBCs) called *macrophages* that have antigen receptors on their surfaces. These antigen receptors steer the antigens to lymphocytes, which have antigen-specific receptors. When a specific antigen is present, it activates the immune response. The lymphocytes begin producing custom-made antibodies against the antigens, at the same time signaling other types of cells in the immune system to attack the invaders. The lymphocytes and the antibodies are unable to destroy the foreign cells independently without the help of phagocytes and complement cells. This group of cells is selective in identifying and destroying foreign protein. Unfortunately, this part of the immune system can become a renegade faction and turn on its own healthy cells. One or more of the autoantibodies listed in Figure 48-1 are present in 85% to 90% of individuals that develop type 1 DM.

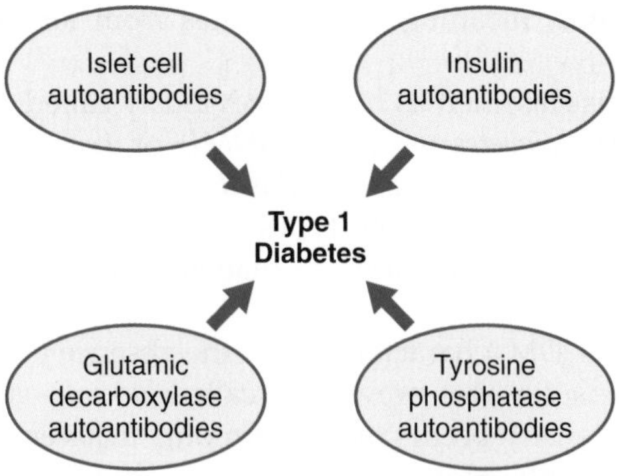

FIGURE 48-1 Possible immunologic causes of diabetes mellitus (DM).

RISK FACTORS

Risk factors for type 1 DM, other than genetic ones, are not known. According to the National Diabetes Information Clearinghouse (NDIC), which is part of the National Institutes of Health (NIH), risk factors for type 2 DM include the following:

- Obesity
- Sedentary lifestyle
- Family history of diabetes
- Age 40 years and older
- History of GDM
- History of delivering infant weighing more than 10 lb
- Ethnicity derived from Alaskan Native, Native American, African American, Latino, Asian American, or Pacific Islander (see *Cultural Considerations* box)
- Polycystic ovary syndrome
- Cardiovascular disease and hypertension
- Presence of acanthosis nigricans or other conditions associated with insulin resistance

Cultural Considerations

What Does Culture Have to Do with Diabetes?

The risk of diabetes mellitus (DM) among Latinos is 300% that of Caucasian Americans. Effective measures to decrease this risk must be sensitive to cultural practices and values.

Pharmacology Capsule

Pharmacologic use of glucocorticoids can elevate the blood glucose level. Although unlikely to cause DM in people with normal pancreatic function, glucocorticoid therapy may unmask latent diabetes. It also complicates management of known DM.

Metabolic Syndrome

Metabolic syndrome is the common name used to describe a syndrome that is thought by many to be a precursor to diabetes. This syndrome is also referred to as *syndrome X, insulin resistance syndrome*, and *cardiovascular dysmetabolic syndrome.* Patients with metabolic syndrome typically have impaired glucose tolerance (IGT), high serum insulin, hypertension, elevated triglycerides, low high-density lipoprotein (HDL) cholesterol, and altered size and density of low-density lipoprotein (LDL) cholesterol. It is believed that metabolic syndrome represents a chronic low-grade inflammatory process affecting endothelial tissue (the lining of the heart, blood and lymph vessels). The long-term effects include atherosclerosis, ischemic heart disease, left ventricular hypertrophy, and sometimes type 2 DM. Research is now directed at learning how to detect this syndrome early and what interventions might slow or arrest the progress.

COMPLICATIONS

Long-Term Complications

The duration of diabetes and poor control of blood glucose are the best predictors of the severity of complications. These complications affect almost every organ of the body. They may be classified as *microvascular, macrovascular*, or *neuropathic.*

Microvascular Complications. **Microvascular** complications result from changes in small blood vessels that are unique to diabetes and occur in both type 1 and type 2 diabetes. The basement membrane of capillaries thickens, which impairs the exchange of nutrients, gases, and wastes. Tissues that are most vulnerable to microvascular complications are the eyes (**retinopathy**) and the kidneys (**nephropathy**). Changes in the capillaries appear to be related to persistent hyperglycemia and are aggravated by hypertension and smoking. Neuropathy is sometimes classified with microvascular complications; it is discussed below.

Retinopathy. Among people ages 25 to 74 years, DM is the leading cause of new-onset blindness. People with diabetes are at increased risk for retinopathy, cataracts, and glaucoma. *Diabetic retinopathy* is a term used to describe pathologic changes in the retina that are associated with DM. Two types of diabetic retinopathy have been identified: (1) nonproliferative and (2) proliferative. Both types may be present at the same time. Manifestations of nonproliferative disease include small hemorrhages and aneurysms in the retina, hard lipid and protein exudates that leak from the blood vessels, infarcted nerve fibers (described as "cotton wool spots"), and changes in retinal veins. Proliferative disease is characterized by the growth of abnormal capillaries on the retina and the optic disc. These fragile vessels can penetrate the vitreous humor and rupture. When hemorrhaging into the vitreous occurs, it becomes cloudy and vision is lost. The blood is eventually reabsorbed but scars may remain, which places traction on the retina and may result in retinal detachment.

Macular edema occurs with both types of diabetic retinopathy. The macula is the center of vision and edema causes loss of central vision. To illustrate the effect, imagine this page with only the outer margins clearly visible. The center would be clouded.

Signs and symptoms that suggest impending eye problems are the presence of spots ("floaters") in the field of vision, seeing "cobwebs," or sudden visual changes. Often no warning signs of retinal changes exist. Therefore patients with diabetes should have an eye examination at least once a year so that early changes in the eye can be detected and measures taken to try to prevent further deterioration and possible blindness. One strategy that may reduce the risk of injury to the eye is control of hypertension. Early laser treatment of macular edema can halt the progression of retinopathy and may even improve vision.

Nephropathy. Diabetes is the most common cause of end-stage renal disease (ESRD) in the United States. Renal disease develops in about 10% to 20% of people with diabetes but individuals with type 1 DM have 12 times the risk for developing ESRD than those with type 2 DM. African Americans, Native Americans, and Mexican Americans have a four to six times greater risk for developing ESRD (see *Cultural Considerations* box). Factors that contribute to the development of nephropathy (i.e., kidney damage) include poor control of blood glucose, hypertension, long-standing diabetes, and genetic susceptibility. High concentrations of **glycosuria** (i.e., glucose in the urine), along with hypertension, gradually destroy the capillaries that supply the renal glomeruli. Increased permeability of the glomeruli permits serum proteins to be lost in the urine. No symptoms are seen in the early stages but rising microalbuminuria signals the onset of kidney damage. When the level of protein in the urine exceeds 300 mg/day of albumin or 500 mg/day of total protein, the condition will likely progress to ESRD. Signs and symptoms of kidney failure include persistent proteinuria, elevated blood pressure (BP) and serum creatinine, hematuria, and oliguria or anuria. Diagnosis is based on laboratory values (see Chapter 42).

Cultural Considerations

What Does Culture Have to Do with Nephropathy?

Genetic factors increase the risk for nephropathy among African Americans, Native Americans, and Mexican Americans.

Measures to reduce the risk of damage to the kidneys include good glycemic control, control of hypertension, use of angiotensin-converting enzyme (ACE) inhibitors or angiotensin receptor blockers (ARBs), maintaining good hydration, and avoiding nephrotoxic chemicals, including drugs. Modest protein restriction may be recommended. Screening for microalbuminuria can detect early renal changes that may be reversible. Early detection and treatment may slow the development and progression of ESRD.

Macrovascular Complications. Atherosclerotic plaque development occurs earlier and is more severe and more extensive in people with diabetes than in other people. Atherosclerosis affects the peripheral, carotid, cerebral, and coronary blood vessels. The accelerated atherosclerotic changes associated with diabetes are called **macrovascular** complications. Individuals with diabetes have a twofold to fourfold increase in risk for heart disease and stroke, which account for 68% of the deaths in people with diabetes.

Chronic hyperglycemia as a result of poor blood glucose control may play an important role in the premature development of atherosclerosis in patients with diabetes. However, evidence indicates that the elevated insulin levels occurring with insulin resistance also play a role in the development of atherosclerosis. This is especially apparent in Caucasian middle-aged men. Hyperinsulinemia damages the endothelium of blood vessels, permitting lipids to be easily deposited on the cell walls of the blood vessels. Other risk factors for macrovascular complications are central obesity, hyperlipidemia, hypertension, genetics, sedentary lifestyle, and smoking.

Macrovascular changes are associated with coronary heart disease (CHD); cerebrovascular accidents (CVAs), or stroke; and peripheral vascular disease (PVD). The risk for heart disease, stroke, and PVD is two to four times higher for individuals with diabetes. Due to these risks, aspirin therapy should be considered for individuals with diabetes. Signs and symptoms of PVD may include diminished pedal pulses and claudication (i.e., pain in the calf, back, or buttocks while walking). When arteries in the lower extremities can no longer deliver oxygen (O_2) and nutrients to peripheral tissues, gangrene may develop, necessitating amputation of affected parts of extremities.

Treatment for macrovascular disease is directed toward weight loss and exercise. Patients who smoke are strongly encouraged to quit because of vasoconstriction caused by nicotine. With weight loss, insulin uptake improves and circulating insulin levels decrease. As a result of aerobic exercise, insulin receptor sites become more sensitive and serum insulin levels decrease. Exercise, in conjunction with weight loss, reduces the amount of exogenous insulin needed. Because it is thought that exogenous insulin may create immune complexes that damage arterial walls, reduced exogenous insulin needs may reduce the risk for macrovascular disease in DM.

For additional information about CHD, CVA, and PVD, see Chapters 36, 28, and 37.

Neuropathic Complications. Pathologic changes in nerve tissue, called **neuropathy**, are related to poor glucose control, ischemic lesions of nerves, and chemical changes in peripheral nerve cells. Almost 30% of individuals with diabetes over age 40 have impaired sensation in at least one area of the foot. Neuropathy affects approximately 13% of all people with diabetes. Patients who have had diabetes for more than 25 years have a 50% chance of experiencing neuropathies. Neuropathy can be classified as *mononeuropathy, polyneuropathy*, or *autonomic neuropathy*.

Mononeuropathy. Mononeuropathy affects a single nerve or group of nerves. It results from inadequate blood supply and is experienced as sharp, stabbing pain. Pain and atrophy occur in muscles enervated by the affected nerve. Sometimes the pain is relieved by walking.

Polyneuropathy. Polyneuropathy involves sensory and autonomic nerves. Sensory polyneuropathy commonly affects both legs symmetrically. Symptoms range from tingling, numbness, and burning sensations to complete loss of sensation. Pain is often worse during the night. Sometimes polyneuropathy resolves spontaneously. All patients with DM should have a comprehensive foot examination annually, including testing for loss of protective sensation.

Autonomic Neuropathy. Autonomic neuropathy affects the sympathetic and parasympathetic nervous systems. It can affect the pupillary response and functions of the cardiovascular, gastrointestinal (GI), and genitourinary systems. Cardiovascular involvement may be manifested as postural hypotension, resting tachycardia, exercise intolerance, and failure of the heart rate to increase with vigorous exercise. Common GI symptoms include constipation or, less commonly, diarrhea as well as anorexia, nausea, vomiting, gastric reflux, and bloating after meals. The stomach may dilate and lose muscle tone so that gastric emptying is delayed, a condition called *gastroparesis*.

The patient may have urinary problems such as an atonic bladder, in which the bladder capacity increases and eventually causes retention with overflow. Sexual problems in men such as erectile dysfunction and retrograde ejaculation are common. Women may have painful intercourse.

Diabetic amyotrophy (i.e., loss of muscle mass) causes pain in the muscles of the pelvic girdle and thighs. This pain may be so severe that it interferes with activity and sleep. The muscles look wasted and fasciculation (i.e., involuntary twitching of muscle fibers) may be visible under the skin. These contractions do not produce movement.

Hypoglycemic Unawareness. Normally, patients recognize signs and symptoms of **hypoglycemia** (i.e., abnormally low level of glucose in the blood) so that they can take corrective action. With hypoglycemic unawareness, the usual symptoms of tachycardia, palpitations, tremor, sweating, and nervousness may be absent. Without this "early warning system," the patient suddenly may have changes in mental status as the first sign of hypoglycemia. This phenomenon has been attributed to autonomic neuropathy but that relationship has not been consistently demonstrated.

Foot Complications of Diabetes. People with diabetes may have foot problems associated with neuropathy, inadequate blood supply, or a combination of both. When neurologic function is impaired but blood flow is adequate, the foot is warm and pink with good pulses but lacks normal sensation. The patient may have a foot injury but fail to recognize it in the absence of pain.

If the blood supply is impaired but neurologic function is adequate, the foot is cold but sensation is normal. When the foot is raised, it turns pale. When the foot is lowered, it becomes red. Pulses are weak or absent.

Neuropathic ulcers can result from injury to the foot caused by the following:

- *Mechanical irritation,* such as that caused from rough shoe linings or amateur attempts at shaving calluses or cutting toenails
- *Thermal injury,* such as burns caused from heat exposure such as heating pads and sitting too close to a fire or radiator
- *Chemical irritation* caused by substances such as salicylic acid, found in many corn plasters

Patients who cannot see or feel their feet may fail to notice injuries or dangerous situations (see *Patient Teaching* box). A neglected callus may become inflamed, allowing blood and fluid to accumulate beneath the lesion, which can create a site for infection. Poor perfusion caused by PVD can make these injuries worse. An abscess may form that ruptures to create an ulcer. Treatment is difficult and not always effective, so the best treatment is prevention.

Patient Teaching

"Dos and Do Nots" Regarding Foot Care

DO

- Check your feet every day. Look for red spots, cuts, swelling, and blisters. Use a mirror if you cannot see the bottom of your feet.
- Be more active.
- Wash your feet every day. Dry them carefully, especially between the toes.
- Keep your skin soft and smooth. Rub a thin coat of lotion over the tops and bottoms of your feet but not between your toes.
- Trim your toenails across and file the edges with an emery board.
- Protect your feet from hot and cold.
- Wear shoes at all times.
- Test the water before putting your feet in to make sure the water is not too hot.
- Inspect the insides of your shoes for foreign objects, torn linings, and rough or sharp points.
- Buy shoes that are comfortable at the time of purchase. Wear shoes that are supportive and flexible and do not create pressure on any area of the feet.
- See your physician regularly and ask him or her to examine your feet at each visit.

DO NOT

- Smoke.
- Use hot water bottles, heating pads, or electric blankets. You can burn your feet before you realize it.
- Soak your feet in hot water.
- Walk barefoot, even in the house.

Patient Teaching—cont'd

- Walk on hot surfaces such as sidewalks or sandy beaches.
- Remove corns or calluses yourself. See a podiatrist for their removal.
- Wear shoes without stockings.

Modified from American Diabetes Association: Clinical practice recommendations, *Diabetes Care* 36(suppl 1):S38–S39, 2013.

Prevention of Long-Term Complications. The landmark Diabetes Control and Complications Trial (DCCT) found that intensive treatment of type 1 DM delayed the onset or slowed the progress of diabetic retinopathy, nephropathy, and neuropathy. The trial evaluated the effects of tight control of blood glucose levels with multiple daily insulin injections or programmable external insulin pumps. Patients were closely monitored and treated by a team of diabetes experts. The outcomes of the United Kingdom Prospective Diabetes Study (UKPDS) demonstrated similar benefits of tight control with type 2 DM. Tight control means that the blood glucose is maintained in the normal range with carefully balanced drugs, diet, and exercise. The risk for hypoglycemia increases when blood glucose levels are kept in tight control, especially if beta-blockers are part of the treatment regimen. Target glucose levels may need to be adjusted if frequent hypoglycemia occurs, which underlines the need for individualized treatment goals for each patient with diabetes. Other studies, such as the Action to Control Cardiovascular Risk in Diabetes (ACCORD); Action in Diabetes and Vascular Disease: Preterax and Diamicron Modified Release Controlled Evaluation (ADVANCE); and the Veterans Affairs Diabetes Trial (VADT), have shown the potential risk of increased cardiovascular complications when intensive glucose control is achieved. Because of these studies, target glucose levels should be individualized for patients with a long duration of diabetes, recurrent hypoglycemia, severe cardiovascular disease, and advanced age.

The American Diabetes Association acknowledges that other factors increase the risk for developing complications. They recommend that individuals with diabetes strive to keep BP readings less than 140 mm Hg systolic and less than 80 mm Hg diastolic. Lipid goals for individuals with diabetes without known cardiovascular disease include total cholesterol less than 200 mg/dL, LDL less than 100 mg/dL, HDL more than 50 mg/dL, and triglycerides less than 150 mg/dL. Lipid goals should be individualized to reflect risk factors and known cardiovascular disease. Individuals with diabetes should be given information regarding smoking cessation. Use of aspirin and ACE inhibitors is recommended for those with increased cardiovascular and renal risk factors.

Recommendations for Glycemic, Blood Pressure, and Lipid Control for Adults with Diabetes

Glycosylated hemoglobin ($HgbA_{1c}$)	<7% (more stringent goals may be appropriate for selected individuals)
Blood pressure (BP)	<140/80 mm Hg
Total cholesterol	<200 mg/dL
Low-density lipoprotein (LDL) cholesterol	<100 mg/dL

Adapted from American Diabetes Association: Standards of medical care in diabetes, *Diabetes Care* 36(suppl 1):S16–S39, 2013.
Note: More stringent lipid control is advised for individuals with multiple risk factors for CVD.

Acute Emergency Complications

Acute Hypoglycemia. Patients being treated with insulin or other hypoglycemics are at risk for acute hypoglycemia. Events that may trigger this dangerous drop in blood glucose include taking too much insulin, not eating enough food, not eating at the right time, and an inconsistent pattern of exercise. Other variables that lower blood glucose are gastroparesis, renal insufficiency, and certain drugs, including aspirin and beta-adrenergic blockers (see *Complementary and Alternative Therapies* box). Glucose levels between 50 and 70 mg/dL are considered moderate hypoglycemia. However, some people with diabetes have been known to have serum glucose levels below 50 mg/dL without signs and symptoms of hypoglycemia (hypoglycemia unawareness).

Complementary and Alternative Therapies

Among the many herbal supplements that may lower blood glucose are dandelion, onion, garlic, and ginseng. Patients should consult with their physician if they consider using these products.

The signs and symptoms of hypoglycemia are classified as *adrenergic* and *neuroglucopenic.* Adrenergic symptoms appear first and reflect the response of the nervous system to inadequate glucose for cell function. These symptoms are shakiness, nervousness, irritability, tachycardia, anxiety, lightheadedness, hunger, tingling or numbness of the lips or tongue, and diaphoresis. Beta-adrenergic blockers may mask the adrenergic symptoms of hypoglycemia, delaying the diagnosis and treatment of hypoglycemia.

If treatment is delayed, a second set of symptoms may appear. These symptoms are called *neuroglucopenia* or neuroglycopenia because they are caused by a shortage of glucose to the brain. If the glucose level falls rapidly, however, these symptoms may be the first signs of hypoglycemia. They include drowsiness, irritability, impaired judgment, blurred vision, slurred speech, headaches, and mood swings progressing to disorientation, seizures, and unconsciousness. Even more severe hypoglycemia progresses to loss of consciousness, convulsions, coma, and death. It is important to remember that individuals who are experiencing severe hypoglycemia may not be able to recognize and treat the hypoglycemia without assistance.

Treatment. To treat hypoglycemia, give the conscious patient 15 to 20 g of quick-acting carbohydrate, such as the following:

- 4 to 6 oz of undiluted orange or apple juice or soft drink (not sugar-free)
- 8 oz of skim milk
- 1 tablespoon of sugar
- 1 tablespoon of honey or syrup
- 6 to 8 Life Savers
- 3 to 4 glucose tablets or 15 g of glucose gel

Repeat every 15 to 30 minutes until the blood glucose is above 70 mg/dL for adults and above 80 to 100 mg/dL for older adults and children. Once the blood glucose level returns to normal, a meal or snack should be consumed to prevent recurrence of hypoglycemia.

Individuals who are taking insulin should always have injectable glucagon on hand. If the patient is unable to swallow, an intramuscular or subcutaneous injection of 1 mg of glucagon or an intravenous dose of 50 mL of 50% dextrose should be given as ordered or per protocol. On regaining consciousness, the patient should be given an additional treatment of some form of glucose. If it will be 1 hour or more until the next meal, give the patient some form of complex carbohydrate and protein, such as a slice of cheese or meat with crackers.

Diabetic Ketoacidosis. Diabetic **ketoacidosis** (DKA) is a life-threatening emergency caused by a relative deficiency (ineffective amount of insulin) or absolute deficiency (lack of insulin) in addition to elevated counterregulatory hormones (glucagon, catecholamines, cortisol and growth hormone [GH]). This results in disorders in the metabolism of carbohydrates, fats, and proteins. The sequence of events is as follows:

1. Tissues cannot use glucose without insulin, resulting in an increase in serum glucose levels.
2. Excess glucose entering the renal tubules increases osmotic pressure. This results in the reabsorption of water, increasing urine output (i.e., osmotic diuresis). As glucose is eliminated in the kidneys, so are large amounts of water and electrolytes.
3. The patient voids large amounts of dilute urine (i.e., polyuria).
4. To make matters worse, the sympathetic nervous system responds to the cellular need for fuel by converting glycogen to glucose and manufacturing additional glucose.
5. As glycogen stores are depleted, the body begins to burn fat and protein for energy.
6. The breakdown of fat and protein for energy produces acidic substances called **ketone bodies.**

As the ketones accumulate, the pH of the blood decreases and results in severe acidosis, which can be fatal.

7. Protein metabolism results in the loss of lean muscle mass and a negative nitrogen balance (the amount of nitrogen being excreted is greater than the amount of nitrogen ingested).

Early signs and symptoms of DKA are anorexia, headache, and fatigue. As the condition progresses, the classic symptoms of polydipsia, polyuria, and polyphagia develop. If untreated, the patient becomes dehydrated, weak, and lethargic with abdominal pain, nausea, vomiting, fruity breath (because of ketone production), increased respiratory rate, tachycardia, blurred vision, and hypothermia. Late signs are air hunger (seen as Kussmaul respirations: rapid and deep), coma, and shock. Death can result if prompt medical care is not instituted.

The patient with ketoacidosis has hyperglycemia (≥300 mg/dL); ketonuria; and acidosis, with a pH of less than 7.3 or a bicarbonate level of less than 15 mEq/L.

The mortality rate is 2% to 5% for DKA and DKA accounts for half of all deaths in diabetes patients younger than 24 years old. It is most likely to occur when diabetes is undiagnosed; when the patient does not take enough insulin; when the patient with uncontrolled type 1 DM exercises too vigorously; or when the patient experiences stress linked to illness, infection, surgery, or emotions. Some drugs such as corticosteroids, sympathomimetics, and thiazide diuretics also can raise serum glucose. In about one quarter of patients with DKA, no cause is identified. Early identification of DKA and prompt treatment is aimed at correction of the three main problems: (1) dehydration, (2) electrolyte imbalance, and (3) acidosis.

Dehydration. The patient with ketoacidosis may have lost a large volume of fluid as the result of vomiting, polyuria, and hyperventilation. Volume deficits may be estimated at 100 mL/kg of body weight. In addition to the risk of shock because of depleted blood volume, the patient is at risk for development of blood clots.

The first need is to replace the fluid, which will aid the kidneys in eliminating excess glucose. The physician usually orders 1000 mL of normal saline to run over the first hour, followed by an additional 2000 to 8000 mL of intravenous fluids for the next 24 hours. If the patient has hypertension or hypernatremia or is at risk for heart failure (HF), the order may be given for 0.45% saline solution instead of normal saline. In addition, the rate and total amount of fluid may be decreased in older patients who may not tolerate rapid changes in fluid volume.

Electrolyte Imbalance. The electrolyte of primary concern in ketoacidosis is potassium. Potassium shifts out of the cells, causing transient (temporary) hyperkalemia. The hyperkalemia associated with hyperglycemia should be treated with fluid replacement and insulin administration. Medications (e.g., cation-exchange resins) should not be used to lower potassium levels. As the patient is rehydrated and normal urine output is reestablished, potassium is lost in the urine. In addition, insulin replacement enhances the movement of potassium from the extracellular compartment back into the cells. During this time, the patient is at risk for developing severe hypokalemia that can cause life-threatening cardiac dysrhythmias.

Replacement of potassium is initiated only after adequate urine output is established. During potassium replacement, you must monitor the patient closely. Large doses of potassium may be required even though the serum potassium level is normal at the onset of treatment, because the plasma level will drop during treatment. Because potassium is irritating to the veins and a potassium drip must be carefully regulated, it is better to run the intravenous fluid containing potassium by the piggyback method at a prescribed rate, which is slower than the hydration rate. Remember that potassium must *always* be diluted before intravenous administration. !

Sodium deficiency is generally corrected by infusion of normal saline. Phosphate, magnesium, and calcium levels also should be monitored. Once therapy begins, phosphate and magnesium may fall and calcium can rise to dangerous levels.

Pharmacology Capsule

When a patient is given insulin to treat diabetic ketoacidosis (DKA), monitor for hypokalemia because insulin causes potassium to move from the extracellular fluid into the cells.

Acidosis. Ketoacidosis is a problem primarily with type 1 DM. It occurs when ketone bodies accumulate as the result of the breakdown of fats for energy associated with inadequate insulin. In addition, ketoacidosis can occur in individuals with type 2 DM when severe hyperglycemia is associated with another acute condition, such as sepsis or a myocardial infarction.

Ketoacidosis is treated with the slow intravenous infusion of insulin. When the serum glucose level reaches 250 to 300 mg/dL, dextrose solution is added. The intravenous insulin is given continuously or as a bolus until subcutaneous insulin can be given or else the patient may become ketoacidotic again. The serum glucose level returns to normal several hours before the serum bicarbonate level. As long as the serum glucose level is normal but the serum bicarbonate level remains abnormal, the insulin drip must be maintained and glucose level corrected. More glucose is added to the intravenous fluid to cover the insulin. Normal levels of glucose *do not* mean that the acidosis has been corrected. The insulin drip must be maintained until the serum bicarbonate is 15 to 18 mEq/L.

When the patient is able to eat and all laboratory values are normal, subcutaneous insulin can be given and the insulin drip discontinued.

Pharmacology Capsule

For continuous intravenous infusion, insulin is usually diluted in a 100-mL bag of solution. Because insulin binds with plastic, flush plastic tubing with the intravenous solution before adding insulin to the solution.

Hyperosmolar Hyperglycemic Nonketotic Syndrome. Hyperosmolar hyperglycemic nonketotic syndrome (HHNS) is a condition in which a patient goes into a coma from extremely high glucose levels (≥600 mg/dL) but no evidence exists of elevated ketones. With HHNS, the patient's pancreas produces just enough insulin to prevent the breakdown of fatty acids and the formation of ketones but not enough insulin to prevent hyperglycemia. Mortality rates for HHNS are as high as 15%.

The basic defect is the lack of effective insulin or the inability to use available insulin. The patient's persistent hyperglycemia causes osmotic diuresis, resulting in the loss of fluid and electrolytes. To maintain osmotic equilibrium, fluid shifts from the intracellular fluid space to the extracellular space. Dehydration and hypernatremia develop. Dehydration and neurologic changes may be more pronounced with HHNS than with DKA. Patients with HHNS do not experience GI symptoms nor do they experience Kussmaul respirations because they lack significant lactic acid levels. These patients often tolerate polyuria and polydipsia for weeks before seeking treatment. For some patients, HHNS is the first sign of diabetes. Others have been previously diagnosed with borderline diabetes.

HHNS may be caused by the same factors that trigger ketoacidosis. It also can be brought about by total parenteral nutrition (TPN) or dialysis. In both of these procedures, intravenous solutions that contain large amounts of glucose are administered to the patient. Because the digestive system is bypassed, no stimulus triggers the pancreas to release insulin. Treatment of HHNS is similar to the treatment of DKA, except for the fact that no ketoacidosis is associated with HHNS. Older patients should be monitored carefully for signs of fluid overload during the rehydration phase of treatment.

MEDICAL DIAGNOSIS

The diagnosis of DM is based on serum glucose levels. Normal fasting serum glucose levels are between 70 and 100 mg/dL. The official criteria for a diagnosis of DM were published in 1997 by the Expert Committee on the Diagnosis and Classification of Diabetes Mellitus and updated in 2013. A patient who meets one or more of the following criteria on two separate occasions is considered to have DM:

1. Fasting serum glucose level ≥126 mg/dl (after at least an 8-hour fast)
2. Hemoglobin A_{1c} ≥6.5%
3. Symptoms of diabetes (polyuria, polydipsia, polyphagia, unexplained weight loss) plus random glucose level ≥200 mg/dL (A random reading is based on a blood sample drawn any time of day without regard to mealtimes.)
4. Two-hour postprandial glucose level ≥200 mg/dL during an oral glucose tolerance test (OGTT) under specific guidelines (The test must use a glucose load of 75 g of anhydrous glucose dissolved in water.)

In the past, the fasting plasma glucose was the preferred diagnostic method because of the cost and poor reproducibility of the OGTT. In June 2009 the International Expert Committee on the Diagnosis of Diabetes (appointed by the American Diabetes Association, the European Association for the Study of Diabetes, and the International Diabetes Federation) presented their recommendations for including the use of A_{1c} levels for the diagnosis of diabetes. This resulted in the addition of the A_{1c} levels to the diagnostic criteria.

Prediabetes

Individuals with impaired fasting glucose (IFG), impaired glucose tolerance (IGT), or both are referred to as having *prediabetes.* IFG and IGT are risk factors for developing diabetes and cardiovascular disease. The individuals should receive education on weight reduction and increasing physical activity. Diagnostic criteria for prediabetes include:

- IFG: fasting plasma glucose level from 100 to 125 mg/dL
- IGT: 2-hour plasma glucose between 140 and 199 mg/dL during OGTT
- A_{1c}: 5.7% to 6.4%

MEDICAL TREATMENT

The goals of managing diabetes are to normalize the blood glucose, serum lipids, and body weight while meeting energy needs and achieving healthy body weight.

Nutritional Management

Medical nutrition therapy (MNT) is an important part of diabetes management and should be included in diabetes self-management education (see *Nutrition Considerations* box). Because of the complexity of nutritional management, a registered dietitian should be part of the diabetes management team and the individual with diabetes should be included in decision making. The goals of MNT are the following:

1. Attain and maintain optimal metabolic outcomes (glucose, lipids, blood pressure [BP]).

2. Prevent or slow the development of the chronic complications of diabetes (obesity, dyslipidemia, cardiovascular disease, hypertension, and nephropathy) by modifying nutrient intake and lifestyle.
3. Address individual nutritional needs while considering lifestyle, personal and cultural preferences, and the willingness to change.
4. Maintain the pleasure of eating by limiting food choices only when indicated by scientific evidence.

Provide self-management training for safe exercise, including prevention and treatment of hypoglycemia and management during acute illness.

Nutrition Considerations

1. Diet is an essential component in the management of type 1 and type 2 diabetes mellitus (DM).
2. The goal of the diabetic diet is to maintain plasma glucose as near to the normal physiologic range as possible.
3. A person who requires insulin to control DM should coordinate insulin administration with mealtime patterns.
4. Distribute food intake throughout the day to avoid large concentrations of calories, carbohydrates, and sugar.
5. Diet plans are individualized based on glucose and lipid levels, weight management goals, medical history, lifestyle, physical activity, and readiness to change.
6. When hypoglycemia is attributed to an overproduction of insulin in response to carbohydrate ingestion, a low-carbohydrate, high-protein diet with smaller meals may control the condition.

To maintain weight, a caloric intake of 28 calories/kg of body weight is required. To reduce weight, the caloric intake is calculated based on 15 to 20 calories/kg body weight. To arrive at a person's weight in kilograms, divide the weight in pounds by 2.2. For example, if a woman weighs 110 lb, her weight in kilograms is 55 kg. To maintain her weight, she needs to consume 1540 calories daily. Diets that advocate extreme reductions in carbohydrates (<130 g/day) are not recommended for individuals with diabetes.

Several nutrition planning approaches are in use. Carbohydrate counting is particularly useful for people who use intensive insulin therapy or pumps In addition to basal insulin requirements, bolus insulin doses are based on the total grams of carbohydrate ingested since carbohydrates have a greater effect on blood glucose levels than fat or protein. An emphasis is placed on maintaining a consistent carbohydrate intake each day but also allowing for insulin adjustments when carbohydrate intake is increased or decreased. Successful carbohydrate counting depends on understanding what foods are considered carbohydrates, how much of the food is considered a serving, reading labels, and knowing how much insulin is required for each serving of carbohydrate. Usually, 15 grams of total carbohydrate is considered a serving. Carbohydrates include starchy vegetables, fruits, bread, cereal, pasta, milk and milk products, and sweets. The amount of rapid-acting insulin required for each carbohydrate serving varies according to an individualized insulin-to-carbohydrate ratio (ICR) that is determined by a physician or diabetes educator. For example, if the ICR is 1 unit of rapid-acting insulin per carbohydrate serving, a carbohydrate intake of 45 grams would require a 3-unit bolus of rapid-acting insulin. The complexities of carbohydrate counting require motivation of the person using the system and thorough self-management education by a registered dietitian and/or a certified diabetes educator.

For most patients, a more simplified meal plan with the emphasis on a well-balanced diet within the prescribed distribution of proteins, fats, and carbohydrates is useful. The American Diabetes Association supports use of the Create Your Plate method. The American Dietetic Association advocates using the MyPlate food guide. For further explanation of these methods, see the *Health Promotion* box.

Health Promotion

Recommended Calorie Distribution for Patients Who Take Insulin

The American Diabetes Association recommends that the daily calorie intake be distributed as a mix of carbohydrates, protein, and fat adjusted to meet the metabolic goals of the individual. Saturated fat (animal fats, egg yolks, coconut oil, palm kernel oil, palm oil, and hydrogenated vegetable oils) intake should be less than 7% of the total calories. Reduction of trans fat is recommended to lower low-density lipoprotein (LDL) cholesterol and increase high-density lipoprotein (HDL) cholesterol.

High-protein diets are not recommended for weight loss because of the increased risk for kidney damage. Increased protein intake may be associated with an increase in the glomerular filtration rate. Sustained increases in the glomerular filtration rate cause renal and retinal vasodilation, leading to renal damage and retinopathy. Protein choices should come from lower fat sources, such as nonfat dairy products, legumes, skinless poultry, fish, and lean meats.

Carbohydrates should come from whole-grain breads, cereals, pasta, beans, brown rice, fruits, and vegetables. Learning to read food labels is essential because carbohydrate sources vary in calorie and fat content. Key strategies for glycemic control include carbohydrate counting, exchanges, and estimation. High-calorie food with low nutritional value should be limited. Foods containing sugar should be substituted for other carbohydrates (e.g., potatoes). Short-term (up to 1 year) use of low-carbohydrate or low-fat diets may be helpful for weight loss but potential health risks should be considered. Monitoring of lipid levels and renal functions is necessary, as is education on the increased risk for hypoglycemia. Sodium intake may be restricted for individuals with hypertension or renal insufficiency.

The addition of water-soluble fibers in the daily diet may lower total cholesterol and LDL levels. In addition, the lower

Continued

Health Promotion—cont'd

fat intake improves lipid levels, resulting in improved insulin sensitivity in skeletal muscle. Foods containing soluble fibers include oatmeal, rice, dried beans, oat bran, lentils, squash, whole wheat breads, and some fruits. Fiber intake should come from soluble and insoluble sources. When fiber is added to the diet, it should be done gradually. A sudden addition of large amounts of fiber to the diet may reduce the amount of glucose available for the exogenous insulin or hypoglycemic agent taken by the patient and may result in hypoglycemic episodes. Foods with a lower glycemic index that are rich in fiber, vitamins, and other nutrients are encouraged.

Limiting saturated fat to less than 7% of the total intake and minimizing trans fat are essential for controlling lipid levels. Elevated serum cholesterol and triglyceride levels are often associated with type 2 DM, increasing the risk of cardiovascular disease. Cholesterol should not exceed 200 mg/day. Research in the past several years has indicated that replacing some of the allotted fat calories with calories from carbohydrates and fiber has a positive effect on the lipid profile.

A simplified method of meal planning for people with diabetes has been designed by the American Diabetes Association. The Create Your Plate plan focuses on reducing starchy foods and meat and increasing intake of nonstarchy vegetables. The plate is divided in half and then one half is divided again into two sections. The largest section is filled with nonstarchy vegetables. One of the smaller sections is for starchy foods and the other smaller section is for protein. This plan is finished off with a serving of milk and a piece of fruit. The American Dietetic Association advocates a similar approach called MyPlate. The plate is divided into 4 sections, each of which represents a different food (protein, whole grains, fruits, and vegetables), with the addition of a serving of milk.

Patient teaching should include sample menus that include as many favorite foods as possible. People with diabetes require considerable education and support to learn to manage the dietary guidelines (see *Complementary and Alternative Therapies* box). It is vital to consider their personal and ethnic choices. Most nursing care situations do not lend themselves to the in-depth teaching, planning, and reinforcement needed. Outpatient education and visits with a certified diabetes educator (CDE) can help to meet this need.

Complementary and Alternative Therapies

Caution patients who take herbal supplements for diabetes that the supplements should not be used to *replace* conventional therapy. Ensure that the physician is aware of supplements being used.

Exercise

Exercise is a very effective treatment adjunct for people with diabetes. It aids in weight loss in obese patients, improves cardiovascular conditioning, improves insulin sensitivity, and promotes a sense of well-being. Exercising muscle uses glucose at 20 times the rate of a muscle at rest and does not require insulin. Much of the morbidity and mortality in patients with type 2 DM occurs because of the atherosclerosis that accompanies long-term uncontrolled diabetes, which places the patient at risk for CVA (stroke) and cardiovascular disease. Exercise is known to improve LDL cholesterol, serum glucose, BP, some blood coagulation parameters, and triglycerides. People with diabetes are advised to perform at least 150 minutes of exercise each week (see *Patient Teaching* box). However, exercise must be accompanied by appropriate nutrition to have long-term beneficial results.

Patient Teaching

Exercise and Diabetes

- Have a complete medical examination before initiating a new exercise program.
- Because circulating insulin may be inadequate to ensure glucose uptake, avoid exercise when your serum glucose is elevated and ketosis is present.
- Exercise with caution if your serum glucose is greater than 300 mg/dL and no ketosis is present.
- Wear comfortable athletic shoes that provide good support.
- Before every exercise session, warm up with 5 to 10 minutes of slow, continuous aerobic exercise and stretching.
- Discuss with your physician whether to alter food or insulin intake before exercise. A general recommendation is to exercise shortly after eating or to have a small snack before exercising if your serum glucose is less than 100 mg/dL.
- Avoid exercise during the peak action of insulin and oral hypoglycemics when hypoglycemia is more likely to occur.
- Carbohydrate snacking may be necessary with prolonged or intense exercise.
- If you take insulin, inject it in the abdomen rather than in an extremity before a workout because the drug is absorbed much more quickly from the abdomen.
- Some people experience hypoglycemia several hours after exercise; have food available for these situations.

The metabolic adjustments that maintain glucose levels during exercise are regulated largely by hormones. A decrease in plasma insulin levels and the presence of glucagons are necessary for hepatic glucose production during physical activity. Increases in plasma glucagon and catecholamine levels are key factors for hepatic glucose release during prolonged exercise. Exercise affects individuals with type 1 DM differently from those with type 2 DM who do not require insulin. Hyperglycemia may occur with exercise in the patient with type 1 DM when insulin levels are inadequate. An excessive release of counterregulatory hormones and mobilization of free fatty acids result in ketone production, which can lead to the development of DKA. In patients with type 2 DM, exercise makes insulin receptor sites more sensitive to insulin and lowers plasma glucose levels, which can result in hypoglycemia.

Because of this, it is important for individuals with diabetes to monitor blood glucose levels before and after exercise. Individuals taking insulin may also need to monitor blood glucose levels during prolonged exercise. Caution should be taken when exercising during peak activity of injected insulin to decrease the risk of hypoglycemia. Additional carbohydrate intake may be necessary during prolonged exercise and any time glucose levels are less than 100 mg/dL. Physical activity should be avoided if the fasting glucose levels are more than 250 mg/dL and ketones are present. Caution should be used if glucose levels are more than 300 mg/dL in the absence of ketones.

An appropriate combination of aerobic and anaerobic exercises should be determined. Aerobic exercise produces the most therapeutic effect. The patient should exercise for 30 to 60 minutes three to four times a week. Warm-up exercises such as stretching and walking are recommended before exercise, followed by cool-down exercises afterward. The best aerobic exercises are walking, swimming, bicycle riding, and jogging. Anaerobic exercises are done to build muscle mass. These include activities such as weight lifting, yoga, and sit-ups. Very strenuous exercises can raise BP, which is undesirable with retinopathy and nephropathy. Eventually, the patient with type 2 disease who adheres to a sound nutritional plan and exercise regimen may be able to decrease the amount of exogenous insulin or oral hypoglycemics needed (see *Health Promotion* box).

Health Promotion

Physical Activity for People with Prediabetes and Diabetes

Research has shown that physical activity has the following benefits for patients with diabetes—and for the rest of us:

- Lowers blood glucose and blood pressure (BP)
- Lowers low-density lipoprotein (LDL) cholesterol and raises high-density lipoprotein (HDL) cholesterol
- Improves the body's ability to use insulin
- Lowers the risk of heart disease and stroke
- Strengthens bones
- Keeps joints flexible
- Lowers the risk of falling
- Aids in weight loss
- Reduces body fat
- Increases energy level and reduces stress

Physical activity also plays an important part in preventing type 2 DM. A major government study, the Diabetes Prevention Program, showed that a healthy diet and a moderate exercise program resulting in a 5% to 7% weight loss can delay and perhaps prevent the onset of type 2 diabetes.

For those who already have diabetes, physical activity offers all of the benefits listed above. However, because some exercises may worsen diabetic complications, care should be taken in starting and maintaining an exercise program. For example, activities that increase the ocular blood pressure (BP), such as lifting heavy weights, can worsen any existing ophthalmologic complications.

Health Promotion—cont'd

To avoid blisters that go unnoticed, leading to a serious infection, patients who walk or engage in other aerobic activities should wear cotton socks and shoes that are designed for the activity. After exercise, the feet should be checked for cuts, sores, bumps, or redness. Patients with numbness in their feet might try swimming instead of walking for aerobic exercise.

Because exercise can cause hypoglycemia, the following precautions are recommended.

BEFORE EXERCISE

- Patients should be careful about exercising after skipping a recent meal.
- Patients who take insulin should ask their health care team whether they should change their dosage before engaging in physical activity.

DURING EXERCISE

- Patients should wear a medical identification bracelet or other form of identification.
- Patients with type 2 DM should always carry food or glucose tablets so that they are prepared to treat hypoglycemia.

If patients exercise for more than 1 hour, blood glucose should be checked at regular intervals.

AFTER EXERCISE

- Patients should check to see how exercise affected their blood glucose level.

Adapted from National Diabetes Information Clearinghouse, National Institute of Diabetes and Digestive and Kidney Diseases: What I need to know about physical activity and diabetes (website): http://diabetes.niddk.nih.gov/dm/pubs/physical_ez/index.htm. Accessed July 1, 2014.

Insulin Therapy

All patients with type 1 DM need insulin injections and some patients with type 2 DM may eventually need insulin. Insulin is classified by onset and duration of action. For many years, all insulin was obtained from beef and pork. However, beef and pork insulin are not identical to human insulin and patients could form antibodies against them. The advent of recombinant deoxyribonucleic acid (rDNA) technology has allowed the manufacture of insulin that is identical to endogenous insulin. This "human" insulin causes fewer problems than that from animal sources.

Insulin can be classified as *rapid acting, short acting, intermediate acting*, and *long acting*. Rapid-acting insulins include insulin lispro (Humalog), insulin aspart (NovoLog), and insulin glulisine (Apidra). Regular insulin (Humulin R, Novolin R) is classified as *short-acting insulin.* Intermediate-acting insulins are NPH (Humulin N, Novolin N). Long-acting insulins are insulin glargine (Lantus) and insulin detemir (Levemir). All rapid-acting and short-acting insulins are clear. Intermediate-acting and long-acting insulins have traditionally been cloudy but Lantus and Levemir are clear. Insulin vial labels should be read carefully to prevent errors. Onset, peak, and duration for various insulin preparations are compared in Table 48-1. The effect of insulin on blood glucose levels is shown in Figure 48-2.

Table 48-1 Drug Therapy: Insulin Preparations: Time Course of Action

INSULIN TYPE	APPEARANCE	ONSET	PEAK	DURATION
Rapid-Acting Insulin				
Insulin lispro (Humalog) Insulin aspart (NovoLog) Insulin glulisine (Apidra)	Clear	15–30 minutes	30–90 minutes	3–5 hours
Short-Acting Insulin				
Regular insulin (Humulin R, Novolin R)	Clear	30 minutes–1 hour	2–4 hours	5–8 hours
Intermediate-Acting (NPH) Insulin				
Humulin N Novolin N	Cloudy	1–3 hours	6–10 hours	12–16 hours
Long-Acting Insulin				
Insulin glargine (Lantus) Insulin detemir (Levemir)	Clear	1 hour	Minimal	Up to 24 hours

Modified from What I Need to Know About Diabetes Medicines. National Diabetes Information Clearinghouse. National Institute of Diabetes and Digestive and Kidney Diseases. NIH. Last updated February 16, 2012. Retrieved October 3, 2014 from http://diabetes.niddk.nih.gov/dm/pubs/medicines_ez/Insert_C.aspx.

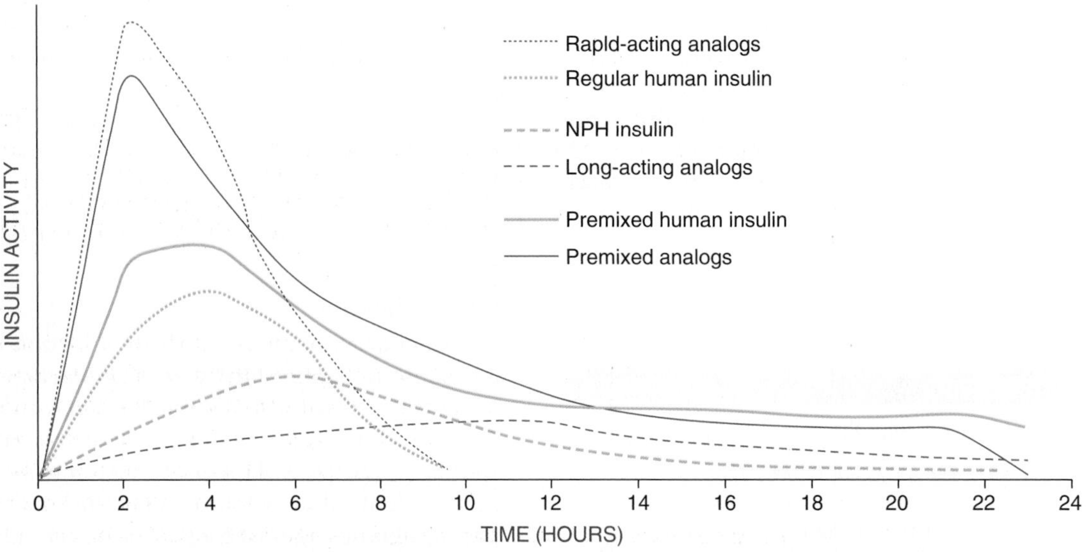

Adapted from product label information approved by the Food and Drug Administration.

FIGURE 48-2 Effect of insulin on blood glucose levels. (Used by permission of the Agency for Healthcare Research and Quality. AHRQ Pub. No. 08(09)-EHC017-3. *Clinician's Guide: Premixed Insulin Analogues, a Comparison with Other Treatments for Type 2 Diabetes*, March 2009.)

Route. Insulin cannot be given orally because it is rendered useless in the GI tract. All insulins can be given subcutaneously. Historically, *only* Regular insulin was given intravenously; however, intravenous administration of rapid-acting insulin has become a common practice. A form of inhaled insulin was on the market briefly; companies continue to work on alternative routes for insulin delivery.

Concentrations. Insulins are available in varying concentrations. U-100 insulin has a concentration of 100 units/mL and U-500 has 500 units/mL. U-100 is most commonly used. U-500 insulin is used only in emergencies and for patients who are extremely insulin resistant.

Premixed Insulin Products. Premixed insulins that contain two types of insulins are available. Four mixtures commonly are used: (1) 70% NPH and 30% Regular insulin (Humulin 70/30, Novolin 70/30), (2) 50% lispro protamine and 50% insulin lispro (Humalog Mix 50/50), (3) 75% lispro protamine and 25% lispro (Humalog Mix 75/25), and (4) 70% aspart protamine and 30% aspart (NovoLog Mix 70/30). Premixed solutions are easier to prepare and they decrease the risk of errors associated with drawing up two types of insulin in the same syringe. The downside to use of premixed insulin is that you cannot adjust each type of insulin individually to fine-tune glucose control.

Dosing Schedules. The pancreas secretes minute amounts of insulin continuously except after the ingestion of a meal, when it secretes a bolus of insulin into the system. Exogenous insulin is administered in an effort to mimic the action of a normal pancreas. Therefore the person with diabetes requires a bolus of rapid-acting or short-acting insulin before meals to prevent too rapid a rise in glucose. A long-acting or intermediate-acting insulin may be prescribed as well in an effort to keep glucose levels even at other times.

Pharmacology Capsule

Insulin lispro, insulin aspart, and insulin glulisine act rapidly. Regular insulin is short acting, NPH is intermediate acting, and insulin glargine and insulin detemir are long acting. Be sure to administer the correct type!

Conventional Therapy. Conventional therapy uses one of several dosage schedules and typically uses a combination of a rapid-acting and an intermediate-acting or long-acting insulin. One example is the one-fifth rule that some physicians use for prescribing insulin. In the morning, the patient takes two fifths of the day's supply in an intermediate-acting insulin such as NPH. In addition, the patient takes one fifth of the daily requirement of insulin as Regular insulin. The latter dose covers breakfast glucose. Because the NPH peaks at lunchtime, the patient does not need Regular insulin for this meal. At suppertime, the patient takes one fifth of the daily insulin requirement in the form of an intermediate-acting insulin and one fifth as rapid-acting insulin to cover supper carbohydrates. For example, a patient who is prescribed 50 units of insulin a day might take it as follows:

- AM: 20 units of NPH insulin
- AM: 10 units of Regular insulin
- PM: 10 units of NPH insulin
- PM: 10 units of Regular insulin

Patients on conventional therapy should monitor their blood glucose before meals at least two times each day. A major problem with conventional therapy is nocturnal hypoglycemia: blood glucose falls between 3 AM and 4 AM. Because of this, intermediate-acting and long-acting insulin may be administered at bedtime.

Basal-Bolus Insulin Therapy. Research supports the use of basal-bolus insulin therapy (also called intensive insulin therapy) for improved glycemic control. This regimen requires the use of:

- Basal insulin (long-acting insulin) to counteract hepatic glucose production. Dosing is based on weight and estimated insulin sensitivity. Basal insulin is usually given once daily, most often at bedtime.
- Rapid-acting insulin before each meal to blunt postprandial glucose spikes. Dosing is based on weight, insulin sensitivity, and carbohydrate intake. The bolus dose can also be adjusted to treat premeal hyperglycemia.

An example of basal-bolus insulin therapy would be the following:

- PREMEAL: Rapid-acting insulin, usually started at 0.05 units/kg/meal (2 to 10 units per meal) plus correctional insulin for hyperglycemia.
- BEDTIME: Long-acting insulin, usually started at 0.2 to 0.3 units/kg/day (20 to 50 units per day) in a single dose at bedtime. Sometimes this basal insulin is divided into two injections.

Home blood glucose monitoring is essential with this regimen. The intensified program permits more flexibility in meal composition and timing. Basal-bolus insulin therapy does increase the risk for hypoglycemia, which underlines the importance of consistent blood glucose monitoring. It is important to note that studies like the RABBIT 2 Trial (Umpierrez, 2011) show that basal-bolus insulin therapy provides better glycemic control in hospitalized patients undergoing surgery when compared to standard sliding scale or PRN insulin. The positive results of this study have led many practitioners to advocate the use of basal-bolus insulin therapy in the outpatient setting.

Continuous Subcutaneous Insulin Infusion. The last dosing schedule uses continuous subcutaneous insulin infusion. The patient has an indwelling subcutaneous catheter connected to an external portable infusion pump. The pump delivers rapid-acting or Regular insulin continuously at basal rates set by the user. Before meals, the patient activates the pump to provide the appropriate amount of insulin bolus for the meal to be consumed. Patients who use pumps also must do self-monitoring of blood glucose (SMBG). Newer versions of insulin pumps allow for multiple settings for basal insulin dosages as well as transmission of blood glucose levels to the insulin pump for more precise insulin dosing. Some insulin pump users can also perform continuous glucose monitoring (CGM) with a separate sensing device that automatically transmits glucose levels to the insulin pump for immediate adjustments in insulin dosages.

Pharmacology Capsule

Remember "clear to cloudy!" When mixing short-acting (clear) and longer-acting (cloudy) insulins, draw the short-acting insulin into the syringe first. Note: Insulin glargine (Lantus) and insulin detemir (Levemir) *cannot be mixed* with other insulin types!

Insulin Injection. The suggested sites for subcutaneous insulin injections are illustrated in Figure 48-3. Site rotation helps to prevent **lipohypertrophy** (i.e., swelling or lumps) or **lipoatrophy** (i.e., hollowing or pitting of the subcutaneous tissue). Patients with the latter problem should see a physician about changing the insulin to human insulin (Humulin). In some cases, injecting these sites with their prescribed daily human insulin has resolved the problem. Because

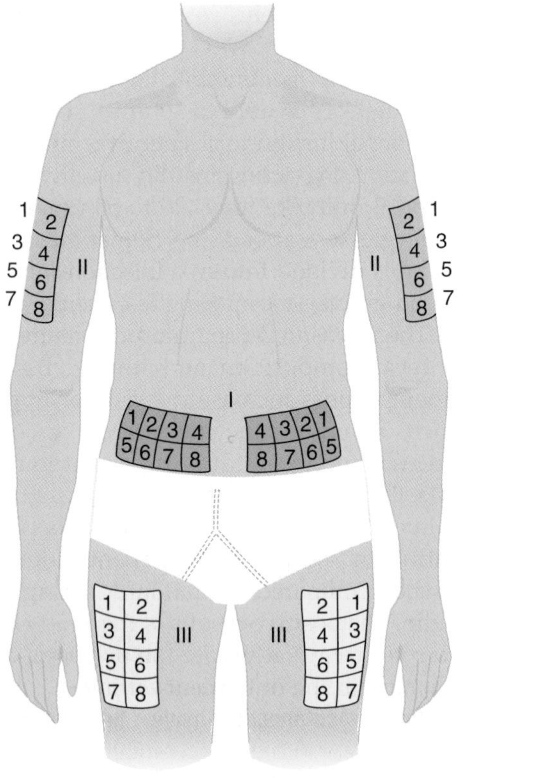

FIGURE 48-3 Insulin injection sites. (From Black JM, Hawks JH: *Medical-surgical nursing: clinical management for positive outcomes*, ed 8, St. Louis, 2009, Saunders.)

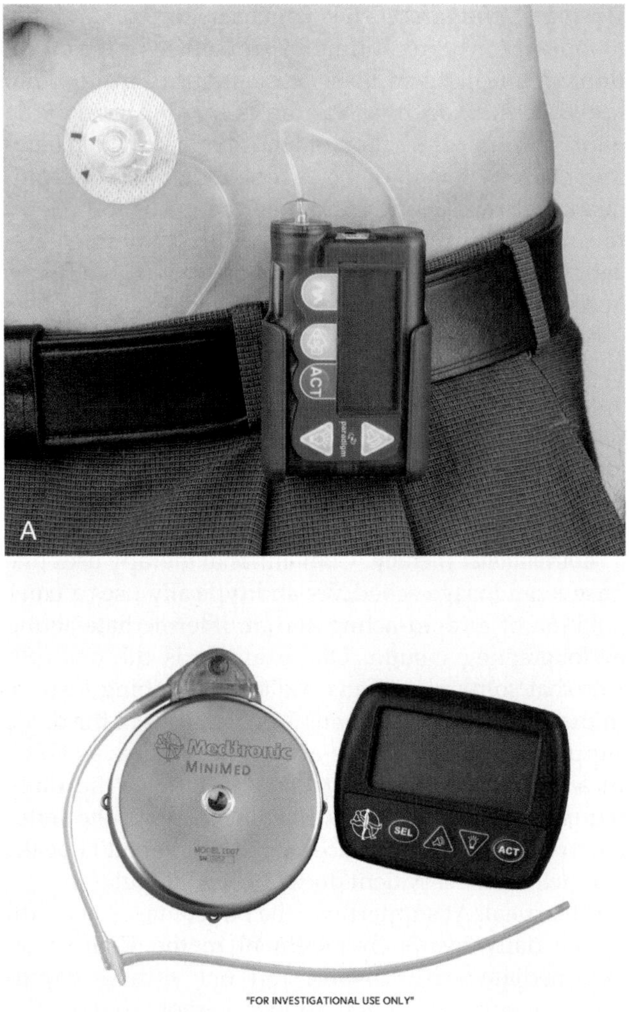

B

FIGURE 48-4 Insulin pumps. **A,** MiniMED 507 Insulin Pump with Quick-Release Infusion Set. *Manufactured by the diabetes division of Medtronic, Inc.* **B,** MiniMed Model 2001 Implantable Insulin Pump and handheld programmer. *Manufactured by the diabetes division of Medtronic, Inc.* (A, B, Courtesy Medtronic Diabetes.)

lipohypertrophy interferes with the absorption of insulin, affected areas should be avoided as injection sites.

The absorption rate of insulin varies with different body sites. The rate of absorption from the abdomen is approximately 50% faster than from the thighs. For this reason, the American Diabetes Association recommends rotating sites within one anatomic area rather than moving among all areas. Heat and massage increase the absorption rate, as does exercise. As mentioned earlier, if insulin is injected into the thigh before exercise such as jogging, the absorption rate is greatly increased.

Insulin Pump. An external insulin pump looks much like a pager. It consists of a battery-driven syringe with a long piece of tubing (usually made of Teflon) that is attached to a small needle. The needle is inserted subcutaneously in an appropriate part of the anatomy (Fig. 48-4). The syringe usually contains a 2- to 3-day supply of insulin. The pump is programmed to deliver a steady trickle of insulin throughout the day and can provide a bolus of insulin at mealtimes. In this manner, the unit mimics the pancreas. The patient calculates the bolus based on self-monitored blood glucose levels. Every 2 to 3 days, the syringe, needle, and tubing are replaced.

One advantage of the external insulin pump is that patients do not have to use intermediate-acting or long-acting insulin, with their uncertain fluctuations in glucose. Other advantages are that it gives the patient more flexibility regarding mealtimes, travel, and exercise. Potential problems with the pump are occlusion of the tubing or the needle and infection at the site of needle insertion. To use the pump, the patient must undergo intensive education and be willing to self-monitor blood glucose levels several times a day if the pump does not monitor blood glucose levels. Some medical insurance companies do not cover the cost of the pump or pump therapy, which makes the cost prohibitive to many. Efforts to develop an "artificial pancreas" are underway. The device would be implanted under the skin and would dispense insulin in response to changing blood glucose levels.

Other less commonly used devices for insulin administration are the jet injector, pen injector, and implanted insulin pump. The jet injector delivers insulin through the skin without a needle. The injection does sting and may bruise thin and older people.

The high cost of the jet injector is a deterrent to its use. The pen injector looks like a fountain pen and holds preloaded cartridges with the prescribed insulin dose. These prefilled insulin pens are very convenient and easy to use because the insulin dose is dialed in. The insulin pens are easy to transport and work well for individuals who are on the go.

Oral Hypoglycemics (Antihyperglycemics or Antidiabetics)

If patients with type 2 DM are unable to control their blood glucose with a nutrition program and exercise, the physician may prescribe one or more oral hypoglycemics. If the serum glucose level stays elevated, insulin may be prescribed temporarily until the blood glucose levels decrease below 200 mg/dL. Oral hypoglycemics include sulfonylureas, alpha-glucosidase inhibitors, biguanides, thiazolidinediones, meglitinides and D-phenylalanines, dipeptidyl peptidase-4 (DPP-4) inhibitors, and sodium glucose cotransporter-2 inhibitors.

Sulfonylureas. Sulfonylureas lower blood sugars by stimulating the pancreas to secrete more insulin and increasing the sensitivity of insulin receptors. First- and second-generation sulfonylureas are equally effective in controlling serum glucose but have some important differences, as shown in Table 48-2. Because of the long duration of action, first-generation sulfonylureas are not often used now.

A significant adverse effect of the sulfonylureas is the risk of hypoglycemia. First-generation sulfonylureas also have the potential for interactions with many other drugs, which is problematic in the patient who is taking multiple medications. First-generation drugs are not recommended in patients with liver or renal disease. Because the sulfonylureas are chemically similar to sulfonamide antibacterials, patients who are allergic to one also may be allergic to the other. Be sure to assess for allergy to sulfonamides before a patient starts taking a sulfonylurea.

The second- and third-generation drugs are more potent (so require lower dosage), pose less risk of hypoglycemia, have fewer other side effects, and have fewer drug interactions. Many older people have diminished renal and liver function, which affects metabolism and elimination of drugs and increases the risk of hypoglycemia. When a sulfonylurea is ordered for the older patient, it is usually glipizide (Glucotrol), which must be taken on an empty stomach; glyburide (DiaBeta, Micronase); or glimepiride (Amaryl). Drugs with long durations of action are more likely to accumulate and cause toxic effects in older patients.

Alpha-Glucosidase Inhibitors. Examples of alpha-glucosidase inhibitors are acarbose (Precose) and

Table 48-2 Drug Therapy: Oral Hypoglycemics for Type 2 Diabetes

DRUG CATEGORY	MEDICATION	ACTION	POSSIBLE SIDE EFFECTS
Sulfonylureas	glipizide (Glucotrol) glyburide (Diabeta, Micronase, Glynase) glimepiride (Amaryl)	Stimulates pancreatic secretion of insulin	Hypoglycemia, weight gain, sulfa allergy
Biguanides	metformin (Glucophage, Fortamet, Riomet)	Inhibits hepatic glucose production, increases insulin sensitivity	Lactic acidosis, hypoglycemia when used with sulfonylurea or meglitinide
Meglitinides/D-phenylalanines	repaglinide (Prandin) nateglinide (Starlix)	Stimulates pancreatic secretion of insulin	Hypoglycemia, weight gain
Thiazolidinediones	pioglitazone (Actos), rosiglitazone (Avandia)	Increases insulin sensitivity in the tissues	Hypoglycemia when used with sulfonylurea or meglitinide, weight gain, decreased effectiveness of oral contraceptives, possible liver dysfunction
Alpha-glucosidase inhibitors	acarbose (Precose), miglitol (Glyset)	Delays absorption of carbohydrates in the intestine	Gastrointestinal (GI) side effects
Dipeptidyl peptidase-4 (DPP-4) inhibitors	sitagliptin (Januvia) saxagliptin (Onglyza)	Increases insulin production and decreases hepatic glucose production	Occasional stomach upset and diarrhea
Sodium glucose cotransporter-2 inhibitor	canagliflozin (Invokana)	Inhibition of SGLT2 reduces renal resorption of glucose resulting in increased urinary glucose excretion	Hypotension, hyperkalemia, renal impairment

Modified from Medicines for Type 2 Diabetes. AHRQ Pub No. 11-EHC038 - A, June 2011. Retrieved Oct. 3, 2014 from http://www.effectivehealthcare.ahrq.gov/index.cfm/search-for-guides-reviews-and-reports/?productid=721&pageaction=displayproduct.

miglitol (Glyset). These drugs delay digestion of complex carbohydrates into glucose and other simple sugars. Sometimes they are given in combination with insulin or a sulfonylurea. Side effects include abdominal cramping and distention, flatulence, and diarrhea. Alpha-glucosidase inhibitors should not be prescribed to individuals with inflammatory bowel disease (IBD) or other intestinal diseases. Acarbose and miglitol do not cause hypoglycemia when used alone. However, if the patient becomes hypoglycemic because of another hypoglycemic agent taken in combination with the alpha-glucosidase inhibitor, oral sucrose will not effectively raise the blood sugar because of the decreased absorption of the sucrose. The patient will instead require treatment with oral glucose.

Biguanides. Metformin (Glucophage, Fortamet) is a biguanide that decreases glucose production by the liver and increases the use of glucose by muscle cells. These medications do not cause hypoglycemia when used alone. Adverse GI effects are fairly common but may be decreased by starting at lower doses and working up to the prescribed dose. Dosing is usually two to three times a day. Glucophage XR is an extended-release form of metformin that is taken only once a day. A rare but potentially fatal adverse effect is lactic acidosis, which usually occurs in the presence of impaired renal function. Biguanides should not be used in the very old or when severe kidney, cardiovascular, or respiratory conditions are present. This medication should also be held after procedures or tests that require the use of intravenous dye.

Thiazolidinediones. Thiazolidinediones include rosiglitazone maleate (Avandia) and pioglitazone HCl (Actos). Classified as *insulin-sensitizing agents*, they increase the uptake of glucose by skeletal muscle and fat tissue. These drugs do not cause hypoglycemia when used alone but may when used with a sulfonylurea. Because the first drug in this class (Rezulin) was found to have serious adverse effects on the liver, liver function must be monitored when this class of drugs is used. To date, Avandia and Actos appear to pose a low risk of liver damage. Side effects include weight gain, edema, and mild transient anemia. Patients should be aware that these drugs decrease the effectiveness of oral contraceptives. They are contraindicated with class III or IV heart failure (HF) and during pregnancy.

Meglitinides and D-Phenylalanines. Repaglinide (Prandin) is a meglitinide and nateglinide (Starlix) is a D-phenylalanine. Because of the similarity of these two types of drugs, called *mealtime insulin secretogogues*, they will be discussed together. Meglitinides and D-phenylalanine stimulate the release of insulin from the pancreas. Taken before each meal, they prevent post-prandial blood glucose elevations and prolonged hypoglycemia. Patients should omit the medications if they skip a meal. Hypoglycemia may occur with strenuous exercise or alcohol consumption. Weight gain is a side effect. They are used cautiously with moderate to severe liver failure.

Dipeptidyl Peptidase-4 Inhibitors. Sitagliptin (Januvia) and saxagliptin (Onglyza) are the newest oral medications to treat diabetes. Januvia and Onglyza stimulate pancreatic release of insulin and inhibit hepatic glucose production. These medications can be taken alone or with other oral diabetes medications. Neither should be taken with insulin. Side effects include stomach upset, diarrhea, and headache. Possible adverse reactions are elevated liver enzymes and inflamed pancreas. Dose adjustments for Januvia and Onglyza are necessary for individuals with moderate to severe renal disease.

Sodium Glucose Cotransporter-2 Inhibitors. Canagliflozin (Invokana) is the first in a new class of glucose-lowering drugs, an oral inhibitor of sodium glucose cotransporter-2 (SGLT2). Inhibition of SGLT2 reduces the resorption of glucose in the kidney, resulting in increased urinary glucose excretion, lowering of plasma glucose levels, and weight loss. Side effects include hypotension, hyperkalemia, yeast infections, urinary tract infections, and decreased urination. These side effects and the link to increased risk for cardiovascular events and strokes may limit the use of this medication.

Combination Oral Medications. With increasing use of combination therapy, patients must take more medication doses—a factor that often reduces compliance. Several combination drugs have been released that help to simplify dosing schedules. These medications include Actoplus Met (pioglitazone and metformin), Avandamet (rosiglitazone and metformin), Avandaryl (rosiglitazone and glimepiride), Glucovance (glyburide and metformin), Metaglip (glipizide and metformin), Janumet (metformin and sitagliptin), PrandiMet (metformin and repaglinide), and Duetact (pioglitazone and glimepiride). The actions and side and adverse effects are the same as for each individual drug.

In 2005 two new injectable medications to treat diabetes were approved by the U.S. Food and Drug Administration (FDA). Pramlintide (Symlin) is a synthetic form of the hormone *amylin*, which plays a role in glucose homeostasis by suppressing postprandial glucagon secretion, slowing gastric emptying, and suppressing appetite. Pramlintide, used to treat type 1 and type 2 diabetes (requiring insulin), increases the risk for hypoglycemia and GI side effects. It is administered by injection before each meal and cannot be mixed with insulin. Exenatide (Byetta, Bydureon) is classified as an *incretin mimetic* that is used only with type 2 diabetes. Exenatide lowers blood glucose levels by increasing insulin secretion, suppressing postprandial glucagon secretion, slowing gastric emptying, and suppressing appetite. Exenatide works only in the presence of elevated glucose levels, so no increased risk for hypoglycemia exists unless the patient is also on sulfonylureas. Most individuals on this medication experience a decreased appetite and weight loss. Both of these new medications have somewhat complex dosing schedules and require injections before each meal. They are also expensive and not covered by many insurance companies. The most recent noninsulin injection that is used to treat diabetes was introduced in 2009. Liraglutide (Victoza) stimulates insulin production while suppressing hepatic glucose output and helps with weight loss. It can initially cause nausea, vomiting, and diarrhea but the side effects usually diminish with time. These injectable medications are detailed in Table 48-3.

Approximately 30% to 40% of patients with type 2 diabetes fail to respond to oral agents. Another 10% cease to respond after a period of successful treatment. To maintain optimal glucose control, it is beneficial for these patients to use insulin. Some of them may have to take one dose of insulin, often at night, and then are able to control serum glucose for the rest of the day with oral drugs. A variety of combination regimens (using oral agents and insulin) are being studied.

Self-Monitoring of Blood Glucose. People with diabetes need to monitor their blood glucose levels so that they can regulate their diet, exercise, and medication regimens to remain euglycemic and lead lifestyles that are as normal as possible. SMBG is seen as the greatest breakthrough in managing diabetes since the advent of insulin. It reduces the complications of long-term diabetes by helping the patient to normalize blood glucose levels. The frequency of blood glucose monitoring depends on individualized treatment plans and patient goals. More frequent monitoring (three to six times a day) is required for patients on insulin or using insulin pumps. Monitoring of postprandial glucose levels may also be appropriate when postmeal glucose targets are not being met. Recent advances in technology also allow for CGM. CGM devices measure the interstitial glucose levels but they must periodically be calibrated to SMBG results.

The use of portable electronic glucose meters has largely replaced other methods of self-monitoring. The patient puts a drop of blood on a special reagent strip and inserts the strip in the meter. In less than 1 minute, the glucose level appears on a monitor. Some meters give plasma glucose values whereas others give whole blood readings. Factors that may affect the use of these meters include cost, comfort with technology, fine-motor coordination, intellectual ability, and willingness to use the meter. SMBG is a useful tool in managing diabetes during pregnancy, when glucose levels may change frequently. It also is a must in managing unstable diabetes and for patients who are prone to sudden hypoglycemic episodes or ketoacidosis or who have abnormal renal glucose thresholds.

Ketone testing is also recommended when symptoms of illness, such as nausea, vomiting, or abdominal pain, are present. Ketones are produced when the body breaks down fat for energy, instead of using carbohydrates. Presence of ketones along with hyperglycemia and illness may indicate the development of DKA. Ketones can be detected in the blood before ketones spill over into the urine, so blood testing is preferred. Some more advance home glucose monitors can also measure ketones. Otherwise, urine ketone testing is recommended.

Goals for glycemic control should be clearly set with consideration to age and comorbidities (i.e., medical conditions in addition to DM). For nonpregnant adults, preprandial plasma glucose levels should be between 70 and 130 mg/dL. Peak postprandial plasma glucose levels should be less than 180 mg/dL. Results falling outside of these recommended parameters warrant alterations in the diabetes regimen. It is important to note that glycemic control during hospitalization must be adjusted. Insulin therapy should be initiated for persistent glucose levels >180 mg/dL with a goal of maintaining glucose levels between 140 and 180 mg/dL. More stringent glucose control during acute illness increases the risk for hypoglycemic episodes.

Glycosylated Glucose Levels

Determination of glycosylated hemoglobin ($HgbA_{1c}$) or fructosamine levels every 2 to 3 months is an essential check of glycemic control. The $HgbA_{1c}$ reflects glucose levels over the past few months whereas the fructosamine levels reflect those over several weeks. When the glucose level is elevated, a certain percentage of the glucose molecules bind to the hemoglobin on the red blood cell (RBC). The glucose stays on the cell for the life of the cell, which is approximately 3 months. By measuring $HgbA_{1c}$ or fructosamine levels, the physician is able to determine how well the blood glucose has been regulated in the recent past. It also allows patients who monitor their own blood glucose levels to evaluate their methods of control. The American Diabetes Association recommends an $HgbA_{1c}$ level less than 7% as a treatment goal—or as close to normal as possible without risking hypoglycemia. Less stringent control is advocated for those with episodes of severe hypoglycemia, those who are very young or very old, and those with increased comorbidities.

Correlation of A_{1c} with Average Glucose

Glycosylated Hemoglobin ($HgbA_{1c}$)	**Mean Plasma Glucose mg/dL**
6	126
7	154
8	183
9	212
10	240
11	269
12	298

Adapted from American Diabetes Association: Standards of medical care in diabetes, *Diabetes Care* 36(suppl 1):S19, 2013.

Table 48-3 Drug Therapy: Additional Drugs Used to Treat Diabetes Mellitus

DRUG	ADMINISTRATION	USE	FEATURES	ACTIONS	MAJOR ADVERSE EFFECTS
pramlintide (Symlin)	Given by injection at mealtimes at same time as insulin but the two cannot be mixed in the same syringe. Slows movement of food through digestive tract, which slows rate of glucose absorption. May decrease amount of insulin needed before meals.	Treats types 1 and 2 diabetes mellitus (DM).	Increases the risk for hypoglycemia and gastrointestinal (GI) side effects (i.e., nausea, vomiting, stomach pain). Complex dosing scheduler. Can delay absorption of other drugs. Expensive.	Decreases glucose production by liver and increases glucose uptake by muscle.	GI symptoms: decreased appetite, nausea, diarrhea, flatulence, cramps, abdominal distention, borborygmus. Lactic acidosis (rarely). Hypoglycemia but only in the presence of excessive insulin.
exenatide (Byetta, Bydureon)	Given by injection within 1 hour before morning and evening meals. Used in addition to metformin or a sulfonylurea. Increases insulin secretion but does not replace the need for insulin in patients who require it. Works only in the presence of elevated glucose levels, so no increased risk for hypoglycemia exists unless the patient is also on sulfonylureas.	Treats type 2 DM.	Can cause hypoglycemia and GI side effects (i.e., decreased appetite and weight loss [common], diarrhea, nausea, and vomiting), dizziness, headache. Complex dosing schedule. Comes in a prefilled pen. Expensive.	Inhibits carbohydrate digestion and absorption, thereby decreasing the postprandial rise in blood glucose. Decreases insulin resistance, thereby increasing glucose uptake by muscle and decreasing glucose production by the liver.	Weight gain, edema, transient anemia. Monitor liver function, even though risk of liver damage is thought to be small.
liraglutide (Victoza)	Given by injection once daily. Doses are not based on glucose levels, meal intake, or activity.	Treats type 2 DM	Easy dosing. Initially can cause nausea, vomiting, and diarrhea.	A glucagon-type peptide 1 (GLP-1) hormone replacement, stimulates insulin production while suppressing hepatic glucose production.	Increases the risk for pancreatitis, pancreatic cancer, and renal failure.

Data from National Diabetes Information Clearing House and the National Institute of Diabetes and Digestive and Kidney Diseases (NIDDK): What I need to know about diabetes medicines (website): http://diabetes.niddk.nih.gov/dm/pubs/medicines_ez/index.htm. Accessed July 1, 2014.

Complications of Therapy

Hypoglycemia. A common complication of diabetes management is hypoglycemia. Hypoglycemia can be the result of excessive insulin or oral hypoglycemic agents, inadequate food intake, delayed or missed meals, and inconsistent or excessive exercise. Treatment of hypoglycemia is discussed in the section titled "Acute Emergency Complications" but the main thing for the nurse to remember is that the patient needs some form of glucose immediately.

Somogyi Phenomenon. Too much insulin can actually cause hyperglycemia. The Somogyi phenomenon is characterized by rebound hyperglycemia that occurs in response to hypoglycemia. The phenomenon begins with an episode of hypoglycemia, often during the night. Hypoglycemia triggers the body's stress response in an attempt to restore homeostasis. Epinephrine is secreted, which stimulates the liver to convert stored glycogen to glucose, thereby raising the blood glucose level to the point of hyperglycemia.

The Somogyi phenomenon should be suspected when a patient reports awakening with a headache and complains of restless sleep, nightmares, enuresis (involuntary voiding during sleep), and nausea and vomiting. The blood glucose records reflect fluctuation between hypoglycemia and hyperglycemia. The patient may have tried without success to correct the hyperglycemia by increasing the insulin.

To confirm suspected Somogyi phenomenon, the patient's blood glucose needs to be measured between 2 and 4 AM and again at 7 AM. The 2 and 4 AM levels below 60 mg/dL and a 7 AM level above 180 mg/dL support the diagnosis of Somogyi phenomenon. This vicious cycle can be broken by gradually decreasing the evening dose of exogenous insulin by 2 or 3 units every 3 or 4 days until the rebound hyperglycemia is brought under control. A bedtime snack also may be helpful.

Dawn Phenomenon. Some people with diabetes who are insulin dependent experience an increase in fasting blood glucose levels between 5 and 9 AM that is not related to a period of hypoglycemia. The most likely cause is the release of GH and cortisol, which increase blood glucose during early-morning rapid eye movement sleep. The blood glucose level is typically normal at 3 AM but elevated at 6 or 7 AM. The condition may be treated with a bedtime snack and delay of the evening intermediate-acting insulin until 10 PM.

❖ NURSING CARE of the Patient with Diabetes Mellitus

■ Assessment

When a person with diabetes seeks medical care in an emergency situation, a complete assessment must be delayed until the patient is stable. The licensed vocational nurse/licensed practical nurse (LVN/LPN) collects data that assist in the management of this situation. If the patient is in ketoacidosis, the assessment is likely to show ketonuria, Kussmaul respirations, orthostatic hypotension, hypertension (at times), nausea, vomiting, and lethargy or change in level of consciousness. In the hypoglycemic patient, expect to find tachycardia, anxiety, trembling, and decreasing level of consciousness. Be alert for indications of HHNS (decreased level of consciousness, polyuria, and polydipsia in the absence of ketosis). In each of these situations, attempt to determine the following:

- Type of diabetes
- Hypoglycemics: name, dosage, when last dose was taken
- Food and fluid intake for the past 3 days
- Relevant laboratory values: blood glucose, blood pH, bicarbonate levels, electrolytes, and serum and urine osmolality

Once the patient is stabilized, a complete health history and physical examination should be done by the registered nurse.

Health History

The health history focuses on the signs and symptoms of chronic hyperglycemia and possible complications. Physical and psychosocial factors that may have an effect on the patient's capacity to learn and perform self-care activities should be documented.

Chief Complaint and History of Present Illness. Ask the patient to describe the signs and symptoms that prompted him or her to seek medical care. The patient might report unexplained weight loss, dryness of skin, vaginal itching, or sores that are slow in healing. Polyphagia, polydipsia, and polyuria, known as the *three Ps,* are classic signs of DM.

Past Medical History. If the patient is known to have DM, note the type and duration. Document the name and dosage of prescribed medications and when they were last taken. If the patient monitors blood glucose, record the type of equipment used, the testing schedule, and recent test results.

The history should note diagnoses of circulatory, cardiac, or renal problems. Previous hospitalizations and surgeries are noted. If the patient is a woman, record an obstetric history, including number of pregnancies (if any), outcomes of all pregnancies, and birth weights of full-term infants. For patients who had GDM, ask whether insulin was required or if diet and exercise maintained adequate control. Other important data to collect are immunization records and allergies.

Family History. A family history of diabetes, heart disease, stroke, hypertension, and hyperlipidemia is significant when a person has or is suspected of having DM.

Review of Systems. The review of symptoms begins with a description of the patient's general health. Note changes in skin moisture or turgor. To detect possible changes in the eyes associated with diabetes, inquire whether the patient has had floaters (i.e., dark spots that cross the field of vision), diplopia (i.e., double vision), or blurred vision or has seen white halos around objects. Document significant abdominal symptoms including diarrhea, abdominal bloating, and gas. Problems passing or holding urine should be noted. If the patient has had any pain in the legs, note when the pain occurs. Describe any numbness, tingling, or burning sensations in the extremities. Last, the patient should be asked if he or she has experienced changes in mental alertness or seizures.

Functional Assessment. The functional assessment explores factors that can affect the patient's ability to perform self-care, including literacy, financial resources such as health insurance, and family support. Ask the patient to describe the usual pattern of activity and rest. A typical 24-hour dietary history is useful in evaluating how well the patient understands and adheres to the prescribed diet. Explore the effect of diabetes on the patient's life, including self-concept, social relationships, and employment.

Physical Examination

In the general survey, note the patient's level of consciousness, posture and gait, and apparent well-being. Record vital signs, including BP, and height and weight. Throughout the examination, note the skin color, warmth, turgor, and lesions.

The trained examiner inspects the eyegrounds for evidence of diabetic retinopathy or cataracts. The vision assessment is important because visual defects may affect the patient's ability to read vital medication instructions or labels. Gross visual acuity may be assessed by having the patient read available print. A Snellen test and other more sophisticated measures also may be used to evaluate the function of the eyes. During the examination of the head and neck, the examiner should be alert for a sweet, fruity odor to the patient's breath that is common with ketoacidosis.

The feet receive special attention. Document blisters, lesions, pallor, discoloration, deformities, and edema. Document the condition of the nails, particularly thickened or ingrown nails. Palpating both ankles and feet simultaneously for warmth and pedal pulses helps to identify poor circulation in either or both extremities. Evaluate strength in the legs by having the patient sit and try to raise and lower each foot while applying pressure to it. Assess range of motion in the ankles and feet.

Testing gait, balance, and motor coordination provides data about neurologic integrity. This is important because patients who have problems walking or feeding themselves have problems manipulating syringes and glucose monitors. In addition, test the lower extremities for the ability to perceive hot, cold, sharp, and dull sensations as well as painful stimuli.

Assessment of the patient with DM is outlined in Box 48-2.

Box 48-2 Assessment of the Patient with Diabetes Mellitus

HEALTH HISTORY

Present Illness
Polydipsia, polyuria, polyphagia, unexplained weight loss, dry skin, vaginal itching, delayed healing, blood glucose, urine ketones

Past Health
Established diagnosis of diabetes mellitus (DM): type, onset; cardiovascular or renal disorders; previous hospitalizations; obstetric history: number of pregnancies, outcomes, birth weights, gestational diabetes mellitus (GDM); immunizations; allergies; and current medications: drug names, dosages, schedules, time last dose of each drug taken

Family History
Diabetes, heart disease, stroke

Review of Systems
Changes in skin moisture or turgor; changes in vision; diarrhea, abdominal bloating, gas; urine retention or incontinence; pain, tingling, or numbness in extremities; changes in mental status; seizures

Functional Assessment
Literacy, financial resources, usual activity and rest pattern, diet, personal effect of diabetes on life; self-monitoring of blood glucose (SMBG): type of equipment used, testing schedule, recent test results

PHYSICAL EXAMINATION

General Survey
Level of consciousness, posture and gait, well-being

Vital Signs
Tachycardia, hypertension, hypotension, Kussmaul respirations

Height and Weight
Current and usual

Skin
Color, warmth, turgor, lesions

Eyes
Changes in eyegrounds, acuity

Mouth
Sweet, fruity breath odor

Lower Extremities
Blisters, lesions, color, edema, pulses, deformities, strength, range of motion

Neurologic
Gait and balance; motor coordination; perception of temperature, touch, and pain

The following diagnoses are not an exhaustive list because many other nursing diagnoses may be made if a patient has complications associated with DM. The nursing care plan must be individualized based on the assessment. Management of emergencies is discussed in the section titled "Acute Emergency Complications."

Interventions

Immediate nursing care of the patient with DM is geared toward urgent needs and complications. After urgent needs are met, nursing care focuses on teaching

Nursing Diagnoses, Goals, and Outcome Criteria: Diabetes

Nursing Diagnoses	Goals and Outcome Criteria
Ineffective Self-Health Management related to lack of knowledge of dietary management of glucose, faulty metabolism, nausea and vomiting, imbalance between food intake and activity expenditure	Effective health maintenance: patient correctly describes self-care measures, maintains blood glucose within limits of 70 and 130 mg/dL, achieves optimal weight
Ineffective Family Therapeutic Regimen Management related to financial, personal, family pattern disruption	Effective management of self-care using prescribed treatment regimen: patient and family verbalize understanding of and intent to adhere to treatment regimen, patient uses resources needed for diabetes mellitus (DM) management
Risk for Deficient Fluid Volume related to hyperglycemia, alterations in urine output	Normal extracellular fluid volume: patient correctly describes fluid needs, recognizes the significance of polyuria and oliguria; pulse and blood pressure (BP) remain within patient norms
Risk for Injury related to adverse effects of drugs, diminished alertness, increased susceptibility to infection	Decreased risk for injury: blood glucose 70 to 130 mg/dL and absence of signs of infection (normal body temperature and white blood cell [WBC] count)
Activity Intolerance related to impaired tissue perfusion, decreased mobility	Stable or improved activity tolerance: patient performs daily activities without excess fatigue
Chronic Pain related to neuropathy	Pain relief: patient states pain is relieved or reduced, appears relaxed
Impaired Skin Integrity related to neurologic and circulatory changes	Absence of injury associated with sensory loss: skin intact, no redness or blisters
Acute Confusion related to abnormal blood glucose, metabolic imbalances	Normal thought processes: patient is alert and oriented to person, place, and time
Ineffective Coping related to diagnosis, dietary restrictions, disturbed body image, sexual dysfunction, anxiety, fear	Effective coping: patient verbalizes feelings about diabetes and expresses willingness to follow plan of care and to use resources as needed

the patient to manage diabetes (see Nursing Care Plan 48-1 and Nursing Care Plan 48-2).

Ineffective Self-Health Management

Patient education requires that the patient understand the physiology of glucose metabolism and the signs and symptoms of hypoglycemia, DKA, and HHNS. Teach the patient how and when to monitor blood glucose and urine ketone levels, how to interpret the results, and the appropriate actions to take based on the results. If the patient is using a glucose meter, explain and demonstrate calibration and operation of the device, collection of blood samples, and disposal of lancets.

The teaching plan also prepares the patient for self-medication as prescribed. Explain drug names, dosages, actions, and adverse effects. If insulin is prescribed, demonstrate proper techniques for drawing up and injecting insulin and explain site rotation. Explain how adjustments in insulin or diet and exercise are used to maintain blood glucose levels between 70 and 130 mg/dL before meals and less than 180 mg/dL after meals. Not only provide verbal instruction but also allow the patient to handle equipment and demonstrate skills multiple times. If the patient cannot correctly draw up insulin, a caregiver can prepare the syringes in advance. If the insulin is refrigerated in prefilled syringes, it is stable for 1 week. The syringes should be stored in a vertical or tilted position (needle up) to reduce clogging of the needle. Before administering, tell the patient to pull back the plunger slightly and gently rock the syringe to remix the solution. Follow manufacturer guidelines for storage of prefilled insulin pens.

Advise the patient to consult the physician or pharmacist before taking new medications because many medications interact with drugs given for diabetes.

Consult the dietitian regarding diet and reinforce nutritional information. During hospitalization, record food intake. Details of medical and dietary management are presented in the section titled "Medical Treatment."

Ideally, you should present small units of content in each teaching session. Unfortunately, there may be time to provide the patient only with "survival skills" during a brief or busy hospitalization. Therefore verbal instructions should be accompanied by other sources of information, such as written materials, compact discs (CDs), or digital video discs (DVDs), as well as by information about local resources such as the hospital's CDE and the local chapter of the American Diabetes Association. Office nurses, community health nurses, and home health nurses also often participate in teaching the patient with diabetes.

Instruct the patient on the importance of having yearly eye examinations. The patient should inform the ophthalmologist of the diagnosis of diabetes. If the patient has impaired vision, audiotapes, CDs, special

Nursing Care Plan 48-1 Patient with Type 1 Diabetes Mellitus

ASSESSMENT

HEALTH HISTORY A 17-year-old woman who has recently been diagnosed with type 1 diabetes mellitus (DM) is hospitalized to begin her insulin therapy and stabilize her blood glucose. She sought medical attention because of persistent thirst and increased urination. She has no other health problems but has had frequent upper respiratory infections the past few years. The review of systems reveals periodic blurred vision, itching, increased appetite, weight loss of 7 lb in 3 months, and fatigue.

PHYSICAL EXAMINATION Vital signs: blood pressure 92/58 mm Hg, pulse 88 bpm, respiration 14 breaths per minute, temperature 98.4°F (36.9°C) measured orally. Height 5′2″, weight 107 lb. Physical findings are all within normal limits (WNL).

Nursing Diagnosis	Goals and Outcome Criteria	Interventions
Ineffective Self-Health Management related to lack of knowledge of diabetes management	The patient will correctly describe type 1 diabetes mellitus (DM) and its treatment. The patient will demonstrate self-medication, meal planning, and understanding of management of exercise and drug effects.	Explain the physiology of glucose metabolism, signs and symptoms of ketoacidosis, and hypoglycemia. Teach the patient to perform self-monitoring of blood glucose (SMBG), urine ketone testing, and how to interpret results. Explain the insulin types, their actions, and their administration. Have the patient practice insulin injection. Explain the relationship between diet, exercise, insulin, and blood glucose. Obtain a dietary consult regarding diet. Monitor food intake and replace food not eaten with a substitute identified by the dietitian.
Ineffective Family Therapeutic Regimen Management related to financial, personal, or family pattern disruption	The patient and family will express intent to adhere to prescribed regimen of care.	Request patient and family education by certified diabetes educator (CDE), if available. If not, present information in a positive manner and in small units. Identify barriers to self-management. Determine resources and sources of support. Have the patient repeat aspects of care and consequences of nonadherence to the program. Acknowledge the difficulty of making major changes in eating and activity patterns and in administering self-injections. Identify community resources such as the local chapter of the American Diabetes Association. Teach the patient and family members to recognize and respond to hypoglycemia and ketoacidosis.
Deficient Fluid Volume related to altered urine output	The patient will maintain normal blood volume, as evidenced by normal tissue turgor, pulse, and blood pressure (BP).	Stress the importance of drinking at least eight glasses of water daily. Point out that excessive urine output may indicate hyperglycemia. Assess hydration, including tissue turgor, mucous membrane moisture, and vital signs.
Risk for Injury related to adverse effects of drugs, increased susceptibility to infection	The patient's blood glucose will remain within goal range established by the physician. The patient will state measures to reduce risk of infection and will identify symptoms that should be reported to the physician.	Teach the patient to recognize the signs and symptoms of hypoglycemia: shakiness, nervousness, irritability, tachycardia, anxiety, lightheadedness, hunger, tingling or numbness of lips and tongue. Instruct the patient to take concentrated sugar if hypoglycemia occurs, followed by a complex carbohydrate (e.g., milk, bread) to prevent rebound hypoglycemia. The patient should contact the physician if ill and unable to take food or fluids. Caution the patient that impaired sensation could develop in the extremities and that healing of injuries may be impaired. Encourage the patient to avoid trauma and to inspect the feet daily to detect any injuries.
Activity Intolerance related to metabolic imbalance	The patient will perform usual activities of daily living (ADL) and carry out planned exercise program without excess fatigue.	An exercise regimen is built into the plan of care. Exercise must be done as part of a regular routine. Tell the patient to avoid injecting insulin into a body area that will be affected by exercise soon after the injection. Patient should not exercise during peak insulin activity and should eat a snack before or during exercise if the blood glucose is <100 mg/dL to avoid hypoglycemia.

Nursing Care Plan 48-1 Patient with Type 1 Diabetes Mellitus—cont'd

Nursing Diagnosis	Goals and Outcome Criteria	Interventions
Risk for Injury related to vision disturbance related to abnormal serum glucose	The patient will report correction of blurred vision.	Advise the patient that blurred vision may be caused by hyperglycemia. Encourage an annual ophthalmologic examination to detect vision changes or problems.
Acute Confusion related to abnormal serum glucose	The patient will continue to be alert and fully oriented.	Monitor the patient's mental status. Recognize confusion as a sign of abnormal serum glucose. Tell the patient and family that mental changes are best treated with carbohydrates. If the patient does not improve, the blood glucose should be measured and medical attention must be sought.
Ineffective Coping related to diagnosis, dietary restrictions, disturbed body image, anxiety, and fear	The patient will identify concerns about living with DM and plan strategies for dealing with it.	Encourage the patient to express feelings about DM and to ask questions. Assure her that most regular activities can be resumed. Identify the patient's strengths and resources. Explore her knowledge about DM and any misconceptions. Tell her that pregnancy must be carefully monitored but is a future option. Offer support groups if available.

Critical Thinking Questions

1. How are type 1 and type 2 DM alike and how are they different?
2. Diagram the mechanisms by which the body tries to adapt to (1) high blood glucose and (2) low blood glucose.
3. Describe the signs and symptoms of ketoacidosis and hypoglycemia.

Nursing Care Plan 48-2 Patient with Type 2 Diabetes Mellitus

ASSESSMENT

HEALTH HISTORY An 80-year-old Latino woman was seen in her physician's office and diagnosed with type 2 diabetes mellitus (DM). A referral has been made to a home health agency. The assessment was done in the patient's home. She lives three blocks from a grocery store, which also has a pharmacy. Her physician prescribed glyburide (Micronase), 2.5 mg daily before breakfast. The patient sought medical treatment for fatigue, weight loss (10 lb in 2 months), and symptoms of a urinary tract infection (UTI). She has a history of hypertension, which is treated with verapamil, and venous insufficiency. When asked, she states that she has had some problems with her vision and vaginal pruritus. She reports that her appetite is very good, so she could not understand why she was losing weight. Her usual diet is primarily Mexican-American food but she reports trying not to eat "too much fat." She expresses concern that a diabetic diet will be too expensive because she has only Social Security income. She says that her father died of a heart attack at age 57; her mother died at age 73 from kidney failure. One of her brothers has DM, one is deceased from heart disease, and a third is alive and well at age 70. The patient says her symptoms have interfered with performance of usual daily activities and that she is getting up frequently during the night to void, which has affected the quality of her rest. She is a widow who lives alone. She has four adult children but only one lives in the same city and visits her on weekends.

PHYSICAL EXAMINATION Vital signs: blood pressure 160/95 mm Hg, pulse 86 bpm, respiration 16 breaths per minute, temperature 97°F (36.1°C) measured orally. Height 5′2″, weight 150 lb. Patient is alert and oriented. Her skin is dry and tissue turgor is poor. She has kyphosis and walks slowly. Heart and breath sounds are normal; 2+ edema in both legs. Popliteal pulses are weak; pedal pulses are not palpable. Skin is dark around the ankles. Feet are cool. Capillary return in toenails is 4 seconds. Toenails are unevenly cut. A reddened area is seen on one heel but the patient says it is not painful.

Nursing Diagnosis	Goals and Outcome Criteria	Interventions
Ineffective Self-Health Management related to lack of knowledge of dietary management of diabetes mellitus (DM), drug therapy, and self-monitoring	The patient will demonstrate the ability to adhere to the prescribed diet and drug therapy and to monitor blood glucose.	Assess the patient's understanding of her condition and treatment and explore her attitude toward managing type 2 DM. Assess gross visual acuity and assist her to get an eye examination and corrective lenses as needed. Contact local Lions Club if she cannot afford prescribed lenses. Design a teaching plan to explain key aspects of care. Emphasize skills needed immediately: how to take medications, what foods to avoid, and how to recognize and treat hypoglycemia. If home blood glucose monitoring is prescribed, practice the process with her and evaluate her ability to perform the test and interpret the results. Develop a plan with her to cover additional topics. Discuss home health referral with physician.

Continued

Nursing Care Plan 48-2 Patient with Type 2 Diabetes Mellitus—cont'd

Nursing Diagnosis	Goals and Outcome Criteria	Interventions
Ineffective Family Therapeutic Regimen Management related to financial limitations and difficulties with transportation for food, drugs, and medical care	The patient will manage her prescribed diet and drug therapy with support from family.	Assess any barriers the patient and family perceive to managing her prescribed diet and drug therapy. If financial problems exist, consult a social worker or determine what assistance is available. If transportation and shopping are difficult, explore how the daughter who lives locally can help or provide information about public transportation available for older adults and the disabled. Provide dietary information that incorporates Mexican-American dishes. Discuss the advantages of using senior nutrition programs or Meals on Wheels to provide some meals and ease the burden of food preparation. Monitor weight and blood glucose to assess effects of treatment.
Risk for Injury related to adverse effects of drugs, circulatory impairment, decreased sensation, and increased susceptibility to infection	The patient will take measures to reduce the risk of injury associated with hypoglycemia, inadequate circulation, and diminished sensation; the patient will remain free of fever.	Explain the importance of eating properly while on oral medications that lower the blood glucose. Describe the related signs and symptoms and advise the patient to consume a glucose source such as sweetened orange juice to reverse hypoglycemia. Stress the importance of contacting the physician if ill and unable to take oral food and fluids. Explain how DM affects the blood vessels and nerves, making the extremities especially vulnerable to injury. Emphasize the importance of protecting the feet from injury by wearing properly fitting shoes and keeping the nails trimmed correctly. She should be told to avoid heating pads and to test bath water with a bath thermometer. Advise her to have foot care done by a physician or other specialist (see *Patient Teaching* box later).
Activity Intolerance related to fatigue, venous insufficiency, and circulatory impairment	The patient will resume her previous level of activity without excessive fatigue.	Assess the patient's energy level. Explore her usual day and discuss ways to conserve energy.
Ineffective Coping related to diagnosis of serious chronic illness that requires alterations in daily life	The patient will demonstrate effective coping with management of diabetes.	Encourage the patient to share her thoughts and feelings about having diabetes and her ability to deal with it. Assure her that many older people learn to manage quite well and that resources are available to help her. Communicate with her frequently until her confidence increases. Let her know how she can reach ready sources of information.

Critical Thinking Questions

1. What effect does nutrition have with regard to blood glucose?
2. What barriers might the patient perceive to managing diet and drug therapy?

reading materials, and special devices for preparing and administering insulin and for testing blood glucose may be needed.

If the patient has a hearing problem, give directions while facing the patient at eye level and speak clearly. Ask the patient to repeat or demonstrate instructions to make sure that they were heard correctly. Supplement verbal information and demonstrations with written material.

Pharmacology Capsule

Many drugs can affect blood glucose. For example, beta-adrenergic blockers lower the blood glucose and hydrochlorothiazides raise it.

Ineffective Family Therapeutic Regimen Management

When a patient has had diabetes education but does not follow the prescribed plan, explore possible barriers to carrying out the plan. Some patients may think that the program is too hard to follow and not even try. Others may think that complications are inevitable and that treatment will not really make a difference. Another reason for noncompliance is lack of financial resources for drugs, supplies, and a balanced diet. Nursing interventions depend on the barriers identified. They are designed to provide practical help, support, and encouragement.

Teach family members how to support and help the family member with diabetes. Treat the family as integral members of the health care team. It is especially important in the nutrition teaching to include the person who does the shopping and cooking. A referral to social services is necessary if the patient cannot afford syringes and insulin. A referral to a diabetes educator, home health nurse, or community health nurse for follow-up teaching and monitoring also is recommended.

Risk for Deficient Fluid Volume

Teach the patient the relationship between blood glucose and urine output. Explain that abnormally increased output may signal hyperglycemia and may eventually lead to dehydration and DKA or HHNS.

Risk for Injury

Advise the patient to keep immunizations current because of increased susceptibility to infection and impaired healing. Teach patients to see a physician promptly if they have signs and symptoms of infection such as fever, cough, painful urination, or lesions with purulent drainage.

On sick days, insulin or oral agents should be taken as usual and blood glucose checked every 2 to 4 hours. If the blood glucose exceeds 250 mg/dL, the blood or urine should be tested for ketones. Glucose levels greater than 300 mg/dL and the presence of ketones in the blood or urine should be reported to the physician. Patients with type 1 DM may need additional insulin. To prevent dehydration and ketoacidosis, the patient should eat 10 to 15 g of carbohydrates every 1 to 2 hours and drink small amounts of fluid every 15 to 30 minutes: 4 oz of orange or apple juice, nondiet soda, or Jell-O provides approximately 15 g of carbohydrates. If nausea and vomiting occur, suggest soft foods or liquids instead of solid foods. Tell the patient to report nausea, vomiting, and diarrhea to the physician at once, because severe fluid loss may occur. The patient who is unable to retain oral fluids may require hospitalization to restore fluid and electrolyte balance.

Activity Intolerance

An exercise regimen can be designed with the hospital rehabilitation department. "All things in moderation" is the best rule of thumb. Lack of exercise or too vigorous activity just before bedtime may contribute to sleeplessness. Details about the effects of exercise on blood glucose and activity recommendations are discussed in the section titled "Exercise."

Chronic Pain

Leg pain as the result of long-term complications may require analgesics. Document pain, administer medications as ordered, and evaluate the effects of interventions. If the patient is taking analgesics at home, explain how the medication is to be taken and any significant side effects such as drowsiness.

Impaired Skin Integrity

Alterations in tactile sensations may result in burns or frostbite. The patient and the family need to be aware of the danger of impaired sensation. Instruct the patient to avoid injury from heat or cold when outdoors in extreme weather. Caution the patient about the possibility of burns when using heating pads or electric blankets, working around a hot stove, or sitting next to a hot radiator. When taking a bath, measure the temperature of the bath water with a bath thermometer. The temperature should not exceed 43°C (109.4°F). Tissue may be burned before the patient is aware of the excessive heat.

The patient or someone else should examine the patient's feet daily for signs of trauma. A physician should see injuries or blisters promptly. Foot care for the diabetic is summarized in the *Patient Teaching* box.

Acute Confusion

Acute confusion may be caused by hypoglycemia, ketoacidosis, or HHNS. Without treatment, the hypoglycemic patient may be irritable at first, then confused, irrational, lethargic, and eventually comatose. In ketoacidosis, the patient becomes drowsy and the level of consciousness decreases and may progress to coma. HHNS also is characterized by altered levels of consciousness, progressing from confusion to coma. Emergency and medical treatments are covered in the section titled "Acute Emergency Complications."

When the patient is confused or disoriented, first initiate actions to determine the cause and seek appropriate medical care. Meanwhile, have someone remain with the patient to ensure safety until the condition improves. Because of the risk of disturbed thought processes, people with diabetes should wear a medical alert tag. The tag identifies the patient as having diabetes so that medical attention will be sought.

Ineffective Coping

Patients may be anxious about the immediate and long-term effects of diabetes and how it will affect their lives. They may be overwhelmed by what they need to learn for self-care. They also may be fearful about lifestyle changes, self-medication, glucose testing, adverse drug effects, and possible complications. Encourage patients to express these concerns so that they can be addressed. Talking with other people who are coping successfully with diabetes can have positive effects.

Encourage patients to express their feelings regarding diabetes and to ask for help or advice when needed. Make every effort to encourage them to resume normal activities and to continue their usual social activities. Help patients to identify their strengths and weaknesses and explore coping strategies for managing areas of concern.

One source of stress to some patients is altered sexual function. Listen to the patient's concerns and encourage consultation with the physician on the matter. Altered sexual function may be the result of diabetes but other causes are possible. Some diagnostic procedures may be done to assess erectile dysfunction. For irreversible erectile dysfunction, the physician can offer the male patient several options (see Chapter 50). Research is ongoing into treatments for female dysfunction. You can explore with the patient the importance of sexual intercourse and his or her willingness to consider alternative means of sexual expression. Patients and their partners may wish to seek counseling from therapists with expertise in sexual dysfunction.

Patient Teaching

Diabetes Mellitus

- Learn the names of your prescribed drugs, dosages, schedule, and (if on insulin) technique for injections.
- Take some form of carbohydrate if you have symptoms of hypoglycemia: nervousness, palpitations, hunger.
- Monitoring your blood glucose helps you to see how well your diabetes is being controlled.
- We will teach you how to check your blood glucose, how to interpret the findings, and what actions, if any, to take.
- Nutrition is an important part of managing your diabetes. The dietitian will discuss dietary guidelines with you.
- Regular exercise helps to control your blood glucose and improves circulation.
- Because your feet are susceptible to injury and may not heal well, wear properly fitting shoes, inspect your feet daily, and immediately seek medical care for wounds, blisters, and calluses.
- When you are sick, monitor your blood glucose and ketones; continue your insulin (if taking), take in carbohydrates that provide 10 to 15 g of carbohydrates every 1 to 2 hours, and take small amounts of fluids every 15 to 30 minutes.
- Although no cure for diabetes exists at this time, you can reduce your risk of complications with good management.

HYPOGLYCEMIA

PATHOPHYSIOLOGY

Hypoglycemia may result from causes other than the pharmacologic treatment for diabetes. Regulation of blood glucose depends on insulin levels, available glucagon, and the secretion of catecholamines, GH, and cortisol. Hypoglycemia may occur if abnormalities in these regulators are noted. Hypoglycemia is defined as a syndrome that develops when the blood glucose level falls to less than 60 mg/dL. Symptoms can occur at different blood levels according to individual tolerances and how rapidly the level falls. The causes of hypoglycemia may be divided into three categories: (1) exogenous, (2) endogenous, and (3) functional. Summaries of each of these three categories are presented in Table 48-4.

Exogenous hypoglycemia results from outside factors acting on the body to produce a low blood glucose. These include insulin, oral hypoglycemic agents, alcohol, or exercise. *Endogenous hypoglycemia* occurs when internal factors cause an excessive secretion of insulin or an increase in glucose metabolism. These conditions may be related to tumors or genetics.

Functional hypoglycemia may result from a variety of causes, including gastric surgery, fasting, or malnutrition. Alimentary hypoglycemia occurs in a patient who has undergone gastric surgery. The gastric contents empty rapidly, resulting in increased glucose absorption. In response to the increased glucose, excessive insulin production occurs, causing the hypoglycemia. In IGT hypoglycemia, an excessive response of insulin to glucose occurs. Spontaneous reactive hypoglycemia has received much publicity by the lay and medical communities alike. Symptoms occur as a result of an extreme insulin response to ingestion of foods containing carbohydrates. Low blood glucose levels need to be verified for the diagnosis to be accepted.

SIGNS AND SYMPTOMS

Signs and symptoms of hypoglycemia vary according to how quickly the blood glucose levels are falling. When the levels fall rapidly, epinephrine, cortisol, glucagon, and GH are secreted by the body in an attempt to increase glucose levels. Adrenergic symptoms that result from these physiologic responses include weakness, hunger, diaphoresis, tremors, anxiety, irritability, headache, pallor, and tachycardia. The symptoms of a blood glucose level that falls over several hours are attributed to lack of essential glucose to brain tissue. These neuroglucopenic symptoms include confusion, weakness, dizziness, blurred or double vision, seizure, and, in severe cases, coma.

MEDICAL DIAGNOSIS

The diagnosis of hypoglycemia not associated with diabetes can be based on fasting blood glucose, OGTT, intravenous glucose tolerance test, and 72-hour inpatient fasting. The diagnosis should be based on three criteria known as *Whipple's triad:* (1) the presence of symptoms, (2) documentation of low blood glucose when symptoms occur, and (3) improvement of these symptoms when blood glucose rises. These criteria must occur in the absence of sulfonylurea treatment or abnormal plasma insulin and C peptide (which indicates levels of endogenous insulin being produced).

MEDICAL TREATMENT

Treatment of hypoglycemia depends on the cause of the problem and the patient's condition. In an unconscious patient who has diabetes, hypoglycemia should be suspected until it is ruled out as a cause of the patient's symptoms. Fifty milliliters of 50% glucose solution should be administered intravenously immediately. The patient with a milder form of hypoglycemia is treated with 15 g of carbohydrate. If the patient's

Table 48-4 Exogenous, Endogenous, and Functional Causes of Hypoglycemia in Adults

CAUSES	PREDISPOSING FACTORS	OCCURRENCE
Exogenous Causes		
Insulin	Intentional or accidental overdose; may be combined with inadequate food intake, usually increased exercise, decrease in insulin requirement, or potentiating medications	Most frequent cause of hypoglycemia
Oral hypoglycemics	Intentional or accidental overdose; may be combined with inadequate food intake, increased exercise, or potentiating medications	Frequent cause of hypoglycemia with sulfonylureas and meglitinides
Alcohol	Particularly likely in chronically malnourished or acutely food-deprived people	Occurs within 6 to 36 hours of ingesting moderate to large amounts of alcohol
Exercise	Increased duration and intensity of exercise increases glucose uptake and normally decreases insulin secretion	Occurs with both insulin sulfonylurea administration and intense exercise but may be unpredictable in onset
Endogenous Causes		
Organic hypoglycemia	Insulinoma (a tumor of the beta cells of the pancreatic islets of Langerhans)	Uncommon neoplasm of beta cells of the islets of Langerhans
Extrapancreatic neoplasms	May be mesenchymal tumors, hepatomas, adrenocortical carcinomas, gastrointestinal (GI) tumors, lymphomas, or leukemias	Rare; most common in adults 40 to 70 years old
Functional Causes		
Alimentary hypoglycemia	Rapid dumping of carbohydrates into upper small intestine	Postgastrectomy
Drug-related (ethanol, haloperidol, pentamidine, salicylates) reactive hypoglycemia	Syndrome with symptoms such as diaphoresis, tachycardia, tremulousness, headache, fatigue, drowsiness, and irritability	Rarely diagnosed throughout the world; widely diagnosed in the United States, prompting American Diabetes Association and Endocrine Society to issue statement that entity is probably overdiagnosed
Abrupt discontinuation of hyperalimentation	Drinking alcohol on an empty stomach	More common with drinks containing saccharin (e.g., beer, gin and tonic, rum and cola, whiskey and ginger ale)
Rapid discontinuation of total parenteral alimentation	Endocrine deficiency states (cortisol, growth hormone [GH], glucagons, epinephrine)	Easily prevented
Glucocorticoid deficiency	Critical illness (cardiac, hepatic, and renal disease)	A danger for any person with adrenal insufficiency
Severe liver deficiency	Insufficient glucose output by liver	Fasting hypoglycemia
Lack of body stores for protein, fat, and carbohydrates	Profound malnutrition	Common; also found with relative frequency in kwashiorkor
Prolonged muscular exercise	Metabolism of energy-producing substances	Occurs if exercise is too prolonged or severe or if nutritional intake and carbohydrate stores are insufficient

Modified from Shamoon H: Hypoglycemia. In Felig P, Baxter JD, Broadus AD, et al., editors: *Endocrinology and metabolism*, ed 4, New York, 2001, McGraw-Hill.

condition does not improve, another 15 g of carbohydrate should be given after 10 minutes. Giving more than 15 g initially may lead to rebound hyperglycemia. In terms of food exchanges, one bread exchange contains 15 g of carbohydrate, one fruit exchange contains 15 g of carbohydrate, and one milk exchange contains 12 g of carbohydrate.

Prevention of hypoglycemia by proper food intake is an important treatment component. The diet is directed by the underlying cause. If the cause is related to an overproduction of insulin after carbohydrate ingestion, a low-carbohydrate, high-protein diet is commonly ordered. Restriction of carbohydrates to no more than 100 g/day is recommended. Simple sugars are avoided and complex carbohydrates are encouraged. Because no significant increase in blood glucose is noted with protein ingestion, a high-protein diet is recommended. The remaining calories in the diet are obtained from fat. Because carbohydrates are restricted, the calories required from fat are high. Patients may tolerate smaller, more frequent meals. Alcohol should be avoided. Remember that hypoglycemia associated with the treatment of diabetes uses different guidelines for treatment.

NURSING CARE of the Patient with Hypoglycemia

Assessment

The health history is especially important in the diagnosis of hypoglycemia. Describe the present illness, which may include the following symptoms: shakiness, nervousness, irritability, tachycardia, anxiety, lightheadedness, hunger, tingling or numbness of the lips or tongue, nightmares, and crying out during sleep. Note when the episodes occur in relation to meals and particular food intake. The past medical history documents diabetes, previous gastric surgery, abdominal cancer, or adrenal insufficiency. Record medications, paying particular attention to hypoglycemic agents. Note the names of hypoglycemic agents, prescribed dose, and the time that the last dose was taken. The functional assessment elicits information about current diet, exercise, alcohol intake, and the effects of symptoms on daily activities. Important aspects of the physical examination include general behavior, appearance, pulse, and BP.

Nursing Diagnoses, Goals, and Outcome Criteria: Hypoglycemia

Nursing Diagnoses	Goals and Outcome Criteria
Deficient Knowledge of management of hypoglycemia	Patient understands and can manage hypoglycemic episodes: patient accurately describes and demonstrates self-care measures
Risk for Injury related to episodes of dizziness and weakness	Absence of injury: no falls or injuries as a result of hypoglycemic episodes
Ineffective Self-Health Management related to effects of illness on lifestyle	Effective management of hypoglycemia: patient describes and practices measures to manage hypoglycemia

Interventions

Deficient Knowledge

Patient education is a priority after a confirmed diagnosis to prevent future occurrences. Teach patients to recognize the signs and symptoms and to treat them promptly. Advise the patient of factors that may trigger hypoglycemic episodes, such as foods, medications, alcohol, fasting, and exercise. Basic concepts of the diet described earlier need to be stressed and reinforced. A referral for a consultation with a registered dietitian may be helpful for the patient. As a patient educator, you are very influential in promoting self-monitoring and treatment of hypoglycemia.

Risk for Injury

The hypoglycemic patient is at risk for injury as a result of weakness and dizziness. Be alert for signs and symptoms of hypoglycemia. Monitor serum glucose levels. Administer carbohydrates as prescribed by the physician. Until the episode passes, keep the patient in bed with the side rails up and the call bell nearby. Advise the patient not to get up unassisted.

Ineffective Self-Health Management

Emotional support for the patient with hypoglycemia is necessary during diagnosis and treatment. Prepare the patient for diagnostic tests and tell the patient what to expect. Once the diagnosis is made, explore the patient's feelings and concerns. Support the patient in learning to incorporate the management of hypoglycemia into his or her lifestyle. Guide the patient to anticipate problem situations and possible solutions.

Get Ready for the NCLEX® Examination!

Key Points

- DM is a condition characterized by impaired metabolism related to tissue resistance to insulin or insulin deficiency.
- DM is managed with diet, exercise, and insulin or oral hypoglycemic agents (or with both).
- The major complications of DM are ketoacidosis, hyperosmolar nonketotic coma, vascular changes, and neuropathy.
- Ketoacidosis causes dehydration, electrolyte imbalance, and metabolic acidosis and is treated with fluid and electrolyte replacement and insulin.
- Hyperosmolar nonketotic coma is loss of consciousness caused by extremely high serum glucose without ketoacidosis.
- The major complications of insulin therapy are hypoglycemia, insulin shock, and hyperglycemia (Somogyi effect).

- Nursing care of the patient with DM focuses on ineffective self-health management, ineffective family therapeutic regimen management, deficient fluid volume, risk for injury, activity intolerance, chronic pain, impaired skin integrity, acute confusion, and ineffective coping.
- Hypoglycemia (low serum glucose) in the absence of DM can be caused by pancreatic tumors, adrenal insufficiency, liver disease, and pituitary disorders but sometimes no specific cause is identified.
- Nursing care of the nondiabetic patient who has hypoglycemia focuses on deficient knowledge, risk for injury, and ineffective self-health management.

Additional Learning Resources

SG Go to your Study Guide for additional learning activities to help you master this chapter content.

evolve Go to your Evolve website (http://evolve.elsevier.com/Linton/medsurg) for the following learning resources and much more:

- Interactive Prioritization Exercises
- Fluid & Electrolyte Tutorial
- Pharmacology Tutorial
- Review Questions for the NCLEX® Examination

Review Questions for the NCLEX® Examination

1. Functions of insulin include which of the following? (Select all that apply.)
   1. Serve as an energy source
   2. Help to transport glucose into cells
   3. Metabolize glucose for energy
   4. Synthesize fatty acids and proteins
   5. Stimulate excretion of excess glucose

   NCLEX Client Need: Health Promotion and Maintenance
2. The incidence of DM is greatest among people of which ethnicity?
   1. Latino
   2. African
   3. European
   4. Asian

   NCLEX Client Need: Physiological Integrity: Reduction of Risk Potential
3. Macrovascular complications of diabetes include which conditions? (Select all that apply.)
   1. Retinopathy
   2. End-stage renal disease
   3. Cerebrovascular accident
   4. Coronary heart disease
   5. Peripheral vascular disease

   NCLEX Client Need: Physiological Integrity: Reduction of Risk Potential
4. You are collecting data from a patient who has had type 2 DM for 10 years. He complains of dizziness when rising to a standing position and increasing fatigue with his usual exercise program. His vital signs are normal except for a heart rate of 108 bpm. You should report these data to the RN because these findings are consistent with which of the following?
   1. CHD
   2. Inadequate control of blood glucose
   3. Autonomic neuropathy
   4. Hyperglycemic episodes

   NCLEX Client Need: Physiological Integrity: Reduction of Risk Potential
5. A patient who has just been diagnosed with diabetes and started on oral medications says, "I feel strange and my mouth feels numb. Something is wrong!" You note that his hands are trembling and that he is perspiring. What is your best response?
   1. "These are common symptoms of diabetes. They will go away soon."
   2. "Let's check your blood sugar. It is probably low."
   3. "Your physician will probably need to increase your medication dose."
   4. "This is very unusual. I will call your physician."

   NCLEX Client Need: Physiological Integrity: Pharmacological Therapies
6. A patient recently diagnosed with DM asks why he should limit his protein intake. The nurse's response should be based on which of the following?
   1. Metabolism of excess protein causes ketoacidosis.
   2. Protein needs are decreased because excess glucose meets metabolic needs.
   3. High protein intake interferes with absorption of other nutrients.
   4. High protein intake indirectly contributes to the development of nephropathy.

   NCLEX Client Need: Physiological Integrity: Reduction of Risk Potential
7. Which of the following is the advantage of human insulin over beef and pork insulin?
   1. Human insulin is less expensive.
   2. People do not form antibodies for human insulin.
   3. Human insulin has a longer duration of action.
   4. Human insulin does not cause hypoglycemia.

   NCLEX Client Need: Physiological Integrity: Pharmacological Therapies
8. Which type of oral DM medication is *least* likely to cause hypoglycemia?
   1. Alpha-glucosidase inhibitors
   2. Sulfonylureas
   3. Meglitinides
   4. D-Phenylalanines

   NCLEX Client Need: Physiological Integrity: Pharmacological Therapies
9. Which of the following comprise the classic signs and symptoms of DM? (Select all that apply.)
   1. Polydipsia
   2. Polyhidrosis
   3. Polyphagia
   4. Polyuria
   5. Polycythemia

   NCLEX Client Need: Physiological Integrity: Physiological Adaptation
10. A patient who was newly diagnosed with diabetes says, "Everyone I know with diabetes has had one or both legs amputated." What is the most appropriate reply?
    1. "Try not to think about that."
    2. "Most people with diabetes eventually have to have amputations."
    3. "The ones who had amputations did not follow their physician's orders."
    4. "You can do many things to reduce your risk of future amputations."

    NCLEX Client Need: Physiological Integrity: Reduction of Risk Potential

chapter 49

Female Reproductive Disorders

http://evolve.elsevier.com/Linton/medsurg

Margit B. Gerardi

Objectives

1. List data to be collected related to the assessment of the female reproductive system.
2. Describe the nursing interventions for women who are undergoing diagnostic tests and procedures for reproductive system disorders.
3. Identify the nursing interventions associated with douche, cauterization, heat therapy, and topical medications used to treat disorders of the female reproductive system.
4. Explain the pathophysiology, signs and symptoms, complications, diagnostic procedures, and medical or surgical treatment for selected disorders of the female reproductive system.
5. Assist in developing a nursing care plan for patients with common disorders of the female reproductive system.
6. Describe the nursing interventions for the patient who is menopausal.

Key Terms

Cystocele (SĬS-tō-sēl)
Dysmenorrhea (dĭs-mĕn-ō-RĒ-ă)
Dyspareunia (dĭs-pă-ROO-nē-ă)
Dysplasia (dĭs-PLĀ-sē-ă)
Endometriosis (ĕn-dō-mē-trē-Ō-sĭs)
Hysterectomy (hĭs-tĕr-ĔK-tō-mē)
Mastitis (măs-TĪ-tĭs)
Menarche (mĕ-NĂR-kē)
Menopause (MĔN-ō-păwz)
Menorrhagia (mĕn-ō-RĀ-jă)
Metrorrhagia (mē-trō-RĀ-jă)
Rectocele (RĔK-tō-sēl)
Retroversion (RĔT-rō-vĕr-zhŭn)
Salpingo-oophorectomy (săl-pĭng-gō-ō-ŎF-ō-RĔK-tō-mē)
Vaginitis (vă-jĭ-NĪ-tĭs)
Vulvitis (vŭl-VĪ-tĭs)

The female reproductive system includes external and internal genitalia and the breasts. The term *vulva* refers to the external genitalia, which comprise the mons pubis, labia majora, labia minora, clitoris, and pudendum (Fig. 49-1). In addition, included in the vulva are mucus-secreting glands. Bartholin glands are located on both sides of the posterior edge of the vaginal opening and Skene glands are located just inside the urethral opening. The perineum is the area between the posterior junction of the labia minora and the anus. The internal genitalia include two ovaries, two fallopian tubes, the uterus, and the vagina (Fig. 49-2).

ANATOMY AND PHYSIOLOGY OF THE FEMALE REPRODUCTIVE SYSTEM

EXTERNAL GENITALIA

The mons pubis is a pad of fatty tissue that covers and protects the symphysis pubis. The labia majora are extensions of the fatty tissue that cover and protect inner vulvar structures. The labia majora extend from the mons pubis to the perineum. The inner folds of the labia majora are smooth and moist.

The labia minora are thin folds of smooth skin that form a hood, called the *prepuce*, over the clitoris. The clitoris is a small structure that corresponds to the male penis. Like the penis, the clitoris is composed of erectile tissue with sensory nerve endings that are responsive to psychologic and physical stimuli. The labia minora are richly endowed with sebaceous glands, nerves, and blood vessels that also respond to psychologic and physical stimulation. The labia minora may be entirely covered by the labia majora or may be visible between the outer labia.

The urethral (urinary) meatus is below the clitoris. The openings of Skene glands are located on both sides of the urinary meatus. The vaginal opening, the introitus, is partially or entirely covered by a thin fold of tissue called the *hymen*. The hymen may be intact, distended, or ruptured. The size of the introitus varies from very small to large and gaping.

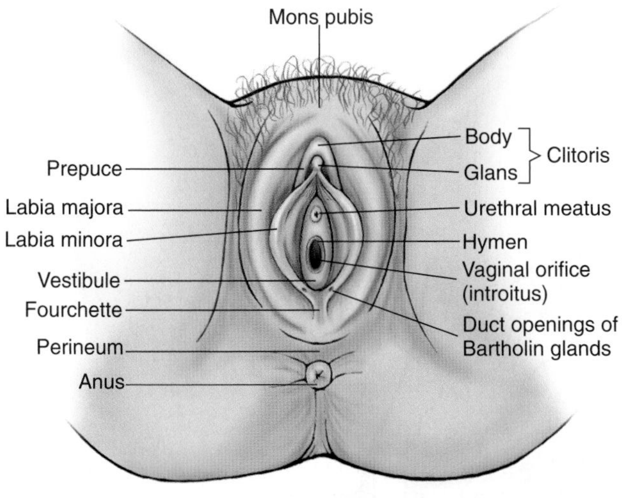

FIGURE 49-1 External female genitalia. (From Monahan FD, Drake DT, Neighbors M, editors: *Medical-surgical nursing: foundations for clinical practice*, ed 2, Philadelphia, 1998, Saunders.)

INTERNAL GENITALIA

The vagina is a canal that extends from the vulva to the uterus. This structure has the ability to expand and lengthen to accept an erect penis and to provide an exit for a term fetus. The mucous membranes of the vaginal walls secrete lubricating fluid that cleanses the vagina and interacts with bacteria to maintain an acid pH.

The uterus is a firm, muscular organ that is pear shaped and hollow. Its lower segment is called the *cervix.* The end of the cervix extends into the upper aspect of the vagina. The os is the opening of the cervix into the vagina. The inner lining of the uterus is called the *endometrium.* The upper segment of the uterine body, or corpus, is called the *fundus.*

The two fallopian tubes are thin, hollow, cilia-lined, tubular structures that extend from the uterine fundus. The fallopian tubes have funnel-shaped ends that partially surround the ovaries and that receive the ovum from the ovary. The fallopian tubes serve as passages for ova from the ovaries and for sperm that travel through the vagina and into the tubes. Fertilization, the union of sperm and ovum, takes place in the fallopian tubes.

The two ovaries are almond-shaped structures located on each side of the uterus. They correspond to the male testes. Ovarian functions include maturation and release of ova (ovulation) and secretion of hormones—estrogens, progesterone, androgens, and relaxin.

It is important to note that the pathway through the female reproductive tract, intended to serve as a route for reproduction, also provides a route for infectious organisms to access the pelvic cavity and its organs.

BREASTS

Although the breasts are not directly involved in the reproductive process, they are addressed as accessories to reproduction because of their function: to nourish the infant after birth. Breast structure is illustrated in Figure 49-3. The inner structure is composed of glandular and ductal tissue, fibrous tissue, and fat. (The fat is responsible for most of the variation in breast size and shape.) The breast is divided into several lobes, each divided into lobules. Lobules contain many hollow, grape-shaped alveoli that produce milk when stimulated by the pituitary hormone *prolactin.* Ducts carry milk from the lobules, through the lobes, to the opening in the nipple.

The nipple with its surrounding areola is a pigmented structure located at the midline of each breast. Breast milk passes through the openings of the lactiferous ducts. Small, round sebaceous glands called *Montgomery tubercles* are visible under the skin of the areolae. These glands produce a lubricating secretion that protects nipple tissue. Except during normal lactation, no discharge from the nipple should occur.

MENSTRUAL CYCLE

The menstrual cycle, or female reproductive cycle, consists of the ovarian cycle and the uterine cycle. It results from a complex interaction of the hypothalamus, anterior pituitary, and ovary (Fig. 49-4). The interaction causes the ovary to release a mature ovum (i.e., ovulation) and prepares the uterine lining to receive and nourish the ovum if it is fertilized. If the ovum is not fertilized, the menstrual cycle begins with the onset of menstruation. Menstruation is the passage through the vagina of a mixture of blood, other fluids, and tissue formed in the lining of the uterus to receive the fertilized ovum.

The length of the menstrual cycle averages 28 to 30 days but the range may be 21 to 40 days and may be affected by various factors such as stress, physical activity, and illness. Regardless of the length of the cycle, the progression is the same:

1. Menstruation (day 1 through days 4 to 7) occurs.
2. Maturation of an ovarian follicle occurs, with subsequent rupture and release of an ovum in response to follicle-stimulating hormone (FSH) and luteinizing hormone (LH) from the anterior pituitary (days 1 to 14 in a 28-day cycle).
3. Estrogen production (days 6 to 14) by the maturing follicle occurs; progesterone production (days 15 to 26) by the corpus luteum that is formed from the ruptured follicle occurs.
4. Preparation of the uterine lining for implantation of the fertilized ovum occurs, stimulated by estrogen and progesterone from the follicle and corpus luteum (days 6 to 26).

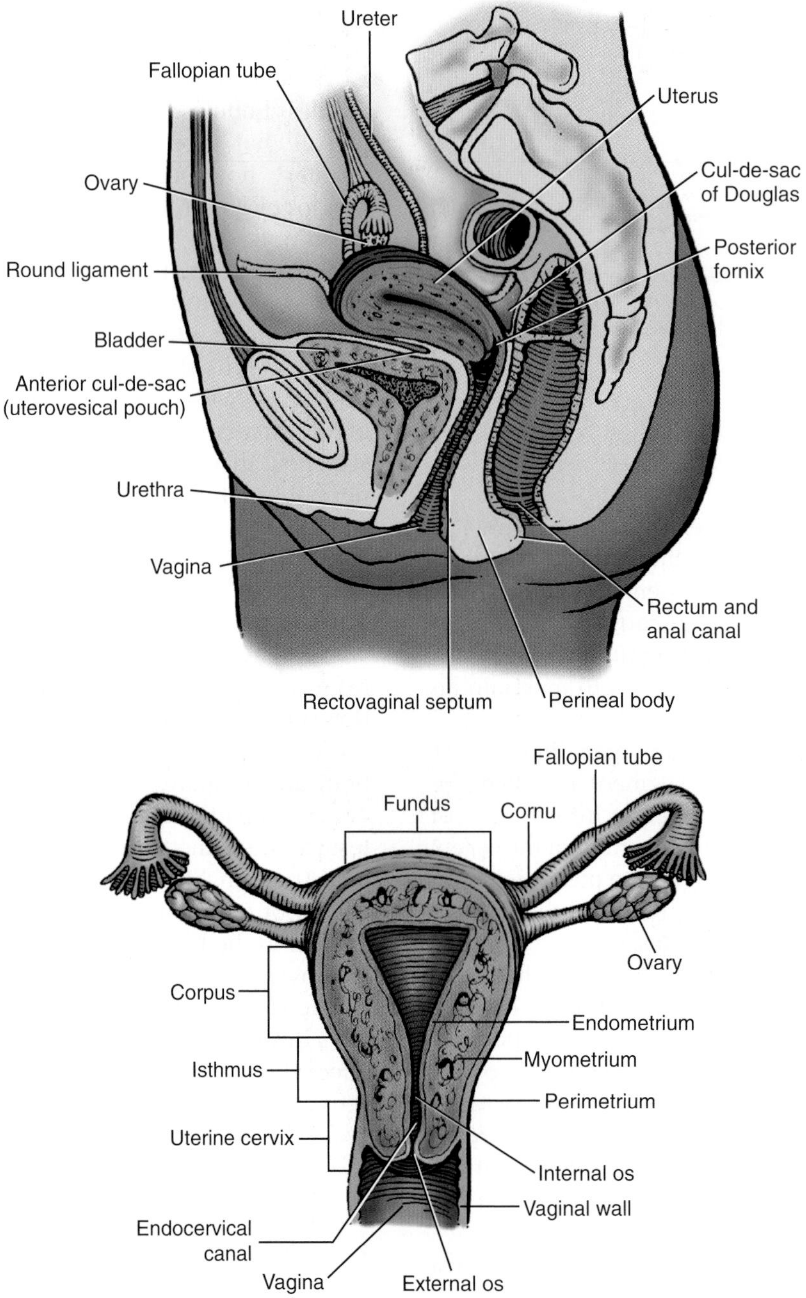

FIGURE 49-2 Internal female genitalia. (From Monahan FD, Drake DT, Neighbors M, editors: *Medical-surgical nursing: foundations for clinical practice*, ed 2, Philadelphia, 1998, Saunders.)

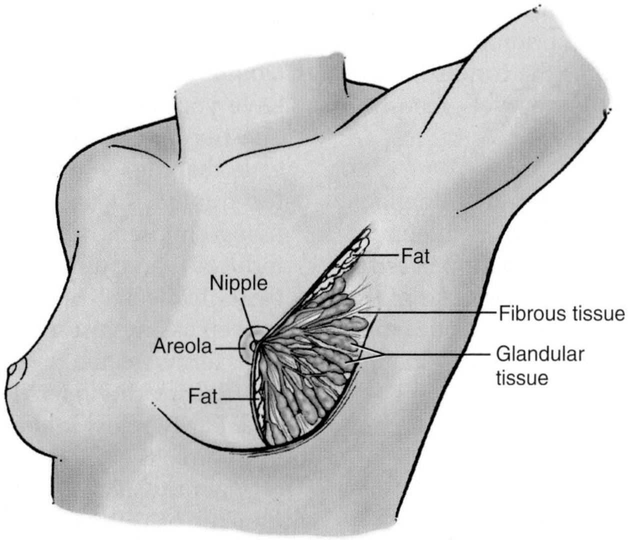

FIGURE 49-3 Structure of the mature female breast. (From Monahan FD, Drake DT, Neighbors M, editors: *Medical-surgical nursing: foundations for clinical practice*, ed 2, Philadelphia, 1998, Saunders.)

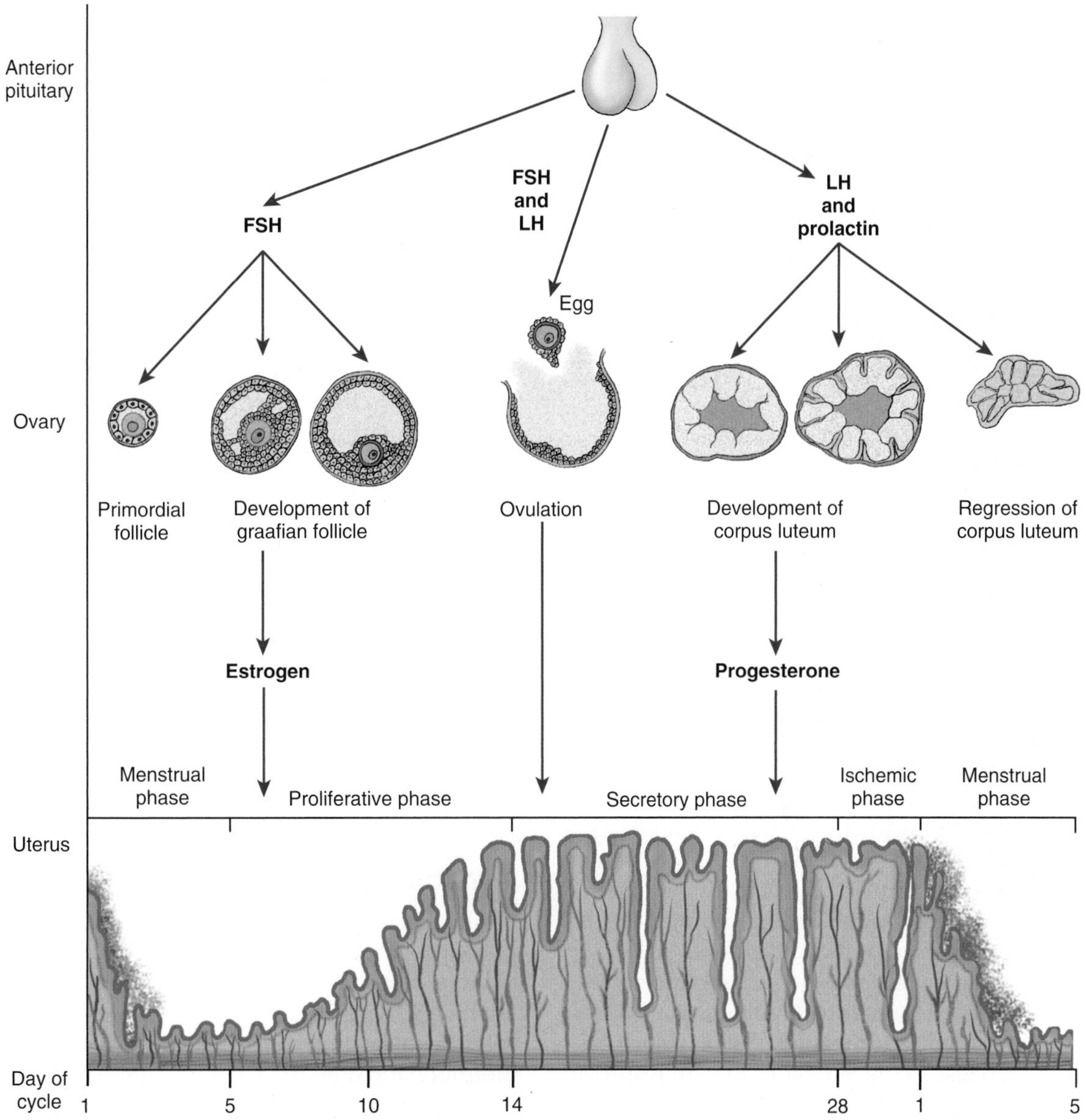

FIGURE 49-4 Female hormonal cycle. *FSH*, Follicle-stimulating hormone; *LH*, luteinizing hormone. (From Monahan FD, Drake DT, Neighbors M, editors: *Medical-surgical nursing: foundations for clinical practice*, ed 2, Philadelphia, 1998, Saunders.)

5. The fertilized ovum implants in the uterine lining and secretes human chorionic gonadotropin (HCG), which maintains the corpus luteum and estrogen and progesterone levels; menstruation does not occur (day 14).

or

6. The unfertilized ovum does not implant. Absence of HCG causes the corpus luteum to degenerate, which in turn causes a drop in estrogen and progesterone levels and necrosis of the uterine lining (days 27 to 28). The necrotic lining is shed as menstrual flow and begins another cycle at day 1.

NURSING ASSESSMENT OF THE FEMALE REPRODUCTIVE SYSTEM

HEALTH HISTORY

The licensed vocational nurse/licensed practical nurse (LVN/LPN) collects data that contribute to the professional nurse's complete assessment. The complete assessment is described here even though the LVN/LPN would not be responsible for all of it.

Chief Complaint and History of Present Illness

The basic assessment begins with the patient's reason for seeking medical care. "What is the reason for your visit?" is an opening question that allows the patient to describe in her own terms the reason for the visit and to include related information that may guide subsequent questions. If the reason for the visit is an existing problem, include related signs and symptoms and their onset, frequency, and effect on normal functioning.

Past Medical History

Menstrual History. Record the age at which menstruation began (**menarche**), the date of the onset of the last menstrual period, the usual number of days between the onset of one period and the onset of the next, the total amount of menstrual flow, the usual number of days of menstrual flow per period, and the use of tampons.

"Many women experience problems with their periods. What problems have you noticed?" is a questioning technique that implies acceptance of a wide variety of problems and invites the patient to provide additional relevant information. Problems commonly reported include spotting or frank bleeding between periods, abdominal pain at the time of ovulation, abdominal cramping or pain before or during periods (or both), and premenstrual mood changes.

For women who have stopped menstruating owing to **menopause**, important data include the age at which menstruation ceased and related details, such as whether menopause occurred naturally or resulted from surgery, chemotherapy, or radiation therapy. Include information about menopausal symptoms and prescribed or over-the-counter (OTC) medications taken to relieve menopausal symptoms.

Obstetric-Gynecologic History. "How many times have you been pregnant?" is an appropriate opening question for the obstetric history. If the response indicates that the woman has been pregnant, inquire about the number of term and preterm births, number of living children, number of abortions (spontaneous or induced), and number of multiple pregnancies (e.g., twins, triplets). Note blood type and Rhesus (Rh) factor as well as any history of rubella or rubella immunization. Terms related to obstetric history are *gravidity* and *parity*. Gravidity refers to the total number of pregnancies. Parity refers to the number of pregnancies reaching 20 weeks of gestation, which is considered the "age of viability." Parity may be recorded according to a number of different codes that use one- to five-digit numbers. Each institution provides direction on how parity is to be coded for obstetric histories.

The gynecologic history addresses such problems as infections and sexually transmitted infections (STIs), cysts and tumors, structural and functional abnormalities, birth control, infertility, sexual trauma and rape, and stress incontinence.

Family History

Record a family history of diabetes mellitus (DM), cancer, heart disease, psychiatric disorders, complications of pregnancy, multiple pregnancies, genetic disorders, or congenital anomalies.

Review of Systems

Information regarding symptoms and any prescribed or self-selected treatments should be recorded. Commonly reported symptoms are pain, itching, burning, vaginal bleeding between periods or after menopause, heavy or prolonged bleeding with periods, vaginal discharge, painful intercourse, lesions, and urinary frequency or urgency.

Functional Assessment

The functional assessment includes a diet history; use of dietary supplements including calcium, iron, and botanical medications; health maintenance to include immunizations; exercise pattern; sexual history; substance use; disabilities; occupational exposure to potential teratogens; and effects of symptoms on usual activities.

PHYSICAL EXAMINATION

In the general survey, important data include the patient's appearance, facial expression, and any obvious signs of distress. Measure vital signs, including height, weight, and blood pressure (BP). Note skin color, texture, and moisture. Examine the breasts for dimpling and abnormal skin texture. With the patient leaning forward, observe for asymmetry in the breasts. Ask the patient about changes from usual contours.

Palpate all breast tissue for thickening or lumps (see the section titled "Breast Self-Examination").

Inspect the abdomen for distention and palpate for tenderness. Inspect the legs for swelling and palpate for tenderness. The pelvic examination may be done by the physician or a nurse with advanced training. Therefore it is discussed in detail with other diagnostic tests and procedures. Basically, the examiner assesses the external genitalia for lesions, lumps, swelling, and discharge. The vagina and uterine cervix are inspected for lesions, growths, discharge, and redness. The vagina, abdomen, and rectum are palpated for abnormalities. Assessment of the female reproductive system is summarized in Box 49-1.

DIAGNOSTIC TESTS AND PROCEDURES

The physician or nurse practitioner performs most diagnostic tests and procedures. The responsibilities of the nurse usually focus on patient instruction regarding the procedure, preparation of the patient, support of the patient throughout the tests and procedures, and assistance to the physician or nurse practitioner. Regardless of the test or procedure to be performed, provide anticipatory guidance by telling the patient what to expect. Check the institution's procedure manual for specific preparations and assistants' responsibilities for each test or procedure.

PELVIC EXAMINATION

The pelvic examination allows inspection and palpation of external and internal reproductive structures to identify deviations from normal, provide information for medical diagnoses, and collect specimens for laboratory analysis.

Slightly elevate the head of the examination table before positioning your patient. The patient assumes the lithotomy position, with her buttocks at the edge of the examination table, her hips and knees flexed, and her feet in stirrups. Many women report that the position is unpleasant because of the sense of vulnerability they experience. To decrease this effect, delay positioning until just before the examination begins, carefully drape to preserve modesty, and provide verbal and nonverbal support. Remember to take care in positioning older patients who have osteoarthritis or have had prior hip surgery to avoid excessive hip rotation and knee movement. To decrease physical discomfort associated with use of the stirrups, cover them with thick footlets or encourage the patient to continue to wear her socks or shoes.

Box 49-1 Assessment of the Female Reproductive System

HEALTH HISTORY

Present Illness

Reason for visit, related signs and symptoms, onset and frequency of symptoms, effects on normal functioning

Past Medical History

Menstrual History

Age at menarche, date of onset of last menstrual period, duration of menstrual period, amount of menstrual flow, use of tampons, pain, bleeding between periods, premenstrual mood changes; for menopausal women: age at which menopause occurred, whether menopause was natural or surgical, related symptoms, medications taken to relieve symptoms

Obstetric and Gynecologic History

Number of pregnancies, number of term and preterm births, number of living children, number of abortions (spontaneous and induced), number of multiple pregnancies, past problems with reproductive organs, fertility, stress incontinence, sexual trauma and rape, history of rubella or rubella immunization, frequency of breast self-examination (BSE), contraception use

Family History

Diabetes, cancer, complications of pregnancy, heart disease, psychiatric disorders, genetic disorders, multiple pregnancies, congenital anomalies

Review of Systems

Pain, itching, burning, vaginal bleeding between periods or after menopause, heavy or prolonged bleeding with periods, vaginal discharge, urinary frequency or urgency

Functional Assessment

Diet; use of dietary supplements including calcium, iron, and botanical medications; health maintenance to include immunizations; exercise pattern; sexual history; substance use; disabilities; occupational exposure to potential teratogens

PHYSICAL EXAMINATION

General Survey

Appearance, facial expression, obvious distress

Vital Signs

Height and Weight

Skin

Texture, moisture, color

Breasts

Dimpling, texture changes in skin, asymmetry when leaning forward, changes from usual contours, changes in texture, vascular pattern changes, lumps, nipple discharge

Extremities

Temperature, rashes, swelling, tenderness

Abdomen

Contour, distention, vascular pattern changes, tenderness

Pelvic Examination

External Genitalia

Appearance, lesions, lumps, swelling, discharge

Vagina and Uterine Cervix

Appearance, lesions, growths, discharge, redness

Rectal Examination

Appearance, lesions, growths

The pelvic examination is divided into three parts: (1) visual inspection and palpation of the external genitalia, (2) visual inspection of the vagina and uterine cervix after introduction of a plastic or metal speculum (Fig. 49-5), and (3) bimanual palpation of the vagina and abdomen. The latter procedure may be performed with two fingers of one gloved hand in the vagina or with one finger in the vagina and one finger in the rectum (Fig. 49-6) and the other hand on the abdomen to allow compression of internal structures between the two hands. The final step is a rectal examination with a gloved finger.

The examiner can do much to decrease the patient's anxiety if this is her first pelvic examination by explaining each step in advance using models or showing equipment before the examination. Discomfort varies among women. Some women report no discomfort other than feelings of pressure; other women report pain. One common discomfort is related to a cold speculum. This can be prevented by warming the speculum in water or by wrapping the packaged speculum in the folds of a heating pad. Supportive measures include talking to the patient and directing breathing and relaxation techniques to relieve pain and tension. After the pelvic examination, assist the patient to sit up and to get off the table. Provide tissues to wipe the perianal area and, if possible, an adhesive panty liner to absorb lubricant as it is expelled from the vagina.

STAINS AND CULTURES

Collection of specimens for laboratory analysis is one of the purposes of the pelvic examination (see Fig. 49-5, *D*). Institutional policy specifies the necessary equipment and the care of slides for each specimen.

Specimens are routinely collected for a Papanicolaou (Pap) test for detection of cervical cancer and other abnormal cervical cells (**dysplasia**). Additional

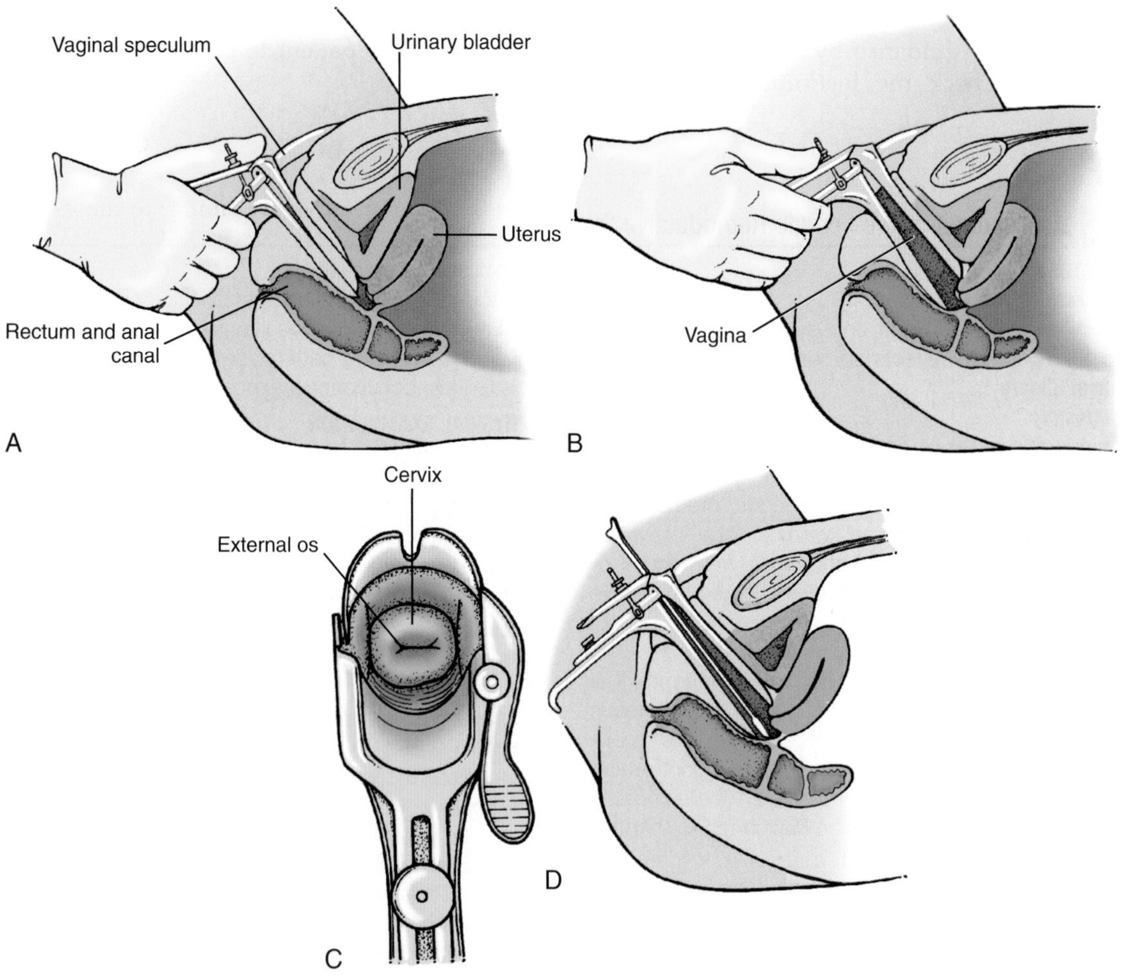

FIGURE 49-5 Internal examination of the cervix. **A,** Insertion of the speculum. **B,** Open speculum within the vagina. **C,** Examiner's view of the cervix through an open speculum. **D,** An instrument called an Ayre spatula is inserted through the speculum to obtain a cervical specimen for a Papanicolaou (Pap) test. (From Monahan FD, Drake DT, Neighbors M, editors: *Medical-surgical nursing: foundations for clinical practice*, ed 2, Philadelphia, 1998, Saunders.)

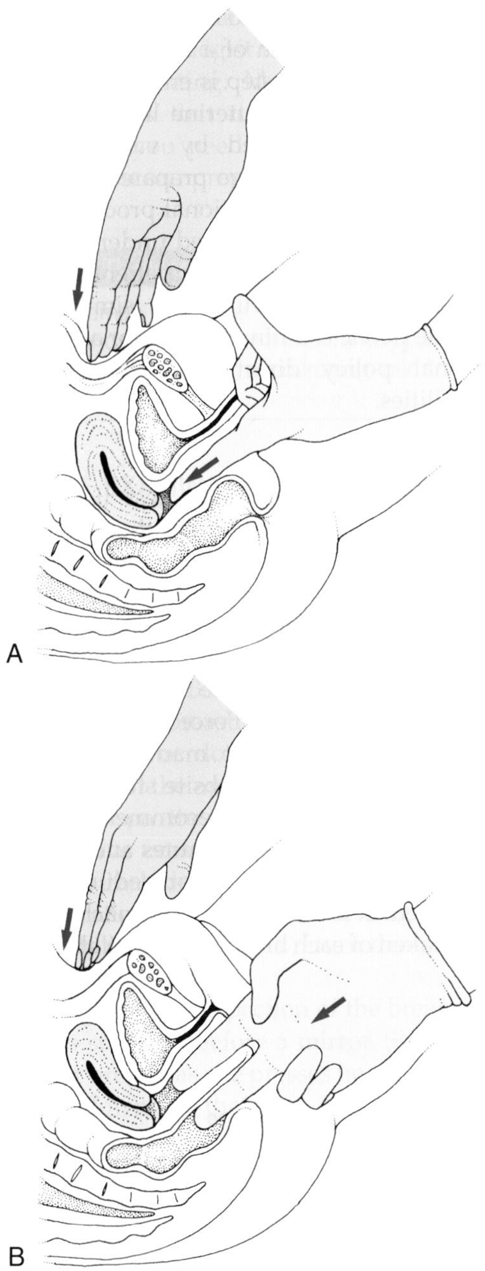

FIGURE 49-6 Bimanual palpation. **A,** Bimanual pelvic examination. **B,** Bimanual rectovaginal examination. (From Ignatavicius DD, Workman ML, Mishler M: *Medical-surgical nursing: a nursing process approach*, ed 2, Philadelphia, 1995, Saunders.)

specimens may be collected for the identification of possible infections such as herpes, *Chlamydia*, and gonorrhea. The examiner may swab vaginal and cervical fluid to identify bacterial-, fungal-, or trichomonal-related infections, as well as to assess pH.

ENDOMETRIAL AND CERVICAL BIOPSIES

Endometrial biopsies generally are performed for four reasons: (1) to assess the endometrium for readiness to accept and nourish a fertilized ovum, (2) to indirectly assess corpus luteum function in cases of possible infertility, (3) to diagnose irregular uterine bleeding patterns, (4) and to diagnosis uterine cancer. The nurse's responsibilities are similar to those for a pelvic examination and collection of specimens for stains and cultures. The physician or nurse practitioner dilates the cervix and scrapes tissue specimens from the endometrium. The procedure may cause cramping so severe that an anesthetic is necessary.

Cervical biopsies are used to remove suspicious tissue and rule out cervical cancer. Two types of biopsy exist: (1) multiple punch and (2) cone. Multiple punch biopsies are done in a physician's office or an outpatient clinic. Because several specimens are obtained by punching out small samples of cervical tissue, the process is usually painful. The nurse's responsibilities are similar to those for endometrial biopsies. You can support the patient by coaching her to use breathing and relaxation techniques to minimize discomfort.

The cone biopsy is invasive surgery and requires admission to an outpatient surgery facility or a hospital. Under general anesthesia, a large amount of cervical tissue is removed. Although the cone biopsy is rarely used to diagnose cancer, its advantage lies in its potential to diagnose and remove cancerous tissue.

COLPOSCOPY

An instrument called a *colposcope* is used to inspect the cervix under magnification and to identify abnormal and potentially cancerous tissue. Colposcopy is commonly done before cervical biopsies. Patient preparation and nursing care are similar to those for a pelvic examination.

CULDOSCOPY

A culdoscopy is an invasive surgical procedure usually performed with light sedation and local anesthetic on an outpatient basis. When performed by a skillful physician, culdoscopy is the simplest way to directly visualize the female pelvic cavity. With the patient in the knee-chest or lithotomy position, the culdoscope is inserted through a small incision in the posterior vagina. The culdoscope permits examination of the patient's uterus, ovaries, and fallopian tubes. It is performed to obtain tissue specimens and to identify ectopic pregnancy, pelvic masses, and causes of infertility or pain.

The nurse's responsibilities are similar to those for other outpatient procedures, with details specified by institutional policies. Scrupulous asepsis must be maintained. Many women consider the knee-chest position physically uncomfortable, embarrassing, and humiliating. Assure the patient that she will be draped throughout the procedure and be conscientious about following through with that assurance. When the procedure is completed, help the patient to get out of the knee-chest position without exposure. Advise her that she may experience shoulder pain caused by air entering the pelvic cavity during the procedure. In addition, reassure her that the incision will close and heal

Table 49-2 Drug Therapy: Drugs Used to Treat Disorders of the Female Reproductive System—cont'd

DRUG	USE AND ACTION	SIDE EFFECTS	NURSING INTERVENTIONS
etonogestrel/ethinyl estradiol (NuvaRing) vaginal contraceptive device		Vaginal ulceration or irritation may occur with NuvaRing.	Should not use with a diaphragm. Expulsion of the ring is possible.
etonogestrel (Nexplanon) subdermal contraceptive	A rod containing a synthetic progesterone is implanted in the upper arm. The drug is slowly dispensed over 3 years. The rod is then removed.	Irregular vaginal bleeding	Implanted contraceptive may be less effective in overweight women. Rod needs to be removed if thromboembolic event or jaundice occurs and after 3 years of use.
intrauterine contraceptive device (IUD)	IUDs used for contraception. Mirena also used for menorrhagia; ParaGard also for emergency contraception.		IUDs are indicated for women in a mutually monogamous/stable relationship. Replaced every 5 years.
levonorgestrel intrauterine device (Mirena, ParaGard)		Risk of PID, especially with STIs. Both can cause cramping and altered menstrual patterns.	
Ovulatory Stimulant and Fertility Drugs			
clomiphene citrate (Clomid)	All stimulate or mimic actions of natural pituitary gonadotropins. All can result in multiple births.	Hot flashes, breast tenderness, nausea, vomiting, visual disturbances, headache, depression, fatigue, reversible hair loss, weight gain, dizziness, ovarian enlargement.	Contraindicated with liver dysfunction, pregnancy, abnormal bleeding. Safety precautions if patient is dizzy or has visual disturbances. Stop drug and contact physician if visual disturbances occur. Tell patient to report vaginal bleeding or weight gain, signifying ovarian hyperstimulation, in which case monitor fluid status, weight, and possible signs of internal bleeding. Tell patient to avoid sexual intercourse with ovarian enlargement because of possible rupture.
menotropins (Repronex, Menopur)	Promotes follicular maturation and ovulation. After follicle matures, hCG is given to promote ovulation.	Ovarian hyper-stimulation with sudden enlargement of ovaries. If severe, ascites, pleural effusion, and pain require hospitalization. Pain and irritation at injection site. Rarely, flulike symptoms: nausea, vomiting, fever.	Reconstitute per directions and administer immediately. Patient should know that menotropin therapy often results in multiple births.
urofollitropin (Metrodin)	Stimulates ovarian follicular growth. Used to treat selected patients who have not responded to clomiphene citrate.	Same as with menotropins.	

Table 49-2 Drug Therapy: Drugs Used to Treat Disorders of the Female Reproductive System—cont'd

DRUG	USE AND ACTION	SIDE EFFECTS	NURSING INTERVENTIONS
Emergency Contraceptive Drugs			
progestin emergency contraception (Plan B) vaginal contraceptives	Plan B used as emergency postcoital contraceptive ("morning-after pill"); taken within 72 hours after unprotected intercourse to prevent implantation of fertilized ovum.	Heavier menstrual bleeding, nausea, abdominal pain, headache, dizziness, vomiting	
selective progesterone receptor modular emergency contraception (ella)	Ella is used within 120 hours (5 days) after unprotected intercourse.	Headache, nausea, dysmenorrhea, abdominal pain.	

Note: Research evidence has revealed increased risks of coronary heart disease and invasive breast cancer when combination estrogen and progestin therapy is used in women with an intact uterus.

DISORDERS OF THE FEMALE REPRODUCTIVE SYSTEM

UTERINE BLEEDING DISORDERS

Pathophysiology

Normal menstrual patterns vary widely in length of cycles (21 to 40 days), duration of menstruation (2 to 8 days), and amount of blood lost (40 to 100 mL). Bleeding patterns that are irregular in the spacing and amount are common in the first 2 years after the onset of menarche and in the 5-year period before menopause. Deviations from the normal cycles are viewed as uterine bleeding disorders. Two of the most common abnormal bleeding patterns, **metrorrhagia** (i.e., bleeding or spotting between menstrual periods) and **menorrhagia** (i.e., menstrual periods characterized by profuse or prolonged bleeding), are addressed in Table 49-3. *Amenorrhea* is the absence of menses.

Cause and Risk Factors

Metrorrhagia and menorrhagia are symptoms of underlying factors rather than being specific definable conditions in themselves. Underlying causes for each vary widely. Common causes include hormonal dysfunction, benign and malignant tumors, coagulation disorders, systemic diseases, use of some contraceptives, endometrial hyperplasia, and inflammatory processes. The amount of blood loss varies with the type of disorder. Causes of amenorrhea include pregnancy; excessive weight gain or loss, physical activity, or stress; pituitary, hypothalamic, thyroid, or adrenal disorders; ovarian failure; and uterine abnormalities.

Medical Diagnosis and Treatment

The diagnosis of uterine bleeding is based on the health history and physical examination as well as on the results of various diagnostic tests and procedures. Colposcopy, biopsy, and ultrasonography as well as laboratory analyses of blood components, hormone levels, and tissue specimens or stains provide diagnostic information. Because anemia may result from excessive bleeding, hemoglobin (Hgb) and hematocrit (Hct) levels are usually measured as well.

The treatment of amenorrhea depends on the cause and whether the patient desires pregnancy. Pharmacologic treatment is often used and can include oral contraceptives or progestins in either oral or intrauterine devices. Surgery is also used if abnormal uterine structures need to be removed. Endometrial ablation is another common procedure often completed as outpatient surgery to treat perimenopausal and postmenopausal menorrhagia.

NURSING CARE of the Patient with Uterine Bleeding

Assessment

Complete assessment of the female patient with a disorder affecting the reproductive system is summarized in Box 49-1. When a patient has metrorrhagia or menorrhagia, the menstrual history is especially important.

Nursing Diagnoses, Goals, and Outcome Criteria: Metrorrhagia or Menorrhagia

Nursing Diagnoses	Goals and Outcome Criteria
Deficient Knowledge of condition and treatment	Patient understands condition and treatment: patient accurately describes condition and treatment
Anxiety related to unknown cause of menorrhagia or metrorrhagia	Reduced anxiety: patient states that she feels less anxious, calm manner

Table 49-3 Uterine Bleeding Disorders

CAUSE	SIGNS AND SYMPTOMS	MEDICAL TREATMENT
Metrorrhagia		
Ovulation	Spotting with regularity 14 days before menses	None—this is regarded as a normal deviation.
Intrauterine contraceptive device	Intermittent spotting between menses	None if bleeding is not severe and if other causes are ruled out. Monitor serum hemoglobin; if low, iron supplements are prescribed. Remove intrauterine device if bleeding is severe.
Oral contraceptive use	Irregular spotting Early cycle spotting Late cycle spotting	Patient is directed to take pill at same time each day. Estrogenic potency of oral contraceptive is increased. Progestational potency of oral contraceptive is increased.
Trauma; introduction of foreign objects	Sudden onset of frank bleeding or spotting	Foreign object is removed. Tissue damage is repaired.
Vaginitis, cervicitis	Spotting combined with vaginal discharge characteristic of infectious organism	Vaginal examination; testing, wet prep, and Papanicolaou test to identify underlying cause; cause treated as warranted.
Ectopic or molar pregnancy	Spotting or frank bleeding in addition to symptoms specific to molar pregnancy, ectopic pregnancy	Ultrasonography and laboratory tests (serum human chorionic gonadotropins level) done. Surgical removal of products of conception. Methotrexate may be used to stop cell growth in an ectopic pregnancy.
Reproductive tract pathology: Endocervical polyps Cervical eversion Cervical dysplasia Endometriosis Salpingitis Ovarian cyst Benign neoplasm Malignant neoplasm	Spotting or frank bleeding in addition to other symptoms characteristic of specific pathology	Diagnostic procedures and treatment specific to identified pathologic condition: hormone therapy, antimicrobial or other drug therapy, surgery.
Menorrhagia		
Intrauterine contraceptive device	For all: By definition, profuse or prolonged bleeding during menstruation in addition to other symptoms characteristic of specific cause	Substitution of intrauterine device discontinuation or removal of intrauterine device, with substitution of alternative contraceptive method. Use of PGSIs may be effective in reducing menstrual blood loss. Treatment for remaining causes is specific for each cause.
Hormonal disturbances		Determination of hormone status is critically important before hormone therapy or other drug therapy is initiated. Treatment may include hormone therapy.
Endometrial hyperplasia		Endometrial hyperplasia may be diagnosed and treated by dilation and curettage. For women past childbearing age, hysterectomy may be performed.
Benign neoplasm		Benign tumors may be left alone and monitored.
Malignant neoplasm		Malignant tumors require a combination of surgical and medical interventions.
Inflammatory process		Specific cause is treated.
Systemic diseases		Specific cause is treated.

PGSI, Prostaglandin synthesis inhibitor.

Interventions

Deficient Knowledge

When the course of treatment has been selected, it may be your responsibility to teach the patient her role in the treatment process and ensure that she is able to follow through appropriately.

Anxiety

You can be a source of emotional support for the patient, who often is fearful or anxious about the unidentified cause of abnormal bleeding. The underlying causes of abnormal uterine bleeding may be relatively simple and easily treatable or complex and life threatening. Therefore you must be prepared to help patients cope with all eventualities. Supportive measures such as encouraging the patient to express her feelings, use of touch, and listening convey concern to the patient. Generally it is your responsibility to provide information regarding procedures to be done. Give explanations in terms the patient can understand.

INFECTIONS

Infections of the female reproductive tract affect patients physiologically and psychologically. The physiologic effects range from short-term reversible changes to long-term changes that result in infertility. The potential psychologic effects are numerous. Changes in relationships, feelings of distrust toward sexual partners, shame, embarrassment, and diminished self-esteem are but a few.

The majority of infections covered in this chapter often are transmitted through unprotected sexual activity (oral, genital, and rectal). In addition, the causative organisms often are those associated with STIs, as discussed in Chapter 51. However, this chapter focuses primarily on the effects of the microorganisms on the female reproductive tract and subsequent medical and nursing interventions rather than on the specific disease processes.

Because of their association with sexuality and sexual function, many women view reproductive tract infections as threats or insults to their self-image. They may react with guilt, embarrassment, denial, defensiveness, or a combination of these reactions that cause them to delay seeking diagnosis and treatment. Others are coping with infertility problems that result from infectious processes. When interacting with women who have reproductive tract infections or their effects, you must be sensitive, tactful, and absolutely nonjudgmental.

Vulvitis and Vaginitis

Pathophysiology. Inflammation of the vulva is called **vulvitis**. Depending on the causative agent, vulvitis may be viewed as an infection, a local manifestation of a general skin disease, a reaction to a chemical irritant or allergen, or a common consequence of the aging process. Regardless of its cause, the most common characteristics of vulvitis are inflammation usually with intense pruritus of the vulva and perianal region.

Like vulvitis, **vaginitis** is characterized by a local inflammatory response to various factors. Vaginitis and vulvitis differ in that a significant vaginal discharge is usually present with vaginitis.

Cause and Risk Factors. Vulvitis and vaginitis are caused by a number of factors that precipitate an inflammatory response. The two common causes of infection are *Candida albicans* (fungus, or yeast infection) and *Trichomonas vaginalis* (protozoal infection). Both most commonly infect the vagina and produce characteristic vaginal discharges that are irritating to the vulva and vagina. The discharge associated with *C. albicans* has a distinctive odor and a cottage cheese–like appearance; the discharge associated with *T. vaginalis* is profuse, frothy, and yellow-gray in color and has a fishy odor. Both can be transmitted sexually, although yeast infections often are associated with disruption of the normal vaginal flora by antibiotic therapy or with DM. Bacterial vaginosis (BV) is also a very common infection caused by an overgrowth of several different species of bacteria, especially anaerobes. The discharge associated with BV is malodorous ("fishy"), white or gray, and of a thin consistency. It takes place when a loss or reduction of protective lactobacilli occurs in the vagina and an increase in concentration of other bacteria commonly found in the gastrointestinal (GI) tract is seen. Although BV is more frequently found in women who are sexually active, the role of sexual activity in the development of this infection is not clear.

Generalized skin diseases that may involve the vulva include psoriasis and inflammation of sweat glands. When these conditions affect the vulva, the constant moist state intensifies the inflammation and subsequent itching.

Vulvar reactions to chemical irritants are common. The vulva is exposed to a wide variety of chemicals that may act as irritants and thus elicit an inflammatory response; the response often extends into the vagina. Perfumed soaps, scented toilet tissue and perineal pads, feminine hygiene sprays, laundry detergent residues, and spermicides are a few examples of common irritants.

Estrogen deficiency associated with the aging process frequently results in nonpathogenic vulvitis and vaginitis because of a combination of tissue atrophy and a decrease in the acid vaginal secretions that normally maintain healthy mucous membranes.

Signs and Symptoms. Regardless of the cause, signs and symptoms include local swelling, redness, and itching. Some infectious agents cause characteristic signs and symptoms that aid in their identification.

Complications. Ascending infection (an infection that moves through the vagina to internal structures) is a potential complication of vulvitis and vaginitis. Infection confined to the lower reproductive tract seldom poses a threat to life or fertility.

Medical Diagnosis. The diagnosis is based on the patient's symptoms and on inspection of the vulva and vagina. Discharge specimens may be collected to aid in identification of specific microbes if microbial infection is suspected.

Medical Treatment. Treatment specific to the causative agent may include topical antifungal creams, oral antiprotozoals or antibiotics, vaginal suppositories to reestablish normal vaginal flora, topical or systemic estrogen replacement therapy (ERT), improved diabetes control, and avoidance of offending chemical agents. Symptoms are managed with frequent cleansing with neutral agents; wearing cotton panties, cotton-crotched pantyhose, and nonconstricting clothing; and heat in the form of sitz baths and perineal irrigations. Advise the patient not to scratch the itching tissues, which can cause further mechanical trauma and infection. During the course of treatment, the patient should avoid sexual intercourse or use of condoms. The woman's sexual partner or partners may be treated for some infections to avoid reinfection.

NURSING CARE of the Patient with Vulvitis or Vaginitis

Vulvitis and vaginitis usually are diagnosed and treated on an outpatient basis. Because patients usually manage their own treatment, you may be responsible for ensuring that the patient understands all self-care instructions and reinforcing other instructions the physician or nurse practitioner provides. General nursing care of patients with reproductive tract infections is addressed in Table 49-4.

Bartholin Gland Abscess (Bartholinitis)

Pathophysiology. Because of their location on either side of the vaginal opening, Bartholin glands are vulnerable to a wide variety of infectious microorganisms. The resultant edema and pus formation occlude the duct of the affected gland and form an abscess.

Cause and Risk Factors. Various microorganisms can be transmitted from the anus, vulva, or vagina to the Bartholin gland duct. Commonly tested organisms include normal intestinal bacterial flora, *Staphylococcus aureus, Streptococcus, Trichomonas vaginalis, Neisseria gonorrhoeae, Chlamydia trachomatis,* and *Mycoplasma hominis.* The organisms are often introduced through improper perineal hygiene (i.e., wiping from the anus toward the vagina).

Signs and Symptoms. Perineal pain is the symptom that most commonly motivates the woman to seek medical assistance. Additional signs and symptoms include fever, labial edema, chills, malaise, and purulent discharge.

Complications. Without proper treatment, bartholinitis may progress from a local infection to a systemic infection.

Medical Diagnosis. Visual inspection reveals a swollen, often reddened mass on the affected side of the vaginal introitus. Gentle palpation causes pain, tenderness, or both. If drainage is seen, a specimen may be obtained for culture and sensitivity testing.

Table 49-4 Care of Patients with Reproductive Tract Infections

PATIENT PROBLEM	NURSING INTERVENTIONS
Denial, embarrassment related to questions about infection	Convey acceptance of the patient. Use tact in eliciting information about hygiene and sexual practices. Relevant data might include the following: • All products applied on or near the vulva or in the vagina, such as feminine hygiene products and "love potions" (i.e., flavored or scented lubricants, massage oils) • Anal contact with penis, fingers, or other objects before contact with vulva or vagina • Number of sexual partners; accessibility to partners if their treatment is indicated
Deficient knowledge regarding treatment and self-care	Explanation of teaching about use of creams, jellies, and suppositories: • Purpose • Position for application or insertion • Application or insertion method • Position after insertion • Care of equipment (i.e., applicator) • Use of tampon or perineal pad to hold medication in place Instructions about perineal hygiene: • Frequent washing with neutral soap • Thorough rinsing • No douching unless specifically ordered • No commercial perineal deodorants • Frequent change of underpants (preferably cotton) • Sitz baths to relieve pain, itching • Wiping perineal-anal area from front to back; one stroke per tissue • Complete full course of prescribed drug therapy

Because causative microorganisms include those responsible for transmission of STIs, the patient is usually screened for these diseases (see Chapter 51).

Medical Treatment. Conservative treatment consists of oral analgesics and moist heat in the form of frequent sitz baths or hot wet packs. The moist heat relieves pain and facilitates spontaneous rupture and drainage of the abscess. The physician or nurse practitioner may do surgical incision and drainage of the abscess. More aggressive treatment with broad-spectrum antibiotics is indicated if symptoms of systemic infection are present.

❖ NURSING CARE of the Patient with Bartholinitis

Basic nursing interventions are outlined in Table 49-2. Provide the appropriate instruction to help the patient comply with the prescribed treatment. Tactful instruction in basic perineal hygiene principles is in order if the evidence indicates that inappropriate or inadequate practices are being followed. Basic practices include soap-and-water cleansing at least once daily and wiping the perineal area with a clean tissue from front to back after urination or defecation.

Cervicitis

Pathophysiology. Cervicitis is inflammation of the cervix. It may be acute or chronic. Although cervicitis is usually the result of an infectious process associated with STIs, the inflammation may be associated with physical or chemical trauma.

Cause and Risk Factors. Cervicitis is caused by a variety of agents: infectious organisms, scraping of cells for diagnostic tests, cryosurgery, use of vaginal tampons or medications, childbirth, neoplasia, and decreased estrogen levels after menopause.

Signs and Symptoms. Cervicitis is usually asymptomatic, although it may cause pain, visible vaginal discharge, bleeding, or dysuria. Unsuspected cervicitis may be detected on pelvic examination or on routine Pap tests. When viewed via a speculum, the cervix appears swollen and reddened; gentle touch may precipitate bleeding. Mucopurulent discharge and vesicular or ulcerated lesions most often are associated with STIs.

Complications. Cervicitis itself is considered to be a relatively benign condition. However, if the causative agent is an infection, the infection may ascend through the reproductive tract and cause pelvic inflammatory disease (PID). Certain microorganisms that cause cervicitis also alter the vaginal pH and exert a spermicidal effect that results in infertility.

Medical Diagnosis and Treatment. Cervicitis may be diagnosed on the basis of the pelvic examination or results of the Pap test. Treatment depends on the causative agent or agents. Infections are treated with systemic or topical antimicrobials. Cervicitis related to menopause is treated with topical or oral estrogen. Additional treatment options include topical application of acidic preparations in the form of douches or jellies, cauterization with silver nitrate, and cryosurgery or laser surgery. Cryosurgery is the use of a cold probe to destroy selected tissue.

Pharmacology Capsule

Instruct patients to complete the full course of antimicrobial therapy to treat infections.

❖ NURSING CARE of the Patient with Cervicitis

Cervicitis usually is diagnosed and treated in outpatient settings. In most cases the physician, the nurse practitioner, or the patient administers treatment. Nursing care is limited to assisting with assessment procedures, patient support, and teaching the patient to carry out the prescribed treatment and posttreatment procedures.

Mastitis

Pathophysiology. **Mastitis** is an infection-induced inflammation of breast tissue most commonly occurring in the lactating woman. Historically, early postpartum mastitis epidemics were common among women who delivered in hospitals and who were hospitalized for the then-usual 10 or more days. With today's short hospital stays, mastitis is associated not with hospitalization but rather with a combination of ineffective breastfeeding techniques that result in poor drainage of mammary ducts and alveoli, lowered resistance to infection because of stress and fatigue, and exposure of breast tissue to infection-causing organisms.

Cause and Risk Factors. *S. aureus* is the microorganism most commonly associated with mastitis; however, *Escherichia coli* and streptococci also may be the agents of infection. The nipple serves as the portal of entry for the organism. Cracked nipples are especially susceptible. A common mechanism of organism transmission is touching the nipples with unclean hands.

Signs and Symptoms. Mastitis is usually confined to one breast and may be asymptomatic except for breast tenderness and low-grade (and often unsuspected) fever. The infection therefore may be undetected if frequent breastfeeding empties breast ducts and alveoli and if the woman's natural immune response prevents spread of the infection. In symptomatic mastitis, the causative organism invades the breast connective tissue or the lobes and ducts and stimulates an inflammatory response that results in localized pain, fever, tachycardia, general malaise, and headache. The affected breast tissue feels hard and warm on palpation; the skin over the infected area is reddened.

Complications. Untreated symptomatic mastitis may result in abscess formation as the sepsis becomes localized. Enlargement of axillary lymph nodes also may result.

Medical Diagnosis and Treatment. The diagnosis is based on presenting symptoms. Symptomatic mastitis is unmistakable. If a purulent discharge from the nipple is noted, a specimen can be collected for culture and sensitivity testing. However, treatment is initiated based on the symptoms alone and consists primarily of immediate and aggressive antibiotic therapy.

Symptoms are managed by frequent emptying of the breast, heat application, rest, and administration of an analgesic. The question of whether to empty the breast by breastfeeding or by artificial pumping is controversial. Many broad-spectrum antibiotics are tolerated well by the mother and the infant. This is significant because antibiotics taken by the mother will be present in her breast milk.

If an abscess forms, surgical excision and drainage of the abscess may be necessary and a longer period of antibiotic therapy will be required.

NURSING CARE of the Patient with Mastitis

The most effective nursing intervention is teaching patients how to prevent mastitis (see *Patient Teaching* box).

Assessment

Explore the breastfeeding woman's knowledge of measures to prevent mastitis. Take the patient's temperature. Palpate the breasts for pain, tenderness, warmth, and hardness and inspect for purulent discharge from the nipple.

Nursing Diagnoses, Goals, and Outcome Criteria: Mastitis

Nursing Diagnoses	Goals and Outcome Criteria
Risk for Injury related to possible abscess formation	Recovery without complications: absence of fever, pain, redness, and purulent drainage
Deficient Knowledge of mastitis prevention and treatment	Patient understands how to treat mastitis and prevent recurrence: patient accurately describes and demonstrates self-care measures

Interventions

Risk for Injury

If mastitis or breast abscess occurs, reinforce the prescribed treatment. If heat treatments or drug therapy are prescribed, ensure that the patient understands the instructions.

Deficient Knowledge

The points commonly addressed in breastfeeding education are those that also prevent the infectious process from occurring.

Patient Teaching

Mastitis

- Be sure to complete your course of antibiotics as prescribed.
- Report continued or additional symptoms.
- Pain usually can be managed with analgesics as prescribed.
- Allow for extra rest periods.
- To prevent recurrence during breastfeeding, do the following:
  - Breast-feed frequently and completely empty the breasts.
  - Wash hands thoroughly before handling breasts.
- To avoid cracked nipples, do the following:
  - Make certain that the infant's lips and gums are around the areola and not on the nipple itself.
  - Break suction before removing the nipple from the infant's mouth.
  - Cleanse with plain water to prevent chemical trauma from soap, alcohol, and other drying agents.
  - Leave milk on nipples and expose them to the air or a heat lamp after breastfeeding.
  - Wear a supportive but nonconstrictive bra.
  - Get adequate rest, nutrition, and fluids.
  - Promptly report early symptoms of breast infection to a health care provider.

FIBROCYSTIC CHANGES

Pathophysiology

Fibrocystic breast changes represent an exaggerated response to hormonal influences. Excess fibrous tissue develops accompanied by overgrowth of the lining of the mammary ducts, proliferation of mammary ducts, and the formation of cysts. Fibrocystic nodules do not "become cancerous" but their presence may make it more difficult to detect malignant tumors by palpation.

Cause and Risk Factors

Fibrocystic changes are more common among women who have never given birth, have had a spontaneous abortion, and had an early menarche and late menopause. The risk also is greater for women who have premenstrual abnormalities and do not use oral contraceptives.

Signs and Symptoms

This painful condition usually affects both breasts. Smooth round lumps that are freely movable may be felt. Sometimes milky yellow or green discharge from the nipple is seen. Symptoms commonly are most apparent during the premenstrual phase of the menstrual cycle and typically improve after the menstrual period.

Medical Diagnosis and Treatment

Diagnosis is based on the physical examination and health history. A mammogram or ultrasound can help to distinguish lumps as fibrocystic changes rather than cancer. If indicated, fluid for study may be aspirated from a mass or the mass may be surgically removed for examination. Women with fibrocystic changes should learn to perform BSE and should have periodic professional breast examinations.

No specific cure exists for fibrocystic changes. Danazol reduces symptoms by decreasing estrogen production. However, the side effects (i.e., acne, edema, excess hair growth) make it unacceptable to many women. Other therapies that lack evidenced-based support but seem to help some women include vitamin E, diuretics, a low-salt diet, wearing a good support bra, stress reduction, and restriction of coffee and chocolate.

❖ NURSING CARE of the Patient with Fibrocystic Changes

Fibrocystic breast changes are treated on an outpatient basis. Therefore the primary role of the nurse is to instruct the patient in self-examination and to encourage scheduled professional examinations.

PELVIC INFLAMMATORY DISEASE

Pathophysiology

PID is an infectious process that may affect any or all structures in the pelvic portion of the reproductive tract and peritoneal cavity. It is called an *ascending infection* because causative organisms migrate upward from the portal of entry, the vulva or vagina.

PID is a major female reproductive health problem and a major cause of infertility in the United States. The infectious process results in scarring and adhesions in the fallopian tubes that can cause total or partial obstruction. Total obstruction results in infertility. Partial obstruction often results in ectopic pregnancy, in which the fertilized ovum implants in a site other than the uterus, usually in the fallopian tube or pelvic cavity. Unfortunately, the incidence of PID is particularly high in adolescent girls.

Cause and Risk Factors

Because the majority of PID cases are caused by sexually transmitted organisms, PID is generally classified as an *STI syndrome. N. gonorrhoeae, C. trachomatis,* and *M. hominis* are recognized as the organisms most associated with PID. *Chlamydia* infection is thought to be the most commonly occurring STI and the one most often responsible for PID. As such, it is often implicated in infection of the fallopian tubes (salpingitis) and is considered to be the primary cause of ectopic pregnancy and infertility associated with tubal obstruction.

However, non-STI organisms also have been identified as causative agents. Staphylococcal, streptococcal, and other organisms have been cultured from women with PID. Sources of non–STI-associated PID include contaminated hands or instruments during gynecologic surgery, childbirth, abortion, and pelvic examinations. Women with compromised resistance to infection and women who are poorly nourished are particularly prone to developing non–STI-associated PID.

The risk of PID increases as the number of sexual partners increases. This factor is most applicable to PID caused by organisms implicated in STIs.

Vaginal douching also is considered to be a possible risk factor for PID. It is thought that the force of the fluid used in douching may propel microorganisms from the vagina through the cervical os (opening) and into the uterus, fallopian tubes, and pelvic cavity.

Signs and Symptoms

PID may be a silent infection with no symptoms. As a result, it may remain untreated while causing damage to pelvic structures. Symptomatic PID may appear with either the gradual onset of dull, steady, low abdominal pain or the sudden onset of severe abdominal pain, chills, and fever. Other symptoms may include dysuria, irregular bleeding, a foul-smelling vaginal discharge that may cause inflammation and skin breakdown of the vulva, and **dyspareunia** (i.e., pain during sexual intercourse).

Symptomatic PID is much more likely to be diagnosed and treated than asymptomatic PID. In many instances, evidence of PID is first discovered during surgery for ectopic pregnancy, blocked fallopian tubes, ovarian abscess, or other pelvic disorders.

Complications

The risk of complications of PID increases with each repeated infection. Common effects of PID include ectopic pregnancy, infertility, and chronic abdominal discomfort. Without prompt diagnosis and aggressive treatment, infection of the entire peritoneal cavity (i.e., peritonitis) and systemic septic shock also are potential complications.

Medical Diagnosis

The diagnosis is based on the presenting symptoms (if any) and the pelvic examination. The definitive diagnosis is based on culture of the causative organism or organisms. Sonography, laparoscopy, and culdocentesis are additional diagnostic procedures that may be used.

Medical Treatment

PID usually can be treated at home. However, very acute symptoms and severe pain may require inpatient care. Treatment includes rest; application of heat via warm compresses, a heating pad, or sitz baths; and a regimen of analgesics and broad-spectrum antibiotics. Depending on the severity and extent of the infection, oral or parenteral antibiotics (or both) are prescribed. Directly observed therapy is generally recommended because some patients do not take prescribed drugs as ordered. The woman should avoid sexual intercourse for at least 3 weeks. If the causative organism is thought to have been transmitted sexually, the woman's sexual partner or partners should be treated to avoid repeated infection. Expedited partner therapy in which the patient is provided with a prescription or additional drugs for her partner has been found to be more effective than referring partners for treatment. Follow-up is recommended to ensure successful treatment.

NURSING CARE of the Patient with Pelvic Inflammatory Disease

Assessment

Nursing assessment of the woman with a disorder of the reproductive system is summarized in Box 49-1. Preparation of the patient for physical examination includes anticipatory guidance, positioning and draping, and emotional support (see Table 49-2). You need to simultaneously assist the examiner and provide support for the patient. Precautions to avoid reproductive tract infections and transmission of infection are summarized in the *Patient Teaching* boxes.

Nursing Diagnoses, Goals, and Outcome Criteria: Pelvic Inflammatory Disease

Nursing Diagnoses	Goals and Outcome Criteria
Acute Pain related to inflammation	Pain relief: patient states that pain is relieved
Impaired Skin Integrity related to infectious drainage	Restored skin integrity: intact skin without excessive redness or edema
Deficient Knowledge of treatment and prevention of reinfection	Patient understands and carries out treatment and preventive measures: patient verbalizes instructions and states intent to follow prescribed measures

Patient Teaching

Precautions to Avoid Reproductive Tract Infection

- Maintain optimum general health: adequate nutrition and sleep, good stress management.
- Cleanse the perianal area daily with neutral soap followed by thorough rinsing; apply no other products unless ordered to do so by your health care provider.
- Wipe the perianal area with one front-to-back swipe per tissue.
- Avoid sharing of any equipment (including washcloths) used for perineal or vaginal hygiene.
- Change perineal pads or tampons frequently during menses even when flow is slight. Increase soap-and-water cleansing to at least twice per day.
- Inspect the genitalia of your partner before intercourse or other contact with the perianal area. Avoid contact if any lesions or discharge is noted. The same precautions should be followed for any part of the partner's anatomy (e.g., mouth, hands, fingers) that will contact the perianal area during a sexual encounter.
- Wash the penis, hands, or other objects that contact the anus with soap and water before contact with the vulva or vagina.
- Use condoms with spermicidal cream or jelly for penis-vulva-vaginal contact when a monogamous relationship is not well established.
- Avoid intercourse during treatment for a reproductive tract infection. Use a condom if intercourse cannot be avoided.

Interventions

Care of the patient with PID includes rest with limited activity, application of heat as ordered, administration of prescribed antibiotics, patient education, and recognizing and reporting signs and symptoms of the side effects of antibiotics.

Acute Pain

Prescribed analgesics are administered for pain control. Additional pain relief measures are discussed in Chapter 15. Monitor and record the efficacy of analgesics.

Impaired Skin Integrity

If perineal pads are needed for collection of vaginal discharge, change them frequently. Note the character, amount, color, and odor of vaginal discharge. Frequent perineal cleansing is done with mild soap and water, followed by rinsing and patting dry. Inspect the vulva for signs of inflammation or excoriation and monitor and record the temperature.

Patient Teaching

Prevention of Pelvic Inflammatory Disease

When teaching prevention of pelvic inflammatory disease (PID) to the sexually active woman with multiple partners or with a single partner with an unknown sexual history, include the following:

- During sexual intercourse, always use protective mechanical or chemical barriers such as a condom, diaphragm, vaginal sponge, and spermicidal vaginal jelly or cream.
- Recognize the signs and symptoms of common sexually transmitted infections (STIs).
- Seek prompt medical diagnosis and treatment of STIs or other possible reproductive tract infections.
- Have a routine yearly pelvic examination by a physician or nurse practitioner, with testing done to detect *Neisseria gonorrhoeae, Chlamydia trachomatis*, and other organisms.
- Routinely inspect the sexual partners' genitalia for signs of infection before each contact for sexual intercourse.

Deficient Knowledge

Nurses play a significant role in the primary prevention of PID and in fostering early diagnosis and treatment of reproductive tract infections so that they do not result in PID. Primary prevention includes measures to reduce risk factors. All women should practice good reproductive tract hygiene habits. The patient with PID needs to understand the importance of taking antibiotics as prescribed. Failure to complete the course of therapy encourages the development of resistant strains of bacteria. Other teaching points include the need to abstain from intercourse for the prescribed period and the need for the sexual partner to be treated if advised.

BENIGN GROWTHS

Endometriosis

Pathophysiology. The cause of endometriosis is uncertain. It may involve retrograde menstruation, metaplasia, or altered function of immune-related cells (or a combination of these conditions). The most popular theory (the Sampson theory) suggests that retrograde menstruation seeds the peritoneal cavity with endometrial cells. Endometrial tissue that lines the uterus responds to hormonal influences during the menstrual cycle. During menstruation, small amounts of menstrual fluid are thought to be ejected through the fallopian tubes into the pelvic cavity rather than through the cervical os into the vagina. In some women, the endometrial cells deposited in the pelvic cavity implant on structures within the cavity; once there they continue to respond to menstrual cycle hormonal stimulation. The result is the periodically painful and potentially destructive condition called **endometriosis**. In women with endometriosis, the ectopic (out of place) endometrial tissue behaves in the pelvic cavity as it does in the uterus: it proliferates and then bleeds if fertilization of the ovum does not occur. As a result, more and more endometrial cells attach to pelvic structures and may form cell clusters called *implants.* When in the ovaries, the implants are sometimes referred to as *chocolate cysts* because of their color and cystic quality. The implants are thought to migrate to other areas of the body, possibly transported by blood or lymph. Bleeding by endometrial tissue causes local inflammation and pain wherever the site of implantation may be located. The number of implants gradually increases, creating multiple sites of inflammation and pain. In response to the inflammation, fibrous tissue that results in scarring and adhesions forms (Fig. 49-9).

Cause and Risk Factors. Although it is known that almost all women experience retrograde menstruation to some degree, it is not known why some women develop endometriosis and others do not. Several theories have been explored; one is that endometriosis may be linked to a defect in the immune system of its victims. The disease is believed to occur in 10% of all women of reproductive age. The incidence and severity are greatest in women with relatives who have endometriosis.

Signs and Symptoms. As noted previously, the major symptom is pain, although some women are asymptomatic. Because the uterine endometrial tissue is bleeding simultaneously, pain appears as

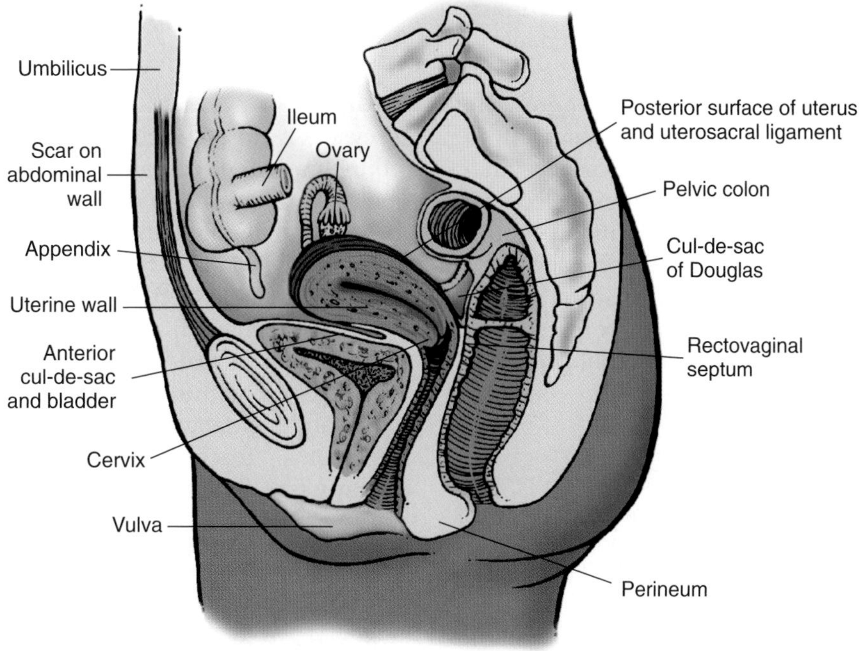

FIGURE 49-9 Common sites of endometriosis. (From Monahan FD, Drake DT, Neighbors M, editors: *Medical-surgical nursing: foundations for clinical practice*, ed 2, Philadelphia, 1998, Saunders.)

dysmenorrhea and may extend to a feeling of general pelvic heaviness. Additional symptoms can include pain with defecation, dyspareunia, and abnormal bleeding. Emotional symptoms, including anger and depression, also are common. Infertility may be a sign of endometriosis when adhesions affect uterine position or fallopian tube patency, movement, or both.

Complications. The most common complication of endometriosis is constriction of pelvic structures by endometriosis-related adhesions. Constriction of the bowel, ureters, or both may cause partial or complete obstruction within the affected structure, creating a medical emergency.

Medical Diagnosis. Visualization and excision of endometrial implants via laparoscopy provide specimens for laboratory analysis and are the primary diagnostic procedures for endometriosis. Ultrasonography may be used as a preliminary diagnostic tool to determine the presence of pelvic masses.

Medical Treatment. Medical management includes the use of nonsteroidal antiinflammatory drugs (NSAIDs) to relieve pain. The most commonly used drugs for pharmacologic treatment of endometriosis are GnRH agonists or a synthetic androgenic steroid. GnRH agonists suppress the secretion of GnRH, causing the estrogen level to fall, which permits endometriosis implants to shrink. Several such drugs exist, including leuprolide acetate (Lupron) or goserelin acetate (Zoladex) and nafarelin acetate (Synarel). Leuprolide therapy requires monthly intramuscular injection. Goserelin is released slowly from a subdermal implant and nafarelin is taken by nasal inhalation. Side effects are similar to those seen with danazol. Danazol (Danocrine), a synthetic androgenic steroid, inhibits gonadotropin excretion, resulting in amenorrhea and atrophy of intrauterine and ectopic endometrial tissue. Many women find the common side effects of danazol to be unacceptable: masculinizing characteristics such as voice deepening, hirsutism (i.e., excess hair growth), clitoral enlargement, and skin changes as well as menopausal symptoms such as hot flashes, vaginal atrophy, and dryness. Both classes of drugs are contraindicated during pregnancy, so the patient should know to use a barrier contraceptive during and for 1 to 3 months after the first normal menstrual period after therapy. Oral contraceptives may be prescribed on a long-term basis to inhibit endometrial proliferation, thereby relieving symptoms.

Pharmacology Capsule

Androgens have masculinizing effects on women. The effects usually resolve when the drugs are discontinued.

Pharmacology Capsule

Oral contraceptives are contraindicated in a woman with a history of cardiovascular disease, cerebrovascular disease, or thrombophlebitis.

Surgical management is commonly used and includes laparoscopy for diagnosis and removal of endometrial implants via resection, electrocauterization, or laser vaporization. Because it is difficult to visualize and remove all implants and because the underlying cause continues to exist, such surgery does not constitute a permanent cure and may need to be repeated at intervals. When fertility is no longer desired or complications develop, total abdominal **hysterectomy** with bilateral **salpingo-oophorectomy** (i.e., excision of the uterus, fallopian tubes, and ovaries) may be performed. Removal of the ovaries prevents the production of estrogen that would stimulate endometrial tissue. However, ERT is not an option to relieve menopausal effects for these women as long as endometrial implants remain because the implants continue to respond to the estrogen and symptoms return.

❖ NURSING CARE of the Patient with Endometriosis

Endometriosis is usually treated on an outpatient basis, so nursing care is limited unless the patient is admitted for surgery. Perhaps the most significant nursing interventions are validating that the pain is real and providing information about pain relief measures (see Chapter 15). The office or clinic nurse may be involved in patient teaching. Specific patient teaching depends on the treatment method selected and includes anticipatory guidance and treatment-specific instructions. Because periodic bleeding of all endometrial sites may cause anemia, teaching should include symptoms of anemia and the need for dietary or supplemental vitamin and mineral therapy. Preoperative and postoperative nursing care of the patient who has had a hysterectomy is addressed in the nursing care plan (see Nursing Care Plan: Patient with a Hysterectomy).

Cysts

A cyst is a closed, saclike structure that is lined with epithelium and contains fluid, semisolid, or solid material. Cysts are classified as *neoplasms* and may be benign or malignant; the majority are benign. The most common ovarian and breast cysts are covered individually in Table 49-5.

For women with ovarian or breast cysts, nursing intervention focuses on teaching. Instruct the patient to keep a diary of symptoms, detailing when they occur and any factors that may be associated with the symptoms. Teaching is specific to the prescribed therapy (see *Cultural Considerations* box).

Cultural Considerations

What Does Culture Have to Do with Uterine Fibroid Tumors?

The incidence of fibroid tumors is increased among African-American women. These women should be advised to report menstrual irregularities and pain so that the condition can be diagnosed early and treatment can be initiated.

Nursing Care Plan — Patient with a Hysterectomy

ASSESSMENT

HEALTH HISTORY A 42-year-old married woman has a diagnosis of uterine fibroid tumors. She has been pregnant three times and has three living children, two boys and one girl, all of whom are teenagers still living at home. Her menstrual periods have been regular, with onset every 30 days and lasting for 6 days. She describes her menstrual flow as heavy. She states that she saturates six to eight heavy-day pads and six to eight super tampons per 24 hours for the first 3 days of each period, after which the flow tapers off and she can manage the remainder of each period with four to six tampons per 24 hours. Her last period ended 6 days ago. She describes her health as excellent, with the exception of the uterine fibroids that were diagnosed when she was 33 years old. She is admitted for a total abdominal hysterectomy with bilateral salpingo-oophorectomy. This will be her first experience with surgery.

PHYSICAL EXAMINATION Vital signs: blood pressure 116/74 mm Hg, pulse 72 bpm, respiration 18 breaths per minute, temperature 97.8°F (36.6°C) measured orally. Height 5′3″, weight 116 lb. Lungs clear on auscultation. Skin color medium tan; nail beds pink with rapid capillary refill. Appears to be in good physical condition: body is firm with little evidence of adipose tissue and with excellent muscle tone; abdomen firm but protruding, appears about 5 months pregnant.

LABORATORY Urinalysis, complete blood count (CBC): All reports indicate no deviation from normal ranges except for hemoglobin (Hgb) concentration 10.4 g/dL (normal: 11 to 16 g/dL) and hematocrit (Hct) 30% (normal: 31% to 44%). She has been typed and crossmatched for 2 U of whole blood "on hold" for surgery.

Nursing Diagnosis	Goals and Outcome Criteria	Interventions
PREOPERATIVE NURSING DIAGNOSES		
Risk for **Situational Low Self-Esteem** related to perceived potential changes in femininity, effect on sexual relationship	The patient will verbalize understanding of expected changes in anatomy and physiology and of ability to resume a satisfying sexual relationship with her husband after recovery from surgery.	Explain the following: 1. The only expected noticeable effects of loss of the uterus and ovaries will be cessation of menstrual periods and ability to become pregnant, in addition to cessation of symptoms for which she is seeking surgery. 2. She may experience vaginal numbness for a short period of time. 3. Many women experience improved libido and sexual satisfaction after hysterectomy; sexual spontaneity may increase with the lack of need for contraception. 4. Although penile or vaginal intercourse should not be resumed until at least 6 weeks after surgery, oral sex and masturbation to orgasm are safe. 5. Positions for sexual intercourse should avoid pressure on the abdominal incision for as long as incisional tenderness persists. 6. Orgasmic contractions of the uterus will no longer be present; this change of uterine sensation is noted by some but not most women. 7. Estrogen replacement therapy (ERT) will prevent atrophy of the vagina and decreased lubrication associated with removal of ovaries.
Deficient Knowledge related to information or misinterpretation of effects of hormone replacement therapy (HRT)	The patient will verbalize understanding of potential side effects of HRT and strategies to minimize side effects.	Explain the following: 1. The dosage of estrogen replacement may be adjusted for optimum therapeutic effect; she should report any concerns to her gynecologist. 2. Estrogen may increase fluid retention, which may make one "feel fat." Dietary control of sodium intake will reduce the tendency for fluid retention. 3. Gradual resumption of presurgical physical activity and a well-balanced diet should maintain weight and fitness at presurgical levels.
POSTOPERATIVE NURSING DIAGNOSES*		
Ineffective Peripheral Tissue Perfusion related to anemia, surgical trauma, effects of anesthesia	The patient will have adequate oxygenation of tissues, as evidenced by a pulse rate of 66 to 80 beats per minute (bpm), respiratory rate of 12 to 20 breaths per minute, stable skin color, alert mental status, and negative Homans sign.	Monitor pulse, respiration, and blood pressure rates and auscultate respirations on schedule according to institutional policy. Assist patient to turn, deep breathe, cough on schedule; assist with incentive spirometer if ordered. Monitor skin color, temperature, and capillary refill, including lower extremities. Instruct and assist with foot and leg exercises while patient is confined to bed; encourage and assist with ambulation when allowed. Assess ability to answer questions appropriately. If elastic hose are ordered, ensure they are applied and removed according to schedule when patient is in bed and at all times when out of bed; instruct patient about self-application. Monitor laboratory reports. Report to appropriate person any deviations from normal ranges. Medicate with analgesics to maximize comfort status.

Continued

Nursing Care Plan — Patient with a Hysterectomy—cont'd

Nursing Diagnosis	Goals and Outcome Criteria	Interventions
Risk for Deficient Fluid Volume related to postoperative bleeding	The patient will maintain adequate fluid volume, balanced fluid intake and output, moist mucous membranes, stable pulse and blood pressure.	Check abdominal dressing and perineal pad at least every hour for the first 12 hours; report any drainage observed on dressing, excessive vaginal bleeding. Should saturate less than one perineal pad per hour. Compare fluid intake (intravenous, oral) with urinary output (indwelling catheter collection bag or voided); report discrepancies. Monitor intravenous infusion; carry out related responsibilities according to institutional policy. Encourage fluid intake when allowed. Check mucous membranes for moisture; offer frequent mouthwashes during nothing-by-mouth status. Monitor pulse and blood pressure; compare with baseline levels; report deviations from acceptable ranges.
Urinary Retention related to surgical manipulation, local tissue edema, temporary sensory or motor impairment	The patient will empty bladder at regular intervals without catheterization.	Assist patient to bathroom or commode; use bedpan only if absolutely necessary. Assist patient to assume comfortable position. Provide privacy but remain within calling distance. If patient is unable to void without assistance, employ assistive measures: run water in sink or shower; pour warm water over perineum. Teach or assist patient to perform perineal hygiene at least every 8 hours: wash vulva with warm, soapy water; rinse with warm water from irrigating apparatus; rinse perineum after every voiding. Measure and record urine output; note color, clarity, and odor of urine. Palpate for bladder fullness above symphysis pubis to assess for urinary retention. If patient is unable to void or is retaining urine, allow her to rest for 30 minutes and repeat attempt for spontaneous voiding. Follow order for intermittent catheterization or repeat insertion of indwelling catheter if patient is unable to void a sufficient quantity. Continue to monitor and to assist with voiding until patient consistently empties her bladder without assistance.
Constipation related to weakening of abdominal musculature, abdominal pain, decreased physical activity, dietary changes, drug side effects	The patient will have bowel movement on or before the fourth day after surgery.	Auscultate abdomen for bowel sounds, palpate for distention. Insert rectal tube as ordered, if appropriate. When oral intake is allowed, administer antiflatulent if ordered; teach patient self-administration if allowed. Encourage early and frequent ambulation. Encourage oral intake of fluids, especially of fruit juices. Assess for nausea and vomiting; administer antiemetic if nausea and vomiting are present. Follow protocol for diet; encourage selection of high-fiber foods when patient is allowed options. Administer stool softener or laxative if ordered. Assist patient to splint abdomen while attempting to pass feces. Report inability to have a bowel movement within the allotted time period.

Critical Thinking Questions

1. How would you explain the effects of HT to a patient who has deficient knowledge related to this intervention?
2. Outline your strategy for helping this patient to deal with the emotional trauma of a hysterectomy.

*See Chapter 17 for general postsurgical diagnoses and care.

Fibroid Tumors (Myomas, Leiomyomas)

Pathophysiology. Uterine fibroid tumors are benign and common. It is predicted that at least 20% to 30% of all women will develop fibroid tumors during their reproductive periods. Fibroid tumors grow slowly during the reproductive years but tend to atrophy after the onset of menopause.

Cause and Risk Factors. Although the exact cause is unknown, it is widely thought that fibroid tumors form and grow in response to stimulation by estrogen, primarily estradiol. Human growth hormone and human placental lactogen may also promote the tumors' development and growth.

Signs and Symptoms. Fibroid tumors may be asymptomatic but the most common symptoms are menstrual irregularities: menorrhagia and dysmenorrhea. Discomfort from pressure on pelvic structures and dyspareunia may be associated with a large tumor. For some women, the initial hint that something is wrong is the gradual enlargement of the lower abdomen, which may be mistaken for pregnancy.

Complications. A very large fibroid tumor may compress the urethra, obstructing urine flow and causing secondary hydronephrosis. More common complications include infertility, crowding and malpositioning of the fetus during pregnancy, and degenerative changes related to interruption of blood supply.

Table 49-5 Common Ovarian and Breast Cysts

TYPE OF CYST	PATHOPHYSIOLOGY	SIGNS AND SYMPTOMS	DIAGNOSIS AND MANAGEMENT
Follicular ovarian cyst	Forms when a dominant follicle fails to rupture and release its ovum and thus continues to grow. Occasionally formed in response to ovarian hyperstimulation by fertility drugs. May rupture and bleed into the pelvic cavity, causing sudden, severe abdominal pain.	Usually asymptomatic unless very large; then pelvic heaviness or congestion and an aching feeling are noted.	Usually detected during a pelvic examination. Most disappear spontaneously in 2–3 months without treatment. If it remains on reexamination after 6–10 weeks, the cyst may be examined by laparoscope and drained or removed via needle aspiration.
Corpus luteum ovarian cyst	Forms after ovulation; characterized by excessive bleeding into the luteal cavity and by increased progesterone secretion. Use of fertility drugs is associated with ovarian hyperstimulation and formation of multiple cysts. Associated with more complications than follicular cysts. May rupture and hemorrhage into the pelvic cavity, causing a degree of pain related to the amount of bleeding.	Initial symptom is delayed onset of the menstrual period, followed by irregularities in menstrual amount and duration of flow. Patient may have dull, aching pelvic pain or cramping.	Is palpable as a small, tender mass on the affected ovary. If severe abdominal pain exists, ectopic pregnancy should be ruled out as a cause. May be visualized via laparoscopic or culdoscopic examination if the diagnosis is questionable. Usually no treatment is indicated. Normally disappears spontaneously.
Dermoid ovarian cyst	Composed of tissue from the three embryonic germ cell layers. May contain remnants of fat, hair, teeth, cartilage, and nerve tissue. Usually arises from the ovary on a pedicle (stalk). A small number (3%–5%) of dermoid cysts become malignant.	Asymptomatic when small. Pelvic aching or heaviness with a large cyst. Moderate pain if pedicle gradually becomes twisted; severe pain with sudden twisting.	Palpated as a dense, firm mass during pelvic examination. With a long pedicle, the mass may be found some distance from the ovary to which it is attached. A pregnancy test is needed to rule out ectopic pregnancy. If radiographs show teeth in the mass, the diagnosis of dermoid cyst is confirmed. Any dermoid cyst should be removed surgically because of the potential for malignancy.
Breast cyst	Most commonly identified cause is ovarian estrogen secretion. Additional contributing factors may be stress and caffeine. Is an exaggerated response to hormonal influence. May enlarge during the premenstrual period and shrink from the onset of menstruation until the next ovulation. Commonly called *fibrocystic disease.* Controversial: Some fibrocystic subtypes are considered precancerous.	Most are round, freely movable, benign cysts. May be soft or firm, depending on the contents. Small cysts are numerous; breasts have lumpy "cottage cheese" consistency. Varying degrees of pain are noted between ovulation and menstruation.	Methods of preliminary diagnosis include the following: palpation, mammography, and ultrasonography (useful for initial study). Contents of fluid-filled cysts may be aspirated for laboratory study or observed over time. Accurate diagnosis of a solid cyst requires surgical biopsy. Treatment includes oral analgesics and heat application. Dietary measures include caffeine restriction, decreased salt intake, and supplementary vitamins and fatty acids. Most aggressive surgical treatment is mastectomy, which occasionally is an option selected by women who undergo repeated surgical biopsies. Hormone therapy: 1. Danazol (Danocrine): Decreases secretion of estrogen. Dosage is generally low enough to avoid serious side effects. 2. Low-dose estrogen with progesterone or progestins.

Medical Diagnosis. On pelvic examination, the uterus is found to be enlarged and distorted. A pregnancy test, Pap stain analysis, and complete blood count (CBC) should be done to rule out other conditions.

Medical Treatment. Many women need no treatment and their tumors atrophy after menopause. Methods of contraception are limited by fibroid tumors: intrauterine devices are contraindicated, the estrogen in oral contraceptives may stimulate growth of the tumors, and diaphragms may be uncomfortable. For women who desire to become pregnant, some gynecologic surgeons perform myomectomy (removal of the tumor alone), usually by laser surgery. Some small tumors can be removed endoscopically or destroyed with cryosurgery. A procedure to block blood flow to the tumor has also been used to destroy the tissue. For tumors that are very large or associated with complications, hysterectomy is the usual surgery of choice. Pregnancy should be delayed for 4 to 6 months after myomectomy. Leuprolide (Lupron), a GnRH agonist, may be ordered to shrink large tumors before surgery. However, concerns exist that this drug causes bone demineralization.

❖ NURSING CARE of the Patient with Fibroid Tumors

Assist the physician or nurse practitioner with diagnostic procedures and provide support to the patient. Women tend to equate the word *tumor* with malignancy. Therefore you may need to give repeated reassurance that the fibroid tumor is benign. If the practitioner elects a conservative approach of monitoring tumor growth, the patient may need reassurance that this approach is commonly used (see Nursing Care Plan: Patient with a Hysterectomy). If the patient with fibroid tumors has heavy bleeding, she should be advised to avoid aspirin and other drugs that enhance bleeding.

UTERINE DISPLACEMENT

Cystocele and Rectocele

Pathophysiology. **Cystocele** and **rectocele** are vaginal disorders caused by weakness of supportive structures between the vagina and bladder (cystocele) or the vagina and rectum (rectocele). They typically occur together. Bulging of the bladder and rectum through the vaginal wall is visible and palpable on vaginal examination. Although small cystoceles and rectoceles may cause no problems, larger herniations may cause problems with emptying of bladder and bowel. Stress incontinence, incomplete bladder emptying, difficulty with expulsion of fecal matter collected in the area of herniation, and incontinence of gas or liquid feces are problems typically reported.

Cause and Risk Factors. During pregnancy and childbirth, the muscles that support the pelvic floor may be weakened. Repeat pregnancies result in further weakening that may eventually allow the bladder and the bowel to press through the vaginal wall.

Signs and Symptoms. Symptoms other than the already described common bladder and bowel problems include dyspareunia, lower back and pelvic discomfort, and recurrent bladder infections.

Medical Diagnosis and Treatment. The diagnosis is made on the basis of inspection and palpation. Treatment of small cystoceles and rectoceles may be limited to pelvic floor (Kegel) exercises, which improve muscle tone. ERT or HT may be prescribed to improve tone and vascularity of supportive tissues. A pessary may be helpful with cystocele. A pessary is a device that is inserted into the vagina to provide support. Surgical intervention via anterior colporrhaphy and posterior colporrhaphy (A&P) repair to tighten the vaginal wall has long been the treatment of choice for larger or symptomatic cystoceles and rectoceles. An anterior colporrhaphy reduces the size of the anterior vaginal wall and is used to treat a cystocele. Posterior colporrhaphy reduces the size of the posterior vaginal wall and is used to treat a rectocele. A risk of vaginal stenosis exists, which results in painful intercourse after posterior repair. These procedures usually are not done during the childbearing years because vaginal delivery would disrupt the repair.

It is interesting to note that nurse researchers who use noninvasive methods based on pelvic floor exercises report long-term success rates comparable to those found with colporrhaphy.

❖ NURSING CARE of the Patient with Cystocele and Rectocele

■ Assessment

Assessment of the patient with a disorder of the reproductive system is outlined in Box 49-1. When a patient has uterine displacement, also record problems related to urinary and bowel function. If surgery is planned, assess the patient's understanding of the procedure, the preoperative and postoperative care, and the patient's concerns.

Nursing Diagnoses, Goals, and Outcome Criteria: Cystocele and Rectocele

Nursing Diagnoses	Goals and Outcome Criteria
Stress Urinary Incontinence related to pelvic muscle weakness	Control of urine elimination: patient reports improved bladder control
Constipation related to collection of feces in herniated bowel	Normal bowel elimination: regular bowel movements without straining
Sexual Dysfunction related to painful intercourse	Satisfying sexual practices without pain: patient's statement of lack of pain during intercourse

Nursing Diagnoses, Goals, and Outcome Criteria: Cystocele and Rectocele—cont'd

Nursing Diagnoses	Goals and Outcome Criteria
Risk for Infection related to incomplete bladder emptying	Absence of urinary tract infections (UTIs): normal body temperature, no pain on urination
After surgical intervention, additional nursing diagnoses and goals are the following.	
Acute Pain related to tissue trauma	Reduced pain: patient states pain is relieved, relaxed manner
Risk for Injury related to infection and stress on surgical incisions	Wound healing without disruption or infection: intact surgical incisions without increasing redness or purulent drainage
Deficient Knowledge of postoperative self-care	Patient understands surgical routines and self-care: patient accurately describes postoperative self-care

Interventions

Nursing interventions vary depending on the medical treatment.

Stress Urinary Incontinence

For conservative treatment, you can teach Kegel exercises (see Chapter 23). The exercise is viewed as a preventive measure that can be adopted in early adulthood to maintain optimum pelvic floor muscle support throughout life.

Constipation

For the patient who reports problems with expelling feces, teaching includes directions to maintain soft stool consistency and regular bowel elimination. Dietary support focuses on frequent ingestion of fluids and a wide variety of high-fiber foods such as fruits, vegetables, and grains. Regular use of bulk stool softeners may be necessary.

Sexual Dysfunction

For the patient who is treated with colporrhaphy, preoperative nursing care includes anticipatory guidance regarding the impending surgery and postsurgical period and carrying out the physician's orders. The patient may fear painful intercourse postoperatively or may be concerned about the effects of surgery on sexual function. Explain that intercourse should be delayed for a prescribed period of time for healing to occur. No permanent impairment of sexual function is expected.

Risk for Infection

Preoperative orders commonly include a vaginal douching with an antibacterial solution, a cleansing enema, and hair removal according to agency procedure. Postsurgical nursing care is directed at prevention of infection and protection of the suture line. Perineal care is provided at regular intervals. In addition to incisional infections, the patient is at risk for urinary tract infections (UTIs). An indwelling urethral or suprapubic catheter commonly is left in place for several days to keep the bladder empty and thus prevent strain on sutures and to let local edema subside. Instruct the patient to report urinary frequency, burning, or foul odor, which suggests infection of the urinary tract.

Acute Pain

Postoperative perineal care includes cleansing of the perineum at regular intervals, initial application of cold to reduce pain and swelling, and subsequent application of heat via sitz baths and heat lamps. Because postoperative pain may be severe, administer analgesics as ordered. Assess the effects of comfort measures and inform the physician if pain is not relieved.

Risk for Injury

A low-residue diet reduces fecal bulk and stool softeners are recommended to prevent straining during defecation after surgery. Encourage adequate fluids and ambulation.

Deficient Knowledge

Discharge teaching focuses on the patient's responsibility for continued self-care as the physician orders. Reinforce instructions regarding diet, medications, activity restrictions, and avoidance of sexual intercourse for the time the physician specifies. Reassure the patient that loss of vaginal sensation is expected and will resolve after a few months. To minimize vaginal stenosis after posterior repair, the surgeon may instruct the patient to use dilators and vaginal lubricants and to resume intercourse 6 weeks after surgery.

Uterine Prolapse

Uterine prolapse is a condition in which the uterus descends into the vagina from its usual position in the pelvis (Fig. 49-10). Descent is rated as *first degree* if the cervix is above the vaginal introitus, *second degree* if the cervix protrudes from the introitus, and *third degree* if the vagina is inverted and the cervix and the body of the uterus protrude from the introitus. If the vagina inverts, it carries with it the adjacent bladder and rectum. Although uterine prolapse can occur in women who have never been pregnant, it is most common in postmenopausal women who have had multiple pregnancies.

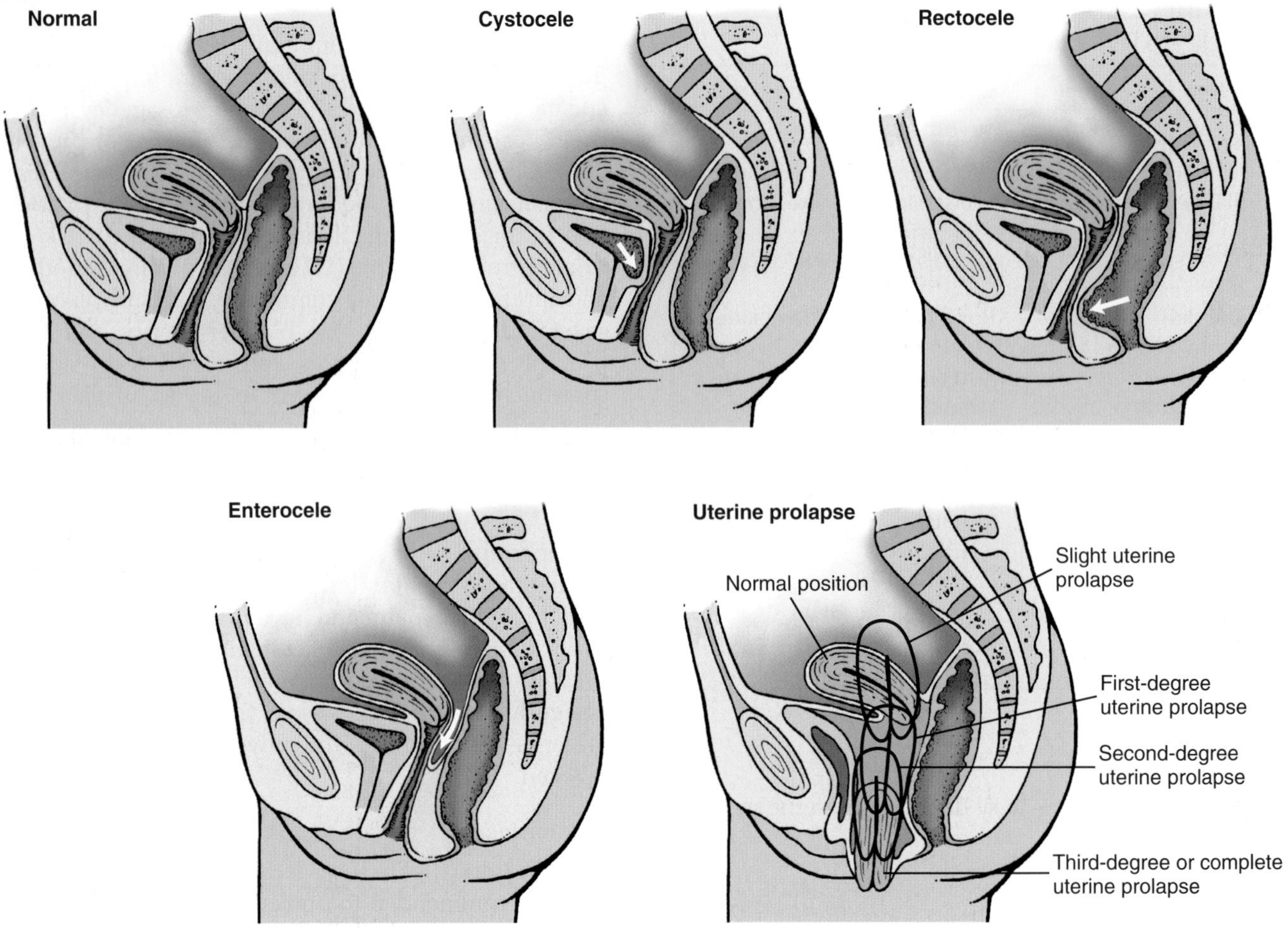

FIGURE 49-10 Types of genital prolapse. (From Monahan FD, Drake DT, Neighbors M, editors: *Medical-surgical nursing: foundations for clinical practice*, ed 2, Philadelphia, 1998, Saunders.)

Cause and Risk Factors. Cardinal and uterosacral ligaments and fascia support the uterus in its anatomic position. The ligaments may be congenitally weak or may become stretched during pregnancy or injured during childbirth, resulting in weakening of support. Pelvic trauma, connective tissue diseases, and medical conditions that increase abdominal pressure (e.g., obesity) are also risk factors. As a woman ages, other supportive structures and uterine walls tend to relax, resulting in some degree of uterine prolapse.

Signs and Symptoms. Dyspareunia, backache, and a feeling of pelvic heaviness and pressure are commonly reported symptoms. Cystocele and rectocele usually accompany uterine prolapse.

Complications. In second-degree and third-degree prolapse, the protruding uterine portion is subject to trauma and may become eroded and necrotic.

Medical Diagnosis. Second-degree and third-degree prolapse are readily detected by visual inspection. First-degree prolapse is diagnosed through pelvic examination, although early first-degree prolapse may escape detection because the uterine descent is not evident when the patient is supine.

Medical Treatment. Vaginal hysterectomy with anterior and posterior colporrhaphy is the most common surgical treatment for uterine prolapse. For the woman who desires to preserve childbearing capability, it is possible to shorten the supportive ligaments surgically and return the uterus to the correct anatomic position.

For women who are poor surgical risks or who refuse surgical treatment, pessaries may be used. Pessaries are instruments that are inserted into the vagina to apply pressure on the vaginal wall, thereby supporting the uterus in the pelvis. Several types of pessaries exist, including ring ("donut") pessary and lever pessary. After placement of a pessary, advise the patient to return within 24 hours for the physician to assess placement, effectiveness, and problems related to pressure on surrounding structures. Pessaries must be removed, cleaned, and replaced periodically. If they are not maintained or are fitted improperly, they may act as irritants and cause tissue erosion, malignant tissue changes, or both. Be sure to document that the patient has a pessary so that it will not be forgotten and neglected. Topical estrogen creams or vaginal tablets may improve the tone of the muscles in the pelvic floor.

NURSING CARE of the Patient with Uterine Prolapse

Assessment

Nursing assessment of the patient with a disorder of the reproductive system is outlined in Box 49-1. When the patient has uterine prolapse, record related symptoms. If the prolapsed uterus is visible, note any signs of trauma or tissue breakdown.

Nursing Diagnoses, Goals, and Outcome Criteria: Second- or Third-Degree Uterine Prolapse

Nursing Diagnoses	Goals and Outcome Criteria
Disturbed Body Image related to interference with daily activities	Improved body image: positive patient remarks about self and ability to manage uterine prolapse
Sexual Dysfunction related to abnormal uterine position	Satisfying sexual function: patient states sexual activity is satisfying and without pain
Risk for Injury related to trauma of the exposed uterus	Absence of uterine trauma: no breaks in tissue integrity of uterus
Deficient Knowledge of self-care	Patient understands and practices self-care: patient accurately describes self-care, keeps follow-up appointments

Interventions

You can serve as a source of emotional support and information for the patient. Nursing care depends on the treatment selected. Proper use of a pessary can reduce the risk of uterine trauma. When a pessary is the treatment of choice, explain the importance of frequent examinations by a physician or nurse practitioner, the need to report pessary-related discomfort to the health care provider, and the need for pessary care. Although some primary health care providers prefer to remove, clean, and replace pessaries, capable patients can be taught to do this themselves.

Put on Your Thinking Cap!

A newly hired nurse in a long-term care facility is surprised to learn that some patients have pessaries. The nurse says, "Nobody uses those things anymore!" How would you explain the use of pessaries in this population?

Retroversion and Retroflexion, Anteversion and Anteflexion

The position of the uterus relative to the vagina has common variation. Positions of the uterus are stable throughout a woman's lifetime unless trauma or disease conditions arise. Displacements are classified as *anteflexion, anteversion, retroflexion,* or *retroversion.* The uterus is commonly positioned at a 45-degree angle anterior to the vagina, with the cervix pointed downward toward the posterior vaginal wall (Fig. 49-11). With anteversion, the entire uterus tilts forward at a sharper angle to the vagina. With anteflexion, the uterus bends forward as if folding on itself. **Retroversion** is a backward tilt of the uterus with the cervix pointed downward toward the anterior vaginal wall. With retroflexion, the body of the uterus bends backward on itself. Displacement from the woman's normal uterine position may be related to a number of other factors (Fig. 49-12). The uterus may become fixed and immobile if trapped by disease or scar tissue.

Cause and Risk Factors. Weakening and stretching of the round, broad, and uterosacral ligaments and weakened pelvic floor musculature related to childbearing are the most common causes of uterine displacement. Other causes include surgical trauma, pelvic tumors, PID, and endometriosis.

Signs and Symptoms. Most uterine displacement is asymptomatic, although dyspareunia and low back pain may occur with retroversion.

Complications. Difficulty with conception has been associated with uterine displacement, particularly with retroversion. However, most complications are now thought to be associated with an underlying pathology (e.g., endometriosis, PID) rather than with displacement itself.

Medical Diagnosis and Treatment. The pelvic examination reveals uterine displacement. Treatment is seldom used, although some women find relief from backache by assuming a knee-chest position. Kegel exercises may be used to strengthen the pelvic floor muscular support system. For patients who are not candidates for surgery, a pessary may be used (see the section titled "Uterine Prolapse").

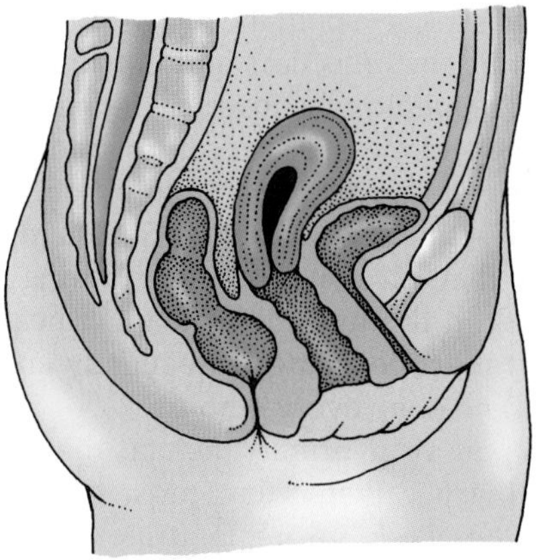

FIGURE 49-11 Normal position of the uterus. (From Ignatavicius DD, Workman ML, Mishler MA: *Medical-surgical nursing across the health care continuum*, ed 3, Philadelphia, 1999, Saunders.)

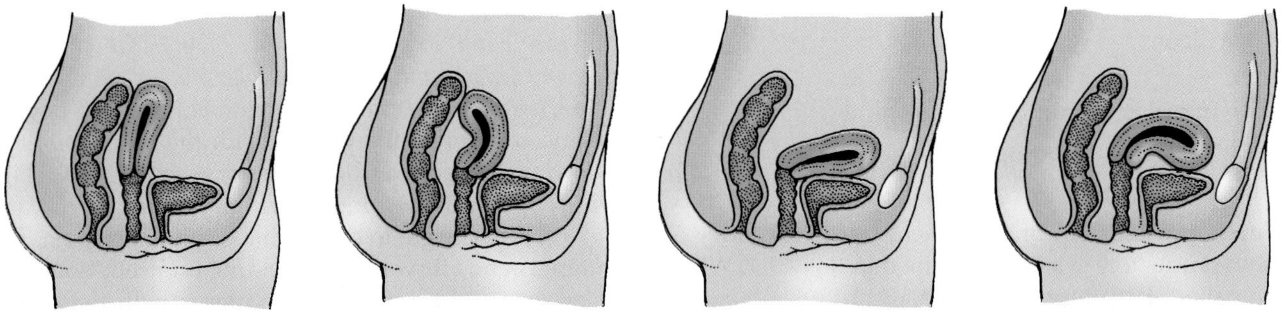

In **retroversion**, the uterus *tilts posteriorly*, and the cervix rotates anteriorly.

In **retroflexion**, the uterus *bends posteriorly.*

In **anteversion**, the uterus *tilts anteriorly.*

In **anteflexion**, the uterus *bends anteriorly.*

FIGURE 49-12 Types of uterine displacement. (From Ignatavicius DD, Workman ML, Mishler MA: *Medical-surgical nursing across the health care continuum*, ed 3, Philadelphia, 1999, Saunders.)

NURSING CARE of the Patient with Retroversion and Retroflexion, Anteversion and Anteflexion

The nurse's role is usually limited to history taking and providing information. If a pessary is inserted, provide instructions similar to those described in the section titled "Uterine Prolapse."

VAGINAL FISTULAS

Vaginal fistulas are abnormal passageways between the vagina and other pelvic organs. A fistula between the vagina and the urinary bladder is called a *vesicovaginal fistula*; a *urethrovaginal fistula* is located between the urethra and the vagina. Both of these fistulas permit urine to flow into the vagina. A *rectovaginal fistula* is located between the vagina and the rectum and permits flatus and feces to pass into the vagina. Urine or fecal matter in the vagina can lead to severe vaginal and vulvar irritation and infection. Vaginal fistulas often can be diagnosed on the basis of the health history and physical examination findings. Dye may be injected into the vagina and radiographs may be made to locate the fistula.

Surgical correction is often needed, although some small fistulas close spontaneously. Surgery may be delayed until the infection and inflammation have subsided. Preoperatively, instruct the patient in perineal hygiene and measures to control odor. Encourage fluid intake to reduce the risk of infection. The physician may prescribe sitz baths and deodorizing douches. Remember that excessive pressure during douching may force fluid through the fistula. Perineal pads are needed but must be changed frequently and perineal care should be done every 4 hours.

After repair of a urinary fistula, the patient will have a urinary catheter that must be kept patent. Encourage fluids to promote urine output and to maintain catheter patency. After repair of a rectovaginal fistula, a liquid, low-residue diet is ordered initially to delay the need for a bowel movement so that the surgical site can heal. After several days, stool softeners and laxatives may be ordered to promote bowel elimination. Enemas are contraindicated because they may disrupt the sutured area. Unfortunately, surgical correction is not always successful.

CANCER

A diagnosis of cancer of the female reproductive system can have profound psychologic effect. For example, cancer implies threats to personal survival, sexual relationships, family integrity, and a woman's concept of herself as a woman. You can play a potentially significant role in helping the patient to cope with decision making, treatment methods and their effects, the inevitable grieving process, and the reactions of family members and friends.

Breast Cancer

Breast cancer is the most prevalent form of cancer in American women; the current prediction is that 1 in every 8 or 9 women will develop breast cancer at some point in her life. It is the second leading cause of cancer deaths in women. Men can have breast cancer also, although it accounts for only 0.22% of all cancer deaths among men. It once was thought that survival rates were poorer for men but that is not true.

For early detection of breast cancer, the ACS recommends periodic mammography and clinical breast examinations. Regular monthly BSE is described as an option for women beginning in their 20s. Although it is estimated that 80% of breast lumps prove to be benign, those that are malignant must be identified and treated aggressively to prevent invasion of surrounding tissue, metastasis to distant structures, and death.

The three major types of breast cancer, according to the type of cells undergoing malignant changes, are (1) ductal, (2) lobular, and (3) nipple. Malignant growths usually are singular and unilateral (affecting only one breast) and they can be found in any part of the breast. However, nearly one half of all malignant breast tumors are located in the upper outer quadrant and nearly one fourth are located in the nipple-areolar complex. Most malignant lumps are painless and are palpated as firm, irregularly shaped, and fixed to underlying structures or skin. However, they sometimes resemble benign lumps: soft or semifirm, symmetric in shape with discrete borders, and freely movable. Therefore no lump should be ignored because it "feels" benign. Prompt evaluation is vital and may include tissue examination of cells obtained by needle aspiration or surgical biopsy.

Cause and Risk Factors. Caucasian, non-Latino women have the highest incidence of breast cancer. African-American women are most likely to die from it (see *Cultural Considerations* box).

Cultural Considerations

What Does Culture Have to Do with Breast Cancer?

Some genetic factors increase the risk of breast cancer. Other potential risk factors, including high-fat diet, obesity, and sedentary lifestyle, may be culturally based. No race or culture is free of breast cancer.

Although no cause has been identified for breast cancer, statistical evidence indicates the existence of several risk factors (Box 49-2). Women who have a mutation of the breast cancer (*BRCA*) genes have a 50% to 85% lifetime risk of developing breast cancer. However, these women account for only 5% to 10% of all breast cancers.

Family history is important. The risk rises if one or more first-degree family members (mother, sister, daughter) have had breast cancer and if that cancer was premenopausal and bilateral. Additional risk factors reported in some studies are radiation exposure, late menopause, obesity, excessive alcohol intake, hormone therapy (HT), sedentary lifestyle, nulliparity, high-fat diet, and oral contraceptives. The risk of developing breast cancer rises as the number of factors rise. However, it is important to remember that most women who are diagnosed with breast cancer have none of these known risk factors (see *Nutrition Considerations* box).

Box 49-2 Established Risk Factors for Breast Cancer

- Female gender
- Family history: mother, sister, or daughter diagnosed with breast cancer
- Age: 50 years or older
- Age at menarche: 11 years or younger
- Age at first childbirth: 30 years or older (or nulliparous)
- Personal medical history: atypical hyperplasia in the breast, breast cancer
- *BRCA1* or *BRCA2* gene mutation

Nutrition Considerations

1. Long-term dieting is associated with amenorrhea and reduced fertility.
2. Factors that may interfere with optimal nutrition for women of childbearing age include lack of resources, lack of nutrition knowledge, self-imposed dietary restrictions, and genetic idiosyncrasies.
3. High dietary fat intake (especially animal fat) has been associated with higher risk for developing breast cancer.

Prognosis. Relative survival rates are determined by comparing survival rates among cancer patients with overall survival rates in similar groups of people who do not have cancer. When cancer is confined to the breast, the 5-year relative survival rate is 96.8%. When cancer has spread to surrounding tissue, the 5-year survival rate is 75.9%; when the disease has metastasized, the 5-year survival rate is 20.6%. See *Cultural Considerations* box.

Cultural Considerations

What Does Culture Have to Do with Breast Cancer Survival?

Low-income African-American women more often have advanced disease when diagnosed and are more likely than Caucasian women to die from breast cancer. This population should be targeted for instruction in breast self-examination (BSE). Resources for evaluation and treatment that are available to these women must be identified.

Signs and Symptoms. Painless breast tissue thickening or lump is the initial sign, palpated during BSE or visualized on a mammogram. Most late symptoms—dimpling of the skin, nipple discharge, nipple or skin retraction, edema, dilated blood vessels, ulceration, and hemorrhage—are associated with the tumor's invasion of surrounding tissues. Dry, patchy nipple skin is suggestive of Paget disease, an uncommon cancer of the nipple and areola. Chest pain may be associated with metastasis to the lung.

Complications. Infiltration of adjacent breast and axillary tissue and metastasis to distant sites are the major complications of advanced breast cancer.

Medical Diagnosis. Routine screening methods for breast cancer follow specific guidelines.

- Clinical breast examination every 3 years until age 40 and every year after age 40.
- ACS recommends a baseline mammogram by age 40, followed by repeat mammograms every 1 to 2 years from ages 40 to 49 and every year beginning at age 50. (Some experts now advocate delaying the first mammogram until age 50 for most women.)
- Breast ultrasound, digital mammography, or magnetic resonance imaging (MRI) for questionable mammogram readings.

- Biopsy of suspicious tissue for histologic analysis: fine-needle aspiration, core-needle aspiration, incisional biopsy, or excisional biopsy.

Medical Treatment. If tissue examination confirms the malignancy, the patient and her physician consider surgical options based on the type, size, and extent of the cancerous growth. Women are playing increasingly active roles in the decision-making process and may "shop" for surgeons with whom they can agree on the selected surgical method. An oncologist may serve as a consultant in the decision-making process. Surgical options include lumpectomy, simple mastectomy, and radical mastectomy. Lumpectomy is removal of the tumor with a margin of surrounding healthy tissue but with preservation of most of the breast. A simple mastectomy is removal of the entire breast. Radical mastectomy is removal of all breast tissue, overlying skin, axillary lymph nodes, and underlying pectoral muscles. A variation of radical mastectomy adds removal of the internal mammary lymphatic chain. Three commonly used options are depicted in Figure 49-13. Lymphatic mapping and sentinel node biopsy uses dye or radioactive material to locate the lymph node that drains first from the site of the tumor. Study of this node enables the surgeon to determine whether and how far the cancer has spread. This procedure may avoid more extensive and unnecessary node dissection. For treatment of early-stage cancer, evidence indicates that lumpectomy plus radiotherapy offers the same long-term survival rate as more extensive surgery with radiotherapy. Additional treatment options depend on staging, which is outlined in Figure 49-14.

Breast cancer is staged according to the American Joint Committee on Cancer (AJCC) tumor-node-metastasis (TNM) classification explained in Chapter 25. The stages are summarized in Figure 49-14. Another critical factor is determined by a test of breast biopsy tissue called the hormone receptor assay. Knowing a patient's hormone receptor assay results provides valuable information for optimal treatment because as much as two thirds of breast cancers are hormone receptor positive. Cancer cells are estrogen receptor positive (ER+) or estrogen receptor negative (ER–). If cells are ER+, indicating that the tumor needs estrogen for growth, the drug *tamoxifen citrate* may be prescribed. Tamoxifen is a SERM. SERMs block circulating estrogen from reaching the receptor cells. The use of SERMs *tamoxifen* and *raloxifene* to prevent initial malignancy in selected women who are at high risk for the development of breast cancer is under study. Additionally, a cancer can be progesterone receptor positive (PR+) if it has progesterone receptors. Cancer cells that are PR+ receive signals from progesterone that can promote tumor growth. Armed with knowledge of hormone receptor assay results, the oncologist will tailor treatment accordingly.

The oncologist plays a critical role in continued management of care. Chemotherapy, hormone therapy, radiation therapy, biologic therapy, or a combination of these may be used before, during, or after surgery. Most physicians routinely follow lumpectomy with radiation therapy, even though evidence indicates that all malignant cells were removed. Radiation therapy is used because studies indicate that small metastases may exist without nodal involvement. See Chapter 25 for a discussion of treatment modalities.

Many women elect to have breast reconstruction after modified radical mastectomy or radical mastectomy. Reconstruction is performed by a plastic surgeon and may be initiated immediately after the mastectomy and before closure of the wound or may be delayed. Reconstruction usually begins with implantation of a tissue expander placed under the pectoralis muscle. Small amounts of normal saline are injected periodically into the expander until it creates a space the size of the prosthesis that will replace the expander in a future surgical procedure. Other reconstruction methods use transfer of tissue from other areas of the patient's own body, including the abdomen and back (Table 49-6). The last stage of breast reconstruction is creation of a natural-appearing nipple. The new nipple is constructed from tissue taken from the other breast or the upper, inner thigh. Permanent pigment may be used to create the appearance of the nipple and areola.

NURSING CARE of the Patient with Breast Cancer

Assessment

Nursing assessments are focused on physical manifestations of disease, physical and psychologic responses to treatments, review of all body systems, presence of pain, psychosocial factors, and level of knowledge. In the immediate postoperative period, the LVN/LPN may monitor the patient's vital signs, the wound dressings and drainage, and the arm on the affected side for edema.

Care of the surgical patient is discussed in Chapter 17 and care of the patient who has cancer is discussed in Chapter 25. Additional specific nursing diagnoses and goals for the mastectomy patient are listed in the following box.

Interventions

Disturbed Body Image

The breasts are an important part of a woman's self-image. To many women, loss of a breast represents loss of femininity. Even with immediate reconstruction, the breasts do not look completely normal. The patient may see herself as sexually unattractive and fear rejection by her sexual partner. These feelings are superimposed on the fear created by a diagnosis of cancer.

Be accepting of the patient, whose feelings may surface in a variety of ways, including anger, denial, and depression. From the early postoperative period, encourage the patient to attend to her appearance.

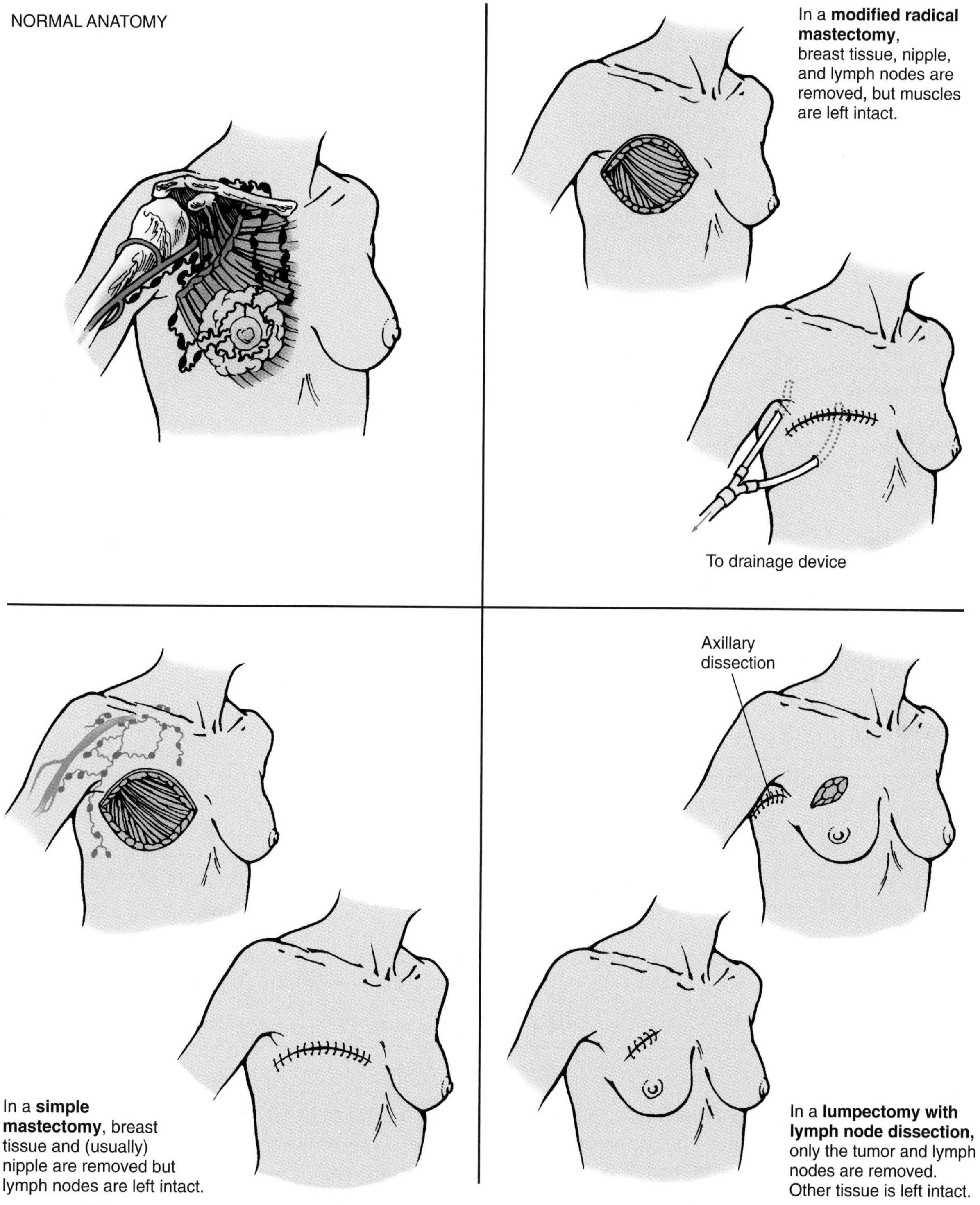
NORMAL ANATOMY
In a **modified radical mastectomy**, breast tissue, nipple, and lymph nodes are removed, but muscles are left intact.
To drainage device
Axillary dissection
In a **simple mastectomy**, breast tissue and (usually) nipple are removed but lymph nodes are left intact.
In a **lumpectomy with lymph node dissection,** only the tumor and lymph nodes are removed. Other tissue is left intact.

FIGURE 49-13 Options in the surgical management of breast cancer. (From Ignatavicius DD, Workman ML: *Medical-surgical nursing: patient-centered collaborative care*, ed 6, St. Louis, 2010, Saunders.)

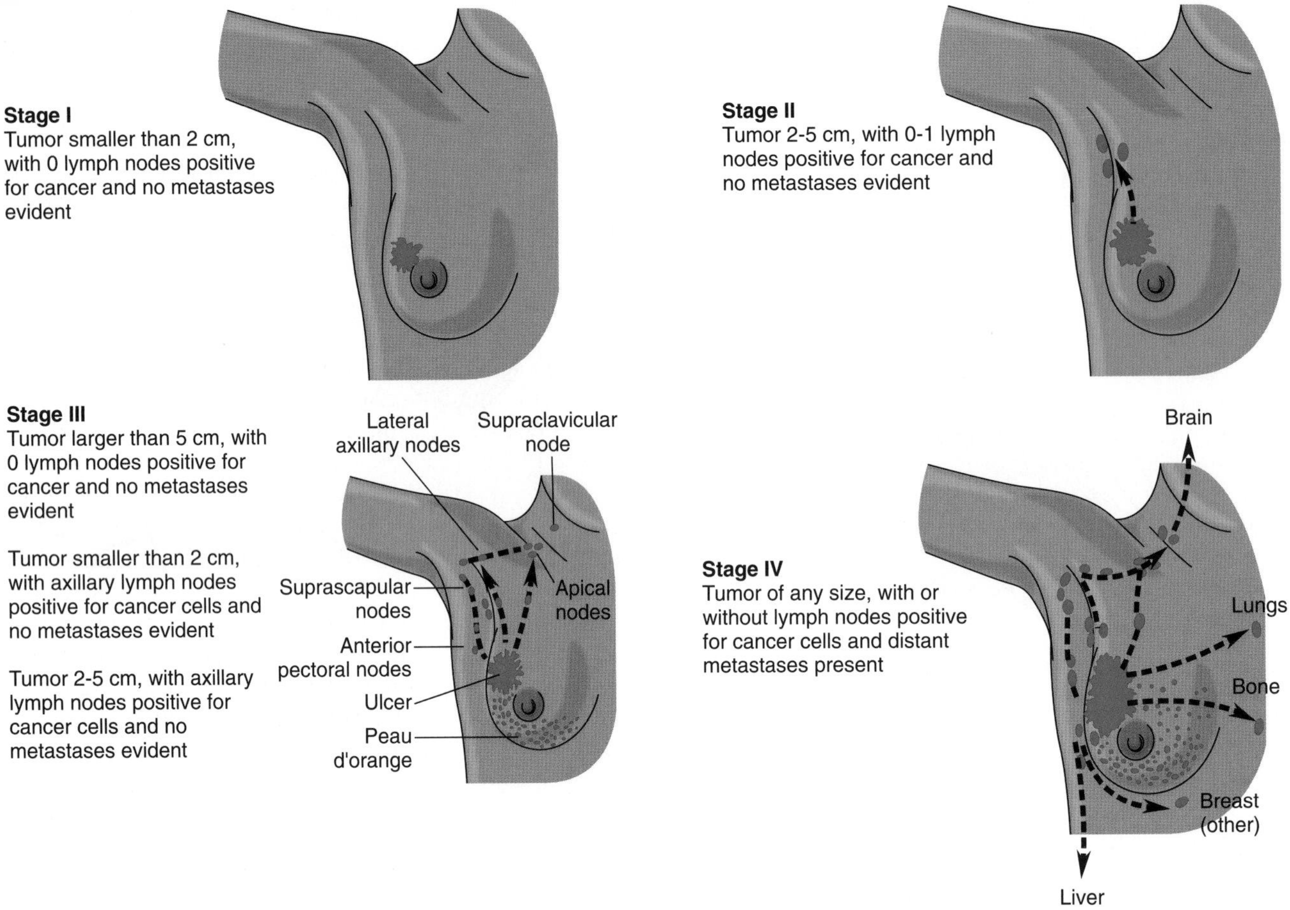

Stage I
Tumor smaller than 2 cm, with 0 lymph nodes positive for cancer and no metastases evident
Stage II
Tumor 2-5 cm, with 0-1 lymph nodes positive for cancer and no metastases evident
Stage III
Tumor larger than 5 cm, with 0 lymph nodes positive for cancer and no metastases evident
Tumor smaller than 2 cm, with axillary lymph nodes positive for cancer cells and no metastases evident
Tumor 2-5 cm, with axillary lymph nodes positive for cancer cells and no metastases evident
Lateral axillary nodes
Supraclavicular node
Suprascapular nodes
Apical nodes
Anterior pectoral nodes
Ulcer
Peau d'orange
Stage IV
Tumor of any size, with or without lymph nodes positive for cancer cells and distant metastases present
Brain
Lungs
Bone
Breast (other)
Liver

FIGURE 49-14 Stages of breast cancer. (From Ignatavicius DD, Workman ML, Mishler MA: *Medical-surgical nursing across the health care continuum*, ed 3, Philadelphia, 1999, Saunders.)

Table 49-6 Examples of Breast Reconstruction Procedures

PROCEDURE	DESCRIPTION
Implantation	An implant matching the size of the other breast is placed under the muscle of the operative side to create a breast mound.
Tissue expansion	A tissue expander is placed under the muscle and gradually expanded with saline to stretch the overlying skin and create a pocket. After several weeks the tissue expander is exchanged for an implant.
Myocutaneous flaps	A flap of skin, fat, and muscle is transferred from the donor site to the operative area. The flap contains an appropriate amount of fat to match the other breast and is similar in appearance to breast tissue. A blood supply is established by reanastomosis of vessels from the operative area to those with the flap when possible. A new nipple may be created with tissue from the other nipple, labia, or thigh. Nipples can also be created by tattooing.

Provide information about breast prostheses and clothing designed for women who have had mastectomies. If the patient has had chemotherapy, hair loss also may contribute to her body image disturbance. Strategies and resources for the cancer patient with a body image disturbance are discussed in Chapter 25 (see *Cultural Considerations* box).

Risk for Injury

A radical mastectomy includes the removal of lymph nodes in the axilla on the affected side. Because lymph nodes normally help to return tissue fluid to the bloodstream, their removal can result in lymphedema (i.e., the accumulation of fluid in the affected area). An important aspect of postoperative care after mastectomy is directed toward preventing and minimizing lymphedema in the arm on the affected side. Interventions to manage lymphedema include the following:

- Elevate the arm to a height above the level of the heart.
- Measure BP on the arm on the unaffected side, *never on the affected side.*

Nursing Diagnoses, Goals, and Outcome Criteria: Mastectomy, Postoperative

Nursing Diagnoses	Goals and Outcome Criteria
Disturbed Body Image related to altered appearance, loss of breast, perceived loss of attractiveness	Improved body image: patient demonstrates comfort with the new body image
Risk for Injury related to lymphedema secondary to excision of lymph nodes	Decreased risk for injury: absent or minimal lymphedema, arm circumference unchanged
Impaired Physical Mobility of affected arm related to axillary lymph node dissection	Normal mobility of affected arm: patient has full range of motion in affected arm within 6 weeks
Deficient Knowledge of self-care and resources	Patient understands self-care: patient demonstrates self-care and identifies resources

Cultural Considerations

What Does Culture Have to Do with Body Image after Mastectomy?

The importance of reproductive capacity as a measure of a woman's value depends on cultural values. In cultures that associate the breasts with sexuality, the loss of a breast can cause a woman to feel undesirable.

- Do not use the affected arm for venipuncture, injections, or parenteral fluid administration.
- Do not apply deodorant to or shave the axilla on the affected side.
- Frequently measure the circumference of the affected arm; immediately report an increase.
- Encourage frequent and progressive exercise of the arm on the affected side.
- Encourage the patient to use the arm for as many activities of daily living (ADL) as possible.

Position the patient alternately on her unaffected side and her back, observing regular postoperative care as described in Chapter 17.

Impaired Physical Mobility

Dissection of the lymph nodes in the axilla may or may not be done with a mastectomy. If the axilla is dissected, the patient is at risk for contractures unless proper positioning is maintained and exercises are begun as soon as the surgeon permits. Postoperatively, place the patient in semi-Fowler position with the affected arm elevated on a pillow. Encourage her to flex and extend her fingers. Offer analgesics 30 minutes ahead of time so that the exercises can be done more comfortably. The exercises should be done three to five times each day until full arm and shoulder range of motion is restored (Fig. 49-15).

Deficient Knowledge

With the patient's permission, arrangements can be made for visits from a representative of the ACS's Reach for Recovery program. The representatives are volunteers who have experienced breast cancer themselves and learned to cope successfully with the diagnosis, treatment, and related stressors. They assist patients by providing information, anticipatory guidance, and emotional support.

Patient teaching should have begun preoperatively but must be reinforced postoperatively. Content to cover includes signs and symptoms of infection, wound care, arm exercises, prevention of lymphedema, resources, and (if appropriate) management of the effects of chemotherapy or radiotherapy. With the patient's permission, include her significant other in the teaching process. This provides an opportunity for the partner to understand the patient's experience, demonstrate support, and participate in her recovery. With simple mastectomies, patients are sometimes discharged in less than 24 hours. This makes patient teaching especially challenging. Be sure to provide written information and resources along with verbal instructions.

Cervical Cancer

Cervical cancer generally grows slowly. For patients who have regular pelvic examinations and Pap tests, cervical cancer is usually diagnosed and treated in its early stage. Advanced cervical cancer may invade such surrounding structures as pelvic walls, bowel, and bladder.

Cause and Risk Factors. Research indicates that the risk for cervical cancer is increased in women who have been infected with the human papillomavirus (HPV) or human immunodeficiency virus (HIV). Additional factors associated with cervical cancer are cigarette smoking, initial sexual intercourse in early adolescence, a compromised immune system, and multiple sexual partners. New vaccines, Gardasil and Cervarix, are available to protect against HPV infection and therefore dramatically reduce cervical cancer. These vaccines are now available for both young men and women. It is hoped that by vaccinating all teens before they start their own families, the rates of cervical cancer will be reduced dramatically in the near future.

In the past, a drug called *diethylstilbestrol* was used to prevent spontaneous abortion. It has since become apparent that this therapy increased the risk of reproductive system cancers in offspring that were exposed to the drug. Diethylstilbestrol is no longer used for this purpose but you may encounter women who have had cancer related to the drugs given to their mothers

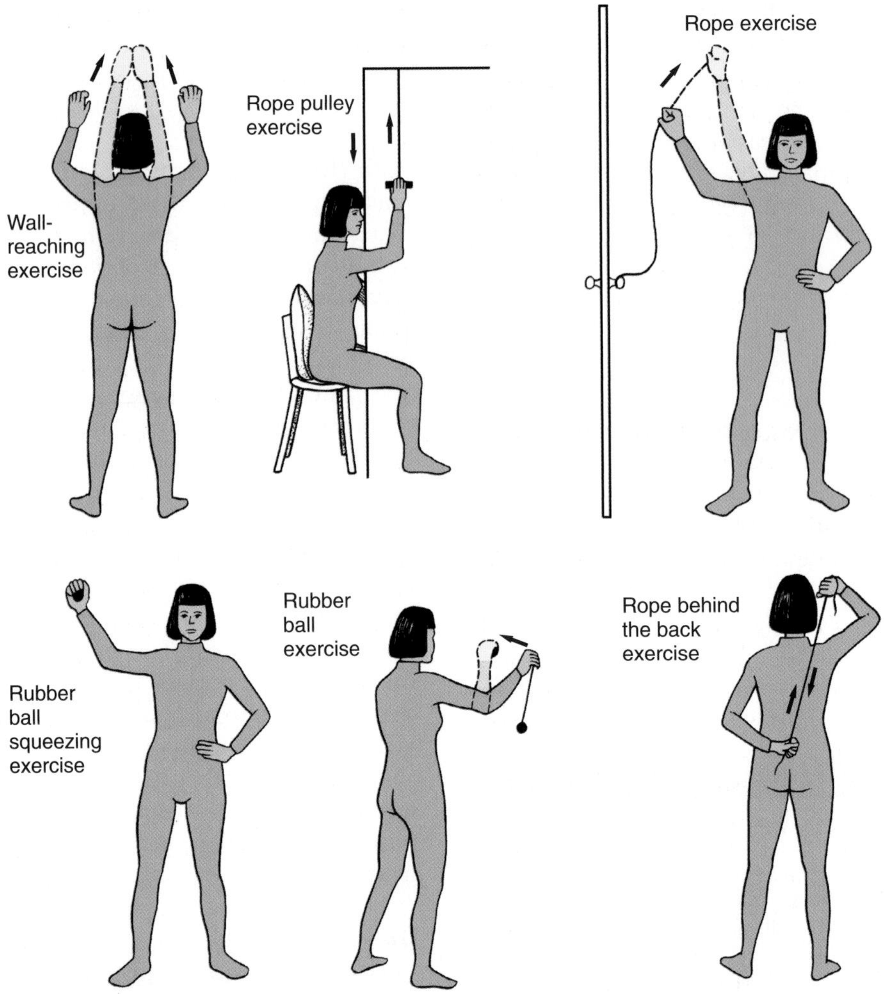

FIGURE 49-15 Arm exercises for mastectomy patients. (From Monahan FD, Drake DT, Neighbors M, editors: *Medical-surgical nursing: foundations for clinical practice*, ed 2, Philadelphia, 1998, Saunders.)

during pregnancy. No evidence indicates that family history or the patient's menstrual history increases the risk of cervical cancer. Although cervical cancer formerly was thought to be linked to sexual intercourse with uncircumcised males, current research does not support this speculation.

Signs and Symptoms. Early cervical cancer is asymptomatic. Advanced cancer also may be asymptomatic or may be associated with blood-tinged or frank bloody vaginal discharge, menstrual irregularities, or bleeding after intercourse.

Complications. Invasion of cervical cancer into adjacent structures causes site-related symptoms such as pain, backache, and bleeding. Anemia because of chronic bleeding may develop.

Medical Diagnosis. Cervical cancer often is first suspected when a positive Pap test result reveals atypical cells. Tissue specimens obtained by multiple punch biopsy, endocervical curettage, or conization are studied for microscopic evidence of malignancy. Cervical cancer is preceded by changes in cells called *dysplasia*.

Cervical cancer is staged according to the extent of invasion, with stage 0 signifying limitation to the cervical epithelium and stage IVb indicating metastasis to distant organs.

Medical Treatment. Treatment depends on the stage of the tumor and on various general health factors. Mild dysplasia may be treated with loop electrosurgical excision. This procedure, which can be done in an outpatient setting, uses electricity to destroy abnormal tissue. Localized carcinoma (in situ) may be treated with laser destruction, cryosurgery, or conization alone; total hysterectomy may be performed if childbearing is not desired.

Invasive cancer is treated with radiation, surgery, or both. Radiotherapy may be external or internal. If the therapy is internal, a sealed source is placed in the vagina for a specified period of time. Because effective treatment requires proper placement, the patient is immobilized as much as possible for the duration of the treatment. Radiotherapy and related nursing care are discussed in detail in Chapter 25.

If surgery is elected, the extent of the surgery depends on the extent of invasion. It ranges from radical hysterectomy (removal of the uterus, fallopian tubes, upper third of the vagina, and usually the ovaries) to total pelvic exenteration (removal of the uterus, ovaries, fallopian tubes, vagina, bladder, urethra, descending colon, rectum, anal canal, and pelvic lymph nodes). Nursing care of the patient with cervical cancer is discussed in the section titled "Nursing Care of the Patient with Cancer of the Cervix, Ovaries, Vulva, or Vagina."

Ovarian Cancer

Ovarian cancer occurs most often in women between the ages of 55 and 65. Although the incidence is relatively low compared with that of other cancers, the mortality rate from ovarian cancer is the highest of all female reproductive system cancers. The high mortality is because ovarian cancer is asymptomatic until it is advanced, so it usually grows for an extended period of time before it is diagnosed. In most cases, abnormal cell growth occurs in both ovaries.

Cause and Risk Factors. No specific causes have been found for ovarian cancer. However, risk factors include a family or personal history of ovarian cancer; a personal history of ovarian dysfunction or of breast, endometrial, or colorectal cancer; high-fat diet; nulliparity (i.e., has not produced a viable offspring); and early menarche and late menopause. Ovarian cancer rarely is found in women who have had children or who have used oral contraceptives. Therefore birth control pills or prophylactic bilateral oophorectomy (i.e., surgical removal of the ovaries) may be suggested for women at high risk for ovarian cancer.

Scientists are now researching how genetic mutations to our deoxyribonucleic acid (DNA) can increase the risk of ovarian and other cancers. They are looking at two possibilities. They believe that mutations can either turn off tumor suppressor cells or allow damaged cells to continue to multiply.

Signs and Symptoms. Ovarian cancer is asymptomatic in its early stage. Symptoms of even advanced ovarian cancer tend to be vague and nonspecific, usually attributed to various other conditions before ovarian cancer is considered. Abdominal pain and bloating, heavy feeling in the pelvis, unexplained and worsening back pain, GI tract symptoms such as flatulence, and urinary tract complaints may be reported. Abnormal uterine bleeding is not common. In extremely advanced cancer, ascites may be noted.

Complications. Ovarian cancer can spread to the peritoneum, omentum, and bowel surface via direct invasion, peritoneal fluid, and the lymphatic and venous systems.

Medical Diagnosis. Palpable tumors may be discovered on pelvic and rectal examinations. Abdominal and vaginal ultrasound with color Doppler imaging may be used as diagnostic tools. Blood may be drawn for a cancer antigen 125 (CA-125) serum marker test, which if elevated may indicate ovarian epithelial cancer. If evidence supports a diagnosis of ovarian cancer, an exploratory laparotomy or laparoscopy is done to visualize the tumor or tumors directly and to obtain tissue for definitive diagnosis and for staging and grading of the malignancy.

Some practitioners advocate routine screening of blood serum for CA-125 for early detection of ovarian cancer. However, elevated CA-125 levels can be caused by other factors in addition to ovarian cancer.

Medical Treatment. Treatment depends on the staging of the tumor or tumors. Options include surgery (usually total abdominal hysterectomy and bilateral salpingo-oophorectomy), systemic or intraperitoneal chemotherapy, intraperitoneal radioisotope instillation, and external radiation therapy. Even with advanced disease, treatment can improve comfort. Regardless of the stage and prognosis for survival, CA-125 levels may be monitored to assess tumor progression or regression. Nursing care of the patient with ovarian cancer is discussed in the section titled "Nursing Care of the Patient with Cancer of the Cervix, Ovaries, Vulva, or Vagina."

Vulvar Cancer

Cancer of the vulva is relatively rare but also one of the most visible of the cancers of the female reproductive system. It may appear as a visible and palpable lump on the vulva or as a deviation from the normally pink, moist mucosa. The lesion may be scaly; red, white, or irregularly pigmented; and edematous. Drainage from the lesion may be pink (serosanguineous) or bloody. The most common site is the labia majora.

Although it is rare, malignant melanoma may occur in the vulva. Its incidence is highest in postmenopausal women. The symptoms are similar to those of the more common vulvar cancers.

Cause and Risk Factors. The cause of vulvar cancer is unknown but it may be related to STIs, particularly HPV. Other risk factors are DM and hypertension.

Signs and Symptoms. The most commonly reported symptom is pruritus (itching). Pain and bleeding are additional symptoms.

Complications. Although cancer of the vulva generally remains localized, it may become invasive if not discovered and treated. It can invade adjacent structures or metastasize via the lymphatic system.

Medical Diagnosis. A preliminary diagnosis is made through palpation of a mass or by visualization of tissue that appears suspicious. Biopsy is necessary for definitive diagnosis.

Medical Treatment. Treatment depends on the extent to which the malignant cells have spread. For localized lesions, conservative removal of the malignant tissue by laser surgery or topical chemotherapy may be used. For wider, deeper, or invasive lesions, radical surgical removal through hemivulvectomy or vulvectomy and bilateral dissection of groin lymph nodes or through pelvic exenteration may be necessary. Radical hemivulvectomy is generally preferred because radical vulvectomy results in greater scarring and loss of function and is more prone to wound breakdown. Pelvic exenteration is the removal of all pelvic organs, including the bladder; the descending colon and anal canal may or may not be removed. Chemotherapy, radiation therapy, or both may follow surgery. Nursing care of the patient with vulvar cancer is discussed in the section titled "Nursing Care of the Patient with Cancer of the Cervix, Ovaries, Vulva, or Vagina."

Vaginal Cancer

The vagina is an extremely rare site for reproductive tract cancer. It seldom is the primary site for cancer; rather, it is the site for the extension of cancer that originates in the vulva, cervix, or endometrium. Except for young women whose vaginal cancers are associated with intrauterine exposure to diethylstilbestrol, vaginal cancer is found most commonly in postmenopausal women. Over one half of all new cases of vaginal cancer occur in women older than age 70.

Cause and Risk Factors. No definite cause has been identified for vaginal cancer. However, researchers have identified the following risk factors: STIs (syphilis, herpes virus type 2, HPV), younger age at initial sexual intercourse, greater number of lifetime sexual partners, smoking, HPV infection, a previous diagnosis of cervical or vulvar cancer, previous radiation therapy, and intrauterine exposure to diethylstilbestrol.

Signs and Symptoms. In its early and most easily treated form, vaginal cancer usually is asymptomatic. Later symptoms include a burning sensation, vaginal discharge that may have a foul odor, dyspareunia, spotting after intercourse, and vaginal bleeding. Pelvic pain usually is associated with invasion of adjacent structures.

Complications. Invasion of adjacent structures and metastasis are the most common complications of epithelial vaginal cancer. The prognosis is poor for vaginal malignant melanoma, with an extremely low 5-year survival rate.

Medical Diagnosis and Treatment. Most cases are detected during inspection of the vagina and from routine Pap tests. A definitive diagnosis is made via colposcopy and biopsy of suspicious areas followed by tissue studies. Treatment of vaginal cancer depends on the extent of invasion. In situ (localized) cancer may be treated relatively simply with local laser surgery or cryosurgery. More radical treatment is indicated if the cancer is more invasive. Possible treatments used either alone or in combination include topical chemotherapy, internal or external radiotherapy, partial or total vaginectomy, and pelvic exenteration.

NURSING CARE of the Patient with Cancer of the Cervix, Ovaries, Vulva, or Vagina

The patient with cancer of the cervix, ovaries, vulva, or vagina presents many challenges. She has a life-threatening condition whose treatment very often threatens not only her self-concept but also her sexual function. Treatments beyond local excision of affected tissue may result in disfigurement or in anatomic changes that hinder penile-vaginal intercourse, or both. The patient's psychosocial needs are as critical as her physical needs.

Assessment

Complete assessment of the patient with a disorder of the female reproductive system is summarized in Box 49-1. When the patient has or may have cancer, the health history documents signs and symptoms and possible risk factors. When reviewing the systems, describe changes or problems that may be related such as fatigue, pain, infection, and bowel or bladder dysfunction. Explore the effects of the symptoms on normal functioning. The patient may react to the diagnosis with anxiety, fear, depression, anger, or withdrawal. A complete physical examination should be done. The physician or nurse practitioner performs a pelvic examination that may reveal lesions, masses, and lymph node enlargement.

Interventions

Anxiety and Fear

The woman needs to be able to express her feelings about her diagnosis and prescribed treatment without being judged. Listen carefully to determine any knowledge deficits or misconceptions. Provide information or sources of information as appropriate. Many women of all ages are computer literate and therefore have access to endless sources. However, patients should be cautioned that not all information on the internet is accurate or appropriate for their situations. National organizations such as the ACS have excellent patient education materials. Community agencies may have a lending library of books and videotapes. Support groups are often helpful because patients learn from others who have had similar experiences. Many patients appreciate follow-up phone calls or the ability to call a resource person when needed.

Disturbed Body Image

The patient may be distressed if a change occurs in appearance or function caused by the cancer or the treatment. Loss of reproductive capacity can be especially painful for women who still wish to bear children. You can listen kindly when the patient wishes to express her thoughts. Patients who are severely disturbed should be offered the benefit of a mental health

Nursing Diagnoses, Goals, and Outcome Criteria: Cancer of the Cervix, Ovaries, Vulva, or Vagina

Nursing Diagnoses	Goals and Outcome Criteria
Anxiety and Fear related to threat to health and lack of knowledge about the cancer and prescribed treatment	Reduced anxiety and fear: patient's statement of reduced anxiety and fear, calm manner
Disturbed Body Image related to change in body appearance or function	Improved body image: positive patient statements about self and efforts to maintain or improve appearance
Ineffective Sexuality Pattern related to physical and emotional effects of cancer of the reproductive system	Satisfactory sexual patterns: patient's discussion of effects of disease or treatment on sexuality and coping strategies
Compromised Family Coping related to lack of knowledge, situational crisis, role changes, or patient preoccupation with self	Appropriate family and patient interactions: family demonstration of support and positive coping
Risk for Injury (to patient and others) related to effects of radiotherapy, chemotherapy	Decreased risk of injury from treatment: maintenance of applicator position and adherence of patient and others to radiation precautions

professional or spiritual counselor. Encourage measures to improve the appearance and praise the patient's positive efforts. Management of alopecia (i.e., hair loss) associated with cancer therapy is discussed in Chapter 25.

Ineffective Sexuality Pattern

The physician should present realistic expectations for future sexual functioning. The patient may be advised to abstain from sexual intercourse during the treatment and healing. Permanent effects of the disease and treatment may require alternative sexual practices. The patient may wish to discuss this topic with you. It is critical that you show an accepting attitude toward sexuality in general and toward any specific sexual practices acceptable to the patient and her partner. A psychiatric nurse practitioner or counselor may be consulted to help the patient adapt.

Compromised Family Coping

Include the family or identified support system in care. The family needs to understand the effects of the cancer and the treatments. They also need to understand the patient's need for support and for assistance during therapy and recovery. Encourage members of the household to consider ways to reduce demands on the patient. In addition, be sensitive to the needs of family members who may fear losing a loved one. Inclusion of the woman's sexual partner is particularly critical if altered sexual expression is expected after treatment.

Risk for Injury

Physical care of the patient varies with the prescribed treatment and is based on physician's orders, institutional policies and procedures, and nursing diagnoses. General guidelines for the care of the patient who is having radiotherapy are discussed in Chapter 25.

Internal radiation poses a nursing challenge. If a sealed radiation source is to be implanted in the vagina, an indwelling urinary catheter is inserted first. An applicator that will contain the radiation source is inserted into the vagina while the patient is in the operating room. The placement is checked on radiographs and is maintained by vaginal packing. The radiation source may be placed in the applicator before the applicator is inserted or after the patient is transferred to her room and positioned in bed. The radiation dosage is determined and ordered by a radiologist; the duration of implantation is based on the total dosage but generally ranges from 24 to 72 hours.

The patient poses a source of radiation exposure to anyone within a radius of several feet, so usual radiation precautions are in force. For each nurse who is allowed to care for the patient, exposure should not exceed a total of 30 minutes per 24 hours. Although not generally used for patient-related radiation exposure less than 30 minutes, the nurse may don a lead apron, which can reduce exposure slightly. Visitors are screened according to protocol; those cleared to visit should be instructed to remain outside a 6-foot radius of the patient and to limit the duration of visits according to policy.

Put on Your Thinking Cap!

A patient with pelvic cancer has had a surgical procedure that includes removal of the vagina. She tearfully says, "I will never be able to make love to my husband again." What are some things you could say or do to show acceptance of her feelings at this time?

The patient is assigned a private room for the duration of internal radiotherapy. Enforce strict bed rest to prevent dislodgment of the applicator. Movement is restricted to cautious turning from side to side. The facts that radiation therapy may precipitate nausea, vomiting, and diarrhea; that movement must be restricted; and that total time for nursing care is restricted make care particularly challenging. You need to be exceptionally well organized and able to anticipate and act efficiently. Administration of antiemetics, sedatives, and antidiarrheal medications may control radiation side effects and thus facilitate patient comfort, maintenance of applicator position, and efficiency of nursing care time.

Effects of radiation on local tissue produce a profuse, foul-smelling vaginal discharge that is largely absorbed by the packing and thus cannot be controlled with cleansing. A room deodorizer may be partially effective in making the odor tolerable. After removal of the packing and applicator at the conclusion of therapy, a cleansing vaginal douche may be ordered. The patient then is no longer a source of radiation and can resume her normal activities. Consider transfer of the patient to another room to remove her from a noxious environment and to allow housekeeping personnel to clean and air the room. External radiation therapy sometimes is used instead of internal treatment. See Chapter 25 for care of the patient having external radiation.

Care of the patient admitted for a pelvic exenteration is exceptionally complex and beyond the scope of this text. An expert nursing staff is essential to provide the emotional support and physical care demanded for this patient.

INFERTILITY

Infertility generally is defined as the inability to conceive within 1 year of regular unprotected sexual intercourse. Infertility is categorized as *primary infertility* if the woman has never conceived or if the man has never impregnated a woman. *Secondary infertility* refers to the woman who has conceived at least one time but is not able to conceive again. An estimated 10% of American females from 15 to 44 years of age (or 15% of couples) are infertile. Treatment enables approximately 60% of those couples to conceive and carry pregnancies to term.

In recent years the entertainment and news media have provided mechanisms for the frank discussion of components of infertility: causes, psychosocial effects, and treatments. Associated problems and treatments have been described by professional health care providers and scientists and personal accounts have been given by affected individuals. For many, the acceptance of infertility as a topic suitable for public discussion has removed the stigma of infertility as a source of shame and embarrassment; myths have been debunked and lay and professional people are becoming more knowledgeable about the subject. As a result, infertility has become a major subspecialty of gynecology and infertility researchers have developed highly sophisticated and effective diagnostic techniques and treatments.

Cause and Risk Factors

Causes of infertility may be related to the woman, the man, or both. Sometimes the cause cannot be determined. Conception depends on a number of factors, broadly categorized as follows:

1. Timing and techniques used for sexual intercourse:
   A. Impregnation of ovum by the sperm must occur within 24 hours after ovulation. Intercourse should be scheduled for every other day around ovulation time to optimize the potential for fertilization of the ovum.
   B. Semen should be deposited deeply in the vagina, in proximity to the cervical os.
2. Production and release of a healthy ovum by the woman and of numerous (approximately 20 million to 150 million per ejaculate) healthy sperm by the man.
3. Anatomically and physiologically correct female and male reproductive systems:
   A. The woman should have patent fallopian tubes with active fimbriated ends and uterine endometrium prepared for reception and implantation of a fertilized ovum.
   B. The man should have an epididymis temperature that maintains sperm viability during storage, patent seminiferous tubules, and a vas deferens with enervated musculature.
4. Biochemical compatibility between female vaginal-cervical-fallopian environment and male ejaculate.

Faulty timing or technique for sexual intercourse is easily corrected through patient education. Many other causes for infertility exist. As mentioned previously, untreated or inadequately treated STIs can impair fertility by altering anatomy, physiology, and patency of the reproductive tracts of either or both partners. Additional identified influences on conception include dysfunction of any part of the hypothalamic-pituitary-endocrine system, malnutrition or obesity, smoking, drug and alcohol use, exposure to toxic chemicals or radiation, nervous system disorders that affect reproductive structures that transfer ova and sperm, and male practices that maintain above-normal epididymal temperature (i.e., wearing tight underwear and pants, frequent and prolonged immersion in hot water or sauna). Causes of infertility are summarized in Box 49-3.

Medical Diagnosis

The diagnosis is based on data obtained from exhaustive psychosocial and physical health and sexual health histories of both partners. If the histories provide clues that may explain possible detriments to fertility, such as poor timing or techniques of sexual intercourse or habitual epididymal exposure to high temperatures, then further diagnostic attempts may be delayed until the couple has had time to remediate the potential problem or problems. If such simple factors are not identified, history taking is followed by systematic, comprehensive physical examinations and laboratory tests.

Box 49-3 Causes of Infertility

FEMALE GENDER
- Developmental: uterine abnormalities
- Endocrine: pituitary, thyroid, and adrenal dysfunctions; ovarian dysfunctions (inhibit maturation and release of ova)
- Diseases: pelvic inflammatory disease (PID), especially from gonococcus; fallopian tube obstructions; diseases of cervix and uterus that inhibit passage of active sperm
- Other: malnutrition, severe anemia, anxiety

MALE GENDER
- Developmental: undescended testes, other congenital anomalies (inhibit development of sperm)
- Endocrine: hormonal deficiencies (pituitary, thyroid, adrenal) (inhibit development of sperm)
- Diseases: testicular destruction from disease, orchitis from mumps, prostatitis
- Other: excessive smoking, fatigue, alcohol, excessive heat (hot baths), marijuana use

BOTH MALE AND FEMALE GENDERS
- Diseases: sexually transmitted diseases (STDs), cancer with obstructions (inhibit transport of ovum or sperm)
- Other: immunologic incompatibility (inhibit sperm penetration of ovum), marital problems
- Diethylstilbestrol exposure in utero (suggested but not proved as a cause of male infertility)

From Phipps WJ, Monahan FD, Sands JK, et al.: *Medical-surgical nursing: health and illness perspectives,* ed 7, St. Louis, 2003, Mosby.

The male partner usually is the initial focus of diagnostic procedures because tests for diagnosis of male-associated infertility problems are generally easier, less invasive, less expensive, and (unlike a complete female fertility workup) not cycle dependent. A semen specimen for analysis is collected by masturbation after a period of sexual abstinence (usually 2 to 3 days) that approximates the man's average frequency interval for intercourse. The specimen is then assessed for volume and for sperm count, morphology (shape), duration of viability, motility, and liquefaction. A second specimen is examined if variations from normal are found. He may be referred to a urologist or endocrinologist for further diagnosis and possible treatment.

Evaluation of the female partner includes a battery of tests. The woman may be instructed to maintain a record of her basal body temperature or monitor for daily symptoms, which are taken each morning on awakening. The basal body temperature rises when ovulation occurs, which suggests the timing of intercourse. She also may assess for cervical mucus changes that occur in response to ovulation. The woman will note the change from cervical mucus that is thick (pre- and postovulatory) to a slippery, stretchy, and thin quality that peaks during ovulation. She also may sense a cramping sensation in the lower abdomen as the ovum ruptures, referred to as *mittelschmerz.*

Another tool is the ovulation prediction kit that measures LH in the urine. Daily measurements detect a rise in LH, which usually is followed by ovulation in 28 to 36 hours. Other diagnostic data are obtained with cervical and vaginal stains, endometrial biopsy, and measurement of plasma progesterone.

Pharmacology Capsule

Ovulatory stimulants can cause ovarian hyperstimulation with possible rupture of the enlarged ovary.

If the diagnostic tests indicate normal hormonal functions, a postcoital test may be done. The couple has intercourse around the expected time of ovulation and 2 to 12 hours before the scheduled test. The physician or nurse practitioner aspirates a specimen of cervical and vaginal secretions from the cervix. The characteristics of the mucus are assessed by gross inspection and microscopic examination. The examiner also inspects the specimen for number and motility of sperm. If a previous test of the male's semen indicated normal motility and viability of sperm but the postcoital test indicates nonviable sperm, this suggests that the cervical mucus is not conducive to sperm survival, perhaps because of an antigen-antibody response to the semen.

Determination of fallopian tube patency usually is accomplished with hysterosalpingography. A radiopaque dye is injected through the cervix. Radiographs are then taken to visualize the uterus and tubes. Physical assessment of the peritoneal cavity, if required, uses laparoscopy or culdoscopy. Ultrasonography may be used for additional assessment.

Women are considered to be sterile and thus are not candidates for infertility diagnosis and treatment if they have congenital reproductive tract anomalies that cannot be corrected by surgery. Absence of one or more reproductive tract structures is also untreatable.

Medical Treatment

Treatment for infertility depends on specific diagnostic findings. A brief overview of specific problems and related treatments is presented in Table 49-7.

NURSING CARE of the Patient with an Infertility Disorder

Assessment

Assessment of the female reproductive system is summarized in Box 49-1. The LVN/LPN assists with data collection for the assessment.

Interventions

Fertility tests and treatments are generally done on an outpatient basis. The woman who undergoes the process usually has a prolonged relationship and frequent contacts with the nurse in the outpatient setting.

Table 49-7 Common Causes of Female Infertility and Related Medical Treatment

CAUSE	MEDICAL TREATMENT
Failure to ovulate, associated with the following: Delayed follicular maturation Hypogonadotropin secretion Hypothalamic-pituitary dysfunction Elevated prolactin level Hypothyroidism Ovarian tumors	Clomid (clomiphene citrate) Letrozole (aromatase inhibitor) Pergonal (menotropins) Gonadotropin-releasing hormone (GnRH) Parlodel (bromocriptine mesylate) Thyroid-stimulating hormone (TSH) Surgical excision
Inadequate endometrial development	Progesterone therapy
Endometriosis	Lupron therapy; surgery Gamete intrafallopian transfer
Reproductive tract infections	Antimicrobial therapy
Tubal construction	Hysterosalpingogram
Sperm-inhospitable cervical mucus	Therapeutic intrauterine insemination In vitro fertilization
Immunologic reaction to sperm	Use of condoms to reduce antibody titer, followed by unprotected intercourse at time of ovulation only In vitro fertilization

Nursing Diagnoses, Goals, and Outcome Criteria: Infertility

Nursing Diagnoses	Goals and Outcome Criteria
Situational Low Self-Esteem related to inability to conceive or feeling of failure	Improved self-esteem: positive expressions about self
Ineffective Sexuality Pattern related to structured efforts to conceive or loss of spontaneity	Acknowledgment of the effects of the situation on one's sexual relationship: patient identifies ways to maintain a satisfying sexual relationship
Ineffective Coping related to unmet expectations or feelings of loss	Effective coping: patient uses healthy coping strategies
Deficient Knowledge of diagnostic and treatment procedures	Patient understands diagnostic and treatment procedures: patient verbalizes diagnostic and treatment procedures

Situational Low Self-Esteem

Invasion of personal privacy is necessarily greater in fertility diagnosis and treatment than in any other condition. Gently explore the feelings of the patient and her partner about their difficulty conceiving. An open, empathetic attitude is vital if the patient is to be open. Support groups or professional counselors may help the couple to maintain self-esteem.

Ineffective Sexuality Pattern

The most intimate details of the patient's sexual relationship with her partner are elicited and diagnostic and treatment procedures repeatedly violate the desire for modesty. Lovemaking becomes scheduled rather than spontaneous.

Ineffective Coping

You may be the only person with whom the woman shares her psychologic reactions to the diagnosis of infertility and her subsequent emotional highs and lows throughout diagnosis and treatment. You therefore play a critical role in assisting the patient to cope with infertility. Give the patient the opportunity to discuss her thoughts and feelings about infertility and to explore coping strategies.

Deficient Knowledge

The needs of the patient's sexual partner must be considered as well and he should be included in patient teaching. Patient teaching includes information about diagnostic procedures, treatments, causes of infertility, and resources.

MENOPAUSE

Menopause is the cessation of menstruation that marks the end of a woman's reproductive capacity. Natural menopause is part of normal aging but surgical menopause results from removal of the ovaries. Natural menopause occurs gradually and may permit better adaptation than surgical menopause, which suddenly eliminates the source of natural estrogen. Diminished ovarian function associated with aging causes ovulation to cease and estrogen production to decline. The onset of menopause may begin as early as age 35 but more commonly occurs between ages 45 and 55 with the average age of menopause being 51. With natural menopause, the woman's first sign may be menstrual irregularity. Menstrual periods tend to be spaced farther apart and the amount of bleeding gradually diminishes. The entire process from earliest signs to complete cessation of menstruation usually is 2 years or less. A woman is said to be *menopausal* when she has not had a menstrual period for 1 year. Some women experience a surgical menopause brought on by the surgical removal of the ovaries. Unless estrogen replacement is begun promptly, the patient develops the signs and symptoms of menopause rapidly.

SIGNS AND SYMPTOMS

The signs and symptoms of menopause may include hot flashes, a warm feeling caused by vasodilation that affects the face, neck, and upper body. Hot flashes are typically accompanied by perspiration and sometimes by a feeling of faintness. Other common symptoms are vaginal dryness, insomnia, joint pain, headache, and nausea. Without estrogen, the uterus becomes smaller, the vagina shortens, and vaginal tissues become drier. Breast tissue may lose its firmness and pubic and axillary hair become sparse. Supporting pelvic structures relax, causing some women to have stress incontinence. Significant loss of bone mass may occur, leading to fragile bones, a condition called *osteoporosis.* Some women report emotional instability, irritability, and depression but the effect of menopause on a woman is very individualized. Some grieve for the loss of reproductive capacity and some feel a loss of femininity and sexual attractiveness. Others welcome the end of menstrual periods and no longer having to worry about the risk of pregnancy.

Complementary and Alternative Therapies

Black cohosh is sometimes used to treat menstrual cramps and as an alternative to estrogen for treatment of menopausal symptoms. Research studies have conflicting results about this botanical medicine's effectiveness in reducing hot flashes. The two most common side effects are headache and gastrointestinal (GI) upset. Patients are advised to limit its use to 6 months because of lack of information about long-term effects.

MEDICAL TREATMENT

Estrogen therapy decreases the risk of osteoporosis but, if taken for more than 5 years, *may* increase the risk of breast cancer. Therefore each woman's health history must be considered so that she and her physician can decide whether HT will be used. Estrogens are contraindicated with estrogen-dependent cancer, undiagnosed abnormal vaginal bleeding, and current or past thromboembolic disorders.

Many drug regimens exist. The patient who still has her uterus and ovaries has typically been treated with estrogens and progestins (compounds that have actions like progesterone). Because progestin decreases the risk of endometrial cancer related to estrogen therapy, it is not needed in women who no longer have a uterus. Findings from the Women's Health Initiative indicate that combination therapy in women with intact uteruses increases the risk of invasive breast cancer and coronary heart disease.

Oral drug therapy is most commonly used but transdermal forms of estrogen are also available. The transdermal drug is delivered by an adhesive bandage–like patch or spray. Estrogen creams, vaginal tablets, and suppositories may be used to relieve vaginal dryness. Drugs used to control "hot flashes" include clonidine patches, gabapentin, Bellergal-S, and several antidepressants such as venlafaxine and paroxetine (see *Complementary and Alternative Therapies* box).

Complementary and Alternative Therapies

Over-the-counter (OTC) options to sustain the patient's well-being in menopause include natural vitamin E with mixed tocopherols (400 to 800 IU PO [by mouth] daily), vitamin B complex (200 mg PO daily), and calcium (1500 mg with vitamin D per manufacturer's instructions).

NURSING CARE of the Menopausal Patient

Assessment

Assessment of the woman with a disorder of the reproductive system is summarized in Box 49-1. When a woman has menopausal symptoms, record them and explore how the patient is coping with this significant life change.

Nursing Diagnoses, Goals, and Outcome Criteria: Menopause

The primary nursing diagnosis for the menopausal patient is usually *ineffective self-health management* related to lack of understanding of the effects and treatment of menopause. The goals of nursing care are effective management of prescribed therapy and decreased signs and symptoms of menopause. The outcome criterion is the patient's report of reduced symptoms.

Interventions

Assess the patient's understanding of menopause and how she feels about it. The patient may need reassurance that her symptoms and responses are normal and common. If drug therapy is used, instruct the patient regarding self-medication. Caution patients on estrogen to report any signs of circulatory disorders (i.e., numbness, pain in calf, shortness of breath) to the physician immediately. Additional information about drug therapy is summarized in Table 49-2. The patient who cannot (or chooses not to) take hormone therapy needs additional assistance to cope with the symptoms of menopause. Women who wish to prevent "menopausal" pregnancy should use a reliable form of contraception for at least 1 year after cessation of menses.

Get Ready for the NCLEX® Examination!

Key Points

- The female reproductive system includes the external and internal genitalia and the breasts.
- Common therapeutic measures for the female reproductive system include douche, cauterization, heat application, and topical medications.
- Two common uterine bleeding disorders are metrorrhagia (bleeding or spotting between menstrual periods) and menorrhagia (menstrual periods characterized by profuse bleeding).
- The primary nursing diagnoses for the patient with a uterine bleeding disorder are deficient knowledge of condition and treatment and anxiety related to unknown cause of bleeding.
- The effects of reproductive tract infections may include infertility, changes in relationships, feelings of distrust toward sexual partners, shame, embarrassment, and diminished self-esteem.
- Because most infections are treated on an outpatient basis, the nurse's primary role is to educate the patient in preventing and treating infections.
- Benign growths of the female reproductive system include cysts of the breasts and ovaries and endometriosis.
- The two primary nursing diagnoses for the patient with endometriosis, a disorder marked by the growth of endometrial tissue outside the uterus, are acute pain and deficient knowledge.
- Cysts are saclike structures that contain fluid, semisolid, or solid material and are usually benign.
- Fibroid tumors are benign but may have to be removed because they can compress abdominal structures and lead to infertility, crowding, and malpositioning of the fetus during pregnancy as well as to degenerative changes related to interruption of blood supply.
- Herniation of the bladder or of the rectum into the vagina can disrupt urinary and bowel function and is often corrected surgically.
- Nursing diagnoses after surgery for correction of a cystocele or rectocele may include impaired urinary elimination, risk for injury, and acute pain.
- Uterine prolapse, the descent of the uterus into the vagina, may be treated with corrective surgery or vaginal hysterectomy.
- Breast cancer is the most common form of cancer in American women. It has a 5-year survival rate of more than 90% when detected early.
- After mastectomy, nursing diagnoses may include risk for injury, impaired physical mobility, risk for infection, disturbed body image, and ineffective sexuality pattern.
- Cervical cancer can be detected early by regular pelvic examinations and Papanicolaou (Pap) tests. Prompt treatment is usually curative.
- Ovarian cancer has the highest mortality rate of all female reproductive system cancers because it is asymptomatic in the early stages.
- Nursing diagnoses for the patient with cancer of the reproductive system may include anxiety, fear, disturbed body image, ineffective sexuality pattern, compromised family coping, and (if treated with radiotherapy) risk for injury.
- Infertility, the inability to produce viable offspring, can sometimes be treated medically or surgically.

Additional Learning Resources

SG Go to your Study Guide for additional learning activities to help you master this chapter content.

evolve Go to your Evolve website (http://evolve.elsevier.com/Linton/medsurg) for the following learning resources and much more:

- Interactive Prioritization Exercises
- Fluid & Electrolyte Tutorial
- Pharmacology Tutorial
- Review Questions for the NCLEX® Examination

Review Questions for the NCLEX® Examination

1. Fertilization occurs in which site?
   1. Uterus
   2. Ovary
   3. Fallopian tube
   4. Vagina

   NCLEX Client Need: Health Promotion and Maintenance
2. Which question collects data about the patient's menarche?
   1. "At what age did you begin menstruating?"
   2. "Would you describe your menstrual flow as light or heavy?"
   3. "What was your age when you first experienced hot flashes?"
   4. "Do you usually have any changes in mood before your menstrual period?"

   NCLEX Client Need: Health Promotion and Maintenance
3. Which of the following statements are appropriate to prepare a patient for culdoscopy? (Select all that apply.)
   1. "You will need to be in a knee-chest or lithotomy position."
   2. "You will have no restrictions after the procedure."
   3. "You will need to return in 1 week to have your sutures removed."
   4. "You may have shoulder pain caused by air entering the pelvic cavity."
   5. "You will be given general anesthesia for this procedure."

   NCLEX Client Need: Reduction of Risk Potential
4. You are teaching a class on BSE to women of various ages. Which of the following should you tell women who no longer menstruate about BSE? (Select all that apply.)
   1. "BSE is not a substitute for professional examinations."
   2. "Perform BSE on the same day of each month."
   3. "Older women should perform BSE every day."
   4. "Mammograms are needed only if you discover a lump."
   5. "Palpate the axilla as well as the breasts."

   NCLEX Client Need: Physiological Integrity: Reduction of Risk Potential

5. A young woman has come to the physician's office for a routine pelvic examination. During the health history, she tells you that her mother says douching is an essential part of feminine hygiene. What is your best response?
   1. "Your body has normal processes to cleanse the vagina, so douching is unnecessary."
   2. "Douching is not really necessary but it is a harmless procedure."
   3. "No medically appropriate reasons exist for douching."
   4. "Douching is safe if sterile solution is used."

   NCLEX Client Need: Health Promotion and Maintenance
6. Which organism is *not* commonly associated with PID?
   1. *Neisseria gonorrhoeae*
   2. *Chlamydia trachomatis*
   3. *Mycoplasma hominis*
   4. *Escherichia coli*

   NCLEX Client Need: Physiological Integrity: Physiological Adaptation
7. A patient completed a 6-month course of danazol (Danocrine) for treatment of endometriosis. She would like to become pregnant. Which of the following is it important for her to understand?
   1. She will begin menstrual bleeding within 1 week after stopping the danazol.
   2. Her best chances of pregnancy are in the first month after completing danazol therapy.
   3. She should not become pregnant for 1 month because danazol can cause birth defects.
   4. She is unlikely to become pregnant for at least 1 year after taking danazol.

   NCLEX Client Need: Physiological Integrity: Pharmacological Therapies
8. An older woman with uterine prolapse is being fitted with a pessary. What information should be included in the teaching plan?
   1. The pessary permanently corrects the uterine prolapse.
   2. Once the pessary is in place, no further care is needed.
   3. No complications are associated with pessaries.
   4. The position of the pessary must be checked in 24 hours.

   NCLEX Client Need: Physiological Integrity: Reduction of Risk Potential
9. Which palpable breast lump is most characteristic of breast cancer?
   1. A single painless lump in the upper, outer quadrant of one breast
   2. A firm, painful lump that feels oval shaped and is freely movable
   3. Bilateral multiple small lumps that are tender just before menstruation
   4. Soft, painless, symmetric lumps in the lower outer quadrant of both breasts

   NCLEX Client Need: Physiological Integrity: Physiological Adaptation
10. A 30-year-old woman who reports menarche at age 12, first sexual intercourse at age 14, and a history of treatment for HPV infection at age 15 is at increased risk for which of the following?
    1. Breast cancer
    2. Uterine prolapse
    3. Cervical cancer
    4. Fibroid tumors

    NCLEX Client Need: Physiological Integrity: Reduction of Risk Potential

chapter 50

Male Reproductive Disorders

http://evolve.elsevier.com/Linton/medsurg

Objectives

1. Describe the major structures and functions of the normal male reproductive system.
2. Identify data to be collected when assessing a male patient with a reproductive system disorder.
3. Explain commonly performed diagnostic tests and procedures and the nursing implications of each.
4. For selected disorders of the male reproductive system, explain the pathophysiology, signs and symptoms, complications, medical diagnosis, and medical treatment.
5. Identify common therapeutic measures used to treat disorders of the male reproductive system and the nursing implications of each.
6. Assist in developing a nursing care plan for a male patient with a reproductive system disorder.

Key Terms

Cryptorchidism
Epididymitis (ĕp-ĭ-dĭd-ĕ-MĪ-tĭs)
Erectile dysfunction (ĕ-RĔK-tīl dĭs-FŬNK-shŭn)
Hematocele (HĔM-ăh-tō-sēl)
Hydrocele (HĪ-drō-sēl)
Infertility (ĭn-fĕr-TĬL-ĭ-tē)
Paraphimosis (păr-ă-phī-MŌ-sĭs)
Phimosis (fī-MŌ-sĭs)
Prostatectomy (prŏs-tă-TĔK-tō-mē)
Prostatitis (prŏs-tă-TĪ-tĭs)
Sterile (STĔR-ĭl)

ANATOMY OF THE MALE REPRODUCTIVE SYSTEM

The male reproductive system consists of the scrotum, testes, epididymis, vas deferens, seminal vesicles, prostate gland, ejaculatory duct, internal urethra, and penis (Fig. 50-1).

SCROTUM

The scrotum is a thin, pendulous sac on the outside of the body that encloses each of the two testicles in separate compartments. Sperm production and survival require a temperature 3°C lower than core body temperature. Therefore the scrotum helps to regulate testicular temperature. The scrotum contracts into thick folds (i.e., rugae) during fear, anger, arousal, or cold, drawing the testes close to the body for protection and insulation. On warm days the scrotal muscles relax and allow the scrotum to hang free of the body. Sweat glands may be activated to cool the testes and maintain a testicular temperature that is below body temperature.

TESTES

The two testes (testicles) are the male reproductive organs. They lie within the scrotum, suspended from the spermatic cord (Fig. 50-2). They are composed of numerous highly coiled seminiferous tubules that produce spermatozoa and the male hormone testosterone. The testicles develop in the embryo at about the seventh week of gestation and begin producing small amounts of testosterone. Secretion of this male hormone results in the development of other male reproductive organs and causes the testes to descend into the scrotum during the last 2 months of gestation. At around 10 to 13 years of age, during puberty, the increased production of testosterone results in the production of sperm and the development of body hair, muscle mass, and other secondary sex characteristics.

EPIDIDYMIS

Newly developed sperm move from each testicle through the epididymis, a coiled tubule almost 20 feet long that rests along the top and side of the testes. This passage may take several days and allows the sperm to mature and develop the capability for motility (movement) and fertilization (see Fig. 50-2).

VAS DEFERENS

As mature sperm leave the epididymis, they enter the vasa deferentia (*sing.*, vas deferens), which are tubes

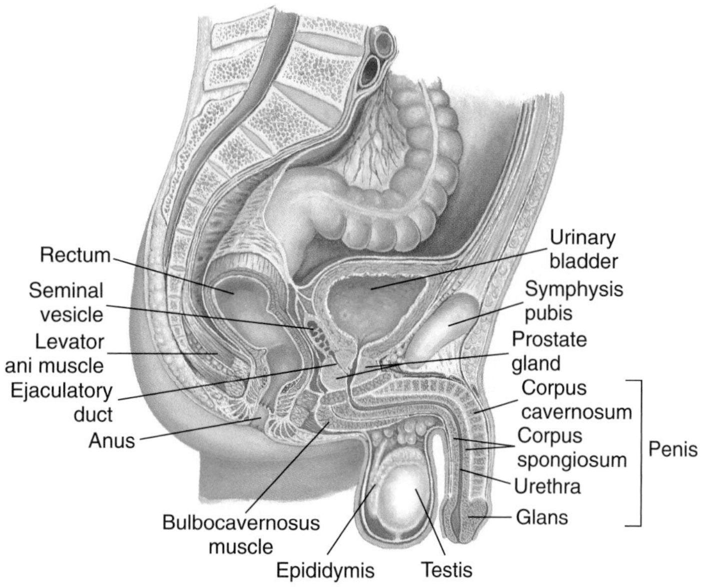

FIGURE 50-1 Male reproductive system. (From Seidel HM, Ball JW, Dains JE, et al.: *Mosby's guide to physical examination*, ed 7, St. Louis, 2010, Mosby.)

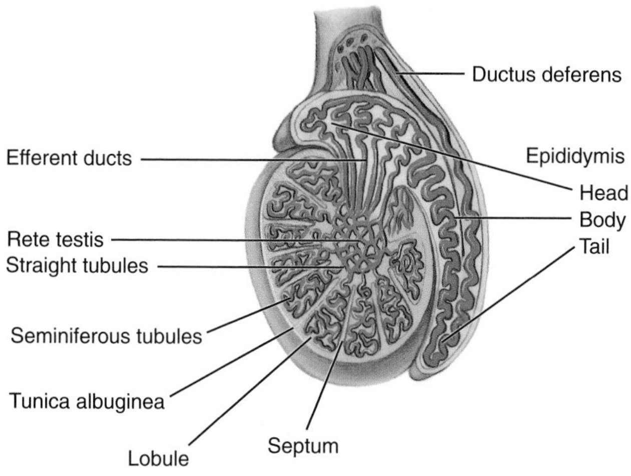

FIGURE 50-2 Basic structures of a testis. (From Applegate EJ: *The anatomy and physiology learning system*, ed 4, St. Louis, 2011, Saunders.)

of secretory ducts that serve as the primary storage sites for sperm, contribute to the fluid content of semen, and contract to help propel the mature sperm into the urethra during ejaculation. The vas deferens is bundled together with the spermatic artery and veins, lymphatic vessels, and nerves by the spermatic cord; the bundle exits the scrotum and enters the pelvic cavity via the inguinal canal (see Figs. 50-1 and 50-2).

SEMINAL VESICLES

The seminal vesicles are hollow, twisted, tubular secretory glands located on the posterior surface of the bladder. They produce a mucoid fluid that constitutes about 60% of the volume of the semen and provides nutrients and hormones important for motility and successful fertilization (see Fig. 50-1; Fig. 50-3).

PROSTATE GLAND

The prostate is a walnut-sized fibromuscular gland that surrounds the neck of the urinary bladder and the first inch of the internal urethra. The prostate produces a thin, milky, alkaline liquid that enhances the motility and fertility of the sperm and contracts to propel semen into the urethra during ejaculation (see Fig. 50-3).

COWPER GLANDS

Cowper glands (bulbourethral glands) are pea-sized structures, located just below the prostate, that secrete a clear mucus into the urethra. The secretion contributes little to semen volume but provides lubrication during sexual arousal.

URETHRA

The urethra extends from the bladder to the urinary meatus at the end of the penis. The vas deferens and the seminal vesicles come together to form the ejaculatory duct, which passes through the prostate and empties into the internal urethra. The sperm and fluids from the vasa deferentia, seminal vesicles, and prostate are propelled through the ejaculatory duct into the penile urethra during ejaculation. The urethra serves to empty urine from the bladder and provide outflow for semen during ejaculation. However, urine and semen are never in the urethra at the same time because the sphincter flap between the bladder and urethra closes during ejaculation.

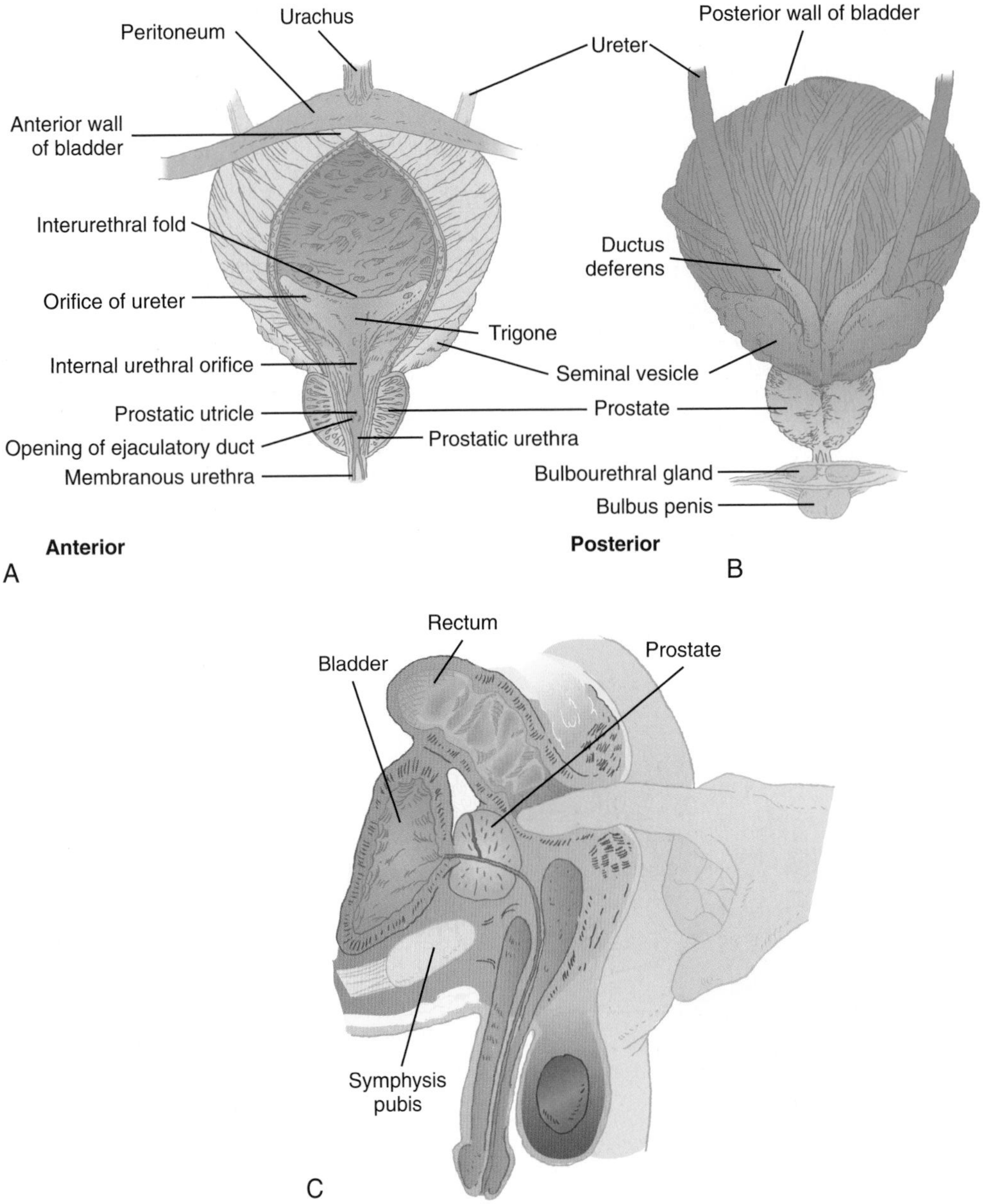

FIGURE 50-3 **A and B,** Anterior and posterior views of the prostate gland. **C,** Diagrammatic representation of the anatomic position of the prostate gland. It surrounds the urethra at the base of the bladder. (From Black JM, Hawks JH, Keene AM: *Medical-surgical nursing: clinical management for continuity of care*, ed 6, Philadelphia, 2001, Saunders.)

PENIS

The external penis in its flaccid state is a soft, round cylinder of spongy tissue ending in an acorn-shaped tip known as the *glans*. The glans has a sensitive ridge at its base called the *corona* that gives rise to a hood or foreskin. In uncircumcised men, the foreskin can be rolled back to expose the glans. About one half of the penis extends within the body toward the anus and attaches to the pelvis. Two corpora cavernosa lie on the upper side of the penis. These erectile chambers provide a huge surface area for the inflow of blood and blood storage, which results in expansion of the penis during sexual arousal, called an erection. The corpus spongiosum on the underside of the penis surrounds the urethra and supplies blood to the glans (Fig. 50-4).

PHYSIOLOGY OF THE MALE REPRODUCTIVE SYSTEM

SPERMATOGENESIS

Sperm are produced in the seminiferous tubules of the testes from about age 13 years throughout the remainder of life. Testosterone is believed to set in motion the division of germinal cells into spermatocytes, which subsequently develop into sperm. The process may take 75 days.

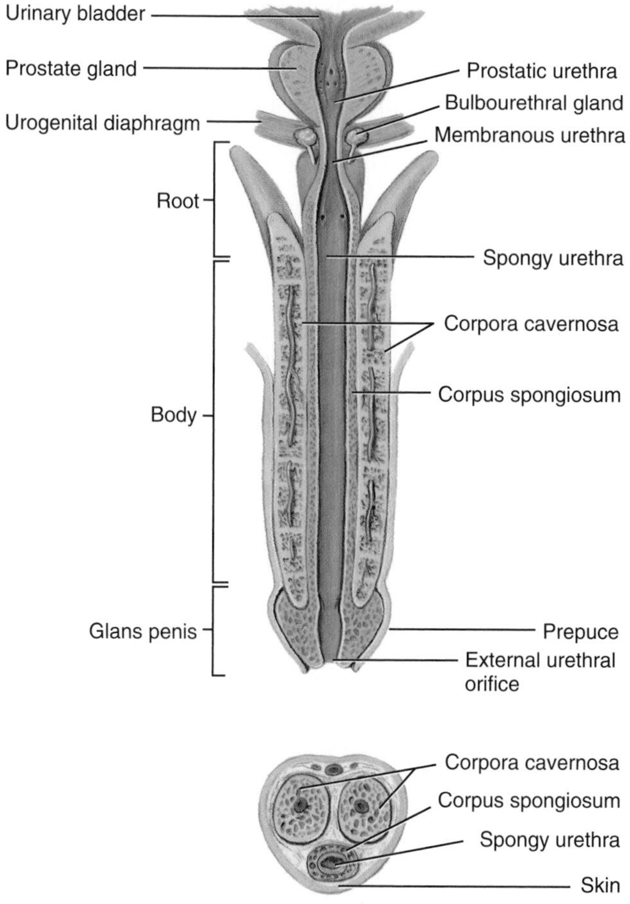

FIGURE 50-4 Cross-section of the penis. (From Applegate EJ: *The anatomy and physiology learning system*, ed 2, Philadelphia, 2000, Saunders.)

The cooling function of the scrotum is essential for spermatogenesis. An increase in testicular temperature may cause degeneration of some of the cells of the seminiferous tubules and may contribute to sterility.

Cryptorchidism, or failure of the testicles to descend from the abdomen into the cooler scrotum, may result in sterility. Incomplete or partial descent of the testicles may be resolved by surgical assistance before maturity but if fetal testes are abnormally formed and do not secrete enough testosterone to cause the testicles to descend into the scrotum, surgical intervention is unlikely to be successful. The tubular epithelium of testes that remains in the warm abdomen degenerates completely and is incapable of producing sperm.

ERECTION

For the penis to become erect, it must have a high-pressure supply of arterial blood, a means of relaxing the smooth muscle tissue of the cavernosal arterioles, and a functioning blood storage mechanism to keep the blood in the penis long enough for sexual function. The blood pressure (BP) in the flaccid corpus cavernosa is about 6 to 8 mm Hg—very low when compared with the 120/90 mm Hg BP in the arm or cavernosal artery.

During sexual arousal, parasympathetic nerves release neurotransmitters that cause the cavernosal arteriole walls to relax. This allows the relatively high-pressure arterial blood to flood the sinuses of the erectile chambers, increasing the blood volume of the penis to eight to ten times the flaccid volume and raising the cavernosal BP to approximately the same as arterial BP.

The blood storage mechanism for the penis is unique. The cavernosal artery is buried deep in the erectile chambers, causing them to fill from the inside. The venules that drain blood from the erectile chambers are near the surface and are compressed against the outer coat of the chambers during engorgement. The elastic limitations of this covering severely decrease the drainage of blood from the chamber sinuses and maintain the erection. After stimulation ceases or ejaculation occurs, sympathetic nerves release constricting neurotransmitters that narrow the arteriole walls and decrease the inflow of blood. As the cavernosal pressure decreases, drainage increases and the penis returns to a flaccid state.

EMISSION AND EJACULATION

The male sex act culminates in emission and ejaculation. Emission is the result of sympathetic stimulation leaving the spinal cord at L1 and L2. The pudendal nerve communicates with the spinal cord at S2 and S3 and affects motor responses for ejaculation. Physical stimulation of internal and external sex organs initiates contractions of the vasa deferentia and prostatic capsule. The contractions move sperm to the ejaculatory ducts and expel them into the internal urethra. There they mix with prostatic and seminal fluids and are propelled forward through the penile urethra. The filling of the urethra excites nerves in the sacral region of the spinal cord to initiate rhythmic muscular contractions of the internal genital organs, pelvis, and body trunk and results in ejaculation (expulsion) of semen.

Although psychic stimulation is not essential to the male sex act, it is an enhancing factor and should be considered in the physiology. Experience, culture, and self-development influence the effect of visual, fantasy, and dream stimulation on sexual sensation and nocturnal erections and emissions.

AGE-RELATED CHANGES IN THE MALE REPRODUCTIVE SYSTEM

Normal aging produces several changes in the male reproductive system. Testosterone production continues throughout life after puberty but decreases rapidly after the age of 50 (Fig. 50-5). This phenomenon has been called the *male climacteric* and may be associated with symptoms of hot flashes, feelings of suffocation, and psychic disorders similar to those of menopause. These symptoms may be relieved by the administration of testosterone and other androgens.

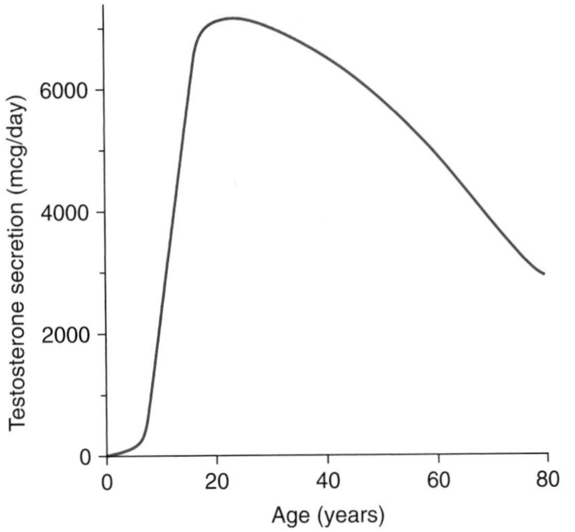

FIGURE 50-5 Testosterone secretion by age. (From Guyton AC, Hall JE: *Textbook of medical physiology*, ed 9, Philadelphia, 1996, Saunders.)

Many men believe that sexual function inevitably ends with aging. When changes in sexual response occur, they may lose interest or become depressed. Men in their late 40s and early 50s may be slower to arouse and have a longer refractory period between erections but in a healthy man spermatogenesis and the ability to have erections last a lifetime. Changes in lifestyle related to alcohol consumption, dietary habits, exercise, and the complexities of managing chronic conditions such as hypertension and diabetes and multiple medication therapies also contribute to loss of function and satisfactory sexual activities.

NURSING ASSESSMENT OF THE MALE REPRODUCTIVE SYSTEM

Assessment of the male reproductive system should include information on changes in the patient's health status, sexual function, and sexual relationships as well as the patient's knowledge level and ability for self-care. The extent of the nursing assessment of the male reproductive system depends on the nurse's education, experience, and role in the setting. This section describes a complete nursing assessment, although some aspects may be performed only by an examiner with advanced training. The licensed vocational nurse/licensed practical nurse (LVN/LPN) contributes data for the overall assessment.

The interview and physical assessment may be particularly difficult for some male patients because of health beliefs, the need for privacy, or defensiveness about behaviors. It is important to allow the patient to tell his own story and maintain as much control over the environment and experience as possible. Establishing a comfortable relationship with the patient is most successful if open-ended questions are used. The examiner should avoid questions beginning with "why?" and leave sensitive questions until later in the interview. Although it is helpful to empathize with the patient and gently press for important details, comments on how he *should* feel or behave are inappropriate. The assessor should not jump to conclusions too early or bias the patient's story by expressing a personal opinion.

HEALTH HISTORY

Present Illness

The health history begins with a detailed description of the current problem. Complaints may include pain, weight loss, infertility, **erectile dysfunction** (impotence), alteration in self-image, scrotal masses, penile discharge, or skin lesions. If the symptoms are acute, include detailed information about the onset and development of the problem and about activities related to the symptoms. If the patient has pain, tools such as pain scales provide objective data.

Past Medical History

The past medical history helps to link the current problem with previous symptoms, injuries, diseases, operations, or allergies and the treatments or medications prescribed for them. Question the patient about his management of chronic health problems such as diabetes, thyroid or pituitary dysfunction, cardiovascular disease, neurologic injury or disease, and addictive behavior. Because trauma to the groin or perineum may be related to disorders of the urethra or penile circulation (or both), document childhood injuries or accidents. Spinal cord injuries are significant because the level of the injury is associated with specific types of sexual dysfunctions.

Patients who are reluctant to discuss what many consider to be the most private part of their lives also may be unwilling to do regular self-examinations or follow recommended self-care regimens. Thoughtfully planned questioning provides clues about knowledge deficits and patient participation in health management. This information is important in developing plans for care that include the patient and his significant other and require their cooperation.

Family History

In the family history, note the age and health or age at death of parents, grandparents, and siblings. In addition, record any family history of cancer, diabetes, hypertension, stroke, and blood disorders such as sickle cell anemia and hemophilia.

Review of Systems

Review of all systems with a focus on male reproductive system disorders begins with an assessment of the patient's general health. Questions focus on changes in appetite, weight, exercise or activity level, and the management of daily self-care. These data may reveal general changes in health status that may affect the reproductive system.

Describe changes in the skin, including lesions, drainage, bleeding, itching, or pain. If the patient has itching or pain, note whether it is intermittent or continuous and whether it has any relationship to specific activities or time. Encourage the patient to use descriptive terms, such as *stinging* or *aching*. When assessing pain, having the patient describe the intensity on a scale from 1 to 10 is helpful.

A review of the circulatory and pulmonary systems provides data about hypertension, cardiac or pulmonary disease, and exercise tolerance.

Symptoms of possible endocrine dysfunction are important because undiagnosed or poorly managed endocrine disorders may have a direct and devastating effect on sexual function, sterility, and self-image for the male patient. Questions about fatigue, nervousness, heat or cold intolerance, polyphagia, polydipsia, polyuria, and medications taken for pituitary or thyroid conditions may yield important clues.

Review of the musculoskeletal and nervous systems should include questions about weakness, paralysis, coordination problems, joint pain or stiffness, mood changes, and depression.

The health history should note medications the patient is taking because many drugs, including a number of antihypertensive agents, can impair sexual function.

Functional Assessment

The functional assessment elicits information about diet, usual activities, sleep and rest, medications, and the use of tobacco, alcohol, and illicit drugs. Record sources of stress and coping strategies. Once you establish a therapeutic relationship with the patient, you also should cover the interest level and satisfaction of sexual relationships. Questions may include the frequency of intercourse, the ability to have and maintain an erection, the desire and ability to have children, and the relationship of sexual function to self-image.

PHYSICAL EXAMINATION

The physical examination of the male reproductive system is usually done by the physician or nurse practitioner. Gloves are always worn to examine the genitals. The LVN/LPN may prepare the patient for the examination, collect some data, and see that specimens are processed properly. Instruct the patient to empty the bladder before the examination and to collect a urine specimen if needed. The patient should be properly draped for privacy.

Record the patient's height, weight, and vital signs and note his general appearance. Inspect the skin for lesions or discolorations and the breasts for gynecomastia (enlargement). For the examination of the genitals, the patient may be standing or supine with the legs slightly spread. The skin of the external organs and perineum should be warm, dry, and free of lesions, edema, and odor. The pubic hair is normally distributed in a diamond-shaped area across the symphysis pubis, covering the base of the penis and spreading along the inner thighs. The lower abdomen and groin are palpated for masses.

Penis

The normal flaccid penis is semisoft and straight. The size, shape, and appearance are noted. The examiner palpates for nodules, swelling, and lesions. If the patient is uncircumcised, the foreskin is retracted to inspect the glans (Fig. 50-6). A small amount of white, thick, odoriferous smegma (sebaceous secretion) may be seen between the glans and the foreskin. The urethral meatus should be at the tip of the penis. If any discharge from lesions or the urethra is seen, a specimen may be collected for culture.

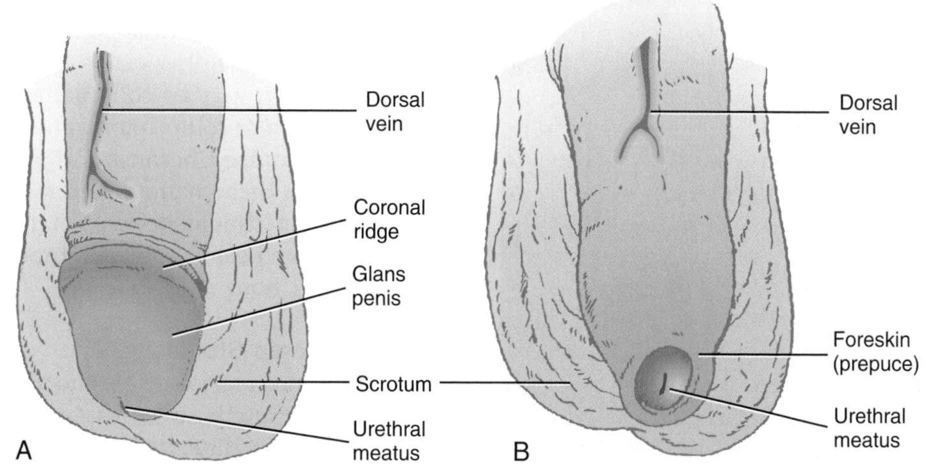

FIGURE 50-6 Appearance of the penis. **A,** Circumcised. **B,** Uncircumcised. (From Black JM, Hawks JH, Keene AM: *Medical-surgical nursing: clinical management for continuity of care*, ed 6, Philadelphia, 2001, Saunders.)

Scrotum

The skin of the scrotum should be slightly darker in color, wrinkled, and loose. Because the scrotum is close to the body and may not be well ventilated, it is susceptible to irritation from heat and moisture, fungal infections, abscesses, and parasites.

Each side of the scrotum should be palpated for the right and left testes, epididymis, and vasa deferentia. It is normal for the testes to retract temporarily when the scrotum is touched or cooled; they will reappear with relaxation or rewarming. The left testicle hangs lower than the right. Both should be oval in shape, smooth, firm, and without masses or tenderness. Older patients may have smaller, softer testes. It is important, especially in the young patient, to note that two testes exist.

The examiner proceeds to palpate the epididymis and the vas deferens. If scrotal thickening, nodules, masses, or asymmetric conditions are discovered, they can be further investigated by shining a light through the scrotum in a darkened room, a technique called *transillumination* (Fig. 50-7). **Hydrocele**, a mass filled with serous fluid, glows red in the light. If the mass is solid (e.g., a **hematocele** or tumor), no light passes through it, making it appear as a dark shadow.

The examiner inspects for hernias, which are protruding segments of the bowel through the abdominal wall. The most common sites for hernia are the lower abdomen, groin, and upper scrotal area. The examination is done first with the patient standing quietly and again when straining as if to have a bowel movement. The practitioner with advanced training is able to palpate inguinal hernias by reaching up through the scrotum into the inguinal canal. Abnormal findings should be noted and referred to a physician.

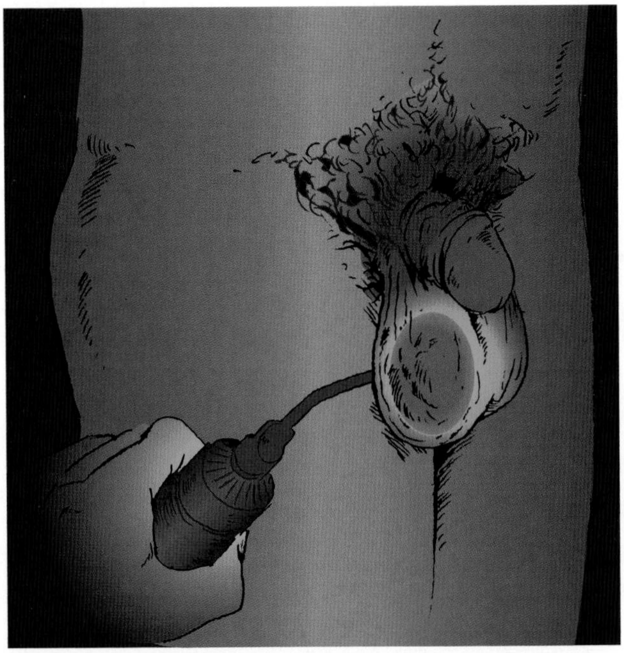

FIGURE 50-7 Transillumination of the scrotum. (From Black JM, Hawks JH: *Medical-surgical nursing: clinical management for positive outcomes*, ed 8, St. Louis, 2009, Saunders.)

The advanced practitioner or physician also examines the prostate gland by inserting the examining finger through the anus toward the anterior wall of the rectum. Variations in the firmness and size of the prostate may be associated with benign hyperplasia, chronic prostatitis, or malignancy.

The skin of the perineum is darker than the skin on the buttocks and should be intact. The anal area has more coarse skin and is moist and without hair. Inspect the area for lesions, irritation, inflammation, fissures, abscesses, and dilated veins (hemorrhoids). With the patient bearing down, the examiner again inspects the anus for rectal prolapse or internal hemorrhoids. The advanced practitioner or physician examines the anal canal with an index finger to assess for resistance, bleeding, sphincter tone, nodules, or polyps. A stool specimen may be tested for occult blood when appropriate.

The assessment of the male reproductive system is summarized in Box 50-1.

DIAGNOSTIC TESTS AND PROCEDURES

Diagnostic tests and procedures for disorders of the male reproductive system include laboratory studies and radiologic imaging procedures.

LABORATORY STUDIES

Semen Analysis

Analysis of the semen may be done to assess male fertility or to document sterilization after a vasectomy. The analysis may include gross evaluation of semen for volume, thickness, color, and pH and microscopic evaluation of the sperm for count, motility, shape, and ability to penetrate cervical mucus. The patient is instructed to abstain from sexual activity for 2 to 3 days and then collect a semen specimen in a clean container. Discourage patients from prolonged abstinence because it may result in diminished quality and motility of the sperm. If the patient is unable to collect the specimen in the physician's office or laboratory by masturbating, it may be collected at home by using a plastic condom or coitus interruptus. Rubber condoms should not be used because the powders and lubricants used in their manufacture may be spermicidal. The specimen should be kept at room temperature, protected from heat or cold, and brought to the laboratory within 1 hour after collection.

Endocrinologic Studies

The endocrine system secretes hormones that regulate metabolism, growth, stress response, and reproduction (gonadotropins) directly into the blood. The serum levels of these hormones can be determined from blood drawn from the patient without special preparation.

Box 50-1 Assessment of the Male Reproductive System

HEALTH HISTORY
Present Illness
Pain, weight loss, infertility, erectile dysfunction (ED), scrotal mass, penile discharge, lesions
Past Medical History
Previous injuries, diseases, or surgeries
Chronic Illnesses
Diabetes mellitus (DM), cardiovascular disease, addictive behavior
Allergies
Current Medications
Family History
Diabetes, hypertension, stroke, blood disorders, cancer
Review of Systems
General Health State
Changes in appetite, weight, activity, self-care
Skin
Lesions, drainage, bleeding, itching, pain
Cardiovascular
Edema
Respiratory
Cough, dyspnea
Endocrine
Fatigue, heat or cold intolerance, nervousness
Nervous
Paralysis
Genitourinary
Changes in urination or urine characteristics
Sexual Function
Interest in sexual relationship, frequency of intercourse, ED, desire to have children, effect of sexual function on self-image
Functional Assessment
Usual Day
Occupation, home roles and responsibilities, diet, rest
Use of Tobacco and Alcohol
Stressors and Coping Strategies
Sexual Relationships

PHYSICAL EXAMINATION
Vital Signs
General Appearance of Genitalia
Skin lesions or discoloration, hair distribution
Penis
Size, shape, skin lesions, discharge, position of urinary meatus, nodules, swelling
Scrotum
Color, edema, irritation, presence of testicles, testicular tenderness or masses
Inguinal Hernia
Prostate
Size, texture, masses
Perineum
Color, lesions
Anus
Lesions, irritation, inflammation, fissures, abscesses, hemorrhoids, rectal prolapse

Testosterone is secreted by Leydig cells in the interstitium of the testes. Below-normal levels of testosterone may be the result of hypothalamic or pituitary dysfunction or seminiferous tubule destruction. Among the causes of increased levels of testosterone in the adult male are testicular tumor, adrenal tumor, adrenal dysfunction, and some drugs (anticonvulsants and barbiturates). Lower serum levels of testosterone may be related to gonad hypofunction, orchidectomy, hepatic cirrhosis, and some drugs (androgens, alcohol, phenothiazines, spironolactone, and corticosteroids). Testosterone levels fall with age, beginning around the age of 30.

Follicle-stimulating hormone (FSH) is secreted by the anterior pituitary gland and causes stimulation of Sertoli cells in the testes to complete the formation and maturation of sperm. The negative-feedback system prevents oversecretion of FSH and maintains a constant level of sperm production. Below-normal levels of sperm result in increased secretion of FSH from the pituitary gland and high serum levels of FSH. Spermatogenesis results in decreased excretion of FSH and normal serum levels.

Luteinizing hormone (LH) is secreted by the anterior pituitary gland and causes stimulation of special cells (i.e., Leydig cells) in the testes to produce testosterone. As testosterone is produced, a negative-feedback system reduces the amount of LH secreted by the pituitary. Low levels of testosterone result in high levels of serum LH. This indicates an effort by the pituitary to stimulate Leydig cell function and return testosterone levels to normal.

Prolactin, another hormone secreted by the anterior pituitary gland, is closely related to LH. It has a potentiating effect on testosterone production. In some patients, when endocrine function is in question, serum prolactin levels may be tested. Secretion of prolactin is controlled by a negative-feedback system. Above-normal levels of prolactin may be caused by a benign pituitary tumor and may result in gynecomastia in the male patient.

Tumor Markers

Tumor markers are substances found in the serum of cancer patients. When used in conjunction with other diagnostic tools, they can be helpful in diagnosing cancer, estimating the degree of cancer development, predicting the effect of treatment, and monitoring the effect of treatment on the cancer or the return of cancer after treatment. Prostate-specific antigen (PSA) is used as a screening tool to detect prostate cancer; however, it can be elevated by many factors other than cancer. Some experts recommend that two PSA confirmatory results should be done before any action is taken. Current recommendations for periodic PSA screening are covered later in this chapter. No special preparation is needed for these tests.

General Laboratory Studies

Urinalysis provides information about infection of the genitourinary tract as well as measures of kidney function. Clean-catch samples usually can be used unless the patient is unable to collect the urine without contamination. If appropriate instruction is given for collection, no other patient preparation is needed. If the patient is unable to clean himself properly, cannot see well enough, or is not able to understand the instructions, it may be necessary to obtain a specimen by catheterization.

Blood studies may include a complete blood count (CBC) to establish baseline data and provide information in forming a diagnosis when anemia or bone metastases are suspected. Alkaline phosphatase and serum calcium levels also may be measured because they increase with metastasis to bone (Table 50-1). Thyroid function studies and tests for diabetes mellitus (DM) may be done in patients with erectile dysfunction. No special preparation for these tests is usually necessary. The venipuncture site should be observed for bleeding and dressed with a small pressure bandage on completion of sample collection.

RADIOLOGIC IMAGING STUDIES

Computed tomography (CT) may be used in assessing metastatic testicular and prostatic tumors. Ultrasound may be used to examine scrotal masses or define prostatic lesions. Examination of the prostate is done via the rectum. Magnetic resonance imaging (MRI) is used to stage prostate cancer.

Radionuclide imaging may be done to assess testicular abnormalities such as torsion, tumors, abscesses, epididymitis, or hydroceles. Radioactive substances are injected intravenously or given orally. After a waiting period to allow for distribution of the substance throughout the body, scans are done to locate organs and tissues that have increased concentrations of the isotopes because of abnormal tissue metabolism. Diagnostic tests and procedures and related nursing care are summarized in Table 50-2.

Ultrasound

Transrectal ultrasound is the most accurate method for obtaining anatomic details of the prostate. A biopsy specimen may be obtained, guided by the transrectal ultrasound image.

DISORDERS OF THE MALE REPRODUCTIVE SYSTEM

INFECTIONS AND INFLAMMATORY CONDITIONS

Infections of the male reproductive system may be caused by bacteria, viruses, protozoa, fungi, and ectoparasites that can be acquired through sexual contact. Sexually transmitted infections (STIs) are discussed in

Table 50-1 Laboratory Tests for Male Reproductive Disorders

TEST	REFERENCE VALUES	CONDITION IN WHICH LEVELS ARE ALTERED
Hematologic Tests (CBC)		
Hemoglobin (Hgb)	14–18 g/dL	↓ In anemia; nonspecific; may indicate malignancy
Hematocrit (Hct)	40%–50%	↓ In anemia; nonspecific; may indicate malignancy
Leukocytes (WBCs)	4800–11,000/mm^3	↓ In metastatic bone disease
Neutrophils	54%–62%	↓ In bone marrow depression
Lymphocytes	25%–30%	↓ In bone marrow depression
Eosinophils	1%–3%	↓ In bone marrow depression
Platelets	150,000–300,000/mm^3	↓ In bone marrow depression
Blood/Serum Tests		
Acid phosphatase	0.11–0.60 mU/mL	↑ In metastatic prostate cancer
Alkaline phosphatase	20–90 mU/mL	↑ In cancer of bone or bone metastases, liver cancer
Calcium	9.0–11.0 mg/dL	↑ In bone metastasis
Tests for Tumor Markers		
AFP	<10 ng/mL	↑ In nonseminomatous testicular cancer
CEA	0–2.5 ng/mL nonsmokers	↑ In prostate cancer
HCG	0.5 IU/L	↑ In germ cell testicular cancer
Prostatic acid phosphatase	0.26–0.83 U/L	↑ In metastatic prostate cancer
PSA	0–4 ng/mL	↑ In prostate cancer

AFP, Alpha-fetoprotein; *CBC,* complete blood count; *CEA,* carcinoembryonic antigen; *HCG,* human chorionic gonadotropin; *PSA,* prostate-specific antigen; *WBC,* white blood cell.

Table 50-2 Diagnostic Tests and Procedures **Male Reproductive System**

TEST AND PURPOSE	PATIENT PREPARATION	POSTPROCEDURE NURSING CARE
Mumps Test: ELISA		
Determines whether a person is susceptible or resistant to the mumps virus. Not commonly used because mumps vaccine can be safely given to patients without knowing their immune status.	Inform the patient that a blood sample will be drawn.	Assess the venipuncture site for bleeding. Apply a small dressing.
Urethral Smears and Stains		
Prepares a small amount of material for microscopic study to detect STIs and identify pathogens. The physician may massage the prostate to increase organisms in the urethra.	Tell the patient a sterile swab will be inserted into the urethra to obtain a specimen. Have the patient lie down because the instrument may trigger a hypotensive episode with fainting. Specimens also may be obtained from the anal canal and pharynx. Use Standard Precautions to handle body fluids and contaminated instruments. Collect the specimen for culture before beginning prescribed antimicrobials.	Assess for hypotension, bradycardia, and pallor before assisting the patient to rise. Prepare specimens and send them to the laboratory.
Cultures of Organisms		
Permit identification of pathogens and susceptibility to various antimicrobials.	Explain the specimen collection process.	Prepare specimens according to laboratory protocol. Send them to the laboratory.
Semen Analysis		
Examines a semen specimen to assess male fertility or to document sterilization after vasectomy.	Instruct the patient to abstain from sexual activity and alcoholic beverages for 2–3 days; then collect the specimen in a clean container. Rubber condoms should not be used. The best specimen is obtained in the office or laboratory by masturbation. If the specimen is collected at home, it should be kept at room temperature and brought to the laboratory within 1 hour. When the specimen will be used to evaluate the effects of vasectomy, the patient should ejaculate several times before the day on which the specimen is collected.	No special care is needed.
Endocrinologic Studies		
Studies include measurement of LH, prolactin, FSH, and testosterone.	Tell the patient that a venous blood sample will be drawn.	Assess the venipuncture site for bleeding. Apply a small dressing.
Assess level of hormones needed for sexual development and function.		
Tumor Markers		
Studies include measurement of markers such as serum PSA and %FPSA.	Tell the patient a venous blood sample will be drawn. Fasting is not necessary.	Assess the venipuncture site for oozing or hematoma. Apply a small dressing. If %FPSA is ordered, handle the sample per specific laboratory guidelines.
Detect increases that may be associated with prostatic cancer, prostatic hyperplasia, cirrhosis, osteoporosis, and a number of other conditions. %FPSA is more helpful in differential diagnosis.		

Continued

Table 50-2 Diagnostic Tests and Procedures Male Reproductive System—cont'd

TEST AND PURPOSE	PATIENT PREPARATION	POSTPROCEDURE NURSING CARE
Cystoscopy		
Uses a lighted instrument inserted through the urethra to visualize the urethra, bladder, and prostatic urethra. May detect prostatic hyperplasia and bladder tumors.	Routine preoperative measures are indicated (i.e., signed consent form, skin scrub, food restriction). Antibiotics may be prescribed. Inform the patient the procedure is done in a special room under sterile conditions. Local anesthetic is instilled in the urethra and a sedative is given intravenously.	Measure the patient's urine output for 24 hours. Urine will be pink tinged. Report excessive bleeding or inability to void promptly. Encourage fluid intake when the patient is voiding well. Burning and hesitancy are common for several days. Give antibiotics as ordered.
Computed Tomography		
Creates images of internal structures to locate or assess testicular and prostatic tumors.	Assess allergy to iodine or previous contrast reactions if contrast dye will be injected. Report allergy to the radiologist. Tell the patient he will lie on a movable table while a machine moves around him. No sensations occur unless dye is injected. Some patients react to dye with nausea, vomiting, flushing, itching, or a bitter taste. Claustrophobic patients may need mild sedation.	No special postprocedure care is required. If dye is injected, the patient is encouraged to drink fluids to flush the dye from the body.
Ultrasonography		
Uses sound waves to create images of internal structures; used to study the prostate for enlargement or lesions.	Tell the patient an instrument will be inserted in the rectum to study the prostate. A full bladder is no longer required. Tell the patient the procedure is uncomfortable.	No special care is needed.
Radionuclide Imaging		
Uses radioactive substances injected intravenously or given orally followed by imaging to assess testicular abnormalities (i.e., torsion, tumors, abscesses, epididymitis, hydrocele).	Assess allergies to radioactive substance and inform the radiologist if allergic. Reassure the patient that the radiation dose is low and does not cause cell destruction.	Fluid intake is encouraged to promote elimination of the isotope.

Data from Pagana KD, Pagana TJ: *Mosby's diagnostic and laboratory test reference,* St. Louis, 2007, Mosby.
%FPSA, Percent free prostate-specific antigen; *ELISA,* enzyme-linked immunosorbent assay; *FSH,* follicle-stimulating hormone; *LH,* luteinizing hormone; *PSA,* prostate-specific antigen; *STI,* sexually transmitted infection.

Chapter 51. The most common inflammatory conditions are prostatitis and epididymitis. Orchitis is rare but important because it can cause sterility.

Prostatitis

Prostatitis is inflammation of the prostate gland. The types of prostatitis are acute bacterial prostatitis, chronic bacterial prostatitis, chronic prostatitis/chronic pelvic pain syndrome, and asymptomatic inflammatory prostatitis.

Signs and symptoms of acute prostatitis are swelling, warmth, and tenderness. The patient also may have dysuria, frequency, hematuria, and foul-smelling urine. Patients with chronic inflammation may have less dramatic pelvic pain, urinary tract symptoms, and sexual dysfunction. Diagnosis is based on the patient's complaints, confirmed by laboratory studies of prostatic secretions. Other diagnostic procedures may include urinalysis, white blood cell (WBC) count, and PSA. Imaging studies using MRI or transabdominal ultrasound may be done to rule out prostate abscess.

Acute bacterial prostatitis and *chronic bacterial prostatitis* are treated with antibiotics, analgesics, muscle relaxants, and sitz baths. A 4-week course of antibiotics usually is prescribed for acute bacterial prostatitis (and up to 16 weeks of therapy for chronic bacterial prostatitis). Chronic prostatitis/chronic pelvic pain syndrome may be treated with a short course of antibiotics but this is often ineffective. Depending on the severity of the pain, antiinflammatory drugs or opioid analgesics may be used. However, opioids must be used cautiously with chronic pain because of the potential for abuse. The patient is advised to increase fluid intake and to rest. Stool softeners may be prescribed to prevent constipation, which is especially painful with prostatitis. Urethral catheterization is contraindicated with urethral inflammation but suprapubic catheterization may be necessary if the patient has difficulty voiding. Prostate massage and ejaculation may be helpful with some types of prostatitis because they drain excess prostatic secretions.

Asymptomatic inflammatory prostatitis may be treated with a single daily dose of an alpha-adrenergic blocker to improve voiding by relaxing the bladder neck and prostate. Symptoms are managed with analgesics, antiinflammatory drugs, and sitz baths.

Most patients with prostatitis are treated as outpatients but hospital admission may be indicated if a high fever is present, the patient has urinary retention, or intravenous antibiotic therapy is needed. Ask the patient about pain and administer analgesics and other treatments as ordered. If the patient is discharged with medications, provide instructions and information about the drugs.

Epididymitis

Epididymitis, inflammation of the epididymis, may be caused by infections, trauma, or the reflux of urine from the urethra through the vas deferens. Signs and symptoms are painful scrotal edema, nausea, vomiting, chills, and fever. Epididymitis is treated with bed rest, ice packs, sitz baths, analgesics, antibiotics, antiinflammatory drugs, and scrotal support. A bridge made of tape and gauze or a rolled towel can be placed across the patient's thighs while in bed to elevate the scrotum and reduce pain. If the condition is associated with a sexually transmitted infection, the patient's sexual partner is treated with antibiotic therapy as well. Nursing care involves monitoring temperature, edema, and comfort. Carry out prescribed treatments and record their effects.

Orchitis

Orchitis is inflammation of one or both testes. It may be related to trauma or to infections such as mumps, pneumonia, or tuberculosis. Signs and symptoms of orchitis include fever, tenderness and swelling of the affected testicle, and scrotal redness. The inflammation can lead to reduced fertility or sterility. Orchitis is treated with analgesics, antipyretics, bed rest, scrotal support, and local heat to the scrotum. Nursing care includes pain management, assistance with activities of daily living (ADL), patient teaching, and anxiety reduction.

BENIGN PROSTATIC HYPERPLASIA (HYPERTROPHY)

Benign prostatic hyperplasia is enlargement of the prostate gland. It is a common age-related change.

Signs and Symptoms

Signs and symptoms of benign prostatic hyperplasia can be described as *obstructive* or *irritative.* Obstructive symptoms include decreasing size and force of the urinary stream, urine retention, and postvoid dribbling. Irritative symptoms include urgency, frequency, dysuria, nocturia, hematuria, and sometimes urge incontinence. Factors that may trigger retention are alcohol, infections, delayed voiding, bed rest, opioids, antihistamines, and chilling.

Medical Diagnosis

A diagnosis of benign prostatic hyperplasia is based on results of the reported symptoms, a voiding diary, rectal examination, laboratory and radiographic studies, endoscopy, ultrasound, catheterization for residual urine, and sometimes urodynamic testing (see Chapter 42). A urine specimen and prostatic secretions are obtained and examined for evidence of infection.

Medical Treatment

Conservative measures can decrease urinary retention. These include maintaining fluid intake of 1500 to 2000 mL/day, fluid restriction for 2 hours before bedtime, avoidance of caffeine and alcohol, and some bladder training exercises (see Chapter 23). Drugs that may be prescribed to treat benign prostatic hyperplasia and related symptoms include 5-alpha reductase inhibitors and alpha$_1$-adrenergic receptor antagonists (alpha$_1$ blockers). 5-Alpha-reductase inhibitors suppress prostatic tissue growth by decreasing testosterone levels. Examples are finasteride (Proscar) and dutasteride (Duagen). Alpha$_1$ blockers such as tamsulosin (Flomax), doxazosin (Cardura), and terazosin (Hytrin) are used to relax smooth muscle in the bladder neck and prostate, thereby reducing obstruction to urinary flow. Combinations of drugs are proving more effective than either type of drug alone (see *Complementary and Alternative Therapies* box).

> **Complementary and Alternative Therapies**
>
> Saw palmetto is an extract from berries of a small tree. Some people take it to relieve urinary symptoms associated with benign prostatic hyperplasia. However, research has not found it to be effective.

Surgical and Invasive Treatments

Surgical or other invasive intervention is usually advised if complete urinary obstruction develops, if evidence of existing or impending renal damage exists, if the patient has repeated urinary tract infections (UTIs), or if significant bleeding occurs. In general, invasive procedures involve surgical removal of all or part of the prostate (**prostatectomy**) or ablation (destruction) of prostate tissue.

Types of Prostatectomy. The most widely used surgical procedure is the transurethral resection of the prostate (TURP). During a TURP, an instrument is inserted into the urethra and an electrode or laser is used to cut away or destroy obstructing portions of the gland. No external incision is made. A triple-lumen urinary catheter commonly is used to maintain continuous irrigation and bladder drainage. Continuous irrigation is intended to clear the bladder of blood and debris. If the catheter output is less than the irrigating fluid delivered, the catheter may be obstructed. Manual irrigation may be needed as ordered to clear the clots and restore drainage. If drainage cannot be restored, the physician should be notified immediately. Pressure in the bladder is one cause of painful bladder spasms. Because only part of the gland is removed, the remaining tissue can continue to grow and obstruction may recur.

A suprapubic prostatectomy is performed through the bladder by way of a low abdominal incision. It may be selected when the prostate is very large or when bladder abnormalities also exist that require surgical correction. Convalescence is longer than with a transurethral prostatectomy and some patients develop incontinence or erectile dysfunction. A retropubic prostatectomy uses a low abdominal incision of the front of the prostate. The bladder is not cut. Although the risk is small, some men develop incontinence, erectile dysfunction, or both. A perineal prostatectomy requires an incision between the scrotum and the anus to gain access to the prostate. Radical prostatectomy is discussed in the section titled "Prostatic Cancer."

Complications. Depending on the type of prostatectomy, the patient is at risk for urinary infection and incontinence, hemorrhage, urinary leakage, inflammation of the pubic bone, and erectile dysfunction. Retrograde ejaculation may occur, meaning that semen enters the bladder instead of being ejected through the urethra. The semen is then voided later with urine. This is not harmful to the patient but does render him **sterile** (infertile).

Alternative Invasive Procedures. Alternative procedures use heat (transurethral microwave thermotherapy or transurethral needle ablation [TUNA]) to destroy selected prostate tissue or laser incision and vaporization of prostate tissue. Stents can be placed to prevent obstruction of urine flow. Balloon dilation is controversial.

❖ NURSING CARE of the Patient with Benign Prostatic Hyperplasia

■ Assessment

Data needed for assessment of the patient with benign prostatic hyperplasia include a complete description of urinary symptoms: frequency, urgency, hesitancy, a change in stream size or force, and nocturia. Record the presence of pain or hematuria and palpate the lower abdomen or use a Doppler to detect bladder distention. If ordered, the patient may be catheterized after voiding to measure residual urine.

■ Interventions

Impaired Urinary Elimination

Instruct the patient to void promptly when the urge is felt and to space fluid intake throughout the day rather than consuming large amounts of liquids at one time. A daily total fluid intake of 1500 to 2000 mL is recommended. Fluid restriction is *not* recommended because it increases the risk of UTI. However, avoiding fluids for 2 hours before bedtime may reduce nighttime voiding.

Notify the physician if the patient is unable to void and the bladder becomes distended. Perform catheterization as ordered. It may be difficult to pass the catheter because of the enlarged prostate. If the catheter does not pass easily, do not force it. Inform the physician. The procedure is usually done by a urologist using special instruments. !

Nursing Diagnoses, Goals, and Outcome Criteria: Benign Prostatic Hyperplasia

Nursing Diagnoses	Goals and Outcome Criteria
Impaired Urinary Elimination related to obstruction	Normal bladder emptying: no distention on palpation, urine output approximately equal to fluid intake
Fear related to invasive diagnostic and therapeutic procedures	Reduced fear: patient states fear is reduced, appears calm
Ineffective Self-Health Management of treatment and self-care related to lack of knowledge, limited resources	Patient understands condition and treatment and follows prescribed plan of care: patient correctly describes condition and treatment, demonstrates self-care

Pharmacology Capsule

Common nonprescription drugs, including many cold remedies, may cause urinary retention in the patient with prostatic hyperplasia.

Put on Your Thinking Cap!

Draw an illustration that you could use to teach a patient the effects of prostate enlargement.

Fear

Explore the patient's fears and provide information about anticipated procedures and effects.

Ineffective Self-Health Management

Because this condition requires long-term management, the patient or a caregiver must understand how to manage the condition. Advise the patient that over-the-counter (OTC) drugs containing antihistamines or pseudoephedrine, which are commonly found in cold remedies, can aggravate urinary symptoms (see *Patient Teaching* box). The patient should avoid caffeine and alcohol, which have a diuretic effect.

Patient Teaching

Prostatic Hyperplasia

- An enlarged prostate compresses the urethra, which interferes with passage of urine.
- To prevent urinary retention, drink fluids throughout the day.
- Consult your physician or pharmacist about nonprescription drugs. Common drugs such as antihistamines can cause urinary retention.
- Report signs and symptoms of infection (i.e., burning on urination, foul urine odor, cloudy urine) and obstruction (i.e., feeling of bladder fullness, inability to empty bladder, lower abdominal pain).
- Take your medications as prescribed and notify your physician of any adverse effects. (Provide the patient with information about specific drugs.)

NURSING CARE of the Patient with a Prostatectomy

Detailed care of the surgical patient is presented in Chapter 17. This section addresses the specific needs of the postoperative prostatectomy patient (see Nursing Care Plan: Patient with a Prostatectomy).

Assessment

When the patient returns to the nursing unit, measure his vital signs and compare them with preoperative measurements. Inspect urine, dressings, and wound drainage for excess bleeding. Maintain careful records of fluid intake and output to avoid overdistention of the bladder; input and output should be balanced. Record the color of the urine and any clots present. Check intravenous fluids and regulate the rate of flow. Monitor the patient's level of comfort for incisional pain and bladder spasms.

Interventions

Risk for Deficient Fluid Volume

Restlessness and an increasing heart rate are early signs of fluid volume deficit. Blood in the urine is expected for several days after a prostatectomy; however, the drainage should be light pink within 24 hours. Bleeding with clots can signal hemorrhage and must be reported to the physician immediately. Bright-red blood may indicate arterial bleeding that requires surgical intervention. Dark blood may require pressure on the surgical area at the neck of the bladder. To apply pressure, the physician may inject additional fluid into the balloon that anchors the indwelling catheter. The catheter is then pulled so that the balloon fits tightly against the neck of the bladder and various forms of traction are used, including taping the catheter to the thigh. This traction may be maintained for several hours or more and then released by the physician.

Continuous bladder irrigation helps to prevent clot formation and subsequent obstruction that can cause bladder spasms and infection. Hang irrigating fluids (usually normal saline) and regulate flow at the prescribed rate.

Nursing Diagnoses, Goals, and Outcome Criteria: Prostatectomy

Nursing Diagnoses	Goals and Outcome Criteria
Risk for Deficient Fluid Volume related to hemorrhage	Normal fluid balance: balanced fluid intake and output, stable vital signs consistent with patient norms
Acute Pain related to tissue trauma and bladder spasms	Pain relief: patient states pain is relieved, relaxed expression
Risk for Infection related to invasive procedures of the urinary tract and surgical incision	Reduced risk of infection: freely flowing, clear urine
Risk for Injury related to obstructed urine flow, excessive absorption of irrigating fluids, trauma to the urinary sphincter	Absence of complications because of obstruction, water intoxication, or sphincter injury
Urge Urinary Incontinence related to poor sphincter control, bladder contractions	Improved control of urine elimination: patient controls urine passage; has decreasing incidents of incontinence
Sexual Dysfunction related to removal of prostate, retrograde ejaculation, possible neurologic injury	Management of sexual dysfunction: patient states he understands sexual dysfunction and identifies appropriate adaptations and resources
Situational Low Self-Esteem related to anticipated alteration in sexual function	Improved self-esteem: patient makes positive statements about self
Deficient Knowledge of postoperative routines and self-care	Patient understands routines and self-care: patient correctly describes limitations and demonstrates self-care activities

Acute Pain

Pain after prostatectomy may be associated with urinary obstruction, bladder spasms, and surgical trauma. If urine is not draining freely, reposition the tubing and irrigate according to agency policy. Antispasmodic agents such as oxybutynin chloride (Ditropan), belladonna and opium suppositories, or propantheline bromide (Pro-Banthine) are usually effective in relieving bladder spasms. Administer

Nursing Care Plan — Patient with a Prostatectomy

ASSESSMENT

HEALTH HISTORY Patient is a 77-year-old retired radio announcer who underwent a transurethral prostatectomy this morning. He returned to the nursing unit 3 hours ago. He complains of genital pain and states that he feels like he needs to empty his bladder. He appears tense and is clenching the side rails.

PHYSICAL ASSESSMENT Vital signs: blood pressure 122/70 mm Hg, pulse 84 bpm, respiration 18 breaths per minute, temperature 98°F (36.7°C) measured orally. Height 5′11″, weight 165 lb. Alert and oriented. Breath sounds clear on auscultation. Intravenous fluids infusing at 100 mL/h. Three-way Foley catheter in place, taped to inner thigh and draining freely into collection bag. Irrigation fluid set at the prescribed flow rate. Urine pink, not viscous. Several clots observed in bag.

Nursing Diagnosis	Goals and Outcome Criteria	Interventions
Risk for Deficient Fluid Volume related to hemorrhage	The patient will have balanced fluid intake and output without signs of hypovolemia (i.e., tachycardia, decreased urine output, hypotension, restlessness).	Monitor the patient's urine for excessive bleeding: thick, bright blood with clots. Assess for signs of hypovolemia. Ensure that traction is maintained on catheter by keeping tape in place until surgeon removes it. Maintain flow of irrigating fluid as ordered. If urine flow decreases or bladder distention is detected, irrigate the catheter manually as ordered. Turn off the irrigating fluid and inform the surgeon if unable to irrigate or urine output remains low.
Acute Pain related to tissue trauma and bladder spasms	The patient will verbalize relief from pain and will appear more relaxed.	Check tubing to ensure that urine is draining freely. If not, reposition the tubing and irrigate it as ordered or per agency policy. Notify the surgeon immediately if unable to clear tubing. Administer analgesics and antispasmodics as ordered. Reposition the patient. Give back rubs. Use distraction. Assess the effects of pain relief interventions.
Risk for Infection related to invasive procedures of the urinary tract or catheterization	The patient will remain free of infection, as evidenced by normal body temperature, normal white blood cell (WBC) count, and absence of confusion or cloudy, foul urine.	Use strict aseptic techniques when handling the urinary drainage system. Keep closed system intact. Monitor temperature and urine characteristics. Report fever (>101°F), confusion, and cloudy or foul urine.
Risk for Injury related to obstructed urine flow or trauma to urinary sphincter	The patient will have no injuries, as evidenced by continuous urine flow.	Maintain flow of isotonic irrigating fluid as ordered. Monitor output and assess bladder for distention. Monitor vital signs. Administer stool softeners as ordered to prevent constipation. Encourage fluid intake when able.
Sexual Dysfunction related to removal of prostate or retrograde ejaculation	The patient will correctly describe the physiologic effects of prostatectomy.	Be open to the patient's questions about the effects of surgery on sexual function. Reinforce preoperative teaching that erectile dysfunction is not common after transurethral prostate resection. Retrograde ejaculation may occur but is not harmful. Offer to include the sex partner in teaching. Be sensitive to possible feelings about loss of masculinity. The patient may demonstrate some anger or sadness related to a sense of loss.
Deficient Knowledge of postoperative routines or self-care	The patient will demonstrate understanding of postoperative exercises and procedures.	Support and encourage the patient to turn and deep breathe at least every 2 hours (q2h). Explain the catheter and the irrigation system. Tell him that some blood is normal the first few days after surgery. Encourage early ambulation as soon as permitted and explain the benefits of activity to recovery. Before discharge, advise the patient to restrict strenuous activity and heavy lifting (no more than 10–20 lb as specified by the physician) for 4–6 weeks. If he will go home with a catheter, discuss catheter care.

Critical Thinking Questions

1. Describe the application of strict aseptic technique in the care of this patient.
2. Why might this surgery affect sexual function?

analgesics as ordered and assess effectiveness (see *Complementary and Alternative Therapies* box).

Complementary and Alternative Therapies

In addition to analgesics, try nonpharmacologic interventions for postoperative pain such as repositioning, back rubs, and relaxation exercises.

Risk for Infection

To reduce the risk of infection, use strict aseptic technique when handling urinary drainage, wound drains, and dressings. Keep closed urinary drainage systems intact to prevent the introduction of pathogens. Following an open prostatectomy, provide wound care in accordance with the physician's orders or the agency's policy. Monitor for signs of infection, including temperature above 101°F (38.3°C), purulent wound drainage, and confusion in older patients.

Risk for Injury

Urinary obstruction and bladder distention can lead to renal complications (i.e., hydronephrosis), infection, and increased bleeding. Therefore it is critical to maintain urine flow. If urine flow ceases, assess the bladder for distention. If the bladder is distended, temporarily turn off the irrigating fluid and manually irrigate the bladder as ordered. If you cannot clear the tubing, notify the surgeon immediately. After the catheters are removed, you must continue to monitor output because edema or scarring may occur and obstruct the urethra.

Urge Urinary Incontinence

Urinary incontinence or dribbling is common immediately after the catheter is removed. In most cases, control can be improved with perineal exercises. Instruct patients to contract and relax the perineal muscles 10 to 20 times each hour. If control does not improve, the physician may recommend biofeedback, a penile clamp, a condom catheter, or incontinence briefs. In severe cases, an artificial sphincter may be surgically implanted. Some patients never regain full control of urination. For additional information, see Chapter 23.

Sexual Dysfunction and Situational Low Self-Esteem

Alterations in sexual function that may distress the patient include sterility, retrograde ejaculation, and erectile dysfunction. The patient should be encouraged to discuss these concerns with the physician before surgery. Erectile dysfunction is not common after surgical treatment of benign prostatic hyperplasia but if it does occur, the patient may need counseling, as described in the section titled "Erectile Dysfunction (Impotence)." No treatment for retrograde ejaculation exists but you can reassure the patient that it is not harmful. All of these alterations can threaten the patient's self-image and self-esteem. Be sensitive to the patient's feelings of loss and need to assert a masculine image. The patient may wish to include his sex partner in teaching and counseling sessions.

Deficient Knowledge

Teaching for postoperative care must begin in the preoperative period because patient hospitalizations are usually short and the patient may be discharged with a catheter. Verbal instructions should be accompanied by written material (see *Patient Teaching* box).

Patient Teaching

Postprostatectomy

- After a prostatectomy, semen may be ejaculated into the bladder (retrograde ejaculation). This is not harmful.
- Signs and symptoms of complications that should be reported include inability to pass urine, bladder distention, renewed bleeding, fever, and cloudy or foul-smelling urine.
- Practice perineal exercises as instructed to reduce the risk of incontinence.
- Walking is encouraged but avoid strenuous activity or heavy lifting until approved by the physician.
- Drink at least eight glasses of fluids each day.
- To prevent constipation and straining, which could cause bleeding, take stool softeners as prescribed and consume a high-fiber diet.
- Keep your urinary drainage system closed except when emptying it. Wash your hands before and after handling the system.
- Do not resume driving or sexual intercourse until directed by the surgeon (usually about 6 weeks).

PROSTATIC CANCER

Cancer of the prostate is found on postmortem examination in 30% of men over the age of 50 and the incidence increases steadily with each decade to 100% of men in the tenth decade. More than 233,000 new cases were expected to be diagnosed in the United States in 2014 and more than 29,000 deaths from prostate cancer were predicted in that year. Although the cause is unknown, the risk factors include age over 50 years, African-American race, family history of prostate cancer, and ingestion of a high-fat diet (see *Cultural Considerations* box).

Cultural Considerations

What Does Culture Have to Do with Prostate Cancer?

The incidence of prostate cancer among African-American men is nearly twice that among Caucasian Americans. High-risk groups should be targeted for education about the importance of early evaluation of urinary symptoms.

Early Detection

Serum PSA increases with prostate cancer but also with a variety of other conditions. Whether PSA should be used as a screening tool is controversial. In 2012 the

U.S. Preventive Services Task Force recommended against PSA-based screening for prostate cancer. The Task Force indicated that elevated PSA often led to cancer treatment with serious complications for many men whose cancer never would have become life threatening. On the other hand, the American Cancer Society (ACS) recommends that at age 50 all men discuss with their physician the pros and cons of periodic screening (PSA with or without rectal examination) so that they can make a decision that is right for them. The ACS recommends that African-American men initiate this discussion by age 45.

Medical Diagnosis

Prostatic lesions are typically slow growing and confined to the prostatic capsule. However, younger men tend to have very aggressive tumors. Prostatic tumors may go undetected until the disease is advanced and has metastasized to bone or liver. Large tumors may cause bladder outlet obstruction, rectal pressure, stool changes, painful defecation, or painful ejaculation. Because early diagnosis may improve treatment results, methods to permit early detection may be advised.

The diagnosis may be based on rectal examination, transrectal ultrasound, PSA level, and needle aspiration and biopsy. If a diagnosis of prostate cancer is made, additional procedures may be done to identify the stage of the disease. These may include radiographs, radionuclide imaging, bone scans, excretory urography, transurethral ultrasound, CT, and MRI.

Medical Treatment

The treatment of prostate cancer is controversial because of the difficulty in staging tumors and the unpredictable biologic behavior of the disease. Treatment options include "watchful waiting," radiotherapy, brachytherapy, cryosurgery, and radical surgery. Chemotherapy is useful in limited cases. Sometimes "watchful waiting" is recommended for patients with a life expectancy of less than 10 years who have small cancers or who are not good surgical risks. The patient is monitored frequently and treatment is initiated if the tumor begins to enlarge.

Radical prostatectomy includes removal of the prostate gland, the outer capsule, the seminal vesicles, sections of the vas deferens, and sometimes a portion of the bladder neck. Most operations include removal of the pelvic lymph nodes to check for metastasis. The surgical approach usually is perineal or retropubic. The latter approach permits an autonomic nerve-sparing technique, which may preserve erectile function. The urinary incontinence that occurs in 10% to 15% of men who undergo radical prostatectomy subsides within 6 months in 85% to 90% of those affected. Minimally invasive radical prostatectomy using a laparoscope and robot-assisted technology is available in some settings. It is believed that less invasive techniques will result in less blood loss and less postoperative pain.

Radiation alone often is effective when the cancer is confined to the prostate. Radiation can be delivered by external beam or by implanting seeds (brachytherapy) of radioactive gold, iodine, or iridium in the prostate through hollow needles inserted under anesthesia. External beam radiation requires only a few minutes, 5 days a week for 6 to 8 weeks. Side effects include skin dryness and irritation; diarrhea, cramping, and gastrointestinal (GI) bleeding; sexual dysfunction; fatigue; bone marrow suppression; and various urinary symptoms such as dysuria, frequency, hesitancy, urgency, and nocturia. The radioactive seeds affect surrounding tissues less than external beam radiation. Patients often have some urinary symptoms of irritation or obstruction after the seeds are implanted. Newer radiation options include three-dimensional conformal radiation therapy or intensity-modulated radiation therapy. The new procedures deliver higher doses to the target tissue with less toxicity.

Prostate cancer growth is influenced by hormones. Therefore hormonal therapy is used to eliminate the androgenic effect by interfering with androgen production or blocking receptors for the androgens. Testosterone production also can be achieved by removing the testicles. Many men elect drug therapy over the surgical option. Types of drugs used in hormonal therapy include luteinizing hormone–releasing hormone (LHRH) agonists and androgen receptor blockers. LHRH analogs include leuprolide (Lupron), goserelin acetate (Zoladex), buserelin (Suprefact), and triptorelin (Trelstar). These agents inhibit the release of pituitary hormones necessary for testosterone production. They are given intramuscularly or subcutaneously. One form is available in pellets that are implanted subcutaneously and deliver medication for 1 year. With initial therapy, patients may experience bone pain, which resolves over time. Drugs that inhibit the action of testosterone include flutamide (Eulexin), bicalutamide (Casodex), and nilutamide (Nilandron). They may be used in combination with LHRH agonists (Table 50-3).

The adverse effects of all of these agents can include hot flashes and erectile dysfunction. When these agents are no longer effective, other drugs may be used that reduce testosterone production in the adrenals. Examples are spironolactone (Aldactone), aminoglutethimide (Cytadren), and glucocorticoids. Hormonal therapy is usually effective for a limited period of time, generally 1 to 3 years. Bone pain and fractures are complications of prostate cancer. Bisphosphonates such as alendronate (Fosamax) may be ordered to help relieve bone symptoms. PSA is a useful tool for the follow-up of patients who have undergone treatment. Persistent or rising PSA levels indicate advancing or recurrent tumor growth.

Table 50-3 Drug Therapy: Disorders of the Male Reproductive System

DRUG	USE AND ACTION	SIDE EFFECTS	NURSING INTERVENTION
Androgens: Testosterone			
Oral preparations: methyltestosterone (Methitest, Testred), fluoxymesterone (Androxy) Intramuscular preparation: testosterone cypionate (Depo-Testosterone) Transdermal patch (Androderm) Transdermal gel (AndroGel, Testim, Fortesta) Transdermal underarm solution (Axiron) Implantable pellets (Testopel) Buccal system (Striant)	Treats hormone deficiency caused by developmental disorders, testicular diseases, or removal of testicles. Increases testosterone level.	Retention of water, sodium, potassium, and chloride. Jaundice, GI distress. Increased effects of anticoagulants and oral hypoglycemics. Androderm patches may irritate skin. Buccal tablets may irritate the mouth and gums. Gels and underarm solution can be transferred to others via intimate contact. Females should not have contact with these.	Assess for hypertension and edema. IM injections should be given deeply in the gluteus muscle using the Z-track technique. Androderm patches are applied to the arm, back, abdomen, or thigh; *NOT to the scrotum.* AndroGel and Testim can be applied to the upper arm and shoulder. AndroGel can also be applied to the abdomen; none should be applied to the scrotum. Axiron is applied to one or both armpits each morning. Pellets are implanted subcutaneously.
Drugs Used to Treat BPH			
5-alpha reductase inhibitors: finasteride (Proscar), dutasteride (Avodart)	Reduce prostate size, which decreases urethral obstruction. Effects not evident for several months.	Decreased ejaculate volume and libido. Decreases PSA, which must be considered in interpreting PSA screening results. Teratogenic for male fetus.	Females who are or might become pregnant should not handle medication with bare hands or be exposed to patient's semen. Tell patient that effects are not immediate.
alpha-1 adrenergic antagonists (blockers): tamsulosin (Flomax), doxazosin (Cardura), terazosin (Hytrin), silodosin (Rapaflo), alfuzosin (Uroxatral)	Relaxes smooth muscle in bladder neck, prostate capsule, and prostatic urethra, which reduces urethral obstruction.	Doxazosin, terazosin, alfuzosin: lower BP, dizziness, sleepiness. Silodosin and tamsulosin: abnormal ejaculation. All: risk of complications of cataract surgery.	Therapy must be continued lifelong to maintain benefit. Monitor BP. Caution with other drugs that lower BP. Tell patient if changes in ejaculation may occur.
Testosterone Inhibitors (Androgen Receptor Blockers)			
flutamide (Eulexin) bicalutamide (Casodex) nilutamide (Nilandron)	Decreases testosterone level. Used with LHRH to treat prostate cancer.	GI distress, hepatotoxicity, gynecomastia, ED, hot flashes, edema, hypertension, anxiety, confusion, mental depression.	Liver function must be monitored. Do not double up if a dose is missed. Be sure patient understands that drug must be taken with LHRH. Advise of effects on sexual function. Tell patient to report GI distress, pain in right side, dark urine, yellowish color of skin or sclera.
abarelix (Plenaxis)	Suppresses testosterone production. Used for palliative therapy for advanced prostate cancer.	Risk of severe immediate allergic reactions with hypotension and fainting, hot flashes, sleep disturbances, gynecomastia, breast pain/ nipple tenderness, pain, constipation, peripheral edema.	IM injection. Monitor blood pressure for 30 minutes after injection.

Continued

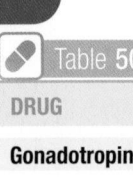

Table 50-3 Drug Therapy: Disorders of the Male Reproductive System—cont'd

DRUG	USE AND ACTION	SIDE EFFECTS	NURSING INTERVENTION
Gonadotropin-Releasing Hormone Agonists (LHRH Analogs)			
leuprolide (Eligard, Lupron, Viadur) triptorelin (Trelstar Depot, Trelstar LA) goserelin (Zoladex)	Leuprolide desensitizes pituitary receptors for GnRH; testosterone release rises at first, then declines. Used for advanced prostate cancer. May be given with an androgen receptor blocker to reduce adverse effects.	Hot flashes, impotence, loss of libido, reduced muscle mass, increased adipose mass. May cause increased pain initially; usually resolves over time.	Leuprolide can be given daily (subcutaneously), monthly or quarterly (IM), or yearly (implant). Triptorelin given IM monthly or quarterly. Goserelin comes as a pellet that is injected into the upper abdominal wall with a 16-gauge needle; a local anesthetic may be given first.
Agents Used to Treat Erectile Dysfunction			
sildenafil (Viagra) vardenafil (Levitra) tadalafil (Cialis)	Relaxes smooth muscle in corpus cavernosum, which increases blood flow with subsequent erection. Tadalafil is available for PRN or daily use.	Headache, dizziness, abnormal vision, diarrhea, dyspepsia, priapism, UTI, flushing, rash. MI, sudden death, cardiovascular collapse, especially if taken with organic nitrate therapy. Numerous other contraindications including MAO inhibitors, severe hepatic or renal impairment, pregnancy or lactation (not recommended for women at this time), history of coronary artery disease, CHF, dysrhythmias, or stroke. Many interactions; refer to a drug handbook when administering.	*Do not* take if taking organic nitrates (e.g., nitroglycerin); combination can be fatal. Drug is only effective with sexual stimulation. Patients over age 65 may be started on the lowest dose and increased if necessary. If on PRN tadalafil, instruct patient to take 1 hour before sexual activity and not to take more than once daily.
papaverine plus phentolamine	Increases arterial blood flow to penis and decreases venous outflow. Produces erection within 10 minutes that lasts 2–4 hours. Sometimes given in combination with alprostadil.	Priapism (erection lasting more than 6 hours), painless fibrotic nodules at injection sites, orthostatic hypotension, transient numbness, bruising at injection site.	Injected directly into the corpus cavernosum. Advise patient to seek medical attention for priapism.
alprostadil injection (Caverject) and intraurethral suppositories (MUSE)	Increase blood flow to penis.	Injection: priapism, fibrotic nodules. Suppository: urethral pain, inflammation.	Teach patient self-administration. Advise to seek treatment for persistent erection.
Other Drugs for Disorders of the Male Reproductive System			
estramustine (Emcyt) (a hybrid of estrogen and an alkylating agent)	Palliative therapy for advanced prostate cancer.	Gynecomastia, heart failure, thrombosis causing stroke or MI, fluid retention, nausea, vomiting, diarrhea, hypercalcemia.	Monitor for heart failure: dyspnea, edema, fatigue. Inform patient not to take with milk or other high-calcium food.

BP, Blood pressure; *BPH,* benign prostatic hyperplasia; *CHF,* congestive heart failure; *ED,* erectile dysfunction; *GI,* gastrointestinal; *GnRH,* gonadotropin-releasing hormone; *IM,* intramuscular; *LHRH,* luteinizing hormone–releasing hormone; *MAO,* monoamine oxidase; *MI,* myocardial infarction; *PRN,* as needed; *PSA,* prostate-specific antigen; *UTI,* urinary tract infection.

NURSING CARE of the Patient with Prostatic Cancer

Details of the assessment of the male reproductive system are summarized in Box 50-1. Nursing care of male patients should include encouragement to discuss whether to have periodic screenings for prostate cancer. If the patient has undergone surgery, nursing care is similar to that described in the section titled "Nursing Care of the Patient with Benign Prostatic Hyperplasia." Nursing care of the patient with cancer is discussed in Chapter 25 and the care of patients having urologic surgery is discussed in Chapter 42. Specific problems that may require special interventions after prostate surgery are bladder spasms, erectile dysfunction, urinary incontinence, and body image disturbances associated with changes in the reproductive system.

ERECTILE DYSFUNCTION (IMPOTENCE)

Erectile dysfunction (ED), which is the inability to produce and maintain an erection for sexual intercourse, can be devastating for a man and his partner. An adequate erection requires intact neurologic function, sufficient inflow of blood to fill the corpus cavernosa, and a leak-proof storage mechanism for maintaining the erection. Factors that contribute to ED and related treatments are summarized in Table 50-4.

Contributing Factors

A number of vascular, endocrine, neurologic, and psychologic factors may cause or contribute to erectile dysfunction.

Vascular Disorders. Systemic or local changes in blood flow can impair the ability to achieve an erection. Generalized atherosclerosis may be a factor in inadequate filling of the corpus cavernosa. Many modifiable factors contribute to the development of atherosclerosis. These include high cholesterol levels, smoking, excessive alcohol consumption, illicit drug use, and inadequate exercise. The cavernosal artery in the perineum between the scrotum and the anus may be damaged by physical injury to the pelvis, falls on the crossbar of a bicycle, horseback riding, or other blows. Significant damage to the artery limits the inflow of blood to the corpus cavernosa.

Endocrine Disorders. Endocrine disorders that affect sexual function include DM and low testosterone. Patients with DM are at risk for erectile dysfunction because of atherosclerosis and autonomic neuropathy. Autonomic neuropathy is the dysfunction of some aspect of the autonomic nervous system, which is essential to normal sexual response.

Approximately 50% of men who have diabetes, regardless of type of treatment, develop erectile dysfunction, making diabetes the most common cause of erectile dysfunction. Diabetes is believed to interfere with blood supply to the penis when arterial walls lose flexibility, or distensibility, as a result of hardening of the arteries (atherosclerosis). Atherosclerosis may be accelerated by diabetes.

Autonomic neuropathy in patients with diabetes affects the ability of nerves to relax the smooth muscle surrounding the tiny sinuses (lacunar spaces) of the erectile chambers. Without relaxed muscle tone and expansion of the sinuses, adequate filling with blood for an erection may not be possible.

Effective management of DM is always desirable for general good health but maintenance of strict blood glucose levels has not been shown to reduce the incidence of ED. Although the primary cause of ED related to DM is physiologic, the psychologic reaction to the problem is an important factor. Cognitive behavioral therapy may be used to teach the patient to manage negative thinking.

Vascular surgery to clear blocked arteries is not usually recommended for people with diabetes because they often have complicating problems with nerves,

Table 50-4 Factors Related to Erectile Dysfunction

FACTOR	DESCRIPTION	TREATMENTS
Psychologic factors	Depression, fear, grief, anxiety, interpersonal problems with partner	Psychotherapy, marital therapy, group therapy, sex therapy
Medical conditions	Cardiovascular disease, diabetes mellitus (DM), stroke, osteoarthritis, Parkinson disease, back pain, chronic obstructive pulmonary disease (COPD)	Management of underlying condition. Erectile dysfunction (ED) drug therapy, vacuum therapy, penile implant Adaptation of sexual practices to accommodate disabilities.
Medical and surgical interventions	Medication side effects Pelvic radiation Perineal surgery, ostomy, mastectomy	Alternative drug therapy. Counseling. ED drug therapy, vacuum therapy, penile implant. Adaptation of sexual practices to accommodate disabilities.
Lifestyle	Tobacco use Excessive alcohol intake Lack of physical conditioning Obesity	Minimize or cease use of tobacco and alcohol. Regular exercise. Weight control.

cells, erectile tissue, and blood vessels throughout the penis.

A penile implant (Fig. 50-8) may be recommended for a patient with failure to initiate (nerve damage) or failure to fill (artery damage), which are related to diabetes. As many as one third of penile implant patients have diabetes.

Phosphodiesterase type 5 inhibitors such as sildenafil (Viagra) and tadalafil (Cialis) are oral drugs that may be effective. Papaverine plus phentolamine self-injection is indicated as a treatment for failure to initiate or fill and has been widely accepted by patients. Alprostadil (prostaglandin E_1) is available in an injectable form and as a pellet that is inserted into the urethra. Patients need training in self-injection and must have hand dexterity and adequate vision.

Neurologic Disorders. Spinal cord injuries and other neurologic disorders may cause ED. If communication between the spinal cord and the penis remains intact, the penis becomes erect with direct stimulation. For the penis to remain erect, smooth muscle relaxation is necessary and in some way relies on communication between the brain and the spinal cord. The more complete the injury and the lower the injury, the more likely it is that erection will be affected, even though higher injuries tend to cause more paralysis and loss of sensation. In addition to spinal cord injuries, perineal and rectal surgery can damage nerves involved in erectile function.

Treatment of ED related to spinal cord injuries or neurologic disorders such as multiple sclerosis (MS) may include phosphodiesterase type 5 inhibitors, papaverine, or alprostadil; vacuum constriction devices; or penile implants.

Medication Side Effects. Medications used to treat a variety of conditions may cause or contribute to ED. Drugs used to reduce high BP (antihypertensive agents) are the most likely to interfere with erection. If systemic hypertension is accompanied by blockages and stiffening in the arterial walls of the penis, antihypertensives that lower the BP in all arteries of the body may reduce the BP in penile arteries to the extent that failure to fill occurs. Digoxin, which is used to treat heart conditions, may increase levels of estrogen and

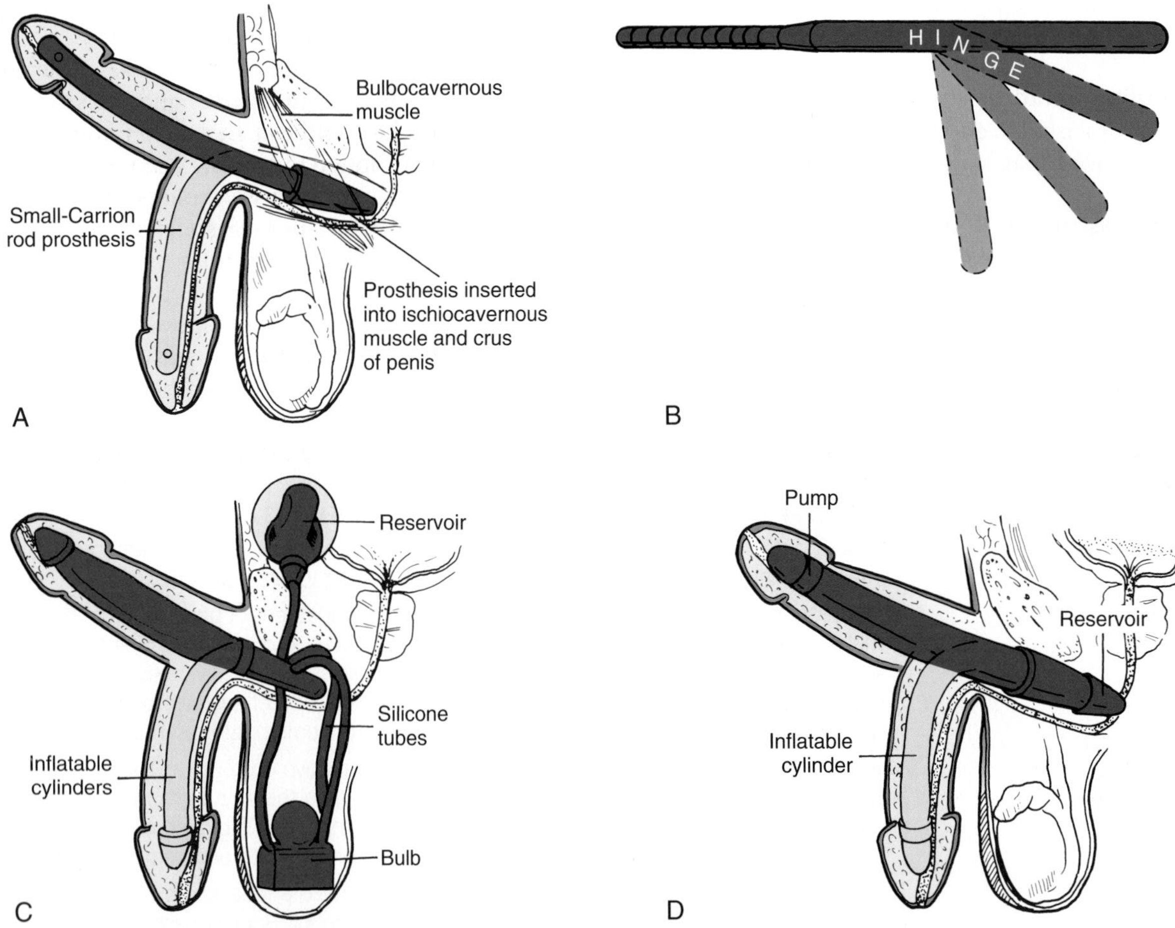

FIGURE 50-8 Penile prostheses. **A,** Small-Carrion prosthesis. **B,** Flexi-rod semirigid implant. **C,** Inflatable prosthesis. **D,** Self-contained prosthesis. (From Black JM, Matassarin-Jacobs E: *Luckmann and Sorenson's medical-surgical nursing: clinical management for continuity of care*, ed 5, Philadelphia, 1997, Saunders.)

decrease levels of testosterone; medications for stomach ulcers, such as cimetidine, and anticancer drugs may decrease libido and anticholinergics and antihistamines may block neurotransmitters that cause relaxation of smooth muscle (see *Complementary and Alternative Therapies* box).

Complementary and Alternative Therapies

Siberian ginseng and *Ginkgo biloba* are herbs that some believe increase penile blood flow. Scientific validation is lacking at this time.

Treatment for ED related to these drugs' side effects may include changes in drugs or dosage but such changes can be made only on a physician's order (see *Complementary and Alternative Therapies* box). Counseling or sex therapy, vacuum constriction devices, drug therapy, or penile implants may be appropriate for these patients.

Complementary and Alternative Therapies

Therapies that may be used alone or with traditional medication to treat erectile dysfunction include acupuncture, aromatherapy (with essential oils of sandalwood, rose, jasmine, and ylang ylang), imagery, biofeedback, and progressive relaxation.

Pharmacology Capsule

Antihypertensive drugs are among those most likely to interfere with erection.

Psychologic Factors. The psychologic aspects of ED are extremely important and should be included in the medical history. Psychogenic ED is often the result of anxiety about performance. Problems may arise with aging, sexual beliefs, or behavior; communication patterns or relationships with sex partners; changes in lifestyle; changes in medications; or chronic or poorly managed disease processes. Anxiety may cause constriction of smooth muscle tissue in the penis and its arteries, reducing inflow and increasing outflow of blood from the penis, leaving it flaccid. Sex therapy that includes behavior modification techniques may be able to restore potency.

Medical Treatment

Drug Therapy

Phosphodiesterase Type 5 Inhibitors. Examples are sildenafil (Viagra), tadalafil (Cialis), and vardenafil (Levitra). These oral vasodilators may be prescribed for failure to fill or store. They must be prescribed with care in patients with cardiovascular disease because of the risk of myocardial infarction and sudden death. They are contraindicated for patients taking nitrate vasodilators or alpha-adrenergic antagonists because of the risk of hypotension and cardiovascular collapse.

Alprostadil. Alprostadil can be used for intracavernosal injection (Caverject) or urethral suppositories (MUSE). It has been successful for some men. It is a vasodilator but produces a more localized effect on arteriole filling and improved storage. Urethral pain and urethritis are possible complications.

Papaverine. Self-injection of intracavernosal papaverine may be recommended for failure to initiate, fill, or store or for psychogenic causes. Papaverine is injected with a small needle into the erectile chambers, with relatively little pain. Erection is achieved within 10 to 15 minutes and lasts 30 to 60 minutes. Papaverine acts on smooth muscles to relax arterial walls and erectile tissue, increasing blood flow into the penis. Papaverine is often mixed with phentolamine, which blocks the constriction of erectile tissue, making it possible to sustain the erection.

Testosterone. Testosterone replacement for men with low hormone levels may improve libido but is unlikely to improve ED (see Table 50-3).

Vacuum Constriction Devices. Vacuum constriction devices may be prescribed for failure to initiate, fill, or store or for psychogenic causes. The flaccid penis is slipped into a cylinder and then the patient squeezes a pump that removes all of the air from the space in the cylinder around the penis, creating a vacuum that draws blood into the penis. When the erection has been achieved, a rubber ring is slipped off the bottom of the cylinder onto the penis near the base, trapping the blood safely for up to about 30 minutes. When air is again allowed into the cylinder, the cylinder can be removed.

Revascularization. Revascularization is a surgical procedure that bypasses blocked arteries, removes or ties off incompetent veins, and tightens the surrounding tissue. This procedure is not commonly done and is generally considered experimental.

Penile Implants. Penile implants (see Fig. 50-8) may be prescribed for patients with failure to initiate or failure to fill or store and for some patients with psychogenic problems that are not appropriate for or responsive to counseling or sex therapy. Semirigid implants are silicon cylinders placed in the erection chambers that keep the penis firm at all times but without increasing circumference. Rigid models can be bent downward but still may not be easily concealed under clothing. Hydraulic implants have cylinders that can be inflated by squeezing a pump in the scrotum or at the end of the penis behind the glans. The pumping action causes the cylinders to fill with fluid from a reservoir in the abdomen or the scrotum. These implants more closely duplicate the natural states of flaccidity and erection.

NURSING CARE of the Patient with Erectile Dysfunction

Assessment

The nursing assessment of a man with ED includes a health history that elicits information about the frequency of intercourse and satisfaction with sexual relations (see *Cultural Considerations* box). The LVN/LPN may collect data that contribute to the complete assessment. The interviewer should not assume that sexual activity is no longer important to older adults. ED may be the first sign of DM, so a complete exploration of the patient's general health and family history to look for diabetes is important. Surgical procedures, injuries, illness, cancer, and medications used regularly should be recorded. The patient's habits and lifestyle, including daily activities, diet, use of alcohol and illicit drugs, exercise habits, lifestyle, health care beliefs, interpersonal relationships, capability for self-care, age, physical condition, and educational needs, should be explored.

Cultural Considerations

What Does Culture Have to Do with Erectile Dysfunction?

Beliefs and values related to sexual function, as well as acceptable forms of sexual expression, are largely learned in one's culture. If a cultural belief is that older adults lose interest in sex as their abilities decline, older adults may try to act accordingly. That is, they may accept erectile dysfunction as "normal" and not seek treatment.

Nursing Diagnoses, Goals, and Outcome Criteria: Erectile Dysfunction

Nursing Diagnoses	Goals and Outcome Criteria
Sexual Dysfunction related to erectile dysfunction	Improved sexual function or satisfying alternatives to sexual intercourse: patient states function has improved or he is satisfied with alternatives
Situational Low Self-Esteem related to impaired sexual function	Improved self-esteem: patient makes more positive comments about self
Ineffective Self-Health Management related to lack of knowledge of factors contributing to erectile dysfunction and measures to improve sexual function or related to reluctance to seek help	Patient understands factors contributing to erectile dysfunction and uses measures to improve sexual function: patient states management is satisfactory

■ Interventions

The management of ED requires sensitivity and knowledge. When a therapeutic relationship has been established with the patient, he may choose to share his concerns with you. Listen and be careful not to dismiss the issue as unimportant. Provide factual information and resources. If you are not well informed about ED, you should refer patients to the physician, advanced practice nurse, or a counselor with training in this area.

PEYRONIE DISEASE

Peyronie disease is the development of a hard, nonelastic, fibrous tissue (plaque) just under the skin on the dorsal surface of the penis. The plaque develops spontaneously or as a result of an injury. It interferes with the ability to fill during an erection. The plaque is usually located on the dorsal midline surface of the penis and results in an upward bending of the penis during erection that may be painful and interfere with successful vaginal penetration (Fig. 50-9). The choice of treatment for Peyronie disease depends on the size of the plaque and the curvature and resultant degree of dysfunction. A variety of drugs have been used with varying degrees of success. Radiation therapy has been used but many experts in the United States do not recommend it. Surgical correction involves excision of the plaque.

PRIAPISM

Priapism is a prolonged, unwanted penile erection that may be classified as low flow or high flow. Low-flow priapism is very painful. It is a medical emergency because it may lead to ischemia of the penis, gangrene, fibrosis, and ED if not treated promptly. Urine flow may be obstructed, causing hydronephrosis. Priapism is associated with many factors, including sickle cell crisis, injury to the penis, leukemia, and malignant tumors. Drugs that may be responsible include cocaine, phosphodiesterase type 5 inhibitors (sildenafil, vardenafil), and papaverine plus phentolamine intracavernosal injections.

Immediate removal of blood may be accomplished by aspirating blood from the erectile chambers or by injecting drugs that cause contraction of smooth muscle, inhibiting inflow of blood and allowing outflow. If these efforts fail, emergency surgery may be needed.

Nursing care must be particularly sensitive to the embarrassment the patient may experience.

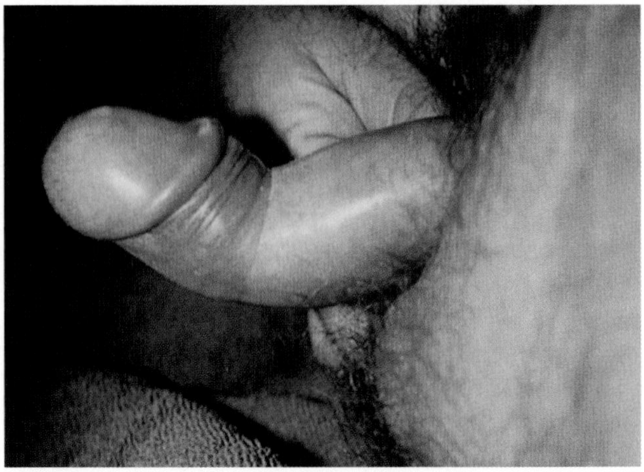

FIGURE 50-9 Peyronie disease. (Courtesy Dr. Hans Stricker, Department of Urology, Henry Ford Hospital, Detroit, Mich.)

Understanding the condition and alleviating pain are important.

PHIMOSIS AND PARAPHIMOSIS

Normally the penile foreskin in the uncircumcised male can be retracted, exposing the glans. Uncircumcised men need to retract the foreskin for cleaning as part of daily hygiene. As a result of poor hygiene, the foreskin may become inflamed and swollen, preventing retraction of the foreskin. This condition, called **phimosis**, is treated with antimicrobial agents and proper cleansing. Circumcision is sometimes recommended to prevent recurrences. **Paraphimosis** is just the opposite in that the foreskin is retracted and cannot be moved over the glans. Constriction of the penis causes the glans to swell. If the foreskin cannot be reduced to cover the glans, surgical intervention is necessary.

INFERTILITY

Infertile is a term used to describe couples who have had unprotected intercourse over a 12-month period and have been unable to become pregnant. **Infertility** may be caused by a reproductive problem in the man, the woman, or both.

Cause and Risk Factors

Male infertility may be related to endocrine disorders, testicular problems, or abnormalities of the ejaculatory system. Correction of endocrine disorders may restore fertility. Infections can affect testicular and ejaculatory function. Structural factors that can affect testicular function are cryptorchidism, testicular torsion, and varicocele (dilation of the veins that drain the testes). Drug therapy, radiation, substance abuse, and environmental hazards also can affect the testes. In addition to infection, the ejaculatory mechanism can be disrupted by obstruction and some surgical procedures.

Infections. Destruction of the seminiferous tubular epithelium results in failure or reduced ability to produce sperm. Mumps may result in acute orchitis and epididymitis, accompanied by fever and debilitating pain, bilateral swelling, and redness of the testicles. If damage to seminiferous epithelium occurs, the size of the testes will be reduced. Other infections such as tuberculosis, pneumonia, and syphilis may affect the testes but less dramatically than mumps.

Genitourinary tract infections can cause infertility in men. *Chlamydia trachomatis* is sexually transmitted and is most prevalent in young adults with multiple sex partners. The infection is most commonly limited to the urethra and causes varying degrees of painful urination and discharge. Progressive infection may include the epididymis and prostate gland. *Neisseria gonorrhoeae* is a common urethral infection in the United States. It is sexually transmitted and may cause extremely painful urination and a purulent discharge. Infections that ascend to the epididymis may result in decreased fertility.

Cryptorchidism. **Cryptorchidism** is defined as any testis located in other than a dependent scrotal position. It is a common congenital condition, being found in approximately 30% of preterm male infants and in 1.0% to 3.4% of full-term male infants (Fig. 50-10). Although genetic disorders can cause cryptorchidism, the cause is usually unknown. Because the abdominal cavity is warmer than the scrotum, excessive warmth can damage the seminiferous epithelium of undescended testes and result in decreased spermatogenesis.

Medical Treatment. Cryptorchidism must be corrected within the first 18 months of life to give the best chance for fertility. Men with undescended testes have a 10 to 30 times higher incidence of testicular cancer than men whose testes descended normally. The risk remains higher even if the condition is subsequently corrected. If the testes are within the normal path but do not descend or cannot be pulled into the scrotum, they usually do not respond to hormonal therapy and surgery is needed. Whether medical or surgical therapy is indicated, it is performed after the first birthday and before the second birthday. Untreated bilateral cryptorchidism results in sterility. Unilateral cryptorchidism may result in a low sperm count but spermatogenesis continues and pregnancies are sometimes initiated without difficulty.

Testicular Torsion. Testicular torsion occurs when the spermatic cord twists, cutting off the blood supply to a testicle (Fig. 50-11). It most commonly occurs in adolescents. Symptoms are intense pain, often accompanied by nausea and vomiting. If it does not resolve spontaneously, emergency surgery is required to untwist the cord and restore blood flow. If the testicle is deprived of blood for more than 4 hours, it may

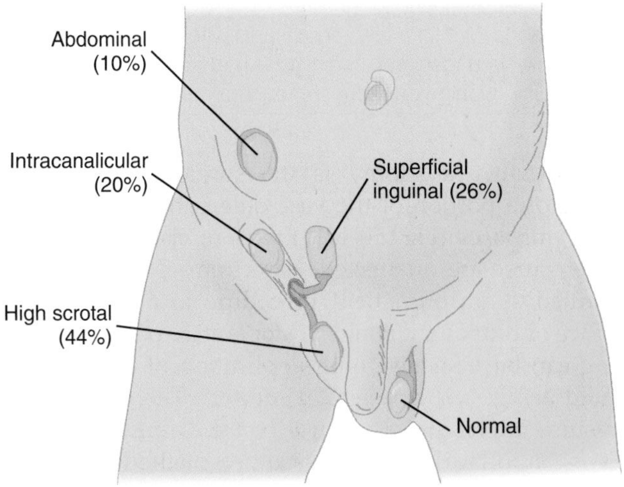

FIGURE 50-10 Common sites of undescended or mispositioned testicles. (From Black JM, Hawks JH: *Medical-surgical nursing: clinical management for positive outcomes*, ed 8, St. Louis, 2009, Saunders.)

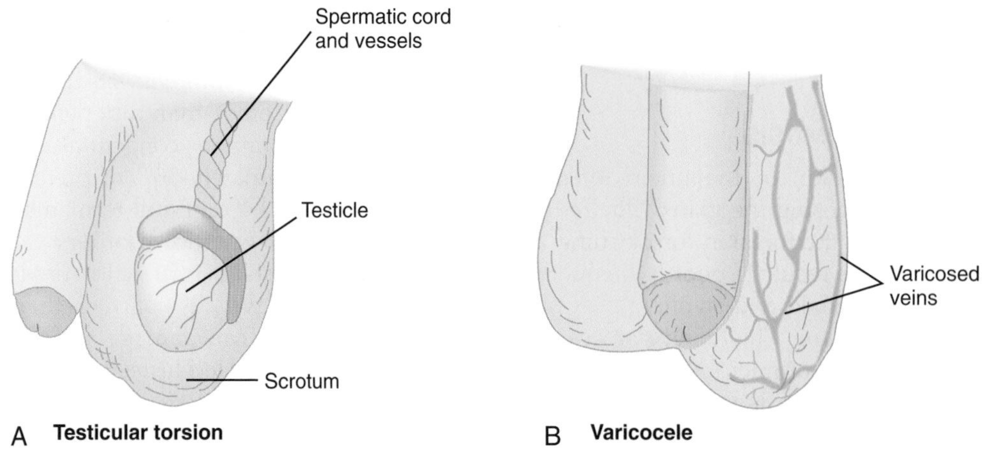

FIGURE 50-11 Disturbances of the testes. **A,** Torsion of the testis. **B,** Varicocele. (From Black JM, Hawks JH: *Medical-surgical nursing: clinical management for positive outcomes*, ed 8, St. Louis, 2009, Saunders.)

become necrotic and require removal. After testicular torsion is corrected, lowered sperm counts and infertility may follow.

Varicocele. A varicocele is a lengthening and enlargement of the scrotal portion of the venous system that drains the testicle (see Fig. 50-11). Varicoceles are caused by incompetent or absent valves in the spermatic venous system, which allows pooled blood and the resulting increased pressure to dilate the veins. Most often, only the left testicle is affected. Affected testicles may be smaller and may have reduced spermatogenesis. Varicoceles are a factor in about half of male infertility cases. Treatment includes surgical ligation or injection of a sclerosing agent into the dilated vein. Varicoceles may reappear after surgery and fertility may or may not improve.

Put on Your Thinking Cap!

A couple visits the clinic seeking help for infertility. During the initial interview, one of them says, "My brother and his wife couldn't get pregnant either. Then he switched from briefs to boxer shorts. Within a few months, his wife was pregnant! Do you think his underwear could have had anything to do with that?" How would you reply appropriately and accurately?

Vasectomy. Vasectomy is the surgical removal or tying of a portion of the vasa deferentia for sterilization purposes (Fig. 50-12). Erection, ejaculation, and intercourse are unaffected. Vasectomy is usually performed as an outpatient procedure in a physician's office or outpatient clinic. Postoperative pain or swelling can be managed with application of an ice bag, mild analgesics, and scrotal support. The patient can resume intercourse as soon as he feels comfortable but it is important that he use other methods of birth control until analysis of the semen determines that a complete absence of sperm exists. The patient can expect the analysis to be done after about 15 ejaculations postvasectomy.

The physician should explain the procedure but the nurse can tell the patient what to expect and reinforce postoperative self-care. Although a vasectomy can sometimes be successfully reversed, it should be considered permanent. The reversal procedure in which the severed ends of the vas deferens are anastomosed (surgically joined) is called a *vasovasectomy.* The nurse should be sensitive to the readiness of the male patient to undergo this procedure. Fears related to postoperative loss of sexual function may cause anxiety in some men, even though they desire the procedure. Acceptance and reassurance are important.

PENILE CANCER

Cancer is a frightening diagnosis for any patient. Cancer of the male reproductive system may arouse the worst fears about sexual dysfunction, disfigurement, and diminished self-esteem. Penile cancer is relatively rare in the United States. Risk factors include not being circumcised in early life, infection with some types of human papillomavirus (HPV) or human immunodeficiency virus (HIV), and smoking. Cancer may appear as a shallow ulcer or dry, painless growth on the penis that is easily confused with a wart. It can be removed surgically if treated in early stages. Growths in advanced stages may ulcerate and involve the foreskin and penile shaft. Extensive resection or amputation as well as resection of nearby lymph nodes may be necessary. Radiotherapy or chemotherapy may be used for advanced cases.

TESTICULAR CANCER

Testicular germ cell carcinoma occurs most often in young men between the ages of 15 and 35 years. Among the risk factors for this type of cancer are cryptorchidism, a genetic abnormality, HIV infection, and acquired immunodeficiency syndrome (AIDS) (see *Cultural Considerations* box). A painless palpable mass or enlargement of one testis is the most common symptom of testicular cancer. A feeling of heaviness

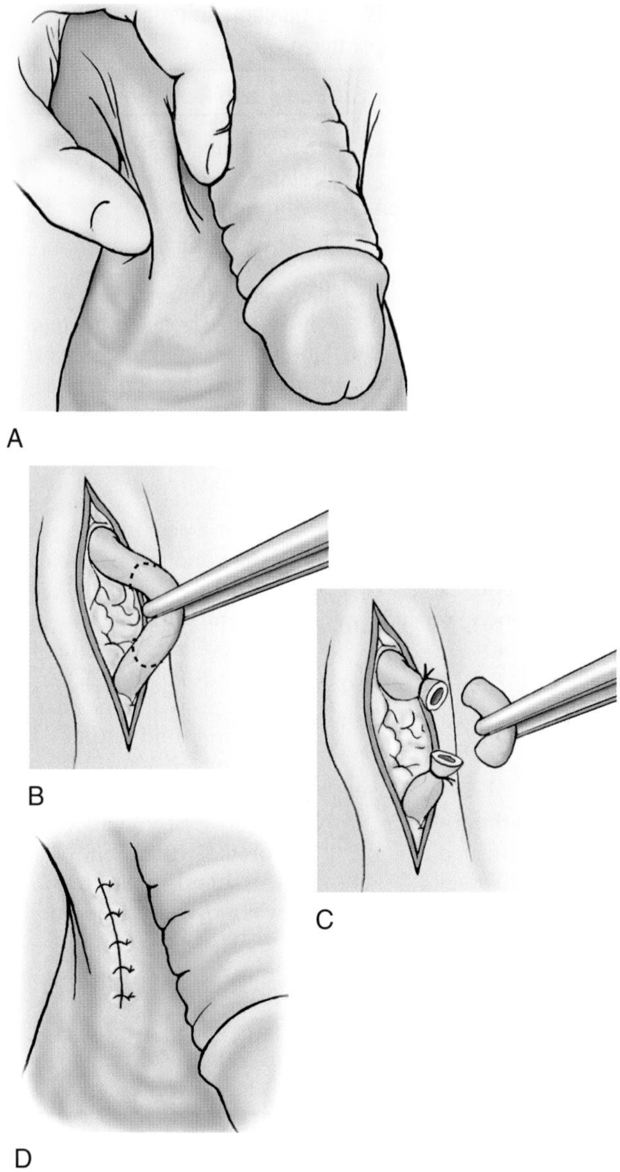
A
B
C
D

FIGURE 50-12 Vasectomy. **A,** Vas deferens located. **B,** Vas deferens exposed. **C,** Small segment of vas deferens removed and severed ends tied. **D,** Scrotal wound closed. (From Monahan FD, Drake DT, Neighbors M, editors: *Medical-surgical nursing: foundations for clinical practice*, ed 2, Philadelphia, 1998, Saunders.)

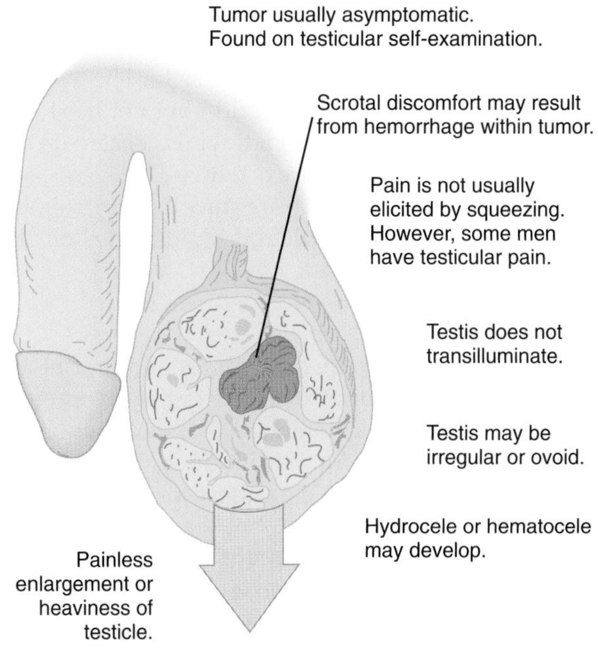
Tumor usually asymptomatic.
Found on testicular self-examination.
Scrotal discomfort may result from hemorrhage within tumor.
Pain is not usually elicited by squeezing. However, some men have testicular pain.
Testis does not transilluminate.
Testis may be irregular or ovoid.
Hydrocele or hematocele may develop.
Painless enlargement or heaviness of testicle.

FIGURE 50-13 Characteristics of testicular tumors. (From Black JM, Hawks JH, Keene AM: *Medical-surgical nursing: clinical management for continuity of care*, ed 6, Philadelphia, 2001, Saunders.)

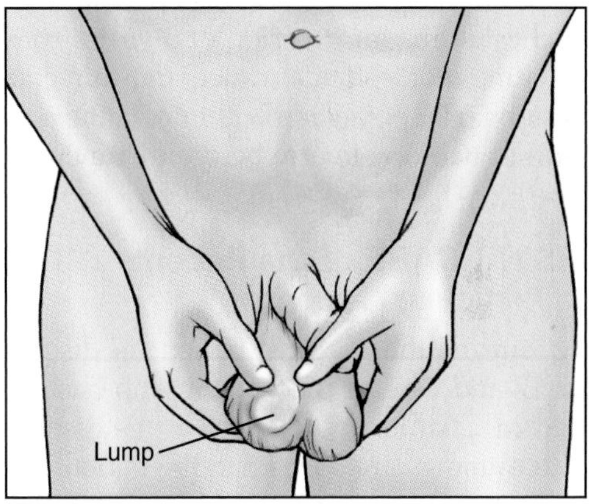
Lump

FIGURE 50-14 Testicular self-examination. (From Monahan FD, Drake DT, Neighbors M, editors: *Medical-surgical nursing: foundations for clinical practice*, ed 2, Philadelphia, 1998, Saunders.)

and pain in the testicle occurs as the tumor grows (Fig. 50-13). The diagnosis is often delayed because patients do not seek medical help.

Cultural Considerations

What Does Culture Have to Do with Testicular Cancer?

Young male Caucasians are at highest risk for testicular cancer. Therefore education in testicular self-examination should target these individuals.

Early Detection

Self-examination and early diagnosis offer the highest chance of finding early-stage disease and subsequent cure. Therefore men need to be educated about the need for self-examination. Although men are used to touching their genitals, they may not feel comfortable examining themselves. Self-examination includes monthly examination of the penis, scrotum, and perineal area. The individual should use a mirror to visualize areas that he cannot see and look for any changes from normal such as swelling, lumps, tenderness, lesions, asymmetry, discoloration, or discharge. The examination is best done after a warm bath or shower, when he is warm and the scrotum is relaxed. The scrotum is held in the palm of his hands with the index and middle fingers on the underside of the testicle and the thumb on top (Fig. 50-14). Each testicle is palpated between the thumbs and forefingers of both hands, with the testicle rolled gently between the fingers. The left testicle usually is lower than the right. The testicles are egg shaped and should feel firm but not hard and smooth without lumps. The epididymis, located on the top and posterior side of each testicle, feels soft and spongy. The spermatic cords are smooth, firm, tubular structures that run upward from the testicles on the back side.

Medical Diagnosis

Diagnostic procedures include ultrasound and blood studies to measure tumor markers: alpha-fetoprotein and human chorionic gonadotropin. If the diagnosis is in doubt, surgical exploration is done. Radiographs and CT scans may be done to assess for metastasis.

Medical and Surgical Treatment

Treatment for testicular cancer is designed according to the type of cancer and the stage. Treatment options are orchiectomy (i.e., surgical excision of the testis), radical orchiectomy, radiation, and chemotherapy. If treated in stage 1, orchiectomy alone is curative for most patients. If desired, a testicular prosthesis may be placed at the time of orchiectomy or later. Follow-up includes monitoring tumor marker levels and abdominal and chest scans for a period of 5 years from diagnosis. Treatment of testicular cancer may affect fertility and erections. The physician will inform the patient of the option of banking sperm before treatment begins.

NURSING CARE of the Patient with Testicular Cancer

Nursing care of the surgical patient is discussed in Chapter 17 and care of the patient who has cancer is discussed in Chapter 25. Therefore this discussion is limited to nursing care specific to the patient with testicular cancer.

Assessment

The nursing assessment of the male reproductive system is outlined in Box 50-1. When a patient has testicular cancer, fears or concerns related to the effects of surgery and other treatment must be assessed.

Interventions

Anxiety

From the time cancer is suspected, the patient faces anxiety-producing threats to self-image and self-esteem. You must be sensitive to the patient's fears of altered sexual function, loss of fertility, stressful treatments, and the threat of a potentially fatal disease. You can help the patient through listening actively, providing information, and referring him for counseling if needed. The patient may wish to have a significant other included in interactions with you and other health professionals.

Nursing Diagnoses, Goals, and Outcome Criteria: Testicular Cancer, Postoperative

Nursing Diagnoses	Goals and Outcome Criteria
Anxiety related to the diagnosis of cancer and the anticipation of side effects of treatments	Reduced anxiety: patient states anxiety is reduced, calm manner
Acute Pain related to surgical incision	Pain relief: patient states pain is relieved, relaxed manner
Impaired Urinary Elimination related to the effects of anesthesia and abdominal or pelvic surgery	Normal urine elimination: no bladder distention
Risk for Injury (shock, infection, fluid and electrolyte imbalances) related to surgery	Absence of excess bleeding or infection and normal fluid balance: vital signs consistent with patient norms, oral temperature less than 101°F (38.3°C), electrolytes within normal ranges and fluid output approximately equal to fluid intake
Constipation related to diminished or absent peristalsis caused by bowel manipulation during surgery (with abdominal procedure)	Normal bowel elimination: no abdominal distention, bowel sounds present, bowel movements resume
Situational Low Self-Esteem and **Disturbed Body Image** related to potential loss of reproductive capacity and loss of one or both testes.	Improved self-esteem: patient makes positive remarks about self
Deficient Knowledge of disease, treatment, and self-care	Patient understands disease, treatment, and self-care: patient accurately describes condition, treatment, side effects, and management of side effects; patient demonstrates self-care

Acute Pain

The amount of postoperative pain will vary with the type of procedure done. Assess pain with each vital sign check and take steps to treat it promptly. In addition to analgesics, you can use other pain control techniques such as mental imagery and relaxation exercises (see Chapter 15).

Impaired Urinary Elimination

Radical orchiectomy usually requires a short hospitalization and has few complications. Nevertheless, monitor the patient's urinary status to confirm normal function before discharge. If the patient has a radical retroperitoneal lymph node dissection, he probably will have a catheter immediately after surgery.

Risk for Injury

Some patients with testicular cancer undergo radical retroperitoneal lymph node dissection. These patients have extensive surgical incisions and usually need intensive nursing care initially. As with any major abdominal surgery, the patient is at risk for shock, infection, bowel and bladder dysfunction, and fluid and electrolyte imbalances. Shock can result from fluid loss and the effects of anesthesia during the lengthy surgery. Measure and evaluate vital signs and fluid intake and output. Monitor the patient's electrolyte levels and administer intravenous fluids as ordered to maintain fluid and electrolyte balance. The patient is likely to have a urinary catheter in place and a nasogastric tube attached to suction.

Constipation

Palpate the abdomen for bowel or bladder distention and auscultate for bowel sounds. When permitted, encourage ambulation, increased fluid intake unless contraindicated, and a diet with adequate fiber to promote bowel elimination. Administer stool softeners as ordered.

Situational Low Self-Esteem and Disturbed Body Image

The patient may or may not be rendered sterile as a result of the treatment used. Radical orchiectomy results in sterility but does not impair erection and orgasm. If radiotherapy is used, the patient's sperm count typically declines at first but usually returns to normal by 2 to 3 years after treatment is completed. The effects of chemotherapy on fertility vary with the drug used. Retroperitoneal lymph node dissection often causes ED and problems with ejaculation. Help the patient to formulate questions for the physician about the effects of specific treatments on sexual function and fertility. If sterility is anticipated, the patient should be counseled preoperatively about the possibility of banking sperm for future use. Because this type of cancer commonly affects young men, the potential to father a child at a later date may be very important to them.

Deficient Knowledge

Teaching is essential to prepare the patient for treatment and to provide the tools needed for him to cope with the diagnosis. The patient teaching plan will vary greatly with the extent of the cancer and the type of treatment given. Include the type of therapy prescribed, the side effects, the management of side effects, and available resources.

Get Ready for the NCLEX® Examination!

Key Points

- The male reproductive system consists of the scrotum, testes, epididymides, vasa deferentia, seminal vesicles, prostate gland, ejaculatory duct, Cowper glands, internal urethra, and penis.
- Prostatitis is an inflammation of the prostate gland that is treated with antimicrobials, analgesics, and sitz baths.
- Epididymitis is an inflammation of the epididymis that is treated with bed rest, cold packs, sitz baths, analgesics, antibiotics, and scrotal support.
- Benign prostatic hyperplasia—enlargement of the prostate gland that may lead to obstruction of the urethra—may be treated with drugs or surgical intervention.
- Nursing care after prostatectomy addresses risk for deficient fluid volume, acute pain, risk for infection, risk for injury, urge urinary incontinence, sexual dysfunction, situational low self-esteem, and deficient knowledge.
- Erectile dysfunction (impotence), the inability to achieve or maintain an erection adequate for sexual intercourse, may be treated with psychologic intervention, oral drug therapy, vacuum constriction devices, self-injection therapy, intraurethral pellets, or penile implants.
- Nursing care of the patient with ED may focus on sexual dysfunction, situational low self-esteem, and ineffective self-health management.
- Peyronie disease is the formation of fibrous tissue in the penis that causes it to bend upward during erection, causing pain and interfering with vaginal penetration.
- Priapism is prolonged penile erection not related to sexual desire that requires emergency treatment to prevent ischemia, gangrene, fibrosis, and future ED.
- Infertility is the inability to impregnate despite unprotected intercourse over a 12-month period.
- Causes of infertility include endocrine or testicular dysfunction and disorders of the ejaculatory system.
- Cancer of the male reproductive system may affect the penis, testicles, or prostate gland.
- Nursing care of the patient with testicular cancer focuses on anxiety, acute pain, risk for injury, impaired urine elimination, constipation, situational low self-esteem, and deficient knowledge.
- Other disorders affecting the male reproductive system are hydrocele, phimosis, and paraphimosis.

Additional Learning Resources

SG Go to your Study Guide for additional learning activities to help you master this chapter content.

evolve Go to your Evolve website (http://evolve.elsevier.com/Linton/medsurg) for the following learning resources and much more:

- Interactive Prioritization Exercises
- Fluid & Electrolyte Tutorial
- Pharmacology Tutorial
- Review Questions for the NCLEX® Examination

Review Questions for the NCLEX® Examination

1. The school nurse is teaching students about normal growth and development. The nurse should inform the students that the hormone responsible for male sexual development is:
   1. LH
   2. Testosterone
   3. Gonadotropin
   4. Progesterone

   NCLEX Client Need: Health Promotion and Maintenance
2. Normal age-related changes in the reproductive system of a healthy man include which of the following? (Select all that apply.)
   1. Decreasing production of testosterone beginning at age 50
   2. Longer refractory period between erections
   3. Loss of ability to maintain an erection by age 70
   4. Increased time needed for sexual arousal
   5. Lack of interest in sexual activity

   NCLEX Client Need: Health Promotion and Maintenance
3. Which of the following should be included when teaching a patient about benign prostatic hyperplasia? (Select all that apply.)
   1. Moderate use of alcohol will promote emptying of the bladder.
   2. Void promptly when you feel the urge to empty your bladder.
   3. Limit your daily fluid intake to six glasses of water.
   4. Medications that contain antihistamines may cause you to retain urine.
   5. Prolonged exposure to warm temperatures promotes bladder spasms.

   NCLEX Client Need: Physiological Integrity: Reduction of Risk Potential
4. Bleeding after a transurethral prostatectomy is *most likely* to be detected by inspection of which of the following?
   1. Abdominal dressing
   2. Perineal drainage
   3. Urine characteristics
   4. Suprapubic drain

   NCLEX Client Need: Physiological Integrity: Reduction of Risk Potential
5. Which of the following is a drug that reduces the size of the prostate without lowering circulating testosterone levels?
   1. Tamsulosin (Flomax)
   2. Flutamide (Eulexin)
   3. Oxybutynin chloride (Ditropan)
   4. Finasteride (Proscar)

   NCLEX Client Need: Physiological Integrity: Pharmacological Therapies
6. When preparing to irrigate a urinary catheter for a patient who had a prostatectomy this morning, the nurse checks to be certain that she has normal saline solution. Why is normal saline preferable for urinary catheter irrigation?
   1. It is isotonic and will not cause water intoxication.
   2. It is less expensive than sterile water for irrigation.
   3. It is absorbed into the bloodstream to maintain blood volume.
   4. Sterile water stings when it comes in contact with the surgical sites.

   NCLEX Client Need: Physiological Integrity: Reduction of Risk Potential
7. A couple has come to the fertility clinic for evaluation. During the health history, the husband reports having had all of the childhood diseases listed below. Which may be significant in relation to infertility in men?
   1. Measles
   2. Chickenpox
   3. Mumps
   4. Diphtheria

   NCLEX Client Need: Physiological Integrity: Physiological Adaptation
8. A nurse in the newborn nursery assesses a newborn male for the presence of the testes in the scrotum. The nurse knows that failure of the testes to descend into the scrotum (cryptorchidism) must be treated early in life to prevent:
   1. Testicular torsion
   2. Varicocele
   3. Chronic infection
   4. Sterility

   NCLEX Client Need: Health Promotion and Maintenance
9. Patient teaching related to vasectomy should include which of the following?
   1. You will be sterile immediately after the procedure.
   2. Vasectomy is easily reversible if you wish to father a child later.
   3. Postoperative problems with erection and ejaculation are common.
   4. You will need to have a semen analysis to determine if sperm are present.

   NCLEX Client Need: Physiological Integrity: Reduction of Risk Potential
10. A patient is undergoing treatment for prostate cancer. The clinic nurse reminds him that he will need to come in periodically for which of the following to determine the effectiveness of his treatment?
    1. Measurement of the PSA level
    2. Periodic biopsies of perineal tissue
    3. Studies of urine flow rates
    4. Radiographs of the abdomen

    NCLEX Client Need: Physiological Integrity: Reduction of Risk Potential

chapter 51

Sexually Transmitted Infections

http://evolve.elsevier.com/Linton/medsurg

Objectives

1. Describe tests used to diagnose sexually transmitted infections and the nursing considerations associated with each.
2. Explain why specific sexually transmitted infections must be reported to the health department.
3. List infectious diseases classified as *sexually transmitted infections.*
4. Describe the pathophysiology, signs and symptoms, complications, and medical treatment for selected sexually transmitted infections.
5. Explain the importance of the nurse's approach when dealing with patients who have sexually transmitted infections.
6. List nursing considerations when a patient is on drug therapy for a sexually transmitted infection.
7. Identify data to be collected when assessing a patient with a sexually transmitted infection.
8. Assist in developing a nursing care plan for a patient with a sexually transmitted infection.
9. Design a teaching plan on the prevention of sexually transmitted infections.

Key Terms

Chancre (SHĂNG-kĕr)
Latent (LĀ-tĕnt)
Opportunistic infections
Pelvic inflammatory disease (PID)
Sexually transmitted infections (STIs)

Sexually transmitted infections (STIs) include a number of conditions that can be transmitted from one person to another during intimate contact. The term *sexually transmitted disease (STD)* is commonly used to describe these same conditions as well. The difference in the two terms is that a disease, by definition, has recognizable signs and symptoms whereas infections may or may not manifest specific signs and symptoms.

Despite medical advances, STIs continue to be a serious public health problem in the United States. Worldwide the incidence of STIs increases every year. Each year, more than 100,000 women are left sterile by STIs. In the United States, an estimated 20 million new infections occur each year. Almost half of these are in persons aged 15 to 24 years. Although STIs are more common in people of lower socioeconomic status and in those with less education and limited access to health care, all segments of the population are represented. Drug abuse and having multiple sexual partners also are risk factors. In the United States, STI rates are highest among African Americans, followed by Latinos and then by non-Latino Caucasians (see *Cultural Considerations* box).

Despite public education efforts, some people resist taking preventive measures. Infected people do not always inform their sexual partners, so the disease continues to be passed on to others. In addition, symptoms are sometimes absent or subtle; thus STIs that go undetected can spread and invade other parts of the body. These infections may have serious and permanent consequences.

Nurses must be aware of their feelings about working with people who have STIs. A stigma is associated with these infections and we must ensure the same quality of care to patients with an STI that we give to patients with any other diagnoses. Judgmental behavior on the part of health care providers discourages people from seeking appropriate medical care. In this chapter, specific diseases are explained, followed by a general discussion of nursing care appropriate for all patients with STIs.

> **Cultural Considerations**
>
> **What Does Culture Have to Do with Sexually Transmitted Infections?**
>
> The incidence of sexually transmitted infections (STIs) varies among races, but poverty, lack of education, and limited access to health care probably play a larger role than race and ethnicity. In addition, cultural beliefs about sexual practices, use of condoms, and educating children about STI prevention may all affect the incidence of STIs in any given population.

DIAGNOSTIC TESTS AND PROCEDURES

Individuals who engage in high-risk sexual behaviors are at increased risk for each of the STIs. Therefore patients diagnosed with one STI should be evaluated for others as well. Infections with some STIs actually appear to increase the risk of human immunodeficiency virus (HIV) infection. The primary measures used to diagnose STIs are serologic tests and studies of smears and cultures. Some over-the-counter (OTC) tests can be purchased for home use or mail service. Concerns with this type of testing include possible false-negative or false-positive results, uncertainty about the reliability of a specific product or lab, and possible delayed treatment of serious infections.

SEROLOGIC TESTS

Serologic tests may be ordered to detect infections with hepatitis A, B, C, D, and E; syphilis; HIV; herpes simplex; and cytomegalovirus. These tests are designed to detect infections by measuring antigens or antibodies in the blood. Many factors can cause inaccurate results, especially with older tests. Agency laboratory procedures specify the patient preparation for specific tests.

SMEARS, SWABS, AND CULTURES

Patients with gonococcal, chlamydial, herpes simplex, *Trichomonas*, or yeast infections often have discharge from the vagina or penis. In addition to this discharge, exudate from lesions can be collected and studied to determine the exact infecting organism. For women, the sample may be collected from the vagina or cervix. The procedure varies with the type of organism suspected. To collect a sample from a male patient, a swab or special loop may be used. The person who collects the sample wears gloves and treats the sample as a potential source of infection. The sample may be submitted for microscopic examination or for culture and sensitivity tests.

Pharmacology Capsule

When you have an order to obtain a specimen for culture and another order to administer antiinfective agents, collect the specimen before giving the first dose of the antiinfective.

DRUG THERAPY

The drugs recommended by the Centers for Disease Control and Prevention (CDC) are noted with the discussion of each specific infection. The CDC also recommends alternate drugs for people who are allergic to the primary drugs, pregnant women, infants and children, and people who are being treated for multiple infections. Details are available at the CDC website: www.cdc.gov/std/treatment/2010/toc.htm. Examples of drugs commonly used to treat STIs are presented in Table 51-1.

REPORTING SEXUALLY TRANSMITTED INFECTIONS

Confirmed cases of HIV, acquired immunodeficiency syndrome (AIDS), gonorrhea, syphilis, chlamydia, chancroid, and viral hepatitis are among the infections that must be reported to the local health department. A current list is posted yearly at http://wwwn.cdc.gov/NNDSS/script/ConditionList.aspx?Type=0&Yr=2014. An investigator asks the patient to name his or her sexual contacts. Those individuals are contacted and advised that they have been exposed to the disease and are encouraged to seek medical evaluation. The purpose of this process is to identify and treat infected individuals so that transmission of the infection can be slowed. Another approach is to provide the patient with a prescription or additional drugs for his or her sexual partner without examination of the partner. This approach, which is legal in some but not all states, is called *expedited partner therapy (EPT)*.

SPECIFIC SEXUALLY TRANSMITTED INFECTIONS

CHLAMYDIAL INFECTION

Chlamydial infection is thought to be the most common bacterial STI in the United States. More than 1 million new cases are reported to the CDC each year. The symptoms are similar to those of gonorrhea. Chlamydia is an intracellular bacterium that comprises multiple genera and species. The specific species that causes the infection classified with STIs is *Chlamydia trachomatis*. This infection is transmitted by contact with the mucous membranes in the mouth, eyes, urethra, vagina, or rectum. Clinical manifestations can include urethritis, epididymitis, cervicitis, pelvic inflammatory disease (PID), proctitis, oropharyngeal infection, reactive arthritis, and conjunctivitis. Newborns of infected women may have eye infections (infant inclusion conjunctivitis) or infant pneumonia. Therefore erythromycin ophthalmic ointment may be ordered for the newborn because it is effective against chlamydial infection as well as gonorrhea.

Lymphogranuloma venereum (LGV) is a more invasive systemic infection caused by the LGV strain of *C. trachomatis*. Lesions may affect the inguinal lymph nodes and the rectal mucosa. Chlamydia facilitates the transmission of HIV.

Signs and Symptoms

One reason chlamydial infection is so common is that most people have no symptoms. Symptoms, if any, are generally noted 1 to 3 weeks after being infected. Symptoms are more noticeable in men and include penile discharge, which is initially thin and becomes creamy later. Another common complaint among men is painful or frequent urination. Women may experience vaginal discharge, painful urination, nausea, fever, painful intercourse, bleeding between menstrual

Table 51-1 Drug Therapy: Drugs Used to Treat Sexually Transmitted Infections

General Considerations

- Always assess for history of allergies before giving any antimicrobial.
- If the patient reports being allergic to the prescribed drug, withhold it and notify the physician.
- Observe all patients for possible allergic responses: rash, difficulty breathing, hypotension.
- Obtain specimens for culture before administering the first dose of the antimicrobial.
- When giving intravenous antimicrobials through a secondary line, check compatibility with primary fluid.
- Tell the patient it is important to complete the full course of treatment to prevent organisms from becoming resistant and to prevent relapse because all organisms had not been killed.
- Tell the patient that the sexual partner or partners should be treated at the same time to prevent infection.
- Assess for drug interactions.

DRUG	USE AND ACTION	SIDE EFFECTS	NURSING INTERVENTIONS
Antibacterial Agents			
Beta-Lactams			
penicillin G (Bicillin, Pfizerpen, Crysticillin, Benzathine)	First choice for treatment of syphilis.	Nausea, vomiting, diarrhea, pain at injection site, anaphylaxis. Jarisch-Herxheimer reaction: headache, fever, chills, diaphoresis, tachycardia, muscle and joint pain. If allergic to cephalosporins, may also be allergic to penicillins.	Scratch test may be ordered to assess allergy. Alternative drugs are available if allergic. Check drug insert for preparation of injection. (Give by deep injection in large muscle. Do not pause during injection; needle may clog. Massage site.) Have patient wait 30 minutes after injection in case there is allergic reaction. Tell patient Jarisch-Herxheimer reaction may occur; resolves within 24 hours.
ceftriaxone sodium (Rocephin)	Effective against organism that causes gonorrhea.	Nausea, vomiting, headache, dizziness, and (rarely) bleeding. Allergic reactions, including anaphylaxis. Patients allergic to penicillin may have cross-sensitivity to cephalosporins. Nephrotoxicity with high doses or renal disease. Superinfections: diarrhea, candidiasis. IV route: pain, thrombophlebitis. Intramuscular (IM) route: pain, induration at injection site.	Notify physician of profuse, watery diarrhea. Report vaginal or anal itching. Assess for bruising, bleeding. IM injection is painful.
Tetracyclines			
doxycycline (Vibramycin)	Effective against organisms that cause gonorrhea (in combination with ceftriaxone), chlamydia, granuloma inguinale, syphilis, and lymphogranuloma venereum.	Anorexia, nausea, vomiting, diarrhea, dysphagia, fungal infections, anaphylaxis, increased intracranial pressure, photosensitivity. Rarely: rash, urticaria, hemolytic anemia.	Assess allergies to tetracycline and to sulfites. Monitor food intake and stools. Assess blood pressure and level of consciousness. Report genital or anal itching. Give with full glass of water.
Macrolides			
erythromycin (E-Mycin, Ilosone, Erythrocin Stearate)	Effective against organisms that cause chlamydial infection, syphilis, and gonorrhea. Ophthalmic ointment used in newborn to prevent eye infection.	Nausea, vomiting, diarrhea, phlebitis at infusion site, allergic reactions, hepatitis, ototoxicity.	Report tinnitus or jaundice. Give oral drug on empty stomach with full glass of water—no fruit juice.

Continued

Table 51-1 Drug Therapy: Drugs Used to Treat Sexually Transmitted Infections—cont'd

DRUG	USE AND ACTION	SIDE EFFECTS	NURSING INTERVENTIONS
azithromycin (Zithromax)	Effective against *Chlamydia* (which causes urethritis and cervicitis). Used in combination with ceftriaxone for gonorrhea.	Diarrhea, nausea, vomiting, abdominal pain, vaginitis.	Caution if patient has liver impairment. Do not give with antacids. Give 1 hour before meals or 2 hours after meals.
Miscellaneous Antiinfectives			
tinidazole (Tindamax) metronidazole (Flagyl)	Tinidazole is first choice for *Trichomonas.* Metronidazole is used to treat bacterial vaginosis and is second choice for treating *Trichomonas.*	Headache, dizziness, nausea, vomiting, abdominal pain, anorexia, diarrhea, skin irritation, peripheral neuropathy, leukopenia.	Give with food or milk. Instruct patient not to take a double dose if a dose is missed. Tell patient to avoid alcohol. Advise patient to follow safety precautions if dizziness occurs. Monitor fluid status because drug contains sodium. Urine may be dark. Monitor blood cell counts. Severe reaction with alcohol
clindamycin vaginal cream	Used to treat bacterial vaginosis.	Headache, dizziness, abdominal pain, nausea, vomiting.	Advise patient that cream weakens latex condoms and diaphragms, which may interfere with their effectiveness. Instruct in use of applicator. Should be used at bedtime. Wash hands after use. Avoid sexual intercourse during treatment. Advise sanitary napkin to prevent stains on clothing.
Antivirals			
acyclovir (Zovirax) valacyclovir (Valtrex) famciclovir (Famvir)	Decreases frequency and severity of genital herpes infections. Is not curative.	Dizziness, headache, diarrhea, nausea, vomiting, renal failure, seizures.	Apply ointment with gloved finger. Do not double up if an oral dose is missed. Tell patient drug is not curative. Condoms should be used during sexual contact and sexual contact should be avoided when lesions are present.
Dermatologic Agents			
podophyllin (Podocon-25)	Topical agent used to remove genital warts.	Highly caustic; can be applied directly on warts. Excessive application can cause kidney damage, neuropathy, blood dyscrasias. Teratogenic; contraindicated during pregnancy.	Should be applied only by physician. Treated area must be washed with alcohol or soap and water within 1–4 hours.
imiquimod (Aldara)		Erythema, erosion, flaking. Local itching, burning, pain. No systemic effects.	Instruct patient to apply at bedtime and wash off in morning. Usual application is 3 times/week for 16 weeks or until warts are gone.

Table 51-1 **Drug Therapy: Drugs Used to Treat Sexually Transmitted Infections—cont'd**

DRUG	USE AND ACTION	SIDE EFFECTS	NURSING INTERVENTIONS
podofilox (Condylox)		Local inflammation, erosion, pain, itching, bleeding. Causes more discomfort than imiquimod but costs less and treatment is shorter.	Instruct patient to apply twice daily for 3 consecutive days, then take 4 days off. The cycle can be repeated if needed for a maximum of 4 cycles until the warts are gone. Does not have to be washed off. Advise patient not to use more than 0.5 mg/day and apply only to warts, not to normal skin.
kunecatechins (Sinecatechins)	Used to treat genital warts.	Erythema, pruritus, burning, pain, ulceration, edema, rash.	Must be applied three times a day or for 16 weeks until warts clear. Advise patient to avoid sexual contact when gel is applied. Do not apply to vagina, rectum, or open wounds.
HAART (Highly Active Antiretroviral Therapy) Agents			
A highly effective strategy to treat human immunodeficiency virus (HIV) infection by using various combinations of nonnucleoside reverse transcriptase inhibitors, nucleoside reverse transcriptase inhibitors, and protease inhibitors. See details in Chapter 35.			

periods, and lower abdominal pain. Rectal infection is characterized by pain, discharge, bleeding (or a combination of these problems). Unlike other forms of chlamydial infection, LGV patients have fever, muscle aches, swollen inguinal lymph nodes, and elevated white blood cell (WBC) count.

Complications

If left untreated, chlamydial infection can result in sterility in men and women. The sperm ducts can become inflamed and blocked. In women, **pelvic inflammatory disease (PID)**, which involves the ovaries, fallopian tubes, and pelvic area, can block the fallopian tubes and damage the uterus. The risk of ectopic pregnancy (i.e., the fertilized ovum develops outside the uterus) is increased in the presence of chlamydial infection. In addition, women with chlamydial infection are approximately five times more likely to become infected with HIV if exposed to it.

Medical Diagnosis and Treatment

The diagnosis is based on the individual's sexual history and the results of laboratory studies. The nucleic acid amplification test (NAAT) is the most effective diagnostic tool; it has largely replaced the cell tissue culture.

The infection usually is treated with a single dose of azithromycin (Zithromax) or a 7-day course of doxycycline (Vibramycin). Review the patient's complete drug profile because azithromycin (Zithromax) interacts with many other common drugs. Other antimicrobials also may be administered because patients with chlamydial infection may have gonorrhea as well. The culture should be repeated 3 to 4 months after treatment to confirm successful treatment. The patient is advised to avoid all sexual contact (genital, oral, anal) until a cure has been achieved. When sexual activity is resumed, condom use is recommended to prevent reinfection.

Nursing care of the patient with chlamydial infection and other STIs is discussed in the section titled "Nursing Care of the Patient with a Sexually Transmitted Infection." Information about chlamydial infection is summarized in Table 51-2.

GONORRHEA

Gonorrhea is one of the most commonly reported STIs in the United States. According to the CDC, 334,826 new cases of gonorrhea were reported in 2012. Gonorrhea is transmitted most often through direct sexual contact. Cases have been reported of transmission to newborn infants by infected mothers and to medical personnel with skin lacerations who have come in contact with infected fluids. The infection is not picked up from toilet seats, doorknobs, or towels.

The bacterium that causes this disease is *Neisseria gonorrhoeae*. This organism lives in warm, moist areas of the body such as the cervix and the urethra. Areas affected by local gonorrhea infections may include the pharynx, rectum, urethra, prostate, epididymis, uterus, and fallopian tubes. A high incidence of rectal gonorrhea exists among men who have sex with men. The presence of bacteria in the throat is common among individuals who perform oral sex (fellatio) on an infected partner. With systemic (disseminated)

Table 51-2 Chlamydial Infection

SIGNS AND SYMPTOMS	POSSIBLE COMPLICATIONS	MEDICAL TREATMENT	NURSING CONSIDERATIONS
Sometimes no signs or symptoms. *Males:* penile discharge (thin at first, then creamy); painful, frequent urination. *Females:* vaginal discharge, lower abdominal pain.	Sterility in both sexes. Transmission to newborn infants, causing eye infections or pneumonia.	azithromycin (Zithromax) or doxycycline (Vibramycin).	Counsel about importance of treatment to prevent complications. Advise of need for follow-up to ensure that infection has been treated successfully. Tell patient to avoid sexual contact until cured.

infection, the heart, joints, skin, and meninges may become involved.

Signs and Symptoms

Many people with gonorrhea have no symptoms. When present, symptoms typically occur 2 to 10 days after exposure and are generally more apparent in men than in women. Men who do have symptoms often have whitish or greenish discharge from the penis and often complain of a burning sensation during urination. Testicular pain and swelling may be present. Women may experience vaginal discharge, bleeding during sexual intercourse, redness and swelling of the external genitalia, a burning sensation during urination, abdominal pain, or abnormal menstruation. A rectal infection may cause discharge, anal itching, soreness, bleeding, or painful bowel movements. Symptoms of rectal infection usually occur 2 to 5 days after infection but may be as long as 30 days later. Throat infections usually have no symptoms but a sore throat may be present. Symptoms generally disappear after a few weeks but if the infection is untreated, the bacteria remain in the body and the person remains highly infectious.

Complications

If untreated, gonorrhea can cause sterility in both sexes and infections that may lead to damage to heart tissue and joints. Men may develop epididymitis and prostatitis. Women may develop PID. People with gonorrhea are at increased risk for HIV; people with HIV *and* gonorrhea are more likely to transmit HIV to another person.

Medical Diagnosis

The diagnosis is based on the individual's health history and physical examination findings as well as on laboratory studies. Although smears and cultures of exudate from infected body parts or urinalysis are still used in some settings, NAATs are now the preferred diagnostic tool.

Medical Treatment

Treatment is usually initiated based on the physical examination without waiting for laboratory results. This is because many patients will not return for follow-up and immediate treatment has been highly effective. Treatment usually consists of a single dose of intramuscular ceftriaxone sodium (Rocephin) and either azithromycin or doxycycline. One of these regimens cures most cases of gonorrhea quickly and safely. Penicillin is not used as much as it once was because many organisms have developed resistance to it. Erythromycin ophthalmic ointment may be ordered for the newborn to prevent eye infection caused by exposure to gonococci during delivery.

Instruct patients to follow up with a physician to ensure that the treatment was effective. Additional information about drug therapy for gonorrhea is provided in Table 51-1.

Nursing care of the patient with gonorrhea and other STIs is discussed in the section titled "Nursing Care of the Patient with a Sexually Transmitted Infection." Table 51-3 summarizes information related to the signs and symptoms of gonorrhea, the possible complications, the medical treatment, and the nursing considerations.

Follow-up examination is essential after antimicrobial therapy for gonorrhea to ensure that the infection has been eradicated.

SYPHILIS

Syphilis is caused by a spirochete (coiled bacterium) called *Treponema pallidum*. The organism is generally transmitted by sexual contact but also can be spread through breaks in the skin. It also can be passed through the placenta, thus causing an infant to be born with the disease (i.e., congenital syphilis). In the United States in 2012, 15,667 new cases of primary and secondary syphilis and 322 cases of congenital syphilis were reported.

Signs and Symptoms

Signs and symptoms change throughout the course of the disease. If untreated, syphilis progresses through four stages: (1) primary, (2) secondary, (3) latent, and (4) late.

Primary Stage. A typical lesion, called a **chancre**, is the first sign of syphilis. The chancre is generally first noticed 1 to 12 weeks after contact. During the primary

Table 51-3 Gonorrhea

SIGNS AND SYMPTOMS	POSSIBLE COMPLICATIONS	MEDICAL TREATMENT	NURSING CONSIDERATIONS
Men: Thick urethral discharge (purulent green or yellow), swelling and redness of the meatus, urinary urgency and dribbling.	Epididymitis, urethritis, infections of Cowper and Tyson glands.	Treated with ceftriaxone (Rocephin) and azithromycin OR doxycycline (Vibramycin).	Send specimen to lab for culture. Instruct the patient that all sexual partners should also be treated. Instruct the patient to take complete prescription of the drug (if receiving ciprofloxacin [Cipro] or tetracycline for self-medication), even if symptoms have disappeared. Stress abstinence or condom use.
Women: Increased, foul-smelling vaginal discharge; dysuria (difficulty urinating); fever; abnormal or painful menstruation; vulval soreness; peritonitis; backache; lower back pain (usually involving only one side).	Infertility, urethral and labial infection, risk of tubal pregnancy, pelvic inflammatory disease (PID), septicemia.	Same as for male patients.	Counsel the patient about potential complications.

stage, a reddish papule appears where the organism entered the body, usually on the genitals, anus, or mouth. Within 1 week, the papule becomes a painless red ulcer. Lymph nodes in the area of the chancre may be enlarged but are not tender. The chancre may last from 1 to 5 weeks. When it disappears, patients may assume that they are cured when in fact the infecting organism has moved into the blood (Fig. 51-1).

Secondary Stage. The secondary stage occurs 1 to 6 months after contact. Symptoms may include a rash on the extremities, chest or back, palms of the hands, and soles of the feet. Pustules that contain highly contagious material often develop. Fever, sore throat, and generalized aching are also seen in this stage. The patient is contagious during the first and second stages.

Latent Stage. The **latent** stage, in which no symptoms exist, follows the secondary stage. Although no symptoms are present, the organisms are invading the major organs. The infection is not spread by sexual contact during the latent stage but may be transmitted by blood exposure.

Late ("Tertiary") Stage. It is generally 3 years after contact before late syphilis develops, although it may be decades. Even without treatment, most patients never advance to this stage. Signs and symptoms of late syphilis include arthritis, numbness of the extremities, lesions of the skin and internal organs (called gummas), and pain because of damage to the heart, blood vessels (especially the aorta), or central nervous system.

Complications

The patient with untreated syphilis may develop severe, potentially fatal complications, including neurosyphilis (meningitis, blindness, paralysis) and cardiovascular disease. An infected woman who becomes pregnant has a greatly increased risk of fetal infection, deformities, or death. The lesions also make it easier for a person to transmit and contract HIV infection.

Medical Diagnosis

The diagnosis is based on physical examination findings and a blood test to detect the presence of antibodies. Tests for syphilis include screening and confirmation tests. Two screening tests are (1) the Venereal Disease Research Laboratory (VDRL) test and (2) the rapid plasma reagin (RPR) test. Both detect a protein that appears in the blood when a person has syphilis. Screening tests can be inaccurate because other factors can cause false-positive reactions. In addition, the tests are not effective until antibodies for *T. pallidum* are present in the blood. This may not occur until 3 to 4 weeks after exposure.

Confirmation tests, those that specifically detect *T. pallidum*, are needed to confirm the disease. They are the fluorescent treponemal antibody absorption (FTA-ABS) test and the microhemagglutination test. Because patients with syphilis often have multiple infections, HIV testing is often recommended as well. Facilities that have the necessary equipment may use dark-field examination of specimens to confirm the presence of spirochetes.

Pharmacology Capsule

About 60% of patients treated for syphilis with penicillin experience the Jarisch-Herxheimer reaction. Patients have headache, fever, and muscle aches that persist for 12 to 24 hours after treatment.

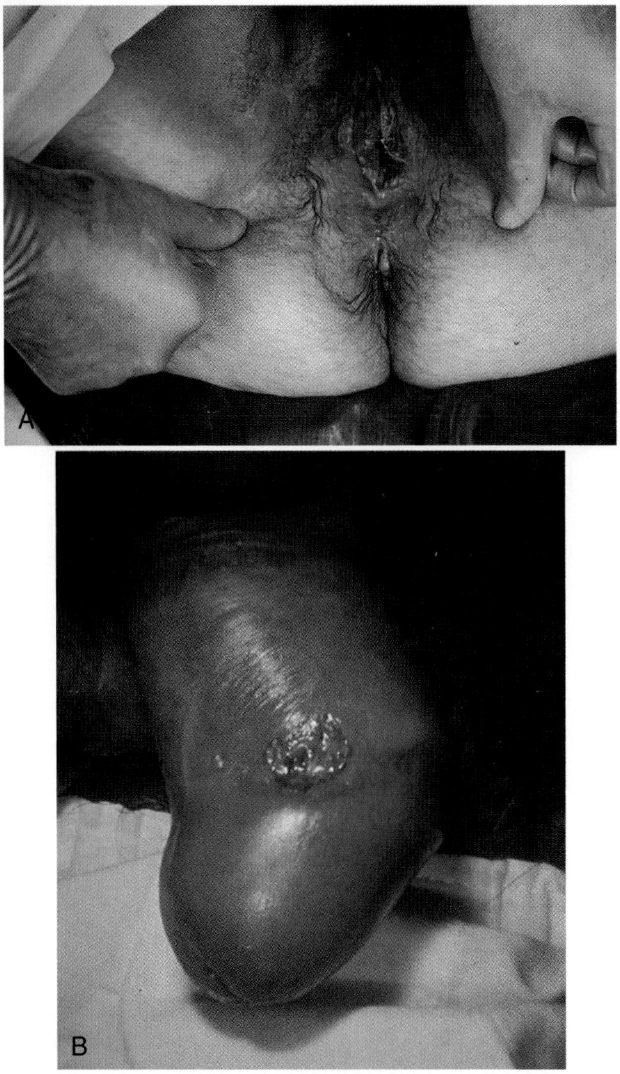

FIGURE 51-1 Chancre typical of primary syphilis. **A,** Chancre typical of primary syphilis (female subject). **B,** Chancre typical of primary syphilis (male subject). (A, Courtesy Leonard Wolf, MD, New York, NY. B, Courtesy New York City Health Department.)

Pharmacology Capsule

Patients who do not complete the prescribed course of anti-infective therapy may not be cured of the infection.

Medical Treatment

The treatment of choice for syphilis is parenteral penicillin G unless contraindicated. For an infection of less than 1 year's duration, a single dose is usually sufficient. For infections of 1 year's duration or longer, a longer course of therapy is indicated. Neurosyphilis and other complications may require other drug therapy. Information about drug therapy for syphilis is presented in Table 51-1. Advise the patient to make a follow-up appointment with a physician to determine whether the treatment was effective. In addition, advise the patient not to engage in sexual activity until 1 month after completing treatment for primary or secondary syphilis.

Nursing care of the patient with syphilis and other STIs is discussed in the section titled "Nursing Care of the Patient with a Sexually Transmitted Infection." Table 51-4 summarizes the signs and symptoms of syphilis, possible complications, medical treatment, and nursing considerations.

HERPES SIMPLEX

The herpes virus has plagued humans for many centuries. Several different types of the virus are passed easily from person to person. The virus that causes cold sores (*herpes febrilis* or herpes simplex virus-1 [HSV-1]) was first described in AD 100 and is transmitted through contact with open lesions, usually on the lips or inside the mouth. Prevention strategies generally focus on avoiding direct contact (kissing). Nurses should use good hand washing technique when caring for infected persons.

The incidence of genital herpes (caused by herpes simplex virus-2 [HSV-2]) has been on the rise since the 1960s. HSV-2 is generally transmitted by sexual contact. Vaginal or anal intercourse and oral-genital contact are the primary transmission modes but HSV-2 can be transferred by hand contact as well.

Although HSV-1 and HSV-2 are similar, type 1 is *usually* nongenital, with lesions typically above the waist. Type 2 is considered an STI because it is *most often* below the waist and is transmitted by genital contact. A characteristic of herpes viruses is the ability to become latent. The virus can remain in the tissues in an inactive state for long periods of time and then be reactivated.

Signs and Symptoms

Symptoms of genital herpes infection include painful, itching sores on or around the genitals approximately 2 to 20 days after infection. These symptoms last about 2 to 3 weeks. A rash may appear first, followed by small blisters that eventually ulcerate. People often complain of flulike symptoms and a burning sensation during urination. Episodes of active symptoms may recur and are frequently precipitated by anxiety (Fig. 51-2).

Complications

An increased risk of cervical cancer exists in women who have genital herpes. An infected woman should be taught to have a Papanicolaou (Pap) test done annually to detect cervical cancer early. If she is pregnant, a physician should supervise her closely. Various guidelines are used to determine whether the patient should have a vaginal delivery or a cesarean section. The goal is to decrease the risk of transmission to the baby. New diagnostic procedures allow the physician to detect active disease more accurately than in the past. Herpes simplex encephalitis is a dangerous complication, usually caused by HSV-1. It has a mortality

Table 51-4 Syphilis

SIGNS AND SYMPTOMS	POSSIBLE COMPLICATIONS	MEDICAL TREATMENT	NURSING CONSIDERATIONS
Primary Syphilis			
Chancre (round ulcer with well-defined margin): lesion thickened, rubbery, and painless. (If untreated, the lesion persists only for 3–6 weeks and heals.) Regional lymphadenopathy: enlarged lymph nodes only in the area of the chancre.	Prompt, effective treatment can result in complete recovery without complications. Otherwise, the infection progresses to the secondary stage.	Parenteral penicillin G is given IM in a single dose. If the patient is unable to take penicillin, PO tetracycline or doxycycline is used.	Ensure that ordered blood studies are done: VDRL, RPR, FTA-ABS. Assess for transient fever, flulike symptoms, and malaise. Provide rest periods. Wear gloves to assess the skin and mucous membranes. Inspect for skin changes and lesions. Provide medications. After administration of parenteral antibiotics, observe the patient for 30 minutes for allergic reactions such as rash, fever, or chills. Have emergency drugs on hand in the event of anaphylaxis.
Secondary Syphilis			
Sore throat, malaise, rash, fever, weight loss, headaches, musculoskeletal pain.	May become latent without further problems or may progress to tertiary stage.	Increased dose of penicillin given IM in 3 doses at 1-week intervals.	
Tertiary Syphilis			
Pain, areas that lack sensation, loss of position sense, abnormal gait, foot deformity and ulcerations.	Irreversible complications: arthritis, bursitis, osteitis, liver enlargement, heart disease, meningitis, CNS disorders.	Same as for secondary syphilis or penicillin IV every 4 hours for 10–14 days.	

CNS, Central nervous system; *FTA-ABS,* fluorescent treponemal antibody absorption; *IM,* intramuscularly; *IV,* intravenously; *PO,* by mouth; *RPR,* rapid plasmin reagin; *VDRL,* Venereal Disease Research Laboratory.

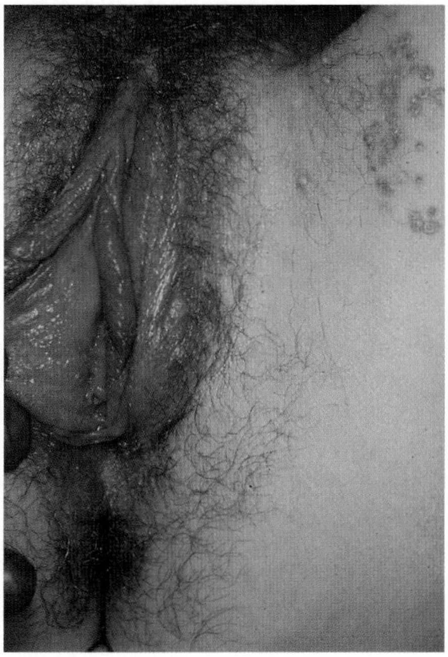

FIGURE 51-2 Genital herpes lesions on the vulva and inner thigh. (Courtesy Leonard Wolf, MD, New York, NY.)

rate of 30% and half of survivors have moderate to severe neurologic impairment.

Medical Diagnosis and Treatment

A diagnosis of HSV-2 may be suspected based on the appearance of genital lesions. Laboratory tests are used to confirm the diagnosis. These include antigen detection tests and NAAT using tissue or fluid specimens. Exudate from lesions can be examined under a microscope and cultured to reveal the virus.

No cure for HSV infection exists but the oral antiviral drugs acyclovir (Zovirax), valacyclovir (Valtrex), and famciclovir (Famvir) help by partially controlling the signs and symptoms during initial and recurrent episodes. Patients should know to start the drug when preliminary (prodromal) symptoms of recurrence are experienced or within 1 day of the outbreak of lesions. Some patients with especially disabling recurrences take one of these drugs continuously to reduce the frequency of outbreaks.

Nursing care of the patient with HSV and other STIs is discussed in the section titled "Nursing Care of the

Table 51-5 Herpes Simplex Infections

SIGNS AND SYMPTOMS	POSSIBLE COMPLICATIONS	MEDICAL TREATMENT	NURSING CONSIDERATIONS
Painful genital lesions, burning during urination.	Localized infections; risk of infecting baby on delivery.	Treatment is basically symptomatic and includes sitz baths. Acyclovir may minimize symptoms; however, no cure for herpes exists. Recurrences may be treated with acyclovir, valacyclovir, or famciclovir.	Ensure that the patient notifies sexual contacts. Inform the patient that the virus can survive on objects such as towels. Assist in decreasing the patient's anxiety by allowing him or her to verbalize feelings. Instruct the patient to avoid sexual contact when lesions are present and to use condoms at other times.

Patient with a Sexually Transmitted Infection." Table 51-5 summarizes the signs and symptoms of HSV infections, possible complications, medical treatment, and nursing considerations.

TRICHOMONIASIS

Trichomoniasis is caused by the protozoan parasite *Trichomonas vaginalis* and is usually sexually transmitted. However, the parasite can survive for hours on damp cloths and clothing. The CDC estimates that more than 7 million new cases occur each year. This infection usually affects the vagina in women and the urethra in men. Trichomoniasis is associated with an increased risk of HIV transmission. During pregnancy, it may cause premature birth or low birth weight.

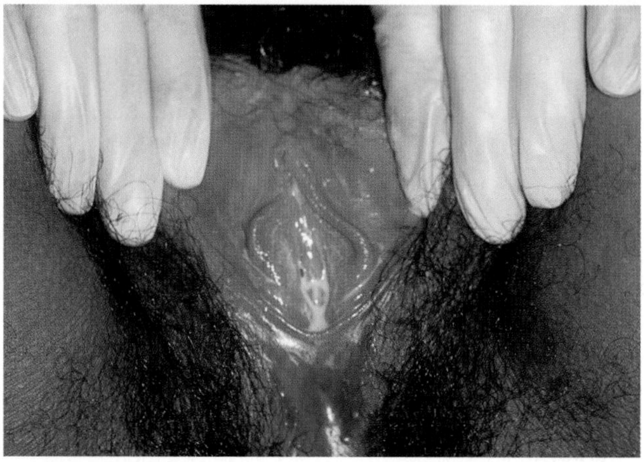

FIGURE 51-3 Trichomoniasis vaginal discharge is profuse and watery and appears purulent. (Courtesy Leonard Wolf, MD, New York, NY.)

Signs and Symptoms

Women typically complain of a frothy, yellowish vaginal discharge that has a foul odor; however, some women have no symptoms. Vaginal irritation and itching also may be present. Urinary frequency and burning suggest that the infection has invaded the urethra (Fig. 51-3). If the infection becomes chronic, bladder and anal involvement are possible. Although the incidence of trichomoniasis is less common in men, it can certainly occur. Men usually have no symptoms, although some have a mild discharge or slight burning after urination or ejaculation.

Medical Diagnosis and Treatment

The organism may be detected by microscopic study of vaginal discharge or urine (in men). The discharge also can be cultured to reveal the organism.

Tinidazole (Tindamax) is the drug of choice for treating trichomoniasis, with metronidazole (Flagyl) as a less expensive option. A single dose is usually effective. It is important that the patient and any sexual partners be treated at the same time to avoid reinfection.

Nursing care of the patient with trichomoniasis and other STIs is discussed in the section titled "Nursing Care of the Patient with a Sexually Transmitted Infection."

HUMAN PAPILLOMAVIRUS

Infection with human papillomavirus (HPV) is the most common STI in the United States, with more than 6 million new cases reported every year. More than 100 types of HPV exist, some classified as *low-risk* types and others as *high-risk* types. High-risk types have been associated with cervical, vulvar, vaginal, anal, and penile cancer whereas low-risk types of HPV are associated with condylomata acuminata, or genital warts. Although not always seen, the presence of genital warts is the most easily recognized sign of HPV infection. They generally affect the genital and anal regions of both men and women. Transmission of the virus is by vaginal, anal, or genital contact with an infected person. Incidents of transmission have been reported from persons who had no visible signs of infection. The incubation period usually ranges from 3 weeks to 8 months.

Fortunately two vaccines are available. Gardasil protects against four types of HPV, including types 6 and 11 that cause genital warts and types 16 and 18 that cause 70% of cervical cancers. Cervarix protects against types 16 and 18 only but is believed to confer protection for a longer period of time.

Signs and Symptoms

Men generally have warts on the glans, foreskin, urethral opening, penile shaft, or scrotum. These lesions may be single or multiple. In women, warts generally appear in or around the vulva, vagina, cervix, perineum, anal canal, and urethra. Less often, the lesions are seen on the labia and deep within the vaginal canal and endocervix. In homosexual and bisexual men and women who engage in anal intercourse, warts are common in the anal area. Oral, pharyngeal, and laryngeal lesions occur as well.

Condylomata warts are generally pink or red and soft, with a cauliflower-like appearance. These lesions may be single or multiple. In women, warts generally appear in or around the vulva, vagina, cervix, perineum, anal canal, and urethra. Less often, the lesions are seen on the labia and deep within the vaginal canal and endocervix. In men who have sex with men and women who engage in anal intercourse, warts are common in the anal area. Oral, pharyngeal, and laryngeal lesions occur as well. Multiple warts can become so large that they obstruct the vaginal opening or rectal canal. Genital warts tend to grow large if they are located in an area that is kept moist by vaginal or urethral discharge. For unknown reasons, pregnancy can stimulate genital warts to grow very large (Fig. 51-4).

Medical Diagnosis

The diagnosis is usually made on the basis of a simple observation of the warts. A biopsy of the lesions is necessary to make a definitive diagnosis. When genital warts are present, the physician usually will screen for cervical cancer as well as for HPV.

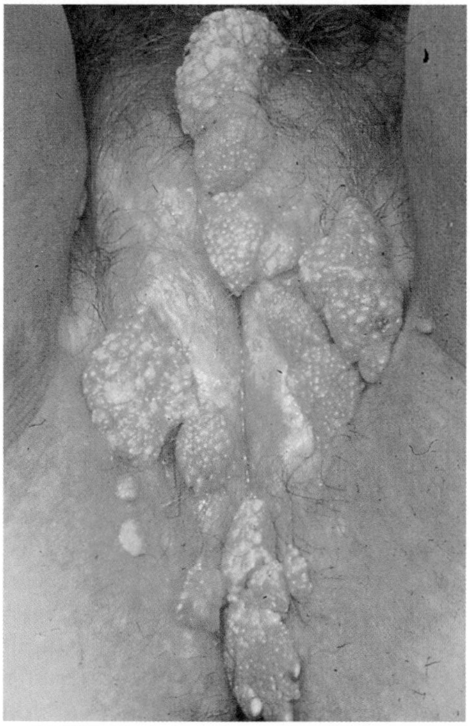

FIGURE 51-4 Condylomata acuminata in a female patient. (Courtesy New York City Health Department.)

Medical Treatment

Genital warts may or may not disappear spontaneously. Although no cure for condylomata acuminata exists, removal of visible warts provides symptomatic relief. Some treatments, such as the application of podofilox, imiquimod, or kunecatechins, can be managed by the patient. Other treatments must be administered by the physician (i.e., cryotherapy, which uses liquid nitrogen or solid carbon dioxide [CO_2] to freeze the warts; topical trichloroacetic acid, bichloroacetic acid, or podophyllin resin; surgical removal; injection of interferon into the lesions). Note that the safety of podofilox and imiquimod and of podophyllin resin during pregnancy has not been established. None of these methods has proven totally effective in all cases. The recurrence rate is very high.

Nursing care of the patient with condylomata warts and other STIs is discussed in the section titled "Nursing Care of the Patient with a Sexually Transmitted Infection."

BACTERIAL VAGINOSIS

Bacterial vaginosis is caused by *Gardnerella vaginalis* and other anaerobic bacteria. The infectious bacteria tend to emerge when the normal bacteria in the vagina are suppressed. It has been associated with having multiple sex partners, douching, and the presence of an intrauterine device (IUD). It is not clear whether it is actually transmitted sexually. The signs and symptoms are genital irritation and itching, painful urination, a thin gray discharge, and a fishy odor; however, some women report no symptoms. The infection is diagnosed by microscopic examination of the discharge fluid and by culture. Some commercially available card tests are also available. The condition is treated with a course of metronidazole (Flagyl) administered orally or vaginally or clindamycin vaginal cream. The patient is advised not to consume alcohol while taking metronidazole. The combination of alcohol and metronidazole may trigger a disulfiram-like reaction, with vomiting, tachycardia, and hypotension. When using clindamycin cream, the patient should know that the cream can weaken latex condoms and diaphragms. Treatment of sex partners has not been found to affect relapse or recurrence. (For a discussion of the potential complications of bacterial vaginosis, see the *Health Promotion* box.)

Health Promotion

Preventing Complications of Bacterial Vaginosis

In most cases, bacterial vaginosis causes no complications. However, an association has been documented between bacterial vaginosis and conditions such as pelvic inflammatory

Continued

Health Promotion—cont'd

disease (PID), gonorrhea, and human immunodeficiency virus (HIV) infection. Bacterial vaginosis can also cause premature birth and low-birth-weight infants. Therefore some health experts recommend that all pregnant women be assessed for bacterial vaginosis if they have previously delivered a premature baby. A pregnant woman who has not delivered a premature baby should be treated if she has symptoms and laboratory evidence of bacterial vaginosis.

No longer considered merely a harmless annoyance, this condition is the object of serious study as research nurses and other scientists try to clarify its role in such conditions as PID and pregnancy-related complications.

HUMAN IMMUNODEFICIENCY VIRUS INFECTION

Many diseases that cause illness or death have plagued Americans but it is likely that none of these has had the profound medical, social, economic, and psychologic effects as has the HIV infection known as *AIDS*. This syndrome is a disorder of the immune system caused by HIV. HIV gradually destroys T4 lymphocytes, which are essential for resisting pathogens. As the number of T4 lymphocytes declines, the patient becomes increasingly susceptible to **opportunistic infections**. An opportunistic infection is one that thrives when the immune system is impaired. HIV is transmitted through exposure to body fluids. No cure for the infection exists, although combination drug therapy can delay progress of the disease. Chapter 35 is devoted to a thorough discussion of HIV infection.

Put on Your Thinking Cap!

Consider this situation: A 30-year-old minister's wife is admitted after being injured in an automobile accident. While hospitalized, she is diagnosed with gonorrhea. You recognize that staff members are treating her differently since the gonorrhea was diagnosed. What behaviors would indicate lack of acceptance of the patient?

Do you think you would feel differently about this patient? What could you do to demonstrate acceptance and caring?

NURSING CARE of the Patient with a Sexually Transmitted Infection

Assessment

Assessment of the female and male reproductive systems is discussed in Chapters 49 and 50 and outlined in Boxes 49-1 and 50-1. When a patient has an STI, certain aspects of that assessment are especially important (see Nursing Care Plan: Patient with Gonorrhea). The licensed vocational nurse/licensed practical nurse (LVN/LPN) may be responsible for collecting important data to contribute to the assessment.

Health History

A thorough history is necessary to identify high-risk behaviors. A discussion of sexual behavior can be awkward for the nurse and the patient. Before nurses can deal with patients' sexuality, they must be aware of their own feelings and values. Privacy is essential for the patient interview. Questions about sexuality should be addressed in a straightforward manner. The interviewer should keep in mind that many patients lack scientific knowledge about the reproductive system and sexual activity. The patient may use some words that are considered crude by professionals but the nurse must be careful not to embarrass or shame the patient.

History of Present Illness. The history begins with an exploration of the patient's reason for seeking medical care. With an STI, common reasons include pain, fever, lesions, or genital discharge. Obtain a thorough description of the signs and symptoms, including onset, duration, and severity.

Past Medical History. In the discussion of past health, document serious conditions or chronic illnesses. The obstetric history may be significant as well. If the patient is of childbearing age, record the date of the last menstrual period. Record recent and current medications and note drug allergies.

Review of Systems. The review of systems elicits potentially significant signs and symptoms, including weight change; fever; weakness; fatigue; skin rashes or lesions; oral lesions; dysuria; whether the patient is sexually active; pain, lesions, or lumps in the genitals; vaginal or penile discharge; and altered sexual functioning. It is important to document a history of blood transfusions.

Functional Assessment. Relevant aspects of the functional assessment include frequency and variety of sexual behaviors, intravenous drug use, past infections with STIs, and sexual contact with a person known to have an STI. In addition, determine whether the patient may be classified as an *at-risk patient* because age (e.g., an adolescent experimenting with sexuality), sexual preference (men who have sex with men), or habits (drug use) place him or her at a higher risk for acquiring an STI. Victims of sexual abuse (of all ages) may have been exposed to STIs. Occupation also may be significant if the patient comes into contact with potentially infected body fluids. Health care providers at risk for exposure include nursing personnel, physicians, emergency medical technicians, operating room technicians, housekeepers in health care facilities, and medical laboratory technicians.

Physical Examination

The physical examination begins with inspection of the patient's skin for rashes and lesions. During the head and neck examination, the mouth is inspected for lesions. Palpate the neck for enlarged lymph nodes. Inspect the abdomen for distention and palpate for tenderness. Depending on the setting and your specialized education, you may examine the genitals or assist the physician or nurse practitioner in the

Nursing Care Plan Patient with Gonorrhea

ASSESSMENT

HEALTH HISTORY A 23-year-old woman comes to the physician's office because of painful urination, abdominal pain, and vaginal discharge of 3 days' duration. She has had no serious illnesses or injuries. She has had two sexual partners in the past 6 months, with her most recent contact 2 weeks ago, when a condom was not used. The patient expresses concern about sexually transmitted infections (STIs) and human immunodeficiency virus (HIV). She states that she cannot believe she was "so stupid" and is very embarrassed about these symptoms.

PHYSICAL EXAMINATION Vital signs: blood pressure 130/82 mm Hg, pulse 84 bpm and regular, respiration 14 breaths per minute. T 98 orally. Height 5′3″, weight 110 lb. The physical examination findings are all normal except for the genital and pelvic examination. The vaginal tissues are red and edematous, with a whitish discharge. A smear is taken for examination. The nurse practitioner makes a preliminary diagnosis of gonorrhea. A single dose of intramuscular ceftriaxone sodium (Rocephin) is ordered. The patient is also given a prescription for 7 days of oral doxycycline calcium (Vibramycin) because chlamydia often accompanies gonorrhea.

Nursing Diagnosis	Goals and Outcome Criteria	Interventions
Impaired Tissue Integrity and Acute Pain related to infection and inflammation	The patient will report decreased pain and redness and discharge will diminish.	Tell the patient that the symptoms should improve with treatment. Mild analgesics may be needed as ordered. Sitz baths may be soothing.
Risk for Injury related to disease process	The patient will report for follow-up examination and remain free of signs and symptoms of complications.	Explain that persistent infection can lead to sterility and affect the heart and joints. Emphasize the importance of completing medications and returning for an examination to ensure successful treatment.
Anxiety related to possible complications of gonorrhea or stigma of sexually transmitted infection (STI)	The patient will express reduced anxiety and will be calm.	Provide opportunity to talk. Help the patient focus on the source of anxiety. For example, if she does not know what to expect, information is needed. If she is trying to decide how to discuss the condition with her sexual partners, help her solve the problem. Assure her that proper treatment is usually effective and prevents complications.
Situational Low Self-Esteem related to diagnosis	The patient's self-image will improve, as evidenced by positive comments about self.	Be accepting and nonjudgmental. Assure the patient that she has done the right thing by seeking medical attention.
Deficient Knowledge of disease process, treatment, or prevention of future infections	The patient will verbalize the importance of treatment, complications of untreated infection, and measures to prevent future infections.	Explore her understanding of gonorrhea. Provide information as needed. Emphasize use of condoms in sexual contacts to reduce risk of future infections with gonorrhea or other STIs. Ask about drug allergies before giving antimicrobials. Explain self-medication dosage, side effects, and adverse effects.

Critical Thinking Questions

1. How can you help this patient to decide how to discuss this condition with her sexual partner?
2. Describe the best approach in addressing the patient's embarrassment about her condition. How might you put her at ease?

examination. The examiner wears gloves to examine the genitals. A good light source is essential for thorough inspection. In the male patient, the examiner notes the general appearance of the penis, scrotum, and anal area. Any skin breaks, rashes, or redness is noted.

The LVN/LPN may prepare the female patient for a pelvic examination. While the patient is on the examination table and properly draped, the genitalia and the perianal area are inspected. The labia are separated and inspected for skin breaks, redness, or rashes. If a vaginal examination is to be done, ensure that the speculum and other supplies are ready. The speculum is warmed and lubricated before insertion in the vagina. Tissue and fluid specimens may be taken, including tissue scrapings for a Pap test. You may be responsible for preparing the specimen and sending it to the laboratory.

In cases of sexual assault, it is especially important that the examiner be specially trained to deal with such situations. Not only does the patient need a great deal of support but the examination may produce evidence that must be preserved for legal purposes.

If a discharge is present, its color, amount, and consistency are recorded. Specimens may be collected for laboratory study. The specimen is handled as infective material, prepared according to agency procedures, labeled, and sent to the laboratory.

Assessment of the patient with an STI is outlined in Box 51-1.

Box 51-1 Assessment of the Patient with a Sexually Transmitted Infection

HEALTH HISTORY

Present Illness

Pain, fever, lesions, genital discharge

Past Medical History

Serious conditions, chronic conditions, hemophilia, obstetric history, date of last menstrual period, recent and current medications

Review of Systems

Weight change, fever, weakness, fatigue, skin rashes or lesions, oral lesions, dysuria, whether sexually active, sexual contact with a person known to have a sexually transmitted infection (STI), sexual dysfunction, history of blood transfusions

Functional Assessment

Frequency and variety of sexual behaviors, intravenous drug use, past STIs, sexual preference, occupational exposure to infective material

PHYSICAL EXAMINATION

General Survey

Distress, lethargy

Skin

Rashes, lesions

Mouth

Lesions

Abdomen

Distention, tenderness

Genitals

General appearance; lesions; rashes; redness; color, amount, odor, and consistency of discharge

Nursing Diagnoses, Goals, and Outcome Criteria: Sexually Transmitted Infection

Nursing Diagnoses	Goals and Outcome Criteria
Impaired Tissue Integrity related to lesions, rash	Restored tissue integrity: healed, intact skin and mucous membranes
Acute Pain related to lesions, inflammation	Pain relief: patient reports pain is relieved, relaxed manner
Risk for Injury related to disease process, potential adverse effects of drugs	Freedom from additional injury: absence of signs and symptoms of complications
Anxiety related to possible effects of sexually transmitted infection (STI), reaction of partner	Reduced anxiety: patient reports anxiety is reduced, calm manner
Situational Low Self-Esteem related to diagnosis of STI	Improved self-esteem: increased positive comments about self, confident manner
Impaired Social Interaction related to presence of communicable disease, social stigma	Resumption of satisfying social interactions: patient states is satisfied with socialization
Sexual Dysfunction related to fear of transmission, impaired tissue integrity	Practices safe sexual behaviors: patient accurately describes safe behaviors, indicates will not engage in unsafe behavior
Ineffective Coping related to stigma associated with STI, shame, anger	Effective coping: patient states is better able to deal with stress of condition
Ineffective Self-Health Management related to denial, embarrassment, lack of understanding of disease process, mode of transmission, treatment, and prevention	Effective management of therapeutic plan: patient seeks medical care and follow-up, accurately describes self-care measures, expresses intent to follow plan of care and preventive measures

Interventions

Impaired Tissue Integrity

If you have daily contact with the patient, assess the patient's skin on a daily basis. Record changes in lesions. Carry out orders for treatments, including topical medications and sitz baths for patients in health care settings. Monitor the patient's temperature at regular intervals to detect fever that may accompany acute infection. Handle soiled clothing and bed linens in accordance with agency policy. Ensure that patients who will treat themselves at home understand the prescribed therapy and how to protect others from infection.

Acute Pain

Some STIs are painless but patients may have pain associated with pelvic infection, oral lesions, or rectal lesions. The lesions of HSV are especially painful. Document the severity of the patient's pain and provide analgesics as ordered. Apply topical medications, ice packs, or warm compresses as ordered or teach the patient how to do so.

Risk for Injury

Untreated STIs can lead to serious complications such as PID and sterility. The patient with AIDS is at high risk for secondary infections (called *opportunistic infections*) because of impaired immune function. Infected patients also pose a threat to their sexual partners. An STI may be passed to the fetus in utero or transmitted during delivery. Therefore it is important for the patient to receive the entire course of prescribed therapy. In addition, stress the importance of notifying sexual contacts so that they can be tested and treated as well, if necessary.

Drug therapy has the potential for injury. Before administering medications, assess the patient's allergies. When injections are given to an outpatient, ask the patient to remain for 30 minutes afterward in case an allergic reaction occurs. Emergency drugs, including epinephrine, corticosteroids, and diphenhydramine hydrochloride (Benadryl), must be readily available. Information about drugs commonly used to treat STIs is presented in Table 51-1.

Anxiety

The patient may be anxious about the outcome of treatment and the potential complications of the disease. Anxiety may be heightened by the stigma associated with having contracted an STI and the patient may feel ashamed. Encourage the patient to verbalize fears and frustrations. Provide accurate information and teach the patient how to avoid reinfection and infecting others. Patients with HIV infections also must deal with a life-threatening illness.

Situational Low Self-Esteem

The patient's self-esteem may suffer because of a diagnosed STI. Provide an opportunity for the patient to talk about the effects of the disease on self-concept. Try to guide the patient to focus on his or her positive attributes. If the patient's self-esteem remains low despite nursing intervention, a referral to a mental health counselor may be suggested.

Impaired Social Interaction

A diagnosis of STI can be very distressing to the patient, who may fear rejection by others. The patient may be angry at the person who transmitted the infection and may be concerned about infecting others. Because STIs must be reported to public health authorities who attempt to trace all sexual contacts, the patient may also fear reprisals. One way you can help is by demonstrating acceptance of the patient through kindness and touch.

Sexual Dysfunction

Patients with STIs may experience sexual dysfunction related to fear of transmission, the presence of lesions, or anxiety. In addition, precautions that should be taken to prevent transmission of the disease may require changes in sexual practices. In general, sexual activity should be avoided until the infection is cured. Chronic infections such as HSV and HIV require permanent alterations in sexual activity. Explore the importance of sexual activity to the patient. Accept the patient's feelings in a nonjudgmental way. Explain that emotions and sexual function are closely related and that dysfunction may be overcome by dealing with the emotional reactions to the disease. For persistent dysfunction, advise the patient to discuss the problem with the physician. Offer to make a referral to a therapist who specializes in sexual dysfunction. Encourage the patient to communicate openly with the sexual partner about the difficulties experienced. Alternative means of sexual expression (other than intercourse) may be suggested. Box 51-2 compares the relative safety of various sexual practices.

Ineffective Coping

Ineffective coping may be related to guilt, shame, anger, actual or anticipated rejection, or a combination of these reactions. Behaviors associated with ineffective coping include failure to adhere to the prescribed treatment, failure to exercise precautions to prevent spread of the disease or reinfection, chronic anxiety or depression, and inability to cope. The patient with an HIV infection also must deal with the potential for developing AIDS, sometimes with inadequate personal support. Show support for the patient by being sensitive, courteous, and nonjudgmental. Point out dangerous behaviors. Encourage the patient to evaluate his or her lifestyle and to identify modifications that could reduce future risks (see *Nutrition Considerations* box). You may refer patients who have HSV and HIV infections to support groups. A spiritual counselor also may be contacted if the patient desires.

Nutrition Considerations

1. Persons with oral lesions may require modified diets.
2. Patients who are taking antibiotics generally are advised to drink at least 2000 mL of fluids each day to prevent harm to the kidneys.

Ineffective Self-Health Management

Patient teaching is essential for effective treatment and prevention of future infections. Explain to the patient what causes the infection, how it is transmitted, how

Box 51-2 Comparative Safety of Various Sexual Practices to Prevent Transmission of Infection

SAFE PRACTICES
- Mutual masturbation
- Closed-mouth kissing
- Body massage
- Use of own sex devices or toys

POSSIBLY SAFE PRACTICES
- Open-mouthed kissing
- Vaginal or anal intercourse with properly used condom
- Oral sex with properly used condom

UNSAFE PRACTICES
- Vaginal or anal intercourse without condom
- Oral sex without condom
- Oral-anal contact
- Insertion of hand into vagina or rectum
- Ingestion of urine or semen
- Contact with blood

Modified from Lewis SM, Rickert BD: Altered immune response. In Lewis SM, Collier IC, editors: *Medical-surgical nursing*, St. Louis, 1992, Mosby.

it can be prevented (including "safe sex" practices), and why treatment and follow-up care are important. (See the *Patient Teaching* box.)

Patient Teaching

Sexually Transmitted Infections

- Be sure to complete the prescribed course of antibiotics and return so that the physician can determine whether the treatment was effective.
- Sexually transmitted infections (STIs) are transmitted by sexual contact. Avoid sexual contact with high-risk individuals: people who have had multiple sex partners, prostitutes, and those with known human immunodeficiency virus (HIV) or hepatitis B virus (HBV).
- Avoid sexual activity until your infection is cured.
- If you engage in sexual activity that involves any genital contact, use condoms.
- If you have sexual contact with high-risk individuals, people you do not know well, or persons who do not use condoms, you should have periodic medical examinations.
- Use condoms if you have condylomata.
- If you have herpes simplex virus (HSV) infection, you should abstain from sexual activity when lesions are present. Use condoms at all times. It is important to realize that although periods of remission are seen, the condition is chronic and transmissible.
- Women with HSV or condylomata are advised to have annual Pap tests because they are at increased risk of cervical cancer.
- If you have HIV infection, medical treatment may prevent or delay the development of acquired immunodeficiency syndrome (AIDS). Precautions must be taken to prevent infecting sexual partners even though you may not have signs and symptoms of disease.
- Because HIV is transmitted through body fluids, you cannot donate blood if you are HIV positive.

Knowledge does not guarantee compliance but patients cannot comply unless they understand what they need to do to care for themselves. Determine what the patient knows about the infection. Provide information about the disease and its treatment in terms the patient can understand. If the patient can read, include supplementary written material. Stress the importance of completing the course of therapy and returning for follow-up to reduce the risk of complications associated with untreated disease. Evaluate the patient's understanding of the material covered and explore any barriers that might prevent the patient from following the instructions.

CONDOM USE

Many people do not know how to use condoms correctly. At this time, only male condoms are in common use, although female condoms are available. (See the *Patient Teaching* box.)

Patient Teaching

Use of a Condom

- Condoms do not provide 100% protection against disease transmission.
- Latex condoms are preferred because some pathogens can pass through natural membrane condoms.
- Protect condoms from heat and sunlight to keep them from deteriorating.
- Do not use condoms that are brittle, discolored, or in damaged packages.
- Use only water-based lubricants because other lubricants can cause the condom to break. Spermicidals may be used.
- To put on a condom, hold it by the tip and unroll it onto the penis. Leave a space of about 1 inch at the tip for semen.
- Withdraw the penis carefully after ejaculation to prevent the condom from slipping off and spilling the contents and to avoid unprotected contact.
- Always discard used condoms for sanitary disposal.

Get Ready for the NCLEX® Examination!

Key Points

- EPT is an approach to treating partners of persons with STIs. The infected patient is provided with a prescription or extra medications to give to the partner.
- Gonorrhea is one of the most commonly reported STIs in the United States but it often has no symptoms.
- Gonorrhea can lead to damage to the heart and joints as well as to PID.
- Chlamydial infection is diagnosed in more than 1 million people in the United States each year; it can result in sterility in both sexes.
- Syphilis, if untreated, progresses through four stages, with eventual damage to the cardiovascular and nervous systems, the skin, and the joints.
- Newborns of women with gonorrhea or chlamydial infection may acquire eye infections during birth.
- HSV can be transmitted by sexual contact; however, it also can be transmitted by hand contact.
- Because HSV increases the risk of cervical cancer in infected women, they are advised to have annual Pap tests.
- Condylomata acuminata (genital warts), is caused by HPV and have a high rate of recurrence despite drug therapy, cryotherapy, cautery, and surgical or laser excision.
- Infection with HIV leaves the patient unable to resist opportunistic infections.

- HIV is transmitted through exposure to body fluids and no cure exists for the infection, although combination drug therapy can delay progress of the disease.
- Most STIs except HSV infection and HIV infection can be cured by antimicrobials.
- HSV infection is minimized but not cured by acyclovir sodium (Zovirax).
- Abstinence from sexual contact is the best way to prevent transmission of STIs but use of condoms during sexual contact also reduces the risk.
- Standard Precautions prescribe specific protective measures for health care providers to take when working with people who have infections that can be transmitted through body fluids.
- The nursing care of patients with STIs may address impaired tissue integrity, acute pain, risk for injury, anxiety, situational low self-esteem, impaired social interactions, sexual dysfunction, ineffective coping, and ineffective self-health management.
- Patient teaching is essential for patients with STIs and should include information about drug therapy and other treatment options, disease transmission, abstinence during treatment, and preventive measures.

Additional Learning Resources

SG Go to your Study Guide for additional learning activities to help you master this chapter content.

evolve Go to your Evolve website (http://evolve.elsevier.com/Linton/medsurg) for the following learning resources and much more:

- Interactive Prioritization Exercises
- Fluid & Electrolyte Tutorial
- Pharmacology Tutorial
- Review Questions for the NCLEX® Examination

Review Questions for the NCLEX® Examination

1. Which of the following is the purpose of reporting STIs?
   1. To prosecute the individuals who are transmitting the disease to others
   2. To emphasize to infected persons the importance of practicing safe sex
   3. To reduce transmission of the infection by treating all infected persons
   4. To teach the general public about measures to prevent STIs

   NCLEX Client Need: Safe and Effective Care Environment: Safety and Infection Control
2. Nurses in the newborn nursery anticipate that erythromycin ophthalmic ointment will be ordered for the newborn of a mother who has: (Select all that apply.)
   1. Genital warts
   2. Chlamydia
   3. Gonorrhea
   4. Hepatitis B
   5. Syphilis

   NCLEX Client Need: Physiological Integrity: Pharmacological Therapies
3. A patient who was diagnosed with gonorrhea did not return for treatment. When contacted, she reported that her symptoms had gone away so she thought she had recovered from the infection. The most appropriate response by the nurse would be which of the following?
   1. "Without treatment, the bacteria remain in your body and you remain highly infectious."
   2. "As long as your symptoms have cleared up, no reason exists to treat you now."
   3. "If you have symptoms in the future, come to the clinic immediately."
   4. "Fortunately, gonorrhea has no serious complications but I must advise you to seek treatment anyway."

   NCLEX Client Need: Health Promotion and Maintenance
4. A patient who was admitted to the hospital after an injury is diagnosed with syphilis in the primary stage. During the nursing assessment, the nurse is likely to find:
   1. A rash on the extremities, chest or back, palms of the hands, and soles of the feet
   2. A reddish papule or painless red ulcer on the genitals, anus, or mouth
   3. Tender lymph nodes in the area of the skin lesion
   4. Fever, sore throat, and generalized aching

   NCLEX Client Need: Physiological Integrity: Physiological Adaptation
5. The patient with untreated syphilis may develop which of the following? (Select all that apply.)
   1. Blindness
   2. Mental illness
   3. Paralysis
   4. Heart disease
   5. Osteoporosis

   NCLEX Client Need: Physiological Integrity: Reduction of Risk Potential
6. In a health education class, the nurse is teaching the students about herpes simplex virus infection. Which statements are true regarding the HSV-1 and HSV-2? (Select all that apply.)
   1. "Type 2 is most often transmitted by genital contact."
   2. "The modes of transmission of both types 1 and 2 are the same."
   3. "Both types 1 and 2 can be treated with antiviral drugs."
   4. "Type 1 *only* affects the genitals and type 2 *only* affects the mouth."
   5. "Vaccines are available to prevent HSV-1 but not HSV-2."

   NCLEX Client Need: Physiological Integrity: Physiological Adaptation

7. A young woman is being treated at the university clinic for a genital HSV-2 infection. The teaching plan for her should include which of the following statements? (Select all that apply.)
   1. "You should have yearly Pap tests because you are at increased risk for cervical cancer."
   2. "You should not become pregnant because the herpes infection causes fetal deformities."
   3. "Once you have finished taking your medicine, you will be cured of the herpes infection."
   4. "Your partner must use a condom for intercourse even when lesions are not present."
   5. "Medications may reduce the frequency and severity of your symptoms."

   NCLEX Client Need: Physiological Integrity: Physiological Adaptation
8. The teaching plan for a patient with genital warts should include which of the following statements?
   1. "This condition cannot be transmitted to a sexual partner."
   2. "Genital warts are caused by poor personal hygiene."
   3. "A topical medication can remove the warts but is not curative."
   4. "Once the warts are removed, they are unlikely to come back."

   NCLEX Client Need: Physiological Integrity: Physiological Adaptation
9. Information for effective use of condoms should include which of the following statements? (Select all that apply.)
   1. "Condoms provide 100% protection against disease transmission."
   2. "Latex condoms are preferred over natural membrane condoms."
   3. "Use only oil-based lubricants to prevent breakage of the condom."
   4. "Leave a space of about 1 inch at the tip for semen."
   5. "Remove the used condom carefully to prevent spillage of contents."

   NCLEX Client Need: Health Promotion and Maintenance
10. Which of the following STIs usually can be cured with antimicrobials? (Select all that apply.)
    1. Gonorrhea
    2. Herpes simplex
    3. Syphilis
    4. Trichomoniasis
    5. Chlamydia

    NCLEX Client Need: Physiological Integrity: Pharmacological Therapies

chapter 52

Skin Disorders

Mary Walker

http://evolve.elsevier.com/Linton/medsurg

Objectives

1. Describe the structure and functions of the skin.
2. Define terms used to describe the skin and skin lesions.
3. List the components of the nursing assessment of the skin.
4. Explain the tests and procedures used to diagnose skin disorders.
5. Explain the nurse's responsibilities regarding the tests and procedures for diagnosing skin disorders.
6. Explain the therapeutic benefits and nursing considerations for patients who receive dressings, soaks and wet wraps, phototherapy, and drug therapy for skin problems.
7. Describe the pathophysiology, signs and symptoms, diagnostic tests, and medical treatment for selected skin disorders.
8. Assist in developing a nursing care plan for the patient with a skin disorder.

Key Terms

Acne (ĂK-nē)
Acrochordons (ăk-rō-KŎR-dŏn)
Angiomas (ăn-jē-Ō-mă)
Debridement (dă-BRĒD-mĕnt)
Dermatitis (dĕr-mă-TĪ-tĭs)
Intertrigo (ĭn-tĕr-TRĪ-gō)
Keratolytics (kĕr-ă-tō-LĬT-ĭk)
Lentigo (*pl.* lentigines) (lĭn-TĒ-gō, lĭn-TĬ-jŭ-nēz)
Nevus (*pl.* nevi) (NĒ-vŭs, NĒ-vī)
Pemphigus (PĔM-fĭ-gŭs)
Pruritus (proo-RĪ-tŭs)
Psoriasis (sō-RĪ-ă-sĭs)

ANATOMY AND PHYSIOLOGY OF THE SKIN

The skin is an organ that covers the body surface. The anatomy of the skin is illustrated in Figure 52-1. It is composed of two distinct layers: (1) the epidermis and (2) the dermis. The epidermis is the outermost layer that covers the dermis. The base of the epidermis continually produces new cells to replace those at the surface. Epidermal cells produce melanin, a dark pigment that helps to determine the color of the skin. Strong ultraviolet light, such as in sunlight, stimulates the production of melanin.

The dermis is strong connective tissue that contains nerve endings, sweat glands, and hair roots. The dermis is well supplied with blood vessels, causing the skin to redden when surface vessels are dilated. Subcutaneous tissue lies beneath the dermis.

The hair, nails, and sebaceous glands are appendages (or derivatives) of the skin. The hair root is located in a tube in the dermis called a *hair follicle.* The arrector muscles of the hair (i.e., arrectores pilorum), located around the hair follicles, can contract, causing the hairs to stand erect and the skin to take on a gooseflesh appearance. Also around the hair follicles are sebaceous glands that secrete an oily substance called *sebum.* Sweat glands, found in most parts of the skin, secrete water through the skin surface that contains salts, ammonia, amino acids, lactic acid, ascorbic acid, uric acid, and urea.

FUNCTIONS OF THE SKIN

The functions of the skin are protection, body temperature regulation, secretion, sensation, and synthesis of vitamin D. In addition, the blood vessels of the skin can serve as a blood reservoir.

Protection

The skin performs its protective function by shielding underlying tissues from trauma and pathogens and by preventing excess loss of fluids from those tissues. A second type of protective function is fulfilled by Langerhans cells, which initiate an immune response when foreign substances invade the epidermis.

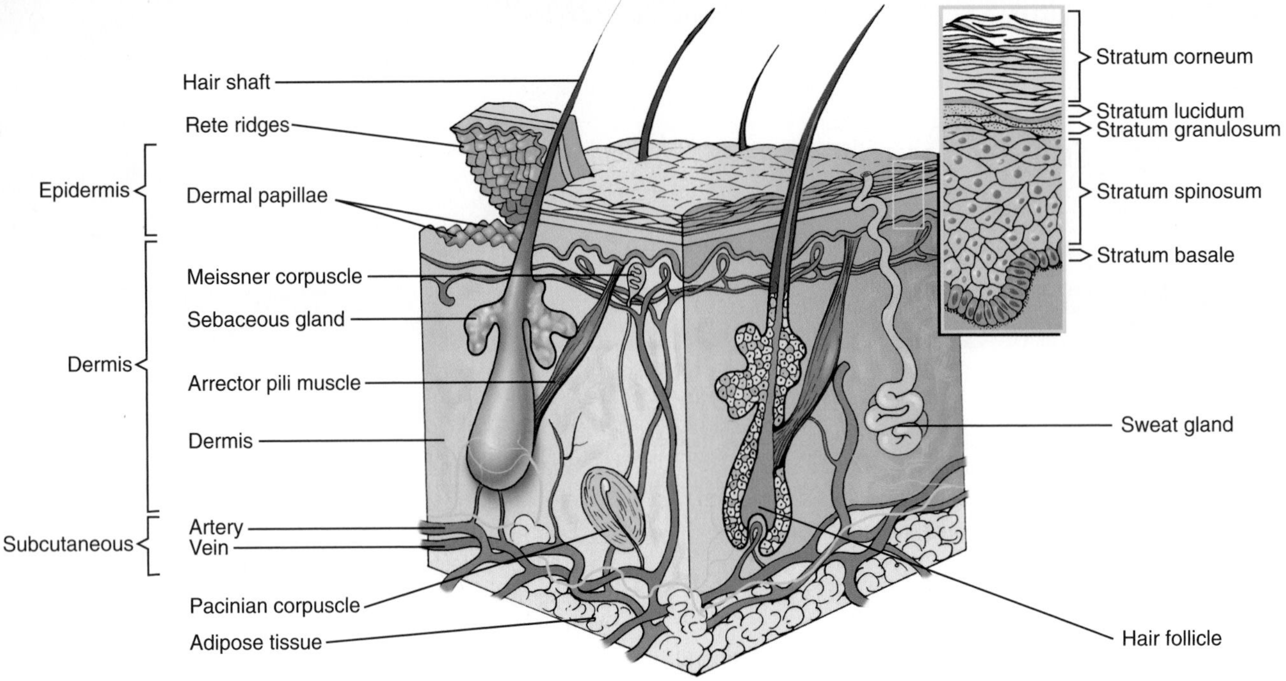

FIGURE 52-1 Anatomy of the skin. (From Monahan FD, Drake DT, Neighbors M, editors: *Medical-surgical nursing: foundations for clinical practice*, ed 2, Philadelphia, 1998, Saunders.)

Temperature Regulation

The skin participates in temperature regulation by altering the diameter of surface blood vessels and through sweating. To dissipate heat, the blood vessels dilate. As the blood flows close to the body surface, heat is lost through the surface. To retain heat, blood vessels constrict and heat loss is minimized. Sweating helps to cool the body because heat is lost as sweat evaporates from the skin.

Secretion

Sweat is one skin secretion; sebum is another. Sebum coats the skin, creating an oily barrier that holds in water. Sweat promotes loss of body heat through evaporation, as noted previously, and plays a role in excretion of wastes.

Sensation

The skin is heavily endowed with sensory receptors for touch, pressure, pain, and temperature. When these sensory receptors are stimulated, nerves convey messages to the brain for interpretation.

Synthesis of Vitamin D

Ultraviolet rays in sunlight activate a substance in the skin called *7-dehydrocholesterol* that undergoes a series of changes that eventually convert it into vitamin D.

Blood Reservoir

The skin contains an extensive blood vessel network that can store as much as 10% of the body's total blood volume. Constriction of these superficial blood vessels shunts blood to vital organs when needed.

AGE-RELATED CHANGES IN THE SKIN

Changes in the skin are probably the most readily recognized of all signs of physical aging. Wrinkling of the skin occurs as a result of thinning of the skin layers and degeneration of elastin fibers. A loss of elasticity and strength occurs. Sweat glands decrease in size and number, although sweat production changes little until advanced age. The production of sebum by sebaceous glands decreases with age, becoming apparent earlier in women than in men. Dryness and **pruritus** (i.e., itching) are common. Skin often becomes paler as people age because the number of cells that produce melanin decreases. Many skin lesions are more common in older adults. They include the following:

1. **Lentigines**: pigmented spots on sun-exposed areas (*sing.* lentigo). They are commonly called *liver spots*, although they have nothing to do with the liver.
2. Senile purpura: large, purplish bruises that resolve very slowly. They can result from minor trauma.
3. Senile **angiomas**: bright-red papules.
4. Seborrheic keratoses: waxy, raised lesions that are flesh colored to dark brown or black and variously sized from small and nearly flat to large and prominent.
5. **Acrochordons** (skin tags): small, soft, raised lesions that are flesh colored or pigmented.

Figure 52-2 illustrates some age-related changes in the skin.

The risk of premalignant and malignant skin lesions also increases with age. These are discussed along with

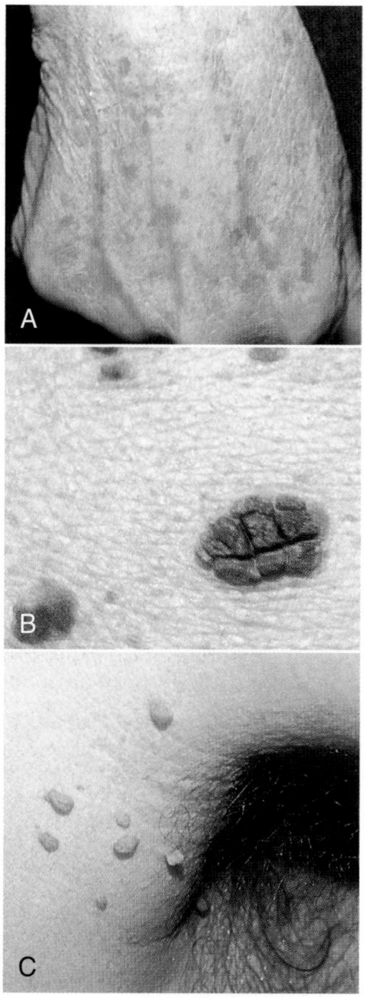

FIGURE 52-2 Common skin changes in the older adult. **A,** Lentigines. **B,** Seborrheic keratoses. **C,** Skin tags. (From Lookingbill DP, Marks JG: *Principles of dermatology*, ed 2, Philadelphia, 1993, Saunders.)

other pathologic conditions in the section titled "Cancer."

By age 50, approximately half of all people have some gray hair. Men commonly begin to lose some hair from the scalp in their fourth decade and by 80 years of age many men are almost bald. Scalp hair thins in women as well but usually is less obvious. Many older women and men have an increase in facial hair. Men also may have increased hair in the nares, eyebrows, or helix of the ear. In addition to aging changes in the skin and hair, the nails flatten and become dry, brittle, and discolored.

Put on Your Thinking Cap!

A patient who has just returned from surgery complains of being cold. Your assessment reveals pale hands and feet, weak pedal pulses, and slight shivering. Both feet and ankles are cold to the touch. Her vital signs are normal and her wound dressing is dry. Explain the basis of each of the assessment findings.

Put on Your Thinking Cap!—cont'd

You obtain a warmed blanket and cover the patient snugly, increase the temperature in the room, and ask her to call you if she does not feel better soon. When you return in 15 minutes, her hands and feet are warm and pedal pulses are palpable. She is resting quietly with no shivering. Explain the physiology behind her condition changes.

NURSING ASSESSMENT OF THE SKIN

HEALTH HISTORY

Chief Complaint and History of Present Illness

When a patient has a skin disorder, the chief complaint may be discomfort, pruritus, color changes, lesions, hair loss, or abnormal hair growth. The history of the present illness should describe the onset of the condition and any precipitating and alleviating factors. Precipitating factors should include any new medications, soaps, laundry detergent, or perfumes that may have been added within the last week. The progression of symptoms and changes in the distribution or appearance of lesions may be helpful in the diagnostic process.

Past Medical History

Document previously diagnosed skin diseases or problems, current and recent medications (including nonprescription drugs), and allergies.

Review of Systems

The review of systems includes additional data that may be related to the skin problem: change in skin color or pigmentation, change in a mole, sores that have been slow to heal, itching, dryness or scaliness, excessive bruising, rashes, lesions, hair loss, unusual hair growth, and changes in nails. The review of systems also may reveal other disorders that cause changes in the skin. Specific signs and symptoms may be associated with circulatory, respiratory, renal, hepatic, gastrointestinal (GI), and endocrine conditions. For example, skin manifestations may occur with diabetes mellitus (DM), cancer, kidney failure, thyroid disease, liver disease, and anemia.

Put on Your Thinking Cap!

Can you think of one change in the skin that might occur with disorders of each of the following: circulatory system, respiratory system, urinary system, and the liver?

Functional Assessment

Because the functional assessment can provide important clues to skin problems, record the patient's past and present occupations, exposure to chemicals or other irritants, skin care habits, and extent of sun exposure. Note recent changes in the work or living environment. Also inquire about current stresses and sources of anxiety.

PHYSICAL EXAMINATION

The licensed vocational nurse/licensed practical nurse (LVN/LPN) has many opportunities to collect data about the skin while providing care. When a complete physical examination is done, the examiner assesses the skin throughout the examination. The skin is inspected with attention to the color and variations in pigmentation. Sun-exposed areas are typically darker than protected areas. Document dilated blood vessels and angiomas (i.e., benign tumors composed of blood vessels). Table 52-1 describes variations in skin color and the significance of each. Carefully inspect **nevi** (i.e., moles) for irregularities in shape, pigmentation, and ulcerations or changes in surrounding skin. Nevi also are palpated for tenderness and measured in centimeters. If a rash is present, describe the location, distribution, and characteristics. If any drainage exists, note the color, amount, and odor. Terms used to describe skin lesions are defined in Table 52-2 and illustrated in Figure 52-3.

Table 52-1 Variations in Skin Color

COLOR CHANGE	DESCRIPTION	CAUSES
Pallor	White or pale in light-skinned people, yellowish-brown in brown-skinned people, ashen in black-skinned people; may be evident in mucous membranes, lips, and nail beds as well as skin	Vasoconstriction because of acute anxiety or fear, cold, some drugs, cigarette smoking; edema.
Erythema	Bright red	Increased local blood flow because of inflammation, fever, or emotions such as embarrassment or anger
Cyanosis	Bluish	Excess deoxygenated blood in the tissue because of anemia, respiratory disorders, or cardiovascular disorders
Jaundice	Golden or greenish yellow	Reflects increased bilirubin in the blood because of liver disease or destruction of red blood cells (RBCs)

Table 52-2 Common Skin Lesions

LESION	CHARACTERISTICS	EXAMPLES
Macule	Distinct flat area with color different from surrounding tissue	Freckle, petechiae, hypopigmentation
Papule	Any raised, solid lesion with clearly defined margins; <1 cm in diameter	Mole, wart
Vesicle	Raised, fluid-filled cavity; <1 cm in diameter	Herpes simplex, herpes zoster
Pustule	Raised, well-defined cavity that contains pus	Acne, impetigo
Patch	Macule >1 cm	Vitiligo
Plaque	Combined papules that form a raised area >1 cm in diameter	Psoriasis
Nodule	Raised, solid lesion >1 cm in diameter; may be hard or soft and may extend deeper into dermis than papule	Fibroma, xanthoma
Wheal	Superficial, irregular swelling caused by fluid accumulation	Allergic response, insect bite
Tumor	Firm or soft lesion that extends deep into dermis; may be firm or soft	Lipoma, hemangioma
Bulla	Thin-walled, fluid-filled chamber >1 cm in diameter	Blister
Crust	Thick, dried exudate remaining after vesicles rupture	Impetigo, weeping eczematous dermatitis
Scale	Dry or greasy skin flakes	Psoriasis, seborrheic dermatitis, eczema
Fissure	Distinct linear crack extending into dermis	Cheilosis, tinea pedis
Erosion	Shallow, superficial depression	Impetigo, herpes zoster, or herpes simplex lesions after vesicles rupture
Ulcer	Depression deeper than erosion; may bleed	Pressure ulcer, chancre
Excoriation	Abrasion caused by scratching	Scratching with insect bites, scabies, dermatitis
Nevus (mole)	Flat or raised; color darker than surrounding skin	
Cyst	Fluid-filled cavity in dermis or subcutaneous tissue	Sebaceous cyst

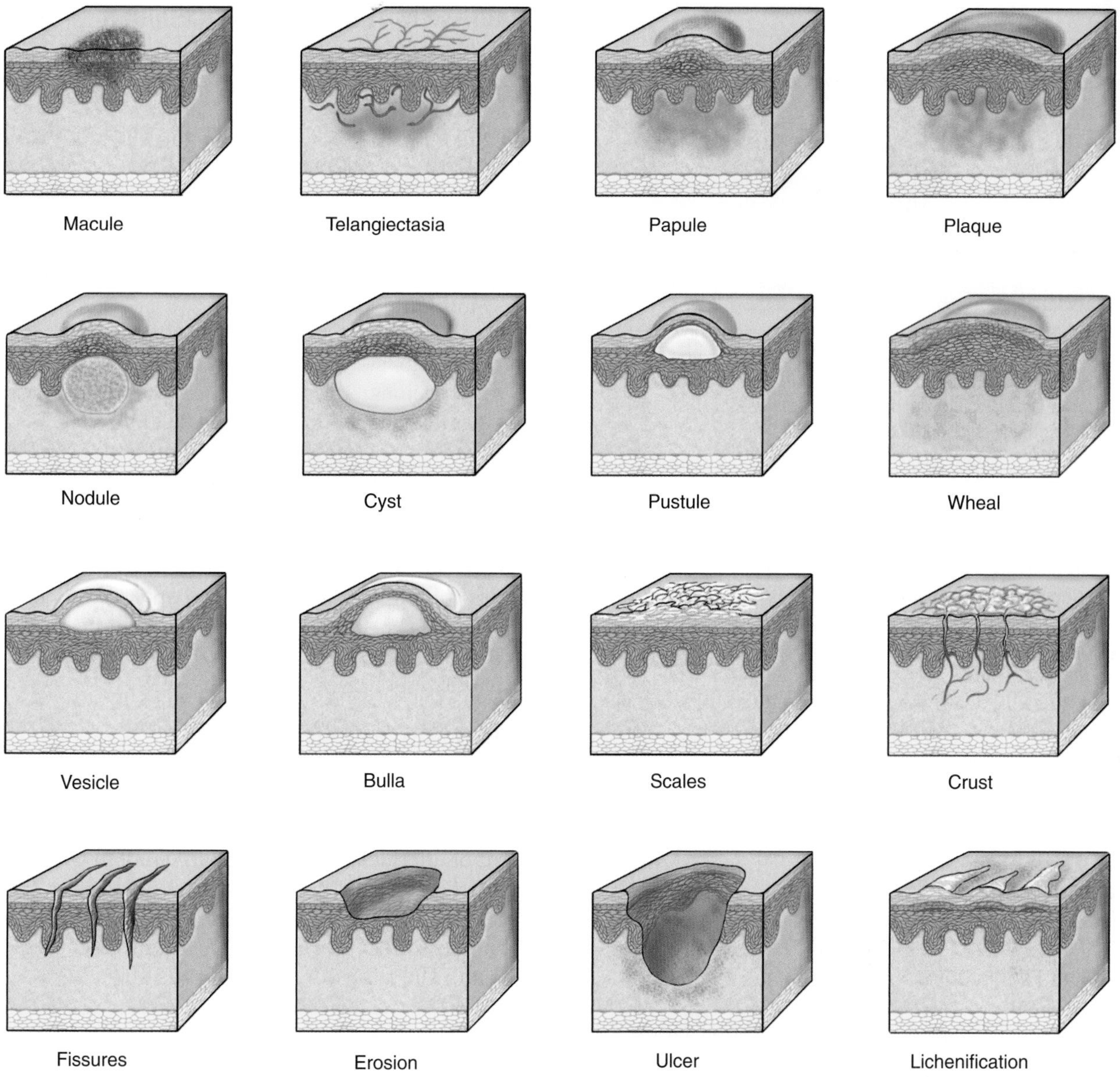

FIGURE 52-3 Skin lesions. (From Monahan FD, Drake DT, Neighbors M, editors: *Medical-surgical nursing: foundations for clinical practice*, ed 2, Philadelphia, 1998, Saunders.)

Palpating the skin is a way to collect data about the temperature, moisture, texture, thickness, edema, mobility, and turgor. Assessment of mobility and turgor is illustrated in Figure 52-4.

Some skin changes are less apparent in dark-skinned people than in light-skinned people (see *Cultural Considerations* box). Healthy black skin has a reddish undertone. A grayish tone may reflect cyanosis, which is best seen around the mouth, over the cheekbones, and on the earlobes. Inflammation may be better detected by areas of abnormal warmth and firmness than by color changes. Rashes are better seen by shining a light at an angle to reveal irregularities in skin surface.

Inspect the hair for color, distribution, and oiliness and palpate to determine the texture. Inspect the scalp for scaliness, infestations, and lesions. The term *lesion* is a general term that applies to wounds, sores, ulcers, tumors, and any other tissue damage. Various lesions are described in this chapter.

Note the shape and contour of the fingernails and toenails and the color of the nail bed. Check capillary refill by applying pressure to the nail to cause blanching and then releasing the pressure. The color should return to normal within 3 to 5 seconds. The angle of the nail base reveals clubbing of the nails (see Fig. 31-4).

Cultural Considerations

What Does Culture Have to Do with Skin Assessment?

It may be more difficult to assess some skin characteristics in dark-skinned people. To inspect for cyanosis, jaundice, and pallor, check the oral mucous membranes, the conjunctivae, the palms of the hands, and the soles of the feet.

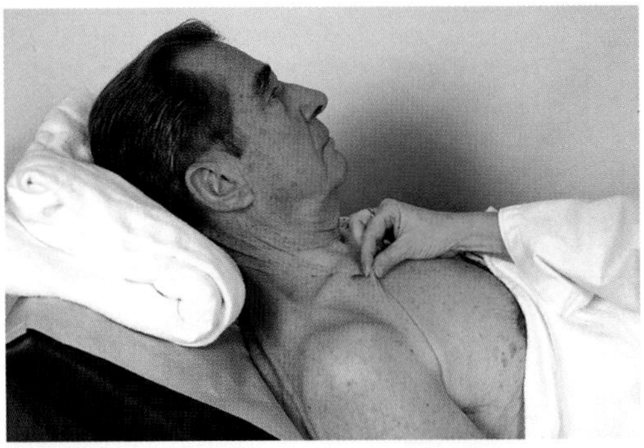

FIGURE 52-4 Skin mobility is determined by assessing how easily a large fold of skin is pinched up. Skin turgor is evaluated by observing how quickly the fold returns to the previous position. (From Jarvis C: *Physical examination and health assessment*, ed 5, Philadelphia, 2008, Saunders.)

Box 52-1 Assessment of the Patient with a Skin Disorder

HEALTH HISTORY

Chief Complaint or History of Present Illness

Pruritus, skin color changes, lesions, hair loss, abnormal hair growth

Past Medical History

Skin diseases or problems; drug therapy; allergies; chronic illnesses: diabetes mellitus (DM), cancer, kidney failure, thyroid disease, liver disease, anemia

Review of Systems

Change in skin color or pigmentation, change in a mole, sores that heal slowly, itching, dryness or scaliness, excessive bruising, changes in nails

Functional Assessment

Occupation, exposure to chemicals or other irritants, skin care habits, extent of sun exposure, dietary habits

PHYSICAL EXAMINATION

Skin

Color, pigmentation, dilated blood vessels, angiomas, nevi, lesions, rash, drainage, temperature, texture, moisture, thickness, edema, mobility, turgor, scars

Hair

Color, distribution, oiliness, texture, nits

Scalp

Scaliness, lesions

Nails

Shape, contour, color of nail bed, blanching with pressure, capillary refill, angle of nail base

The nursing assessment of the patient with a skin disorder is outlined in Box 52-1. The link between nutrition and skin health is discussed in the *Nutrition Considerations* box.

Nutrition Considerations

1. Vitamin A is essential for healthy skin.
2. Food sources of vitamin A are liver, pumpkin, sweet potatoes, carrots, spinach, broccoli, cantaloupe, and apricots.
3. Food allergies can cause atopic dermatitis.
4. Skin changes associated with malnutrition include cracked skin, dermatitis, xerosis (i.e., dry skin), purpura, and petechiae (i.e., purple or red spots).

DIAGNOSTIC TESTS AND PROCEDURES

CULTURE AND MICROSCOPIC EXAMINATION OF SKIN SPECIMENS

Studies of skin specimens that are used to diagnose skin conditions include the following:

- A potassium hydroxide (KOH) examination is done to diagnose fungal infections of the skin, hair, or nails by studying a skin specimen. For a culture, the skin scraping or a nail clipping is implanted in medium.
- A Tzanck test is used to diagnose viral skin infections.
- A scabies scraping is used to detect scabies (mites), eggs, or feces excreted by mites.
- Skin specimens may be cultured to identify fungal, bacterial, and viral infections.

WOOD'S LIGHT EXAMINATION

In a Wood's light examination, a black light is used to assess for pigmentation changes and superficial skin infections. It also may be used to examine the vulva after a sexual assault because it may reveal traces of saliva or semen.

PATCH TESTING FOR ALLERGY

To identify allergens, very small amounts of common irritants are applied to the skin, covered, and later examined for allergic reactions. Assessment and treatment of allergies are discussed in detail in Chapter 13.

BIOPSY

A biopsy is the removal of tissue for microscopic examination. The types of skin biopsies (Fig. 52-5) are as follows:

- *Shave biopsy:* A specimen no deeper than the dermis is obtained with a scalpel or other specialized instrument. Bleeding is usually minimal and controlled with pressure, cautery, or chemicals.
- *Punch biopsy:* A circular tool cuts around the lesion, which is then lifted up and severed. Pressure or chemicals usually control bleeding but suturing may be needed to close the site. The excision is relatively shallow.
- *Incisional biopsy:* A wedge of tissue is removed from the lesion.
- *Excisional biopsy:* For deep specimens, surgical excision biopsy is indicated. The entire lesion is removed. Sutures are required to close the defect left by the procedure.

Table 52-3 presents additional details and nursing interventions for patients undergoing diagnostic procedures.

COMMON THERAPEUTIC MEASURES

DRESSINGS

Dressings are used to protect healing wounds and to retain surface moisture to promote healing. Many

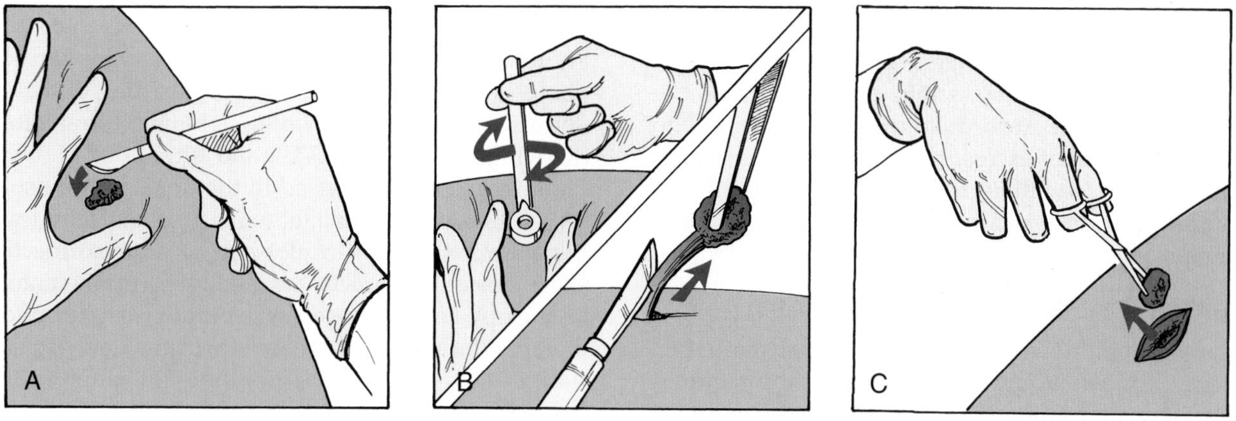

FIGURE 52-5 Types of biopsy procedures. **A,** Shave. **B,** Punch. **C,** Surgical excision. (From Black JM, Matassarin-Jacobs E: *Luckmann and Sorenson's medical-surgical nursing: clinical management for continuity of care*, ed 5, Philadelphia, 1997, Saunders.)

Table 52-3 Diagnostic Tests and Procedures Skin Disorders

TEST AND PURPOSE	PATIENT PREPARATION	POSTPROCEDURE CARE
Potassium hydroxide (KOH) examination is used along with a culture to diagnose fungal infections of the skin and nails.	Inform the patient that a small scraping of skin will be taken from the affected area for microscopic examination. The skin scrapings and a nail clipping are used for cultures to determine the exact cause of the lesion. The procedure is painless.	Inform the patient when results will be available.
Tzanck test is used to diagnose viral infections.	Tell the patient the lesion will be washed and opened to obtain a fluid sample, which will be examined microscopically. The procedure may cause mild discomfort. The results may be available immediately.	No special care is required.
Scabies scraping is used to assess skin lesions for the presence of scabies (i.e., mites), eggs, or feces excreted by the mites.	Inform the patient that the top of a lesion will be taken off for microscopic examination. The procedure is briefly uncomfortable but requires no anesthesia.	No special care is required.
Wood's light examination uses black light to reveal superficial skin infections and changes in pigmentation.	Tell the patient the procedure is done in a dark room. The skin will be inspected carefully under black light. The procedure is noninvasive and painless.	No special care is required.
Patch testing is used to identify substances to which patients are allergic.	Inform the patient that various common irritants are applied to the skin and covered with special patches or tape. The patches must be left in place and examined ("read") after 48, 72, and 96 hours and sometimes after 1 week. Skin reactions that indicate allergy include redness, swelling, and blisters. Patch testing is painless.	No special care is required.
Biopsy is the removal of tissue for microscopic examination.	Tell the patient the physician will remove some tissue for diagnostic evaluation. Small, shallow biopsies usually require only a dressing. Deeper biopsies require sutures. Patients are usually advised to avoid aspirin or other nonsteroidal antiinflammatory drugs (NSAIDs) for 48 hours before the biopsy to prevent excessive bleeding.	Inspect the site for bleeding. Apply direct pressure if necessary to control bleeding. If sutures are used, instruct the patient to return on a specified date for suture removal. Tell the patient how to care for the biopsy site (protocols vary) and when results are expected.

types of dressings exist, including wet, dry, absorptive, and occlusive dressings. Dry dressings protect wounds and absorb drainage. Wet dressings are used to decrease inflammation, soften crusts, and promote tissue granulation. Absorptive dressings are used to promote removal of excess exudate and are especially useful in wounds with necrotic tissue. Occlusive dressings protect wounds and maintain moisture to promote healing.

NEGATIVE PRESSURE WOUND THERAPY

Negative pressure wound therapy, such as the V.A.C. systems, appears to greatly reduce the time required for healing of traumatic wounds, dehisced surgical wounds, skin grafts, pressure ulcers, and chronic ulcers. To use this approach, the wound is first cleansed with normal saline. Then a skin preparation product is applied around the wound to receive the adhesive dressing. The wound is then filled with one of two types of sponges, depending on the wound characteristics. A tube in the sponges is used to exert negative pressure. A transparent adhesive dressing is applied over the sponges and around the tubing so that the wound closure is airtight. The tubing is connected to suction that is set at a prescribed negative pressure. Suction may be applied intermittently or continuously as ordered. Continuous suction is less painful than intermittent suction. A small suction canister attached to the machine collects drainage from the wound. This suction canister needs to be checked periodically, as once the container is full the suction will not function. Notify the enterostomal therapist, wound care specialist, or physician if the pain is distressing. The pressure may have to be reduced or converted from intermittent to continuous suction. Because dressing changes are painful, give the patient an analgesic about 1 hour before the procedure. The suction is discontinued and the sponges are moistened with normal saline before removal. This prevents the sponge from adhering to the wound.

SOAKS AND WET WRAPS

Soaks and wet wraps are used to soothe, soften, and remove crusts, debris, and necrotic tissue. Warm water is used and various agents may be added for specific skin conditions. After a soak, gently dry the treated area. A wet wrap may be applied to a single affected area or to the entire body. It is usually covered by a dry dressing and left in place for 15 to 20 minutes. Moisten the wet dressing again before removal. Otherwise, healthy tissue may adhere to the dry material and be traumatized. If debridement is intended, the gauze is not moistened before removal because the purpose of a wet-to-dry dressing is to remove debris and drainage. Once a wound is clean, wet-to-dry dressing is no longer appropriate. After various soaks and dressings, topical medications are applied if ordered.

PHOTOTHERAPY

Phototherapy is the use of light in combination with photosensitive drugs to promote shedding of the epidermis. Types of ultraviolet light are ultraviolet A (UVA), ultraviolet B (UVB), and ultraviolet C (UVC). Phototherapy may be used in the treatment of psoriasis, vitiligo, and chronic eczema. It is contraindicated in patients with a history of herpes simplex infection, skin cancer, cataracts, and lupus erythematosus because it aggravates these conditions. After phototherapy, the patient may have pruritus and dry skin. Assess for signs and symptoms of phototoxicity (redness, vesicles, pain).

Phototherapy with a psoralen and UVA (PUVA) is a treatment that uses a combination of oral or topical 8-methoxypsoralen and UVA (long-wave ultraviolet light). It is used to treat vitiligo, psoriasis, and cutaneous T-cell lymphoma. For 8 hours before and after the treatment, the patient is instructed to wear sunscreen, protective clothing, and dark glasses to decrease exposure to other sources of ultraviolet light. The Goeckerman regimen is a type of phototherapy specifically used to treat psoriasis and atopic dermatitis. The patient first bathes in a tar emulsion bath. Then a topical tar product is applied and the patient is exposed to ultraviolet light.

DRUG THERAPY

A number of topical and oral drugs are used to treat skin disorders and skin manifestations of other conditions. Topical drugs include **keratolytics** (capable of dissolving keratin), antipruritic agents, emollients, lubricants, sunscreens, tars, antiinfectives, glucocorticoids, antimetabolite agents, antihistamines, antiseborrheic agents, and vitamin A derivatives. Examples of selected drug classifications and their actions, side effects, and nursing interventions are presented in Table 52-4.

For topical application, drugs are combined with various substances in forms called *vehicles*. Topical medication vehicles include powders, lotions, aerosols, gels, creams, and ointments (see *Complementary and Alternative Therapies* box).

> **Complementary and Alternative Therapies**
>
> Topical herbal preparations that are used as emollients include balm of Gilead, coltsfoot, and comfrey.

DISORDERS OF THE SKIN

PRURITUS

Pruritus is simply itching. It is a symptom rather than a disease but is very common with many skin and systemic disorders. Therefore an overview of pruritus is presented here.

Table 52-4 **Drug Therapy: Skin Disorders**

DRUG	USE AND ACTION	SIDE EFFECTS	NURSING INTERVENTIONS
Keratolytics			
benzoyl peroxide (also an antimicrobial) salicylic acid sulfur coal tar	Dissolve keratin and slow bacterial growth. Used to treat dandruff, acne, and psoriasis.	Excessive dryness, irritation, scaling, edema, photosensitivity.	Advise patient to avoid excessive sun exposure. Assess effects.
Topical Antibacterials			
bacitracin Polysporin (bacitracin and polymixin B)	Destroy microorganisms. Used to treat skin infections. Also used on partial-thickness (first-degree) burns.	Contact dermatitis. Allergy (rare): itching, burning, anaphylaxis.	Ask about allergies before applying. Apply as prescribed after allergy ruled out. Report itching, burning, rash, redness.
silver sulfadiazine (Silvadene)	Bactericidal. Used to prevent and treat wound infection with serious burns.	Rash, pruritus, burning, pain. Rare: nephritis, anorexia. Can cause blood dyscrasias, hepatitis, nephrosis, hypoglycemia.	Apply to clean burn surface with gloved hands. Use a 4 × 4 or a tongue blade to remove the cream from the jar. Do not reinsert 4 × 4 in the jar. Cover burn completely and continuously. Monitor renal and GI distress, headache, joint pain, hepatic function. Monitor vital signs, CBC, serum glucose.
Antivirals			
acyclovir (Zovirax) famciclovir valacyclovir foscarnet	Interfere with viral replication. Used to treat infections caused by herpes simplex virus types 1 and 2 and herpes zoster. Not curative but may reduce severity and duration of symptoms.	Topical form: burning, stinging, pruritus. Oral form: nausea and vomiting. IV form: phlebitis, rash, urticaria, hypotension, hematuria, diaphoresis. Rare: confusion, agitation, seizures. Nephrotoxicity with high IV doses.	Ask about allergies. Monitor closely if patient has renal impairment. Measure I&O. Monitor infusion site for redness. Monitor neurologic status. Use gloved finger to apply ointment. Encourage adequate fluid intake.
Topical Antifungals			
nystatin clotrimazole (Mycostatin, Mycelex) oxiconazole (Oxistat) naftifine (Naftin) terbinafine (Lamisil)	Effective against fungi. Used to treat fungal infections.	Irritation, erythema, burning, rash. Abdominal cramps and cystitis with vaginal preparations.	Apply as directed. Do not apply occlusive dressings without order
Oral Antifungals			
terbinafine (Lamisil) griseofulvin (Fulvicin P/G) ketoconazole (Nizoral)	Used to treat fungal infections that do not respond to topicals. Common use: nail infections.	Terbinafine: hepatotoxicity, headache, diarrhea, GI distress. Griseofulvin: headache, rash, insomnia, GI distress. Ketoconazole: hepatotoxicity.	Give ketoconazole with food or milk to minimize GI effects and 2 hours apart from any drugs that reduce gastric acidity. Monitor liver function with ketoconazole and terbinafine. Griseofulvin decreases effects of warfarin.
Topical Antiinflammatory Agents			
hydrocortisone (Cortizone et al.) triamcinolone (Aristocort et al.) fluocinolone (Bio-Syn et al.)	Reduce inflammation in various skin disorders.	Itching, erythema, irritation. Severe allergic reactions rare. Systemic absorption varies with specific drug preparation and size of area treated.	Do not apply occlusive dressing without order. Apply sparingly and rub in thoroughly.

Continued

Table 52-4 Drug Therapy: Skin Disorders—cont'd

DRUG	USE AND ACTION	SIDE EFFECTS	NURSING INTERVENTIONS
Topical Antimicrobials			
azelaic acid (Azelex) clindamycin (Cleocin et al.) erythromycin (Eryderm et al.)	Antimicrobial against *Propionibacterium acnes* and *Staphylococcus epidermides.*	Pruritus, burning, stinging, tingling. Allergy: mild to moderate inflammatory acne vulgaris.	Avoid occlusive dressings. Keep away from mouth, eyes. Temporary skin irritation common. Two antiinfectives needed to prevent *P. acnes* resistance.
Vitamin A Derivative			
Topical: tretinoin (Retin-A) Oral: isotretinoin (Accutane)	Reduces formation of comedones. Increases mitosis of epithelial cells. Used to treat acne. Decreases size of sebaceous glands. Decreases sebum production. Used to treat severe acne. May decrease risk of skin cancer and PUVA.	Stinging, erythema, scaling expected. Allergy rare. Occasionally severe erythema, blistering. Excessive dryness of skin, nose, mouth. Conjunctivitis, vomiting, elevated serum triglycerides, bone or joint pain, muscle aches. Rare: hepatitis, IBD, depression. Cases of suicide have been reported in people on isotretinoin. Risk for major fetal deformities with isotretinoin. See www.ipledgeprogram.com for details of a program intended to ensure that pregnant women never take isotretinoin.	Tell patient not to use with keratolytics or other topical antiacne drugs. Do not apply tretinoin to eyes, mouth, angles of nose. Patient should avoid sun exposure, use sunscreen. If dryness is excessive, decrease frequency of use. Tell patient to expect symptoms to worsen at first, then improve. Report severe GI symptoms. Avoid sun exposure because of photosensitivity. With isotretinoin: Promptly notify prescriber if symptoms of depression occur. Because the drug is teratogenic, two negative serum pregnancy tests must be obtained before starting therapy. Explain importance of testing for pregnancy every month when taking therapy. Two reliable forms of contraception must be used simultaneously beginning 1 month before starting therapy and continuing for 1 month after therapy is completed.
tazarotene (Tazorac) adapalene (Differin)	Tazarotene and adapalene both are topical agents used to treat acne. Tazarotene is also used to treat psoriasis.	Both can cause itching, burning, and stinging. More serious skin reactions sometimes occur.	Advise patients to avoid direct sunlight and use sunscreens because of photosensitivity. Acne may worsen before beneficial results occur. Instruct patient in correct application (see instructions for each drug).
Pediculicides and Scabicides			
crotamiton (Eurax) permethrin (Nix)	Kill parasites and their eggs. Used to treat pediculosis (lice) and scabies (mite) infestations.	Skin and eye irritation. Systemic effects with excessive use.	Follow directions specifically. Avoid contact with eyes. Most products are effective with one application but a repeat treatment may be recommended. Clothing and bed linens must be treated to prevent reinfestation.
Antipsoriatics			
anthralin and tar (Estar gel)	Used to treat psoriasis.	Anthralin: erythema, inflamed eyes, staining. Tar: skin irritation, photosensitivity, staining.	Protect skin and clothing from preparations that stain. Most have unpleasant odor.

Table 52-4 Drug Therapy: Skin Disorders—cont'd

DRUG	USE AND ACTION	SIDE EFFECTS	NURSING INTERVENTIONS
Retinoid Antipsoriatic			
acitretin (Soriatane)	Decreases proliferation of epidermal cells; antiinflammatory, immunomodulatory. For severe psoriasis only.	Hair loss, skin peeling, dry mouth, rhinitis, gingivitis, elevated liver enzymes and triglycerides. Many other side and adverse effects.	*Contraindicated during pregnancy!* Ensure that patient understands risk to fetus and uses contraception if sexually active for at least 3 years after therapy is completed. Should be taken with meals. Monitor for all side effects.
Photosensitivity Drug			
methoxsalen (Oxsoralen)	Decreases proliferation of epidermal cells in psoriasis.	Nausea, headache, vertigo, rash, pruritus, burning and peeling of skin. Can cause anemia, leukopenia, thrombocytopenia, ulcerative stomatitis, bleeding, alopecia, cystitis.	Encourage patient to return for periodic blood tests as ordered and to report easy bruising or excessive bleeding.
Biologic Agents			
etanercept (Enbrel)	Used in the treatment of rheumatoid arthritis, psoriatis arthritis, plaque psoriasis. Neutralizes tumor necrosis factor.	Infection, Stevens-Johnson syndrome, heart failure, cancer, neutropenia, tuberculosis, thrombocytopenia, liver failure	

CBC, Complete blood count; *GI,* gastrointestinal; *I&O,* intake and output; *IBD,* inflammatory bowel disease; *IV,* intravenous; *PUVA,* psoralen and ultraviolet A.

Cause and Risk Factors

The sensation of itching is not completely understood but it may be triggered by touch; temperature changes; emotional stress; and chemical, mechanical, and electrical stimuli. The severity of the response to stimulation is enhanced by emotional stress, anxiety, and fear.

Pruritus is a prominent symptom with psoriasis, dermatitis, eczema, and insect bites. It also may be seen with the following systemic conditions: urticaria, some cancers, renal failure, DM, thyroid disorders, liver disease, and anemia. Among the drugs that can cause pruritus are opiates and phenothiazines.

Medical Treatment

When the cause of pruritus is known, treatment is directed at correcting the cause. Measures that may help to control pruritus include stress management and avoidance of known irritants; sudden temperature changes; and alcohol, tea, and coffee. Lubricants in the bath water and emollients applied after bathing also may help. Medications that often are ordered for pruritus include corticosteroids, antihistamines, and local anesthetics. In some situations, antidepressant and antiserotonin drugs may be ordered.

❖ NURSING CARE of the Patient with Pruritus

■ Assessment

When a patient has pruritus, collect data about his or her symptoms that may help to determine the cause. The history of the current illness is important because pruritus may be just one symptom of a condition that requires attention. Possible contributing factors to be documented include exposure to irritants, drug therapy, and past medical history.

Nursing Diagnoses, Goals, and Outcome Criteria: Pruritus

Nursing Diagnoses	Goals and Outcome Criteria
Impaired Skin Integrity related to scratching	Intact skin: absence of abrasions
Ineffective Self-Health Management related to lack of understanding of prevention or management of pruritus	Patient adheres to prescribed measures to prevent or treat condition: patient correctly states correct measures, demonstrates self-care

■ Interventions

The specific interventions vary with the cause of pruritus. If the patient has dry skin, application of lubricants or emollients may be helpful. The addition of oils to bath water is often recommended but could create an unsafe situation in the bathtub. Advise patients to avoid bathing in very hot water. In most cases, lotion can be applied to unbroken skin without a physician's order. If topical or systemic drugs are ordered, administer them or instruct the patient in their use. Inspect the skin daily to determine the effects of the treatments. Explain possible causes of pruritus and encourage the patient to avoid them (see *Patient Teaching* box).

Patient Teaching

Pruritus

- Avoid factors that aggravate itching such as temperature extremes, extremely dry air, irritating fabrics, chemicals, frequent hot baths, sweating, and stress.
- To prevent itching, avoid extreme temperatures, humidify room air, take less frequent and cooler baths, apply emollients, avoid irritating fabrics and chemicals, and practice stress management.
- Use therapeutic measures as prescribed.
  - Topical agents: lotions, creams
  - Systemic agents: antihistamines (i.e., dosage, side effects)
  - Treatment of underlying conditions

INFLAMMATORY CONDITIONS AND INFECTIONS

Atopic Dermatitis (Eczema)

Pathophysiology. Atopic **dermatitis** is one of several disorders referred to as *eczema.* Eczema has three stages. The acute stage is characterized by a red, oozing, crusty rash and intense pruritus. Manifestations of the subacute stage include redness, excoriations, and scaling plaques or pustules. Fine scales may give the patient's skin a silvery appearance. In the chronic stage, the skin becomes dry, thickened, scaly, and brownish-gray in color (Fig. 52-6). Open lesions invite infection and scarring may occur. Multiple stages may be present at the same time.

Cause and Risk Factors. Most patients with atopic dermatitis have a personal or family history of asthma, hay fever, eczema, or food allergies. People with atopic dermatitis have an immune dysfunction but it is not known whether that dysfunction is a cause or an effect of the disorder.

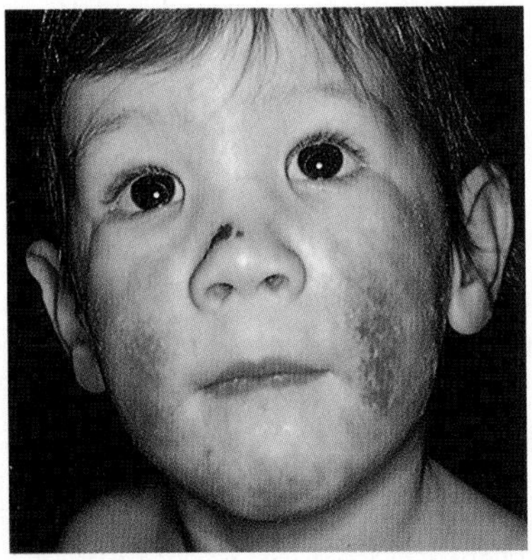

FIGURE 52-6 Atopic dermatitis. (From Hurwitz S: *Clinical pediatric dermatology: a textbook of skin disorders of childhood and adolescence*, ed 2, Philadelphia, 1993, Saunders.)

Medical Diagnosis. A medical diagnosis of atopic dermatitis is based primarily on the health history and physical examination. Other procedures that might be done to confirm the diagnosis are skin biopsy, serum immunoglobulin E levels, and cultures to diagnose secondary infections. If allergy is suspected as a cause of dermatitis, the physician may perform allergy tests to identify allergens.

Medical Treatment. Topical corticosteroids and moisturizers provide the best control of inflammation. However, steroids can cause skin atrophy, loss of pigmentation, permanent red lesions, and, with high doses, adrenal suppression. Soaks, occlusive dressings, and emollients help to keep the skin moist. Systemic antihistamines may be ordered to relieve itching and inflammation. In severe cases that do not respond to topical agents, a short course of systemic corticosteroids may be ordered. Patients who do not respond to safer therapies may be treated with the immunosuppressants tacrolimus ointment (Protopic) or pimecrolimus cream (Elidel). These drugs may increase the risk of skin cancer and lymphoma. Treatment of allergic disorders is discussed in Chapter 13.

NURSING CARE of the Patient with Atopic Dermatitis

Assessment

Assessment of the patient with a skin disorder is summarized in Box 52-1. When the patient has atopic dermatitis, specifically inquire about known allergies, bathing practices (i.e., frequency, water temperature, use of soaps), and current medications to identify possible contributing factors. The physical examination includes inspection and palpation of the skin for lesions, moisture, and abrasions.

Nursing Diagnoses, Goals, and Outcome Criteria: Atopic Dermatitis

Nursing Diagnoses	Goals and Outcome Criteria
Impaired Skin Integrity related to plaques, open lesions, and pustules	Improved skin integrity: intact, moist skin
Risk for Infection related to break in skin, decreased resistance to infection	Absence of infection: no fever, decreasing redness and drainage
Disturbed Body Image related to lesions	Improved body image: positive patient statements about self

Interventions

Impaired Skin Integrity

Measures that decrease itching and moisturize the skin help to maintain skin integrity. Encourage the patient to maintain the room temperature at 68°F to 75°F with

45% to 55% humidity. Advise the patient to avoid possible irritants. New clothing should be washed before it is worn. Mild detergent should be used for laundry and clothes should be rinsed twice. Recommend open-weave fabrics and loose clothing. Advise the use of moisturizers and sunscreens. If drugs are ordered for pruritus, administer them or instruct the patient in self-medication. Evaluate skin integrity and hydration on an ongoing basis (see *Complementary and Alternative Therapies* box).

Complementary and Alternative Therapies

When a patient has an allergic skin reaction, be sure to assess for topical use of herbal products. For example, aloe can cause allergic dermatitis in susceptible persons and angelica can cause a skin rash if a patient is exposed to sunlight.

Risk for Infection

Any break in the skin presents an entry for pathogens. Inspect the skin and report new lesions to the physician. Monitor the temperature for elevation that may reflect a systemic infection. Teach the patient the importance of protecting the skin from trauma. If scratching is a problem, the fingernails need to be cut short and kept smooth (see *Patient Teaching* box). Gloves or mittens may help to prevent traumatic scratching during sleep or in the confused person. Administer antibiotics as ordered.

Patient Teaching

Atopic Dermatitis

- Avoid known irritants and constrictive clothing.
- Use moisturizers and sunscreens.
- Take drugs as prescribed: name, dosage or application instructions, adverse effects.
- After swimming in chlorinated water, shampoo and bathe or shower using a mild soap. Then apply a moisturizer.

Disturbed Body Image

Demonstrate acceptance of the patient's appearance through attentive care and touch. Teach the patient and family that dermatitis is not contagious and is not caused by poor hygiene. Explore the patient's concerns about the skin disorder. If the patient is very stressed, the nurse can discuss coping strategies or request a referral for professional counseling.

Contact Dermatitis

Contact dermatitis is an inflammatory condition caused by contact with a substance that triggers an allergic response. Allergic and immune disorders are discussed in Chapter 13.

Seborrheic Dermatitis

Pathophysiology. Seborrheic dermatitis is a chronic inflammatory disease of the skin. It usually affects the scalp, eyebrows, eyelids, lips, ears, sternal area, axillae, umbilicus, groin, gluteal crease, and area under the breasts. Seborrheic dermatitis of the scalp is called *dandruff*. Areas affected by this condition may have fine, powdery scales; thick crusts; or oily patches. Scales may be white, yellowish, or reddish. Pruritus is common.

Cause and Risk Factors. The cause of seborrheic dermatitis is unknown. It may be an inflammatory reaction to infection with the yeast *Malassezia*. Because the condition is aggravated by emotional stress and neurologic disease, some researchers think there may be a central nervous system (CNS) influence.

Medical Diagnosis. Diagnosis of seborrheic dermatitis is based on the health history and physical examination.

Medical Treatment. Initial treatment of seborrheic dermatitis uses topical ketoconazole (Nizoral), sometimes with topical corticosteroids. Dandruff is treated with medicated shampoos used two or three times a week. Appropriate shampoos are those that contain selenium sulfide (Selsun), ketoconazole, tar, zinc pyrithione, salicylic acid, or resorcin. Some corticosteroid solutions also may be prescribed.

NURSING CARE of the Patient with Seborrheic Dermatitis

Although seborrheic dermatitis does not require inpatient treatment, it is a common condition encountered among patients in the community and long-term care and among those hospitalized for other reasons.

Assessment

Relevant data include symptoms and identification of treatments being used. Inspect and describe the affected areas.

Nursing Diagnoses, Goals, and Outcome Criteria: Seborrheic Dermatitis

Nursing Diagnoses	Goals and Outcome Criteria
Ineffective Self-Health Management related to lack of knowledge about disease process	Patient implements the prescribed treatment plan: correctly describes plan and self-care treatment
Disturbed Body Image related to altered appearance (lesions)	Improved body image: decreasing signs of the condition, patient's statements reflect a positive view of self

Interventions

Explain the condition and reinforce the physician's instructions for treatment. Suggest measures to relieve pruritus, as described earlier under "Disorders of the Skin." Discuss the patient's concerns about the condition and emphasize that seborrheic dermatitis can be controlled with treatment. Demonstrate acceptance of the patient through genuine interest and use of touch.

Psoriasis

Pathophysiology. Psoriasis is an autoimmune disorder characterized by abnormal proliferation of skin cells. The classic sign of **psoriasis** is the appearance of bright-red lesions that may be covered with silvery scales (Fig. 52-7). Although the onset is common in young adulthood, it can appear at any age. Psoriasis may affect a limited body area or may be extensive. Some people have systemic effects of the disease, such as psoriatic arthritis. Patients should be educated about the signs and symptoms of arthritis during the initial education session on psoriasis.

Cause and Risk Factors. Psoriasis is a condition caused by rapid proliferation of epidermal cells. It is usually chronic with cycles of exacerbations and remissions. Multiple factors acting on a genetically predisposed person are thought to cause this disorder. Factors that aggravate psoriasis are stress; streptococcal infections; overuse of alcohol; and drugs such as lithium, antimalarials, angiotensin-converting enzyme (ACE) inhibitors, and beta-blockers.

Medical Diagnosis. Psoriasis is diagnosed based on the health history and the physical examination.

Medical Treatment. No cure for psoriasis exists but it can be treated topically or systemically. Patients with mild psoriasis are usually treated with topical medications: corticosteroids, tazarotene, Estar, and vitamin D derivatives (calcipotriene [Dovonex]). Topical salicylic acid may be used with the corticosteroids. Tazarotene (Tazorac) is a topical retinoid agent that stays in the skin longer, leading to longer remissions. Anthralin (Anthra-Derm) may be used to remove heavy scales. With a gloved hand, it is applied only to the lesions. After a specified period, anthralin is removed with tissues. The patient removes the residue by showering or bathing. The medication must be handled carefully because it stains hair, skin, fingernails, furniture, and bathroom fixtures. Newer preparations that may not stain (e.g., Estar gel) are now available. UVB may be used to enhance topical therapy with tar and anthralin.

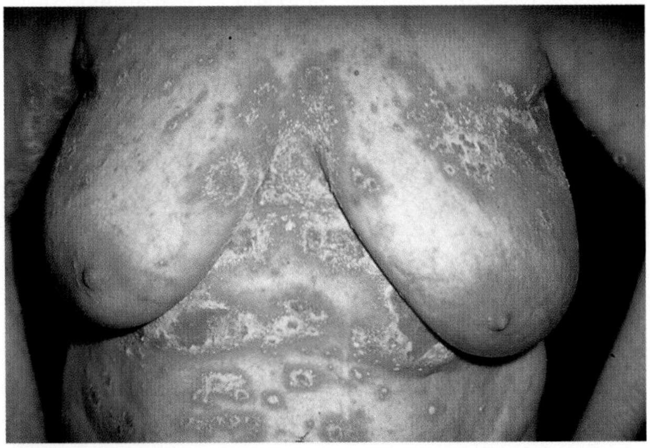

FIGURE 52-7 Psoriasis. (Courtesy Columbia Presbyterian Dermatology Associates, New York, NY.)

Moderate to severe psoriasis may be treated with PUVA, a combination of methotrexate and UVA. Other oral drugs include oral retinoids (acitretin [Soriatane]) and biologic agents (etanercept [Enbrel]). Patients receiving biologic agents should be monitored closely for infections, as these agents tend to decrease the number of circulating T cells. Oral retinoids may reduce the risk of skin cancers associated with PUVA. Systemic corticosteroids may be used on a short-term basis. Patients on most forms of systemic therapy require periodic liver testing and blood studies because of the adverse effects. Methotrexate and oral retinoids are contraindicated during pregnancy because of the risk of fetal harm.

Pharmacology Capsule

If a woman of childbearing age is taking methotrexate or oral retinoids, ensure that she understands that these drugs are harmful to a fetus. If the patient suspects she is pregnant, she should inform her physician immediately if taking either of these drugs. Instruct women of childbearing age to use appropriate methods to prevent pregnancy while on these drugs.

Pharmacology Capsule

Because of risks to the fetus, women should use reliable contraception during and for 3 years after therapy with Soriatane.

NURSING CARE of the Patient with Psoriasis

Assessment

Relevant data for the patient with psoriasis include a description of symptoms and identification of treatments being used (see Nursing Care Plan: Patient with Psoriasis). Inspect the affected areas for lesions and scales. Document joint pain or stiffness because the condition may cause arthritis. Explore the effect of psoriasis on the patient's everyday life and the coping strategies used.

Nursing Diagnoses, Goals, and Outcome Criteria: Psoriasis

Nursing Diagnoses	Goals and Outcome Criteria
Ineffective Self-Health Management related to lack of knowledge about the skin condition and treatment	Effective management of treatment regimen: patient correctly describes and demonstrates self-care
Disturbed Body Image related to lesions and scales on skin	Improved body image: patient makes effort to improve appearance and makes positive remarks about self
Social Isolation related to embarrassment about skin lesions	Decreased social isolation: patient shows continued involvement in social activities

Nursing Care Plan — Patient with Psoriasis

ASSESSMENT

HEALTH HISTORY A 45-year-old police officer came to the physician's office because of a "rash" on his trunk. He reports that he is in good health and has had no major injuries or illnesses except a left knee injury sustained in a fall as a teenager. He is taking no medications but is allergic to penicillin. He is alarmed by the rash and is afraid it might spread and be something serious. The physician diagnoses psoriasis. The patient is divorced and enjoys socializing, especially dancing. He is concerned about how people might react to his condition.

PHYSICAL EXAMINATION Vital signs: blood pressure 144/88 mm Hg, pulse 84 bpm, respiration 16 breaths per minute, temperature 98.2°F (36.8°C) measured orally. Height 5′10″, weight 164 lb. He is alert and oriented but mildly anxious. The skin on the face, arms, and legs is normal. Bright-red lesions with silvery scales are distributed over the anterior and posterior chest, abdomen, buttocks, and hands. Heart and breath sounds are normal. The abdomen is soft, with bowel sounds present in all four quadrants. Full range of motion of all joints is possible, with crepitation in the left knee. Peripheral pulses are strong and symmetric. The extremities are warm and dry.

Nursing Diagnosis	Goals and Outcome Criteria	Interventions
Ineffective Self-Health Management related to lack of understanding of psoriasis and its treatment	The patient will correctly describe psoriasis and prescribed treatment measures.	Explain that psoriasis typically has periods of exacerbation and remission, that it is not contagious, and that symptoms can be improved with treatment. Explain the prescribed treatment, including proper application of topical medications and side and adverse effects of drug therapy. For oral drugs, provide information about the schedule as well as adverse and side effects. Tell the patient signs of secondary infection (i.e., fever, purulent drainage, increased redness) that should be reported to the physician. Encourage the patient to plan for adequate rest and eat a balanced diet. Explore stress management strategies. Refer the patient to a mental health counselor if needed. Supplement verbal teaching with written material.
Disturbed Body Image related to lesions and scales on skin	The patient's body image will improve, as evidenced by positive statements about self.	Demonstrate acceptance of the patient through eye contact and touch. Be aware of personal reaction to lesions. Encourage the patient to share feelings about the condition. Help the patient to feel "in control" by providing information about the management of psoriasis.
Social Isolation related to embarrassment about skin lesions	The patient will continue social activities and identify strategies to deal with social situations.	Explore how the patient thinks others will react to his condition. Role-play strategies to use in social situations. Encourage continued activity. Emphasize expected improvement.

Critical Thinking Questions

1. Why is stress management important in the treatment of psoriasis?
2. What are the psychosocial effects of a diagnosis of psoriasis?

Interventions

Ineffective Self-Health Management

The focus of nursing care for the patient with psoriasis is patient education that enables the patient to manage the prescribed regimen. The patient and family need to know that the condition is chronic but not contagious and usually responds to treatment. Teach the patient about the prescribed medications and treatments. Tell the patient to report signs of secondary infection (i.e., fever, purulent discharge, increased redness) to the physician. In addition, encourage adequate rest, good nutrition, and stress management. If taking drugs that suppress the immune system, the patient should avoid crowds and people with infections and practice good hand washing.

Disturbed Body Image

Give the patient the opportunity to express feelings about psoriasis and the effects on his or her life. Demonstrate acceptance of the patient's appearance and the feelings that are expressed. Learning to manage the condition can help the patient to feel more hopeful, realizing that remission will occur.

Social Isolation

Encourage the patient to maintain social contacts and plan strategies to deal with exacerbations without undue stress.

Intertrigo

Pathophysiology. **Intertrigo** is inflammation of the skin where two skin surfaces touch: axillae, abdominal skinfolds, and the area under the breasts. The affected area is usually red and "weeping," with clear margins. The area may be surrounded by vesicles and pustules.

Cause and Risk Factors. The inflammation of intertrigo results from heat, friction, and moisture between two touching body surfaces. These factors create the perfect environment for infection by *Candida albicans* (yeast) or bacteria.

Medical Diagnosis and Treatment. The medical diagnosis is based on the site and appearance of the inflamed skin and the presence of *C. albicans* as confirmed by KOH examination and culture of skin scrapings. If the skin is not broken, it can be washed with water twice daily. The area is then rinsed and patted dry. Soft gauze may be used to separate layers of body tissue and absorb moisture. Cornstarch is contraindicated because it supports the growth of *C. albicans*. For severe inflammation or fungal infection, treatment may include a topical corticosteroid or antifungal. Examples of topical antifungals are nystatin, ketoconazole, clotrimazole, and terbinafine. Vytone 1% is a combination corticosteroid, antibacterial, and antifungal preparation. Wet soaks with tap water or Burow solution are sometimes ordered to remove exudate if an infection is present.

NURSING CARE of the Patient with Intertrigo

Assessment

Intertrigo is fairly common among patients in long-term care facilities. Investigate complaints of pain, irritation, or redness in body folds. Monitor body temperature to detect possible infection. Inspect susceptible areas (i.e., axillae, groin, beneath breasts, abdominal skinfolds) on a daily basis.

Nursing Diagnoses, Goals, and Outcome Criteria: Intertrigo

Nursing Diagnoses	Goals and Outcome Criteria
Impaired Skin Integrity related to inflammation	Improved skin integrity: intact skin without redness
Risk for Infection related to moist environment, broken skin, and medications	Absence of infection: no fever, pain, or redness

Interventions

Areas where skin surfaces are in close contact must be kept clean and dry. Apply topical medications (antifungals and corticosteroids) as ordered. Report increasing redness and tenderness, fever, and broken skin to the physician. Encourage women with pendulous breasts to wear a soft, supportive bra. If incontinence has contributed to perineal intertrigo, positioning the patient with the legs apart allows moisture to evaporate. Encourage clients to keep nails short and to report excessive scratching to the health care provider so that additional medication can be provided to decrease pruritis.

Fungal Infections

Pathophysiology. Humans are susceptible to a number of fungal infections. Superficial infections of the skin and mucous membranes caused by fungi include tinea pedis (athlete's foot), tinea manus (hand), tinea cruris (groin), tinea capitis (scalp), tinea corporis (body), tinea barbae (beard), and candidiasis, which can affect the skin, mouth, vagina, GI tract, and lungs.

Cause and Risk Factors. The organisms that cause tinea infections take advantage of trauma in moist, warm tissue. Some organisms can be spread through direct contact or by inanimate objects. Lesions vary but may be scaly patches with raised borders. The lay term *ringworm* is sometimes used to describe these circular lesions. Pruritus is a common symptom of tinea. Scratching that breaks the skin may lead to a secondary bacterial infection. Tinea capitis, tinea corporis, and tinea pedis are rather easily spread by sharing contaminated objects.

Candidiasis, commonly called a *yeast infection*, is caused by *C. albicans*. Patients at risk for candidiasis include those who are pregnant, malnourished, immunosuppressed, or taking antibiotics or oral contraceptives. People with DM are also at risk for this disease. Common sites affected are the mouth, vagina, and skin. The skin around an ostomy site also is susceptible to candidiasis because of the constant moisture there. Infections of the mucous membranes are manifested as red lesions with white plaques. Skin infections with *C. albicans* are seen as moist, red lesions (Fig. 52-8). The lesions often are found in folds of body tissue (see section titled "Intertrigo").

Pharmacology Capsule

Antibiotic therapy eliminates the microorganisms that normally control fungal growth, making the patient susceptible to fungal infections.

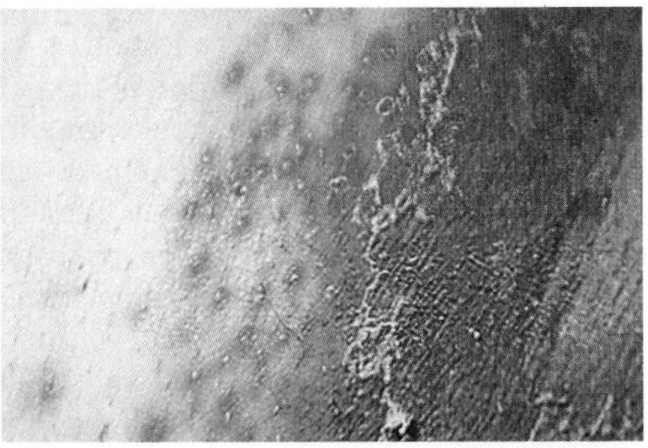

FIGURE 52-8 Candidiasis. (From Lookingbill DP, Marks JG: *Principles of dermatology*, ed 2, Philadelphia, 1993, Saunders.)

Medical Diagnosis. Fungal infections are usually diagnosed on the basis of the history and physical examination but may be confirmed by microscopic examination of scrapings from a lesion using a KOH wet mount preparation.

Medical Treatment. Fungal infections of the skin and mucous membranes are usually treated with antifungal powders and creams. Wet compresses and keratolytics may be ordered to soften scales with some tinea infections. Butenafine (Lotrimin) is used for tinea pedis, tinea corporis, tinea cruris, and tinea versicolor. Oral candidiasis is treated with clotrimazole troches, nystatin mouthwash or lozenges, or oral amphotericin B. For acquired immunodeficiency syndrome (AIDS) patients, clotrimazole is superior to nystatin. Candidiasis of the vulva and vagina may be treated with topical azoles (e.g. clotrimazole, miconazole, tioconazole) or oral fluconazole (Diflucan). Systemic fungal infections require intravenous amphotericin B, an effective but very toxic drug. Patients receiving amphotericin B usually are pretreated with an antihistamine and a nonopioid analgesic to reduce the risk of chills, fever, and headache. Patients with severe adverse effects may be given a glucocorticoid and either meperidine or dantrolene for rigors (i.e., shaking chills).

Pharmacology Capsule

Systemic amphotericin B is highly toxic to the kidneys. An infusion of 1 L of saline on the day of treatment helps to reduce renal damage.

NURSING CARE of the Patient with a Fungal Infection

Assessment

The nursing assessment identifies conditions that might make a person susceptible to fungal infections, including DM, malnutrition, and immunosuppression. Note antibiotic therapy, another risk factor. During the physical examination, inspect the skin and mucous membranes for lesions. Creamy white lesions that can be scraped off easily are characteristic of oral candidiasis.

Nursing Diagnoses, Goals, and Outcome Criteria: Fungal Infection

Nursing Diagnoses	Goals and Outcome Criteria
Disturbed Body Image related to skin lesions	Improved body image: absence of skin lesions, patient's positive statements about appearance
Impaired Oral Mucous Membrane related to oral candidiasis	Healthy oral mucous membranes: absence of oral lesions, infection
Risk for Injury related to reinfection	Decreased risk of recurrent infection: patient correctly describes and demonstrates self-care

Interventions

Disturbed Body Image

Be sensitive to the patient's reaction to a skin infection. Visible lesions may be embarrassing to the patient. If the genitalia are affected, the patient may think that the symptoms are due to a sexually transmitted infection (STI). Explain the cause of the infection, how it is treated, whether it is contagious, and how transmission and reinfection can be avoided. If medication is prescribed, instruct the patient in proper use of the agent. Tell the patient to keep the affected areas of the skin as clean and dry as possible. A cool environment helps by reducing perspiration.

Eradication of candidiasis infections in bedridden patients can be especially challenging. Frequently reposition the patient to permit evaporation of moisture. The thighs can be separated by using a pillow between the knees and a folded cloth may be placed beneath pendulous breasts.

Impaired Oral Mucous Membranes

Instruct the patient with oral candidiasis in the proper use of prescribed medications. Mouthwashes may be swished to coat all oral surfaces before swallowing. Lozenges should be dissolved in the mouth. If the patient wears dentures, they should be soaked in an antifungal solution.

Risk for Injury

Advise patients with tinea infections to avoid sharing personal items such as hairbrushes and clothing. They also should dry thoroughly after bathing and wear absorbent underwear and socks.

Acne

Pathophysiology. **Acne** is a skin condition that affects the hair follicles and sebaceous glands. It is characterized by comedones (whiteheads and blackheads), pustules, and cysts. These lesions most often develop on the face, neck, and upper trunk. Acne commonly begins in adolescence and may last into adulthood. Most cases are mild but serious cases with extensive inflammation can cause permanent scarring.

Cause and Risk Factors. Acne lesions develop when androgenic hormones cause increased sebum production and bacteria *(Propionibacterium acnes)* proliferate, causing sebaceous follicles to become blocked and inflamed. Despite popular opinion, acne is not caused by fatty foods, chocolate, or poor hygiene. In addition to androgenic hormones, exacerbations of acne can be triggered by high levels of progestin in birth control pills, oil-based cosmetics, high doses of systemic corticosteroids, hormonal changes associated with the menstrual period, and some endocrine disorders.

Medical Diagnosis. Acne is diagnosed on the basis of the health history and physical examination findings.

Medical Treatment. Treatment varies with the severity of the condition. Mild cases may respond very well

Pharmacology Capsule

Accutane can cause mental depression, possibly leading to suicidal ideation. Should depression develop, contact the physician immediately to have the drug discontinued. Depression should resolve once the drug is stopped. Should depression continue, the patient should be referred for additional counseling. The parents and the child should be taught the signs and symptoms of depression to report immediately to a parent or health care provider.

to topical antimicrobials or retinoids (vitamin A preparations). Topical antimicrobials include azelaic acid (Azelex) and benzoyl peroxide; topical retinoids include tretinoin (Retin-A) or tazarotene (Tazorac). If these agents do not adequately control acne, oral antibiotics (i.e., tetracycline, azithromycin, erythromycin) may be given over a period of several months. Estrogen also may be prescribed to counteract the effects of androgenic hormones. Spironolactone may be used for its antiandrogenic effects. If acne is severe and unresponsive to all of these treatments, isotretinoin (Accutane) may be prescribed.

Nonpharmacologic treatment may include comedone extraction or cryotherapy. Dermabrasion may be used to reduce scarring.

Pharmacology Capsule

Isotretinoin (Accutane) can cause severe fetal deformities. Therefore women who take the drug must prevent pregnancy until at least 1 month after therapy has been completed.

NURSING CARE of the Patient with Acne

Assessment

Explore the patient's concerns and knowledge about acne. Document any treatments being used. Note all medical conditions and medications because some contribute to or aggravate acne. Inspect the skin to determine the extent and severity of the condition.

Nursing Diagnoses, Goals, and Outcome Criteria: Acne

Nursing Diagnoses	Goals and Outcome Criteria
Disturbed Body Image related to comedones, pustules, and cysts	Improved body image: decreased lesions and patient's expression of improved body image
Ineffective Self-Health Management related to lack of understanding of causes and treatment of acne	Effective treatment management: patient correctly describes and demonstrates prescribed skin care and self-medication

Interventions

Disturbed Body Image

When working with a person who has acne, provide support and information. Because acne almost always affects the face, most patients with moderate or severe acne suffer body image disturbances. Be sensitive to this concern and encourage the patient to see a dermatologist for treatment. This condition can be very harmful to the patient's self-esteem and should not be dismissed as a minor problem.

Ineffective Self-Health Management

Explain the causes of acne as well as the many myths about the disease. Assure the patient that acne does not reflect poor hygiene but that cleanliness does reduce the risk of infections. Dietary interventions are no longer thought to be useful. Discourage picking or squeezing lesions because it may force infected material deeper into the follicle. Advise the patient that harsh cleansers and vigorous scrubbing have no therapeutic value.

Explain prescribed drugs and discuss any adverse effects. Patient teaching is especially important if isotretinoin is used. Isotretinoin is an oral medication that has a drying effect on the skin. Tell the patient to expect the condition to worsen initially and then begin to improve. Advise the patient that the drug is teratogenic, meaning that it is harmful to a developing fetus. Therefore two forms of effective contraception must be used if the patient is sexually active while taking the drug. When isotretinoin is prescribed for females, the patient must have two negative pregnancy tests within 2 weeks of starting therapy and one negative test before each monthly refill. The drug should be started on the third or fourth day of the next normal menstrual period. Because of the very high risk of fetal deformity, patients must agree to the terms of the iPLEDGE program to receive the drug. See www.ipledgeprogram.com for detailed information about this program.

Herpes Simplex

Cause and Risk Factors. The herpes simplex virus (HSV) causes an infection that begins with itching and burning and progresses to the development of vesicles that rupture and form crusts (Fig. 52-9). Sites most often infected by the virus are the nose, lips, cheeks, ears, and genitalia. Oral HSV lesions are commonly

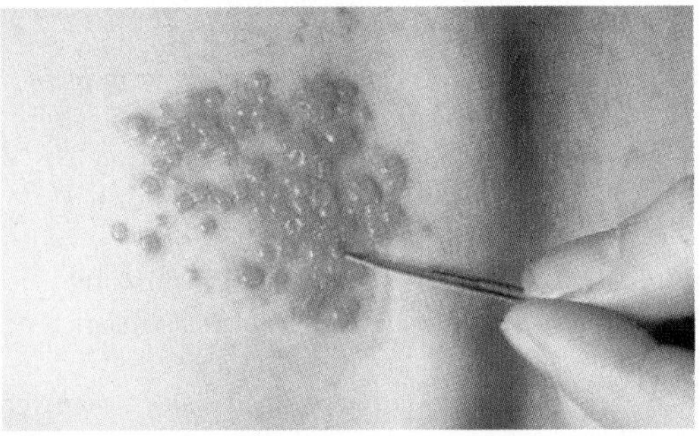

FIGURE 52-9 Herpes simplex lesions. (From Lookingbill DP, Marks JG: *Principles of dermatology*, ed 2, Philadelphia, 1993, Saunders.)

called *cold sores* or *fever blisters.* Two types of HSV exist. Infections on the face and upper body are usually caused by HSV-1; genital infections are usually caused by HSV-2. However, either type may cause oral or genital infections. Patients typically have repeated outbreaks and remissions. HSV can be transmitted by direct contact. Genital infection is therefore considered an STI and is discussed in detail in Chapter 51.

Medical Diagnosis. Diagnostic tests used to identify herpes infections include laboratory studies of exudate from a lesion and blood studies to detect specific antibodies.

Medical Treatment. Herpes simplex infections are treated with acyclovir (Zovirax) or, for cold sores, docosanol (Abreva). Antiviral drugs are not curative but may reduce the severity and frequency of outbreaks. Oral acyclovir is more effective than the topical preparation for initial and recurrent infections. Analgesics and topical anesthetics may be prescribed for pain.

❖ NURSING CARE of the Patient with Herpes Simplex

Nursing care consists primarily of patient education about the nature of the herpes simplex infection and its treatment and prevention. Emphasize that the condition is contagious and tends to recur. Prevention of sexually transmitted herpes simplex is discussed in Chapter 51. This section focuses on HSV-1.

■ Assessment

The health history describes the development of the herpetic lesions. Sexual contacts are documented so that those persons can be advised of the need for medical evaluation. A complete medical history is taken with particular attention to disorders or medications that might suppress the immune response. The physical examination includes a careful inspection of the lesions. The examiner should wear gloves to avoid direct contact with lesions.

Nursing Diagnoses, Goals, and Outcome Criteria: Herpes Simplex

Nursing Diagnoses	Goals and Outcome Criteria
Acute Pain related to lesions	Pain relief: patient statement of pain relief, relaxed expression
Ineffective Coping related to anticipated recurrent lesions, embarrassment	Effective coping: patient statement of ability to cope with condition
Ineffective Self-Health Management related to inadequate knowledge of disease, treatment, and risk of transmission	Effective management: patient describes self-care, follows plan of care, takes precautions to protect partner

■ Interventions

Acute Pain

Document patient reports of pain. Administer analgesics and topical anesthetics as ordered or instruct the patient in self-medication. Compresses saturated with astringent solutions such as Burow solution are sometimes ordered.

Ineffective Coping

Explore the patient's knowledge and concerns about HSV-1. Lesions on the face may be especially distressing because they are so obvious. Demonstrate acceptance of the patient's feelings and provide factual information to enable the patient to cope with the condition.

Ineffective Self-Health Management

Topical and oral drugs may be ordered. Instruct the patient in use of the drugs. Stress that HSV remains in a dormant state in the body after the initial infection. Periodic recurrences are expected and may be triggered by stresses, including emotional distress, fever, trauma, sunburn, or fatigue. The patient may be able to identify personal triggers and try to avoid or minimize them. Recurrent episodes are typically less severe than the initial one.

To prevent transmission of the infection to others, advise the patient to avoid oral contact while the lesions are present. The patient should exercise good hand washing and avoid touching the lesions. Immunosuppressed patients are especially susceptible to herpes infections and must be protected from infected people. Patients who do not follow adequate self-management practices may experience secondary skin infections that may require additional treatment. Most of these infections occur secondary to scratching. Advise the patient to keep nails short, bathe daily, and use medications as prescribed. The health care provider may prescribe medication to decrease itching.

Pharmacology Capsule

Acyclovir (Zovirax) does not cure herpes simplex virus (HSV) infections. Patients still can transmit the infection to others despite antiviral therapy and the absence of lesions.

Herpes Zoster

Cause and Risk Factors. Herpes zoster infection is commonly called *shingles.* It is caused by the varicella-zoster virus, the same organism that causes chickenpox. In some people who have had chickenpox, the virus remains latent (alive but inactive) in nerve tissue until the infection is activated in the form of shingles. The first symptoms are pain, itching, and heightened sensitivity along a nerve pathway, followed by the formation of vesicles in the area. When the skin is affected, crusts form (Fig. 52-10). When the mucous membranes

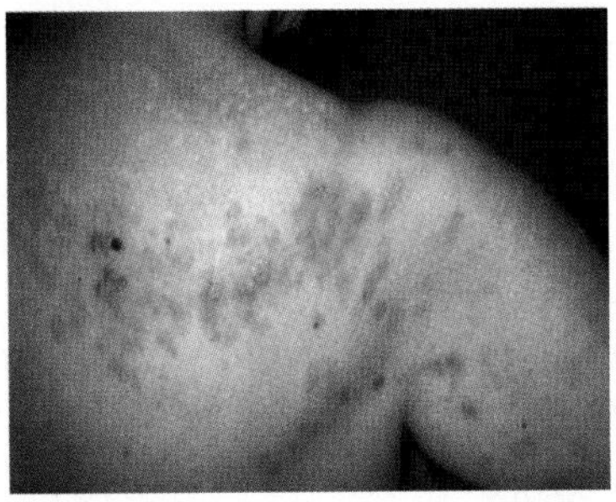

FIGURE 52-10 Herpes zoster lesions (i.e., shingles). (From Lookingbill DP, Marks JG: *Principles of dermatology*, ed 2, Philadelphia, 1993, Saunders.)

are affected, ulcers develop. The lesions typically last approximately 2 weeks. The infection is contagious to people who have not had previous exposure to the virus. Home health providers and nurses working in the clinic may be the first to recognize herpes zoster and should report their findings immediately to the client's health care provider.

Older adults are especially susceptible to complications, which include postherpetic neuralgia, trigeminal herpes zoster (affecting the facial and acoustic nerves), and ophthalmic involvement. With postherpetic neuralgia, pain and itching may persist for years. Immunosuppressed people are at increased risk for herpes zoster infections and may have very serious systemic complications.

Medical Diagnosis. A diagnosis of herpes zoster infection usually can be made on the basis of the health history and physical examination findings. The diagnosis can be confirmed by a Tzanck test or a viral culture of material from a lesion.

Medical Treatment. Herpes zoster infection is treated with antivirals. Topical agents are available but are used primarily to treat herpes simplex. The most commonly prescribed drugs include acyclovir, famciclovir, valacyclovir, and foscarnet. Oral treatment is effective for most patients. However, the intravenous route is used for persons who have impaired immune system function. Treatment is most effective if initiated within 72 hours of the onset of the rash. Wet dressings soaked in Burow solution may be ordered to loosen crusts, decrease oozing, and soothe the affected areas. Pain may be treated with analgesics and sedatives. After crusts form, a topical antibiotic ointment may be ordered two or three times a day. Systemic corticosteroids seem to be helpful in reducing pain and may or may not decrease the risk of herpetic neuralgia.

Postherpetic neuralgia is treated with a variety of analgesics, anticonvulsants, and antidepressants. Topical antiinflammatory and anesthetic drugs may be applied. Other methods that may be tried to relieve pain are transcutaneous electrical nerve stimulation (TENS), nerve blocks, and acupuncture.

Individuals 60 years of age and older may receive a vaccine for herpes zoster. Anyone younger than 60 years who has herpes zoster can also be given the vaccine. The initial patient assessment should note whether the individual has been given this vaccine.

❖ NURSING CARE of the Patient with Herpes Zoster

■ Assessment

Describe the patient's present illness. A complete medical history is needed to identify conditions or treatments that might cause the patient to have a reduced immune response. Explore the effect of the symptoms on the patient's life. If this is a recurrent infection, evaluate the patient's understanding of the condition. In the physical examination, document the distribution and appearance of the lesions.

Nursing Diagnoses, Goals, and Outcome Criteria: Herpes Zoster

Nursing Diagnoses	Goals and Outcome Criteria
Impaired Skin Integrity related to lesions	Improved skin integrity: absence of vesicles and pruritus
Acute Pain related to lesions, inflammation, or postherpetic neuralgia	Pain relief: patient statement of pain relief, relaxed manner
Ineffective Coping related to long-term pain associated with postherpetic neuralgia	Effective coping: patient uses strategies to cope with acute and chronic symptoms

■ Interventions

Impaired Skin Integrity

Inspect the lesions each day. Apply cool medicated compresses and administer antipruritics as ordered. Individuals who have not had chickenpox are susceptible to herpes simplex infection. They should avoid contact with the lesions.

Acute Pain

Administer prescribed analgesics and antiviral medications or instruct the patient in self-medication. Follow up to determine the effectiveness of the drugs in relieving pain. Inform the physician if the patient's pain persists despite medication.

Ineffective Coping

Emotional support is especially important for the patient who has chronic pain. Management of chronic pain is discussed in detail in Chapter 15. To promote healing, prevent transmission, and support coping, provide information about herpes zoster: cause, course, treatment, and communicability. Advise the patient that the condition is communicable to people who have never been exposed to chickenpox.

Necrotizing Fasciitis

Necrotizing fasciitis is an infection of the deep fascial structures under the skin. Aerobic and anaerobic organisms may be present, including *Streptococcus, Staphylococcus, Peptostreptococcus, Bacteroides,* and *Clostridium* species. The organisms excrete enzymes that destroy tissue, including blood vessels that supply the affected area. Deprived of blood flow, tissue necrosis occurs.

Necrotizing fasciitis should be suspected when a patient has a small external wound with evidence of larger underlying inflammation. The infection may progress rapidly with loss of large amounts of tissue and can result in death. Treatment involves extensive debridement, intravenous and topical antibiotics, and eventual skin grafting. Amputations may occur depending on response to therapy. Patients and family need to be aware of the severity of the disease process and nursing staff need to collaborate with other members of the health care team in providing emotional, spiritual, and psychological support.

Other Infections

A number of skin infections can occur in addition to those discussed in this chapter. Some of the more common conditions (i.e., impetigo, folliculitis, furuncles, carbuncles, erysipelas, cellulitis, warts) are presented in Figure 52-11 and Table 52-5.

Infestations

Lice and scabies infestations are described in Table 52-6. Pediculosis is illustrated in Figure 52-12.

Pemphigus

Pemphigus is a chronic autoimmune condition in which bullae (blisters) develop on the face, back, chest, groin, and umbilicus. The blisters rupture easily, releasing a foul-smelling drainage. Potassium permanganate baths, Domeboro solution, and oatmeal products with

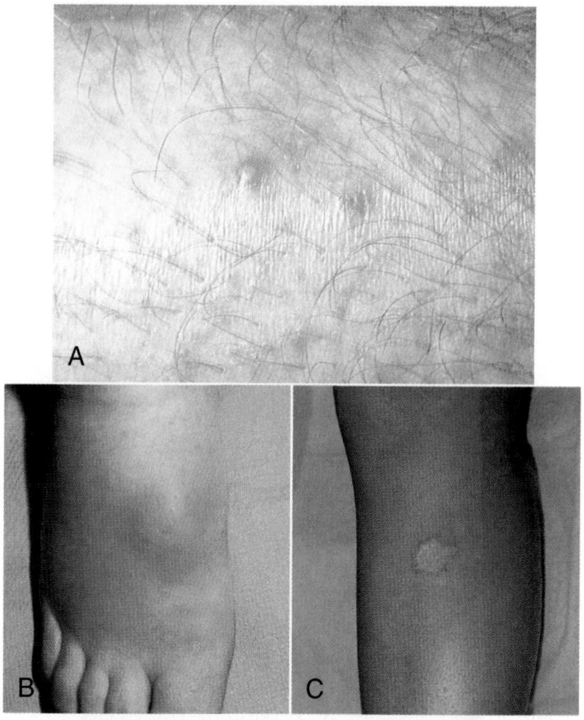

FIGURE 52-11 **A,** Folliculitis. **B,** Furuncle and abscess. **C,** Tinea corporis. (From Lookingbill DP, Marks JG: *Principles of dermatology*, ed 2, Philadelphia, 1993, Saunders.)

Table 52-5 Additional Skin Infections

INFECTION	CAUSE	SIGNS AND SYMPTOMS	TREATMENT
Impetigo	Group A streptococci	Vesicle or pustule that ruptures, leaving a thick crust	Antibiotic therapy: erythromycin or dicloxacillin
Folliculitis	*Staphylococcus aureus*	Inflamed hair follicles with white pustules	Warm compresses, topical antibiotics
Furuncle (boil)	*Staphylococcus aureus*	Inflamed skin and subcutaneous tissue with deep, inflamed nodules	Warm compresses, topical antibiotics
Carbuncle	*Staphylococcus aureus*	Clustered, interconnected furuncles	Systemic antibiotics, incision and drainage
Erysipelas	Beta-hemolytic group A streptococci	Round or oval patches that enlarge and spread; redness, swelling, tenderness, warmth	Systemic antibiotics, usually penicillin
Cellulitis	Usually *Streptococcus pyogenes*	Local tenderness and redness at first, then malaise, chills, and fever; site becomes more erythematous; nodules and vesicles may form; vesicles may rupture, releasing purulent material identified by culture	For *S. pyogenes*: penicillin, a cephalosporin, or vancomycin; other antibiotics for other organisms
Verruca (wart)	Human papillomavirus	At first, small shiny lesions; they enlarge and become rough	Electrical current to destroy lesion followed by removal with curette, cryotherapy (freezing), topical medications

Table 52-6 **Infestations of the Skin**

INFECTION	CAUSE	SIGNS AND SYMPTOMS	TREATMENT
Scabies	*Sarcoptes scabiei*, sometimes called *itch mite*	Thin, red lines on skin; itching	Topical scabicide applied and repeated 1 week later; clothing and bed linens washed in hot water or dry-cleaned
Lice	*Pediculus humanus* or *Phthirus pubis*	Itching of hairy areas of body (head, pubis); nits (eggs) seen as tiny white particles attached to hair shafts	Head lice: pediculicide shampoo applied to dry hair, then hair combed with fine-toothed comb to remove nits and dead lice; also treat brushes and combs Body or pubic lice: apply pediculicide lotion as directed For both sites: wash clothing and bed linens in hot water or have dry-cleaned; usually need to treat all members of household Assure patient that infestations are common and not caused by unsanitary living

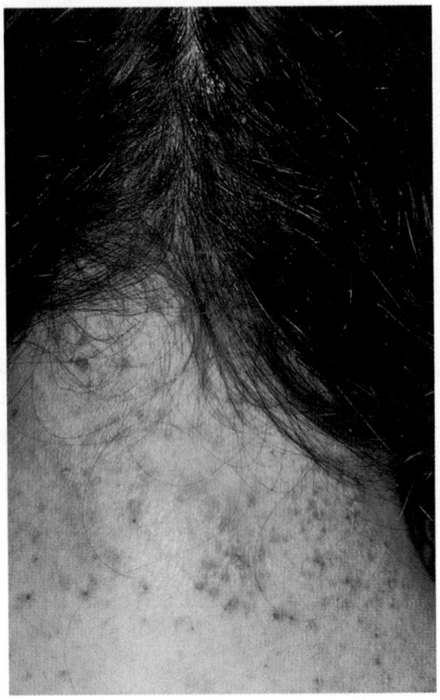

FIGURE 52-12 Pediculosis. (From Lookingbill DP, Marks JG: *Principles of dermatology*, ed 2, Philadelphia, 1993, Saunders.)

oil may be ordered to soothe the affected areas, reduce odor, and decrease the risk of infection. Treatments may include corticosteroids, other immunosuppressants, and oral or topical antibiotics. Patients with extensive skin loss require the same care as burn patients (see the section titled "Nursing Care of the Patient with Burn Injury").

CANCER

Skin cancers are classified as *nonmelanoma* or *melanoma*. Nonmelanoma skin cancers include basal cell carcinoma and squamous cell carcinoma. Risk factors for skin cancer are sun exposure, fair skin with freckling, light-colored hair and eyes, male gender, cigarette smoking, tanning beds, and a tendency to sunburn easily (see *Cultural Considerations* box). Tanning beds were specifically labeled *carcinogenic to humans* after years of controversy and study. The risk of melanoma increases by 75% among people who begin using them before age 30 years. The risk of nonmelanoma skin cancers increases with the total amount of sun exposure. The risk of melanoma increases with the severity of sunburn.

Cultural Considerations

What Does Culture Have to Do with Skin Cancer?

Caucasians have an increased incidence of skin cancer compared to either African Americans or Native Americans. Patients with light skin who live in sunny climates should protect themselves from excessive exposure and routinely assess for skin changes.

A discussion of skin cancers begins with actinic keratosis, which is actually considered a precancerous condition. Cutaneous T-cell lymphoma (Fig. 52-13) and Kaposi sarcoma are mentioned here as well because they are manifested by skin lesions. See Chapter 25 for detailed nursing care of the patient with cancer.

Skin cancers may be suspected because of the lesion's appearance and location. The diagnosis is confirmed by microscopic examination of cells obtained from the excised lesion or a tissue sample obtained by biopsy.

Actinic Keratosis

Actinic keratoses are precancerous lesions most often found on the face, neck, forearms, and backs of the hands—all areas exposed to sunlight. They may become malignant if not treated. Actinic keratoses are most common among Caucasian older adults. They typically appear as papules or plaques of irregular shape. The hard scale on the lesion may shed and reappear (see Fig. 52-13, A).

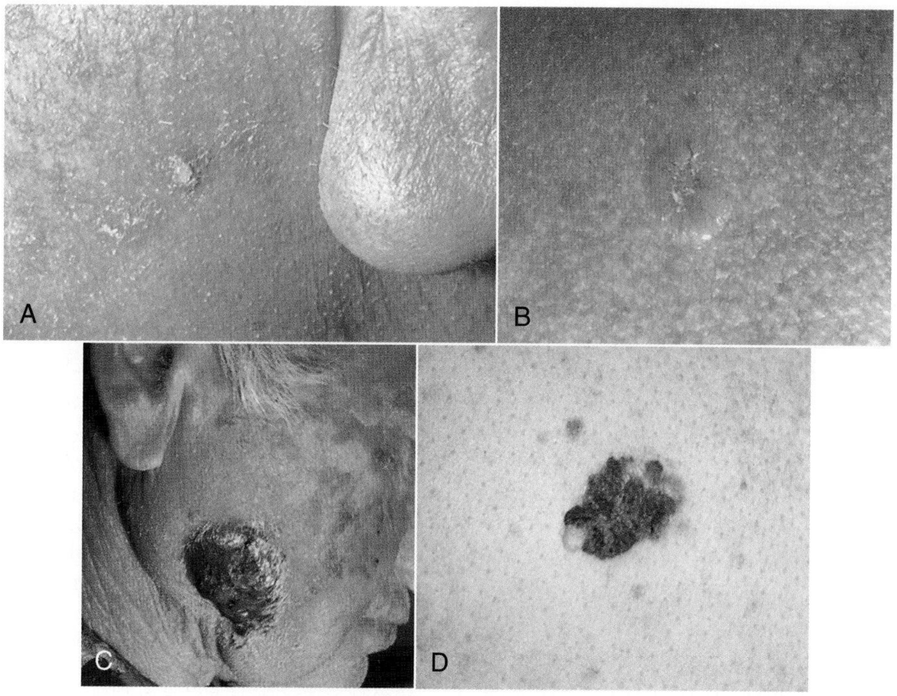

FIGURE 52-13 Skin cancers. **A,** Actinic keratosis (a premalignant lesion). **B,** Basal cell carcinoma. **C,** Squamous cell carcinoma. **D,** Malignant melanoma. (A to C, From Lookingbill DP, Marks JG: *Principles of dermatology*, ed 2, Philadelphia, 1993, Saunders. D, From Jarvis C: *Physical examination and health assessment*, ed 3, Philadelphia, 1999, Saunders.)

A number of treatments for actinic keratosis exist, including drug therapy, cryotherapy, electrodesiccation, and surgical excision. Drugs used to treat actinic keratosis include topical 5-fluorouracil and diclofenac sodium. Another choice is topical aminolevulinic acid with blue light photoactivation after 14 to 18 hours. Topical treatments cause irritation and photosensitivity. Therefore patients should be cautioned to avoid direct sun exposure during treatment. Cryotherapy is the use of liquid nitrogen to freeze and destroy the lesion. The procedure may cause a blister to form. Electrodesiccation is the use of electrical current to destroy the lesion, which is then scraped off. The patient is given a local anesthetic. Surgical excision may be done in several ways and the patient may or may not have sutures.

Nonmelanoma Skin Cancer

Basal Cell Carcinoma. Basal cell carcinomas usually begin as painless, nodular lesions that have a pearly appearance (see Fig. 52-13, B). They are thought to be related to sun exposure. Basal cell carcinomas grow slowly and rarely metastasize. Nevertheless, they should be removed because they can cause local tissue destruction. Basal cell carcinomas are treated with surgical excision, Mohs micrographic excision, electrodissection and curettage, cryotherapy, radiation, or drugs that are applied topically or injected into the lesion. Mohs surgery is a technique in which microscopic tissue samples are studied to determine the margins of the malignancy.

Squamous Cell Carcinoma. Squamous cell carcinomas may appear as scaly ulcers or raised lesions. Usually no clear lesion margins exist (see Fig. 52-13, C). Like basal cell carcinomas, they most often develop on sun-exposed areas, including the lips and in the oral cavity. Squamous cell carcinomas are most often associated with overuse of tobacco and alcohol. Unlike basal cell carcinomas, they grow rapidly and metastasize. Treatment may include surgical excision, cryotherapy, and radiation therapy.

Melanoma

A malignant melanoma arises from the pigment-producing cells in the skin. It is the most serious form of skin cancer because it can be fatal if it metastasizes. Melanomas can be found anywhere on the body, not just on sun-exposed areas. Typical melanomas have irregular borders and uneven coloration (see Fig. 52-13, D). Many are very dark but some are light in color. They usually begin as a tan macule that enlarges. Malignant melanomas are removed surgically, with Mohs technique often used. This approach is meant to avoid leaving malignant tissue around the excised lesion. A wide area around a melanoma is usually excised. Chemotherapy and immunotherapy also may be used.

Cutaneous T-Cell Lymphoma

Cutaneous T-cell lymphoma is characterized by the migration of malignant T cells to the skin. Several manifestations of cutaneous T-cell lymphoma exist, including mycosis fungoides and Sézary syndrome. At first, cutaneous T-cell lymphoma may resemble eczema, with macular lesions appearing on areas that are protected from the sun. They form tumors, enlarge, and can spread to distant sites. When confined to the skin, this type of lymphoma can be cured with topical chemotherapy, systemic PUVA, or superficial radiotherapy (or a combination of these treatments).

Kaposi Sarcoma

Kaposi sarcoma is a malignancy of the blood vessels. It is manifested by red, blue, or purple macules accompanied by pain, itching, and swelling. The lesions appear first on the legs and then on the upper body, face, and mouth. They enlarge to form large plaques that may drain. Kaposi sarcoma may be seen in patients with human immunodeficiency virus (HIV) infection but it is not confined to this group. Local lesions may be excised or injected with intralesional chemotherapy. Systemic lesions are treated with chemotherapy, immune therapy, and radiotherapy. Unfortunately, treatment results have been discouraging (see Chapter 35).

DISORDERS OF THE NAILS

The two major conditions affecting the nails are (1) infections (fungal or bacterial) and (2) inflammation caused by ingrown nails. Infections are usually indicated by redness, swelling, and pain around the margin of the nail. They are treated with warm soaks and topical or systemic antiinfective agents. The most effective treatment of fungal infections of the nail, called *onychomycosis*, is a 3- to 6-month course of oral terbinafine (Lamisil) and itraconazole (Sporanox). Incision and drainage may be necessary.

An ingrown toenail causes painful inflammation at the distal corner of the nail. It is usually caused by trimming the nail too short at the corners or wearing shoes that are too tight on the toes. The ingrown nail should be protected from pressure as it grows out. Warm soaks may be soothing. Sometimes surgical excision of the ingrown portion of the nail is needed.

❖ NURSING CARE of the Patient with a Nail Disorder

Nail disorders do not often require inpatient care unless complications exist. However, nurses may be the first to detect nail problems and often teach patients how to prevent or treat them.

■ Assessment

The health history should document the diagnoses of DM or peripheral vascular disease (PVD). In the physical examination, inspect around the nails for redness, swelling, or pain. Inquire about the use of artificial nails and professional manicures and pedicures. Artificial nails carry a high incidence of fungal infections and some nail salons do not follow aseptic practices. Inspect the extremities for lesions and abnormal color and palpate for warmth and peripheral pulses. It is important to teach the diabetic patient the importance of seeing a podiatrist on a regular basis. It is also important to teach the diabetic client to have his or her nails trimmed by a podiatrist and not to cut the nails at home.

Nursing Diagnoses, Goals, and Outcome Criteria: Nail Disorder

Nursing Diagnoses	Goals and Outcome Criteria
Risk for Injury related to improper nail trimming, poor peripheral circulation	Decreased risk of injury: properly trimmed nails Absence of injury: no evidence of inflammation (e.g., redness, swelling, pain, excess warmth)
Ineffective Self-Health Management related to lack of understanding of proper nail care and treatment of nail disorders	Effective management of therapeutic measures: patient demonstrates correct nail care and prescribed treatments

■ Interventions

Teach patients how to trim their nails correctly and the importance of wearing properly fitting shoes. Toenails should be cut straight across and even with the end of the toe. Show patients with PVD or DM how to inspect their feet daily and advise them to seek medical attention for any abnormality. A seemingly minor foot infection can have drastic consequences, including amputation, for the patient with poor circulation. If the patient cannot care for the feet adequately, seek a referral to a podiatrist. It is also important to teach the patient with DM, PVD, or both the importance of bathing the feet daily; wearing clean, dry socks; and wearing shoes that fit properly. These patients should be discouraged from going barefoot.

BURNS

Burns are tissue injuries caused by heat. Depending on the source of the injury, the burn is described as thermal (i.e., flame, flash, scalding liquids, hot objects), chemical, electrical, radiation, or inhalation. Burns are a leading cause of accidental death despite improved survival rates attributed to tremendous advances in the care of burn patients. Sadly, 75% of all burn injuries could have been prevented. Educating the public about ways to prevent burns is essential.

Emergency treatment of the burn patient is discussed in Chapter 16. Acute care of seriously burned patients is an advanced specialty that is beyond the scope of this book; therefore this section provides a limited discussion of nursing care of the patient after he or she reaches a medical facility.

CLASSIFICATION OF BURNS

Burns are classified by the size and depth of the tissue injury. It is important to reevaluate the burn periodically because evidence of the extent of the injury can change over time. Size is often defined as the percentage of body surface area affected. To describe depth, a burn is classified as *partial thickness* or *full thickness*, depending on the layers of tissue injured.

Burn Size

Burn size may be estimated using the *rule of nines* or the Lund and Browder method. The rule of nines estimates the percentage of body surface area burned. Areas of the body are assigned percentage values of nine or multiples of nine (Fig. 52-14). The percentages are totaled to estimate burn size. For example, in an adult, if one arm and hand are burned, the burn size is estimated as 9.5%.

The Lund and Browder method also estimates the percentage of body surface burned but the body is divided into smaller segments. Different percentages are assigned to body parts depending on the patient's age. This is more accurate than the rule of nines because it accounts for differences in body proportions. For example, the head of an infant is 19% of the total body surface area whereas the head of an adult is only 7% of the total body surface area. Figure 52-15 is an

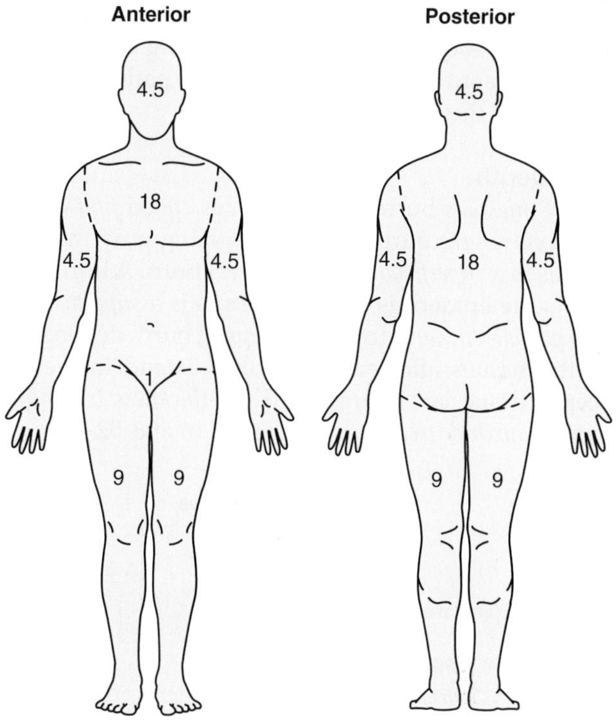

FIGURE 52-14 Rule of nines. (From Monahan F, Sands J, Neighbors M, et al.: *Phipps' medical-surgical nursing: health and illness perspectives*, ed 8, St. Louis, 2007, Mosby.)

Body area	0-1 Years	1-4 Years	5-9 Years	10-14 Years	15 Years	Adult
Head	19	17	13	11	9	7
Neck	2	2	2	2	2	2
Ant. trunk	13	13	13	13	13	13
Post. trunk	13	13	13	13	13	13
R. buttock	2.5	2.5	2.5	2.5	2.5	2.5
L. buttock	2.5	2.5	2.5	2.5	2.5	2.5
Genitalia	1	1	1	1	1	1
R. u. arm	4	4	4	4	4	4
L. u. arm	4	4	4	4	4	4
R. l. arm	3	3	3	3	3	3
L. l. arm	3	3	3	3	3	3
R. hand	2.5	2.5	2.5	2.5	2.5	2.5
L. hand	2.5	2.5	2.5	2.5	2.5	2.5
R. thigh	5.5	6.5	8	8.5	9	9.5
L. thigh	5.5	6.5	8	8.5	9	9.5
R. l. leg	5	5	5.5	6	6.5	7
L. l. leg	5	5	5.5	6	6.5	7
R. foot	3.5	3.5	3.5	3.5	3.5	3.5
L. foot	3.5	3.5	3.5	3.5	3.5	3.5

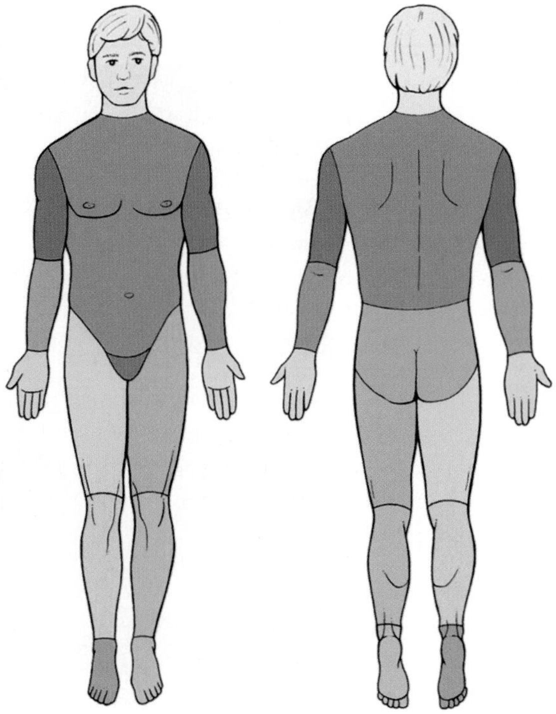

FIGURE 52-15 Berkow's adaptation of the Lund and Browder method of estimating body surface area burned. (From Monahan FD, Drake DT, Neighbors M, editors: *Medical-surgical nursing: foundations for clinical practice*, ed 2, Philadelphia, 1998, Saunders.)

example of the Lund and Browder chart as modified by Berkow. A quick method of estimating the percentage of body surface burned is to use the patient's palm. The size of the palm represents 1%.

Burn Depth

Partial-thickness burns are sometimes called *first-degree* or *second-degree* burns. A burn affecting only the epidermis is a *superficial* (or *first-degree*) burn. A burn that affects the epidermis and the dermis is a *superficial* or *deep partial-thickness* (or *second-degree*) burn, depending on the tissues affected. Burns that extend into even deeper tissue layers are called *full-thickness* (or *third-degree, fourth-degree*) burns (Figs. 52-16 and 52-17).

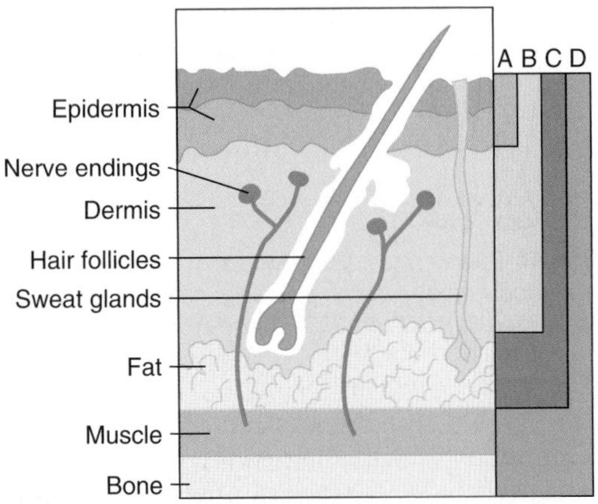

FIGURE 52-16 Burn classification by depth. **A,** First-degree. **B,** Second-degree (partial-thickness). **C,** Third-degree (full-thickness). **D,** Fourth-degree. (From Monahan F, Sands J, Neighbors M, et al.: *Phipps' medical-surgical nursing: health and illness perspectives*, ed 8, St. Louis, 2006, Mosby.)

Superficial Burns. A superficial burn, like a sunburn, is pink to red and painful.

Superficial Partial-Thickness Burns. Superficial partial-thickness burns are painful and usually appear blistered or weepy and pale to red or pink. A severe sunburn can be a superficial partial-thickness burn.

Deep Partial-Thickness Burns. A deep partial-thickness burn is characterized by large, thick-walled blisters or by edema and weeping, cherry-red, exposed dermis. It is painful and sensitive to cold air.

Full-Thickness Burns. Full-thickness burns involve the epidermis, dermis, and underlying tissues, including fat, muscle, and bone. Full-thickness burns typically appear dry, feel leathery, and may be red, white, brown, or black. The burned tissue usually lacks sensation.

Burn Severity

Burn severity is based on size, depth, location, age, general health status, and mechanism of injury. Various criteria are used to define major burns. The American Burn Association criteria for a major burn in an adult are the following:

1. Burn size: 25% or more body surface area for people younger than 40 years; 20% or more body surface area for people older than 40 years
2. Disfiguring or disabling injuries to the face, eyes, ears, hands, feet, or perineum
3. High-voltage electrical burn injury
4. Inhalation injury (any time you see black soot around the mouth and nose, an inhalation injury should be suspected)
5. Major trauma in addition to the burn

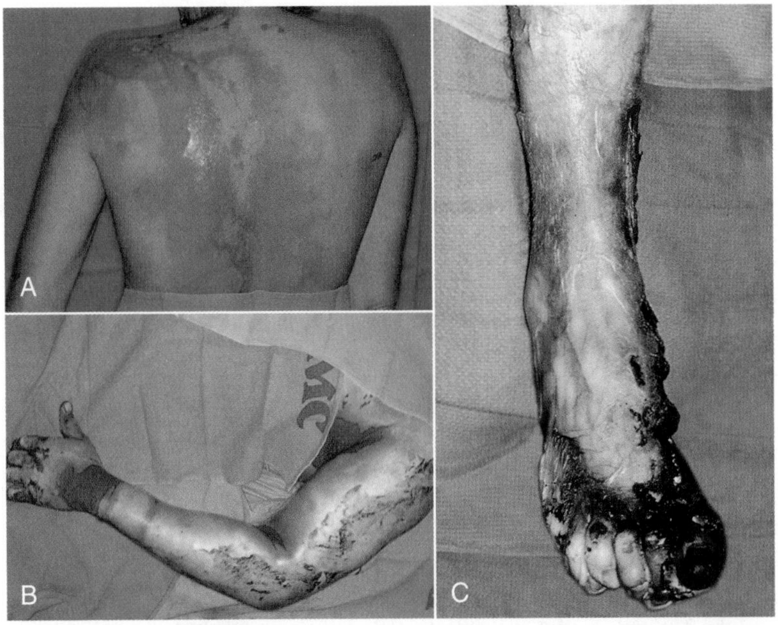

FIGURE 52-17 Burn depth. **A,** Partial-thickness (i.e., second-degree). **B,** Full-thickness (i.e., third-degree). **C,** Full-thickness (i.e., fourth-degree). (A-B, From Black JM, Hawks JH: Medical-surgical nursing: Clinical management for positive outcomes, ed 8, St Louis, 2009, Saunders. C, From Black JM, Hawks JH, Keene AM: *Medical-surgical nursing: Clinical management for continuity of care,* ed 6, Philadelphia, 2001, Saunders.)

PATHOPHYSIOLOGY OF BURN INJURY

Local Effects

Burn-injured tissue releases chemicals that cause increased capillary permeability, which permits plasma to leak into the tissues. Injury to cell membranes permits excess sodium to enter the cell and allows potassium to escape into the extracellular compartment. These shifts in fluids and electrolytes cause local edema and a decrease in cardiac output. Fluid evaporates through the wound surface, further contributing to the declining blood volume. Eighteen to 36 hours after a burn injury, capillary permeability begins to normalize and reabsorption of edema fluid begins. Cardiac output returns to normal and then increases to meet increased metabolic demands.

Systemic Effects

Fluid Balance. The shift of plasma proteins from the capillaries may result in hypoproteinemia, which causes fluid to shift from the bloodstream to the extracellular tissue. This shift decreases blood volume and causes generalized edema in the early postburn period. Blood is shunted from the kidneys to compensate for the fluid volume deficit and urine output falls. These fluid shifts, if not corrected, result in decreased tissue perfusion and decreased cardiac output that may lead to hypovolemic shock. Fluid resuscitation is critical during the first 24 to 48 hours. Intake and output should be strictly monitored to prevent shock.

As the capillaries recover and edema fluid is reabsorbed, the patient's blood volume increases. If kidney function is adequate, urine output increases to prevent hypervolemia.

Gastrointestinal Function. Blood flow to the intestines decreases and an ileus may develop. Some patients have stress ulcers, sometimes called *Curling ulcers*, after severe burns. Therefore they are routinely treated with antacids to neutralize gastric acid and H2 receptor blockers to reduce gastric acid secretion.

Immune System. Because immunity is depressed after a serious burn, the patient is less able to resist infection. The loss of the protective skin barrier also puts the patient at risk for life-threatening infection. Burn patients are monitored closely for signs of infection. The most common are methicillin-resistant *Staphylococcus aureus* (MRSA) and vancomycin-resistant *Enterococcus* (VRE). Because of military commitments, a threat also exists for infections related to organisms that are not routinely seen in the United States. The most common organism that may be seen in burn patients that come from overseas is *Acinetobacter*. Members of the military who return to the United States for burn treatment should be routinely cultured on admission to rule out any of the mentioned infections.

Respiratory System. The burn patient may suffer inhalation injuries, including carbon monoxide poisoning, smoke poisoning, and thermal damage. Inhalation injury occurs with flame burns or from being trapped in an enclosed space filled with smoke. Suspect inhalation injury if the patient has facial burns, redness and swelling of the pharynx, restlessness, cough, dyspnea, or sooty sputum. Carbon monoxide displaces oxygen (O_2) on hemoglobin (Hgb), so the blood is unable to transport O_2 to the tissues. The patient will show signs of hypoxia and die if the condition is not corrected (see Chapter 16 for additional discussion of carbon monoxide poisoning).

Smoke poisoning is the result of inhaling combustion by-products. Thermal damage to the lower airway is rare but can happen if the patient was unconscious or inhaled live steam. With inhalation injury, pulmonary edema develops and may progress to adult respiratory distress syndrome. Anyone suspected of having an inhalation injury needs to have the airway protected and should be evaluated immediately for any signs of respiratory distress. Before being discharged from the hospital, anyone with an inhalation injury should have pulmonary function studies completed to evaluate lung function.

Myocardial Depression. Evidence exists of myocardial depression in the early postburn period. Laboratory studies are usually done to evaluate the effects of burns on the myocardium. Patients should be evaluated for the need for beta-blockers.

Psychological Effects. Psychological responses to burn injuries are highly individual. A psychologist, psychiatric nurse practitioner, or psychiatric clinical nurse specialist should be involved with the care of the patient and the family from the beginning. Four stages of psychologic response have been identified: (1) impact, (2) retreat or withdrawal, (3) acknowledgment, and (4) reconstruction. Because of the effects that burns have on the patient and his or her return to home and community, the burn patient may need a psychological evaluation to determine the need for further counseling and support. Psychosocial support may be needed for months and years after the burn because the patient may experience long-term effects such as posttraumatic stress disorder.

STAGES OF BURN INJURY

Care of the burn patient is often described in terms of three stages: (1) emergent, (2) acute, and (3) rehabilitation. The emergent stage begins with the injury and ends when fluid shifts have stabilized. The acute stage begins with fluid stabilization. Some sources mark the end of the acute stage when all but 10% of the burn wounds are closed but others define the acute stage as extending until all wounds are closed. The rehabilitation stage follows the acute stage and lasts as long as efforts continue to promote improvement or adjustment. Some overlap exists between the acute and rehabilitation stages because nursing care in the acute stage can significantly affect the potential for rehabilitation.

In reality, rehabilitation starts as soon as the patient stabilizes. Physical therapy and occupational therapy should be consulted immediately when the patient is admitted.

MEDICAL TREATMENT IN THE EMERGENT STAGE

In the emergency department, the staff first assesses airway, breathing, and circulation and then determines whether the patient has injuries in addition to the burn. If inhalation injury is suspected, O_2 therapy is started. The patient may require intubation if the airway is compromised. Intravenous lines are established to begin fluid resuscitation and to provide emergency vascular access. An indwelling urinary catheter and a nasogastric tube are usually inserted. Blood is drawn for baseline laboratory studies (hematocrit, electrolytes, and blood gases, if indicated). Tetanus prophylaxis may be administered. Pain is assessed and analgesics are ordered. The wound is then cleaned, debrided, and inspected. Unless the patient is at a major burn center, the burns may not be debrided immediately. If the patient is to be transported, the burns are covered with clean sheets.

Once the initial care is completed, the patient with serious burns is transferred to a burn specialty care unit or a critical care unit. Intravenous fluid therapy is an essential aspect of care during the first few days of burn treatment. Several formulas are used to select the volumes and solutions to be administered. Volume is based on the patient's weight and extent of injury. For the first 24 hours, intravenous fluids may consist of various combinations of electrolyte, colloid, and dextrose solutions. However, specific formulas vary among specialty care units. For example, some formulas prescribe *only* electrolyte solutions in the first 24 hours.

For the second 24 hours, volume is usually decreased based on urine output. Fluids then consist of different combinations of electrolyte, colloid, and dextrose solutions. Some formulas omit electrolyte solutions in the second 24 hours.

In addition to fluids, medical care may include antibiotic therapy and surgical procedures.

WOUND CARE

Wound care after a burn injury is intended to promote healing, prevent infection, control heat loss, retain function, and minimize disfigurement. Burn wounds may be treated by the open or closed method. The method of wound care is based in part on the state of the wound. The open method involves the use of topical antimicrobials but no dressings. Open care is less restrictive and simpler than closed care but provides increased opportunity for loss of fluid and heat through the wound surface. Closed care uses topical medications covered by dressings. Because some areas of the wound may be deeper than other areas, it is not unusual to see open care for some of the patient's wounds and closed care for others. Examples of topical medications that may be used are silver sulfadiazine (Silvadene) and mafenide acetate (Sulfamylon). To prevent tetanus, a tetanus toxoid booster is usually given if the patient has not been immunized within the past 5 years. Patients who have never been immunized are given tetanus immune globulin and the first in a series of tetanus toxoid.

For clean partial-thickness wounds that will heal without grafting, temporary wound coverings often are used. Temporary wound coverings include amniotic membranes, grafts from cadavers or pigs, and a number of synthetic materials that promote wound healing or protect donor or graft sites. Grafted areas in need of protection are often covered by temporary wound coverings that prevent grafts from shifting during the first 72 hours. Graft sites are also treated with negative pressure wound therapy. Donor sites also are treated with a variety of products, including fine-mesh gauze and synthetic and biosynthetic products. Donor sites are more painful than graft sites because of the exposure of nerve endings.

Debridement

A partial-thickness burn may blister, peel, and heal with minimal long-term effects. A full-thickness burn, however, is often covered by a thick, leathery layer of burned tissue (eschar) that shelters microorganisms and inhibits healing. Eschar must be removed before healing can take place. Further, if eschar encircles a limb, it may need to be incised to permit tissue swelling without compromising circulation. **Debridement** is the removal of debris and necrotic (dead) tissue from a wound. In the case of a burn wound, debridement includes removal of eschar. Debridement may be accomplished by mechanical means (using scissors and forceps), surgical excision, or the use of enzymes. Enzymatic debridement is the use of topical medications containing enzymes capable of dissolving necrotic tissue. These substances are applied directly to the wound but should not be applied to wounds that communicate with major body cavities or to exposed nerves. Enzymatics may cause pain and bleeding.

Skin Grafting

A burn wound may be covered using the patient's own skin, called an *autograft*. The graft is usually taken from the thigh or buttocks using a tool called a *dermatome.* The thickness of the graft determines whether it is a split-thickness or a full-thickness graft. If a thin layer of skin is used, it is considered a split-thickness graft. A split-thickness graft may be a sheet graft (an intact section of skin) or a meshed graft. A meshed graft has multiple tiny slits that allow the skin to be stretched to cover a larger area. The slits also allow for wound exudate to be absorbed by the cover dressing. Grafts vary in size, with the smallest being pinch and postage stamp grafts. Larger grafts may be needed to cover all or part of the burn.

For very deep burns and burns of the face, neck, or hands, a full-thickness graft may be preferred. A full-thickness graft includes skin and subcutaneous tissue and provides better cosmetic results. Another type of full-thickness graft is a pedicle or flap graft, in which one end of a section or tube of donor tissue is sutured to the recipient site while another section remains attached to the donor site. This type of graft continues to receive blood from the donor site. Once the graft "takes" or attaches to the recipient site, the pedicle or flap is cut free from the donor site.

After grafting, the recipient site is inspected for bleeding under the graft that could interfere with survival of the graft. The area is immobilized for 3 to 7 days to permit attachment of the graft to the wound base. Splints, traction, and restraints may be used for immobilization. This will vary with the institution. In most burn centers, the grafts are inspected on day 3 to assess the degree of attachment. The graft is inspected again on day 5 and a determination is made about removal of staples. By day 7, all staples should be removed. After an autograft, the patient's donor site requires care as well. The donor site is usually covered with fine-mesh gauze or synthetic dressings and bandages. The dressings are usually removed 24 hours after surgery to allow the site to air dry. If the donor site is still wet, a heat lamp may be used to assist in the drying process. As the donor site dries, the fine-mesh gauze or Xeroform will begin to lift off the skin. The excess material is trimmed as it lifts off the treated area.

Scarring

The formation of burn scars can be minimized by the use of pressure dressings in the early stages of care, followed by the use of custom-fitted garments that apply continuous pressure. These garments are worn 23 hours a day and may be prescribed for as long as 2 years (Fig. 52-18). Explain to the patient that the garments need to be tight in order to be effective. Massage of the area either by hand or with a battery-operated device also helps to reduce the appearance of scars.

Patients with facial burns need to be encouraged to do facial exercises that will decrease the appearance of scar tissue.

❖ NURSING CARE of the Patient with Burn Injury

■ Assessment

When the patient is stabilized, a complete assessment should be done. As priorities change, additional relevant data will be needed.

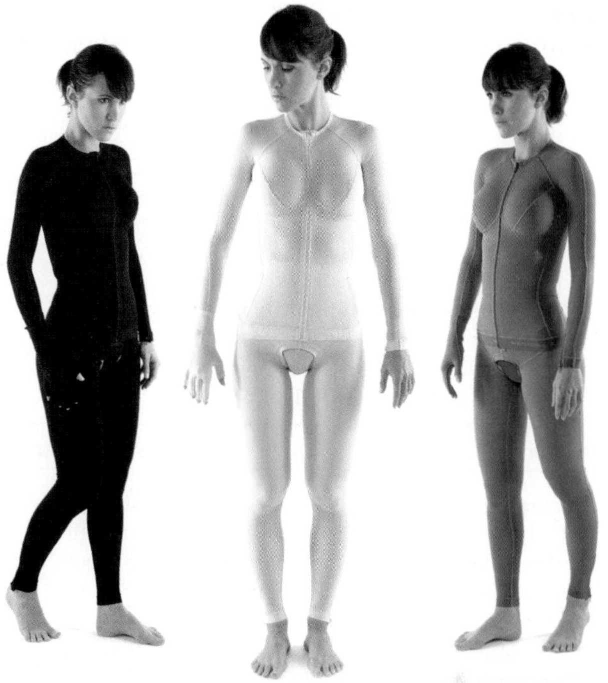

FIGURE 52-18 A pressure garment minimizes the hypertrophic scarring that is common after burn injuries. (Courtesy Medical Z.)

Health History

The history of the present illness describes the circumstances surrounding the burn injury. The past medical history documents any chronic diseases, surgeries, or hospitalizations. Identify medications and allergies. Take a family history even though it is not specific to burn injuries because it may alert the staff to other problems. The review of systems detects current problems with each body system. In the functional assessment, the patient's habits and lifestyle, roles and responsibilities, stressors, and coping strategies are described.

Physical Examination

The physical examination begins with vital signs. The examiner should be alert for abnormalities that suggest hypoxia (i.e., restlessness, tachypnea), excess fluid volume (i.e., bounding pulse, hypertension), deficient fluid volume (i.e., tachycardia, hypotension), hypovolemia (i.e., hypotension, tachycardia), or infection (i.e., fever, tachycardia). Measure the patient's height and weight as soon as possible, if the patient is stable enough to do so.

Throughout the examination, inspect the skin for burn wounds and other lesions. Note wound color and the presence of any eschar. Palpate intact skin for temperature and turgor. Observe chest expansion and auscultate the lungs for wheezing, stridor, or atelectasis. Auscultate the apical pulse for rate and rhythm. Assess the abdomen for active bowel sounds and distention.

Inspect the extremities for injury and deformity. Delay range-of-motion assessment if an extremity is immobilized.

Nursing Diagnoses, Goals, and Outcome Criteria: Burn Injury

Depending on the severity and type of burn, nursing diagnoses for the patient with burn injury may include those listed in this table. The first two diagnoses are most likely to occur in the emergent stage; the remaining diagnoses may be made in the emergent, acute, or rehabilitation stages.

Nursing Diagnoses	Goals and Outcome Criteria
Decreased Cardiac Output related to hypovolemia secondary to shift of fluid from vascular to extracellular compartment	Normal cardiac output: pulse and blood pressure (BP) consistent with patient norms
Excess Fluid Volume related to changes in capillary permeability and accumulation of fluid in body tissues	Normal fluid balance: edema decreasing or absent, increased urine output
Acute Pain related to tissue trauma of burn injury	Pain relief: patient statement of pain relief, more relaxed manner
Risk for Infection related to loss of protective skin barrier	Absence of infection: normal body temperature and white blood cell (WBC) count, negative wound cultures
Hypothermia related to impaired heat-regulating ability of injured skin	Normal body temperature: temperature within patient norms
Imbalanced Nutrition: Less Than Body Requirements related to high metabolic demands	Adequate nutrition: stable body weight
Impaired Physical Mobility related to contractures, therapeutic immobilization, pain	Adaptation to physical limitations: minimal contractures, clear breath sounds, bowel movement at least every 2 to 3 days
Ineffective Coping related to possible disfigurement, dysfunction, fear of death	Effective patient coping: positive patient statements about future, participates in rehabilitation efforts
Compromised Family Coping related to uncertain outcome, fear of patient death, and altered family function	Effective family coping: positive family statements about the future, family interest in ways to help patient's recovery

Interventions

Decreased Cardiac Output

The risk of decreased cardiac output is greatest in the emergent stage when fluid has shifted from the blood to the extracellular compartment. If blood volume is not maintained, the patient's blood pressure (BP) falls and tissue perfusion is impaired. To monitor cardiac output, record the patient's vital signs and fluid intake and output. Signs of decreased cardiac output include hypotension, tachycardia, and decreased urine output. Inadequate tissue perfusion may be manifested by cool, pale, or cyanotic skin; restlessness; and confusion. Administer intravenous fluids as ordered with close, continuous monitoring of fluid status. Strict monitoring of intake and output is essential. The patient may also need invasive lines, such as a pulmonary artery catheter, to monitor cardiac output.

Excess Fluid Volume

Excess fluid volume may result from the retention of fluid in the extracellular compartment. As capillary permeability returns to normal and fluid is reabsorbed, the patient's blood volume increases. If the patient's kidneys can eliminate the excess fluid efficiently, the patient suffers no ill effects from the increasing blood volume. However, a risk exists that the patient's circulatory system may be unable to adapt to the increased volume. This puts the patient at risk for heart failure (HF).

Monitor the patient's vital signs for hypertension; dyspnea; and full, bounding pulse. Measure urine output and compare it with fluid intake. Administer intravenous fluids as ordered and monitor the patient closely. Document data collected for the assessments.

Acute Pain

Partial-thickness wounds are typically very painful. Full-thickness burns lack sensation because of the destruction of the superficial nerves. However, burns are often uneven in depth, so patients with full-thickness burns often have pain as well. The burn patient is given opioid analgesics such as morphine as ordered. An opioid agonist such as fentanyl (Sublimaze) may be given intravenously or orally before performing painful wound care. If given orally, administer the medication 45 minutes before the procedure. If given intravenously, administer the drug 5 to 10 minutes ahead of time. The intramuscular route is not routinely used until fluid shifts have stabilized because absorption is less reliable. Nonsteroidal anti-inflammatory drugs (NSAIDs) also may be prescribed. Pain is aggravated by anxiety, so use measures to reduce fear and anxiety in the management of pain. Document the patient's response to interventions. Additional nursing measures for pain are described in Chapter 15.

Risk for Infection

The burn patient, without protective skin, is at great risk for infection. Routinely monitor for signs of local infection (i.e., pus, foul odor, increased redness) and systemic infection (i.e., fever, increased white blood cell [WBC] count). Infection can come from the staff, visitors, the environment, and the patient's own body. Specific infection control measures vary with the agency. Strict hand washing should be practiced by the patient and all who enter the room. Body hair around wounds is usually shaved or cut to prevent wound contamination. However, *do not shave the eyebrows*—if shaved, they tend to grow back in a disorganized pattern. Carry out wound care as ordered or according to routines of the specialty care unit.

Hypothermia

Loss of heat through the burn wound surface places the patient at risk for hypothermia (i.e., low body temperature). This is especially problematic for older adults whose ability to maintain body temperature is already compromised because of various age-related changes.

Monitor the patient's tympanic or rectal temperature to detect declining body temperature. Keep the room warm and use external heat sources as needed. The room temperature should be above 76°F. In a burn intensive care unit, the temperature may be above 85°F. Attempt to limit body surface area exposure during wound care. Body heat loss may be increased if the patient is on an air-fluidized bed, so carefully monitor the temperature of the bed.

Imbalanced Nutrition: Less Than Body Requirements

Healing of a large burn wound requires considerable energy. Therefore it is critical that adequate nutrition be provided to meet the increased metabolic demands. Consult with the dietitian about the patient's nutritional needs and preferences. Calorie needs may be as much as twice the patient's baseline needs. Regular meals may need to be supplemented with between-meal feedings. Stress to the patient the need for increased intake during the recovery period. Try to create an environment conducive to eating and encourage the patient to eat all food served. Provide assistance with meals, if needed. Some patients require tube feedings or total parenteral nutrition (TPN) to meet their calorie needs. Encourage the patient to drink protein drinks rather than water. Calorie counts may be done at the bedside to ensure that the patient is consuming enough calories to meet the increased metabolic needs associated with burns.

Impaired Physical Mobility

Patients with burns may have mobility restrictions imposed by the injury or the treatment. The hazards

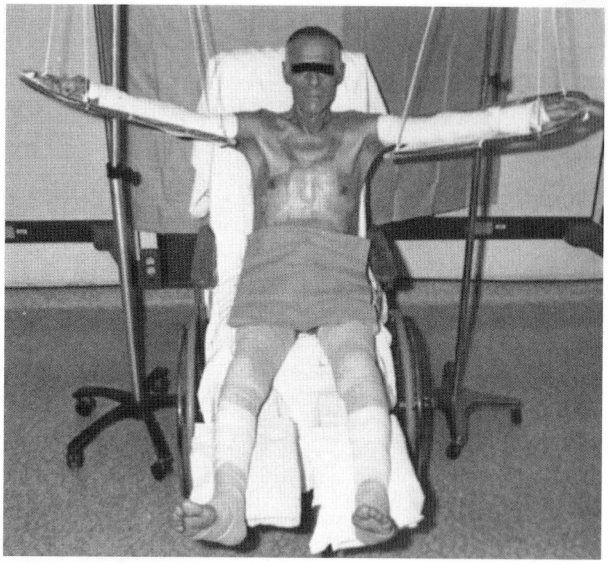

FIGURE 52-19 Therapeutic positioning. This patient's arms are extended to prevent flexion contractures. Pressure dressings on legs prevent edema and minimize scarring. (From Black JM, Matassarin-Jacobs E: *Luckmann and Sorenson's medical-surgical nursing: clinical management for continuity of care*, ed 5, Philadelphia, 1997, Saunders.)

of immobility, including pressure sores, joint contractures, pneumonia and atelectasis, constipation, and urinary infections, are discussed in Chapter 21. Monitor range of motion in affected joints and perform passive or active exercises unless contraindicated. Keep injured limbs in functional positions as much as possible (Fig. 52-19). In addition, exercise unaffected joints to maintain flexibility and strength. Impaired mobility may interfere with the patient's ability to participate in his or her own care. Evaluate the ability to provide self-care and provide assistance as needed. As the patient moves toward recovery, the rehabilitation team helps the patient to adapt self-care activities for permanent injuries.

Ineffective Coping

Severe burns can result in disfigurement and loss of function. The patient faces a long and difficult recovery period. The emotional responses of the burn patient are often like those of any grieving person: shock, disbelief, withdrawal, denial, regression, depression, and anger. Demonstrate acceptance of the patient regardless of the emotional state. Provide opportunities for the patient to express his or her thoughts and feelings. The patient may find it helpful to talk to a clinical nurse specialist, counselor, or spiritual adviser. Some patients find support groups helpful in learning to live with their injuries. Encourage the patient to identify and use coping strategies that have been effective in the past. If effective coping strategies are used, the patient eventually incorporates the physical and functional changes into a new body image (see *Patient Teaching* box).

Patient Teaching

Burns

When the patient is acutely ill, patient teaching consists of telling the patient what is being done, why, and what to expect. As the patient stabilizes, the teaching plan should include the following points:

- You can help to prevent wound infection by practicing good hygiene and avoiding others with infections.
- Because your nutritional needs are greatly increased as a result of the healing that needs to occur, you must eat all food provided, including meal supplements. You should try to eat six small meals plus supplements while you are healing.
- Positioning, exercise, and splints help to prevent stiffening of joints, skin breakdown, and blood clots in your legs.
- Pain management is possible, so tell the nurse or physician if your pain is not controlled.
- Protect grafts from pressure and shearing force so they can heal.
- Clothing, makeup, hairpieces, and prostheses can be used to conceal scars and improve appearance.
- Adaptive devices are available to compensate for disabilities.
- Rehabilitation resources will be provided once the acute phase has passed.

Compromised Family Coping

A serious burn injury that may require months or years of therapy has a tremendous effect on the family. Significant others must be included in the patient's care. When the family arrives after the injury, the physician or clinical nurse specialist advises them of the patient's injuries, what to expect when they see the patient, and what is being done for the patient. The family should be offered an opportunity to talk with a social worker, clinical nurse specialist, counselor, or spiritual adviser. A social worker or case manager should be assigned to the patient soon after admission.

CONDITIONS TREATED WITH PLASTIC SURGERY

Plastic surgery includes aesthetic (cosmetic) and reconstructive procedures. Aesthetic surgical procedures are performed to improve appearance whereas reconstructive procedures are done to correct abnormalities. In addition to usual surgical approaches, plastic surgery may include use of flaps and grafts, skin expansion, implants, liposuction, and microvascular surgery.

AESTHETIC SURGERY

In general, aesthetic surgery alters a body feature that is structurally normal but perceived by the patient as unattractive. Examples of aesthetic surgery are rhytidectomy, blepharoplasty, chin implants, rhinoplasty, abdominoplasty, breast augmentation, and breast reduction. A rhytidectomy, commonly called *a facelift*, is done to remove facial wrinkles and tighten sagging tissue (see *Complementary and Alternative Therapies* box). A blepharoplasty is the removal of excess tissue around the eyes. It is usually an aesthetic procedure but may be done to improve function if droopy eyelids impair vision. Chin implants are done by placing a prosthesis to correct a receding chin. A rhinoplasty alters the shape or size, or both, of the nose. In an abdominoplasty, excess skin and adipose tissue are removed and the abdominal muscles are tightened.

Breast augmentation is breast enlargement, which may be performed to increase the size of both breasts or to improve breast symmetry. A variety of techniques have been used for breast augmentation. The most common procedure has been to implant a silicone rubber implant filled with saline. Silicone implants are being used again after a 14-year ban because of concerns about possible adverse effects of silicone leakage. Breast reduction decreases breast size and may be requested to improve appearance or body proportion or to eliminate discomfort associated with excessively large breasts. Liposuction is the removal of excess adipose tissue with a suction device, most commonly used on the thighs, abdomen, arms, and buttocks.

RECONSTRUCTIVE SURGERY

A number of procedures may be classified as *reconstructive*. Reconstructive surgery may be done to repair disfiguring scars, to restore body contours after radical surgery such as mastectomy, to eliminate benign lesions such as birthmarks, to restore features damaged by trauma or disease, and to correct developmental defects.

❖ NURSING CARE of the Patient Having Plastic Surgery

When working with people who are having plastic surgery, you must be aware of your own biases and feelings. If you view cosmetic procedures as vain or frivolous, you may have difficulty being supportive of patients who choose to have these procedures done. Many factors may motivate people to have aesthetic surgery. Physical appearance is a component of body image and may affect self-esteem. Some people believe that a change in appearance will benefit their personal or professional lives. A person who is very self-conscious about a physical feature can benefit immensely from aesthetic surgery. It is important not to judge the patient's motivation for seeking surgery. It is also important to be alert to the patient's unrealistic expectations for the surgical outcome.

Although each procedure may require some specific nursing interventions, this section addresses general nursing care for the patient having plastic surgery. Some specific procedures are presented in Table 52-7.

❖ PREOPERATIVE NURSING CARE

Many of these procedures may be done in day surgery or short-stay surgical units. Therefore patient

Table 52-7 Complications of Common Plastic Surgery Procedures

PROCEDURE	DESCRIPTION	COMPLICATIONS
Rhytidectomy (facelift)	Removal of excess skin and tissue from face	Hematoma, hemorrhage, temporary or permanent facial nerve damage, wound infection, bruising, edema, skin necrosis, hair loss
Blepharoplasty	Removal of bulging fat and excess skin around eye	Hematoma, ectropion, corneal injury, visual loss (rare), wound infection (rare)
Rhinoplasty	Removal of excess cartilage and tissue from nose with correction of septal defects if indicated	Hematoma, hemorrhage, temporary bruising and edema, wound infection, septal perforation, minor skin irritation
Augmentation mammoplasty	Insertion of breast-shaped synthetic implants	Hematoma, hemorrhage, wound infection, phlebitis, capsule formation and contraction
Reduction mammoplasty	Excision of excessive breast tissue and skin	Hematoma; hemorrhage; infection; fat necrosis; wound dehiscence; necrosis of nipple, areola, and skin flap

Modified from Ignatavicius DD, Workman MS, Mishler MA, editors: *Medical-surgical nursing across the health care continuum*, ed 3, Philadelphia, 1999, Saunders.

preparation emphasizes teaching for self-care. Initial teaching may be done by the physician, office nurse, or staff nurse.

Assessment

Health History

Document the patient's description of the problem being treated with plastic surgery and what the patient expects the procedure to accomplish. The past medical history may elicit conditions that might affect wound healing, such as DM, circulatory disorders, and impaired blood coagulation. In the review of systems, the surgical area should receive special attention. For example, if a blepharoplasty is being done, visual acuity should be tested and documented. The functional assessment describes the patient's lifestyle and usual activities, which may require some temporary modification after plastic surgery.

Physical Examination

The routine preoperative physical examination is performed as described in Chapter 17. The condition that is being treated is described. Most plastic surgeons have preoperative photographs made to document the condition. If the nurse takes the photograph, he or she should be sensitive to the patient's discomfort or embarrassment.

Interventions

Anxiety

Note whether the patient seems anxious by observing for nervousness, trembling, increased pulse, and difficulty concentrating. Share such observations and ask how the patient feels about the planned surgery. Anxiety may be reduced by encouraging the patient to express concerns, acknowledging that these feelings are normal, and providing information about what to expect.

Nursing Diagnoses, Goals, and Outcome Criteria: Plastic Surgery, Preoperative

Nursing Diagnoses	Goals and Outcome Criteria
Anxiety related to uncertain outcome, anticipated change in appearance, surgical procedure	Reduced anxiety: patient's statement of less anxiety, absence of trembling or tachycardia, relaxed expression
Deficient Knowledge related to unfamiliarity with surgical routines	Understanding of surgical routines: patient correctly describes routines, identifies any actions to be carried out before admission and postoperatively

Deficient Knowledge

Determine the patient's perception of the procedure and its outcome. Discuss surgical preoperative and postoperative procedures and self-care. Advise the patient if swelling, bruising, and scars are expected in the immediate postoperative period. Usually patients have been told not to take drugs that prolong bleeding time, including aspirin and herbal products, before surgery. Smoking is discouraged because nicotine causes vasoconstriction, which can interfere with healing. The patient may be instructed to scrub the surgical area at intervals before the procedure. Specific teaching depends on the exact procedure and the surgeon's orders or agency's protocol.

POSTOPERATIVE NURSING CARE

Routine postoperative nursing care is detailed in Chapter 17. This section emphasizes special considerations when a patient has plastic surgery.

Assessment

The patient may have had general, regional, or local anesthesia. Monitor vital signs and level of consciousness. Inspect dressings for drainage or bleeding but do not remove them without specific orders. Some dressings, such as those used after rhinoplasty, may serve as splints, so they must not be disturbed. Observe flaps and grafts for color and evidence of fluid accumulation; palpate for warmth. If drains are present, inspect and measure the contents each shift. The fluid should gradually lighten from sanguineous (red) to serosanguineous (pink) to serous (pale yellow). Remember that it is important to monitor the patient's comfort level.

Nursing Diagnoses, Goals, and Outcome Criteria: Plastic Surgery, Postoperative

Nursing Diagnoses	Goals and Outcome Criteria
Acute Pain related to tissue trauma	Reduced pain: patient states pain is relieved, relaxed manner
Risk for Infection related to surgical incision	Absence of infection: no fever or foul drainage, decreasing redness and edema
Risk for Injury related to inadequate circulation to grafted tissue, pressure created by edema or implants, nerve damage	Adequate tissue perfusion: normal tissue warmth and color, normal neuromuscular function (i.e., sensation, movement, reflexes)
Risk for Deficient Fluid Volume related to effects of liposuction	Normal fluid balance: vital signs consistent with patient norms, fluid intake equal to output
Disturbed Body Image related to altered appearance	Healthy body image: patient expresses understanding of temporary appearance, expresses satisfaction with outcome
Ineffective Self-Health Management related to lack of information about postoperative care	Appropriate postoperative self-care: patient describes and demonstrates self-care correctly

Interventions

Acute Pain

Minor procedures such as blepharoplasty usually cause minimal pain but major procedures such as grafting or abdominoplasty can be very painful. Pain is treated with analgesics as ordered. Aspirin usually is not ordered because it prolongs bleeding time. After surgery on the face or head, the head of the bed usually is elevated and cold compresses are ordered to decrease swelling. Document the effects of interventions. Notify the physician if the patient reports increasing pain or if pain is not responsive to treatment.

Complementary and Alternative Therapies

In addition to analgesics, recommend comfort measures, such as positioning, relaxation, and imagery, to decrease pain.

Risk for Infection

Monitor for signs and symptoms of infection (although these are unlikely to be seen during a brief hospitalization). Instruct the patient to report increasing redness, swelling, drainage, or fever. The nurse and patient must exercise good hand washing before any contact with the incisions, flaps, or grafts. Give antimicrobial drugs as ordered. Some plastic surgeons order topical antimicrobials applied to the incisions. After rhytidectomy, the patient is usually not permitted to shampoo the hair for several days to avoid contamination of the incisions.

Risk for Injury

After plastic surgery, inspect the affected tissues for evidence of adequate circulation. Grafts rely on blood flow in underlying tissue to supply nutrients and O_2 and to remove wastes. Therefore grafts must be protected from trauma and pressure. Pallor, cyanosis, and coolness in a graft suggest inadequate circulation and must be reported to the surgeon immediately. If fluid accumulates under the graft, it separates the graft from the underlying tissue, depriving it of O_2 and nutrients. Therefore swelling or blisters must be reported to the surgeon, who may remove the accumulated fluid with a small-gauge needle and syringe.

Rhytidectomy poses a risk of injury to the facial nerve, which is manifested by facial asymmetry. If asymmetry is observed, notify the surgeon immediately. The patient may be returned to surgery in an effort to relieve the pressure on the nerve and prevent permanent damage.

After blepharoplasty, monitor the patient's visual status. Although the risk is slight, the eye could be injured during the procedure.

After abdominoplasty, the patient may be required to protect the operative site by remaining in a flexed position for a specified period of time. Familiarize yourself with specific postoperative orders of your patient's surgeon. Position the bed so that the patient's head and knees are elevated to reduce stress on the suture line. When out of bed, the patient may be required to continue the flexed position. The patient is gradually permitted to straighten up; however, again, such directions vary with different surgeons.

After breast augmentation, monitor the patient for bleeding, infection, and altered sensation. The patient is also at risk for capsule formation, in which scar tissue gradually encloses the implant, causing the breast to become hard and misshaped. The surgeon may advise the patient to massage the breast to reduce the risk of capsule formation. This procedure involves pushing each breast up, to the side, and toward the center of the chest, holding each position to the count of 10. For a period specified by the surgeon, the patient should avoid raising the arms above the head.

Risk for Deficient Fluid Volume

Patients who have liposuction are at risk for hypovolemia because of excessive fluid loss. Intravenous fluids may be ordered after surgery and oral fluids are usually encouraged when the patient is fully alert. Monitor vital signs for tachycardia and hypotension associated with fluid volume deficit. Use caution when assisting patients out of bed. If the blood volume is low, the patient may feel dizzy or faint.

Disturbed Body Image

In the immediate postoperative period, the patient often has edema and bruising as well as visible incisions. Assure the patient that these effects will gradually resolve. You can explore measures to conceal the evidence of trauma but no makeup should be applied to surgical incisions until they are well healed.

Ineffective Self-Health Management

In preparing for discharge, provide verbal and written instructions for self-care. The following topics must be included: drug therapy (names of drugs ordered, schedule), wound care, signs and symptoms of infection, activity restrictions, and measures to prevent complications.

Get Ready for the NCLEX® Examination!

Key Points

- The functions of the skin are protection, body temperature regulation, secretion, sensation, synthesis of vitamin D, and blood storage.
- The skin assessment may detect skin disorders and systemic disorders that affect the skin.
- Pruritus (itching) is a symptom rather than a disease. It is treated by correction or removal of the underlying cause, by skin moisturizers, and by drugs such as antihistamines, corticosteroids, and local anesthetics.
- Atopic dermatitis, one type of eczema, is abnormally dry, itchy skin that is treated with moisturizers, antihistamines, antibiotics, and corticosteroids.
- Seborrheic dermatitis is a chronic inflammatory disease of the skin caused by increased sebum production. It is treated with medicated shampoos for the scalp and topical corticosteroids and antibiotics for other body sites.
- Psoriasis, characterized by bright-red lesions with silvery scales, may require treatment with topical corticosteroids, keratolytics, vitamin A derivatives, antipsoriatics, oral retinoids, biologic agents, ultraviolet light, and vitamin D derivatives (calcipotriene [Dovonex]).
- Fungal infections, including tinea pedis, tinea manus, tinea cruris, tinea corporis, tinea barbae, and candidiasis, are usually treated with antifungal drugs.
- Necrotizing fasciitis, a very serious infection that affects the fascia under the skin, is treated with antibiotics, debridement, and skin grafting.
- Acne, which is characterized by comedones, pustules, and cysts primarily on the face, neck, and upper trunk, may be treated with topical medications, oral antibiotics, estrogen, spironolactone, and retinoids.
- HSV-1 and HSV-2, which cause outbreaks of vesicles that rupture and form crusts, is treated with antiviral drugs that reduce the frequency and severity of outbreaks but are not curative.
- Herpes zoster infection (shingles) causes pain and itching along a nerve pathway and may respond to antiviral drugs such as acyclovir.
- Common nursing diagnoses for the patient with an infectious or inflammatory skin disorder include impaired skin integrity, acute pain, risk for (secondary) infection, disturbed body image, social isolation, and ineffective self-health management.
- Lice and scabies are tiny parasites that may infest the hair and skin, causing intense itching.
- Pemphigus is a chronic autoimmune condition in which fragile bullae develop and rupture, spilling a foul drainage.
- Skin cancers include basal cell carcinoma, squamous cell carcinoma, melanoma, cutaneous T-cell lymphoma, and Kaposi sarcoma; actinic keratosis is a premalignant lesion.
- The two major conditions affecting the nails are (1) infections and (2) inflammation caused by ingrown nails.
- Burns are classified by size and depth of the tissue injury.
- Serious burns affect not only the skin but also fluid balance, GI function, respiratory function, and the immune system.
- The three stages of burn injury are (1) emergent, (2) acute, and (3) rehabilitation.
- Wound care after burn injury is intended to promote healing, prevent infection, control heat loss, retain function, and minimize disfigurement.
- Nursing care of the burn patient may address decreased cardiac output; excess fluid volume; acute pain; risk for infection; hypothermia; imbalanced nutrition: less than body requirements; impaired physical mobility; ineffective coping; compromised family coping; and ineffective self-health management.

Additional Learning Resources

SG Go to your Study Guide for additional learning activities to help you master this chapter content.

evolve Go to your Evolve website (http://evolve.elsevier.com/Linton/medsurg) for the following learning resources and much more:

- Interactive Prioritization Exercises
- Fluid & Electrolyte Tutorial
- Pharmacology Tutorial
- Review Questions for the NCLEX® Examination

Review Questions for the NCLEX® Examination

1. You are caring for several clients with skin disorders. You understand that the skin regulates body temperature by which of the following?
   1. Reacting to foreign substances that invade the epidermis
   2. Dilating and constricting surface blood vessels
   3. Secreting sebum to insulate the outer layers of skin
   4. Reacting to sunlight by producing vitamin C

   NCLEX Client Need: Physiological Integrity: Reduction of Risk Potential
2. When inspecting the skin of an older adult, you observe flat, pigmented spots on the backs of both hands. You should recognize these as ____________________.

   NCLEX Client Need: Health Promotion and Maintenance
3. You are caring for a client who is experiencing severe itching secondary to atopic dermatitis. Which of the following measures should be recommended to help prevent scratching and skin injury? (Select all that apply.)
   1. Maintain the room temperature around 70°F
   2. Apply keratolytic agents liberally to affected areas
   3. Wash new clothing before wearing it
   4. Take daily hot baths
   5. Wear loose clothing

   NCLEX Client Need: Physiological Integrity: Reduction of Risk Potential
4. You are caring for a client who asks you about the causes of contact dermatitis. You understand that contact dermatitis is caused by which of the following?
   1. Infestations of parasites
   2. Reactions to drugs
   3. Excessive skin dryness
   4. An allergic response

   NCLEX Client Need: Physiological Integrity: Physiological Adaptation
5. You are giving a lecture to a group of clients who have psoriasis. Your discussion should include which of the following? (Select all that apply.)
   1. Psoriasis usually can be cured with drug therapy.
   2. Direct contact with others can transmit psoriasis.
   3. Anthralin must be kept on the skin continuously.
   4. Psoriasis can be aggravated by stress.
   5. Treatment may include methotrexate and ultraviolet light (UVA).

   NCLEX Client Need: Physiological Integrity: Physiological Adaptation
6. While assessing an obese older patient in a long-term care facility, you notice that the patient has intertrigo in body folds (axilla, beneath the breasts). Which measure is *most* appropriate to reduce the risk of a recurrence?
   1. Keep body folds clean and dry
   2. Reduce bathing to three times each week
   3. Liberally sprinkle cornstarch on body creases
   4. Scrub affected areas with topical antiseptics

   NCLEX Client Need: Health Promotion and Maintenance
7. You are caring for a female patient who is being treated with isotretinoin (Accutane) at the clinic for severe acne after other treatments have failed. All of the following statements should be included in the teaching plan. Which of the following statements is *most* important?
   1. "Your skin may become very dry and peel."
   2. "It may take several months to see improvement."
   3. "You will sunburn very easily while on this drug."
   4. "If sexually active, you must use reliable contraception."

   NCLEX Client Need: Physiological Integrity: Reduction of Risk Potential
8. Which of the following is a drug used to treat HSV-1?
   1. Hydrocortisone (Cortizone)
   2. Isotretinoin (Accutane)
   3. Acyclovir (Zovirax)
   4. Methoxsalen (Oxsoralen)

   NCLEX Client Need: Physiological Integrity: Pharmacological Therapies
9. What is the *best* way to prevent skin cancer?

   NCLEX Client Need: Health Promotion and Maintenance
10. Characteristics of typical melanomas include which of the following?
    1. Nodular lesion with a pearly appearance
    2. Irregular lesion with uneven coloration
    3. Scaly ulcer with no clear margins
    4. Painful red, blue, or purple macules

    NCLEX Client Need: Physiological Integrity: Physiological Adaptation

chapter 53

Eye and Vision Disorders

http://evolve.elsevier.com/Linton/medsurg

Objectives

1. Identify the data to be collected in the nursing assessment of the eye and vision.
2. Identify the nursing responsibilities for patients having diagnostic tests or procedures to diagnose eye disorders.
3. Describe the nursing care of patients who require common therapeutic measures for eye disorders: irrigation, application of ophthalmic drugs, and surgery.
4. List measures to reduce the risk of eye injuries.
5. Describe the pathophysiology, signs and symptoms, diagnosis, and treatment of selected eye conditions.
6. Assist in developing a nursing care plan for the patient with an eye disorder.

Key Terms

Astigmatism (ă-STĬG-mă-tĭzm)
Blepharitis (BLĔF-ă-RĪ-tĭs)
Cataract (KĂT-ă-răkt)
Chalazion (kă-LĀ-zē-ŭn)
Conjunctivitis (kŏn-jŭnk-tĭ-VĪ-tĭs)
Cycloplegic (sī-klō-PLĒ-jĭk)
Ectropion (ĕk-TRŌ-pē-ŏn)
Entropion (ĕn-TRŌ-pē-ŏn)
Enucleation (ē-nū-klē-Ā-shŭn)
Hordeolum (hŏr-DĒ-ŭh-lūm)
Hyperopia (hī-pĕr-Ō-pē-ă)
Keratitis (kĕr-ă-TĪ-tĭs)
Miotic (mī-ŎT-ĭk)
Mydriatic (mĭd-rē-ĂT-ĭk)
Myopia (mī-Ō-pē-ă)
Presbyopia (prĕz-bē-Ō-pē-ă)
Refraction (rē-FRĂK-shŭn)
Scotomata (skō-TŌ-mă-tă)
Tonometry (tō-NŌM-ĕ-trē)

It could be said that the eye is the window to the world. Indeed, vision plays an extremely important part in everyday life. It enables people to move about freely, to avoid danger, and to appreciate physical beauty. The eyes also are credited with conveying (or betraying!) one's emotions and communicating trust. Romantics speak of gazing into the eyes of a loved one.

In the United States, an estimated 21 million people have some vision impairment even when wearing glasses or contact lenses. For most people, loss of vision is perceived as a most tragic event. Nurses can play important roles in the prevention of vision loss, treatment of disorders of the eye, and rehabilitation of people with vision disturbances.

ANATOMY AND PHYSIOLOGY OF THE EYE

The eyeball is the primary structure involved in seeing. Several structures in addition to the eyeball serve to make up the visual system. The external structures of the visual system include the eyelids, eyelashes, conjunctiva, cornea, sclera, and extraocular muscles.

EXTERNAL STRUCTURES

The external structures of the visual system serve to protect and move the eyeball. The eyelids and eyelashes protect the eye by keeping it moist and shielding it from foreign substances. The lids are lined with a mucous membrane called the *palpebral conjunctiva.* The membrane continues from the inner eyelid margins to form a pocket around the eye and then covers the sclera up to the margin of the iris. The portion of the membrane that covers the anterior sclera is the *bulbar conjunctiva*.

Lacrimal glands located above the eyes secrete tears into the eyes through lacrimal ducts in the upper eyelids. Spontaneous blinking (approximately 15 times a minute) bathes the eyeballs in tear fluid. Tear fluid provides oxygen (O_2) and some nutrients to the cornea. Normally, the fluid drains from the eye through the lacrimal sac into the nose. With excessive tear production, tears run from the eyes. Increased tear production occurs with trauma, irritation, or emotional distress. Decreased tear production occurs to some extent with aging. It should be noted that the passage of tear fluid through the lacrimal sac is the route by which eye drops can be absorbed into the system. That is why eye drops can have systemic effects and explains the need to apply pressure to the lacrimal sac after instilling eye drops. Severe deficiencies in tear fluid cause dry eyes, making the cornea susceptible to injury (Fig. 53-1).

Normal vision requires the eyes to move together. The simultaneous movement of both eyes in the same direction is called *conjugate movement.* Eye movements are coordinated by three cranial nerves and six extra-ocular muscles.

EYEBALL

The eyeball consists of three layers of tissue: (1) the sclera, (2) the choroid, and (3) the retina (Fig. 53-2).

Sclera

The sclera is the tough outer layer of the eyeball. It is mostly white except for the clear cornea over the iris.

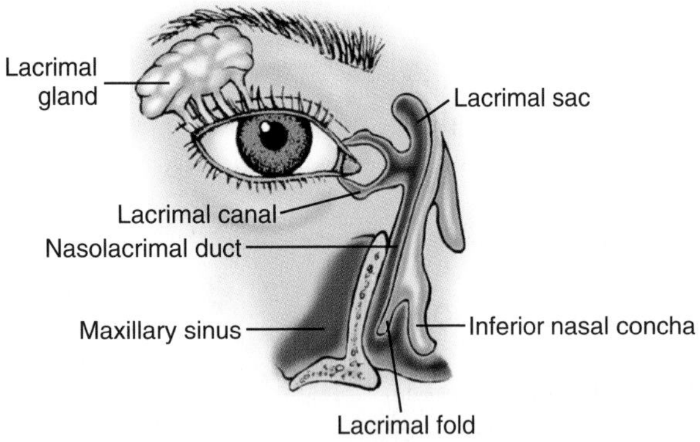

FIGURE 53-1 Lacrimal structures. (From Monahan FD, Drake DT, Neighbors M, editors: *Medical-surgical nursing: foundations for clinical practice*, ed 2, Philadelphia, 1998, Saunders.)

The cornea is covered by a protective membrane called the *conjunctiva.*

Choroid

The choroid or middle layer makes up the iris and ciliary muscle at the front of the eye. The colored part of the eye, the iris, is actually a muscle. The hole in the center of the iris is the pupil. The iris contracts and relaxes to control the amount of light entering the eye through the pupil. Dim light or severe stress causes the iris to contract. This makes the pupil dilate, or enlarge. Bright light causes the iris to relax, leaving the pupil constricted. The choroid is rich in blood vessels that deliver nourishment to the retina in the back of the eye.

Retina

The retina is the inner lining of the eyeball. It is composed of two layers. The pigmented layer is between the choroid and the sensory layer; it receives nutrients and O_2 from the choroid and supplies the sensory layer.

The area at the back of the eye contains light-sensitive receptors called *rods* and *cones.* Rods are most important for vision in dim light. Cones are used for daylight vision and color perception. The area of sharpest vision on the retina is the *macula.* Because the macula has no blood vessels, it depends on the choroid for nourishment.

Optic Nerve

The optic nerve enters the back of the eyeball. This nerve sends visual messages to the brain for interpretation. When the eye is examined with an ophthalmoscope, the part of the optic nerve that can be seen is referred to as the *optic disc.*

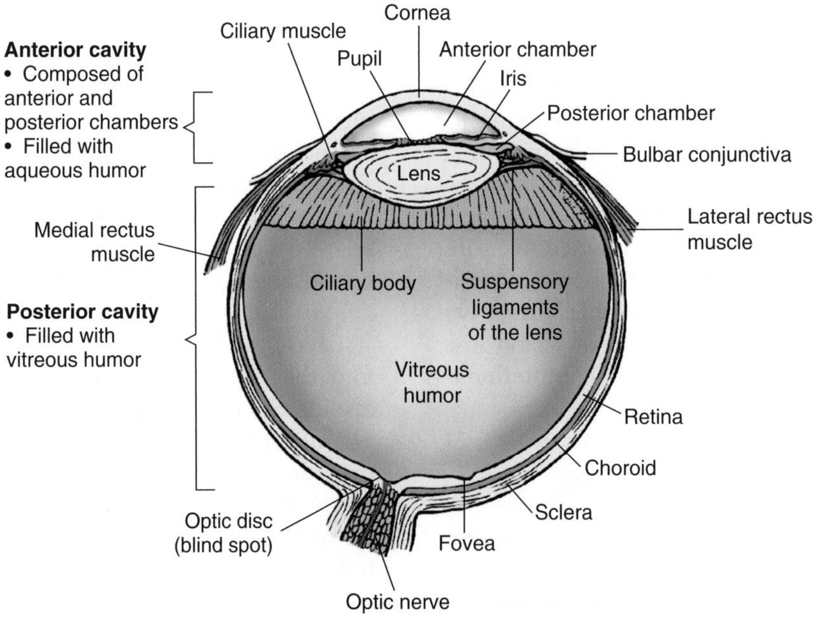

FIGURE 53-2 Internal structures of the eye. (From Monahan FD, Drake DT, Neighbors M, editors: *Medical-surgical nursing: foundations for clinical practice*, ed 2, Philadelphia, 1998, Saunders.)

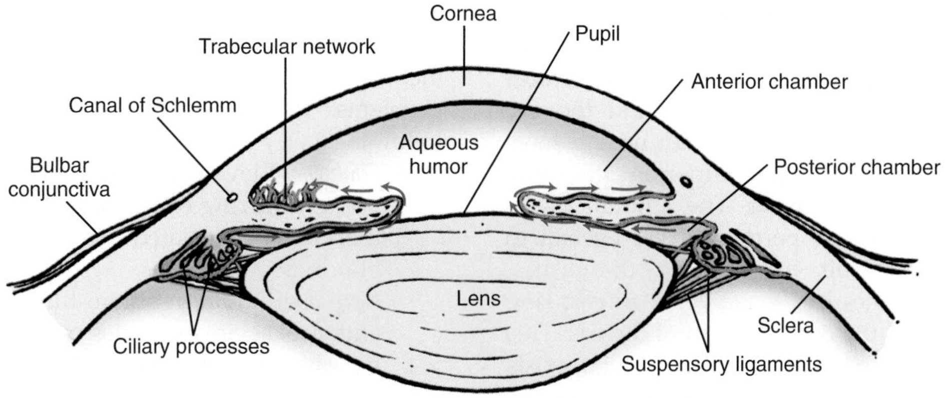

FIGURE 53-3 The flow of aqueous humor through the eye. Fluid is produced by the ciliary body. It flows through the pupil into the anterior chamber and out through the trabecular meshwork and the canal of Schlemm. (From Monahan FD, Drake DT, Neighbors M, editors: *Medical-surgical nursing: foundations for clinical practice*, ed 2, Philadelphia, 1998, Saunders.)

Fluid Chambers

Anterior Chamber. Within the eyeball are two chambers separated by the lens. The anterior chamber is located between the iris and the cornea. It is filled with aqueous humor, a clear, watery fluid. Aqueous humor is produced in the ciliary body. It flows over the lens, through the pupil, and out through the trabecular meshwork into the canal of Schlemm. The canal of Schlemm returns the fluid to the venous circulation. The flow of aqueous humor is illustrated in Figure 53-3.

The function of aqueous humor is to moisturize and nourish the lens and cornea. The production and drainage of the fluid from the eye must be balanced to maintain normal pressure within the eye.

Posterior Chamber. The larger posterior chamber behind the lens is filled with vitreous humor. Vitreous humor is a clear, gelatinous material that helps to hold the retina in place.

Lens

The lens is a transparent structure behind the iris. It is attached to the ciliary muscle. The ciliary muscle relaxes and contracts to change the shape of the lens. This process, called *accommodation*, permits the eye to focus on objects at different distances. To focus on a near object, the ciliary muscle contracts, making the lens curve. For distance, the muscle relaxes, making the lens flatter.

VISUAL PATHWAY

As light enters the eye, it passes through the transparent cornea, aqueous humor, lens, and vitreous humor. These structures are called *refractive media.* They refract (bend) horizontal and vertical light rays so that the light rays focus on the retina.

On the retina, the light rays reflected from the image are reversed and upside down. Images are carried as impulses through the optic nerve. At the optic chiasm, fibers from the left field from each eye join to form the left optic tract. Fibers from the right field of each eye join to form the right optic tract. Images are transmitted to the brain by way of the optic tracts (Fig. 53-4).

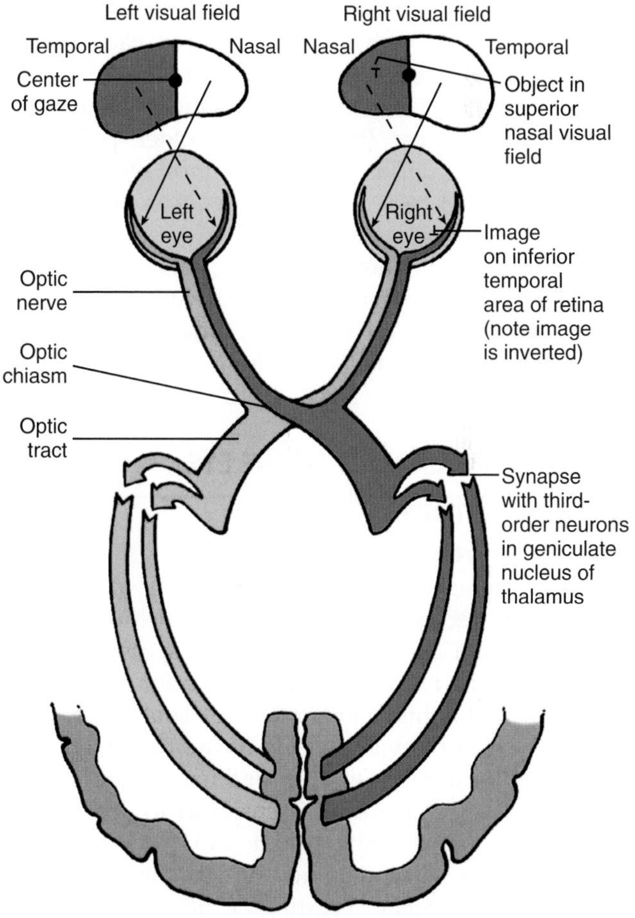

FIGURE 53-4 The visual pathway. (From Monahan FD, Drake DT, Neighbors M, editors: *Medical-surgical nursing: foundations for clinical practice*, ed 2, Philadelphia, 1998, Saunders.)

AGE-RELATED CHANGES IN THE EYE

As people age, typical changes occur in the structures and function of the eye. The skin around the eye becomes wrinkled and looser. The eyelids usually have some excess tissue; this is not important clinically unless it interferes with vision. The amount of fat around the eye decreases, permitting the eyeball to sink deeper into the orbit. Tear secretion diminishes, and the cornea becomes less sensitive. A grayish ring may be seen around the outer margin of the iris. This ring is called the *arcus senilis.* Some disagreement exists about the significance of the arcus senilis. It may be related to elevated serum lipid levels; it does not affect vision. The pupil is usually smaller in the older person and responds somewhat more slowly to light.

Vision changes associated with age are related to changes in the lens and the ciliary muscle. The lens becomes less elastic, more dense, opaque, and yellow. These changes have several significant effects. First, light passing through the lens scatters, causing the patient to be sensitive to glare. The second, more important, effect is that the ability to focus is impaired. This farsightedness (**hyperopia**) in older people is called **presbyopia**. This is the reason most older people have to wear glasses for reading or other close work. Some older people report seeing specks moving across the field of vision. These dark spots, called *floaters*, are actually bits of debris in the vitreous. Despite the age-related changes in the eye, most older people retain adequate vision for daily activities.

NURSING ASSESSMENT OF THE EYE

HEALTH HISTORY

History of Present Illness

When collecting data for the assessment of specific eye complaints, record changes in vision, including blurring, diplopia (i.e., double vision), spots, floaters, flashes of light, tunnel vision, altered color perception, halos around lights, blind spots (i.e., **scotomata**), and loss of part of the visual fields. If the patient reports pain, inquire about its location and nature (e.g., sharp, stabbing, aching). Document sensitivity to light, called *photophobia.* Ask the patient to describe any discharge from the eyes. Drainage might be described as tears, purulent discharge, or crusting of the eyelids or eyelashes. In addition, note complaints that the eyes feel dry and irritated. Other complaints that might prompt the patient to seek medical attention are redness or swelling of the lids, eyes, or periorbital area (around the eyes).

Past Medical History

People tend to assume that changes in vision are caused by problems in the eye or related structures. Although this is often true, visual disturbances also can be associated with many other conditions. Therefore it is important to obtain a good history of past medical problems from the patient who reports vision problems. Conditions to be alert for include the following:

- *Diabetes.* Elevated blood glucose can cause temporary blurring of vision. Permanent changes in the retina associated with diabetes can cause blindness.
- *Neurologic disorders.* Brain tumors, head injuries, and strokes are examples of conditions that may impair vision. Effects may be blurred vision, diplopia, inability to move eyes, or loss of part of the visual fields.
- *Thyroid disease.* Hyperthyroidism may cause exophthalmos (i.e., bulging eyes).
- *Hypertension.* Hypertension can cause changes in the blood vessels of the eye, eventually leading to vision loss.

Note any eye injury or previously diagnosed eye disease, including date of last examination and treatment.

A current medication history also is important in assessing vision problems. Some drugs can cause temporary or permanent changes in visual acuity and color vision. Others may contribute to the development of cataracts or glaucoma.

> **Pharmacology Capsule**
>
> Drugs that are especially likely to be related to vision disturbances are digitalis, corticosteroids, indomethacin, and sulfisoxazole. Patients taking thioridazine, chlorpromazine, or ethambutol also should be monitored for ocular toxicity.

Family History

The family history includes any known eye diseases as well as a history of arteriosclerosis, diabetes, and thyroid disease.

Functional Assessment

The functional assessment documents the patient's occupation, roles, and usual activities. Be alert for activities that might pose a risk to the eyes.

PHYSICAL EXAMINATION

The physician performs a complete examination, including inspection of the inner eye. However, the nurse can inspect the external eye, assess response of the pupil to light, and evaluate gross visual acuity. If abnormalities are suspected, inform the physician or advise the patient to seek medical evaluation.

> **Put on Your Thinking Cap!**
>
> What are some ways you could assess gross visual acuity when diagnostic charts are not available or not practical?

In the eye examination, first inspect the eyelids for redness, drainage, and position. The lids should cover the eyeball completely when closed. When the eyes are open, the lower lid should be at the level of the iris. The upper lid should barely cover the upper margin of the iris. The lids should fit closely to the eyeball and the eyelashes should not turn toward the eye. Describe any crusting or drainage on the lids or the lashes.

Inspect the eyeball for color and moisture. The sclera should be clear white. Excessive redness may be caused by irritation or inflammation. A yellow color, called *icterus*, is associated with liver dysfunction.

Observe the pupils for size, equality, and reaction to light. Pupils that are unequal or dilated or do not respond to light suggest neurologic problems. Some medications also can affect pupil characteristics. Accommodation is tested by having the patient focus on the examiner's finger held at a distance and then having the patient watch the finger as it is slowly moves toward the patient's nose. The pupils should constrict and the eyes converge, meaning that the pupils become smaller and both eyes move to fix on the same point. The abbreviation PERRLA is commonly used to document that pupils are equal, regular, react to light, and accommodate.

Visual acuity is commonly tested using the Snellen chart (Fig. 53-5). The Snellen chart has rows of progressively smaller letters. From a distance of 20 feet, the patient is instructed to read down the chart until more than two mistakes are made on a single line. Each eye is tested separately and then together. The lines are numbered 20 over 200, 100, 70, 50, 40, 30, 25, 20, and 15. The findings are reported as the last line the person could read with no more than two errors. That is, if the person read the 20/30 line with one error but made three errors on the 20/25 line, the vision would be recorded as 20/30 in the eye tested. This means that the person could read at 20 feet what a person with normal vision could read at 30 feet. The Snellen chart may be used for vision screening in clinic and office settings. In the hospital, it may be more practical simply to ask the patient to read available print. This provides some practical measure of visual acuity.

Some nurses learn to assess visual fields, extraocular movements, and the corneal reflex. In addition, several tests are used to detect strabismus.

When assessing the eyes, be alert for the signs of trouble listed in Box 53-1. If any of these are present, refer the patient to the physician for evaluation. The nursing assessment of the patient with an eye disorder is summarized in Box 53-2.

DIAGNOSTIC TESTS AND PROCEDURES

Several professionals are trained to assess and treat conditions of the eye. An ophthalmologist is a physician with specialized training in diagnosing and treating eye conditions. The ophthalmologist prescribes corrective lenses for refractive errors and treats other eye conditions with medications and surgery. An optometrist is trained to diagnose errors of refraction and to prescribe corrective lenses. An optician fills prescriptions written by an ophthalmologist or optometrist and fits the prescribed lenses.

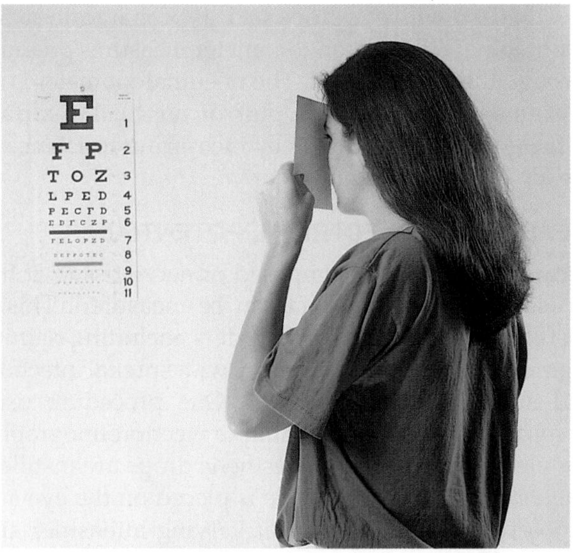

FIGURE 53-5 The Snellen chart is used to measure visual acuity. (From Jarvis C: *Physical examination and health assessment*, ed 5, Philadelphia, 2008, Saunders.)

Box 53-1 Signs of Eye Problems in Adults

If you notice any of these signs of possible eye problems, see an eye doctor for a complete eye examination:

- Unusual trouble adjusting to dark rooms
- Difficulty focusing on near or distant objects
- Squinting or blinking due to unusual sensitivity to light or glare
- Change in color of iris
- Red-rimmed, encrusted, or swollen lids
- Recurrent pain in or around eyes
- Double vision
- Dark spots in the center of viewing
- Lines and edges appear distorted or wavy
- Excess tearing or "watery eyes"
- Dry eyes with itching or burning
- See spots, ghost-like images

The following may be indications of potentially serious problems that might require emergency medical attention:

- Sudden loss of vision in one eye
- Sudden hazy or blurred vision
- Flashes of light or black spots
- Halos or rainbows around light
- Curtain-like blotting out of vision
- Loss of peripheral (side) vision

From Prevent Blindness America: *Signs of eye problems in adults* (website): www.preventblindness.org/signs-eye-problems-adults. Accessed December 24, 2013.

Box 53-2 Assessment of the Patient with an Eye Disorder

HEALTH HISTORY

Present Illness

Changes in vision; symptoms of eye disorders: pain, photophobia, drainage, dryness, irritation, redness, swelling

Past Medical History

Diabetes, neurologic disorders, thyroid disease, hypertension, previously diagnosed eye disease or injury, date of last eye examination, current medications (specifically, digitalis, corticosteroids, indomethacin, sulfonamides)

Family History

Known eye diseases, arteriosclerosis, diabetes, thyroid disease, arthritis

Functional Assessment

Occupation, roles, usual activities, changes required by eye problems

PHYSICAL EXAMINATION

Eyelids

Redness, drainage, position, closure, crusting, inversion, or eversion

Eyeball

Color, moisture

Sclera

Color, redness, jaundice

Pupils

Size, equality, reaction to light, accommodation

Visual Acuity

Measured with Snellen chart, gross acuity

Visual Fields

Extraocular Movements

Corneal Reflex

Inner Eye

Ophthalmoscopic examination of anterior chamber, lens, vitreous, and fundus (inner surface of retina)

Nursing care related to diagnostic tests and procedures for disorders of the eye is described in Table 53-1.

OPHTHALMOSCOPIC EXAMINATION

The ophthalmoscopic examination involves using an ophthalmoscope (Fig. 53-6) to examine the lens, vitreous humor, retina, and optic disc. A solution such as phenylephrine ophthalmic preparation may be instilled in the eye first to dilate the pupil. This permits a better view of the inner eye. A darkened room also causes the pupil to dilate.

The examiner studies the cornea, lens, and vitreous for opacities. The blood vessels at the back of the eye (called the *fundus*) are inspected for evidence of disease. Degenerative changes of the retina may be observed.

REFRACTOMETRY

As light enters the eye, it passes through the aqueous humor, lens, and vitreous humor. The light rays bend so that they focus on the retina. This bending is called **refraction**. Refractive errors occur when the light does not bend properly. This causes alterations in vision, which are discussed in the section titled "Errors of Refraction." Refraction is assessed by dilating the pupil and having the patient read a chart through a series of lenses. The patient identifies which lens permits the clearest image. This procedure, called *refractometry*, enables the examiner to detect refractive errors. The procedure requires no special preparation or aftercare. In patients who cannot cooperate, retinoscopy may be done to measure refractive error.

VISUAL FIELDS

Visual fields include the area a person can see while looking straight ahead without moving the head. Some conditions, such as glaucoma, retinal detachment, and certain neurologic abnormalities, cause loss of parts of the visual fields. Visual fields are assessed by comparing the patient's field of vision with that of a normal examiner (Fig. 53-7). The patient and examiner sit facing each other. The examiner moves his or her hand out of the line of vision and then brings it into the expected line of vision in a specific pattern. The patient states when the examiner's fingers are seen. No special preparation, equipment, or postprocedure care is needed.

TONOMETRY

Tonometry is the measurement of pressure in the anterior chamber of the eye. Normal intraocular pressure (IOP) is 10 to 20 mm Hg. Routine measurement of IOP is important to detect high pressures that damage the retina if untreated.

Several procedures are used to measure IOP. The most accurate procedure is called *applanation.* It is done with a slit lamp microscope. The Tono-Pen is a handheld instrument that is touched to the surface of the eye several times; the resulting pressure measurements are averaged (Fig. 53-8). Procedures in which the instrument touches the eye require that the cornea be anesthetized with eye drops such as proparacaine 0.5% (Ophthaine). The Diaton tonometer measures pressure through the closed eyelid. The pneumatonometer is an instrument that directs a puff of air to the surface of the eye. It measures IOP by measuring resistance to the air.

MEASURE OF ELECTRICAL POTENTIAL

Because the retina is composed of nerve tissue, it has an electrical potential that can be measured. This is useful in detecting retinal disorders, including retinitis pigmentosa, massive ischemia, widespread infection, and some chemical toxicities. One procedure used to measure electrical potential is electroretinography. For electroretinography, anesthetic drops are instilled. Then a contact lens electrode is placed on the eye and exposed to flashes of light at varying intensities and speeds. The response of the retina is recorded. The patient must fix his or her gaze on a target and remain very still.

Table 53-1 Diagnostic Tests and Procedures **The Eye**

TEST AND PURPOSE	PATIENT PREPARATION	POSTPROCEDURE NURSING CARE
Ophthalmologic examination: Examines the inner eye through the pupil to diagnose abnormalities of retina, optic disc, and blood vessels.	Administer mydriatic medication if ordered to dilate pupil. Room is darkened during examination. Visual acuity may be reduced because of pupil dilation.	If pupils are dilated, eyes will be sensitive to light. Clinics usually have inexpensive disposable "sunglasses" that can be given to the patient. If visual acuity is poor, patient will need someone else to drive home.
Refractometry: Identifies refractive errors and corrective lens needed.	No special preparation. If pupils are dilated, eyes will be sensitive to light.	If pupils are dilated, patient will need sunglasses until pupils return to normal.
Tonometry: One of several instruments used to measure intraocular pressure (IOP).	For procedures in which an instrument touches cornea, anesthetic drops are ordered. Inform patient of need to remain still during procedure.	Advise patient not to rub eyes for 15 min after the procedure because injury could occur when eye is anesthetized.
Fluorescein angiography: Pictures of blood vessels in the eye are taken after a dye is injected into a vein in the hand or arm. Permits diagnosis of abnormalities of vessels and retina.	Signed consent required. Administer mydriatic or cycloplegic medication as ordered to dilate the pupil. Assess allergies to iodine and seafood. Notify physician if patient is allergic. Diphenhydramine (Benadryl) may be ordered to reduce risk of allergic reaction to dye; have emergency supplies available in case of severe allergic reaction. Tell patient a dye will be given intravenously, then photographs taken through the pupil. A blue light that will flash when photos are taken may cause temporary vision disturbance. Flashing light can trigger seizure activity in patients with epilepsy.	Dye may cause a yellowish skin color for 6–24 h. Urine may be greenish as dye is eliminated. Visual acuity may be reduced because of pupil dilation. Advise patient to wear sunglasses. May need someone to drive patient home.
Visual fields: Identifies the area a person can see while looking straight ahead. Assessed by comparing the fields the patient can see with those of an examiner with normal visual fields. Patient and examiner sit facing each other. They cover opposite eyes. Examiner moves his or her hand out of line of vision, then brings it into expected line of vision in a specific pattern. Patient states when examiner's fingers are seen.	No preparation needed.	No postprocedure care needed.
Electroretinography: Used to detect some retinal disorders. A contact lens electrode is placed and the eye is exposed to flashes of light. The retinal response is recorded.	Anesthetic eye drops will be administered. The patient will need to remain still and focus on a target.	Advise patient not to rub eye because of risk for injury while anesthetized.

FLUORESCEIN ANGIOGRAPHY AND CORNEAL STAINING

To detect abnormal blood vessels or blood flow, fluorescein is injected intravenously and the retina is observed and photographed as the dye circulates (Fig. 53-9). Preparation for fluorescein angiography includes (1) the use of mydriatic drops to dilate the pupil and (2) initiation of intravenous access. The patient should be asked about allergies to dyes. A signed consent form is required. The dye will cause the patient's skin to appear yellow for several hours after the test. Encourage the patient to drink fluids to promote elimination of the dye. As the dye is excreted, the urine will appear bright green. It is common for patients to feel nauseated after the procedure.

Fluorescein also can be used to detect abrasions of the cornea. Fluorescein is applied to the surface of the

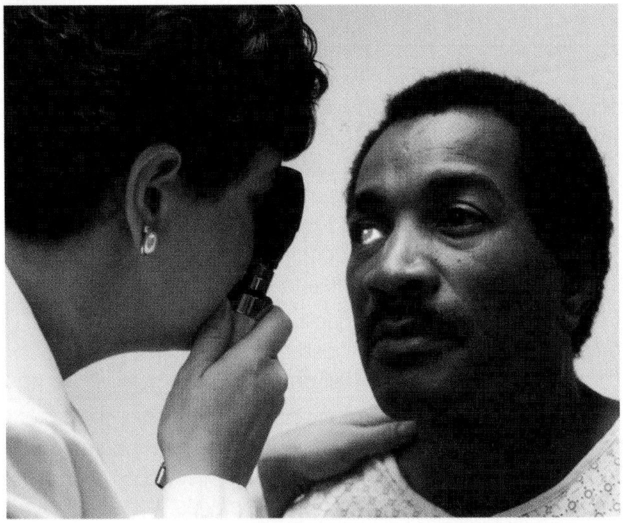

FIGURE 53-6 An ophthalmoscope is used to examine the inner structure of the eye. (From Ignatavicius DD, Workman ML: *Medical-surgical nursing: patient-centered collaborative care*, ed 6, St. Louis, 2010, Saunders.)

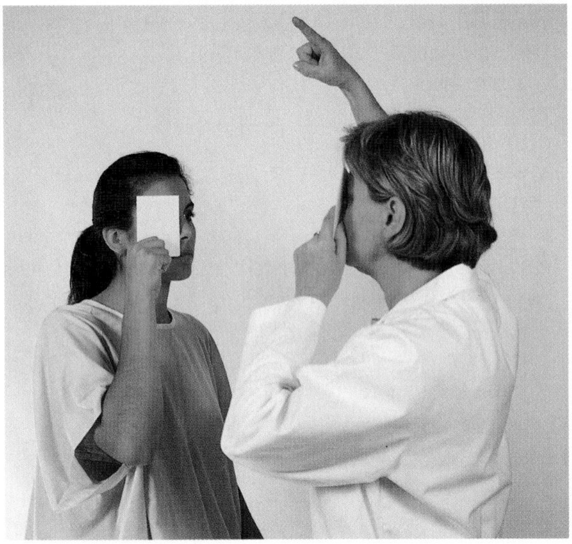

FIGURE 53-7 Assessment of visual fields. (From Jarvis C: *Physical examination and health assessment*, ed 5, Philadelphia, 2008, Saunders.)

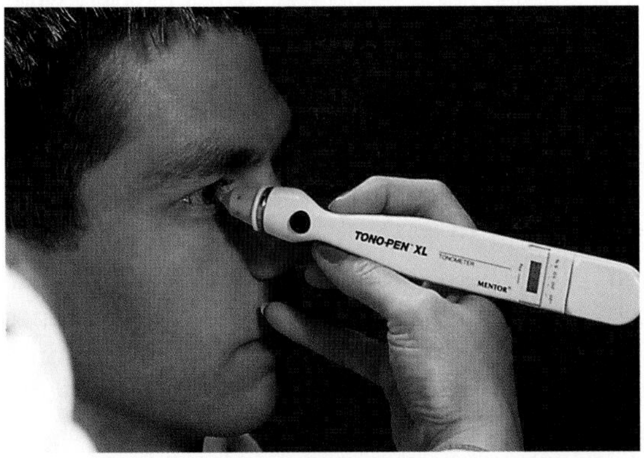

FIGURE 53-8 Tono-Pen tonometry. (From Monahan F, Sands J, Neighbors M, et al.: *Phipps' medical-surgical nursing: health and illness perspectives*, ed 8, St. Louis, 2006, Mosby.)

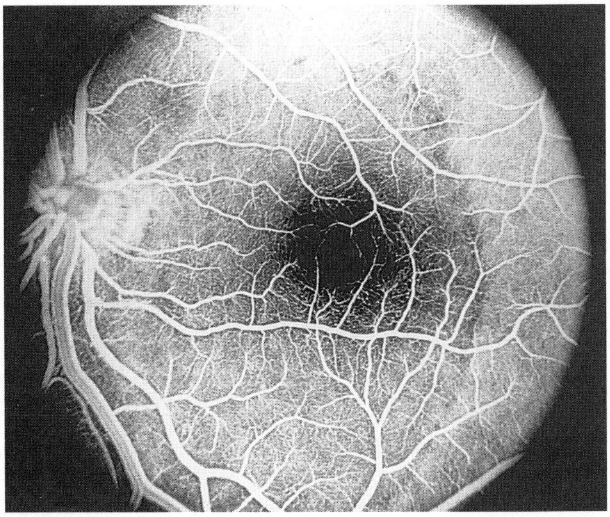

FIGURE 53-9 Fluorescein angiography permits visualization of the blood vessels of the eye to examine the inner structure of the eye. (From Black JM, Hawks JH, Keene AM: *Medical-surgical nursing: clinical management for continuity of care*, ed 6, Philadelphia, 2001, Saunders.)

eye, followed by a saline rinse. The cornea is then examined through a blue filter. Dye permits scratches to be seen more readily.

IMAGING PROCEDURES

Ultrasonography may be used to obtain images of the eye for diagnostic purposes.

AMSLER GRID TEST

This test is used to monitor for changes in vision with macular disease. A card with grid lines that has a dot in the center is provided to the patient. The patient is asked to fixate on the dot and identify anything abnormal in the shape, clarity, or completeness of the grid.

COMMON THERAPEUTIC MEASURES

EYE IRRIGATION

Irrigations are done to remove irritating chemicals from the eye. Sterile normal saline is the best solution to use. Plain water also is acceptable, especially in emergencies. In the hospital or clinic setting, the physician sometimes orders irrigations with ophthalmic medications. Key points in irrigating the eye include the following:

1. While wearing gloves, cleanse the eyelids and eyelashes.
2. Position the patient with the affected eye down so that contaminated fluid does not run into the unaffected eye.
3. Place a basin and waterproof pad to collect the fluid.
4. Gently direct the fluid into the lower conjunctival sac from the inner canthus (corner of the eye) to the outer canthus.

5. Do not touch the eye with the tip of the irrigating syringe.
6. Have the patient blink occasionally to move particles toward the lower conjunctival sac.
7. If extended irrigation is needed, special irrigation systems may be used.

TOPICAL MEDICATIONS

A number of medications are available for application directly to the eye. These include **miotics**, **mydriatics**, anesthetics, **cycloplegics**, antibiotics, and antiinflammatory drugs. Mydriatics dilate the pupils, miotics constrict the pupils, and cycloplegics prevent accommodation. Some drug manufacturers color code the caps and labels of topical ophthalmic drugs to help you select the correct drug. The caps and labels of mydriatics are red; miotics are green; nonsteroidal antiinflammatory drugs (NSAIDs) are gray; antiinfectives are brown or tan; and beta-blockers are yellow or blue. Nevertheless, you must always read the drug label carefully and compare it to the physician's order. Some systemic drugs, such as diuretics to reduce pressure in the eye, also may be ordered. Examples of ophthalmic drugs are included in Table 53-2.

Table 53-2 Drug Therapy: Disorders of the Eye

General Nursing Considerations

1. Advise the patient to follow directions exactly.
2. If the condition worsens or does not improve, notify the physician.
3. If multiple ophthalmic drugs are ordered, wait 5 minutes between them.
4. After administering ophthalmic solutions, apply gentle pressure to inner canthus for approximately 1 minute to decrease absorption and systemic effects.
5. Teach the patient or family member the correct technique for drug administration.
6. Emphasize that patients should never share eye medication.

DRUG	USE AND ACTION	SIDE EFFECTS	NURSING INTERVENTIONS
Adrenergics			
epinephrine bitartrate (Epitrate) dipivefrin HCl (Propine) phenylephrine (Neo-Synephrine), oxymetazoline (Visine L. R., OcuClear)	Dilate pupil. Used in open-angle (chronic) glaucoma. Decrease corneal congestion. Control hemorrhage.	Cardiac stimulation, headache, brow pain, insomnia, nervousness, allergy, worsening of acute (narrow-angle) glaucoma. Rebound redness.	Sunglasses needed for 6 h. Tell patient to report eye pain immediately; may be caused by increased intraocular pressure (IOP).
alpha-2 adrenergic agonists: apraclonidine, brimonidine	Alpha-2 agonists decrease aqueous formation to lower IOP in open-angle glaucoma.	Headache, dry mouth, dry nose, altered taste, conjunctivitis, lid reactions, pruritus.	
Anticholinergics (Antimuscarinics)			
atropine (Isopto Atropine) homatropine (Isopto Homatropine) scopolamine (Isopto Hyoscine) cyclopentolate (Cyclogyl) tropicamide (Mydriacyl)	Dilate pupil. Used before eye examinations and for uveitis. Decrease lacrimal gland secretion. Cyclopentolate and tropicamide have shorter duration of action.	Photophobia, inability to accommodate, corneal dryness and irritation.	Apply at ordered time before eye examination. If eye pain occurs, may indicate undetected glaucoma. Safety measures while pupils dilated because vision is blurred. Artificial tears may be needed.
Antibacterials			
gentamicin sulfate (Garamycin Ophthalmic) erythromycin (Ilotycin) polymyxin B sulfate (neomycin sulfate, bacitracin) sulfonamides (Sulamyd Ophthalmic) ciprofloxacin (Ciloxan)	Treatment or prevention of eye infections.	Allergic reaction, conjunctivitis.	Screen for previous allergic reactions; withhold drug and notify physician if allergic. Inspect eyes and lids for increasing redness.

Continued

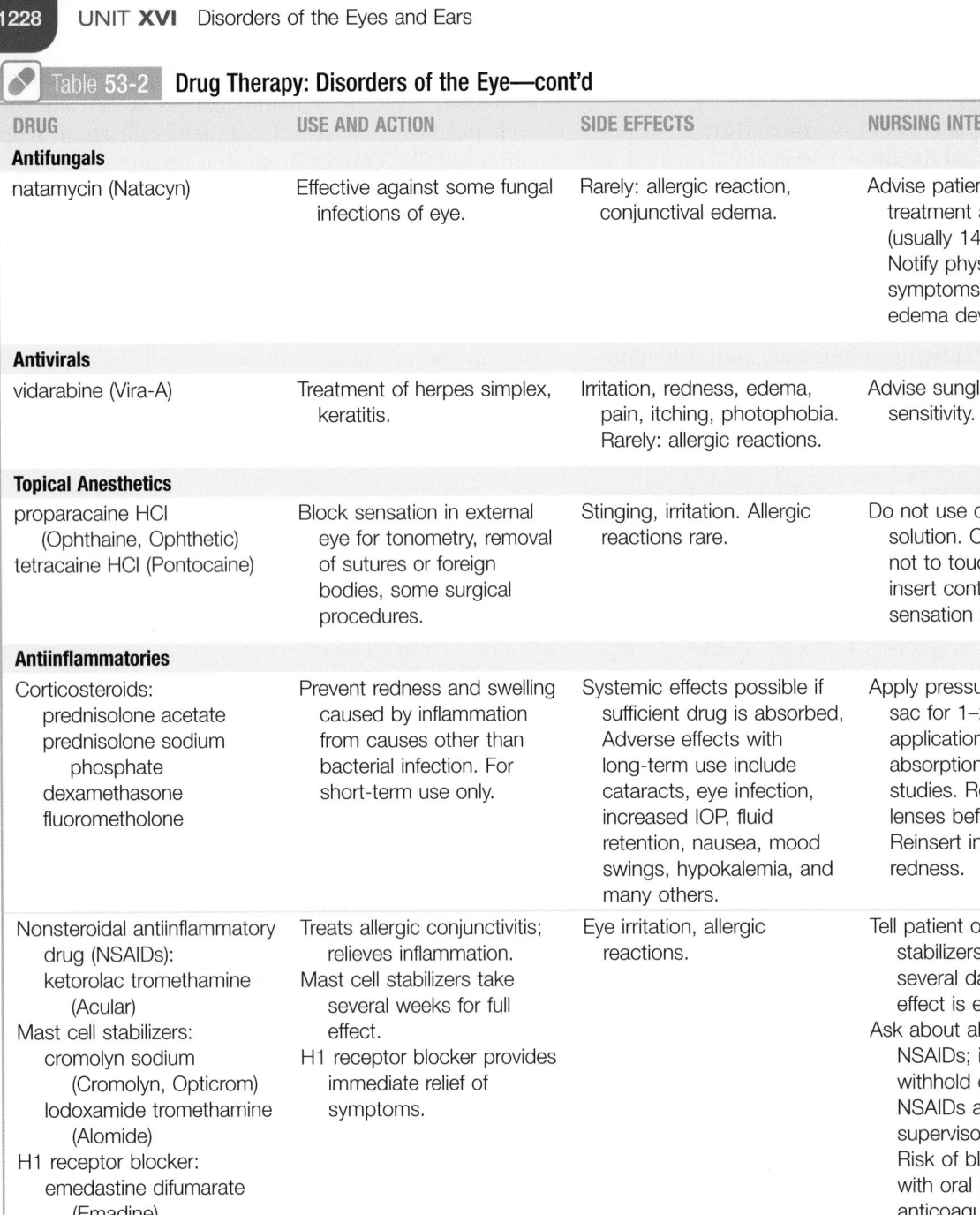

Table 53-2 Drug Therapy: Disorders of the Eye—cont'd

DRUG	USE AND ACTION	SIDE EFFECTS	NURSING INTERVENTIONS
Antifungals			
natamycin (Natacyn)	Effective against some fungal infections of eye.	Rarely: allergic reaction, conjunctival edema.	Advise patient to continue treatment as prescribed (usually 14–21 days). Notify physician if symptoms continue or if edema develops.
Antivirals			
vidarabine (Vira-A)	Treatment of herpes simplex, keratitis.	Irritation, redness, edema, pain, itching, photophobia. Rarely: allergic reactions.	Advise sunglasses for sensitivity. Refrigerate.
Topical Anesthetics			
proparacaine HCl (Ophthaine, Ophthetic) tetracaine HCl (Pontocaine)	Block sensation in external eye for tonometry, removal of sutures or foreign bodies, some surgical procedures.	Stinging, irritation. Allergic reactions rare.	Do not use discolored solution. Caution patient not to touch or rub eye or insert contact lens until sensation returns.
Antiinflammatories			
Corticosteroids: prednisolone acetate prednisolone sodium phosphate dexamethasone fluorometholone	Prevent redness and swelling caused by inflammation from causes other than bacterial infection. For short-term use only.	Systemic effects possible if sufficient drug is absorbed, Adverse effects with long-term use include cataracts, eye infection, increased IOP, fluid retention, nausea, mood swings, hypokalemia, and many others.	Apply pressure to lacrimal sac for 1–2 min after application to reduce absorption. Monitor blood studies. Remove contact lenses before using. Reinsert in 10 min if no redness.
Nonsteroidal antiinflammatory drug (NSAIDs): ketorolac tromethamine (Acular) Mast cell stabilizers: cromolyn sodium (Cromolyn, Opticrom) lodoxamide tromethamine (Alomide) H1 receptor blocker: emedastine difumarate (Emadine) Decongestant: phenylephrine (Neo-Synephrine)	Treats allergic conjunctivitis; relieves inflammation. Mast cell stabilizers take several weeks for full effect. H1 receptor blocker provides immediate relief of symptoms.	Eye irritation, allergic reactions.	Tell patient on mast cell stabilizers it will be several days before full effect is evident. Ask about allergies to NSAIDs; if allergic, withhold ophthalmic NSAIDs and notify supervisor or physician. Risk of bleeding if taken with oral NSAIDS or anticoagulants.
Angiotensin Inhibitors			
ranibizumab (Lucentis) aflibercept (Eylea) bevacizumab (Avastin)	Injected into the vitreous humor to slow progression of wet macular degeneration. May improve vision. Repeated every 1–2 months.	Inflammation in the eye, blurred vision, corneal edema, conjunctival hemorrhage, increased IOP, "floaters," eye discomfort.	Advise patient to notify physician immediately if pain, light sensitivity, or redness occur (may have inflammation). Reinforce need for follow-up and repeat treatments.

The following are key points to remember when administering topical eye medications:

!

1. Be *very* careful that only medications labeled for *ophthalmic* use are put in the eye!
2. Drops should be room temperature when administered. Rolling the bottle between the palms is a good way to warm the medication.
3. Tell the patient to tilt his or her head back and look at the ceiling. The head can be turned slightly so that excess medication runs out the outer canthus of the eyes and does not contaminate the opposite eye.
4. Place your finger below the lower lid and gently pull the eyelid down to expose the conjunctival sac and create a pouch.
5. Brace the hand holding the medication and then drop the medication into the conjunctival sac without touching the eyelid with the container to avoid contaminating the medication container.
6. Tell the patient to close his or her eyes and move them as if looking around. This distributes the medication over the eye.
7. You or the patient should apply gentle pressure to the lacrimal sac at the inner canthus of the eye for approximately 1 minute. This reduces the amount of the medication entering body fluids, thereby reducing systemic effects.
8. If more than one medication is being given, *wait 5 minutes* between each medication administration.

EYE SURGERY

A number of eye conditions are treated or corrected with surgery. Eye surgery may involve surgical incisions, the use of lasers, and application of heat (thermal therapy) or cold (cryotherapy). Individualized care plans must be developed based on the specific type of procedure done. However, some general considerations apply to most patients having eye surgery.

❖ PREOPERATIVE NURSING CARE

■ Assessment

Preoperative assessment and care are discussed in detail in Chapter 17. Before eye surgery, the assessment specifically focuses on the patient's emotional state, ability to perform self-care, and knowledge of surgical routines and outcomes. Most patients awaiting eye surgery are somewhat anxious. They may be fearful that the procedure will not be successful or that some complication will lead to further loss of vision. Determine whether any current or future activity limitations exist. If the patient has poor vision, document the type of help needed. In addition, note the physician's orders for intravenous fluids and/or preoperative medications. Food and fluid intake is usually restricted from the evening before surgery to reduce the risk of nausea, vomiting, and aspiration after surgery. Because many procedures on the eye are done in day surgery facilities, ensure that the patient understands the preoperative routine. Document who will take the patient home after the procedure because the patient will not be able to drive until cleared to do so by the physician.

Nursing Diagnoses, Goals, and Outcome Criteria: Eye Surgery, Preoperative

Nursing Diagnoses	Goals and Outcome Criteria
Anxiety related to uncertain outcome, lack of knowledge about surgery and surgical routines	Reduced anxiety: patient states anxiety is reduced, relaxed manner
Bathing, Dressing, Feeding Self-Care Deficit related to visual impairment	Achievement of activities of daily living (ADL): daily activities completed successfully

■ Interventions

Anxiety

Explore the patient's feelings about the surgery and provide information. Refer specific questions about the surgical procedure, risks, complications, or outcomes to the physician. Explain general surgical and postoperative routines.

Bathing, Dressing, Feeding, Self-Care Deficit

On admission, orient the visually impaired patient to the room. Keep objects in one place and advise the patient of any new equipment or articles in the environment. Follow agency policy for obtaining consent for surgery. Offer to read any written material to the patient.

❖ POSTOPERATIVE NURSING CARE

■ Assessment

After surgery, check the patient's vital signs and level of consciousness during recovery from anesthesia. Inspect the dressing or the operative eye for bleeding or drainage. In addition, ask about pain and nausea. If vision is impaired, inspect the environment for safety hazards. Before discharge, determine the patient's understanding of and ability to administer prescribed medications by having the patient or caregiver demonstrate self-medication.

■ Interventions

Risk for Injury

The physician may prescribe limitations on activity, position, or both. The head of the bed is usually elevated. The patient may be wearing a bulky dressing or a small eye patch. Either may be covered with a

Nursing Diagnoses, Goals, and Outcome Criteria: Eye Surgery, Postoperative

Nursing Diagnoses	Goals and Outcome Criteria
Risk for Injury related to pressure or trauma	Decreased risk of injury: patient avoids potentially harmful activities (e.g., rubbing eye, bending forward)
Readiness for Enhanced Coping	Adaptation to impaired vision: patient makes adjustments in lifestyle to accommodate vision change
Acute Pain related to tissue trauma	Pain relief: patient states pain is reduced or absent, relaxed manner
Anxiety related to temporary vision impairment	Decreased anxiety: patient states is less anxious, calm demeanor
Ineffective Self-Health Management related to lack of understanding of self-care measures and usual postoperative course	Effective self-health management: patient adheres to plan of care, demonstrates appropriate self-care

lightweight metal or plastic shield (Fig. 53-10). The dressing absorbs any drainage and the shield protects the eye from rubbing. Instruct the patient not to rub the eye. Check the physician's orders to determine whether the dressing can be changed. Eye drops or ointments may be ordered and may be different from those used before surgery. When an eye is patched, take safety precautions to prevent injury. !

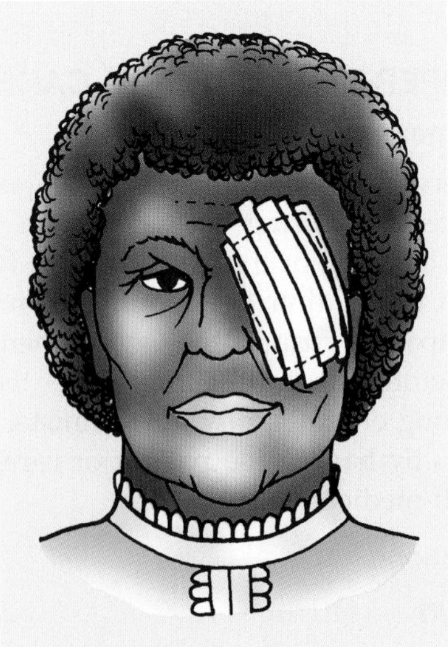

FIGURE 53-10 The shield protects the operative eye from pressure or rubbing. (From Ignatavicius DD, Workman ML, Mishler MA: *Medical-surgical nursing across the health care continuum*, ed 3, Philadelphia, 1999, Saunders.)

An important aspect of the postoperative care of patients having eye surgery is to prevent increased IOP. Caution the patient against activities that increase pressure, including straining, leaning forward, lifting, and lying on the affected side. The physician will specify how long restrictions are necessary. Because vomiting and retching raise IOP, treat nausea promptly. !

Put on Your Thinking Cap!

After eye surgery, patients often go home on the same day. Considering the usual restrictions imposed to prevent increased intraocular pressure (IOP), what are some obstacles the patient might encounter? What strategies might you suggest to the patient?

Readiness for Enhanced Coping

Measures to help the patient adapt to visual impairment are discussed in detail in the section titled "Nursing Care of the Visually Impaired Patient."

Acute Pain

Although one might expect eye surgery to be painful, postoperative pain is usually mild to moderate. Give mild analgesics as ordered. If a patient reports severe pain, notify the physician.

Anxiety

To reduce anxiety, explain what is being done and why and encourage the patient to express concerns and ask questions.

Ineffective Self-Health Management

Patients who have had eye surgery often are discharged with some medications. Provide careful directions and a written schedule for the medications. To determine the patient's ability to self-administer eye medications, have the patient demonstrate the procedure before discharge. If necessary, instruct a family member in administering the medications.

Put on Your Thinking Cap!

An 80-year-old patient is being discharged after ocular surgery. He has several topical ophthalmic drugs that must be applied twice daily. One eye is to remain patched until he sees the physician in 1 week. What information would you want to gather to determine whether he will be able to manage at home?

PROTECTION OF THE EYES AND VISION

Maintaining adequate vision involves the prevention of injuries and the treatment of abnormalities. Nurses must be knowledgeable about the protection and care of the eyes.

PATIENT TEACHING

Nurses can teach people how to care for their eyes to protect vision. Adults younger than 40 years should have their eyes examined every 3 to 5 years. After the age of 40 years, eye examinations should be done every 2 years and should include testing for glaucoma. This permits early detection and treatment of eye disorders.

Tell patients to report sharp, stabbing eye pain or deep, throbbing eye pain. Other symptoms that should be reported to a physician are photophobia (i.e., sensitivity to light), blurred or double vision, loss of part of the visual fields, halos around lights, and floaters. Floaters are spots that appear to move across the field of vision. Some patients describe floaters as being like birds swooping past one's face. Other symptoms that require medical evaluation are burning sensations, itching, excessive tearing, and the presence of drainage from the eyes.

When symptoms of eye problems exist, patients should seek medical advice rather than try home remedies. First aid for eye injuries is explained in Chapter 16.

Sometimes nurses have the opportunity to correct misconceptions that people have about vision. The following are some examples of misconceptions:

- Watching too much television or sitting too close to the television injures the eyes.
- Eating foods that contain large amounts of vitamin A improves vision. However, it is true that vitamin A deficiency can cause vision impairment (see *Nutrition Considerations* box).
- Eyes need to be rinsed regularly.

Nutrition Considerations

1. Vitamin A is essential for normal vision.
2. An early symptom of vitamin A deficiency is night blindness.
3. Severe vitamin A deficiency causes clinical eye disease that leads to blindness.
4. The AREDS formulation is a combination of vitamins and minerals that may reduce the risk of developing age-related macular degeneration.

Prevention of Injuries

Injuries caused by foreign objects are a major cause of vision loss. Teach young children the danger of throwing or poking objects at the faces of playmates. Assess toys for safety. Adult activities that produce sparks or cause fragments to be dispersed also cause injuries. Advise protective eyewear for such potentially dangerous activities.

Basic Eye Care

Gently cleanse the eyelids each time the face is washed. Use a clean cloth without soap. Wash the eye from the inner canthus (near the nose) toward the outer canthus. Dry crusts on the eyelids and eyelashes usually can be wiped off them. If necessary, place a warm, damp cloth on the lids for several minutes to soften the crusts.

Routine eye rinses and drops are unnecessary for most people. Exceptions are people with inadequate tear production and those whose eyes do not close completely. Lubricating drops called *artificial tears* are available for those people. Sometimes, eye patches are applied or the lids are taped shut to prevent drying of the cornea.

EFFECT OF VISUAL IMPAIRMENT

Vision loss usually has significant effects on all areas of a person's life. Mild losses may require only some adaptations. More serious losses affect independence, mobility, employment, and interpersonal relationships. In addition, pleasure in seeing the people and things a person treasures is lost.

The loss of vision triggers a grief response. People grieve for the lost function just as they might grieve after the death of a loved one. Reactions that are likely to follow loss of vision include shock, denial, anger, bargaining, and depression.

Factors that affect a person's response to this loss include personality, usual coping style, effect of vision loss on the person's life, and the circumstances of the loss. If grief is resolved in a healthy manner, adaptation and acceptance eventually occur. People who have progressive loss of vision may experience anticipatory grief. Nursing care to help the person who is grieving is discussed in Chapter 24.

NURSING CARE of the Visually Impaired Patient

When people hear the word *blind*, they think of someone who is unable to see. However, degrees of visual impairment exist. Although some visually impaired people are unable to see at all, many others have partial vision. Therefore medical literature is more likely to use terms such as *visual impairment* or *visually handicapped* rather than *blind*. In addition, a stigma may be attached to the word *blind*, as some people automatically associate blindness with helplessness.

Trauma, disease, and some congenital defects account for visual handicaps throughout the life span. Some types of visual disturbances are more common in older people.

To work with the visually impaired, you need to be aware of their thoughts and feelings about visual handicaps. You should assume that people with visual impairments can be independent and productive. Pity has no place in this situation because it encourages hopelessness and helplessness. The person needs help with some tasks but should still be treated as an adult.

The extent of vision loss determines the types of assistance that might be needed. Many people have visual problems that can be corrected with eyeglasses, drug therapy, or surgical treatment. Many products are available to enable visually impaired people to function more independently. When planning care, consider whether the patient's condition is temporary, permanent, correctable, treatable, or progressive.

Assessment

The nursing assessment of the patient with an eye disorder is summarized in Box 53-2.

Nursing Diagnoses, Goals, and Outcome Criteria: Impaired Vision

Nursing Diagnoses	Goals and Outcome Criteria
Knowledge Deficit related to strategies to adapt to altered reception, transmission, and interpretation of visual stimuli	Adaptation to vision impairment: patient has no falls or other traumatic injuries, uses assistive devices and techniques to maintain as much independence as possible
Ineffective Coping related to decreased independence, threat to body image, denial	Effective coping: patient makes efforts to adapt, participates in self-care to maximum degree possible
Feeding Self-Care Deficit related to visual impairment	Appropriate self-feeding: patient feeds self with minimal assistance
Impaired Walking related to impaired vision, anxiety	Safe walking: patient walks safely; uses strategies to move about safely
Ineffective Self-Health Management related to lack of understanding of treatment of vision impairment	Effective self-health management: prescribed plan of care is managed appropriately, patient carries out plan of care and participates in rehabilitation programs if indicated

Interventions

Knowledge Deficit

When a visually impaired person is admitted to a health care facility, provide an orientation to the environment. The fact that the patient has visual impairment should be reflected on the nursing care plan. In addition, a sign may be posted to alert other caregivers and employees. Safety is a primary consideration for these patients. Measures to support the patient with impaired vision and to prevent injury include the following:

1. When you enter the room, announce your presence and introduce yourself to avoid startling or embarrassing the patient.
2. Speak before touching the patient to avoid startling him or her.
3. Speak in a normal tone of voice. People tend to act as if those who cannot see cannot hear, so a tendency exists to raise one's voice when talking to the visually impaired.

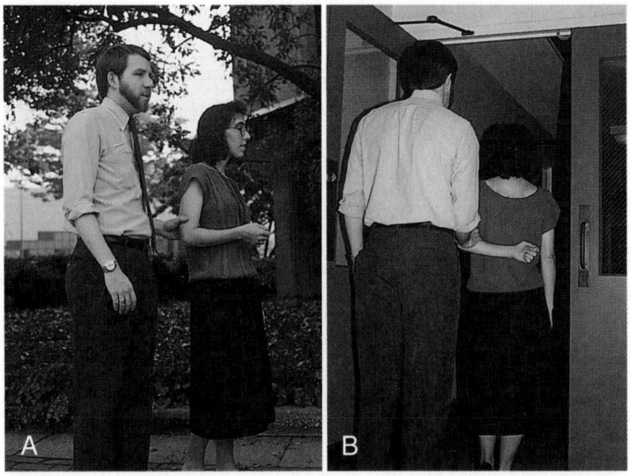

FIGURE 53-11 **A,** To escort a visually impaired person, allow the person to grasp your upper arm. **B,** To enter a narrow passage or doorway, bring your arm behind your back to alert the person. (Courtesy Cleveland Sight Center, Cleveland, Ohio. www.clevelandsightcenter.org.)

4. Address the patient in the appropriate manner for his or her age and intellectual ability. Visual impairment is not associated with mental impairment.
5. Advise the patient what to expect during procedures.
6. Tell the patient when you leave the room.
7. Leave the bed in low position.
8. Place the call bell within reach and ensure that the patient knows how to use it.
9. Keep doors either open or closed so that the ambulatory patient does not run into a partially closed door.
10. Do not rearrange the room after orienting the patient.
11. Eliminate meaningless noise from the environment as much as possible.
12. To lead a blind person, have him or her take your arm (Fig. 53-11).

The environment significantly influences the visually impaired patient's ability to function. It should be safe and promote maximal independence. As mentioned, orientation to the setting is especially important. Ensure that the patient can use the call system, locate personal items, and use the bathroom. Tell the patient if any new equipment or furniture is brought into the room. Keep pathways in the room free of clutter.

For patients who are partially sighted, lighting is very important. Glare must be reduced because it actually interferes with vision. Windows should have adjustable shades, blinds, or sheers. Floors should not be highly polished (Fig. 53-12). Color can provide important cues to enable the partially sighted person to function. This is especially true of the older person whose color perception may have changed. Older people perceive warm colors (e.g., red, orange, yellow) more accurately than cool colors (e.g., blue, green). Furniture color should be distinctly different from the

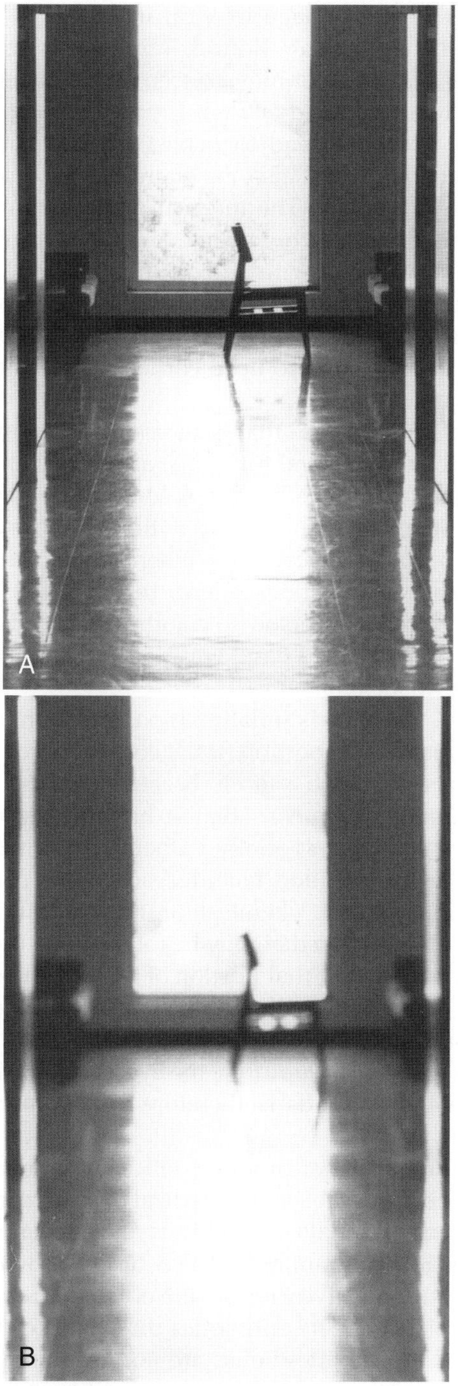

FIGURE 53-12 Glare perceived by **(A)** a person with normal vision and **(B)** an older person whose eyes have undergone age-related changes. (From Linton AD, Lach H: *Matteson and McConnell's gerontological nursing*, ed 3, Philadelphia, 2007, Saunders.)

color of floors and walls. Light switches, handrails, and steps marked with contrasting colors are easier to locate. Dishes and cups with colored rims facilitate self-feeding and reduce spills.

Ineffective Coping

People who have lived with vision impairment usually have developed routines and strategies to cope with the situation. Ask about such routines and maintain them as much as possible. If the patient uses assistive devices such as eyeglasses or magnifying glasses, make sure they are available and encourage their use. The older person who becomes confused during hospitalization may show dramatic improvement when eyeglasses are provided.

Encourage diversional activities when appropriate. The patient with some vision may be able to enjoy reading with magnifiers or large-print reading material. Talking books are available without charge through the American Foundation for the Blind. Many bookstores stock audio books (i.e., books recorded on compact disks [CDs]). Braille reading material and typewriters can be used by those who have been trained in this method. Braille uses arrangements of raised dots to represent letters. The reader reads the material by moving the fingertips over the characters. Not everyone is able to master reading Braille because of the sensitive touch needed. Special telescopic lenses and magnifiers can enable some patients to read, write, and use a computer. Canes and guide dogs permit independent ambulation. Voice recognition programs permit computer use without typing.

Feeding Self-Care Deficit

Ask the patient what assistance is required instead of assuming that help is needed. Many patients are quite independent despite impaired vision. Do not encourage dependence during hospitalization. To orient the patient to the location of foods, fluids, or other objects, think of their arrangement as a clock face (e.g., "your meat is at 3 o'clock").

Impaired Walking

A consistent environment enables the patient to be more independent with less risk of injury. Do not move furniture, personal effects, and equipment without patient consent. Rehabilitation experts teach patients techniques and adaptive equipment to facilitate physical mobility.

Some visually impaired people have guide dogs that enable them to move about more independently. These dogs are trained to guide their owners inside and outside the home. They usually can go anywhere their owners go. Laws that restrict pets in public places usually do not apply to guide dogs. When the dogs are wearing their harnesses, they are working and should not be distracted by friendly strangers.

Ineffective Self-Health Management

Patients with severe impairment should be referred to specialists in rehabilitation. They need to learn self-care activities, safe mobility, and strategies to carry out usual roles such as child care and occupational skills. Teach patients with diseases of the eye any prescribed measures to cure or slow the progression of the disease.

DISORDERS AFFECTING THE EYE OR VISION

EXTERNAL EYE DISORDERS

Inflammation and Infection

The eye is a potential site for infectious and inflammatory conditions. Because of the sensitivity of the eye, such disorders can cause considerable discomfort. Some may even threaten vision if not treated. These are typically treated on an outpatient basis but the clinic nurse or long-term care nurse may interact with patients affected by these disorders.

Eyelid Infection and Inflammation. **Blepharitis** is an inflammation of the hair follicles along the eyelid margin. It can be caused by bacteria, most often by staphylococci. Seborrheic blepharitis is often found with seborrhea of the scalp and eyebrows. Symptoms include itching, burning, and photophobia. Scales or crusts may be seen on the lid margins. The patient may complain that the eyelids are sealed shut by dried crusts on awakening.

Untreated blepharitis could lead to inflammation of the cornea or hordeolum (i.e., stye). The physician may prescribe an antibiotic ointment for the condition. Be certain that any medication applied to the eye is an *ophthalmic* preparation. The eyelids also can be gently cleansed with baby shampoo solution.

Hordeolum is commonly called a *stye.* It is a common acute staphylococcal infection of the eyelid margin that originates in a lash follicle. The affected area of the lid is red, swollen, and tender. If a person has repeated infections, these may be related to staphylococcal infections at some other location on the body. The primary treatment is the application of warm, moist compresses several times a day. The physician may order ophthalmic antibiotics or may incise and drain the stye.

Chalazion is an inflammation of the glands in the eyelids. Swelling prevents fluid from leaving the glands, causing them to become enlarged and tender. Warm compresses may bring some relief. Treatment may include a corticosteroid injection into the chalazion to reduce inflammation or incision and drainage of the lesion.

Conjunctivitis. **Conjunctivitis** is an inflammation of the conjunctiva caused by bacteria, viruses, allergy, or chemical irritants. Warm or cool compresses, antiinflammatory eye drops, and topical vasoconstrictors may be ordered. Mast cell stabilizers with or without antihistamines may be ordered for long-term management of allergic conjunctivitis.

Bacterial conjunctivitis is commonly called *pinkeye.* It is characterized by redness of the conjunctiva, mild irritation, and purulent drainage. The condition usually clears up spontaneously but topical antibiotics may be prescribed.

Viral conjunctivitis can be caused by adenoviruses, herpes simplex virus type 1 (HSV-1), and herpes zoster virus. Viral infections are characterized by redness and drainage. The drainage in viral infections is watery rather than purulent. Round, raised areas that are white or gray in color may be seen on the conjunctiva. These areas are called *follicles.*

Viral infections tend to persist longer than bacterial infections. They also are more likely to produce severe eye damage. The medical management varies with the causative organism. Infections caused by HSV-1 are treated with idoxuridine (HerpEX) ointment or other topical medications. Corticosteroids are contraindicated with viral conjunctivitis because they may contribute to deep corneal ulcers and other complications.

Other organisms that can cause conjunctivitis include chlamydia and fungi that are more common in developing countries but are seen occasionally in the United States. They are treated with topical or systemic antimicrobial medications. When conjunctivitis is caused by an infectious agent, the infection can be passed from one person to another. Infected people should practice good hand washing and should avoid sharing washcloths.

Keratitis. **Keratitis** is inflammation, infection, or both of the cornea. The portion of the cornea in front of the pupil has no blood vessels because it must remain transparent. This means that it has no direct blood supply, making it especially vulnerable to infections.

Sources of infection include bacteria, viruses, and fungi. In addition, chemical or mechanical injuries cause inflammation that may be followed by infection. If scar tissue forms, that portion of the cornea becomes cloudy and vision is impaired. In addition, the infection can extend to the inner structures of the eye. Serious lesions can rupture if the eye is rubbed. Prompt treatment of keratitis is therefore very important to preserve vision.

Keratitis does not produce noticeable drainage but it causes considerable pain. Medical treatment includes topical antibacterials or antivirals and topical corticosteroids. Systemic antibiotics also may be ordered after culture and sensitivity results are obtained. Sometimes the physician injects antibiotics directly into the conjunctiva. Topical anesthetics are not used because the patient might accidentally cause additional injury to the anesthetized cornea. Eye pads are not used with keratitis because they provide a dark, damp environment for microorganisms to grow.

Entropion and Ectropion

Proper closure of the eyelids is important to protect the eye and keep the cornea moist. **Entropion** is a condition in which the lower lid turns inward. Eyelashes rub against the eye, causing pain and possibly scratching the cornea. Surgical correction usually is recommended.

Ectropion is a condition in which the lower lid droops and turns outward. The eye does not close completely, causing it to become dry and irritated. The dry cornea is easily injured. Ectropion may be treated symptomatically or surgically.

Foreign Body

Everyone has experienced the discomfort of having a foreign body in the eye. Blinking and tearing usually will wash small irritants from the eye. If the foreign body remains in the eye, evert the upper and lower lids as illustrated in Figure 53-13. If the object is clearly visible and does not appear to be embedded in the eye, you may attempt to remove it. Use a sterile cotton swab to touch the object gently. If the object is not embedded, it usually clings to the swab and can be removed. A physician should remove foreign bodies that are embedded in the eye.

Chemical Spills and Splashes

Chemical spills and splashes are discussed in Chapter 16.

Corneal Opacity

A healthy cornea is clear, allowing light to enter the pupil. When the cornea is injured by infection or trauma, scar tissue may form. In some cases a rigid contact lens can correct the uneven corneal surface. If scar tissue prevents light from entering the eye, varying degrees of vision impairment occur. Phototherapeutic keratectomy (PTK) uses the excimer laser to destroy corneal abnormalities. The procedure has a high rate of success and a recovery period of only a few days. If PTK fails or is not an option, the only other treatment for corneal opacity is removal of the scarred cornea and replacement with a healthy cornea. The surgical procedure is called a *keratoplasty.*

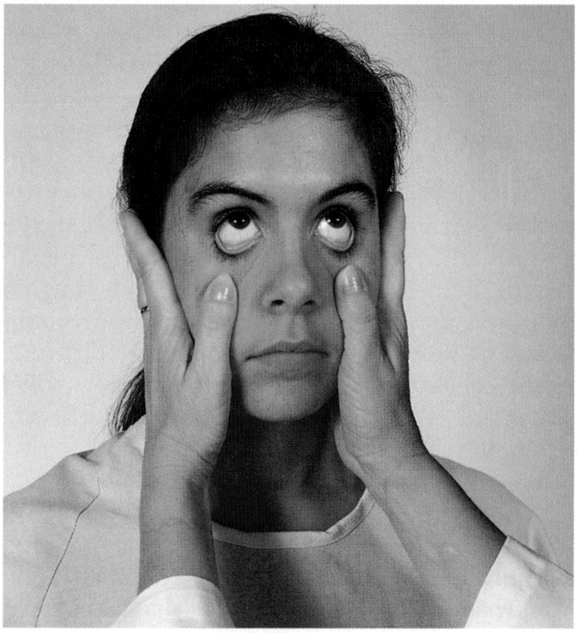

FIGURE 53-13 Eversion of the eyelids for inspection of the sclera and conjunctiva. (From Jarvis C: *Physical examination and health assessment*, ed 5, Philadelphia, 2008, Saunders.)

Healthy corneas are obtained from donors shortly after death. This may be authorized by the donor before death or by the family. The donated tissue is removed and preserved, preferably within 4 hours of death. Eye tissue is easier to preserve than other body tissues. This permits keratoplasty to be done as a scheduled procedure rather than as an emergency on-call procedure. It can be done under local anesthesia. Before surgery, eye drops may be ordered to either dilate or constrict the pupil. Usually, drops are used that constrict the pupil (miotics). Constriction of the pupil pulls the iris over the lens like a curtain and protects the lens during surgery. Sometimes, however, it is necessary to remove the lens as well as the cornea. Lens extraction is necessary if the lens is cloudy because of injury or age-related changes. In this case, preoperative mydriatic drops are ordered to allow access to the lens.

The types of grafts used in keratoplasty vary in depth. A penetrating graft consists of all layers of the cornea. If the graft is not full depth, it is called a lamellar graft. Precise techniques that attempt to replace only the layer of the cornea that is scarred include Descemet's membrane endothelial keratoplasty (DMEK), Descemet's stripping endothelial keratoplasty (DSEK), and deep lamellar endothelial keratoplasty (DLEK). The type of graft used depends on the extent of injury to the recipient's cornea.

During a keratoplasty, the surgeon first removes the patient's damaged cornea. An identically sized graft is then taken from the donor eye and secured to the recipient's eye with very fine sutures, as shown in Figures 53-14 and 53-15. When a penetrating keratoplasty is done, the aqueous humor is lost from the anterior chamber of the eye. The surgeon replaces the fluid with a saline solution.

❖ NURSING CARE of the Patient Having Keratoplasty

Preoperative nursing care of the patient having eye surgery is discussed in the section titled "Preoperative Nursing Care." After surgery, the keratoplasty patient has an eye pad and a metal shield over the operative eye. Sometimes the other eye is temporarily patched as well, because the eyes normally track together. This reduces eye movement until the operative eye heals. Corticosteroid eye drops may be ordered to reduce inflammation. Unlike other tissue transplants, corneal transplants do not require immunosuppressant therapy to prevent tissue rejection.

■ Assessment

Inspect the dressing for drainage and ask if the patient is having any pain or nausea. After the dressing is removed, inspect the eye for corneal opacity. In addition, evaluate the patient's visual acuity. It is common for vision to be blurry for the first few weeks followed

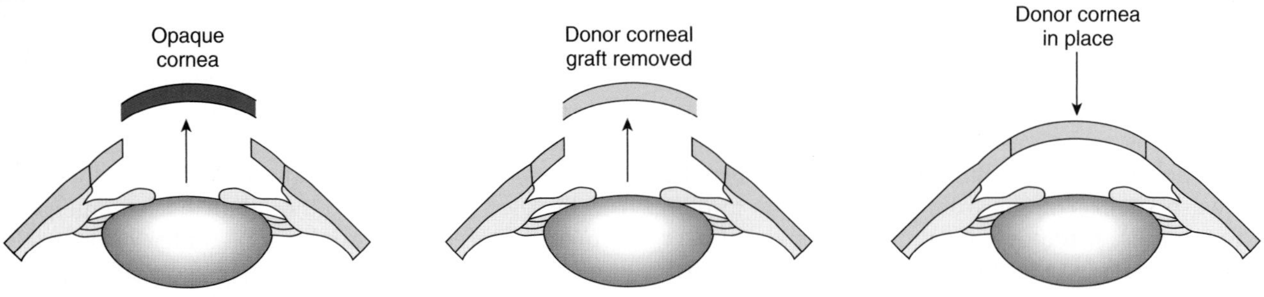

FIGURE 53-14 Keratoplasty. The damaged cornea is removed and then replaced with a corneal graft from a donor eye.

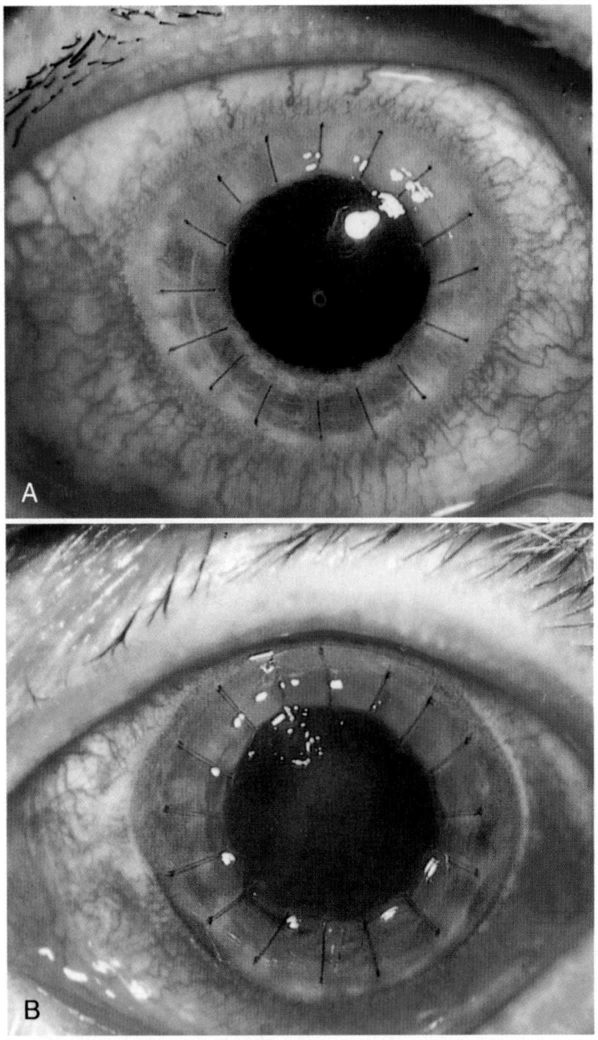

FIGURE 53-15 Keratoplasty. **A,** Appearance of the eye soon after keratoplasty. **B,** Acute corneal rejection. (Courtesy Ophthalmic Photography at the University of Michigan, W.K. Kellogg Eye Center, Ann Arbor, Mich.)

by gradual improvement. Complete recovery may take as long as 6 to 12 months.

The normal appearance of the eye soon after keratoplasty is shown in Figure 53-15, *A.*

In addition to routine postoperative care after eye surgery, the following specific care may apply after keratoplasty.

Nursing Diagnoses, Goals, and Outcome Criteria: Keratoplasty, Postoperative

Nursing Diagnoses	Goals and Outcome Criteria
Risk for Injury related to activities that increase intraocular pressure (IOP)	Decreased risk for injury: patient avoids activities that increase IOP (e.g., bending forward, lifting, straining)
Acute Pain related to tissue trauma	Pain relief: patient states pain is relieved, relaxed manner
Impaired Tissue Integrity related to inflammation or rejection of transplanted tissue	Adaptation to temporary vision impairment: patient performs usual activities with minimal assistance Gradual improvement in visual acuity: patient report, improved visual acuity scores
Ineffective Self-Health Management related to lack of understanding of usual postoperative course	Effective management of prescribed plan of care: patient correctly describes and demonstrates self-care measures

Interventions

Risk for Injury

Caution the patient to avoid any activities that increase pressure in the eye, including rubbing the eye, bending forward, lifting, straining at stool, and coughing. Report and promptly treat nausea because vomiting raises IOP. Administer stool softeners as ordered to prevent constipation. The patient probably will be instructed to wear the shield for several weeks while sleeping to prevent accidental trauma.

Acute Pain

Only mild to moderate pain is expected after keratoplasty. The physician usually orders analgesics such as acetaminophen to be given as needed. Notify the physician of severe or increasing pain because it suggests increased IOP or infection.

Impaired Tissue Integrity

Rejection of corneal grafts is not common but it can happen. When rejection occurs, blood vessels appear in the cornea and the cornea becomes cloudy (see Figure 53-15, *B*). Corticosteroid drops are ordered to reduce inflammation and the risk of rejection. Patients should know that symptoms of rejection include redness, swelling, decreased vision, and pain. Other topical medications that usually are ordered are antibiotics to prevent infection and mydriatics to dilate the pupil.

Ineffective Self-Health Management

Nurses and patients should realize that the grafted eye must heal just like any other body part that has undergone surgery. In the movies, the physician removes the dressing dramatically. The patient blinks a few times and the world comes into focus. In reality, it takes a while before the patient's vision clears. Reassure the patient that this is normal.

Before discharge, determine what medications the patient will be taking at home. Review the medications with the patient, demonstrate proper self-administration, and have the patient return the demonstration. Instruct the patient to promptly report symptoms of graft rejection, which include unusual redness in the eye, eye pain, sudden change in visual acuity, and increased light sensitivity.

ERRORS OF REFRACTION

Light must pass through the cornea, aqueous humor, lens, and vitreous humor to reach the retina. These structures through which light passes are called *refractive media.* The term *refraction* refers to the bending of light rays—in the case of the eye, so that they focus on the retina. Abnormalities, called *errors of refraction,* occur when refractive media do not bend light rays correctly. Myopia, hyperopia, and astigmatism are common problems caused by variations in the structure of the eyeball. Figure 53-16 illustrates these variations and the type of correction required.

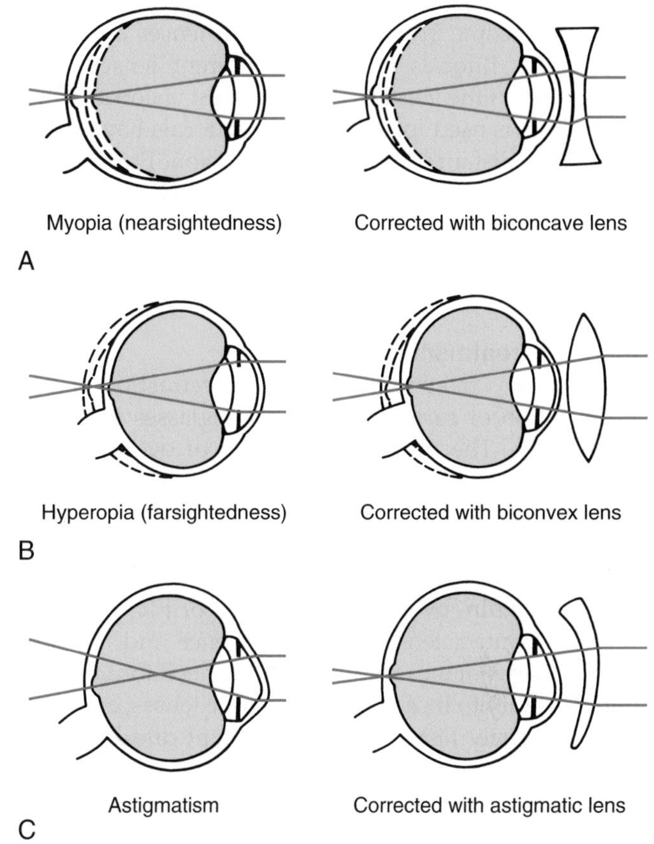

FIGURE 53-16 Refraction. **A,** Myopia: Light rays converge before they reach the retina because the lens is too far from the retina. **B,** Hyperopia: Light rays converge beyond the retina because the lens is too close to the retina. **C,** Astigmatism: Uneven surfaces of the cornea bend light rays in a way that causes distortion of the image. (From Black JM, Hawks JH, Keene AM: *Medical-surgical nursing: clinical management for continuity of care*, ed 6, Philadelphia, 2001, Saunders.)

Types of Errors of Refraction

Myopia and Hyperopia. **Myopia** is the medical term for *nearsightedness.* In myopia, the lens is situated too far from the retina. Light rays come together to focus in front of the retina. People with myopia have difficulty seeing distant images clearly. It is often recognized in the early school years. Typically, the condition progresses slowly until adolescence. New glasses usually are needed approximately every 2 years.

When the lens is too close to the retina, light rays come together behind the retina. This condition creates *hyperopia,* commonly known as *farsightedness.* The hyperopic person sees clearly in the distance but has difficulty focusing on close objects. Convex corrective lenses are needed for correction.

Astigmatism. When irregularities in the cornea or lens exist, **astigmatism** results. Most people have some degree of astigmatism. If the condition is mild, the natural lens can correct for the abnormality. If it is severe, however, then vision is distorted and corrective lenses are needed. A person can have astigmatism with myopia or hyperopia.

Presbyopia. Presbyopia is another disorder that is classified with errors of refraction. Presbyopia is poor accommodation that is due to loss of elasticity of the ciliary muscles. Accommodation is the adjustment of the lens for near and distant vision. It is accomplished by contraction or relaxation of the ciliary muscles, which causes the lens to change shape.

Presbyopia is usually considered a normal age-related change. It most often develops after age 40. As it progresses, people may be observed holding reading material at arm's length. People who are already hyperopic tend to have presbyopia at an earlier age than other people. Myopic people are usually able to read small print by holding it close.

Corrective lenses are needed when the visual changes become bothersome. Bifocal lenses are often prescribed. Bifocals have two different lenses. The upper part of the lens is used for distant vision and the lower part is used for near vision. Trifocals have three lenses, for distant, closer, and near vision. Progressive lenses gradually blend the lens needed for seeing various distances. The wearer scans the lens to find the area needed for a particular task. Reading lenses usually must be changed every 2 to 3 years.

Medical Treatment

The primary treatment of errors of refraction is the prescription of corrective lenses. Eyeglasses are used most often. The obvious advantage of eyeglasses is that they require no special skills to use. Disadvantages are heavy frames and dirty lenses.

Contact lenses are tiny plastic and silicone disks made to fit over the patient's cornea. The lenses float on the tear film over the cornea. The primary advantages of contact lenses are convenience and appearance. Disadvantages include cost, the need for training and dexterity to insert and remove the lenses, and that they are easily lost. Another important disadvantage is the risk of corneal injury.

Contact lenses are either rigid or soft. Rigid lenses are standard or gas permeable. Gas-permeable lenses are made of materials that allow O_2 and carbon dioxide (CO_2) to pass through them. This is important because the cornea exchanges gasses through the tear film beneath the contact lens. Hard lenses must be removed from the eye at the end of the day to prevent damage to the cornea.

Soft lenses include several variations: standard, high water content, toric, disposable, and daily disposable. Standard and daily disposable lenses must be removed at night. The other varieties may be used for daily or extended wear. Disposable extended-wear contact lenses can be worn for as long as 2 weeks. For this reason, they may be prescribed for older patients who have cataract surgery. The patient is cautioned to follow the prescribed cleaning routine for the type of lenses worn.

Surgical Treatment

Surgical correction of refractive errors has advanced dramatically in recent years. *Photorefractive keratectomy* (PRK) uses an excimer laser to reshape the cornea for treatment of myopia, hyperopia, and astigmatism. An alternative procedure to correct those problems is the *laser-assisted in situ keratomileusis* (LASIK) procedure. LASIK involves peeling back a thin layer of the cornea and using a laser to reshape the middle layer of the cornea. Intracorneal ring segments (ICRS) are implanted between layers of the cornea to treat mild myopia. Intraocular lenses (IOLs) can correct both myopia and hyperopia. Phakic IOLs are implanted in front of the natural lenses. Refractive IOLs actually replace the patient's natural lens, making it a more invasive procedure with a higher risk of complications.

These procedures are done under local anesthesia in outpatient facilities. The outcomes cannot be evaluated immediately because refraction stabilizes slowly after surgery.

❖ NURSING CARE of the Patient with Errors of Refraction

Nursing responsibilities for the patient with errors of refraction are limited to encouraging periodic examinations and knowing if the patient uses corrective lenses. In emergency situations, the nurse may have to remove contact lenses for the patient. When caring for patients who have laser surgery, it may be your responsibility to teach postoperative care to the patient. You should include proper use of any prescribed eye drops, measures to protect the eye, and symptoms to be reported to the surgeon.

INTERNAL EYE DISORDERS

Cataract

The lens is a clear, flexible structure encased in an elastic capsule. It is located behind the iris and changes shape to focus on images of various sizes. When the lens becomes opaque (i.e., cloudy) so that it is no longer transparent, the condition is called a **cataract**.

Causes. Cataracts may be congenital, traumatic, or degenerative. Congenital cataracts are those that are present at birth. Traumatic cataracts are caused by chemical, mechanical, heat, or radiation injury. Degenerative cataracts are more common with aging but they occur earlier in people with diabetes or Down syndrome.

Pathophysiology. The lens may become opaque (i.e., cloudy) quickly or slowly. Injuries tend to cause opacity rapidly whereas age-related opacity progresses slowly. As opacity increases, light is unable to enter the eye and vision becomes cloudy. Blindness eventually results if a cataract is untreated. With age, both eyes are usually affected, although they may not change at the same rate.

Signs and Symptoms. Signs and symptoms of cataracts include cloudy vision, seeing spots or ghost images, and floaters. The pattern of vision changes depends on the location of the developing cataract. A central cataract is located in the center of the lens. Patients with central cataracts may have fairly good peripheral vision. They may actually see better in dim light because the pupil dilates, allowing them to see around the cloudy center of the lens. Conversely, patients who have peripheral cataracts can see straight ahead but not to the side. As cataracts develop, people who initially were hyperopic may have temporary improvements in near vision. This is called *second sight*.

Medical Treatment. The only curative treatment for cataract is removal of the lens, although mydriatics may be helpful in the early stages. Cataract extraction is the most frequently performed eye operation in the United States. Several types of cataract extraction exist, as illustrated in Figure 53-17. If the lens and capsule are removed, it is called an *intracapsular cataract extraction.* The preferred procedure is the *extracapsular cataract extraction* in which the lens is removed, leaving the capsule in place. A small incision is made in the eye. Then the surgeon extracts the lens or uses sound waves to break up the lens (phacoemulsification) followed by aspiration of the fragments out of the eye. Cataract extraction typically is accompanied by placement of an artificial lens behind the iris. Sometimes the remaining capsule becomes cloudy, causing vision to become blurred again. This usually can be corrected easily with laser treatment.

Cataract extraction is commonly done on an outpatient basis. Most patients tolerate the procedure well with just a mild sedative and local anesthesia. In some cases, general anesthesia may be preferred. Cataract surgery is usually considered safe, even for those who are very old.

Complications. Complications that sometimes occur include leakage of vitreous humor, hemorrhage into the eye, and opening of the incision.

Lens Replacement. Once the lens has been removed, the eye is said to be *aphakic.* The patient is extra farsighted and unable to accommodate for changes in object size. Some type of artificial lens is needed for correction.

Contact Lenses. Whereas contact lenses have many advantages over eyeglasses, they have drawbacks as well. Considerable dexterity is required to insert, remove, and care for contact lenses. This makes them impractical for some older patients. The main complication of contact lens use is corneal injury.

Intraocular Lenses. The invention of plastic lenses (see Fig. 53-17) that can be implanted in the eye has been a tremendous advance for many cataract patients. This type of lens is called an *intraocular lens.* The intraocular lens is almost always implanted immediately after removal of the natural lens. Complications of insertion include corneal edema, secondary glaucoma, lens displacement, and retinal detachment. Although some new intraocular lenses accommodate for near and far vision, the patient may still require reading glasses for close work.

❖ NURSING CARE of the Patient with Cataracts

Cataract extractions often are done in day surgery clinics. You may have limited opportunity for patient and family teaching. Care of the patient having eye surgery is presented earlier under "Common Therapeutic Measures: Eye Surgery." This section emphasizes additional care specific to cataract surgery.

❖ PREOPERATIVE NURSING CARE

Eye drops often are ordered at frequent intervals before cataract surgery. The orders must be followed exactly.

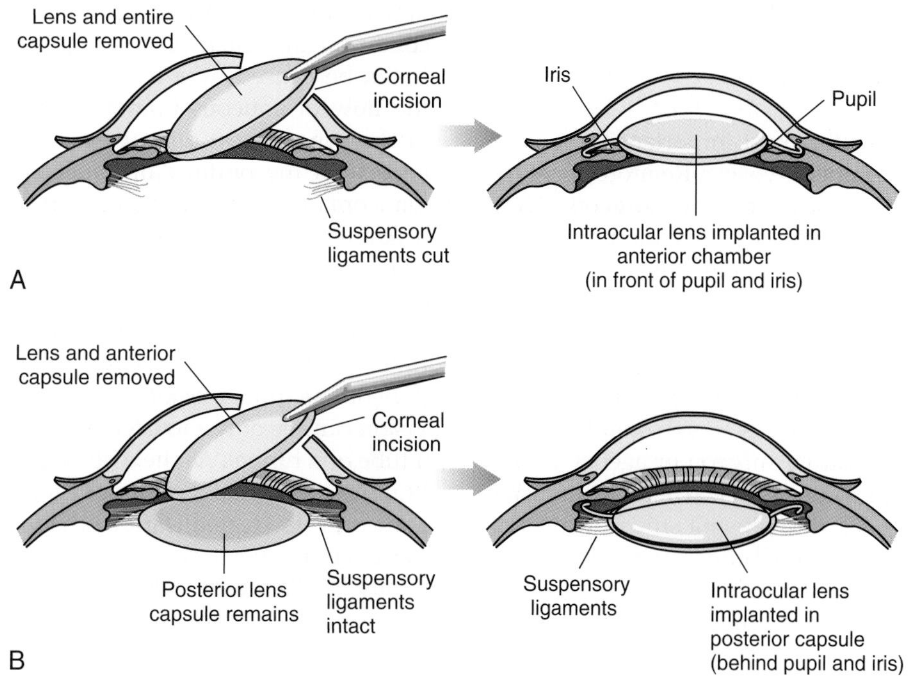

FIGURE 53-17 Methods of cataract extraction. **A,** Intracapsular cataract extraction with removal of entire lens and capsule. **B,** Extracapsular cataract extraction leaving the posterior lens capsule intact. (From Monahan F, Sands J, Neighbors M, et al.: *Phipps' medical-surgical nursing: health and illness perspectives*, ed 8, St. Louis, 2006, Mosby.)

Common drops used before cataract surgery are mydriatics, cycloplegics, antibiotics, and NSAIDs. Mydriatics dilate the pupil, making it easier for the surgeon to access the lens. Cycloplegics temporarily paralyze the muscles of accommodation, keeping the eye still during the procedure. Antibiotics reduce the risk of infection and NSAIDs reduce inflammation. A sedative may be given to decrease anxiety.

❖ POSTOPERATIVE NURSING CARE

■ Assessment

After cataract surgery, ask about pain and nausea. The patient is likely to return from surgery wearing a patch and shield over the operative eye. Note the presence of the patch and any apparent drainage. In addition, note the patient's level of consciousness and orientation (see Nursing Care Plan: Patient Having Cataract Surgery, Postoperative).

Nursing Diagnoses, Goals, and Outcome Criteria: Cataract Surgery: Postoperative

Nursing Diagnoses	Goals and Outcome Criteria
Risk for Injury related to increased intraocular pressure (IOP), vision impairment	Reduced risk for injury: patient avoids activities that increase IOP, IOP remains 12 to 20 mm Hg. Patient demonstrates self-care, maneuvers in environment without injury, administers medications properly

■ Interventions

Risk for Injury

After cataract surgery the most important thing is to prevent strain on the operative eye. Reinforce postoperative limitations specified by the surgeon. They might include the following. Caution the patient not to rub the eye. Examples of restrictions intended to decrease strain are to sleep on the unaffected side, not to lift more than 5 lb, and to avoid bending forward. You may see less restrictive postoperative care in some settings because researchers are questioning some of the traditional practices. However, you should follow the orders of the individual surgeon or agency protocols until newer guidelines are issued. Administer stool softeners as ordered to prevent straining at stool or instruct the patient in self-medication. If nausea occurs, promptly administer an antiemetic as ordered.

Always be aware of safety precautions after cataract surgery. When one eye is patched, the patient has limited peripheral vision. The unoperated eye often has some degree of impairment as well. Medications may be ordered that cause blurred vision. To prevent injury, ensure that the patient is familiar with the environment and knows how to use the call bell. Keep the bed in low position and the environment free of obstacles. Outpatient surgery allows the patient to return to a familiar setting on the same day. If the patient resides in a long-term care facility, ensure that the environment is uncluttered and personal items are conveniently placed.

Confusion sometimes occurs in the postoperative period, especially in those who are very old. The confused person may fail to follow safety precautions or may place strain on the operative eye. Therefore monitor mental status until the person returns to his or her preoperative mental state.

Medications prescribed after cataract surgery usually include antibiotics and corticosteroids or NSAIDs. You may need to teach a family member or friend how to give the medications until the patient is able to administer them.

A mild analgesic is usually ordered as needed. Postoperative patients with cataract surgery should not have severe pain. If a patient complains of severe pain, notify the physician. Severe pain may indicate hemorrhage or rising pressure within the eye.

Glaucoma

Glaucoma is one of the leading causes of blindness in the United States. It occurs in infants, children, and adults. It is thought to affect 2.2 million Americans, with only half of those having been diagnosed. Blindness from glaucoma is six to eight times more common among African Americans than Caucasians.

Pathophysiology. Normally, aqueous humor enters and leaves the anterior chamber so that IOP is maintained between 10 and 20 mm Hg. Glaucoma is a condition in which IOP is increased above normal. It can be caused by a number of changes that affect the flow of aqueous humor in the anterior chamber of the eye. It most often is caused by some interference with the outflow of aqueous humor. Although glaucoma may follow trauma, the exact cause is often unknown.

Excess pressure damages the back portion of the eye. It impairs blood flow to the optic nerve and retina, resulting in vision impairment. Peripheral vision is lost first. The field of vision gradually narrows until the patient has tunnel vision. The patient who has tunnel vision can see only a small circle, as if looking through a tube or a tunnel. As the disease progresses, complete blindness eventually occurs. Vision may be restored if glaucoma is treated early; otherwise, vision loss is permanent.

Types of Glaucoma. The two most common types of glaucoma are (1) open-angle glaucoma and (2) angle-closure glaucoma. They are similar in that increased IOP is present in both but they have some important differences. The main adverse effect of increased IOP is damage to the optic nerve with subsequent vision loss. Both chronic open-angle and acute angle-closure

Nursing Care Plan: Patient Having Cataract Surgery, Postoperative

ASSESSMENT

HEALTH HISTORY A 72-year-old retired welder is seeking medical care because of cloudy vision that has become increasingly worse. He reports spots moving across his field of vision. Cataracts were diagnosed, with the right lens affected more severely than the left. He had a right extracapsular cataract extraction under local anesthesia this morning in the outpatient surgery department. He says that he has mild pain in the eye area at this time. His record reveals a history of myocardial infarction 5 years ago and surgery for prostate enlargement 6 months ago. Although he is retired, he works every day on his small farm. He lives with his wife and an adult daughter.

PHYSICAL EXAMINATION Vital signs: blood pressure 142/68 mm Hg, pulse 88 bpm, respiration 18 breaths per minute, temperature 98°F (36.7°C) measured orally. Height 5′7″, weight 155 lb. Is alert, oriented, and in semi-Fowler position. An eye pad is in place over the right eye, protected with a metal shield. A small amount of clear drainage is noted seeping below the dressing.

Nursing Diagnosis	Goals and Outcome Criteria	Interventions
Risk for Injury related to increased intraocular pressure (IOP), trauma	Decreased risk for injury: patient avoids activities that increase IOP. IOP remains 12 to 21 mm Hg.	Keep head of bed elevated. Instruct the patient not to impose stress on operative eye, rub the operative eye, strain, lean forward, or lie on the affected side. Administer antiemetics immediately as ordered for nausea and vomiting. Change damp pad as allowed. Administer eye drops (antimicrobials and corticosteroids) as ordered. Encourage patient to take stool softeners as ordered to prevent constipation.
Knowledge Deficit about postoperative care	The patient will adapt to visual impairment and function in environment without injury.	The patient will probably go home several hours after surgery. Until then, keep the bed in low position. Approach the left side. Place the call bell on the left and instruct in use. When the patient returns home, some assistance with activities of daily living (ADL) may be needed for a day or two.
Acute Pain related to tissue trauma	The patient will report that pain has decreased, will appear relaxed.	Assess pain. Notify the surgeon if severe (may indicate increased IOP). Administer analgesics as ordered and evaluate effects.
Anxiety related to temporary vision impairment, activity restrictions	The patient will report decreased anxiety and will appear calm.	Explain what is being done and why. Be sensitive to concerns about surgery. Answer questions. Respond promptly to needs.
Ineffective Self-Health Management related to lack of understanding of condition, self-care, and limitations	Effective self-health management: the patient (and family member) will demonstrate instillation of medications and state activity limitations.	Explain postoperative limitations. No lifting over 5 lb, bending forward, or straining until cleared by physician. Review procedure for eye drops and have patient or family member demonstrate instillation. Supplement verbal instructions with written information.

Critical Thinking Questions

1. Why is it important to prevent constipation in a patient who has had cataract surgery?
2. Explain why activities that increase IOP must be avoided postoperatively.

glaucoma are considered *primary glaucomas.* Increased IOP because of other conditions is called *secondary glaucoma.*

Chronic Open-Angle Glaucoma. Open-angle glaucoma is more common than angle-closure glaucoma. Chronic open-angle glaucoma results from some alteration that prevents the normal passage of aqueous humor through the trabecular meshwork. It is more common among African Americans on corticosteroid therapy and those with a parent or sibling who has the condition.

Usually no signs and symptoms appear at first. Some patients complain of tired eyes, occasional blurred vision, and halos around lights. Another clue may be the need for frequent changes in eyeglass prescriptions.

Open-angle glaucoma usually is treated first with drug therapy. The types of medications used include beta-adrenergic blockers, adrenergics, cholinergics, carbonic anhydrase inhibitors, and hyperosmotic agents. Drugs work either by decreasing the production of aqueous humor or by improving the outflow of aqueous humor.

Beta-blockers often are the first drug used in the treatment of glaucoma. These drugs probably lower IOP by decreasing the production of aqueous humor. Adrenergics decrease IOP by decreasing the formation of aqueous humor. Cholinergic miotics facilitate the outflow of aqueous humor. These drugs constrict the pupil, which permits fluid to flow more easily through the angle where the iris meets the cornea and into the trabecular meshwork. A disadvantage of many currently used miotic agents is that they must be administered frequently. Some new preparations, including ocular inserts, are effective for a longer period of time. Carbonic anhydrase inhibitors reduce IOP by decreasing the production of aqueous humor. Various forms are available for oral, topical, and parenteral use. Hyperosmotic agents, including oral glycerin and intravenous mannitol, promote movement of fluid from the intraocular structures.

Examples of each classification of drugs used to treat glaucoma as well as additional details are provided in Table 53-3.

Surgical intervention may be recommended when drugs do not reduce pressure adequately, the patient does not use prescribed drugs properly, or adverse reactions interfere with drug therapy. Surgical procedures for glaucoma include trabeculoplasty, trabeculectomy, and cyclocryotherapy. Trabeculoplasty may be tried first because it can be done under local anesthesia in an outpatient setting. A laser is used to create multiple holes in the trabecular meshwork, which improves drainage of aqueous humor from the anterior chamber. If the procedure is successful, IOP falls over a period of time. Meanwhile, the physician usually has the patient continue using glaucoma medications.

A trabeculectomy is one of several surgical procedures that create a channel to allow aqueous humor to drain under the conjunctiva. If this procedure is not effective, cyclocryotherapy may be done. A cold probe, called a *cryoprobe*, is used to freeze part of the ciliary body. Freezing destroys some of the tissue, resulting in decreased production of aqueous humor.

Angle-Closure Glaucoma. Angle-closure glaucoma is also called *acute glaucoma*. It accounts for only approximately 10% of all glaucomas. With angle-closure glaucoma, the flow of aqueous humor through the pupil is blocked. Pressure forces the iris forward, causing it to block the trabecular meshwork. A rapid rise in IOP exists. Pressure is often greater than 50 mm Hg. If the pressure is not lowered promptly, permanent blindness can result. Therefore angle-closure glaucoma is considered a medical emergency. Unlike open-angle glaucoma, angle-closure glaucoma causes sudden, acute pain. Other signs and symptoms are blurred vision, halos around lights, nausea and vomiting, and headache on the affected side.

The goal of medical treatment is to reduce the intraocular pressure quickly. Drugs used initially to treat angle-closure glaucoma include miotics and oral or intravenous carbonic anhydrase inhibitors (see Table 53-3). After the pressure has been lowered, iridotomy or iridectomy is usually recommended to prevent recurrence. These procedures create an opening in the iris to permit aqueous humor to flow through the pupil normally. The procedure may be done on both eyes because the healthy eye is likely to experience similar problems in the future. Two types of iridotomy exist: (1) peripheral and (2) keyhole.

One other procedure is cyclodialysis, a procedure that involves opening the angle in the anterior chamber with a special instrument inserted through a small incision in the sclera.

NURSING CARE of the Patient with Glaucoma

Nurses who work in acute care settings are most concerned with preserving vision with drug therapy and patient teaching for self-care. Patients with chronic glaucoma who are hospitalized for other reasons still require management of their glaucoma.

Assessment

General assessment of the patient with an eye disorder is outlined in Box 53-2. Nurses who work in special clinics or units may also be trained to measure IOP. When a patient has glaucoma, you must collect data about the patient's knowledge of the disease and treatment as well as about the patient's ability to carry out self-care.

If the patient has impaired vision, additional diagnoses may be appropriate. These are discussed in detail in the section titled "Nursing Care of the Visually Impaired Patient."

Interventions

Risk for Injury

One of the most important things you can do to prevent damage to the optic nerve is to keep IOP within normal limits by administering prescribed medications. Be extremely cautious in selecting and administering ophthalmic medications. Different medications are often ordered for the affected and the unaffected eye. The procedure for applying eye drops and ointments is described in the section titled "Topical Medications."

Fear and Ineffective Self-Health Management

You must be sensitive to the patient's fears about glaucoma leading to blindness (see *Patient Teaching* box). Emphasize that adherence to prescribed drug therapy

Table 53-3 **Drug Therapy: Glaucoma**

General Nursing Considerations

1. Teach patient or caregivers, or both, proper way to administer eye drops.
2. Recognize that failure to control IOP can result in permanent blindness.
3. Avoid corticosteroids, succinylcholine, and anticholinergics in glaucoma patients.
4. Ophthalmic solutions should be tightly capped and protected from light.
5. Ophthalmic solutions should not be used if they change color or other characteristics.
6. Be alert for systemic effects of ophthalmic drugs.

DRUG	USE AND ACTION	SIDE EFFECTS	NURSING INTERVENTIONS
Beta-Adrenergic Blockers			
timolol (Timoptic) metipranolol (OptiPranolol) carteolol (Ocupress) levobunolol (Betagan Liquifilm) betaxolol (Betoptic)	Treatment of chronic open-angle glaucoma. Decreases aqueous formation. Often used in combination with other drugs.	Eye irritation. Possible systemic effects of beta-blockers: bronchospasm, heart failure. All contraindicated with asthma except betaxolol, which is beta-1 selective. See drug handbook for individual beta-blocker adverse effects.	Monitor pulse, BP, and respiration. Assess for wheezing, bronchospasm, bradycardia, hypotension, dysrhythmias. Question order for nonselective beta-blocker in patient with asthma.
Cholinergics			
pilocarpine (Pilipine HS) carbachol (Isopto Carbachol)	All cholinergics increase aqueous outflow. Constrict pupil.	Myopia. Poor vision in dim light. Lacrimation (tearing). Systemic effects (i.e., change in pulse rate or rhythm, bronchospasm, decreased BP, nausea, diarrhea, headache).	Advise patient to use caution for tasks requiring distant vision or vision in dim light. Antidote: atropine. Minimize side effects by applying pressure over lacrimal duct after administering drug.
pilocarpine (Ocusert ocular system)		Few side effects.	Ocusert therapeutic system lasts 1 week. More costly.
echothiophate iodide (Phospholine Iodide)		Blurred vision, brow ache, eyelid twitching, watering eyes, nausea, diarrhea, tachycardia.	Assess pulse.
Adrenergics			
apraclonidine (Iopidine)	Short-term use only.	Headache, dry mouth, conjunctivitis, ocular itching.	Oral hygiene. Assess conjunctiva for redness, itching.
brimonidine (Alphagan)	Long-term use with open-angle glaucoma or ocular hypertension.	Hypertension with Alphagan but not with Iopidine. Headache, dry mouth and nose, altered taste, conjunctivitis.	Monitor BP. Oral hygiene. Assess conjunctiva for redness, itching.
Prostaglandin Analogs			
latanoprost (Xalatan) travoprost, bimatoprost	Increases aqueous outflow in open-angle glaucoma and ocular hypertension.	Permanent darkening of green-brown, yellow-brown, and blue/gray/brown irides of the eyes. Also blurred vision, burning, headache, sensation of having foreign body in eye.	Inform patient of possible sensation of having foreign body in eye.
Carbonic Anhydrase Inhibitors			
Oral: acetazolamide (Diamox) dichlorphenamide methazolamide (Neptazane)	Treatment of acute and chronic glaucoma. Decreases aqueous formation. Used less now than in past.	Increased urinary output, potential hypokalemia. Possible allergic response in people who are allergic to sulfonamides. Tingling of fingers and toes (paresthesia). Itching. Sore throat, skin rash, and fever may suggest serious blood disorders.	Monitor intake and output. Withhold and notify physician if patient is allergic. Assess for hypokalemia (pulse changes, mental status changes, muscle weakness, abdominal distention). Expect increased urine output. Provide access and assistance to toilet. Do not give at bedtime.

Continued

Table 53-3 **Drug Therapy: Glaucoma—cont'd**

DRUG	USE AND ACTION	SIDE EFFECTS	NURSING INTERVENTIONS
Topical Carbonic Anhydrase Eye Drops			
brinzolamide (Azopt) dorzolamide (Trusopt)	Open-angle glaucoma.	Irritation, bitter taste.	Monitor for local and systemic allergic reactions.
Osmotic Diuretics			
	Preoperative preparation for acute angle-closure glaucoma surgery.	Increased urinary output. Potential hypokalemia. Elevated blood glucose. Headache. Tissue necrosis because of infiltration of IV solution.	Record intake and output. Assess for hypokalemia (pulse changes, muscle weakness, mental status changes, abdominal distention). Monitor patients with diabetes for elevated glucose. Monitor IV infusion. Stop infusion if infiltration is suspected and notify RN.
mannitol (Osmitrol)		Mannitol reserved for crisis situations because of risk of circulatory overload.	Mannitol may form crystals if cooled. If this happens, place vial in warm water until crystals dissolve. Cool to body temperature before administration.
glycerin (Osmoglyn)			Synthetic glycerin available for people with diabetes to reduce effects on blood glucose.
Combination Agent			
dorzolamide (Cosopt)	Combined action of beta-blocker and carbonic anhydrase inhibitor.	See each type.	See each type. Contraindicated with asthma.

BP, Blood pressure; *IOP,* intraocular pressure; *IV,* intravenous; *RN,* registered nurse.

Nursing Diagnoses, Goals, and Outcome Criteria: Glaucoma

Nursing Diagnoses	Goals and Outcome Criteria
Risk for Injury related to increased intraocular pressure (IOP)	Decreased risk for injury: adherence to prescribed measures to reduce IOP, normal IOP readings
Fear related to actual or potential loss of vision	Decreased fear: patient states feeling less fearful
Ineffective Self-Health Management related to lack of understanding of disease, treatment, and complications	Effective management of condition: patient correctly describes and adheres to prescribed drug therapy
Acute Pain related to acute increase in IOP, inflammation caused by corrective procedures	Pain relief: patient states pain is reduced or relieved, relaxed manner

usually can control IOP and reduce the risk of complications. Because open-angle glaucoma is painless, the patient may not appreciate the need for ongoing treatment. Stress the importance of keeping regular appointments for evaluation of IOP. Unfortunately, noncompliance with drug therapy is a frequent nursing diagnosis with glaucoma. Remember (and teach the patient) that any drugs that dilate the pupil are contraindicated. Patients may not be aware that many nonprescription cold and allergy remedies contain drugs that dilate the pupil. The physician or pharmacist should be consulted before taking any additional drugs.

Patient Teaching

Glaucoma

- Glaucoma usually responds to treatment but it can lead to blindness if untreated.
- Regular checkups are essential to monitor intraocular pressure (IOP) because glaucoma is usually painless.
- Consult with a pharmacist or physician before taking any new medication.
- Wear a medical alert tag.
- Take along spare medication when traveling.
- Notify your physician if visual acuity or peripheral vision decreases.

Patients who have glaucoma should wear a bracelet to alert health care providers to the condition. They should keep their medications on hand at all times. When traveling, the patient with glaucoma should keep spare medications in separate locations in case one is lost. It is helpful to have a wallet card stating the exact medication schedule in case the patient becomes ill and is unable to give this information.

Acute Pain

Pain in acute glaucoma attacks is treated with drugs that reduce IOP. Analgesics may be given as ordered. If the patient has surgery for glaucoma, postoperative care is similar to the general care after eye surgery, described in the section titled "Postoperative Nursing Care." Monitoring IOP is especially important after glaucoma surgery. Postoperative pain usually can be treated with nonopioid analgesics. Report increasing or unrelieved pain to the surgeon.

Many drugs are contraindicated with glaucoma (see *Complementary and Alternative Therapies* box). Caution patients not to take nonprescription drugs without consulting their pharmacist or physician.

Complementary and Alternative Therapies

Caution patients not to take over-the-counter (OTC) drug products without consulting with the physician or pharmacist. Many OTC drugs, including herbal medications, can raise intraocular pressure (IOP).

Retinal Detachment

Pathophysiology. Retinal detachment is a separation of the sensory layer of the eyeball from the pigmented layer. It begins when a tear in the retina allows fluid to collect between the sensory and pigmented layers. The fluid causes the two layers to separate. Separation deprives the sensory layers of nutrients and O_2 that normally are supplied by the blood vessels in the choroid. This leads to damage to the nerve tissue in the sensory layer and resultant partial or complete loss of vision. Retinal tears may occur spontaneously or as a result of trauma. They are more common in older people and in people with myopia.

Signs and Symptoms. Signs and symptoms of retinal detachment depend on the location and extent of the detachment. Patients may report seeing flashes of light or floaters. Vision may be cloudy. If the area of detachment is large, vision may be lost completely. Some patients say that it seems as if a curtain has come down or across the line of vision (Fig. 53-18). This is very frightening to the patient.

Medical and Surgical Treatment. Special procedures are required to repair retinal detachments. Most holes or tears must be sealed promptly. Laser photocoagulation is one method commonly used to do this. The intense light burns the detached portion of the retina. As the area heals, scar tissue forms that seals the tear. Cryotherapy also causes scar tissue to form but it uses a cold probe applied to the eyeball behind the tear. The cold radiates through the layers of tissue, freezing the torn tissue. Another procedure that may be used is retinopexy, in which gas is injected into the eye to apply pressure to the tear.

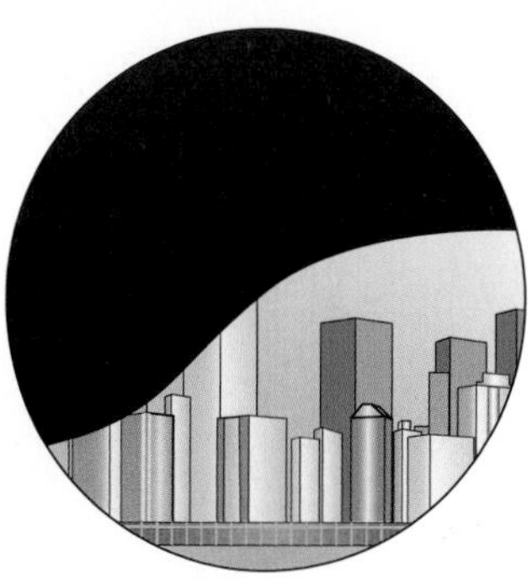

FIGURE 53-18 Loss of partial field of vision because of retinal detachment. (Courtesy National Industries for the Blind, Alexandria, Va.)

Scleral buckling is often done along with laser treatment or cryotherapy. The scleral buckle is a silastic band that is secured around the eyeball under the sclera. Small silicone implants are sutured under the band opposite the area of detachment. This procedure brings the layers of tissue back together by pressing from the outside. The band is left in place permanently (Fig. 53-19). The physician may inject an air bubble or some normal saline into the vitreous humor after the surgical procedure. The purpose of this is to apply internal pressure to the detached portion of the retina.

Sometimes tears cause bleeding into the vitreous. Significant amounts of blood in the vitreous interfere with vision. When this occurs, the physician may do a vitrectomy to remove the bloody tissue. Vitrectomy also is indicated when the vitreous is creating traction on the retina.

NURSING CARE of the Patient with Retinal Detachment

Before corrective measures are taken, the patient usually is placed on strict bed rest with the head elevated. In the preoperative period, many patients are very anxious. Encourage them to talk about their fears and to ask questions. Even though the procedure may be done under local anesthesia, oral intake may be restricted to reduce the risk of postoperative vomiting. Intravenous fluids may be ordered.

Postoperative care is essentially the same as for other patients undergoing eye surgery, as described in the section titled "Postoperative Nursing Care." Positioning orders may be very specific for these patients. If an air bubble has been injected, it will rise to the top of the eye. If the patient's detachment is in the back of the eye, a face-down position is necessary to keep the bubble in the right place. Saline travels down rather than up, so the same patient would need to stay face up if saline had been injected. The surgeon prescribes any activity limitations. The length of hospitalization varies depending on the location and severity of the tear, the type of repair, and the surgeon's routines.

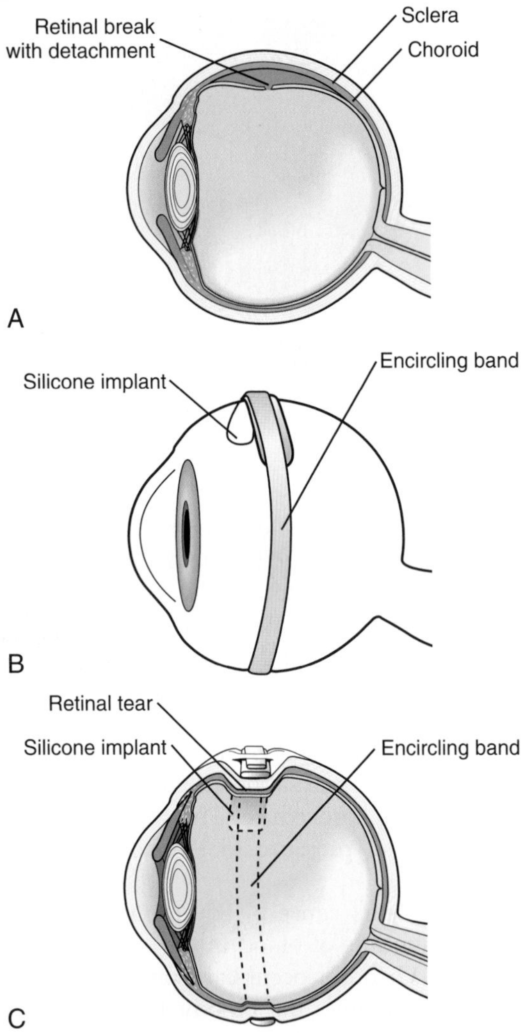

FIGURE 53-19 A, Retinal detachment. **B and C,** Scleral buckle and silicone implant in place to treat retinal detachment. (From Lewis SM, Heitkemper MM, Dirksen SR, et al.: *Medical-surgical nursing: assessment and management of clinical problems*, ed 8, St. Louis, 2011, Mosby.)

Senile Macular Degeneration

The macula is the part of the retina that is responsible for central vision. As people age, changes in the eye cause the macula to degenerate. Both eyes are usually affected. The two types of macular degeneration are dry (strophic) and wet (exudative). The dry type occurs first and may or may not progress to the wet form. In the wet form, abnormal blood vessels develop in or near the macula, resulting in loss of vision in a specific area. In the dry form, central vision gradually gets worse (Fig. 53-20). Patients often report difficulty reading or doing close work. Both types are progressive. Peripheral vision remains intact. It is usually adequate to allow mobility in familiar settings.

Regular eyeglasses do not improve vision with macular degeneration. Special telescopic lenses may be helpful. Laser treatments or vitrectomy may offer hope to some patients with macular degeneration. The most promising treatment is a series of intraocular injections of an angiogenesis inhibitor (a drug that inhibits the growth of new blood vessels) such as ranibizumab (Lucentis). This procedure is done in a clinic setting and is relatively painless. At best, the patient actually has some improvement in vision. For others, the progression of the condition is slowed. The nurse needs to help the patient and family members to learn to cope with the level of vision impairment the patient experiences. The nursing care is like that described in the section titled "Nursing Care of the Visually Impaired Patient" (see *Complementary and Alternative Therapies* box).

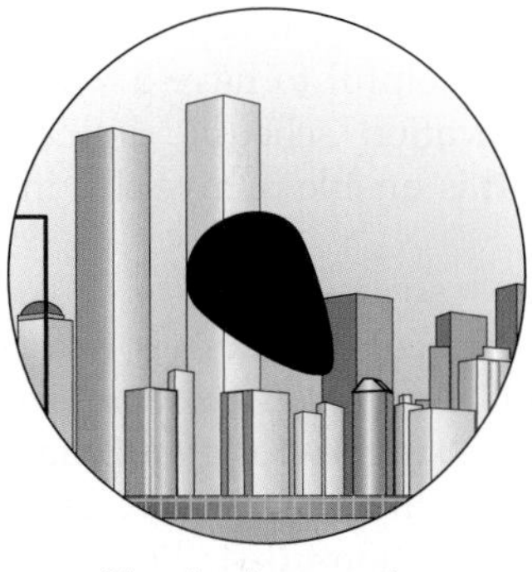

FIGURE 53-20 Vision of the patient with macular degeneration. (Courtesy of the National Industries for the Blind, Alexandria, Va.)

Complementary and Alternative Therapies

Some practitioners believe that high doses of vitamins C and E, beta-carotene, and zinc may slow the progression of age-related dry macular degeneration. Note that smokers should not take large doses of beta-carotene.

Enucleation

Some eye conditions are so serious that removal of the eyeball is the only treatment. **Enucleation** is the term used for removal of the eyeball. Conditions that may result in enucleation include injury, infection, sympathetic ophthalmia, and some glaucomas and malignancies.

During the surgical procedure, the eyeball is removed. A round device is placed in the cavity, and muscles are sutured over it. The conjunctiva is then sutured over the muscle. This procedure creates a foundation for the future placement of a prosthesis. The patient returns from surgery with a temporary shell called a *conformer* in the prosthesis base, which is covered with a pressure dressing. Observe for excessive bleeding or increasing pain. Report any temperature elevation. After the pressure dressing is removed, the physician may order wound care and topical medications.

Approximately 1 month after the enucleation, an optician can fit a prosthesis. The prosthesis is carefully made to look like the patient's natural eye. The patient

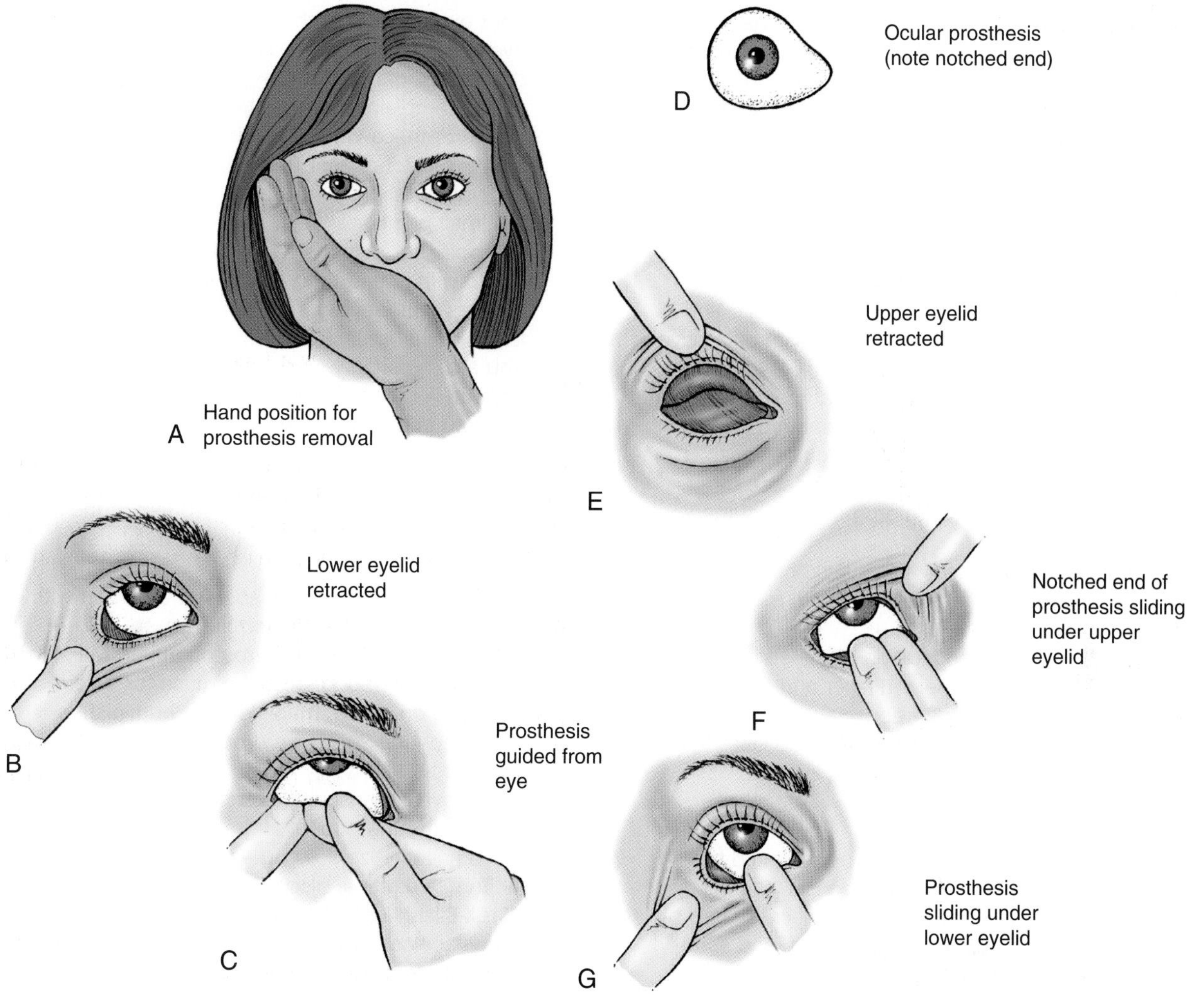

FIGURE 53-21 Removal **(A to C)** and insertion **(D to G)** of an eye prosthesis. (From Monahan FD, Drake DT, Neighbors M, editors: *Medical-surgical nursing: foundations for clinical practice*, ed 2, Philadelphia, 1998, Saunders.)

must learn to insert, remove, and clean the prosthesis. Nurses also should know how to care for an eye prosthesis as illustrated in Figure 53-21. The steps to remove and clean a prosthesis are the following:

1. Wash hands thoroughly.
2. Gently depress and pull the lower lid down.
3. Allow the prosthesis to slip out over the lower lid.
4. Wash the prosthesis under running water, using the fingers to remove any debris.

If the prosthesis is to be stored, it should be placed in a container with normal saline or water.

To reinsert the prosthesis, do the following:

1. Raise the upper lid by pressing it up against the orbit.
2. Slip the top of the prosthesis under the orbit.
3. Pull the lower lid down so that the prosthesis can slip into place.

The patient's nursing care plan should always inform staff that the patient has a prosthesis.

Get Ready for the NCLEX® Examination!

Key Points

- An estimated 21 million people in the United States have some vision impairment.
- After eye surgery, nursing care addresses risk for injury, disturbed sensory perception, acute pain, anxiety, and ineffective self-health management.
- Increased IOP must be controlled to prevent permanent vision loss.
- Vision loss affects all aspects of a person's life: independence, mobility, employment, communication, and interpersonal relationships.
- Common nursing diagnoses for patients with impaired vision include knowledge deficit, readiness for enhanced coping, anxiety, ineffective coping, self-care deficit (feeding, dressing, bathing), impaired walking, and ineffective self-health management.

- Infectious and inflammatory conditions of the eye include blepharitis, hordeolum, chalazion, conjunctivitis, and keratitis.
- Entropion is inversion of the lower lid; ectropion is eversion of the lower lid.
- Only a physician should remove a foreign body embedded in the eye.
- Corneal opacity is treated with removal of the scarred cornea and replacement with a healthy donor cornea in a procedure called *keratoplasty*.
- Errors of refraction include myopia, hyperopia, and astigmatism and are often correctable with corrective lenses.
- An opaque lens, called a *cataract*, can be removed and vision restored with a lens replacement in the form of eyeglasses, contact lenses, or intraocular lenses.
- Glaucoma, increased IOP, is a leading cause of blindness and is treated with drug therapy, surgery, or both.
- Nursing care of the patient with glaucoma focuses on risk for injury, fear, ineffective self-health management, and acute pain.
- Retinal detachment is separation of the sensory layer of the eyeball from the pigmented layer and can result in partial or complete loss of vision.
- Treatments for retinal detachment include laser therapy, cryotherapy, retinopexy, scleral buckling, and vitrectomy.
- Senile macular degeneration causes progressive loss of central vision but may be slowed or improved by intraocular injections of an angiogenesis inhibitor.
- Enucleation is removal of the eyeball necessitated by injury, infection, sympathetic ophthalmia, and some glaucomas and malignancies.
- After enucleation, a prosthesis can be used to restore the patient's normal appearance.

Additional Learning Resources

SG Go to your Study Guide for additional learning activities to help you master this chapter content.

evolve Go to your Evolve website (http://evolve.elsevier.com/Linton/medsurg) for the following learning resources and much more:

- Interactive Prioritization Exercises
- Fluid & Electrolyte Tutorial
- Pharmacology Tutorial
- Review Questions for the NCLEX® Examination

Review Questions for the NCLEX® Examination

1. Which of the following is the fluid that fills the anterior chamber of the eye?
   1. Aqueous humor
   2. Ciliary fluid
   3. Vitreous humor
   4. Refractive fluid

   NCLEX Client Need: Physiological Integrity: Physiological Adaptation
2. Your examination of the eyes of an older adult reveals eyeballs slightly sunken in the orbits, small pupils that do not respond to light, a grayish ring around the iris, and a complaint that the eyes feel dry sometimes. Which of these would you consider *normal* in an older adult? (Select all that apply.)
   1. Eyeballs slightly sunken
   2. Small pupils
   3. Pupils not responsive to light
   4. Grayish ring around iris
   5. Eyes that feel dry sometimes

   NCLEX Client Need: Health Promotion and Maintenance
3. You are assisting with a community vision screening project. A participant says, "The nurse says my vision is 20/40 in both eyes. What does that mean?" Your response should be:
   1. "You see best at 20 to 40 feet from objects."
   2. "You cannot see more than 40 feet in the distance."
   3. "At 40 feet, you can read what most people can read at 20 feet."
   4. "At 20 feet, you can read what a person with normal vision could read at 40 feet."

   NCLEX Client Need: Health Promotion and Maintenance
4. When a patient comes to the office for an eye examination, the ophthalmologist administers phenylephrine 2.5% eye drops for which of the following reasons?
   1. To reveal any scratches on the cornea
   2. To dilate the pupil
   3. To anesthetize the cornea
   4. To dilate retinal blood vessels

   NCLEX Client Need: Physiological Integrity: Pharmacological Therapies
5. A patient is being discharged after cataract surgery. Discharge instructions should include which of the following statements? (Select all that apply.)
   1. "Always lie on the unaffected side."
   2. "Avoid pressure on the operative eye."
   3. "Moderate to severe pain is expected."
   4. "Resume usual activities immediately."
   5. "Expect a small amount of bleeding."

   NCLEX Client Need: Physiological Integrity: Reduction of Risk Potential
6. You are teaching a new nurse's aide how to assist a visually impaired resident to walk to the dining room. You should instruct her to:
   1. Stand side by side and hold the person's hand
   2. Let the person hold your upper arm
   3. Walk behind the patient and advise of obstacles
   4. Have the person walk behind you with hands on your shoulders

   NCLEX Client Need: Safe and Effective Care Environment: Safety and Infection Control
7. After keratoplasty, you observe that the patient's cornea is cloudy. What should you do?
   1. Reassure the patient that cloudiness is normal for several weeks after surgery.
   2. Elevate the patient's head and encourage increased fluid intake.
   3. Report signs of corneal rejection to the physician.
   4. Prepare the patient for emergency surgery.

   NCLEX Client Need: Physiological Integrity: Reduction of Risk Potential

8. Drugs used to treat open-angle glaucoma act by which of the following mechanisms? (Select all that apply.)
   1. Increasing aqueous outflow
   2. Dilating the canal of Schlemm
   3. Relaxing the trabecular meshwork
   4. Decreasing aqueous formation
   5. Reducing systemic blood pressure

   NCLEX Client Need: Physiological Integrity: Pharmacological Therapies
9. A patient came to the clinic complaining of severe eye pain. The physician diagnosed acute angle-closure glaucoma. The nurse understands that the most serious complication of angle-closure glaucoma is:
   1. Rupture of the eyeball
   2. Permanent blindness
   3. Nausea and vomiting
   4. Increased intracranial pressure

   NCLEX Client Need: Physiological Integrity: Reduction of Risk Potential
10. Two patients had surgery for retinal detachments this morning. Postoperatively, one is positioned on the left side with the head of the bed flat. The other is in Fowler position. What factors determined the best postoperative position for these patients? (Select all that apply.)
   1. Patient preference
   2. Intraocular pressure
   3. Location of the repaired tear
   4. Use of air or saline to support the repair
   5. Whether or not a scleral buckle was applied

   NCLEX Client Need: Physiological Integrity: Physiological Adaptation

chapter

54 Ear and Hearing Disorders

http://evolve.elsevier.com/Linton/medsurg

Objectives

1. Identify the data to be collected for the assessment of a patient with a disorder affecting the ear, hearing, or balance.
2. Describe the tests and procedures used to diagnose disorders of the ear, hearing, or balance.
3. Explain the nursing considerations for each of the tests and procedures.
4. Explain the nursing care for patients receiving common therapeutic measures for disorders of the ear, hearing, or balance.
5. Describe the pathophysiology, signs and symptoms, complications, and medical or surgical treatment for selected disorders.
6. Identify measures the nurse can take to reduce the risk of hearing impairment and to detect problems early.
7. Assist in the development of a nursing care plan for a patient with a disorder of the ear, hearing, or balance.

Key Terms

Cerumen (sĕ-ROO-mĕn)
Dizziness
Equilibrium (ē-kwĭ-LĬB-rē-ŭm)
Otalgia (ō-TĂL-jē-ă)
Otic (Ō-tĭk)
Ototoxic (ō-tō-TŎK-sĭk)
Presbycusis (prĕz-bē-KŪ-sĭs)
Tinnitus (tĭ-NĪ-tĭs)
Tympanic membrane (tĭm-PĂN-ĭk MĔM-brān)
Vertigo (VĔR-tĭ-gō)

Approximately 17% of Americans (37 million) report some degree of hearing loss. Of those older than 85 years, 80% have some hearing loss. Loss of hearing can have significant impact on most aspects of an individual's life. Health care providers can reduce disability by teaching people how to prevent hearing loss and by helping to rehabilitate those who are impaired.

ANATOMY AND PHYSIOLOGY OF THE EAR

The ears are essential organs for hearing and for position sense. Position sense enables a person to know the position of body parts without looking. It is also necessary for **equilibrium** (i.e., the state of balance needed for walking, standing, and sitting).

ANATOMY

The ear has three major sections: (1) the external ear, (2) the middle ear, and (3) the inner ear (Fig. 54-1).

External Ear

Auricle. The external ear includes the auricle and the external auditory canal. The auricle, also called the *pinna*, is the visible part of the ear.

Innervation. Many nerves innervate the ear. This is the reason why pain in the ear can sometimes be traced to disorders of the nose, mouth, or neck. Of special importance is the facial nerve (the seventh cranial nerve), which lies alongside the auditory canal. The facial nerve is protected in the canal by a thin bony covering. It exits from the skull just in front of the ear and branches across the face to control muscle movement.

Lymph Drainage. Lymph nodes located in front of, behind, and below the auricle drain the ear. In the presence of ear infections, they may become enlarged.

External Auditory Canal. The external auditory canal extends from the external opening of the ear to the tympanic membrane. The **tympanic membrane** is commonly called the *eardrum*. The canal is lined with cells that secrete **cerumen** (i.e., earwax). The waxy secretion coats and protects the canal.

Tympanic Membrane. The tympanic membrane at the end of the external auditory canal is shiny and pearl gray. Sound waves entering the external auditory canal cause the membrane to vibrate.

Middle Ear

Bones. The middle ear is an air-filled space in the temporal bone. It contains three small bones (i.e., ossicles): (1) the malleus (hammer), (2) the incus (anvil), and (3) the stapes (stirrup). The function of these bones

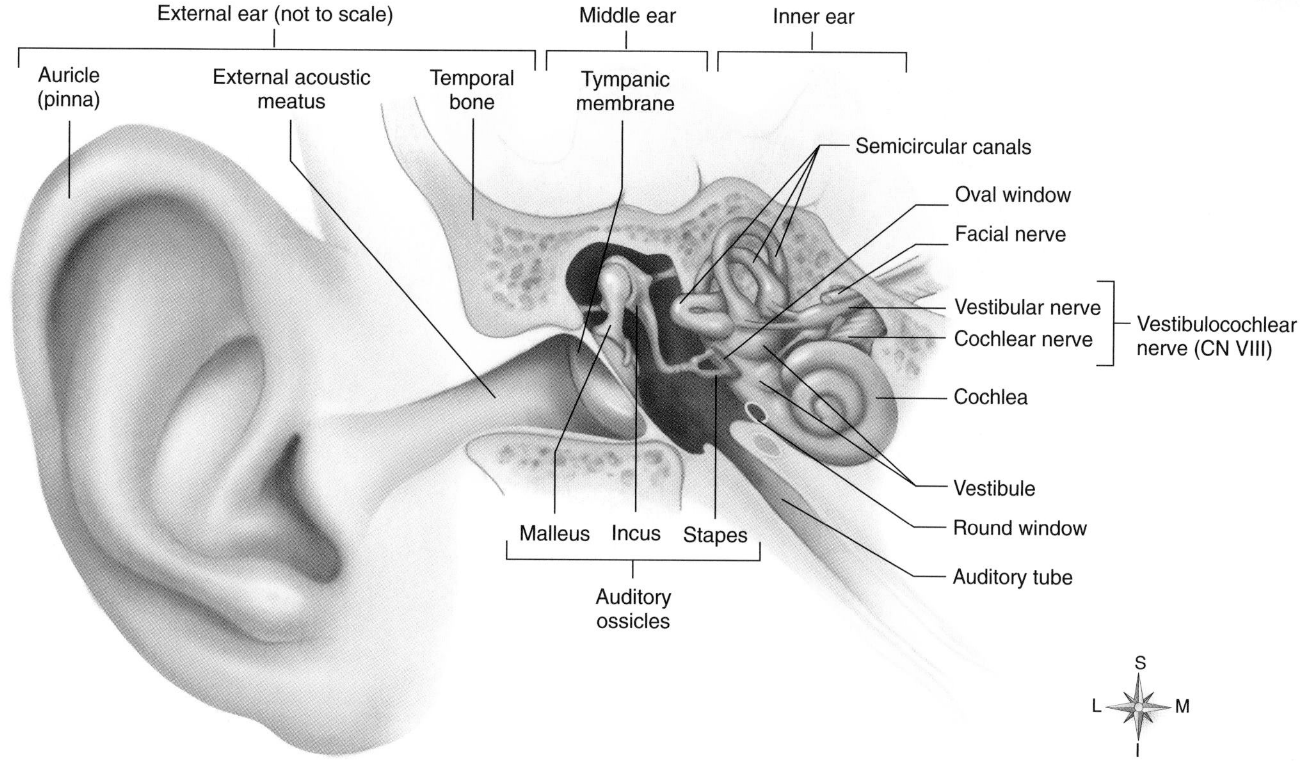

FIGURE 54-1 Anatomic structure of the ear illustrating the three major sections: (1) the external ear, (2) the middle ear, and (3) the inner ear. *CN*, Cranial nerve. (From Patton KT, Thibodeau GA: *Anatomy and physiology*, ed 8, St. Louis, 2013, Mosby.)

is to forward the sound waves transmitted by the tympanic membrane to the inner ear.

The malleus lies directly under the tympanic membrane. One portion of the malleus is attached to the membrane and another portion is connected to the incus. The incus is connected to the stapes. The stapes has a footplate that fits into the oval window. The oval window, which opens into the vestibule, separates the middle ear from the inner ear. Sound waves are transmitted from the tympanic membrane to the malleus, the incus, the stapes, and then the oval window.

Eustachian Tube. An important structure in the middle ear is the eustachian tube. The eustachian tube extends from the middle ear to the nasopharynx, as illustrated in Figure 54-2. It creates an air passage to the middle ear so that air pressure remains the same on both sides of the tympanic membrane.

Mastoid Process. The mastoid process is the bony structure behind the auricle. The interior is made up of air cells that are directly connected to the middle ear. The mastoid process is very close to the brain.

Inner Ear

The inner ear consists of the membranous labyrinth and the bony labyrinth. The membranous labyrinth contains fluid called *endolymph*. Endolymph moves with changes in body position.

The parts of the bony labyrinth are the vestibule, semicircular canals, and cochlea. The oval window opens into the vestibule. Receptors in the vestibule monitor the position of the head to maintain posture balance. Receptors in the semicircular canals monitor changes in rate or direction of movement to maintain balance during movement. The cochlea is a coiled tube that looks like a snail. It contains the organ of Corti, which is the receptor end-organ of hearing. The organ of Corti transmits stimuli from the oval window to the acoustic (auditory) nerve.

PHYSIOLOGY OF HEARING

The perception and interpretation of sound depend on a complex series of steps. A malfunction at any step can result in some type of hearing impairment. Figure 54-3 illustrates the steps involved in the hearing process.

AGE-RELATED CHANGES IN THE EAR

Changes occur in the external, middle, and inner ear with aging. Some changes have no functional significance but others can lead to serious problems with hearing or balance.

The skin of the auricle may become dry and wrinkled. Dryness of the external canal causes itching. Cerumen production declines and the protective wax is drier. Hairs in the canal become coarser and longer, especially in men. The combination of dry cerumen and coarse hairs sometimes leads to obstruction of the

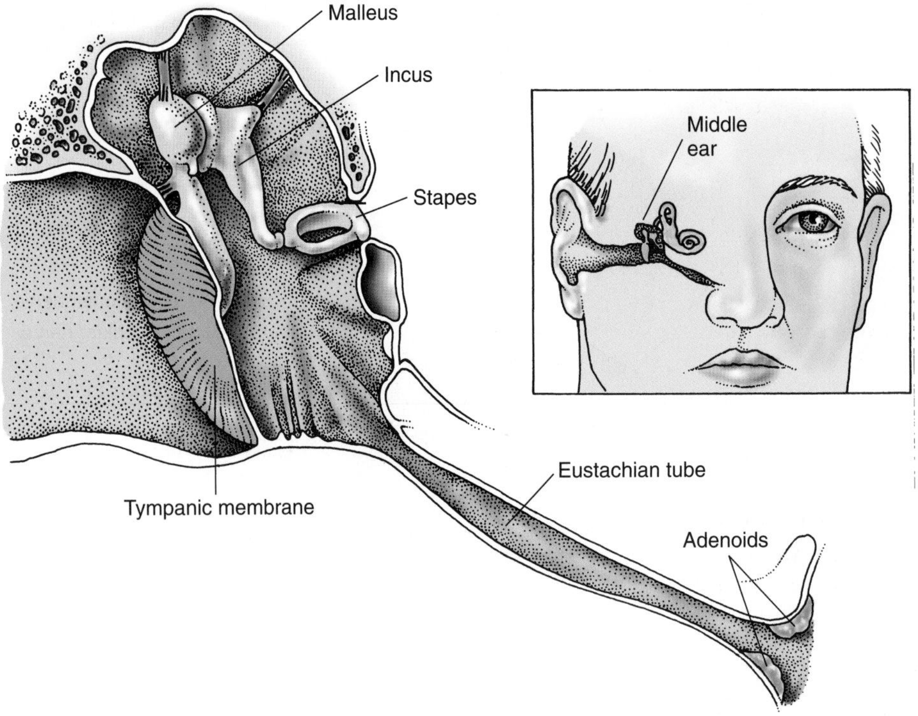

FIGURE 54-2 The eustachian tube extends from the middle ear to the nasopharynx. (From Ignatavicius DD, Workman ML: *Medical-surgical nursing: patient-centered collaborative care*, ed 6, St. Louis, 2010, Saunders.)

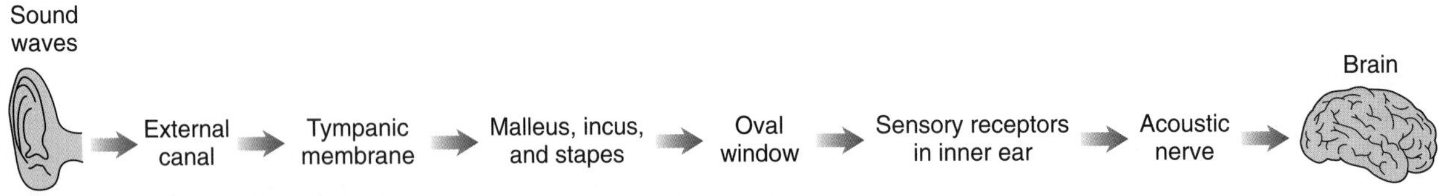

FIGURE 54-3 Physiology of hearing.

canal. The eardrum thickens and the bony joints in the middle ear degenerate somewhat. Surprisingly, these changes are not thought to impair hearing significantly.

However, changes in the inner ear affect sensitivity to sound, understanding of speech, and balance. Degenerative changes include atrophy of the cochlea, the cochlear nerve cells, and the organ of Corti. The result is that many older people have some degree of hearing loss and some have problems with balance. The type of hearing loss most often associated with age is called **presbycusis**. Presbycusis is discussed later under "Nursing Care of the Patient with Presbycusis."

NURSING ASSESSMENT OF THE EXTERNAL EAR, HEARING, AND BALANCE

The nursing assessment of the ear includes inspection of the external ear and evaluation of hearing and balance. In addition to collecting data about the patient's hearing and balance, the licensed vocational nurse/licensed practical nurse (LVN/LPN) may be trained to perform some specific diagnostic procedures to evaluate hearing. To collect data from the patient, the assessor must first determine if the patient has a hearing impairment that interferes with verbal communication. If the patient's hearing impairment is severe, determine the usual means of communication. It may be necessary to call on a family member or a sign language interpreter or to use written communication during the assessment.

HEALTH HISTORY

History of Present Illness

The health history begins with a full description of any symptoms that may reflect problems with the ear, including changes in hearing acuity, pain, tinnitus, dizziness, vertigo, nausea, vomiting, and problems with balance. Describe changes in hearing acuity to include the kind of change that occurred and whether it was sudden or gradual. Ask the patient to describe the nature of the pain (e.g., sharp, throbbing, dull) and when it occurs. Pain in the ear is called **otalgia**. If

tinnitus (i.e., ringing in the ears) is present, ask if the sound heard is continuous or intermittent. Document dizziness, vertigo, nausea, vomiting, or problems with balance and the circumstances under which they occur.

Past Medical History

Ask about any previous acute or chronic ear problems. Acute conditions that may affect hearing or balance include sinus infections, dental problems, allergies, and upper respiratory infections. Chronic conditions that may be significant are hypertension, diabetes mellitus (DM), and hypothyroidism. Note recent surgical procedures on the ear or throat or a recent head injury.

Hearing impairments are often congenital (present at birth). One cause of hearing loss in an infant is rubella during the mother's pregnancy. Therefore it is significant to note whether female patients have had rubella or have been immunized for the infection.

The medication history is important to identify any drugs taken that might be ototoxic. The term **ototoxic** means that a drug can damage the eighth cranial nerve or the organs of hearing and balance. Examples of drugs that can have ototoxic effects are aspirin and aminoglycoside antibiotics. Ototoxicity is discussed more fully in the section titled "Nursing Care of the Patient with Ototoxicity." Document a family history of hearing loss.

Pharmacology Capsule

Some drugs, including aspirin, are ototoxic. Signs and symptoms of ototoxicity are tinnitus, hearing loss, dizziness, and ataxia.

Functional Assessment

In the functional assessment, describe exposure to excessively loud noise such as amplified music, firearms being used, or noisy machinery. Note the use of any assistive hearing devices.

PHYSICAL EXAMINATION

Some general observations of the patient give important clues about hearing and balance. Observe how the patient responds to a normal voice. Patients who do not hear well use many adaptive behaviors. They may turn a good ear toward the speaker, ask people to repeat things, ask "what?" frequently, or watch the speaker's mouth closely. Note the presence of a visible hearing aid. The patient's posture and balance while walking and sitting alert the examiner to possible inner ear problems.

External Ear

The position of the auricles is significant. Normally, the top of the auricle is at approximately the level of the eye. The ears should be positioned symmetrically. The auricles should be examined for shape, lesions, and nodules. The auricles and the mastoid process are palpated for tenderness. Palpation in front of, below, and behind the ear may locate enlarged lymph nodes.

Box 54-1 Assessment of Patients with Disorders of the Ear, Hearing, and Balance

HEALTH HISTORY

Present Illness
Changes in the external ear, hearing acuity, or balance

Past Medical History
Sinus infections, dental problems, allergies, upper respiratory infections, hypertension, diabetes mellitus (DM), hypothyroidism, surgery on ear or throat, recent head injury, rubella and rubella immunization, recent and current medications

Family History
Hearing impairments

Review of Systems
Pain in ear or throat, tinnitus, dizziness, vertigo, nausea, vomiting

Functional Assessment
Exposure to excessively loud noise, use of hearing aid

PHYSICAL EXAMINATION

General Survey
Response to normal voice, gait, posture, and balance

External Ear
Position of auricles; lesions, tenderness, or nodules

Lymph Nodes
Enlargement of lymph nodes in front of or behind ear

Mastoid
Tenderness

External Auditory Canal
Obstruction, lesions, drainage

Tympanic Membrane
Redness, bulging

External Auditory Canal

Use a penlight to inspect the outer portion of the external auditory canal for any obvious obstructions or drainage. The only normal secretion in the canal is cerumen. It should be golden to brown in color and should not block the opening to the canal. If any drainage is seen, record the color, amount, and odor.

Some nurses are taught to use an otoscope to inspect the external canal and the tympanic membrane. The tympanic membrane should be shiny and pearl gray. The nursing assessment is outlined in Box 54-1.

DIAGNOSTIC TESTS AND PROCEDURES

Several specialists handle different aspects of the diagnosis and treatment of hearing disorders. An otologist is trained to diagnose types of hearing loss. An audiologist carries out tests to determine whether a hearing aid will help a particular patient. If it is thought that a patient would benefit from a hearing aid, the audiologist also identifies the best kind of hearing aid. An otolaryngologist is a physician who specializes in diseases of the ears and throat.

The otoscopic examination and tuning fork tests for gross hearing acuity are usually part of the general physical examination. Various procedures and tests may be used to assess auditory and vestibular function. Auditory function tests include pure tone audiometry, speech audiometry, auditory evoked potential (AEP), electrocochleography, auditory brainstem response (ABR), and tympanometry. Tests of vestibular function are the caloric test stimulus, electronystagmography (ENG), posturography, and rotary chair testing.

Diagnostic tests and procedures for patients with disorders of the ear, hearing, and balance are described in Table 54-1.

Table 54-1 Diagnostic Tests and Procedures Disorders of the Ear, Hearing, and Balance

TEST AND PURPOSE	PATIENT PREPARATION	POSTPROCEDURE NURSING CARE
Audiometry		
Pure tone audiometry tests: detect hearing impairment by assessing the patient's ability to hear a range of sounds.	Tell the patient the test will be conducted in a sound-isolated room. The examiner will place earphones on the patient and introduce tones. The patient will be asked to identify when sounds are heard and when they disappear. A tuning fork will be placed near the patient's ear and the patient will be asked when vibrating sound is heard and when it ceases. No other preparation is needed.	No special postprocedure care.
Speech audiometry: measures the ability to hear spoken words.	The patient will listen to simple words through earphones and repeat the words that are understood. No special preparation is needed.	No special postprocedure care.
Auditory brainstem evoked potentials (ADEPs): used to estimate magnitude of hearing loss and determine whether a lesion is in the cochlea, eighth cranial nerve, or brainstem. Useful in assessing infants or others who cannot communicate.	Electrodes are placed on the scalp and earlobes. The patient is exposed to a series of clicks via earphones.	The scalp should be clean before electrodes are placed. After the test, remove electrode gel.
Electrocochleography: used to measure electrical activity in cochlea and auditory nerve in patients who cannot cooperate.	The nurse is not usually directly involved in the test but can inform the patient that electrodes will be placed on the head and a tiny microphone and earphone will be placed in the outer ear canal. The patient will be instructed to relax while a series of clicking sounds are made. No patient response is required.	No specific nursing interventions.
Auditory brainstem response (ABR): measures electrical activity along auditory pathway to detect certain tumors, brainstem problems, and stroke.	Although the nurse does not usually participate in this test, tell the patient electrodes will be applied to the head (like those applied to the chest for an EKG) and brain wave activity recorded in response to sound. The patient is encouraged to rest or sleep during the test because no response is required.	No specific nursing interventions.
Tympanometry: assesses response of middle ear to pressure changes.	Although the nurse is not likely to participate in the test, tell the patient that a device that creates pressure will be placed in the external ear canal. Loud noises may be heard. The patient needs to remain still and quiet and not swallow during the test.	No specific nursing interventions.
Vestibular Tests		
Caloric test: the ears are irrigated with warm or cool water to assess for dizziness. Dizziness is consistent with a diagnosis of Meniere disease.	Tell the patient that the ears will be irrigated to assess for dizziness. Tell the examiner if the patient has had central nervous system depressants, alcohol, or barbiturates because they alter test response. The examiner will then observe the patient for nystagmus, nausea, vomiting, or dizziness.	Assess for nausea. Offer small amounts of clear liquids at first. Safety measures if dizzy.

Table 54-1 Diagnostic Tests and Procedures Disorders of the Ear, Hearing, and Balance—cont'd

TEST AND PURPOSE	PATIENT PREPARATION	POSTPROCEDURE NURSING CARE
Electronystagmography: used to detect lesions in the vestibule.	Nothing by mouth for 3 h before the test. No alcohol or caffeine for 24–48 h before the test. Take eyeglasses to the test. Withhold medications as ordered. Tell the patient electrodes will be placed around the eyes and he or she will be asked to focus on specific targets. The ears are irrigated and the patient is turned in various positions in a special chair.	Assess for nausea. Offer small amounts of clear fluids at first. Safety precautions if dizzy.
Posturography assesses for lesions affecting balance.	Inform the patient that he or she will be placed in a box with a floor that moves to assess balance. Inform patient that test is uncomfortable and can be stopped at any time if patient requests.	Assess for nausea. Offer small amounts of clear fluids at first. Safety precautions if dizzy.
Rotary chair testing: assesses balance.	Tell patient the room will be darkened. A light meal before the test is advised. Patient will sit in a chair that is rotated by a motor. Sedatives are best withheld for 24 hours before test.	Assess for nausea. Offer small amounts of clear fluids at first. Safety precautions if dizzy.

OTOSCOPIC EXAMINATION

The otoscope is the instrument used to examine the external auditory canal. The purpose of the otoscopic examination is to inspect the external auditory canal and tympanic membrane. The examination permits diagnosis of inflammatory and infectious processes as well as obstructions of the external canal. When using an otoscope, you should do the following:

1. Use the largest speculum that fits the ear canal easily.
2. For adult patients, pull the auricle up and back to straighten the canal; then guide the speculum gently into the canal.
3. Steady the otoscope by resting the little finger against the patient's cheek, as illustrated in Figure 54-4.
4. Never force the speculum into the ear.
5. If the patient is unable to cooperate, have someone hold the head still during the examination.
6. Clean the speculum between patients and between ears on each patient.

The appearance of the normal tympanic membrane is illustrated in Figure 54-5.

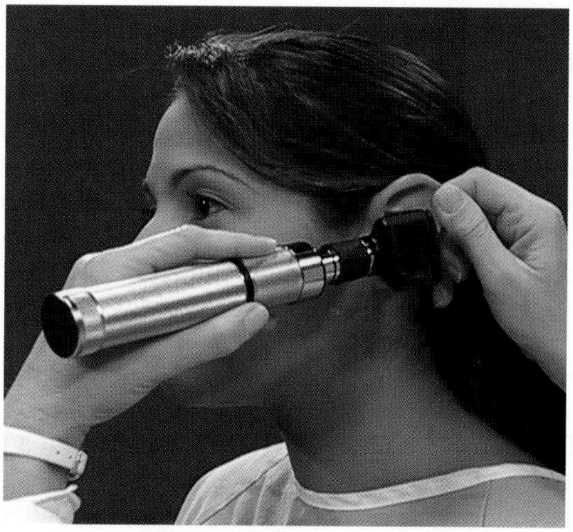

FIGURE 54-4 Correct technique for using an otoscope to examine the external auditory canal and the tympanic membrane. The adult auricle is pulled up and back; the examiner's hand is stabilized against the patient's face. (From Seidel HM, Ball JW, Dains JE, et al.: *Mosby's guide to physical examination*, ed 7, St. Louis, 2010, Mosby.)

TUNING FORK TESTS

Rinne and Weber tests use a tuning fork to assess the conduction of sound by air and by bone. These are useful in determining the nature of the hearing loss and in selecting the best treatment. Some nurses are taught to perform these tests. The procedures are described here in case you need to be able to use these skills.

Rinne Test

For the Rinne test, tap the tuning fork on the hand to activate it. Then place the base of the tuning fork on the patient's mastoid bone. If the vibration is conducted through the bone, the patient hears a humming sound. When the sound is no longer heard, move the fork so that the tines of the tuning fork are near but not touching the ear canal. Ask the patient if he or she can hear the sound and, if so, to report when the sound disappears. This assesses the patient's ability to hear sound waves conducted through the air.

Normally, air conduction is better than bone conduction. Therefore the patient should be able to hear the sound transmitted through air even after it can no longer be heard through bone. This normal finding is recorded as "AC > BC" (air conduction is greater than bone conduction). If bone conduction is greater than air conduction, the patient has a conductive hearing loss.

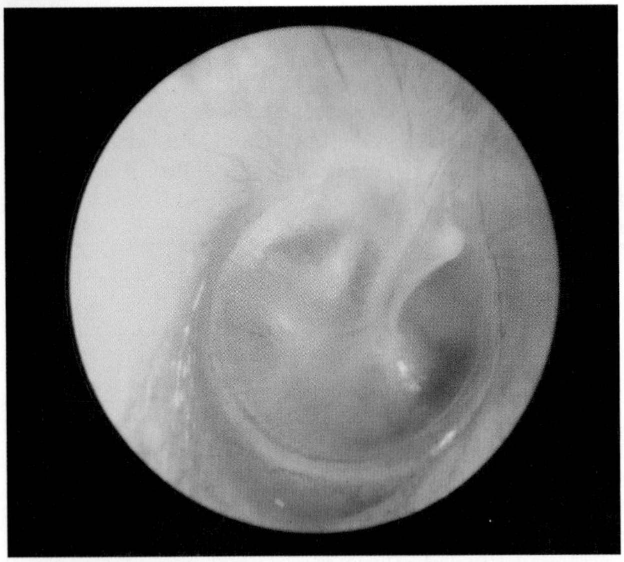

FIGURE 54-5 Normal appearance of the tympanic membrane through the otoscope. (From Ignatavicius DD, Workman ML, Mishler MA: *Medical-surgical nursing across the health care continuum*, ed 3, Philadelphia, 1999, Saunders.)

Weber Test

For the Weber test, place the base of an activated tuning fork on the midline of the skull. Ask the patient to identify the side in which the sound is loudest. With normal hearing in both ears, the sound is heard equally on each side. The sound is louder in an ear with conductive hearing loss and softer in an ear with sensorineural hearing loss.

AUDIOMETRY

Pure tone audiometry is the assessment of the ability to hear simple sound waves. It requires a machine called an *audiometer*. Special training is needed to use the audiometer and to interpret test results. Nurses in some work settings learn to do these tests. Speech audiometry, which the nurse may do, evaluates the patient's ability to hear simple words correctly. The patient needs no special preparation for these tests.

Audiometry gives a precise measurement of hearing acuity. The nurse can do other simple tests for a gross assessment of hearing. The whisper test can be done easily in any setting. Stand 1 to 2 feet from the patient, facing away from him or her. Have the patient occlude the ear on the opposite side. Exhale and then speak in a low whisper. Ask the patient to tell you what was whispered. The words can be repeated louder until the patient is able to hear them. After assessing one ear, change sides and assess the other ear. This simple test gives you an idea about the patient's general hearing ability.

CALORIC TEST

The caloric test is used to diagnose disorders in the vestibular system or its central nervous system (CNS) connections. The ear is irrigated with warm or cold water and the patient is observed for reactions that suggest vestibular problems. A person with a labyrinth disorder responds with specific abnormal eye movements (i.e., nystagmus), vertigo, and nausea and vomiting. A person with vestibular disease has a decreased or absent response to the test.

Test results are altered by CNS depressants, barbiturates, and alcohol. Inform the examiner if the patient has had any of these drugs before the examination.

ELECTRONYSTAGMOGRAPHY

Electronystagmography is used to detect lesions in the vestibule. Electrodes are placed around the eyes and eye movements are measured as the patient focuses on specific targets as the ears are irrigated with water, as air is blown into the ears, and as the head position is changed. A normal response is involuntary rapid eye movements, called *nystagmus*.

The patient is usually allowed nothing by mouth (NPO) for 3 hours before the test. No caffeine or alcoholic beverages should be consumed for 24 to 48 hours before the test. Medications may be withheld on the physician's directions. Patients who normally wear eyeglasses are instructed to bring them to the test. After the test, the patient may report nausea and may vomit. If the patient is dizzy, take appropriate safety precautions.

OTHER AUDITORY AND VESTIBULAR TESTS

Electrocochleography, tympanometry, posturography, and rotary chair testing are described in Table 54-1. Computed tomography (CT) and magnetic resonance imaging (MRI) scans may be used to locate lesions that affect hearing and balance.

COMMON THERAPEUTIC MEASURES

Problems of the ear and related structures sometimes require medications or surgery. Other therapeutic measures for problems of the ear include irrigations and the use of hearing aids. You may encounter patients who are being treated by any of these measures.

EAR DROPS

Medications intended to be placed directly into the external ear canal are called **otic** drops or simply *ear drops*. Ear drops may be ordered to treat infection or inflammation, to reduce pain, or to soften earwax. When administering ear drops, keep the following points in mind:

1. Be sure to use an *otic* solution.
2. Warm the drops to body temperature by rolling the bottle between the palms.
3. Have the patient tilt the head so that the ear to be treated is positioned toward you.
4. Straighten the external auditory canal of an adult by pulling the auricle up and back. For a child, the auricle is pulled down and back.

5. Hold the dropper at the opening of the canal but do not contaminate the tip by touching the skin.
6. Instruct the patient to keep the treated ear up for several minutes to keep the medication from leaking from the ear. Sometimes the physician orders that a cotton ball be placed loosely in the canal to keep the medicine in place.

Examples of commonly used otic medications are listed in Table 54-2.

Pharmacology Capsule

Medications intended to be administered into the external ear are called *otic drugs*.

IRRIGATION

Irrigation is the use of a solution to cleanse the external ear canal or to remove something from the canal. A common indication for irrigation is impacted cerumen. Impacted cerumen is dried earwax that blocks the canal. The nurse may perform the irrigation, if agency policy permits, or may assist with the procedure. If the tympanic membrane (i.e., eardrum) is ruptured, the canal should *not* be irrigated because fluid could be forced into the middle ear.

The following key points should be remembered when irrigating an ear:

1. Select the correct solution as ordered by the physician.
2. Warm the solution to body temperature (95°F to 105°F).
3. Have the patient sit up and hold an emesis basin under the ear to be irrigated.
4. Drape the shoulder under the basin.
5. Straighten the external canal of an adult by pulling the auricle up and back. For a child, pull the auricle down and back.
6. Select an irrigating syringe or bulb syringe with a tip that is smaller than the canal.
7. Do not allow the syringe tip to completely block the canal.
8. Direct the solution toward the top of the canal in a steady stream, not toward the eardrum.

Table 54-2 Drug Therapy: Otic Medications

DRUG	USE AND ACTION	SIDE EFFECTS	NURSING INTERVENTIONS
Antibiotics			
chloramphenicol (Chloromycetin otic)	Broad-spectrum antibiotic used to treat infections of lining of external auditory canal.	Hypersensitivity: redness, rash, swelling, burning, pain.	If patient shows signs of hypersensitivity, withhold drug and notify physician.
Topical Corticosteroids			
Cipro HC (ciprofloxacin and hydrocortisone) Ciprodex (ciprofloxacin and dexamethasone) Floxin otic (ofloxacin alone)	Treat inflammation, pruritus, and allergic response. Usually combined with antibacterial or antifungal.	Can encourage microbial resistance to fluoroquinolones.	Do not put in ear if tympanic membrane is perforated. Caution to avoid eye contact.
Antibacterials and Softening Agents			
carbamide peroxide with glycerin (Debrox, Murine ear drops)	Soften earwax. Treat aphthous ulcers.	Redness, irritation, superinfection.	Contraindications: ear surgery, perforated tympanic membrane; ear drainage, redness, pain, or tenderness. Teach patient not to clean ear with cotton swabs, which force wax deeper into ear.
Drying Agents			
Boric acid in isopropyl alcohol (Ear-Dry, Swim-Ear)	Dry external canal after swimming or bathing. Decrease risk of infection.	Local irritation.	Instilled in external canal immediately after swimming or bathing. Contraindicated with perforated tympanic membrane.
Antiemetics			
scopolamine (Transderm Scop) dimenhydrinate (Dramamine) meclizine (Antivert) chlorpromazine (Thorazine)	Prevent or treat nausea, vomiting, motion sickness.	Sedation, drowsiness, tremor, fever, tachycardia, hypotension, constipation, dry mouth.	Safety precautions for drowsiness. Monitor pulse and blood pressure. Monitor stools and urinary output. Mouth care.

9. The procedure can be repeated several times if needed.
10. Sometimes ear drops are ordered to soften impacted cerumen before irrigating.
11. Describe any substances flushed out of the ear.
12. If the impacted cerumen or foreign body does not wash out, inform the physician.

HEARING AIDS

Following an evaluation, the audiologist can inform the patient what, if any, technology is most likely to be beneficial. Technological options include assisted listening devices, hearing aids, and cochlear implants. Assisted listening devices include such options as an amplified telephone receiver or a personal television listening device.

A hearing aid is a device that amplifies sound; that is, it makes sound louder. All hearing aids have four components: (1) a microphone to receive sound waves and convert them to electrical signals, (2) an amplifier to strengthen the signals, (3) a receiver to convert signals to sound waves, and (4) a battery to power the device. Various aids are designed to be worn in the ear, behind the ear, or in the middle of the chest. The device worn in the middle of the chest (i.e., "body hearing aid") is the most powerful. It consists of a wire that connects the ear speaker to an amplifier and battery worn on the body (Fig. 54-6). Technology is advancing so that modern hearing aids have overcome many limitations of older models. Features such as directional microphones and improved background noise filters have made a significant difference in acceptability. The hearing aid requires some care. Wash the ear mold (the part that fits into the ear) daily with soap and water and then dry it. When it is not being worn, turn the aid off and store it in a protective case with the battery compartment open. Ensure that the case is labeled with the patient's name. Keep extra batteries on hand.

If the hearing aid is not working, first check to ensure that it is turned to the on position. If it is on, check the ear mold to see if it needs cleaning. The next step is to check battery placement. If the battery is not inserted correctly, the hearing aid will not work. If the hearing aid has a cord, check it to see if it is broken or unplugged. If these checks fail to locate the problem, change the battery. If a new battery does not correct the problem, the cord can be changed. Should the hearing aid still not work, return it to the dealer for service.

Nurses and other health care providers need to be familiar with hearing aids and how they work. The patient's nursing care plan should indicate that the patient usually wears a hearing aid. Confusion in some older patients might be avoided if the hearing aid were kept in place. The cost of hearing aids can range from several hundred to several thousand dollars if both ears are involved. When patients are hospitalized, take care to prevent loss of these devices.

It may take considerable persuasion from family members and health care providers to get a hearing-impaired person to try a hearing aid. It may be helpful to point out the benefits of improved hearing in the patient's everyday life.

Hearing aids amplify all sounds, including background noise. This is especially annoying when a person first tries to use an aid. Patients are advised to wear the aid first in quiet settings. Once they learn to adjust the volume and tone comfortably, they can try it in noisy settings. It may take several months before a hearing aid feels comfortable.

Pharmacology Capsule

Among the drugs that can cause hearing impairment are salicylates, furosemide, ethacrynic acid, aminoglycoside antibiotics, and some chemotherapeutic drugs.

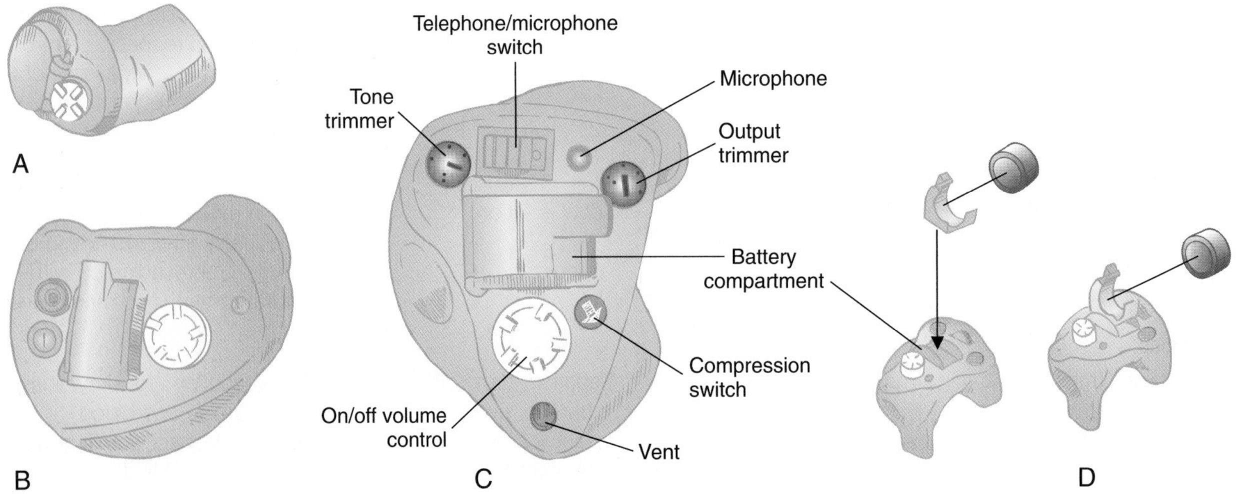

FIGURE 54-6 Types of hearing aids and components. **A,** In-the-canal aid. **B,** In-the-ear aid. **C,** Hearing aid components. **D,** Battery compartment. (Courtesy Arnold G. Schuring, MD.)

COCHLEAR IMPLANTS

A cochlear implant may be recommended for people who cannot benefit from regular hearing aids. A cochlear implant has variable results for the profoundly deaf. Some can hear well enough to understand speech on a telephone; others can hear only environmental sounds, such as sirens, doorbells, and ringing telephones.

The cochlear implant consists of a microphone, a processor, a transmitter, and a receiver. The microphone, at ear level, picks up sounds that are then amplified by the processor (Fig. 54-7). The sound, in the form of magnetic signals, is transmitted electronically to the receiver. The receiver is surgically implanted behind the ear. Electrodes attached to the receiver stimulate nerve fibers in the cochlea to produce sound. Several months of training are needed to learn to tell sounds apart. Therefore candidates for the cochlear implant must be highly motivated and carefully screened. Current efforts to improve cochlear implants include the use of bilateral implants and development of a totally implantable device. Some controversy exists in the deaf community as to whether individuals should be accepted as nonhearing rather than attempting to introduce them to sound.

SURGERY ON THE EAR AND RELATED STRUCTURES

Many ear disorders are treated surgically. Nursing care of patients having specific surgical procedures is discussed with the appropriate pathophysiologic process. However, some general measures apply to most patients after surgery on the ear.

NURSING CARE of the Patient Having Ear Surgery

Before surgery, determine what the patient understands about the procedure and surgical routine. Ask whether the patient is feeling nervous or anxious. *Deficient knowledge* and *anxiety* are typical nursing diagnoses. Supply needed information about the preoperative and postoperative routines. If the patient is anxious, explore the specific concerns. Sometimes patient teaching and reassurance are sufficient to reduce anxiety. Notify the physician if the patient is very anxious.

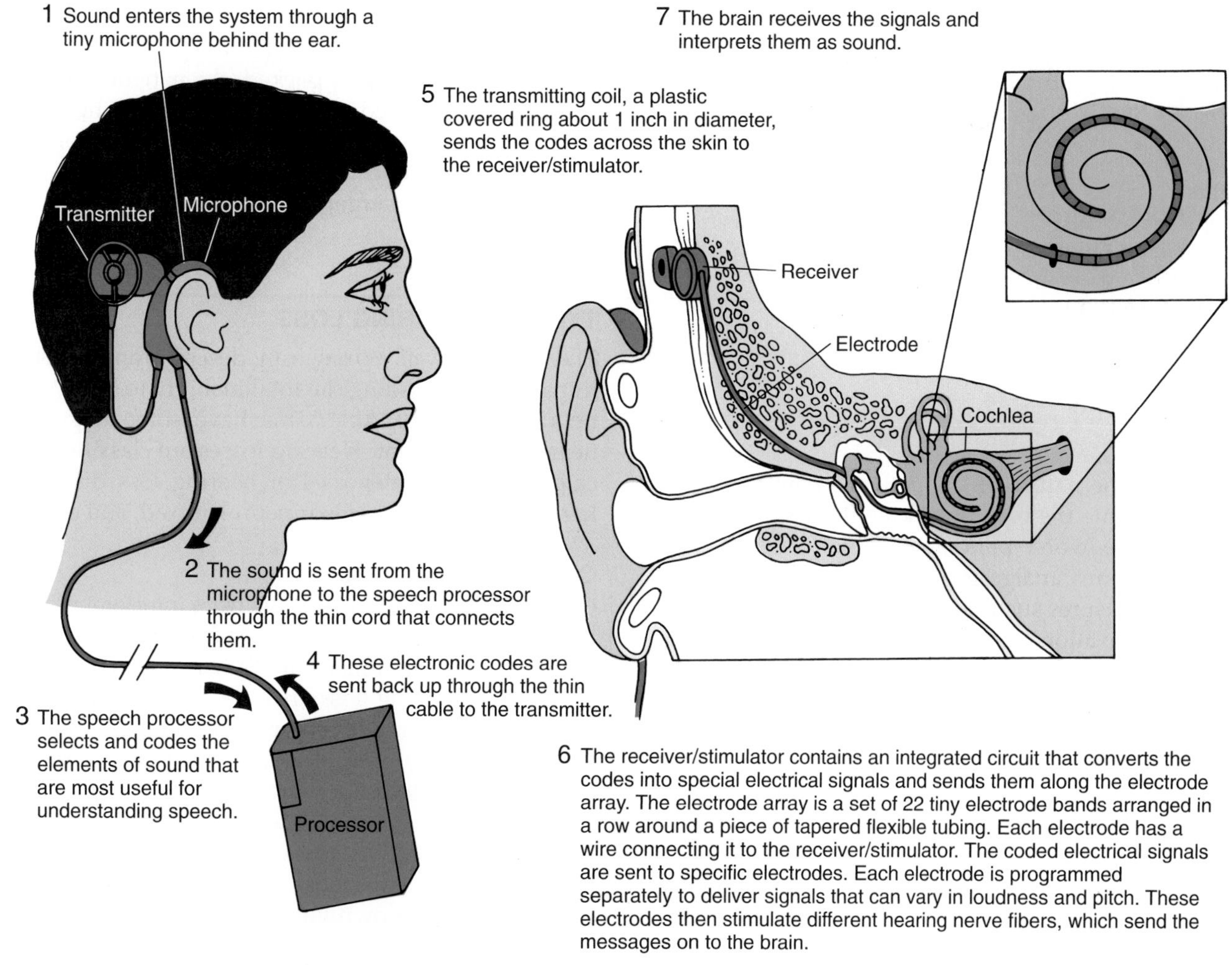

1 Sound enters the system through a tiny microphone behind the ear.
Transmitter
Microphone
2 The sound is sent from the microphone to the speech processor through the thin cord that connects them.
3 The speech processor selects and codes the elements of sound that are most useful for understanding speech.
Processor
4 These electronic codes are sent back up through the thin cable to the transmitter.
5 The transmitting coil, a plastic covered ring about 1 inch in diameter, sends the codes across the skin to the receiver/stimulator.
Receiver
Electrode
Cochlea
6 The receiver/stimulator contains an integrated circuit that converts the codes into special electrical signals and sends them along the electrode array. The electrode array is a set of 22 tiny electrode bands arranged in a row around a piece of tapered flexible tubing. Each electrode has a wire connecting it to the receiver/stimulator. The coded electrical signals are sent to specific electrodes. Each electrode is programmed separately to deliver signals that can vary in loudness and pitch. These electrodes then stimulate different hearing nerve fibers, which send the messages on to the brain.
7 The brain receives the signals and interprets them as sound.

FIGURE 54-7 Cochlear implant to restore hearing. (Modified from Black JM, Hawks JH: *Medical-surgical nursing: clinical management for positive outcomes*, ed 8, St. Louis, 2009, Saunders.)

Immediate preoperative care usually includes having the patient remove any articles such as eyeglasses or hearing aids. The hearing-impaired person going to surgery may feel very helpless without the hearing aid. Notify the operating room staff and ask if the patient can wear the hearing aid to the surgical suite. Place a note on the front of the chart to alert caregivers to the patient's hearing impairment and to the presence of a hearing aid.

Assessment

In the postoperative period, monitor the patient for pain, nausea, dizziness, and fever. Inspect the wound dressing for drainage. Document drainage color, odor, and amount.

Nursing Diagnoses, Goals, and Outcome Criteria: Ear Surgery, Postoperative

Nursing Diagnoses	Goals and Outcome Criteria
Acute Pain related to tissue trauma or edema	Pain relief: patient states pain is relieved, relaxed manner
Risk for Injury related to dizziness or vertigo, fluid accumulation, pressure in the ear	Decreased risk for injury: maintains prescribed position, avoids behavior that increases pressure Absence of injury: patient does not fall
Risk for Infection related to surgical incision	Healing without infection: normal body temperature and white blood cell (WBC) count
Impaired Verbal Communication related to packing and edema in affected ear	Effective communication: patient and nurse use effective strategies to facilitate verbal communication

Interventions

Acute Pain

Determine the nature of the patient's pain and have the patient rate the pain on a scale from 1 to 10, with 10 being the worst pain imaginable. Surgical pain usually requires analgesics for several days. In addition, use measures such as positioning and massage to promote relaxation.

Risk for Injury

Dizziness and vertigo are common after surgery on the ear. **Dizziness** is a feeling of unsteadiness whereas **vertigo** is the sensation that one's body or the room is spinning.

Vertigo is often triggered by sudden movements, so advise the patient to move slowly and carefully. Instruct the patient to call for help when getting up the first few times. Assist the patient for as long as dizziness is a problem. Raise side rails and leave the bed in low position.

The ear is commonly packed and covered with a dressing. A drain may be in place; only the physician can remove the packing. A specific position may be ordered after surgery. If drainage is being encouraged, the patient is most likely positioned on the affected side. However, if the procedure includes a graft on the tympanic membrane, the patient is usually positioned on the unaffected side.

Straining is contraindicated because it increases pressure in the ear. The patient should avoid nose blowing, coughing, and sneezing; however, if these are unavoidable, the mouth should be kept open to relieve pressure. Stool softeners may be ordered to prevent constipation and straining. Ear surgery, like any other type of surgery, creates a wound that must heal. Healing requires a balanced diet with adequate protein and vitamin C.

Risk for Infection

Take measures to reduce the risk of postoperative infection. Advise the patient to avoid crowds and people with colds for several weeks. The ear canal should be kept dry for 2 to 4 weeks as instructed by the physician. Shampooing usually is not allowed for 2 weeks, although it is restricted longer in some cases.

Impaired Verbal Communication

While the affected ear is packed, the patient's hearing in that ear is impaired. If the patient does not hear well in the unaffected ear, you must devise appropriate means of communication. It is best to plan this with the patient before surgery.

HEARING LOSS

TYPES OF HEARING LOSS

The term *hard of hearing* can describe any level of impairment, including the total inability to hear (deafness). Millions of Americans have some degree of hearing impairment. Hearing losses are classified into categories. The categories of hearing loss discussed here are conductive, sensorineural, mixed, and central.

Conductive Hearing Loss

Conductive hearing loss results from interference with the transmission of sound waves from the external or middle ear to the inner ear. Factors that may cause conductive hearing loss include obstruction of the external canal or eustachian tube and otosclerosis. Otosclerosis is a condition in which the stapes in the middle ear does not vibrate.

Patients who have conductive hearing loss hear better in noisy settings than in quiet settings. They do not speak loudly because bone conduction allows them to hear their own voices.

Most conditions that cause conductive hearing loss are treatable. Obstructions usually can be removed. Otosclerosis can be treated surgically with a procedure called a *stapedectomy*. This condition is discussed in more detail in the section titled "Nursing Care of the Patient Having Stapedectomy." Hearing aids are usually helpful for patients with conductive hearing loss.

Sensorineural Hearing Loss

Sensorineural hearing loss is sometimes called *nerve deafness*. It is a disturbance of the neural structures in the inner ear or the nerve pathways to the brain. Sensorineural hearing loss may be congenital but it also can be caused by noise, trauma, aging, Meniere disease, ototoxicity, diabetes, and syphilis.

Patients with sensorineural hearing loss can hear sounds but have difficulty understanding speech. They often complain that speech sounds muffled. This type of hearing loss is not as easily corrected. Hearing aids may help by amplifying the sound but it will still be muffled.

Mixed Hearing Loss

Mixed hearing loss is a combination of conductive and sensorineural losses. Treatment of any reversible problems often results in improvement of mixed hearing loss.

Central Hearing Loss

Central hearing loss is due to some problem in the CNS. The patient either cannot perceive or cannot interpret sounds that are heard.

SIGNS AND SYMPTOMS

Most hearing loss progresses over time. Patients may not readily recognize the loss. They may complain that their hearing is fine but that others are mumbling. Many behaviors should lead the nurse to suspect hearing loss. The patient may lean toward the speaker or turn one ear toward the speaker. The patient with a hearing loss may fail to follow directions, speak while others are speaking, or turn the radio or television up very loud. Irritability and even hostility are not unusual. Some people become very suspicious of others because they cannot hear what others are saying. Hearing loss often has no other symptoms. Otalgia (i.e., ear pain), dizziness, and tinnitus (i.e., ringing in the ears) may be present with certain types of disorders.

EFFECT OF HEARING IMPAIRMENT

People with obvious physical disabilities usually receive some consideration and understanding from strangers. People who have hearing impairments may not be treated as well.

Those who had impairments in early childhood usually have speech difficulties. If speech is not clear, others may assume that the person is intellectually impaired. Sadly, the phrase *deaf and dumb* has been used to refer to people who neither hear nor speak. This term is understandably offensive to the hearing-impaired person. The term *deaf* is not offensive but suggests a total inability to hear. *Hearing impairment*, on the other hand, implies a range of abilities.

It is interesting that most adults accept the use of eyeglasses fairly easily but often are resistant to using a hearing aid. A tendency exists to deny one's hearing loss. When a person refuses to admit to a hearing loss, family members and others may stop trying to communicate. The hearing-impaired person may alienate those who would like to be close and supportive.

People with severe hearing impairment probably suffer the most severe social isolation of those with sensory disorders. Nurses can help by educating the public about hearing loss.

ADAPTATIONS TO HEARING LOSS

Some hearing impairments can be corrected. If not, the patient and family need to learn to cope with the loss. For many people, hearing aids produce at least some improvement in hearing. Many patients read lips and observe body language closely to enhance understanding of spoken messages.

Sign language uses a universal set of hand signals. It provides a very effective means of communicating as long as others know how to use it. Unfortunately, most nurses are not trained in this skill.

Several electronic devices are available to serve the hard of hearing. Telephones can be adapted to send and receive written messages. Earphones are readily available for use with radios, stereos, and televisions. These allow the hearing-impaired person to adjust the volume as needed. They also reduce environmental noises. Some television channels provide closed-captioned programming, in which a written script is shown on the bottom of the screen. A portable telecommunication device for the deaf makes telephone communication possible. In the home, flashing lights can be used to alert the person to doorbells, telephone rings, and alarm clocks. For the person who does not speak, small handheld computers called *personal communicators* print out messages typed by the user.

For many years, guide dogs have been used to help people with visual impairments. A similar intervention is being used with dogs trained to assist the hard of hearing. These dogs are taught to recognize common sounds (e.g., doorbell, telephone, smoke alarm, crying baby) and to get the attention of the owner.

NURSING CARE of the Patient with a Hearing Impairment

Assessment

Assessment of the patient with a hearing impairment is summarized in Box 54-1.

Interventions

Impaired Verbal Communication

Many techniques are available to improve communication with the hard of hearing. You can use these

Nursing Diagnoses, Goals, and Outcome Criteria: Hearing Impairments

Nursing Diagnoses	Goals and Outcome Criteria
Impaired Verbal Communication related to inability to hear	Effective communication: patient and others use alternative means of communication
Social Isolation related to inability to communicate verbally	Reduced social isolation: participation in social activities
Ineffective Coping related to change in social interaction, threat to body image, or denial	Effective coping with permanent hearing impairment: patient has satisfying social interactions, makes positive statements about self, plans realistically
Deficient Knowledge of prevention, diagnosis, and treatment of hearing impairment	Patient knowledge of prevention and treatment: patient correctly practices preventive measures and describes treatments and resources for adaptation

approaches and teach others to use them. When working with a hearing-impaired patient, follow these guidelines:

1. Ensure that the patient knows you are present. Try to move into the patient's line of vision before touching him or her.
2. Find out the patient's usual means of communication and ensure that he or she has access to any assistive devices.
3. Speak slowly and distinctly.
4. Ensure that the patient can see your face clearly. Do not turn away while speaking.
5. Do not eat, smoke, or chew gum if the patient reads lips.
6. Provide adequate lighting directed *toward* your face. A strong light behind you creates a glare and makes it hard to see your features.
7. Lower your voice tone.
8. Assess the patient's ability to hear a normal voice tone. The volume can be increased a little if needed but shouting simply distorts the message. People who wear hearing aids often complain that everyone shouts at them.
9. If the patient has a good ear, speak toward that side.
10. Amplify your voice, if necessary, by using a rolled-up sheet of paper or a stethoscope. To use the stethoscope, put the earpieces in the patient's ears and speak into the bell.
11. Help patients to follow spoken messages by informing them of the topic to be addressed.
12. Use short sentences or phrases.
13. Use body language to support the verbal message.
14. Have a writing pad or Magic Slate available. Use it if the patient cannot understand you or if you do not understand the patient.
15. Try to validate patient understanding by encouraging feedback and assessing whether directions are followed.
16. When a hearing-impaired patient is hospitalized, ensure that a call bell is provided but remind staff that the patient cannot use the intercom.

Social Isolation

The preceding guidelines may improve communication with the hearing-impaired person. However, the most important thing you can do is to have a positive attitude toward trying to communicate with the patient. Genuine interest and attention encourage the patient to express himself or herself in whatever way is possible.

When other people seem hurried or annoyed, they discourage the patient's attempts to communicate. Some patients withdraw from social interactions. They may become isolated and depressed. Encourage the patient to learn new communication methods. Teach the patient how to use assistive devices. Provide information about community resources for the hard of hearing. Explore the type of activities that are satisfying to the patient and encourage continued involvement. Advise the physician if the patient becomes increasingly sad or withdrawn. Counseling with a mental health professional may be suggested.

Ineffective Coping

The way people cope with hearing loss varies with the individual. Some deny the problem for as long as possible; others deliberately learn everything they can about treatments and adaptive strategies. Recognize that both of these behaviors are responses to a stressful situation. It is important to explore the patient's feelings about hearing loss. If the patient is anxious, you may use stress reduction techniques (e.g., relaxation exercises, massage, meditation). The patient who denies hearing loss is often resistant to teaching, so he or she may not take advantage of opportunities to deal with the problem effectively.

Deficient Knowledge

Most people with hearing impairment have some hearing ability. Emphasize measures to reduce the risk of additional impairment. Advise the patient to seek prompt treatment of any symptoms of infection (i.e., fever, pain in the ear, drainage). Hearing protection is recommended in excessively noisy settings. Patients who are taking ototoxic drugs (e.g., aspirin) are told to contact the physician if hearing acuity worsens or tinnitus develops (see *Patient Teaching* box). If ear drops or irrigations are ordered, demonstrate the procedure and reinforce the physician's orders. Patients also need instruction in the use of hearing aids, as described in the section titled "Hearing Aids."

Patient Teaching

Hearing Impairments

- Many types of hearing loss are correctable or at least capable of being improved.
- Hearing is not related to intelligence.
- No reason exists to be ashamed of a hearing impairment.
- Some measures can be taken to reduce the risk of certain types of hearing loss.
- All women of childbearing age should be immunized for rubella to prevent one form of congenital hearing impairment.

DISORDERS AFFECTING HEARING AND BALANCE

EXTERNAL EAR AND CANAL

Foreign Bodies and Cerumen

Occasionally, foreign bodies get into the external ear canal. Most small objects can be flushed from the ear by gentle irrigation. Insects can be killed by instilling a small amount of mineral oil. They can then be flushed from the canal. An alternative method is to hold a flashlight near the auricle. Because insects are often attracted to light, they may move out of the canal.

One of the most common causes of obstruction of the external ear canal is impacted cerumen. The patient is not always aware of the obstruction but may complain of hearing loss, ear pain, or tinnitus. When a large amount of hardened cerumen is present, the physician may order ear drops to soften the cerumen before irrigation. It may be necessary to repeat the procedure several times before all cerumen is removed. If the foreign body or cerumen is not removed by irrigation, the physician can use ear forceps or a cerumen spoon to remove it.

NURSING CARE of the Patient with Impacted Cerumen

Nurses, especially in long-term care facilities, need to inspect the ear canal routinely for impacted cerumen. The dry cerumen may be gold to dark brown. Sometimes it fills the entire canal. If both ears are affected, the patient has some degree of hearing impairment.

In this situation, the primary nursing diagnosis is *impaired verbal communication* related to obstruction of the external auditory canal. The nursing goal is restored hearing. Report the findings to the physician and carry out orders for ear drops. The physician or nurse may do irrigations depending on the agency's policy. Successful interventions are evaluated by examining the canal and documenting the absence of obstructions. Educate patients to avoid trying to remove cerumen with cotton-tipped applicators or other tools. These efforts can harm the ear canal or the tympanic membrane in addition to forcing cerumen or foreign bodies further into the canal. In long-term care settings, patients should be assessed for impacted cerumen on a regular basis.

Infection and Inflammation

Infection or inflammation of the lining of the external ear canal is called *external otitis* or *swimmer's ear*. It may be caused by scratching or cleaning the ear with sharp objects. Swimming can lead to otitis by washing out protective cerumen, which leaves the lining of the external canal susceptible to infectious agents. When infection is present, it often is caused by staphylococci or streptococci but may also be fungal in origin.

Signs and Symptoms. The most characteristic symptom of external otitis is pain that increases when the auricle is pulled. Other symptoms can include dizziness, fever, and drainage. Drainage may be purulent or blood tinged.

Medical Treatment. Topical antibacterial or antifungal drugs are ordered to treat external otitis. Corticosteroid drops may be ordered to reduce inflammation unless the infection is caused by a fungus. In that case, corticosteroids are contraindicated. Ensure that drops are at room temperature; cold could trigger dizziness. If the external canal is obstructed by edema, the physician may insert an ear wick through the blocked canal. An ear wick is a long piece of gauze that extends out of the ear canal. Medication placed on the external portion of the ear wick soaks the gauze and distributes the medication in the canal. Moist heat, topical anesthetic drops, and mild analgesics may be ordered for pain. Any drainage from the ear should be treated as infected material and handled carefully.

NURSING CARE of the Patient with External Otitis

External otitis is typically treated on an outpatient basis, so nursing care is limited. Assessment includes inspection of the external canal and evaluation of pain. Nursing diagnoses are *acute pain* related to inflammation and *deficient knowledge* of preventive practices and treatment of external otitis. Goals of nursing care are pain relief, patient knowledge of prevention, and patient management of treatment plan.

Oral analgesics and topical corticosteroids and antibiotics are given as ordered to treat pain and to reduce inflammation and infection. Administer the prescribed drops or teach the patient to do so. Because it is awkward to put drops into one's own ear, you also may need to teach a family member how to do it. Teach patients to prevent external otitis by not using sharp instruments to clean the auditory canal and by avoiding suspected irritants such as hair spray and earphones. Advise the use of ear plugs while swimming. The physician may instruct the patient to use a drying agent (e.g., Ear-Dry) after swimming or bathing.

Criteria for effective nursing interventions are patient statement of pain relief and the patient's correct description of preventive measures and appropriate administration of prescribed medication.

MIDDLE EAR

Conditions of the middle ear are serious because of the risk for complications, including permanent hearing loss and involvement of the inner ear.

Otitis Media

Otitis media is an infection of the middle ear. Several types of otitis media exist. Acute otitis media and chronic otitis media are sometimes called *suppurant* or *purulent otitis media* because of the presence of purulent material. In serous otitis media, sterile fluid accumulates behind the tympanic membrane. It can precede or follow acute otitis media. Adhesive otitis media may develop if fluid remains in the middle ear. It is characterized by thickening and scarring in the middle ear structures.

Acute Otitis Media. Acute otitis media usually develops with colds. Edema leads to blockage of the eustachian tubes. Fluid accumulates in the middle ear, causing painful pressure on the tympanic membrane. The tympanic membrane may rupture, resulting in scarring and subsequent hearing loss. The patient often has a fever and complains of headache. Acute otitis media is more common in children than in adults.

Medical Treatment. Although acute otitis media often resolves without intervention, oral antibiotics may be prescribed in some circumstances. Another option is topical ear drops, usually combinations of antibacterials and corticosteroids, that are given for 1 week. Before the drops are administered, the canal should be cleared of debris. Have the patient lie on the unaffected side for a few minutes after instilling the drops to promote flow of the medication into the canal. If a wick has been placed in the canal because of swelling, apply the ear drops directly to the wick. Antihistamines may be ordered if allergies are thought to be contributing to the problem. Sometimes myringotomy is performed. Myringotomy is the creation of a small opening in the tympanic membrane to reduce pressure and allow fluid to drain. If infection is eliminated, the tympanic membrane should heal without permanent damage. A tympanostomy tube may be placed to allow for continuous drainage.

Chronic Otitis Media. Chronic otitis media is characterized by hearing loss and continuous or intermittent drainage. The condition usually is not painful. On examination, the eardrum is usually perforated (i.e., ruptured) or shows signs of a healed perforation. An audiogram may detect some conductive hearing loss if the bones in the middle ear have been damaged by the chronic infection.

Possible complications of chronic otitis media include mastoiditis, meningitis, labyrinthitis, cholesteatoma, and hearing impairment.

Mastoiditis. Because the middle ear is directly connected to the air cells in the mastoid bone, infection in the middle ear can extend into the mastoid bone. In addition, because the brain lies next to the mastoid bone, the infection can spread there as well. Signs and symptoms of mastoiditis include mastoid swelling (directly behind the ear) and soreness, headache, malaise, and an elevated white blood cell (WBC) count. Thick, purulent drainage from the ear may be seen. Mastoiditis is very serious because it can lead to a brain abscess, meningitis (i.e., inflammation of the covering of the brain), or paralysis of the facial muscles.

Cholesteatoma. A cholesteatoma is a growth in the middle ear. When the tympanic membrane is perforated around the margin where it attaches to the ear canal, epithelial cells grow into the middle ear. The cells form a ball of tissue that grows and that may damage the facial nerve, the ossicles, and the labyrinth. A cholesteatoma must be removed surgically.

Medical Treatment. Chronic otitis media is treated with systemic antibiotics and, if the eardrum is intact, irrigations to remove debris. If the tympanic membrane does not heal, tympanoplasty may be done to repair it. The procedure may be done through the ear canal or through an incision behind the auricle. Sometimes grafts of the patient's tissue are used to repair the tear. Tissue may be taken from the external canal or the temporalis muscle. After the graft is placed, the middle ear is filled with Gelfoam and a cotton ball is put in the external ear to hold the graft in place. If the ossicles (bones) in the middle ear are diseased, they may be replaced with prostheses.

If the infection has extended to the mastoid bone, a mastoidectomy is often done at the same time. A mastoidectomy can be modified (simple) or radical. In a modified procedure, infected mastoid tissue is removed but the middle ear is left intact. In a radical mastoidectomy, all structures in the middle ear are removed. The radical procedure is not done as often now as it was in the past.

❖ NURSING CARE of the Patient Having a Mastoidectomy

General care of the patient having surgery on the ear is discussed earlier in the section titled "Nursing Care of the Patient Having Ear Surgery." Before mastoid surgery, the emphasis is on patient teaching and reduction of anxiety. Primary considerations after surgery on the middle ear include comfort, safety, prevention of infection, and prevention of pressure on the tympanic membrane. Nausea is another common problem after middle ear surgery. Keep an emesis receptacle nearby. The physician usually orders antiemetics to be given as needed for nausea. If the patient vomits frequently, a risk of deficient fluid volume exists. Monitor intake and output and give intravenous fluids if ordered.

The type of dressing varies. It may be small and placed over the auricle. However, if the surgeon entered through the mastoid bone, expect a large head dressing with a drain. Inspect the dressing and describe any drainage but *do not disturb or remove the dressing*. Assist the patient the first time out of bed in case dizziness is a problem. The patient should avoid any activity that creates pressure on the tympanic membrane (e.g., blowing the nose, coughing, sneezing, straining). If the patient needs to cough or sneeze, advise him or her to do so with the mouth open.

Otosclerosis

Otosclerosis is a hereditary condition in which an abnormal growth causes the footplate of the stapes to become fixed. The fixed stapes cannot vibrate, so sound waves cannot be transmitted to the inner ear. The effect of this abnormality is a conductive hearing loss. If the disease also involves the inner ear, the patient has sensorineural hearing loss as well. The condition affects both ears but may progress faster in one ear than in the other.

Otosclerosis is most common in young Caucasian women. The onset is usually in the late teens or early 20s. During pregnancy, it progresses at a faster rate.

Signs and Symptoms. The primary symptom of otosclerosis is slowly progressive hearing loss in the absence of infection. In the early stages, the patient may report tinnitus. The Rinne test reveals bone conduction to be greater than air conduction.

Medical Treatment. The most common treatment for otosclerosis is a surgical procedure called *stapedectomy*. The physician advises the patient of the surgical risks, including complete hearing loss, infection, prolonged vertigo, and damage to the facial nerve. Stapedectomy is done under local anesthesia. The stapes is removed and replaced with a prosthesis. A tissue graft taken from the patient is placed over the oval window. The physician puts packing in the ear canal at the completion of the stapedectomy. A small dressing is then placed over the ear. When the graft heals, hearing is restored in most patients (Fig. 54-8).

After surgery, bed rest may be ordered for several days; drugs are prescribed to control nausea and vertigo. Usually the patient is allowed to lie on the back or the unaffected side but specific position restrictions may be ordered.

❖ NURSING CARE of the Patient Having Stapedectomy

Care of the patient having ear surgery is detailed in the section titled "Nursing Care of the Patient Having Ear Surgery." In addition to the usual preoperative teaching, tell the patient having stapedectomy that hearing usually is worse immediately after surgery but improves gradually over approximately 6 weeks.

After surgery you should be concerned with pain relief, safety, prevention of infection, and avoidance of pressure in the ear. Because pressure can cause the graft to separate, it is especially important that the patient not do anything that increases pressure in the ear. After stapedectomy, nausea, vomiting, and vertigo are common.

The packing in the ear should not be disturbed. The physician removes it approximately 1 week after the surgery. After the dressing and packing are removed, the patient usually is advised to keep the ear dry for

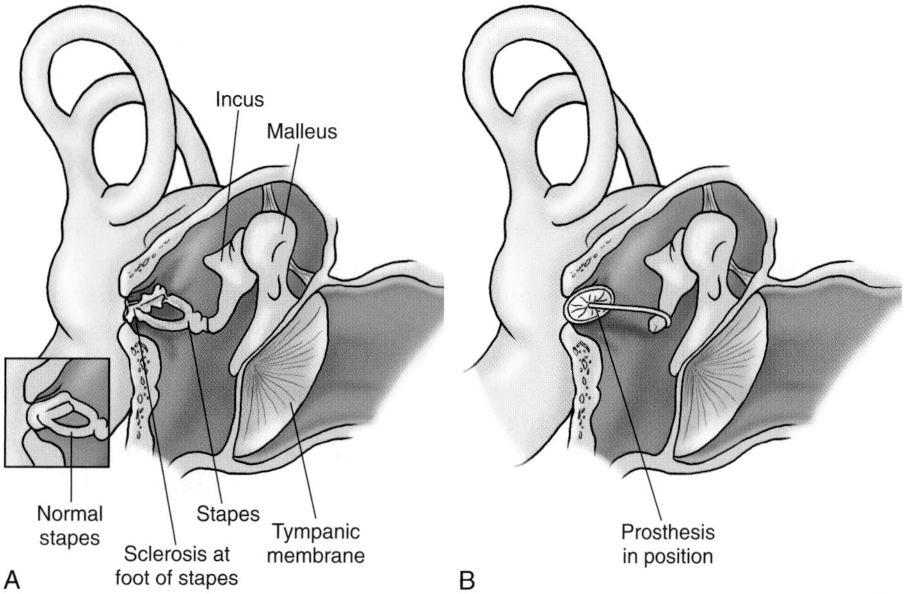

FIGURE 54-8 Otosclerosis: **(A)** Before and **(B)** after stapedectomy. (From Monahan FD, Drake DT, Neighbors M, editors: *Medical-surgical nursing: foundations for clinical practice*, ed 2, Philadelphia, 1998, Saunders.)

at least 2 weeks. Swimming and showering usually are not permitted for approximately 6 weeks.

The patient should avoid contact with people who have colds. A balanced diet and adequate rest are needed for tissue healing and resistance to infection. Vertigo may persist after discharge and you must help the patient to plan for assistance with activities of daily living (ADL). It is important to reinforce that hearing improvement is gradual.

INNER EAR

Labyrinthitis

Labyrinthitis is inflammation of the labyrinth. It may be acute or chronic. Acute labyrinthitis usually follows an acute upper respiratory infection, acute otitis media, pneumonia, or influenza. It also can be an adverse effect of some drugs (see *Complementary and Alternative Therapies* box). One type of labyrinthitis is suppurative labyrinthitis. It is an inner ear infection that usually follows an upper respiratory infection, ear infection, or ear surgery. The effects can destroy the labyrinth and cochlea, causing permanent deafness.

Complementary and Alternative Therapies

Caution patients who have inner ear disorders that many herbal products can cause dizziness, nausea, and vomiting. Drowsiness is another side effect of many herbals, which may enhance the sedative effects of drugs used to manage vertigo.

Signs and Symptoms. Signs and symptoms of labyrinthitis include vertigo, nausea, vomiting, headache, anorexia, nystagmus, and sensorineural hearing loss on the affected side. A typical episode lasts 3 to 6 weeks. Nystagmus is an abnormal, rhythmic jerking movement of the eyes. Additional symptoms of suppurative labyrinthitis are tinnitus and hearing loss.

Medical Treatment. Labyrinthitis is treated with antiemetics and supportive care until it resolves. Antibiotics are prescribed if infection is present.

NURSING CARE of the Patient with Labyrinthitis

Assessment

During an acute episode of labyrinthitis, describe the patient's symptoms. Monitor intake and output, daily weights if possible, and food intake if persistent vomiting occurs.

Interventions

Safety is a major concern for the patient with vertigo. Assist and supervise the patient when he or she is out of bed. Give antiemetics as prescribed for nausea and vomiting. If vomiting persists, the patient is at risk for development of fluid and electrolyte imbalances (i.e., hypokalemia, fluid volume deficit) and intravenous fluids may be needed. The patient needs reassurance that the condition resolves in time.

Nursing Diagnoses, Goals, and Outcome Criteria: Labyrinthitis

Nursing Diagnoses	Goals and Outcome Criteria
Risk for Injury related to vertigo	Safety: absence of injury or falls
Imbalanced Nutrition: Less Than Body Requirements related to anorexia and nausea	Adequate nutrition: stable body weight
Risk for Deficient Fluid Volume related to vomiting	Adequate hydration: equal fluid intake and output, moist mucous membranes, vital signs consistent with patient norms
Anxiety related to acute illness	Reduced anxiety: patient states anxiety is reduced, calm manner

Meniere Disease

Meniere disease (endolymphatic hydrops) is a disorder of the labyrinth. More than 2 million Americans are thought to have attacks of Meniere disease. The onset is usually in people ages 30 to 60 years. It usually affects only the ear. The cause is unknown but the symptoms are related to an accumulation of fluid in the inner ear. Some things that have been found to trigger attacks include alcohol, nicotine, stress, and certain stimuli such as bright lights and sudden movements of the head.

Signs and Symptoms. Some patients with Meniere disease have more serious symptoms than others. Acute attacks occur at intervals and last for hours to days. The frequency of attacks often can be reduced with medical treatment. During an acute attack, the classic symptoms are hearing loss and vertigo accompanied by pallor, sweating, nausea, and vomiting. The hearing loss is unilateral, meaning that only one ear is affected. Tinnitus accompanies acute attacks. It is heard as a low buzzing sound that sometimes becomes a roar. Hearing usually improves between attacks but some loss of low-frequency sounds may remain. Patients who have had many attacks may eventually have permanent sensorineural hearing loss.

Vertigo is a sensation of movement that causes dizziness and nausea. Patients may say that the room seems to be spinning or that they feel like they are spinning. A feeling of fullness and pressure in the ear often precedes a vertigo attack. Attacks may last several minutes to several hours. Sudden movement during an attack of vertigo can cause vomiting.

Medical Diagnosis. Diagnosis of Meniere disease is based on the history and physical findings. The patient describes hearing and balance disturbances as described earlier. An audiogram often reveals a loss of the ability to hear low-frequency sounds. If the caloric test or electronystagmography is done, the patient with Meniere disease has a severe attack of vertigo. A glycerol test involves audiometry testing before and after giving the patient oral glycerol (a diuretic that draws fluid from the inner ear). Improved hearing after glycerol is given suggests Meniere disease.

Meniere disease is actually diagnosed by ruling out other conditions that can cause similar symptoms. Therefore the physician is likely to order a number of radiographs and other tests to detect any neurologic, allergic, or endocrine disorders.

Medical Treatment. Meniere disease may be treated medically or surgically (see *Complementary and Alternative Therapies* box). Drugs prescribed during an acute attack include atropine, epinephrine, benzodiazepines such as diazepam (Valium), antihistamines, antiemetics, anticholinergics, vasodilators, and diuretics. Drugs that may be prescribed between attacks in an attempt to reduce their frequency and severity are diuretics and drugs that help to control vertigo. Meclizine and transdermal scopolamine are less sedating than many other agents and may allow the patient to maintain a more normal life.

Complementary and Alternative Therapies

Biofeedback, self-hypnosis, and relaxation techniques may be recommended to help the patient learn to live with Meniere disease.

A low-sodium diet and diuretics seem to increase the length of time between attacks by reducing edema in the inner ear. If moderate sodium restriction is not effective, the patient may be put on a strict sodium-free diet (see *Nutritional Considerations* box). Caffeine, nicotine, and alcohol are discouraged. Vestibular rehabilitation is a series of exercises performed to help the patient develop a tolerance for vertigo. It begins with moving the eyes and the head up and down and side to side and progresses to more vigorous activity. Usually the physical therapist teaches vestibular rehabilitation. Most patients respond positively to conservative medical treatment. Pressure pulse treatment is a more recent development that reduces dizziness and tinnitus for some people. It is a device that fits into the external ear and delivers pressure to the middle ear intermittently. Patients use it at home three times a day for 5 minutes each time.

Nutrition Considerations

A low-salt diet is sometimes prescribed for people with Meniere disease. Caffeine, alcohol, chocolate, and nicotine may aggravate or trigger an attack.

Surgical Treatment. Surgery is usually advised only when all other measures have failed. Surgical procedures drain excess fluid from the inner ear (endolymphatic shunt) or cut the part of the acoustic nerve that controls balance (vestibular nerve section). The incision may be inside or behind the ear. In general, these surgical procedures pose some risk for permanent hearing loss. More destructive surgical procedures are labyrinthotomy and labyrinthectomy. These procedures are reserved for conditions that have not responded to other measures. They are only done if the affected ear already has profound hearing loss.

Potential complications of surgery for Meniere disease include infection, hearing loss, loss of cerebrospinal fluid (CSF), and damage to the seventh cranial nerve. The leakage of CSF may occur with procedures that require opening the skull. The seventh cranial nerve is the facial nerve that is located very close to the ear canal. It controls the movement of certain muscles of the face. Surgical procedures in and around the ear can result in trauma to the facial nerve.

❖ NURSING CARE of the Patient with Meniere Disease

■ Assessment

The pattern of acute attacks should be documented (see Nursing Care Plan: Patient with Meniere Disease). Note substances or stimuli that trigger the episodes. Document specific symptoms, including nausea, vomiting, vertigo, and tinnitus. Determine how the condition affects the patient's life, what the patient knows about the disease, and what coping mechanisms are used.

Nursing Diagnoses, Goals, and Outcome Criteria: Meniere Disease

Nursing Diagnoses	Goals and Outcome Criteria
Risk for Injury related to vertigo	Safety: absence of falls and injuries
Risk for Deficient Fluid Volume related to vomiting	Normal hydration: equal fluid intake and output, normal vital signs, moist mucous membranes
Anxiety related to acute illness or disruption of usual lifestyle	Reduced anxiety: patient states anxiety is reduced, calm manner
Ineffective Self-Health Management related to lack of knowledge about management of Meniere disease	Effective self-health management: appropriate self-care, patient correctly describes and demonstrates self-care measures

■ Interventions

Risk for Injury

Safety is a major concern. Attacks come on suddenly and can be dangerous in many circumstances. Fortunately, many people can recognize an aura, or peculiar feeling, that precedes an attack. They should know to seek safety promptly when an aura occurs. If driving, the patient should pull over and stop the car as soon as possible.

Nursing Care Plan Patient with Meniere Disease

ASSESSMENT

HEALTH HISTORY A 62-year-old man has had repeated episodes of nausea, hearing loss, and vertigo over the past year. His attacks last 2 to 3 hours, during which he is completely incapacitated. His wife brought him to the emergency department after he vomited repeatedly and seemed very weak. His health history reveals repeated urinary tract infections (UTIs) but no other serious illness or injuries. He is an accountant who owns his own business.

PHYSICAL EXAMINATION Vital signs: blood pressure 136/82 mm Hg, pulse 88 bpm, respiration 16 breaths per minute, temperature 98°F (36.7°C) measured orally. Height 5′4″, weight 200 lb. Patient appears acutely ill and unable to sit or stand. Physical findings are normal except for mild hearing loss. The physician's diagnosis is probable Meniere disease.

Nursing Diagnosis	Goals and Outcome Criteria	Interventions
Risk for Injury related to vertigo	A safe environment is provided: The patient will have no injuries during acute episodes.	Assist the patient to bed and allow him to remain still. Raise the side rails and put the bed in low position. Place the call bell within reach and caution him not to try to get up unassisted. Darken the room and keep it quiet. Postpone nonessential care. Provide a urinal for voiding. When the attack subsides, assist the patient out of bed until he is no longer dizzy.
Risk for Deficient Fluid Volume related to vomiting	The patient will be adequately hydrated, as evidenced by vital signs consistent with patient's norms, moist mucous membranes, and fluid intake equal to output.	Give antiemetics and antihistamines as ordered. Provide an emesis basin. If the patient vomits, promptly empty, clean, and return the emesis basin. Administer intravenous fluids as ordered.
Anxiety related to acute illness, disruption of usual lifestyle	The patient will state that anxiety is reduced and will appear more relaxed.	Be available but let patient lie quietly. When the patient is able to talk, explore how the condition affects his life and how he can deal with it. Tell him that the condition usually can be improved with treatment.
Ineffective Self-Health Management related to lack of knowledge of condition and treatment	The patient will describe measures to manage acute attacks and to reduce frequency of attacks.	Explain drugs to patient, including dosage, schedule, side and adverse effects, and information that should be reported to the physician. If sodium restriction is prescribed, explain that some patients benefit from the restriction. Request dietary consult if special diet is ordered.

Critical Thinking Questions

1. Why is it important to let the patient lie still and remain undisturbed as much as possible?
2. Why do some patients with Meniere disease benefit from sodium restriction?

Risk for Deficient Fluid Volume

During an acute attack in the hospitalized patient, allow the patient to remain still because movement may trigger vomiting. Keep the room dark and quiet. Postpone nonessential care such as bathing. Promptly give medications for nausea and vomiting and keep an emesis basin close to the patient. An intravenous infusion probably will be ordered to provide fluids, medications, or both. After the symptoms subside, assist the patient when getting up until dizziness goes away.

Anxiety

Patients with Meniere disease may be anxious about the condition and the limitations it imposes. Encourage the patient to share concerns and help the patient to learn how to manage the condition (see *Patient Teaching* box).

Ineffective Self-Health Management

Interventions involve patient teaching as presented in the *Patient Teaching* box.

Patient Teaching

Meniere Disease

- You need to know prescribed medications and how to manage their side effects (provide specifics).
- Alcohol, caffeine, and tobacco may make your symptoms worse.

Put on Your Thinking Cap!

Think about a routine day. Consider how a person's life might be affected by frequent attacks of Meniere disease.

POSTOPERATIVE NURSING CARE

If the patient has surgery for Meniere disease, postoperative care depends on the exact procedure. Carefully check the physician's orders for position and activity limitations. General nursing care is concerned with safety, comfort, and detection of complications. On the first few days after surgery, the patient's symptoms are usually severe. Antiemetics are ordered to control nausea and vomiting. Delay nonessential care until the patient tolerates movement. Assist patients when getting up and walking until they are able to walk steadily. The call bell should always be within reach. It is not unusual for these patients to be dizzy for several days and unsteady for several weeks.

Observe for facial nerve damage by having the patient smile and show his or her teeth. If the facial nerve is damaged, the muscles on the affected side do not respond and the patient's face is not symmetric. Immediately notify the surgeon of any evidence of facial nerve damage. Nerve damage may be reversible if treated promptly.

Put on Your Thinking Cap!

Explain why patients with inner ear disorders often have problems with balance as well as with hearing.

Presbycusis

Although many older people hear very well, approximately half of those older than 75 years have some difficulty hearing. *Presbycusis* is the term used to describe hearing loss associated with aging. It is the result of changes in one or more parts of the cochlea. The extent of the disability depends on the location of the changes in the cochlea.

Signs and Symptoms. People with presbycusis may hear well in quiet surroundings but hear poorly in noisy places. Some patients deny that they do not hear well. Instead they may blame others for not speaking clearly.

Medical Diagnosis and Treatment. A thorough hearing evaluation is indicated for the older person whose hearing seems to be declining. Many people have the mistaken idea that hearing loss in older adults is inevitable and not treatable. In fact, many patients with presbycusis do benefit from hearing aids. If a hearing aid is recommended, the patient needs to learn how to use and care for it, as described in the section titled "Hearing Aids." Hearing aids are helpful but are not the only way to improve communication. The patient needs to be willing to tell others how they can be understood more easily. The patient also can practice and improve listening skills.

In addition to hearing aids, other electronic devices are available to improve hearing. These are described in the section titled "Adaptations to Hearing Loss" and include phone amplifiers and personal earphones for radios and televisions.

NURSING CARE of the Patient with Presbycusis

Nursing assessment, diagnosis, goals, and interventions for the patient with impaired hearing are described earlier under "Nursing Care of the Patient with Impaired Hearing." In addition, nurses need to educate people about hearing loss and aging. They can also work to overcome the resistance that many people have to admitting hearing loss. Once the problem has been diagnosed, nurses can help the patient to adapt and learn to use supportive devices.

Ototoxicity

Ototoxicity is damage to the ear or eighth cranial nerve caused by specific chemicals, including some drugs. Common ototoxic drugs are salicylates (i.e., aspirin) and aminoglycoside antibiotics. These and other ototoxic drugs that pose a threat to hearing are listed in Box 54-2. Ototoxicity can range from reversible tinnitus to permanent hearing loss. Hearing, balance, or both may be affected. The primary symptom of ototoxicity with salicylates is tinnitus, which disappears when the drug is discontinued. Aminoglycosides, on the other hand, can cause permanent hearing loss. The extent depends on the drug dosage and how long it was given. Patients who have poor renal function are at special risk for ototoxicity because drugs are excreted more slowly. This increases the likelihood of toxicity.

Box 54-2 Ototoxic Drugs

ANTIBIOTICS

AMINOGLYCOSIDES
- amikacin sulfate (Amikin)
- gentamicin sulfate (Garamycin)
- kanamycin sulfate (Kantrex)
- neomycin sulfate
- streptomycin sulfate
- tobramycin sulfate (Nebcin)

ERYTHROMYCINS
- erythromycin estolate (Ilosone)
- erythromycin ethylsuccinate (Pediamycin)
- erythromycin stearate (Erythrocin)
- erythromycin lactobionate (Erythrocin)

TETRACYCLINE
- minocycline (Minocin)

MISCELLANEOUS AGENT
- vancomycin

DIURETICS
- furosemide (Lasix)
- ethacrynic acid (Edecrin)

ANTIDYSRHYTHMIC AGENTS
- quinidine

ANTIINFLAMMATORIES/ANALGESICS
- aspirin
- ibuprofen (Motrin)
- indomethacin (Indocin)

ANTINEOPLASTIC AGENTS
- bleomycin (Blenoxane)
- cisplatin (Platinol, CDDP)
- dactinomycin (Cosmegen)
- mechlorethamine (nitrogen mustard, Mustargen)

NURSING CARE of the Patient with Ototoxicity

The primary nursing responsibilities are early detection and prevention of progressive hearing loss caused by ototoxic drugs. To reduce the risk of ototoxicity, be familiar with these drugs. Instruct patients to report hearing loss, tinnitus, or problems with balance. Promptly report such symptoms to the physician. In addition, teach patients that aspirin is not a harmless drug. Monitor the urine output of patients on ototoxic drugs because low urine output may mean that the potentially toxic drug is excreted slowly, increasing the risk of toxicity. Report low urine output to the physician. The nursing care plan should alert all staff to the potential for ototoxicity.

Disorders that impair hearing or balance can have a profound effect on a person's life and well-being. The nurse plays an important role in the prevention, early detection, and treatment of hearing and balance disturbances.

Get Ready for the NCLEX® Examination!

Key Points

- Approximately half of all adults older than 75 years have some hearing loss.
- Common nursing diagnoses after ear surgery include acute pain, risk for injury, risk for infection, and impaired verbal communication.
- Hearing losses are classified as *conductive, sensorineural, mixed*, or *central*.
- Adaptations for the hard of hearing include sign language, electronic devices, television closed captioning, personal communicators, telephones for the deaf, and trained dogs.
- Nursing care of the patient with hearing impairment addresses impaired verbal communication, social isolation, ineffective coping, and deficient knowledge.
- Cerumen (earwax) can become impacted and obstruct the external ear canal, causing pain and hearing impairment.
- External otitis, infection and inflammation of the external ear canal, is treated with topical antibiotics and corticosteroids.
- Otitis media, infection of the middle ear, can cause permanent hearing loss and inner ear problems.
- Otosclerosis is a condition in which the stapes becomes fixed, causing a conductive and sometimes sensorineural hearing loss.
- Hearing aids are useful if the patient has only conductive hearing loss.
- The results of cochlear implants range from minimal to marked improvement.
- Labyrinthitis, which is inflammation of the labyrinth, causes vertigo and nausea and may be treated with antiemetics and antibiotics.
- Meniere disease, characterized by attacks of hearing loss and vertigo, may be treated with drug therapy, low-sodium diet, surgical intervention, or a combination of these.
- Nursing care of the patient with Meniere disease may address risk for injury, risk for deficient fluid volume, anxiety, and ineffective self-health management.
- Presbycusis is hearing loss associated with aging that may be improved with a hearing aid.
- Ototoxicity is damage to the eighth cranial nerve producing effects that may range from tinnitus to permanent hearing loss.

Additional Learning Resources

SG Go to your Study Guide for additional learning activities to help you master this chapter content.

evolve Go to your Evolve website (http://evolve.elsevier.com/Linton/medsurg) for the following learning resources and much more:

- Interactive Prioritization Exercises
- Fluid & Electrolyte Tutorial
- Pharmacology Tutorial
- Review Questions for the NCLEX® Examination

Review Questions for the NCLEX® Examination

1. For an otoscopic examination of the external auditory canal of an adult, the examiner should do which of the following?
   1. Pull the auricle straight up
   2. Pull the earlobe down
   3. Pull the auricle up and back
   4. Pull the auricle straight back

   NCLEX Client Need: Physiological Integrity: Reduction of Risk Potential
2. During the Rinne test, a patient reports hearing the tuning fork when it is placed on the mastoid bone and when the tines are then positioned near the ear canal. How should this information be interpreted?
   1. The patient probably has an obstruction in the ear canal.
   2. The patient probably has a conductive hearing loss.
   3. The patient's response to this test is normal.
   4. The patient probably has a sensorineural hearing loss.

   NCLEX Client Need: Physiological Integrity: Reduction of Risk Potential
3. Normal age-related changes in the ears of the older adult include which of the following?
   1. Increased cerumen secretion
   2. Coarser hair in the ear canal
   3. Progressive hearing loss
   4. Thinning of the eardrum

   NCLEX Client Need: Health Promotion and Maintenance

4. A resident in a long-term care facility points to her ear and loudly says, "I can't hear!" The patient's hearing aid appears to be positioned correctly in her ear canal. What is the *first* thing you should do?
   1. Remove the aid and clean it
   2. Replace the battery
   3. Turn up the volume
   4. See if it is set to the on position

   NCLEX Client Need: Health Promotion and Maintenance
5. During shift change, it is noted that a new patient is severely hard of hearing. What is the most important question for you to ask about this patient initially?
   1. What means of communication does the patient use?
   2. Is the patient aware of the latest technology to assist the hard of hearing?
   3. Has the patient ever been hospitalized before?
   4. Can a family member stay with the patient to interpret?

   NCLEX Client Need: Health Promotion and Maintenance
6. You are preparing to administer otic drops when you notice that the patient has gauze in the affected ear with a piece of narrow gauze extending from the ear. What should you do?
   1. Gently remove the packing, instill the drops, and replace the packing.
   2. Apply the drops to the narrow piece of gauze for transport into the ear.
   3. Trim the gauze so that the packing is not accidentally pulled out of the ear.
   4. Inform the registered nurse (RN) that the drops cannot be given at this time.

   NCLEX Client Need: Physiological Integrity: Reduction of Risk Potential
7. Which nursing measures are appropriate for the patient who is having an acute attack of Meniere disease? (Select all that apply.)
   1. Keep the room quiet and dark
   2. Advise the patient to drink additional fluids
   3. Delay routine care until the patient is no longer dizzy
   4. Monitor vitals every hour until stable and then every 4 hours
   5. Assist the patient to sit up in the bedside chair for 1 hour twice a day

   NCLEX Client Need: Physiological Integrity: Reduction of Risk Potential
8. When a patient is taking an aminoglycoside antibiotic, instructions should include which of the following?
   1. "Let me know if you have any 'ringing' in your ears."
   2. "Check the white part of your eyes for a color change."
   3. "Restrict your fluid intake to 1 L each day."
   4. "Change position slowly in case your blood pressure (BP) drops."

   NCLEX Client Need: Physiological Integrity: Pharmacological Therapies
9. Stapedectomy is used to correct which of the following?
   1. Sensorineural hearing loss
   2. Meniere disease
   3. Otosclerosis
   4. Otitis media

   NCLEX Client Need: Physiological Integrity: Reduction of Risk Potential
10. Patients who are considering having a cochlear implant should be told which of the following?
    1. "This procedure restores perfect hearing in 99% of patients."
    2. "Complications of cochlear implant are often disabling."
    3. "Results vary from minimal to excellent improvement in hearing."
    4. "Cochlear implants cannot enable you to discriminate speech."

    NCLEX Client Need: Physiological Integrity: Reduction of Risk Potential

chapter 55

Psychologic Responses to Illness

http://evolve.elsevier.com/Linton/medsurg

Mary Ann Matteson

Objectives

1. Define mental health.
2. Discuss the concepts of stress, anxiety, adaptation, and homeostasis.
3. Discuss how age and cultural and spiritual beliefs affect an individual's ability to cope with illness.
4. Identify some basic coping strategies (defense mechanisms).
5. Discuss the concepts of anxiety, fear, stress, loss, grief, helplessness, and powerlessness in relation to illness.
6. Describe several factors that may precipitate adaptive or maladaptive coping behaviors in response to illness.
7. Discuss implementation of the nursing process to enhance a patient's mental health as the patient deals with the stresses of illness.

Key Terms

Adaptation
Anxiety (ăng-ZĪ-ĭ-tē)
Conflicts
Coping
Crisis
Defense mechanisms
Feelings
Helplessness
Maladaptive coping (măl-ă-DĂP-tĭv)
Personality
Self-esteem
Stress
Stressor

Part of being human is the need to cope with different types of stressors at different times of life. Individual coping strategies are influenced by many factors, such as personal beliefs and values as well as one's family, cultural practices, and community resources. Patients and their families may experience a wide range of feelings and emotions in response to illness. To promote adaptation to illness and to minimize maladaptive behaviors, you need to be well acquainted with the range of responses that individuals can experience during illness. The nursing process provides a systematic approach to individualized care based on careful assessment and understanding of human behavior.

DEFINITION OF MENTAL HEALTH

A person is a living being with physical, cognitive, affective, behavioral, and social dimensions who interacts with the environment to achieve a chosen life purpose. The *physical dimension* includes the biologic and physiologic aspects of a person. The *physical dimension* refers to the person's internal environment and how it is integrated with cognitive, affective, behavioral, and social dimensions. The *cognitive dimension* involves an individual's ability to formulate thoughts, process information, and solve problems. The *affective dimension* involves an individual's ability to experience and express feelings and emotions. The *behavioral dimension* reflects a person's individuality and involves integration of the physical, cognitive, and affective dimensions. The *social dimension* involves an individual's skills in living as a member of a family and community. Together these dimensions form a complete or total person.

Environment typically refers to everything outside a person; however, it is more accurate to think of environment as having two dimensions: (1) the external environment and (2) the internal environment. The external environment includes the physical and social elements that are external to and interactive with an individual. In a health care setting, you are a part of the external environment. Environment can also refer to the internal environment of a person. An individual's internal environment refers to physical, biologic states inside the individual, such as fluid and electrolyte balance, body temperature, and nutritional status. Because all of these elements affect an individual's overall health, they also affect a person's mental health.

Mental health is a dynamic process in which a person's physical (internal environment), cognitive, affective, behavioral, and social dimensions interact functionally with one another and the external environment. Mentally healthy individuals are able to perceive reality accurately, manage the way that emotions are experienced and expressed, think clearly and logically, communicate effectively, anticipate events and solve problems, initiate and maintain meaningful relationships, develop a positive self-concept, and generally behave in ways that promote personal growth and development. The understanding of human needs, both psychologic and physical, is central to all aspects of the nursing process because nurses seek to promote or restore personal growth and development. The American psychologist Abraham Maslow was among the first to describe and define human needs in the form of a hierarchy. Maslow's theory evolved to be known as *Maslow's hierarchy of needs* (see Fig. 8-2).

Maslow first described his theory of human motivation and related needs in 1943. His theory identifies a hierarchical set of five basic human needs that motivate the human person and allow for growth toward what Maslow describes as *self-actualization*. Maslow points out that the human consciousness is able to reach toward attaining higher goals once more basic goals, or needs, are met. The most basic of the five needs includes physiologic needs such as food, water, air, shelter, sex, and other basic needs for general survival. Once met, the individual may seek to satisfy safety needs such as security; stability; protection; and freedom from fear, anxiety, and chaos. Safety needs also include the need for order, structure, and limits. The third set of needs is grouped as belongingness and love needs, including the need for love; affection; a sense of belongingness; and family, friends, groups, and community. Esteem needs follow as the fourth set and include the need for self-esteem, self-confidence, esteem of others, achievement, recognition, appreciation, and dignity and mastery over one's self and one's environment. Self-actualization is achieved when one meets the needs of self-mastery, gains a desire to help others, has the ability to direct one's own life, has rich emotional experiences, and develops a sense of meaning to one's life.

Nursing has a unique appreciation of Maslow's hierarchy of needs because threats to homeostasis as the result of stress and illness can impair an individual's ability to satisfy even the most basic of needs. Throughout the nursing process, you will apply Maslow's hierarchy of needs to understand your patient's needs and develop the most appropriate interventions designed to meet these needs based on your assessment of unmet needs along the hierarchy. Disturbances in health, or homeostasis, represent potential threats to the patient's ability to meet his or her needs across the hierarchy.

According to Maslow, healthy, self-actualized individuals possess several characteristics:

- An accurate perception of reality
- The ability to accept oneself and others
- The ability to be spontaneous
- The ability to solve problems
- A need for privacy
- Independence or autonomy
- The ability to express the self emotionally
- A frequency of "peak experiences" (i.e., happy moments that produce a sense of worth, hope, and love of life)
- Identification with humankind
- The ability to maintain satisfactory relationships
- A sense of ethics
- Some sense of resistance to conformity

STRESS

The word *stress* has different meanings depending on the context or science in which it is used. In the science of physics, for example, **stress** refers to the internal distribution of forces exerted on a material body or structure. Think of a bridge crossing over a river. The bridge must be able to bear weight (i.e., stress) sufficiently to maintain its structural integrity. The word *stress* was first used in biology by the endocrinologist Hans Selye, who investigated the physiologic responses of living organisms to changes in the internal environment (physical) and external environment. The term *stress* was later broadened to refer to real and perceived challenges (i.e., stressors) and responses experienced by human beings.

Stressors can originate in any or all of the dimensions of the self. At any given moment, individuals are adapting to a variety of stressors from each of the five dimensions. Thus a person's level of health is directly related to the ability to adjust to a variety of internal and external stressors. A **stressor** can be anything, positive or negative, that necessitates an adaptive response on the part of the individual. Stress is necessary for growth and development. Mild stress produces mild anxiety and enables people to use energy focused exclusively on the problem. The result can be successful problem solving, which in turn promotes self-esteem. However, stress can also be perceived as harmful. Examples of potentially harmful stressors are the loss of a job or the death of a family member.

Adaptation refers to a person's biologic and psychologic efforts to respond to a stressor and affects the whole organism. For example, the normal stress associated with physical activity and exercise results in maintaining or building muscle mass, circulation, and joint flexibility. If a person becomes immobilized, the lack of stress (i.e., exercise) may result in the muscles beginning to atrophy, joints becoming rigid and inflexible, and so on, until all systems of the body are affected. So it is with mental health. The dimensions of the person—physical, cognitive, affective, behavioral, and social—are not separate entities. These dimensions interact, resulting in the development of a unique human being.

HOMEOSTASIS

Stress, response, and adaptation can be thought of as a process aimed at maintaining homeostasis or equilibrium. If stressors are relatively mild and the person is able to respond and adapt, mental health is maintained. However, if the person is overwhelmed by many stressors or does not have sufficient coping behaviors or problem-solving strategies to maintain equilibrium, illness or crisis may ensue. A **crisis** results in inner tension and anxiety, which may affect an individual's ability to function.

PERSONALITY

Individuals' personalities affect their reactions to stress and illness. Although there are many different theories of **personality**, it is generally accepted that personality consists of the characteristic patterns of thoughts, feelings, and behaviors that make a person unique. Personality is made up of permanent traits that give consistency and individuality to a person's behavior. Thus people generally respond to and act in the same or similar ways in a variety of situations.

GROWTH AND DEVELOPMENT

Growth refers to an individual's gradual process of evolution from conception until death. As human beings move through sequential stages of development, they become increasingly complex. Each individual is shaped throughout life by all of the events and perceived interactions with individuals, the community, and the environment. Growth, then, refers not only to a change in physical size and structure but also to an increasingly complex process of development.

Development is usually divided into stages that correspond to a specific age group. Developmental tasks are a part of the work of moving through each of these stages. In part, successful development depends on how individuals negotiate through each stage. Individual experiences influence how people respond to illness.

Infancy and early childhood are times when nurturing is critical and exploration of the world begins. As children grow and progress through school, they must learn the rules of society. Preschoolers must learn to handle joint decision making and interpersonal **conflicts**. Middle childhood is a time for learning to deal with frustration and unfavorable events, while also learning to celebrate good things and feeling pleasure. During adolescence, teenagers learn to develop as individuals, become independent, and begin to think for themselves. They have to learn how to delay gratification, relax, and interact with peers of both genders. In early adulthood, most people find a life partner and life work and may begin a family. Adults progressing through middle age begin to look at the effect their lives have had or could have had on the world around them. Older age is often a time of introspection, when older adults look back on their lives, accept what has been, and attempt to face increasing frailty with grace. Throughout life, individuals strive to make sense of the world by searching for meaning.

BEHAVIORAL THEORY

Behavioral theory is based on the idea that all behaviors are learned responses. Conditioning is one type of learning. A conditioned response was demonstrated by Pavlov, who rang a bell (i.e., stimulus) when feeding (i.e., reinforcement) his dog. The dog would salivate when the food was presented. The reflex response of salivation eventually occurred with the ringing of the bell only. Theorists such as B.F. Skinner, Albert Bandura, and Joseph Wolpe have based their theories on the idea that all behavior is learned and is a series of habitual responses to familiar stimuli.

PSYCHOLOGIC RESPONSES TO ILLNESS

Responses to illness are as unique as patients themselves. Individual responses to illness are related to the individual's personality, life experiences, self-concept, perceptions, values, cultural perspectives, and spiritual beliefs, to name a few. The individual's ability to adapt to stress (i.e., adaptation) is also an important factor in how they will respond to illness.

COPING WITH ILLNESS

Most people see illness as a distressing, abnormal state of being. This state of distress demands that individuals draw from their inner resources to cope. These resources may come from any or all of the following dimensions: physical, cognitive, affective, behavioral, social, and spiritual. For some, the inner strengths drawn from these various dimensions may be sufficient to cope effectively with illness. For others, however, attempts to cope may be ineffective or maladaptive. Nursing intervention is essential in fostering healthy adaptation and coping during times of illness.

A caring attitude is basic to helping a patient cope with illness. Through the trust developed in a therapeutic nurse-patient relationship, the nurse can help the patient to cope with stressors precipitated by illness (see *Patient Teaching* box).

Patient Teaching

Helping Patients and Their Families to Cope with a Serious Diagnosis

Share with patients the following steps to help them deal effectively with the initial diagnosis and make the best possible decisions for themselves and their families:

- *Step 1: Take the time you need.* Do not rush important decisions about your health. In most cases you will have time to carefully examine your options and decide what is best for you.
- *Step 2: Get the support you need.* Look for support from family and friends, people who are going through the same thing you are, and those who have "been there." They can help you to cope with your situation and make informed decisions.
- *Step 3: Talk with members of your health care team.* Good communication with your health care team can help you to feel more satisfied with the care you receive. Research shows it can even have a positive effect on things such as symptoms and pain. Getting a second opinion may help you to feel more confident about your care.
- *Step 4: Seek out information.* When learning about your health problem and its treatment, look for information that is based on a careful review of the latest scientific findings published in medical journals. Be skeptical of websites and other sources that stand to make a profit by influencing your decision.
- *Step 5: Decide on a treatment plan.* Work with your physician and other members of the health care team to decide on a treatment plan that best meets your needs. Research shows that patients who are more involved in their health care tend to get better results and be more satisfied.

Adapted from Agency for Healthcare Research and Quality, Department of Health and Human Services: *Next steps after your diagnosis* (website): www.ahrq.gov/consumer/diaginfo.htm. Accessed November 2, 2014.

To assess an individual's potential for coping with an illness effectively, you need to understand that the ability to cope is affected by various factors. Among these factors are age, cultural beliefs, spirituality, self-concept, family and community resources, emotions, stress, fear, anxiety, loss, grief, and mourning.

Factors That Affect Coping with Illness

Age. Age affects the coping ability of children and adults alike. The developmental process continues throughout the life span. Illness can interfere with developmental progress and the patient's developmental stage can influence how he or she responds to illness. Much stress may be experienced when illness interferes with development. Illness can interfere with a number of adult roles. New or existing relationships, careers, family responsibilities, and a host of other roles may be affected by the onset of illness. An illness can be especially traumatic if a family breadwinner is self-employed or has insufficient health insurance.

When collecting data about the patient's ability to cope with illness, you need to understand that illness is a stressful, disruptive experience regardless of age. It not only disrupts the developmental process of the individual but also has a traumatic effect on spouses, children, and other loved ones. You will play an essential role in helping patients and their loved ones to cope with an illness and the changes that result.

Cultural Beliefs. Culture is a system of symbols shared by a group of humans. Culture is transmitted from each generation to the next and is influenced by other social contexts as well. Culture brings organization and security to people's lives. It provides many of the underlying values and beliefs on which behavior is based. Culture can affect attitudes toward health and illness, diet and eating practices, reaction to pain, and values concerning death and dying. *Ethnicity* is a broader term that denotes a group's affiliation because of shared language, race, and cultural values.

For individuals to be seen as unique, their cultural and ethnic backgrounds must be considered (see *Cultural Considerations* box). This becomes especially important when trying to determine whether patients need assistance in coping with the stresses of illness. Remember, however, that not all people who look as if they belong to a specific cultural or ethnic group because of language, surname, or physical characteristics necessarily identify with any specific group. Effective nursing interventions can be determined only when we understand the patient as a unique individual, not only as Caucasian, African American, or Latino; man or woman; gay or straight.

Cultural Considerations

What Does Culture Have to Do with Illness?

Culture shapes attitudes toward health and illness, nutrition, pain, and death and dying.

When helping patients to cope with illness, you need to recognize that your own racial and cultural background may affect your ability to intervene effectively. This is especially true if the patient's cultural values and your own values differ greatly. It is important to respect the patient, regardless of your own personal beliefs, values, and culture. A judgmental attitude on your part interferes with delivering the best nursing care possible.

In the nursing plan of care, you should consider whether the nursing approach being suggested is relevant to the patient's individual needs. Does the nursing care help patients to deal with stress or does it contribute to stress? Effective care is individualized according to the patient's needs, values, and beliefs.

Spirituality. During the crisis of illness, patients often turn to their spiritual beliefs and values to find meaning in the experience. Patients who perhaps had not thought of themselves as being religious may suddenly have a need to visit with a spiritual counselor. Many patients experience spiritual distress when under the stress of an illness. They may feel that the illness is unfair and that God has betrayed or abandoned them. Sometimes people feel that the illness is a punishment from God for some transgression they believe they have made.

Spiritual distress can be characterized by the following: (1) patients question the meaning of suffering or existence; (2) patients experience a sense of conflict between their personal beliefs (or desires) and their relationship with their God; or (3) patients experience symptoms such as nightmares, sleep disturbances, and alterations in behavior and mood.

To determine whether spirituality is an asset or a liability to the patient's ability to cope with illness, you must understand that all individuals are experts on their own spiritual needs and paths. Patients need an opportunity to express their feelings in a therapeutic and nonjudgmental environment. Simply put, your role is to listen, support, and care. Effective therapeutic nursing interventions enhance the healing process by supporting patients as they work through their spiritual distress and by shoring up their relationship with their spiritual connectedness.

Self-Concept. Self-concept refers to the notions, beliefs, and convictions that persons hold about themselves. It is related to self-esteem and influences a person's relationship with others. **Self-esteem** develops from individuals' own evaluations of their competence and of the value others place on them. Body image refers to the combination of conscious and unconscious attitudes that people have about their own bodies. Past and present perceptions of the body and the person's feelings about their body's size, shape, function, appearance, and potential make up the body image.

Self-concept can be affected by changes in self-esteem and body image. Patients' perception of these changes and their ability or inability to cope with the changes may result in stress, fear, and anxiety. Age and developmental levels may directly affect the patient's self-esteem and body image. Adolescents are especially vulnerable to changes in body image because they have a strong need to look like their peers. Certain changes in body image can be quite traumatic at this developmental stage. Adults also can be vulnerable.

People such as actors, models, or professional football players, who rely on their physical characteristics to make a living, may not be able to cope well with an illness or injury that affects body image. A disfiguring or disabling injury could have a devastating effect on body image and self-esteem. Their personal strengths and weaknesses would determine how well they are able to cope with the threat that illness imposes on the self-concept.

Some patients, through their life experiences, have developed coping styles that allow them to confront problems effectively. Others may require more external resources such as friends, family, and the community to cope with the stress of illness.

Family and Community Resources. The basic functions of the family include providing for physical needs, giving love, providing a sense of belonging, and strengthening the self-esteem of its members. Functional families may provide optimal support for a patient facing the stress of illness. However, the family's ability to provide support for the patient depends on many factors, including the quality of relationships among family members and the family's ability to access needed resources.

Because of increasing stresses on the family unit, many families are not able to provide as much support as the patient may need. The stress of illness in a family member may overburden a family that was already only marginally coping. Illness may have precipitated such stressors as changes in family roles, economic pressures, and geographic isolation that may make it difficult to access medical and other needed resources.

Many of the functions once provided by families increasingly are assumed by social institutions within the community. Like families, communities vary in their ability to assist their members. Some communities are well equipped to assist the family with many challenges that it may face (e.g., financial, physical, legal, spiritual, emotional). Other communities are less able to meet those same needs. This is especially true if the patient lives in an impoverished, underserved, or rural community. Your knowledge of available resources can be invaluable to patients and families. Throughout the hospital stay, you must anticipate the patient's needs before discharge. Providing contact information and creating links for patients in the community to help meet the needs of the patient outside the institution are essential parts of preparing the patient and his or her family for discharge. Local, state, and national organizations can be very helpful resources that may keep a family from succumbing to the pressures of a catastrophic illness.

Emotions. When a serious illness occurs, patients and their families must adapt to many changes. Some of these changes may involve permanent alterations in lifestyle, frequent visits to health care providers, frequent hospitalizations, financial problems, and increased social isolation. For those in crisis, coping can be difficult at best and seemingly impossible at worst.

This section discusses a broad range of feelings and emotions that people may experience. Many of these **feelings** are normal and to be anticipated. However, times exist when the coping methods being used by patients and families are maladaptive. It is important for you to differentiate adaptive from maladaptive coping mechanisms.

Stress. The term *stress* is derived from the Latin word *stringer*, which means *to draw tight*. Stress is any physiologic or psychologic tension that threatens a person's total equilibrium. Stress affects all dimensions of the individual. If prolonged or chronic, it poses a serious threat to physical and emotional health. As the duration or intensity of stress or the number of stressors increases, a person's ability to adapt effectively decreases.

Perceptions of stress and coping mechanisms are highly individualized. People subjected to prolonged stressors eventually became totally exhausted. Individuals who cannot cope adequately with stress may experience a threat to their emotional well-being. They may find their perceptions of reality skewed, their ability to solve problems considerably compromised, and their stress consequently increased. In other words, without effective coping strategies, individuals can be caught in a vicious cycle of ineffective coping and increased stress that will stop only at the point of total exhaustion and may result in death.

You must learn to recognize individuals whose coping skills are ineffective and who consequently are caught in a downward spiral of debilitating exhaustion. Without effective nursing interventions to reverse this downward spiral, serious impairment will result.

Fear. The words *fear* and *anxiety* often are used interchangeably. However, fear generally denotes a response to a specific threat and anxiety is often a response to a nonspecific threat. The body's physiologic reaction to fear is similar to its response to anxiety. The person experiencing the crisis of illness has much to fear: pain, financial ruin, disfigurement, loss of self-esteem, and not being able to return to a previous lifestyle.

Fears vary according to the developmental status and age of the individual. For example, toddlers may fear separation from their mothers whereas adolescents may fear threats to their body image. Terminally ill patients may be struggling with fears of death and dying.

You can be very helpful in assisting patients and families to cope with fear. Sometimes just allowing an opportunity to express fear helps to lessen the stress caused by fear. Providing information about tests or surgical procedures may empower clients to begin to cope with fear. However, too much information also can be very stressful. In deciding how much information to provide, you must assess the patient's current understanding of the situation and any anticipated procedures he or she may be about to face. Providing basic information and then following up by answering the patient's questions is usually best.

Anxiety. **Anxiety** is a vague and sometimes intense sense of impending doom or apprehension that may appear to have no clearly identifiable cause. Anxiety is often an early response to illness. The degree of anxiety may vary with the severity of the illness. Anxiety may lead to physical and psychologic stress and may be caused by real or imagined fear resulting from loss. As people develop, they learn to cope with this painful emotion. The fight-or-flight response actually provides the physiologic ability for one to either fight or flee. Individuals continually regulate their behavior based on their level of perceived anxiety. When anxiety intensifies to an excessive level, the perception of reality becomes focused solely on the crisis.

Loss. Loss is an experience usually related to the involuntary separation of the self from someone or something loved or treasured. It may involve a separation from a person or object, relationship, personal attribute, hope, dream, desire, role, functional ability, or potential. Perceived loss of control, sense of worth, and loss of health are also types of loss.

Actual loss can be recognized by others as well as by the patients. Examples of actual loss include the loss of a spouse or the loss of a limb. *Anticipatory loss* is a sense of loss experienced before the actual loss occurs. Families may experience anticipatory loss during the terminal stages of a loved one's illness.

Loss can be a significant stressor that precipitates feelings of fear and anxiety. The fears associated with loss can be stressful enough to compromise the ability of an individual to recover from illness. One of the first psychologic steps that must be taken to begin the process of coping is to permit oneself to experience the full emotional effect of the loss. This emotional response is known as *grief* or *mourning*.

The experience of loss is related to the individual's self-concept. The extent of loss depends on how strongly the individual's sense of self was connected to that which was lost.

Grief and Mourning. Grief is the subjective, emotional response that evolves from a sense of loss. Mourning is the process through which grief is faced and ultimately resolved or altered over time. Mourning occurs when a person is forced to relinquish original hopes. The process of mourning prepares the individual to reappraise values and to accept substitutions for hope.

Individuals who are experiencing grief may be under a great deal of stress and that stress may make them even more vulnerable to disease. They may become irritable and difficult to get along with; sometimes they may experience a sense of guilt. Some people blame themselves for whatever they have lost. They may perceive their illness and subsequent loss as a punishment from God for not having been a better person, a better parent, or a better spouse.

To alter the loss that grief causes, the self must change. The process of change is unique to each individual and each circumstance. One individual's need for change may require only a change in exercise and dietary habits. Another person's need for change may encompass a career, a lifestyle, or the development of better strategies to cope with stress. Most changes in a person's life are stressful. The greater the change, the greater the resulting stress. To cope with stress, the individual may mobilize psychologic resources known as *coping mechanisms*. Adaptive coping mechanisms can be effective, therapeutic ways of dealing with stress. **Maladaptive coping** behaviors, however, can be detrimental and decrease the ability to cope with illness. Chapter 24 addresses loss and grief in detail.

COPING MECHANISMS AND STRATEGIES

Coping is the process of responding to stress or a potential stressor. Coping with stress is a self-regulatory process by which people manage their responses to stress and thus relieve the tension related to the stressor. Coping strategies can be conscious or unconscious behaviors. Unconscious coping strategies are referred to as **defense mechanisms**.

Defense Mechanisms

According to Freud, the ego may devise strategies or defense mechanisms to cope with stress or anxiety. Defense mechanisms are used in an effort to diminish anxiety; however, when used excessively or inappropriately, they can hinder the developing personality. Defense mechanisms used to protect against anxiety include the following:

- *Compensation*—an attempt to make up for real or imagined weakness. For example, an adolescent perceived as unattractive becomes an outstanding athlete.
- *Denial*—a refusal to acknowledge a real situation. For example, a woman who finds a suspicious lump in her breast does not keep an appointment for a breast biopsy.
- *Displacement*—transferring the associated feelings from one source to another that is considered less threatening. For example, a boy who is angry with a teacher comes home and yells at his dog.
- *Identification*—the emulation of admirable qualities in another to enhance one's self-esteem. For example, a child dresses and uses mannerisms similar to those of a famous rock star.
- *Rationalization* or *intellectualization*—the use of logic, reasoning, and analysis to avoid unacceptable feelings. For example, a student fails to complete an assignment correctly and rationalizes subsequent feelings of incompetence by complaining about the teacher's expectations for the assignment.
- *Introjection*—internalizing or taking on the values and beliefs of another person. For example, a child takes on the values and beliefs of a parent.
- *Isolation*—the separation of emotion from an associated thought or memory. For example, a man appears apathetic as he discusses a firefight in which he participated in Vietnam.
- *Projection*—transferring unacceptable feelings or impulses to another. For example, a partner who is jealous of her significant other accuses the partner of being jealous.
- *Reaction formation*—avoiding unacceptable thoughts and behaviors by expressing opposing thoughts or behaviors. For example, a patient who unconsciously hates his father continuously says how great his father is.
- *Regression*—withdrawing to an earlier level of development to benefit from the associated comfort levels of the previous level. For example, a child starts sucking her thumb when her new brother comes home from the hospital.
- *Repression*—an unconscious defense mechanism in which unacceptable ideas, impulses, and memories are kept out of consciousness. For example, a woman cannot remember a sexual assault.
- *Somatization*—the transfer of painful feelings to body parts, so that the person's feelings are expressed in the form of a physical symptom. For example, a woman who has experienced intolerable internal conflict develops a physical complaint of pain in the wrist that cannot be explained by diagnostic means.
- *Sublimation*—the transformation of unacceptable impulses or drives (e.g., aggressiveness, anger, sexuality) into constructive or more acceptable behavior. For example, a person who has aggressive tendencies becomes a jackhammer operator.
- *Suppression*—(a conscious mechanism) a conscious or voluntary inhibition of unacceptable ideas, impulses, and memories. For example, a child who fails an algebra class puts that event out of his or her mind.
- *Undoing*—actually or symbolically attempting to cancel out an action that was unacceptable. An example is sprinkling salt over one's left shoulder to prevent bad luck after spilling salt on the table.
- *Substitution*—replacing a highly valued, unattainable object with a less-valued, attainable object. For example, the person who has a strong unconscious sexual attraction to a parent marries someone who resembles that parent.
- *Conversion*—turning an emotional conflict into a physical symptom, which provides the individual with some sort of benefit (secondary gain). For example, the individual who witnesses a murder then experiences sudden blindness without an organic cause.

Individuals adapt defense mechanisms as protective measures to allow the ego relief from anxiety. One factor that enhances the development of ego is an environment with experiences that match the child's capacity to adapt. Ideally, unhealthy defense mechanisms are shed and replaced by more realistic and efficient methods of adaptation as the individual matures.

Conscious Coping Strategies

Conscious coping strategies are purposeful behaviors that are used to make an unfamiliar situation into one that is perceived as more controllable and predictable. Coping strategies and mechanisms vary from

Put on Your Thinking Cap!

Recall two incidents when you recognized a defense mechanism being used to cope. Describe the behavior, label the mechanism, and indicate the positive and negative outcomes of the mechanism. Share and discuss this with your classmates.

individual to individual. What all these behaviors have in common is that they are attempts to help people feel less stressed and anxious about their illness. Some of these methods provide only temporary relief while others provide more permanent results. It is important for you to identify and evaluate the effectiveness of coping mechanisms used by the patient.

Some techniques that can be used to help patients cope are known as *relaxation techniques*. Relaxation techniques include interventions such as imagery, relaxation strategies, therapeutic touch, and music therapy. Relaxation techniques elicit the relaxation response that reduces the effects of stress and decreases anxiety. These techniques can provide clients with self-control during moments of stress. Relaxation techniques are taught only when patients are not in acute discomfort because the exercise will be ineffective if the patient cannot concentrate. *Imagery* is the use of the imagination to develop sensory images that focus the mind away from the stressful experience and emphasize other sensory experiences and pleasant memories. *Relaxation strategies* include biofeedback, meditation, deep-breathing exercises, yoga, and Zen practices. *Therapeutic touch* is a process by which the therapist acts as a channel for environmental and universal energy through the therapist's mental concentration.

Music therapy is another relaxation technique that may help the patient to cope by enhancing the relaxation response and facilitating positive imagery. Musical selections should match a patient's mood and musical taste. Earphones with audio CDs or cassettes help the patient to avoid annoying others and allow him or her to concentrate on the music. This coping method provides only temporary relief of stress; however, use of such techniques can help to establish a therapeutic environment in which you can begin to discuss the real sources of the patient's concerns, fears, and anxieties.

Tapping into the spiritual dimension also can be a very effective way of coping with the stress of illness. You can talk with patients about their spiritual needs without relying on traditional religious language. The opportunity to discuss beliefs about a higher power or the search for meaning in suffering proves to be an effective way of coping for many patients.

MALADAPTIVE COPING MECHANISMS AND STRATEGIES

In an effort to reduce the stress and anxiety that is precipitated by the crisis of an illness, an individual may sometimes engage in thinking patterns or behaviors that are ineffective or even self-destructive. These ineffective coping mechanisms may evolve from a sense of helplessness or powerlessness.

Helplessness

Helplessness typically occurs when individuals have had repeated exposure to events they perceive as being uncontrollable. This leads to loss of motivation, feelings of despair or anxiety, and cognitive impairment. The individual may begin to express anger as a means of diminishing feelings of helplessness. This anger may take the form of a personal attack on you and other caregivers. The expression of anger is really not aimed at you but is simply an attempt to cope with feelings of loss of control. Helplessness can be prevented by allowing individuals to control as many events as possible within the constraints imposed by treatment and their energy level.

Powerlessness

Powerlessness is a feeling that one's actions cannot affect an outcome or that one lacks personal control over certain events or situations. Characteristics of powerlessness include nonparticipation in care of decision making when opportunities are provided, reluctance to express feelings, passivity, submissiveness, apathy, feelings of hopelessness, and expressions of having no control or influence over a situation or outcome (Gulanick, Myers, Klopp, Galanes, Gradishar, & Puzas, 2009). When people are not ready to cope with the threat of illness, unconscious defense mechanisms of avoidance, such as denial, may be used. These avoidance defense mechanisms protect individuals from having to confront and deal with the threat of illness.

Denial

Denial is the subconscious blocking out of emotional experiences. Denial can take several forms: (1) verbal denial, (2) minimizing the severity of the illness, (3) displacing symptoms onto another organ system, and (4) engaging in behaviors contrary to medical advice. The outcome of denial may be positive or negative. Denial can lead to negative consequences if people fail to engage in appropriate problem-focused behaviors. Patients who claim that they were never afraid or insist that nothing is wrong with them are engaging in denial. Denial is maladaptive when the patient's behavior interferes significantly with obtaining appropriate care. Arguing with patients about their denial only reinforces the inappropriate behavior.

When working with people in denial, make a special effort to accept them even though it may be uncomfortable to care for individuals who deny their illnesses. You may need to allow the individual to deny the illness and at the same time ask for cooperation. Once an effective therapeutic nurse-patient relationship has been established, patients may be better able to lower unconscious defenses and begin to discuss true feelings of fear and anxiety.

NURSING PROCESS IN ILLNESS

In this section the various steps of the nursing process are discussed to help you collect relevant data and help to plan nursing interventions that will facilitate the patient's task of dealing with the crisis of illness.

ASSESSMENT

An individual's ability to cope with an illness varies from moment to moment and from situation to situation. Therefore assessment must be an ongoing process. To determine the effectiveness of individual coping strategies, seek answers to the following questions:

- Do individuals see themselves as effective in coping with their illness?
- What efforts have individuals made to seek information about their situation?
- How skillful are individuals in caring for themselves?
- What resources do individuals believe are available to them in dealing with their illness?
- Do individuals effectively adhere to their medical regimen?
- Do individuals feel that they have been able to keep a sense of normalcy in their lives despite their illness?
- How have individuals and their families been able to cope with any role modification that the illness has brought about?
- Have individuals been able to maintain a sense of hope in spite of the demands of the illness?
- Do individuals feel that the important relationships in their life remain intact?

Data collected by the licensed vocational nurse/licensed practical nurse (LVN/LPN) can help to answer these questions. After problem areas have been identified, meaningful nursing diagnoses can be formulated.

NURSING DIAGNOSIS

The purpose of a nursing diagnosis is to clearly identify and frame patient problems. The nursing diagnosis leads to the formulation of a plan of care that includes nursing interventions to help patients achieve their desired goals. Patients and their families must be included in the process so that nursing care plans are based on patients' values and perceptions of the problems. The following are a few nursing diagnoses often identified in persons with inadequate coping:

- Anxiety
- Caregiver role strain
- Chronic sorrow
- Complicated grieving
- Compromised family coping
- Decisional conflict
- Defensive coping
- Delayed growth and development
- Disturbed body image
- Disturbed personal identity
- Fatigue
- Fear
- Ineffective coping
- Ineffective denial
- Ineffective role performance
- Ineffective sexuality pattern
- Interrupted family processes
- Powerlessness
- Readiness for enhanced sleep
- Risk for loneliness
- Sexual dysfunction
- Situational low self-esteem
- Social isolation
- Spiritual distress

These serve only as examples of nursing diagnoses that could be identified for patients and their families. Appropriate nursing diagnoses follow a careful nursing assessment and are formulated once the patient and the family have had a chance to contribute by sharing their perception of the problem or problems. Patients or family members need to agree that the identified problems are important ones if effective coping is to take place. This is especially true if a patient has a long-term or chronic illness.

NURSING GOALS, OUTCOME CRITERIA, AND INTERVENTIONS

The goal of nursing care is to help people manage and successfully cope with their illness. When effective coping strategies are used, patients can manage their illness and adapt to a new lifestyle that incorporates healthy behaviors and realistic goals. In addition, patients should emerge from the process with a positive self-concept and self-esteem.

People with chronic, debilitating illnesses may have difficulty acquiring and maintaining coping skills for long periods of time. Individuals may be able to cope with their illness today but tomorrow may bring a whole new set of challenges. This is especially true in terminal stages of illness, when physical deterioration is on an accelerated course and every day brings new losses that need to be mourned and coped with by the patient and family.

Nursing interventions are based on identified nursing diagnoses (see the Sample Nursing Care Plan: Patient Coping with Illness Ineffectively).

Sample Nursing Care Plan **Patient Coping with Illness Ineffectively**

Nursing Diagnosis	Goal and Outcome Criteria	Interventions
Ineffective Coping related to feelings of powerlessness, as evidenced by the patient's verbalization, "I don't know if I can live through this."	Patient will demonstrate more effective coping, as evidenced by verbalization that he or she feels more capable of dealing with the demands of the illness.	1. Give the patient an opportunity to verbalize feelings of powerlessness by approaching patient care in an unhurried manner. 2. Determine the patient's and family's current coping strategies and behaviors. 3. Conduct teaching sessions with the patient and family to enhance their coping skills and empower the patient to begin self-care. 4. Provide community resource information and encourage the patient to ask for help from others. 5. Implement stress reduction strategies (e.g., music therapy) to help the patient cope with stressful moments.

Get Ready for the NCLEX® Examination!

Key Points

- Individuals' level of health is directly related to their ability to adjust to a variety of internal and external stressors.
- Stress is necessary for growth and development.
- A stressor is anything that causes the individual stress and adaptation to stress affects the entire organism.
- Illness or crisis may ensue if individuals are overwhelmed by many stressors or do not have the coping behaviors or problem-solving strategies necessary to maintain equilibrium.
- A crisis is the point at which the individual may move toward illness on the continuum between illness and health; it can result in inner tension and anxiety, which may affect an individual's ability to function.
- Growth refers to a process of development that becomes increasingly complex.
- Anxiety is a painful emotion that results from one's perception of danger and individuals continually regulate their behavior based on the level of perceived anxiety.
- Defense mechanisms are strategies used in an effort to diminish anxiety; however, when unconscious defense mechanisms are used excessively, they can hinder the developing personality.
- Behavioral theory is based on the idea that all behavior is a learned response.
- Each person's response to illness is unique and is based on such subjective experiences as self-concept, perception of threat to body image, and spiritual and cultural values.
- Illness produces a stressful state that requires individuals to draw on their innate resources or inner strengths.
- Some people have enough inner strength to cope effectively with illness; others may have ineffective or maladaptive coping abilities.
- Factors that influence an individual's ability to cope with illness are age, cultural beliefs, spirituality, self-concept, family and community resources, and emotional responses to illness.
- Specific emotional responses to illness include stress, fear, anxiety, loss, and grief and mourning.
- Coping is the process of responding to stress or a potential stressor.
- Coping strategies are conscious, purposeful behaviors that are used to make an unfamiliar situation into one that is perceived as more controllable and predictable.
- Ineffective coping mechanisms may evolve from a sense of helplessness or powerlessness.
- A nurse's caring and nonjudgmental attitude is basic to helping a client cope with illness.

Additional Learning Resources

SG Go to your Study Guide for additional learning activities to help you master this chapter content.

evolve Go to your Evolve website (http://evolve.elsevier.com/Linton/medsurg) for the following learning resources and much more:

- Interactive Prioritization Exercises
- Fluid & Electrolyte Tutorial
- Pharmacology Tutorial
- Review Questions for the NCLEX® Examination

Review Questions for the NCLEX® Examination

1. The statement "Sometimes I feel so overwhelmed and sad" reflects which dimension of a human being?
   1. Cognitive
   2. Affective
   3. Behavioral
   4. Social

   NCLEX CLIENT NEED: Psychosocial Integrity
2. Which of the following are characteristic of stress? (Select all that apply.)
   1. Requires the individual to adapt
   2. May be a negative or positive experience
   3. Increases with ineffective coping
   4. Affects all dimensions of the individual

   NCLEX CLIENT NEED: Psychosocial Integrity

3. Developmental tasks of old age include which of the following? (Select all that apply.)
   1. Learn how to delay gratification
   2. Find a life partner and life work
   3. Face increasing frailty with grace
   4. Accept what has been

   NCLEX CLIENT NEED: Health Promotion and Maintenance
4. Which of the following is the primary difference between fear and anxiety?
   1. Anxiety is much more disabling than fear.
   2. Anxiety indicates that the patient has poor coping skills.
   3. Anxiety interferes with effective problem solving more than fear does.
   4. Anxiety is evoked by a nonspecific threat rather than a specific threat.

   NCLEX CLIENT NEED: Psychosocial Integrity
5. Which statement suggests that the patient is experiencing spiritual distress?
   1. "The medication that you gave me is not relieving my pain."
   2. "I think my cancer is punishment for the bad things I have done."
   3. "I will never be able to perform again with these terrible scars."
   4. "My family is too busy to come see me and do things for me."

   NCLEX CLIENT NEED: Psychosocial Integrity
6. Which data best support a nursing diagnosis of disturbed body image?
   1. The patient states that he is just glad to be alive, despite some paralysis.
   2. Although the burns have healed well, the patient refuses to go out in public.
   3. The patient dresses every morning, brushes her hair, and applies her makeup.
   4. During the dressing change, the patient carefully examines her incision.

   NCLEX CLIENT NEED: Psychosocial Integrity
7. Which of the following is the basic function of defense mechanisms?
   1. To enhance self-esteem
   2. To avoid reality
   3. To disguise true feelings
   4. To reduce anxiety

   NCLEX CLIENT NEED: Psychosocial Integrity
8. A 9-year-old girl likes to wear her 14-year-old sister's nail polish and tries to fix her hair like the older sister's. Of which of the following is this an example?
   1. Regression
   2. Introjection
   3. Identification
   4. Projection

   NCLEX CLIENT NEED: Psychosocial Integrity
9. The benefits of relaxation strategies include reduced effects of stress and decreased ______________.
   1. Anxiety
   2. Cholesterol
   3. Denial
   4. Avoidance

   NCLEX CLIENT NEED: Psychosocial Integrity and Health Promotion and Maintenance
10. Mrs. A has been in a long-term care facility for 6 months. She has given up participation in group activities, rarely leaves her room, and is fretful and irritable. Her behavior is characteristic of which of the following?
    1. Denial
    2. Isolation
    3. Helplessness
    4. Regression

    NCLEX CLIENT NEED: Psychosocial Integrity
11. What term is used to refer to a person's biologic and psychologic efforts to respond to a stressor?
    1. Adaptation
    2. Accommodation
    3. Acclimation
    4. Acquiescence

    NCLEX CLIENT NEED: Psychosocial Integrity

chapter 56

Psychiatric Disorders

Mary Ann Matteson

http://evolve.elsevier.com/Linton/medsurg

Objectives

1. Describe the differences between social relationships and therapeutic relationships.
2. Describe key strategies in communicating therapeutically.
3. Describe the components of the mental status examination.
4. Identify target symptoms, behaviors, and potential side effects for the following types of medications: antianxiety (anxiolytic), antipsychotic, and antidepressant drugs.
5. Summarize current thinking about the cause of schizophrenia and major depressive and bipolar disorders.
6. Identify key features of the mental status examination and their relevance in anxiety disorders, schizophrenia, major depressive and bipolar disorders, cognitive disorders, and personality disorders.
7. Identify common nursing diagnoses, goals, and interventions for persons with anxiety disorders, schizophrenia and schizoaffective disorders, major depressive and bipolar disorders, cognitive disorders, and personality disorders.

Key Terms

Biologic approach (bī-ō-LŎ-jĭk)
Cognitive-behavioral approach
Denial (dē-NĪ-ăl)
Depersonalization (dē-PĔR-sŭn-ŭl-ĭ-ZĀ-shŭn)
Extrapyramidal side effects (EPS) (ĕks-tră-pĭ-RĂM-ĭ-dăl)
Interpersonal approach
Parkinsonian syndrome
Projection
Psychoanalytic approach (sī-kō-ăn-ă-LĬT-ĭk)
Psychosis (sī-KŌ-sĭs)
Repression
Schizoaffective disorder
Schizophrenia (skĭ-zō-FRĔN-ē-ŭh)
Sensorium (sĕn-SŌ-rē-ŭm)
Tardive dyskinesia (TĂR-dĭv dĭs-kĭ-NĒ-zē-ă)

How people think about and explain mental health and mental illness has varied from one geographic location and culture to another and from one time period to another. In early cultures, people believed that supernatural forces were responsible for mental illness. People used rituals to appeal to these supernatural forces to cure mental illnesses. It is now understood that many factors contribute to the development of a mental illness and many strategies are available for helping people with psychiatric disorders. Treatment settings include outpatient, intensive outpatient, partial hospitalization, and inpatient hospitalization as well as residential settings. Within these settings, treatment methods include milieu therapy, individual psychotherapy, group or family psychotherapy, educational groups, and treatment with medications. New and safer medications allow treatment primarily on an outpatient basis. Nursing interventions are diverse and geared toward helping patients and families to cope with the mental illness, manage their lives, and enhance quality of life. Mental illness and mental health exist along a continuum. Some people who are experiencing a psychiatric disorder may experience acute symptoms and require hospitalization. Others may have chronic and persistent mental illnesses. Therefore nursing interventions are delivered in many settings, including the hospital and the community.

Nurses who work with patients in other health care settings such as medical clinics, medical and surgical inpatient units, or intensive care units also see patients who have psychiatric difficulties along with their other health problems. Therefore the ability to provide a high quality of nursing care to patients with mental illness in any work setting is important.

Nursing interventions are based on a number of theoretic approaches, which are described according to biologic, psychoanalytic, interpersonal, cognitive-behavioral, and other theories.

The **biologic approach** assumes that mental disorders are related to physiologic changes within the central nervous system (CNS). In this approach, mental illness is managed with medications, much as any other acute or chronic illness—such as diabetes—is managed. The biologic approach dominates much of the current thinking about psychiatric disorders but is only one aspect of treatment.

The **psychoanalytic approach** is based on the theory that (1) humans function at different levels of awareness, ranging from conscious to unconscious; and (2) people use ego defense mechanisms, such as **repression, denial,** and **projection,** to prevent or minimize anxiety.

The **interpersonal approach** has three components: (1) anxiety is often communicated interpersonally, (2) the patient learns new ways of coping or maturing in a therapeutic relationship, and (3) the establishment of trust is an important first step in working with patients.

Key ideas from the **cognitive-behavioral approach** are that (1) behavior is learned, (2) behavior increases as a result of a response to that behavior from the environment (i.e., reinforcement), and (3) the way a person thinks about things (his or her thoughts) influences emotional states and behavior.

Put on Your Thinking Cap!

Four patients are receiving different treatments for mental illness. An aspect of each type of treatment is listed below. Can you identify the theoretic approach behind each treatment?

- A patient is helped to develop new coping skills through a therapeutic relationship.
- A patient is guided to recall events that could be related to her present illness.
- A patient is helped to understand the consequences of his behavioral patterns.
- A patient is prescribed an antianxiety (anxiolytic) drug.

ESTABLISHING THERAPEUTIC RELATIONSHIPS

In caring for a patient with a psychiatric disorder, you must first establish a therapeutic (rather than a social) relationship (Table 56-1). A range of interpersonal strategies has been found to be particularly helpful in promoting the patient's level of comfort with the nurse. They include being available, listening, clarifying, sharing observations, and accepting silence. Therapeutic use of self is key to providing good care to patients with psychiatric illness, avoiding advice giving, and assisting patients at their level of comprehension.

Table 56-1 Therapeutic Relationships versus Social Relationships

THERAPEUTIC	SOCIAL
• Purpose is to benefit the patient.	• Purpose is to benefit both participants in the relationship.
• Relationship develops purposefully.	• Relationship develops spontaneously.
• Focus is on personal and emotional needs of patient.	• Focus is on personal and emotional needs of both participants.
• Helper has responsibility for evaluating the interaction and the changing behavior.	• Participants are not formally responsible for evaluating their interaction.
• Relationship has some boundaries (i.e., purpose, place, time) and a clear ending.	• Relationship may or may not have clear boundaries and a clear ending.

BEING AVAILABLE

When you are working with a patient, direct all of your attention completely toward that person. Avoid involvement in any other activity, such as reading a newspaper or watching television, that might be interpreted by the patient as lack of availability. Avoid interruptions in your conversation with the patient as much as possible.

LISTENING

Use empathy when you are listening to the patient. Concentrate on what the patient is saying and remember that you are trying to hear how he or she experiences and describes his or her life. When listening therapeutically, make every effort to avoid cutting the patient off or jumping to conclusions. You are trying to get the essence of how the patient perceives his or her situation, experiences certain symptoms, and describes his or her circumstances.

To listen well, you must be aware of your own thoughts and feelings. These feelings are an important source of data for you because you may experience a wide range of feelings while interacting with patients. If you are aware of your own feelings, you will be able to manage your physical (body language) and verbal responses. Listening is done by concentrating on the patient and by refraining from thinking of responses while the patient is speaking.

CLARIFYING

Clarifying is one way of validating that you understand what the patient is saying. For example, you might ask, "So what you are saying is that you are feeling very sad right now?" Asking questions also may help patients to clarify their thoughts. For example, if a patient says, "I have problems at home," you might ask, "What is happening at home that is troubling you?" If a patient states, "My world is falling apart," you might say, "Tell me more about what you mean when you say, 'My world is falling apart.'" It is helpful to avoid the word *why* when asking questions. For example, instead of asking, "Why do you feel that way?" try asking "How did you come to feel that way?"

SHARING OBSERVATIONS

Patients benefit from knowing what you see and hear while listening. For example, you might say, "You are saying that your life is falling apart and I notice that you are fidgeting and tapping your foot. It looks like this is really difficult for you." This statement provides the patient with input that he or she is heard and that you are really listening.

ACCEPTING SILENCE

Sometimes it is therapeutic to allow moments of silence between you and the patient. This is called *therapeutic silence.* It is important that you feel comfortable with silence because silence enables patients to consider their own thoughts as well as what you are communicating to them. Although they may feel strange at first, silences allow patients to sort through their feelings and organize their thinking.

NURSING ASSESSMENT OF THE PSYCHIATRIC PATIENT

The nursing assessment of a patient with mental illness provides the foundation for nursing diagnoses and development of the plan of care. The observations of the licensed vocational nurse/licensed practical nurse (LVN/LPN) contribute important data to the assessment. In addition to the usual data for the physical assessment, you will want to understand what brings the patient to the care setting where you are practicing. This is often called the *chief complaint.* Ask the patient to tell you what has been happening recently that has caused him or her to seek treatment. The next section of the assessment is sometimes referred to as the *history of the present illness.* In contrast to the chief complaint, which is typically brief, the history of the present illness is a narrative description of the symptoms and acuity, onset, duration, and length of time each symptom has been present. These data elements provide clues to determine nursing diagnoses. After the patient has explained these factors, inquire about the person's past psychiatric history by asking the patient if he or she has ever felt like this before. You should also ask if the patient has been treated in the past for anxiety, depression, or other mental health problems. Included in the past psychiatric history are past hospitalizations and outpatient treatment. This information adds to the nursing assessment and will assist in developing the proper plan of care.

Another component of the assessment is listing medications the patient has been taking, including both medications taken to treat psychiatric problems and all other medications and over-the-counter (OTC) medications, herbal remedies, and vitamin supplements. A family and social history is collected to document family history of mental illness, substance abuse, current family configuration, employment or school activities, and resources available to the patient. Collecting information on current and recent use of tobacco, alcohol, prescription drugs, and abused drugs is also essential to determine if the patient is at risk for substance-related problems such as withdrawal (see *Complementary and Alternative Therapies* box). This also provides information on how the patient may attempt to cope with stressors.

Complementary and Alternative Therapies

Be aware of any herbal supplements the patient is taking. Some can interact with drugs used for mental illness.

Another major feature of a complete health assessment of a psychiatric patient is the mental status examination. This examination is usually conducted as part of the admission process and is an ongoing assessment tool throughout the course of treatment. It consists of observations regarding appearance, psychomotor activity, mood and affect, speech and language, thought content, perceptual disturbances, insight and judgment, sensorium, memory, attention, and general intellectual level. Suicidal thoughts, intentions, and plans are also assessed in the mental status examination. Each of these components is evaluated by collecting the data detailed in Table 56-2.

Nursing diagnoses commonly identified in persons with major psychiatric disorders are derived from the health assessment. Causes, related factors, or both for each diagnosis are quite specific depending on the individual and his or her unique presentation.

Table 56-2 Components of the Mental Status Examination

COMPONENT	RELEVANT DATA
Appearance	Age, clothing, personal hygiene, unusual physical characteristics
Activity	Recent change in activity level, hyperactivity, agitation, psychomotor retardation, repetitive mannerisms, stereotypes
Mood and affect	Happiness, sadness, worry; constricted or expanded feelings; intensity; lability; appropriateness
Speech and language	Mutism, paucity, pressured speech, tangential speech, blocking, loose associations, word salad
Thought content	Obsessions, compulsions, phobias, delusions
Perceptual disturbances	Illusions, hallucinations
Insight and judgment	Potential for suicide
Sensorium	Orientation to time, place, person; level of consciousness
Memory and attention	Remote and recent memory, attention, calculation
General intellectual level	Vocabulary, knowledge of current events, abstract thinking

Therefore you should consult a text specific to nursing diagnoses common to psychiatric and mental health nursing.

MENTAL STATUS EXAMINATION

Appearance

The first step in a mental status examination is to observe how a person looks. Specific data include the following:

- Appearance in relation to stated age (Does the patient look his or her stated age?)
- Appropriateness of clothing in relation to the patient's particular peer group or subculture
- Personal grooming and hygiene
- Unique physical characteristics
- Motor activity

Note any recent change in the patient's activity level (increase or decrease). Other types of activity that are observed include the following:

- Hyperactivity or activity at a level considerably above average purposeful activity
- Agitation or purposeless activity, such as wringing of hands, pacing, picking at clothing, foot tapping
- Psychomotor retardation or a decrease in movement; slowness; delayed actions, thoughts, and speech
- Repetitive movements that are part of a purposeful activity (mannerisms)
- Repetitive movements that are not part of purposeful activity (stereotypy)

Mood and Affect

Mood is a sustained feeling state or emotion that a person experiences in several aspects of life. Mood is assessed in terms of its intensity, depth, duration, and fluctuation. Words that often are used to describe mood include *irritable, anxious, depressed, euphoric, labile* (up and down), and *despairing.*

Affect describes a person's external presentation of a feeling state and emotional responsiveness. Affect ranges from blunted, flat, and constricted to euphoric, expansive, and intense. A normal affect exists when the person's body language, mannerisms, and verbal responses are consistent with the person's mood and within an average range of emotional intensity. Affect is also described according to its appropriateness and congruence. Appropriate affect exists when the person's outward emotional expression matches what he or she is saying or doing. For example, a patient who is discussing sadness and despair may be tearful and look sad. An example of inappropriate affect is when someone tells you that he or she is sad and feeling guilty about something that happened but at the same time is smiling, laughing, and very animated. In the latter example, the affect is considered incongruent with mood.

The intensity of feelings may be increased or decreased (diminished). Feelings also may be stable or consistent rather than labile or rapidly changing.

Speech and Language

Assessment includes characteristics of speech and language. Normally, speech is of appropriate rate, rhythm, and volume. Unusual findings in the assessment of speech include mutism (i.e., not speaking), long pauses before responding, minimal or very little speech (i.e., paucity), and pressured speech (i.e., loud and insistent). Some clues to problems of thought, described in the following section, are evidenced in a person's speech.

Thought Content

Tangential speech may be noted, which means that a patient starts out toward a particular point but veers away and never reaches the point. Tangential speech is commonly an indicator of disorganized thinking. When the person stops speaking before reaching the point, it is called *thought blocking.* Loose associations—continual shifting from topic to topic—and shifting between topics to the point of incoherence ("word salad") also may be noted. Tangential thinking, thought blocking, looseness of associations, and word salad are all noteworthy findings that are related to thought content in speech. Further assessment of thought content includes identifying the following:

- *Obsessions*—repetitious, unwanted thoughts
- *Compulsions*—actions repeatedly carried out in a specific manner; they typically include washing, counting, or checking (Obsessions and compulsions are often closely related.)
- *Phobias*—unrealistic fears of specific objects or situations
- *Delusions*—fixed beliefs that cannot be changed even when there is conflicting evidence
- *Suicidal ideations*—thoughts or plans (or both) of killing oneself

This area must be assessed with clear and direct questions such as "Do you have any thoughts of harming yourself or killing yourself?" Further assessment includes determining whether the patient has constructed any plans to hurt himself or herself. If the patient endorses suicidal ideations, you must ask whether the patient has made any plans to commit suicide. If yes, ask him or her to describe the plans. This information is useful in assessing the lethality of the plans. Another part of the assessment includes determining whether the patient has any means available to carry out a suicide plan. For example, if a patient has planned to shoot himself or herself, is a gun available at home? If the patient has thoughts of overdosing on medication, does the patient have available supplies of medications?

Perceptual Disturbances

Perceptual disturbances may involve any one of the senses such as vision, hearing, taste, touch, and smell. One type of perceptual disturbance is an illusion, in which a specific stimulus, such as a spot on the wall, is misinterpreted (e.g., a spot is perceived as a bug). Another is hallucination, which is a sensory experience that occurs without an external stimulus (e.g., a person sees nonexistent bugs crawling on the floor or feels nonexistent bugs crawling on the skin). Sometimes this is referred to as *internal stimuli.* Evidence of this may include a person sitting alone, talking as if someone were present, or looking around as if someone were talking to or calling the patient.

Insight and Judgment

Insight is the ability of a person to understand the correct cause or meaning of a situation and judgment is the ability to assess a situation accurately and determine the appropriate course of action. Insight and judgment are often considered in relation to suicide potential.

Sensorium

Sensorium focuses on orientation in terms of time, place, person, and self. These data are obtained by asking the patient direct questions (e.g., "What time is it now?" "What day is today?" "Where are we now?" "Can you tell me your name?"). The patient's level of consciousness also is noted. The four levels of consciousness are (1) comatose, (2) stuporous, (3) drowsy, and (4) alert.

Memory and Attention

Remote memory (i.e., memory of the distant past) is assessed by comparing the patient's memory of past events with what is recalled by other reliable historians. If you are collecting data related to recent memory or the ability to recall new information, ask the patient to learn three unrelated words and to recall these words 5 minutes later. A quick way to determine recent memory is to ask what was eaten at the previous meal. Asking the patient to subtract 7s from 100 or 3s from 20 or to spell a word like *world* backward can test the patient's attention as well as his or her ability to calculate (as an aspect of general intellectual level).

General Intellectual Level

General intellectual level is estimated by determining the patient's vocabulary and knowledge of current events. For example, ask the patient to name the president of the United States and the name of the previous president. Abstract thinking is another area of general intellectual level. Data that provide evidence of the intellectual level can be collected by asking the patient to identify the common element of two objects, such as a banana and an apple (e.g., "What do a banana and an apple have in common?"), or asking the patient to interpret proverbs (e.g., "What does the phrase *a rolling stone gathers no moss* mean?").

Suicide Risk Assessment

Assess suicide risk by asking the patient if he or she has had or is currently having any thoughts or ideas about suicide (suicidal ideation). Ask if the patient has ever attempted suicide (past suicide attempts). Asking the patient if he or she ever had or currently has any ideas about how to commit suicide provides information about suicide plans (plans). Finally, ask the patient if he or she ever had or currently has any intention to carry out a plan to commit suicide (intention). The three main elements of suicide risk assessment in the mental status examination are (1) suicidal ideations (thoughts), (2) suicide plans (plans or means of committing suicide), and (3) intent to follow through with a suicide plan (intention).

TYPES OF PSYCHIATRIC DISORDERS

The American Psychiatric Association defines psychiatric disorders in the *Diagnostic and Statistical Manual of Mental Disorders,* Fifth Edition (DSM-V), authored in part by a task force and various work groups consisting of more than 1000 experts. The DSM-V is organized by diagnostic categories (e.g., anxiety disorders, personality disorders). Each disorder is diagnosed according to specific signs and symptoms.

ANXIETY DISORDERS

An anxiety disorder is characterized by excessive fear and anxiety and related behavioral disturbances. According to DSM-V, fear is a response to a real or perceived imminent threat while anxiety is an anticipation of a future threat. Responses to fear are characterized by fight-or-flight and escape behaviors to avoid imminent danger whereas anxiety is associated with cautious and avoidance behaviors in preparation for future danger. Common physical signs and symptoms of anxiety are increased heart rate, elevated blood pressure (BP), sweaty palms, trembling, urinary frequency, diarrhea, a tight sensation in the chest, and difficulty breathing. Psychologic manifestations often include irritability, restlessness, tearfulness, thought blocking, and lack of concentration.

Anxiety is experienced on various levels, ranging from mild to panic stages, depending on each person's subjective experience and ability to cope. Mild anxiety can be useful. It may motivate a person to take constructive action or focus attention on a particular task (e.g., concentrating on an examination). Moderate anxiety often is considered the optimal level for learning to take place. As anxiety progresses to severe or panic levels, however, an individual's ability to think clearly and to solve problems becomes progressively impaired. A person in a panic state may misperceive surrounding events altogether and may react impulsively by running or striking out at others. This may explain instances in which individuals jump from burning buildings despite imminent rescue.

All people experience anxiety. For most people, it is episodic and does not interfere greatly with day-to-day functioning. Even normally well-adjusted people can experience anxiety of panic proportions under significant stress. If anxiety persists at a high level for an extended period and causes significant interference with daily functioning, the person usually is determined to have an anxiety disorder. Examples of anxiety disorders are panic disorder, agoraphobia, obsessive-compulsive disorder (OCD), and posttraumatic stress disorder (PTSD). In general, drugs used for anxiety disorders are benzodiazepines and selective serotonin reuptake inhibitors (SSRIs).

Panic Disorder

In panic disorder the person experiences recurrent panic attacks, which are episodes of intense fear or discomfort that reach a peak within minutes. Panic attacks vary in length, may progress to the point of terror, and are often accompanied by feelings of impending doom. They may be *unexpected,* in which there is no obvious trigger and they seem to occur out of the blue, or *expected,* where there is an obvious trigger that consistently provokes attacks. Physical symptoms of severe anxiety—such as increased pulse, elevated BP, trembling, diaphoresis, shortness of breath, chest pain, nausea, dizziness, and fear of losing control or "going crazy" also are present. All four categories of antidepressants are effective in treating panic disorder.

Specific Phobia

A phobia is a disorder in which the patient experiences a marked and persistent, fear that is excessive, unreasonable, or both. The fear is precipitated by the presence or anticipation of a particular object or situation (e.g., the presence of a spider, as is the case with arachnophobia). The phobia is specific in that it pertains to a specific object or situation (e.g., animals, flying, heights, other people). Patients with specific phobias typically recognize the fear as disproportionate to the object or situation but they may have anxiety or panic when encountering or anticipating the object or situation, resulting in significant distress. These patients work hard at avoiding the object or situation that precipitates these symptoms.

Agoraphobia

The person with agoraphobia is extremely fearful of situations outside the home. This often includes fearfulness that the person may be in a place from which quick escape would be difficult (e.g., a grocery store) or a place where help may be unavailable. The person typically copes by avoiding the anxiety-producing place or situation, often becoming progressively reclusive and very dependent on family and friends. Agoraphobia may occur by itself or together with panic disorder.

Obsessive-Compulsive Disorder

OCD consists of recurrent obsessions (i.e., thoughts), compulsions (i.e., behaviors), or both that produce distress, are time-consuming, and interfere with functioning. Obsessions frequently involve intrusive thoughts about unpleasant or even violent acts that a person cannot stop. For example, a person may be obsessed with the idea of being dirty and needing to wash. Compulsive behaviors typically evolve as a way to reduce the anxiety experienced as a result of obsessive thoughts. Examples of compulsions are hand washing, counting, and checking (e.g., repeated checking to see whether the door is locked). The person experiencing obsessions and compulsions knows that these thoughts and behaviors are not "normal" and may be embarrassed by them. However, if the compulsion is resisted, the internal anxiety may become too overwhelming to handle.

Research has found that neurophysiology plays a role in the origin of this disorder. Some studies have shown that changes in electroencephalography findings are seen in people with OCD. Many people with OCD have considerably reduced their symptoms with a tricyclic antidepressant (TCA) or an SSRI. This phenomenon also suggests that the cause of this disorder may be physiologic rather than a response to some unresolved unconscious conflict as was previously proposed.

Posttraumatic Stress Disorder

PTSD is a cluster of symptoms experienced after a distressing event that is outside the range of normal events (e.g., watching one's family being murdered) and in which the person experienced intense fear, helplessness, horror, or a combination of these feelings. Examples of symptoms include reexperiencing the trauma through repeated and intrusive recall of the event (at times as a flashback); avoiding situations that in some way remind the person of the event; feeling detached from other people; and having a heightened sense of arousal, which is experienced as difficulty falling asleep, hypervigilance, an exaggerated startle response, or a combination of these. Recommended treatment employs psychotherapy and drug therapy. Preferred drugs are SSRIs (fluoxetine, paroxetine, sertraline) and a serotonin–norepinephrine reuptake inhibitor (SRNI) (venlafaxine).

The case of a subject named Patrick provides a clinical example of PTSD with nursing interventions:

> Patrick was admitted to the psychiatric inpatient unit with the diagnosis of PTSD. Two months before admission, he and his co-worker friend were in a truck accident on an overpass. Patrick watched in horror as his friend fell out of the truck, which was hanging over the edge.

The fall killed his friend instantly. Patrick was able to climb out of the passenger side and sustained injuries to his back and legs. He received physical therapy for his injuries. For the past 2 weeks he has been continually preoccupied by the event, has had persistent insomnia and nightmares, repeatedly says that he should have been the one to die, becomes easily irritable, does not show feelings when with others, and jumps whenever he hears a loud noise or someone touches him unexpectedly. The nurse assigned to work with Patrick found him pacing. She remained with him as he paced. The following nursing diagnoses were immediately relevant: anxiety, disturbed sleep pattern, posttrauma syndrome, and complicated grieving. Patrick and the nurse decided together that the priorities were to decrease his anxiety and to improve his sleep. Patrick was willing to learn a progressive relaxation exercise (which involves relaxing one group of muscles at a time until the body is relaxed). After learning the exercise, Patrick worked on deep abdominal breathing and agreed to use this strategy when he found himself preoccupied with the accident. The nurse did not purposefully probe the details of the event but if Patrick had brought it up, she would have listened attentively and offered support and empathy.

Acute Stress Disorder

As in PTSD, the person with acute stress disorder has been exposed to a distressing event that is outside the range of normal events. The event or events have happened recently. The symptoms last from 3 days to 1 month. This disorder is characterized by the following:

- *Intrusion symptoms*—recurrent distressing dreams, recurrent memories of the traumatic event, or flashbacks of the event that in serious cases may occur with complete loss of awareness of present surroundings
- *Negative mood*—persistent inability to experience feelings of happiness, satisfaction, or love
- *Dissociative symptoms*—feeling a sense of detachment; having a reduced awareness of one's surroundings; inability to remember aspects of the traumatic event
- *Avoidance symptoms*—avoiding distressing memories or external reminders of the traumatic event
- *Arousal symptoms*—sleep disturbances, irritability, angry outbursts, problems with concentration, or exaggerated startle response

SOMATIC SYMPTOM DISORDER

Individuals with somatic symptom disorder experience multiple, current physical symptoms that are distressing or result in significant disruption of daily life. The disorder is usually persistent and the symptoms may involve pain predominately. These individuals tend to worry excessively about illness and often think the worst about their health. Some people may fear that their condition is serious even when there is no evidence to support that fear. Excessive time and energy may be devoted to symptoms and health concerns.

Conversion Disorder (Functional Neurologic Symptom Disorder)

In conversion disorder, symptoms may include blindness, deafness, or paralysis of the legs without a physiologic cause. Usually the symptoms are neurologic and occur in response to some threatening or traumatic event. The symptoms are real and not created; they can cause significant distress or impairment in social, occupational, or other important areas of functioning. In some cases a true physiologic cause for the symptoms has been discovered years later; therefore a diagnosis of conversion disorder is usually tentative and provisional.

Illness Anxiety Disorder

In illness anxiety disorder, formerly known as *hypochondriasis*, individuals are preoccupied with having or acquiring a serious, undiagnosed illness. They are convinced that they have a serious medical problem despite the absence of any concrete medical findings. They will seek other opinions if one physician does not validate their concerns and they often take multiple prescription medications from various health care providers. Concern about the feared illness often becomes a central part of people's lives and may impair social, occupational, or other important areas of functioning. In some cases of hypochondriasis, the person does not recognize that the concern about having a serious illness is excessive or unreasonable.

DISSOCIATIVE DISORDERS

Dissociative disorders involve a change in identity, memory, consciousness, motor control, and behavior. The change may be sudden or gradual, may be transient or occur over a long period, and is thought to be an escape from anxiety. In a sense, persons unconsciously dissociate or remove themselves psychologically from anxiety-provoking situations because the situations are too much to bear. Even normal persons may experience **depersonalization** under severe stress. In this case, individuals feel that they are outside of themselves or floating overhead watching what is happening, as if it were happening to someone else. Examples of dissociative disorders are amnesia or dissociative identity disorder (formerly multiple personality disorder).

Dissociative amnesia is characterized by a gap in memory, usually of a traumatic or stressful nature, that is too extensive to be explained by normal forgetfulness. Five major types of amnesia exist: (1) localized amnesia, or difficulty remembering anything about the first few hours after a profoundly disturbing event; (2) selective amnesia, or the ability to remember some but not all of the events surrounding a traumatic experience; (3) generalized amnesia, or failure to remember one's entire life; (4) continuous amnesia, or inability to recall events after a specific time up to and including the present; and (5) systematized amnesia, or loss of memory for certain categories of information, such as all memories related to one's family or to a particular person.

Dissociative identity disorder is a relatively rare dissociative disorder with two major components: (1) presence of two or more distinct personality states and (2) possession. In the first, two or more distinct personalities exist within the person and at least two personalities repeatedly take control of the person's behavior. Legal identity is retained by the "host personality." Other personalities within the body are called *alter personalities*. Individuals with this disorder experience frequent gaps in memory for personal history, both remote and recent. Most patients with dissociative identity disorders report severe childhood abuse, including physical, sexual, or ritual cult abuse; however, these experiences are difficult to verify. In the second, possession-form identities appear as though a spirit, supernatural being, or outside person has taken control so that the individual begins speaking or acting in a distinctly different manner. For example, a person who appears to be possessed by the devil may take on the characteristics of a satanic entity. The identities that are present are recurrent, unwanted, and involuntary; cause significant distress or impairment; and are not a normal part of cultural or religious practice.

Medical Treatment

Drug Therapy. The category of medications used to treat the acute symptoms of anxiety is the anxiolytic category. The primary anxiolytic (antianxiety) medications are the benzodiazepines (e.g., diazepam [Valium], chlordiazepoxide hydrochloride [Librium], lorazepam [Ativan], alprazolam [Xanax], and clonazepam [Klonopin]). (The nursing implications and patient teaching needs related to drug therapy are described in Table 56-3.) These medications usually are prescribed for brief periods. Side effects are those associated with sedation, such as drowsiness, fatigue, dizziness, and confusion. Because physical and psychologic dependence occur, withdrawal from these medications must be medically supervised. Abrupt cessation of benzodiazepines may result in withdrawal symptoms, including seizures and even death. Thus these medications are typically used at the initial phase of treatment to reduce symptoms until other medications can take effect.

Antidepressants are used much more commonly to treat anxiety disorders, either alone or in combination with anxiolytics. Antidepressants, such as the SSRIs and some of the newer antidepressants such as venlafaxine (Effexor), nefazodone (Dutonin, Nefadar [formerly Serzone]), and duloxetine (Cymbalta), are often very useful in reducing anxiety, decreasing distress, and improving overall functioning. This is especially true when the patient suffers from depression as well as anxiety.

Pharmacology Capsule

Anxiolytic medications, which are given for anxiety disorders or as an adjunct medication for treating schizophrenia, may have side effects such as drowsiness, loss of coordination, fatigue, confusion, blurred vision, and psychologic dependence.

Table 56-3 Drug Therapy: Common Anxiolytics (Antianxiety Medications) in the Benzodiazepine Class

DRUG NAME	NURSING IMPLICATIONS	PATIENT TEACHING
alprazolam (Xanax) chlordiazepoxide (Librium) clonazepam (Klonopin) clorazepate (Tranxene) diazepam (Valium) halazepam (Paxipam) lorazepam (Ativan)	Effective in the treatment of anxiety and panic disorders. However, the short half-life may lead to rebound anxiety. Sometimes used to treat acute alcohol withdrawal. Depresses the central nervous system (CNS). The long half-life allows for once- or twice-a-day dosing. May potentiate other CNS depressants; therefore administer these drugs with caution with other CNS depressants. Administer with extreme caution in older adults and those who are frail because these patients may be more sensitive to the effects of these medications and more prone to confusion or falls. Abrupt cessation after prolonged or excessive use may result in withdrawal, including seizures and death. An intermediate half-life allows dosing at three or four times per day.	Avoid alcohol when taking medications in this class because alcohol will intensify their effects. Rebound anxiety may result when medication wears off, especially when taking those with short half-lives. If this happens, report it to your practitioner. Do not take more medication at one time than prescribed or use medication more frequently in a day than prescribed. May impair driving, decrease attention and concentration, and cause drowsiness. May impair the ability to drive safely. Avoid driving or operating dangerous machinery until the effects of the medicine on coordination, reaction time, motor control, and judgment are known. Do not abruptly stop taking this medication without consulting with your practitioner.

❖ NURSING CARE of the Patient with an Anxiety Disorder, Somatic Symptom Disorder, or Dissociative Disorder

■ Assessment

The patient's self-report of symptoms and his or her objective observations help to determine the presence and level of anxiety (i.e., mild, moderate, severe, or panic). Particularly relevant mental status examination categories include motor activity, speech and language, and thought content.

Nursing Diagnoses, Goals, and Outcome Criteria: Anxiety, Somatic Symptom Disorder, and Dissociative Disorders

Nursing Diagnoses	Goals and Outcome Criteria
Anxiety related to severe stress, as evidenced by patient's self-report, wringing and trembling of hands, and fearful appearance	Reduced anxiety: patient able to solve problems, labels symptoms as those of anxiety, appears calm and relaxed
Ineffective Coping related to dissociation, amnesia in stressful situations	More effective coping with anxiety: patient recognizes ineffective ways of coping; identifies and implements new ways of coping with anxiety, stress, and their precipitants; learns and implements relaxation techniques, guided imagery, and other coping strategies

■ Interventions

Strategies to help patients reduce anxiety from a panic state or from a severe level to a mild level center on remaining calm; speaking firmly with short, simple instructions (e.g., "Sit down with me here"); and walking to a less stimulating area of the unit. Once the anxiety is reduced to a manageable level, assist patients in exploring what happened, clarifying their usual ways of relieving anxiety (e.g., by expressing anger or experiencing somatic symptoms instead of more typical anxiety symptoms), and identifying what triggered the anxiety (e.g., feelings of self-doubt regarding finding employment after discharge). You can assist clients in problem-solving decisions and can teach ways to prevent and manage heightened anxiety in the future (see *Complementary and Alternative Therapies* box).

Complementary and Alternative Therapies

Useful techniques to manage anxiety include relaxation techniques, warm baths, positive self-talk, and physical exercise.

SCHIZOPHRENIA AND SCHIZOAFFECTIVE DISORDERS

Schizophrenia is a term used to refer to a group of very serious, usually chronic thought disorders in which psychotic symptoms primarily impair the affected person's ability to interpret the world accurately. Schizophrenia is characterized by disturbances in thinking, mood, and behavior. **Psychosis** is a state in which a person has distorted perceptions of reality. Psychotic symptoms include delusions, hallucinations, disorganized thinking (speech), grossly disorganized or abnormal motor behavior, and negative symptoms. The symptoms are characterized as either *positive* or *negative.* Positive symptoms appear to reflect an excess or distortion of normal functions and include delusions, hallucinations, problems with communication, and bizarre behavior. Negative symptoms appear to reflect a decrease or loss of normal functions and include diminished emotional expression (i.e., flattened affect), slowed thinking and speech, and difficulty initiating goal-directed behavior.

Typically, patients with schizophrenia have functioned normally in early life; they often are very intelligent and well educated before the onset of the first symptoms. The symptoms usually begin in adolescence or early adulthood; however, some types of schizophrenic disorders are more often diagnosed in later life. The schizophrenic patient's ability to function in the areas of work, interpersonal relationships, or self-care deteriorates significantly during acute episodes and may not return to baseline after the first psychotic episode. With each subsequent episode, the ability to function independently continues to deteriorate, intelligence quotient (IQ) levels drop, and thinking becomes very concrete. Patients are unable to tolerate even the typical stressors of daily living. However, newer medications have been very successful in helping people to return to their previous activities.

Cause and Risk Factors

The cause of schizophrenia disorder is not certain. The model that integrates diverse potential causes states that patients who are most vulnerable to acquiring the disorder encounter factors (stress) that precipitate the disorder. The model is called the *stress-diathesis model.* Researchers have established that people with schizophrenia probably were genetically vulnerable to the disorder. The range of biologic factors being investigated includes (1) neurotransmitters (e.g., dopamine, norepinephrine, and gamma-aminobutyric acid) and their receptors; (2) structural abnormalities such as degeneration of the limbic system, enlargement of the lateral and third ventricles, and loss of neurons in the temporal lobe; (3) infectious agents; and (4) hormonal deregulation.

In males the disorder usually first occurs in the early to mid-20s whereas in females the age of onset is generally in late 20s. The incidence is between 0.3% and 0.7%, although there is variation by race/ethnicity and country of origin and in various countries. Psychotic symptoms tend to decrease as people age, possibly due to age-related declines in dopamine activity. Twenty percent of people with schizophrenia attempt suicide on one or more occasions; 5% to 6% die by suicide.

Medical Treatment

Drug Therapy. The most commonly administered medications for people with schizophrenia are antipsychotic (neuroleptic) medications and antiparkinsonism medications, which are at times administered to prevent or relieve some of the side effects of the antipsychotics. (The nursing implications and patient teaching needs related to drug therapy are described in Table 56-4.) Anxiolytic medications also may be administered in conjunction with the antipsychotics to decrease agitation and akathisia (a potential side effect of antipsychotics in which the patient is restless and unable to sit still). Two broad categories of antipsychotics exist: (1) first-generation agents (FGAs) and (2) second-generation agents (SGAs). FGAs are also referred to as conventional or typical agents. They are the older agents that were very useful in treating the positive symptoms of schizophrenia such as auditory and visual hallucinations; however, they were not particularly useful in treating the negative symptoms, such as poverty of thought, delayed thinking, and decreased function. The SGAs are known to help with both positive and negative symptoms and have a reduced incidence of side effects compared to the older FGAs.

When working with patients who are receiving antipsychotics, you are responsible for observing and recording accurately all data relevant to the target behaviors and symptoms of the medications as well as the potential side effects. A variety of potential side effects exists, some of which have rapid onset and require immediate treatment.

One side effect that can be managed with nursing interventions and patient teaching is orthostatic hypotension (or postural hypotension), which is a drop in BP when a person changes position from lying down to sitting or from sitting to standing. This problem, which creates a risk for falls, occurs most frequently in the early weeks of treatment and is more common in the morning, after the patient has been in bed during the night, as well as after a large meal. Older adults and those in poor physical health are at particular risk for this side effect. See Chapter 38 for details on the assessment and management of orthostatic hypotension.

Another group of side effects are referred to as **extrapyramidal side effects (EPS)** and stem from the effect of the antipsychotic agents on the extrapyramidal tracts of the CNS. These tracts play a role in the control of involuntary movements. Different EPS may occur at different periods in the course of medication therapy and are described as follows.

Acute dystonic reactions may occur after one dose of medication or during the first few days of treatment. The reactions consist of severe muscle contractions involving the tongue, face, neck (i.e., torticollis), and back (i.e., opisthotonos). The larynx also may be constricted (i.e., laryngospasm), which compromises the patient's airway. The reaction is reversed with benztropine mesylate (Cogentin), given intramuscularly or intravenously as ordered, or with diphenhydramine hydrochloride (Benadryl), administered intravenously as ordered. Acute dystonia is a medical emergency and must be treated immediately. It is important to note that certain antiemetics such as promethazine (Phenergan) and prochlorperazine (Compazine) may also cause dystonic reactions.

After 1 to 2 weeks of treatment with antipsychotic medications, the **parkinsonian syndrome**—consisting of masklike face, rigid posture, shuffling gait, and resting tremor—may occur. Other extrapyramidal syndromes that may occur later in treatment are akathisia, a reversible restlessness manifested as an urge to pace and difficulty sitting still. Some references state that akathisia is the most common side effect of neuroleptic medications.

Tardive dyskinesia is usually an irreversible syndrome that may occur after prolonged use of antipsychotic drug therapy. It consists of persistent involuntary movements of the face, jaw, and tongue that lead to grimacing, jerky movements of the upper extremities, and tonic contractions of the neck and back. Treatment includes discontinuing the causative agent; however, the symptoms usually continue.

Neuroleptic malignant syndrome occurs in 1% of people receiving antipsychotic (neuroleptic) agents and certain antiemetics such as prochlorperazine (Compazine). Mortality rates reported for people with this condition range from 14% to 30%. The first symptom is usually muscular rigidity accompanied by akinesia (i.e., emotional unresponsiveness and blunted affect) and respiratory distress and may include involuntary muscle movements but the cardinal sign is hyperthermia (a temperature of 101°F to 103°F or higher). Neuroleptic malignant syndrome is a medical emergency that requires immediate intervention and intensive care because it may result in permanent impairment or even death.

One antipsychotic drug, clozapine (Clozaril), presents a risk for the blood disorder known as *agranulocytosis*, an extreme decrease in granulated white blood cells (WBCs), which frequently manifests as a sore throat and fever. Patients receiving this medication require close supervision and frequent WBC counts. If the WBC drops significantly or if the patient experiences sore throat, fever, and flulike symptoms (or a combination of these symptoms), the medication must

Table 56-4 Drug Therapy: Selected Antipsychotics (Neuroleptics)

DRUG NAME	NURSING IMPLICATIONS	PATIENT TEACHING
First-Generation (Conventional) Antipsychotics		
chlorpromazine (Thorazine) fluphenazine (Prolixin) haloperidol (Haldol) loxapine (Loxitane) mesoridazine (Serentil) perphenazine (Trilafon) thioridazine (Mellaril) thiothixene (Navane) trifluoperazine (Stelazine)	These agents are helpful in the treatment of positive symptoms of schizophrenia and other psychotic processes. They may cause drowsiness and sedation, postural hypotension, dry mouth, and blurred vision (especially in frail and older people). Watch for extrapyramidal side effects (EPS), such as Parkinson syndrome–like involuntary movements, muscle rigidity, dystonia, akathisia, and oculogyric crisis. Long-term administration may result in tardive dyskinesia.	Caution the patient to rise slowly from a lying position to a sitting position and from sitting to standing to avoid a sudden drop in blood pressure (BP). Caution patients to avoid driving or operating dangerous machinery until the effects of the medicine on coordination, reaction time, motor control, and judgment are known. Assess the patient for abnormal, involuntary movements and report these to the prescribing practitioner. Administer medications to treat motor movement side effects as ordered. Provide the patient with hard candy or sugarless chewing gum to help with dry mouth. Provide dietary teaching to help the patient avoid or manage weight gain and diabetes associated with these and other neuroleptics.
Second-Generation (Atypical) Antipsychotics		
aripiprazole (Abilify) clozapine (Clozaril) olanzapine (Zyprexa) quetiapine (Seroquel) risperidone (Risperdal) ziprasidone (Geodon)	These agents treat both the positive and the negative symptoms of schizophrenia and other psychotic disorders. They may cause drowsiness and sedation, postural hypotension, dry mouth, and blurred vision (especially in frail and older people). Watch for EPS, such as Parkinson syndrome–like movements, muscle rigidity, dystonia, akathisia, and oculogyric crisis. Although these side effects are less common with second-generation agents, they are still seen in patients taking these drugs. Long-term administration also may result in tardive dyskinesia, although this may be less likely.	Caution the patient to rise slowly from a lying position to a sitting position and from sitting to standing to avoid a sudden drop in BP. Caution patients to avoid driving or operating dangerous machinery until the effects of the medicine on coordination, reaction time, motor control, and judgment are known. Assess the patient for abnormal, involuntary movements and report these to the prescribing practitioner. Administer medications to treat motor movement side effects as ordered. Provide the patient with hard candy or sugarless chewing gum to help with dry mouth. Provide dietary teaching to help the patient avoid or manage weight gain and diabetes associated with these and other antipsychotics.
	In addition to the implications mentioned above, the patient taking clozapine may experience a significant drop in white blood cell (WBC) count. Routine blood count monitoring must be done to identify any drop in WBC count. If this happens, the medication is withheld (and usually discontinued).	In addition to the other side effects associated with taking clozapine, teach the patient taking atypical neuroleptics to watch for and report immediately to the prescribing practitioner a sore throat, fever, chills, and any other signs of infection.

be held and the physician must be notified at once. Severe infection may result when the WBC counts drop below acceptable levels.

It is clear that in monitoring a patient for drug side effects, a wide range of data is relevant (from vital signs to facial expression). Pay close attention to all patient descriptions of symptoms.

After a period of time, patients taking FGAs almost always experience EPS such as akathisia and pseudoparkinsonism. Tardive dyskinesia also is a significant risk when patients are taking FGAs; thus SGAs are now considered first-line agents.

Weight gain, hyperglycemia, and onset of type 2 diabetes have all been associated with the use of SGAs. Therefore it is important that you teach patients taking these medications about proper diet, exercise, and the need for regular checkups. A few of the SGAs may cause an abnormal increase in serum progesterone (i.e., hyperprolactinemia), which can lead to an enlargement of the breasts (i.e., gynecomastia) and production of milk (i.e., galactorrhea) in both men and women.

NURSING CARE of the Patient with Schizophrenia

Assessment

The following data contribute to the mental status examination of the person with schizophrenia:

- *Appearance*—may have poor grooming and failure to bathe
- *Activity*—may exhibit agitation, bizarre postures, catatonic excitement or stupor, mannerisms or stereotypes, or stiff body movements
- *Mood and affect*—may have flat affect or inappropriate rage or happiness
- *Speech and language*—mutism, tangential speech, blocking, or loose associations
- *Thought content*—delusions that may be persecutory, grandiose, religious, or somatic
- *Perceptual disturbances*—auditory hallucinations (most common) and visual hallucinations (next most common)
- *Insight and judgment*—usually little insight into illness
- *Sensorium*—oriented to person, place, and time
- *Memory*—usually intact (but difficulties with attention make assessment difficult)

Nursing Diagnoses, Goals, and Outcome Criteria: Schizophrenia

Nursing Diagnoses	Goals and Outcome Criteria
Acute Confusion related to delusions (i.e., false beliefs), loose associations, concrete thinking, and symbolism, as evidenced by patient statements such as that the president is out to get him or her	Orientation: patient differentiates illusions from reality, fewer loose associations, more logical thinking
Disturbed Personal Identity related to hallucinations, illusions, and heightened response to irrelevant stimuli, as evidenced by patient's inability to tolerate group therapy, talking to himself or herself, and looking for something when nothing is there	Improved sensory perceptual function: reduced frequency of hallucinations, less response to irrelevant environmental and other stimuli
Impaired Verbal Communication related to delayed thinking as evidenced by very slow and delayed speech	Improved verbal communication: patient expresses thoughts clearly
Self-Neglect related to withdrawal and loss of motivation and judgment, as evidenced by poor hygiene, poor grooming, and avoiding others	Improved self-care: patient performs activities of daily living (ADL) with maximum independence in relation to level of ability

Interventions

Acute Confusion

Nursing interventions include speaking in a gentle and nonconfrontational manner, decreasing unwanted environmental stimuli, focusing on reality (i.e., real events, real people), letting the patient know that you do not share the delusion without directly confronting the delusion (do not argue or try to disprove the delusion), encouraging the patient to express feelings and anxiety, and connecting delusions with anxiety-provoking situations (see interventions for anxiety, discussed earlier under "Nursing Care of the Patient with an Anxiety Disorder, Somatic Symptom Disorder, or Dissociative Disorder.")

Disturbed Personal Identity

Interventions include making brief, frequent contacts with the patient (to interrupt hallucinatory experiences); encouraging the patient to pay attention to what is occurring in the environment (instead of internal stimuli); encouraging involvement in quiet activities; and informing patients that hallucinations are part of the disease process.

Impaired Verbal Communication

Interventions may include seeking clarification and verbalizing the implied, which may be useful if the patient is not speaking (e.g., "It must have been difficult for you when your father didn't come after he told you he would"). You will also want to provide regular contact with the patient and use gentle encouragement, understanding that the patient's thinking may be slowed.

Self-Neglect

Possible interventions include providing recognition for all constructive self-care actions (e.g., "I see you've bathed and washed your hair"), demonstrating how to perform an activity if necessary, intervening to assist when necessary, offering finger foods or cans of food for the patient to open, or serving meals family style if the patient believes that food has been poisoned.

Schizoaffective Disorder

Schizoaffective disorder has similar features to schizophrenia with the additional symptoms of a major mood disorder throughout the illness. An individual may have impaired occupational functioning, restricted social contact, and difficulties with self-care but negative symptoms are usually less severe and persistent than in schizophrenia. The disorder is about one third as common as schizophrenia and the age of onset is usually in young adulthood. Treatment and nursing care are similar for patients with schizophrenia and those with mood disorders.

MAJOR DEPRESSIVE AND BIPOLAR DISORDERS

People with major depressive and bipolar disorders experience significantly elevated or depressed moods. Some people experience cycles of elevated mood and depressed mood. An episode of persistent depressed mood is referred to as a *major depressive disorder.* An episode of elevated mood is called a *manic episode.* Alternation between significantly depressed mood and significantly elevated mood over time is termed *bipolar disorder.*

Major depressive disorder is one of the most common psychiatric disorders, with a 12-month prevalence of 7%. The occurrence is three times higher in people ages 18 to 29 years than in people over age 60. Beginning in adolescence, one and a half to three times as many women as men are diagnosed with major depression. There is a greater risk for family members with major depressive disorder and people with depressive personality traits. Stress is also related to the onset of major depressive disorder.

For bipolar disorder, the lifetime prevalence is 1%, with the mean age at onset being 30 years. Rates are similar for men and women and are higher among single and divorced people than among married people. People in higher socioeconomic groups and those with lower levels of education have higher rates of bipolar disorder.

Cause and Risk Factors

Definite causes of major depressive and bipolar disorders have not been established. Probable causes include neurotransmitter dysregulation, neuroreceptor deficits, neuroendocrine dysfunctions, genetic factors, loss of significant others, learned helplessness, and negative thoughts about life experiences.

Medical Treatment

Drug Therapy. Several types of antidepressant medications exist: SSRIs; newer antidepressants such as nefazodone (Dutonin, Nefodar), venlafaxine (Effexor), and duloxetine (Cymbalta); TCAs; and monoamine oxidase inhibitors (MAOIs). (Important considerations related to drug therapy are listed in Table 56-5.)

The manic phase of bipolar disease is usually treated with lithium or divalproex (Depakote). (Nursing implications and patient teaching needs are described in Table 56-6.) When administering medications, you are responsible for ensuring that medication has been swallowed and not held in the mouth and later discarded or saved for an overdose (see *Complementary and Alternative Therapies* box). As the patient responds to antidepressant medication and the energy level increases, the risk of suicide also increases.

Complementary and Alternative Therapies

Many people use the herbal preparation St. John's wort to relieve depression. However, additional study is needed before it can be recommended as a replacement for conventional drugs used to treat major mental illnesses.

Pharmacology Capsule

The side effects of tricyclic antidepressants (TCAs) are drowsiness, fatigue, orthostatic hypotension, dry mouth, blurred vision, urinary retention, and constipation.

MAOIs sometimes are prescribed for patients with a depression that is resistant to the SSRIs, TCAs, and other antidepressants. A 2-week period should elapse between ending most antidepressants and beginning an MAOI. The very serious side effect of a hypertensive crisis occurs if the patient taking an MAOI ingests tyramine-containing food or drink, such as avocados, bananas, beer, bologna, canned figs, chocolate, cheese (except cottage cheese), liver, papaya products, pâté, herring, fava beans, raisins, salami, sausage, sour cream, soy sauce, some wines, and yogurt. These foods also must be avoided for 3 weeks after stopping treatment with an MAOI. Symptoms of a hypertensive crisis, which requires immediate treatment, include headache, palpitations, visual changes, neck stiffness, nausea, vomiting, sweating, sensitivity to light, pupil changes, and bradycardia or tachycardia. A "washout" period of about 4 weeks must elapse when discontinuing a MAOI before starting most other antidepressants.

Sexual dysfunction (i.e., anorgasmia, delayed or absent ejaculation, decreased libido) may occur with

Table 56-5 Drug Therapy: Antidepressant Drugs

DRUG	CONSIDERATIONS
SSRIs	
citalopram (Celexa) escitalopram (Lexapro) fluoxetine (Prozac) fluvoxamine (Luvox) paroxetine (Paxil) sertraline (Zoloft)	SSRIs can be taken once a day, making adherence to a prescribed treatment easier for the patient. SSRIs are not considered cardiotoxic; thus an overdose is unlikely to cause life-threatening dysrhythmias. Besides depression, SSRIs may be useful in panic disorder and OCD. Most patients tolerate the medications in the morning whereas others may feel tired and thus should take the SSRIs in the evening. Can cause weight gain. Fluoxetine causes sexual dysfunction.
Tricyclics	
amitriptyline (Elavil) clomipramine (Anafranil) desipramine (Norpramin) doxepin (Sinequan) imipramine (Tofranil) nortriptyline (Pamelor) trimipramine (Surmontil)	TCAs affect not only serotonin but also epinephrine and norepinephrine. As such, they may cause cardiac complications. Severe and life-threatening dysrhythmias may result from an overdose. Side effects may be more problematic in this group of medications than with SSRIs. Many of these medicines cannot be taken once a day; bid or tid dosing must be used to reach the total daily dose.
Tetracyclics	
maprotiline (Ludiomil) mirtazapine (Remeron)	These agents are at least as potentially dangerous as TCAs; significant sedation may occur. May be given in single or divided doses.
Other Agents	
bupropion (Wellbutrin) duloxetine (Cymbalta) nefazodone (Dutonin, Nefadar) trazodone (Desyrel) venlafaxine (Effexor)	Dosing schedules vary. Bupropion can cause seizures; does not cause weight gain or sexual dysfunction—unlike SSRIs. Duloxetine also used for diabetic peripheral neuropathy, generalized anxiety disorder, chronic musculoskeletal pain, and fibromyalgia, Though not common, nefazodone can cause severe liver injury. Trazodone is sedating; often used to relieve anti-depressant induced insomnia.
MAOIs	
phenelzine (Nardil) tranylcypromine (Parnate)	Phenelzine (Nardil) is not a first-line (i.e., first choice) drug. Strict diet restrictions are necessary for patients taking these medications. Interactions with foods containing tyramine, other antidepressants, and many other drugs can lead to life-threatening hypertensive crisis. Must be given in divided doses. Warn patients to avoid OTC medications until approved by prescriber of MAOI.

bid, Twice a day; *MAOI,* monoamine oxidase inhibitor; *OCD,* obsessive-compulsive disorder; *OTC,* over-the-counter; *SSRI,* selective serotonin reuptake inhibitor; *TCA,* tricyclic antidepressant; *tid,* three times a day.

any antidepressant but seems to be more commonly related to SSRIs. Some antidepressants such as nefazodone (Dutonin, Nefadar), and bupropion (Wellbutrin) are much less likely to cause this troublesome side effect.

Put on Your Thinking Cap!

A patient with bipolar disorder is being treated for severe depression in an inpatient facility with bupropion (Wellbutrin) and divalproex sodium (Depakote). Identify the nursing implications related to these medications.

Electroconvulsive Therapy. Electroconvulsive therapy (ECT) is a form of therapy in which an electrical current is introduced to the brain through electrodes placed on the temples. The electrical current produces a grand mal seizure; however, drugs are administered to minimize the manifestations of a seizure. This type of therapy most often is prescribed when other forms of therapy have failed with people who are severely depressed. Its advantage is that it acts more quickly than medications and may have fewer side effects in older people.

Key nursing interventions include patient and family teaching, making certain that the patient takes nothing by mouth (NPO) after midnight on the day of a treatment, asking the patient to void and to remove eyeglasses or contact lenses and dentures, administering atropine sulfate as ordered (to decrease secretions), positioning the patient on the side after the procedure to prevent aspiration, monitoring vital signs, remaining with the patient until he or she is awake, and providing orienting information as needed (e.g., "It's 10 AM on Wednesday and you just finished your treatment"). Temporary memory loss and confusion are common side effects of ECT and instances of prolonged memory loss have occurred. You must take appropriate safety precautions and be patient with the person who has undergone this procedure.

Table 56-6 **Drug Therapy: Mood Stabilizers**

DRUG NAME	NURSING IMPLICATIONS	PATIENT TEACHING
carbamazepine (Tegretol)	Used in the treatment of bipolar mood disorder as well as in seizure disorders. Requires careful monitoring of liver enzymes and drug levels. May cause anemia. May cause life-threatening allergic skin reactions (Stevens-Johnson syndrome), watch for development of rash, hold medication if rash develops and notify prescriber immediately. May cause dizziness, drowsiness, unsteady gait. May result in fetal abnormalities if used during pregnancy.	Take exactly as prescribed, notify prescriber at once if rash develops, and hold medication until further advice from a health care provider. Keep all medical appointments and have blood work done as ordered. Notify your prescriber immediately if you suspect you are pregnant. Do not breast-feed while taking this medication.
lamotrigine (Lamictal)	Used in the treatment of bipolar disorders as well as seizure disorders. May cause life-threatening allergic skin reactions (Stevens-Johnson syndrome), watch for development of rash, hold medication if rash develops and notify prescriber immediately. May cause dizziness, drowsiness, unsteady gait. Must be started at a low dose and titrated up slowly not more than once every 1 to 2 weeks. May result in fetal abnormalities if used during pregnancy.	Take exactly as prescribed. Do not double up for missed dosages. Swallow the regular tablets whole; do not split, chew, or crush them. Tell your doctor if you are pregnant, plan to become pregnant, or are breastfeeding. If you become pregnant while taking lamotrigine, call your doctor.
lithium (Lithium Carbonate, Lithobid, Lithium SR)	Used in the treatment of bipolar disorders; occasionally used as adjunct treatment for depression. Narrow therapeutic range of 0.5 to 1.5 mEq/L (check your local lab reference range). Watch for signs of lithium toxicity (tremulousness, nausea, vomiting, diarrhea, changes in level of consciousness). Maintain adequate hydration. Monitor renal function (serum creatinine and BUN) and report abnormal findings. Monitor serum level of lithium. Do not change from immediate release to sustained release or vice versa unless directed by prescriber because this may alter serum levels unexpectedly.	Take exactly as prescribed. Drug must be taken regularly to achieve and maintain adequate blood level. Do not alter salt intake. Do not double up on doses if one is missed. Maintain adequate fluid intake, especially in hot weather. Avoid excessive use of caffeinated beverages. Keep follow-up appointments and have blood levels drawn as directed. Report signs of toxicity at once.
valproic acid, divalproex sodium (Depakote, Depakene)	Used in the treatment of bipolar disorders. Serum levels must be monitored for therapeutic range (50 to 100 mcg/mL). Metabolized by the liver, so periodic monitoring of liver enzymes is necessary. May cause some sedation. May cause hair loss; if moderate to severe, notify prescribing practitioner. Report moderate to severe abdominal pain immediately to prescriber (may cause pancreatitis).	Take medication exactly as prescribed. Drug must be taken regularly to achieve and maintain adequate blood level. Do not double up on medication if a dose is missed. Avoid driving or operating dangerous machinery until exact effects of medication are known. Keep follow-up appointments and have blood levels drawn as directed. Report moderate to severe abdominal pain immediately to prescriber (may cause pancreatitis).

BUN, Blood urea nitrogen.

NURSING CARE of the Patient with Major Depression

Assessment

Data that are relevant to the mental status assessment of a patient who has depression include the following:

- *Activity*—The patient is likely to exhibit psychomotor retardation and possibly no spontaneous movements, with a downcast gaze, although he or she may exhibit agitation (e.g., hand wringing and hair pulling), especially if an older adult.
- *Mood and affect*—The patient may or may not have depressed feelings and may not appear depressed.
- *Speech and language*—The patient's speech volume and rate may be decreased. In addition, his or her response to questions may be delayed and mutism may be present.
- *Thought content*—The patient expresses a generally negative view of self and world. He or she may ruminate about loss, guilt, suicide, and depression. If the patient is psychotic, he or she may have delusions of guilt, failure, worthlessness, or terminal illnesses.
- *Insight and judgment*—The possibility of suicidal ideation occurs at all times during major depressive episodes. Risk factors include past history of suicide attempts or threats, male gender, being single or living alone, and feeling hopeless. Insight into illness may be impaired because of negative perceptions of reality.
- *Sensorium*—The patient is oriented but may not have energy to answer questions.
- *Memory and attention*—The patient often complains of impaired concentration and forgetfulness.

Nursing Diagnoses, Goals, and Outcome Criteria: Major Depression

Nursing Diagnoses	Goals and Outcome Criteria
Risk for Self-Directed Violence related to hopelessness and increased energy level associated with treatment, as evidenced by patient endorsing suicidal ideations	Reduced risk of harm to self: patient seeks out staff member if an urge to harm self is experienced; develops coping skills to replace self-destructive behavior and displays acceptable ways of expressing anger, rage, and hostility; mobilizes social support systems
Chronic Low Self-Esteem or **Situational Low Self-Esteem** related to negative feelings about self	Improved self-esteem: patient accepts own body, has positive feelings about self, identifies aspects of self he or she likes; identifies thoughts about self
Imbalanced Nutrition: Less Than Body Requirements related to anorexia	Adequate nutrition: achieves and maintains ideal weight and has more energy
Disturbed Sleep Pattern related to anxiety	Improved sleep pattern: patient sleeps within 30 minutes of retiring and remains asleep for 6 to 8 uninterrupted hours

Interventions

Risk for Self-Directed Violence

Interventions may include establishing a no-harm contract; frequently assessing a patient's suicidal potential (see the section titled "Nursing Assessment of the Psychiatric Patient"); taking necessary suicide precautions; removing dangerous objects such as pantyhose, belts, and any sharp objects; maintaining continuous one-to-one contact if indicated; encouraging honest expression of feelings; assisting in identifying symbols of hope in the patient's life; identifying community resources for times of crisis; and communicating the message that the patient is worthwhile.

Chronic Low Self-Esteem or Situational Low Self-Esteem

Interventions may include helping the patient to identify positive aspects and limitations regarding his or her body; to like the body despite its imperfections; to improve hygiene, grooming, and posture, which makes positive affirmations about self; to limit self-criticism; to be aware of negative self-statements; to learn to give and receive compliments; and to develop social skills.

Imbalanced Nutrition: Less Than Body Requirements

Possible interventions include involving a dietitian in planning an adequate diet for the patient; directly assisting patients to make healthy choices regarding their menu and eating choices; documenting intake; determining food preferences and attempting to satisfy those preferences; and offering small, frequent meals.

Disturbed Sleep Pattern

For patients with sleep disturbances, discourage sleep during the day; provide sleep-producing measures such as a light, small snack and warm bath; and teach relaxation exercises that can be used before retiring. The patient should avoid exercising before bedtime, watching television in bed, and ingesting caffeine after 2 PM. The patient may be asked to keep a sleep diary (see Nursing Care Plan: Patient with Major Depression).

Nursing Care Plan — Patient with Major Depression

ASSESSMENT

HEALTH HISTORY A 53-year-old woman is admitted to a psychiatric hospital with a diagnosis of major depression. During the past few weeks, she has become increasingly listless, apathetic, and disinterested in anyone or anything. She cries frequently and says that her life has not seemed to be worth living. She complains that she cannot sleep and has no appetite. She frequently talks about wanting to commit suicide. She was referred to a psychiatrist, who recommended that she be admitted to the hospital for treatment.

PHYSICAL EXAMINATION Vital signs: blood pressure 110/70 mm Hg, pulse 78 bpm, respiration 22 breaths per minute, temperature 98.8°F (37.1°C) measured orally. Height 5′4″, weight 120 lb. Appears apathetic, sad, and cries frequently. Somewhat disheveled. Gaunt and tired looking.

Nursing Diagnosis	Goals and Outcome Criteria	Interventions
Risk for Self-Directed Violence related to suicidal feelings	The patient will not harm herself, as evidenced by seeking out nursing staff if she experiences the urge to harm herself; developing coping skills to replace self-destructive behavior; and developing acceptable ways to express anger, rage, and hostility.	Establish a no-harm contract (e.g., ask the patient to state or write that she will not harm herself and will inform a nurse if she has thoughts of harming herself while in the hospital). Frequently assess her suicidal potential and take necessary suicide precautions; remove dangerous objects from the environment; maintain continuous one-to-one contact; encourage honest expression of feelings; and assist in identifying symbols of hope in the patient's life, such as recognizing personal strengths or setting small, realistic goals.
Chronic Low Self-Esteem or **Situational Low Self-Esteem** related to depression	The patient will maintain or enhance self-esteem, as evidenced by acceptance of her own body and sense of self, identification of negative thoughts about herself, and identification of aspects of herself she likes.	Help the patient to identify positive aspects and limitations regarding her body and to accept her body regardless of limitations. Encourage the patient to improve her hygiene. Assist the patient to accept compliments and to limit self-criticism.
Imbalanced Nutrition: Less Than Body Requirements related to anorexia or lack of interest in food	The patient will gain weight and experience a higher energy level, as evidenced by more participation and interaction in activities with others.	Involve the dietitian in planning an adequate diet. Determine food preferences and attempt to satisfy those preferences. Offer small, frequent meals.
Disturbed Sleep Pattern related to depression relapse	The patient will sleep within 30 minutes of retiring and remain asleep for 6 to 8 uninterrupted hours.	Provide sleep-producing measures such as small snacks, warm baths, and relaxation exercises before the patient retires.

Critical Thinking Questions

1. Explain why the patient requires close monitoring when she begins to feel more energetic.
2. What are some examples of symbols of hope in a person's life?

NURSING CARE of the Patient with Bipolar Disorder with Manic Episodes

Assessment

The nurse may observe the following:

- *Appearance*—The patient's form of dress is often inappropriate (e.g., bright, nonmatching colors; excessive makeup and jewelry).
- *Activity*—The patient is hyperactive and has a decreased need for sleep.
- *Mood, affect, and feelings*—Although frequently euphoric, the patient also may be very irritable, angry, and hostile (based on low frustration tolerance) as well as emotionally labile.
- *Speech and language*—The patient is talkative and uses pressured speech that is difficult to interrupt. In addition, he or she has a flight of ideas (i.e., continuous, rapid shift from one topic to another), and the rate and volume of speech is increased.
- *Thought content*—Themes of self-confidence, self-aggrandizement, and possibly delusions of grandeur (e.g., a false belief that one has great wealth or power) or delusions of persecution are noted.
- *Sensory perception*—The patient may experience hallucinations.
- *Judgment and insight*—The patient often has little insight regarding his or her illness. In addition, the patient's judgment is impaired, as evidenced by actions such as large spending sprees, sexual activities incongruent with usual behavior, suicide attempts, and homicide attempts.

Nursing Diagnoses, Goals, and Outcome Criteria: Bipolar Disorder with Manic Episodes

Nursing Diagnoses	Goals and Outcome Criteria
Risk for Injury related to impaired judgment	Reduced risk for injury: patient does not exhibit potentially injurious activities
Risk for Other-Directed Violence related to impaired judgment, low frustration tolerance, and emotional lability	Reduced risk of violence toward others: patient does not harm others, verbalizes anger appropriately
Imbalanced Nutrition: Less Than Body Requirements related to hyperactivity	Balanced nutrition: patient consumes necessary daily nutrients in appropriate form for manic state, maintains body weight
Disturbed Sleep Pattern related to hyperactivity	Improved sleep pattern: patient sleeps at least 6 uninterrupted hours

Interventions

Risk for Injury

Interventions include decreasing environmental stimuli (e.g., providing a quiet, simply decorated room), discouraging group activities, encouraging a few one-to-one contacts, removing hazardous objects and substances from the environment, and providing a structure that includes physical activities such as brisk walks.

Risk for Other-Directed Violence

Interventions include decreasing environmental stimuli, observing the patient frequently, removing harmful objects, finding physical outlets, demonstrating a show of strength if necessary, administering prescribed medications, and restraining the patient if other measures have failed to calm him or her. Restraints should be applied following an established protocol by staff who have been educated to restrain patients in a safe and humane manner. The patient in restraints should be checked at least every 15 minutes to make certain that circulation to extremities is satisfactory and to assess needs regarding nutrition and elimination.

Imbalanced Nutrition: Less Than Body Requirements

Interventions include providing foods that can be consumed on the run, attempting to have the patient's favorite foods and easy-to-eat and finger foods available, and educating the patient on the importance of satisfactory nutrition (see *Nutrition Considerations* box).

Nutrition Considerations

- During manic episodes, patients may not meet nutritional needs because of increased physical activity and difficulty sitting down to complete a meal.
- Anorexia may be a problem for depressed patients.

Disturbed Sleep Pattern

Interventions may include ensuring that the environment has low stimuli; observing closely for signs of fatigue, such as fine tremor and puffy, dark circles below the eyes; and encouraging warm baths and soft music at bedtime.

The key medications for people with manic episodes are divalproex sodium (Depakote) or lithium carbonate. Because relief from symptoms may take up to 3 weeks, the patient also may receive an antipsychotic (neuroleptic) medication.

The therapeutic level of divalproex sodium in the blood is 50 to 100 μg/mL (depending on the laboratory). The patient may develop toxicity if the blood level exceeds the therapeutic range. Therefore a valproic acid level is done at intervals to assess blood levels. Because divalproex is metabolized by the liver, patients with liver disorders may receive lower dosages.

Lithium is excreted by the kidneys and has a narrow therapeutic range. The therapeutic blood level for acute mania is 0.5 to 1.5 mEq/L (depending on the laboratory). If the level is greater than 1.5 mEq/L, symptoms of toxicity occur. It is critical for the patient taking lithium to stay well hydrated. If a patient taking lithium becomes dehydrated, he or she can easily become lithium toxic. Signs and symptoms of lithium toxicity include tremor, nausea, vomiting, diarrhea, and changes in level of consciousness.

Pharmacology Capsule

Older adults and medically compromised patients are exceptionally vulnerable to experiencing the side effects of all psychotropic medications, especially postural hypotension, falls, and confusion.

NEUROCOGNITIVE DISORDERS

The key problems for people with cognitive disorders stem from impairments in cognition or memory. The term *neurocognitive disorders* replaced the term *organic mental disorders* because the latter incorrectly implied that "nonorganic" mental disorders do not have a biologic basis. Delirium and dementia are two different disorders that involve deficits in orientation, memory, language comprehension, and judgment. Delirium is potentially reversible whereas dementia usually is not. Delirium is usually fairly rapid in onset. Dementia is slow in its onset.

Common causes of delirium are meningitis, neoplasms, drugs ranging from alcohol to steroids, electrolyte imbalance, endocrine dysfunction, liver abnormalities, renal failure, thiamine deficiency, and postoperative states. Common types of dementia are dementia of the Alzheimer type, vascular dementia, Pick disease, and Parkinson disease. Delirium and dementia are discussed in greater detail in Chapter 22.

PERSONALITY DISORDERS

Every individual exhibits particular personality traits. A person may be shy, aggressive, dependent, or manipulative. When personality traits become inflexible and dysfunctional, a person may have a personality disorder. The essential features of a personality disorder are that it is pervasive (it concerns all aspects of one's life), chronic, and maladaptive. Examples of personality disorders are as follows:

- *Antisocial personality disorder*—a pattern of disregard for and violation of the rights of others (The individual repeatedly breaks the law; lies; fails to plan ahead; shows a reckless disregard for the safety of self and others; is irresponsible; and lacks remorse for having hurt, mistreated, or stolen from another.)
- *Avoidant personality disorder*—a pattern of social inhibition accompanied by feelings of inadequacy and hypersensitivity to negative evaluation (The individual avoids occupational activities that involve interpersonal activities because of fear of criticism, disapproval, or rejection. In addition, he or she is unwilling to get involved with people unless certain of being liked, is preoccupied with being criticized or rejected in social situations, views self as inferior to others, and is unusually reluctant to take personal risks.)
- *Borderline personality disorder*—a pattern of instability in interpersonal relationships, self-image, and affect as well as marked impulsivity (The individual makes frantic efforts to avoid real or imagined abandonment; has chronic feelings of emptiness; shows inappropriate, intense anger or has difficulty controlling anger; has an unstable self-image or sense of self; and exhibits recurrent suicidal behavior, gestures, or threats.)
- *Narcissistic personality disorder*—a pattern of grandiosity, need for admiration, and lack of empathy (The individual has an exaggerated sense of self-importance; requires excessive admiration; takes advantage of others to achieve his or her own ends; is often envious of others; and exhibits arrogant, haughty behaviors or attitudes. *Note:* People with antisocial, borderline, histrionic, or narcissistic personality disorder often appear dramatic, highly emotional, or erratic.)
- *Obsessive-compulsive personality disorder*—difficulty establishing and sustaining close relationships associated with a pattern of preoccupation with orderliness, perfectionism, and control (The individual is preoccupied with details, rules, lists, order, organization, or schedules to the extent that the major part of the activity is lost. In addition, he or she shows perfectionism, rigidity, stubbornness, and restricted emotional expression.)
- *Schizotypal personality disorder*—a pattern of difficulties in social and interpersonal relationships in which the person suffers from acute discomfort with close relationships and therefore has a decreased capacity for such relationships (The individual also has cognitive and perceptual distortions as well as eccentricities of behavior that make close relationships difficult.)

BORDERLINE PERSONALITY DISORDER

The person with borderline personality disorder has patterns involving unstable relationships, unstable self-image, and unstable mood. Two theories offer explanations for the cause of this disorder. First, because families of patients with this disorder have a greater history of alcoholism, a genetic influence is thought to exist. The second explanation is related to particular developmental experiences. Some theorists view an essential component of psychosocial development as separation-individuation. Some feel that problems with attachment exist. It is thought that between 2 and 3 years of age, the child separates from the parents as a unique self. If the parents are nonaccepting or ambivalent about the child's increasing autonomy and if the parents reinforce dependent behavior, the child does not fully experience self as separate. This problem with separation-individuation is thought to form the basis of *splitting*, a frequently used mechanism in borderline personality disorder. Persons who are splitting view others as all good or all bad and may shift their views of a particular other from all good to all bad. A person who has a clearly developed sense of self and who does not split views others as having a mix of good qualities and negative qualities. The case of a patient named Bonnie provides a clinical example of borderline personality disorder:

> Nora, an LVN, worked part-time on a psychiatric unit. She reported to work at 11 PM one night after 5 days of not working to discover that Bonnie had been readmitted after opening the suture line on her wrists with a steak knife. One year ago Bonnie had cut this wrist, saying that she was trying to feel something. Bonnie told Nora that she had missed her terribly and she hoped Nora would work with her that night. Nora said that Susan (the full-time registered nurse [RN]) would work with her that night. Bonnie swore and returned to her room. When Nora made rounds, Bonnie said that she was sure something was wrong and began walking around the room with a staggering gait. Bonnie said that she had not taken anything to create this problem. Her vital signs were stable and her pupils were normal in size and reaction to light. Nora reported the situation to Susan and reflected on her responses to Bonnie. Initially she felt anger, telling herself that Bonnie was manipulative when she did not have her way. She thought about how Bonnie

manipulates others when she feels helpless (she has no idea of how to meet her own needs). She also thought about Bonnie's splitting (seeing Nora as good nurse and Susan as a bad nurse). Nora felt less angry as she considered the reasons for Bonnie's behavior. When Susan entered Bonnie's bedroom, Bonnie's gait was normal. Susan conversed with Bonnie for two 10-minute periods (at the beginning and end of her shift), during which time Bonnie could share whatever was on her mind and discuss her goals and plans for the following day.

NURSING CARE of the Patient with Borderline Personality Disorder

Assessment

The most relevant aspects of the mental status examination are the following:

- *Mood, affect, feelings*—The patient may experience mood swings or chronic feelings of emptiness and boredom or intense anger.
- *Insight and judgment*—The patient makes repeated suicidal threats and gestures and exhibits self-mutilating behavior.

Nursing Diagnoses, Goals, and Outcome Criteria: Borderline Personality Disorder

Nursing Diagnoses	Goals and Outcome Criteria
Risk for Self-Directed Violence and **Risk for Self-Mutilation** related to episodes of anger and impaired judgment	Absence of self-directed violence: patient does not harm self
Impaired Social Interaction related to unstable relationships	Improved social interaction: patient maintains relationships
Disturbed Personal Identity related to splitting	Improved sense of personal identity: patient clarifies own unique characteristics; differentiates thoughts and feelings of self and others; less splitting, clinging, and disturbing behaviors

Interventions

Risk for Self-Directed Violence and Risk for Self-Mutilation

In addition to the interventions identified in the section titled "Major Depressive and Bipolar Disorders," various interventions are more specific to the issues of borderline personality disorder. It is important to be aware of your own feelings to refrain from any automatic responses that are not helpful (e.g., avoiding the patient who has cut himself or herself). If patients mutilate themselves, it is important to care for wounds without acting in a way that might reinforce the self-mutilation (e.g., offering sympathy). Conversely, it is not appropriate to express disgust or in any way denigrate the patient. Ask patients to talk about feelings that occurred just before the self-mutilation. You can act as a role model for constructive expression of angry feelings and acknowledge the patient's positive expressions of negative feelings.

Impaired Social Interaction

Interventions include assisting patients in examining their own behaviors in relationships, communicating availability, acknowledging (reinforcing) independent behavior, and setting limits as appropriate.

Disturbed Personal Identity

Interventions include helping the patient to discuss and take ownership of his or her own thoughts and feelings, clarifying values while being cautious not to impose one's own values, and avoiding empathetic responses that may be viewed as mind reading (e.g., "I know how you feel").

SUMMARY

Nurses work with patients with psychiatric disorders in a variety of settings, including psychiatric inpatient units. Treatment for psychiatric disorders is influenced by the particular culture, place, and acuity of the present illness. You can use various strategies in communicating therapeutically with patients. The mental status examination is one aspect of the assessment of patients and is particularly relevant on a psychiatric unit. Systematically use the mental status examination with patients on admission and on an ongoing basis. For each of the major psychiatric disorders, possible observations for the relevant mental status examination categories are presented. Possible nursing diagnoses, goals, and interventions have been suggested for each disorder.

Get Ready for the NCLEX® Examination!

Key Points

- According to current thinking, mental illnesses are related to specific physiologic changes in the CNS.
- The psychoanalytic approach to mental illness is based on the theory that human beings function at different levels of awareness, ranging from conscious to unconscious, and that people use ego defense mechanisms to prevent anxiety.
- The interpersonal approach to mental illness has three components: (1) anxiety is often communicated interpersonally, (2) the patient learns new ways of

coping or maturing in a therapeutic relationship, and (3) establishing trust is an important first step in the nurse's work with patients.

- Key ideas from the cognitive behavioral approach to mental illness are that behavior is learned, that behavior changes in response to positive consequences (positive reinforcement) or in response to the removal of negative stimuli (negative reinforcement), and that particular thoughts influence emotional states.
- In caring for a patient with a psychiatric disorder, nurses establish therapeutic (as opposed to social) relationships.
- The mental status examination consists of observations regarding appearance, activity, mood and affect, speech and language, thought content, perceptual disturbances, insight and judgment, sensorium, and memory and attention.
- A patient with an anxiety disorder experiences either the highly uncomfortable feeling of anxiety directly or a symptom such as compulsive hand washing that prevents or reduces the occurrence of anxiety.
- In panic disorder a patient experiences recurrent panic attacks, which are intense episodes of apprehension, at times to the point of terror; often these attacks are accompanied by the feeling of impending doom.
- A person with agoraphobia is extremely fearful of situations outside the home from which escape may be difficult or in which help may be unavailable.
- OCD involves recurrent obsessions (thoughts), compulsions (behaviors), or both that produce distress and interfere with functioning.
- PTSD is a cluster of symptoms experienced after a distressing event that is outside the range of normal events.
- Individuals with a somatic symptom disorder, such as conversion disorder or illness anxiety disorder, are convinced that they have serious medical problems despite the absence of concrete medical findings.
- Dissociative disorders involve a change in identity, memory, or consciousness, usually to escape from anxiety.
- Goals for the nursing care of patients with anxiety, somatic symptom disorders, and dissociative disorders are to decrease anxiety to a point at which problem solving can occur and to teach methods such as relaxation techniques to interrupt anxiety as it escalates.
- The term *schizophrenia* refers to a highly problematic group of biologic disorders in which symptoms of psychosis exist, including delusions, hallucinations, marked loosening of associations, catatonia, and flat or inappropriate affect.
- People with major depressive and bipolar disorders experience a significantly elevated mood, a significantly depressed mood, or both.
- Dementia is a group of disorders characterized by cognitive deficits sufficiently severe enough to impair social or occupational functioning.
- Personality disorders occur when personality traits become inflexible and dysfunctional and are pervasive, chronic, and maladaptive.
- Drug therapy for people with psychiatric disorders employs anxiolytics, antidepressants, antipsychotics, and mood stabilizers.

Additional Learning Resources

SG Go to your Study Guide for additional learning activities to help you master this chapter content.

evolve Go to your Evolve website (http://evolve.elsevier.com/Linton/medsurg) for the following learning resources and much more:

- Interactive Prioritization Exercises
- Fluid & Electrolyte Tutorial
- Pharmacology Tutorial
- Review Questions for the NCLEX® Examination

Review Questions for the NCLEX® Examination

1. Which of the following is the primary focus of nursing care for patients with mental illness and their families?
   1. Helping them to cope with and manage mental illness
   2. Administering medications
   3. Protecting other people from the patient
   4. Controlling the patient's behavior

   NCLEX Client Need: Psychosocial Integrity
2. Which of the following are important characteristics of a therapeutic relationship? (Select all that apply.)
   1. The purpose is to benefit both the patient and the nurse.
   2. The relationship has a clear purpose and ending.
   3. The relationship has no clear boundaries.
   4. The relationship develops purposefully.
   5. The nurse's emotional needs are met.

   NCLEX Client Need: Psychosocial Integrity
3. Which statement best illustrates the strategy of *clarifying* in a nurse-patient interaction?
   1. "When you mention your son, you look very sad."
   2. "What were you saying while I was on the telephone?"
   3. "Why do you get quiet when I ask about your husband?"
   4. "Are you saying that you are afraid of him?"

   NCLEX Client Need: Psychosocial Integrity
4. In the mental status examination, the nurse collects data on multiple areas, including which of the following? (Select all that apply.)
   1. Thought content
   2. Mood and affect
   3. Appearance
   4. Reaction time
   5. Memory and attention

   NCLEX Client Need: Psychosocial Integrity
5. Mr. Brooks was hospitalized after a major automobile accident in which another person died. Mr. Brooks reports having no sensation in his legs and is unable to move them. Diagnostic studies reveal no physical basis for his symptoms. The patient's symptoms are typical of which of the following?
   1. Illness anxiety disorder
   2. Posttraumatic stress disorder
   3. Conversion disorder
   4. Panic disorder

   NCLEX Client Need: Psychosocial Integrity

6. John is a young college student who has just been diagnosed with schizophrenia. His concerned parents ask for information about his diagnosis. Which reply would be correct and appropriate?
   1. "Schizophrenia is a mental illness that affects a person's thinking and distorts his or her view of reality."
   2. "Most people with schizophrenia eventually require permanent care in a psychiatric facility."
   3. "At this time no medications or treatments are available for schizophrenia."
   4. "Most episodes of schizophrenia resolve within 1 or 2 weeks."

   NCLEX Client Need: Psychosocial Integrity
7. Nursing interventions to promote communication with the person who has schizophrenia include which of the following? (Select all that apply.)
   1. Let the patient know that you do not share his or her delusions
   2. Encourage the patient to attend to activities in the environment
   3. Point out the flaws in the patient's illogical statements
   4. Inform the patient that hallucinations are part of the disease
   5. Ask the patient to explain why he or she behaves as he or she does

   NCLEX Client Need: Psychosocial Integrity
8. Several residents in a long-term care facility have been taking a first-generation antipsychotic for a prolonged period of time. Which data should the LVN/LPN collect related to this drug therapy? (Select all that apply.)
   1. Dry mouth
   2. Shuffling gait
   3. Muscle rigidity
   4. Abnormal movements
   5. Faintness upon changing from a sitting to a standing position

   NCLEX Client Need: Physiological Integrity: Pharmacological Therapies
9. People who are arrogant, need excessive admiration, and take advantage of others for their own gain may have which type of personality disorder?

   NCLEX Client Need: Psychosocial Integrity
10. A patient with bipolar disorder who is taking divalproex (Depakote) is advised that blood samples will be taken periodically to monitor for which adverse effect?
    1. Liver damage
    2. Dystonic reactions
    3. Kidney damage
    4. Extrapyramidal syndromes

    NCLEX Client Need: Physiological Integrity: Pharmacological Therapies

chapter

57

Substance-Related and Addictive Disorders

Mary Ann Matteson

http://evolve.elsevier.com/Linton/medsurg

Objectives

1. Apply the biologic, environmental, and behavioral theories to the risks of substance-related and addictive disorders.
2. Discuss prevention and treatment for substance-related and addictive disorders.
3. Describe the development, course, and outcomes of substance-related disorders.
4. Describe the development, course, and outcomes of gambling addiction.
5. Describe the data to be collected for the nursing assessment of a patient with substance-related and addictive disorders.
6. Describe the nursing diagnoses and interventions associated with substance-related and addictive disorders.
7. Discuss populations that present special problems in relation to substance use and gambling addiction.

Key Terms

Addiction (Ă-DĬK-shŭn)
Codependent
Delirium tremens
Comorbidity and dual diagnosis (dī-ăg-NŌ-sĭs)
Tolerance (TŎL-ĕr-ăns)
12-step program
Withdrawal

THE SCIENCE OF ADDICTION

Addiction has become a problem of such worldwide significance over the past 50 years that a large amount of energy and financial resources have been targeted toward a better understanding of the disorder. The consequences of addiction affect people of all ages and the cost in the United States is upward of half a trillion dollars a year, when calculated considering their combined medical, economic, criminal, and social impact. Drug and alcohol use disorders contribute to the death of more than 100,000 Americans and tobacco is associated with an estimated 400,000 deaths per year. Researchers are attempting to discover the specific causes of *substance-related disorders* and *addiction* to prevent and treat them more effectively.

According to the National Institute on Drug Abuse (NIDA), addiction is a "chronic, relapsing brain disease that is characterized by compulsive drug seeking and use, despite harmful consequences." A person with a substance use disorder continues to use a substance in spite of significant cognitive, behavioral, and physiologic symptoms associated with its use. Research has shown that drugs change the structure of the brain and how they work and the effects may be long lasting and sometimes irreversible. Addiction also affects behavior to the degree that judgment, decision making, learning, memory, and self-control are impaired.

The *Diagnostic and Statistical Manual of Mental Disorders,* Fifth Edition (DSM-V), describes drug use and addictive disorders as mental illnesses because addiction changes the brain in the same way that mental illness does. The diagnosis of the disorder is grouped into four different categories: (1) impaired control, (2) social impairment, (3) risky use, and (4) pharmacologic criteria. *Impaired control* features the need to increase the amount of substance over a period of time; multiple unsuccessful attempts to decrease or discontinue use; an inordinate amount of time spent obtaining, using, or recovering from the effects of the substance; and an intense craving for the substance. *Social impairment* consists of a failure to fulfill major role obligations at work, school, or home; continued use of the substance despite social or interpersonal problems; reduced social or recreational activities; and withdrawal from family activities and hobbies in order to use the substance. *Risky use* is characterized by continued use despite physically hazardous conditions and despite physical or psychologic problems associated with use. *Pharmacologic criteria* include increased **tolerance** to the degree that more of the substance is needed to gain the same effect and **withdrawal** that occurs when blood and tissue levels of the drug decline after prolonged use.

The DSM-V no longer uses the terms *dependence* and *abuse* in association with substance-related disorders. Rather, the conditions are described in terms of severity based on the number of symptom criteria an individual demonstrates. For example, a mild disorder is indicated by the presence of two to three symptoms, a moderate disorder by four to five symptoms, and a severe disorder by six or more symptoms. It takes time for new terminology to be widely accepted. Therefore many practitioners may still use the more familiar terms *drug abuse* and *addiction* when diagnosing and treating substance-related and addictive disorders.

CAUSE AND RISK FACTORS

In recent years, scientists have studied the effects that drugs have on the brain and behavior and have found that many factors combine to influence whether a person becomes addicted. The biologic makeup of an individual, which can be influenced by gender, ethnicity, developmental stage, and the surrounding environment, may be a major risk factor (Fig. 57-1). Predisposition to addiction differs among individuals and the more risk factors a person has, the greater the chance for the disease of addiction.

Initially, people may take drugs to feel good or achieve a sense of euphoria, to relieve stress or anxiety, to enhance performance, or—especially among adolescents—in response to peer pressure. Most addictions begin with casual or social use of a drug, leading to habitual and more frequent use. Gradually there may be a need for larger doses to get high, followed by the need for the drug just to feel good. Finally, it may be increasingly difficult to go without the drug and individuals may reach the point where they seek and take the drugs despite the problems caused to themselves and loved ones. Stopping may cause intense cravings and withdrawal symptoms.

BIOLOGY AND GENES

Genetic factors account for 40% to 60% of an individual's vulnerability to addiction; in addition, people with mental disorders are at greater risk for substance use disorder and addiction than the general population. Substance use disorders and mental disorders often coexist; mental illnesses may precede addiction or addiction may worsen the mental illness.

Scientists have identified specific areas of the brain where every major drug that is associated with substance use disorders, including opiates, methamphetamine, cocaine, tobacco, alcohol, and marijuana, has its initial effects. With repeated drug exposure, significant disruptions in these brain circuits cause the circuits to "reset," leading to compulsive behavior to seek and use drugs. Thus the medical community considers addiction to be a chronic medical illness, similar to those that have the following characteristics: (1) incurability, (2) a genetic predisposition to develop under the right conditions, and (3) a potential to be treated effectively only by total abstinence from the substance that the body cannot handle.

ENVIRONMENTAL FACTORS

Major environmental factors that may play a role in the process of becoming addicted are the home environment and peer and school influences. Children who live in a home where older adults have substance or alcohol use disorders or who engage in criminal behavior may be at increased risk for addiction; in addition, at-risk children may have been subjects of verbal or

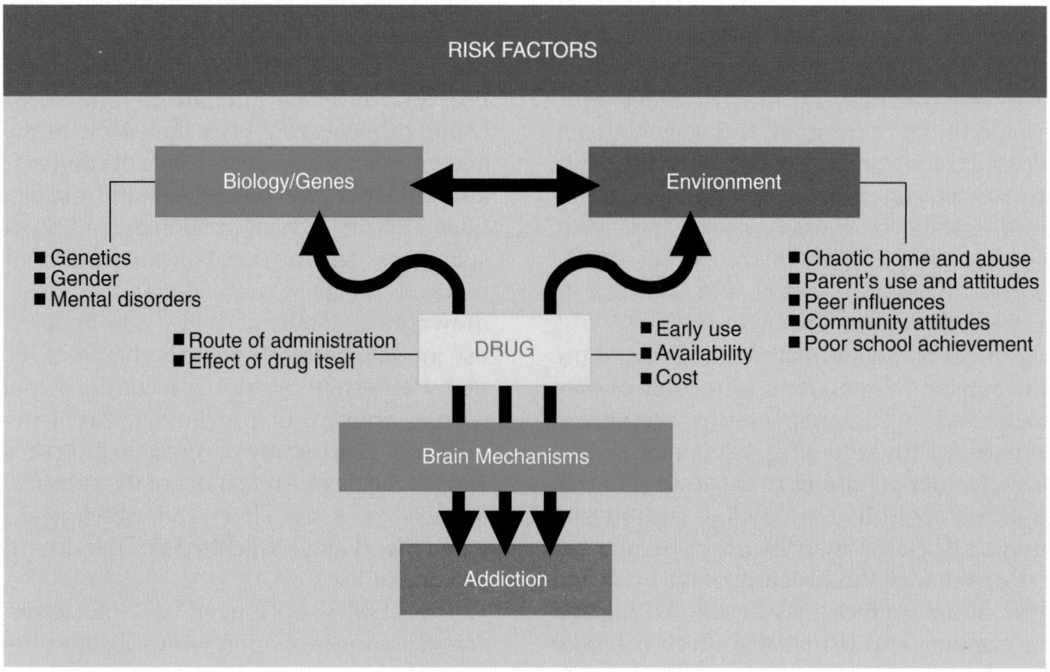

FIGURE 57-1 The overall risk for addiction is affected by the biologic makeup of the individual and his or her surrounding social environment. (Adapted from National Institute on Drug Abuse, National Institutes of Health: *Drugs, brain and behavior: the science of addiction*, Washington, DC, 2010, U.S. Department of Health & Human Services.)

physical abuse. In adolescence, friends and schoolmates can influence even teens without risk factors to try drugs for the first time. Academic failure and poor social skills also can put a teen at risk for developing an addiction.

The ways in which biologic sex and gender interact with each other and with substance use are complex. Drugs, reasons for use, and consequences frequently vary by sex and gender. Gender is influenced by sociocultural factors, such as expected social roles and behaviors that often differ according to race and class and that can change over time. In general, the overall rate of substance use is greater in males than in females; however, some studies have shown that females demonstrate different reactions to drugs than males in brain responses, risk factors, reasons for abusing prescription drugs, benefits of treatment, and reasons for relapsing.

Many people who live in poverty and in crime-ridden areas use drugs to relieve the stress inherent in these environments. In contrast, it can be observed that individuals with strong religious values that prohibit the excessive use of drugs have lower rates of addiction. Among certain subcultures, the use of certain drugs can be a rite of entry into a gang or a badge of honor proving that one has "made it." In college, students may be exposed to alcohol and other drugs in ways they have not been previously. Binge drinking, for example, is not an uncommon phenomenon in college dorms, fraternities, and sororities, sometimes starting as a rite of initiation. Even among middle-class Americans, the average person often parties to excess on New Year's Eve, for example. Certain cultural groups, such as the Irish, are commonly stereotyped as heavy drinkers. Among country music fans, "crying in your beer" is often portrayed as the typical means of coping with loss and rejection.

OTHER FACTORS

Other factors that increase the risk of addiction are early use, availability, cost, and method of administration. Research has shown that the earlier individuals begin to use substances, the more likely they are to develop more serious use disorders. This may be explained by the harmful effect on the developing brain, genetic susceptibility, mental illness, unstable family relationships, and exposure to physical or sexual abuse.

Smoking or injecting a substance into a vein increases its addictive potential. The drug enters the brain within seconds, producing a powerful rush of pleasure or "high" that lasts only a few minutes, followed by a "low" after the drug has worn off. It is thought that addiction results from the need to continually achieve the high associated with the substance used.

Cost and availability of substances also affect predisposition to addiction. The lower the cost and the easier it is to obtain drugs, the more likely a person will become addicted.

COMORBIDITY

Comorbidity, sometimes called **dual diagnosis**, is a term used to describe a situation in which two disorders or illnesses occur in the same person at the same time or when one follows the other. This may result in interactions between the illnesses that affect the course and prognosis of both.

Many people who are addicted to drugs are also diagnosed with mental illnesses and vice versa. Surveys have found that individuals diagnosed with mood or anxiety disorders are almost twice as likely to suffer from a drug use disorder and that individuals diagnosed with drug use disorders are twice as likely to suffer from mood and anxiety disorders. In addition, there is a higher prevalence of smoking among patients with mental disorders. Three possibilities for comorbidity exist: (1) drug use can cause abusers to experience one or more symptoms of another mental illness; (2) mental illness can lead to drug use, particularly as a form of self-medication to relieve symptoms; and (3) both drug use disorders and other mental illnesses are caused by combined biologic and environmental factors. Because there is a high incidence of comorbidity between drug use disorders and mental illness, a comprehensive approach to diagnosis and treatment should be used.

PRESCRIPTION DRUGS

The nonmedical use of prescription drugs, particularly opioid pain relievers, attention deficit hyperactivity disorder (ADHD) stimulants, and antianxiety drugs, is highest among young adults (ages 18 to 25 years). They may use these substances to get high or because the stimulants may help them to study better. In 2010, almost 3000 young adults died from prescription drug (mainly opioid) overdoses, a 250% increase from 1999. More males than females use prescription drugs nonmedically.

PREVENTION AND TREATMENT

Prevention

Because early use of drugs increases a person's risk for addiction, prevention is the best strategy to reduce the possibility of developing a substance use disorder. National drug use surveys indicate that some children are already addicted to drugs by age 12 or 13 years. Therefore adolescence is a critical time for preventing drug addiction. Teenagers are still developing judgment and decision-making skills, which limits their ability to assess risks accurately and make sound decisions about drugs. Although alcohol use has decreased among teens, marijuana use has increased, especially among boys. Several principles of prevention can be applied to most substances (see *Health Promotion* box).

Health Promotion

Preventing Alcohol Use among Children

- Alcohol use often begins at an early age and the proportion of young people who drink frequently or heavily is alarming. The Leadership to Keep Children Alcohol Free initiative is a coalition of federal government agencies and private foundations dedicated to mobilizing resources to combat this public health problem.
- Research has shown that adolescents who abuse alcohol recall 10% less of what they have learned than those who do not drink. Alcohol use also may lead to increased sexual activity, unplanned pregnancy, sexually transmitted infections, criminal activity (including drunk driving), suicide attempts, and other destructive or violent behavior.
- The age at which a person first uses alcohol is a powerful predictor of lifetime alcohol abuse and dependence. An epidemiologic study published in the *Journal of Substance Abuse* found that more than 40% of those who begin drinking before age 15 will develop alcohol abuse or alcohol dependence at some time in their lives.

As a health professional, talking to people about this issue will help to keep it high on the public agenda. Here are some suggestions:

- Talk to children about the dangers of early alcohol use. As appropriate, encourage your patients, friends, and neighbors to talk to their children. Some organizations, such as Mothers Against Drunk Driving (MADD) and Students Against Drunk Driving (SADD), provide speakers free of charge.
- Ask other health care professionals, such as pediatric nurses, to discuss alcohol use during children's annual physicals.
- Share literature about preventing alcohol abuse with members of your community.
- Support recreational alternatives to drinking in your community.
- Encourage parents to learn about their responsibilities regarding alcohol access and serving alcohol to minors in their homes.
- Talk to teachers, counselors, school administrators, and school board members to ensure that school prevention programs put equal emphasis on alcohol and illicit drug use.
- Place the issue of alcohol use by children on agendas for meetings of the Parent-Teacher Association, the city council, faith groups, the Rotary Club, the local chamber of commerce, and other community groups and organizations.
- Involve young people in your community's prevention efforts.
- Write letters to the editors of your local newspapers asking them to print articles about the dangers of early alcohol use.
- Contact elected and appointed officials at local and state levels to inform them about the problem and what can be done to solve it.
- Enlist support for immediate and consistent enforcement of underage alcohol-related drinking laws in your community.

Adapted from National Institute on Alcohol Abuse and Alcoholism, National Institutes of Health: Leadership to keep children alcohol free. In *Keep kids alcohol free: strategies for action.* Available at https://roar.nevadaprc.org/system/documents/145/original/Keep_Kids_alc_Free.pdf?1294418582.

Treatment

Addiction is a treatable disease that can be managed successfully like other chronic illnesses. According to NIDA, key principles have emerged based on scientific research since the 1970s, as follows:

- Addiction is a complex but treatable disease that affects brain function and behavior.
- No single treatment is appropriate for everyone.
- Treatment needs to be readily available.
- Effective treatment attends to multiple needs of the individual, not just to his or her drug abuse.
- Remaining in treatment for an adequate period of time is critical.
- Counseling—individual and/or group—and other behavioral therapies are the most commonly used forms of addiction therapy.
- Medications are an important element of treatment for many patients, especially when combined with counseling and other behavioral therapies.
- An individual's treatment and service plan must be assessed continually and modified as necessary to ensure that it meets his or her changing needs.
- Many drug-addicted individuals also have other mental disorders.
- Medically assisted detoxification is only the first stage of addiction treatment and by itself does little to change long-term drug abuse.
- Treatment does not need to be voluntary to be effective.
- Drug use during treatment must be monitored continuously, as lapses during treatment do occur.
- Treatment programs should assess patients for the presence of human immunodeficiency virus/acquired immunodeficiency syndrome (HIV/AIDS), hepatitis B and C, tuberculosis, and other infectious diseases as well as provide targeted risk-reduction counseling to help patients modify or change behaviors that place them at risk of contracting or spreading infection.

GAMBLING DISORDER

Gambling disorder was added to the DSM-V list of mental illnesses related to addiction. A gambling disorder is a persistent and recurrent problematic gambling behavior leading to a clinically significant impairment or distress. Gambling involves risking something of value in the hopes of gaining something of greater value, causing disruptions in personal, family, and/or vocational pursuits. An individual needs to gamble with increasing amounts of money to achieve the desired excitement but, after losing the money, often returns on another day to get even ("chasing" one's losses). The person lies to conceal the extent of involvement with gambling and may rely on others to provide money to relieve desperate financial situations caused by the gambling.

The prevalence of gambling disorder is higher in males and African Americans and is more common among young and middle-aged adults than older adults. The addiction usually develops over a course of years, gradually increasing in frequency and amount. Only about 10% of those with a gambling addiction seek treatment.

NURSING ASSESSMENT OF THE PERSON WITH AN ADDICTION

HEALTH HISTORY

Thorough data collection is essential to initiate the nursing process effectively when working with patients with substance use and addictive disorders. Information can be gathered from a variety of sources, including an interview with the patient, family members, and significant others; a social assessment; medical records; and school or military records. The licensed vocational nurse/licensed practical nurse (LVN/LPN) may participate in the collection of data from these sources. Many people with substance use and addictive disorders have sustained major losses—of jobs, relationships, property, self-esteem, and health. They may face legal charges. Often they will not seek professional help until they have "hit bottom." Even then, they may seek help only when given an ultimatum of some type, often from their family, employer, or a court of law.

Questioning the patient produces the most reliable data when the questioning is nonjudgmental, direct, and specific and the answers are verified by more than one source when possible. For example, if the patient reports drinking a couple of beers after work each night, you should ask exactly how many were ingested, how many ounces each contained, or how big the bottle or glass used actually was. It also is important to know when the patient ingested the drug last and how much was taken to predict the possibility and timing of physical withdrawal symptoms. A nonjudgmental and matter-of-fact manner is the least likely to alienate an already defensive patient. At the same time, do not be so supportive and nurturing that clients can avoid facing the negative effect that substance use has had on their lives. Finding the most appropriate balance of support and reality-based confrontation is a highly developed skill that increases the likelihood that patients will continue in the treatment process. Many team members who work in substance use disorder treatment centers are recovering from addiction themselves, which often helps the client to be more honest and less defensive and feel less hopeless and alone.

Patterns and Consequences of Substance Use and Addictive Disorders

The patient who has been abusing one or more substances will describe typical patterns of behavior and a combination of physical or psychologic withdrawal symptoms characteristic of the substances used. A few patients may not experience any physical withdrawal symptoms despite a history of prolonged, frequent, and heavy use, even of some substances that usually are physically addicting. Much depends on the stage of addiction, the habitual patterns of use, the patient's baseline physical status, and the combinations and interactions of the drugs used.

Many people with substance use and addictive disorders experience erratic and unprovoked mood swings. They may describe a lifestyle revolving almost totally around obtaining and using the substance of choice, starting early in the day, often alone, and requiring more of the substance over time to get the desired effects. Many with substance abuse disorders make efforts to hide the extent of their habit from others and, despite their best efforts, have been unsuccessful in limiting use of the substance. Blackouts may have occurred when under the influence of a particular substance (especially alcohol). Blackouts are episodes of amnesia in which the individual does not remember what happened during a period of time. Patients often have significant work problems or damaged relationships as a result of being unable to meet the expectations placed on them.

Defense Mechanisms

Typical defense mechanisms used by individuals with substance use and addictive disorders include denial, rationalization, intellectualization, and projection. Denial is readily apparent when patients state that they do not have a problem with drug use despite evidence to the contrary. Individuals also may initially minimize the problems they have had with using drugs. Some deny that they need help in staying clean and sober. Some insist that they do not need to change friends or attend a 12-step program meeting such as Alcoholics Anonymous (AA) regularly.

Rationalization is a defense mechanism in which addicts attempt to justify the reasons for substance use. This is an "excuse" for addiction. An example is the individual who insists that he or she *had* to use heroin because no other way to cope with the pain of a physical injury was available: "The drugs my doctor gave me weren't working."

Intellectualization is closely related to rationalization but differs in that the person focuses only on objective facts as a way of avoiding dealing with unconscious conflicts and the emotions they evoke. For example, an alcoholic who killed someone while driving under the influence of alcohol would be intellectualizing if he or she stated that it was better that the victim die suddenly rather than have to live as a paraplegic.

Projection in persons with substance use and addictive disorders involves shifting the blame for their behavior onto someone or something else. Drug users using projection might insist that they became addicted to alcohol as a result of the pressure to drink at work-related social functions to keep colleagues from thinking they were prudes. They also may blame a spouse or loved one.

PHYSICAL EXAMINATION

On physical examination, many people with substance abuse disorders appear malnourished and poorly cared for. Evidence of physical trauma from falls, abrasions, or fights may be present. Jaundice or discolored sclera of the eyes may suggest cirrhosis or other liver problems. Hypertension is a critical sign of withdrawal and is often accompanied by the physical signs of fluid retention in the legs or a protuberant abdomen swollen by liver ascites. Changes in mental status such as anxiety, confusion, irritability, memory loss, tremors, lack of coordination, and other neurologic signs are significant and may be associated with a number of causes, including nutritional deficits (see *Nutrition Considerations* box). It is important for you to recognize and report these findings because they may indicate that the patient is entering physical withdrawal and may be at risk for **delirium tremens** (or "DTs") and seizures if the drug being used is alcohol, a benzodiazepine, or both. Be alert for needle tracks in unexpected parts of the body (e.g., between the toes, in tattoos) in an individual who is believed to have been using substances intravenously. The atypical client may not have any obvious signs of physical problems but abnormalities may be found on laboratory tests done when the client enters a treatment program.

Nutrition Considerations

1. Heavy drug or alcohol intake has a negative effect on nutrition because it displaces foods in the diet that are more nutritious and impairs absorption and metabolism of nutrients in the body.
2. The nutritional goals for persons with alcoholism are to support them in avoiding alcohol and to correct nutritional deficits.
3. Individuals with chronic alcoholism may need supplements of folate and vitamin B_6.
4. Stimulants may induce anorexia; however, as the effects of the stimulants subside, hunger develops.

DIAGNOSTIC TESTS

To assess the patient's physical status, a thorough physical examination is done on initiation of treatment, along with a basic laboratory screen chosen to identify problems in any of the major organ systems. Abnormalities are often seen on liver function tests, in electrolyte values, and on tests reflecting nutritional status and gastric function. Diseases such as hepatitis B and hepatitis C that can be spread through blood and body fluids may be identified, especially among intravenous drug users. Syphilis rates are increasing and the escalating rate of HIV infection in this population is of national concern. Infections of various kinds are common. Special neurologic, neuropsychologic, and imaging studies may disclose brain damage.

BLOOD ALCOHOL STUDY

A blood alcohol study is the most accurate type of test available to measure the degree of intoxication on initiation of treatment for alcohol use. A blood alcohol level greater than 0.3% requires treatment for overdose; at concentrations greater than 0.4%, death is likely. Legal intoxication definitions vary from state to state but commonly are determined when a person's blood alcohol level is greater than 0.05%.

URINE DRUG SCREENING

Urine drug screening is the preferred way to screen for the recent use of an unknown drug and is commonly done along with the initial laboratory work. Drugs that are most likely to be identified in this way include amphetamines, barbiturates, benzodiazepines, cocaine, "crack," opiates, marijuana, phencyclidine (PCP), lysergic acid diethylamide (LSD), opioid analgesics, sedatives, and stimulants. With this test, drug metabolites can be identified for days or weeks after use, depending on the drug used. A special screen is necessary when looking for methadone. Typically, to ensure that tampering with the specimens or substitution of another person's urine has not occurred, a staff member of the same sex witnesses the collection of a urine specimen. After collection, the sample is kept under chain of custody (i.e., each person handling the sample signs a special document that accompanies the sample until it can be analyzed). Any temporary storage of the sample is maintained under secure conditions.

HAIR ANALYSIS

Hair analysis is a recent addition to the methods for detection of substance use. It requires sensitive technology but may be very helpful in monitoring patients for relapse. Depending on the length of the hair, a substance can be detected for up to 1 year after only 2 or 3 days of use. However, the presence of addiction or whether the person is currently under the influence of the substance cannot be inferred from a positive finding. The evidence that this test provides regarding long-term substance use may be a valuable tool in the diagnosis and follow-up of substance use disorders.

SUBSTANCE-RELATED DISORDERS

In DSM-V, 10 separate classes of drugs associated with substance-related disorders are identified: (1) alcohol, (2) caffeine, (3) cannabis (marijuana), (4) hallucinogens, (5) inhalants, (6) opioids, (7) sedatives, (8) hypnotics and anxiolytics, (9) stimulants, and (10) tobacco and other or unknown substances (Table 57-1).

Table 57-1 Common Mood-Altering Chemicals

DRUG NAME	EFFECTS	SITE OF ACTION	LENGTH OF EFFECT
Alcohol			
Alcohol, beer, wine (as beverages)	Relaxation, sedation, release of inhibitions, objective signs (i.e., incoordination, nausea, vomiting, slurred speech)	Central nervous system (CNS), respiratory system	Onset: 20 minutes to 1 hour Duration: dose-related
Caffeine			
Coffee, tea, chocolate, caffeinated drinks	Stimulation, restlessness, anxiety, objective signs (i.e., increased heart and respiratory rates, diarrhea, gastric disorder, insomnia, tremors)	CNS	Onset: 10–30 minutes Duration: 3–7 hours
Cannabis			
Marijuana, hashish	Failure in judgment and memory, euphoria, mild intoxication, relaxation, sexual arousal, panic states, visual hallucinations, objective signs (i.e., reddened eyes, dry mouth, incoordination, heart rate to 140 beats/min)	CNS, cardiovascular system, respiratory system	Onset: 20–30 minutes Duration: 3–7 hours (Administration- and dose-dependent)
Hallucinogens			
Psilocybin ("magic" mushrooms), lysergic acid diethylamide (LSD), mescaline (from peyote cactus), dimethoxymethamphetamine (DOM), STP (no chemical name), 3,4-methylenedioxyamphetamine (MDMA, ecstasy)	Altered body image, euphoria, sharpened perceptions, somatic effects (i.e., dizziness, tremors, weakness, nausea), psychosis-like symptoms, emotional swings, suspiciousness, bizarre behavior, increased blood pressure (BP), increased temperature, objective signs (i.e., dilated pupils, flushing, tremors)	CNS	Onset: 40–60 minutes Duration: 6–12 hours
Hallucinogens			
Phencyclidine (PCP, "angel dust")	Detachment from surroundings, decreased sensory awareness, illusions of superhuman strength, acute intoxication, objective signs (i.e., flushing, fever, sweating, coma, agitation, confusion, hallucinations, paranoia, violence)	CNS	Onset: 2–3 minutes up to 45 minutes (rapid onset) Duration: drug- and dose-related
Inhalants			
Benzene (paint thinner, cleaning fluid, glue), nitrites, nitrous oxide	Euphoria, giddiness, headache, fatigue, drowsiness, objective signs (i.e., dysrhythmias, damage to kidneys, liver abnormalities)	CNS, cardiac effect	Onset: immediate Duration: 20–45 minutes
Opioids, Semisynthetics, and Synthetic Analgesics			
Codeine, morphine, heroin, hydromorphone (Dilaudid), methadone, meperidine (Demerol), propoxyphene (Darvon), designer drugs	Analgesia, euphoria, escape, reduced sexual and aggressive drives, respiratory depression, sedation, sleepiness, objective signs (i.e., hypertension, pupillary constriction, constipation)	CNS (opioid receptors), respiratory system	Onset: 20–30 minutes Duration: 4–8 hours

Continued

Table 57-1 Common Mood-Altering Chemicals—cont'd

DRUG NAME	EFFECTS	SITE OF ACTION	LENGTH OF EFFECT
Sedatives, Hypnotics, and Anxiolytics			
Barbiturates (secobarbital [Seconal], phenobarbital [Nembutal], amobarbital [Amytal], amobarbital/secobarbital [Tuinal]) Barbiturate-like agents (methaqualone [Quaalude]) Benzodiazepines (alprazolam [Xanax], chlordiazepoxide [Librium], diazepam [Valium], lorazepam [Ativan])	Drowsiness, sedation, euphoria, escape, loss of aggressive and sexual drives, emotional lability, poor judgment	CNS, cardiovascular system, respiratory system	Onset: 30–40 minutes Duration: varies with each drug (Barbiturates may have longer half-life than benzodiazepines, depending on the drug.)
Stimulants			
Amphetamine (methamphetamine, Dexedrine, Benzedrine), methylphenidate (Ritalin), cocaine, crack	Euphoria, grandiosity, wakefulness, relief of fatigue, stimulation, energy, anxiety, depression, suppression of appetite, aggressive feelings, paranoia, objective signs (i.e., sweating, dilated pupils, increased BP, rapid heart and respiratory rates, tremors, seizures)	CNS, peripheral nervous system, cardiovascular system	Onset: 10–30 minutes (route-related) Duration: drug-related
Nicotine			
Cigarettes, smokeless tobacco	Stimulation, enhanced performance	CNS, respiratory system, cardiovascular system, endocrine system	Onset: immediate Duration: 5–15 minutes

Data from Naegle MA: Substance-related disorders. In Haber J, Krainovich B, McMahon AL, et al, editors: *Comprehensive psychiatric nursing,* ed 5, St. Louis, 1997, Mosby.

ALCOHOL AND ALCOHOLISM

Alcoholism is the most common drug-related disorder in the United States. According to the American Society of Addiction Medicine, alcoholism is:

> a primary, chronic disease with psychosocial and environmental factors influencing its development and manifestations. The disease is often progressive and fatal. It is characterized by continuous or periodic impaired control over drinking, preoccupation with the drug alcohol, use of alcohol despite adverse consequences, and distortions in thinking, most notably denial.

Environmental risks for the disease are cultural attitudes toward drinking, availability, peer pressure, and ineffective coping with stress. Genetic predisposition accounts for 40% to 60% of the risk for alcoholism and males have higher rates of alcohol-related disorders than females. However, females may develop higher blood alcohol levels per drink than males because they have more fat and less water in their bodies and metabolize less alcohol in their esophagus and stomach.

Pharmacology Capsule

The American Society of Addiction Medicine defines alcohol as a *drug* because it has addictive qualities similar to those associated with other drug-related disorders. Simple intoxication from alcohol usually lasts less than 12 hours and is followed by the unpleasant experience of a hangover beginning about 4 to 6 hours after the last drink. Typical symptoms include headache, upset stomach, vomiting, sweating, thirst, fatigue, and blurred vision or "seeing stars." The cause of these symptoms has not been pinpointed; however, it is believed to be a result of hypoglycemia, dehydration, and the buildup of acetaldehyde and lactic acid in the blood.

Chronic use involves the regular daily ingestion of large quantities of alcohol, regular heavy drinking only on weekends, or binges of heavy drinking followed by long periods of abstinence. Physical **addiction** occurs when alcohol becomes integrated into physiologic processes at the cellular level. The cell becomes dependent on the alcohol to carry on certain metabolic processes; if alcohol is no longer available, the cell goes into "shock" and is unable to compensate for the loss quickly. Thus alcohol withdrawal syndrome begins after the individual stops or decreases the amount ingested. Heavy chronic drinkers may experience the onset of withdrawal without actually stopping drinking simply because they are no longer able to ingest enough alcohol to meet the body's demands for the substance to function.

Alcohol withdrawal syndrome involves physiologic and behavioral symptoms that begin when the individual's blood alcohol level drops. It is divided into two stages, depending on the onset and severity of symptoms. The first stage usually occurs within 6 to 12 hours after the last drink and is called *early withdrawal*. Symptoms begin with anxiety, agitation, and irritability. If the patient does not drink, tremors may be observed. Blood pressure (BP), pulse, and temperature all begin to rise. Sweating, nausea, vomiting, and diarrhea are typical.

The second stage, *major withdrawal*, begins with the onset of seizures and hallucinations and can advance to life-threatening delirium tremens. This stage usually occurs after approximately 3 days (sometimes less) without alcohol or treatment and can be predicted from extreme elevations in temperature, pulse, and BP. The patient typically becomes disoriented and confused. Hallucinations are often visual and "animal" in nature. Bugs, snakes, and rats are commonly described, sometimes perceived to be crawling on the person. Familiar jokes about seeing "pink elephants" probably evolved out of this type of withdrawal experience.

Alcohol withdrawal is the *most* life-threatening withdrawal syndrome compared with those associated with other types of drugs, even heroin. (Withdrawal from barbiturates and benzodiazepines also can result in delirium tremens; both types of drugs have similar central nervous system [CNS] depressant effects.) Thus it is critical to counsel alcoholics never to attempt to withdraw on their own or "go cold turkey." They always should seek medical treatment. Most require inpatient hospitalization and administration of medications such as lorazepam (Ativan) or chlordiazepoxide (Librium) to prevent the severe consequences of withdrawal and to ensure early detection and treatment of symptoms.

Medical Complications

Common medical complications of chronic alcoholism include cirrhosis of the liver, pancreatitis, gastrointestinal (GI) bleeding (often from esophageal varices), Wernicke encephalopathy, Korsakoff psychosis, and fetal alcohol syndrome.

Wernicke Encephalopathy. Wernicke encephalopathy is due to vitamin B_1 (thiamine) deficiency. Its symptoms include delirium, confabulation because of memory loss, unsteady gait, a sense of apprehension, and altered levels of consciousness that can proceed to coma. If it is not properly treated with vitamin supplementation, Korsakoff psychosis may develop.

Korsakoff Psychosis. In this disorder, both thiamine and niacin deficiencies contribute to the degeneration of the cerebrum and the peripheral nervous system. Symptoms include amnesia, confabulation, disorientation, and peripheral neuropathies. Despite treatment, some residual problems persist in both Wernicke encephalopathy and Korsakoff psychosis. However, dementia is permanent if the patient progresses to Korsakoff psychosis. Both of these disorders are classified as *alcohol amnesic disorders*.

Fetal Alcohol Syndrome. Fetal alcohol syndrome is a medical complication that is of great concern in many countries. If a woman drinks alcohol during pregnancy, the unborn child is at risk for symptoms such as low birth weight, mental retardation, growth deficiencies, heart defects, facial malformations, learning disabilities, and hyperactivity. Recent controversy has arisen over whether maternal alcoholism constitutes child abuse and is thus reportable under child protection statutes.

Treatment for Alcohol Addiction

Because alcoholism affects everyone in the family system, active family involvement in the treatment of an alcohol-related disorder has come to be seen as a critical factor in the success of treatment outcomes. Alcoholism often produces predictable patterns of individual behavior or changes in roles that may significantly handicap various family members in getting their needs met. Examples of some of the labels given to these atypical roles are the hero, the mascot, the lost child, and the scapegoat. Adult children of alcoholics may struggle with issues throughout their lives as a result of dysfunctional patterns of thoughts and behaviors learned in childhood through the enactment of these types of roles. Spouses of alcoholics frequently struggle with "enabling" behaviors. These are described as any behavior that "covers up" or protects alcoholics from the consequences of their drinking behaviors. For example, a woman might lie to her husband's boss about why he will not be at work, when in reality the husband is too "hung over" to perform adequately. Those who enable are sometimes considered **codependent**, in that their behavior is highly structured around managing and adapting to the alcoholic's dysfunctional behavior.

Family, peer pressure, and confrontation can be critical factors in inducing the alcoholic to seek treatment. Through participation in a 12-step self-help support group for the significant others of persons with a substance use disorders, called *Al-Anon* and *Alateen*, spouses, children, friends, and co-workers can learn new ways of coping with issues and how to avoid enabling the alcoholic so that it becomes harder for him or her to continue the destructive pattern of drinking.

Intervention. An intervention is a planned, structured meeting by family and friends to confront the alcoholic with the effect that the person's alcohol use has on each member of the group. Often the alcoholic or substance user is brought into the meeting without prior notification about the intervention. The intervention is led by a specially trained interventionist who helps those involved in the process to prepare by writing down the ways in which the person's alcohol use affects them personally. The interventionist offers suggestions on how to word ideas in ways less likely to evoke defensiveness and how to focus on the issues to reject the problem drinking but not the person. During the intervention, all of the participants have an opportunity to read their letters aloud to the alcohol user. At the end of each letter, the reader requests that the alcoholic go into treatment to get help. Usually, after experiencing a confrontation from a roomful of significant people, users will go unhappily, but voluntarily, directly from the intervention into a treatment program that has been arranged for in advance.

The use of this strategy has come under criticism because the user confronted in this way often feels coerced into treatment. After the intervention, the user may harbor angry feelings directed at members of the family for being critical, pushy, and having "tricked" him or her. Ideally, for treatment to be most effective, individuals should choose to go voluntarily. Proponents of the use of intervention respond that the user may die or suffer terrible consequences of the disease before seeking help on a totally voluntary basis and thus the end justifies the means.

Detoxification. Detoxification is usually done in an inpatient hospital or rehabilitation center. During detoxification, the patient's vital signs are monitored frequently. Initially, patients do not participate in group therapy because of their physical status. Rest and nutrition are emphasized. Drugs from the anxiolytic (benzodiazepine) group most often are used in detoxification of the alcohol-dependent patient. The two most common benzodiazepines used to treat acute alcohol withdrawal are lorazepam (Ativan) and diazepam (Valium). Intravenous magnesium sulfate may be used to prevent seizures in rare cases. Scheduled anticonvulsant agents are prescribed if seizures occur. Fluids are encouraged to combat dehydration and vitamin replacement therapy is instituted.

Rehabilitation. Once patients are medically stable, they are referred to either an inpatient or an outpatient treatment program, depending on individual needs and resources. The traditional inpatient program, or Minnesota model, lasts about 28 days and includes highly structured scheduling of drug education films and presentations; increasingly confrontational individual, group, and family therapy; recreational and occupational therapy; milieu therapy; and introduction to AA, a self-help support group. However, the availability of third-party reimbursement for an inpatient rehabilitation stay has all but disappeared. More commonly, patients are referred to partial hospitalization programs (day treatment programs) and outpatient therapy as well as to other community resources. Less common is an extended residential program that may last 1 to 2 years.

Alcoholics Anonymous. AA is a nonprofit, worldwide organization of alcoholics who meet together anonymously in small groups at various times during the day throughout the year to assist each other in staying sober. The organization uses a strong spiritual base, which is controversial, and a **12-step program** (Box 57-1) involving discussions and written exercises designed around each of the 12 steps as a means of keeping the alcoholic from relapsing. Members identify another participant of the same sex who is seasoned in the recovery process, and to whom they can relate, to act as their sponsor. The sponsor agrees to be available to the person for support and advice in staying sober. Service work in the community also is seen as integral to focusing outside oneself.

Members use regular readings from *The Big Book of Alcoholic Anonymous*, written by founding members to

Box 57-1 Twelve Steps of Alcoholics Anonymous

1. We admit we were powerless over alcohol—our lives had become unmanageable.
2. Came to believe that a Power greater than ourselves could restore us to sanity.
3. Made a decision to turn our will and lives over to the care of God, as we understood Him.
4. Made a searching and fearless moral inventory of ourselves.
5. Admitted to God, to ourselves, and to another human being the exact nature of our wrongs.
6. Were entirely ready to have God remove all these defects of character.
7. Humbly asked Him to remove our shortcomings.
8. Listed all persons we had harmed and became willing to make amends to them all.
9. Made direct amends whenever possible, except when to do so would injure them or others.
10. Continued to make personal inventory and when we were wrong promptly admitted it.
11. Sought through prayer and meditation to improve our conscious contact with God, as we understood Him, praying only for knowledge of His will for us and the power to carry it out.
12. Having had a spiritual awakening as the result of these steps, we tried to carry this message to alcoholics and to practice these principles in all our affairs.

keep themselves on track (Box 57-2 lists the 12 traditions of AA). No dues are required from AA members; instead the organization relies on donations. In addition, AA has no political affiliations and makes no endorsements of candidates or products. Everyone involved participates on a voluntary basis. Even group leaders are volunteers and are not professional counselors. Meetings may be advertised in the community using the title "Friends of Bill W." as a means of maintaining the anonymity of participants (Bill W. was one of two originators of the organization). Before discharge from an inpatient treatment program, alcoholics have the opportunity to attend various community AA meetings to increase the odds of continued outpatient participation and to begin the process of finding a "home group" to which they can connect.

Recently, research has begun to question what actually works in alcohol rehabilitation. Actual outcomes of the traditional types of treatment approaches have not been documented clearly. As a result, many insurance companies no longer fund 28-day inpatient treatment. Many 28-day inpatient treatment programs have been forced to close because of a lack of clients able to afford the cost of this intensive treatment. Treatment facilities have been forced to provide brief and creative inpatient rehabilitation with rapid referral to an outpatient program and aftercare.

One trend is toward using more nontraditional treatment approaches that have produced successful outcomes. Some components of alcohol rehabilitation that have been shown to be very useful in maintaining continued sobriety are the teaching of stress management, social skills training, behavioral approaches, marital therapy, and matching clients with a therapist who uses a style most likely to benefit their personality type. A move also is underway in which treatment programs are attempting to group patients with similar lifestyles and characteristics together rather than to group everyone together. Other factors being considered in developing more homogeneous small groups are styles of thinking (abstract versus concrete thinkers), sex role–related issues, ethnicity, and age. The current trend is away from a "recipe card" approach to treatment that is expected to work for anyone who is an alcoholic (see Nursing Care Plan: Patient Who Is Abusing Alcohol).

Cost containment has stimulated the development of many new types of outpatient programs for the treatment of alcoholism. Most day treatment or partial hospitalization programs are very similar to the traditional inpatient milieu and offer similar types of therapies but they allow patients to return to their own homes at night. In this case the risk of relapse often requires the use of medication such as disulfiram (Antabuse) or metronidazole (Flagyl), which makes the user ill if mixed with alcohol. Usually, involvement in the program is intensive but does not last for the traditional 30 days.

Other individuals use active involvement in AA as the primary means for recovery by attending at least 90 meetings in 90 days. Other community programs also are available to assist the alcoholic in the recovery process and should not be overlooked. Some are church related; some are focused on getting the recovering user back to work by providing job placement or an opportunity to return to school. One example of a community recovery program that exists in various parts of the country is the Patrician Movement. In addition, halfway houses may be available in the local area as a service of community mental health organizations.

Relapse Prevention. Relapse prevention is a key component in the treatment of persons with substance use disorder. Relapse prevention involves assisting patients to identify triggers to their substance use. For example, a person may identify friends who consistently use the abused substance or may identify places where

Box 57-2 Twelve Traditions of Alcoholics Anonymous

1. Our common welfare should come first; personal recovery depends on AA unity.
2. For our group purpose, there is but one ultimate authority—a loving God as He may express Himself in our group conscience. Our leaders are but trusted servants; they do not govern.
3. The only requirement for AA membership is a desire to stop drinking.
4. Each group should be autonomous except in matters affecting other groups or AA as a whole.
5. Each group has but one primary purpose—to carry its message to the alcoholic who still suffers.
6. An AA group ought never endorse, finance, or lend the AA name to any related facility or outside enterprise, lest problems of money, property, and prestige divert us from our primary purpose.
7. Every AA group ought to be fully self-supporting, declining outside contributions.
8. AA should remain forever nonprofessional, but our service centers may employ special workers.
9. AA, as such, ought never be organized; but we may create service boards or committees directly responsible to those they serve.
10. AA has no opinion on outside issues; hence the AA name ought never be drawn into public controversy.
11. Our public relations policy is based on attraction rather than promotion; we need always maintain personal anonymity at the level of press, radio, and films.
12. Anonymity is the spiritual foundation of all our traditions, ever reminding us to place principles before personalities.

Nursing Care Plan: Patient Who Is Abusing Alcohol

ASSESSMENT

HEALTH HISTORY A 37-year-old man was admitted for alcohol detoxification. He was found lying on the floor at home, unconscious, and appeared to have vomited and been incontinent of urine and feces. He has a long history of alcohol use but claims that he does not have a problem because he drinks only beer. He recently lost his job because he was not reporting for work on time and his wife has threatened to leave him if he does not stop drinking. His two children, ages 8 and 10 years, are afraid of him when he drinks. His usual intake of alcohol is two six-packs of beer a day. He has been detoxified in the hospital and is now ready for the rehabilitation phase of his treatment.

PHYSICAL EXAMINATION Vital signs: blood pressure 128/72 mm Hg, pulse 80 bpm, respiration 20 breaths per minute, temperature 97.6°F (36.4°C), measured orally. Height 5′10″, weight 160 lb. The patient's skin and eyes have a slightly yellowish tinge. There is a cast is on his left arm from below the elbow to the fingers. He appears thin and wasted.

Nursing Diagnosis	Goals and Outcome Criteria	Interventions
Ineffective Denial related to continued alcohol use	The patient will acknowledge that he has a problem, stop ingesting alcohol, and attend Alcoholics Anonymous (AA) meetings on a regular basis.	Use confrontational techniques to help the patient accept the diagnosis of alcoholism and support his 12-step program of rehabilitation.
Ineffective Coping related to alcohol ingestion as a means of coping with stressors	The patient will overcome his impulse to drink alcohol until intoxicated and to use alcohol as a coping mechanism, as evidenced by stopping ingestion of alcohol and substituting other coping mechanisms.	Help the patient to overcome cravings by introducing new coping mechanisms such as exercise and stress management skills. Encourage him to attend his treatment program and AA meetings on a regular basis.
Chronic Low Self-Esteem related to loss of control, guilty feelings	The patient will maintain an adequate self-concept, as evidenced by lessened self-criticism, good hygiene, and positive interactions with others. The patient will develop a realistic sense of self, verbalize positive aspects of self and begin to forgive himself, and express his true feelings.	Help the patient to maintain self-esteem after confrontational therapy sessions by allowing him to vent his feelings and acting as a role model for dealing with others. Allow the patient to vent his feelings about his illness and to explore his feelings about his past behaviors. Support the patient in his 12-step program of rehabilitation.
Risk for Injury related to excessive use of alcohol and high risk for relapse	The patient will not injure himself or others as a result of excessive ingestion of alcohol.	Encourage the patient to abstain from drinking by supporting his participation in rehabilitation activities. Intervene at the first signs of impending relapse.

Critical Thinking Questions

1. Describe two techniques you might use to help the patient vent his feelings.
2. Describe in detail two coping mechanisms that may help the patient to overcome cravings for alcohol.

drinking or using occurs. The person then recognizes that being with those friends or in those places sets him or her up to drink or use. As part of the relapse prevention strategy, the person then actively avoids those people and places. Other coping strategies are developed that can be used if the person encounters a trigger.

Aftercare and Recovery. One of the newer aspects of the recovery process involves various types of aftercare services to assist alcoholics who have completed a treatment program successfully to make a gradual transition back into the community with the support necessary to prevent relapses. Many inpatient substance disorder use programs now provide aftercare groups to discharged patients as a supplement to continued involvement in AA and other 12-step support groups such as Adult Children of Alcoholics and Co-Dependents Anonymous.

Medications. The treatment team may recommend the use of disulfiram (Antabuse) to assist the alcoholic who is highly motivated to remain sober but who recognizes that poor impulse control may increase the odds of relapse. This particular drug inhibits the metabolism of alcohol in the body, producing an uncomfortable, potentially life-threatening reaction to exposure to alcohol. Disulfiram is taken daily and lasts in the body for up to 2 weeks. If the alcoholic gets the urge to drink, the presence of the drug in the system usually provides the necessary negative reinforcement to resist that impulse. Signs and symptoms of a disulfiram-alcohol reaction include flushing, headache, nausea, vomiting, dizziness, rapid heart rate, difficulty breathing, sweating, confusion, and hypotension that may lead to coma, convulsions, and death. The severity of the symptoms varies from person to person and symptoms can last for 30 to 60 minutes or more.

Naltrexone (Revia, Depade) is a newer medication used to treat cravings or desires for alcohol once the individual has quit drinking. It is believed that this medication helps to reduce the desire to drink by blocking receptors in the brain responsible for taking up opiates and resulting in euphoria. Naltrexone is an opioid antagonist that acts at opiate receptors to competitively inhibit the effects of opiate agonists. It has no analgesic activity of its own. This medication is not a cure for alcoholism; however, clinical trials have demonstrated an increase in the number of days sober after quitting alcohol compared with those who attempted to abstain from alcohol without this medication. Studies have demonstrated the effectiveness of treatment with this medication combined with psychosocial treatments such as individual psychotherapy. Side effects may include nausea, headache, constipation, dizziness, nervousness, insomnia, drowsiness, or anxiety. Patients should be warned to avoid opioid analgesics such as codeine, hydrocodone, oxycodone, morphine, hydromorphone, and heroin. Patients must wait 7 to 10 days after taking opioids before taking naltrexone or risk acute withdrawal symptoms.

Pharmacology Capsule

Disulfiram (Antabuse) is sometimes used to assist a recovering alcoholic who is highly motivated to remain sober but who recognizes that poor impulse control may increase the odds of relapse.

Pharmacology Capsule

Naltrexone (Revia, Depade) does not cure alcoholism but may help to decrease the desire to drink, thereby extending the length of time an individual maintains sobriety. Patients must wait 7 to 10 days after discontinuing opioids before starting this medication and may not use opioids of any kind while on naltrexone.

Pharmacology Capsule

To avoid a disulfiram-alcohol reaction, patients who are taking disulfiram (Antabuse) must be instructed to avoid alcohol in foods (e.g., sauces, candies), topical preparations (e.g., cologne, aftershave), mouthwashes, and medications (e.g., over-the-counter [OTC] cold preparations, cough syrup).

The danger of giving disulfiram to a person who is poorly motivated to stop drinking is that he or she might either stop taking the medication or drink despite taking the medication and become seriously ill. As a result, careful patient teaching is essential. The patient must be taught to avoid alcohol in foods (e.g., salad dressings, sauces, candies, chocolate prepared with liqueurs), topical preparations (e.g., cologne, aftershave, liniments), medications (e.g., over-the-counter [OTC] cold preparations or cough syrups), and mouthwashes containing alcohol. Alcohol wipes cannot be used by the nurse to cleanse the skin in preparation for an injection without a topical reaction. Because of the risks of accidental exposure to a substance containing alcohol, patients are encouraged to wear a medical alert bracelet or carry a card in their wallets to alert emergency care personnel to a possible disulfiram-alcohol reaction in the event that they are found unconscious. Patients also are asked to sign a consent form for the use of the drug before it is prescribed to document that proper instructions about diet, risks, precautions, and type of emergency care needed in the event of exposure to alcohol have been offered and are understood. It is important for the nurse to be alert for patient attempts to bypass the prohibitive effects of disulfiram by ingesting large doses of vitamin C to have a drink on occasion. Patients who are addicted are often very knowledgeable about drug treatment and can easily find out that massive doses of vitamin C are given intravenously for the treatment of overdose or disulfiram-alcohol reaction.

Pharmacology Capsule

Do not use alcohol to cleanse injection sites if the patient is taking disulfiram (Antabuse).

The use of disulfiram is contraindicated in individuals with impaired liver function, heart problems, or significant debilitation. Obviously, safe use of the drug also requires that the person have no memory impairments, self-destructive intentions, or poor judgment.

Sometimes, metronidazole (Flagyl) is used for similar purposes because it also produces an uncomfortable reaction when combined with alcohol but does not produce the severe life-threatening reactions described for disulfiram. In addition, it does not remain in the system for an extended period and can be given in the event of many medical problems for which disulfiram is contraindicated.

Research efforts continue to attempt to identify other types of drugs that could assist alcoholics to go through withdrawal more comfortably and avoid relapse. Medications currently under scrutiny for this purpose include naltrexone hydrochloride (Trexan); antidepressants such as amitriptyline hydrochloride (Elavil), desipramine hydrochloride (Norpramin), and fluoxetine hydrochloride (Prozac); and angiotensin-converting enzyme (ACE) inhibitors such as enalapril maleate (Vasotec).

CAFFEINE

Caffeine is derived from coffee, tea leaves, kola nuts, and cocoa beans and the content varies among varieties of food. OTC pain relievers, cold medications, and diet pills and even decaffeinated coffee may contain caffeine. Because caffeine is a central nervous system stimulant, regular use may cause mild physical dependence, altering mood and behavior; however, there are few health and adverse social consequences as with other addictive substances. Withdrawal occurs within 12 to 24 hours after stopping caffeine intake and may lead to mild to moderate withdrawal symptoms, including headache, fatigue, anxiety, irritability, depressed mood, and difficulty concentrating.

CANNABIS (MARIJUANA)

Marijuana, "pot," "weed," "grass," or "hemp" is a mixture of dried leaves, stems, seeds, and flowers of the *Cannabis* or hemp plant. The drug is smoked or taken orally in capsules or food. Individuals experience heightened awareness; euphoria, followed by drowsiness or relaxation; impaired short-term memory, attention, judgment, coordination, and balance; increased heart rate; and increased appetite. Marijuana is psychologically addicting in about 9% of its users. Controversy persists about the negative effects of chronic use of this drug. Long-term use in vulnerable individuals is associated with mental disorders such as schizophrenia, depression, and anxiety. In the medical community, derivatives of marijuana show promise as medication for the treatment of glaucoma, asthma, and nausea and vomiting as a result of chemotherapy and as an appetite stimulant.

HALLUCINOGENS

Hallucinogens include LSD (lysergic acid diethylamide, or "acid"), PCP (phencyclidine, or "angel dust"), and MDMA (3,4-methylenedioxymethamphetamine, or "ecstasy" and "Adam").

LSD

LSD is not physically addicting but can produce physical symptoms of altered perceptions that are dreamlike, often with an altered sense of time and feelings that one has attained special insight. Emotions are intensified and labile. Individuals often experience depersonalization, in which they feel as if they are floating outside of themselves or in unreal surroundings. The drugs typically are used to enhance self-awareness and usually are taken episodically (approximately twice a week). Acute adverse reactions are most often described as a "bad trip" involving paranoia, depression, frightening hallucinations, and confusion. The person experiencing a bad trip is responsive to verbal support and reassurance. The primary danger of the use of these drugs is accidental death as a result of perceptual distortions (e.g., attempting to fly off a building) or seizures related to the cutting agent used. Cutting agents are chemicals that may be quite toxic, which are used in the manufacturing or dilution of the final drug product. Chronic long-term adverse reactions include psychosis, depression, paranoia, and flashbacks. LSD use is regaining popularity.

PCP

PCP differs from other hallucinogens in that users experience a psychotic state similar to that observed in schizophrenics. Brain reward areas are stimulated so that users can stimulate themselves mentally in a pleasurable way. Studies also suggest that this drug is strongly physically addictive, with a severe withdrawal reaction occurring after binge use. Unexpected sensory stimuli that interrupt the individual's internal experience may provoke unpredictable violence. The person may possess enormous strength and may feel no pain. The risks of use thus involve serious injury to oneself or others, in addition to severely elevated temperature, hypertensive crisis, and renal failure. Under acute intoxication, patients are best managed by reducing stimuli as much as possible, often by seclusion, even to the point of avoiding talking or performing routine treatments until the patient is stabilized. If violent, mechanical restraint is necessary.

INHALANTS

A very dangerous type of substance use is that involving inhalant misuse. Examples of chemicals often inhaled for the mind-altering response include paint, glue, aerosol sprays, Wite-Out correction fluid, and gasoline. These products are usually inhaled after being placed in a plastic bag or other container that is placed over the nose and mouth, a process also known as *huffing*. Symptoms appearing in the individual under the influence of the drug depend on the substance inhaled and include nosebleeds, bloodshot eyes, infected lesions around the nose and mouth, and severe disorientation or unconsciousness. The risks include progressive brain damage, asphyxiation, seizures, depressed bone marrow leading to aplastic anemia, liver or kidney damage, or cardiac dysrhythmias. No physical withdrawal syndrome is seen.

This particular group of drugs often is misused among teenagers because of its easy availability and low cost. The cumulative brain damage from chronic use is a very serious problem among poor and minority adolescents.

OPIOIDS

The opioids most often misused are heroin, morphine, oxycodone (Oxycontin), hydrocodone, pentazocine (Talwin), methadone, and meperidine (Demerol).

Heroin

Heroin is a highly addictive opioid that produces euphoria on intravenous use. The person experiences a "rush" and then gradually nods off to sleep. On awakening, the person feels immune to stressors until the withdrawal symptoms begin to trigger the need to "cop a fix" again. This usually occurs 8 to 12 hours after the last use. Risks of chronic use of heroin include overdose, malnutrition, and respiratory arrest as well as hepatitis B, hepatitis C, and HIV infections from shared needle use.

Symptoms of withdrawal include tearing of the eyes, runny nose, gooseflesh, sweating, alternating fever and chills, muscle and joint pain, upset stomach, diarrhea, loss of appetite, restlessness, and irritability. Individuals usually are in such subjective distress that they inappropriately seek medications from the staff while in treatment. It is very challenging to work with these patients and sometimes difficult to remain nonjudgmental.

To support their ever-increasing habit, many people addicted to heroin resort to crime, such as stealing. Sometimes they seek detoxification only to reduce the level of the dose needed to experience the pleasurable response to the drug, since a lower dose is less expensive to obtain.

SEDATIVES, HYPNOTICS, AND ANXIOLYTICS

Sedatives, hypnotics, and anxiolytics are drugs that generally are obtained by prescription for anxiety or insomnia or are purchased illegally. They are typically taken orally and can become addictive. Symptoms of overdose include oversedation, respiratory depression, impaired coordination, and brain damage. Intoxication with barbiturates is even more dangerous than with benzodiazepines. Although benzodiazepines and barbiturates are similar to alcohol in terms of dangerous physical withdrawal reactions (e.g., delirium tremens, seizures), barbiturate overdose induces an anesthesia-like state. Symptoms of barbiturate withdrawal usually occur somewhat later, sometimes days after the last use, depending on the half-life of the particular drug. Once a person is addicted, abruptly stopping any of these drugs may trigger psychosis.

STIMULANTS

Stimulants include amphetamines ("speed"), methamphetamine ("meth" and "crystal meth") and similar drugs, and cocaine or "crack."

Amphetamines

Amphetamines usually are used orally or intravenously on a daily basis or on binges. They are very psychologically addictive; the dose is gradually increased over time to produce the euphoria (or "high") that is extremely pleasurable. Symptoms often include hyperactivity, irritability, combativeness, and paranoia after extended use. A person intoxicated by amphetamines may be very dangerous. No physical withdrawal symptoms are noted but the user typically experiences a profound depression and sense of exhaustion called *crashing*. Selective serotonin reuptake inhibitors (SSRIs) and other types of antidepressants such as bupropion (Wellbutrin) are commonly used to treat the depression, which may persist in chronic users for up to 2 years after the last amphetamine use. Toxic psychosis may occur in approximately 90% of chronic users up to 1 year past the last use. Unfortunately, 5% to 15% of these individuals never fully recover. Neuroleptics may be used to treat toxic psychosis.

Methamphetamine. Methamphetamine is an illegal drug sold on the streets that also may be known as meth, crank, speed, crystal meth, and ice. The substance is a white, odorless, bitter-tasting crystalline powder that easily dissolves in water or alcohol. This drug is taken orally, intranasally (snorting the drug powder into the nose), by injecting the drug through a needle, or by smoking. Methamphetamine causes rapid release of the neurotransmitter dopamine while also blocking dopamine's natural reuptake into the neuron. This rapid release of dopamine occurs in reward regions of the brain, causing intense euphoria or a "rush" in the user. Over time, chronic methamphetamine use causes several alterations in brain function, with actual changes in structure and neuronal function. Effects last as long as 14 hours; the user often will do anything to obtain the drug and also is considered at risk for being very dangerous while under the influence. Long-term use may lead to symptoms such as insomnia, major mood swings, delusional behavior, and extreme paranoia; in addition, users may display repeated infections, missing and rotted teeth (called "meth mouth"), severe weight loss, skin sores, and heart attack or stroke. Large doses can result in agitation, chest pain, heart attack, difficulty breathing, kidney damage or failure, paranoia, seizures, and (in extreme cases) cardiac arrest or coma.

Cocaine

Cocaine is a highly addictive alkaloid of the plant *Erythroxylum coca*, which grows mainly in Peru and Bolivia. Cocaine produces an intense feeling of euphoria that usually lasts only 30 to 60 minutes; however, the substance remains in the brain for about 10 days after use. Pure forms of cocaine are quite expensive. The drug is typically inhaled nasally or mixed with other drugs, such as heroin, and injected intravenously ("speedballs"). Symptoms of chronic inhalation include runny nose, sniffles, frequent colds, weight loss, hyperactivity, and damage to the nasal mucosa or septum that may be severe enough to require surgical repair. In instances when the drug is injected, severe allergic reactions may result and there is increased risk for HIV, hepatitis C, and other bloodborne diseases from contaminated needles.

Cocaine is very psychologically addicting, which is thought to be the result of overstimulation of the pleasure centers of the brain. Users may lose interest in their usual activities and demonstrate abrupt mood swings, poor judgment, impatience, and ultimately suspiciousness and hallucinations. Cocaine constricts blood vessels; dilates pupils; increases body temperature, heart rate, and blood pressure; and causes headaches, abdominal pain and nausea, and decreased appetite. Cocaine is a very dangerous drug in that strokes, seizures, and heart attacks that are sometimes fatal can occur even in first-time users.

Withdrawal occurs when heavy cocaine users decrease or stop use of the drug and experience a "crash." Treatment often consists of diazepam (Valium) or phenobarbital for their sedative effects. Neuroleptics may be used in the event of psychosis. Many clients are severely depressed for up to 2 years after quitting. Studies have shown that damage to the brain may impair the patient's ability to experience pleasure. Antidepressants such as bupropion (Wellbutrin), beta-blockers such as propranolol hydrochloride (Inderal), or calcium channel blockers may be helpful in this event.

Crack

Crack is a hardened form of cocaine that is smoked. It presents major problems in many urban areas of the United States because it is readily available and inexpensive compared with other drugs. It produces a tremendously addicting, short-acting euphoria that is quickly followed by "crashing," which stimulates continued cravings and use. The cravings are so intense that, as with "ice," the user will do almost anything to obtain more of the drug and often resorts to violence if thwarted. Overdose of this drug is life threatening because no drug is available to counteract the overstimulation, which results in respiratory failure.

TOBACCO

Nicotine, the addictive substance in tobacco, increases the level of dopamine, a neurotransmitter that acts on the reward centers of the brain. Within 10 seconds of inhaling a cigarette, the drug level peaks in the brain. However, the effects decrease rapidly so that the smoker must continue dosing to maintain the drug's pleasurable effects and prevent withdrawal. Pharmacologic effects of withdrawal produce symptoms including irritability, craving, depression, anxiety, cognitive and attention deficits, sleep disturbances, and increased appetite. These symptoms may occur within the first few days after smoking cessation and usually subside within a few weeks; however, symptoms can last for months. Behavioral factors related to the actual activity associated with smoking such as handling, lighting, and smoking the cigarette can also influence the severity of symptoms and difficulty in stopping tobacco use.

Nearly half of all smokers try to quit each year. Success is greatest when counseling is used along with smoking cessation aids. First-line pharmacologic aids are nicotine-based products that deliver nicotine via a patch, chewing gum, lozenge, nasal spray, or inhaler and the nicotine-free products varenicline (Chantix) and bupropion (Wellbutrin). Electronic cigarettes ("e-cigarettes") are battery-operated products that deliver nicotine, flavor, and other chemicals. The chemicals are converted into an aerosol that the user inhales. The benefits and potential adverse effects of electronic cigarettes have not yet been fully evaluated.

OTHER OR UNKNOWN SUBSTANCES

A new group of used drugs on the illegal market includes synthetic drugs especially designed to sidestep categorization with any of the drugs identified as illegal in the United States. Although use of these drugs may not be technically illegal, their misuse presents unique hazards. Ecstasy is an example of a synthetic drug generally grouped with the hallucinogens; it is also called Adam. A very similar second-generation designer drug is called Eve. China White is an example of a synthetic type of heroin that acts in much the same way as heroin. Major risks are present when the user mixes these drugs with those from the other groups because the results are unpredictable.

CONDITIONS ASSOCIATED WITH SUBSTANCE USE DISORDERS

The risk of human immunodeficiency virus disease (HIVD), the illness that precedes AIDS, continues to present the greatest danger for patients with substance use disorders who are using intravenous drugs because of the common practice of sharing needles. The Centers for Disease Control and Prevention (CDC) indicate an alarming number of new cases of HIV-positive diagnoses among intravenous drug users and their sexual partners. Nursing care for these patients now includes teaching them how to clean their "works" with bleach and how to use condoms correctly.

Individuals who have or are predisposed to a serious psychiatric illness may have an active case of the mental disorder. By altering levels of brain chemicals that control emotions, thought processes, and behavior, misuse of these chemicals can trigger an exacerbation of an existing illness.

Another major area of concern is the effect of intrauterine exposure to these chemicals on the fetus. Fetuses carried by mothers who are physically addicted to an opioid are born addicted and also may experience developmental delays and a prolonged lack of the capacity to feel pleasure even after they have been successfully weaned from the substance used. "Cocaine babies" are currently being studied for clues to the consequences of prenatal exposure to the drug. Findings suggest that attention deficit disorder (with or without hyperactivity) occurs more often in this population, along with dyslexia, other neurologic problems, and learning disabilities.

Clients with chronic pain disorders also are very vulnerable to the substance use disorders, especially those of the opioid and depressant groups, because of their frequent frustration over an inability to manage their pain effectively. In addition, many lack knowledge of the risks of regular use of pain medication. They often feel betrayed by their physician and other caregivers because they were not informed about prescribed analgesics and pain management (e.g., the importance of temperate use along with the use of exercise and other types of supportive techniques to manage pain and avoid addiction).

TREATMENT FOR SUBSTANCE USE DISORDERS

Treatment of substance use disorders is very similar to alcohol detoxification and rehabilitation. Narcotics Anonymous (NA) is structured much like AA but focuses on drugs other than alcohol. Often inpatient treatment programs place recovering addicts with persons with alcohol use disorder for educational and therapy groups. However, the rate of relapse is much higher for most drug abuse patients, especially those who use highly addicting intravenous drugs. A booming area of research is the identification of alternative treatments and medications that will help drug users to detoxify more comfortably from the chemicals that they are addicted to and reduce the risks of relapse. Currently, some support exists for treating drug use disorders separately from alcohol use disorder.

As with treatment for alcohol use disorder, family involvement in the process is very important. Al-Anon is the support group for family members or significant others of a substance-abusing person. It is recommended that members of the family begin attending meetings as soon as they realize that the person is using some type of drug. The intervention process described earlier under "Treatment for Alcohol Abuse" may be used in an attempt to get the person into treatment.

Many patients who use drugs have legal problems, which may provide the catalyst for seeking help. Sometimes they are mandated by the courts to go into treatment; at other times their attorney recommends treatment before the case goes to court to influence the judge favorably before sentencing. In the past, many individuals were involuntarily committed to state hospital drug treatment programs for 30 days. However, many state hospital systems across the country are closing their drug and alcohol treatment units because of the program expense and the need to provide additional services to the seriously mentally ill, which often is judged more of a priority.

DETOXIFICATION

Detoxification from physically addicting drugs is very complex because of the likelihood of polysubstance use and the uncertainty of what to expect when two or more drugs are mixed together. Usually, inpatient hospitalization is recommended for safety. However, some individuals who have been using drugs that are primarily psychologically addicting may not demonstrate many physical symptoms but rather experience intense psychologic cravings. For example, if a conversation about past drug use occurs within the recovering addict's hearing or if something in the environment triggers memories of the "high" sensation that he or she experienced while using, the person may experience cravings that stimulate feelings of restlessness, itching, hives, flushing, and elevated BP and pulse, which are believed to be psychogenic in origin. These patients need a great deal of support to help them overcome the profound urge to use. This experience puts the patient at very high risk for relapse.

MEDICATIONS

Methadone

Methadone is one drug used in the treatment of heroin addicts. However, some controversy exists about using this medication because the drug is a synthetic opioid analgesic that also may be prescribed appropriately for chronic severe pain. Given orally (in diskette or liquid form), it is absorbed slowly and does not produce the "rush" normally experienced with the intravenous use of heroin. It also alleviates the cravings for more opioids for a short period of time, depending on the dose given. In detoxification, the dose of the drug is gradually reduced without telling patients exactly what dose they are getting. Although this process is one of substituting another addictive drug for the one misused by the client, some believe it to be justified in that withdrawal from methadone is less uncomfortable for the patient. The patient also risks severe respiratory depression in the event that heroin is injected while methadone is in the system. The most typical problematic side effects of methadone include severe constipation and profound sweating.

Pharmacology Capsule

Methadone is a synthetic opioid analgesic that may be used in the detoxification of heroin-related opioid addiction.

Clonidine

Clonidine hydrochloride (Catapres) has become a more popular means of assisting the substance user through detoxification. It is a nonopiate antihypertensive drug that partially blocks withdrawal symptoms. Clonidine does not completely remove the unpleasant feelings that accompany heroin withdrawal (see *Complementary and Alternative Therapies* box). Unfortunately, some may leave treatment because of the inherent discomfort and unrealistic expectations that they should not feel sick at all while using the drug to withdraw.

Complementary and Alternative Therapies

Some herbal remedies are being studied for use as agents to reduce withdrawal symptoms.

Put on Your Thinking Cap!

Can you explain why Narcan would cause a person who is addicted to an opioid to experience acute withdrawal symptoms?

Naloxone

Naloxone hydrochloride (Narcan) and nalmefene (Revex) are opioid antagonists that counteract the dangerous respiratory depressant effects of heroin or other opiate overdose. When Narcan is given to a person who is addicted and under the influence of an opiate, the person may experience acute withdrawal symptoms.

Many other drugs are currently under investigation to determine whether they could assist the person with a substance use disorder by reducing the cravings for the drug used reducing the cravings for the drug abused or by counteracting the long-term psychologic consequences of use of certain drugs. Examples of these include some of the antidepressants, anticonvulsants, and various herbal agents.

Still other medications may be used in the supportive treatment of those undergoing opiate withdrawal to control symptoms such as diarrhea; abdominal cramping; and generalized, diffuse pain.

REHABILITATION

In most cases, the process of rehabilitation for substance use disorder is very similar to that for alcohol use disorder. Instead of attendance at AA meetings, the client often participates in NA at least some of the time. This support group is based on the 12 steps of AA, except that the word *drugs* replaces the word *alcohol* in all of the literature. In addition, the case histories used for reading assignments are about other addicts in recovery related specifically to the use of drugs other than alcohol; this is to help the client identify with people with similar struggles. Relapse rates for individuals abusing drugs other than alcohol alone are much higher and present unique issues. Trends suggest that future treatment programs will be more likely to separate clients into small groups of people facing similar issues and having similar characteristics; this is to individualize the recovery process much more than is done in most settings today. Most current settings may advertise more than one "track" for substance abuse treatment. However, in reality, clients share the same facilities and participate in most of the traditional programming mixed together despite different learning styles and other issues. It has been suggested that this practice may actually place clients who do not fit the traditional mold at higher risk for relapse.

On an outpatient basis, these clients are encouraged to participate in NA on a regular basis (90 meetings in the first 90 days), just as do those recovering from alcoholism. Attempts are usually made to allow the client to experience different group locations and times before discharge from the inpatient setting to increase the likelihood that the client will participate as recommended. Various other community programs may be available, such as the Patrician Movement, which provides outpatient treatment on an ongoing basis for those who cannot afford more costly inpatient rehabilitation. Many private health care systems are opening day treatment programs for people with substance use disorders as insurance reimbursement for long-term inpatient programs becomes less available.

AFTERCARE AND RECOVERY

Individuals recovering from substance use disorders may be offered an opportunity to participate in a support group provided by the hospital at which they received treatment. Many of the same people who went through treatment at the same time participate together. Because the relationships built during this time of crisis are often intense, the groups can be very helpful in preventing relapse. It is hoped that clients also will continue regular participation in NA groups on an ongoing basis. Some individuals do well in halfway houses, which allow for a new living environment surrounded by other recovering addicts during the difficult transition back into the community. Sometimes it is recommended that patients do not return to work until their ability to cope with stress is more developed.

METHADONE MAINTENANCE

Some patients who have experienced multiple relapses into heroin use after treatment may have sustained permanent damage to chemical receptor sites in the brain, which decreases their ability to resist relapse. As a result, methadone maintenance is not uncommon. In this process, the person goes to a methadone clinic on a daily or three-times-a-week basis to receive a dose or doses of the medication to cover the next 24 to 72 hours. A single dose may be administered in liquid form or in a diskette dissolved in juice and the person is carefully observed by clinic staff members to ensure that the medication is actually taken and not hoarded in any way. The patient may continue this process indefinitely, often for many years. Sometimes the dose of the methadone is maintained at the same level without attempts to reduce it while at other times gradual titration is attempted.

Methadone maintenance programs have been criticized across the United States because the process is often viewed as exchanging one addiction for another without attempts to detoxify the patient. In addition, clinic records and security have been lax in many instances, resulting in clinic methadone thefts and illegal sales on the street. Supporters of the programs counter these arguments by pointing out that criteria for involvement in these programs require that patients have been unsuccessful in remaining "clean" after detoxification on more than one occasion and that patients no longer are "forced" into crime to support their habits. In addition, methadone is administered in such a way that no rush is experienced, allowing the person to return to school or work and reintegrate into society without the risk of losing everything to relapse. Methadone maintenance programs also are more cost effective than residential treatment or incarceration.

The controversy over methadone maintenance has resulted in the frequent use of naltrexone (Trexan) as an alternative. This drug is related to naloxone (Narcan) and is a pure opioid antagonist. This means that the drug reduces or completely blocks the effects of any intravenous opioids in the patient's system. The detoxified patient is placed on this drug to help prevent use of heroin. If the patient takes small doses of heroin while on naltrexone, no effect is experienced; however, if the patient injects large doses, he or she will become very physically ill and may die or sustain serious injury such as a coma. An addicted person taking naltrexone soon after regular use of heroin will experience withdrawal symptoms because of the antagonist actions of the drug.

Pharmacology Capsule

Methadone maintenance is used for patients who have experienced multiple relapses into heroin use after standard treatment and rehabilitation efforts.

Research is underway to evaluate the use of various types of other psychotropic medications to stabilize neurochemical and neurophysiologic alterations in the brains of addicted persons. This may eventually provide an answer to the high rates of relapse in individuals with substance use disorder involving opioids.

NURSING CARE of the Person with a Substance Use Disorder

Assessment

The initial step in developing a nursing plan of care for the patient with a substance use disorder is always a thorough assessment. The data you collect on first contact with the patient can help to identify and prioritize problems that must be addressed to maximize the likelihood that the patient will remain sober. Examples of the types of problems often seen in substance use disorders of any kind are denial, poor impulse control, high risk for injury, high risk for relapse, guilt, and low self-esteem. Detailed assessment of the person with a substance disorder is detailed earlier in the section titled "Nursing Assessment of the Person with Addiction."

Interventions

Nursing interventions for persons with substance use disorders in detoxification involve regular physical assessment (with the frequency determined by the severity of symptoms), administration of appropriate medications, and teaching the patients about their actions and consequences. Providing adequate nutrition is critical because the patient may have been eating very irregularly and also may be quite dehydrated. High levels of anxiety during detoxification also require a great deal of reassurance and support, providing the opportunity to help the patient begin to process the impending decision to continue in rehabilitation.

Once the patient has agreed to participate in rehabilitation, the focus of nursing care changes from one of primarily attending to the physical concerns of the patient to assisting the client in processing the meaning of his or her substance use disorder and planning for a future without continued use of that substance. The biggest issue to be addressed at first is the heavily entrenched denial that most substance users possess. Often they minimize the severity of the use, perhaps

Nursing Diagnoses, Goals, and Outcome Criteria: Substance Use Disorder

Nursing Diagnoses	Goals and Outcome Criteria
Ineffective Coping related to substance use, as evidenced by using substances to deal with anxiety, emotional discomfort, and stress	Improved coping: identifies and uses healthy alternative coping strategies to deal with anxiety, emotional discomfort, and stress; patient verbalizes strategies to prevent relapse
Ineffective Denial related to substance use and refusal to acknowledge actual consequences of substance use	Verbalizes an internalized sense that the substance use is unhealthy and out of control and that the treatment is required
Risk for Injury related to excessive use of the drug and high risk for relapse, manifested by a history of falls, driving while under the influence, combining the substance used with other substances, being aggressive while under the influence, reduced attendance at Alcoholics Anonymous (AA) or Narcotics Anonymous (NA) meetings, frequent dreams of drug use, returning to places where one used drugs, and not seeking relief for high stress	Decreased risk for injury to self and others: patient does not engage in dangerous activities when under drug's influence

lying outright about how much they actually were using. You must work toward penetrating this denial without further damaging the individual's self-esteem. This has traditionally demanded more confrontational techniques than appropriate in other types of psychiatric treatment. In many "substance use only" treatment programs, the style of confrontation used was often overly hostile and critical. This approach is no longer seen as the most helpful to the patient. Studies now show that patients who were treated in this way were far more likely to leave treatment early to return to their "drugging and drinking." This is of great concern because the person may never return to treatment and may die or be seriously injured as a result of the continued substance abuse.

You also can be very helpful in assisting the patient to work through the 12-step process. After intense educational AA or NA meetings and group therapy sessions during most of the day, patients often want to ventilate feelings and process thoughts about what they are learning. Conflicts with family members, bosses, friends, or parents often are overwhelming. Patients usually lack the skills to handle these types of interpersonal stressors because of habitual avoidance of issues through past substance use. You can act as an ally in helping patients to cope and begin to practice new ways of reacting. Teaching stress management and practicing these new skills with patients can greatly increase the odds that they will not relapse after discharge.

Relapse prevention is a critical area to attend to in dealing with each patient. The patient must be taught to recognize symptoms that often lead to relapse. Examples of these include overtiredness or poor health, being unnecessarily dishonest with others, impatience, argumentativeness, depression, self-pity, cockiness, forgetting or minimizing the risk of relapse, unreasonable expectations of self and others, decreased or irregular participation in AA or NA meetings or daily meditation and self-inventory, use of a chemical other than those previously abused, forgetting to be thankful that their lives are better, and feeling all-powerful.

Another effective means of intervention is to act as a good role model in handling feelings, participating appropriately in meetings, and communicating to the patient in a way that supports the program. For example, telling patients that participation in AA meetings is not necessary for recovery could undermine their struggle to initiate the profound changes in lifestyle necessary to stay drug free.

SPECIAL PROBLEMS FOR POPULATIONS OF PEOPLE WITH SUBSTANCE USE DISORDERS

The unique characteristics of many groups of individuals influence the process of recovery and contribute to a high risk for relapse into chronic use of whatever substance the person has used. Recent research in addressing these problems has proved very promising. As mentioned earlier, the trend is to provide specially designed treatment approaches for groups of individuals who have common traits and problems that may contribute to their dependency on alcohol or other drugs.

OLDER ADULTS

Although older adults use approximately 25% of the medications used in the United States, only about 2% to 5% of men and fewer than 1% of women older than 65 years have alcohol use disorder. Substance use disorder among older adults is more likely to involve use OTC and prescription sleeping pills, pain medications, or tranquilizers than illegal drugs such as cocaine. Misuse is seldom for recreational purposes among this age group.

Because of a decreased ability to metabolize and eliminate alcohol or drugs from the body, older adults with substance use disorders over extended periods of time may experience significant medical problems as a result. The most typical physical consequences of alcohol use disorder among older adults include malnutrition, cirrhosis of the liver, bone thinning, gastritis, poor memory, and decreased cognitive ability to process new information. If the person combines alcohol with any other medication that has CNS depressant effects, the danger of oversedation, impaired responses, or respiratory depression is very great.

Most older adults with alcohol use disorder have maintained a regular pattern of use over many years without obvious problems. As their bodies age, their ability to tolerate the same quantities decreases, putting them at risk for falls or other injuries as a result of intoxication. Others turn to first-time or heavier patterns of use to cope with anxiety produced by the typical stressors of aging such as retirement, losses of significant others, family conflict, health problems, social isolation, and loss of self-worth. Among older adults who move to more affluent retirement communities, a rise in alcoholism has been noted. This may be because of involvement in cocktail parties, regular drinking with meals, and peer pressure to participate to be accepted.

Problems of substance use disorder in the older population are usually diagnosed by the family physician as a result of complaints related to the psychologic or physical effects of alcohol use disorder, such as memory impairment or insomnia. Older adults often deny that they have a substance use problem and may resist treatment without the support and pressure of their family.

Treatment of alcoholism in older adults is similar to that of younger individuals, except that the period of withdrawal must be monitored more closely and must occur more slowly because of the older person's physical frailty. Rehabilitation groups and educational programs ideally should be structured to permit processing information more slowly to allow for the cognitive slowing that is normal for this age group. In addition, cognitive changes may be more pronounced because of the neurologic effects of chronic use of alcohol or other drugs, or of both. Involvement in AA is critical and can be difficult if patients do not have easy access to a "home group" with other older adults who can relate to their problems and issues.

ADOLESCENTS

Substance use disorders among adolescents has received much attention in recent years. It is estimated that 1 in 4 adolescents becomes involved in substance abuse. It also has become apparent that children are experimenting with drugs at younger ages than ever before. The younger the age at onset of drug use, the greater is the risk for significant interference in the physical and psychologic development of the individual.

The developmental issues of this age group also contribute to the adolescent's vulnerability. This is a stage of establishing one's identity, experimenting with newly developed abilities to think abstractly, egocentricity, limited impulse control, and poor judgment. Identification with one's peer group is an important aspect of feeling accepted. Average adolescents view themselves as omnipotent and deny the likelihood of negative consequences of their behaviors. This is the age of rebellion.

Substance use disorders in this population also is viewed as a symptom of family issues. The family is often dysfunctional—patterns of communication may be ineffective and children in the family may be emotionally or physically neglected, abused, or subject to rigid and unrealistic expectations for their behavior. A family history of substance use disorders may exist or the adolescent may fall in with the "wrong crowd" of other young people who are already involved in the drug culture.

The progression of physical consequences of substance use disorders in the adolescent population is correlated with the risks related to the substance used and the likelihood of polysubstance use. The risks of accidental overdose or suicide are significant. Intravenous drug use and the likelihood of sexual activity without the use of precautions have been linked to an increased risk of HIV infection among adolescents.

Entry into treatment usually occurs as a result of a crisis situation revealing the severity of drug use as well as parental insistence. Breaking through adolescents' denial is the most difficult aspect of treatment, especially because they seldom want to be in treatment and do not see the potential negative consequences of their behaviors. It also may be difficult to distinguish the substance use disorder from the adolescent who is still in the early stages of experimentation and unlikely to persist in chronic substance use. Most adolescents do not reach the point of believing it when they say, "Hi, I'm an alcoholic" (or drug user) at the beginning of each AA or NA meeting.

Rehabilitation of the adolescent with substance use disorder requires that the approach to treatment be modified to meet the needs of this age group more effectively. It remains very controversial to mix adolescents with adults in treatment programs because of adolescents' vulnerability to being influenced by the more experienced and usually charismatic adult substance user. Obviously, careful supervision is necessary if mixing age groups for treatment is the only option. In addition, many of the abstract concepts addressed in the 12 steps of AA may need to be adapted to the level of understanding of the individual adolescent.

Successful rehabilitation usually involves regular involvement in an AA group made up of younger people to whom the adolescent can relate; successful development of a new, nondrug-using peer group; and reentry into school with the support of other recovering classmates. AA group meetings may be held at high schools in some cities.

COMORBIDITY OR DUAL DIAGNOSIS

Patients who already have been diagnosed with a serious psychiatric illness and also have a substance use disorder (comorbidity or dual diagnosis) have special concerns for rehabilitation. Dually diagnosed patients usually have psychiatric illnesses of depression, schizophrenia, or bipolar illness. Often mental retardation and organic brain disease also are included in the group of medical problems identified as presenting special concerns in the event of a concurrent substance abuse problem. (Many times, individuals with a substance use disorder have a personality disorder, although this group of psychiatric disorders is generally not considered to be the result of some physiologic process and usually is not included under dual diagnosis.)

In some individuals, chronic drug or alcohol use may exacerbate an already fragile neurophysiology, producing psychiatric symptoms. This is seen in cases of young adolescents who use marijuana or some other type of drug before their first psychotic break in schizophrenia. Toxic psychosis may occur more frequently with the use of cocaine or amphetamines mixed with alcohol. In other cases, people may use a mind-altering drug to treat psychiatric symptoms without understanding the reason. They just know that they feel better.

People with chronic psychiatric problems require special teaching and supervision in the event of substance relapse. Antipsychotic medications do not mix with alcohol. For example, if a patient with bipolar disorder is on lithium, the fluid losses as a result of drinking alcohol could precipitate lithium toxicity. Patients who take anxiolytics or antidepressants with alcohol could risk accidental overdose as a result of additive effects on the CNS or could be deliberately attempting to harm themselves.

The approach to rehabilitation must be modified to adapt to this special population. Each patient's ability to comprehend the abstract ideas from the 12-step process of AA will vary. In addition, traditionalists in the recovery process often frown on the use of any mind-altering chemical and may subtly pressure dually diagnosed clients to stop their prescribed medications. This lack of knowledge and rigid approach to recovery could contribute to exacerbation of the underlying psychiatric illness.

PEER ASSISTANCE PROGRAMS

Substance use disorder is expected to be one of the most widespread problems of the next 20 years. People from all walks of life are at risk, including health care professionals, who are at high risk because of easier access to addictive drugs. As a result, many professional groups have developed peer assistance programs. These programs are designed to offer a supportive alternative to health professionals (physicians, dentists, nurses, and others) who become addicted to a substance instead of taking immediate disciplinary action against their licenses. Peer assistance programs for nurses exist in most states. Referrals may be made by the nurses or by their employers and peers who have reason to believe that the nursing practice is impaired by the use of a substance. With the help of representatives of the program, usually volunteers, information is gathered to support an intervention in hopes of getting the nurse into treatment and recovery.

The goals of an intervention for a nurse whose practice is impaired are as follows:

- Assist the nurse whose practice is impaired to receive treatment
- Protect the public from an untreated nurse
- Help the recovering nurse to reenter nursing in a systematic, planned, and safe way
- Assist in monitoring the continued recovery of the nurse for a period of time

Usually at least a 2-year period exists after diagnosis and onset of treatment in which the nurse is required to attend AA or NA groups regularly, to participate in peer support groups, to meet routinely with an identified support person representing the peer assistance program, and to undergo random urine drug screens to ensure that he or she has not relapsed. If nurses are unable to comply with the process, information regarding their substance use and how that has impaired their practice can be turned over to the Board of Nursing for that state. Until that point, however, the information regarding each nurse involved is kept confidential and, if they successfully complete the requirements of the program, will never become part of the licensing board's records. Many peer assistance programs also work with nurses whose practices have become impaired as a result of mental illness.

Substance abuse will continue to be a major health care problem in the future. Nurses who work in this field are presented with difficult challenges and must be able to be nonjudgmental and supportive of the patients with whom they work. The knowledge base for this specialty area is growing quickly as a result of the widespread research being done. No matter where nurses work, they will come in contact with patients whose health status is compromised by substance use. The opportunity to play a powerful role in promoting healthier lifestyles is one that can be very fulfilling.

Put on Your Thinking Cap!

Is there a peer assistance program for nurses in the state where you live?

Get Ready for the NCLEX® Examination!

Key Points

- The majority of experts in substance-related disorders subscribe to the biologic theory that proposes that faulty physiologic processes contribute to addiction to a specific substance and that addiction is a physical illness.
- Some theorists contend that sociocultural factors contribute to the development of substance-related disorders.
- According to behavioral and learning theories, a substance-related disorder is a learned maladaptive way of coping with stress and anxiety.
- Although the specific causes of addiction have not been established, it is most likely that the true cause involves a combination of biologic, cultural, and behavioral factors.
- To obtain reliable data when questioning a person about a substance-related disorder, the nurse must be nonjudgmental, direct, and specific. More than one person should verify the information obtained when possible.
- The lifestyle of an addict may focus entirely on obtaining and using the substance of choice, with an increasing need for more and more to get the desired effects.
- Individuals with substance-related disorders often have erratic and unprovoked mood swings, blackouts, significant work problems, and damaged relationships.

- Typical defense mechanisms used by addicts include denial, rationalization, intellectualization, and projection.
- Many alcoholics appear malnourished and poorly cared for, have evidence of physical trauma from falls or violence, appear jaundiced, and when in withdrawal may be hypertensive with signs of fluid retention.
- Tests for detecting substance use include a blood alcohol study, a urine drug screen, and hair analysis.
- Chronic alcoholism involves the regular daily ingestion of large amounts of alcohol, regular heavy drinking only on weekends, or binges of heavy drinking followed by long periods of abstinence.
- Physical addiction occurs when the cells of the body are dependent on alcohol to carry out certain metabolic processes; without the alcohol, the cells go into shock.
- Alcohol withdrawal syndrome begins after an individual stops or decreases the amount of alcohol ingested and involves physiologic and behavioral symptoms that begin when the individual's blood alcohol level drops.
- Alcoholism has an effect on the entire family. Family and peer pressure can be critical factors in inducing an alcoholic to seek treatment.
- Strategies that have been successful in alcohol rehabilitation are 12-step programs, stress management, social skills training, behavioral approaches to marital therapy, and matching clients with therapists who use a style most likely to benefit their personality type.
- Substance-related disorders encompass the following classes of drugs: (1) alcohol; (2) caffeine; (3) cannabis; (4) hallucinogens; (5) inhalants; (6) opioids; (7) sedatives, hypnotics, and anxiolytics; (8) stimulants; (9) tobacco; and (10) other or unknown substances.
- Treatment for drug addiction is similar to alcohol detoxification and rehabilitation; however, relapse rates are higher and treatment may need to be more individualized.
- Methadone maintenance may be used for long-term heroin users who have sustained permanent damage to chemical receptor sites in the brain and therefore have a decreased ability to resist relapses or who have failed multiple attempts at rehabilitation.

Additional Learning Resources

SG Go to your Study Guide for additional learning activities to help you master this chapter content.

evolve Go to your Evolve website (http://evolve.elsevier.com/Linton/medsurg) for the following learning resources and much more:

- Interactive Prioritization Exercises
- Fluid & Electrolyte Tutorial
- Pharmacology Tutorial
- Review Questions for the NCLEX® Examination

Review Questions for the NCLEX® Examination

1. The theory that substance dependence is caused by faulty physiologic processes is the ___________ theory.
   NCLEX Client Need: Psychosocial Integrity
2. Mr. White was arrested for public intoxication and was advised by his attorney to enroll in an alcohol treatment program. A nurse interviews him when he comes to a mental health center. He tells the nurse that he really does not have a problem with alcohol and that he just had a few too many drinks while celebrating with a friend. This is an example of which defense mechanism?
   NCLEX Client Need: Psychosocial Integrity
3. What is the chief advantage of using hair analysis to detect drug use?
   1. Hair samples can be taken without patient permission.
   2. Hair samples will reveal drug use as long as 1 year later.
   3. It is not possible for a patient to substitute someone else's hair.
   4. The chain of custody is unnecessary with hair samples.

   NCLEX Client Need: Physiological Integrity: Reduction of Risk Potential
4. An alcoholic patient was injured in an automobile accident. She said that she had her last drink 2 hours before the accident. About 8 hours after admission, she developed symptoms of early alcohol withdrawal. You should anticipate delirium tremens by _____ hours after her last drink.
   NCLEX Client Need: Psychosocial Integrity
5. Mr. Jones calls the hospital to report that his wife, a dietitian, cannot come to work because she has the "flu." In reality, she consumed a large amount of alcohol the previous evening and has a hangover. This has happened several times in the past. Mr. Jones' behavior is an example of which of the following?
   1. Support
   2. Enabling
   3. Rationalization
   4. Compensation

   NCLEX Client Need: Psychosocial Integrity
6. When a patient who is taking disulfiram (Antabuse) consumes alcohol, expected outcomes include which of the following? (Select all that apply.)
   1. Hypotension
   2. Tachycardia
   3. Confusion
   4. Nausea and vomiting
   5. Pallor

   NCLEX Client Need: Physiological Integrity: Pharmacological Therapies
7. Young people should be warned that inhalants can cause which of the following?
   1. Progressive brain damage
   2. Sexual dysfunction
   3. Schizophrenia
   4. Aggressive behavior

   NCLEX Client Need: Psychosocial Integrity

8. A patient being treated for an overdose of opioids is given Narcan. Narcan is given for which of the following reasons?
   1. To stimulate the heart
   2. To raise BP
   3. To treat respiratory depression
   4. To sedate the patient and prevent seizures

   NCLEX Client Need: Physiological Integrity: Pharmacological Therapies
9. Which of the following are among the drugs most commonly used by older adults with substance use disorder? (Select all that apply.)
   1. Cocaine
   2. Pain medications
   3. Sleeping aids
   4. Alcohol
   5. Marijuana

   NCLEX Client Need: Physiological Integrity: Pharmacological Therapies
10. Which statement most accurately describes drug use among adolescents?
    1. Only 1 in 10 adolescents have problems with substance use.
    2. Adolescents tend to deny any possible negative outcomes of drug use.
    3. Most adolescents seek treatment for substance use on their own.
    4. Adolescents should be treated with adults who can model mature behavior.

    NCLEX Client Need: Psychosocial Integrity

Glossary

A

Abdominal thrusts Technique for ejecting a foreign body from the airway by using abdominal thrusts.
acid Solution containing a high number of hydrogen ions.
acid–base balance Homeostasis of the hydrogen ion (H^+) concentration in body fluids.
acidosis Abnormal pH of body fluids caused by excess acid in relation to bicarbonate.
acne Inflammatory skin disorder characterized by comedones, pustules, and cysts.
acquired immunity Antibody- or cell-mediated response that is specific to a particular pathogen and is activated when needed.
acrochordon Small, soft, raised lesion (skin tag).
acromegaly Disease of middle-aged adults resulting from overproduction of growth hormone by the anterior pituitary.
action Ability to respond to others with genuineness, compassion, sensitivity, and self-disclosure to promote their well-being.
active acquired immunity Immunity developed after direct contact with an antigen through illness or vaccination.
active exercise Exercise carried out by the patient.
active transport Movement of solutes across membranes; requires the expenditure of energy.
acute illness Illness or disease that has a relatively rapid onset and a short duration.
acute pain Occurs after injury to tissues from surgery, trauma, or disease and is usually sudden in onset, temporary, easily localized, and decreases as healing takes place.
adaptation Organism's attempts to return to homeostasis.
addiction "Chronic, relapsing brain disease that is characterized by compulsive drug seeking and use, despite harmful consequences" (National Institute on Drug Abuse [NIDA]).
Addison disease Deviation resulting from a deficiency of adrenocorticotropic hormone caused by the destruction or dysfunction of the adrenal glands.
ADL Abbreviation for activities of daily living.
adrenaline Epinephrine; a powerful vasoactive substance produced by the adrenal medulla in times of stress or danger.
adrenocorticotropic hormone (ACTH) Pituitary hormone that stimulates the cortex of the adrenal glands to produce adrenal hormones.
advance directive Written statement of a person's wishes regarding medical treatment.
advanced cardiac life support Use of drugs and equipment while providing continued care for the person who has suffered cardiac or respiratory arrest.
aerosol Solid or liquid particles suspended in a gas.
affect Feelings such as happiness, sadness, or worry. An inappropriate affect is incongruence between the thought and feeling expressed.
afterload Amount of resistance the left ventricle must overcome to eject the blood volume.
ageism Process of systematic stereotyping and discrimination against people because of their age; usually directed against older people.
aging Process of growing older or more mature.
agoraphobia Fear of situations outside the home.
AICD Abbreviation for automatic implantable cardioverter defibrillator.
AIDS Abbreviation for acquired immunodeficiency syndrome; an advanced stage of human immunodeficiency virus (HIV) infection that weakens the body's immune system, progressively destroying the body's ability to fight pathogens and certain cancers. The condition is clinically diagnosed in HIV-positive individuals who have a T cell count below 200 and one or more of the opportunistic viral, fungal, or bacterial infections associated with the disease.
akathisia Reversible condition of restlessness that is manifested as an urge to pace.
algor mortis Cooling of the body after death.
alkaline (base) Solution containing a low number of hydrogen ions.
alkalosis Abnormal pH level of body fluids caused by an excess of bicarbonate in relation to acid.
ALL Abbreviation for acute lymphocytic leukemia.
allergen Antigen that causes a hypersensitive (allergic) reaction.
alopecia Loss of hair.
ALS Abbreviation for amyotrophic lateral sclerosis.
AMI Abbreviation for acute myocardial infarction.
amino acids Group of 22 substances that can be bonded in different ways to make a variety of proteins. The body can manufacture sufficient amounts of amino acids if the 9 essential amino acids are provided in the diet.
AML Abbreviation for acute myelogenous leukemia.
amputation Removal of a limb, part of a limb, or an organ; may be performed by surgical means or through an accident.
amputee Individual who has undergone an amputation.
amyopathy (amyotonia) Loss of muscle tone.
analgesia State of not feeling pain.
analgesic Drug that acts to relieve or reduce the suffering or intensity of pain.
anaphylactic shock Severe, potentially fatal, allergic reaction characterized by hypotension and bronchial constriction.
anastomosis Communication or connection between two organs or parts of organs.
androgens Hormones produced by the adrenal cortex, testes, and ovaries that stimulate the development of male characteristics.
anemia Reduction in the number of red blood cells or in the quantity of hemoglobin in the blood.
anesthesia Partial or complete loss of sensation with or without loss of consciousness.
anesthesiologist Physician who specializes in the administration of anesthetics and monitors patients while they are under anesthesia.
anesthetic Agent that abolishes the pain sensation.
angioma Benign tumor composed of blood vessels.
ankylosis Joint immobility.
anorectal incontinence Fecal incontinence caused by weak perineal muscles, loss of anal reflexes, loss of anal sphincter tone, or rectal prolapse.
anorexia Loss of appetite for food.
anteflexion Bending forward of the top of an organ.

anteversion Bending forward of an entire organ.
antibody Protein that is created in response to a specific antigen.
antibody-mediated acquired immunity Defensive response by B cells assisted by TH cells that is aimed at invading microorganisms such as bacteria.
antidiuretic hormone (ADH) Hormone released by the posterior pituitary gland that causes the reabsorption of water in the distal tubules and collecting ducts of the kidney.
antigen Substance, usually a protein, that is capable of stimulating a response from the immune system.
antihistamine Drug that blocks the effects of histamine, which is a body chemical that causes allergic symptoms.
antineoplastic Agent that inhibits the maturation or reproduction of malignant cells.
antithrombotic Capability of preventing the formation of blood clots.
anuria Absence of urine production.
anxiety Vague sense of impending doom or an apprehension that appears to have no clearly identifiable cause.
aphasia Inability to understand words or to respond with words or both.
apical Pointed end of a structure.
apnea Cessation of breathing.
ARDS Abbreviation for adult respiratory distress syndrome.
Arrhythmia Disturbance in cardiac rhythm; dysrhythmia.
arteriosclerosis Abnormal thickening, hardening, and loss of elasticity of the arterial walls.
arthralgia Pain in a joint.
arthritis Inflammation of a joint.
arthroplasty Plastic repair of a joint; joint replacement.
asbestosis Interstitial fibrosis of the lungs caused by inhalation of asbestos fibers.
ascites Accumulation of excess fluid in the peritoneal cavity.
aspiration Regurgitation and passage of fluids into the respiratory tract.
assessment Collection of data about the health status of a patient or client.
assignment "The distribution of work that each staff member is to accomplish in a given work period" (NCSBN, 2005, p. 1); what a person is asked to do.
assimilation Process of replacing or giving up values, beliefs, and practices for those of another culture.
asthma Potentially reversible obstructive airway disorder characterized by airway inflammation, hyperresponsiveness, and obstruction.
astigmatism Error of refraction caused by an uneven curvature of the cornea or lens; causes visual distortion.
ATC Abbreviation for around the clock.
atelectasis Collapsed lung or part of a lung.
atherosclerosis Abnormal thickening and hardening of the arterial walls caused by fat and fibrin deposits.
aura Peculiar sensation that precedes a set of symptoms.
auscultation Listening to sounds produced by the body, such as heart, lung, and intestinal sounds.
autocratic leadership Authoritative, directive, or bureaucratic type of leadership.
autoimmunity Condition in which the body is unable to distinguish self from nonself, which causes the immune system to react and destroy its own tissues.
automaticity Ability of a cell to generate an impulse without external stimulation.
automatism Aimless behavior performed without conscious control or knowledge.
autonomic dysreflexia (AD) Abnormally exaggerated response of the autonomic nervous system to a stimulus.
autonomy Freedom from external authority to make decisions about one's own health and health care.
autopsy Examination of a body after death to determine or confirm the cause of death.
avulsion Tearing away of tissue.
azotemia Accumulation of nitrogenous compounds in the blood.

B

bacteria One-celled microorganisms that are capable of multiplying rapidly within a susceptible host.
basal metabolic rate (BMR) Energy expended in the resting state; measured with the body at complete mental and physical rest but not asleep.
basic life support Immediate care given to prevent cardiac or respiratory arrest or to support the circulation and respiration of a person who is in cardiac arrest until advanced medical support is available.
Behçet syndrome Chronic syndrome with oral, gastrointestinal, and genital ulcerations and uveitis—arthritis, vasculitis, synovitis, meningitis, and phlebitis.
beneficence Act of doing good; behavior of a health care provider that is in the best interest of the patient's.
benign Not malignant.
bid Abbreviation for twice a day.
bioethics Ethics of biologic science, medicine, and health care.
biologic age Functional capabilities of various organ systems in the body.
biologic approach Assumes that mental disorders are related to physiologic changes within the central nervous system.
biopsy Excision of a small piece of tissue for microscopic examination; usually performed to determine a specific diagnosis.
bipolar disorder Characterized by alternating periods of elevated mood (manic episodes) and depression.
blepharitis Inflammation of the hair follicles and glands on the margins of the eyelids.
body image One's perception of one's own body.
bone marrow Spongy center of bones in which the white blood cells, red blood cells, and platelets are made.
bone remodeling Process in which immature bone cells are gradually replaced by mature bone cells.
borderline personality disorder A pattern of instability in interpersonal relationships, self-image, and unstable mood.
botulism Food poisoning caused by *Clostridium botulinum*.
Bouchard nodes Enlarged proximal interphalangeal joints of the fingers.
Bowel incontinence Inability to control the passage of feces; fecal incontinence.
BPH Abbreviation for benign prostatic hypertrophy.
brachytherapy Placement of a radiation source in the body to treat a malignancy.
bradycardia Slow heart rate, usually defined as fewer than 60 beats per minute.
BRM Abbreviation for biologic response modifier.
bronchiectasis Permanent dilation of a portion of the bronchi or bronchioles.
bronchitis Bronchial inflammation.
bruit Murmur detected by auscultation.
BSE Abbreviation for breast self-examination.
bulla Blister.
BUN Abbreviation for blood urea nitrogen.

C

cachexia Profound wasting and a loss of body mass; is usually related to malnutrition.
CAD Abbreviation for coronary artery disease.
CAL Abbreviation for chronic airflow limitation.
calculus (*pl.* calculi) Hard inorganic mass (e.g., "concretion") that is commonly called a *stone*; is formed of mineral salts and found in hollow organs or their passages.

calorie Standard unit for measuring energy; the amount of heat needed to raise the temperature of 1 gram of water at a standard temperature by 1°C.
cannula Tube that can be inserted into a body cavity or duct; needle or catheter used for intravenous therapy.
capitation Accepting a fixed amount of money to provide health care services to all health care plan members with no additional billing.
carcinogen Substance that can cause cancer.
cardiac output Amount of blood (in liters) ejected by the heart per minute.
cardiac tamponade Presence of blood in the pericardial sac that causes decreased cardiac output.
cardiopulmonary arrest Absence of heartbeat and breathing.
cardioversion Delivery of an electrical shock to the myocardium to restore normal sinus rhythm.
caries Destructive process of tooth decay.
caring Process characterized by understanding, action, and concern.
cataract Clouding or opacity of the normally transparent lens within the eye; causes vision to blur and objects to take on a yellowish hue.
catecholamines Chemicals (e.g., dopamine, epinephrine, norepinephrine) released at sympathetic nerve endings in response to stress.
cathartic Agent that stimulates bowel evacuation; is usually rapid in effect and produces a watery stool.
CBC Abbreviation for complete blood count.
cell-mediated acquired immunity Defensive response by Tc cells aimed at intracellular defects such as viruses and cancer.
cerebral death Absence of cerebral cortex functioning.
cerumen Waxy secretion in the external auditory canal; earwax.
cervicitis Inflammation of the cervix (i.e., narrow, lower end of the uterus).
chalazion Inflamed, enlarged meibomian (sebaceous) gland on the eyelid.
chancre Papule that breaks down into a painless ulcer at the site of entry of the spirochete organism.
CHD Abbreviation for coronary heart disease.
cheilitis Inflammation of the lips.
cheilosis Cracking of the lips and corners of the mouth.
chemical restraints Psychotropic medications given to subdue the agitated or confused patient.
chemotherapy Use of chemicals to treat illness.
CHF Abbreviation for congestive heart failure.
choking Airway obstruction caused by a foreign body in the airway.
cholangitis Inflammation of the biliary ducts.
cholecystectomy Removal of the gallbladder.
cholecystitis Inflammation of the gallbladder.
choledocholithiasis Obstruction of the common bile duct by a gallstone.
cholelithiasis Presence of gallstones in the gallbladder.
chronic illness Permanent impairment or disability that requires long-term rehabilitation and medical or nursing treatment.
chronic pain Pain that persists or recurs for more than 3 to 6 months; is most often neuropathic pain that results from nerve damage and follows an abnormal pathway for processing pain; may include abnormal sensations that occur in the absence of painful stimulus. Cause is often unknown and may or may not respond to treatment.
Chvostek sign Spasm of the facial muscles when the facial nerve is tapped; indicative of hypocalcemia.
cirrhosis Chronic, progressive liver disease.
client Consumers of nursing services; denotes a feeling of partnership or working with someone
CLL Abbreviation for chronic lymphocytic leukemia.
closed amputation Limb or part of a limb is removed and the wound is surgically closed.
closed or simple fracture Fracture in which the broken bone does not break through the skin.
closed reduction or manipulation Nonsurgical realignment of the bones to their previous anatomic position using traction, angulation, or rotation or a combination of these realignment procedures.
clotting factors Substances in the blood that help the blood to clot; are numbered I through XII.
CML Abbreviation for chronic myelogenous leukemia.
CNS Abbreviation for central nervous system.
CO Abbreviation for cardiac output.
codependency Exaggerated dependent pattern of self-defeating behaviors, beliefs, and feelings that are learned as a result of a pathologic relationship with a chemically dependent or otherwise dysfunctional person.
cognition Workings of the mind—language, memory, intellect, and reasoning.
cognitive behavioral approach Approach to therapy that uses behavior modification (e.g., positive and negative reinforcement) and recognizes that particular thoughts influence emotional states.
cognitive developmental approach Management of behavioral symptoms of dementia in which the environment and interactions are adapted to the patient's cognitive abilities.
collateral Accessory; side branch.
colostomy Surgically created opening in the colon.
colporrhaphy Operative technique that narrows the vagina by suturing the vaginal wall.
comminuted fracture Fracture in which the bone is broken or crushed into small pieces.
communicable disease Illness caused by infectious organisms or their toxins that can be transmitted either directly or indirectly from one person to another.
community-acquired infections Infections that are acquired in day-to-day contact with the public.
compartment syndrome Serious complication of a fracture caused by internal or external pressure on the affected area, resulting in decreased blood flow, pain, and tissue damage.
compensation Adaptations made by the heart and circulation to maintain normal cardiac output.
complement One of a series of proteins that enhance the inflammatory process and immune response.
complementary proteins Combination of incomplete proteins that provide all nine essential amino acids when consumed together.
complete fracture Fracture in which the break extends across the entire bone, dividing it into two separate pieces.
complete protein Protein that contains all nine essential amino acids; is usually of animal origin (e.g., meat, eggs).
compliance Elasticity.
compromised host precautions Actions taken to help protect patients with low white blood cell counts from infection.
compulsions Actions repeatedly carried out in a specific manner; typically include washing, counting, or checking.
conduction deafness Hearing impairment as a result of a blockage of the ear canal caused by excessive wax buildup, abnormal structures, or infection.
conductivity Ability of the cell to transmit electrical impulses rapidly and efficiently to distant regions of the heart.
confidentiality Assurance that private information is accessible only to authorized parties for specific, limited, and clearly defined purposes.
conflict Psychologic struggle that results when two incompatible possibilities occur at the same time.
confusion Disordered consciousness; lack of orientation in relation to person, place, and/or time.
congenital amputation Deformity or absence of a limb or limbs occurring during fetal development.

conjunctivitis Inflammation of the membrane that lines the eyelids and eyeball.
constipation Infrequent bowel movements with hard stools that are passed with difficulty.
contamination Presence of an infectious organism on a body surface or an object.
continent Capable of controlling natural impulses. In relation to an ostomy, the ability to retain feces or urine.
contractility Capacity for shortening in response to stimuli.
contracture Shortening of the muscles and tendons.
contralateral Opposite side.
conversion disorder Neurologic symptoms, such as blindness, deafness, or paralysis without physiologic causes, that occur in response to some threatening or traumatic event.
COPD Abbreviation for chronic obstructive pulmonary disease.
coping Any behavioral or cognitive activity used to deal with stress.
coping strategy Adaptive or maladaptive mental attitude, behavior, or both that is consciously or unconsciously perceived as helping to reduce stress, anxiety, or fear.
cor pulmonale Right-sided heart failure associated with pulmonary disease.
corpus cavernosum (*pl.* corpora cavernosa) Erectile chamber of the penis.
coryza Discharge from the nasal mucous membranes; acute rhinitis.
CP Abbreviation for cerebral palsy.
CPK Abbreviation for creatine phosphokinase.
crackles Abnormal lung sounds heard on auscultation; discrete single sounds heard on inspiration and occurring in brief bursts; may be fine (i.e., high pitched and soft) or coarse (i.e., low pitched and loud); "rales."
Credé method Expression of urine from the bladder by applying pressure over the lower abdomen.
crepitus Crackling sound or sensation.
CREST syndrome Form of a systemic scleroderma less severe than other forms, consisting of calcinosis cutis, Raynaud phenomenon, esophageal dysfunction, sclerodactyly, and telangiectasia.
cretinism Permanent mental and physical retardation caused by congenital deficiency of thyroid hormones.
crisis The point at which the individual moves toward illness and disequilibrium.
CSF Abbreviation for cerebrospinal fluid.
CT Abbreviation for computed tomography.
cultural diversity Existence of many cultures in a society.
culture Integrated system of learned values, beliefs, and practices that is characteristic of a society and that guides individual behavior.
Cushing disease Caused by the hypersecretion of glucocorticoids as a result of the excessive release of adrenocorticotropic hormone by the pituitary.
Cushing syndrome Resulting from excessive glucocorticoids in the body as a result of a tumor or the hypersecretion of the pituitary gland or by the prolonged administration of large doses of exogenous steroids.
cusp Cup-shaped structure. Semilunar heart valves have three cusps.
CVA Abbreviation for cerebrovascular accident.
CVP Abbreviation for central venous pressure.
cycloplegic Agent that paralyzes the ciliary muscle so that the eye does not accommodate.
cystectomy Removal or resection of the urinary bladder or of a cyst.
cystocele Herniation of the urinary bladder into the vagina.
cystotomy Creation of a surgical opening into the bladder.
cytologic Related to cells or the study of cells.

D

D&C Abbreviation for dilation and curettage.
DC Abbreviation for dilated cardiomyopathy.
debride Removal of debris, including necrotic tissue.
decerebrate posturing Abnormal extension of the upper extremities with extension of the lower extremities; accompanies increased pressure on the entire cerebrum and the motor tract structures of the brainstem.
decongestant Agent that reduces swelling, especially of the nasal mucous membranes.
decorticate posturing Abnormal flexion of the upper extremities with the extension of the lower extremities; is accompanied by increased pressure on the frontal lobes.
deep partial thickness burn Involves the epidermis and dermis.
defense mechanism Unconscious mechanism that is used to relieve anxiety; excessive or inappropriate use can hinder personality development.
defibrillation Termination of cardiac fibrillation, usually by electric shock.
dehiscence Separation of previously joined edges; reopening of a surgical wound.
delayed union Fracture healing that does not occur in the normally expected time.
delegation "The act of transferring to a competent individual the authority to perform a selected nursing task in a selected situation" (NCSBN, 2004).
delirium Disturbance of consciousness and a change in cognition that develops over a short period.
dementia Clinical syndrome or a collection of symptoms that is chronic in nature and is characterized by the impairment of intellectual function, problem-solving ability, judgment, memory, orientation, and appropriate behavior.
democratic leadership Achievement of goals through the participation by all group members.
denial Defense mechanism in which the individual refuses to acknowledge a real situation.
deontology Theory that defines right and wrong, based on how a person accomplishes goals rather than on what is accomplished; an act (i.e., means) can be wrong even if it produces a result (i.e., end) that is the best possible outcome.
depersonalization State of feeling outside of oneself, watching what is happening as if it were happening to someone else.
depression Mood of sadness; a withdrawal from usual commitments.
dermatitis Inflammation of the skin.
dermatome Area of skin supplied by sensory nerve fibers from a single posterior spinal root.
dermatomyositis Acute, subacute, or chronic disease marked by nonsuppurative inflammation of the skin, subcutaneous tissue, and muscles, with necrosis of muscle fibers.
DES Abbreviation for diethylstilbestrol.
diabetes insipidus (DI) Disease caused by the inadequate secretion of the antidiuretic hormone by the posterior portion of the pituitary gland.
diagnosis-related group (DRG) System of reimbursement standards for care in hospitals. The reimbursement is based on a fixed fee for a diagnostic category, regardless of cost.
dialysis Passage of molecules through a semipermeable membrane into a special solution.
diaphoresis Excessive perspiration.
diaphoretic Wet with excessive perspiration.
diarrhea Passage of frequent watery stools.
diffusion Random movement of particles in all directions through a solution.
diplopia Double vision.
disability Measurable loss of function; is usually delineated to indicate a diminished capacity for work (see *handicap*).
discoid lupus Circular, scaly lesions with erythematous raised rims; occurs over scalp, ears, face, and areas exposed to sun.

disorder Term used when a definite organic cause is established for behaviors and symptoms (see *syndrome*).
dissociative disorder Change in identity, memory, or consciousness that allows persons to remove themselves from anxiety-provoking situations; for example, multiple personality disorder and amnesias.
distress Stress that is perceived as harmful.
diuresis Increased production of urine.
dizziness Feeling of unsteadiness.
DM Abbreviation for diabetes mellitus.
DNR order Abbreviation for "do not resuscitate" order. Written order from a patient or primary decision maker, in consultation with the health care team, that resuscitation is not to be attempted in the event of cardiac or respiratory arrest.
dual diagnosis Simultaneous existence of a major psychiatric condition and a substance use disorder.
dysarthria Inability to speak clearly because of neurologic damage that impairs normal muscle control.
dysfunctional communication Unclear transmission of a message or information that prohibits the receiver from understanding the intent or meaning of what the sender transmits.
dysmenorrhea Painful menstruation.
dyspareunia Difficult or painful sexual intercourse in women.
dyspepsia Epigastric discomfort after meals; is caused by impaired digestion.
dysphagia Difficulty swallowing.
dysphasia Difficulty speaking.
dysplasia Abnormal cells.
dyspnea Difficulty breathing.
dyspraxia Partial inability to initiate coordinated voluntary motor acts.
dysreflexia Disordered response to stimuli; North American Nursing Diagnosis Association (NANDA) diagnosis for person with spinal cord injury at or above the seventh thoracic vertebra who experiences or is at risk for experiencing autonomic dysreflexia.
dysrhythmia Disturbance of rhythm; arrhythmia.
dysuria Difficult or painful urination.

E

ecchymosis Purplish skin lesions resulting from blood leaking out of the blood vessels.
ECF Abbreviation for extracellular fluid.
ECG Abbreviation for electrocardiogram.
ectropion In relation to the eyelid, the outward turning of the lid.
EEG Abbreviation for electroencephalogram.
ego In psychoanalytic theory, the "rational self" or "reality" principle of personality; mediates between *id* and *superego*.
egocentric Belief that one is the center of the universe.
eicosanoid Class of fatty acids that regulate blood vessel vasodilation, temperature elevation, white blood cell activation, and other physiologic processes involved in immunity.
ejaculation Reflexive expulsion of semen from the male urethra.
ejection fraction Percentage of ventricular end–diastolic volume ejected with each contraction of the left ventricle.
electroconvulsive therapy Uses electrical current to the brain to evoke a grand mal seizure in patients with depression. Seizure manifestations are controlled with drugs.
electrolyte Substance that develops an electrical charge when dissolved in water.
electromyography Diagnostic procedure in which needle electrodes are used to detect electrical impulses in muscle tissue. Impulses are recorded and information is provided about function of the nerves that supply muscles.
embolism Sudden obstruction of an artery by a floating clot or foreign material.
embolus (*pl.* emboli) Unattached blood clot or other substance in the circulatory system.
emesis Vomiting.
emission Delivery of semen into the internal urethra by rhythmic smooth muscle contractions of the epididymis, vas deferens, seminal vesicles, and prostate.
emotional lability Instability; episodes of unexplained and uncontrollable happiness and sadness.
empathy Ability to identify with and understand another person's situation, feelings, and motives.
emphysema Abnormal accumulation of air in body tissue. In the lung, a disorder characterized by loss of lung elasticity with trapping of air, retained carbon dioxide, and dyspnea.
empowerment Giving patients the information they need to be active participants in their care.
encephalitis Inflammation of brain tissue.
enculturation Process of learning to be part of a culture.
endocrine gland Gland that secretes a substance directly into the blood.
endogenous Internally produced or caused by internal factors.
endometriosis Condition in which endometrial tissue is located outside the uterus.
energy Capacity to do work; the way the body uses nutrients received through food consumption.
entropion In relation to the eyelid, the inward turning of the lid.
enucleation Removal of an intact organ, such as the eyeball.
enuresis Involuntary passage of urine, usually during sleep.
epididymitis Inflammation of the epididymis.
epidural On or outside the dura mater (i.e., outer membrane covering the spinal cord); opioids may be administered epidurally for pain relief.
epistaxis Nosebleed.
equianalgesic Having approximately the same degree of pain relief effect.
equilibrium State of balance needed for walking, standing, and sitting.
erection Swelling and rigidity of the penis.
eructation Expulsion of gas from the stomach through the mouth; belching.
erythema Redness of the skin; usually a sign that capillaries have become congested because of impaired blood flow.
ESR Abbreviation for erythrocyte sedimentation rate.
estrogen Hormone produced by the ovaries, adrenal glands, and fetoplacental unit in women; it is responsible for the sexual development and maturation of women.
ET Abbreviation for enterostomal therapist.
ethical dilemma Situation in which an apparent conflict between moral imperatives exists and in which obeying one results in transgressing the other.
ethics Values, codes, and principles related to what is right that influence decisions in nursing practice.
ethics of care Theory that sees care as a "central activity of human behavior"; it places emphasis on relationships.
ethnic group Group of individuals with a unique identity based on shared traditions, national origin, physical characteristics, and customs.
ethnocentrism Tendency to view the world from the perspective of one's own culture or ethnicity.
ETT Abbreviation for exercise tolerance test.
euglycemia Normal blood glucose level.
eustress Stress that is perceived as helpful (e.g., graduation, vacation).
evisceration Protrusion of internal organs through a wound.
excitability Ability of a cell to respond to an electrochemical stimulus.
exocrine gland Gland that secretes substances externally through ducts.
exogenous Developed outside the organism.

exophthalmos Protrusion of the eyeballs; is associated with hyperthyroidism.
expressive aphasia Difficulty speaking, reading, and writing; is characterized as nonfluent; caused by a lesion in the Broca area.
external fixation Use of rods, pins, nails, screws, or metal plates to align bone fragments and keep them in place for healing; similar to internal fixation but the devices in the bone are attached to an external frame.
extracellular fluid (ECF) Fluid outside the cell.
extrapyramidal effects Side effects of antipsychotic drugs on the portion of the central nervous system controlling involuntary movements.
extravasation Escape of fluid or blood from a blood vessel into body tissue.
extrinsic factors Factors in the environment.

F

fall Circumstance in which one unintentionally comes to rest on a lower level.
family Two or more persons who are joined together by bonds of sharing and emotional closeness and who identify themselves as being part of a family.
fasciculation Small involuntary muscle contraction.
fat embolism Condition in which fat globules are released from the marrow of the broken bone into the bloodstream, migrate to the lungs, and cause pulmonary hypertension.
fat-soluble vitamins Vitamins that are soluble in fat solvents, are absorbed into the body with other lipids, and build up in fat cells; they include vitamins A, D, E, and K.
fear Analogous to anxiety but related to the dread of a specific or real occurrence.
fecal incontinence Inability to control the passage of feces; bowel incontinence.
fee for service Established amount set by physicians or health care providers for services or procedures actually provided.
feelings All emotional and physical responses and sensations.
feminist ethics Branch of ethical study that focuses on gender inequalities and other disparities between and among individuals and groups of people. Feminist ethics places a particularly high value on relationships.
FEV Abbreviation for forced expiratory volume.
FFP Abbreviation for fresh frozen plasma.
filtration Transfer of water and solutes through a membrane from a region of high pressure to a region of low pressure.
fixation Performed during the open reduction surgical procedure to attach the fragments of the broken bone together when reduction alone is not feasible.
flaccid Soft; in relation to muscles, lacking tone.
flaccidity Diminished muscle tone.
flail chest Loss of support in the chest wall where several adjacent ribs are broken in more than one place.
flatulence Formation of excessive gas in the stomach or intestines.
flatus Gas in the digestive tract that is expelled through the rectum.
fluent aphasia Ability to speak clearly but without meaning.
fluid Any liquid or gas.
fluid volume deficit Abnormally decreased volume of body water; types are (1) isotonic extracellular fluid deficit (hypovolemia) and (2) hypertonic extracellular fluid deficit (dehydration); deficient fluid volume.
fluid volume excess Abnormally increased volume of body water; types are (1) extracellular fluid excess (isotonic fluid excess) and (2) intracellular water excess (hypotonic fluid excess); excess fluid volume.
fracture Break or disruption in the continuity of a bone.
FRC Abbreviation for functional residual capacity.
frostbite Serious tissue damage caused by cold.
frostnip Mild tissue damage caused by cold.
full-thickness burn Involves the epidermis, dermis, and underlying tissues such as fat, muscle, and bone.
functional communication Clear transmission of a message or information that enables the receiver to understand the intent or meaning of what the sender transmits.
functional incontinence Inappropriate voiding in the presence of normal bladder and urethral function.
fungi Vegetable-like organisms that feed on organic matter and are capable of producing disease.
FVC Abbreviation for forced vital capacity.

G

gangrene Necrosis or death of tissue, usually as a result of a deficient or absent blood supply; may result from inflammatory processes, injury, arteriosclerosis, frostbite, or diabetes mellitus.
gastrectomy Removal of all or part of the stomach.
gastritis Inflammation of the stomach.
gastrostomy Surgically created opening in the stomach.
GBS Abbreviation for Guillain-Barré syndrome.
gerontologic nurses Professional and advanced level of practitioners such as nurse practitioners, clinical specialists, and nurses holding national certification in the specialty of gerontologic nursing.
gerontology Study of aging.
GI Abbreviation for gastrointestinal.
gigantism Disease caused by excessive growth hormone in children and young adolescents resulting in excessive proportional growth.
gingivitis Inflammation of the gums.
gland Organ or structure that secretes substances used in other areas of the body.
glaucoma Condition in which high fluid pressure in the eye causes damage to the optic nerve.
glucocorticoids Class of adrenocortical hormones that affect protein and carbohydrate metabolism and help protect the body against stress.
glucometer Electronic device used to measure blood glucose.
gluconeogenesis Synthesis of glucose from sources other than carbohydrates.
glycogenesis Formation of glycogen from glucose.
glycogenolysis Splitting of glycogen into glucose.
glycosuria Presence of glucose in the urine.
goiter Enlargement of the thyroid gland.
goitrogen Substance that suppresses thyroid function.
goniometer Instrument used to measure joint range of motion.
granuloma Collection of inflammatory cells commonly surrounded by fibrotic tissue that represents a chronic inflammatory response to infectious or noninfectious agents.
gratification Sense of comfort and satisfaction derived from the fulfillment of one's needs.
gravidity State of a woman with respect to the total number of pregnancies.
greenstick fracture Fracture in which the bone is broken on one side but only bent on the other; most common in children.
grief Emotional response to a loss.
growth and development Physical, cognitive, and psychologic development that is predictable and sequential.
guillotine amputation Limb or portion of a limb is severed from the body and the wound is left open; a type of open amputation.

H

HAART Abbreviation for highly active antiretroviral therapy. Combination of antiretroviral drugs that may be prescribed when the human immunodeficiency virus (HIV) viral load reaches certain levels.

handicap Inability to perform one or more normal daily activities because of mental or physical disability (see *disability*).
HDL Abbreviation for high-density lipoprotein.
Health care associated infection Infection that occurs within a health care facility and may affect both the patient and the health care worker; previously called nosocomial infection.
health maintenance organization (HMO) Organization responsible for both financing and delivering comprehensive health services to an enrolled population for a prepaid fixed fee.
heartburn (pyrosis) Burning or tight sensation rising from the lower sternum to the throat.
heat stroke Body core temperature of 106°F or higher.
Heberden nodes Protrusions of the distal interphalangeal finger joints associated with osteoarthritis.
helminth Parasitic worm found in the soil and water that is transmitted to humans from hand to mouth.
hematocele Accumulation of blood in the scrotum, usually as a result of blunt trauma.
hematocrit (Hct) Percentage of red blood cells in whole blood.
hematuria Blood in the urine.
hemiparesis Weakness on one side of the body.
hemiplegia Paralysis on one side of the body.
hemoconcentration Concentration of the blood.
hemodynamics Study of the movement of blood and the forces that affect it.
hemoglobin (Hgb) Protein of the red blood cell that carries oxygen.
hemorrhage Loss of a large amount of blood.
hemostasis Control of bleeding.
hemothorax Presence of blood in the pleural cavity, causing the lung on the affected side to collapse.
hepatic Pertaining to the liver.
hepatitis Inflammation of the liver.
hepatomegaly Enlargement of the liver.
HIV Abbreviation for human immunodeficiency virus.
HIV positive Condition in which the blood has antibodies for human immunodeficiency virus (HIV), meaning that the individual has been infected with this virus.
holism Way of viewing people as whole individuals.
homeostasis Tendency of the biologic system to maintain stability of the internal environment while continually adjusting to changes necessary for survival.
homonymous hemianopsia Loss of half of the field of vision; loss is on the side opposite the brain lesion.
hopelessness Condition of a lack of hope, which may hinder action.
hordeolum Inflammation of a sebaceous gland of the eyelid; commonly called a *sty*; also spelled *stye*.
humoral immunity Immediate response to specific antigens involving B lymphocytes and the production of antibodies.
hydrocele Accumulation of clear fluid in the tunica vaginalis of the testicle or along the spermatic cord.
hypercalcemia Abnormally high serum calcium.
hypercapnia Excessive level of carbon dioxide in the blood.
hyperglycemia Abnormally high level of serum glucose.
hyperkalemia Abnormally high level of serum potassium.
hyperlipidemia Excess insoluble fats in the blood.
hypernatremia Abnormally high level of serum sodium.
hyperopia Farsightedness; ability to see distant objects better than near objects.
hypertension Persistent elevation of arterial blood pressure of 140/90 mm Hg or greater.
hyperthermia Elevation of body core temperature above 99°F.
hypertonic solution Solution with a higher concentration of electrolytes than normal body fluids.
hypertrophy Enlargement of existing cells resulting in increased size of an organ or tissue.
hyperuricemia Elevated level of uric acid in the blood.
hyperventilation Abnormally fast and deep breathing.
hypervolemia Increased circulating blood volume.
hypocalcemia Abnormally low level of serum calcium.
hypochondriasis Belief that a serious medical condition exists when medical findings are absent.
hypoglycemia Abnormally low level of glucose in the blood.
hypokalemia Abnormally low level of serum potassium.
hyponatremia Abnormally low level of serum sodium.
hypophysectomy Surgical removal of all or part of the pituitary gland.
hypotension Abnormally low blood pressure.
hypothermia Decrease in body core temperature below 95°F.
hypotonic solution Solution that has a lower concentration of electrolytes than normal body fluids.
hypoventilation Reduced movement of air into the alveoli.
hypovolemia Reduced circulating blood volume.
hypoxemia Low level of oxygen in the blood.
hypoxia Low oxygen level; decreased availability of oxygen to body tissues.
hysterectomy Surgical removal of the uterus.

I

IADL Abbreviation for instrumental activities of daily living.
iatrogenic infections Infections caused by a treatment (e.g., superinfection related to antimicrobial therapy).
IBD Abbreviation for inflammatory bowel disease.
IC Abbreviation for inspiratory capacity.
icterus Jaundice; golden-yellow skin color caused by the deposition of bile pigments.
id In psychoanalytic theory, the *pleasure principle* of the personality.
IE Abbreviation for infective endocarditis.
ileostomy Surgically created opening in the ileum.
IM Abbreviation for intramuscular or intramuscularly.
immobility Inability to move; imposed restriction on the entire body.
immunity Resistance to or protection from a disease.
immunodeficiency Condition in which the immune system is unable to defend the body against a foreign invasion of antigens.
immunoglobulin Membrane-bound, Y-shaped binding proteins produced by B lymphocytes; when immunoglobulins are released from the cell membrane, they are called *antibodies*.
immunosuppressant Agent that reduces immune response.
impaction (fecal) Accumulation of stool in the intestines that is not readily eliminated.
impairment Physical or psychologic disturbance in functioning.
impotence (erectile dysfunction) Inability to achieve and maintain an erection for sexual intercourse.
incomplete fracture Fracture in which the bone breaks only partly across, leaving some portion of the bone intact.
incomplete protein Protein lacking one or more essential amino acids.
incontinence Inability to hold urine or feces.
infarct Area of ischemic necrosis caused by the disruption of circulation.
infection Condition in which the body is invaded by infectious organisms that multiply, causing injury and a local inflammatory response that may progress to a systemic response.
infertility Inability to conceive and produce viable offspring.
infiltration Collection of infused fluid in tissues surrounding a cannula inserted for intravenous therapy.
inflammation Nonspecific immune response that occurs in response to bodily injury.
informed consent Patient's ability to make an independent health care decision after being given sufficient information and advice regarding the risks, benefits, and alternatives as well as the consequences of accepting or refusing treatment.

innate immunity Defensive system that is operational at all times, consisting of anatomic and physiologic barriers, the inflammatory response, and the ability of certain cells to phagocytose invaders.
inspection Purposeful observation or scrutiny of the person as a whole and then of each body system.
inspissated Thickened and dried; often used to describe pulmonary secretions.
instinct Inborn source of bodily need or impulse.
interferon Biologic response modifier secreted by virus-infected cells; natural and synthetic forms are used to treat cancer and to boost the immune system.
intermediate care facility Nursing homes that provide custodial care for people who are unable to care for themselves because of mental or physical infirmity.
internal fixation Use of rods, pins, nails, screws, or metal plates to align bone fragments and to keep them in place for healing.
interpersonal approach Patient learns new ways to behave in a therapeutic relationship built on trust.
intertrigo Skin inflammation where two skin surfaces touch.
intracellular fluid Fluid within the cell.
intracerebral Within the cerebrum.
intracranial Within the skull.
intracranial pressure (ICP) Pressure within the cranium or skull.
intrinsic factors Factors related to the internal functioning of an individual, such as the aging process or physical illness.
ipsilateral Same side.
ischemia Deficient blood flow as a result of an obstruction or constriction of blood vessels.
isolation technique Strategies employed to separate infected patients from other patients and health care workers in order to prevent spread of the infection.
isometric exercise Muscle contraction without movement used to maintain muscle tone.
isotonic Solution that has the same concentration of electrolytes as normal body fluids.
isotonic solution Solution that has the same concentration of electrolytes as normal body fluids.
IV Abbreviation for intravenous.

J

jaundice Golden-yellow color of the skin, sclerae, and mucous membranes caused by deposition of bile pigments; is associated with liver dysfunction or bile obstruction, causing hyperbilirubinemia.
justice Concept of fairness, equity, and appropriateness of treatment.

K

keratitis Inflammation of the cornea.
keratolytic Capability of dissolving keratin, the outer surface of the epidermis.
ketoacidosis Metabolic acidosis related to accumulated ketone bodies in the blood.
ketone bodies Products of fatty acid metabolism.
kyphosis Abnormal curvature of the thoracic spine as viewed from the side.

L

LA Abbreviation for left atrium.
laissez-faire leadership Nondirective type of leadership.
laryngectomy Surgical removal of the larynx.
laryngitis Inflammation of the larynx.
laryngospasm Spasmodic closure of the larynx.
latent Dormant; during the latency period of a disease, no signs or symptoms of the disease are present.
lavage Irrigation.
laxative Agent that promotes bowel evacuation.
LDH Abbreviation for lactic dehydrogenase.
LDL Abbreviation for low-density lipoprotein.
leadership Guidance or showing the way to others.
lentigo (*pl.* lentigines) Pigmented spot on sun-exposed skin.
LES Abbreviation for lower esophageal sphincter.
leukemia Cancer of the blood-forming tissue in which the bone marrow produces too many immature white blood cells.
leukocytes White blood cells that play a key role in immune responses to infectious organisms and other antigens. Also spelled leucocytes.
leukocytosis Part of the inflammatory process that causes an increase in white blood cells.
leukopenia Reduced number of leukocytes (white blood cells) in the blood.
leukoplakia Hard white patches on the gums, oral mucosa, or tongue that may become malignant.
libido In psychoanalytic theory, psychic energy is used to operate the id, ego, and superego.
lipids Fats in solid or liquid form that store energy, carry fat-soluble vitamins, and maintain healthy skin and hair. They supply essential fatty acids and promote a feeling of fullness (satiety).
lipoatrophy Decreased subcutaneous fat mass.
lipohypertrophy Increased subcutaneous fat mass.
lipoproteins Lipid-wrapped proteins carried into the bloodstream; they include high-density and low-density lipoproteins, which carry cholesterol.
lithotomy Removal of calculi through an incision in a duct or organ.
lithotripsy Crushing or disintegration of calculi.
livor mortis Discoloration of the body after death.
LOC Abbreviation for level of consciousness.
long-term care facility Nursing home that provides intermediate and nonskilled or custodial care for people who are unable to care for themselves because of mental or physical disabilities.
loss Real or potential absence of someone or something that is valued.
LSD Abbreviation for lysergic acid diethylamide; a hallucinogenic drug.
LV Abbreviation for left ventricle.
lymphocytopenia Reduced number of lymphocytes in the blood; also called *lymphopenia*.
lymphoma Cancer of the lymph system.
lymphopenia Lymphocytopenia; reduced number of lymphocytes in the blood.

M

macrovascular Pertaining to the large blood vessels.
macule Flat, colored lesion such as a freckle.
maladaptive Attempts to cope using strategies that ultimately do not return the individual to homeostasis.
malaise Vague feeling of discomfort.
malignant Tending to progress in virulence; has the characteristics of becoming increasingly undifferentiated, invasive of surrounding tissues, and colonizing distant sites.
malpractice Professional negligence by a health care provider that causes patient injury.
managed health care Provision of comprehensive health care at a reasonable cost through enrollment in a health maintenance organization (HMO), preferred provider organization (PPO), or similar plan with incentives to save costs.
management Effective use of selected methods to achieve desired outcomes.
mastitis Inflammation of breast tissue.
matrix Intercellular substance of a tissue.

Medicaid Program that provides health care services for needy, lower-income, and disabled individuals through funds distributed at the state level.
medical asepsis Limiting the spread of microorganisms; often called the *clean technique*.
Medicare Health insurance program administered by the federal government that is funded by Social Security payments.
menarche Onset of menstrual function.
menopause Cessation of menstruation.
menorrhagia Menstrual periods characterized by profuse or prolonged bleeding.
menstruation Vaginal discharge of a mixture of blood and other fluids and tissue that are formed in the uterus to receive a fertilized ovum.
mental health continuum Model used to demonstrate the range of mental health on a line between health at one end and illness at the opposite extreme.
mental status examination Observations and descriptions regarding appearance, mood and affect, speech and language, thought content, perceptual disturbances, insight and judgment, sensorium and memory, and attention.
metastasis Process by which cancer spreads to distant sites.
metrorrhagia Bleeding or spotting between menstrual periods.
MG Abbreviation for myasthenia gravis.
MI Abbreviation for myocardial infarction.
microvascular Pertaining to the small blood vessels (e.g., arterioles, capillaries, venules).
micturition Urination.
mineralocorticoid Type of hormone secreted by the adrenal cortex and involved in the regulation of fluid and electrolyte levels in the body.
minerals Small amounts of metals (e.g., calcium, sodium, potassium) and nonmetals (e.g., chloride, phosphate) that are essential to the body; can build up.
miotic agent Agent that causes the pupil to constrict.
monoamine oxidase inhibitor (MAOI) Class of antidepressant drugs; patients on MAOIs must be careful to avoid life-threatening food and drug interactions.
mood Feeling state experienced by the patient over a period; can be constricted (i.e., not experiencing a variety of feelings) or expanded (i.e., experiencing more than usual feelings).
moral distress Feeling of powerlessness that occurs when institutional barriers prevent a health care provider from acting in accordance with his or her own moral beliefs.
moral outrage Feeling of being powerless to intervene after witnessing an immoral act by another health care provider.
morality Shared concept in society of what is right or wrong.
morals Ethical habits of a person.
mourning The outward part of coping with grief. It represents a period of grieving marked by social customs.
MRI Abbreviation for magnetic resonance imaging.
MS Abbreviation for multiple sclerosis.
multiple personality disorder Exhibition by one person of two or more distinct personalities.
murmur Sound heard on auscultation of the heart that usually indicates turbulent blood flow across heart valves.
MV Abbreviation for minute volume.
myalgia Muscle pain.
mycoplasmas Gram-negative organisms that usually cause infections in the respiratory tract.
mydriatic agent Causes the pupil to dilate.
myelinated Surrounded with a sheath.
myopathy Muscle disease (*adj.* myopathic).
myopia Nearsightedness; the ability to see near objects better than distant objects.
myxedema Facial edema that develops with severe, long-term hypothyroidism; sometimes used as a synonym for *hypothyroidism*.

N

natural immunity Present at birth (innate) and not dependent on a specific immune response or previous contact with an infectious agent
necrotizing vasculitis Any of a group of disorders characterized by inflammation and necrosis of blood vessels occurring in a broad spectrum of cutaneous and systemic disorders.
neoplasm Tumor; may be benign or malignant.
nephropathy Kidney disease.
nephrostomy Surgically created opening in the kidney to drain urine.
nephrotoxic Having a harmful effect on kidney tissue.
neuralgia Pain in a nerve or along the course of a nerve.
neurogenic bladder Condition in which the bladder does not function normally because of a disorder affecting the nerves of the bladder.
neurogenic (bowel) incontinence Reflexive uncontrolled bowel movement, usually seen in those with dementia.
neurohypophysis Posterior portion of the pituitary gland.
neuroleptic malignant syndrome Effect of medication that can develop after one dose or after years of drug therapy; the first symptoms are usually muscular rigidity, accompanied by akinesia and respiratory distress; the cardinal sign is hyperthermia (body temperature 101°F to 103°F or higher).
neuropathic pain Pain that arises from a damaged nerve.
neuropathy Pathologic changes in the peripheral nervous system.
neurotoxin Substance that poisons or impairs nerve tissue.
neurotransmitter Biochemical messenger at nerve endings that activates receptors and stimulates or inhibits a response.
nevus (*pl.* nevi) Mole.
NG Abbreviation for nasogastric.
nociception Process of pain transmission; is usually related to pain sensation, resulting from the stimulation of pain receptors and transmission of stimuli to the pain fibers, spinal cord, and brain.
nocturia Urination during the night.
nodule Small mass of tissue that can be palpated.
nonfluent aphasia Difficulty initiating speech.
nonmaleficence Concept in health care of first doing no harm; in end-of-life issues, this concept involves providing treatment to control pain but not necessarily to heal.
nonsteroidal antiinflammatory drug (NSAID) Nonopioid drug that reduces pain and inflammation.
nonunion Failure of a fracture to heal.
nosocomial infection Infection that occurs within a health care facility and may affect both the patient and the health care worker. Health-care associated infection is the preferred term.
NPO Abbreviation for nothing by mouth.
NSAID Abbreviation for nonsteroidal antiinflammatory drug.
NTG Abbreviation for nitroglycerin.
nurse anesthetist Registered nurse who specializes in the administration of anesthetics and monitors the condition of patients receiving anesthetics.
nursing diagnosis Actual or potential health problems derived from data gathered during the assessment of a patient.
nursing process Systematic, problem-solving approach to providing nursing care in an organized, scientific manner.
OA Abbreviation for osteoarthritis.
object permanence Idea that an object or person continues to exist even though no longer in sight; object permanence does not develop until about 2 years of age, according to Piaget.
objective data Information about the patient that can be detected with the senses.
obsessions Recurrent intrusive thoughts that interfere with normal functioning.

obsessive-compulsive disorder Recurrent obsessions, compulsions, or both that produce distress and interfere with daily functions.
Oedipus complex Occurs during the phallic stage in psychoanalytic theory; the child unconsciously desires the parent of the opposite sex; this conflict is resolved when the child identifies with the parent of the same sex.
Older Americans Act Act passed in 1965 to ensure that older individuals have an adequate income and suitable housing, physical and mental health services, community services, and the opportunity to pursue meaningful activities.
oliguria Decreased urine output.
Omnibus Budget Reconciliation Act (OBRA) Law enacted in 1987 to protect patients in long-term care facilities.
oncofetal antigen Gene product that normally is suppressed in adult tissues but reappears in the presence of some types of cancer.
OOB Abbreviation for out of bed.
open amputation Amputation that is left open; usually performed in cases of infection or necrosis.
open or compound fracture Fracture in which the fragments of the broken bone break through the skin.
open reduction Surgical procedure in which an incision is made at the fracture site to cleanse the area of fragments and debris; is usually performed on patients with open (compound) or comminuted fractures.
opioid agonist Any morphine-like drug that produces bodily effects including pain relief.
opportunistic infection Infection caused by an organism that usually does not cause a disease but becomes pathogenic when body defenses are impaired.
orthopnea Difficulty breathing when lying down.
orthostatic hypotension Sudden drop in systolic blood pressure when changing from a lying or sitting position to a standing position.
orthostatic vital sign changes Changes in the vital signs as a person moves from lying to sitting to standing positions in which the pulse increases by 20 beats per minute and the blood pressure decreases by 20 mm Hg, indicating that the patient is hypovolemic.
osmolality Concentration of a solution; is measured as the number of dissolved particles per kilogram of water.
osmolarity Concentration of a solution; is measured as the number of dissolved particles per liter of solution.
osmosis Movement of water across a membrane from a less concentrated solution to a more concentrated solution.
osteoarthritis Noninflammatory degenerative joint disease marked by degeneration of the articular cartilage, hypertrophy of bone at the margins, and changes in the synovial membrane.
osteomyelitis Infection of the bone.
osteoporosis Decreased bone mass.
ostomy Surgical procedure that creates an opening into a body structure.
otalgia Pain in the ear.
otic Pertaining to the ear.
ototoxic Capable of injuring the eighth cranial (acoustic) nerve or other structures involved in hearing and balance.
overflow incontinence (bowel/fecal) Uncontrolled passage of stool associated with constipation.
overflow incontinence (urine) Involuntary loss of urine associated with a full bladder.
oximeter Device that uses a photoelectric sensor to measure the oxygen saturation of the blood.
oxygenation Transport of oxygen from the lungs to the tissues.

P

PACU Abbreviation for postanesthesia care unit (i.e., recovery room).
pain Unpleasant sensory and emotional experience associated with actual or potential tissue damage existing whenever the person says it does; a unique, private experience involving the whole person in a time dimension of past, present, and future and influenced by internal and external environments.
pain threshold Level of intensity that causes the sensation or feeling of pain.
pain tolerance Amount of pain a person is willing to endure before taking action to relieve pain.
palliative Relieves symptoms or improves function without correcting the basic problem.
palpation Method of physical examination that uses touch to assess various parts of the body.
palpitation Heartbeat that is strong, rapid, or irregular enough that the person is aware of it.
pancreatitis Inflammation of the pancreas.
panic disorder Experience of intense episodes of apprehension to the point of terror.
papule Raised area on the skin that is less than 1 cm in diameter.
paracentesis Removal of ascitic fluid from the peritoneal cavity.
paraphimosis Retraction of phimotic foreskin, causing painful swelling of the glans.
paraplegia Loss of motor and sensory function as a result of damage to the spinal cord that spares the upper extremities but, depending on the level of the damage, affects the trunk, pelvis, and lower extremities.
paresthesia Abnormal sensation.
parity Describes the state of a woman with respect to the number of pregnancies carried 20 or more weeks.
parkinsonian syndrome Adverse effect of long-term antipsychotic drug therapy; patient exhibits masklike face, shuffling gait, resting tremor, and rigid posture.
parotiditis Inflammation of the parotid (salivary) gland; most commonly called *parotitis*.
parotitis Inflammation of the parotid gland.
paroxysmal nocturnal dyspnea Sudden difficulty breathing when asleep.
participative leadership Mixture of autocratic and democratic leadership; feedback from group members is used by the leader to make a final decision.
passive acquired immunity Temporary immunity acquired after receiving antibodies or lymphocytes produced by another individual.
passive exercise Exercise of the patient that is carried out by the therapist or nurse without the assistance of the patient.
pathogen Disease-causing microorganism.
pathologic fracture Fracture that occurs because of a pathologic condition in the bone, such as a tumor or disease process, which causes a spontaneous break.
patient Person for whom the nurse provides care; denotes a feeling of doing to or for.
patient-centered care Care that supports active involvement of patients, maximizing outcomes and client satisfaction.
patient-controlled analgesia Self-administration of an analgesic by a patient instructed in doing so; usually refers to self-dosing with intravenous opioids through a programmable pump.
PCA Abbreviation for patient-controlled analgesia.
PCP Abbreviation for phencyclidine.
PE Abbreviation for pulmonary embolism.
peer group Group of people with which the individual identifies and derives a sense of belonging.
pelvic inflammatory disease Infection of the ovaries, fallopian tubes, and pelvic area.
pemphigus Chronic autoimmune condition characterized by blisters on the face, back, chest, groin, and umbilicus.
percussion Tapping on the skin to assess the underlying tissues.

perforation Hole or break in a structure.
perfusion Passage of blood through the vessels of an organ.
periarteritis nodosa Inflammatory disease of the outer coats of small- and medium-sized arteries and of surrounding tissue.
periarticular Around the joint.
periorbital edema Accumulation of excess fluid around the eye.
peristalsis Circular, wavelike contractions of the muscles of the digestive tract propel food down the tract.
peritoneum Membrane that lines the walls of the abdominal and pelvic cavities.
peritonitis Inflammation of the peritoneum.
personality Deeply ingrained patterns of behavior that include the way an individual relates to, perceives, and thinks about the environment and self.
personality disorders Pervasive, chronic, and maladaptive personality characteristics that interfere with normal functioning; examples are paranoid, schizoid, antisocial, borderline, avoidant, obsessive-compulsive, and passive-aggressive.
pessary Device inserted into the vagina to support the uterus.
PET Abbreviation for positron emission tomography.
petechiae Small (1 to 3 mm) red or reddish purple spots on the skin resulting from capillaries breaking and leaking small amounts of blood into the tissues.
pH Symbol used to indicate hydrogen ion concentration. A solution with a low pH (<7) is an acid; a solution with a high pH (>7) is alkaline or base. A pH of 7 is neutral. The normal pH of body fluids is between 7.35 and 7.45.
phagocytes Certain white blood cells (e.g., neutrophils, monocytes, macrophages) that engulf and destroy invading pathogens, dead cells, and cellular debris.
phantom limb sensation Feeling that a limb still exists after an amputation; the perception that pain exists in a removed limb is called *phantom limb pain*.
phimosis Constriction of the opening in the prepuce to ensure that the prepuce cannot be retracted back over the glans.
phlebitis Inflammation of a vein.
phlebothrombosis Development of venous thrombi without venous inflammation.
photophobia Excessive sensitivity to light.
physical assessment Physical examination that is a systematic, thorough way of obtaining objective data.
physical dependence Physical need for a substance on which an individual is dependent to avoid unpleasant physical withdrawal symptoms.
physical restraint Anything that restricts movement and cannot be removed by the individual.
PICC Abbreviation for peripherally inserted catheter.
PID Abbreviation for pelvic inflammatory disease.
plasma Clear, straw-colored fluid that carries red blood cells, white blood cells, and platelets through the circulatory system.
platelet Small, disk-shaped blood component responsible for activating the blood clotting system.
pneumoconiosis One of many occupational diseases caused by the inhalation of particles of industrial substances.
pneumonitis Inflammation of the lung.
pneumothorax Presence of air in the pleural cavity that causes the lung on the affected side to collapse.
PO Abbreviation for by mouth.
poikilothermy Coolness in an area of the body as a result of decreased blood flow.
poison Any substance that, in small quantities, is capable of causing harm after ingestion, inhalation, injection, or contact with the skin.
polydipsia Excessive thirst.
polymyalgia rheumatica Connective tissue disorder characterized by stiffness and pain in the shoulders and hips.
polymyositis Chronic, progressive inflammatory disease of skeletal muscle.
polyp Growth that protrudes from a mucous membrane.
polyphagia Excessive hunger; food ingestion.
polyuria Excessive urine output.
postictal After a seizure.
posttraumatic stress disorder Symptoms experienced after a traumatic event; examples are flashbacks, detachment, and sleep difficulties.
powerlessness Feeling that an individual's action will not affect an outcome or that an individual lacks personal control over certain events or situations.
preferred provider organization (PPO) System that uses a network of independent physicians, hospitals, and other providers who provide services to a pool of patients for a discounted fee.
preload Amount of blood in the left ventricle at the end of diastole; the pressure generated at the end of diastole.
presbycusis Hearing loss associated with old age.
presbyopia Visual impairment associated with older age in which the lens becomes more rigid and less able to change shape, resulting in a decreased ability to focus on near objects.
pressure ulcer Open wound caused by pressure on a bony prominence; also called a *pressure sore*.
primary prevention First level of prevention; includes steps taken to improve health and prevent disease and injury.
PRN Abbreviation for as needed.
problem-oriented medical record Method of record keeping that focuses on patient problems rather than on medical diagnoses.
progressive systemic sclerosis (PSS) Scleroderma; multisystem autoimmune disorder characterized by a hardening of the skin and affecting blood vessels, gastrointestinal tract, lungs, heart, and kidneys.
projection Defense mechanism in which individuals see others as a source of their own unacceptable thoughts, feelings, or impulses.
prolapse Downward displacement.
prostatectomy Removal of all or part of the prostate gland.
prostatitis Inflammation of the prostate gland.
prostatodynia Prostatic and pelvic pain in the absence of infection or inflammation.
protease inhibitor Class of medications used to treat or prevent such viral infections as human immunodeficiency virus (HIV) and hepatitis C. These medications prevent viral replication by inhibiting the activity of protease.
proteins Large organic compounds made of various combinations of amino acids; found in meat, milk, fish, and eggs.
protozoa One-celled organisms capable of producing disease that usually is spread by contaminated food and water.
pruritus Itching.
psoriasis Skin condition characterized by scaly lesions and caused by rapid proliferation of epidermal cells.
psychoanalytic approach Based on the theory that people function at different levels of awareness (i.e., conscious to unconscious) and that ego defense mechanisms such as denial and repression are used to prevent anxiety.
psychologic age Behavioral capacity of a person to adapt to changing environmental demands.
psychosis State in which an individual's perception of reality is impaired, thereby interfering with the capacity to function and relate to others.
ptosis Drooping of the upper eyelid.
PTT Abbreviation for partial thromboplastin time.
Public Health Service Branch of the Department of Health and Human Services of the U.S. government whose chief purpose is to provide better health services for the American people.

purpura Red or reddish purple skin lesions measuring 3 mm or more, resulting from blood leaking outside the blood vessels.
PVD Abbreviation for peripheral vascular disease.
pyrogen Substance released in inflammation that causes body temperature to increase.

Q

q Abbreviation for every. (See inside back cover for cautions pertaining to this abbreviation.)
quadriplegia Loss of motor and sensory function in all four extremities due to damage to the spinal cord.

R

RA Abbreviation for right atrium.
radiotherapy Use of radiation in the treatment of cancer and other diseases.
range-of-motion (ROM) exercise Exercise in which each joint is moved in various directions to the farthest possible extreme without producing pain.
RAP Abbreviation for right atrial pressure.
receptive aphasia Inability to comprehend words; characterized as fluent; lesion in Wernicke area.
recovery Lifelong process of maintaining abstinence from the substance to which an individual is addicted; a return to moderate substance use is never the end result of recovery.
rectocele Herniation of part of the rectum into the vagina.
red blood cell Biconcave, disk-shaped blood component responsible for carrying oxygen to the tissues and removing waste carbon dioxide from the tissues.
red blood cell (RBC) count Total number of RBCs found in 1 cubic millimeter of blood.
reduction Process of bringing the ends of the broken bone into proper alignment.
reflex training Technique to stimulate defecation using the Valsalva maneuver and rectal stretching.
reflux Backward flow.
refraction Bending of light rays.
regeneration Replacement of damaged cells by cells of their own kind during the wound healing process.
regurgitation Backward flow (cardiovascular system); gentle ejection of the stomach contents into the mouth without nausea or retching (digestive tract).
rehabilitation Process of restoring individuals to the best possible health and functioning after physical or mental impairment.
Reiter syndrome Connective tissue disease characterized by a triad of arthritis, urethritis, and conjunctivitis.
relaxation State of decreased anxiety and muscle tension.
repair Replacement of damaged cells by connective tissue and then eventually by scar tissue during the wound healing process.
replantation Surgical reattachment of a limb to its original site.
residual limb Stump; partial limb remaining after amputation.
resources Persons, items, concepts, or organizations that can be drawn on for a sense of support (e.g., family, money, skills, beliefs).
respiration Exchange of oxygen and carbon dioxide in the alveoli (external respiration) and in the tissues and cells (internal respiration).
respiratory arrest Absence of breathing.
resting metabolic rate (RMR) Measurement of energy expenditure made at any time of the day and 3 to 4 hours after the last meal.
retinopathy Disease of the retina of the eye.
retroflexion Bending backward of the upper portion of an organ.
retroversion Bending backward of an entire organ.
reverse isolation Protection of severely compromised patients from other patients and health care workers.
reversible ischemic neurologic deficit Neurologic deficit that lasts longer than 24 hours but resolves completely; is caused by diminished cerebral blood flow.
rheumatoid arthritis (RA) Chronic systemic disease characterized by inflammatory changes occurring throughout the body's connective tissues; is most apparent in diarthroses (synovial joints).
rhinitis Inflammation of the nasal mucous membrane.
rhonchus (*pl.* rhonchi) Dry, rattling sound caused by partial bronchial obstruction.
rickettsiae Microorganisms that are usually transmitted to humans through flea and tick bites.
rigor mortis Stiffening of the body after death.
role Expectation of how an individual is to behave in a situation or what is expected of an individual in a certain position.
RV Abbreviation for right ventricle.

S

salpingo-oophorectomy Surgical excision of a fallopian tube and ovary.
sanguineous Bloody.
saturated fatty acids Compounds that come chiefly from animal sources and are usually solid at room temperature; also includes coconut and palm oils.
SCD Abbreviation for sudden cardiac death.
scheduled toileting Encouraging patients to use the toilet at specific times based on their usual patterns.
schizophrenia Very serious, usually chronic thought disorders in which psychotic symptoms primarily impair the affected person's ability to interpret the world accurately; characterized by disturbances in thinking, mood, and behavior.
sclerodactyly Hardening and shrinking of connective tissue of fingers and toes; scleroderma of fingers and toes.
scleroderma Chronic multisystem autoimmune disease characterized by a hardening of the skin and affecting the blood vessels, gastrointestinal tract, lungs, heart, and kidneys.
sclerotherapy Injection of hardening agents into blood vessels.
scotoma Blind spots.
secondary prevention Second level of prevention; includes steps taken to detect disease early and begin treatment as soon as possible.
seizure Convulsion; series of involuntary contractions of voluntary muscles.
selectively permeable membranes Membranes that separate fluid compartments of the body and regulate movement of water and certain solutes from one compartment to another.
self Individual's personhood.
self-concept Individual's mental image or picture of self.
self-esteem Perception of self as having worth.
sensorineural deafness Hearing impairment resulting from damage to the nerve centers within the brain as a result of exposure to loud noises, disease, and certain drugs.
sensorium Level of consciousness and orientation to time, place, person, and self.
septum Wall that divides a body cavity.
serosanguineous Made up of blood and serum.
serous Containing serum.
sexually transmitted infection (STI) Disease that can be transmitted by intimate genital, oral, or rectal contact.
shearing forces Caused by two contacting parts sliding on each other.
shock Acute circulatory failure that can lead to death; is caused by blood loss, heart failure, overwhelming infection, severe allergic reactions, or extreme pain or fright.
shroud Wrap in which the body is placed after death for transport to the morgue or mortuary.

sinusitis Inflammation of the paranasal sinuses.
Sjögren syndrome Symptom complex of unknown cause marked by the triad of keratoconjunctivitis, xerostomia, and the presence of a connective tissue disease.
skilled nursing facility Type of long-term care facility that provides rehabilitative care for people who need nursing care that consists of observation during illness, administration of medications and treatments, bowel or bladder retraining, and changing of sterile dressings.
skilled observation and assessment Used to determine adequacy of home environment, knowledge level of the patient and family regarding care procedures, side effects of treatment, and family's level of comfort in performing specific procedures.
skilled procedures Certain nursing procedures, such as dressing changes, Foley catheter insertions, and venipuncture.
SLE Abbreviation for systemic lupus erythematosus.
smegma Sebaceous secretion found beneath the foreskin.
social age Roles and habits of an individual in relation to other members of society.
soluble fiber Partially digestible roughage found in plant cells; helps to soften stool and works chemically to reduce absorption of certain substances in the bloodstream.
solution Liquid containing one or more dissolved substances.
somatoform disorder Characterized by vague, multiple, recurring physical complaints that are not caused by real physical illness.
Somogyi effect Rebound response to excess insulin, causing hyperglycemia.
spastic Increased muscle tone, characterized by sudden, involuntary muscle spasms.
spasticity Abnormally increased muscle tone.
spermatocele Cystic mass on the epididymis.
sprain Injury to a ligament.
sputum Mucous secretion from the respiratory tract.
staged amputation Amputation that is performed over the course of several operations, usually to control the spread of infection or necrosis.
statutory law Written laws (statutes) legislated by government in response to a perceived need to clarify the functioning of government, improve civil order, provide for a public need, or codify existing law.
steatorrhea Excess fat in the stools.
stenosis Narrowing of a passage or opening.
sterile Free of microorganisms; infertile.
sterility State of being free of microorganisms; unable to reproduce.
stoma Opening created to drain contents of an organ.
stomatitis Inflammation of the oral mucosa.
strain Injury to muscle tissues or the tendons that attach them to bones or both.
stress Physical and emotional state always present in individuals, which is intensified when an internal or external environmental change or threat to which the individuals must respond occurs.
stress fracture Fracture caused by either sudden force or prolonged stress.
stress incontinence Involuntary loss of urine during physical exertion.
stressor Factor that causes stress.
stump Distal portion of an amputated limb; residual limb.
subarachnoid Between the arachnoid and pia mater layers of the membranes covering the brain.
subculture Group of individuals within a culture whose members share different beliefs, values, and attitudes from those of the dominant culture.
subjective data Information reported by patients or family members.
substance use disorder Continued use of a substance in spite of significant cognitive, behavioral, and physiologic symptoms associated with its use.
substance dependence Ingestion of substances in gradually increasing amounts in response to a physical need; is used interchangeably with the terms *chemical dependence* and *drug dependence*.
superficial partial thickness burn Burn that affects the epidermis.
support system Resources that are used to cope with stress.
surgical asepsis Elimination of microorganisms from any object that comes in contact with the patient; is often called *sterile technique*.
SVR Abbreviation for systemic vascular resistance.
symptomatic incontinence Bowel/fecal incontinence associated with colorectal disease.
syncope Fainting.
syndrome Behaviors and symptoms.
syndrome of inappropriate antidiuretic hormone Disorder caused by excess antidiuretic hormone production; symptoms include decreased urination, edema, and fluid overload.
systemic Related to the body as a whole.
systole Contraction phase of the cardiac cycle.

T

tachycardia Rapid heart rate; is usually defined as greater than 100 beats per minute.
tachypnea Rapid respiratory rate.
tardive dyskinesia Frequently irreversible side effect of antipsychotic medication that develops after years of use; symptoms include involuntary movements of face, jaw, and tongue, leading to grimacing, jerky movements of upper extremities, and tonic contractions of neck and back.
telangiectasis Vascular lesion created by the dilation of a group of small blood vessels.
tertiary prevention Third level of prevention; includes steps taken to prevent disease recurrence or complications of diagnosed disease or injury.
testis (*pl.* testes) Male reproductive organs.
tetany Steady muscle contraction; is caused by hypocalcemia.
TGV Abbreviation for thoracic gas volume.
theory X Management by autocratic rule with little participation in decision making by workers.
theory Y Democratic style of management with some participation in decision making by workers.
theory Z Management with full participation in decision making by workers.
thoracentesis Insertion of a needle through the chest wall into the pleural space to remove fluid, blood, or air or to administer medication.
thoracotomy Surgical opening of the chest wall.
thrombocytopenia Abnormally reduced number of platelets in the blood.
thromboembolism Obstruction of a blood vessel with a blood clot transported through the bloodstream.
thrombophlebitis Development of venous thrombi in the presence of venous inflammation.
thrombosis Development or presence of a thrombus.
thrombus (*pl.* thrombi) Stationary blood clot.
thyroiditis Inflammation of the thyroid gland.
thyrotoxicosis Excessive metabolic stimulation caused by an elevated level of the thyroid hormone.
tinnitus Ringing, buzzing, or roaring noise in the ears.
tissue perfusion Blood flow through the blood vessels of tissue.
TLC Abbreviation for total lung capacity.
tolerance Physiologic result of repeated doses of an opioid in which the same dose is no longer effective in achieving the same analgesic effect; a larger dose of the opioid is required to achieve the same analgesic effect.

tonicity Measure of the concentration of electrolytes in a fluid.
tonometry Measurement of pressure such as intraocular pressure.
tonsillitis Inflammation of the tonsils.
tophus (*pl.* tophi) Deposit of sodium urate crystals under the skin.
tort Civil wrong against a person that is recognized as grounds for a lawsuit.
TPN Abbreviation for total parenteral nutrition.
transcultural nursing Integration of cultural considerations into all aspects of nursing care.
transcutaneous electrical nerve stimulation (TENS) Method of producing analgesia through electrical impulses applied to the skin.
transient incontinence Temporary loss of control over voiding.
transient ischemic attack (TIA) Diminished cerebral blood flow producing neurologic deficits that last less than 24 hours.
triglycerides Lipids composed of three fatty acid chains and a glycerol molecule.
Trousseau sign Carpopedal spasm after compression of the nerves in the upper arm; is a sign of hypocalcemia.
12-step program Self-help support process outlining 12 steps to overcoming a physical or psychologic dependence on something outside of a person that has a destructive effect on the person's life.
tympanic membrane Eardrum; the membrane that separates the external and middle portions of the ear.

U

understanding Ability to listen to and relate to others to perceive their feelings and the meaning of their words.
unipolar depression Depressed mood.
universal donor Person with type O–negative blood who can donate blood to anyone because the individual does not have any of the common antigens present in the blood.
universal recipient Person with type AB–positive blood who can receive transfusions with any type of blood because the individual has all of the common antigens (A, B, and Rh) present in the blood.
unsaturated fatty acids Compounds that come from plants or fish and are generally liquid at room temperature; can be monounsaturated (e.g., olive, peanut, canola, avocado) oils or polyunsaturated (e.g., corn, safflower, sesame) oils.
uremia Azotemia; the signs and symptoms typical of chronic renal failure.
ureterostomy Surgically created opening in the ureter.
urethritis Inflammation of the urethra.
urge incontinence Involuntary loss of urine; usually occurs shortly after a strong urge to void.
urinary incontinence Inability to control the passage of urine.
UTI Abbreviation for urinary tract infection.
utilitarianism Ethical doctrine that holds that the moral worth of an action is determined by its contribution to its overall utility in society; that is, the best course of action is the one that will produce the greatest good for the greatest number of individuals.
uveitis Usually refers to inflammation of the iris, ciliary body, and/or choroid of the eye; is also used to indicate inflammation of sclera, cornea, and/or retina.

V

vaginitis Inflammation of the vagina.
value system Personal standards for decision making.
values Principles or standards that determine the worth an individual gives to an idea or action.
values clarification Process by which a person learns to make choices from alternatives that may be morally ambiguous.
varices Enlarged, tortuous blood or lymphatic vessels.
VAS Abbreviation for visual analog scale.
vasculitis Inflammation of blood vessels.
vasoconstriction Decrease in blood vessel diameter.
vasodilation Increase in blood vessel diameter.
VC Abbreviation for vital capacity.
ventilation Movement of air in and out of the lungs.
veracity In the health care setting, truth and honesty in discussions with patients, in documentation of care, and in communication with colleagues.
vertigo Sensation that an individual's body or surroundings are rotating.
vesicle Small fluid-filled bladder or sac; blister.
vesicostomy Surgically created opening into the urinary bladder.
viruses Infectious microorganisms that can live and reproduce only within living cells; are capable of causing illness, inflammation, and cell destruction.
viscosity Resistance to flow related to the friction between two components; thickness.
vitamins Organic compounds supplied by food that the body needs for normal growth and development.
VLDL Abbreviation for very-low-density lipoprotein.
void Act of urinating.
vulvitis Inflammation of the vulva.

W

water-soluble vitamins Vitamins that are soluble in water; are not as potentially toxic as fat-soluble vitamins and are readily excreted by the body; they include vitamins except for A, D, E, and K.
WBC Abbreviation for white blood cell.
wheeze High-pitched sound heard as air passes through constricted airways.
withdrawal Unpleasant and sometimes life-threatening physical substance-specific syndrome occurring after stopping or reducing the habitual dose or frequency of a drug.

X

xerostomia Dry mouth caused by inadequate production of saliva.

Index

Page numbers followed by f indicate figures; t, tables; b, boxes.

B

T

U

W